Pain Management

Pain
Management

SECOND EDITION

Steven D. Waldman, MD, JD
Clinical Professor of Anesthesiology
Professor of Medical Humanities and Bioethics
University of Missouri–Kansas City School of Medicine
Kansas City, Missouri

ELSEVIER
SAUNDERS

ELSEVIER
SAUNDERS

1600 John F. Kennedy Blvd.
Ste 1800
Philadelphia, PA 19103-2899

PAIN MANAGEMENT   ISBN: 978-1-4377-0721-2

Notices

Knowledge and best practice in this field are constantly changing. As new research and experience broaden our understanding, changes in research methods, professional practices, or medical treatment may become necessary.
   Practitioners and researchers must always rely on their own experience and knowledge in evaluating and using any information, methods, compounds, or experiments described herein. In using such information or methods, they should be mindful of their own safety and the safety of others, including parties for whom they have a professional responsibility.
   With respect to any drug or pharmaceutical products identified, readers are advised to check the most current information provided (i) on procedures featured or (ii) by the manufacturer of each product to be administered, to verify the recommended dose or formula, the method and duration of administration, and contraindications. It is the responsibility of practitioners, relying on their own experience and knowledge of their patients, to make diagnoses, to determine dosages and the best treatment for each individual patient and to take all appropriate safety precautions.
   To the fullest extent of the law, neither the Publisher nor the authors, contributors, or editors assume any liability for any injury and/or damage to persons or property as a matter of products liability, negligence, or otherwise, or from any use or operation of any methods, products, instructions, or ideas contained in the material herein.

Library of Congress Cataloging-in-Publication Data
Pain management / [edited by] Steven D. Waldman. – 2nd ed.
     p. cm.
Includes bibliographical references and index.
ISBN 978-1-4377-0721-2 (hardcover : alk. paper) 1. Pain–Treatment. I. Waldman, Steven D.
RB127.P332284 2011
616'.0472–dc22

                                                                    2011009894

Acquisitions Editor: Pamela Hetherington
Senior Developmental Editor: Lucia Gunzel
Publishing Services Manager: Anne Altepeter
Team Manager: Radhika Pallamparthy
Senior Project Manager: Doug Turner
Project Manager: Vijay Vincent
Designer: Louis Forgione
Producer: Kitty Lasinski

Printed in the United States of America

Last digit is the print number: 9 8 7 6 5 4 3 2 1

To my children:
David for his caring nature and amazing work ethic,
Corey for his integrity and determination,
Jennifer for her intellect and compassion,
and Reid for his ambition and unabashed joie de vivre.

Steven D. Waldman
Summer 2010

Contributors

Salahadin Abdi, MD, PhD
Vice Chair and Chief of Pain Medicine
Department of Anesthesia, Critical Care,
    and Pain Medicine
Beth Israel Deaconess Medical Center;
Associate Professor
Harvard Medical School
Boston, Massachusetts

Bernard M. Abrams, MD, BS
Clinical Professor
Department of Neurology
University of Missouri–Kansas City School
    of Medicine
Kansas City, Missouri;
Medical Director
Dannemiller, San Antonio, Texas

Vimal Akhouri, MD, MBBS
Instructor
Department of Anesthesia
Harvard Medical School;
Staff
Department of Anesthesia, Critical Care,
    and Pain Medicine
Beth Israel Deaconess Medical Center
Boston, Massachusetts

J. Antonio Aldrete, MD, MS
Professor Emeritus
Department of Anesthesiology
University of Alabama at Birmingham;
President and Founder
Arachnoiditis Foundation, Inc.
Birmingham, Alabama

Frank Andrasik, PhD
Distinguished Professor and Chair
Department of Psychology
University of Memphis
Memphis, Tennessee

Sanjib Das Adhikary, MD
Assistant Professor
Department of Anesthesiology
Penn State College of Medicine
Milton S. Hershey Medical Center
Hershey, Pennsylvania

Hifz Aniq, MBBS, FRCR
Honorary Lecturer
Mersey School of Radiology
University of Liverpool;
Consultant Radiologist
Radiology Department
Royal Liverpool University Hospitals Trust
Liverpool, United Kingdom

Bassem Asaad, MD
Assistant Professor
Department of Anesthesiology
Stony Brook University
Stony Brook, New York

Sairam L. Atluri, MD
Director
Tri-State Spine Care Institute
Cincinnati, Ohio

Zahid H. Bajwa, MD
Secretary
American Academy of Pain Medicine;
Director
Education and Clinical Pain Research
Beth Israel Deaconess Medical Center;
Assistant Professor
Department of Anesthesia
Harvard Medical School
Boston, Massachusetts

Samir K. Ballas, MD, FACP
Professor
Departments of Medicine and Pediatrics
Thomas Jefferson University
Philadelphia, Pennsylvania

David P. Bankston, MD
Consultant in Pain Management
Overland Park, Kansas

Ralf Baron, MD
Head
Division of Neurological Pain Research
    and Therapy
Department of Neurology
University Hospital Schleswig-Holstein,
    Campus Kiel
Kiel, Germany

Andreas Binder, MD
Consultant Neurologist
Division of Neurological Pain Research
    and Therapy
Department of Neurology
University Hospital Schleswig-Holstein,
    Campus Kiel
Kiel, Germany

**Nikolai Bogduk, MD, PhD, DSc,
    FAFRM, FFPM (ANZCA)**
(Conjoint) Professor of Pain Medicine
University of Newcastle;
Director
Department of Clinical Research
Newcastle Bone and Joint Institute
Royal Newcastle Centre
Newcastle, Australia

David Borenstein, MD
Clinical Professor of Medicine
George Washington University Medical Center
Washington, District of Columbia

Mark V. Boswell, MD, PhD, MBA
Professor and Chair
Department of Anesthesiology
University of Louisville School of Medicine
Louisville, Kentucky

Geoffrey M. Bove, DC, PhD
Associate Professor
College of Osteopathic Medicine
University of New England
Biddeford, Maine

Fadi Braiteh, MD
Director, Phase I Program
Medical Oncology
Comprehensive Cancer Centers of Nevada
Las Vegas, Nevada

Eduardo Bruera, MD
Professor and Chair
Department of Palliative Care and Rehabilitation
    Medicine
The University of Texas M.D. Anderson Cancer
    Center
Houston, Texas

Allen Burton, MD
Professor and Chair
Department of Pain Medicine
The University of Texas M.D. Anderson Cancer
    Center
Houston, Texas

Roger Cady, MD
Founder
Primary Care Network and Headache Care
    Center;
Adjunct Professor
Missouri State University
Springfield, Missouri;
Associate Executive Chair
National Headache Foundation
Chicago, Illinois

Robert Campbell, MB, ChB, FRCR
Honorary Clinical Lecturer
University of Liverpool;
Consultant Musculoskeletal Radiologist
Department of Radiology
Royal Liverpool University Hospitals Trust
Liverpool, United Kingdom

Kenneth D. Candido, MD
Chairman
Department of Anesthesiology
Advocate Illinois Masonic Medical Center;
Professor of Clinical Anesthesiology
University of Illinois College of Medicine
Chicago, Illinois

Joseph S. Chiang, MD
Professor
Department of Anesthesiology
The University of Texas M.D. Anderson Cancer
    Center
Houston, Texas

Martin K. Childers, DO, PhD
Professor
Department of Neurology
Wake Forest University Health Sciences;
Investigator
Institute for Regenerative Medicine
Wake Forest University School of Medicine
Winston-Salem, North Carolina

Saima Chohan, MD
Assistant Professor
Department of Medicine
Section of Rheumatology
University of Chicago
Chicago, Illinois

**Philip G. Conaghan, MB, BS, PhD,
    FRACP, FRCP**
Professor
Department of Musculoskeletal Medicine
Section of Musculoskeletal Disease
University of Leeds;
Deputy Director
NIHR Leeds Musculoskeletal Biomedical
    Research Unit
Leeds Teaching Hospitals NHS Trust
Leeds, United Kingdom

Darin J. Correll, MD
Assistant Professor
Department of Anesthesia
Harvard Medical School;
Director
Acute Postoperative Pain Management Service;
Administrative Director of Resident Education
Department of Anesthesiology, Perioperative,
    and Pain Medicine
Brigham and Women's Hospital
Boston, Massachusetts

Scott C. Cozad, MD
Radiation Oncologist
Liberty Radiation Oncology Center;
Clinical Assistant Professor
University of Kansas Medical Center
Kansas City, Missouri

Edward V. Craig, MD
Attending Surgeon
Hospital for Special Surgery;
Professor of Clinical Orthopedic Surgery
Cornell Medical School
New York, New York

Paul Creamer, MD, FRCP
Senior Clinical Lecturer
University of Bristol Medical School;
Consultant Rheumatologist
Department of Rheumatology
Southmead Hospital
North Bristol NHS Healthcare Trust
Bristol, United Kingdom

**Sukded Datta, MD, DABPM, FIPP,
    DABIPP**
Director
Vanderbilt University Interventional Pain
    Program;
Assistant Professor
Department of Anesthesiology
Vanderbilt University Medical Center
Nashville, Tennessee

Miles R. Day, MD
Professor and Medical Director
International Pain Center
Department of Anesthesiology and Pain
    Management
Texas Tech University Health Sciences Center
Lubbock, Texas

Timothy R. Deer, MD
President and Chief Executive Officer
Center for Pain Relief;
Clinical Professor
Department of Anesthesiology
West Virginia University School of Medicine
Charleston, West Virginia

Seymour Diamond, MD
Director Emeritus and Founder
Diamond Headache Clinic
Chicago, Illinois;
Adjunct Professor
Department of Cellular and Molecular
    Pharmacology;
Clinical Professor
Department of Family Medicine
Chicago Medical School
Rosalind Franklin University of Medicine
    and Science
North Chicago, Illinois;
Lecturer
Department of Family Medicine (Neurology)
Stritch School of Medicine
Loyola University Chicago
Maywood, Illinois

Anthony Dickenson, PhD, BSc
Professor
Department of Neuroscience, Physiology,
    Pharmacology
University College London
London, United Kingdom

Charles D. Donohoe, MD
Associate Clinical Professor
Department of Neurology
University of Missouri–Kansas City School
    of Medicine
Kansas City, Missouri

Maxim Savillion Eckmann, MD
Assistant Professor
Director of Acute Pain Service
Department of Anesthesiology
The University of Texas Health Science Center
    at San Antonio
San Antonio, Texas

James J. Evans, MD
Assistant Professor
Department of Neurological Surgery
Division of Neuro-oncologic Neurosurgery
    and Stereotactic Radiosurgery;
Co-Director
Center for Minimally Invasive Cranial Base
    Surgery and Endoscopic Neurosurgery
Thomas Jefferson University
Philadelphia, Pennsylvania

Frank J.E. Falco, MD
Clinical Assistant Professor
Temple University Medical School
Philadelphia, Pennsylvania;
Medical Director
Midatlantic Spine
Newark, Delaware

Kathleen Farmer, PsyD
Co-Founder and Psychologist
Headache Care Center
Springfield, Missouri

Colleen M. Fitzgerald, MD
Physical Medicine and Rehabilitation
    Specialist
Rehabilitation Institute of Chicago
Chicago, Illinois

Frederick G. Freitag, DO
Co-Director
Diamond Headache Clinic
Chicago, Illinois;
Clinical Assistant Professor
Department of Family Medicine
Chicago Medical School
Rosalind Franklin University of Medicine
    and Science
North Chicago, Illinois;
Director
Headache Medicine Research
Baylor University Medical Center;
Clinical Director
Department of Headache Medicine
Baylor Neuroscience Center
Baylor University Medical Center
Dallas, Texas

M. Kay Garcia, MSN, MSOM, DrPH
Adjunct Associate Professor
American College of Acupuncture and Oriental
    Medicine;
Advanced Practice Nurse/Acupuncturist
Department of Integrative Medicine
The University of Texas M.D. Anderson Cancer
    Center
Houston, Texas

F. Michael Gloth III, MD
Corporate Medical Director
Mid-Atlantic Healthcare
Timonium, Maryland;
Associate Professor
Department of Medicine
Johns Hopkins University School
   of Medicine;
Adjunct Associate Professor
Department of Epidemiology and Preventive
   Medicine
University of Maryland School of Epidemiology
   and Preventive Medicine
Baltimore, Maryland

Vitaly Gordin, MD
Associate Professor
Department of Anesthesiology
Director
Pain Medicine Clinic;
Medical Director
Spine Center;
Co-Director
Pain Medicine Fellowship Program
Penn State College of Medicine
Milton S. Hershey Medical Center
Hershey, Pennsylvania

Martin Grabois, MD
Professor and Chair
Department of Physical Medicine
   and Rehabilitation
Baylor College of Medicine;
Adjunct Professor
Department of Physical Medicine
   and Rehabilitation
University of Texas Health Science Center
   at Houston;
Professor
Department of Anesthesiology
Baylor College of Medicine
Houston, Texas

Mark A. Greenfield, MD
The Headache and Pain Center
Leawood, Kansas

H. Michael Guo, MD, PhD
Assistant Professor
Director, Neurorehabilitation Fellowship
   Program
Section of Physical Medicine
   and Rehabilitation
Wake Forest University Baptist Medical Center
Winston-Salem, North Carolina

Brian Hainline, MD
Clinical Associate Professor
Department of Neurology
New York University School of Medicine
New York, New York;
Chief
Department of Neurology and Integrative Pain
   Medicine
ProHEALTH Care Associates
Lake Success, New York

Howard Hall, PhD, PsyD, BCB
Associate Professor
Department of Pediatrics
Case Medical Center
Rainbow Babies and Children's Hospital
Cleveland, Ohio

Brian L. Hazleman, MA, MB, FRCP
Associate Lecturer
Department of Medicine;
Fellow
Corpus Christi College
University of Cambridge;
Visiting Consultant
Rheumatology Research Unit
Addenbrooke's Hospital
Cambridge, United Kingdom

James E. Heavner, DVM, PhD
Professor
Department of Anesthesiology and Cell
   Physiology and Molecular Biophysics
School of Medicine
Anesthesiology and Pain Research
Texas Tech University Health Sciences Center
Lubbock, Texas

D. Ross Henshaw, MD
Director
Sports Medicine Program
Section of Orthopedic Surgery
Danbury Hospital
Danbury, Connecticut

Bernard H. Hsu, MD
Assistant Clinical Professor
Department of Anesthesiology
School of Medicine and Biomedical Sciences
State University of New York at Buffalo
Buffalo, New York

Takashi Igarashi, MD
Associate Professor
Department of Anesthesiology and Critical
   Care Medicine
Jichi Medical University School of Medicine
Shimotsuke, Japan

Jeffrey W. Janata, PhD
Associate Professor
Departments of Psychiatry
   and Anesthesiology
University Hospitals Case Medical Center;
Director
Behavioral Medicine Program
Case Western Reserve University School
   of Medicine
Cleveland, Ohio

Ravish Kapoor, MD
Resident
Department of Anesthesiology
Penn State College of Medicine
Milton S. Hershey Medical Center
Hershey, Pennsylvania

Joel Katz, PhD
Professor and Canada Research Chair in Health
   Psychology
Department of Psychology
York University;
Professor
Department of Anesthesia
University of Toronto;
Director
Acute Pain Research Unit
Department of Anesthesia and Pain Management
Toronto General Hospital
Toronto, Canada

Yoshiharu Kawaguchi, MD, PhD
Associate Professor
Department of Orthopaedic Surgery
University of Toyama
Toyama City, Japan

Richard M. Keating, MD
Professor
Department of Medicine
Section of Rheumatology
University of Chicago
Pritzker School of Medicine
Chicago, Illinois

Bruce L. Kidd, MD, DM
Professor
William Harvey Research Institute
Bart's and the London Queen Mary School
   of Medicine and Dentistry
London, United Kingdom

Katherine A. Kidder, OT, MBA
Executive Director
Society for Pain Practice Management
Leawood, Kansas

Paul T. King, MD, PhD, FRACP
Respiratory Physician
Department of Respiratory and Sleep Medicine;
Senior Lecturer
Department of Medicine
Monash University
Monash Medical Centre
Melbourne, Australia

Nicholas Kormylo, MD
Assistant Clinical Professor
Department of Anesthesiology
University of California, San Diego
La Jolla, California

Dhanalakshmi Koyyalagunta, MD
Associate Professor
Department of Pain Medicine
The University of Texas M.D. Anderson Cancer
   Center
Houston, Texas

Milton H. Landers, DO, PhD
Associate Clinical Professor
Department of Anesthesiology
University of Kansas–Wichita School of Medicine;
Pain Clinician
Pain Management Associates
Wichita, Kansas

Erin F. Lawson, MD
Assistant Professor
Department of Anesthesiology
Division of Pain Medicine
University of California, San Diego
La Jolla, California

Mark J. Lema, MD, PhD
Professor and Chair
Department of Anesthesiology
School of Medicine and Biomedical Sciences
State University of New York at Buffalo;
Chair
Division of Anesthesiology
Roswell Park Cancer Institute
Buffalo, New York

Jennifer B. Levin, PhD
Assistant Professor
Department of Psychiatry
Case Western Reserve School of Medicine;
Clinical Psychologist
University Hospitals Case Medical Center
Cleveland, Ohio

John Liu, MD
Associate Professor
Department of Neurosurgery
Northwestern University Feinberg School
of Medicine
Chicago, Illinois

Mirjana Lovrincevic, MD
Associate Professor
Department of Clinical Anesthesiology
and Oncology
Roswell Park Cancer Institute;
Clinical Assistant Professor
Department of Anesthesiology
School of Medicine and Biomedical Sciences
State University of New York at Buffalo
Buffalo, New York

Z. David Luo, MD
Associate Professor
Department of Anesthesiology
School of Medicine
University of California, Irvine
Irvine, California

John A. Lyftogt, MD, MRNZCGP
Senior Medical Officer
Active Health Clinic
QEII Sports Stadium
Christchurch, New Zealand

James A. MacDonald, MD
Assistant Professor
Department of Neurology
Wake Forest University Baptist Medical Center
Winston-Salem, North Carolina

Mark N. Malinowski, DO, DABA
Medical Director
Center for Pain Management
Wood County Hospital
Bowling Green, Ohio

Laxmaiah Manchikanti, MD
Medical Director
Pain Management Center
Paducah, Kentucky;
Associate Clinical Professor
Department of Anesthesiology and Perioperative
Medicine
University of Louisville
Louisville, Kentucky

Danesh Mazloomdoost, MD
Medical Director
Paradigm Pain Management Medicine
Lexington, Kentucky

†Brian McGuirk, MB, BS, DPH, FAFOEM
Senior Staff Specialist
Occupational and Musculoskeletal Medicine
Newcastle Bone and Joint Institute
Royal Newcastle Centre
Newcastle, Australia

Ronald Melzack, PhD
Professor Emeritus
Department of Psychology
McGill University
Montreal, Canada

Jeffrey P. Meyer, MD
President and Chief Executive Officer
Midwest Pain Consultants
Oklahoma City, Oklahoma

George R. Nissan, DO
Clinical Assistant Professor
Department of Medicine
Chicago Medical School
Rosalind Franklin University of Medicine
and Science
North Chicago, Illinois;
Co-Director
Diamond Headache Clinic
Chicago, Illinois

John L. Pappas, MD
Chief
Department of Anesthesiology
Beaumont Hospital;
Medical Director
Division of Pain Medicine
Department of Anesthesiology
Beaumont Hospitals
Troy, Michigan

Winston C.V. Parris, MD, CMG, FACPM, DABPM
Professor
Department of Anesthesiology;
Chief
Division of Pain Medicine
Duke University Medical Center
Durham, North Carolina

Divya J. Patel, MD
Director
Carolina Regional Orthopedics
Rocky Mount, North Carolina

Richard B. Patt, MD
President and Chief Medical Officer
Patt Center for Pain Management
Houston, Texas

David R. Patterson, PhD, ABPP, ABPH
Professor
Department of Rehabilitation Medicine
University of Washington School of Medicine
Seattle, Washington

Marco R. Perez-Toro, MD

David Petersen, MD
Department of Orthopaedic Surgery
Minsurg Corporation
Clearwater, Florida

Brett T. Quave, MD
Medical Director
Water's Edge
Memorial's Pain Relief Institute
Yakima, Washington

Gabor B. Racz, MD, ABA, FIPP, ABIPP
Grover Murray Professor
Professor and Chair Emeritus
Department of Anesthesiology and Pain
Medicine
Texas Tech University Health Sciences Center
Lubbock, Texas

P. Prithvi Raj, MD
Professor Emeritus
Department of Anesthesiology and Pain Medicine
Texas Tech University Health Sciences Center
Lubbock, Texas

Somayaji Ramamurthy, MD
Professor
Department of Anesthesiology;
Director
Pain Medicine Fellowship Program
Department of Anesthesiology
The University of Texas Health Science Center
at San Antonio
San Antonio, Texas

Matthew T. Ranson, MD
Attending Physician
The Center for Pain Relief
Charleston, West Virginia

K. Dean Reeves, MD
Clinical Associate Professor
Department of Physical Medicine and Rehabilitation
University of Kansas Medical Center
Kansas City, Kansas

Lowell W. Reynolds, MD
Professor
Department of Anesthesiology
Loma Linda University School of Medicine;
Director of Acute Pain
Department of Anesthesiology;
Program Director
Regional Anesthesia Fellowship
Loma Linda University Medical Center
Loma Linda, California

†Deceased.

Carla Rime, MA
Counselor and Biofeedback Technician
Intermountain Children's Home
Helena, Montana

Richard M. Rosenthal, MD, DABPM, FIPP
Medical Director
Nexus Pain Care
Fellowship Director;
Utah Center for Pain Management and Research
Provo, Utah

Matthew P. Rupert, MD, MS, FIPP, DABIPP
Director
Integrative Pain Solutions
Franklin, Tennessee

Lloyd R. Saberski, MD
Medical Director
Advanced Diagnostic Pain Treatment Center
Yale-New Haven at Long Wharf
Yale-New Haven Hospital
New Haven, Connecticut

Jörn Schattschneider, MD
Consultant
Division of Neurological Pain Research and Therapy
Department of Neurology
University Hospital of Schleswig-Holstein,
    Campus Kiel
Kiel, Germany

Thomas Schrattenholzer, MD
Medical Director
Legacy Pain Management Center
Portland, Oregon

Curtis P. Schreiber, MD
Neurologist
Headache Care Center Primary Care Network
Springfield, Missouri

David M. Schultz, MD
Medical Director
Medical Advanced Pain Specialists
Minneapolis, Minnesota

Jared Scott, MD
Physician
Advanced Pain Medicine Associates
Wichita, Kansas;
Pain Fellowship at Texas Tech University
    of Health Sciences
Lubbock, Texas

Mehul Sekhadia, DO
Assistant Professor
Department of Anesthesiology
Northwestern University Feinberg School
    of Medicine
Chicago, Illinois

Sam R. Sharar, MD
Professor
Department of Anesthesiology and Pain
    Medicine
University of Washington School of Medicine;
Head, Pediatric Anesthesia Section
Harborview Medical Center
Seattle, Washington

Khuram A. Sial, MD
Medical Director
PainMedGroup, Inc.
Murrieta, California

Shawn M. Sills, MD
Medical Director
Interventional Pain Consultants, LLC
Medford, Oregon

Steven Simon, MD, RPh
Assistant Clinical Professor
Department of Physical Medicine
    and Rehabilitation
University of Kansas;
Clinical Associate Professor
Department of Family Medicine
Kansas City University of Medicine and Biosciences
Kansas City, Missouri;
Medical Director
Department of Pain Management
Pain Management Institute
Leawood, Kansas

Thomas T. Simopoulos, MD, MA
Assistant Professor
Department of Anesthesia
Harvard Medical School;
Director
Interventional Pain Management
Arnold Pain Management Center
Department of Anesthesia, Critical Care,
    and Pain Medicine
Beth Israel Deaconess Medical Center
Boston, Massachusetts

Vijay Singh, MD
Medical Director
Pain Diagnostics Associates
Niagara, Wisconsin

Daneshvari Solanki, FRCA (Eng)
Laura B. McDaniel Distinguished Professor
Department of Anesthesiology
University of Texas Medical Branch
Galveston, Texas

David A. Soto-Quijano, MD
Staff Physician
Department of Physical Medicine and
    Rehabilitation
Veterans Affairs Caribbean Healthcare System;
Assistant Professor
Department of Physical Medicine, Rehabilitation
    and Sports Medicine
University of Puerto Rico School of Medicine
San Juan, Puerto Rico

C.R. Sridhara, MD
Director
MossRehab Electrodiagnostic Center
Department of Pain Management
    and Rehabilitation
Albert Einstein Medical Center
Elkins Park, Pennsylvania;
Clinical Professor
Department of Rehabilitation Medicine
Thomas Jefferson University;
Associate Chair
Department of Pain Management
    and Rehabilitation
Albert Einstein Medical Center;
Adjunct Clinical Professor
Department of Pain Management
    and Rehabilitation
Temple University School of Medicine
Philadelphia, Pennsylvania

Michael Stanton-Hicks, MB, BS, DrMed, FRCA, ABPM, FIPP
Staff Member
Department of Pain Management
Cleveland Clinic;
Consulting Staff Member
Pediatric Pain Rehabilitation Program
Cleveland Clinic Children's Hospital Shaker
    Campus;
Joint Appointment to Outcomes and Research
    Department
Anesthesiology Institute;
Joint Appointment to Center for Neurological
    Restoration Imaging Institute
Cleveland Clinic;
Professor of Anesthesiology
Lerner College of Medicine
Case Medical School
Case Western Reserve University
Cleveland, Ohio

M. Alan Stiles, DMD
Clinical Professor
Facial Pain Management
Department of Oral Maxillofacial Surgery
Thomas Jefferson University
Philadelphia, Pennsylvania

Robert B. Supernaw, PharmD
Professor and Dean
School of Pharmacy
Wingate University
Wingate, North Carolina

Rand S. Swenson, MD, PhD, DC
Professor and Chair
Department of Anatomy;
Professor
Department of Anatomy and Neurology
Dartmouth Medical School
Hanover, New Hampshire

Victor M. Taylor, MD
President and Medical Director
Amarillo Interventional Pain Management;
Pain Management Fellowship
Department of Anesthesiology
Texas Tech University School of Medicine
Lubbock, Texas

Kevin D. Treffer, DO
Associate Professor
Departments of Family Medicine
    and Osteopathic Manipulative Medicine
College of Osteopathic Medicine
Kansas City University of Medicine
    and Biosciences
Kansas City, Missouri

Robert Trout, MD
Consultant in Physical Medicine
    and Rehabilitation
Headache and Pain Center
Leawood, Kansas

George J. Urban, MD
Co-Director
Diamond Headache Clinic
Chicago, Illinois;
Clinical Instructor of Medicine
Chicago Medical School
Rosalind Franklin University of Medicine
    and Science
North Chicago, Illinois;
Lecturer
Department of Medicine (Neurology)
Stritch School of Medicine
Loyola University of Chicago
Maywood, Illinois

Sobhan Vinjamuri, MD, MSc, FRCP
Professor
Department of Nuclear Medicine
Royal Liverpool University Hospitals Trust
Liverpool, United Kingdom

Corey W. Waldman
Red 2 Docent Unit
University of Missouri–Kansas City School
    of Medicine
Kansas City, Missouri

Howard J. Waldman, MD
Consultant in Physical Medicine and
    Rehabilitation
The Headache and Pain Center;
Director of Neurophysiology Laboratory
Doctors Hospital
Leawood, Kansas

Jennifer E. Waldman
Neuroscience Brain Tissue Bank and Research
    Laboratory
University of Missouri–Kansas City School
    of Medicine
Kansas City, Missouri

Steven D. Waldman, MD, JD
Clinical Professor of Anesthesiology
Professor of Medical Humanities
    and Bioethics
University of Missouri–Kansas City School
    of Medicine
Kansas City, Missouri

Mark S. Wallace, MD
Professor
Department of Clinical Anesthesiology;
Chair
Division of Pain Medicine
Department of Anesthesiology
University of California, San Diego
La Jolla, California

Carol A. Warfield, MD
Lowenstein Professor
Department of Anesthesia
Harvard Medical School
Boston, Massachusetts

Michael L. Whitworth, MD
Pain Management Specialist
Pain Center
Columbus Regional Hospital
Columbus, Indiana

Shelley A. Wiechman, PhD
Associate Professor
Rehabilitation Medicine
University of Washington School of Medicine;
Attending Psychologist
Harborview Medical Center
Seattle, Washington

Alon P. Winnie, MD
Clinical Professor
Department of Anesthesiology
Northwestern University Feinberg School
    of Medicine
Chicago, Illinois

Cynthia A. Wong, MD
Professor
Department of Anesthesiology
Northwestern University Feinberg School
    of Medicine;
Section Chief,
Obstetric Anesthesiology
Northwestern Memorial Hospital
Chicago, Illinois

Tony L. Yaksh, PhD
Professor
Department of Anesthesiology
    and Pharmacology;
Vice Chair for Research
Department of Anesthesiology
University of California, San Diego
La Jolla, California

Manuel Ybarra, MD
Assistant Professor
Department of Anesthesiology
The University of Texas Health Science Center
    at San Antonio
San Antonio, Texas

Preface

It is hard to believe that 5 years have passed since the publication of the first edition of *Pain Management*. Even at that time, when we had no knowledge of where electronic publishing would be in 2011, the conventional wisdom was that large, comprehensive textbooks were dinosaurs and that the future of medical books would be in smaller, more manageable, more specialized texts. Fortunately, this bit of conventional wisdom was off the mark. The first edition of *Pain Management* was published and has established itself as a popular reference among pain management practitioners across a variety of specialties.

Electronic publishing has changed the face of the publishing business and has revolutionized the way in which we, as practitioners, consume content and learn new things. The explosion in the use of smart phones, e-readers and, more recently, tablets have made some of us hard-core readers wonder whether the printed book would go the way of the handwritten illuminated scroll. Actually, the challenge for publishers now is to deliver valuable content more quickly and in many different formats. In response to the changing times, this edition will also be published online at www.expertconsult.com, where you will find fully searchable text and images, as well as all the references hyperlinked to PubMed.

It is with great pride, and a sigh of relief, that I give you *Pain Management*, Second Edition!

Steven D. Waldman, MD, JD

Acknowledgments

Many thanks to the dedicated clinicians and scientists who took time from their already busy schedules to contribute chapters to the second edition of *Pain Management*. I'd like to extend a special note of thanks to Milton H. Landers, DO, PhD; Mark A. Greenfield, MD; Mauricio Garcia, MD; Robert Campbell, MD; and Frank Judilla, MD, for their generosity in sharing their knowledge, experience, and images for this edition. I'd also like to thank the staff at Elsevier for their advice and expertise—Pamela Hetherington, acquisitions editor; Lucia Gunzel, developmental editor; and Doug Turner, project manager.

Steven D. Waldman, MD, JD

Contents

Section V
Specific Treatment Modalities for Pain and Symptom Management

Section I

The Basic Science of Pain

Chapter 1

A Conceptual Framework for Understanding Pain in the Human

Joel Katz and Ronald Melzack

Theories of pain, like all scientific theories, evolve as result of the accumulation of new facts as well as leaps of the imagination.[1] The gate control theory's most revolutionary contribution to understanding pain was its emphasis on central neural mechanisms.[2] The theory forced the medical and biologic sciences to accept the brain as an active system that filters, selects, and modulates inputs. The dorsal horns, too, are not merely passive transmission stations but sites at which dynamic activities—inhibition, excitation, and modulation—occur. The great challenge ahead of us is to understand how the brain functions.

A Brief History of Pain in the 20th Century

The theory of pain we inherited in the 20th century was proposed by Descartes 3 centuries earlier. The impact of Descartes' specificity theory was enormous. It influenced experiments on the anatomy and physiology of pain up to the first half of the 20th century (reviewed in Melzack and Wall[3]). This body of research is marked by a search for specific pain fibers and pathways and a pain center in the brain. The result was a concept of pain as a specific, straight-through sensory projection system. This rigid anatomy of pain in the 1950s led to attempts to treat severe chronic pain by a variety of neurosurgical lesions. Descartes' specificity theory, then, determined the "facts" as they were known up to the middle of the 20th century and even determined therapy.

Specificity theory proposed that injury activates specific pain receptors and fibers that, in turn, project pain impulses through a spinal pain pathway to a pain center in the brain. The psychological experience of pain, therefore, was virtually equated with peripheral injury. In the 1950s, there was no room for psychological contributions to pain, such as attention, past experience, anxiety, depression, and the meaning of the situation. Instead, pain experience was held to be proportional to peripheral injury or disease. Patients who suffered back pain without presenting signs of organic disease were often labeled as psychologically disturbed and were sent to psychiatrists. The concept, in short, was simple and, not surprisingly, often failed to help patients who suffered severe chronic pain. To thoughtful clinical observers, specificity theory was clearly wrong.

Several attempts were made to find a new theory. The major opponent to specificity was labeled "pattern theory," but several different pattern theories were put forth, and they were generally vague and inadequate (see Melzack and Wall[3]). However, seen in retrospect, pattern theories gradually evolved (**Fig. 1.1**) and set the stage for the gate control theory. Goldscheider[4] proposed that central summation in the dorsal horns is one of the critical determinants of pain. Livingston's[5] theory postulated a reverberatory circuit in the dorsal horns to explain summation, referred pain, and pain that persisted long after healing was completed. Noordenbos'[6] theory proposed that large-diameter fibers inhibited small-diameter fibers, and he even suggested that the substantia gelatinosa in the dorsal horns plays a major role in the summation and other dynamic processes described by Livingston. However, none of these theories had an explicit

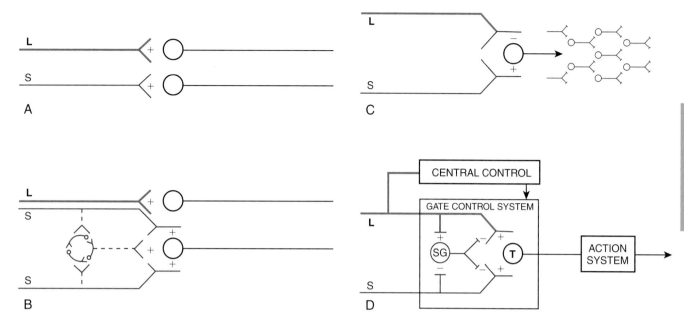

Fig. 1.1 **Schematic representation of conceptual models of pain mechanisms.** **A,** Specificity theory. Large (L) and small (S) fibers are assumed to transmit touch and pain impulses, respectively, in separate, specific, straight-through pathways to touch and pain centers in the brain. **B,** Goldscheider's[4] summation theory, showing convergence of small fibers onto a dorsal horn cell. The central network projecting to the central cell represents Livingston's[5] conceptual model of reverberatory circuits underlying pathologic pain states. Touch is assumed to be carried by large fibers. **C,** Sensory interaction theory, in which large (L) fibers inhibit (−) and small (S) fibers excite (+) central transmission neurons. The output projects to spinal cord neurons, which are conceived by Noordenbos[6] to comprise a multisynaptic afferent system. **D,** Gate control theory. The large (L) and small (S) fibers project to the substantia gelatinosa (SG) and first central transmission (T) cells. The central control trigger is represented by a line running from the large fiber system to central control mechanisms, which in turn project back to the gate control system. The T cells project to the entry cells of the action system. +, excitation; −, inhibition. *(From Melzack R: The gate control theory 25 years later: new perspectives on phantom limb pain. In Bond MR, Charlton JE, Woolf CJ, editors: Pain research and therapy: proceedings of the VIth World Congress on Pain, Amsterdam, 1991, Elsevier, pp 9–21.)*

role for the brain other than as a passive receiver of messages. Nevertheless, the successive theoretical concepts moved the field in the right direction: into the spinal cord and away from the periphery as the exclusive answer to pain. At least the field of pain was making its way up toward the brain.

The Gate Control Theory of Pain

In 1965, Melzack and Wall[2] proposed the gate control theory of pain. The final model, depicted in Figure 1.1D in the context of earlier theories of pain, is the first theory of pain that incorporated the central control processes of the brain.

The gate control theory of pain[2] proposed that the transmission of nerve impulses from afferent fibers to spinal cord transmission (T) cells is modulated by a gating mechanism in the spinal dorsal horn. This gating mechanism is influenced by the relative amount of activity in large- and small-diameter fibers, so that large fibers tend to inhibit transmission (close the gate), whereas small fibers tend to facilitate transmission (open the gate). In addition, the spinal gating mechanism is influenced by nerve impulses that descend from the brain. When the output of the spinal T cells exceeds a critical level, it activates the Action System—those neural areas that underlie the complex, sequential patterns of behavior and experience characteristic of pain.

The theory's emphasis on the modulation of inputs in the spinal dorsal horns and the dynamic role of the brain in pain processes had a clinical as well as a scientific impact. Psychological factors, which were previously dismissed as

"reactions to pain," were now seen to be an integral part of pain processing, and new avenues for pain control by psychological therapies were opened. Similarly, cutting of nerves and pathways was gradually replaced by a host of methods to modulate the input. Physical therapists and other health care professionals who use a multitude of modulation techniques were brought into the picture, and transcutaneous electrical nerve stimulation became an important modality for the treatment of chronic and acute pain. The current status of pain research and therapy indicates that, despite the addition of a massive amount of detail, the conceptual components of the theory remain basically intact up to the present.

Beyond the Gate

The great challenge ahead of us is to understand brain function. Melzack and Casey[7] made a start by proposing that specialized systems in the brain are involved in the sensory-discriminative, motivational-affective, and cognitive-evaluative dimensions of subjective pain experience (**Fig. 1.2**). These names for the dimensions of subjective experience seemed strange when they were coined, but they are now used so frequently and seem so "logical" that they have become part of our language. So, too, the McGill Pain Questionnaire, which taps into subjective experience—one of the functions of the brain—is the most widely used instrument to measure pain.[8–10] The newest version, the Short-Form McGill Pain Questionnaire-2,[10] was designed to measure the qualities of both neuropathic and non-neuropathic pain in research and clinical settings.

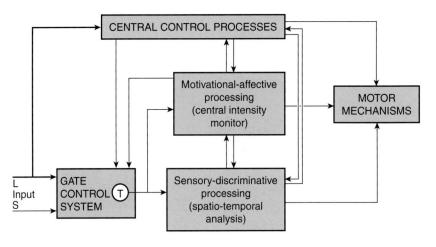

Fig. 1.2 Conceptual model of the sensory, motivational, and central control determinants of pain. The output of the T (transmission) cells of the gate control system projects to the sensory-discriminative system and the motivational-affective system. The central control trigger is represented by a line running from the large fiber system to central control processes; these, in turn, project back to the gate control system, and to the sensory-discriminative and motivational-affective systems. All three systems interact with one another and project to the motor system. L, large fiber; S, small fiber. *(From Melzack R, Casey KL: Sensory, motivational, and central control determinants of pain. In Kenshalo D, editor:* The skin senses, *Springfield, Ill, 1968, Charles C Thomas, pp 423–443.)*

In 1978, Melzack and Loeser[11] described severe pains in the phantom body of paraplegic patients with verified total sections of the spinal cord and proposed a central "pattern generating mechanism" above the level of the section. This concept, generally ignored for more than 2 decades, is now beginning to be accepted. It represents a revolutionary advance: it did not merely extend the gate; it said that pain could be generated by brain mechanisms in paraplegic patients in the absence of a spinal gate because the brain is completely disconnected from the spinal cord. Psychophysical specificity, in such a concept, makes no sense; instead we must explore how patterns of nerve impulses generated in the brain can give rise to somesthetic experience.

Phantom Limbs and the Concept of a Neuromatrix

It is evident that the gate control theory has taken us a long way. Yet, as historians of science have pointed out, good theories are instrumental in producing facts that eventually require a new theory to incorporate them, and this is what has happened. It is possible to make adjustments to the gate theory so that, for example, it includes long-lasting activity of the sort Wall has described (see Melzack and Wall[3]). However, one set of observations on pain in paraplegic patients just does not fit the theory. This does not negate the gate theory, of course. Peripheral and spinal processes are obviously an important part of pain, and we need to know more about the mechanisms of peripheral inflammation, spinal modulation, midbrain descending control, and so forth. However, the data on painful phantoms below the level of total spinal section[12,13] indicate that we need to go above the spinal cord and into the brain.

Note that more than the spinal projection areas in the thalamus and cortex are meant. These areas are important, of course, but they are only part of the neural processes that underlie perception. The cortex, Gybels and Tasker[14] made amply clear, is not the pain center, and neither is the thalamus. The areas of the brain involved in pain experience and behavior must include somatosensory projections as well as the limbic system. Furthermore, cognitive processes are known to involve widespread areas of the brain. Despite this increased knowledge, we do not yet have an adequate theory of how the brain works.

Melzack's[13] analysis of phantom limb phenomena, particularly the astonishing reports of a phantom body and severe phantom limb pain in people with a total thoracic spinal cord section,[11] has led to four conclusions that point to a newer conceptual model of the nervous system. First, because the phantom limb (or other body part) feels so real, it is reasonable to conclude that the body we normally feel is subserved by the same neural processes in the brain as the phantom; these brain processes are normally activated and modulated by inputs from the body, but they can act in the absence of any inputs. Second, all the qualities we normally feel from the body, including pain, are also felt in the absence of inputs from the body; from this we may conclude that the origins of the patterns that underlie the qualities of experience lie in neural networks in the brain; stimuli may trigger the patterns but do not produce them. Third, the body is perceived as a unity and is identified as the "self," distinct from other people and the surrounding world. The experience of a unity of such diverse feelings, including the self as the point of orientation in the surrounding environment, is produced by central neural processes and cannot derive from the peripheral nervous system or the spinal cord. Fourth, the brain processes that underlie the body-self are "built in" by genetic specification, although this built-in substrate must, of course, be modified by experience. These conclusions provide the basis of the newer conceptual model[12,13,15] depicted in **Figure 1.3**.

Outline of the Theory

Melzack[12,13,15] proposed that the anatomic substrate of the body-self is a large, widespread network of neurons that consists of loops between the thalamus and cortex as well as between the cortex and limbic system. He labeled the entire network, whose spatial distribution and synaptic links are initially determined genetically and are later sculpted by sensory inputs, a *neuromatrix*. The loops diverge to permit parallel processing in different components of the neuromatrix and converge repeatedly to permit interactions among the output products of processing. The repeated *cyclical processing and synthesis* of nerve impulses through the neuromatrix imparts a characteristic pattern: the *neurosignature*. The neurosignature of the neuromatrix is imparted on all nerve impulse patterns that flow through it; the neurosignature is produced by the patterns of synaptic connections in the entire neuromatrix. All inputs from the body undergo cyclical

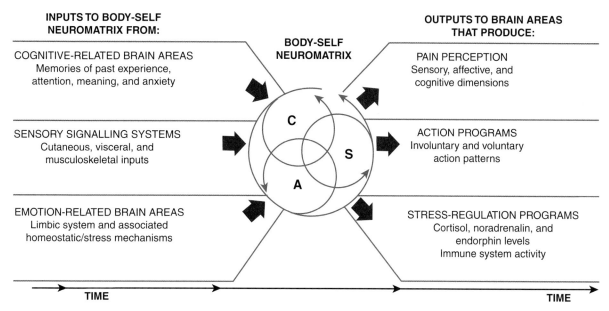

Fig. 1.3 Factors that contribute to the patterns of activity generated by the body-self neuromatrix, which is composed of sensory, affective, and cognitive neuromodules. The output patterns from the neuromatrix produce the multiple dimensions of pain experience, as well as concurrent homeostatic and behavioral responses. *(From Melzack R: Pain and the neuromatrix in the brain,* J Dent Educ 65:1378–1382, 2001.)

processing and synthesis so that characteristic patterns are impressed on them in the neuromatrix. Portions of the neuromatrix are specialized to process information related to major sensory events (e.g., injury, temperature change, and stimulation of erogenous tissue) and may be labeled neuromodules that impress subsignatures on the larger neurosignature.

The neurosignature, which is a continuous output from the body-self neuromatrix, is projected to areas in the brain—the *sentient neural hub*—in which the stream of nerve impulses (the neurosignature modulated by ongoing inputs) is converted into a continually changing stream of awareness. Furthermore, the neurosignature patterns may also activate a neuromatrix to produce movement. That is, the signature patterns bifurcate so that a pattern proceeds to the sentient neural hub (where the pattern is transformed into the experience of movement), and a similar pattern proceeds through a neuromatrix that eventually activates spinal cord neurons to produce muscle patterns for complex actions.

The Body-Self Neuromatrix

The body is felt as a unity, with different qualities at different times. Melzack[12,13,15] proposed that the brain mechanism that underlies the experience also comprises a unified system that acts as a whole and produces a neurosignature pattern of a whole body. The conceptualization of this unified brain mechanism lies at the heart of this theory, and the word "neuromatrix" best characterizes it. The neuromatrix (not the stimulus, peripheral nerves, or "brain center") is the origin of the neurosignature; the neurosignature originates and takes form in the neuromatrix. Although the neurosignature may be triggered or modulated by input, the input is only a "trigger" and does not produce the neurosignature itself. The neuromatrix "casts" its distinctive signature on all inputs (nerve impulse patterns) that flow through it. Finally, the array of neurons in a neuromatrix is genetically programmed to perform the specific function of producing the signature pattern. The final,

integrated neurosignature pattern for the body-self ultimately produces awareness and action.

The neuromatrix, distributed throughout many areas of the brain, comprises a widespread network of neurons that generates patterns, processes information that flows through it, and ultimately produces the pattern that is felt as a whole body. The stream of neurosignature output with constantly varying patterns riding on the main signature pattern produces the feelings of the whole body with constantly changing qualities.

Conceptual Reasons for a Neuromatrix

It is difficult to comprehend how individual bits of information from skin, joints, or muscles can all come together to produce the experience of a coherent, articulated body. At any instant in time, millions of nerve impulses arrive at the brain from all the body's sensory systems, including the proprioceptive and vestibular systems. How can all this be integrated in a constantly changing unity of experience? Where does it all come together?

Melzack[12,13,15] conceptualized a genetically built-in neuromatrix for the whole body. This neuromatrix produces a characteristic neurosignature for the body that carries with it patterns for the myriad qualities we feel. The neuromatrix, as Melzack conceived of it, produces a continuous message that represents the whole body in which details are differentiated within the whole as inputs come into it. We start from the top, with the experience of a unity of the body, and look for differentiation of detail within the whole. The neuromatrix, then, is a template of the whole, which provides the characteristic neural pattern for the whole body (the body's neurosignature), as well as subsets of signature patterns (from neuromodules) that relate to events at (or in) different parts of the body.

These views are in sharp contrast to the classical specificity theory in which the qualities of experience are presumed to be inherent in peripheral nerve fibers. Pain is not injury; the *quality of pain experiences* must not be confused with the physical event of breaking skin or bone. Warmth and cold are not "out there"; temperature changes occur "out there," but the *qualities of experience* must be generated by structures in the brain. Stinging, smarting, tickling, and itch have no external equivalents; the *qualities* are produced by built-in neuromodules whose neurosignatures innately produce the qualities.

We do not learn to feel qualities of experience: our brains are built to produce them. The inadequacy of the traditional peripheralist view becomes especially evident when we consider paraplegic patients with high-level complete spinal breaks. In spite of the absence of inputs from the body, virtually every quality of sensation and affect is experienced. It is known that the absence of input produces hyperactivity and abnormal firing patterns in spinal cells above the level of the break,[11] but how, from this jumble of activity, do we get the meaningful experience of movement, the coordination of limbs with other limbs, cramping pain in specific (nonexistent) muscle groups, and so on? This must occur in the brain, in which neurosignatures are produced by neuromatrixes that are triggered by the output of hyperactive cells.

When all sensory systems are intact, inputs modulate the continuous neuromatrix output to produce the wide variety of experiences we feel. We may feel position, warmth, and several kinds of pain and pressure all at once. It is a single unitary feeling, just as an orchestra produces a single unitary sound at any moment even though the sound comprises violins, cellos, horns, and so forth. Similarly, at a particular moment in time we feel complex qualities from all of the body. In addition, our experience of the body includes visual images, affect, and "knowledge" of the self (versus not-self), as well as the meaning of body parts in terms of social norms and values. It is hard to conceive of all of these bits and pieces coming together to produce a unitary body-self, but we can visualize a neuromatrix that impresses a characteristic signature on all the inputs that converge on it and thereby produces the never-ending stream of feeling from the body.

The experience of the body-self involves multiple dimensions—sensory, affective, evaluative, postural, and many others. The sensory dimensions are subserved, in part at least, by portions of the neuromatrix that lie in the sensory projection areas of the brain; the affective dimensions, Melzack assumed, are subserved by areas in the brainstem and limbic system. Each major psychological dimension (or quality) of experience, Melzack[12,13,15] proposed, is subserved by a particular portion of the neuromatrix that contributes a distinct portion of the total neurosignature. To use a musical analogy once again, it is like the strings, tympani, woodwinds, and brasses of a symphony orchestra that each make up a part of the whole; each instrument makes its unique contribution yet is an integral part of a single symphony that varies continually from beginning to end.

The neuromatrix resembles Hebb's "cell assembly" by being a widespread network of cells that subserves a particular psychological function. However, Hebb[16] conceived of the cell assembly as a network developed by gradual sensory learning, whereas Melzack proposed that the structure of the neuromatrix is predominantly determined by genetic factors, although its eventual synaptic architecture is influenced by sensory inputs. This emphasis on the genetic contribution to the brain does not diminish the importance of sensory inputs. The neuromatrix is a psychologically meaningful unit, developed by both heredity and learning, that represents an entire unified entity.[12,13,15]

Action Patterns: The Action-Neuromatrix

The output of the body neuromatrix, Melzack[12,13,15] proposed, is directed at two systems: (1) the neuromatrix that produces awareness of the output and (2) a neuromatrix involved in overt action patterns. In this discussion, it is important to keep in mind that just as there is a steady stream of awareness, there is also a steady output of behavior (including movements during sleep).

Behavior occurs only after the input has been at least partially synthesized and recognized. For example, when we respond to the experience of pain or itch, it is evident that the experience has been synthesized by the body-self neuromatrix (or relevant neuromodules) sufficiently for the neuromatrix to have imparted the neurosignature patterns that underlie the quality of experience, affect, and meaning. Apart from a few reflexes (e.g., withdrawal of a limb and eye blink), behavior occurs only after inputs have been analyzed and synthesized sufficiently to produce meaningful experience. When we reach for an apple, the visual input has clearly been synthesized by a neuromatrix so that it has three-dimensional shape, color, and meaning as an edible, desirable object, all of which are produced by the brain and are not in the object "out there." When we respond to pain (by withdrawal or even by telephoning for an ambulance), we respond to an experience that has sensory qualities, affect, and meaning as a dangerous (or potentially dangerous) event to the body.

Melzack[12,13,15] proposed that after inputs from the body undergo transformation in the body-neuromatrix, the appropriate action patterns are activated concurrently (or nearly so) with the neuromatrix for experience. Thus, in the action-neuromatrix, cyclical processing and synthesis produce activation of several possible patterns and their successive elimination until one particular pattern emerges as the most appropriate for the circumstances at the moment. In this way, input and output are synthesized simultaneously, in parallel, not in series. This permits a smooth, continuous stream of action patterns.

The command, which originates in the brain, to perform a pattern such as running activates the neuromodule, which then produces firing in sequences of neurons that send precise messages through ventral horn neuron pools to appropriate sets of muscles. At the same time, the output patterns from the body-neuromatrix that engage the neuromodules for particular actions are also projected to the sentient neural hub and produce experience. In this way, the brain commands may produce the experience of movement of phantom limbs even though the patient has no limbs to move and no proprioceptive feedback. Indeed, reports by paraplegic patients of terrible fatigue resulting from persistent bicycling movements[17] and the painful fatigue in a tightly clenched phantom fist in arm amputees[18] indicate that feelings of effort and fatigue are produced by the signature of a neuromodule rather than by particular input patterns from muscles and joints.

The phenomenon of phantom limbs has allowed researchers to examine some fundamental assumptions in psychology. Among these assumptions are that sensations are produced only by stimuli and perceptions in the absence of stimuli are psychologically abnormal. Yet phantom limbs, as well as phantom seeing,[19] indicate that this notion is wrong. The brain does more than detect and analyze inputs; it generates perceptual experience even when no external inputs occur.

Another entrenched assumption is that perception of one's body results from sensory inputs that leave a memory in the brain; the total of these signals becomes the body image. However, the existence of phantoms in people born without a limb or who lost a limb at an early age suggests that the neural networks for perceiving the body and its parts are built into the brain.[12,13,20,21] The absence of inputs does not stop the networks from generating messages about missing body parts; the networks continue to produce such messages throughout life. In short, phantom limbs are a mystery only if we assume that the body sends sensory messages to a passively receiving brain. Phantoms become comprehensible once we recognize that the brain generates the experience of the body. Sensory inputs merely modulate that experience; they do not directly cause it.

Pain and Neuroplasticity

The specificity concept of the nervous system for had no place for "plasticity," in which neuronal and synaptic functions are capable of being molded or shaped so that they influence subsequent perceptual experiences. Plasticity related to pain represents persistent functional changes, or "somatic memories,"[22,23] produced in the nervous system by injuries or other pathologic events. The recognition that such changes can occur is essential to understanding the chronic pain syndromes, such as low back pain and phantom limb pain, that persist and often destroy the lives of the people who suffer them.

Denervation Hypersensitivity and Neuronal Hyperactivity

Sensory disturbances associated with nerve injury have been closely linked to alterations in central nervous system (CNS) function. Markus, Pomerantz and Krushelnyky[24] demonstrated that the development of hypersensitivity in a rat's hind paw following sciatic nerve section occurs concurrently with the expansion of the saphenous nerve's somatotopic projection in the spinal cord. Nerve injury may also lead to the development of increased neuronal activity at various levels of the somatosensory system (see review by Coderre et al[25]). In addition to spontaneous activity generated from the neuroma, peripheral neurectomy also leads to increased spontaneous activity in the dorsal root ganglion and the spinal cord. Furthermore, after dorsal rhizotomy, increases in spontaneous neural activity occur in the dorsal horn, the spinal trigeminal nucleus, and the thalamus.

Clinical neurosurgery studies reveal a similar relationship between denervation and CNS hyperactivity. Neurons in the somatosensory thalamus of patients with neuropathic pain display high spontaneous firing rates, abnormal bursting activity, and evoked responses to stimulation of body areas that normally do not activate these neurons.[26,27] The site of abnormality in thalamic function appears to be somatotopically related to the painful region. In patients with complete spinal cord transection and dysesthesias referred below the level of the break, neuronal hyperactivity was observed in thalamic regions that had lost their normal sensory input, but not in

regions with apparently normal afferent input.[26] Furthermore, in patients with neuropathic pain, electrical stimulation of subthalamic, thalamic, and capsular regions may evoke pain,[28] and in some instances it may even reproduce the patient's pain.[29–31]

Direct electrical stimulation of spontaneously hyperactive cells evokes pain in some but not all patients with pain; this finding raises the possibility that in certain patients the observed changes in neuronal activity may contribute to the perception of pain.[26] Studies of patients undergoing electrical brain stimulation during brain surgery reveal that pain is rarely elicited by test stimuli unless the patient suffers from a chronic pain problem. However, brain stimulation can elicit pain responses in patients with chronic pain that does not involve extensive nerve injury or deafferentation. Lenz et al[30] described the case of a woman with unstable angina who, during electrical stimulation of the thalamus, reported "heart pain like what I took nitroglycerin for" except that "it starts and stops suddenly". The possibility that the patient's angina was the result of myocardial strain, and not the activation of a somatosensory pain memory, was ruled out by demonstrating that electrocardiograms, blood pressure, and cardiac enzymes remained unchanged over the course of stimulation.

It is possible that receptive field expansions and spontaneous activity generated in the CNS following peripheral nerve injury are, in part, mediated by alterations in normal inhibitory processes in the dorsal horn. Within 4 days of a peripheral nerve section, one notes a reduction in the dorsal root potential and, therefore, in the presynaptic inhibition it represents.[32] Nerve section also induces a reduction in the inhibitory effect of A-fiber stimulation on activity in dorsal horn neurons.[33] Furthermore, nerve injury affects descending inhibitory controls from brainstem nuclei. In the intact nervous system, stimulation of the locus ceruleus[34] or the nucleus raphe magnus[35] produces inhibition of dorsal horn neurons. Following dorsal rhizotomy, however, stimulation of these areas produces excitation, rather than inhibition, in half the cells studied.[36]

Advances in our understanding of the mechanisms that underlie pathologic pain have important implications for the treatment of both acute and chronic pain. Because it has been established that intense noxious stimulation produces sensitization of CNS neurons, it is possible to direct treatments not only at the site of peripheral tissue damage, but also at the site of central changes (see review by Coderre and Katz[37]). Furthermore, it may be possible in some instances to prevent the development of central sensitization, which contributes to pathologic pain states. The evidence that acute postoperative pain intensity and the amount of pain medication patients require after surgery are reduced by preoperative administration of variety of agents administered by the epidural[38–40] or systemic route[41–43] suggests that the surgically induced afferent injury barrage arriving within the CNS, and the central sensitization it induces, can be prevented or at least obtunded significantly (see review by Katz[44]). The reduction in acute pain intensity associated with preoperative epidural anesthesia may even translate into reduced pain[45] and pain disability[46] weeks after patients have left the hospital and returned home.

The finding that amputees are more likely to develop phantom limb pain if they had pain in the limb before amputation[23] raises the possibility that the development of longer-term neuropathic pain also can be prevented by reducing the potential for central sensitization at the time of amputation (see Katz and Melzack[47]). Whether chronic postoperative problems such as painful scars, postthoracotomy chest wall pain, and phantom limb and stump pain can be reduced by blocking perioperative nociceptive inputs awaits additional well-controlled clinical trials (see Katz and Seltzer[48]). Furthermore, research is required to determine whether multiple-treatment approaches (involving local and epidural anesthesia, as well as pretreatment with opiates and anti-inflammatory drugs) that produce effective blockade of afferent input may also prevent or relieve other forms of severe chronic pain such as postherpetic neuralgia[49] and complete regional pain syndrome. It is hoped that a combination of new pharmacologic developments, careful clinical trials, and an increased understanding of the contribution and mechanisms of noxious stimulus–induced neuroplasticity will lead to improved clinical treatment and prevention of pathologic pain.

Pain and Psychopathology

Pains that do not conform to present day anatomic and neurophysiologic knowledge are often attributed to psychological dysfunction.

There are many pains whose cause is not known. If a diligent search has been made in the periphery and no cause is found, we have seen that clinicians act as though there was only one alternative. They blame faulty thinking, which for many classically thinking doctors is the same thing as saying that there is no cause and even no disease. They ignore a century's work on disorders of the spinal cord and brainstem and target the mind....These are the doctors who repeat again and again to a Second World War amputee in pain that there is nothing wrong with him and that it is all in his head.[50, p. 107]

This view of the role of psychological generation in pain persists to this day notwithstanding evidence to the contrary. Psychopathology has been proposed to underlie phantom limb pain,[18] dyspareunia,[51] orofacial pain,[52] and a host of others including pelvic pain, abdominal pain, chest pain, and headache.[53] However, the complexity of the pain transmission circuitry described in the previous sections means that many pains that defy our current understanding will ultimately be explained without having to resort to a psychopathologic etiology. Pain that is "nonanatomic" in distribution, spread of pain to noninjured territory, pain that is said to be out of proportion to the degree of injury, and pain in the absence of injury have all, at one time or another, been used as evidence to support the idea that psychological disturbance underlies the pain. Yet each of these features of supposed psychopathology can now be explained by neurophysiologic mechanisms that involve an interplay between peripheral and central neural activity.[3,52]

Data linking the immune system and the CNS have provided an explanation for another heretofore medically unexplained pain problem. Mirror-image pain, or *allochiria,* has puzzled clinicians and basic scientists ever since it was first documented in the late 1800s.[54] Injury to one side of the body is experienced as pain at the site of injury as well as at the contralateral, mirror-image point.[55,56] Animal studies show that induction of sciatic inflammatory neuritis by perisciatic microinjection of immune system activators results in both ipsilateral hyperalgesia and hyperalgesia at the mirror-image point on the opposite side in the territory of the contralateral healthy sciatic nerve.[57] Moreover, both ipsilateral hyperalgesia and contralateral hyperalgesia are prevented or reversed by intrathecal injection of a variety of proinflammatory cytokine antagonists.[58]

Mirror-image pain is likely not a unitary phenomenon, and other nonimmune mechanisms may also be involved.[59] For example, human[60] and animal[61] evidence points to a potential combination of central and peripheral contributions to mirror-image pain because nerve injury to one side of the body has been shown to result in a 50% reduction in the innervation of the territory of the same nerve on the opposite side of the body in uninjured skin.[61] Although documented contralateral neurite loss can occur in the absence of contralateral pain or hyperalgesia, pain intensity at the site of the injury correlates significantly with the extent of contralateral neurite loss.[60] This finding raises the intriguing possibility that the intensity of pain at the site of an injury may be facilitated by contralateral neurite loss induced by the ipsilateral injury,[61] a situation that most clinicians would never have imagined possible.

Taken together, these novel mechanisms that explain some of the most puzzling pain symptoms must keep us mindful that emotional distress and psychological disturbance in our patients are not at the root of the pain. Attributing pain to a psychological disturbance is damaging to the patient and provider alike; it poisons the patient-provider relationship by introducing an element of mutual distrust and implicit (and at times, explicit) blame. It is devastating to the patient, who feels at fault, disbelieved, and alone.

Conclusion: The Multiple Determinants of Pain

The neuromatrix theory of pain proposes that the neurosignature for pain experience is determined by the synaptic architecture of the neuromatrix, which is produced by genetic and sensory influences. The neurosignature pattern is also modulated by sensory inputs and by cognitive events, such as psychological stress.[62] Furthermore, stressors, physical as well as psychological, act on stress regulation systems, which may produce lesions of muscle, bone, and nerve tissue and thereby contribute to the neurosignature patterns that give rise to chronic pain. In short, the neuromatrix, as a result of homeostasis regulation patterns that have failed, may produce the destructive conditions that give rise to many of the chronic pains that so far have been resistant to treatments developed primarily to manage pains that are triggered by sensory inputs. The stress regulation system, with its complex, delicately balanced interactions, is an integral part of the multiple contributions that give rise to chronic pain.

The neuromatrix theory guides us away from the Cartesian concept of pain as a sensation produced by injury or other tissue disease and toward the concept of pain as a multidimensional experience produced by multiple influences. These influences range from the existing synaptic architecture of the neuromatrix to influences from within the body and from other areas in the brain. Genetic influences on synaptic architecture may determine—or predispose to—the development of chronic pain syndromes. Figure 1.3 summarizes the factors that contribute to the output pattern from the neuromatrix that produce the sensory, affective, and cognitive dimensions of pain experience and the resultant behavior.

Multiple inputs act on the neuromatrix programs and contribute to the *output* neurosignature. They include the following: (1) sensory inputs (cutaneous, visceral, and other somatic receptors); (2) visual and other sensory inputs that influence the cognitive interpretation of the situation; (3) phasic and tonic cognitive and emotional inputs from other areas of the brain; (4) intrinsic neural inhibitory modulation inherent in all brain function; and (5) the activity of the body's stress regulation systems, including cytokines as well as the endocrine, autonomic, immune, and opioid systems. We have traveled a long way from the psychophysical concept that seeks a simple one-to-one relationship between injury and pain. We now have a theoretical framework in which a genetically determined template for the body-self is modulated by the powerful stress system and the cognitive functions of the brain, in addition to the traditional sensory inputs.

References

Full references for this chapter can be found on www.expertconsult.com.

Chapter **2**

Anatomy of the Pain Processing System

Tony L. Yaksh and Z. David Luo

Anatomic Systems Associated with Pain Processing*

Extreme mechanical distortion, thermal stimuli (>42°C [108°F]), or changes in the chemical milieu (plasma products, pH, potassium) at the peripheral sensory terminal will evoke the verbal report of pain in humans and efforts to escape in animals, as well as the elicitation of activity in the adrenal-pituitary axis. This chapter provides a broad overview of the circuitry that serves in the transduction and encoding of this information. First, the stimuli already mentioned evoke activity in specific groups of small myelinated or unmyelinated primary afferents of ganglionic sensory neurons, which make their synaptic contact with several distinct populations of dorsal horn neurons. By long spinal tracts and through a variety of intersegmental systems, the information gains access to supraspinal centers that lie in the brainstem and in the thalamus. These rostrally projecting systems represent the substrate by which unconditioned, high-intensity somatic and visceral stimuli give rise to escape behavior and verbal report of pain. This circuitry constitutes the afferent limb of the pain pathway.

Primary Afferents†

Fiber Classes

Sensory neurons in dorsal root ganglia have a single process (glomerulus) that bifurcates into a peripheral (nerve) and central (root) axon. The peripheral axon collects sensory input originating from the environment of the innervated tissue. The central axon relays sensory input to the spinal cord or brainstem. Sensory axons are classified according to their diameter, state of myelination, and conduction velocity, as outlined in **Table 2.1**. In general, conduction velocity varies directly with axon diameter and the presence of myelination. Thus, Aβ axons are large and myelinated, and they conduct rapidly; A∂ axons are smaller in diameter and myelinated, and they conduct more slowly; and C fibers are small and unmyelinated, and they conduct very slowly.

Properties of Primary Afferent Function

Recording from single peripheral afferent fibers reveals three important characteristics. First, in the absence of stimulation, minimal, if any, "spontaneous" afferent traffic occurs. Accordingly,

---

*For a more detailed discussion of the material in this section, see Reference 1.

†For more detailed discussions of the material in this section, see References 2 to 4.

the system operates on a very high signal-to-noise ratio. Second, regardless of the fiber type examined, with increasing intensities of the appropriate stimulus, a monotonic increase in the discharge frequency for that axon is observed (**Fig. 2.1**). This finding reflects the fact that the more intense the stimulus, the greater is the depolarization of the terminal and the more frequently will the axon discharge. Third, different axons may respond most efficiently to a particular stimulus modality. This modality specificity reflects the nature of the terminal properties of the particular afferent axon that transduces the physical or chemical stimulus into a depolarization of the axon. These nerve endings may be morphologically specialized, as with the pacinian corpuscle that is found on the terminals of large afferents. The specialized structure translates the mechanical distortion of the structure

Table 2.1 **Classification of Primary Afferents by Physical Characteristics, Conduction Velocity, and Effective Stimuli**

Fiber Class*	Velocity Group*	Effective Stimuli
A-beta	Group II (>40–50 m/sec)	Low-threshold Specialized nerve endings (pacinian corpuscles)
A-delta	Group III (>10 and <40 m/sec)	Low-threshold mechanical or thermal High-threshold mechanical or thermal Specialized nerve endings
C	Group IV (<2 m/sec)	High-threshold thermal, mechanical, or chemical Free nerve endings

*The Erlanger-Gasser A-beta/A-delta/C classification scheme is based on anatomic characteristics. The Lloyd-Hunt group II/III/IV classification scheme is based on conduction velocity in muscle afferents.

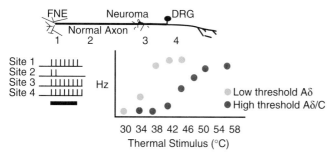

Fig. 2.1 *Top:* Schema of C fiber with peripheral free nerve ending (FNE; a region of normal axon and a local injury [neuroma] and the dorsal root ganglion [DRG]). In this schema, a pressure stimulus is applied to the axon at the four sites (FNE, normal axon, neuroma, and DRG), and the characteristic response is displayed in the *lower left* drawing. The normal axon does not transduce the continued mechanical distortion, whereas such transduction does occur at sites 1, 3, and 4. On the *lower right*, low-threshold A-delta (Aδ) and high-threshold A-delta/C fibers typically show little if any spontaneous activity; both will show a monotonic increase in response to increasing stimulus intensities. The low-threshold axon shows a monotonic increase over a range of intensities that are not aversive. This would be a "warmth" detector. The C fiber, however, does not begin to discharge until a temperature is reached that would correspond with the behavioral report of increasing pain. This response pattern would describe that of a nociceptor.

into a transient opening of sodium channels in that axon, thus generating a brief burst of action potential.

At the other extreme, the axon terminal may display no evident physical structure and be classified as a "free nerve ending." Such endings are commonly associated with small, unmyelinated C fibers. The simplicity of the nerve ending as implied by this name is misleading. Such a terminal is often able to transduce a variety of stimuli including mechanical, thermal, and chemical. As indicated in Table 2.1, A-beta (group II) fibers are activated by low-threshold mechanical stimuli (i.e., mechanoreceptors). Fibers that conduct at A-delta velocity (group III fibers) may belong to populations that are low or high threshold, and mechanical or thermal. Low-threshold afferents may begin firing at temperatures that are not noxious (30°C [86°F]) and increase their firing rate monotonically, although in this range, we perceive the stimulus as warm but not noxious. Other populations of A-delta fibers may begin to show activation at temperatures that are mildly noxious and increase their firing rates up to very high temperatures (52°C to 55°C [126°F to 131°F]). Slowly conducting afferents constitute the largest population of afferent axons. Most of these afferents are activated by high-threshold thermal, mechanical, and chemical stimuli and are called *C-polymodal nociceptors* (see Fig. 2.1). For these axons, the nature of the stimuli, which will evoke activity, is endowed by the nature of the specialized transduction proteins that are present in these terminals. Many of these transducer proteins are particularly sensitive to a range of hot or cold, but in addition they may respond to particular chemicals. One such well-characterized channel is TRPV1, which responds to noxious temperatures and to the molecule capsaicin (which evokes a sensation of intense heat when it is applied to the skin) (**Fig. 2.2**).

An important characteristic of these polymodal nociceptors is that they are also readily activated in a concentration-dependent fashion by specific agents released into the chemical milieu. Such agents, released from local injured cells or inflammatory cells, include a variety of amines (5-hydroxytryptamine, histamine), lipid mediators (prostaglandins), kinins (bradykinin), acidic pH, cytokines (interleukin-1ß) and enzymes (trypsin). Such products can evoke direct activation of the fibers and facilitate

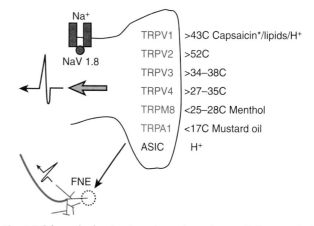

Fig. 2.2 Schematic showing transducer channels on a C-fiber terminal. The range of optimal temperature activation and agents that can activate these channels are shown. Different terminals may express different combinations of transducers, and this would define the thermal response properties of that sensory axon. Channel activation depolarizes voltage sensitive sodium (NaV) channels in the axon. Nav1.8 channels are often found in C fibers.

their activity though their eponymous receptors located on the terminals of these C fibers. This process probably represents the principal mechanism of activating afferents after the acute injury. The nature of these products and their effects on the sensory terminals are discussed in Chapter 3.

Afferents with High Thresholds and Pain Behavior

Electrophysiologic and correlated behavioral evidence indicates that information that can generate a pain event enters the central nervous system by the activation of small-diameter, myelinated (group III-A or A-delta) or unmyelinated (group IV or C) afferents. Thus, single-unit recording in nerve fascicles in humans reveals a close correlation between the dull pain induced by a focal high-intensity thermal stimulus (second pain) and activity in fibers conducting at velocities of less than 1 m/second. Similarly, local anesthetics at low concentrations transiently block conduction in small, but not large, afferents, thus blocking the sensation evoked by high-threshold stimuli and leaving light touch intact. The afferent axons, particularly those derived from unmyelinated fibers, show extensive branching as they proceed distally, and most peripheral terminals of small afferents show little evidence of specialization and terminate as "free" nerve endings. Ample evidence indicates that these "free" nerve endings, commonly designated *polymodal nociceptors,* are characteristically activated only by high-intensity physical stimuli, and this property accounts for the peripheral specificity associating A-delta/C-fiber activity with pain. This transduction specificity is best exemplified in tooth pulp and cornea, in which "free" nerve endings predominate, and local stimulation is painful.

Under certain conditions, low-intensity tactile or thermal stimuli may, in fact, generate a pain state. This anomalous linkage between noninjurious stimuli and pain is referred to as *hyperalgesia.* More specifically, when it involves light mechanical stimuli, it is referred to as *tactile allodynia.* Three practical examples may be cited: (1) local tissue injury such as after a local sunburn leading to increased thermal and tactile sensitivity; (2) inflammation such as in rheumatoid arthritis leading to a state in which normal joint movement is painful; and (3) injury to the peripheral nerve leading to states in which light touch is aversive.

Spinal Dorsal Horn*

Afferent Projections

In the peripheral nerve, large and small afferents are anatomically intermixed in collections of fascicles. As the nerve root approaches the spinal cord, the tendency is for the large myelinated afferents to move medially and to displace the small, unmyelinated afferents laterally. Thus, although this pattern is not absolute, large and small afferent axons enter the dorsal horn by the medial and lateral aspects of the dorsal root entry zone (DREZ), respectively. Some unmyelinated afferent fibers that arise from dorsal root ganglion cells also pass into the spinal cord by the *ventral* roots, and these *ventral root afferents* likely account for pain reports evoked by ventral root stimulation in classic clinical studies.

The sensory innervation of the body projects in a rostrocaudal distribution to the ipsilateral spinal dorsal horn.

Table 2.2 Principal Aspects of Dorsal Horn Organization

Anatomic Region	Rexed Lamina(e)	Afferent Terminals	Nociceptive Cells
Marginal layer	I	A-delta/CA-beta	Marginal
Substantia gelatinosa	II	A-beta/A-delta/C	SG
Nucleus proprius	III/IV/V/VI	A-beta/A-delta	WDR
Central canal	X	A-delta/C	SG-type
Motor horn	VII/VIII/IX	A-beta	

SG, substantia gelatinosa; WDR, wide dynamic range.

Innervation of the head and neck is mediated by a variety of cranial nerves that project into the brainstem.

Anatomy of the Dorsal Horn

In the rostrocaudal axis, the spinal cord is broadly divided into the sacral, lumbar, thoracic, and cervical segments. At each spinal level, in the transverse plane, the spinal cord is further divided on the basis of descriptive anatomy into several laminae (*Rexed laminae*) (**Table 2.2** and **Fig. 2.3**).

On entering the spinal cord, the central processes of the primary afferents send their projections into the dorsal horn. In general, terminals from the small myelinated fibers (A-delta) terminate in the marginal zone or lamina I of Rexed, the ventral portion of lamina II (II inner), and throughout lamina V. Larger myelinated fibers (A-beta) terminate in lamina IV and the deep dorsal horn (laminae V to VI). Fine-caliber, unmyelinated C fibers generally terminate throughout laminae I and II and in lamina X around the central canal.

In addition to sending their axons into the dorsal horn at the segment of entry, primary afferents also collateralize sending axons rostrally and caudally into the tract of Lissauer (small unmyelinated fibers) and into the dorsal columns (large myelinated axons). These afferents collateralize at intervals to send projections into increasingly distal segments. This organizational property emphasizes that input from a single root may primarily activate cells in the segment of entry but can also influence the excitability of neurons in segments distal to the segment of entry (**Fig. 2.4**).

Dorsal Horn Neurons†

Although exceedingly complex, the second-order nociresponsive elements in the dorsal horn may be considered in several principal classes on the basis of their approximate anatomic location and their response properties.

Anatomic Localization
Marginal Zone (Lamina I)

These large neurons are oriented transversely across the cap of the dorsal gray matter (**Fig. 2.5**). Consistent with their locations, they receive input from mainly A-delta and C fibers and respond to intense cutaneous and muscle stimulation. Marginal neurons project to the contralateral

---

*For a more detailed discussion of the material in this section, see Reference 5.

†For more detailed discussions of the material in this section, see References 4 and 6.

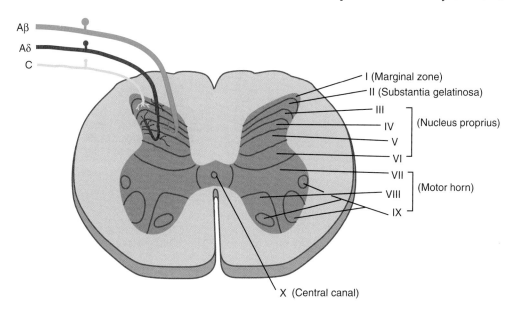

Fig. 2.3 Schematic showing the Rexed lamination *(right)* and the approximate organization of the afferents to the spinal cord *(left)* as they enter at the dorsal root entry zone and then penetrate into the dorsal horn to terminate in the laminae I and II (A-delta [Aδ]/C) or penetrate more deeply to loop upward and terminate as high as lamina III (A-beta [Aβ]). *Photo inset* shows a left dorsal horn with the root entry zone.

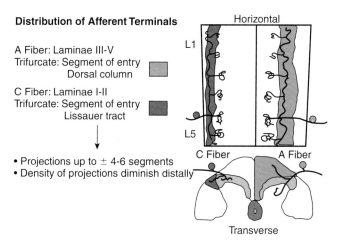

Fig. 2.4 Schematic displaying the ramification of C fibers *(left)* into the dorsal horn and collateralization into the tract of Lissauer *(stippled area)* and of A fibers *(right)* into the dorsal columns *(striped area)* and into the dorsal horn. The most dense terminations are within the segment of entry, and collateralizations into the dorsal horns at the more distal spinal segments are less dense. This density of collateralization corresponds to the potency of the excitatory drive into these distal segments.

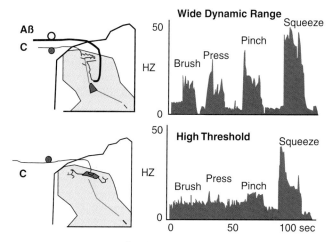

Fig. 2.5 Firing patterns of a dorsal horn wide dynamic range (WDR) neuron and a high-threshold spinothalamic neuron. Graphs present the neuronal responses to graded intensities of mechanical stimulation applied to the receptive fields.

thalamus and to the parabrachial region through the contralateral ventrolateral tracts (see later) of ascending pathways. Other marginal neurons project intrasegmentally and intersegmentally along the dorsal and dorsolateral white matter.

Substantia Gelatinosa (Lamina II)

The substantia gelatinosa contains numerous cell types. Many cells are local interneurons and likely play an important role as inhibitory and excitatory interneurons that regulate local excitability; however, some of these cells clearly project rostrally. Significant proportions of the substantia gelatinosa neurons receive direct input from C fibers and indirect input from A-delta fibers from lamina I and deep dorsal horn. These neurons are frequently excited by activation of thermal receptive or mechanical nociceptive afferents. Many of these cells exhibit complex response patterns with prolonged periods

of excitation and inhibition following afferent activation and reflect the complicated network that regulates local excitability by local interneurons.

Nucleus Proprius (Laminae III, IV, and V)

These magnocellular neurons send their dendritic tree up into the overlying laminae (see Fig. 2.5). Consistent with this organization, many cells in this region receive large afferent (Aß) input onto its cell body and dendrites. In addition, these neurons receive input either directly or through excitatory interneurons, from small afferents (Aδ and C), which terminate in the superficial dorsal horn.

Central Canal (Lamina X)

Branches of small primary afferent fibers enter the region. This area is a peptide-rich area, and cells respond primarily to high-threshold temperature stimuli and noxious pinch with small receptive fields. Cells in this region also receive significant visceral input.

Functional Properties

Two important functional classes of neurons are frequently described: nociceptive specific and wide dynamic range (WDR).

Nociceptive Specific

Lamina I neurons tend to receive primarily high-threshold (small afferent) input. Accordingly, starting at relatively high stimulus intensities, these cells begin to show a threshold increase in discharge that is increased over the increasingly aversive range of stimulus intensities (see Fig. 2.5). In that manner, many of these cells are nociceptive specific.

Wide Dynamic Range Neurons

Many cells in the nucleus proprius have three interesting functional characteristics:

1. Given their connectivity (high threshold small afferents on the distal terminals and low threshold large afferents on their ascending dendrites and soma), these neurons display excitation driven by low- and high-threshold afferent input. This gives the WDR neurons the property of responding with increased frequency as the stimulus intensity is elevated from a very low intensity to a very high intensity (e.g., they have a *wide dynamic response* range). Thus, stimuli ranging from light innocuous touch evoke activity that increases as the intensity of pressure or pinch is increased (see Fig. 2.5). In addition to this property, the WDR neurons have two other characteristics.

2. Organ convergence: Depending on the spinal level, a neuron in the nucleus proprius may be activated by both somatic stimuli and activation of visceral afferent. This convergence results in a comingling of excitation for a visceral organ and a specific area of the body surface and leads to referral of input from that visceral organ to that area of the body surface. A given population of WDR neurons is excited by cutaneous or deep (muscle and joint) input applied within the dermatome coinciding with the segmental location of the cell. Thus, T1 and T5 root stimulation activates WDR neurons that are also excited by coronary artery occlusion. These viscerosomatic and musculosomatic convergences onto dorsal horn neurons underlie the phenomenon of referred visceral or deep muscle or bone pain to particular body surfaces (**Fig. 2.6**).

3. Low-frequency ($>\approx 0.33$ Hz) repetitive stimulation of C fibers, but not A fibers, produces a gradual increase in the frequency discharge until the neuron is in a state of virtually continuous discharge ("wind-up"). This property is discussed later.

Ascending Spinal Tracts[*]

Activity evoked in the spinal cord by high-threshold stimuli reaches supraspinal sites by several long and intersegmental tract systems that travel within the ventrolateral cord and to a lesser degree in the dorsal quadrant.

Ventral Funicular Projection Systems

Within the ventrolateral quadrant of the spinal cord, several systems have been identified, on the basis of their

[*]For more detailed discussions of the material in this section, see References 5 and 7.

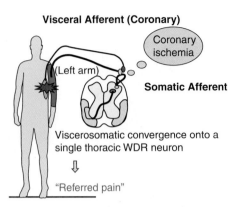

Fig. 2.6 Example of organ convergence: T1 and T5 root stimulation activates wide dynamic range (WDR) neurons that are also excited by coronary artery occlusion. These results indicate that the phenomenon of referred visceral pain has its substrate in the viscerosomatic and musculosomatic convergence onto dorsal horn neurons.

supraspinal projections. These include the spinoreticular, spinomesencephalic, spinoparabrachial, and spinothalamic tracts, which constitute the anterolateral system. These systems originate primarily from the dorsal horn neurons that are postsynaptic to primary afferents. These cells may project either ipsilaterally or contralaterally in the spinal cord. Classic studies showed that unilateral section of the ventrolateral quadrant yields a contralateral loss in pain and temperature sense in dermatomes below the spinal level of the section, a finding indicating that the ascending tracts may travel rostrally several segments before crossing. These findings led to the surgical ventrolateral cordotomy that was used in the early 20th century as an important method of pain control. Conversely, stimulation of the ventrolateral tracts in awake subjects undergoing percutaneous cordotomies results in reports of contralateral warmth and pain. Midline myelotomies that destroy fibers crossing the midline at the levels of the cut (as well as the cells in lamina X) produce bilateral pain deficits. As first described by William Gower in the 1890s, these observations suggest that predominantly crossed pathways in the ventrolateral quadrant are important for nociception.

Dorsal Funicular Projection Systems

The dorsal column medial lemniscal system is a major ascending pathway transmitting sensory information. This system is mainly composed of the collaterals of larger-diameter primary afferents transmitting tactile sensation and limb proprioception, Most fibers in the medial lemniscal system ascend from the spinal cord *ipsilaterally* to the medulla, where they synapse on neurons in the caudal brainstem dorsal column nuclei, which send axons across the medulla to form the medial lemniscus.

Intersegmental Systems

Early studies showed that alternating hemisections poorly modify the behavioral or the autonomic responses to strong stimuli. Systems that project for short distances ipsilaterally may contribute to the rostrad transmission of nociceptive information. Several segmental pathways relevant to the rostrad transmission of nociceptive information are the lateral

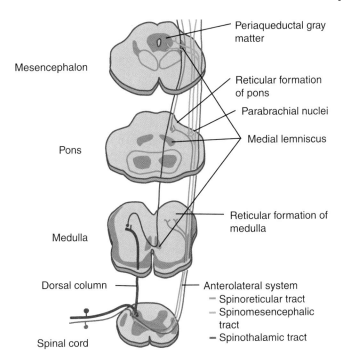

Fig. 2.7 Schematic demonstrating the brainstem projections of spinal neurons into the medulla and mesencephalon. Third-order projections arising from the medullary and mesencephalic neurons project into the intralaminar and ventrobasal thalamus.

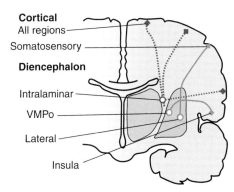

Fig. 2.8 Schematic displaying projections from thalamic neurons to various cortical regions. See text for further discussion. VMPo, posterior portion of the ventral medial nucleus.

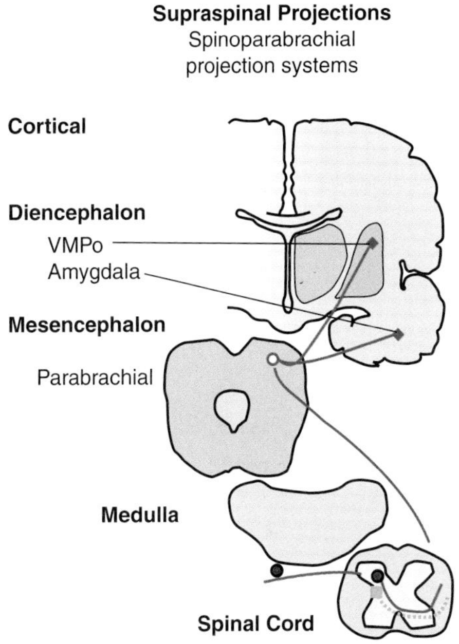

Fig. 2.9 Schematic demonstrating the spinal neuron projections into the parabrachial region and third-order parabrachial neurons projecting into the thalamus and amygdala. VMPo, posterior portion of the ventral medial nucleus.

tract of Lissauer, the dorsolateral propriospinal system, and the dorsal intracornual tract. Selective destruction of the dorsal gray matter (e.g., in the vicinity of the DREZ) has proved to be a possible method of pain management. This finding suggests the relevance of nonfunicular pathways traveling in the spinal gray matter.

Supraspinal Projections*

Spinofugal tracts traveling in the ventrolateral quadrant project principally into three brainstem regions: the medulla, the mesencephalon, and the diencephalon. Neurons in these regions then project further rostrally to the diencephalon and cortex or directly to cortical structures.

Spinoreticulothalamic Projections

This tract represents axons that are largely ipsilateral to the cell of origin. The tract terminates throughout the brainstem reticular formation. Spinomedullary input is believed to play an important role in initiating cardiovascular reflexes. The medullary reticular formation also performs as a relay station for the rostrad transmission of nociceptive information. These medullary neurons project into the intralaminar thalamic nucleus. This nucleus forms a shell around the medial dorsal aspects of the thalamus (**Fig. 2.7**). The intralaminar nucleus projects diffusely to wide areas of the cerebral cortex, including the frontal, parietal, and limbic regions. This forms part of the classic ascending reticular activating system and relates to mechanisms leading to increased global cortical activation (**Fig. 2.8**).

Spinomesencephalic Projections

Ipsilateral projections to this region terminate in periaqueductal gray and mesencephalic reticular formation. Stimulation of the mesencephalic central gray and adjacent mesencephalic reticular formation can evoke signs of intense discomfort in animals, whereas in humans autonomic responses are elicited along with reports of dysphoria. As with more caudal medullary sites, periaqueductal gray and reticular neurons project rostrally into the lateral thalamus (see Figs. 2.7 and 2.8; **Fig. 2.9**).

Spinoparabrachial Projections

These ascending nociceptive fibers originate predominantly from neurons in contralateral laminae. Projections of these neurons terminate in a group of neurons in the parabrachial area that send out axons to the central nucleus of the amygdala and the posterior portion of the ventral medial nucleus (VMpo) in the thalamus. The VMpo projects primarily to the insula (**Fig. 2.10**).

*For more detailed discussions of the material in this section, see References 8 and 9.

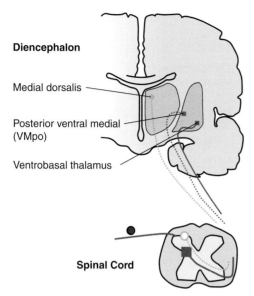

Fig. 2.10 Schematic demonstrating spinal lamina V wide dynamic range neurons projecting into the ventrobasal thalamus and lamina I neurons (high threshold) projecting into the posterior ventral medial nucleus (VMpo) and medial dorsalis neurons.

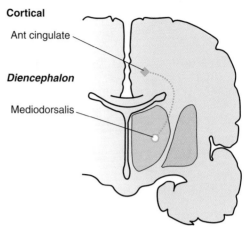

Fig. 2.11 Schematic demonstrating mediodorsalis neurons projecting into the anterior cingulate gyrus.

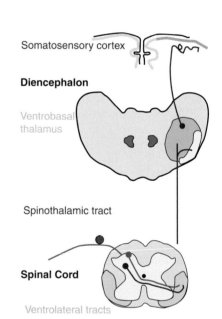

Cortical
SS cortex: Precise map
   (place/intensity/modality)

Thalamocortical projections
VBL -> Somatosensory cortex

Ascending thalamic projections
Lam V-> Ventrobasal (VBL)
           Precise anatomical mapping

Ascending axons in VLT
Spinothalamic

Spinofugal projections
Lam V: WDR-intensity encoded
           High degree of localization

Fig. 2.12 Schematic of an overview of the characteristics of the projections of wide dynamic range (WDR) lamina V (Lam V) neurons in to the somatotopically mapped ventrobasal (VBL) thalamus and from there to the somatosensory (SS) cortex. As described in the text, this organization suggests the properties that would mediate the sensory-discriminative aspects of pain. VLT, ventrolateral tract.

Spinothalamic Projections

This predominantly crossed system displays the following three principal targets of termination (**Fig. 2.11**):

1. The ventrobasal thalamus represents the classic somatosensory thalamic nucleus. Input is distributed in a strict somatotopic pattern. This region projects in a strict somatotopic organization to the somatosensory cortex (see Fig. 2.8).
2. The VMpo then projects into the insula.
3. The media thalamus receives primary input from lamina I (high-threshold nociceptive specific cells). Cells in this region then project to the anterior cingulate cortex (**Fig. 2.12**).

Functional Overview of Pain Processing Systems*

The preceding discussion considers various elements that constitute linkages whereby information generated by a high-intensity stimulus activates small high-threshold afferents and activates brainstem and cortical systems. With a broad perspective, several salient features of this system activated by high-threshold input can be emphasized.

---

*For more detailed discussions of the material in this section, see References 10 to 12.

Frequency Encoding

It appears evident that stimulus intensity in a given system is encoded in terms of frequency of discharge. This holds true for any given link at the level of the primary afferent for both high- and low-threshold axons, in the spinal dorsal horn for WDR, marginal neurons, and at brainstem and cortical loci. The relationship between stimulus intensity and the neuronal response is in the form of a monotonic increase in discharge frequency.

Afferent Line Labeling

Although frequency of discharge covaries with intensity, it is evident that the nature of the connectivity also defines the content of the afferent activity. As indicated, the biologic significance of a high-frequency burst of an Aß versus a high-threshold A-delta or C fiber for pain is evident.

Functionally Distinct Pathways

At the spinal level, it is possible to characterize two functionally distinct families of response. In one spinofugal projection system (see Fig. 2.11), WDR neurons encode information over a wide range of non-noxious to severely aversive intensities consistent with the convergence of low- and high-threshold afferent neurons (either directly or through interneurons) onto their dendrites and soma. These cells project heavily into a variety of brainstem and diencephalic sites to the somatosensory cortex. At every level, the map of the body surface is precisely preserved, as is the broad range of intensity-frequency encoding. In the second spinofugal projection system (see Fig. 2.12), populations of superficial marginal cells display a strong nociceptive-specific encoding property, as defined by the high-threshold afferent input that they receive. These marginal cells project heavily to the parabrachial nuclei, to the amygdala, to the VMpo, the insula, medial thalamic nuclei, and then to the anterior cingulate cortex.

The WDR system is uniquely able to preserve spatial localization information and information regarding the stimulus over a range of intensities from modest to extreme, as initially provided by the frequency response characteristics of the WDR neurons. This type of system is able to provide the information needed for mapping the "sensory-discriminative" dimension of pain. The nociceptive-specific pathway arising from the marginal cells appears less well organized in terms of its ability to encode precise place and response intensity until it is, by definition, potentially tissue injuring. These systems project heavily through the medial thalamic region and VMpo to the anterior cingulate and the insula/amygdala, respectively. These regions are classically appreciated to be associated with emotionality and affect. Accordingly, this type of circuitry would provide an important substrate for systems underlying the affective-motivational components of the pain experience. Functional magnetic resonance imaging and positron emission tomography have demonstrated that although non-noxious stimuli often have little effect, strong somatic and visceral stimuli initiate activation within the anterior cingulate cortex. This substrate involving a precise somatosensory map represents a system capable of mapping a sensory-discriminative dimension of pain. In contrast, the other system involving the limbic forebrain suggests a circuit that can mediate an "affective-motivational" component of the pain pathway. These dimensions were first formally described by Ronald Melzack and Ken Casey.

Plasticity of Ascending Projections

Whereas the pathways outlined are clearly pertinent to the nature of the message generated by a high-intensity stimulus, the encoding of a pain message depends not only on the physical characteristics of the otherwise effective stimulus but also on the properties of associated systems that can modulate (either up or down) the excitability of each of these synaptic linkages. Thus, local interneurons releasing γ-aminobutyric acid and glycine at the level of the spinal dorsal horn commonly regulate the frequency of discharge of second-order neurons excited by large afferent input. Pharmacologically blocking that local spinal inhibition can profoundly change the nature of the sensory experience to become highly aversive. This afferent plasticity is further considered in Chapter 3. In another dimension, such plasticity may also be seen at supraspinal levels. Thus, the potential role of this plasticity is reflected by the finding, in work by Pierre Rainville et al, hypnotic suggestions leading to an enhanced pain report in response to a given experimental stimulus resulted in greater activity in the anterior cingulate. Numerous lesions in humans and animals have been shown to dissociate the reported stimulus intensity psychophysically from its affective component. Such disconnection syndromes are produced by prefrontal lobectomies, cingulotomies, and temporal lobe–amygdala lesions.

Pharmacology of Afferent Transmitter Systems in Nociception[*]

An important question relates to the nature of the neurotransmitters and receptors that link the afferent projection systems. Such transmitter-receptor systems have several defining characteristics. First, the linkages between the primary afferent and second-order spinal neurons, the linkages between the spinofugal axon and the third-order axon, and so on, have as a common property that the interaction leads to the excitation of the proximate neurons. Thus, the neurotransmitters mediating that synaptic transmission are excitatory. For example, at the spinal level, no "monosynaptic inhibition driven by primary afferents" occurs. Although powerful inhibitory events occur in the dorsal horn (and at every synaptic link), such inhibition must take place because of the excitation of a second neuron that releases an inhibitory transmitter. Second, it is increasingly evident that neurotransmission at any given synaptic link may consist not of one transmitter but of several cocontained and coreleased transmitters. At the small primary afferent, an excitatory amino acid (glutamate) and a peptide (e.g., substance P [sP]) are typically released. Third, although not discussed further here, each synaptic link is subject to modifications because of a dynamic regulation of the presynaptic transmitter content and the postsynaptic receptor and its linkages (e.g., with repetitive stimulation, the glutamate receptor undergoes phosphorylation, which serves to accentuate its excitatory response to a given amount of glutamate).

Primary Afferent Transmitters

Considerable effort has been directed at establishing the identity of the excitatory transmitters in the primary afferent transmitters. Currently, excitatory amino acids, such as glutamate and certain peptides, including sP, vasoactive intestinal peptide (VIP),

---

[*]For more detailed discussions of the material in this section, see References 3 and 13 to 17.

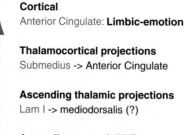

Cortical
Anterior Cingulate: **Limbic-emotion**

Thalamocortical projections
Submedius -> Anterior Cingulate

Ascending thalamic projections
Lam I -> mediodorsalis (?)

Ascending axons in VLT
Spinothalamic

Spinofugal projections
Lam I: Marginal-nociceptive specific
          Poor spatial encoding

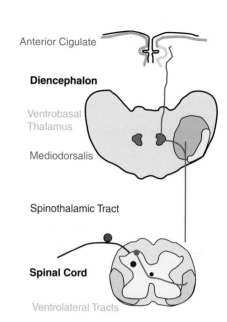

Fig. 2.13 Schematic of an overview of the characteristics of the projections of nociceptive-specific lamina I (Lam I) neurons into the mediodorsalis and from there to the anterior cingulate (Ant cingulate) cortex. As described in the text, this organization suggests the properties that would mediate the affective-motivational aspects of pain. VLT, ventrolateral tract.

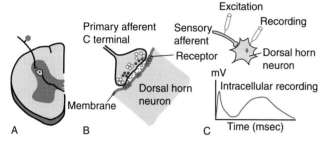

Fig. 2.14 Schematic displays the general characteristics of the primary afferent transmitters released from small, capsaicin-sensitive, primary afferents: C fibers. A, Small afferents terminate in laminae I and II of the dorsal horn and make synaptic contact with second-order spinal neurons. B, Peptides and excitatory amino acids are cocontained in small primary afferent ganglion cells (type B) and in dorsal horn terminals in dense core and clear core vesicles, respectively. C, On release, the excitatory amino acids are able to produce a rapid, early depolarization, whereas the peptides tend to evoke a long and prolonged depolarization of the second-order membrane. mV: transmembrane potential.

somatostatin, calcitonin gene–related peptide (CGRP), bombesin, and related peptides have been observed. C fibers possess the following characteristics (**Figs. 2.13** and **2.14**):

- Peptides have been shown to exist within subpopulations of small type B dorsal root ganglion cells.
- Peptides are in the dorsal horn of the spinal cord (where most primary afferent terminals are found), and these levels in the dorsal horn are reduced by rhizotomy or ganglionectomy or by treatment with the small afferent neurotoxin capsaicin (acting on the TRPV1 receptor).
- Many peptides are cocontained (e.g., sP and CGRP in the same C-fiber terminal) as well as contained with excitatory amino acids (e.g., sP and glutamate).
- Release of peptides is reduced by the spinal action of agents known to be analgesic, such as opiates (see later).
- Iontophoretic application onto the dorsal horn of the several amino acids and peptides found in primary afferents has been shown to produce excitatory effects. Amino acids produce very rapid, short-lasting depolarization. The peptides tend to produce delayed and long-lasting discharge.

- Local spinal administration of several agents such as sP and glutamate does yield pain behavior, a finding suggesting the possible role of these agents as transmitters in the pain process.

Receptor antagonists exist for the receptors acted on by many of these agents (sP, VIP, glutamate). By using such agents, it has been possible to demonstrate that the primary charge carrier for depolarization of the second-order neurons is the α-amino-3-hydroxyl-5-methyl-4-isoxazole-propionate (AMPA) subtype of the glutamate receptor. Block of other glutamate receptors (e.g., the *N*-methyl-D-aspartate [NMDA] receptor) or the peptidergic transmitter receptors such as for sP (neurokinin-1) typically have a modest effect on the acute excitability of the second-order neuron and appear to reflect their role in augmenting the excitability of the neuron. Given the plethora of excitatory transmitter receptors that decorate the second-order neuron, nociceptive-evoked excitation of the second-order neuron may be poorly modified by the block of a single receptor type.

Ascending Projection System Transmitters

Dorsal horn neurons projecting to brainstem sites have been shown to contain numerous peptides (including cholecystokinin, dynorphin, somatostatin, bombesin, VIPs, and sP). Glutamate has also been identified in spinothalamic projections, a finding suggesting the probable role of that excitatory amino acid. sP-containing fibers arising from brainstem sites have been shown to project to the parafascicular and central medial nuclei of the thalamus. In unanesthetized animals, the microinjection of glutamate in the vicinity of the terminals of ascending pathways, notably within the mesencephalic central gray area, evokes spontaneous painlike behavior with vocalization and vigorous efforts to escape, a finding emphasizing the presence of at least an NMDA site mediating the behavioral effects produced by NMDA in this region. Other systems will no doubt be identified as these supraspinal systems are studied in detail.

References

Full references for this chapter can be found on www.expertconsult.com.

Chapter 3

Dynamics of the Pain Processing System

Tony L. Yaksh and Z. David Luo

Primary afferent input results in the activation of numerous circuits at the spinal and supraspinal levels. As reviewed in Chapter 2, there are multiple linkages in these systems. An important consequence of research since the 1990s has been the appreciation that afferent input at each synaptic link is subject to modulation by a variety of specific inputs. The net result is that the response evoked by a given stimulus is subject to well-defined influences that can serve to attenuate or enhance the excitation produced by a given physical stimulus. Specifically, these interactive systems alter the encoding of the afferent message and thereby change the perceived characteristics of the stimulus.

For the sake of discussion, the processing of nociceptive information may be considered in terms of the pain behavior that arises from the following three conditions: (1) the behavior evoked by an acute activation of a high-threshold, slowly conducting afferent, (2) the exaggerated pain behavior (hyperalgesia/hyperesthesia) generated following local tissue injury or inflammation, and (3) the hyperalgesia that results secondary to a local peripheral nerve injury. Current work

suggests some convergence of these underlying mechanisms in the presence of certain persistent inflammatory states. An overview of the pharmacology and physiology of these dynamic states is provided subsequently.

Acute Activation of Afferent Pain Processing[*]

Acute activation of small afferents by a transient, noninjurious stimulus results in clearly defined pain behavior in humans and animals. This event is mediated by the local stimulus-evoked activation of small, high-threshold afferents leading to the release of excitatory afferent transmitters outlined previously (see Chapter 2) and, consequently, the depolarization of spinal projection neurons. The organization of this acutely driven system is typically modeled in terms

---

[*]For a more detailed discussion of the material in this section, see Reference 1.

of linear relationships among stimulus intensity, activity in the peripheral afferent, the magnitude of spinal transmitter release, and the activity of neurons that project out of the spinal cord to the brain. In its most straightforward rendition, this organization resembles the classic "pain pathway" that appears in most texts (**Fig. 3.1**).

Tissue Injury–Induced Hyperalgesia

Psychophysics of Tissue Injury*

With tissue injury, a triad of events is noted shortly after the initiation of the injury: (1) a dull throbbing, aching sensation; (2) an exaggerated response to a moderate intense stimulus (primary hyperalgesia); and (3) an enlarged area around the

*For more detailed discussions of the material in this section, see References 2 and 3.

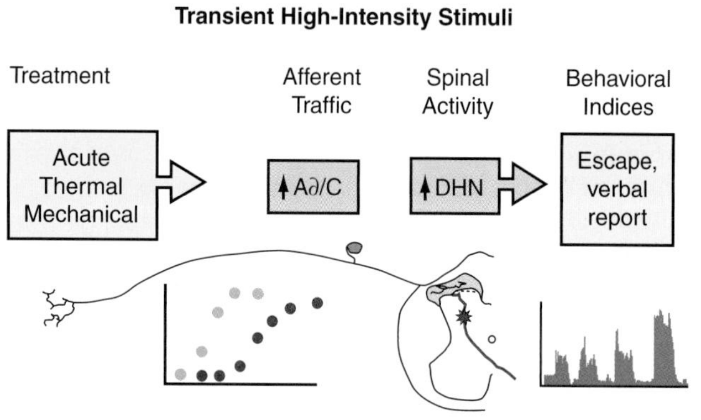

Transient High-Intensity Stimuli

Fig. 3.1 Schematic depicting the principal components of the afferent spinal cord response to an acute high-intensity afferent stimulus. A stimulus intensity–dependent increase in discharge frequency in specific populations of high-threshold primary afferents initiates a stimulus intensity–dependent increase in the firing of dorsal horn neurons (DHN) that projects to higher centers (a wide dynamic range [WDR] neuron is shown here). The outflow of the spinal cord projects to higher centers, as described in Chapter 2.

injury site where a moderate stimulus applied to uninjured tissue generates an aversive sensation (secondary hyperalgesia). It is important to understand what initiates these pain components. As discussed later, it is evident that these events reflect both peripheral and central consequences of the injury and the stimulus presented.

Peripheral Afferent Terminal and Tissue Injury†

Afferent Response Properties

Injury and inflammation in the vicinity of the sensory terminals increase the excitability of C-polymodal nociceptors innervating the injured site. This enhanced excitability is reflected by the appearance of spontaneous afferent activity and a left shift in the stimulus-response curve of the afferent (**Fig. 3.2**). These events underlie the "triple response": a red flush around the site of the stimulus (local arterial dilation), local edema (capillary permeability), and a regional reduction in the magnitude of the stimulus required to elicit a pain response (i.e., hyperalgesia). This local response is in part neurogenic in that it results from local antidromic activity in the peripheral collaterals of the sensory terminal. Here activity initiated in the branch proceeds orthodromically. At a local branch point, the action potential proceeds centrally and antidromically, back toward the periphery. At the peripheral terminal, the action potential results in the local release of the content of the afferent terminal for C fibers, such as substance P (SP) and calcitonin gene–related peptide (CGRP), which lead, respectively, to vasodilation (reddening) and plasma extravasation (swelling).

Pharmacology of Peripheral Sensitization‡

After local tissue injury and inflammation, the milieu of the peripheral terminal is altered secondary to tissue damage and the accompanying extravasation of plasma. These effects result

†For more detailed discussions of the material in this section, see References 3 and 4.
‡For more detailed discussions of the material in this section, see References 5 and 6.

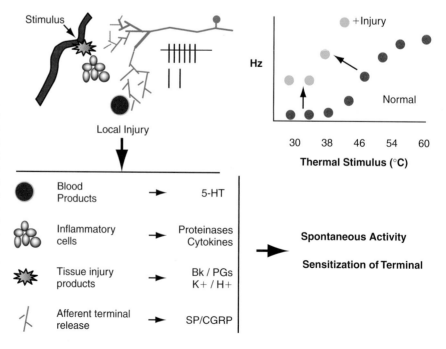

Fig. 3.2 *Left top panel*, Primary afferent terminal. Local tissue-damaging stimulus leads to firing of the fine afferents and local activation of inflammatory cells. *Right top panel*, This injury causes the response profile of a high-threshold afferent to shift up and to the left, thus indicating the appearance of spontaneous activity at non-noxious stimulus intensities and an inflection of the stimulus response curve at a lower stimulus intensity. *Lower panel*, In response to the stimulus, afferent fibers display antidromic release of neuropeptides (substance P/calcitonin gene–related peptide [SP/CGRP]). Hormones, such as bradykinin (Bk), prostaglandins (PGs), and cytokines, or potassium and hydrogen ions (K^+/H^+) released from inflammatory cells and plasma extravasation products result in stimulation and sensitization of free nerve endings. 5-HT, 5-hydroxytryptamine (serotonin).

in the concurrent release of a variety of algogenic agents from damaged tissue and from the peripheral terminals of sensory afferents activated by local C-fiber axon reflexes (**Table 3.1**). These chemical intermediaries have two distinct effects: (1) direct excitation of afferent C fibers; and (2) facilitation of C-fiber activation, resulting in a left shift and increasing slope of the frequency response curve of the C-fiber axon. These

peripheral events likely contribute to the ongoing pain and the increase in the reported magnitude of the pain response evoked by a given stimulus (hyperalgesia).

Central Sensitization and Tissue Injury[*]
Dorsal Horn Response Properties

As reviewed in Chapter 2, a close linkage exists between stimulus intensity and frequency of dorsal horn discharge and pain magnitude. In the presence of tissue injury, there is the onset of a persistent discharge of small afferents. It is now appreciated that this persistent discharge can lead to a facilitation of dorsal horn reactivity. In animal studies, dorsal horn wide dynamic range (WDR) in the deep dorsal horn displays a stimulus-dependent response to low-frequency (0.1-Hz) activation of afferent C fibers. Repetitive stimulation of C (but not A) fibers at a moderately faster rate (>0.5 Hz) results in a progressively facilitated discharge. This exaggerated discharge was named *wind-up* by Lorne Mendell and Pat Wall in 1966 (**Fig. 3.3**). Intracellular recording has indicated that the facilitated state is represented by a progressive, long-sustained, partial depolarization of the cell that renders the membrane increasingly susceptible to afferent input. Given the likelihood that WDR discharge frequency is part of the encoding of the intensity of a high-threshold stimulus, and that many of these WDR neurons project in the ventrolateral quadrant of the spinal cord (i.e., spinobulbar projections), this augmented response is believed to be an important component of the pain message.

Protracted pain states such as those that occur with inflamed or injured tissue would routinely result in such an augmented afferent drive of the WDR neuron and then to the ongoing facilitation. Thus, there would be an enhanced response to a given stimulus (leading to a left shift in the stimulus response curve for the dorsal horn WDR neuron). This sensitization also provides a probable mechanism for the otherwise puzzling change in the size of the receptive field where a stimulus applied to a dermatome adjacent to the injury may yield a pain sensation. As reviewed in Chapter 2, primary afferents entering through a given root make synaptic contact in the spinal level of entry, but they also send collaterals rostrally and caudally to more distant segments, where they can activate these distant neurons (although with less

---

Table 3.1 Representative Classes of Agents Released by Tissue Injury: Activity and Sensitivity of Primary Afferent Fibers
1. **Amines:** Histamine (mast cells) and serotonin (platelets) are released by a variety of stimuli, including trauma, and many are released by chemical products of tissue damage.
2. **Kinin:** Bradykinin is synthesized by a cascade that is triggered by the activation of the clotting cascade. Bradykinin acts by specific bradykinin receptors (B1/B2) to activate free nerve endings.
3. **Lipidic acids:** Lipids such as prostanoids and leukotrienes are synthesized by cyclooxygenases and lipoxygenases. Many prostanoids, such as prostaglandin E_2 can directly activate C fibers and facilitate the excitability of C fibers through specific membrane receptors.
4. **Cytokines:** Cytokines, such as the interleukins or tumor necrosis factor, are formed as part of the inflammatory reaction involving macrophages and powerfully sensitize C-fiber terminals.
5. **Primary afferent peptides:** Calcitonin gene–related peptide and substance P are found in and released from the peripheral terminals of C fibers and produce local cutaneous vasodilation, plasma extravasation, and sensitization in the region of skin innervated by the stimulated sensory nerve.
6. **Hydrogen ion/potassium ion ([H⁺]/[K⁺]):** Elevated H^+ (low pH) and high K^+ are found in injured tissue. These ions directly stimulate C fibers and evoke the local release of various vasodilatory peptides. Various receptors of triglyceride-rich lipoprotein particles are activated by increased H^+.
7. **Proteinases:** Proteinases, such as thrombin or trypsin, are released from inflammatory cells and can cleave tethered peptide ligands that exist on the surface of small primary afferents. These tethered peptides act on adjacent receptors, proteinase-activated receptors, that can depolarize the terminal.

---

[*]For more detailed discussions of the material in this section, see References 7 to 12.

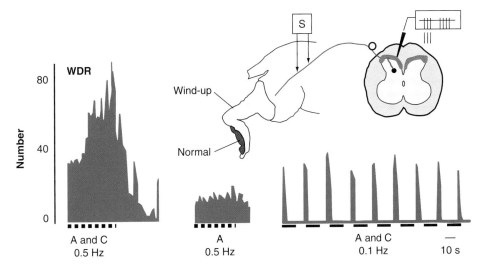

Afferent Stimulation Parameters

Fig. 3.3 *Right,* Single-unit recording from a wide dynamic range (WDR) neuron in response to an electrical stimulus delivered at 0.1 Hz. A very reliable, stimulus-linked response is evoked at this frequency. *Left,* In contrast, when the stimulation rate is increased to 0.5 Hz, there is a progressive increase in the magnitude of the response generated by the stimulation. *Middle,* This facilitation, which results from the C-fiber input and not from A-fiber input, is called wind-up.

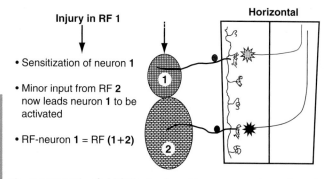

Injury in RF 1

- Sensitization of neuron **1**

- Minor input from RF **2** now leads neuron **1** to be activated

- RF-neuron **1** = RF **(1+2)**

Fig. 3.4 Receptive field (RF) of a dorsal horn neuron depends on its segmental input and the input from other segments that can activate it. After injury in RF 1, neuron 1 becomes "sensitized." Collateral input from RF 2 normally is unable to initiate sufficient excitatory activity to activate neuron 1, but after sensitization, RF 2 input is sufficient. Now the RF of neuron 1 is effectively RF1 + RF2. Thus, local injury by spinal mechanisms can lead acutely to increased receptive fields such that stimuli applied to a noninjured RF can contribute to the post–tissue injury sensation.

security than at the segment of entry). However, as schematically defined in **Figure 3.4**, current thinking suggests that, in the presence of a conditioning injury stimulus, the distant second-order neuron may become sensitized by the high-frequency activity such that input from that proximal dermatome will lead to an intense activation of the distant neuron that provides a "pain signal" referred to the proximal dermatome.

The preceding observations regarding this dorsal horn system have been shown to have behavioral consequences. Psychophysical studies have shown that a discrete injury to the skin of the volar surface of the arm or the direct activation of small afferents by the focal injection of a C-fiber stimulant (capsaicin) results in a small area of primary hyperesthesia surrounded by a much larger area of secondary hyperesthesia. If a local anesthetic block is placed proximal to the injection site before the insult, the onset of the secondary hyperesthesia is prevented. Moreover, WDR wind-up studies are typically carried out in animals under 1 MAC (i.e., minimum alveolar concentration) anesthesia. One would speculate that in patients, the processes considered in the following discussion that lead to spinal facilitation would occur even with such MAC anesthesia. The implication of the afferent-evoked facilitation is that it is better to prevent small afferent input than to deal with its sequelae. This observation is believed to represent the basis for the consideration of the use of preemptive analgesics (e.g., agents and modalities that block small afferent input).

Pharmacology of Central Facilitation[*]

Based on the foregoing commentary and the discussion in Chapter 2, a reduction in C-fiber–evoked excitation in the dorsal horn by blocking axon transmission (sodium channel blockers), by blocking release of small afferent transmitter (as with opiates), or by blocking the postsynaptic receptor (e.g., NK1 for SP or α-amino-3-hydroxy-5-methyl-4-isoxazolepropionic acid [AMPA] for glutamate) will diminish the magnitude of the afferent drive and, accordingly, the facilitated processing evoked by protracted small afferent input. However, the wind-up state reflects more than the repetitive activation of a simple excitatory system. The following is a review of systems that are part of the afferent pathway and other systems that particularly contribute to facilitated processing at the spinal level.

Glutamate Receptors and Spinal Facilitation

The first real demonstration that spinal facilitation represented unique pharmacology was presented by showing that the phenomenon was prevented by the spinal delivery of antagonists for the N-methyl-D-aspartate (NMDA) receptor. Importantly, these antagonists had no effect on acute evoked activity in dorsal horn neurons, but they reduced wind-up. Behavioral work demonstrated that such drugs had no effect on acute pain thresholds but reduced the facilitated states induced after tissue injury and inflammation. As noted, the NMDA receptor does not appear to mediate acute excitation. This finding reflects an important property of this receptor. Under normal resting membrane potentials, the NMDA receptor is in a state referred to as a *magnesium block*. In this condition, occupancy by glutamate will not activate the ionophore. If a modest depolarization of the membrane (as produced during repetitive stimulation secondary to the activation of AMPA and SP receptors) occurs, the magnesium block is removed, permitting glutamate to activate the NMDA receptor. When this happens, the NMDA channel permits the passage of calcium (**Fig. 3.5**). This increase in intracellular calcium then serves to initiate the downstream components of the excitatory and facilitatory cascade. The excitation generated by small primary afferent input has been found to lead to many distinct biochemical events that can serve to enhance the response of dorsal horn neurons and lead to phenomena such as wind-up. Although the activation of the NMDA receptor is an important element of that facilitatory process, it is only one of many. Several representative examples of cascades leading to spinal sensitization are considered here.

Lipid Mediators

In the presence of repetitive afferent stimulation, increased intracellular calcium in spinal neurons leads to the activation of a cascade that releases prostaglandins. These prostanoids act on specific receptors that are presynaptic and postsynaptic to the primary afferent and serve to enhance primary afferent transmitter release and to facilitate the discharge of the postsynaptic dorsal horn neuron (**Fig. 3.6**). The presynaptic effect is believed to be through a facilitation of the opening of the voltage-sensitive calcium channel that is necessary for transmitter release. The postsynaptic action is mediated by the inactivation of a glycine receptor, which is otherwise acted on by glycine released from an inhibitory interneuron. This glycinergic inhibitor interneuron reflexively regulates the magnitude of the firing of the second-order neuron. Loss of the glycinergic inhibition is believed to result in an enhanced response to the afferent input. Cyclooxygenase (COX) inhibitors inhibiting the COX-2 enzyme have been shown to act spinally to block spinal prostanoid release and to diminish injury-evoked hyperalgesia. These results are consistent with the demonstration of the constitutive expression of the several synthetic enzymes, including several phospholipases (PLA_2) and the two COX isoforms.

Nitric Oxide

Nitric oxide (NO) is released following spinal afferent activation through several constitutively expressed NO synthases. NO has been shown to play a role in central facilitation phenomena by increasing transmitter release (see Fig. 3.6). Similarly, in the spinal cord, NO synthase inhibitors have been shown to prevent hyperalgesia.

---

[*]For a more detailed discussion of the material in this section, see Reference 13.

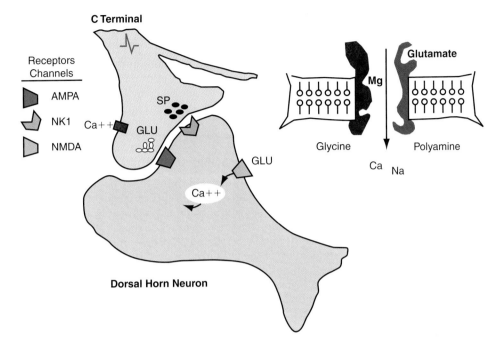

Fig. 3.5 *Left*, Schematic showing the synapse between a C fiber and a second-order dendrite I in the superficial dorsal horn. The synaptic linkage is composed of multiple excitatory transmitters acting on several receptors on the second-order neuron. *Right*, Schematic of an *N*-methyl-d-aspartate (NMDA) ionophore. As indicated in the text, the NMDA receptor is a calcium (Ca^{++}) ionophore that, when activated, results in an influx of Ca. To be activated, the receptor requires the occupancy by glutamate (GLU), the removal of the magnesium (Mg) block by a mild membrane depolarization, the occupancy of the "glycine site," and several allosterically coupled elements, including the "polyamine site." Together, these events permit the ionophore to be activated. AMPA, α-amino-3-hydroxy-5-methyl-4-isoxazolepropionic acid; Na, sodium; NK1, neurokinin 1 receptor; SP, substance P.

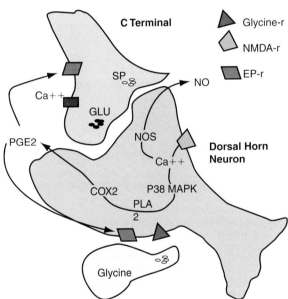

Fig. 3.6 Schematic of primary afferent synapse with second-order neuron in the superficial dorsal horn. On depolarization, multiple transmitters are released. In the presence of persistent depolarization, the glutamate (GLU) receptor is activated, and this leads to increased intracellular calcium (Ca^{++}). This process initiates a variety of cascades, including the activation of nitric oxide synthase (NOS) and the release of nitric oxide. Through P38 mitogen–activated kinase (P38 MAPK), phospholipase A₂ (PLA₂) and cyclooxygenase (COX) lead to the formation and release of prostaglandins (PGE₂). Prostaglandins can act presynaptically to increase the opening of voltage-sensitive calcium channels and postsynaptically to inhibit the activation of a glycinergic inhibitory interneuron. These combined effects are believed to facilitate the activation of the second-order neuron by an afferent input. EP-r, prostaglandin receptor; NMDA-r, *N*-methyl-D-aspartate receptor; SP, substance P.

Phosphorylating Enzymes

Many enzymes found in neurons can phosphorylate specific sites on various enzyme channels, receptors, and channels. Several of these protein kinases in spinal neurons have been shown to be activated by high-frequency small afferent input.

Two examples of this effect are provided by the role of protein kinase C (PKC) and P38 mitogen–activated protein kinase (P38 MAPK). PKC is activated in the presence of increased intracellular calcium and has been shown to phosphorylate certain proteins, including the NMDA receptor. This NMDA receptor phosphorylation has been demonstrated to enhance the functionality of that channel and to lead to increased calcium passage when the channel is activated. This process enhances the postsynaptic effect of any given amount of glutamate release. P38 MAPK is known to be one of the kinases that serve to activate PLA₂. Thus, the formation of prostaglandins dependent on the freeing of arachidonic acid by this enzyme is activated by that kinase. Importantly, activation of P38 MAPK is also known to increase the transcription of specific proteins. In the case of P38 MAPK, one such protein whose expression is increased by P38 MAPK activation is COX-2. Therefore, in the presence of persistent afferent stimulation, activation of this isoform initiates downstream events that change the expression of several proteins relevant to pain processing. This recitation is meant to provide an insight into the types of events that can be mediated by these kinases and is not exhaustive.

Bulbospinal Systems

It is known that afferent input particularly arising from the lamina I marginal cells (see Chapter 2) will activate ascending pathways and lead to excitatory input into the brainstem. At the medullary level, norepinephrine- and serotonin-containing cells have been identified that project into the spinal dorsal horn (e.g., bulbospinal projections). Although these descending pathways have long been considered to be inhibitory, this inhibitory effect is likely the result of the noradrenergic systems. Of particular interest, the serotonergic systems have been shown to play an important *facilitatory* role in the wind-up observed in WDR neurons evoked by small afferent input. Thus, small afferent input activates lamina I projections into the medulla. These activate descending 5-hydroxytryptamine (serotonin; 5-HT) projections, which are excitatory, facilitate the discharge of WDR neurons (**Fig. 3.7**).

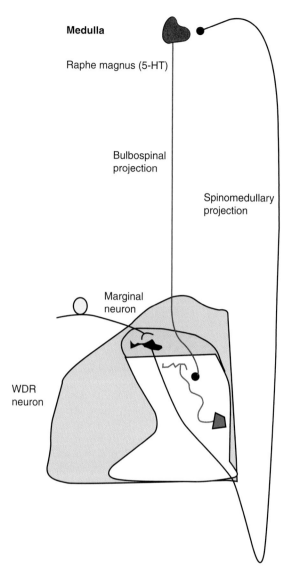

Medulla

Raphe magnus (5-HT)

Bulbospinal
projection

Spinomedullary
projection

Marginal
neuron

WDR
neuron

Fig. 3.7 Schematic showing the linkage whereby small afferent input activates a lamina I cell that projects to the medulla. This projection has been shown to activate a raphe spinal serotonergic projection into the dorsal horn. This input, although an excitatory serotonin receptor, will augment the discharge of the wide dynamic range (WDR) neuron. 5-HT, 5-hydroxytryptamine (serotonin).

Nonneuronal Cells

At the spinal level, large populations of astrocytes and microglia are present. Although these cell systems play an important trophic role, it is increasingly evident that they are also able to regulate the excitability of local neuronal circuits effectively. Thus, astrocytes can regulate extracellular glutamate levels by active reuptake and secretion. These cells also are potent releasers of a variety of active factors such as adenosine triphosphate, lipid mediators, and cytokines. By gap junctions, activation of one astrocyte can lead to a spread of activation that can influence cells over a spatially extended volume. Microglia are similarly interactive by their ability to be activated by a variety of products released from primary afferents and from other neuronal and non-neuronal cells. Spinal agents known to block the activation of astrocytes (fluorocitrate) and microglia (minocycline) have been shown to diminish excitatory states initiated by peripheral

injury and tissue injury rapidly and significantly. In addition to their ability to be influenced by local neuronal circuitry, circulating cytokines (interleukin-1ß [IL-1ß]/tumor necrosis factor-α [TNFα]) released by injury and inflammation can activate perivascular astrocytes and microglia. Accordingly, these cells provide an avenue whereby circulating products can influence neuraxial excitability (**Fig. 3.8**).

Nerve Injury–Induced Hyperalgesia

Psychophysics of Nerve Injury Pain[*]

Over time, after a variety of injuries to the peripheral nerve, a constellation of pain events will appear. Frequent components of this evolving syndrome are as follows: (1) incidences of sharp, shooting sensations referred to the peripheral distribution of the injured nerve; and (2) pain secondary to light tactile stimulation of the peripheral body surface (tactile allodynia). This composite of sensory events was formally recognized by Silas Weir Mitchell in the 1860s. This pain state emphasizes the anomalous role of low-threshold mechanoreceptors (Aß afferents). The ability of light touch to evoke this anomalous pain state indicates that the injury has led to a reorganization of central processing (i.e., it is not necessarily the result of a peripheral sensitization of high-threshold afferents). In addition to these behavioral changes, the neuropathic pain condition may display other contrasting anomalies, including, on occasion, an ameliorating effect of sympathectomy of the afflicted limb and an attenuated responsiveness to analgesics, such as opiates. As an overview, the spontaneous pain and the miscoding of low-threshold afferent nerves are believed to reflect (1) an increase in spontaneous activity in axons in the injured afferent nerve and/or the dorsal horn neurons and (2) an exaggerated response of dorsal horn neurons to normally innocuous afferent input.

Morphologic Correlates of Nerve Injury Pain

Following peripheral nerve ligation or section, several events occur that signal long-term changes in peripheral and central processing. Thus, in the periphery after an acute mechanical injury of the peripheral afferent axon, an initial dying back (retrograde chromatolysis) proceeds for some interval, at which time the axon begins to sprout and to send growth cones forward. The growth cone frequently fails to make contact with the original target and displays significant proliferation. Collections of these proliferated growth cones form structures called *neuromas.*

As reviewed in the following sections, the peripheral injury leads not only to changes at the injury site but also to a very prominent reorganization of the nature of the proteins that are expressed in the dorsal root ganglion (DRG) and spinal cord, as well as the activation of a variety of circuits and cascades involving neuronal and non-neuronal cells.

Spontaneous Pain State[†]

Peripheral and Central Activity Generation

Under normal conditions, primary afferents show little if any spontaneous activity. After peripheral nerve ligation or section, several events are noted to occur: (1) persistent small afferent

---

[*]For more detailed discussions of the material in this section, see References 14 and 15.
[†]For more detailed discussions of the material in this section, see References 16 to 18.

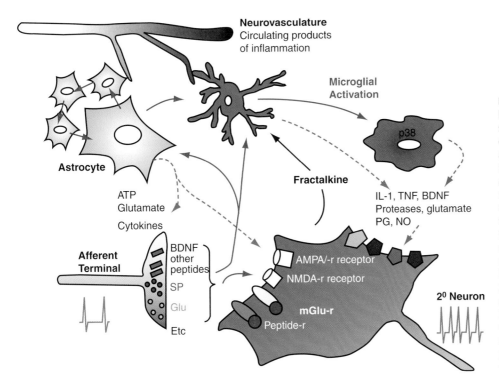

Fig. 3.8 Schematic displays the linkage between the primary afferent and the second-order neuron. The illustration also emphasizes the presence of astrocytes and microglia, which are activated by various products released from activated neurons and from the non-neuronal cells. In addition, the microglia are able to sample the content of the vasculature and these products, such as interleukin-1ß (IL-1ß), can activate these cells. The net effect is that these non-neuronal cells can alter the excitability of local neuronal circuits. AMPA-r, α-amino-3-hydroxy-5-methyl-4-isoxazolepropionic acid receptor; ATP, adenosine triphosphate; BDNF, brain-derived neurotrophic factor; Glu, glutamate; NMDA-r, N-methyl-D-aspartate receptor; NO, nitric oxide; PG, prostaglandin; SP, substance P; TNF, tumor necrosis factor.

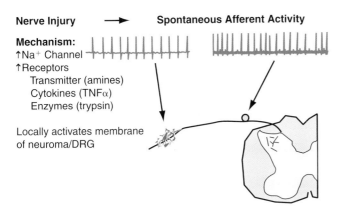

Fig. 3.9 Following nerve injury over an interval of days to weeks, the neuroma of the injured afferent and its dorsal root ganglion (DRG) cell begin to display ectopic activity. Na, sodium; TNFα, tumor necrosis factor-α.

fiber activity originating after a period from the lesioned nerve in both myelinated and unmyelinated axons and (2) spontaneous activity developing from the DRG of the injured nerve. Accordingly, the spontaneous pain sensation may be related to this ongoing afferent traffic. An important question is the source of this afferent traffic. One cannot exclude the likelihood of a spinal generator. Early work indeed demonstrated that after rhizotomy, an increase in activity over time was observed in WDR neurons. With regard to the peripheral generator, several mechanisms have become likely (**Fig. 3.9**).

INCREASED EXPRESSION OF CHANNELS

The events occurring following nerve injury have shown major changes in the proteomics of the DRGs and associated injured axon. Several families of protein that are of particular interest are those associated with the several classes of voltage-gated channels.

Sodium Channels Multiple sodium channels have been identified, based on structure (NaV 1.1 to NaV 1.9), tetrodotoxin sensitivity (TTX), and their activation kinetics. Based on these designations, some of the subtypes are limited in their expression to small primary afferents (NaV 1.8 and 1.9), and some are limited to large myelinated afferents as well as to the central nervous system (NaV 1.3). After nerve injury, there is significant up-regulation of a variety of sodium channels in the neuroma and in the DRG of the injured large and small axons (e.g., NaV 1.3, 1.8, and 1.9). Consistent with the role of sodium channels is that the spontaneous activity originating from the neuromas and from the DRG is blocked by intravenous lidocaine at plasma concentrations lower than those that block conduction in the nerve.

Potassium Channels Potassium channels regulate the terminal and soma polarization state. In the action potential, increased potassium channel activity leads to repolarization of the membrane and thus reduces the probability of repetitive discharge. Decreasing membrane expression on a variety of potassium channels has been observed. This down-regulation of potassium channels leads to enhanced axonal activity.

Calcium Channels Calcium channels serve as charge carriers and as vehicles by which depolarization may lead to increased influx of calcium. For transmitter release, this influx serves to mobilize synaptic vesicles for transmitter release. Various calcium channels (CaV) are expressed in the DRG, and their up-regulation has been reported. Of particular interest is that a component of the N-type calcium channel expressed on the extracellular lumen, which is prominently up-regulated after nerve injury, is the alpha$_2$ delta subunit. As noted later, this is the probable binding site for a family of agents that have efficacy in nerve injury pain states. Many of these changes represent a reversion of the DRG to a neonatal phenotype that is associated with increased excitability.

Changes in Afferent Terminal Sensitivity

The sprouted terminals of the injured afferent axon display a characteristic growth cone that has transduction properties that were not possessed by the original axon. These properties include significant mechanical and chemical sensitivity. Thus, these spouted endings may have sensitivity to numerous humoral factors, such as prostanoids, catecholamines, and cytokines such as TNFα. This evolving sensitivity is of particular importance given that current data suggest that after local nerve injury there is the release of a variety of cytokines, particularly TNFα, that can directly activate the nerve and neuroma. In addition, after nerve injury, an important sprouting of postganglionic sympathetic efferents can lead to the local release of catecholamines. This situation is consistent with the observation that after nerve injury, the postganglionic axons can initiate excitation in the injured axon (see later). These events are believed to contribute to the development of spontaneous afferent traffic after peripheral nerve injury.

Evoked Hyperpathia*

The observation that low-threshold tactile stimulation yields a pain state has been the subject of considerable interest. As noted, most investigators agree that these effects are often mediated by low-threshold afferent stimulation. Several underlying mechanisms have been proposed to account for this seemingly anomalous linkage.

Dorsal Root Ganglion Cell Cross-Talk

Following nerve injury, evidence suggests that "cross-talk" develops between afferents in the DRG and those in the neuroma. Depolarizing currents in one axon would generate a depolarizing voltage in an adjacent quiescent axon. This depolarization would permit activity arising in one axon to drive activity in a second. In this manner, it is hypothesized that a large low-threshold afferent would drive activity in an adjacent high-threshold afferent.

Afferent Sprouting

Under normal circumstances, large myelinated (Aß) afferents project into the spinal Rexed laminae III and deeper. Small afferents (C fibers) tend to project into spinal laminae II and I, a region consisting mostly of nociceptor-responsive neurons. Following peripheral nerve injury, it has been argued that the central terminals of these myelinated afferents (A fibers) sprout into lamina II of the spinal cord. With this synaptic reorganization, stimulation of low-threshold mechanoreceptors (Aß fibers) could produce excitation of these neurons and could be perceived as painful. The degree to which this sprouting occurs is a point of current discussion, and although it appears to occur, it is considerably less prominent than originally proposed.

Dorsal Horn Reorganization

Following peripheral nerve injury, numerous events occur in the dorsal horn. This finding suggests altered processing wherein the response to low-threshold afferent traffic can be exaggerated.

SPINAL GLUTAMATE RELEASE

The post–nerve injury pain state is dependent on spinal glutamate release. After nerve injury, a significant enhancement in resting spinal glutamate secretion occurs. This release is in accord with (1) an increased spontaneous activity in the primary afferent and (2) the loss of intrinsic inhibition that may serve to modulate resting glutamate secretion (see later). The physiologic significance of this release is emphasized by the following convergent observations: (1) intrathecally delivered glutamate evokes powerful tactile allodynia and thermal hyperalgesia through the activation of spinal NMDA and non-NMDA receptors and (2) the spinal delivery of NMDA antagonists attenuates the hyperpathic states arising in animal models of nerve injury. As reviewed earlier in this chapter, NMDA receptor activation mediates neuronal excitability. In addition, the NMDA receptor is a calcium ionophore that, when activated, leads to prominent increases in intracellular calcium. This increased calcium initiates a cascade of events that includes the activation of a variety of enzymes (kinases), some of which phosphorylate membrane proteins (e.g., calcium channels and the NMDA receptors), whereas others (e.g., the mitogen-activated kinases [MAP kinases]) mediate intracellular signaling that leads to the altered expression of a variety of proteins and peptides (e.g., COXe and dynorphin). This downstream nuclear action is believed to herald long-term and persistent changes in function. Various factors have been shown to enhance glutamate release. Two examples are discussed further here.

NONNEURONAL CELLS

Following nerve injury, investigators have shown a significant increase in activation of spinal microglia and astrocytes in the spinal segments receiving input from the injured nerves. Of particular interest is that, in the presence of diseases such as bone cancer, such up-regulation has also been clearly shown. As reviewed earlier, microglia and astrocytes are activated by a variety of neurotransmitters and growth factors. Although the origin of this activation is not clear, when it occurs, it leads to increased spinal expression of COX, NO synthase, glutamate transporters, and proteinases. Such biochemical components have been shown to play important roles in the facilitated state.

LOSS OF INTRINSIC GABAERGIC/GLYCINERGIC CONTROL

In the spinal dorsal horn, large numbers of small interneurons contain and release γ-aminobutyric acid (GABA) and glycine. GABA/glycinergic terminals are frequently presynaptic to the large central afferent terminal complexes and form reciprocal synapses, whereas GABAergic axosomatic connections on spinothalamic cells have also been identified. Accordingly, these amino acids normally exert an important tonic or evoked inhibitory control over the activity of Aß primary afferent terminals and second-order neurons in the spinal dorsal horn. The relevance of this intrinsic inhibition to pain processing is provided by the observation that simple intrathecal delivery of GABA-A receptor or glycine receptor antagonists will lead to powerful, behaviorally defined tactile allodynia. Similarly, animals genetically lacking glycine-binding sites often display a high level of spinal hyperexcitability. These observations lead to consideration that following nerve injury, loss of GABAergic neurons may occur. Although data do support a loss of such GABAergic neurons, the loss appears to be minimal. A second alternative is that after nerve injury, spinal neurons regress to a neonatal phenotype in which GABA-A activation becomes excitatory. This excitatory effect is secondary to reduced activity of the membrane chloride (Cl^-) transporter, which changes the reversal current for the Cl^- conductance. Increasing membrane Cl^- conductance, as occurs with GABA-A receptor activation, results in membrane depolarization.

---

*For more detailed discussions of the material in this section, see References 13 and 19 to 21.

DYNORPHIN

The peptide dynorphin has been identified within the spinal cord. Following peripheral nerve injury, spinal dorsal horn expression of dynorphin is increased. Intrathecal delivery of dynorphin can initiate the concurrent release of spinal glutamate and potent tactile allodynia. This allodynia is reversed by NMDA antagonists.

SYMPATHETIC INPUT

Following peripheral tissue injury, spontaneous discharge appears in otherwise silent small axons. This spontaneous activity is blocked by lidocaine, the sodium channel blocker, at concentrations that do not block the conducted potential. After peripheral nerve injury, innervation of the peripheral neuroma by postganglionic sympathetic terminals is increased. Investigators have shown that an ingrowth of postganglionic sympathetic terminals occurs in the DRGs of the injured axons. These postganglionic fibers form baskets of terminals around the ganglion cells. Several properties of this innervation are interesting: (1) they invest all sizes of ganglion cells, but particularly type A (large ganglion cells); (2) the innervation occurs principally in the DRG ipsilateral to the lesion, but in addition, there is innervation of the contralateral ganglion cell; and (3) stimulation of the ventral roots of the segments containing the preganglionic efferents will produce activity in the sensory axon by an interaction either at the peripheral terminal at the site of injury or by an interaction at the level of the DRG. This excitation is blocked by intravenous phentolamine, a finding emphasizing an adrenergic effect (**Fig. 3.10**).

The observations that sympathetic innervation increases in the ganglion after nerve injury and that afferent activity can be driven by sympathetic stimulation provide some linkage between these efferent and afferent systems and suggest that an overall increase in sympathetic activity per se is not necessary to evoke the activity. These observations also provide a mechanism for the action of alpha antagonists (phentolamine) and alpha$_2$ agonists (clonidine), agents that have been reported to be effective after topical or intrathecal delivery. Thus, alpha$_2$ receptors may act presynaptically to reduce sympathetic terminal release. Spinally, alpha$_2$ agonists are known to depress preganglionic sympathetic outflow. In either case, to the extent that pain states are driven by sympathetic input, these states would be diminished accordingly. This consideration provides some explanation of why opiates do not exert a potent effect on the allodynia observed after nerve injury. As summarized earlier,

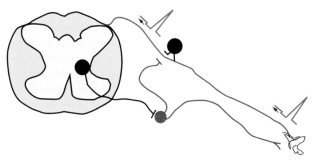

Fig. 3.10 After injury to the peripheral nerve, postganglionic sympathetic afferents sprout into the neuroma. Similar sprouting occurs to the dorsal root ganglion (DRG) of the injured axon. Importantly, electrophysiologic studies have shown that the activation of preganglionic sympathetic outflow to the neuroma or the DRG initiates ectopic activity.

neither microagonists nor alpha$_2$ agonists alter large afferent input, yet alpha$_2$ agonists may reduce allodynia. This differential action may result from the fact that opiates, unlike the alpha$_2$ agonist agents, do not alter sympathetic outflow (as indicated by the lack of effect of spinal opiates on resting blood pressure).

Convergence Between Inflammatory and Nerve Injury Pain States

In the preceding section, the discussion emphasized that several sets of mechanisms underlie the altered processing that arises after tissue and nerve injury. In the presence of persistent injury and inflammation, signs suggesting of a systems response engendered by nerve injury may appear. Thus, with nerve injury, activation of satellite cells and the appearance of cyclic adenosine monophosphate–dependent transcription factor (ATF-3) are commonly observed in the DRG. Investigations have suggested that such changes may also be observed in the presence of persistent inflammatory states. This property suggests that a component of the effects (e.g., observed in rheumatoid disease in which the pain state persists in spite of a significant resolution of the inflammatory signs) may reflect a transition from acute inflammatory mechanisms to a condition representing nerve injury.

Overview of Mechanisms of Action of Several Common Pharmacologic Agents That Modify Pain Processing

Earlier, the discussion considered the various aspects of the pharmacology of the systems that underlie the dynamic aspects of pain processing. The following text briefly considers mechanisms whereby certain pharmacologic modalities exert their action to produce a change in pain processing.

Opioids*

Systemic opioids have been shown to produce a powerful and selective reduction in the human and animal response to a strong and otherwise noxious stimulus. Current data emphasize that these agents may interact with one or a combination of three receptors: mu, delta, and kappa. Given the widespread use of this class of drugs, the site through which these effects are mediated and the mechanisms of those actions are points of interest. Direct assessment of the locus of action can be addressed initially by the focal application of the agent to the various purported sites of action, and the effects of such injections on behavior and the pharmacology of those local effects (to ensure a receptor-mediated effect) can be examined.

Sites of Action

SUPRASPINAL SITES

Microinjection mapping in animals prepared with stereotactically placed guide cannulae revealed that opioid receptors are functionally coupled to the regulation of the animal's response to strong and otherwise noxious mechanical, thermal, and chemical stimuli, which excite small primary afferents. Of the sites that have been principally identified, the most potent is the mesencephalic periaqueductal gray matter (PAG). Here, the local action of morphine blocks nociceptive responses in

---

*For more detailed discussions of the material in this section, see References 22 and 23.

a variety of species. Other sites identified to modulate pain behavior in the presence of an opiate are the mesencephalic reticular formation (MRF), medial medulla, substantia nigra, nucleus accumbens and ventral forebrain, and amygdala.

SPINAL CORD

Intrathecal opiates produce a powerful effect on nociceptive thresholds in all species.

PERIPHERAL SITES

Early studies suggested a possible action of morphine at the site of peripheral injury. Investigators emphasized that the peripheral injection of opiates following the initiation of an inflammation would reduce the hyperalgesic component at doses that did not redistribute centrally.

Mechanisms of Opioid Analgesia

Given the diversity of sites, it is unlikely that all the mechanisms whereby opiates act within the brain to alter nociceptive transmission are identical. Several mechanisms through which opiates may act to alter nociceptive transmission have been identified.

Supraspinal Action of Opioids

Several specific mechanisms are recognized. Two are discussed here (**Fig. 3.11**).

BULBOSPINAL PROJECTIONS

Morphine in the brainstem inhibits spinal nociceptive reflexes. Microinjection of morphine into various brainstem sites reduces the spinal neuronal activity evoked by noxious stimuli.

These effects are in accord with a variety of studies in which (1) activation of bulbospinal pathways known to contain norepinephrine or 5-HT inhibit spinal nociceptive activity; (2) pharmacologic enhancement of spinal monoamine activity (by the delivery of alpha agonists) leads to an inhibition of spinal activity; (3) microinjection of morphine into the brainstem increases the spinal release of norepinephrine; and (4) the spinal delivery of alpha$_2$ antagonists reverses the effects of brainstem opiates on spinal reflexes and analgesia. These observations are in accord with the effects produced when the bulbospinal pathways are directly stimulated and emphasize that the actions of opiates in the PAG are, in fact, associated with an increase in spinifugal outflow.

FOREBRAIN MECHANISMS MODULATING AFFERENT INPUT

Although ample evidence suggests that opiates interact with the mesencephalon to alter input by a variety of direct and indirect systems, the behavioral sequelae of opioids possess a significant component that reflects the affective component of the organism's response to the pain state. Significant rostral projections from the dorsal raphe nucleus (5-HT) and the locus ceruleus (norepinephrine) connect the PAG with forebrain systems and are known to influence motivational and affective components of behavior.

Spinal Action of Opiates

At the spinal level, opioid receptors are present presynaptically on the terminals of small primary afferents and postsynaptically on the second-order neurons. The presynaptic action of morphine

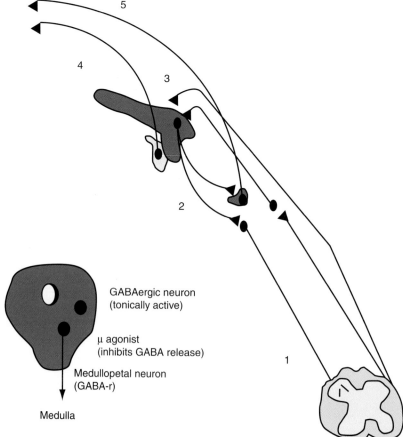

Fig. 3.11 **Schematic of organization of opiate action within the periaqueductal gray matter (PAG).** In this schema, mu (μ) opiate actions block the release of γ-aminobutyric acid (GABA) from tonically active systems that otherwise regulate the projections to the medulla, thus leading to an activation of PAG outflow. The overall organization of the mechanisms whereby a PAG mu opiate agonist can alter nociceptive processing is presented in the adjacent schematic. The following mechanisms are hypothesized: (1) PAG projection to the medulla, which serves to activate bulbospinal projections releasing serotonin and/or norepinephrine at the spinal level; (2) PAG outflow to the medulla, where local inhibitory interaction results in an inhibition of ascending medullary projections to higher centers; (3) opiate binding within the PAG may be preterminal on the ascending spinofugal projection; this preterminal action would inhibit input into the medullary care and mesencephalic core; outflow from the PAG can modulate excitability of dorsal raphe (4) and locus ceruleus (5), from which ascending serotonergic and noradrenergic projections originate to project to the limbic system and forebrain.

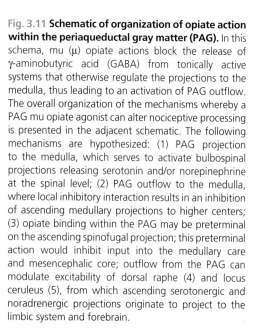

GABAergic neuron
(tonically active)

μ agonist
(inhibits GABA release)

Medullopetal neuron
(GABA-r)

Medulla

through the G-protein–coupled receptor reduces the opening of voltage-sensitive calcium channels and thereby reduces the release of small afferent transmitters. The postsynaptic action reflects a facilitating linkage to voltage-sensitive potassium channels, which then hyperpolarize the second-order neuron and render it resistant to depolarization. These joint effects are believed to underlie the primary regulatory effects of spinal opiates on spinal nociceptive input (**Fig. 3.12**).

Peripheral Action of Opioids

Opioid binding sites are transported in the peripheral sensory axon, but there is no evidence that these sites are coupled to mechanisms governing the excitability of the membrane. High doses of agents, such as sufentanil, can block the compound action potential, but this effect is not naloxone reversible and is thought to reflect a local anesthetic action of the lipid-soluble agent. It is certain that opiate receptors exist on the distant peripheral terminals. Opioid receptors have been shown to be present on the distal terminals of C fibers, and agonist occupancy of these sites can block antidromic release of C-fiber transmitters (e.g., SP/CGRP, "axon reflex"; see the discussion of pharmacology of peripheral sensitization). Importantly, the models in which peripheral opiates appear to work are those that possess a significant degree of inflammation and are characterized by a hyperalgesic component. This finding raises the possibility that these peripheral actions normalize a process leading to an increased sensitivity to the local stimulus environment but do not alter normal transduction. The mechanisms of the antihyperalgesic effects of opiates applied to the inflamed regions (e.g., in the knee joint) are, at present, unexplained. It is possible, for example, that opiates may act on inflammatory cells that are releasing cytokines and products that activate or sensitize the nerve terminal.

Interactions Between Supraspinal and Spinal Systems

As discussed earlier, opioids with an action limited to the spinal cord and to the brainstem are able to produce a powerful alteration in nociceptive processing. Ample evidence indicates that the effects of opiate receptor occupancy in the brain synergize with the effects produced by the concurrent occupancy of spinal receptors. Various studies have shown that the concurrent administration of morphine spinally and supraspinally leads to prominent synergy (i.e., maximal effect with a minimal combination dose).

Nonsteroidal Anti-Inflammatory Drugs*

Nonsteroidal anti-inflammatory drugs (NSAIDs) are widely prescribed agents that have been shown to have significant utility in a variety of acute (postoperative) as well as chronic (cancer, arthritis) pain states. Although NSAIDs may differ in potency, all are believed to have the same efficacy. Importantly, human and animal studies have emphasized that these agents serve not to alter pain thresholds under normal conditions but to reduce a hyperalgesic component of the underlying pain state. NSAIDs are structurally diverse but have a common feature in their ability to function as inhibitors of the enzyme COX, the essential enzyme in the synthesis of prostaglandins. Current thinking emphasizes both peripheral and central mechanisms of action.

Peripheral Action of Nonsteroidal Anti-Inflammatory Drugs

Prostanoids are synthesized at the site of injury and can act on the peripheral afferent terminal to facilitate afferent transduction and augment the inflammatory state. To that degree, inhibition of prostaglandin synthesis by blocking COX can diminish that hyperalgesic state and can reduce the magnitude of inflammation. The analgesic potency of the NSAIDs, however, does not co-vary uniquely with the potency of these agents as inhibitors of inflammation.

Spinal Action of Nonsteroidal Anti-Inflammatory Drugs

Intrathecal injection of NSAIDs, at doses that are inactive with systemic administration, attenuates the behavioral response to certain types of noxious stimuli, a finding that indicates a central action of the agent. As reviewed earlier, the repetitive activation of spinal neurons or the direct excitation of dorsal horn glutamate or SP receptors evokes a facilitated state of processing and the release of prostaglandins. The direct application of several prostanoids to the spinal cord leads to a facilitated state of processing (hyperalgesia). Accordingly, it is currently considered that COX inhibitors can, by their effect on COX-2, exert an acute action that prevents the initiation of the hyperalgesic state otherwise produced by the local spinal action of prostaglandins (see Fig. 3.6).

---

*For more detailed discussions of the material in this section, see References 24 and 25.

Wide Dynamic Range

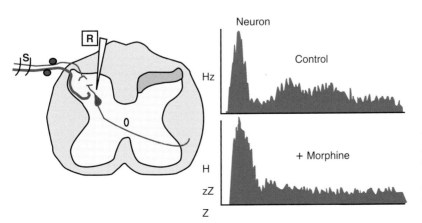

Fig. 3.12 Poststimulus histogram showing the effects of intravenous morphine on the firing of a single dorsal horn wide dynamic range neuron after single activation of A- and C-fiber input. As indicated, early (A-mediated) and late (A/C) activation of the cell occurs. The later-phase activation is preferentially sensitive to morphine (5 mg/kg intravenously) compared with the early component. These effects are readily reversed by naloxone. R, reording; S, stimulating.

Fig. 3.13 **Gabapentinoid agents.** GABA, γ-aminobutyric acid.

N-Methyl-D-Aspartate Receptor Antagonists*

Ketamine is classified as a dissociative anesthetic, but there is a clinical appreciation that ketamine can provide a significant degree of "analgesia." The current thinking is that ketamine acts as an antagonist at the glutamate receptor of the NMDA subtype. As reviewed earlier, the NMDA site is thought to be essential in evoking a hyperalgesic state following repetitive small afferent (C-fiber) input (see Fig. 3.5). In addition, some investigators believe that certain states of allodynia may be mediated by a separate spinal NMDA receptor system, and NMDA antagonists have been shown to diminish the dysesthetic component of the causalgic pain states.

Alpha₂-Adrenergic Agonists†

Systemic alpha₂ -adrenoceptor agonists have been shown to produce significant sedation and mild analgesia. As reviewed earlier, bulbospinal noradrenergic pathways can regulate dorsal horn nociceptive processing by the release of norepinephrine and the subsequent activation of alpha₂-adrenergic receptors. Consequently, the spinal delivery of alpha₂ agonists can produce powerful analgesia in humans and animal models. This spinal action of alpha₂ is mediated by a distinct receptor but with a mechanism similar to that employed by spinal opiates: (1) alpha₂ binding is presynaptic on C fibers and postsynaptic on dorsal horn neurons, (2) alpha₂ receptors can depress the release of C-fiber transmitters, and (3) alpha₂ agonists can hyperpolarize dorsal horn neurons through a Gi-coupled potassium channel. There is growing appreciation that clonidine may be useful in neuropathic pain states. The mechanism is not clear, but the ability of alpha₂ agonists to diminish sympathetic outflow, either by a direct preterminal action on the postganglionic fiber, thereby directly blocking catecholamine release, or by action spinally on preganglionic sympathetic outflow, has been suggested.

Gabapentinoid Agents (Fig. 3.13)‡

Several molecules with a similar structural motif were synthesized to be GABA mimetics with anticonvulsant activity. Their activity in a variety of neuropathic conditions was defined, and subsequent work emphasized that these agents had no affinity for GABA sites. Mechanistically, these molecules show high affinity for a neuronal membrane site that corresponds to the alpha₂delta subunit. This subunit is associated with the extracellular component of the voltage-sensitive calcium channel family. At the spinal level, this binding site is densely present in the superficial dorsal horn in the substantia gelatinosa The importance of the alpha₂delta binding is strongly supported by the observation that point mutations of the alpha₂delta sequence leads to a loss of binding of gabapentin and a parallel loss of anti-hyperalgesic activity. At present, it can be stated that although the mechanism

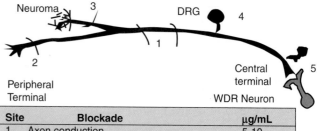

Site	Blockade	µg/mL
1.	Axon conduction	5-10
2.	Spontaneous activity in injured fiber	5
3.	Neuroma firing	3-5
4.	DRG firing	1-3
5.	Glutamate evoked excitation	1-3

Fig. 3.14 Schematic showing sites of generation of spontaneous activity (1-5, *top*); the table (*below*) indicates the sites at which systemically administered lidocaine has been hypothesized to reduce spontaneous or evoked activity. Note that axonal and peripheral nerve terminal blockade has not been demonstrated in whole animal preparations at sublethal systemic lidocaine concentrations, whereas abnormal activity in neuromas, dorsal root ganglia (DRG), and dorsal horn is suppressed by nontoxic lidocaine plasma concentrations. WDR, wide dynamic range.

of action of this family of agents is not fully understood, this family of agents exerts a potent action on facilitated processing, as evoked in the postinjury pain state in the changes in spinal function that occur after peripheral nerve injury.

Intravenous Local Anesthetics§

The systemic delivery of sodium channel blockers has been shown to have analgesic efficacy in a variety of neuropathies (diabetic), nerve injury pain states (causalgia), and late-stage cancer, as well as in lowering intraoperative anesthetic requirements. Importantly, these effects occur at plasma concentrations lower than those required to produce frank block of nerve conduction; for lidocaine, effective concentrations may be on the order of 1 to 3 µg/mL. As reviewed earlier, the mechanism of this action is believed to reflect the importance of the up-regulation of the sodium channel that occurs in the injured axon and DRG. This increase is believed to underlie, in part, the ectopic activity arising from the injured nerve. **Figure 3.14** indicates the potential sites where local anesthetics may interfere with impulse generation that leads to a pain state.

Conclusion

The discussions of the mechanism of nociceptive processing in Chapter 2 and in this chapter only touch on a complex organized substrate. The common threads connecting these comments are that the complexity emphasizes that pain is not a monolithic entity and that, as with other organ systems (e.g., cardiovascular regulation and hypertension), multiple causes lead to the pain report. Because many approaches to regulating elevated blood pressure are available, and the selection of the appropriate therapy depends on the mechanism in the disorder, so too is it likely that a single approach will not be appropriate for all pain states. Improving insight into the pharmacology and physiology of these multiple components should continue to provide new tools for the management of nociception.

References

Full references for this chapter can be found on www.expertconsult.com.

---

*For a more detailed discussion of the material in this section, see Reference 26.
† For a more detailed discussion of the material in this section, see Reference 27.
‡For more detailed discussions of the material in this section, see References 28 and 29.

§ For a more detailed discussion of the material in this section, see Reference 30.

Central Pain Modulation

Anthony Dickenson

Pain provides a model for the study of how the central nervous system (CNS) deals with inputs from the outside world in the context of a system with enormous functional implications for human health and suffering. Plasticity is inherent in the sensory pathways in that the peripheral and central neuronal systems alter in different pain states. The aim of this overview is to summarize the potential targets at central levels in terms of both pain modulation and analgesic therapy. Pain can be acute, but persistent pains can be caused by inflammation and tissue damage, operative procedures, trauma, and diseases such as osteoarthritis and cancer. In addition, pain from nerve damage, neuropathic pain, can be produced by trauma, viral factors, diabetes, and tumors invading nervous tissue. The mechanisms of inflammatory and neuropathic pain are very different from those of acute pain in terms of peripheral origins, and marked changes occur in both the transmission and modulating systems in these prolonged pain states. Finally, some diffuse pains, such as those experienced in irritable bowel syndrome and fibromyalgia, have no clear peripheral pathologic process. In these conditions, central mechanisms may drive the pain state.

Spinal Excitatory Systems

The arrival of sensory information from nociceptors in the dorsal horn of the spinal cord adds considerable complexity to the study of pain and analgesia because most of the receptors found in the CNS are also present in the areas where the C fibers terminate. The density of neurons in these areas is equal to or exceeds that seen elsewhere in the CNS so complex pain syndromes are not unexpected.

As peripheral fibers enter the spinal cord, interactions between peptides and excitatory amino acids become critical for setting the level of pain transmission from the spinal cord to the brain and through local connections to motoneurons (**Fig. 4.1**). L-, N- and P-type calcium channels responsible for the release of these transmitters are differentially and temporally changed by neuropathic and inflammatory nociception (**Fig. 4.2**). In terms of therapy, the N-type channel blocker ziconotide is effective but has secondary effects even with spinal delivery because of the ubiquitous role of this channel. The calcium channels have associated subunits, and

the $alpha_2$delta subunit is the site of action of gabapentin and pregabalin. The subunit is up-regulated after nerve injury. These drugs appear to prevent the trafficking of the subunit so the channels are not in the membrane and are unable to release transmitter. In addition, the actions of the drugs are regulated by descending monoamine systems perhaps linking pain with mood disorders and sleep disturbances.[1,2]

The α-amino-3-hydroxy-5-methyl-4-isoxazolepropionic acid (AMPA) receptor for the excitatory amino acids sets the baseline response of the spinal neurons and is active during both noxious and innocuous responses. Kainate receptors on terminal and neurons may also be important in the generation of neuronal activity. Release of substance P and its actions on the neurokinin-1 receptor removes the magnesium (Mg^{++}) block of the N-methyl-D-aspartate (NMDA) receptor and allows this receptor to operate. Other peptides may also contribute. Activation of the NMDA receptor underlies wind-up and long term potentiation, whereby the baseline response is amplified and prolonged even though the peripheral input remains the same. This increased responsivity of dorsal horn neurons is probably a major basis for central hypersensitivity whereby neurons show enhanced responses and expanded receptive fields. The NMDA receptor does not participate in responses to acute stimuli but is involved in persistent inflammatory and neuropathic pains in which peripheral sensitization in the former and altered ion channel activity in the latter favor enhanced activity. Here the NMDA receptor is critical for both the induction and subsequent maintenance of the enhanced pain state.[1,2] Both volunteer and clinical studies support the ideas that have come from basic research in that the NMDA receptor appears to underlie the hyperalgesia and allodynia seen in inflammatory, postoperative, and neuropathic pains. Ketamine effectively blocks the NMDA receptor but with cognitive and other side effects, so novel antagonists are eagerly awaited.

Induction of certain early genes in spinal neurons may result in prolongation of the excitable state or contribute to its maintenance. Numerous intracellular events downstream of the receptor are subsequently changed, and the gas nitric oxide contributes to wind-up. Spinal generation of prostanoids also occurs after noxious stimuli, and this may be the target for the central actions of nonsteroidal anti-inflammatory drugs (NSAIDs) and cyclooxygenase-2 (COX-2) inhibitors.

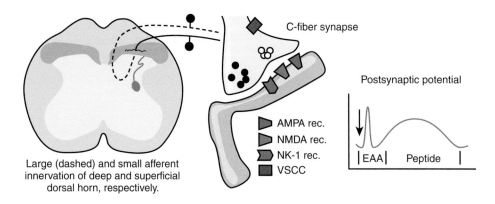

Large (dashed) and small afferent innervation of deep and superficial dorsal horn, respectively.

C-fiber synapse

Postsynaptic potential

AMPA rec.
NMDA rec.
NK-1 rec.
VSCC

| EAA | Peptide |

PRIMARY AFFERENT TRANSMITTER	RECEPTOR	POSTSYNAPTIC ACTION
Peptides		
Substance P	Neurokinin 1 (NK-1)	G protein–coupled; slow, long-lasting depolarization
CGRP	CGRP1	
Growth factors		
BDNF	TRK B	Depolarizes, activates tyrosine kinase (TRK) cascade
Purine		
Adenosine triphosphate (ATP)	P2X receptor (P2X1-7)	Ligand-gated ion channels that differ in ion selectivity, gating properties
	P2Y receptor (P2Y1-14)	Metabotropic G protein–coupled receptors
Excitatory amino acids		
Aspartate, glutamate	AMPA receptor	Sodium ionophore; rapid, short-lasting depolarization; gates sodium A subtype of the AMPA receptor; can also gate calcium
	NMDA receptor	Calcium ionophore; slow onset, long-lasting; gates calcium

AMPA, DL-α-amino-3-hydroxy-5-methyl-4-isoxazole propionic acid; BDNF, brain-derived nerve growth factor; CGRP, calcitonin gene-related peptide; EAA, excitatory amino acids; NMDA, N-methyl-D-aspartate; VSCC, voltage-sensitive calcium channel.

Fig. 4.1 **Summary of primary afferent transmitter organization.** *(From Benzon H: Raj's practical management of pain, ed 4, St Louis, 2008, Mosby.)*

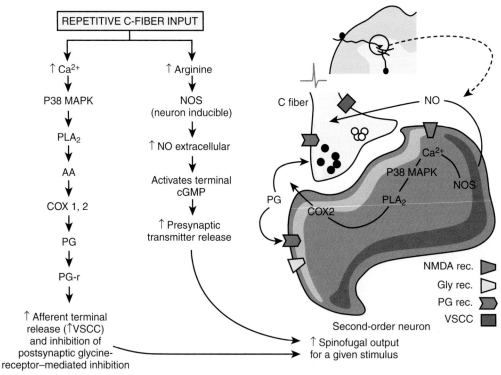

Fig. 4.2 Small-afferent input actives second-order neurons and leads to increased intracellular calcium (Ca^{2+}) concentration, which initiates several intracellular cascades. In the *left column*, activation of phospholipase A_2 (PLA_2) increases free arachidonic acid (AA). This serves as a substrate for cyclooxygenase (COX1 and COX2), which leads to prostaglandin (PG) release. These substances act on eponymous prostanoid receptors located presynaptically on the primary afferent terminal and postsynaptically on the higher-order neurons. In the *right column*, activation of nitric oxide synthase (NOS) in the presence of arginine leads to nitric oxide (NO), which diffuses to enhance transmitter release (e.g., glutamate). These events can serve to increase terminal release and increase postsynaptic excitability. cGMP, cyclic guanine monophosphate; Gly, glycine; NMDA, N-methyl-D-aspartate; P38 MAPK, P38 mitogen-activated protein kinase; rec., receptor; VSCC, voltage-sensitive calcium channel. *(From Benzon H: Raj's practical management of pain, ed 4, St Louis, 2008, Mosby.)*

Spinal Modulatory Systems

The roles of the mu, delta, and kappa opioid receptors have been established with actions at spinal and supraspinal sites.[3] Most clinically used drugs act on the mu receptor, whereas the delta receptor may provide a target for opioids with fewer side effects than morphine that have not yet reached the clinic. The more recently discovered ORL-1 receptor appears to produce spinal analgesia but may well function as an antiopioid at supraspinal sites. The endogenous opioid peptides, the enkephalins, have clear controlling influences on the spinal transmission of pain, whereas the dynorphins have complex actions. Inhibitors of the degradation of the enkephalins have been produced in an attempt to enhance endogenous opioid controls. Because the mu receptor is remarkably similar in structure and function in all species studied, basic research studies will be good predictors for human applications. The detailed structure of these receptors has been described, and some polymorphisms in the receptor appear to relate to opioid efficacy.

The best described central sites of action of morphine are at spinal, brainstem, and midbrain loci. Other actions certainly occur at the highest centers of the brain, but these are poorly understood in terms of their contribution to analgesia.

The spinal actions of opioids and their mechanisms of analgesia involve the following: (1) reduced transmitter release from nociceptive C–fibers, so that spinal neurons are less excited by incoming painful messages; and (2) postsynaptic inhibitions of neurons conveying information from the spinal cord to the brain. This dual action of opioids can result in total block of sensory inputs as the drugs arrive in the spinal cord, but obviously this effect may not be achievable at therapeutic systemic doses. Because spinal neurons project to both cortical (sensory-discriminative aspects of pain) and limbic areas (affective components of pain), block of their spinal inputs has a powerful effect on the pain experience.

Some opioids, such as methadone, may have additional NMDA blocking actions and so may be valuable in cases where morphine effectiveness is reduced, such as in neuropathic pain. However, it not clear that this extra action contributes to clinical effects.

Certain pathologic factors can influence the degree of opioid analgesia and are relevant to pain after nerve injury. Nerve damage can cause a loss of the presynaptic opioid receptors that would be expected to contribute to a reduction in opioid sensitivity. In addition, levels of the peptide cholecystokinin in the spinal cord can also determine the potency of morphine. Changes after nerve damage can result in overexcitability of spinal neurons so that a hypersensitive state is induced, against which opioid controls are insufficiently efficacious. The transmission of painful messages through the normally innocuous A-fiber population can occur after neuropathy as a result of pathologic changes in peripheral or central processes. No opioid receptors are present on the central terminals of these fibers.[3]

Tonic γ-aminobutyric acid (GABA$_A$) and GABA$_B$ receptor controls are important endogenous inhibitory systems in terms of controlling acute, inflammatory, and neuropathic pain states. The GABA$_A$ receptor appears to prevent low-threshold inputs from triggering nociception. GABA levels are reduced after nerve damage yet are increased in the presence of inflammation. Clinically, the widespread roles of this major inhibitory receptor obviate therapy with present drugs acting on this transmitter system.

Supraspinal Modulatory Systems

As pain messages ascend to the brain, inputs into the midbrain can trigger reciprocal projections back to the spinal cord through descending controls. Thus, monoamine systems, originating in the midbrain and brainstem, can modulate the spinal transmission of pain. Early ideas suggested that the descending controls were inhibitory and formed the basis for deep brain stimulation for pain control. However, it is now clear that the balance between descending controls, both excitatory and inhibitory, can be altered in various pain states. Good evidence indicates a prominent noradrenergic alpha$_2$-adrenoceptor–mediated inhibitory system originating from the locus ceruleus in the brain and mimicked by drugs such as clonidine and dexmedetomidine that directly activate the spinal receptors. However, the multiple 5-hydroxytryptamine (5-HT) receptors lead to both inhibitory and excitatory effects of this transmitter. 5-HT$_3$-receptor and likely also 5-HT$_2$-receptor–mediated excitatory controls have been described, as well as 5-HT$_1$ inhibitions, exemplified by the use of the triptans, agonists at this receptor, in headaches. 5-HT in the descending pathways originates from complex networks within the rostroventral medial medulla (RVM) where both on and off cells exist and dually control spinal functions.[1,2]

The ability of cortical function, through these descending controls, to influence spinal function allows for "top-down" processing by these monoamines and so may be one the links between pain and the comorbidities of sleep problems, anxiety, and depression. Evidence from patient studies indicates that diffuse noxious inhibitory controls have reduced inhibitory modulation in several pain states. By contrast, in the case of peripheral neuropathy, spinal injury, and cancer-induced bone pain, the excitatory descending controls appear to be enhanced and further enhance states of increased spinal neuronal hypersensitivity. At least in animals, descending drives can be observed to occur without any alteration in peripheral processes. Possibly, in pain states in which fatigue, mood changes, and diffuse pain occur, such as fibromyalgia and irritable bowel syndrome, there could be altered balances between descending facilitations and inhibitions caused by shifts in central monoamine function.

Drugs that are most effective in neuropathy are the older tricyclic antidepressants and the newer serotonin-norepinephrine reuptake inhibitors. The lesser efficacy of selective serotonin reuptake inhibitors leads credence to the idea that norepinephrine inhibition is a key part of the analgesic effects of these drugs.[4] The antidepressant drugs in clinical use block the uptake of both norepinephrine and 5-HT. Therefore, these drugs alter function within these descending monoamine pathways and so have efficacy in both neuropathic patients and those with fibromyalgia.

Opioids have long been known to have both spinal actions and supraspinal effects. With regard to supraspinal effects, opioids activate the off cells and switch off on cells and thus move RVM output toward descending inhibition. Finally, other drugs may also interact with these systems. Tramadol, a weak opioid with both norepinephrine and 5-HT uptake block, has some efficacy in pain, but the newer molecule, tapentadol, is a mu opioid with norepinephrine reuptake inhibition only. The actions of gabapentin and pregabalin can be governed by supraspinal processes. The spinal actions of these drugs on calcium channel function by their binding to the $alpha_2delta$ subunit depends on descending facilitatory $5\text{-}HT_3$ mediated influences from the RVM. Other studies have implicated increases in descending $alpha_2$-adrenoceptor–mediated inhibitions through supraspinal actions of these drugs. These studies illustrate the interplay between spinal and supraspinal processes and how these relate not only to the pain condition but also to the efficacy of drugs.

Thus, the central modulation of pain involves multiple sites and mechanisms. If a single agent or approach is not sufficiently effective in controlling pain, then combination therapy is a logical option.

References

Full references for this chapter can be found on www.expertconsult.com.

Section II

The Evaluation of the Patient in Pain

Chapter **5**

History and Physical Examination of the Pain Patient

Charles D. Donohoe

The cornerstone of clinical success in the practice of pain management is a correct diagnosis. Unfortunately, in this era of increasing reliance on technology and constant pressure on the physician to become more efficient, the core elements in achieving the correct diagnosis—namely, a targeted history and physical examination—are sadly regarded as less critical in the care of the patient. Proceeding without a concise history often leads to clinical errors that not only squander our limited health care resources but also compromise the patient's opportunity to obtain pain relief.

Indeed, shortcuts taken in obtaining old records, personally reviewing imaging studies, contacting prior treating physicians, calling family members of a confused patient, and most importantly just sitting and listening to what the patient believes to be important frequently lead to misdiagnosis and an unsatisfactory outcome for the patient and pain specialist alike. Frequently, the most cost-effective use of technology is a telephone call to a family member or prior treating physician. Often the discipline to engage in several minutes of conversation with a knowledgeable party can yield countless benefits both in cost saving and in added medical and psychological insight into the patient's predicament.

The bond of trust that is so integral to the relationship between patient and pain specialist is often determined by the care and thoroughness with which the initial historical material is obtained. Experience has shown that when physicians are rushed for time, the intake interview becomes abbreviated, thereby setting the stage for medical errors and interpersonal dissatisfaction.

Many of the chapters that follow highlight the utility of highly sophisticated technology, invasive testing modalities, and diagnostic and therapeutic nerve blocks. Although these clinical interventions may be extremely important in the evaluation of a given patient, they do not replace the preeminent role of the history and physical examination in the diagnosis of the patient in pain. Most, if not all, of what a pain specialist needs to know can be gleaned from simply taking the time to take a concise history and perform a targeted physical examination. By far, the most cost-effective endeavor in the evaluation of the patient in pain is to be thorough in the initial targeted history taking and physical examination. If this initial consultation ends without a clear direction regarding the underlying pathologic process, the likelihood that technology will "save the day" is very remote. It has been said, with varying degrees of conviction, that "one magnetic resonance scanner (MRI) scanner is worth 100 neurologists (or pain specialists)." In this 21st century with an MRI on every other street, this adage can be restated as follows: "One physician (of any specialty) willing to sit and actually listen to patients can be of more practical benefit than 100 magnets (of any Tesla strength)."

The Targeted Pain History

Obtaining a history is a skill. Practice and repetition improve our skills, reduce the tendency to omit important material, and ultimately enable us to focus our questions to conserve time without sacrificing accuracy. As a starting point, the search should be directed to answer two questions[1]: "Where is the disease causing the pain—in the brain, spinal cord, plexus, muscle, tendon, or bone?" and "What is the nature of the disease?" It is the trademark of an experienced clinician to formulate an efficient line of questioning that deals with both these issues simultaneously. Highlights of the critical elements in that process follow. The goal is to keep the process brief, simple, and workable.

The secret of becoming skilled at taking a history is being a good listener. The physician should put the patient at ease. The patient should never be given the impression that the physician is rushed or overworked and that only limited time is available to get the story across. The physician must remember that the patient in pain is usually anxious, if not overtly frightened, and may be inadequate in presenting the situation and having his or her plight properly perceived. Experience teaches us that the physician cannot force the pace of the interview without losing vital information and valuable mutual trust and insight. The following discussion describes the elements of the targeted history that not only define pain in a context useful for proper identification, localization, and source but also enable the physician to determine priorities about the urgency of care.

The Pain Litany

The *pain litany*—a formulaic exploration of the patient's pain history—enables the physician to identify the signature of the specific pain syndrome from its usual manifesting characteristics.[2,3]

The pain litany takes the following form[3]:

1. Mode of onset
2. Location
3. Chronicity
4. Tempo (duration and frequency)
5. Character and severity
6. Associated factors:
   - Premonitory symptoms and aura
   - Precipitating factors
   - Environmental factors (occupation)
   - Family history
   - Age at onset
   - Pregnancy and menstruation
   - Gender
   - Past medical and surgical history
   - Socioeconomic considerations
   - Psychiatric history
   - Medications and drug and alcohol use

The targeted history also allows physicians to distinguish sick patients from well ones. If it is determined that in all probability the patient is well (i.e., has no life-threatening illness), the workup and treatment plan may proceed at a more conservative pace. From the outset, the interviewer proceeds in an orderly fashion but remains vigilant for signals of an urgent situation. Pain of uncertain origin should always be regarded as a potential emergency.

Mode of Onset and Location

The mode of onset of the pain sets the direction of the initial history and carries much weight in distinguishing sick from well patients. For example, the sudden, explosive presentation of a subarachnoid hemorrhage secondary to a ruptured intracranial aneurysm, manifested by severe headache, neck pain, and a sense of impending doom, contrasts sharply with the chronic diffuse headache and vague neck tightness of tension-type cephalalgia.

The location of pain provides additional diagnostic information. The pain in trigeminal neuralgia, for instance, is usually limited to one or more branches of cranial nerve (CN) V and does not spread beyond the distribution of the nerve.[4] The V2 and V3 divisions of this nerve are much more frequently involved than is V1 (**Fig. 5.1**). The pain is rarely bilateral except in certain cases of multiple sclerosis, brainstem neoplasms and skull base tumors, and infections.[5]

Another example of the importance of pain location is the burning, prickling dysesthesias of meralgia paresthetica. The unilateral involvement of the lateral femoral cutaneous nerve produces painful dysesthesias in the anterior thigh, more commonly in men, who notice the disturbance when they put a hand in a trouser pocket.

The physician must find out how and where the pain started. The patient should be asked to identify the site of maximum pain.

Chronicity

The duration of awareness of a painful illness targets the initial history and heavily influences the sick from well distinction. For this reason, it often serves as a starting point. "How long have you had this pain?" is an essential question. The patient should be asked to try to date the pain in relation to other medical events, such as trauma, surgery, and other illnesses.

In general, back pain that has been present for 30 years and is not associated with any progression is strong evidence of a self-limited pain syndrome, hence the "well" determination.

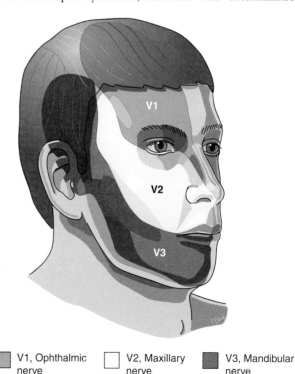

V1, Ophthalmic nerve   V2, Maxillary nerve   V3, Mandibular nerve

Fig. 5.1 **Sensory distribution of the trigeminal nerve.** *(From Waldman SD: Atlas of interventional pain management, ed 2, Philadelphia, 2004, Saunders, 34.)*

Conversely, a patient with severe low back pain of sudden onset or pain that suddenly changes in character must be assigned to the category of "sick until proved otherwise." This type of accentuated pain presentation has often been called the *first or worst syndrome*. It applies to both spinal pain and headache. Patients in this category deserve serious concern, and their pain should be viewed with medical urgency. Equating the concept of chronicity with benign disease has its pitfalls; the physician must beware of failing to

- Identify ominous changes in a long-standing, stable pain syndrome (e.g., when a patient with chronic low back pain suddenly becomes incontinent).
- Attribute the onset of symptoms to a benign cause without adequate evaluation (e.g., dismissing a sudden increase in low back pain in the postoperative patient as muscle spasm without considering diskitis and bacterial epidural abscess).
- Recognize new symptoms superimposed on chronic complaints (e.g., attributing an increase in headache with cough to chronic cervical spondylitis disease rather than considering that because the patient has a known breast malignancy, silent metastasis may be causing increased intracranial pressure).

Indeed, the characteristics of thoroughness, experience, insight into the patient's personality, and constant resistance to being lulled into false security prevent such diagnostic disasters. As Mark Twain observed, "Good decisions come from experience and experience comes from making bad decisions."[6]

Tempo (Duration and Frequency)

The tempo of a disorder may provide one of the best clues to the diagnosis of the pain. In facial pain, trigeminal neuralgia (tic douloureux) is described as brief electric shocks or stabbing pain. Onset and termination of attacks are abrupt, and affected patients are usually pain free between episodes. Attacks last only a few seconds. It is not unusual for a series of attacks to occur in rapid succession over several hours. In contrast, the pain of temporal (giant cell) arteritis is usually described as a dull, persistent, gnawing pain that is exacerbated by chewing.[3]

In migraine, the pain is frequently throbbing and may last for hours to days. Cluster headaches, by contrast, are named for their periodicity: they occur once or more often each day, last about 30 minutes, and often appear shortly after the onset of sleep. They may occur in clusters for weeks to months with headache-free intervals. In short, the concept of pain tempo is another feature of the targeted history that is helpful in differentiating pain syndromes.

Character and Severity

Although considerable overlap exists between character and severity of pain, some generalization can be made when taking a targeted history. Vascular headaches tend to be throbbing and pulsatile, and the pain intensity is often described as severe.[3] Cluster headaches may have a deeper, boring, burning, wrenching quality. This pain is reputed to be among the worst known to humans.

Trigeminal neuralgia is typically described as paroxysmal, jabbing, or shocklike, in contrast to non-neuralgic pain such as experienced in temporomandibular joint (TMJ) dysfunction, which is often described as a unilateral, dull, aching pain in the periauricular region. TMJ pain is exacerbated by bruxism, eating, and yawning but may be patternless. The characteristic pain of postherpetic neuralgia usually includes both burning and aching superimposed on paroxysms of shocks and jabs. It usually occurs in association with dysesthesias, resulting in an unpleasant sensation even with the slightest touch over the skin (allodynia).

Many of the more common pain syndromes have a distinctive character and level of severity that is helpful in properly identifying them. Clinical insight into these characteristics comes with time and through listening to many patients describe their pain. Certain patients with cluster headaches or trigeminal neuralgia have a frantic, almost desperate demeanor that is proportionate to the severity of their pain. The patient with acute lumbar disk herniation often writhes before the physician and is essentially unable to sit in a chair. The body language and facial expressions associated with true excruciating pain are difficult to feign, and exaggerated behaviors often immediately become suspect almost on a visceral level.

Associated Factors

Multiple associated factors round out the targeted pain history. The subtle differences among painful conditions allow clinicians to use these factors to complete the various parts of the puzzle. For example, intermittent throbbing pain behind the eye is consistent with cluster headache. If the patient is a young woman, however, the diagnosis of cluster headache is improbable because of the known male preponderance of this condition.[3] Accordingly, the combination of associated factors such as age and sex aid in the diagnosis. A dull, persistent pain over one temple in a young African American male patient probably is not giant cell or temporal arteritis, a disease most often seen in white women older than 50 years.

Table 5.1 describes various pain syndromes according to patient age, sex, family history, precipitating factors, and occupational issues. As Osler said, "Medicine is a science of uncertainty and an art of probability."[2] Matching our knowledge about the natural history and characteristics of the various diseases that cause pain with information derived from the patient's history is the physician's most powerful diagnostic tool. It is through this process that the physician develops confidence in the diagnosis that often exceeds that based on information from ancillary tests. An autoworker who uses an impact wrench 10 hours a day, complains of numbness in the first three digits of his right hand, and wakes up four times a night "shaking his hand out" has carpal tunnel syndrome, regardless of the results of nerve conduction studies and electromyography.

General Aspects of the Targeted Pain History

An old clinical maxim states, "Healing begins with the history!"[2] The clinician should be able to put the patient at ease and should then ask open-ended questions that will give the patient an opportunity to describe the pain in his or her own words. "Now, tell me about your pain" is an excellent prompt. This approach allows the patient to describe what he or she believes is most important. It is therapeutic in itself. Physicians are often wary of the open-ended question,

Table 5.1 Demographics of Some Common Pain Syndromes

Pain Syndrome	Sex Preponderance (Ratio)	Family History	Age of Onset (yr)	Associated Features and Comments
Migraine				
Childhood (<10 yr)	M (1.5:1)	Positive	3	Abdominal pain, episodic vertigo, mood changes
Adult (> 10 yr)	F (3:1)	Positive	15–20	Decrease by third month of pregnancy, increase with menstruation and oral contraceptives
Cluster headache	M (8:1)	Not positive	25–40	Common at night, precipitated by alcohol and nitrates
Multiple sclerosis	F (2:1)	Positive	20–40	Trigeminal neuralgia, tonic spasms, dysesthesia, extremity pain
Temporal arteritis	F (3:1)	Not positive	>60	Increased erythrocyte sedimentation rate, anemia, low-grade fever, jaw claudication
Trigeminal neuralgia	F (2:1)	Not positive	>55	V2 (45%) > V3 (35%) > V1 (20%); triggered by jaw movement, heat, and cold
Ankylosing spondylitis	M (5:1)	Positive	20–30	Pain forces patient out of bed at night, is not relieved by lying flat
Rheumatoid arthritis	F (3:1)	Positive	35–50	Higher rate in nulliparous women not exposed to oral contraceptives
Thromboangiitis obliterans	M (8:1)	Not positive	20–40	Smoking
Carpal tunnel syndrome	F (2:1)	Not positive	30–60	Certain occupations, pregnancy, diabetes, hypothyroidism

Data from references 1, 3, 4, 9, and 10.

because they are afraid that the patient will ramble. Although this can occur, a far more common problem is that the physician narrows the line of questioning after jumping to a premature conclusion.

The patient's past medical history and family history are often as important as the current complaints. Medications, surgical procedures, and prior imaging studies are not explored in adequate detail. Many patients have been subjected to thousands of dollars of imaging, blood work and neurodiagnostic studies but often remain in the dark not only about their test results but also about the modality or even the actual body part interrogated.

When a patient without records who complains of chronic headaches states that all the "scans" were normal, the physician must be careful. These "scans" may be an MRI image of the brain but could also refer to a computed tomography (CT) scan of the paranasal sinuses or even plain radiographs of the skull. The best policy is to review all pertinent imaging studies and not just the reports. Radiologists truly do a remarkable job of interpreting studies, often with very limited clinical information. In difficult cases, however, review of prior imaging studies in light of a newly derived specific historical or physical finding can be particularly helpful and may even "save the day."

When the pain is chronic, other doctors may already have been consulted. They probably have ordered diagnostic tests and tried therapies; indeed, it is always wise to obtain previous records or, preferably, to contact the other physicians directly. If a diagnosis seems obvious but previous doctors missed it, the physician should be cautious. When nothing has worked before, there is usually a good reason for the treatment failures. Under these circumstances, it is prudent and wise to assume that the other physicians were competent. Physicians are frequent violators of the maxim, "Do unto others as you would have them do unto you." Frank or subtle criticism of a colleague's efforts is pointless, upsets the patient, and may even initiate litigation.

One other impulse that should be resisted is the tendency to ascribe pain to psychogenic causes. Learning to believe patients who have pain averts many awkward and potentially costly errors. Once the physician projects the belief that a patient's pain is based mainly on psychogenic mechanisms, it is an extremely difficult position to recant. At all costs, the pain specialist should remain nonjudgmental, should believe in the patient's pain, and should gain the patient's confidence. The only proven "cure" for having dismissed a patients' pain as psychogenic is to learn that serious organic disease was uncovered by another physician who saw the patient later in the course of the disease. Like everyone in medicine, pain specialists should be humble and careful with their words.

Medication History

The importance of a thorough drug history cannot be overstated, particularly in the setting of chronic benign pain. It is not unusual for a patient to relate a very involved history of pain and multiple operations, diagnostic studies, and consultations. At the end of the interview, not uncommonly as the patient is preparing to leave, he or she will casually mention needing to have a prescription renewed and will add that it is "just a pain pill." It is at this very point that an otherwise pleasant consultation can become confrontational.

Confusion among physicians about the differences among narcotics and opioids is widespread. Many physicians also fail to recognize that the relative analgesic, euphoric, and anxiolytic properties of a given compound are not equivalent. For example, the analgesic strength of propoxyphene (Darvon) may be equivalent to one or two aspirins, but the magnitude of its anxiolytic effects in a given patient can be considerable. Not only opioids pose a problem. Carisoprodol (Soma, Rela) is a noncontrolled skeletal muscle relaxant that is also available through veterinary supply catalogs.[7] Its active metabolite is meprobamate (Equanil, Miltown), an anxiolytic-sedative agent popular in the late 1950s. Patients using carisoprodol may be at risk (frequently unrecognized) for meprobamate dependency.

Triptans, ergots, aspirin, acetaminophen, nonsteroidal anti-inflammatory drugs (NSAIDs), minor tranquilizers, and barbiturate-containing compounds (Fiorinal, Esgic, and Phrenilin) taken in varying doses can contribute to rebound-type headache. In this setting, the daily use of headache-abortive drugs enhances and increases the frequency of daily headaches. The scope of this problem is difficult to assess, but in certain headache clinics, the use of such drugs is the single most common reason for chronic refractory daily headaches.[8] Although every pharmacologic agent has some inherent risk, two practical considerations may be crucial in the targeted pain history. The first involves many individuals, particularly older persons, who are taking anticoagulants (warfarin, heparin) or antiplatelet agents (aspirin, clopidogrel [Plavix], and ticlopidine [Ticlid]) for any of a variety of reasons. Many disasters can occur in this setting. Inadvertent overdosing of an older, confused patient can cause intracerebral bleeding (headache) or back and radicular pain (secondary to retroperitoneal hemorrhage). Second, the physician evaluating headache symptoms should keep in mind that estrogen, progesterone, and nitrates can play major roles as headache-provocative agents and that simply discontinuing these drugs can provide almost immediate improvement.

Both the scope and the frequency of problems related to chemical dependency have been underrecognized in many clinical settings. Some patients are willing to subject themselves to expensive diagnostic studies, multiple nerve blocks, and even surgery to ensure an uninterrupted supply of specific medications (frequently opioids). The specialist in pain management is uniquely positioned to recognize these problems and to offer suggestions in a compassionate, nonjudgmental fashion that may ultimately extricate patients from both their chemical dependency and their convoluted relationship with the medical system. Until drug dependency issues are addressed, effective inroads into the management of chronic pain will be thwarted.

Certain clinicians have described a satisfactory experience administering opioids for chronic benign pain.[9,10] Their positive experience (along with aggressive pharmaceutical company marketing) has promoted liberal prescribing policies among primary care physicians and specialists treating common conditions such as back pain, arthritis, and fibromyalgia. The long-term use of opioids in these diseases is not supported by strong scientific evidence and remains controversial.[11] Such an ambiguous situation only accentuates the importance of obtaining a thorough drug history and assessing the true impact of drug use on the individual patient's pain problems. **Table 5.2** lists the "red flag" agents that, when used by a patient in pain, should alert the physician to consider possible drug abuse or exacerbation of pain by medication. Information on dosage and duration of use is important.

Pain specialists should make it policy to insist that patients bring all their medications at the time of the consultation. If you as a physician believe that a patient has a drug dependency problem, face the problem openly and with kindness. Resist the all too common practice of writing a prescription for that magical minimal amount of the drug being abused, an amount that can end the consultation without a dreaded angry confrontation. For those of us in clinical practice, this is an all too familiar "end of consult" strategy of providing what we know to be part of the problem. Prepare to assume your share of the guilt, Dr. Feelgood, in this major public health disaster.

General Aspects of the Patient Interview

The following general but significant points enhance the patient interview process:

- The surroundings are professional, comfortable, and private.
- The patient is appropriately gowned, is chaperoned if appropriate, and is sitting upright and at eye level with the interviewer, if possible.
- Old records, scans, radiographs, and consultations have been obtained and reviewed before the consultation.
- The physician listens to and does not interrupt the patient or allow outside interruptions.
- The physician remains nonjudgmental; moral, religious, and political beliefs of the physician are irrelevant to this process.
- The physician is honest and open with the patient; keeping information from the patient at the family's request is usually a bad decision.
- Both the patient and the physician can trust in the confidentiality of both the consultation and the medical records.

The specialty of pain management is practiced by physicians from numerous disciplines. In particular, physicians trained in operating room anesthesia may not be as sensitive to some certain issues. From the standpoint of neurologists, for whom interviewing patients is a major component of practice, these basic rules of common etiquette are frequently ignored. First, the office should be both professional and comfortable. For reasons of economy, pain clinics are frequently placed in noisy and crowded additions to either the operating room suite or the emergency department. This atmosphere may not be conducive to dealing with patients with acute and chronic pain, who are often extremely apprehensive and easily frustrated.

It is important that patients have a private place where they undress and are examined. Although this may appear to be a small point, a chaotic examining site can inspire a patient's resentment, even if the medical care is of high quality. One other point that needs reinforcing is that physician and patient should always be properly chaperoned. It is not unusual, because of the hectic schedules of both physicians and ancillary personnel, for a patient and physician to be left alone in situations in which this arrangement is at best uncomfortable and at worst compromising and dangerous. Strict adherence to standardized protocol for chaperoning is really the best way of averting serious problems in this area. The keys to obtaining a complete and effective targeted pain history are listed here The examiner should use the following protocol:

1. Build rapport with the patient by introducing self properly, taking an initial social history, and simultaneously assessing the patient's mood, anxiety level, and capability of giving a history on his or her own.
2. *Most importantly:* Establish the chief complaint at the outset of the history. Why is the patient here? Open-ended questions allow the patient to tell his or her own story.

Table 5.2 "Red Flag" Drugs in the Targeted Pain History

Drug Class	Drug
CONTROLLED ABUSED SUBSTANCES*	
Schedule II narcotics	Morphine (Roxanol, MS Contin) Codeine, fentanyl (Sublimaze) Sufentanil (Sufenta) Hydromorphone (Dilaudid) Meperidine (Demerol) Methadone (Dolophine) Oxycodone (Percodan, Tylox, OxyContin, Roxicodone) Opium Cocaine
Non-narcotic agents	Dextroamphetamine (Dexedrine, Adderall) Methamphetamine (Desoxyn) Methylphenidate (Ritalin) Phenmetrazine (Preludin) Amobarbital (Amytal) Pentobarbital (Nembutal) Secobarbital (Seconal) Glutethimide (Doriden) Secobarbital-amobarbital (Tuinal)
Schedule III narcotics	Codeine (Tylenol with codeine, Fiorinal with codeine) Dihydrocodeine (Synalgos-DC) Hydrocodone (Tussionex, Hycodan, Vicodin, Lortab, Lorcet) Butalbital (Fiorinal, Esgic, Phrenilin, Medigesic)
Schedule IV narcotics	Propoxyphene (Darvon, Darvocet, Wygesic) Butorphanol (Stadol) Pentazocine (Talwin) Alprazolam (Xanax) Chlordiazepoxide (Librium) Clonazepam (Klonopin) Clorazepate (Tranxene) Diazepam (Valium) Eszopiclone (Lunesta) Flurazepam (Dalmane) Lorazepam (Ativan) Midazolam (Versed) Oxazepam (Serax) Quazepam (Doral) Temazepam (Restoril) Triazolam (Halcion) Zaleplon (Sonata) Zolpidem (Ambien)
Non-narcotic agents	Phenobarbital Mephobarbital (Mebaral) Chloral hydrate Ethchlorvynol (Placidyl) Meprobamate (Equanil, Equagesic) Carisoprodol (Soma, Rela)
Schedule V	Buprenorphine (Buprenex) Diphenoxylate (Lomotil) Pregabalin (Lyrica)
NONCONTROLLED ABUSED SUBSTANCES	Triptans (Imitrex, Zomig, Relpax, Amerge, Frova, Treximet, Maxalt, Axert) Ergotamine (Cafergot, Wigraine, Ergostat) Dihydoergotamine (Migranal nasal spray, D.H.E.45) Chlordiazepoxide (Librax) Tramadol (Ultram, Ultracet) (nonscheduled opioid) Nalbuphine (Nubain) (nonscheduled opioid) Caffeine (Excedrin, Anacin)
NONABUSED DRUGS IMPORTANT IN A TARGETED PAIN HISTORY	Oral contraceptives Anticoagulants (heparin, warfarin, clopidogrel [Plavix]) Antiplatelet agents (aspirin, ticlopidine) Antianginals (nitrates)

Narcotic is a nonspecific term still used by state boards to describe a drug that induces sleep or dependence. It is not interchangeable with *opioid*. This table lists many (but not all) drugs that may be abused by patients with pain.

Data from Brust JC: *Neurological aspects of substance abuse,* Boston, 1993, Butterworth-Heinemann, and Missouri Taskforce on the Misuse, Abuse, and Diversion of Prescription Drugs, 1994.

3. Use the framework of the pain litany (discussed earlier) to investigate the pain further. Where is the pain? What is its nature?
4. Do not jump to conclusions. This is the most common cause of error because the interview too soon becomes narrowly focused, and important associations are not pursued or are ignored. The examiner should ask about other doctors whom the patient has seen and their treatments.
5. Determine the impact of the pain on the patient's life—psychological fears, family issues (marriage), compensation, and work record.
6. Explore past medical and family history. Using a timeline approach to establish continuity, the current pain should be placed in context with other major medical events: previous surgery, hospitalizations, cancer, and medical and paramedical relationships.
7. Obtain a thorough drug history (see Table 5.2). Information on duration, frequency, amount, and source of medication should be sought. The importance of this information cannot be overemphasized.

The examination should begin with the physician's introducing himself or herself to the patient and putting the patient at ease. A routine social history, such as occupation, place of employment, marital status, and number of children, should be obtained. During this interchange, the physician should be assessing the verbal and nonverbal cues that ultimately determine the caliber of the historical information. This social introduction affords the physician insight into what type of person the patient is. Over time and with the refinements of experience, this portion of the interview assumes diagnostic importance equal to that of the data-gathering portion of the consultation.

It seems obvious that the patient's chief complaint would be the logical starting point of any history. Unfortunately, too much time can be spent taking a history without ever addressing the chief complaint. Coming to grips with the patient's primary reason for seeking medical attention is really the crucial piece of data. Is it the pain? Is it questions about disability or worker's compensation? Is it a morbid fear of cancer? Is it that the physician who prescribed the patient's pain medications has retired and the patient is concerned about prescription renewal? Until the physician has a strong sense of the principal reason for the consultation, the history is often both misguided and aimless. Sitting in front of the patient, the physician should always ask himself or herself, "Why has this patient come to see me?" Sometimes, the patient's motives are not what they first appear to be.

Summary of the Targeted History

The value of the targeted history cannot be overstated. It affords the physician the greatest chance of understanding the nature of the pain and, more important, its effects on the patient. Diagnostic tests, laboratory reports, and other consultants' opinions often introduce error when they are interpreted from a perspective detached from the patient. The physician should remember that, no matter how many physicians have seen the patient earlier, historical facts critical to the diagnosis may have been overlooked or not properly sought.

Taking the targeted history is a social interaction. Courtesy, professionalism, and kindness consistently result in patient satisfaction. Issues related to compensation, returning to work, and concurrent drug use should be dealt with openly and directly, without imposing the physician's personal, political, or religious value judgments.

The Targeted Physical Examination

If, after obtaining the targeted historical information, the pain specialist is lost, the chance that the situation may be suddenly illuminated by the physical examination findings is extremely remote. As a basic point, the physical examination should follow the history and, indeed, be specifically directed by clues obtained during the patient interview. For example, it makes little sense to concentrate on a detailed examination of sensory function and individual muscle testing in the lower extremities of a patient who has diplopia, facial pain, and a family history of multiple sclerosis.[12] The physical examination is an extension of the history. The examination provides objective support and is performed efficiently and systematically so that important findings are not overlooked. The problem with the neurologic examination has been selecting those elements that are truly critical. In 2009, Canadian neurologists and medical students reached a helpful consensus (**Table 5.3**). It is compact, yet an excellent screening tool.[13]

The examination should not consume a great deal of time. Basic aspects, such as taking blood pressure, performing a screening mental status examination, and checking visual acuity, strength, and deep tendon reflexes, however, pay multiple dividends. On occasion, certain important diseases, such as unrecognized hypertension, diabetic retinopathy, and skin cancer, can be uncovered.

The very physical aspect of examining the patient imparts a reassuring sense of personal caring to the entire consultation. The benefits of this experience are considerable. Pain patients want to be examined, expect to be examined, and ultimately derive benefit from the process. As Goethe said, "We see only what we know."[14] The facility with which we examine patients is ultimately a function of our knowledge, experience, and willingness to learn. The neurologic examination is not difficult and should not intimidate physicians in training or non-neurologists. It can be performed effectively in most cases in less than 10 minutes. The physician should develop a routine and keep it simple.

Table 5.3 Neurologic Examination

Key Elements of the Neurologic Examination	Time to Complete
1. Mental status	90 seconds
2. Cranial nerves/funduscopic examination	90 seconds
3. Power arms/legs	60 seconds
4. Pinprick, vibratory sensation	60 seconds
5. Reflexes, gait, Romberg's sign, tandem walking	90 seconds
	Total time: 6–7 minutes

Data from Heyman CH, Rossman HS: A multimodal approach to managing the symptoms of multiple sclerosis, *Neurology* 14:63:S12, 2004.

General Aspects

The patient's temperature, pulse, and blood pressure should always be recorded, as should height and weight. The patient should be undressed and properly gowned. It is a constant source of amazement how frequently examinations are performed to evaluate painful conditions, even disorders involving the neck and low back, while patients are fully clothed. The pain specialist should do the following: examine the patient's entire body for skin lesions such as hemangiomas, areas of hyperpigmentation, and café au lait spots (neurofibromatosis); document scars from previous operations; and inquire into other scars not mentioned in the initial history. Needle marks, skin ulcerations, and tattoos (which sometimes betray drug culture orientation) may be surprising findings.

The spine should be examined for kyphosis, lordosis, scoliosis, and focal areas of tenderness. Dimpling of the skin or excessive hair growth may suggest spina bifida or meningocele. The motility of the spine should also be evaluated in flexion, extension, and lateral rotation. During this period of the examination, an overall assessment of multiple joints can be done for deformities, arthritic change, trauma, and prior surgical procedures. Clearly, much can be learned just by having the patient stand before the physician and asking the patient about abnormalities that become noticeable. No matter how inconvenient or uncomfortable it is, the physician should try not to omit this portion of the examination. Particularly in patients with chronic pain, this part of the examination may yield crucial and unexpected revelations.

Assessment of Mental Status

Most major intellectual and psychiatric problems become apparent during the history taking. The frequency with which serious intellectual deficits are missed is surprising, however. For example, subtle aspects of memory, comprehension, and language may not be caught unless they are specifically sought. In my experience, aphasia (a general term for all disturbances of language not the result of faulty articulation) is frequently mistaken for an organic mental syndrome or dementia. Recognition of this point not only is critical in diagnostic evaluation but also has important implications for obtaining informed consent for testing, nerve blocks, and surgical procedures.

Table 5.4 summarizes an approach to rapid assessment of the patient's mental status. Each practitioner should develop a personal set of standard questions to gain a sense of the normal versus the abnormal. Attention to these details in assessing mental status helps to avoid the embarrassment of overlooking receptive aphasia, Alzheimer's disease, or Korsakoff's syndrome. **Table 5.5** is the classic Folstein Mini-Mental State Examination with age-adjusted normative data. A score of 24 or higher is considered normal. Although this examination is effective in detecting clinically significant defects in speech and cognitive function, the average practitioner will find it overly tedious for use in routine pain management evaluation. In many of these situations, patients exhibit an unusual capacity to disguise underlying deficits by reverting to evasions or generalities or by filling in gaps with stereotypical responses that they have used before to escape the embarrassment of the discovery of major problems in language, memory, and other spheres of cognitive function.[15]

One final point relates to the patient's emotional state. The examiner must remain vigilant about the patient's mood and displays of emotion. An unusually silly, euphoric, or grandiose presentation may be seen in manic states. Similarly, a discouraged, hopeless, or self-deprecating presentation may signal serious depression. As highlighted in the discussion on the targeted history, the physician must remain alert for clinical manifestations of drug use, such as slurred speech, motor hyperactivity, sweating, flushing, and distractibility. In short, the physician should get to know the patient but, in the end, should vigorously resist any early impulse to suggest that stress or anxiety alone is the principal cause of the patient's pain.

Cranial Nerves

To return to the theme of keeping the targeted physical examination simple so that important points are not missed, the evaluation of CN function often overwhelms practitioners not trained in clinical neurology. It remains an important area, particularly in the evaluation of headache and facial pain. Rapid recognition of CN dysfunction may have profound significance for localizing a cerebral lesion or identifying increased intracranial pressure. In combination with the history, CN dysfunction may also be a strong indicator of a specific disease (e.g., the combined presence of explosive headache and CN III palsy implies a ruptured aneurysm until that diagnosis is excluded).

Table 5.6 highlights an efficient approach to the clinical evaluation of the CNs. Certainly, when headache and facial

Table 5.4 The "Quick and Dirty" Mental Status Examination*

Orientation	Ask the following questions: What is your full name? What is today's date? What is the year? Who is the president? Who is the vice president?
Calculations	Ask the following questions: How many nickels are in a dollar? How many dollars do 60 nickels make?
Memory	Ask the following questions: What was your mother's maiden name? Who was President before George W. Bush? Give the patient three items to remember (examples: a red ball, a blue telephone, and address 66 Hill Street). After several minutes of conversation, ask the patient to repeat the list.
Speech	Have the patient repeat two simple sentences, such as the following: Today is a lovely day. The weather this weekend is expected to be excellent. Have the patient name several objects in the room. Ask the patient to rhyme simple words, such as ball, pat, and can.
Comprehension	Ask the patient to do the following: Put the right hand on the left hand. Point to the ceiling with the left index finger.

*This simple screening mental status examination uncovers many (but not all) cognitive deficits. It can be performed in less than 3 minutes and is useful in evaluating basic aspects of memory, language, and general intellectual capacity.

Table 5.5 Folstein Mini-Mental State Examination

Task	Instructions	Scoring	
Date orientation	"Tell me the date." Ask for omitted items.	One point each for year, season, date, day of week, and month	5
Place orientation	"Where are you?" Ask for omitted items.	One point each for state, county, town, building, and floor or room	5
Register three objects	Name three objects slowly and clearly. Ask the patient to repeat them.	One point for each item correctly repeated	3
Serial 7s	Ask the patient to count backward from 100 by 7. Stop after 5 answers. (Or ask the patient to spell "world" backward.)	One point for each correct answer (or letter)	5
Recall three objects	Ask the patient to recall the objects mentioned earlier.	One point for each item correctly remembered	3
Naming	Point to your watch and ask the patient, "What is this?" Repeat with a pencil.	One point for each correct answer	2
Repeating a phrase	Ask the patient to say, "No ifs, ands, or buts."	One point if successful on first try	1
Verbal commands	Give the patient a plain piece of paper and say, "Take this paper in your right hand, fold it in half, and put it on the floor."	One point for each correct action	3
Written commands	Show the patient a piece of paper with "CLOSE YOUR EYES" printed on it.	One point if the patient's eyes close	1
Writing	Ask the patient to write a sentence.	One point if sentence has a subject, a verb, and makes sense	1
Drawing	Ask the patient to copy a pair of intersecting pentagons onto a piece of paper.	One point if the figure has 10 corners and 2 intersecting lines	1
Scoring		A score of 24 or above is considered normal.	30

Adapted from Folstein et al: Mini Mental State, *J Psych Res* 12:196–198, 1975.

Table 5.6 Clinical Evaluations of Cranial Nerve Function

Cranial Nerves		
Number	**Name**	**Evaluation Procedures**
I	Olfactory	Test ability to identify familiar aromatic odors, one naris at a time with eyes closed (not routinely tested)
II	Optic	Test vision with Snellen chart or Rosenbaum near-vision chart Perform ophthalmoscopic examination of fundi Be able to recognize papilledema Test fields of vision using confrontation and double simultaneous stimulation
III, IV, VI	Oculomotor, trochlear, abducens	Inspect eyelids for drooping (ptosis) Inspect pupil size for equality (direct and consensual response) Check for nystagmus Assess basic fields of gaze Note asymmetrical extraocular movements
V	Trigeminal	Palpate jaw muscles for tone and strength while patient clenches teeth Test superficial pain and touch sensation in each branch: V1, V2, V3
VII	Facial	Test corneal reflex Inspect symmetry of facial features Have patient smile, frown, puff cheeks, wrinkle forehead Watch for spasmodic, jerking movements of face
VIII	Acoustic	Test sense of hearing with watch or tuning fork Compare bone and air conduction of sound
IX	Glossopharyngeal	Test gag reflex and ability to swallow
X	Vagus	Inspect palate and uvula for symmetry with gag reflex Observe for swallowing difficulty Have patient take small sip of water Watch for nasal or hoarse quality of speech
XI	Spinal accessory	Test trapezius strength (have patient shrug shoulders against resistance) Test sternocleidomastoid muscle strength (have patient turn head to each side against resistance)
XII	Hypoglossal	Inspect tongue in mouth and while protruded for symmetry, fasciculations, and atrophy Test tongue strength with index fingers when tongue is pressed against cheek

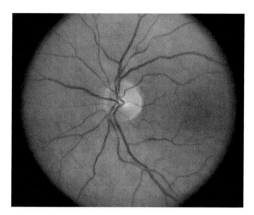

Fig. 5.2 **Normal optic disc.**

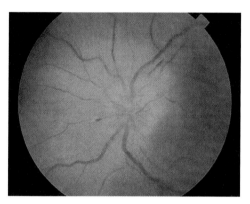

Fig. 5.3 **Early papilledema.**

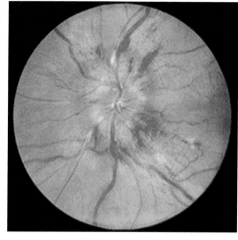

Fig. 5.4 **Advanced papilledema.**

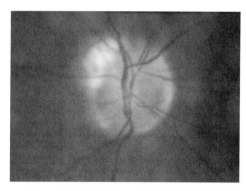

Fig. 5.5 **Optic nerve drusen.** These globules of calcified mucoproteins accumulate at the optic disc.

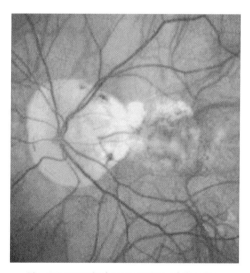

Fig. 5.6 **Myopic degeneration of the disc.**

pain are the basic issues, particular attention should be given to this portion of the examination. The key, once again, is developing a routine that, with practice, becomes thorough. It is far beyond the scope of this chapter to describe all the nuances of CN function.[16] Anyone evaluating patients for headache or facial pain must be able to recognize papilledema and abnormalities of ocular motor nerve function, must be familiar with the sensory division of the trigeminal nerve, and must be able to recognize isolated CN palsies. More complex problems, such as diplopia, cavernous sinus disease, and complex brainstem lesions, are best left to specialists in neuro-ophthalmology and neurology.

The importance of developing the ability to recognize papilledema cannot be overstated. Physicians who evaluate patients with headache who do not examine the patients' fundi are doing substandard work. Using an ophthalmoscope, the physician should turn down the lights and, if the fundus is still not visualized clearly, not hesitate to dilate the patient's eyes. The use of 0.5% tropicamide (Mydriacyl) is helpful for this purpose. Plate 1 demonstrates a few commonly encountered funduscopic findings. It is but a start as the physician begins to gain confidence in this aspect of physical diagnosis. The normal optic disc (**Fig. 5.2**) can be compared with discs seen in early (**Fig. 5.3**) and advanced papilledema (**Fig. 5.4**). Pseudopapilledema can be encountered both with optic nerve drusen (**Fig. 5.5**), which are globules of calcified mucoproteins that accumulate at the optic disc, and with myopic degeneration of the disc (**Fig. 5.6**). Central retinal vein occlusion (**Fig. 5.7**) frequently manifests with loss of central visual acuity with retinal hemorrhages, disc edema, and tortuous dilated veins. Finally, the color of the disc and the configuration and size of the optic cup should be

assessed. **Figure 5.8** demonstrates the pallor of optic atrophy as a result of inadequately treated papilledema. **Figure 5.9** is an example of an enlarged deep optic cup seen in glaucoma. Getting started is always the hard part, but learning to examine an optic fundus is well worth the effort.

This point is emphasized because Donohoe has four young women in his practice who are blind because their papilledema and increased intracranial pressure resulting from pseudotumor cerebri (idiopathic intracranial hypertension) were discovered far too late. Their stories were basically the same. They were all overweight, all had headaches, all were seen by multiple physicians, all had normal MRI brain imaging, and all had lost most of their vision before the correct diagnosis was made and proper therapy was instituted. This diagnosis rests on the ability to maintain a high index of suspicion and properly perform a funduscopic examination.

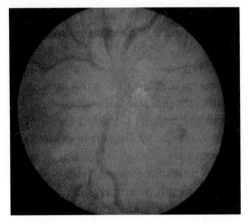

Fig. 5.7 **Central retinal vein occlusion.**

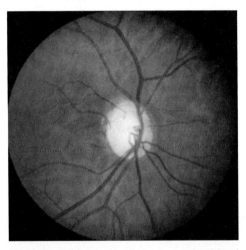

Fig. 5.8 **The pallor of optic atrophy as a result of inadequately treated papilledema.**

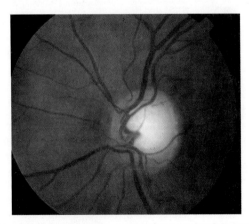

Fig. 5.9 **An enlarged deep optic cup seen in glaucoma.**

In general, the pain specialist, even one whose basic training has been in anesthesia or psychiatry, can, with proper effort, become familiar with the basics of common disorders. Ultimately, the physician who does make the effort to learn this material and incorporate it into clinical pain management practice will not have to deal constantly with feeling uneasy about a weakness in clinical aptitude. Such a physician will also avoid losing precious time in developing experience with these key physical findings associated with a variety of headache and facial pain problems.

Motor Examination

Motor examination should begin with inspection of muscle volume and contour. The physician should pay particular attention to atrophy and hypertrophy. The patient should be properly gowned so that these observations can be made without invading the patient's privacy. During this examination, fasciculations, contractures, alterations in posture, and adventitious movements may be identified. Strength is measured both proximally and distally in the upper and lower extremities and is graded according to the scale shown in **Table 5.7.** Detailed individual muscle testing is not carried out unless a specific nerve root or plexopathy is under investigation.

Tone is best tested by passive manipulation, with note made of the resistance of muscle when voluntary control is absent. Changes in tone are more readily detected in muscles of the arms and legs than in muscles of the trunk. Relaxation is critical to proper evaluation. Hypertonicity is usually seen with lesions rostral to the anterior horn cells, including brain, brainstem, and spinal cord. Hypotonicity is associated with diseases affecting the neuraxis below this level, involving nerve root, peripheral nerve, neuromuscular junction, and muscle. Study of the motor system should be integrated with evaluation of the sensory examination and deep tendon reflexes, to provide cumulative information critical to identifying the site of the lesion—brain, brainstem, spinal cord, root, plexus, nerve, or muscle.

Table 5.7 Grading of Muscle Strength

Clinical Finding	Grade	Percentage of Normal Response
No evidence of contractility	0	0
Slight contractility, no movement	1	10
Full range of motion, gravity eliminated	2	25
Full range of motion with gravity	3	50
Full range of motion against gravity, some resistance	4	75
Full range of motion against gravity, full resistance	5	100

From Chipps EM, Clanin NJ, Campbell VG: *Neurologic disorder,* St Louis, 1992, Mosby-Year Book.

Sensory Examination

The sensory examination should be kept simple and should be targeted by clues obtained through the history. Certainly, time spent in defining sensory loss in the lower extremities would be justified in a patient who complains of pain, weakness, and numbness in the foot but not in a patient who has double vision and facial pain. Note in **Figure 5.10** the difference between the skin areas innervated by dermatomes—specific segments of the cord, roots, or dorsal root ganglia—and the corresponding peripheral nerve cutaneous sensory distribution. These specific differences and changes in motor function and reflexes clinically define a nerve root from a peripheral nerve abnormality. **Tables 5.8** and **5.9** highlight comparisons between specific spinal root and peripheral nerve lesions of the upper and lower

extremities. With time, experience, and persistence, the pain specialist can become confident in the evaluation of peripheral nerve root lesions. So many of the common pain syndromes (cervical radiculopathies, lumbar radiculopathies, carpal tunnel syndrome, femoral neuropathy, peroneal neuropathy) may be rapidly and accurately diagnosed without expensive and uncomfortable neurodiagnostic testing. Being persistent and resisting the fear that the task is overwhelming result in the ability to evaluate patients in pain efficiently.

For pain syndromes of the upper extremity, the examiner should be able to differentiate sensory involvement of the radial, median, and ulnar nerves from that of specific roots (C5-T1) (see Table 5.8). For pain syndromes of the lower extremities, the examiner should be able to differentiate the

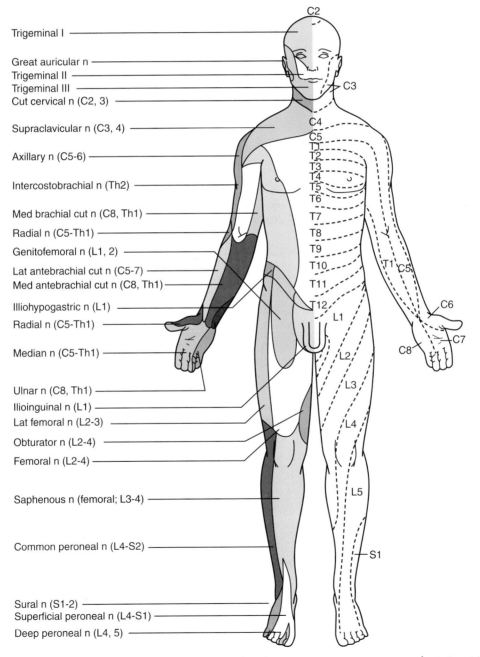

Fig. 5.10 **Comparison of spinal segmental (dermatomal) and peripheral nerve cutaneous sensory supply.** *(Adapted from Haerer AF, editor: DeJong's the neurologic examination, ed 5, Philadelphia, 1992, Lippincott.)*

Table 5.8 Clinical Manifestations of Root Versus Nerve Lesions in the Arm

Roots	C5	C6	C7	C8	T1
Sensory supply	Lateral border upper arm	Lateral forearm, including finger I	Over triceps, midforearm, and finger III	Medial forearm to finger V	Axilla to elbow
Reflex affected	Biceps reflex	None	Triceps reflex	None	None
Motor loss	Deltoid Infraspinatus Rhomboids Supraspinatus	Biceps Brachialis Brachioradialis	Latissimus dorsi Pectoralis major Triceps Wrist extensors Wrist flexors	Finger extensors Finger flexors Flexor carpi ulnaris	Intrinsic hand muscles (in some thenar muscles through C8)

Nerves	Axillary (C5, C6)	Musculotaneous (C5, C6)	Radial (C5–C8)	Median (C6–C8, T1)	Ulnar (C8, T1)
Sensory supply	Over deltoid	Lateral forearm to wrist	Lateral dorsal forearm and back of thumb and finger II	Lateral palm and lateral finger I, II, III, and half of IV	Medial palm and finger V and medial half of finger IV
Reflex affected	None	Biceps reflex	Triceps reflex	None	None
Motor loss	Deltoid	Biceps Brachialis	Brachioradialis Finger extensors Forearm supinator Triceps wrist extensors	Abductor pollicis brevis Long flexors of fingers I, II, III Pronators of forearm Wrist flexors	Intrinsic hand muscles Flexor carpi ulnaris Flexors of fingers IV, V

From Patten J: *Neurological differential diagnosis,* New York, 1977, Springer-Verlag.

Table 5.9 Clinical Manifestations of Root Versus Nerve Lesions in the Leg

Roots	L2	L3	L4	L5	S1
Sensory supply	Across upper thigh	Across lower thigh	Across knee to medial malleolus	Side of leg to dorsum and sole of foot	Behind lateral malleolus to lateral foot
Reflex affected	None	None	Patellar reflex	None	Achilles reflex
Motor loss	Hip flexion	Knee extension	Inversion of foot	Dorsiflexion of toes and foot	Plantar flexion and eversion of foot

Nerves	Obturator (L2–L4)	Femoral (L2–L4)	Peroneal Division of Sciatic (L4, L5, S1–S3)	Tibial Division of Sciatic (L4, L5, S1–S3)
Sensory supply	Medial thigh	Anterior thigh to medial malleolus	Anterior leg to dorsum of foot	Posterior leg to sole and lateral aspect of foot
Reflex affected	None	Patellar reflex	None	Achilles reflex
Motor loss	Adduction of thigh	Extension of knee	Dorsiflexion, inversion, and eversion of foot	Plantar flexion and inversion of foot

From Patten J: *Neurological differential diagnosis,* New York, 1977, Springer-Verlag.

peroneal and tibial nerve sensory distribution from that of the L4, L5, and S1 roots (see Table 5.9). Such distinctions elucidate most of the common problems. Over time, the pain specialist can increase confidence in the examination and may develop a stronger foundation in peripheral neurology than many neurologists, neurosurgeons, and orthopedists possess.

Deep Tendon Reflexes

Deep tendon reflexes are actually muscle stretch reflexes mediated through neuromuscular spindles. This are the one facet of the clinical examination that is objective (**Table 5.10**). Responses to mental status testing and motor examination, performance

Table 5.10 Deep Tendon Reflex Scale

Grade	Deep Tendon Reflex Response
0+	No response
1+	Sluggish
2+	Active or normal
3+	More brisk than expected, slightly hyperactive
4+	Abnormally hyperactive, with intermittent clonus

From Seidel HM, Ball J, Daines J, et al: *Mosby's guide to physical examination,* ed 7. St Louis, 2010, Mosby.

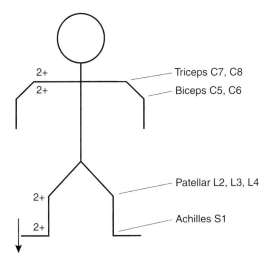

Fig. 5.11 **Diagram of a deep tendon reflex examination.** *(From Waldman SD, editor:* Interventional pain management, *ed 2, Philadelphia, 2001, Saunders, 95.)*

on sensory testing, and even gait can be consciously altered by the patient for any of a variety of reasons. Guillain-Barré syndrome (acute inflammatory polyneuropathy), however, a condition that in its initial stages may be misdiagnosed as anxiety related, characteristically shows absence of all the deep tendon reflexes, an important early clue to the organic nature of the disorder.

A deep tendon reflex examination can be graded using the numerals 1 through 4 (**Fig. 5.11**). Testing of the superficial reflexes, such as the abdominal or cremasteric reflexes, is not particularly valuable in clinical assessment. The only superficial reflex worth evaluating is the plantar reflex (a superficial reflex innervated by the tibial nerve, L4-S2). The response to stroking the plantar surface of the foot is usually flexion of both the foot and the toes. In diseases of the cortical spinal system, dorsiflexion of the toes occurs, especially the great toe, with separation or fanning of the others; this finding, Babinski's sign of upper motoneuron involvement (brain, brainstem, and spinal cord), is often paired with increased deep tendon reflexes and clonus (i.e., sustained muscular contractions following a stretch stimulus noted frequently in the ankle).

Unilateral absence of a deep tendon reflex implies disease at the peripheral nerve or root level. Diffuse reduction or absence of deep tendon reflexes suggests a more generalized process affecting the peripheral nerve, seen frequently in peripheral neuropathies secondary to diabetes, alcohol abuse, or inflammation. The objective data obtained quite rapidly from testing deep tendon reflexes are correlated with motor and sensory findings to determine whether a problem lies in a specific peripheral nerve, a specific nerve root, a diffuse peripheral nerve, or the spinal cord. It should take less than 30 seconds to complete this part of the examination.

Examination of Gait

Walking is an intricate process influenced by mechanical factors such as muscles, bones, tendons, and joints and, more importantly, dependent on nervous system integration. Just watching the patient walk during the examination is an extremely valuable exercise. The patient should be asked to walk with eyes open and closed and to stand with eyes open and closed (Romberg's sign). Gaits associated with parkinsonism (small, short steps with a stooped posture), normal-pressure hydrocephalus (magnetic gait, as if the patient were walking in magnetic shoes across a metal floor), muscular dystrophy, stroke, peripheral nerve injury, cerebellar ataxia, Huntington's chorea, and hysteria (astasia-abasia) are but a few characteristic patterns of disturbed locomotion. In short, a strong measure of neuro-orthopedic well-being is implied by the patient who walks well with eyes open and closed.

Conclusion

The basic point of this chapter is simple. A targeted and well-organized pain history is the foundation of proper diagnosis. Advances in diagnostic technology, no matter how sophisticated, cannot replace listening to the patient's own story of the illness. It is through this process that physicians most effectively gain insight, not only into the nature of the illness but also, and more importantly, into the personality of the patient who is in pain. The professionalism and sensitivity with which physicians obtain this information do much to establish the relationship with the patient and the ultimate success of therapies. If any room exists for shortcuts, it is not in this portion of the evaluation.

The targeted physical examination should be viewed as an extension of the insights derived from the history. It should be performed in a professional, thorough, but not laborious fashion. As the calling of pain management becomes more popular, physicians of various disciplines should avoid faddish technologic advances and opportunism made possible by inequities in reimbursement and should commit themselves to the very basics: obtaining historical data and eliciting physical findings. Energy expended to this end will reduce costs, enhance patient satisfaction, and foster lasting credibility in the evolving field of pain management.

References

Full references for this chapter can be found on www.expertconsult.com.

Chapter 6

Patterns of Common Pain Syndromes

Bernard M. Abrams

Discussions of patterns of pain syndromes form a large portion of this comprehensive book. The text is divided into sections on generalized pain syndromes, including acute pain syndromes, neuropathic pain syndromes, malignant pain syndromes, pain of dermatologic origin, and pain of musculoskeletal origin, and regional pain syndromes, encompassing virtually every part of the body. This chapter does not reiterate material that is discussed in detail in appropriate chapters, but rather outlines the general features and underlying principles of patterns in pain-producing syndromes.

Pain is defined by the International Association for the Study of Pain as an unpleasant sensory and emotional experience associated with actual or potential tissue damage or described in terms of such damage. Several types of pain are recognized.

Nociceptive pain is caused by the ongoing activation of nociceptors (pain receptors) in response to noxious or potentially noxious stimuli. It may be cutaneous, deep somatic, or visceral. It is associated with "proper functioning" of the nervous system, and generally the severity of the pain corresponds closely to the intensity of the stimulus. Although its characteristics may vary with the part of the body involved, the tissues under attack, or the intensity, acuteness, or chronicity of the process, nociceptive pain is familiar, expected, recognizable, and attributable to a source. In short, "it makes sense," or, in modern parlance, it "computes." Many different pain types and patterns emerge.

Neuropathic pain is caused by aberrant signal processing in the peripheral or central nervous system and reflects nervous system damage or dysfunction. It has an unexpected aspect, detached from an obvious stimulus intensity or putative tissue damage. It is characterized by burning, tingling, or shooting sensations, which may be spontaneous or evoked, steady, or intermittent. This pain may be associated with other clear-cut neurologic phenomena, such as sensory loss, allodynia (pain elicited by a non-noxious stimulus, such as clothing, air movement, touch, or an ordinarily nonpainful cold or warm stimulus), or hyperalgesia (exaggerated painful response to a mildly noxious, mechanical, or thermal stimulus). Common sources of neuropathic pain include trauma, metabolic disease (e.g., diabetes mellitus), infection (e.g., herpes zoster), tumors, toxins, side effects of medications (especially chemotherapeutic and antiviral agents used to treat human immunodeficiency virus [HIV] infections), and primary neurologic diseases. Central pain may arise in the setting of stroke, tumor, spinal cord injury, or multiple sclerosis. Neuropathic pain has the characteristic of unfamiliarity, is often inexplicable, is hard to believe (even for the experienced observer), and, in short, "doesn't compute."

Another caveat concerns "what is common." This depends on the patient or physician setting (e.g., whether it is an emergency department, cancer center, or pain clinic). Physician specialty and interests also play an important role. The painful manifestations of rheumatoid arthritis or multiple sclerosis and painful peripheral neuropathies are rarely seen at an average pain clinic, which is more concerned with problems of the axial spine, complex regional pain syndrome, and postherpetic neuralgia. Conditions seen on a daily basis by podiatrists, rheumatologists, or orthopedists may be *terra incognita* to the pain physician.

Several universals are noted in pain patterns. Pain patterns have the following: a temporal and spatial distribution; characteristic pain types (e.g., burning, tearing, gnawing, deep, superficial); and often associated medical diagnoses, other symptoms, and other features that offer important clues to the diagnosis and management. One of the most commonly overlooked features of pain patterns is the occurrence of a secondary or tertiary type of pain pattern. This feature is clearly apparent in radiculopathies, which often manifest as a sharp (and sharply delineated) pain ("epicritic pain") and tend to obscure a deeper, less well-delineated gnawing-type pain ("protopathic pain"). The two types of pain originate in the same relative area of the body (e.g., cervical or lumbar region) and often at the same axial spinal level (e.g., C6-7 or L4-5), but stem from different tissues or structures (e.g., nerve root versus vertebral body or facet joints). Careful inquiry for a secondary or tertiary type of pain (rarely volunteered by the patient) produces a much greater understanding of the pathologic process involved.

Temporal Pattern

It is a well-shown principle of pain management that the temporal pattern of the pain complaint is derived largely from the patient's history and sheds light on the possible cause of the problem. A relentlessly progressive course suggests serious underlying disease and warrants further inquiry (additional comprehensive history, physical examination, appropriate associated laboratory studies, and imaging techniques) for malignancy or infection. A rapid onset and rapid relief of pain are characteristic of neuropathies or neuralgia (e.g., trigeminal neuralgia).

Spatial Pattern

The spatial distribution of the pain in conjunction with physical examination, laboratory tests, and imaging procedures suggests the localization of the problem (e.g., cervical radiculopathy or lumbosacral plexus disease) and tends to limit the diagnostic possibilities. All physicians with even a brief exposure to pain problems recognize the syndromic approach to pain management. This approach is familiar in the example of cervical radiculopathy, with neck pain accompanied by radiation in a dermatopic nerve root distribution down into the thumb, index finger, or both. More detailed questioning may reveal a deep gnawing pain extending into the root of the neck, shoulder, or intrascapular area. This approach may serve well if alternative situations, such as referred pain (e.g., from a distal nerve lesion such as an ulnar nerve palsy or from an internal viscus) and the possibility of a tumor rather than a cervical disk disorder or spondylosis, are not forgotten.

Symptomatic/Anatomic/Etiologic Diagnostic Approach to Pain Problems

It is good practice to form a *symptomatic/anatomic/etiologic diagnosis* for each pain problem. This practice eliminates jumping to a syndromic conclusion and serves as framework for an orderly approach to the problem. This approach is demonstrated by the following cases.

Case 1

A 36-year-old woman developed diffuse neck pain without an antecedent history of illness or injury. The pain was deep and gnawing and was accompanied by sharp pain down the radial aspect of her arm and forearm to the thumb, index, and middle fingers. It was accompanied by a deep, boring (worse at night) intrascapular pain and mild weakness of the right biceps muscle. She had mild numbness of the thumb. Examination revealed limited range of motion of the cervical spine to the right and a right Spurling sign (pain reproduced by extension and lateral rotation to the right). She had mild weakness of the right biceps and brachialis, a diminished right biceps reflex, and hyperesthesia in the right C6 distribution.

The symptomatic diagnosis in this case is pain in the neck and down the right arm with mild C6 motor and sensory signs. This diagnosis is arrived at by a combination of the history and the physical examination. Syndromically, it could be referred to as "cervical radiculopathy without evidence of myelopathy." For reasons that become clear in the next case presentation, the syndromic diagnosis should be made cautiously. The anatomic diagnosis in this case is C6 radiculopathy as a result of physical examination findings. The anatomic diagnosis may be augmented by electromyography, which is an extension of physical examination because it is based on physiologic examination of nerve, nerve root, and muscle. It is *not* based on imaging technique at this point because imaging technique may give irrelevant information and *always* requires clinical correlation. The etiologic diagnosis is cervical radiculopathy resulting from herniated nucleus pulposus at C5-6, based on magnetic resonance imaging (MRI) of the cervical spine that showed a herniated disk at C5-6 *correlated* with the history and physical examination and not *negated* by any more plausible diagnosis. This may seem a convoluted method of diagnosis, but its merits are better illustrated by the following cases.

Case 2

A 56-year-old, right-handed man developed pain in the right supraclavicular region with associated neck pain of boring quality, worse at night, with radiation of fairly sharp pain down the ulnar border of the arm. Neck turning and shoulder movements exacerbated the pain, which was particularly bad at night. Examination revealed that the right pupil was slightly smaller than the left, but fully reactive. The patient had some weakness of the intrinsic hand muscles and hyperesthesia along the ulnar border of the right forearm. No reflex changes were noted. MRI revealed diffuse ridging at all levels, but worst at C7-T1. No long tract signs (signs of spinal cord involvement) were noted.

Syndromic diagnosis would be lower cervical radiculopathy secondary to spondylosis. This diagnosis conceivably could lead to inappropriate therapeutic measures. The symptomatic diagnosis is neck, shoulder, and arm pain in a lower cervical distribution. The anatomic diagnosis is C8-T1 root or brachial plexus involvement (>90% of all cervical nerve root disorders involve the C5-6 or C6-7 levels emanating from the C6 or the C7 nerve roots). The etiologic differential diagnosis includes involvement of the brachial plexus by Pancoast's tumor of the lung, C8-T1 disease or acute brachial plexitis (Parsonage-Turner syndrome), or primary tumor of the nerve roots (meningioma or neurofibroma). In this case, a chest radiograph and computed tomography (CT) scan revealed a malignant tumor of the right upper lobe of the lung, and MRI of the brachial plexus showed erosion by the tumor. In this case, keeping an open mind and using the symptomatic/anatomic/etiologic approach averted a significant error in diagnosis and treatment.

Case 3

A 64-year-old man presented with sharp and aching pain in the left shoulder blade, neck, and elbow. The sharp pain was referred from the elbow into the forearm, and the aching pain in the elbow (occasionally) was referred to the neck and the forearm, related to exertion, although the association was unclear. Some association (again unclear) existed with flexion-extension of the left elbow that produced the sharp and the aching pain. The patient had intermittent numbness of the ulnar portion of the left hand and forearm, as well as weakness of the left abductor digiti, first dorsal interosseous muscle, and adductor pollicis brevis. No cranial nerve, long tract, or sphincteric signs were observed.

In this case, the symptomatic diagnosis is sharp and aching elbow pain and shoulder and forearm pain potentially related to exertion or flexion-extension, or both, of the elbow. The anatomic diagnosis is unclear and requires further elucidation by electromyography for possible ulnar neuropathy at the elbow, brachial plexus lesion, and a cardiology workup for atypical angina pectoris. The anatomic differential diagnosis includes such diverse possibilities as visceral (cardiac or pulmonary), musculoskeletal (scapulocostal syndrome or other chest wall syndrome), or peripheral nervous system (ulnar entrapment at the elbow with radiation to the chest wall or lower brachial plexus or cervical spine pathology) conditions. The etiologic diagnosis is in doubt at this point because numerous possibilities largely depend on the anatomic location of the problem.

Any attempt at syndromic diagnosis is fraught with hazard because it forces the examiner prematurely into identifying an organ system as the cause of the pain with little or no evidence to support any one possibility. The symptomatic/anatomic/etiologic approach serves as a "holding area" while each of the diagnostic possibilities is explored, without the examiner's having to jump to conclusions.

The symptomatic diagnosis seems self-evident, although the tendency is to try to fit it into a defined syndrome, such as cervical radiculopathy, complex regional pain syndrome, or migraine, in clear-cut circumstances. The anatomic diagnosis requires careful analysis of findings from physical examination, electromyography (when applicable), and imaging techniques. The physical examination and imaging findings must be concordant (match), and in case of a discrepancy, especially in spinal imaging in which abnormalities abound in asymptomatic patients, greater weight must be given to the physical examination findings, especially when they explain the clinical history. The etiologic diagnosis should include, at least preliminarily, a checklist of all possible types of pathologic processes. It is useful to review the list in **Table 6.1** or at least give it brief consideration no matter how obvious the apparent cause may be. The putative anatomic site may be subdivided as shown in **Table 6.2**.

Referred Pain Patterns

Physicians become familiar with the patterns of intrathoracic and intra-abdominal pain referral from internal viscera in the earliest years of training in clinical medicine. Referral patterns are particularly well discussed and illustrated in Wiener's classic text.[1] A potential pitfall in referred pain diagnosis is the less well recognized referral of myofascial pain (e.g., referral of pain from the levator scapulae to the chest wall simulating

Table 6.1 Partial List of Etiologic Causes of Pain

Etiology	Examples
Vascular	Claudication, hemorrhage, space-occupying vascular malformations impinging on pain-sensitive structures
Tumor	Primary (e.g., meningioma or neurofibroma) and metastatic
Osseous	Primary bone disorders (e.g., Paget's disease, fibrous dysplasia, leontiasis ossea), DISH syndrome, focal spinal overgrowth (ridging)
Degenerative	Various arthritides, degenerative spine disease (spondylosis, spinal stenosis, spondylolisthesis, degenerated intervertebral disks)
Trauma	Herniated intervertebral disks, compression fractures, microtrauma
Metabolic	Diabetes mellitus, thyroid disorders, parathyroid disorders
Infectious	HIV infection, viral, bacterial, fungal, rickettsial infections
Collagen vascular disorders	Rheumatoid arthritis, systemic lupus erythematosus, polymyalgia rheumatica, temporal arteritis
Toxic	Exogenous and endogenous toxicities
Psychiatric	Substance abuse, depression, psychosis, personality disorders

DISH, disseminated idiopathic skeletal hyperostosis; HIV, human immunodeficiency virus.

Table 6.2 Possible Generalized Sites of Anatomic Pathology Causing Pain

Skin
Subcutaneous tissues, including fat and connective tissue
Ligaments and tendons
Skeletal muscles
Nerves, nerve roots, and plexus
Central nervous system structures, including spinal cord
Vascular structures, including arteries and veins
Lymphatics
Viscera

angina or cholecystitis). So-called trigger points frequently simulate the pain of internal organs, thus raising the possibility of misdiagnosis and mistreatment.[2] The concept of trigger point referral is most closely associated with Simons and Travell, who wrote the classic two-volume work on pain referral patterns.[3] Volume 1 addresses referral patterns in the upper half of body (head, neck, thorax, and abdomen), and volume 2 addresses the lower extremities.

Spinal Pain Patterns

Vertebral Pain Syndromes

Vertebral pain tends to be deep and boring and present at rest. When associated with an aggressive process, the pain tends to increase stepwise and may spread to a radicular distribution,

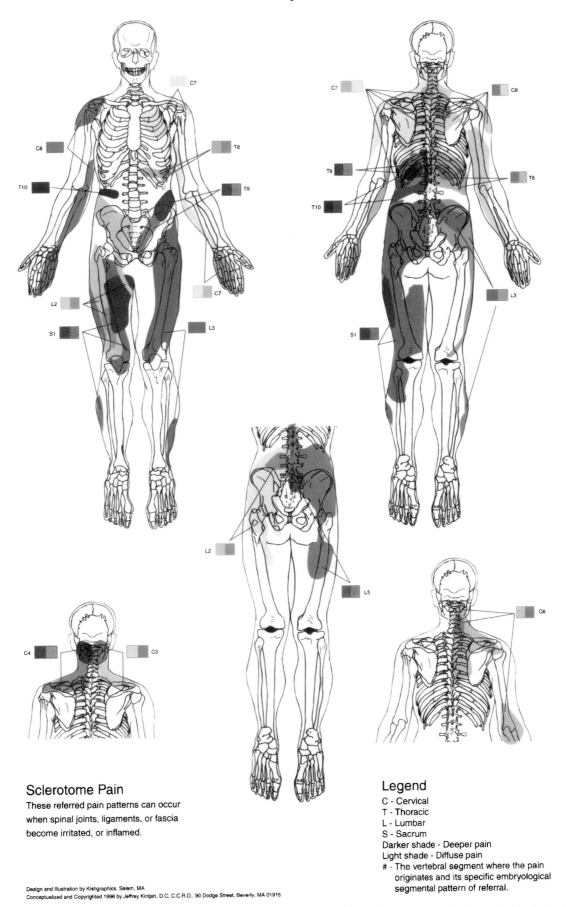

Sclerotome Pain

These referred pain patterns can occur when spinal joints, ligaments, or fascia become irritated, or inflamed.

Legend

C - Cervical
T - Thoracic
L - Lumbar
S - Sacrum
Darker shade - Deeper pain
Light shade - Diffuse pain
\# - The vertebral segment where the pain originates and its specific embryological segmental pattern of referral.

Design and Illustration by Kishgraphics, Salem, MA
Conceptualized and Copyrighted 1996 by Jeffrey Kintish, D.C, C.C.R.D., 90 Dodge Street, Beverly, MA 01915

Fig. 6.1 **Sclerotogenous pain pathways.** This illustration is useful for pinpointing referred sclerotogenous pain from spinal levels C1 through S3. *(From Clinical Charts & Supplies, Beverly, Mass.)*

Continued

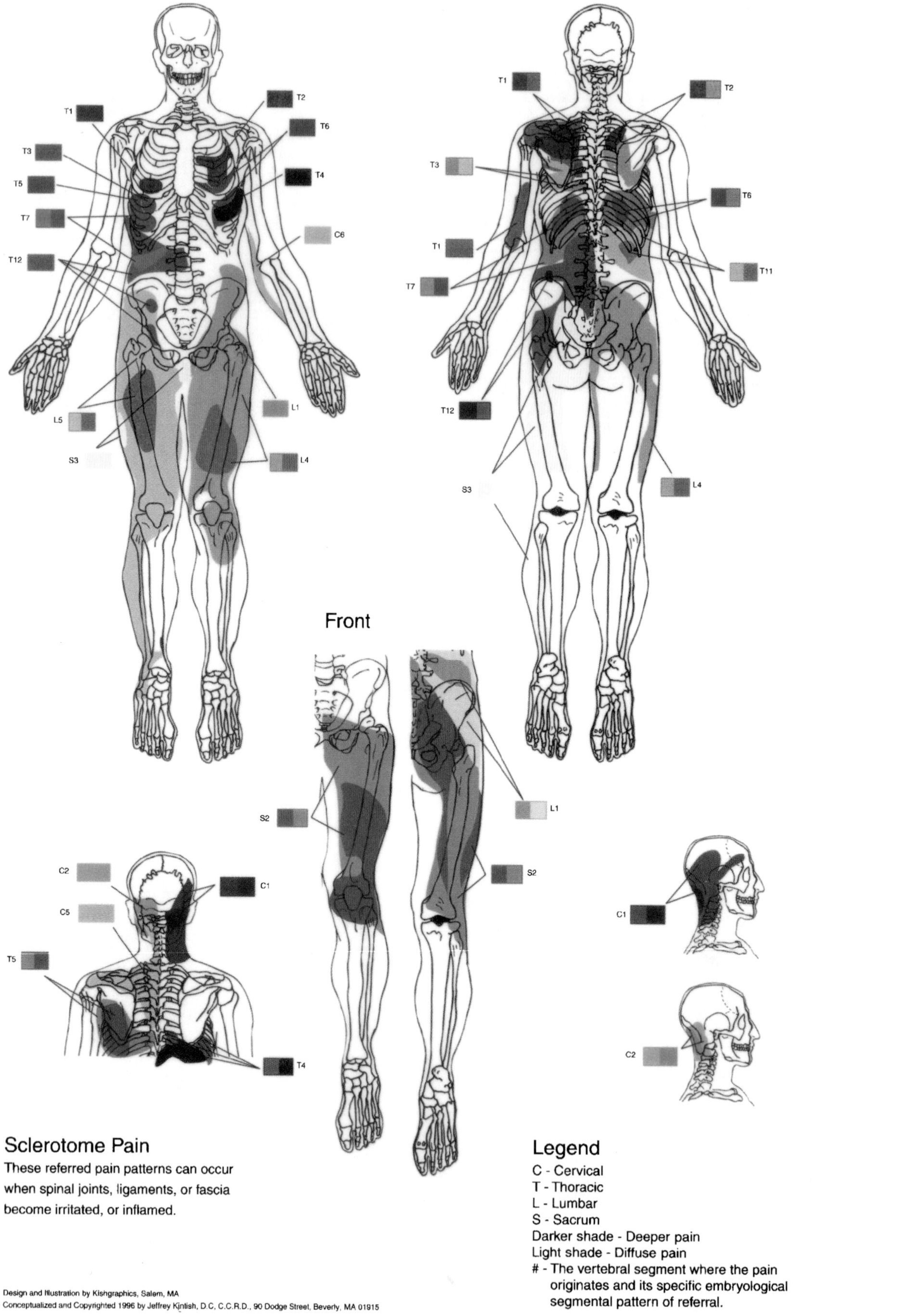
T1
T2
T3
T6
T5
T4
T7
C6
T12
L1
L5
S3
L4
T11
Front
S2
C2
C1
C5
Sclerotome Pain
These referred pain patterns can occur when spinal joints, ligaments, or fascia become irritated, or inflamed.
Legend
C - Cervical
T - Thoracic
L - Lumbar
S - Sacrum
Darker shade - Deeper pain
Light shade - Diffuse pain
- The vertebral segment where the pain originates and its specific embryological segmental pattern of referral.
Design and Illustration by Kishgraphics, Salem, MA
Conceptualized and Copyrighted 1996 by Jeffrey Kintish, D.C, C.C.R.D., 90 Dodge Street, Beverly, MA 01915

Fig. 6.1–cont'd. **Sclerotogenous pain pathways.** This illustration is useful for pinpointing referred sclerotogenous pain from spinal levels C1 through S3. *(From Clinical Charts & Supplies, Beverly, Mass.)*

which may be "girdling" if it is in the abdomen or thorax. Jarring, movement, or percussion may exacerbate the pain. Although the pain characteristics may vary from condition to condition and from individual to individual, the presence at rest is highly suggestive and clearly different from radiculopathies, which tend to be ameliorated by rest and recumbency.

Spinal Radiculopathies

The pain of spinal radiculopathies tends to be quite sharp and well delineated, with the proviso that patients often have an associated deep, gnawing pain that is usually more proximal and less well defined than the sharp pain. This pain is attributable to irritation of nonradicular structures, such as bones and tendinous attachments, and follows a sclerotogenous pattern (**Fig. 6.1**). Radicular pain usually follows well-understood and familiar patterns.[4,5] Pain distribution, sensory changes, motor weakness, and reflex changes in the cervical region are summarized in **Table 6.3**, and changes corresponding to the lumbar region are summarized in **Table 6.4**. Clinical syndromes associated with cervical spondylosis include acute stiff neck, radiculopathy, myelopathy, myeloradiculopathy, vertebrobasilar insufficiency, cervicogenic headache, and Barre-Lieou syndrome (cervical sympathetic syndrome).

Cervical Facet Syndrome

Cervical facet syndrome is a syndrome of head, neck, shoulder, and proximal upper extremity pain largely in a nondermatomal distribution. The pain is usually dull and ill defined; it is worsened by flexion, extension, and lateral flexion of the neck (unilateral or bilateral) and is unaccompanied by motor or sensory deficits. Referral patterns are presented in **Figure 6.2**.

Lumbar Radiculopathy

Patients complain of pain, numbness, tingling, and paresthesias in the appropriate nerve root distribution. The pain may be sharp and lancinating, but it is accompanied by a more vaguely, localized, proximally distributed sclerotogenous pain. Relative contributions of dorsal and ventral roots influence the character of the pain, and the ventral root pain is often duller and less well localized as a result of the predominately motor distribution. Involvement of the sinuvertebral nerve (recurrent nerve of Luschka) ensures at least some painful involvement of the axial structures, whereas a laterally placed process may result in pain purely localized to the limb and confusing because of the absence of the axial pain usually present in radiculopathies.

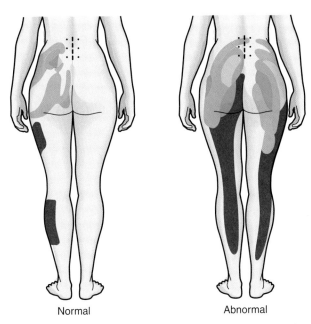

Normal   Abnormal

Fig. 6.2 **Pain referral patterns from lumbar L4-5 and L5-S1 facet joint injections.** On the *left* are areas of pain drawn by asymptomatic subjects following injection of hypertonic saline into the facet joints. On the *right* are areas of pain drawn by patients with chronic back and leg pain who had similar injections. The different methods of shading indicate different patients. *(Redrawn from Renfrew DL. Facet joint procedures. In* Atlas of spine injection, *Philadelphia, 2004, Saunders, 73.)*

Table 6.3 Characteristics of Cervical Radicular Pain

Cervical Root	Pain	Sensory Changes	Weakness	Reflex Changes
C5	Neck, shoulder, anterolateral arm	Numbness in deltoid area	Deltoid and biceps	Biceps reflex
C6	Neck, shoulder, lateral aspect of arm	Dorsolateral aspect of thumb and index finger	Biceps, wrist extensors, pollicis longus	Brachioradialis reflex
C7	Neck, shoulder, lateral aspect of arm, dorsal forearm	Index and middle finger, dorsum of hand	Triceps	Triceps reflex

Table 6.4 Characteristics of Lumbar Radicular Pain

Lumbar Root	Pain	Sensory Changes	Weakness	Reflex Changes
L4	Back, shin, thigh, leg	Shin numbness	Ankle dorsiflexors	Knee
L5	Back, posterior thigh, leg	Numbness at top of foot and first web space	Extensor hallucis longus	None
S1	Back, posterior calf, leg	Numbness at lateral aspect of foot	Gastrocnemius and soleus	Ankle jerk

Lumbar Facet Syndrome

Patients usually are more than 65 years old, and the pain, which is less well localized than radicular pain, is deeper and duller. The pain is exacerbated by standing or lumbar extension and is improved by sitting and forward flexion. Pain is not exacerbated by coughing or other Valsalva-related maneuvers, it may be referred to the buttocks or ipsilateral thigh, and it generally presents in a more proximal distribution than radicular pain.

Lumbar Spondylolisthesis

Dull or sharp back pain is exacerbated with lifting, twisting, or bending. Patients often complain about a "catch" in their back. Rising from a sitting to standing position often reproduces the pain.

Lumbar Spinal Stenosis

Pseudoclaudication of the lower extremities is the characteristic pattern. Multiple roots are typically involved. The pain may disappear with spinal flexion (e.g., riding a stationary bicycle), but it results in fatigue with prolonged walking or standing (**Table 6.5**). Pain is characteristically present in the calf, and it simulates vascular claudication. Pain, numbness, and weakness are seen in the affected segments. Muscle spasms and vague pains are commonly seen, including (paradoxically) pains in the intrascapular region.

Arachnoiditis

Arachnoiditis is characterized by pain (generally duller and less well defined than radiculopathy, but may be severe and excruciating), numbness, tingling, paresthesias, and weakness, often in multiple nerve roots. Muscle spasm in the lumbar region with referral into the buttocks is common. Bladder and bowel symptoms are more frequent than expected with radiculopathy.

Table 6.5 Spinal Stenosis versus Disk Protrusion (Radiculopathy)

	Spinal Stenosis	Disk Protrusion (Radiculopathy)
Pain pattern	Insidious, less well localized, duller Worse with walking or standing Worse with extension	Acute, sharper, better localized Worse with sitting Worse with flexion
Age at onset (yr)	Most commonly 30–50	Most commonly >60
Response to conservative therapy (%)	50	>90

References

Full references for this chapter can be found on www.expertconsult.com.

Rational Use of Laboratory Testing

Charles D. Donohoe

The targeted history and physical examination remain the most cost-effective tools aiding the clinician in the proper diagnosis of a patient's pain. The rational use of laboratory testing is often the next reasonable step to assist the clinician to confirm his or her clinical impression, as well as to help the clinician implement and refine a treatment plan. Unfortunately, the logical use of laboratory tests is too often ignored in favor of expensive radiologic and neurophysiologic studies that, at the very least, add to the cost of a patient's care and, at the very worst, lead to an incorrect diagnosis and subsequent inappropriate therapeutic interventions.

Findings such as pyuria, profound anemia, hyperglycemia and elevation of acute phase proteins are often crucial in identifying the cause of pain and in assessing the general medical status of the patient. Although clinical laboratory medicine is a massive and rapidly evolving discipline that truly defies condensation, it is hoped that this chapter will provide the reader with a guide to the laboratory evaluation of the patient in pain.

Pitfalls of Clinical Practice

Mistakes are commonly made in several areas of clinical practice. The first involves failure to contact the family members of a confused patient who is obviously unable to give a coherent history. The second is failure to obtain old records. Third, and equally serious, is the mistaken supposition that

because the patient has seen multiple physicians in the past, basic laboratory work has been ordered.

The ability to avoid these mistakes demands a discipline that emphasizes that the clinician always consider the critical details of the targeted history and physical examination as well as assess the adequacy of the patient's earlier diagnostic workup. This effort is extremely effective in containing costs, conserving physicians' time, and ultimately arriving at an accurate diagnosis. In difficult patients who have seen several physicians, quality control of earlier historical data and diagnostic workup is often ignored, and each additional consultation simply compounds the sloppy imprecision of the preceding evaluations. Although these basic steps are laborious and time consuming, it almost always rewards the clinician to take time, at the beginning of the patient interaction, to get them right. Frequently, the best use of technology is a telephone call to a concerned family member or a former treating physician. Yet, often in the heat of the moment, this simple act is avoided, thereby instituting a cascade of errors.

The Basics

Table 7.1 lists a basic battery of laboratory tests commonly used to evaluate pain. The clinician can use this table as a starting point for the laboratory evaluation of the patient in pain while realizing that the selection of specific tests depends on multiple factors, including age, gender, duration and location

Table 7.1 **The Basic Pain Laboratory Battery**
Complete blood count (CBC)
Acute phase proteins: erythrocyte sedimentation rate (ESR), C-reactive protein (CRP)
Blood chemistry: glucose, hemoglobin A-1 C, sodium, potassium, chloride, carbon dioxide, calcium, phosphorus, urea nitrogen, creatinine, uric acid, total protein, albumin, globulin, bilirubin
Enzymes: alkaline phosphatase, creatine kinase, lactate dehydrogenase, aspartate aminotransferase, alanine aminotransferase
Thyroid-stimulating hormone (TSH)
Vitamin B_{12}: measure methylmalonic acid if B_{12} level is below 400 pg/mL.
Human immunodeficiency virus (HIV) infection, hepatitis B and C
Serum and urine protein electrophoresis with immunofixation

of pain, coexisting medical problems, and results of other laboratory studies. One preliminary tenet of pain practice management is that, once a physician orders laboratory tests, he or she is responsible not only for seeing that the tests are performed but also for personally reviewing the results. Failure to do both can have serious medical-legal implications and, more importantly, can harm the patient.

Acute Phase Proteins

The erythrocyte sedimentation rate (ESR) and the C-reactive protein (CRP) value are the most commonly used indicators of the acute phase response. This response includes numerous protein changes, including increases in the complement system, fibrinogen, serum amyloid, and acute phase phenomena including fever, thrombocytosis, leukocytosis, and anemia. A reduction in serum albumin concentration is characteristic of the acute phase response. These complex changes are induced by inflammation-associated cytokines, particularly interleukin-1, interleukin-6, and tumor necrosis factor-α (TNFα) and are seen in response to infection, trauma, surgery, burns, cancer, inflammatory conditions, and psychological stress.[1]

The ESR, the rate at which erythrocytes fall through plasma, is actually an indirect measure of plasma acute phase protein concentration and depends mainly on the plasma concentration of fibrinogen. Unfortunately, the ESR can be influenced by other factors, including the size, shape, and number of erythrocytes, as well as by other plasma protein constituents such as immunoglobulins. CRP is a glycoprotein produced during acute inflammation and derives its name from its ability to react and precipitate pneumococcus C polysaccharide. The CRP test has fewer associated technical problems and is resistant to the interference of anemia, pregnancy, hypercholesterolemia, or alterations of plasma protein concentrations, as well as exogenous substances such as heparin that can alter the ESR. The CRP test is easy to perform, and its overall use has increased.

The ESR increases steadily with age, whereas the CRP value does not. The ESR changes relatively slowly (over several days) in response to the onset of inflammation. In contrast, the CRP responds rapidly (several hours). The CRP test has certain advantages over the ESR, and both can be used in concert.

Like the CRP, the ESR determination is used to detect inflammatory disease, to follow its course, and, at times in a more general fashion, to suggest the presence of occult organic disease in patients who have symptoms but no definitive physical or laboratory findings. The ESR is not a specific test. The Westergren ESR method is generally more resistant to the effects of anemia than the Wintrobe method. ESR values greater than 100 mm/hour generally imply infectious disease, neoplasia, inflammatory conditions, or chronic renal disease. While realizing that the ESR is affected by age, a rough index for determining the upper limits of normal can be derived by the following formula:

$$(\text{Age in years} + 5) \div 2 = \text{Age-related upper limit of ESR}$$

For an 85-year-old patient, this would place the upper range of normal of a Westergren ESR at roughly 45 mm/hour. In painful conditions affecting older patients such as temporal arteritis, use of both ESR and CRP tests is encouraged.

Complete Blood Count

The complete blood count (CBC) is a good starting point for laboratory testing in that it provides a cost-effective glimpse into a person's general health. The major emphasis in hematology is placed on cellular elements, including red blood cells (RBCs), white blood cells (WBCs), and platelets. Several tests form the backbone of laboratory diagnosis and can be very useful in the evaluation of both acute and chronic pain. Hemoglobin is the oxygen-carrying compound contained in RBCs and, in association with the RBC count and hematocrit, signals anemia.

Anemia is defined as a hemoglobin value of less than 13 g/dL for men and less than 11 g/dL for women. Conditions that result in pseudoanemia include overhydration, obtaining of blood specimens from an intravenous line, hypoalbuminemia, and pregnancy. Heavy smoking, dehydration, and states of extreme leukocytosis may produce elevated hemoglobin and hematocrit levels.[2] The RBC indices—mean corpuscular volume (MCV), mean corpuscular hemoglobin (MCH), mean corpuscular hemoglobin concentration (MCHC), and RBC distribution width (RDW)—aid in the diagnosis of a variety of conditions, including anemia, hemoglobinopathies, and spherocytosis.

The peripheral blood smear examines size, color, and other morphologic characteristics of RBCs and WBCs important in the evaluation of hematologic disease. Reticulocyte count, serum ferritin level, serum iron, and total iron-binding capacity (TIBC) enhance the evaluation of anemia. The reticulocyte can be viewed as an intermediate between a nucleated RBC in the bone marrow and a mature, non-nucleated RBC. The reticulocyte count is an index of bone marrow activity. Hemolytic anemia, acute bleeding, and the treatment of deficiency states related to vitamin B_{12}, folate, and iron result in reticulocytosis. Anemia associated with bone marrow failure is reflected in a low reticulocyte count.[3]

Because it is the major storage compound of iron, serum ferritin is a very sensitive measure for iron deficiency. Reductions in both serum iron and ferritin have been associated with restless legs syndrome. Serum TIBC is an approximation of the serum transferrin level and is elevated in iron deficiency anemia slightly before a decrease in serum iron becomes evident. Transferrin saturation (the percentage of transferrin bound to iron) declines in classic iron deficiency anemia. In hemochromatosis, a common genetic disorder of iron overload, persistent elevations of ferritin and transferrin saturation are effective screening tools in early recognition of this disorder.[4] The reduction in serum haptoglobin, a plasma glycoprotein that binds to oxyhemoglobin and delivers it to the reticuloendothelial system, is a useful test for evaluating intravascular hemolysis.

At birth, 80% of hemoglobin is fetal-type hemoglobin (HbF), which is replaced by the adult type (HbA) by age 6 months. An abnormal type of hemoglobin common in the Western Hemisphere is sickle hemoglobin (HbS). The heterozygous state, sickle trait (SA), is present in approximately 8% of African Americans. These persons are not anemic and are otherwise healthy. They rarely experience hematuria but may develop splenic infarcts during exposure to hypoxic conditions (e.g., nonpressurized airplanes). Homozygous sickle cell disease (SS) produces moderate to severe anemia. Crises secondary to small vessel occlusion with infarction often manifest with abdominal pain or bone pain. The disease does not become apparent until after age 6 months, with the disappearance of HbF, which has high affinity for oxygen.

Screening tests (sickle cell preparation) rely on the tendency of HbS to become insoluble when oxygen tension is low, a process that ultimately crystallizes and distorts the RBC into a sickle shape. A common screening method (Sickledex) avoids coverslip methods that use chemical (dithionite) deoxygenation and precipitation of HbS. This test is not useful before 6 months of age and does not distinguish between sickle cell disease and the trait. Definitive diagnosis requires hemoglobin electrophoresis. All African Americans with unexplained anemia, hematuria, arthralgias, or abdominal pain should be screened for sickle cell disease.[5]

White Blood Cells

WBCs are the body's first line of defense against infection. Lymphocytes and plasma cells produce antibodies, whereas neutrophils and monocytes respond by phagocytosis. Alterations in the WBC provide a clue to a variety of diseases, both benign and malignant. Most individuals have WBC counts between 5,000 and 10,000/mm³. The mean WBC count in African Americans may be at least 500/mm³ less than that in Europeans, and some individuals have counts as much as 3000/mm³ lower. Diurnal variations also occur in neutrophils and eosinophil counts. Neutrophil levels peak at about 4 PM at values almost 30% higher than values at 7 AM. Eosinophils more consistently parallel cortisol levels and are highest early in the morning and 40% lower later in the afternoon.

The classic picture of acute bacterial infection includes leukocytosis with an associated increased percentage of neutrophils and bands (immature forms); however, the leukocytosis and increased number of bands (shift to the left) may be absent in as many as 30% of acute bacterial infections. Overwhelming infection, particularly in debilitated older persons, may fail to produce leukocytosis. Heavy cigarette smoking has been associated with total WBC counts that average 1000/mm³ higher than those for nonsmokers. Other causes of neutrophilic leukocytosis include metabolic abnormalities such as uremia, diabetic acidosis, acute gouty attacks, seizures, and pregnancy.

Adrenal corticosteroids, even in low doses, can produce considerable increases in segmented neutrophils and total WBC count. Medications such as lithium carbonate (for bipolar disorder) and epinephrine (for asthma) and the toxic effects of lead can result in leukocytosis.

Eosinophilia is most often associated with acute allergic reactions such as asthma, hay fever, and drug allergy. It is also seen in parasitic diseases, skin disorders such as pemphigus and psoriasis, and miscellaneous conditions such as connective tissue disorders, particularly polyarteritis nodosa, Churg-Strauss vasculitis, and sarcoidosis. Eosinophilia may also be a nonspecific indicator of occult malignant disease.

Viral infection is most often manifested by lymphocytosis with an elevated (or relatively elevated) lymphocyte count in a person with a normal or decreased total WBC count. The usual lymphocytosis identified in viral infection is relative: granulocytes are reduced, whereas the total lymphocyte number remains constant. Infectious mononucleosis is associated with absolute lymphocytosis and atypical lymphocytes. The leukemoid reaction is defined as a nonleukemic elevation in the WBC count greater than 50,000/mm³. It is an exaggerated form of the non-neoplastic granulocyte reaction associated with severe bacterial infections, burns, tissue necrosis, hemolytic anemia, and juvenile rheumatoid arthritis.

Neutropenia is defined as a WBC count less than 4000/mm³. Drug-induced agranulocytosis is a major clinical issue in pain management, particularly its association with commonly used medications, including phenytoin (Dilantin), carbamazepine (Carbatrol, Tegretol), nonsteroidal anti-inflammatory drugs (NSAIDs), and many other medications used in pain management. Neutropenia should prompt an immediate review of all medications. Other conditions associated with neutropenia include aplastic anemia, aleukemic leukemia, hypersplenism, viral infections, and cyclic and chronic idiopathic neutropenia. Severe neutropenia (<1500 WBC/mm³) should be regarded as an acute emergency: careful follow-up and hematology consultation are mandatory.

In the area of hematopoietic malignancy, cells of lymphocyte origin predominate. For purposes of simplification, most lymphocytes arise from precursors in bone marrow. Of peripheral blood lymphocytes, approximately 75% are T cells (those lymphocytes that mature in the thymus), and 15% are B cells (those that have matured in the bone marrow, and later in the spleen or lymph nodes). All T lymphocytes develop an antigenic marker for the T-cell family called CD2. The CD (cluster designation classification) applies a single CD number to all antibodies that appear to react with the same or very similar WBC antigens. Of the T cells, approximately 75% are of the CD4 helper-inducer type and approximately 25% are of the CD8 cytotoxic-suppressor type.

B cells are characterized by having a surface immunoglobulin antibody rather than the CD3 antigen receptor characteristic of mature T cells. B cells are parents of plasma cells, which can secrete specific antibodies to antigens initially recognized by the parent B lymphocyte. Initially, these antibodies are immunoglobulin M (IgM); later, the immunoglobulin changes type to IgG (or less commonly to IgA or IgE). Finally, a group of lymphocyte-like cells known as natural killer cells (NKCs) possesses neither a T-lymphocyte marker antigen A nor B lymphocyte surface immunoglobulin. NKCs account for the remaining 10% of peripheral blood lymphocytes.[6]

Platelets and Blood Coagulation

An important aspect of any pain history is the identification of medications that influence coagulation. Heparin, aspirin, NSAIDs, warfarin (Coumadin), ticlopidine (Ticlid), and clopidogrel (Plavix) fall into this category. Any history of easy bleeding or bruising should prompt further evaluation.

Normal human platelet count generally ranges from 150,000 to 400,000 platelets/mm³. Platelet counts lower than 50,000/mm³ indicate severe thrombocytopenia. Platelet counts greater than 900,000/mm³ indicate thrombocytosis and a resultant hypercoagulable state. The most common causes of thrombocytopenia are immune mediated, drug induced, and related to blood transfusions. Many cases have no demonstrable cause. Other factors include hypersplenism, bone marrow deficiency, microangiopathic hemolytic anemia, infection, thyrotoxicosis, uremia, and preeclampsia. Drug-induced thrombocytopenia is common. Intravenous administration of heparin causes thrombocytopenia with platelet counts lower than 100,000/mm³ in as many as 15% of patients.[7] This effect has even been seen with heparin flushes. Other medications commonly implicated include cimetidine (Tagamet), quinine, quinidine, and furosemide (Lasix).

Thrombocytosis with platelet counts greater than 1 million are associated with myeloproliferative disorders, idiopathic thrombocythemia, and severe hemolytic anemia. Other common causes are occult malignancy, postsplenectomy status, and acute and chronic infection or inflammatory disease. Both arterial and venous thrombosis can occur.

Coagulation Parameters

The prothrombin time (PT) evaluates mainly defects in the extrinsic coagulation system. It is used as a liver function test (LFT) and as a general screening tool for coagulation disorders. When PT is used to monitor anticoagulation therapy with warfarin, the international normalized ratio (INR) is preferred because of its ability to standardize varied thromboplastin reagents.[8] The INR is a monitoring value for warfarin after the patient has been stabilized, but it is not useful as a general marker of coagulation or liver function. Awareness that a patient is taking warfarin or antiplatelet agents and of the patient's coagulation status is critical. For example, patients inadequately monitored while on warfarin may develop protracted flank pain secondary to an occult retroperitoneal hemorrhage with marked elevations of PT and INR that went unrecognized for months.

Glucose

Diabetes is a common disorder that affects 6 million persons in the United States. Approximately 1 million of these patients are classified as having type 1 diabetes, their disease ascribed to an autoimmune process that ultimately leads to beta-cell destruction. Insulin resistance, obesity, and a strong genetic predisposition characterize the more prevalent form, type 2 diabetes. The myriad painful complications of diabetes include neuropathy, foot ulceration, and Charcot joints (**Fig. 7.1**).

The American Diabetes Association criteria for the diagnosis of diabetes mellitus are the following (**Table 7.2**):

1. The classic symptoms of diabetes, including polydipsia, polyuria, and weight loss, in addition to a casual

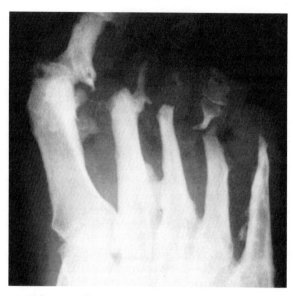

Fig. 7.1 Diabetes mellitus: metatarsophalangeal and interphalangeal joints. Neuropathic osteoarthropathy and infection in the forefoot of a diabetic patient combine to produce bizarre abnormalities consisting of osteolysis of the distal metatarsals and proximal phalanges, with tapering of the osseous contours. *(From Resnick D, Kransdorf M, editors:* Bone and joint imaging, *ed 3, Philadelphia, 2005, Saunders, 1062.)*

Table 7.2 American Diabetes Association Criteria for the Diagnosis of Diabetes Mellitus

Symptoms of diabetes (polydipsia, polyuria, and weight loss) plus a casual glucose ≥200 mg/dL: Casual is defined as any time of the day without regard to time since last meal.

Fasting glucose ≥126 mg/dL: Fasting is defined as no caloric intake for ≤8 hours.

2-hour postload glucose ≥200 mg/dL on an oral glucose tolerance test: Oral glucose tolerance test is not recommended as a first-line test because the fasting glucose is easier to perform, more acceptable to patients, and less expensive.

In the absence of unequivocal hyperglycemia with acute metabolic decompensation, these criteria should be confirmed by repeat testing on a different day. For example, an abnormal casual glucose >200 mg/dL without symptoms should be confirmed on a different day with a fasting glucose determination.

3-Hemoglobin A-1 C of 6.5% or greater

glucose concentration of 200 mg/dL or higher. (Casual is defined as a measurement taken at any time of day, without regard for the time of the last meal.)

2. A fasting plasma glucose value of 126 mg/dL or higher. (Fasting is defined as no caloric intake for at least 8 hours).

3. An oral glucose tolerance test value, 2 hours after load, of 200 mg/dL or higher.

When the diagnosis is based purely on blood glucose measurements—either the fasting blood glucose or the oral glucose tolerance test—in the absence of clinical symptoms, abnormalities must be found on 2 different days rather than on a single occasion only.[9]

The hemoglobin A1c (HbA1c) determination is a valuable tool for monitoring blood glucose, and in 2010 it was also recommended for the initial diagnosis of diabetes. In adults, HbA constitutes approximately 98% of normal hemoglobin. HbH consists of molecules that have been partially modified by the attachment of glucose. HbA1c is the major component of this glycosylated hemoglobin. Levels of HbA1c lower than 5% indicate the absence of diabetes, levels between 5.7% and 6.4% suggest prediabetic status, and levels higher than 6.5% indicate frank diabetes. HbA1c has most often been used as an effective index for monitoring diabetes therapy and patient compliance, and it generally reflects the average blood glucose level during the preceding 2 to 3 months.[10] Because this test does not require fasting, the American Diabetes Association revised their guidelines in 2010 and encouraged the use of the HbA1c test as a more convenient screening tool that will ultimately identify more patients with undiagnosed diabetes.[11]

Clinicians must be aware that medications such as glucocorticoids, nicotinic acid, and phenytoin (Dilantin) can impair insulin activity and elevate blood glucose. Another consideration is misdiagnosis of hypoglycemia. This overused label has been sensationalized in the popular press, arbitrarily defined, and applied in situations in which patients have vague protean symptoms but no objective abnormality of glucose metabolism. Those rather rare diseases in which hypoglycemia is actually a valid issue include insulinoma, nonpancreatic tumors such as fibrosarcoma and hepatoma, hepatic disease (including chronic alcoholism), and insulin overdose.[12]

Electrolytes

The most frequent electrolyte abnormality involves sodium, the most important cation of the body. Hyponatremia is the most common abnormality. Symptoms related to hyponatremia, such as nausea, malaise, lethargy, psychosis, and seizures, generally do not occur until the plasma sodium value falls to less than 120 mEq/L. Diuretics are often implicated. Carbamazepine (Tegretol, Carbatrol), a medication commonly used in pain management, can be associated with persistent hyponatremia. The other major categories of hyponatremia include conditions of general sodium and water depletion (including gastrointestinal loss from vomiting, diarrhea, or tube drainage), losses through skin associated with burns or sweating, endocrine loss associated with Addison's disease, and sudden withdrawal of long-term steroid therapy. Dilutional hyponatremia is associated with congestive heart failure, hyperhidrosis, nephrotic syndrome, cirrhosis, hypoalbuminemia, and acute renal failure.[13]

The syndrome of inappropriate antidiuretic hormone secretion (SIADH) is characterized by hyponatremia with reduced plasma osmolality in the presence of an elevated urinary sodium value but normal extracellular volume and renal, thyroid, and adrenal function. Factitious (but actually dilutional) hyponatremia can be seen when patients have marked hypertriglyceridemia, marked hyperproteinemia, or severe hyperglycemia.

Hypernatremia is much less common than hyponatremia and is usually associated with severe systemic disease in a person whose impaired mental status or physical disability prevents access to water. Other associated conditions include high-protein tube feedings, severe and protracted vomiting and diarrhea, and excessive water output resulting from diabetes insipidus (DI) or osmotic diuresis. Sodium overload can be caused by administration of hypertonic sodium solutions or can have an endogenous origin such as primary hyperaldosteronism (Cushing's syndrome).

DI results from deficiency of antidiuretic hormone (ADH) or from renal resistance to ADH. Central DI results from hypothalamic or pituitary damage secondary to trauma, neoplasm, or intracranial surgery.[14] Nephrogenic DI can be seen in patients with chronic renal failure or hyperglycemia or in patients taking medications such as lithium, chlorpromazine, and demeclocycline. To put hypernatremia in perspective, a serum sodium value more than 160 mEq/L that persists longer than 48 hours carries a 60% risk of death.

Abnormalities in serum potassium concentration are very common. Laboratory determinations can be spuriously increased by a hemolyzed specimen. Potassium values are also altered by acid-base abnormalities, increased extracellular osmolality, and insulin deficiency. A fall in plasma pH of 0.1 likely corresponds to an increased plasma potassium value of 0.5 mEq/L. A rise in pH causes a similar decrease in serum potassium concentration. Hypokalemia may be associated with inadequate potassium intake seen in alcoholism, malabsorption syndrome, and severe illness. Losses can result from diarrhea, diuretic use, vomiting, trauma, cirrhosis, and both primary (Conn's syndrome) and secondary aldosteronism (cirrhosis), renal artery stenosis, and malignant hypertension.

Hyperkalemia is associated with renal failure, dehydration, thrombocythemia, tumor lysis syndrome, and multiple medications, including beta-adrenergic blockers such as propranolol, potassium-sparing diuretics (spironolactone triamterene), several NSAIDs, and cyclosporine. Overlapping clinical symptoms, including weakness, nausea, anorexia, and organic mental changes, are associated with low-sodium, low-potassium, and high-potassium states.[15]

Chloride, the most abundant extracellular anion, is influences by the same conditions that affect sodium. When the serum sodium level is low, chloride concentration is also low, with the exception of the hyperchloremic alkalosis of prolonged vomiting. When carbon dioxide is included in a serum electrolyte panel, bicarbonate accounts for most of what is actually measured. Many clinicians believe that neither chloride nor carbon dioxide determination is a cost-effective routine assay. Most patients with abnormal serum bicarbonate values have a metabolic disturbance that would be better evaluated by blood gas determinations.

Connective Tissue Diseases and Vasculitis

The connective tissues diseases and vasculitides are immune-mediated diseases frequently marked by pain. These disorders are often difficult to diagnose in their early stages, and a basic understanding of laboratory serologic studies is essential. The connective tissue diseases (**Table 7.3**) are multisystem disorders that share the central feature of inflammation—whether of joints, muscles, or skin. Vasculitis is a multiorgan or organ-specific disease whose central feature is blood vessel inflammation (**Fig. 7.2**).

Almost all patients with systemic lupus erythematosus (SLE) develop autoantibodies.[16] The immunofluorescence test for antinuclear antibodies (ANAs) is the most sensitive laboratory test for detecting this disease. It has replaced the LE (lupus erythematosus) cell test and is positive in most patients with SLE. A negative ANA result is strong evidence against SLE. Many different factors that react to either nuclear or cytoplasmic constituents have been demonstrated. **Table 7.4** lists a variety of antibodies and their associated diseases. **Table 7.5** lists the laboratory test abnormalities of SLE, a prototype of autoimmune disease.

The ANA is generally reported in terms of a titer and the pattern of nuclear fluorescence. Nuclear fluorescence patterns can be homogeneous (solid), peripheral (rim), speckled, nucleolar, anticentromere, or nonreactive (normal). For example, an ANA directed against nucleolar RNA suggests progressive systemic sclerosis (scleroderma), particularly when the titer is high.

ANA titers greater than 1:80 are considered positive, but because test results are positive in many conditions, correlation with the history and with other clinical findings is mandatory. A positive ANA result alone is not sufficient to diagnose SLE. SLE can also be associated with a biologic false-positive test result for syphilis. Elevations of ANA titers can be seen in multiple conditions besides SLE, including infections (hepatitis, mononucleosis, malaria, subacute bacterial endocarditis), other connective tissue disorders (scleroderma, Sjögren's syndrome, rheumatoid arthritis), and thyroid disease.[17]

The ANA can be weakly positive in almost 20% of healthy adults, but a titer of 1:320 or higher has specificity of 97% for SLE and other connective tissue diseases. Patients can demonstrate a positive ANA result because they are taking a variety of drugs, including hydralazine, isoniazid (INH), and chlorpromazine (Thorazine).

Additional testing for the specific autoantibody responsible for the positive ANA result can help to identify a particular autoimmune disease. For example, antibodies to the DNA-histone complex suggest drug-induced lupus, whereas antibodies to double-stranded DNA (dsDNA) and to Smith (SM) antigen help to confirm SLE. Wegener's granulomatosis is associated with a

Table 7.3 Common Connective Tissue Diseases and Vasculitides

Systemic lupus erythematosus

Mixed connective tissue disease

Primary Sjögren's syndrome

Rheumatoid arthritis

Progressive systemic sclerosis (scleroderma)

Polymyositis and dermatomyositis

Vasculitides

Polyarteritis nodosa

Churg-Strauss angiitis

Wegener's granulomatosis

Temporal arteritis

Behçet's disease

Primary central nervous system vasculitis

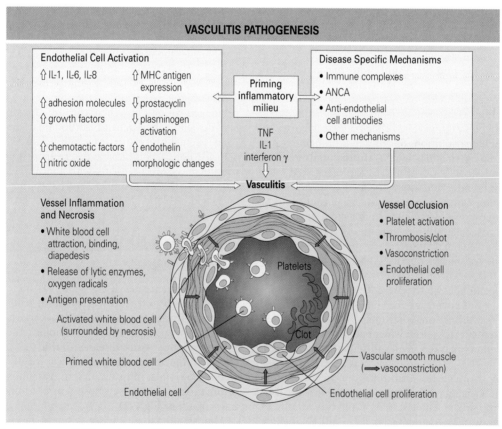

Fig. 7.2 Vasculitis syndromes. ANCA, antineutrophilic cytoplasmic antibody; IL, interleukin; MHC, major histocompatibility complex; TNF, tumor necrosis factor. *(From Klippel J, Dieppe P, editors: Rheumatology, ed 2, London, 1997, Mosby, p 7.20.7.)*

positive antineutrophilic cytoplasmic antibody (ANCA) test.[18] Antibodies directed against nuclear antigens to RO (SS-A) are found frequently in Sjögren's syndrome.

Serum complement is an important component of the immune system that comprises 10% of serum globulins. Total complement (CH50) and complement fractions C3 and C4 are often reduced in patients with SLE who have lupus nephritis.

Rheumatoid arthritis, a common condition in patients in pain clinic, is associated with the production of immunoglobulins, including IgG, IgM, and IgA, known as rheumatoid factors (RFs). From the laboratory standpoint, the most important of the RF is an IgM macroglobulin that combines with altered IgG antigen accompanied by complement. The average sensitivity of RFs (70% to 95%) in rheumatoid arthritis is well established.

Positive RFs can be found in SLE, scleroderma, dermatomyositis, and a variety of diseases associated with increased gamma globulin production—collagen vascular disorders, sarcoidosis, viral hepatitis, cirrhosis, and subacute bacterial endocarditis. As many as 20% of persons older than age 70 years have a positive RF titer.

A striking example of the diagnostic cross-over in autoimmune vasculitis is polyarteritis nodosa. This disease is manifested as painful peripheral neuropathy in as many as 70% of patients. Arthritic complaints involving multiple joints have been reported in as many as 50%. These patients often exhibit various autoantibodies. The ANA test result is positive in some 25% of cases, and the RF test result is positive in approximately 15%. Although sorting out the intricacies of these diseases is certainly the province of rheumatologists, pain specialists are uniquely positioned to entertain the possibility of connective tissue diseases and to initiate appropriate laboratory investigation.

Thyroid Dysfunction

Thyroid dysfunction is a clinical problem often overlooked because of its diverse manifestations. Older hypothyroid patients have a high incidence of gastrointestinal symptoms and atrial fibrillation and even an apathetic, listless appearance that may be confused with dementia. After drug-induced encephalopathy, hypothyroidism ranks as the second most treatable metabolic cause of dementia.[19] The American College of Pathologists recommends thyroid evaluation for all women older than the age of 50 years who seek medical attention, all adults with newly diagnosed dyslipidemia, and all patients entering a geriatric unit, on admission and at least every 5 years thereafter.

The American Thyroid Association recommends the combination of thyroid-stimulating hormone (TSH) and free thyroxine (T_4) tests as the most efficient blood testing regimen for the diagnosis and management of thyroid disease. The preferred method of testing for thyroid disease is a cascade starting with the TSH assay. If the TSH concentration is normal, no further tests are performed. If TSH is abnormal, free T_4 is automatically determined. TSH usually becomes abnormal before free T_4. Decreased TSH values suggest hyperthyroidism, exogenous thyroid hormone replacement, or glucocorticoid effects. Increased TSH levels usually suggest primary hypothyroidism—and only rarely a TSH-secreting pituitary adenoma or a state of thyroid resistance.

Testing of free T_4 should be ordered only when the TSH value is abnormal. In a large series of patients, no thyroid disease was detected in any patient who had normal TSH and low free T_4 levels. Accordingly, in persons with normal TSH and high free T_4 levels, almost all were monitored for thyroid replacement, thyroid suppression, or amiodarone therapy. None of the elevated T_4 levels led to a new diagnosis. Eliminating unnecessary testing can realize substantial savings.[20]

Table 7.4 Serologic Tests for Collagen Vascular Disorders

Rheumatoid factor: 80% sensitive in rheumatoid arthritis

Antinuclear antibodies: titers ≥1:320 have 95% specificity for systemic lupus erythematosus

Antineutrophil cytoplasmic antibody: 90% positive in Wegener granulomatosis

Anti-Ro: antibodies to nuclear antigens extracted from human B lymphocytes present in 70% of patients with Sjögren's syndrome

Antinuclear (nuclear RNA): 60%–90% positive in scleroderma

Anti-SM: highly specific for systemic lupus erythematosus

Anti-centromere: suggests CREST syndrome (calcinosis cutis, *Raynaud phenomenon, esophageal dysmotility, sclerodactyly, telangiectasias*)

SM, Smith antigen.

Table 7.5 Laboratory Findings in Systemic Lupus Erythematosus

Hemolytic anemia

Leukopenia (<14000 leukocytes/mm³)

Thrombocytopenia (<100,000 platelets/mm³)

Antinuclear antibody positivity

Lupus erythematosus cells

Antibodies to double-stranded DNA

Antibodies to SM antigen

False-positive test result for syphilis

SM, Smith antigen.

Prostate-Specific Antigen

Cancer of the prostate is the second most common malignant disease in men and the third most common cause of cancer death in men after 55 years of age. Unfortunately, carcinoma of the prostate may remain asymptomatic even until advanced stages. Pain is a common manifesting symptom of advanced prostate cancer—dysuria and hip and back pain. Prostate-specific antigen (PSA, a glycoprotein enzyme) testing can often detect prostate cancer 3 to 5 years before clinical symptoms appear.[21]

The American Cancer Society and the American Urologic Association recommend annual screening for all men older than 50 years of age with PSA and a digital rectal examination. The PSA value is specific for prostate disease, but not necessarily for prostate cancer. Many conditions other than prostate cancer can increase the PSA level, such as benign prostatic hypertrophy, acute bacterial prostatitis, cystoscopy, and even use of exercise bicycles. The upper limit of normal for PSA is 4 ng/mL. Some advocate age-related cutoffs such as 2.5 ng/mL for the fifth decade, 3.5 ng/mL for the six decade, and 4.5 ng/mL for the seventh decade of life. PSA velocity is also an important concept. A PSA that increases at a rate greater than 0.6 ng/mL/year may be an appropriate marker to trigger a prostate biopsy.

An additional measurement is that of the bound and free PSA, which can help differentiate levels due to cancer from levels due to benign prostatic hyperplasia, particularly in individuals with borderline elevations from 4 to 10 ng/mL. The lower the ratio of free to total PSA, the higher the likelihood of cancer. For example, when the level of free PSA is below 10% of the total, more than half of men were found to have biopsies consistent with cancer.

PSA is more sensitive than biochemical measurement of acid phosphatase, which was previously the accepted test. Annual PSA screening in combination with digital rectal examination has enhanced the detection of early localized cancer. Digital rectal examination and transrectal ultrasound generally do not have a significant effect on PSA measurements. Some 70% of men identified by PSA to have prostate cancer have organ-confined disease. In contrast, in the pre-PSA era, only one third of men diagnosed by digital rectal examination had organ-confined disease. PSA is one of the best tumor markers currently available.[22]

Human Immunodeficiency Virus 1 Infection

Pain is common in human immunodeficiency virus-1 (HIV-1) disease, an RNA retroviral disorder that attacks T-lymphocyte helper (CD4) cells. Common painful conditions associated with HIV-1 disease include abdominal pain, painful neuropathies, oral cavity pain, headache, reactive arthritis, and neuropathic pain associated with herpes zoster. For multiple reasons, not the least of which is squeamishness in dealing with this disease directly, physicians are reluctant to suggest laboratory testing for HIV-1. This observation is supported by the finding that many persons who are HIV-1 positive are unaware of the disease. Acquired immunodeficiency syndrome (AIDS) is a state of advanced infection marked by serologic evidence of HIV-1 antigen in addition to opportunistic infections or neoplasms associated with immunodeficiency.

Enzyme immunoassay testing for HIV-1 has been available since 1985. Specimens that are reactive in this initial screening test are subject to confirmatory Western blot analysis, an immunochromatographic technique that separates the virus into its major components by electrophoresis and exposes it to the patient's serum. Seroconversion generally occurs 6 to 10 weeks after infective exposure and persists for life. Antibody detection methods and a urine test have been developed, and their sensitivity is comparable to that of serum testing.

A quantitative polymerase chain reaction (PCR) assay for HIV-1 has been available since 1996. This test, commonly referred to as the viral load, is used for disease monitoring. An ultrasensitive version of this analysis can detect as few as 50 copies of viral RNA in 1 mL of plasma. The patient whose HIV-1 viral load is greater than 100,000 copies/mL within 6 months of serum conversion is 10 times more likely to progress to AIDS within the first 5 years than is a patient with fewer than 10,000 copies/mL. Maintaining low HIV viral loads (<than 50 copies/mL after 6 months of therapy) is currently the recommended goal of therapy.[23]

Monitoring lymphocytes is one way to assess immune system deficiency. Lymphocytes are divided into three main groups: B cells, T cells (including CD4 and CD8 cells), and NKCs. B cells function through antibody-mediated immunity. T cells are involved in cell-mediated immunity. HIV-1 selectively infects and reduces the number of CD4 (helper-inducer) T lymphocytes. CD8 (suppressive cytotoxic) T-cell numbers remain normal or are increased.

Normal CD4 cell counts range between 600 and 1500 cells/mm^3. Reduction in the CD4 cell count is a good indicator of when to start preventive therapy for numerous opportunistic HIV-associated infections. Generally, levels higher than 500 CD4 cells/mm^3 are not associated with significant problems. Levels between 200 and 500/mm^3 signal an increased risk for herpes zoster, candidiasis, sinus and pulmonary infections, and tuberculosis. When cell counts fall to 50 to 200/mm^3, the risk of *Mycobacterium avium* complex or cytomegalovirus infection and of Kaposi's sarcoma increases dramatically. Levels lower than 50 CD4 cells/mm^3 indicate profound cellular immunodeficiency.

As CD4 counts decline, the possibility of opportunistic infections increases. A ubiquitous organism that can affect the central nervous system is *Toxoplasma*. Toxoplasmosis serologic testing (IgG) is available and is usually performed when a person is found to be HIV-1 positive. Initial positive toxoplasmosis serology results identify a potential candidate for preventive medication. Serologic tests for hepatitis should also be performed, particularly if the patient has abnormalities in the routine chemistry screen, such as an elevated serum transaminase level.

In summary, HIV-related disease is extremely complex. Both patients and physicians consistently exhibit a tendency to ignore HIV-1 infection as a possibility. Enzyme immunoassay testing for HIV-1 antibody has been the initial screening test, followed by Western blot for confirmation. The best predictor of disease progression is not likely to be a single test but rather a combination of studies, including those for both viral load and CD4 cell count.

Spirochetal Diseases

Two spirochetal diseases that have distinguished themselves as "great imitators" because of their various manifestations are syphilis and Lyme disease. Syphilis is a sexually transmitted disease caused by *Treponema pallidum,* and Lyme disease is the most common vector-borne infection in the United States, the vector being the spirochete *Borrelia burgdorferi,* which infects *Ixodes dammini* ticks (**Fig. 7.3**).

Serologic tests currently are the mainstay of syphilis diagnosis and management. Nontreponemal tests, including the Venereal Disease Research Laboratory (VDRL) and rapid plasma reagin (RPR), are used most often. In early primary syphilis, when antibody levels may be too low to detect, the sensitivity of nontreponemal tests ranges from 62% to 76%. As antibody levels rise in the secondary stage of syphilis, the

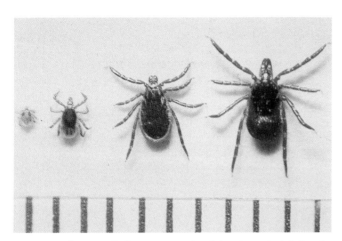

Fig. 7.3 *Ixodes scapularis*. Larva, nymph, adult male, and adult female, on a millimeter scale. *(Courtesy of Pfizer Central Research, Groton, Conn. From Klippel J, Dieppe P, editors:* Rheumatology, *ed 2, London, 1997, Mosby, p 6.5.3.)*

sensitivity of nontreponemal tests approaches 100%; however, in late-stage syphilis, about one fourth of treated patients have negative VDRL results. Therefore, the combination of VDRL and RPR alone cannot be relied on for conclusive diagnosis during the very early or very late stages of syphilis.[24]

Many false-positive nontreponemal test results occur and are caused by collagen vascular disorders, advanced malignant disease, pregnancy, hepatitis, tuberculosis, Lyme disease, intravenous drug use, and multiple transfusions, among others. Because of the high frequency of false-positive results in nontreponemal serodiagnostic testing, all positive results in asymptomatic patients should be confirmed with a more specific treponemal test such as the microhemagglutination assay for *T. pallidum* and the fluorescent treponemal antibody absorption (FTA-ABS) tests. The FTA-ABS test has sensitivity of 84% in primary syphilis and of almost 100% for the other stages and specificity of 96%.

Titers of treponemal tests do not correlate with disease activity, whereas nontreponemal tests (VDRL and RPR) are quite useful for monitoring response to treatment. Treponemal tests should not be used for initial screening because they are expensive and because patients with previously treated infection usually remain reactive for life. Following antibiotic treatment for syphilis, VDRL and RPR values should be checked once each at 6 and 12 months. Successful treatment should produce a fourfold decline in titer, although only approximately 60% of patients will eventually test completely negative.

The other great imitator is Lyme disease, which manifests with multiple painful complaints, including headache, joint pain, cranial neuritis, unilateral or bilateral Bell's palsy, or a particularly painful syndrome of radiculitis with shooting electric pains and focal extremity weakness (Bannwarth's syndrome). Public awareness of Lyme disease has frequently prompted serologic testing of persons who have no clinical signs or symptoms of the disease. The pathogen, *B. burgdorferi*, is a spirochete named after Willy Burgdorfer, Ph.D., a public health researcher who identified it in 1982. A diagnosis of Lyme disease should be based primarily on the patient's symptoms and the probability of exposure to the Lyme organism (**Fig. 7.4**). The mainstays of clinical diagnosis of Lyme disease are a strong history suggesting potential exposure to the causative agent and the physical finding of erythema migrans,

which is present in more than 60% of patients who are ultimately proved to have Lyme disease (**Fig. 7.5**). Laboratory evaluation is appropriate for patients who have characteristic arthritic, neurologic, or cardiac symptoms. It is not warranted for patients who have nonspecific symptoms such as those frequently classified under the vague rubrics of chronic fatigue syndrome or fibromyalgia.

A true-positive result consists of a positive enzyme-linked immunosorbent assay (ELISA) or immunofluorescence assay (IFA) confirmed by a Western blot. Positive results do not prove the diagnosis of Lyme disease and have little predictive value in the absence of clinical symptoms.[25]

False-positive Lyme disease test results caused by cross-reactive antibodies are associated with autoimmune disease or with infections secondary to other spirochetes such as *T. pallidum* and *Leptospira* species, and to bacteria such as *Helicobacter pylori*. Finally, because assays for antibody to *B. burgdorferi* should be used only for supporting a clinical diagnosis of Lyme disease, these tests are unsuitable as screening tools in evaluating asymptomatic persons or patients with nebulous complaints not characteristic of Lyme disease. Evidence suggests that many persons who do not actually have Lyme disease are receiving inappropriate treatment solely because of serologic test results.

Neuropathy

A frequent issue in the evaluation of pain, particularly when the cause is not obvious, involves peripheral neuropathy. Pain, sensory loss, weakness, and dysesthesias are common clinical complaints. Even after exhaustive evaluation, the cause of as many as 50% of peripheral neuropathies remains unknown. The more common causes are diabetes, alcoholism, toxins, nutritional deficits, drugs, and renal and other metabolic disorders. Less familiar disorders include the immune-mediated hereditary neuropathies. It is important to remain aware of the immune-mediated syndromes, not only to enhance diagnostic accuracy but also because these patients often respond to immunomodulatory treatments with dramatic improvements in neurologic function and quality of life.[26]

It is far beyond the scope of this chapter to discuss this rapidly evolving topic in detail. This discussion attempts to introduce the pain specialist to this aspect of neuropathy evaluation, particularly when specific laboratory tests can be critical to diagnostic accuracy. Vitamin B_{12} deficiency is characterized by macrocytic anemia, peripheral neuropathy, and ataxia, and it may be associated with cognitive deficits. Vitamin B_{12} levels higher than 300 ng/L are normal. Levels between 200 and 300 ng/L are borderline. Measurement of methylmalonic acid, a substrate that requires cobalamin for its metabolism, is elevated (>0.4 mmol/L) in states of true vitamin B_{12} deficiency.

Levels of vitamin B_{12} lower than 200 ng/L are abnormal. Serum gastrin concentration is elevated in gastric atrophy, which is usually associated with pernicious anemia. A normal serum gastrin level effectively rules out pernicious anemia, whereas intrinsic factor–blocking antibodies are detectable in only 50% of patients with pernicious anemia. The expensive and time-consuming Shilling test should be reserved for those patients with a low level of vitamin B_{12} who test negative for intrinsic factor–blocking antibodies and who have an elevated serum gastrin level.

LYME DISEASE: U.S. NATIONAL SURVEILLANCE CASE DEFINITION	
Definition	A systemic, tick-borne disease with protean manifestations: dermatologic, rheumatologic, neurologic and cardiac abnormalities. The initial skin lesion, erythema migrans, is the best clinical marker (occurs in 60%-80% of patients)
Case definition	I. Erythema migrans present *or* 2. At least one late manifestation and laboratory confirmation of infection
General Definitions	
1. Erythema migrans (EM)	• Skin lesion typically beginning as a red macule/papule and expanding over days or weeks to form a large round lesion, often with partial central clearing • A solitary lesion must measure at least 5 cm; secondary lesions may also occur • An annular erythematous lesion developing within several hours of a tick bite represents a hypersensitivity reaction and does not qualify as erythema migrans • The expanding EM lesion is usually accompanied by other acute symptoms, particularly fatigue, fever, headache, mildly stiff neck, arthralgias, and myalgias, which are typically intermittent • Diagnosis of EM must be made by a physician • Laboratory confirmation is recommended for patients with no known exposure
2. Late manifestations These include any of the opposite *when an alternative explanation is not found*	**Musculoskeletal system** • Recurrent, brief attacks (lasting weeks or months) of objective joint swelling in one or a few joints, sometimes followed by chronic arthritis in one or a few joints • Manifestations not considered to be criteria for diagnosis include chronic progressive arthritis not preceded by brief attacks, chronic symmetric polyarthritis, or arthralgias, myalgias, or fibromyalgia syndromes alone **Nervous system** • Lymphocytic meningitis, cranial neuritis, particularly facial palsy (may be bilateral), radiculoneuropathy or, rarely, encephalomyelitis alone or in combination • Encephalomyelitis must be confirmed by evidence of antibody production against *Borrelia burgdorferi* in cerebrospinal fluid (CSF), shown by a higher titer of antibody in the CSF than in serum • Headache, fatigue, paresthesias or mildly stiff neck alone are not accepted as criteria for neurologic involvement **Cardiovascular system** • Acute-onset, high-grade (2nd- or 3rd-degree) atrioventricular conduction defects that resolve in days to weeks and are sometimes associated with myocarditis • Palpitations, bradycardia, bundle-branch block or myocarditis alone are not accepted as criteria for cardiovascular involvement
3. Exposure	• Exposure to wooded, brushy or grassy areas (potential tick habitats) in an endemic county no more than 30 days before the onset of erythema migrans • A history of tick bite is not required
4. Endemic county	• A county in which at least two definite cases have been previously acquired or in which a tick vector has been shown to be infected with *B. burgdorferi*
5. Laboratory confirmation	• Isolation of the spirochete from tissue or body fluid *or* • Detection of diagnostic levels of immunoglobulin M or immunoglobulin G antibodies to the spirochete in the serum or the CSF *or* • Detection of an important change in antibody levels in paired acute and convalescent serum samples • States may separately determine the criteria for laboratory confirmation and diagnostic levels of antibody • Syphilis and other known biological causes of false-positive serologic test results should be excluded, when laboratory confirmation is based on serologic testing alone

Fig. 7.4 Lyme disease. A summary of the U.S. National Surveillance Case Definition. *(From Klippel J, Dieppe P, editors: Rheumatology, ed 2, London, 1997, Mosby, p 6.5.2.)*

Immune-mediated neuropathy, acute or chronic, can be associated with pain and may even manifest as a life-threatening emergency. The prototype of acute inflammatory demyelinating neuropathy, Guillain-Barré syndrome, may appear after any of a number of infections, surgery, vaccinations, or immune system perturbations. Chronic inflammatory demyelinating polyneuropathy may be associated with illicit drug use, vaccination, infections, autoimmune disorders, or monoclonal gammopathy. Demyelinating neuropathy associated with anti–myelin-associated glycoprotein (anti-MAG) manifests

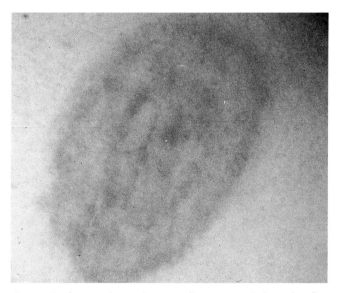

Fig. 7.5 Erythema migrans in Lyme disease. A typical annular, flat, erythematous lesion with a sharply demarcated border and partial central healing. *(Courtesy of Dr. Steven Luger, Olde Lyme, Conn. From Klippel J, Dieppe P, editors:* Rheumatology, *ed 2, London, 1997, Mosby, p 6.5.4.)*

as distal weakness and sensory loss, particularly in the legs. Measurement of IgM anti-MAG antibodies in the serum by the Western blot method detects this clinical disorder.[27]

Small myelinated and unmyelinated axons subserve pain and temperature. Diabetes and alcoholism, the most common causes of peripheral neuropathy in the United States, often manifest as painful small-fiber neuropathy. Leprosy (Hansen's disease) is the principal cause of treatable neuropathy worldwide. Other disorders are amyloidosis, AIDS, and ischemic lesions such as polyarteritis nodosa, SLE, and Sjögren's syndrome. These small-fiber neuropathies often occur with burning, electric shock–like or lancinating pain, and uncomfortable dysesthesias. The patient may also complain of intense pain with only minimal stimulus (allodynia), such as when sheets rub over the feet.

Persons with a characteristic syndrome that is often dismissed as anxiety complain that "my whole body is numb and I feel tingling, painful numbness all over." In middle-aged patients, particularly those who are heavy cigarette smokers, paraneoplastic neuropathy should be considered. One indicator is serum antineuronal nuclear antibodies type I (ANNA: anti-HU). This malignant inflammatory sensory neuropathy is most often associated with small cell lung cancer, although it may be associated with Hodgkin's lymphoma, epidermoid cancer, or colon or breast carcinoma. As in all areas of pain diagnosis, the clinician must resist any impulse to ascribe pain hastily to psychogenic mechanisms: Once the psychogenic arrow has been fired, it is almost impossible to retrieve it gracefully.

Nonmalignant inflammatory sensory neuropathy is a disorder that commonly affects women. It can manifest as distal painful dysesthesias or as ataxia. Serologic markers such as ANAs, RFs, or ANCAs may suggest specific connective tissue disorders, such as, respectively, SLE, rheumatoid arthritis, and Wegener's granulomatosis. Certain patients with nonmalignant inflammatory neuropathy and Sjögren's syndrome test positive for extractable nuclear antigens such as Ro (SS-A) and LA (SS-P). Hereditary conditions, drugs, and toxins are also part of this differential diagnosis.[28]

Immune-mediated neuropathies are always worth remembering because they can respond to immunomodulating treatments. These diagnoses are often overlooked or missed; sometimes patients suffer symptoms for years without a specific diagnosis. Frequently, pain specialists see these persons, and, not uncommonly, the patients' initial workup was fragmented and far from thorough.

A search for serum factors associated with the immune-mediated neuropathies includes testing for monoclonal antibodies (proteins with definite antigenic targets) and for monoclonal and polyclonal antibodies that bind to specific neural components. Measurement of anti-MAG, antisulfatide, and anti-HU antibodies should be considered, as should serum and urine tests for monoclonal antibodies by immunofixation methods. Other elements of the workup are testing serum for cryoglobulins and markers for connective tissue disorders. **Table 7.6** includes a listing of specific laboratory tests that can be helpful in the evaluation of painful neuropathies. Once again, the pain specialist is in a unique position to develop expertise and knowledge, not only in the treatment of pain but also in the evaluation and diagnosis of conditions that frequently escape proper identification, even by experienced subspecialists.[29]

Serum Proteins

Laboratory tests involving the various components of serum proteins can be valuable adjuncts to the evaluation of pain. Abnormalities of the various components of serum proteins may be helpful in investigating connective tissue disorders and several malignant diseases. A lack of familiarity with this area of diagnosis creates a common reticence on the part of the pain specialist in ordering these studies.

Serum protein is composed of albumin and globulin. The word *globulin* is actually an old term that refers to the non-albumin portion of serum protein, a substance that has been found to contain a varied group of proteins, such as glycoproteins, lipoproteins, and immunoglobulins. The total quantity of albumin is about three times that of globulin, and albumin acts to maintain serum oncotic pressure. Globulins tend to have more varied functions, including antibodies, clotting proteins, complement, acute phase proteins, and transport systems for various substances. Serum protein electrophoresis is used to screen for serum protein abnormalities. Various bands are identified that correspond to albumin, alpha$_1$ and alpha$_2$ globulins, beta globulins, and gamma globulins (**Fig. 7.6**).

Acute phase proteins are seen in response to acute inflammation, trauma, necrosis, infarction, burns, and psychological stress. Increases are noted in fibrinogen, alpha$_1$-antitrypsin, haptoglobin, and complement. Albumin and transferrin are often decreased in an acute stress pattern. These changes in serum proteins during acute inflammatory responses are accompanied by polymorphonuclear leukocytosis, an increased ESR, and an increase in CRP that responds very rapidly after the onset of acute inflammation.

Significant changes in albumin are usually reductions rather than elevations. These can be associated with pregnancy, malnutrition, liver disease, cachexia or wasting states (e.g., those of tuberculosis, AIDS, or advanced cancer). Serum albumin may also be lost directly from the vascular compartment secondary to hemorrhage, burns, exudates, or protein-losing enteropathy.

Table 7.6 Clinical and Laboratory Features of Common Neuropathies

Neuropathic Conditions	Clinical Features	Useful Laboratory Tests (Findings)
Diabetic neuropathy	Distal symmetrical polyneuropathy Mononeuritis multiplex Diabetic amyotrophy	Fasting blood glucose HgA1c Glucose tolerance test
Alcohol neuropathy	Burning feet, ataxia Distal areflexia	γ-Glutamyltransferase$\uparrow$ Aspartate transaminase$\uparrow$ Mean corpuscular volume (RBC macrocytosis)$\uparrow$
Neuropathy due to renal disease	60% of dialysis patients have dysesthesias, pain, and cramps in legs	Blood urea nitrogen$\uparrow$ Creatinine$\uparrow$
INFECTIOUS NEUROPATHY		
Leprosy	10 million cases worldwide	Skin biopsy+
Lyme disease	Radiculoneuritis Bell's palsy	Lyme test with Western blot confirmation+
Human immunodeficiency virus 1 (HIV-1)	Guillain-Barré like (acute) Mononeuritis (late) Distal painful sensory neuropathy (late)	HIV test with Western blot confirmation+
NEUROPATHY ASSOCIATED WITH MALIGNANCY		
Lung cancer	Painful sensory neuropathy	Anti-HU antibodies+
Myeloma	Osteosclerotic myeloma	Immunoglobulins G, A, monoclonal gammopathy
Amyloidosis	Distal painful sensory neuropathy associated with plasma cell dyscrasia	Urine Bence Jones protein monoclonal gammopathy
IgM monoclonal gammopathy	Waldenström's macroglobulinemia, chronic lymphocytic leukemia	IgM antibody to MAG, GM1, sulfatide
VASCULITIC NEUROPATHY		
Wegener's granulomatosis		P-ANCA+
Systemic lupus erythematosus		Antinuclear antibodies+
Hepatitis B, C		Serology cryoglobulins+
Sarcoid		Angiotensin-converting enzyme$\uparrow$
Sjögren's syndrome		Anti-SSA-LA, anti-SSB-Ro antibodies
TOXIC NEUROPATHY		
Arsenic	Painful stocking and glove polyneuropathy	Urine levels >25 mg/day unless seafood was eaten recently
Lead	Abdominal pain, fatigue, wrist drop, diffuse weakness	Anemia Urine coproporphyrin$\uparrow$ Urine lead level >0.2 mg/L Blood lead levels can be misleading
Vitamin B$_{12}$ deficiency	Burning hands and feet Cognitive impairment Posterior column loss Ataxias	Low serum B$_{12}$ Homocysteine$\uparrow$ Methylmalonic acid$\uparrow$

+, Positive; $\uparrow$, elevated; HgA1c, glycosylated hemoglobin; IgM, immunoglobulin M; MAG, myelin-associated glycoprotein; P-ANCA, perinuclear antineutrophil cytoplasmic antibody; RBC, red blood cell.

Gamma globulin is composed predominantly of antibodies of the IgG, IgA, IgM, IgD, and IgE types. Marked reduction of the gamma fraction is seen in hypogammaglobulinemia and agammaglobulinemia. Secondary varieties of gamma globulin reduction may be found in patients with nephrotic syndrome, overwhelming infection, chronic lymphocytic leukemia, lymphoma, or myeloma, as well as in patient receiving long-term corticosteroid treatment. Patients with rheumatic and collagen vascular diseases usually demonstrate elevations in gamma globulin. Patients with multiple myeloma and Waldenström's macroglobulinemia have a homogeneous spike or peak in a localized region of the gamma area.

Immunoglobulins are a heterogeneous group of molecules. IgG constitutes approximately 75% of serum immunoglobulins and the majority of antibodies. IgM represents the earliest antibodies formed and accounts for approximately 7% of the total immunoglobulin. The IgM class includes cold agglutinins, ABO blood groups, and RFs. IgA constitutes about 15% of immunoglobulins. IgA deficiency, the most common primary immunodeficiency, is associated with upper respiratory tract and gastrointestinal infections. Phenytoin (Dilantin) is reported to decrease IgA levels in approximately 50% of patients who receive long-term therapy. IgE is elevated in certain allergic and especially atopic disorders.

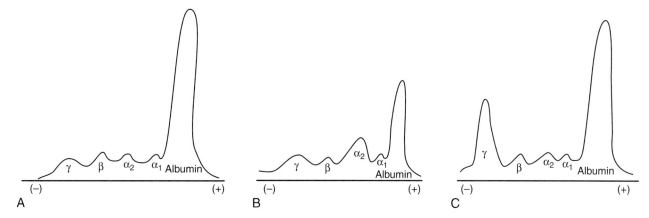

Fig. 7.6 Characteristic serum protein electrophoresis patterns. A, Normal pattern. B, Acute phase response pattern. Note decreased albumin peak and increased alpha$_2$ (α_2)-globulin level, which is associated with burns, rheumatoid disease, and acute stress. C, Monoclonal gammopathy spike. Note the M protein spike in the gamma (α) area. This pattern is associated with myeloma, Waldenström's macroglobulinemia, and idiopathic monoclonal gammopathy. *(From Waldman SD, editor:* Interventional pain management, *ed 2, Philadelphia, 2001, Saunders, 2001, p 95.)*

Multiple myeloma is a malignant disease of plasma cells derived from B-type lymphocytes. The disease is most common in middle-aged men and frequently manifests as bone pain. Anemia is present in nearly 75% of patients, and RBC rouleaux formation (cells stacked like coins) can be identified in peripheral blood smears. Elevated ESR is common, and significant hypercalcemia occurs in approximately one third of patients. A monoclonal gammopathy spike (M protein) is seen in approximately 80% of patients with myeloma. Of all patients who have monoclonal protein, approximately two thirds have myeloma. Roughly 70% have monoclonal protein characterized as IgG; most of the others have IgA.[30]

A normal immunoglobulin molecule is composed of two heavy chains and two light chains (kappa and lambda) connected by a disulfide bridge. IgM is a pentameric configuration of five complete immunoglobulin units. In addition to normal-weight serum monoclonal protein, many patients with myeloma excrete a low-molecular weight protein known as Bence Jones protein, which is composed only of immunoglobulin light chains. Unlike normal-weight monoclonal proteins, it can pass into the urine and, generally, is not demonstrable in the serum. Another condition associated with Bence Jones protein include Waldenström's macroglobulinemia, a lymphoproliferative disorder associated with monoclonal IgM production, lymphadenopathy, hepatosplenomegaly, and hyperglobulinemia. Bence Jones proteinuria is seen in monoclonal gammopathies associated with malignant diseases, and significant quantities (>60 mg/L) are identified. In monoclonal gammopathies of non-neoplastic origins such as rheumatic or collagen vascular disease, cirrhosis, and chronic infection, Bence Jones protein excretion is generally less than 60 mg/L.[31]

Cryoglobulins are immunoglobulins that precipitate reversibly in serum or at least partially gel at cold temperatures. The most common associated symptoms are purpura, Raynaud's phenomenon, and arthralgias. Cryoglobulins usually do not appear as discrete bands on serum protein electrophoresis. The conditions most often associated with cryoglobulins are rheumatoid and collagen vascular disease, leukemia, lymphomas, myeloma, and Waldenström's macroglobulinemia. Cryoglobulins are also associated with a variety of infections and hepatic disease.

Renal Function Tests

Routine urinalysis is an indispensable part of basic clinical laboratory evaluation. Dysuria is extremely common in women; 30% of women experience at least one episode of cystitis during their lifetime. The differential diagnosis of painful urination includes cystitis, pyelonephritis, urethritis, vaginitis, and genital herpes. The most sensitive laboratory indicator for urinary tract infection is pyuria. The basic urinalysis should include specific gravity, albumin, hemoglobin, and microscopic evaluation for casts, crystals, and RBCs and WBCs.[32]

If no vaginal contamination occurs during urine collection, vaginitis generally does not produce pyuria. The presence of WBC casts suggests pyelonephritis. A positive leukocyte esterase test is approximately 90% sensitive in detecting pyuria secondary to infection. Many bacteria produce an enzyme called reductase that converts urinary nitrates to nitrites. The nitrite test enhances the sensitivity of the leukocyte esterase test in defining urinary tract infection. A positive nitrite test result is 90% specific for urinary tract infections. The sensitivity of this test is low but can be improved by obtaining a first-voided morning urine sample.

Urinary tract infection is defined as 100,000 colony-forming units/mL on urine culture. The microscopic examination of the urine must proceed promptly, generally within 1 hour after voiding. Various studies report that as many as 50% of specimens that contained abnormal numbers of WBCs were considered normal after standing at room temperature for several hours.[33]

Urea is a waste product of protein metabolism that is synthesized in the liver and that contains nitrogen (BUN). Creatinine is a metabolic product of creatine phosphate in muscle. Serum levels of BUN and creatinine change only with severe renal disease. Creatinine clearance rate (the amount of creatinine that can be completely eliminated into the urine in a given time) is a much more sensitive measure of mild to moderate glomerular damage. In addition to being sensitive to function, creatinine clearance is one of the more sensitive tests available to warn of impending renal failure.

Elevations of serum BUN and creatinine generally reflect severe glomerular damage, renal tubular damage, or both. An elevated BUN level (azotemia) is not specific for renal disease. Prerenal azotemia may result from decreased renal circulation secondary to shock, hemorrhage, or dehydration. It can also be caused by increased protein catabolism like that associated with overwhelming infections or toxemia. Renal azotemia usually accompanies bilateral chronic pyelonephritis, glomerular nephritis, acute tubular necrosis, and other forms of severe glomerular damage. Postrenal or obstructive azotemia can result from any external compression of the ureter, urethra, or bladder, or, in older men, from benign or malignant prostatic hypertrophy. The studies that test predominantly renal tubular function include specific gravity, osmolality, and urinary excretion of electrolytes.

Osmolality

Although the very term *osmolality* evokes an imposing and esoteric image, it has practical clinical value. Serum osmolality is an indicator of total body water and generally ranges between 280 and 300 mOsm/kg of water. The principal determinants of serum osmolality are sodium, chloride, glucose, and urea. A simplified formula with excellent clinical utility is as follows:

$$\text{Serum osmolality} = 2 \times \text{Sodium} + \text{Glucose} \div 20 + \text{BUN} \div 3$$

Urine osmolality depends on an individual's state of hydration. Under normal conditions, urine osmolality ranges from 400 to 800 mOsm/kg. Profound dehydration is associated with levels greater than 1100 mOsm/kg, and fluid overload produces values lower than 100 mOsm/kg. Simultaneous measurement of urine and serum osmolality is useful in diagnosing SIADH, a condition that can be induced by a variety of causes, including central nervous system tumors, infections, trauma, undifferentiated small cell lung cancer, pneumonia, and various medications, among them opiates, barbiturates, and carbamazepine (Tegretol, Carbatrol). A typical patient with SIADH has a serum osmolality of less than 270 mOsm/kg and a urine osmolality higher than the serum value. In contrast, a patient with DI has a serum osmolality greater than 320 mOsm/kg and a urine osmolality of less than 100 mOsm/kg.

The osmolal gap can be used to screen for low-molecular-weight toxins. The gap is determined by subtracting the calculated osmolality (see the formula cited earlier) from the actual serum osmolality. The calculated and measured values usually fall within 10 units of each other. If the measured value exceeds the calculated value by more than 10 units, other osmotically active substances that can manifest in an emergency room setting should be considered. These include ethanol, methanol, ethylene glycol, propylene glycol, acetone, paraldehyde, and other toxins.

Calcium, Phosphorus, and Magnesium

Symptoms related to hypercalcemia are varied but include vomiting, constipation, polydipsia, polyuria, and encephalopathy. Hypercalcemia is often detected on routine laboratory panels in an otherwise healthy person. Primary hyperparathyroidism accounts for approximately 60% of outpatient abnormalities. In hospitalized patients, malignancy-associated hypercalcemia accounts for the majority of cases. Tumors most often associated with hypercalcemia are breast, renal, and lung cancers and

myeloma. Regulation of serum calcium occurs through a negative feedback loop mediated by the secretion of parathyroid hormone (PTH). A decrease in serum calcium increases secretion of PTH, whereas an increase in serum calcium reduces it. PTH also has a direct action on bone, by increasing bone resorption and the release of bone calcium and phosphorus.

Other causes of hypercalcemia include Dyazide diuretics, lithium therapy, sarcoidosis, hyperthyroidism, and vitamin D intoxication. The effects of PTH, vitamin D, and phosphate produce a reciprocal relationship between the serum calcium and phosphate levels, with elevation of one ultimately leading to reduction of the other. Vitamin D deficiency results in low levels of both calcium and phosphorus but an elevated level of PTH.

Hypophosphatemia is seen in association with hypercalcemia as a manifestation of hyperparathyroidism. Severe hypophosphatemia can cause muscle weakness, bone pain, tremor, seizures, hypercalciuria, and decreased platelet function. Hyperventilation and respiratory alkalosis are major causes of hypophosphatemia in patients with pain, anxiety, sepsis, alcoholism, hepatic disease, heat stroke, or salicylate toxicity. Respiratory alkalosis causes plasma phosphate to shift into the cells. Life-threatening hypophosphatemia can occur if malnourished patients are administered carbohydrates rapidly.

Primary hyperparathyroidism reduces phosphate secondary to increased urinary excretion. Vitamin D deficiency causes hypocalcemia, secondary hyperparathyroidism, and increased urinary phosphate excretion in the presence of decreased intestinal phosphate absorption.

Hypocalcemia and hyperphosphatemia are often seen in tandem. Renal failure accounts for more than 90% of cases of hyperphosphatemia. Plasma phosphate levels rise when the glomerular filtration rate falls to less than 25% of normal. Rhabdomyolysis, hemolysis, and tumor lysis syndrome may produce severe hyperphosphatemia by releasing large amounts of intracellular phosphate. Hypoparathyroidism, acromegaly, and thyrotoxicosis reduce urinary phosphate excretion. Enemas with a high phosphate content can cause hyperphosphatemia, hypocalcemia, and, ultimately, tetany. The ill-advised practice of prolonged storage of blood samples can cause an artificial elevation in phosphate levels.

Routine serum calcium measures address total serum calcium, approximately 50% of which is bound calcium and approximately 50% of which is ionized or free (dialyzable). Most of the bound calcium is complexed with albumin. The most common cause of "bound hypocalcemia" is a decrease in serum albumin. Although laboratory evidence of hypocalcemia is fairly common in hospitalized patients, true decreases of ionized calcium are less prevalent. Symptoms include neuromuscular irritability, mental status changes, and seizures. Causes of true hypocalcemia include primary hypoparathyroidism, pseudohypoparathyroidism secondary to diminished responsiveness of the kidney or skeleton to PTH, vitamin D deficiency, malabsorption, renal failure, chronic alcoholism, rhabdomyolysis, alkalosis, and certain drugs (large amounts of magnesium sulfate, anticonvulsant medication, or cimetidine).

After sodium, potassium, and calcium, magnesium is the fourth most common cation. It is often overlooked in patients with neuromuscular abnormalities. Symptoms of neuromuscular abnormalities include tremor, muscle cramping, seizures, confusion, anxiety, and hallucinations. Magnesium deficiency has been reported in as many as 10% of hospitalized patients. It is often associated with alcoholism, malabsorption, malnutrition, diarrhea, dialysis, diuretic use, and congestive heart failure. The most common cause of elevated serum magnesium is renal failure or a hemolyzed specimen.

Uric Acid

Hyperuricemia is defined by a serum uric acid concentration greater than 7 mg/dL. Gout, principally a disease of middle-aged men, results from the deposition of monosodium urate crystals, typically in a joint in a lower extremity, often the first metatarsophalangeal joint (a lesion called *podagra*). At a physiologic pH, more than 90% of uric acid exists as monosodium urate, but at levels greater than 8 mg/dL, monosodium urate is likely to precipitate into tissues.

Although patients with gout generally have elevated serum uric acid levels, 10% may have levels that fall within normal range. Conversely, many patients with hyperuricemia never experience an attack of gouty arthritis, and by far the most frequent cause of hyperuricemia, particularly in hospitalized patients, is renal disease with azotemia.

Serum uric acid levels may become elevated in any disorder that results in proliferation of cells or excessive turnover of nucleoproteins. Hemolytic processes, lymphoproliferative and myeloproliferative diseases, polycythemia vera, and rhabdomyolysis may result in high uric acid levels. Obesity, alcohol abuse, and ingestion of purine-rich foods such as bacon, salmon, scallops, and turkey can also result in an overproduction of urate.

Approximately 97% of all uric acid the human body produces daily is excreted through the kidneys. In approximately 90% of patients with gout, the primary defect is underexcretion of uric acid. This situation occurs with renal insufficiency, hypertension, diabetes, and various drugs, including cyclosporine, nicotinic acid, and salicylates.

In summary, although patients with gout generally have elevated serum uric acid levels, an isolated elevation in uric acid is not diagnostic for gout, nor does a normal level conclusively rule out the diagnosis. A most accurate and readily available test for gout is the demonstration of uric acid crystals in the synovial fluid of an acutely inflamed joint.

Liver Function Tests

Considerable confusion can be encountered in the interpretation of the many aspects of common LFTs. Many of the routine tests assess liver injury rather than liver function. Of the LFTs, only serum albumin, bilirubin, and PT provide useful information on how efficiently the liver is actually working. Certain of these findings may reflect problems arising outside the liver, such as an elevated bilirubin value, seen with hemolysis, or elevations in alkaline phosphatase associated with skeletal disorders. Normal LFTs do not ensure a normal liver: patients with cirrhosis or bleeding esophageal varices can have normal LFTs.[34]

The most commonly used markers of hepatic injury are the enzymes aspartate aminotransferase (AST) (formerly SGOT) and alanine aminotransferase (ALT) (formerly SGPT). AST and ALT values are higher in healthy obese patients and in men. ALT levels generally decline with weight loss. Slight elevations of the AST or ALT, within 150% of the upper range of normal, may not, in fact, indicate liver disease but rather a skewed (non–bell-shaped) distribution curve, with a higher representation on the far end of the scale (seen in black and Hispanic patients).

The highest ALT levels, often more than 10,000 units/L, are found in patients with acute toxic injury such as acetaminophen overdose or acute ischemic insult to the liver. With typical viral hepatitis or toxic injury, the serum ALT rises higher than the AST value, whereas an AST/ALT ratio greater than 2:1 is more common in alcoholic hepatitis or cirrhosis. Causes of elevated ALT or AST values in asymptomatic patients include autoimmune hepatitis, hepatitis B, hepatitis C, drugs, toxins, alcohol, fatty liver, congestive heart failure, and hemochromatosis.

Lactate dehydrogenase (LDH) is a less specific marker than AST or ALT but is disproportionately elevated after ischemic hepatic injury. AST elevations greater than 500 units/L and ALT values greater than 300 units/L are unlikely to be caused by alcohol intake alone and in a heavy drinker should prompt consideration of acetaminophen toxicity. AST and ALT are found in skeletal muscle and may be elevated to several times the normal value in conditions such as severe muscular exertion, polymyositis, and hypothyroidism.

Stoppage of bile flow (cholestasis) results from blockage of the bile ducts or from a disease that impairs bile function. Alkaline phosphatase (ALP) and γ-glutamyltransferase (GGT) levels typically rise to several times normal after bile duct obstruction or intrahepatic cholestasis. Diagnosis can be confounded during the first few hours after acute bile duct obstruction secondary to a gallstone, when AST and ALT levels rise 500 units/L or more but ALP and GGT can take several days to rise.

Serum ALP originates from both the liver and bone. Bony metastasis, Paget's disease, recent fracture, and placental production during the third trimester of pregnancy can all cause ALP elevations. ALP, like GGT, can be elevated in patients taking phenytoin (Dilantin), and this does not constitute an absolute indication for discontinuing the medication. ALP levels can be persistently elevated in asymptomatic women with primary biliary cirrhosis, a chronic inflammatory disease of small bile ducts associated with the presence of serum antimitochondrial antibodies.

The elevation of GGT alone with no other liver function abnormalities often results from enzyme induction caused by either alcohol or aromatic medications such as phenytoin or phenobarbital. The GGT level is often elevated in asymptomatic persons who take more than three alcohol-containing drinks per day. A mildly elevated GGT level in a person taking anticonvulsant medication does not indicate either liver disease or an absolute need to discontinue the medication.

Bilirubin, an indicator of liver function, is formed from the enzymatic breakdown of the hemoglobin molecule. The unconjugated bilirubin is carried to the liver, where it is rapidly transported into bile. The serum conjugated bilirubin level does not become elevated until the liver has lost half of its excretory capacity. A patient could thus have total left or right hepatic obstruction without a rise in bilirubin.[35]

Unconjugated hyperbilirubinemia is associated with increased bilirubin production as in hemolytic anemia, resorption of a large hematoma or defective hepatic unconjugated bilirubin clearance secondary to severe liver disease, drug-induced inhibition, congestive failure, portacaval shunting, or Gilbert's syndrome. Gilbert's syndrome occurs in many healthy persons whose serum unconjugated bilirubin is mildly elevated (2 to 3 mg/dL). That is the only liver function abnormality: both the conjugated bilirubin value and the CBC remain normal. Gilbert's syndrome has been linked to an enzymatic defect in the conjugation of bilirubin.

Visible staining of tissue with bile is called *jaundice*. The three major causes are extrahepatic and intrahepatic biliary tract obstruction and hemolysis. With hemolysis, unconjugated bilirubin increases, whereas the conjugated fraction remains normal or is only slightly elevated. In the case of extrahepatic biliary obstruction, usually in the common bile duct secondary to either a stone or carcinoma, initially one sees an increase in conjugated bilirubin but no change in the unconjugated level. After several days, however, conjugated bilirubin in the blood breaks down to unconjugated bilirubin and eventually arrives at a ratio of 1:1.

Intrahepatic biliary obstruction is usually caused by liver cell injury from any of a variety of causes, including alcohol abuse, drugs, hepatitis, cirrhosis, passive congestion, or primary or metastatic tumors. Both conjugated and unconjugated fractions may increase, in varying proportions, in this type of obstruction. Hemolysis can be identified by measuring markers such as haptoglobin and reticulocyte count. A final word on jaundice relates to age. In persons younger than 30 years, viral infections account for 80% of cases. After age 60 years, cancer accounts for approximately 50% and gallstones for approximately 25% of cases.

Another marker of hepatic synthetic capacity is serum albumin, which changes quite slowly in response to alterations in synthesis owing to its protracted plasma half-life of 3 weeks. Elevation of serum albumin usually implies dehydration. Patients with low serum albumin levels and no other LFT abnormalities are likely to have other, extrahepatic causes, such as proteinuria, trauma, sepsis, active rheumatic disease, cancer, and severe malnutrition. During pregnancy, albumin levels progressively decrease until parturition and do not return to normal until about 3 months postpartum.[36]

The PT is useful for following hepatic function during acute liver failure. The liver synthesizes clotting factors II, V, VII, IX, and X. Because factor VII has a short half-life (only 6 hours), it is sensitive to rapid changes in hepatic synthetic function. The PT does not become abnormal until more than 80% of hepatic function is lost. Vitamin K deficiency resulting from chronic cholestasis or fat malabsorption can prolong the PT. A therapeutic trial of vitamin K injections (5 mg/day subcutaneously for 3 days) is a reasonable option to exclude vitamin K deficiency.[37]

The measurement of blood ammonia provides a somewhat inexact marker for hepatic encephalopathy. Concentrations of ammonia correlate poorly with the degree of confusion. Although ammonia contributes to the encephalopathy, concentrations are often much higher in the brain than in the blood. Levels are best measured in arterial blood, because venous concentrations can be elevated as a result of muscle metabolism of amino acids. Blood ammonia determinations are more useful in evaluating encephalopathy of unknown origin, rather than for monitoring therapy in a person with known hepatic encephalopathic disease.[38]

The pancreas is another vital organ that, when diseased, may cause pain. Acute pancreatitis manifests with severe epigastric pain, vomiting, and abdominal distention. Two useful tests are serum amylase and lipase determinations. alpha-Amylase is derived from both the pancreas and the salivary glands. Its sensitivity in acute pancreatitis is approximately 90%. Other causes of amylase elevation include biliary tract disease, peritonitis, pregnancy, peptic ulcers, diabetic ketoacidosis, and salivary gland disorders. False-normal results may be seen with lipemic serum.

The serum lipase concentration is slightly less sensitive, but it is probably more specific in acute pancreatitis. The extrapancreatic disorder that most consistently elevates serum lipase is renal failure. Chronic pancreatitis is not generally a painful condition, but it reflects the end stage of acute pancreatitis, hemochromatosis, or cystic fibrosis. Diabetes, steatorrhea, and pancreatic calcification on radiographs are the signature features.

Creatine Kinase

Creatine kinase (CK) is found in cardiac muscle, skeletal muscle, and brain. Total CK can be separated into three major isoenzymes: CK-BB, found predominantly in brain and lung; CK-MM, found in skeletal muscle; and CK-MB, found predominantly in heart muscle. Total CK elevation is seen in certain conditions associated with acute muscle injury or severe muscular exertion. Total CK is also elevated after muscle trauma, myositis, muscular dystrophy, long distance running, or delirium tremens or seizures. Elevated levels can often be noted after intramuscular injections.

In evaluating chest pain, and particularly myocardial ischemia and infarction, total CK elevation is too often false positive, owing principally to skeletal muscle injury. Troponin I is a regulatory protein that is specific for myocardial injury. It becomes elevated in approximately 4 to 6 hours, peaks at approximately 10 hours, and returns to reference range in approximately 4 days. Its major advantage is that it is highly specific for cardiac injury.

The CK-MB level begins to rise 3 to 4 hours after acute myocardial infarction, reaches a peak in 12 to 24 hours, and returns to normal in approximately 36 to 48 hours. The most rapid elevation after cardiac injury is that of serum myoglobin. Unfortunately, myoglobin is found in both cardiac and skeletal muscle. Elevations are noted as early as 90 minutes after cardiac injury. An analysis of myoglobin in conjunction with troponin I can be performed at intervals after the onset of myocardial infarction symptoms. Myoglobin may be viewed as a very early but not particularly specific marker for cardiac injury, whereas troponin is an extremely specific but not as rapidly responsive marker.

Therapeutic Drug Monitoring and Testing for Drugs of Abuse

Particularly when the clinical information seems perplexing and contradictory, it is wise to consider the effects of prescription medications, toxic substances, and drugs of abuse. The practice of pain management inherently attracts patients prone to chemical dependency. They sometimes possess rather sophisticated pharmacologic information and present with detailed histories ultimately aimed at obtaining a specific controlled substance. The treating physician often has a visceral warning about the integrity of these patients but is hampered by an overwhelming sense of social squeamishness or frank denial that ultimately misleads him or her to avoid drug screening and rightfully pursue a valid clinical impression.

It is puzzling that many emergency room physicians faced with patients who exhibit erratic or agitated behavior fail to include toxicology screening in their evaluation. The effects of specific prescription medications or drug interactions in patients taking multiple medications should always be primary concerns.[39]

Therapeutic drug monitoring can be helpful in establishing compliance and therapeutic adequacy and avoiding toxic doses. Medications such as phenobarbital, valproic acid (Depakote), carbamazepine (Tegretol, Carbatrol), primidone (Mysoline), phenytoin (Dilantin), lithium carbonate, and the tricyclic antidepressants have readily available assays. Particularly in older persons, who sometimes exhibit dramatic changes in protein binding, toxicity may occur at levels normally considered therapeutic. With phenytoin, a medication that is approximately 90% bound to protein and that exhibits nonlinear kinetics, it is not unusual for toxicity to cause a variety of symptoms, including ataxia, personality change, nystagmus, dysarthria, tremor, nausea, vomiting, and somnolence. Discovery of a toxic phenytoin level in an older patient with confusion and ataxia of several months' duration may not only suggest a rapid therapeutic course of action but may also save several thousand dollars in unnecessary neurodiagnostic imaging studies.

Selective therapeutic drug monitoring can be very useful in patients taking phenytoin, primidone, phenobarbital, valproic acid, and carbamazepine. Valproic acid may be used for migraine prophylaxis. Carbamazepine and phenytoin are useful for trigeminal neuralgia and for neuropathic pain in general. Many of these compounds have narrow therapeutic windows, and, again particularly in older persons, toxicity may go unnoticed and may be attributed to other causes such as cerebrovascular disease or dementia. It is not unusual to find patients with elevated medication levels who receive an incorrect diagnosis of stroke and whose drug levels consequently are allowed to remain in a protracted state of toxicity.

Lithium carbonate, used for both bipolar disorder and cluster headache management, has a distinctly narrow therapeutic window. Adverse effects include nausea, vomiting, tremor, and hypothyroidism. Lithium is excreted by the kidneys, whereas the anticonvulsant medications mentioned earlier are metabolized in the liver and interact with other drugs that are also metabolized there. Acetaminophen is a commonly used analgesic. Hepatic injury can occur with ingestion of 10 g, and ingestion of 25 g has been known to be fatal. A serum level greater than 200 µg/mL is considered toxic. A pattern of acute hepatocellular injury similar to that of acute hepatitis is noted, with distinct elevations of AST and ALT.[40]

Testing for drugs of abuse is more difficult. Although certain health care professionals incorrectly believe that testing blood is more accurate, urine is clearly the preferred biologic sample. Urine is superior for many reasons including its lower cost, its noninvasive mode of collection, and the increased window of detection (1 to 3 days for most drugs) in urine compared with several hours in serum. A urine drug test (UDT) is helpful in documenting patient adherence to a treatment plan and in identifying illicit or nonprescribed substances, and it may even aid in uncovering illegal diversion. However, it is critical to be aware of the many technical issues that are essential to the proper interpretation of a UDT. Ignorance of these technical factors can result in multiple medical mistakes and can even unfairly damage a patient's reputation.

A UDT usually consists of an initial class-specific immunoassay followed by gas chromatography (used to separate various components within a specimen) and mass spectrometry (a procedure that specifically identifies the individual components) (GC/MS). High-performance liquid chromatography (HPLC) is also used to separate and quantitate various substances in solution. Immunoassay uses the principle of competitive antibody binding and can simultaneously and rapidly test for specific drugs or classes of drugs. Immunoassays use a cutoff above which the test is positive and below which is reported as negative. For example, the cutoff opioid concentration used in federally regulated testing for the Department of Transportation (DOT) is set at 2000 ng/mL, a level far too high to be of value in clinical practice, where it is set at 300 ng/mL.

In addition to the problems with cutoffs, immunoassays suffer from cross-reactivity. Tests for amphetamine and methamphetamine are notoriously cross-reactive with other sympathomimetic amines used in over-the-counter (OTC) preparations such as ephedrine, pseudoephedrine, and desoxyephedrine in the OTC Vicks Inhaler. The clinically ordered UDT should not be used legally against a patient, nor should it damage the patient's employment potential. All positive results should be reviewed with the patient to explore possible explanations. All unexpected results should be verified by the laboratory to ensure technical accuracy. Our current society places greater trust in technology than in fellow human beings. In the end, medicine is about mutual trust and kindness.

A UDT panel should include the following: cocaine, amphetamines, opiates, methadone, marijuana, and benzodiazepines. Immunoassay has its strengths and weaknesses. Although immunoassay for benzodiazepines may not reliably detect clonazepam, a positive result for cocaine and its primary metabolite, benzoylecgonine, is highly predictive for cocaine use and is not subject to cross-reactivity with other compounds.

Immunoassay is often very responsive to morphine and codeine but has a much lower sensitivity for the semisynthetic (hydrocodone, oxycodone, hydromorphone, oxymorphone, and buprenorphine) and synthetic opioids (meperidine, fentanyl, propoxyphene, and methadone). If the purpose of testing is to identify a specific drug (adherence testing) such as oxycodone, one must make certain that the laboratory can reliably identify that specific medication and adjust the cutoff concentration so that lower concentrations can be documented. No reliable relationships exist among the dose of an opioid, its analgesic effect, and the urine drug concentration. The varied issues related to drug testing highlight the special training, experience, and diligence required in dealing with a large practice of patients who are taking opioids on a long-term basis. It is truly a specialized area in clinical medicine.[41]

In addition to problems with specificity and sensitivity, persistence of a drug or its metabolites in the urine varies much among individual agents and among abusers. For example, the urine can be positive for cannabinoids several days after a single casual use of marijuana. Passive smoke inhalation does not explain positive marijuana results at clinically available cutoffs

(50 ng/mL). After cessation in long-term heavy users, the urine may remain positive for as long as a month. All initially positive test results obtained by screening procedures should be confirmed by GC/MS.

The different sensitivity levels of different tests must be kept in mind, as must the effect of urine concentration or dilution. Detection of cannabinoids in the urine indicates that the patient has used marijuana in the past but provides no clear evidence that marijuana is the cause of current cognitive impairment or a behavioral problem. Of equal importance is the concept of chain of custody, which demands strict accountability for a specimen from its collection to its ultimate analysis. A patient could be tragically stigmatized if erroneous results were obtained in a process that was technically flawed.

Cocaine is another popular drug of abuse. Its major metabolite, benzoylecgonine, remains detectable considerably longer than does cocaine and in heavy users may be detectable for several weeks. Amphetamines, usually methamphetamine, are detectable in the urine within 3 hours after a single dose. A positive result for amphetamines in the urine usually implies use within the last 24 to 48 hours, but one should recall the problems with cross-reactivity and the need to confirm initial results with GC/MS. As an overview, the most common classes of drugs found when screening trauma patients, in order of frequency, are ethanol, amphetamines, opiates, and cocaine.[42]

Opioid abuse is particularly problematic in the "pain population." Morphine and codeine are made from the seeds of the opium poppy, whereas heroin is synthesized directly from morphine. Ingestion of moderate amounts of culinary poppy seeds can result in detectable concentrations of morphine in the urine that may last as long as 3 days. A speedball (a combination of cocaine and heroin) remains popular for prolonging cocaine's effects while blunting postcocaine depression. Finally, the easy access to opioids afforded to medical personnel also make this subgroup particularly susceptible to abuse. Medicine is a stressful profession, and the powerful anxiolytic effects of opioids have historically lured many physicians and nurses into self-medication, often with devastating personal and professional consequences.

Toxicology

Mercury, arsenic, bismuth, and antimony are best screened by urine sampling. Hair and nails are preferred for documenting long-term exposure to arsenic or mercury. Occupational lead exposure and lead poisoning remain serious public health problems in the United States. Most exposure is in industry—battery manufacturing, the chemical industry, smelting, soldering, and welding. Symptoms include abdominal pain, myalgias, paresthesias, general fatigue, and, ultimately, encephalopathy and death.

Arriving at the diagnosis requires a constant high index of suspicion. At present, the blood level of lead is the single best indicator of recent absorption of a large dose of lead. The blood lead level rises rapidly within hours of an acute exposure and remains elevated for several weeks. Consecutive measurements averaging 50 μg/dL or higher indicate the necessity to remove an employee from that toxic environment. A blood lead level and a zinc protoporphyrin level provide sufficient information to quantitate the severity and approximate chronology of the lead exposure.

Zinc protoporphyrin reflects the toxic effects of lead on an erythrocyte enzyme system. Levels usually begin to rise when the blood lead level exceeds 40 μg/100 mL. Once elevated, zinc protoporphyrin tends to remain above background levels for several months (the 120-day life span of RBCs). The combination of an elevated blood lead level and an elevated zinc protoporphyrin value suggests that exposure must have lasted longer than several days.[43]

Every year in the United States, the deaths of more than 100,000 persons are associated with the use of alcohol. Intoxication is so common that physicians frequently forget that it can be fatal. Levels higher than 400 mg/dL are suggested lethal, but levels lower than 400 mg/dL have been fatal, and levels of 800 mg/dL have been documented in alert patients. Most states define legal intoxication as a blood alcohol level of 100 mg/dL, although driving skills have been shown to become impaired at levels as low as 50 mg/dL. Alcohol is often ingested with other medications, and, in combination, intoxicating levels or otherwise lethal doses may be strikingly lower. A combination of ethanol with chloral hydrate (a Mickey Finn) has a particularly nasty reputation.

Various tests have been used to screen for chronic alcoholism, including elevated GGT and AST levels, MCV elevation, hyperuricemia and hypomagnesemia, hyponatremia, and hypophosphatemia.[44] These indices correlate to some degree but cannot be taken as specific indicators of alcohol abuse. As in all cases with toxicology, the results should not be accepted without question. Laboratory errors do occur, and any tendency to be judgmental or punitive is strongly discouraged.

Conclusion

The proper use of laboratory testing can be very valuable in evaluating pain. This chapter highlights only the essentials. It is presented as a starting point from which readers can expand their knowledge and attempt to keep up to date with almost constant technologic advances. In clinical experience, laboratory testing is often overlooked, with embarrassing—and sometimes tragic—consequences.

These tests, along with findings of the history and physical examination, form the foundation of clinical diagnosis. The pain specialist should embrace a primary care role in accurate diagnosis by ensuring thoroughness through methodical attention to detail. This approach is much preferred to the all too common one where patients are immediately referred for expensive procedures with a blind hope that advanced technology alone will illuminate the darkness and substitute for a careful history and physical examination.

References

Full references for this chapter can be found on www.expertconsult.com.

Radiography

Hifz Aniq and Robert Campbell

X-rays are produced when highly energetic electrons interact with matter and convert their kinetic energy into electromagnetic radiation. The x-ray tube contains the electron source in the form of a cathode tube filament, as well as a tungsten target in a copper anode. Collimators are used to define the x-ray field. With varying voltage, current, and exposure time, x-ray beams of varying penetrability and spatial distribution can be created.

Radiography depends on differences in radiographic density. A radiograph is a two-dimensional image of a three-dimensional object. This is known as a projection imaging technique, in contradistinction to cross-sectional modalities. The difficulty of interpreting these images results from this superimposition of structures, and thus pathologic processes may appear less clearly defined.

Traditional radiography systems use a film-screen combination consisting of a cassette, one or two intensifying screens, and a sheet of film. The film is simply thin plastic with a photosensitive emulsion coated onto one or both sides. The cassette is designed to protect the film from ambient light before the film is exposed with x-rays. For routine radiography, double-screen, double-emulsion film-screen combinations are often used to improve sensitivity and to reduce radiation exposure. Radiographic views are named by the direction of the x-ray beam from the source to the imaging recording device.

Several different systems are currently available for the acquisition of digital radiographs: the ones most commonly seen in clinical use are computed radiography (CR), charged-coupled devices (CCDs), direct detection flat panel systems, and indirect detection flat panel systems.

The workflow of CR systems is similar to that of conventional screen-film radiography. The CR imaging plate is made of barium fluorobromide or barium fluoride (barium fluorohalide). The CR imaging plate traps the x-ray beam (the electron) within the phosphor layer, and this electromagnetic energy is stored until processing. The CR plate is inserted into a reader that contains a laser that scans across the imaging plate, releases the stored energy, and causes the emission of light. These light emissions are read by a photodiode scanning the imaging plate. The imaging plate is then "cleaned" with a flood of light. The prime advantage of CR over film-screen radiography is the increase in dynamic range. The system can tolerate a wider exposure range, and the result is a smaller number of diagnostically inadequate films. However, the raw data require processing algorithms to produce clinically useful images. CCD detectors form images from visible light. The surface of a CCD chip is photosensitive, and when a pixel is exposed to light, electrons are produced and are built up within the pixel. This technology is used in modern video and digital cameras.

Cervical Spine

Neck pain is a common human experience, although less common than that of low back pain. Neck pain may be a result of local noxious stimulation, or it may be referred from distant structures supplied by the cervical spinal nerves. Although somatic pain is typically referred distally, the acromioclavicular joint and sternoclavicular joints are two sites that may have neck pain by proximal referral. Most cases of neck pain are self-limiting, resulting from mechanical problems; however, in a small percentage of cases, the pain becomes chronic.

The standard cervical spinal radiographic series consists of anteroposterior, lateral, and odontoid views. If the cervicothoracic junction is not demonstrated on the lateral view, one may obtain a swimmer's view, taken while the patient's arm is extended over the head. Plain radiographs are appropriate when the patient has a history of trauma likely to have produced a fracture or severe subluxation or when concern exists regarding instability. To assess for subluxation, four lines are traced along the lateral radiograph. Lines joining the anterior aspect of the vertebral body, the posterior aspect of the vertebral body, the laminae, and the spinous processes should appear as smooth arcs (**Fig. 8.1**). Oblique views of the cervical spine demonstrate the neural foramina, pedicles, articular masses, and apophyseal joints. In the setting of trauma, oblique views have been used in identifying fractures and subluxations of the articular process. Currently, oblique views are rarely performed because computed tomography (CT) is easily available.

Atlantoaxial instability should be specifically assessed. This is performed by evaluating the distance between the posterior aspect of the anterior arch of the atlas and the anterior aspect of the odontoid as seen on a lateral view (**Fig. 8.2**). This measurement normally is less than 3 mm. Atlantoaxial instability can be seen in disease processes that may result in destruction of the transverse ligament complex, such as inflammatory arthropathies (most commonly, rheumatoid arthritis).

Radiography for the evaluation of mechanical neck pain is limited and can be used to document the degree of cervical spondylosis. The term *spondylosis* is often used synonymously with *degeneration,* which includes both the nucleus pulposus and anulus fibrosus processes. Freidenburg and Miller,[1] however, demonstrated no correlation between the presence of degenerative or spondylitic changes in the cervical spine and symptoms of neck pain. Oblique views of the cervical spine have been replaced by magnetic resonance imaging (MRI) scan, which can show the neural foramen much more clearly and does not involve any radiation.

The ligament between the vertebrae and the spinal dura is called the posterior longitudinal ligament. Ossification of the posterior longitudinal ligament (OPLL) is more common in the cervical spine (70%), followed by the thoracic (15%) and lumbar (15%) regions. This entity was originally reported in a large number of Japanese patients with a genetic linkage. Although OPLL is typically asymptomatic, patients may present with symptoms of cervical myelopathy.[2] The typical radiographic appearance is

that of a linear band of ossification along the posterior margin of the vertebral body with a separating sharp, thin radiolucent line. OPLL may be apparent in as many as 50% of cases of diffuse idiopathic skeletal hyperostosis (DISH); conversely, DISH has been observed in more than 20% of cases of OPLL (**Fig. 8.3**).[3]

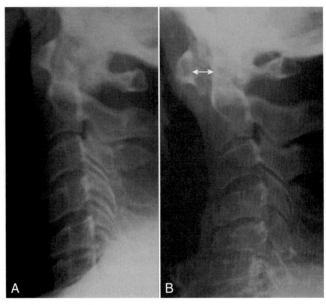

Fig. 8.2 **Lateral cervical spine: two images of a known case of rheumatoid arthritis 8 years apart.** A, Normal atlantoaxial joint. B, Atlantoaxial subluxation. The gap between the arch of the atlas and the odontoid process is wider than 3 mm *(arrow).*

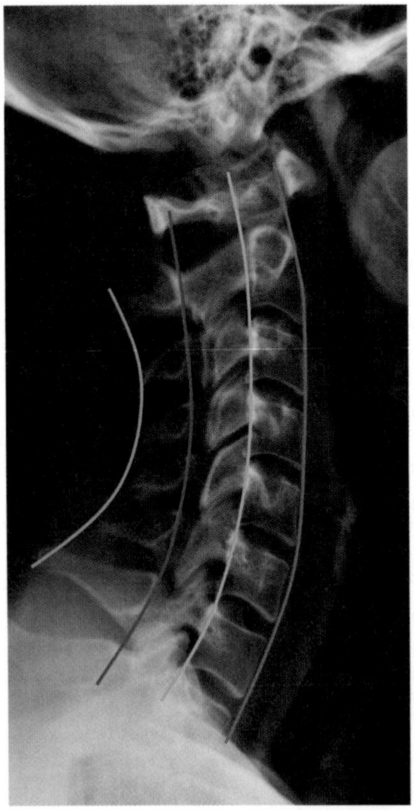

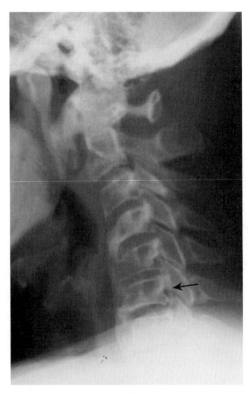

Fig. 8.3 **Ossification of the posterior longitudinal ligament (OPLL) and diffuse idiopathic skeletal hyperostosis (DISH).** The lateral view of the cervical spine shows prominent flowing ossification along the anterior margin of four continuous vertebrae compatible with DISH. A dense vertical band of ossification is seen posterior to the vertebral margin *(arrow)* with a separating radiolucent line consistent with OPLL.

Fig. 8.1 **Lateral radiograph of a normal cervical spine.** From anterior to posterior, these four parallel lines should be observed in every lateral cervical spine examination (anterior spinal line, posterior spinal line, spinolaminar line, spinous process line).

Thoracic Spine

The standard thoracic spinal radiographic series consists of anteroposterior and lateral views. Symptomatic degenerative disk disease is much less common in the thoracic spine than in the cervical and lumbar regions. Thoracic disk herniations are relatively uncommon when compared with cervical and lumbar disk disease. Commonly, thoracic disk herniations manifest as pain, numbness, tingling, and occasionally lower extremity weakness. If the herniation is large enough, bowel or bladder function may be affected.

Scheuermann's disease is a type of thoracic kyphosis defined by anterior wedging of at least 5 degrees of three adjacent thoracic vertebral bodies. Secondary changes of Scheuermann's kyphosis are characterized by irregularities of the vertebral end plates, disk space narrowing, and the presence of intervertebral disk herniations known as Schmorl's nodes. The thoracic spine is most commonly affected, although the lumbar spine may also be involved. This disorder of the spine is often discovered initially in adolescents and was formerly thought to be secondary to osteonecrosis but is now believed to be the result of a congenital weakness in the end plates. For diagnosis, three adjacent vertebral bodies must be involved with 5 degrees or more of anterior wedging.

DISH is a common cause of regional pain syndromes in patients more than 40 years old. The peak incidence is in the sixth and seventh decades of life, and the disorder is more common in men than in women. Although common in the lower thoracic spine, DISH also can be seen in the lumbar and cervical spine. Patients typically present with localized pain and stiffness with decreased range of motion of the affected area. Radiographs of the spine demonstrate the presence of flowing, nonmarginal syndesmophytes along the anterolateral margins of at least four contiguous vertebrae (**Fig. 8.4**). Some patients with DISH also have OPLL (see earlier).

Lumbar Spine

Low back pain is the most common musculoskeletal impairment reported and the second most common complaint to primary physicians after the common cold. Most instances of back pain are benign and self-limiting. More than 50% of all patients improve after 1 week, whereas more than 90% are better at 8 weeks. Careful clinical evaluation is necessary to separate patients with mechanical (no primary inflammatory or neoplastic cause) back pain from those with nonmechanical back pain.

Radiography is stated to have limited use in the evaluation of low back pain. Patients with mechanical back pain often have normal radiographs. Conversely and more commonly, many individuals with radiographic abnormalities are asymptomatic.[4] Evaluation of the lumbar spine includes the anteroposterior and lateral views. The anteroposterior and lateral views demonstrate alignment, disk and vertebral body height, and gross assessment of bone mineral density. The use of lumbar radiography should be limited because it exposes the gonads to significant ionizing radiation. The radiation exposure of oblique views is double the exposure of standard views, which alone are equivalent to the radiation exposure of more than 30 routine chest x-rays.[5]

Radiography is often used as an initial screening tool for patients with unrelenting back pain. Congenital abnormalities or developmental defects such as scoliosis, spina bifida, or anomalous lumbosacral transitional vertebral bodies may be visualized. Spondylolysis, a break in the pars interarticularis, is a common radiographic abnormality associated with low back pain. Spondylolysis may or may not result in spondylolisthesis. However, the combination of spondylolysis and spondylolisthesis frequently distorts the associated neural foramina and leads to compromise of the exiting nerve. Spondylolysis does not necessarily produce back pain. Oblique views of the lumbar spine are particularly useful for the evaluation of spondylolysis because they demonstrate the pars interarticularis in profile (**Fig. 8.5**).

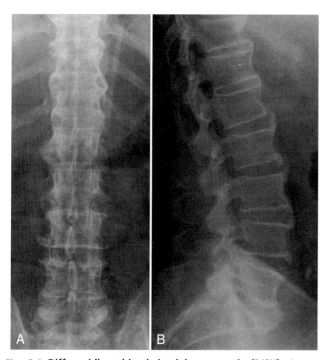

Fig. 8.4 **Diffuse idiopathic skeletal hyperostosis (DISH).** Anteroposterior (A) and lateral (B) views of the thoracic spine show large flowing bony excrescences along at least four vertebral bodies.

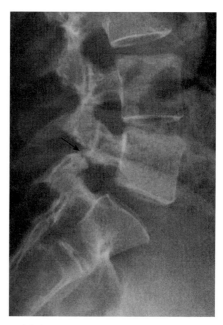

Fig. 8.5 **Spondylolysis.** The lateral radiograph demonstrates discontinuity of the "Scottie dog" neck compatible with a pars defect.

Disorders of the intervertebral disks and zygapophyseal joints may also result in low back pain. Lumbar radiographs may not directly demonstrate findings of disk herniation or spinal stenosis. However, it is unusual for lumbar radiographs to be absolutely normal in these conditions. Acute disk herniation may result in loss of intervertebral disk height. Normal lumbar intervertebral disk height demonstrates an interval increase up to the lumbosacral junction. Plain film findings that may be associated with stenosis include narrowing of the intervertebral disk spaces with diskogenic vertebral sclerosis, zygapophyseal joint osteoarthritis, and spondylolisthesis.[6] Because these findings are nonspecific and are common in asymptomatic older individuals, they have limited predictive value. Congenital stenosis may result from developmentally narrow spinal canal dimensions (developmentally short pedicles) or bone dysplasias such as achondroplasia (dwarfism).

Signs of disk degeneration include loss of disk height, sclerosis of the end plates, and osteophytic ridging. In addition, spondylolisthesis can be diagnosed and the degree of forward slip visualized easily on lateral images. Spondylolisthesis as a result of degenerative changes should never be greater than 25%. Meyerding proposed a grading system for spondylolisthesis that is still used today. The degree of slippage is measured as the percentage of distance the anteriorly translated vertebral body has moved forward relative to the superior end plate of the vertebra below. Grade 1 denotes up to 25% forward slip; grade 2, up to 50%; grade 3, up to 75%; grade 4, up to 100%; and grade 5, greater than 100% slippage (**Fig. 8.6**).

In older individuals with low back pain, more ominous causes need to be considered. Patients with fever or weight loss may have an infection or tumor as the cause of their pain. Radiographs may be normal at the initial onset of disk space infection but will demonstrate increasing destruction with prolonged duration. Infections are generally hematogenous in adults and begin at the vertebral end plate. Radiographic evidence of disk infection includes loss of disk height, erosions or destruction of adjacent vertebral end plates, and reactive new bone formation with sclerosis in chronic cases. If clinical suspicion persists despite normal radiographs, cross-sectional imaging with CT or MRI may be performed. Both modalities demonstrate increased sensitivity for the detection of vertebral osteomyelitis. Numerous neoplastic lesions, both benign and malignant, may be associated with the lumbar spine. Neoplastic lesions may be lytic (radiolucent), blastic (radiodense), or mixed. From 30% to 50% of trabecular bone must be lost before the loss can be visualized on a radiograph.

Osteoporotic patients are at increased risk for developing compression fractures. New or incompletely healed fractures are commonly associated with pain. Although radiographs may be able to distinguish between acute and chronic compression deformities through comparison with prior radiographs, it may be impossible to assess the degree of healing. Scintigraphy and MRI are more useful in this context because they demonstrate increased bone activity and bone marrow edema, respectively, of incompletely healed fractures.

Inflammatory arthropathies that affect the axial skeleton may manifest as low back pain. Radiographs of the sacroiliac joints are often obtained in patients suspected of having inflammatory arthropathy of the axial skeleton. Sacroiliitis can be detected early with radiography. Angled views of the sacroiliac joints by 30 degrees (Ferguson's view) provide greater sensitivity than do routine anteroposterior views.[7] In patients with ankylosing spondylitis, sacroiliitis begins as erosions, followed by sclerosis

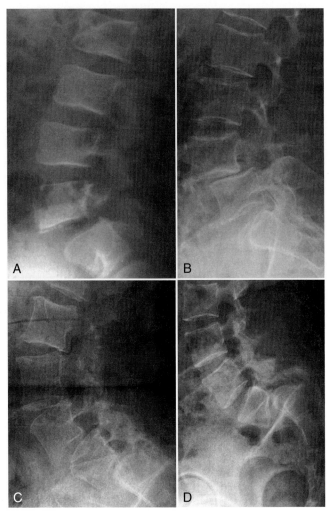

Fig. 8.6 Grading of spondylolisthesis. Lateral views of the lumbar spine demonstrate varying degrees of spondylolisthesis in the lower lumbar spine. **A,** Grade 1: 1% to 25% slippage. **B,** Grade 2: 26% to 50% slippage. **C,** Grade 3: 51% to 75% slippage. **D,** Grade 4: 76% to 100% slippage.

and eventual ankylosis. Sacroiliitis may be unilateral (i.e., infectious), bilaterally symmetrical (i.e., ankylosing spondylitis, enteropathic arthropathy), or bilateral and asymmetrical (i.e., seronegative spondyloarthropathies) (**Fig. 8.7**). CT or MRI is more sensitive and may show early involvement of the sacroiliac joint when the findings of plain radiographs are equivocal.

Kummel's disease, aseptic vertebral osteonecrosis, is an entity that may manifest with localized pain. Although patients may be asymptomatic, local pain and progressive angular kyphotic deformity are clinical hallmarks. Radiographic diagnosis is based on vertebral body collapse or flattening with an associated intranuclear vacuum cleft. Kummel's disease is often associated with a history of trauma, severe osteoporosis, or long-term use of corticosteroids, and it manifests most commonly at the thoracolumbar junction (**Fig. 8.8**).

Shoulder

The shoulder is a complex joint with numerous bony articulations as well as multiple ligamentous and musculotendinous attachments. Shoulder pain may be a result of local trauma or referred pain or may be seen in association with other medical conditions.

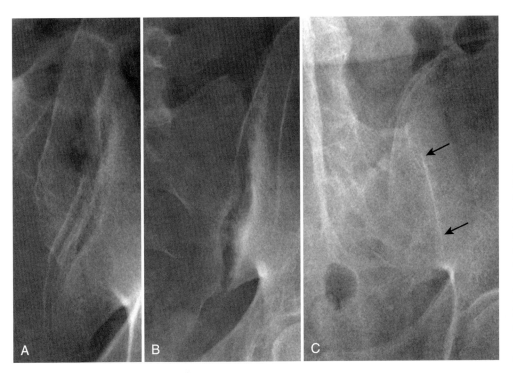

Fig. 8.7 **Normal sacroiliac joint and sacroiliitis.** Magnified views of the sacroiliac (SI) joints of three different patients. A, Normal anteroposterior view of the left SI joint demonstrates sharply defined sacral and iliac sides of the joint without evidence of sclerosis or erosion. B, Sacroiliitis: Posteroanterior view demonstrates erosions and sclerosis predominantly on the iliac side. C, Fusion of the left SI joint *(arrows)* that was also evident on the right in this patient with late-stage ankylosing spondylitis.

Radiographs may demonstrate chronic rotator cuff arthropathy that may be evidenced by calcific tendinitis (**Fig. 8.9**). In these long-standing cases, cystic and sclerotic changes may be seen at the greater tuberosity insertion. Superior migration of the humeral head against the undersurface of the acromion with narrowing of the subacromial space (<6 mm) is another secondary sign of rotator cuff incompetence. Over time, this results in degenerative changes at the subacromial joint and eventual secondary osteoarthritis at the glenohumeral joint.

Acromioclavicular pain is commonly a result of acute or chronic repetitious trauma. Injuries to this joint are graded according to the degree of disruption of the joint capsule and supporting ligaments. Sage and Salvatore proposed a three-grade classification that Rockwood further classified into six types:

Type I: Normal
Type II: Subluxation of acromioclavicular joint space less than 1 cm; normal coracoclavicular space
Type III: Subluxation of acromioclavicular joint space more than 1 cm; widening of the coracoclavicular space more than 50%
Types IV to VI: Subluxation of acromioclavicular joint space more than 1 cm, widening of the coracoclavicular space more than 50%; associated displacement of the clavicle

Grade I injury involves a sprain of the joint capsule without ligamentous disruption. Radiographs of both shoulders may be obtained with stress views (the addition of 10-lb weights) to see whether abnormal or asymmetrical widening of the acromioclavicular space (normal <4 mm) is present.

Osteolysis of the distal clavicle may be seen as a result of acute injury or repetitive stress (i.e., weight lifting) to the shoulder. These changes are typically seen predominantly on the clavicular side. Inflammatory arthritis such as rheumatoid arthritis may also manifest with similar radiographic findings. Patients may present with aching and pain at the limits of flexion and abduction. Radiographs demonstrate resorption of the distal clavicle, often with osteophyte formation, osteoporosis, or tapering. The differential diagnosis of distal clavicular resorption includes postoperative changes, post-traumatic osteolysis, hyperparathyroidism, or changes secondary to inflammatory arthropathy.

Elbow

Pain at the elbow may be related to local disease, or it may be referred pain from cervical or shoulder disease. Generally, fully extended frontal and 90-degree flexed lateral views of the elbow are adequate for evaluation of arthritis; oblique views in full extension can be helpful for further visualization of the joint margins and the radioulnar articulation. An axial view obtained with the elbow in flexion is useful to evaluate the cubital tunnel for marginal osteophytes, which can impinge on the ulnar nerve.

Local processes include both articular (arthritis, osteochondritis, loose bodies, subluxation) and periarticular (epicondylitis, olecranon bursitis, ligamentous lesions, entrapment neuropathy) disorders. Primary osteoarthritis of the elbow is unusual, but involvement frequently occurs in more generalized inflammatory arthritis. Lateral epicondylitis, the most frequent periarticular lesion, affects 1% to 3% of the population.

Osteochondritis dissecans of the elbow usually affects adolescents and young adults. The area of the elbow most frequently affected is the anterolateral surface of the humeral capitellum. In an adolescent with elbow pain, particularly if he or she is a throwing athlete, the diagnosis of osteochondritis dissecans may be considered.[8] Initial investigations include plain radiographs, which may demonstrate radiolucency or rarefaction of the lateral or central portion of the capitellum (**Fig. 8.10**). In advanced stages, loose bodies, radial head hypertrophy, and osteophyte formation may be present. Radiographs may be diagnostic, but bone scan is a more sensitive diagnostic tool, and MRI offers information for staging and characterization of lesions.

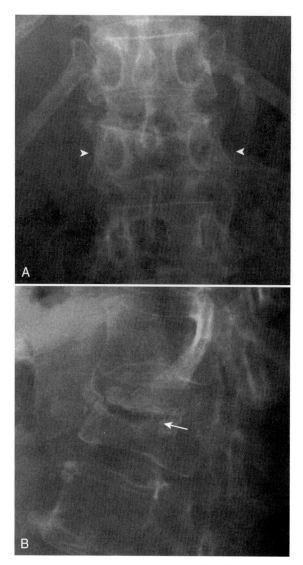

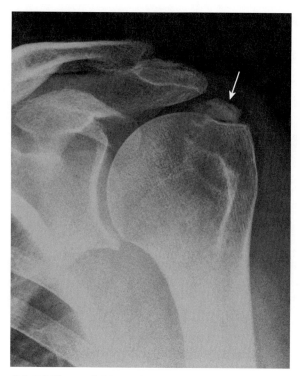

Fig. 8.9 **Calcific tendinitis.** In this anteroposterior view of the right shoulder, irregular calcification is noted in the supraspinatus tendon in keeping with calcific tendinosis.

Fig. 8.8 **Kummel's disease.** Anteroposterior (A) and lateral (B) views at the thoracolumbar junction show vertebral body collapse (arrowheads) with an associated vacuum phenomenon (white arrow).

A second process that also involves the capitellum and should be distinguished from osteochondritis dissecans is Panner's disease, which is osteochondrosis of the capitellum. Panner's disease is thought to be caused by interference in blood supply to the growing epiphysis that results in resorption and eventual repair and replacement of the ossification center. Inciting causes include repetitive trauma, congenital and hereditary factors, and endocrine disturbances. Initial radiographs demonstrate irregularity with areas of radiolucency involving the capitellum. Progressive radiographs demonstrate deformity of the capitellum with eventual collapse and fragmentation.

Wrist and Hand

Radiographs of the hands are the most informative part of any screening series for arthritis. Two views are suggested for evaluation: a posteroanterior view and a "ball catcher's" view of both hands and wrists. Mineralization and soft tissue swelling

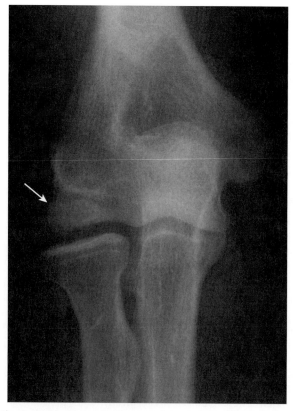

Fig. 8.10 Osteochondritis dissecans (arrow) of the right capitellum.

are clearly imaged by the posteroanterior view. The ball catcher's view profiles the radial aspect of the base of the proximal phalanges in the hand and the triquetrum and pisiform in the wrist. This view is particularly useful for imaging early erosive changes. The hand is not rigidly positioned by the technician for this view, and thus subtle subluxations as seen in inflammatory arthropathies and systemic lupus erythematous may be identified. Soft tissue swelling, subluxation or dislocation, mineralization, calcification, joint space narrowing, erosion, and bone production must all be considered in the examination. Each type of arthropathy has its own characteristic set of changes.

The distribution of primary osteoarthritis in the hands and wrists is characteristic, affecting the scaphoid-trapezium-trapezoid, first carpometacarpal, and first metacarpophalangeal joints, as well as the interphalangeal joints. The second to fifth metacarpophalangeal joints are less often involved. Large osteophytes at the interphalangeal joints can produce deformity and loss of range of motion and are referred to clinically as *Heberden's nodes* at the distal interphalangeal joints and *Bouchard's nodes* at the proximal interphalangeal joints. Secondary osteoarthritis is also common in the wrist in patients with chronic inflammatory arthropathy, especially rheumatoid arthritis, who have suffered severe cartilage damage and ligament tears as a result of their primary disease.

Positive ulnar variance, a situation in which the distal ulna projects farther than the end of the radius, can also result in wrist pain. Positive ulnar variance can cause impaction of the distal ulna or ulnar styloid on the lunate or triquetrum (ulnocarpal impaction syndrome). This situation causes tearing of the triangular fibrocartilage complex, which is caught between these structures, and subsequent osteoarthritis, with pain at the ulnar aspect of the wrist, especially during activities requiring ulnar deviation.

Chondrocalcinosis, which is deposition of calcium pyrophosphate dihydrate (CPPD) crystal, can occur in both hyaline and fibrous cartilage. When this condition seen in two or more joints, the radiographic diagnosis of CPPD deposition disease can be made. Idiopathic CPPD crystal deposition disease, hyperparathyroidism, and hemochromatosis are all known to cause actual deposition of CPPD crystals in cartilage. Soft tissue calcification of hydroxyapatite crystals can be seen in various systemic diseases. Classically seen in shoulder tendinosis or over the greater trochanter, CPPD deposition within the soft tissues of the hand can be related to scleroderma, dermatomyositis, and renal osteodystrophy.

De Quervain's stenosing tenosynovitis is most commonly seen in women between 30 and 50 years of age as a result of occupation-related cumulative microtrauma. Secondary causes include rheumatoid arthritis, systemic lupus erythematosus, scleroderma, psoriatic arthritis, infection, microcrystalline amyloid deposition, sarcoidosis, and pigmented villonodular synovitis. Clinically, De Quervain's tenosynovitis is often confused with osteoarthritis of the first carpometacarpal joint or with the intersection syndrome. Radiographs may demonstrate the changes of osteoarthritis, but ultrasound or MRI is necessary for identification of tenosynovitis. Typically, radiographs are unable to demonstrate changes related to tenosynovitis or ganglion, which are two common causes of wrist pain.

Pelvis and Hip

Clinically, numerous conditions can account for the patient with hip pain. Hip pain may be related to the hip itself, to the periarticular soft tissues, or to the adjacent bones. Referred pain from the lumbar spine may also manifest as hip pain. Anteroposterior (with the leg internally rotated) and frog-leg lateral (hip abducted and externally rotated) views of the hips are the only views typically required for evaluation. Joint narrowing is best assessed on the anteroposterior view; most normal hip joints are wider medially than superiorly by a ratio of approximately 2:1. However, it is useful to add to the protocol an anteroposterior view of the pelvis because this permits comparison with the contralateral side, as well as assessment of the sacroiliac joints.

Primary hip osteoarthritis is readily diagnosed by radiography, as demonstrated by cartilage space narrowing, marginal osteophytes, and subchondral sclerosis. Normal hips should have 4 mm of cartilage space with a difference of less than 1 mm from side to side.[9] In the hips, osteoarthritis is typically associated with asymmetrical joint narrowing; usually, the cartilage loss is most noticeable at the superior weight-bearing aspect of the joint. Osteophytes form at the junction of the femoral head and neck. They are often broad and flat, form a "collar" around the head, and are seen more clearly on the frog-leg lateral view (**Fig. 8.11**). Subchondral cysts can become large and can be mistaken for a lytic lesion when they occur at the acetabulum. Other cystic-appearing foci are common at the femoral neck and may represent synovial herniation pits; these are often seen in asymptomatic individuals without osteoarthritis. Buttressing is seen at the medial aspect of the femoral neck and is a response to the abnormal stresses placed on the joint margins.

Pain is also a presenting complaint in many inflammatory arthritides, including seronegative spondyloarthropathies (ankylosing spondylitis, Reiter's syndrome, psoriatic arthropathy, and enteropathic arthropathy), crystalline arthropathies (gout and pseudogout) and rheumatoid, viral, and septic arthritis. Two different causes of osteonecrosis of the hip are described: traumatic and atraumatic. Traumatic osteonecrosis is secondary to direct injury to the femoral head with resultant damage to its blood supply. Fracture of the femoral head or neck and hip dislocation are the two primary mechanisms of injury. The two most common causes of atraumatic osteonecrosis are corticosteroid use and alcohol abuse. In early osteonecrosis, radiographs are typically normal. Early findings include ill-defined mottling or sclerosis of the trabecular pattern followed by a discontinuity in the subchondral bone, the "crescent sign," which represents a fracture between the subchondral line and the adjacent necrotic bone. As the disease progresses, subchondral collapse and eventual degenerative joint disease result (**Fig. 8.12**).

Several radiographic staging systems are used. The Ficat classification is as follows:

Stage 0: No pain, normal radiographic findings, abnormal bone scan or MRI findings

Stage I: Pain, normal radiographic findings, abnormal bone scan or MRI findings

Stage II: Pain, cysts, or sclerosis visible on radiographs, abnormal bone scan or MRI findings, without subchondral fracture

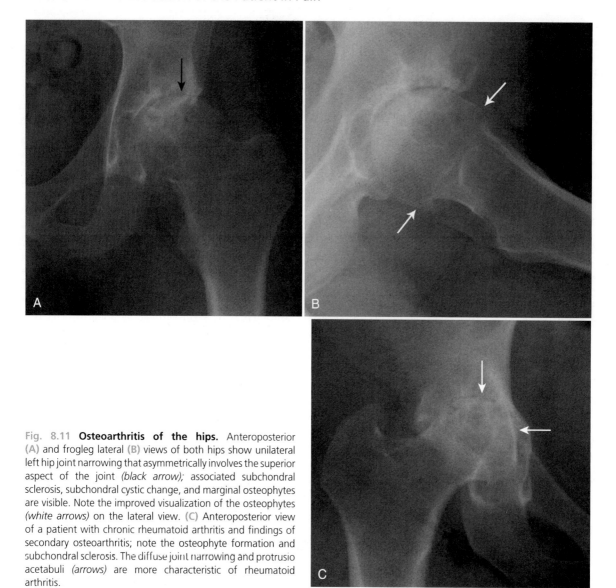

Fig. 8.11 **Osteoarthritis of the hips.** Anteroposterior (A) and frogleg lateral (B) views of both hips show unilateral left hip joint narrowing that asymmetrically involves the superior aspect of the joint *(black arrow)*; associated subchondral sclerosis, subchondral cystic change, and marginal osteophytes are visible. Note the improved visualization of the osteophytes *(white arrows)* on the lateral view. (C) Anteroposterior view of a patient with chronic rheumatoid arthritis and findings of secondary osteoarthritis; note the osteophyte formation and subchondral sclerosis. The diffuse joint narrowing and protrusio acetabuli *(arrows)* are more characteristic of rheumatoid arthritis.

Stage III: Pain, femoral head collapse visible on radiographs, abnormal bone scan or MRI findings, crescent sign (subchondral collapse), or step-off in contour of subchondral bone

Stage IV: Pain, acetabular disease with joint space narrowing and arthritis (osteoarthrosis) visible on radiographs, abnormal MRI or bone scan findings

Osteitis pubis is a syndrome characterized by pain and bony erosion of the symphysis pubis. Radiographs may demonstrate symphysis widening, cystic changes, and sclerotic changes (a later finding). Bone scanning, which is more sensitive than radiography, often demonstrates increased uptake over the symphysis and pubic rami.

Pain in the trochanteric region is another common entity in adults. The cause is either gluteus medius and minimus tendinosis or trochanteric bursitis. This entity is much better defined by clinical examination or MRI. Radiographic findings may include calcification in the gluteus medius or minimus tendons adjacent to the trochanter or bony irregularity. Infectious arthropathy of the hip may manifest radiographically as joint space narrowing,

marked osteopenia, and destruction. Aspiration and evaluation of the aspirate are necessary for diagnosis.

Knee

The initial imaging studies for nontraumatic knee pain are the anteroposterior and lateral radiographs. On the lateral view with the knee flexed 20 to 35 degrees, effusion can be detected; the medial and lateral compartments can be distinguished by matching condyles to their corresponding tibial surface (medial tibial plateau concave, lateral convex). If symptoms are localized to the patellofemoral joint, an axial (skyline) view of the patellofemoral joint is recommended.

In older patients, the most common cause of nontraumatic knee pain is osteoarthritis. Radiographic diagnosis includes indirect evaluation of the articular cartilage by joint space narrowing, as well as the formation of osteophytes, subchondral cysts, and bony sclerosis (**Fig. 8.13**). Standing radiographs have been reported to demonstrate cartilage space narrowing more accurately than supine radiographs.

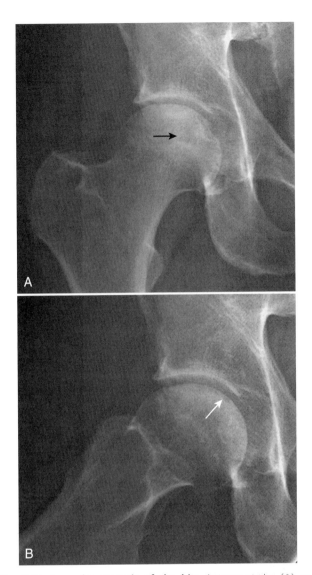

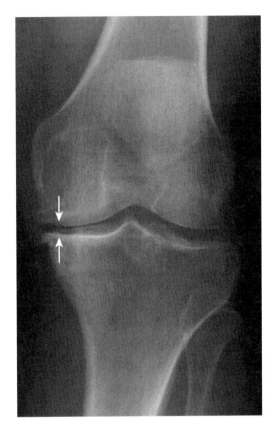

Fig. 8.13 **Osteoarthritis of the knee.** The anteroposterior view shows medial compartment narrowing *(arrows)*, subchondral sclerosis, cystic change at the medial tibial plateau, and large marginal osteophytes.

Fig. 8.12 **Avascular necrosis of the hip.** Anteroposterior (A) and lateral (B) views of the right hip demonstrate sclerosis of the femoral head *(arrow)* with visualization of the "crescent sign" *(white arrow)* representing subchondral bone collapse.

Although the patellofemoral joint is not a weight-bearing joint, patellofemoral joint osteoarthritis is commonly seen in older individuals in conjunction with involvement of the medial and lateral compartments (tricompartmental). The potential causes of patellofemoral joint osteoarthritis include patellar tracking abnormalities, a developmentally shallow patellar sulcus, a high-riding patella (patella alta), and prior patellar dislocation. CPPD arthropathy may also manifest as predominant patellofemoral osteoarthritis with findings of chondrocalcinosis.

Synovial osteochondromatosis is a benign condition characterized by synovial villus proliferation and metaplasia. As the synovial lining undergoes nodular proliferation, fragments may break off from the synovial surface and into the joint. Over time, these fragments may grow, calcify, or ossify. Synovial osteochondromatosis results in joint deterioration with secondary osteoarthritis. Patients are typically between the third and fifth decades, although any age group may be involved. Male patients are more commonly involved than

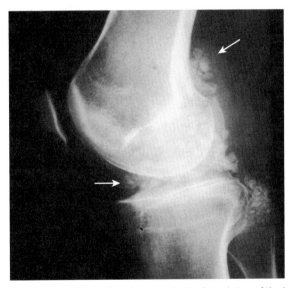

Fig. 8.14 **Synovial osteochondromatosis.** The lateral view of the knee shows numerous round ossific bodies *(arrows)* within the knee joint, all of similar shape and size.

female patients. These patients typically report years of monoarticular joint pain and swelling with limited range of motion. The large joints are more commonly affected; more than 50% of cases occur within the knee, followed by the elbow.[10] Radiographs demonstrate multiple calcified or ossified bodies within the joint or bursa (**Fig. 8.14**). When these fragments are not calcified, intrasynovial fragments may not be seen on radiographs.

Ankle and Foot

Radiographic evaluation of the ankle includes the anteroposterior, lateral, and mortise views. The mortise view is obtained by taking a frontal view with 15 degrees of lateral rotation of the foot to remove the superimposition of the distal fibula from the talar dome, or mortise. This view is best for evaluation of subtle joint narrowing, osteochondral defects, subchondral cysts, and marginal osteophytes. The anteroposterior and mortise views together provide a look at the anterior and posterior aspects of the distal tibiofibular syndesmosis, which contains a synovial recess between the syndesmotic ligaments; erosions from synovial proliferation or widening related to instability can be assessed on these views.

Anteroposterior and lateral images of the foot are generally all that is required for evaluation of arthritis of the foot, but it is recommended that they be obtained while the patient is bearing weight because some deformities are present only on standing views; in addition, this approach aids standard positioning of the foot. Frontal views with slight obliquity are useful for detection of subtle erosions at the metatarsophalangeal joints and interphalangeal joints. They are also helpful to visualize the intertarsal and Lisfranc articulations, which have complex surfaces and various degrees of obliquity and are often obscured on the anteroposterior view. The lateral view is not only useful for evaluation of anterior and posterior osteophytes or erosions but also provides soft tissue information such as distention of the ankle joint capsule by fluid or pannus and retrocalcaneal

bursitis. Calcaneal enthesophytes at the insertion of the Achilles tendon and at the origin of the plantar fascia and long plantar ligament can be evaluated for "fuzzy" margins, as seen in psoriatic arthritis and Reiter's disease. The subtalar joint can also be evaluated on a well-positioned lateral film, but the beam must not be tilted or else the angle will be so oblique that the joint will be out of view. Evaluation of the subtalar joint can also be obtained with a Harris-Beath view in which the ankle is dorsiflexed and an anteriorly tilted axial view of the calcaneus is taken. This view, if properly taken, is tangential to both posterior and middle facets of the subtalar joint.

Tarsal coalition is a congenital abnormality resulting from fibrous, cartilaginous, or osseous union of two or more tarsal bones. The two most common are calcaneonavicular and talocalcaneal coalitions. Lateral radiographs of the foot demonstrate secondary signs of talocalcaneal coalition, including talar beaking, flattening and broadening of the lateral talar process, and a positive C-sign. A Harris-Beath view may be helpful to evaluate the subtalar joint, but a CT scan is often obtained to rule out subtalar coalition. Calcaneonavicular bony bridges can be seen on the lateral view, with the classic "anteater nose" coming from the calcaneus.

References

Full references for this chapter can be found on www.expertconsult.com.

Fluoroscopy

Hifz Aniq and Robert Campbell

Fluoroscopy produces a continuous beam of x-rays to view an organ and part of body in real time. The ability of fluoroscopy to display motion is provided by a continuous series of images produced at a maximum rate of 25 to 30 complete images per second. These images are displayed on the monitor or television screen. With newer advances, digital fluoroscopy is being used with the C-arm or multiplanar imaging. Currently, the major role of fluoroscopy is for guidance of diagnostic and interventional procedures. Fluoroscopy is used for selective nerve root and facet joint injections and for epidural blocks for spinal pain. Fluoroscopically guided injections are also performed in different joints of the appendicular skeleton for magnetic resonance (MR) arthrography and therapeutic steroid injections.

In the appendicular skeleton, imaging-guided injections are performed for diagnostic as well as therapeutic purposes. Many studies have proved that, even in expert hands, a significant proportion of blind injections will end up in an extra-articular location.[1,2] Ultrasound or fluoroscopy can be used for needle guidance. Shoulder injections are more commonly performed under fluoroscopic guidance for needle positioning, and many different techniques and approaches have been described.[3] Intra-articular position of the needle can be confirmed with the injection of a small amount of nonionic contrast. When the needle is intra-articular in position, contrast material will flow away from the needle tip into the joint (**Fig. 9.1**). In the case of an extra-articular location, a blob of contrast material will form around the needle tip. Shoulder injections are performed as a part of MR arthrography when diluted gadolinium is injected into the affected shoulder. However, shoulder joint injections are also performed for therapeutic purposes in conditions such as inflammatory arthritis or adhesive capsulitis.[4]

Fluoroscopically guided arthrography is also performed in other joints of the body such as the elbow, wrist, hip, knee, and ankle (**Fig. 9.2**). In the wrist joint, multicompartment injections are sometimes performed to visualize ligament or triangular fibrocartilage tear. At times, fluoroscopy is coupled with digital subtraction, which shows the flow of contrast material during active injection. Fluoroscopy is used in wrist arthrography not only for needle positioning but also to help in diagnosis, because leakage of contrast material into other compartments can be seen in cases of ligament tear.

Osteoarthritis of the subtalar joint and small joints of the foot can be debilitating. Accurate needle positioning for the subtalar joint is difficult without any imaging assistance. Fluoroscopy is helpful for precise intra-articular injection of steroids in these joints.

Spinal Procedures

Back pain is a complex, multifactorial condition affecting millions of people worldwide. Many factors contribute to back pain, including neuromuscular imbalance, disk disease, lumbar compression fractures, ligamentous disorders, and infections of the vertebrae and disks. Most cases are successfully treated with conservative therapy and analgesics. However, a small percentage of patients may require surgical treatment. Imaging-guided minimally invasive techniques are suggested before surgery to localize pain.[5] These procedures are successfully used to treat patients who are not fit for surgery. By using imaging guidance, accuracy is increased, and the complication rate is reduced.

In spinal imaging, fluoroscopy is used for different types of diagnostic and therapeutic procedures. These procedures include nerve root blocks, epidural injection, vertebroplasty, and median nerve block. Most of these procedures can also be performed under computed tomography (CT) guidance. However, fluoroscopy has advantages of being more easily available and of allowing real-time visualization of the needle during the procedure.

Facet Joint Block

The facet joint is a synovial joint that helps the spine to flex, extend, and rotate. Osteoarthritis is the most common cause of facet joint disease characterized by loss of articular cartilage, marginal osteophyte formation, and bony erosions. Like other degenerative diseases, facet joint osteoarthritis is not limited to one facet. Degenerative change, such as disk disease, occurs in the other parts of the spine. Therefore, localization of the source of pain can be quite challenging.

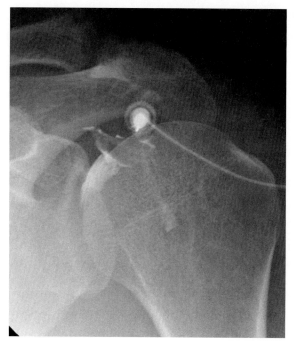

Fig. 9.1 **Shoulder arthrogram.** The needle is placed through the anterior approach, and contrast material is injected to confirm the intra-articular position of the needle.

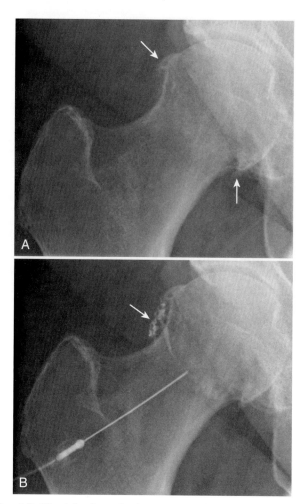

Fig. 9.2 **Hip injection.** A, Degenerative changes with marginal osteophytes *(arrows)* are seen at the femoral head and neck junction. B, A 22-gauge needle is placed along the femoral neck. Contrast material *(arrow)* confirms the intra-articular position.

Imaging modalities such as plain radiography, CT, and MR imaging (MRI) are very helpful in the evaluation of back pain and in localizing the source of pain such as a disk lesion. Facet joint degenerative change can also be identified by these modalities; however, this pathologic finding is not a helpful indicator of facet pain. Many patients with significant facet joint degenerative changes noted on CT and MRI are relatively asymptomatic. Because imaging cannot be relied on for the diagnosis of facet-related pain, history, and clinical examination are the most important components of evaluation. The lumbar spine is the most commonly affected part of the spine in facet joint osteoarthritis. Clinical diagnosis is usually made by finding the area of maximum tenderness on palpation. Facet joint pain typically manifests with bilateral paravertebral lower back pain. Pain is accentuated by twisting or rotational motion, increases on extension, and is relieved by flexion.

The facet block is a block of nerve endings in a richly innervated joint capsule. The sensory nerve endings connect with the sensory fibers of the medial branch of the dorsal primary ramus. The medial branch of the dorsal ramus lies in a small groove at the junction of the superior articular facet and transverse process.

The protocol for lumbar and thoracic facet blocks is as follows. The patient's informed consent is obtained before the procedure. The patient is placed prone on the fluoroscopy table. The C-arm or fluoroscopy tube is placed at 10 to 40 degrees of lateral tilt until the posterior part of the facet joint opens up. The posteroinferior part of the joint should be selected as the joint has the maximum space in this region. After preparing the skin, 1% lidocaine is administered subcutaneously. A 22-gauge needle is advanced, and its tip is

placed within the joint. The position of the needle may be confirmed by injecting 0.25 to 0.5 mL of nonionic contrast (**Fig. 9.3**). Extra-articular injection can also be performed by injecting a relatively large volume (4 to 6 mL) of steroid mixture into the extracapsular soft tissues behind the facet joint. However, intra-articular facet joint block is more effective because the local anesthetic and steroid mixture is administered directly into the joint.[6] Median branch block can be performed by directly injecting a small amount of anesthetic and steroid mixture adjacent to the medial branch of the dorsal ramus. The results are similar to those of an intra-articular facet joint injection.

Cervical facet block can be performed by a direct lateral or posterolateral approach. For a direct lateral approach, the patient is placed on the side in a lateral decubitus position with a pillow under the head to keep it parallel to the table. After skin preparation and marking of the area, a 22-gauge needle is advanced to the facet joint. The needle can easily be seen on biplane fluoroscopy. With single-plane fluoroscopy, the needle should be advanced slowly, and the tip position should be assessed in the anteroposterior and lateral planes. A tiny amount of nonionic contrast material can be

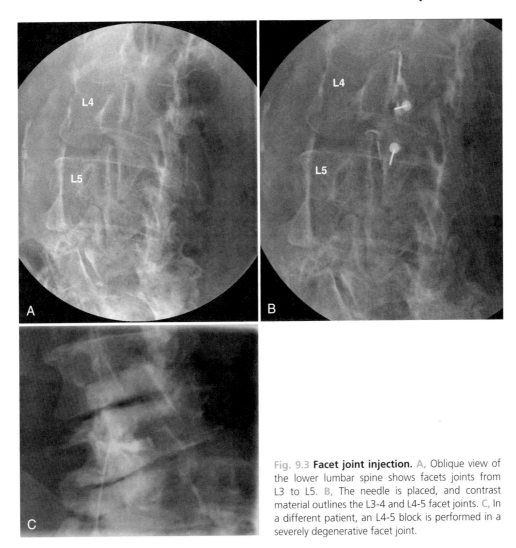

Fig. 9.3 **Facet joint injection.** A, Oblique view of the lower lumbar spine shows facets joints from L3 to L5. B, The needle is placed, and contrast material outlines the L3-4 and L4-5 facet joints. C, In a different patient, an L4-5 block is performed in a severely degenerative facet joint.

administered to confirm the position, but this is not essential. For diagnostic block, 0.5 to 1 mL of long-acting anesthetic is injected into the joint. A pain diary is given to the patient to assess the pain response. For therapeutic block, local anesthetic is mixed with 0.5 to 1 mL of dexamethasone or triamcinolone.

A medial branch block is mainly performed in the thoracolumbar region. A needle is advanced just superior to the transverse process and lateral to the medial border of the superior articulating process.[7] The bevel of the needle is directed downward so that steroid and anesthetic are deposited on the medial branch rather than superiorly into the foramen. Injections are performed above and below the affected facet joint because these joints have a dual nerve supply from the median branches of the level above and below. Results are similar to those of an intra-articular facet joint injection. In the cervical region, medial branch blocks can be more easily performed than facet intra-articular blocks. The midportion of the articular pillar is targeted for injections that are performed above and below the affected facet. If the patient has a significant response to facet joint or median branch block and other causes of back pain have been excluded, radiofrequency denervation is thought to be effective for long-term relief from facet joint pain.

Facet blocks may also be performed using CT scan for needle guidance. Orientation of the facet joints can be identified precisely on CT, and the needle is placed into the joint with much ease. CT-guided facet blocks are especially useful in cases of severe degeneration and bony overgrowth, which obscure the posterior approach on fluoroscopy. Because the needle tip can be localized into the joint, injection of contrast material is not required to confirm the needle position.

Sacroiliac Joint Injection

The sacroiliac joint is a complex joint with both fibrous and synovial parts. The inferior one half to two thirds of the joint is the synovial portion. The joint is oblique in orientation, and obliquity varies among different individuals.[8] Sacroiliac pain can have many different causes, most commonly degenerative or inflammatory disease. Patients with chronic low back pain without any radicular symptoms are candidates for sacroiliac joint injection. Sacroiliac joint injection can be used for both diagnostic and therapeutic purposes. The patient is placed prone on the fluoroscopy table. The tube is angled medially to laterally and in a cephalocaudal direction, which opens up the inferior part of the joint. After skin disinfection and local anesthetic injection, a 22-gauge needle is advanced into the posteroinferior part of the joint. The needle position is confirmed by injecting a small amount of nonionic contrast material, followed by injection of anesthetic and steroid mixture (**Fig. 9.4**).[9]

Selective Nerve Root Block

Selective nerve root block (SNRB) is most appropriately used in patients with radicular pain that is resistant to conventional medical therapy or in patients with postdiskectomy syndrome. In most of these patients, the sources of pain can be identified by MRI. However, in a small percentage of cases, neurologic examination may be equivocal, and imaging studies may show nonspecific findings. In these cases, SNRB can be used to find the exact nerve root level.[10] Most patients with radicular pain, without any neurologic deficit, recover in 4 to 6 weeks. Clinical symptoms are caused by chemical or mechanical irritation of the nerve root. Chemical irritation is produced by the release of phospholipase A_2 resulting from anulus rupture. The nerve root may be mechanically irritated by disk herniation or osteophyte formation in the exiting foramen. In these cases, SNRB can be helpful in the acute phase to control the symptoms until natural recovery occurs.

Cervical nerve root injections are routinely performed under CT guidance. However, if the injection must be performed under fluoroscopy, the patient is placed in the supine oblique position with the side to be injected facing upward. The patient's head is turned slightly to the opposite side. Obliquity is adjusted until the foramina are clearly seen. A 22- or 25-gauge spinal needle is advanced toward the foramen. Anteroposterior and lateral views are obtained to confirm the needle position. The needle should not project medial to the medial margin of the pedicle on the frontal view. The patient often reports reproduction of pain along the nerve distribution when the needle touches the nerve. For C1 and C2 nerve root injections, the patient is placed in the prone position, and the needle is advanced under frontal and lateral fluoroscopic guidance. Once the needle is in position, the stylet is then removed, and absence of cerebrospinal fluid or blood flow is verified with aspiration. Then, 0.25 to 0.5 mL of nonionic contrast material is injected to confirm the needle position in the nerve root sheath. A mixture of local anesthetic and steroid is injected. If the dura mater is perforated, the procedure is terminated and subsequently rescheduled.

Cervical nerve root blocks are usually performed under CT guidance to avoid puncture of the vertebral artery.[11,12] The patient is placed on the side on the CT table, and the needle is advanced posterior to the vertebral artery into the foramen. Once the needle is in place, a mixture of steroid and local anesthetic is injected.

Similarly, for fluoroscopically guided selective thoracic nerve root injections, the patient is placed in the prone position, and the needle is advanced under anteroposterior and lateral fluoroscopic guidance. The tip of the needle should be kept posterior and medial to avoid the pleural space. CT guidance is safe and reliable because it minimizes the risk of pneumothorax. Injections are the same as for cervical nerve roots.

Lumbar nerve root blocks can be performed under fluoroscopy. The patient is placed prone on the fluoroscopy table. The C-arm is rotated so that the "Scotty dog" is formed and the superior articular process projects into the center of vertebral body.[13] The superior end plate of the vertebral body should also appear superimposed on fluoroscopy. A 22-gauge needle is advanced until is it comes in contact with the vertebral body. The tip of the needle should be placed a few millimeters below the pedicle (eye of the Scotty dog). This position should be confirmed on lateral projection. Once the needle tip comes in contact with the nerve root, radicular pain is elicited. If the

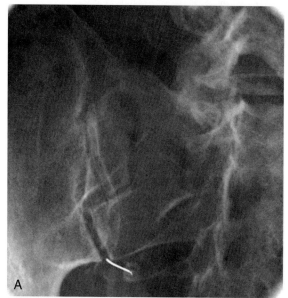

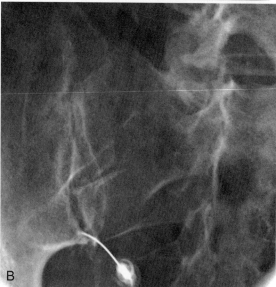

Fig. 9.4 **Sacroiliac injection. A,** The joint line is well seen in the inferior part of the sacroiliac joint. **B,** The needle is in place, and contrast injection confirms the accurate position of the needle.

pain is concordant with the patient's typical pain distribution, 0.5 to 1 mL of nonionic contrast material is injected to confirm needle position in the nerve root sheath (**Fig. 9.5**). Intermittent negative aspiration is performed to check that the needle is not in any vascular structure. Once the needle position has been established a combination of steroid and local anesthetic can be injected. For S1 nerve roots, the C-arm is angled in a caudocranial (angled toward the head) direction until the S1 foramen appears as a round lucency in the upper sacrum. After the procedure, the patient may have some numbness in the

distribution of the nerve injected and, caution should be taken because temporary weakness of the leg may occur.

Vertebroplasty

Vertebroplasty was first performed in 1987 by Gilbert et al[14] for treatment of vertebral angioma. Since then, vertebroplasty has become an established procedure for the treatment of painful osteoporotic fractures. It is also effective for the treatment of painful vertebral metastases, myeloma, and vertebral hemangiomas. Patients who have central intractable back pain at or around the level of vertebral fracture and in whom conservative therapy has failed are suitable candidates for vertebroplasty.[15]

Polymethylmethacrylate (PMMA), also called bone cement, is injected into the vertebral body under imaging guidance. Contraindications include unstable fracture, retropulsed fragment, poorly localized pain that does not correlate with the fracture site, and anticoagulation treatment. For lumbar and thoracic spine vertebrae, a transpedicular or extrapedicular unilateral approach is used (**Fig. 9.6**).[16] The main purpose of vertebroplasty is to achieve pain relief, but the procedure also provides strength and stability to the collapsed vertebra. When PMMA polymerizes, it produces thermal energy resulting in a temperature of up to 100°C [212°F] that destroys nerve endings and coagulates tumor cells. Imaging guidance is required not only for safe placement of the needle but also during the PMMA injection to avoid complications related to extravasation. Cement may leak into the epidural space, a complication for which urgent surgical intervention may be required. Extravasation into the disk or into the venous plexus may also occur, and this complication has the potential to cause pulmonary embolism.[17]

Vertebroplasty can be performed under fluoroscopy or CT guidance. Single-plane or biplane fluoroscopy or CT fluoroscopy can be used, as well as a combination of single-plane fluoroscopy and CT scanning. Fluoroscopy is mainly used for this procedure because it is easier to implement, cost effective, and a reliable image guide. Conversely, CT scan involves more radiation exposure and a small working space for the operator. Cement leakage is best seen on biplane fluoroscopy. CT guidance for vertebroplasty is especially useful for the intercostovertebral and posterolateral approach at the thoracic level when the pedicles are too small. For postprocedural assessment, CT scan is considered the standard technique because it can detect small leakages, which can be missed on fluoroscopy and plain radiographs.

Kyphoplasty is a newer technique used to restore vertebral height in fractures less than 3 months old. Expandable balloons are introduced into the vertebral body through the pedicles and, once in place, are dilated to restore vertebral height.[18] However, the use of kyphoplasty is controversial, and opinion varies among different groups.

Fluoroscopy provides the real-time image guidance for needle placement that is essential for successful diagnostic and therapeutic procedures. Radiation exposure from one

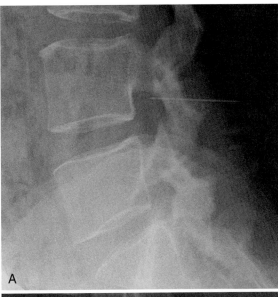
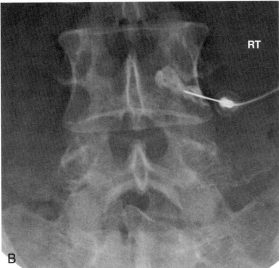

Fig. 9.5 Fluoroscopically guided therapeutic nerve root block. A, In the lateral view, the needle tip is placed in the L4 exiting foramen. B, In the anteroposterior view, the needle tip has been placed below the L4 pedicle, and contrast material is injected to confirm the position of the needle in the L4 nerve root sheath. RT, right side of the patient (as procedure is performed in the prone position).

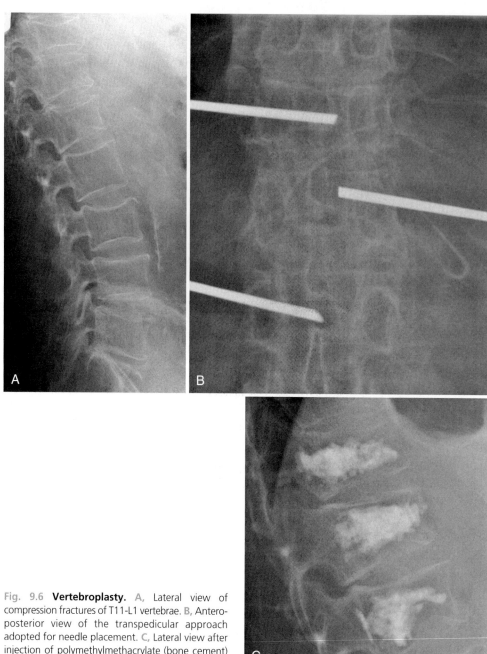

Fig. 9.6 **Vertebroplasty.** **A,** Lateral view of compression fractures of T11-L1 vertebrae. **B,** Anteroposterior view of the transpedicular approach adopted for needle placement. **C,** Lateral view after injection of polymethylmethacrylate (bone cement) in the vertebral bodies.

fluoroscopic image is less as compared with radiography. In fluoroscopy, however, a large series of images is produced, and that may lead to a high radiation dose to the patient. Every attempt should be made to keep the fluoroscopy time as short as possible.

References

Full references for this chapter can be found on www.expertconsult.com.

Nuclear Medicine Techniques for Pain Management

Hifz Aniq, Robert Campbell, and Sobhan Vinjamuri

Nuclear medicine techniques involve the use of radioactive isotopes for diagnosis and treatment of clearly identified medical conditions. Although there is an instant association of radioactivity and either diagnosis or treatment of cancer, these techniques are also frequently used in various nonmalignant conditions such as thyroid disease, arthritis, unstable angina, and dementias.

The diagnostic dimension of nuclear medicine techniques relies on the property of some radioactive isotopes that emit gamma rays. These are essentially "pockets of energy" that are emitted from the site of localization of the radiotracer, and these emissions are then detected using gamma cameras. The localization of radiotracers into particular tissue is determined by the physiologic process that needs characterization. For instance, a radiotracer of glomerular function of the kidneys would selectively localize to the glomeruli and be cleared by them, thereby providing a dynamic picture of the functional activity. When the radioisotopes concurrently emit other types of radiation such as alpha rays or beta rays, these can cause ionization or destruction of the tissue they are applied to and only serve to increase the radiation burden to the individual.[1]

The therapeutic dimension of nuclear medicine techniques, on the other hand, relies on the local destructive property of alpha or beta emissions. Alpha emitters typically have a short range of 50 to 90 μm and transfer most of their energy to the targeted cells, thereby increasing their biologic effectiveness. Alpha emitters have largely remained in the experimental domain because of the possibility of significant damage to adjacent local normal tissue. Beta emitters cover a wide range of energies and long-range radionuclides are considered appropriate for large solid tumors, whereas short-range beta emitters may be preferred for smaller tissues such as small joints. When beta emitters conjointly emit gamma rays, imaging techniques can be applied to localize the target tissues. The advantage of using beta emitters is that there is little danger of irradiating other people and patients can therefore be treated in outpatient clinics.[2,3]

In the setting of pain management, both diagnostic and therapeutic nuclear medicine procedures are considered useful. Since most nuclear medicine techniques rely on specialist expertise and therefore are limited in availability, a careful protocol-led multidisciplinary approach to referrals is considered useful.

Diagnostic Nuclear Medicine

The mechanisms of localization of commonly used radioisotopes such as bone-seeking radiopharmaceuticals include increased vascularity and an enhanced inflammatory response of the tissue to the stimulus, as well as more bone-specific functions such as increased osteoblastic activity, and adsorption onto hydroxyapatite crystals on mineralizing bone surfaces. Bone pain and uncontrolled pain are also mediated through similar cellular responses. From a diagnostic perspective, bone-seeking radiopharmaceuticals have been used to identify areas of occult fractures such as scaphoid fractures or long bone fractures where conventional imaging implies absence of fractures while clinical assessment suggests a fracture (**Fig. 10.1**). These scans are also useful to identify high-grade arthritic activity in a patient with proven arthritis on clinical and biochemical grounds. The site with the highest uptake of radiotracer can be identified for intra-articular injection with steroids or other pain controlling medications that are effective locally **Fig. 10.2**.

In a small number of patients, radiolabeled white blood cells can be used to identify an inflammatory focus and this localization enhances the ability to plan for further surgery in deep-seated bone infections of the foot or the spine (**Fig. 10.3**).

Therapeutic Nuclear Medicine

To gain some therapeutic benefit, radiopharmaceuticals (i.e., radioactive tracers labeled with chemical ligands) need to gain access to the target tissue. Although some tissues such as joints

Thoracic Spine

Seated Pelvis

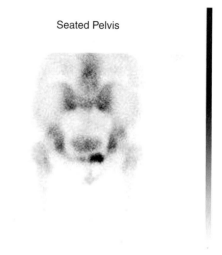

Fig. 10.1 ^{99m}Tc-MDP bone scan showing linearly increased tracer uptake in a midthoracic vertebra probably due to osteoporotic vertebral collapse. On the right there is a focus of intensely increased tracer uptake in the left inferior pubic ramus. Both of these sites represent fractures unseen on conventional radiologic imaging.

R lat foot

Plantar feet

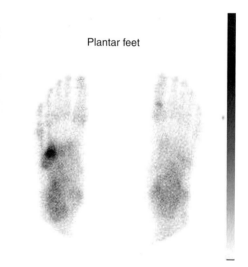

Fig. 10.2 ^{99m}Tc-MDP bone scan of the feet shows an area of intensely increased tracer uptake in the proximal aspect of the fourth metatarsophalangeal joint on the right side. This site is likely to represent the site of most intense symptomatology, and this image can be used to inject anti-inflammatory drugs such as steroids for symptom relief.

ANT ABDO 3 hours

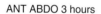

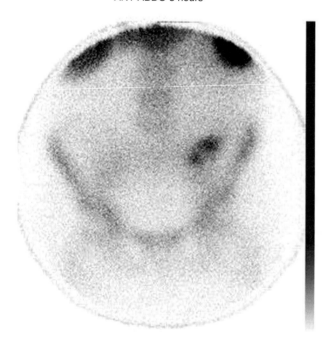

Fig. 10.3 An indium-111 white blood cell (WBC) scan showing focal accumulation of WBCs in the left iliac fossa representing a site of abscess with intense abdominal pain as the main symptom.

respond better to direct injection, some respond better when administered by the intra-arterial route and the vast majority are administered systemically by the intravenous route.

At a cellular level, the best target is the cell itself. Some radiopharmaceuticals rely on internal localization using the chemical component, and then the radioactive component destroys the cell and some adjacent tissue. Some radiopharmaceuticals bind to cell membranes using receptor targeting of specific antigens expressed by the cell membrane and the radioactive component performs the same function.[4]

Painful Bone Metastases

Secondary cancer tumors or metastases located in bone tissue can cause high levels of pain and distress in patients with terminal cancer. Usually the pain is uncontrolled even with higher doses of painkillers, and the aim of treatment is targeted at obtaining relief from pain rather than treating the bone metastases. External beam radiotherapy is considered suitable where the metastatic disease is clearly localized to one anatomic area such as the sacrum, a long bone, or a part of the thoracic spine. When the metastatic disease is extensive and involves many bones and anatomic areas, systemic therapies with bone-seeking radiopharmaceuticals can be considered[5] (**Fig. 10.4**). Strontium-89 is widely used in this setting. It has a long physical half-life of 50.5 days and pure beta emission. The lack of gamma emissions enables outpatient administration of the radiopharmaceutical. It is handled in the body like calcium and is taken up by metabolically active bone with prolonged retention in abnormal

ANT   POS

Whole body scan Tc–99m

Fig. 10.4 ^{99m}Tc-MDP bone scan showing widespread skeletal secondaries in the skull, sternum, rib cage, spine, and pelvis. This patient is likely to benefit from bone-seeking radionuclides such as strontium-89 for symptom relief of refractory pain.

bone.[6] Recently, samarium-153–labeled ethylene diamine tetramethylene phosphonate and rhenium-186 HEDP have also been used with good results.[7,8]

Painful Arthropathy

Arthropathy (involvement of joints in inflammatory processes such as arthritis) is a common medical condition affecting a significant majority of the adult and older population. Arthritis is associated with swelling of joints and the commonest compliant of patients is pain. The synovial membrane lining the joints becomes involved in the inflammation and this can result in a debilitating triad of stiffness, pain, and immobilization.[9] Rheumatoid arthritis and psoriatic arthritis are common examples of inflammatory arthropathy whereas osteoarthritis is considered a noninflammatory pathology in which severe pain and joint damage can be seen in (usually) older patients.

Treatment for these conditions includes nonsteroidal anti-inflammatory drugs, systemic corticosteroids, disease-modifying antirheumatic drugs such as gold, penicillamine, antimalarials, and antimetabolites and sometimes by intra-articular corticosteroid injections. People who do not benefit from standard medications may benefit from synovectomy, which could be surgical, chemical, or radionuclide.

Radionuclide synovectomy involves the direct injection of a beta-emitting radiopharmaceutical into the joint cavity. The fluid concentrates in the inflamed tissue, and because of its close proximity to the synovial membrane an "ablation" or destruction of the synovial tissue can be expected. The adjacent cartilage is frequently unharmed. Yttrium-90 silicate or citrate colloid is used for large joints such as the knee joint[10] (**Fig. 10.5**). Rhenium-186 sulfide can be used for medium-sized joints such as the elbow, ankles, and wrists, and erbium-169 citrate colloid can be used for small inflamed joints such as the interphalangeal and metatarsophalangeal joints, as well as the metacarpophalangeal joints.

Neuroendocrine Tumors

Neuroendocrine tumors are a rare diverse group of cancers that can have a variable rate of progression, but are frequently

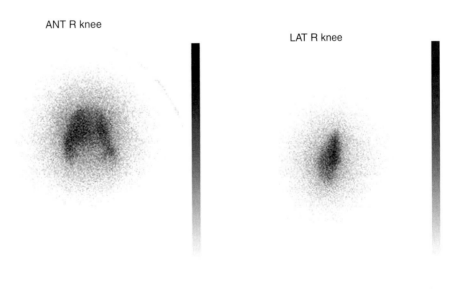

ANT R knee   LAT R knee

Fig. 10.5 Y90 images of the right knee showing localization of radiotracer within the knee joint with no extravasation.

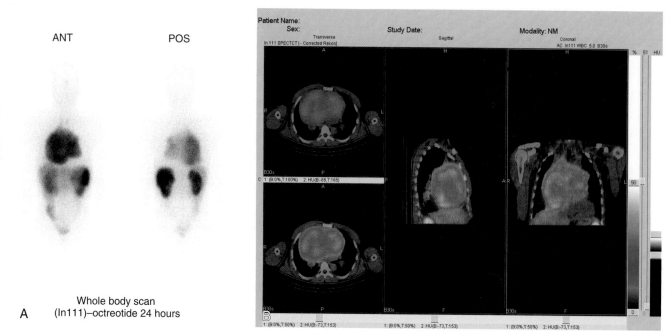

ANT   POS

Whole body scan
A   (In111)–octreotide 24 hours

Fig. 10.6 A, Indium-111 octroetide images of the whole body show a large thymic tumor in the mediastinum that expresses somatostatin receptors. Elsewhere there is normal physiologic distribution in the liver, spleen, kidneys, and gut. B, The same tumor in three dimensions with the background anatomic template of a low-dose single-photon emission computed tomography image.

considered slow-growing. Most of these tumors arise in the gastro-entero-pancreatic region. They usually secrete a host of hormones and physiologically active peptides that can generate disabling symptoms such as nausea, vomiting, abdominal pain, diarrhea, and fatigue.[11]

The initial diagnosis of these tumors is often biochemical and the main screening marker is chromogranin A (CgA), which is a glycoprotein present in almost all neuroendocrine cells. Elevated plasma CgA levels are found in almost all patients with neuroendocrine tumors. Sometimes incidental findings of liver metastases on computed tomography, abdominal ultrasound, or magnetic resonance imaging may eventually be confirmed as neuroendocrine tumors on the basis of confirmative histology.

Imaging of the somatostatin receptors with indium-111 octreotide, which is a somatostatin analog, is a useful technique to identify the extent of the tumor spread and also to plan future therapies (**Fig. 10.6**). Radiolabeled analogs of octreotide have been used to target the somatostatin receptors on tumor cells and thereby render them nonfunctional. The primary aim with these essentially palliative treatments is essentially symptom control, with abdominal pain one of the frequent complaints that needs to be addressed.

References

Full references for this chapter can be found on www.expertconsult.com.

Computed Tomography

Hifz Aniq and Robert Campbell

Since the introduction of the computed tomography (CT) scanner in 1972, the technology has been continually evolving. The main advantages that CT holds over conventional radiography relate to the absence of superimposed tissues on the images and markedly superior contrast resolution brought about by the elimination of scatter. As a result of advances in CT and software technology, the role of CT in musculoskeletal imaging has increased substantially in recent years. Although early scanners were slow and had relatively poor spatial resolution, modern multi-detector row helical scanners can now achieve nearly isotropic resolution while scanning large-volume lengths in just a few seconds.

Imaging Principles

Modern CT still uses this same basic principle of acquiring and reconstructing images by measurement of tissue attenuation in thin, axially oriented cross sections. Attenuation of the tissue that the x-ray beam travels through is measured from multiple angles and is related to the atomic number and density of the material being examined, as well as the energy spectrum of the x-ray beam being emitted. Depending on the matrix size (x- and z-axis) of the scan and the thickness (z-axis) of each axial slice, the area being scanned is partitioned into a number of small boxes. Each small box-like volume of tissue, or *voxel*, is assigned a mean density number that corresponds to a scale ranging from −1024 to +3071, known as the Hounsfield scale. The actual number allotted a given voxel is calculated from data provided by multiple measured *ray projections* and is reconstructed by the computer. The pixel itself is displayed on the screen according to the mean attenuation of the tissue in its corresponding voxel, with water having an attenuation of 0 Hounsfield units (HU) and air measuring −1000 HU. Fat is usually around −100 HU, bone typically measures +400 HU or greater, and metal implants are more than +1000.[1] The exact CT numbers for a given tissue type vary from manufacturer to manufacturer and with changes in x-ray tube potential with the exception of water and air. Because radiologists were accustomed to interpreting images in which black objects were composed of less dense materials (e.g., air and fat) and white objects were more dense (e.g., bone and metal), CT was set up to display its images in similar fashion.[2] CT images are in essence two-dimensional (2D) gray-scale representations of the relative density of the tissues imaged in a "stack" consisting of multiple axial slices. Each picture element, or *pixel*, shown on the monitor represents a certain density within a preselected *window* of densities—set to maximize the contrast between tissues in the area of interest. CT is able to discern a much broader range of densities than radiography and is able to do this primarily because of elimination of scatter.

A variety of system designs have been used to acquire the x-ray data needed for image reconstruction. These different architectural geometries are commonly known as generations. Advancement in CT technology has come in the form of faster acquisition times, higher spatial resolution, and faster computers able to perform larger and more complex data reconstructions.

First-Generation Computed Tomography Scanners

The first commercial scanner produced was the EMI Mark I. It used an x-ray beam that was collimated to a narrow beam directed through the patient to a single detector. A single projection was acquired by translating the x-ray tube and the detector in a straight line on opposite sides of the patient. The next projection was obtained by rotating the frame 1 degree and scanning in the opposite direction. This process was repeated until 180 ray projections were obtained. Such scanning was very time consuming and yielded poor spatial resolution (about 3 mm in a 25 cm field of view) and extremely poor z-axis resolution (about 13 mm thickness in each axial section obtained).[2]

Second-Generation Computed Tomography Scanners

Scan times were improved by adding additional detectors. The extra detectors were placed at angles so that multiple projections could be obtained in each translation. Originally, this method tripled imaging speed and thereby allowed a scan to be performed in 60 translations instead of 180. The number of detectors continued to increase until scanners were fast enough to allow acquisition during a single breath hold. This improvement opened the door for scanning of the chest and abdomen without the images being rendered useless by motion artefact.[3]

Third-Generation Computed Tomography Scanners

The next advance came in the form of higher-power rotating-anode x-ray tubes. These scanners use a fan-shaped x-ray beam that passes through the patient to an arc-shaped row of detectors behind. During the scan both the x-ray source and the detectors rotate around the patient. Rotation of the x-ray tube allows a more powerful tube to be used and thereby increases the speed of scanning through thicker body parts. In addition, because the x-ray beams were no longer parallel to each other but instead divergent, new reconstruction algorithms had to be developed. This system is known as a rotate-rotate design, and nearly all modern helical scanners are versions of this geometry.[3]

Fourth-Generation Computed Tomography Scanners

This design differs from third-generation scanners in that just the x-ray tube rotates within a stationary ring of detectors. Though labeled fourth generation, these scanners were developed almost at the same time as third-generation scanners and, with the exception of some special-purpose applications, are not commercially available. Fourth-generation scanners are not able to use anti-scatter collimators and are much more prone to scatter artifacts than third-generation scanners are.[3]

Spiral/Helical Computed Tomography Scanners

Before the late 1980s, all CT scanners acquired data in individual axial slices regardless of the generation of scanner. Every time that the x-ray tube revolved around the patient a single axial "slice" of data was obtained. The invention of slip-ring technology allowed the table to be translated through the gantry while the x-ray tube and detectors rotated continuously around the patient to create a volume of data. With new reconstruction algorithms this allowed an image to be reconstructed at any point along the path traced by the tube. This advance in technology ultimately reduced patient doses, minimized motion artifacts, and enhanced multiplanar reconstructions.[4,5]

Multi–Detector Row Computed Tomography Scanners

What vendors call *latest-generation* CT scanners are offset from the third-generation architecture in their use of spiral CT with the addition of multiple detector row arrays. Multi–detector row CT (MDCT; also known as multislice CT) is a major improvement in helical CT technology wherein simultaneous activation of multiple detector rows positioned along the z-axis allows the acquisition of interweaving helical sections. The principal difference between MDCT and the preceding generations of CT is improved resolution in the longitudinal or z-axis (direction of the table or gantry).

More of the x-rays generated by the tube are ultimately used to produce imaging data. With this design, section thickness is determined by detector size and not by the collimator itself. Rapid data acquisition is possible because of short gantry rotation intervals combined with multiple detectors providing increased coverage along the z-axis.

The data from an MDCT scanner can be used to generate images of different thicknesses from the same acquisition. In MDCT, the user selects a specific beam collimation but does not need to choose a particular section thickness in advance. This parameter can be implemented after the completion of data acquisition (but cannot be changed after the original acquisition data are purged from the scanner hard drive). The minimum section thickness is reduced to approximately 0.5 mm, and images can be reconstructed at this 0.5 mm interval. Isotropic (equal dimension) voxels measuring 0.5 mm in the x, y, and z directions greatly improve spatial resolution and the quality of reconstructing algorithms and thereby allow the generation of exquisite multiplanar reformats and three-dimensional (3D) images.[3]

MDCT's increased speed of imaging allows fast imaging of large volumes of tissue without compromise in image quality. A single-pass, whole-body protocol is now easily achieved with modern scanners, which can image from the vertex of the head to below the hips in less than a minute. In the setting of hardware (joint implants), there is an improved ability to acquire high-quality images. Metal artifacts are due to photopenic defects in the back-projection and are displayed on CT images as streak artifact. With MDCT the holes in the filtered back-projection are not as pronounced, and a less severe streak artifact results. This improvement is at the expense of excess tissue radiation along the penumbra of the beam, which is then picked up by adjacent detector channels filling in these photopenic defects in the projection. This technology has forced radiologists into redefining the image-viewing process to a *volumetric* paradigm rather than a simple tile mode or section-by-section viewing.

To keep up with this paradigm shift, CT protocols had to be reformulated. Along with the recent deployment of MDCT has come a significantly expanded range of CT applications and indications. The challenges that face imagers using MDCT include selecting optimal imaging sequences, controlling patient radiation exposure, and efficiently managing the large amount of data generated. Some disadvantages of MDCT are high radiation doses to the tissue and potentially noisy images. High radiation dose is an issue, especially in children. Introduction of x-ray current modulation in the transverse (x and y) and longitudinal (z) directions in new scanners can reduce radiation dose significantly.[6] Noise is inversely related to the number of photons per voxel, and because smaller voxels tend to have fewer photons, the result is noisier images. To keep the noise level reasonable, the exposure (and thus the radiation dose) must be increased. Another limitation of CT scanning is inability to visualize ligaments and supporting soft tissues, which can be problem in trauma; however, recent studies in cervical trauma have suggested that MDCT has a 99% negative predictive value for clearing ligamentous injuries and a 100% negative predictive value for clearing unstable spine injuries.[7]

Three-Dimensional Imaging

In tandem with the explosion of MDCT scanners recently placed in clinical practice, powerful new 3D applications have been fielded and have led to an increase in the interpretation and creation of images in planes other than the traditional axial. Though a powerful tool, especially for surgical planning, it can create confusion among radiologists, technologists, and clinicians when trying to describe a particular method or type of image. Protocols need to be designed to optimize image quality and minimize patient radiation exposure. This requires an understanding of beam collimation and section collimation as they apply to MDCT while keeping in mind the time-limited nature of projection data and the need of thin axial sections to perform 3D reconstructions that will be effective in clinical practice.[8]

Multiplanar images can be thickened into slabs with projectional techniques such as average, maximum, and minimum intensity projection, ray sum, and volume rendering. Volume rendering provides versatility and manipulability in the dataset for advanced imaging applications by assigning a range of colors to distinguish different tissue types and by integrating a full spectrum of opacity values within the image (**Fig. 11.1**). Using the data from axial CT images to reconstruct nonaxial, 2D images is known as multiplanar reformation (MPR). MPR images are created by transecting a set or "stack" of axial images that are only 1 voxel thick. Sagittal, oblique, or curved plane images can be generated in this way (see **Fig. 11.3A–C**). MPR images have been found to be more sensitive in detecting and characterizing spinal fractures than radiography or axial CT images.[9] This technique is extremely useful in musculoskeletal examinations because fracture lines and joint alignment are not always easily seen in the axial plane.[10]

Orthopedic Traumatology

One of the most recently evident benefits of MDCT imaging occurs in the setting of appendicular and axial trauma.

Since the introduction of MDCT into emergency departments, there has been a radical change in imaging of cervical spine trauma. Radiography is disappearing as a screening tool and many departments have adopted MDCT as a screening tool. Radiography is still used for monitoring treatment and healing of spinal fractures. When compared with projectional radiography, CT greatly improves the anatomic depiction of spinal injury. However, when compared with single-detector helical CT scanners, MDCT scanners have increased tube-heating capacity and run at a higher table speed, which allows an increased volume of coverage in the same amount of scanning time. This advantage makes screening examination of a portion of the spine or the entire spine feasible and may eliminate screening radiographs in certain settings. Examinations of the thorax and the lumbar spine can be extracted from a CT examination of the chest, abdomen, and pelvis. However, the routine protocols should be modified to optimize the appropriate protocol for screening both skeletal and visceral injuries. In emergency departments, rapid imaging of multiple trauma is absolutely essential to reduce morbidity and mortality rates. Currently, 16-slice or greater detectors are used in emergency departments to scan from the head to below the hips using the "whole body single pass" technique. For the extremities, dedicated imaging is needed.[11] For routine interpretation of a cervical spine examination, bone (high spatial frequency) algorithm images are made with 2.5 mm images. In addition, standard-algorithm (soft tissue), 1.25-mm-thick images are obtained and used for MPR but are not viewed as a stack or in tile mode. MDCT sagittal and coronal reformatted images are of sufficient quality to allow volumetric interpretation and perhaps obviate the need to review every single transverse image unless needed for clarification. However, thin transverse sections are paramount for obtaining optimal reformatted images. Considering the balance between obtaining optimal reformatted images, patient radiation dose, and resource utilization, the following guiding principles may be useful:

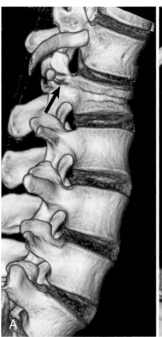 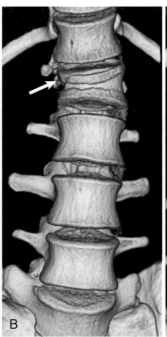 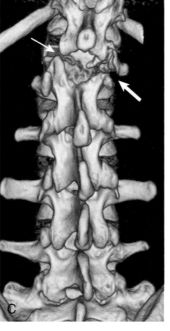

Fig. 11.1 Multi-detector computed tomography (MDCT) three-dimensional (3D) volume rendering of the lumbar spine demonstrates the extent of a "chance" fracture through the posterior elements of L1 (*black arrow*). **A,** Sagittal projection. **B,** Coronal projection in which a buckle in the cortex is seen. **C,** Posterior coronal view. This 3D image can be rotated in space to view the fracture through the right pedicle (*white arrow*) and dislocation of left facet joint (*small arrow*).

- Use the thinnest transverse images feasible.
- Use overlapping transverse images for the MPR images.
- Use standard algorithm (soft tissue) axial images for reformatting.

Bone algorithm images have increased noise and are not useful in terms of a smooth-appearing MPR. As previously stated, this presents a new paradigm (volumetric and 3D viewing) for interpretation related to image processing and viewing software capabilities.

Pelvis and acetabular fractures are usually associated with high-impact road traffic accidents and falls from heights. Hemorrhagic shock is the leading cause of death in pelvis injuries. Plain radiographs are limited in showing the full extent of fracture, number and position of fragments, and intra-articular bony fragments. Bowel gas often obscures sacral fractures, which are associated with neurologic injuries, vascular trauma, and pelvis instability. MDCT not only shows the extent of the fracture and number and position fragments, but contrast-enhanced CT also gives information about the pelvis hemorrhage and any arterial bleeding (**Fig. 11.2**). Modified advanced trauma guidelines omit anteroposterior (AP) pelvis radiographs in polytrauma in patients with a clinically stable pelvis. Coronal reformats have been suggested as a substitute for AP pelvis radiographs.[12]

Plain radiographs are the first investigation for extremity trauma. Indications for CT scanning in these cases include fracture when its presence will alter the management and evaluation of fracture for preoperative planning, and assessment of reduction and healing. Tibial plateau, ankle, calcaneal, and multipart shoulder fractures are routinely scanned for assessment.[13] CT scanning with MPR has revolutionized the understanding of mechanism of injury of these complex fractures and provides guidance in the management of these cases. Complex fractures of the wrist, elbow, and scapula are also assessed by CT. In postreduction scanning, orientation of fracture fragments and their healing is best assessed with the help of MPR.

Several pitfalls may exist, but the most important image artifacts are not unique to MDCT. Such artifacts include metal-induced streak artifacts and patient motion. Because of the higher spatial resolution, the vascular channels of the vertebral bodies are better appreciated and may be mistaken

for abnormal structures. MDCT has some risk, predominantly related to the radiation dose to the individual patient and to the population. The patient's radiation dose increases as the volume of coverage increases and, as always, is most weighed against the potential information needed and the clinical context of ordering the examination.

MDCT allows imaging of very thin sections quickly, much faster than previously possible, thereby allowing for effective screening of spinal injuries and evaluation of extremity injuries. Screening CT of the entire cervical spine is cost-effective if certain high-risk criteria are met, including focal neurologic deficit referable to the cervical spine, head injury (skull fracture, intracranial hemorrhage), unconsciousness at the time of examination, and a high-energy mechanism (motor vehicle accident at a speed greater than 35 miles per hour, pedestrian struck by a car, or a fall greater than 10 feet).

Spine Imaging

CT imaging can detect 0.5% differences in x-ray attenuation with respect to water, the reference standard (the Hounsfield unit [HU] of water is calibrated to zero). The physical interaction is based on the linear attenuation coefficient, which is roughly proportional to density (which is why ligamentous structures such as the anulus fibrosus are hyper-attenuating and subcutaneous fat is hypo-attenuating). Therefore, for CT imaging, contrast is best between very dense structures (bone), highly compact soft tissue (tendons, ligaments, anulus fibrosus), water-containing tissue (muscle, thecal sac), low-density tissue (fat), and gas. This is an improvement over projectional radiography, which requires an approximately 10% change in full scale to detect differences in contrast. One mechanism to improve contrast resolution is to administer a "contrast" agent, which can be done through several different routes. The most commonly used routes for spine imaging are intravenous, intrathecal, and intradiskal. CT diskography and CT myelography are used in certain specific indications and will be discussed in separate chapters of this book.

Magnetic resonance imaging (MRI) has become the mainstay for advanced imaging of the spine and offers features complementary to radiography, so most patients with chronic symptoms will undergo these two imaging modalities. MRI

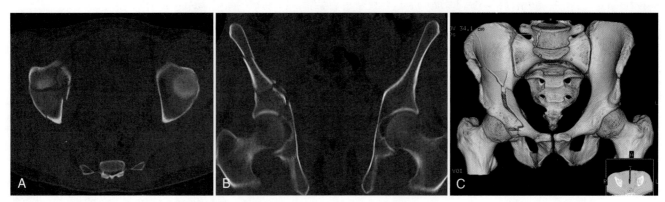

Fig. 11.2 Pelvis fracture: axial (**A**) and coronal (**B**) reformats show comminuted fracture of right acetabulum and iliac bone. **C,** Three-dimensional volume rendering of pelvis shows the extent of fracture lines and position of fragments.

and CT are more sensitive than radiography for the detection of early spinal infections, cancer, herniated disks, and spinal stenosis. The role of imaging in other situations is limited because of the poor association between low back pain symptoms and anatomic findings.[14] In isolation, an imaging finding of disk degeneration may represent part of the aging process and, in the absence of extrusion, is of only modest value in diagnosis or treatment decisions. The most common indication for the use of advanced cross-sectional imaging procedures such as MRI or CT is the clinical context of low back pain complicated by radiating pain (radiculopathy, sciatica) or cauda equina syndrome (bilateral leg weakness, urinary retention, saddle anesthesia), which is usually due to a herniated disk or canal stenosis (or both).

Spinal stenosis has characteristic symptomatology, but accurate localization of the affected level requires radiologic investigation. It has been shown that degenerative structural narrowing can compress the cauda equina even in the absence of a herniated intervertebral disk. Hypertrophic articular processes, marginal vertebral body osteophytes, spondylolisthesis, and subluxation of the zygapophyseal joints with concomitant soft tissue changes can all contribute to impingement. Evaluation of these bony degenerative changes is the forte of CT.[15]

Although MRI generally remains the first-line choice in an advanced imaging workup of low back pain, CT is a capable investigational tool. CT has been asserted to be able to provide reliable diagnosis of intervertebral disk herniation (**Fig. 11.3**). Exacerbation of spinal stenosis from degenerative bone changes can occur in the form of hypertrophic facet capsules, thickening of the ligamentum flavum, or superimposed degenerative disk disease. Neural compression from a bulge in the anulus fibrosus is also more likely in the presence of spinal stenosis produced by bony changes. CT can be an excellent adjunct to other radiologic modalities for evaluating degenerative lumbar spinal stenosis because it directly images both bone and soft tissue (**Fig. 11.4**). MPR provides precise 3D analysis of pathology.[16]

In spondylytic spondylolisthesis, a defect in the pars interarticularis is present that allows the vertebral body to slip forward while the posterior elements remain in anatomic position (**Fig. 11.5**). This most often leads to foraminal stenosis, but rarely can result in spinal stenosis. In spondylolisthesis caused by degenerative changes in the facet joints, the pars interarticularis remains intact and the whole vertebra slips forward. In these cases spinal stenosis commonly occurs. Degenerative spondylolisthesis can be reliably characterized by CT and distinguished from spondylolytic forms of spondylolisthesis.[17]

Computed Tomography Diagnostic Strengths

Because MDCT uses x-rays to generate images, it maintains the strengths of projectional radiography with regard to exquisite bone and joint imaging and at the same time is able to supersede radiography with its improved contrast and 3D imaging. As such, MDCT can be useful in the evaluation of pain sources that might have previously been evaluated with radiographs alone. CT can be useful in evaluation of the appendicular skeleton for fractures, subluxations, and sclerotic and cystic bone lesions, as well as for both presurgical and postsurgical evaluation of hardware implantation.[18] CT can be used to assess bone mineral density, which has been shown to relate to bone strength in the evaluation of osteoporosis. CT excels in evaluation of the spine for fractures, spondylolisthesis, degenerative changes, and disk disease. It can also be useful in conjunction with arthrography in the evaluation of postoperative recurrent tear of a meniscus and cartilage defects, such as those commonly seen in the knee. This modality can be used to assess the stability of osteochondritis dissecans in the knee and ankle joints and is sometimes superior to MRI because of its high spatial resolution. Intra-articular loose bodies can be a source of chronic pain and locking, and CT or magnetic resonance arthrography is extremely helpful to identify their exact

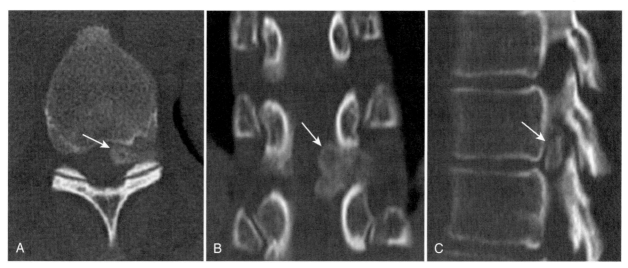

Fig. 11.3 Disk herniation. Chronic disk herniation denoted by a calcified disk *(arrows)* is easily identified on axial **(A)**, coronal **(B)**, and sagittal **(C)** multiplanar reconstructions.

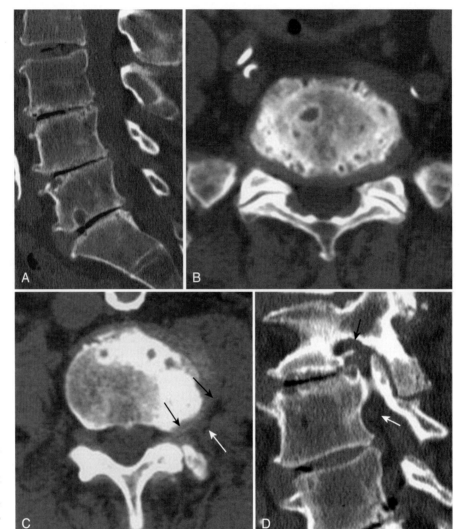

Fig. 11.4 Degenerative disk lesions. A, Sagittal reformat: degenerative disk disease in the lumbar spine with loss of disk heights and vacuum phenomenon. B, Axial L5/S1 level, soft tissue window: disk bulges beyond the outline of vertebral body producing mild spinal stenosis. C, Axial L3/4 level, soft tissue window: left foraminal and extraforaminal broadbase disk protrusion *(black arrows)* stretching the L3 nerve root *(white arrow)*. D, Left parasagittal reformat: narrowing of left L3 foramen due to osteophyte and disk and L3 nerve root *(black arrow)* is displaced superiorly against the pedicle. Left L4 nerve root *(white arrow)* is normal.

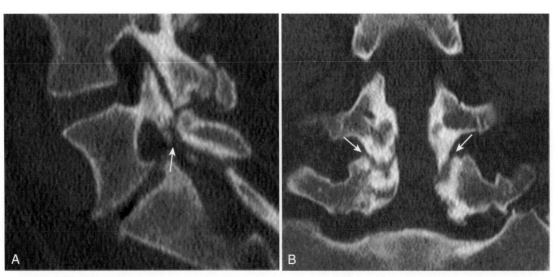

Fig. 11.5 Pars defect. A, Sagittal oblique MPR demonstrates a pars interarticularis defect at L5 *(arrow)* with grade 1 spondylolisthesis of L5 on S1. B, Coronal reformat shows bilateral pars defects *(arrows)*.

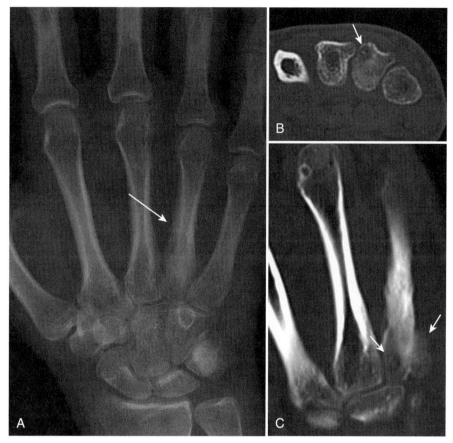

Fig. 11.6 Osteoid osteoma. A, Plain x-ray of hand shows irregular periosteal reaction around the base of the fourth metacarpal. B **and** C, Coronal and axial reformats show lucent nidus with calcification *(arrows)*. Periosteal reaction on coronal reformat *(white arrow)*.

location and confirm whether these are loose or embedded in the soft tissues. In these cases one must weigh the increased radiation exposure to the patient against the potential benefit of an accurate diagnosis.

Currently, the availability of many imaging options for evaluation of the spine has contributed to the quandary of how to best use them. CT is used predominantly for trauma, when MRI is not available or is contraindicated, or for a specific problem-solving application related to osseous integrity. CT is better than MRI in demonstrating cortical bone destruction and more sensitive in identifying calcified tumor matrix to help characterize and diagnose both benign and malignant bone lesions.[19] As an example, CT is commonly considered to be the most important imaging modality for the diagnosis and localization of osteoid osteoma. Specifically, CT is more accurate than MRI in the detection of an osteoid osteoma nidus (**Fig. 11.6**).[20] MRI is better at showing intramedullary and soft tissue changes. However, in some cases this increased sensitivity for detection of edema can produce a misleading aggressive appearance on MRI.[17]

Conclusion

The addition of CT to the clinician's diagnostic armamentarium has been an evolutionary as well as a revolutionary advance in imaging technology. CT shares many of the strengths of conventional radiography with the added advantages of elimination of superimposed tissues on the images and markedly superior contrast resolution. The ability to display both bone and soft tissue in the transaxial plane with MPR techniques allows accurate 3D examination of the spine. CT is particularly valuable in investigating bony abnormalities, including trauma, bony degenerative changes, cortically destructive lesions, spinal stenosis (with or without intrathecal contrast), and anular tears (with the introduction of intradiskal contrast).

References

Full references for this chapter can be found on www.expertconsult.com.

A Practical Approach to Radiation Protection

Hifz Aniq and Robert Campbell

In 1895, Wilhelm Roentgen discovered x-rays. The behavior and physical characteristics of the newly discovered rays were established within a short period. However, it took about 30 years before radiation protection measures and the concept of limit to exposure dose were established. This is because the effects of low-level radiation exposure to patients during diagnostic procedures appeared much later. This led to the radiation protection regulations of today that are based on the concern of late effects of radiation to both patients and health care workers.

Potentially harmful effects of ionizing radiation are divided into deterministic and stochastic effects. Deterministic effects of ionizing radiation result in killing of cells and tissues. This takes place only when the cells or tissues are exposed to doses above a certain threshold. Radiation doses from medical exposures are far below this threshold. However, deterministic effects such as skin burns have been observed in people who have been involved in procedures involving excessive radiation exposure such as interventional procedures. Stochastic radiation effects occur when an irradiated cell is modified rather than killed. Modified cells may become cancerous after a certain latent period (generally several years). In principle, stochastic effects do not have any threshold. These may not occur with certainty, but the exposed individual statistically has a high chance of developing cancer. Radiation exposure of diagnostic investigations might cause stochastic effects, and probability increases as dose of radiation increases.[1] There is no evidence of a threshold below which no damage occurs. Genetic effects of radiation occur in individuals who have not been exposed to radiation directly. It is difficult to determine whether genetic change or malignancy is due to radiation exposure. This linear dose-response relationship suggests that any radiation exposure, however small it may be, can be considered safe. Stochastic effects of radiation include skin malignancy, leukemia, and hereditary effects.

The biologic influences of ionizing radiation are related to the energy absorbed per unit mass in the given tissue or organ. This is termed the *absorbed dose* and is measured in units of Gray (Gy). Body tissues differ in their sensitivity to radiation and this is taken into consideration when calculating the radiation risk after radiation exposure. This is termed the *effective dose* and is based on the average radiosensitivity of the different organs for partial or full-body exposure to members of the public and radiation workers. The unit of this quantity is called Sievert (Sv).[2] The effective dose of various radiologic procedures is shown in **Table 12.1**.

Organizations such as the International Atomic Energy Agency (IAEA), the World Health Organization (WHO), the European Commission (EC), and the International Commission on Radiological Protection (ICRP) provide guidance and recommendations on radiation protection matters. Although radiation exposure of radiology investigations is quite low and the chance of radiation effect is minimal, it is generally agreed that radiation exposure of workers and patients should be "as low as reasonably achievable (ALARA)" or "as low as reasonably practicable" (ALARP) in the United Kingdom.[3] This means that no medical radiation exposure should be made unless it produces sufficient benefits to the exposed individual to offset the radiation damage it causes. This includes correct assessment of the requested examination, knowledge of expected yield, and the way in which results would influence the diagnosis and management.[4] In cases of radiation exposure to patients of reproductive age, it should be kept in mind that the risk of inducing severe hereditary disease is estimated at 2% per Gy to the gonads of either parent.

ICRP has an established system for limitation of radiation with three basic principles.[5]

Justification—no procedure should be adopted unless its benefits outweigh the detrimental effects of radiation.
Optimization—all exposures should be kept as low as reasonably achievable in view of the social and economic factors.
Dose limitation—dose of procedure should not exceed the limits recommended for appropriate circumstances.

Table 12.1 Typical Values of Effective Radiation Dose for a Patient

Procedure	Effective Dose
Chest x-ray	0.02 mSv
Thoracic spine x-ray	0.4 mSv
Lumbar spine x-ray	0.7 mSv
Pelvic x-ray	0.07 mSv
Abdominal CT	8 mSv
Fluoroscopy	1 mSv/min

However, the equipment operator should adjust the quality of the x-ray beam to optimize the critical balance between image quality and exposure to the patient.

Protection of Patient

New x-ray machines have many features and accessories for radiation protection. Factors that can be controlled by a radiographer/technician are field size, choice of image receptors, and source-to-skin distance (SSD). All x-ray machines should have collimators to reduce the field size and the patient's radiation dose. These are rectangular, variable apertures that should be light localized. The x-ray and light beam should not have a discrepancy greater than 2% of the source-to-image receptor distance. Intensifying screens act as image amplifiers for x-ray films. These have been classified into high-speed screens, which require less exposure, and slow-speed screens to provide a given image density. Rare earths (fast screens) are used to reduce patient exposure without loss of diagnostic information. Low-attenuation material (e.g., carbon fiber) should be used for cassette front, grid interspacing, and tabletop.

Staff training and competence are essential both to produce high-quality images and to minimize patient radiation exposure. Repeat x-rays are most often caused by technical errors, including positioning and immobilization. With digital radiography, the issue of repeat x-rays due to exposure factors has been almost completely resolved. Dynamic wide-range receptors are used in digital radiography to produce images with appropriate contrast and a wide range of exposures, unlike x-ray films in which overexposure will produce a black image. For this reason, staff training becomes important to monitor exposure factors and indicators that may lead to increased patient dose. Appropriate use of a properly calibrated automatic exposure control (AEC) is helpful in minimizing unnecessary exposure. However, equipment should be properly calibrated and regularly adjusted to avoid any unnecessary radiation dose. Radiographers can alter the beam quality by adjusting the kilovolt peak (KvP), which means speed of beam, and beam quantity, which means number of photons in the primary beam, by adjusting the mA (tube current). High KvP means that electrons move faster, resulting in a high-quality x-ray image and a lower dose of absorbed radiation (as a result of the greater penetration power of the electrons).[2] Low KvP will result in more absorption of electrons in the body and a higher radiation exposure. SSD should be as large as possible because this will result in a more penetrating x-ray beam and less radiation exposure. Field size is the most important factor

in reducing the dose to the gonads. Radiographers should keep the field as small as possible at all times during the examination. Patients should be positioned carefully to reduce the dose to breasts and gonads. Breasts, eyes, and gonads can be shielded unless the area of interest would be masked. This will halve the radiation to the ovaries, and that to the testes is reduced by a factor of 20. Children up to age 10 are two to four times as sensitive to radiation. Medical radiation doses should be kept to the absolute minimum for adequate quality of images in children.[6]

Fluoroscopy provides real-time x-ray imaging, which is useful in guided diagnostic and therapeutic procedures. Like conventional television, 25 to 30 images are produced per second and provide live imaging of the body. Although exposure per fluoroscopic image is low as compared with x-rays, high patient exposure can result because of the large series of images during fluoroscopic procedures. Therefore the total exposure time is one of the major factors that determine the exposure to the patient during the procedure.[7] The shortest fluoroscopic time should be used that is consistent with the requirements of the procedure. Pulsed fluoroscopy produces fewer images per second and should be used appropriately without affecting image quality during the procedure. Intermittent screening for short periods should be performed to reduce the absorbed dose.[8] Fluoroscopic units should have a cumulative timer and an audible warning system that rings after a preset fluoroscopy time has elapsed. As an x-ray beam moves to different parts of the body, there is a greater chance of radiation exposure to sensitive organs such as the gonads, thyroid, and breasts. Careful positioning of the x-ray beam and shielding of these organs will minimize radiation effects. Magnification should only be used where necessary because this will lead to increased radiation dose rate.[9] In high-dose examinations such as computed tomography, exposure to eyes and other radiosensitive organs should be avoided. Low-dose computed scanning (e.g., chest) should be performed where possible.

Quality assurance plays a major role in reducing the patient dose. Equipment should be tested regularly, including x-ray tube outputs, collimator accuracy, and automatic exposure control performance.[10] Resolution of image intensifiers should be assessed regularly. Reject analysis should be performed regularly, and radiograph rejection rate should be kept below 5%.

All of these measures are taken to ensure that the patient receives the lowest possible radiation dose necessary for diagnosis. Patient radiation dose can be measured using a thermoluminescent dosimeter (TLD) directly on the patient's skin. During fluoroscopy, a dose-area product meter is absolutely essential as the direction of the beam changes during the examination. An ionizing chamber can also be used to measure air kerma dose at a given distance from the known exposure factors. However, effective radiation doses for different examinations fall in a wide range. The absorbed dose for a given examination may vary in different hospitals or even in the same hospital.

Protection of Staff

For staff working with radiation, radiation exposure can be from the direct beam, from scatter, and from leaked radiation. No one other than the patient should be exposed to the direct radiation beam.[11] The hands, forearms, and head should be kept out of the path of the direct beam, especially during fluoroscopy. In mobile radiography, no one other than the patient should be exposed to radiation. The x-ray tube is incorporated in the lead shielding to stop radiation traveling in any direction apart from a useful beam. The leakage of radiation should be as minimal as possible and should not be more than 1 mSv at a distance of 1 meter. X-rays scatter in all directions when the x-ray beam strikes the patient. The radiologist, radiographer, and any other staff in the room should stay as far as practicable for any given procedure. Computed tomography (CT) scanning is a high-KV examination that results in more scatter close to the aperture. Lead gloves and aprons should be used for any procedure during CT fluoroscopy or contrast injection during scanning.

No one should stay in the room when the patient is being exposed to the x-ray beam. The exposure switch should be fixed on the control panel to prevent the radiographer from leaving the protective cubicle during the exposure. Mobile radiography should be as minimal as possible. If an x-ray must be performed in the ward, no one should be near the patient at the time of exposure. The exposure switch cable should be 2 meters long so that the radiographer can stay as far away as possible. In nuclear medicine, radionuclide treatment, and after injection, the patient becomes the source of radiation exposure. Waiting areas should be designed to avoid exposure to staff and other people. Staff should be able to image and expose the patient without any unnecessary exposure to themselves or to the other patients.

During exposure, protective barriers should be used. The protective screen around the control panel should have 2.5 mm of lead and a glass screen through which to view the patient. This should reduce the dose without any protective clothing to the public dose limit. If this is not available, distance should be maintained and protective clothing should be used. Protective gloves should be 0.25 to 0.35 lead equivalent. (Lead equivalent refers to the thickness of lead required to achieve the same shielding against the radiation as provided by the given material.) Protective clothing is designed to protect from scatter radiation only. Hands should be outside the direct beam at all the times. Lead aprons cover 75% of red bone marrow and are generally 0.25 mm lead equivalent. During interventional procedures in which large and prolonged exposure is expected, 0.35 to 0.50 lead equivalent should be used. Lead aprons should be available in all x-ray rooms and with mobile x-ray machines and should be checked periodically for any cracks. Thyroid protective shielding and lead glass spectacles should be worn during fluoroscopic procedures.[12] Thin lead aprons are sufficient for x-rays, but these are inadequate for high-energy gamma radiation. Distance and time of exposure are important in cases when the patient is the source of radiation after radionuclide injection.

In the x-ray room entrance, there should be a warning sign to indicate "controlled area" and a warning light should come on when exposure is being made or fluoroscopy is being performed. In the x-ray room, walls, doors, and windows should be shielded in such a way to reduce the dose to surrounding areas below 0.1 mSv per week under normal workloads. Protection is more important in the floor and areas of wall where the direct beam may fall. The rest of the walls, windows, and doors only receive scatter radiation, and 0.25 mm lead equivalent should be enough.

Many different personal dosimetry systems are available to monitor radiation exposure. Film badges are most commonly used. These should be acquired from a single manufacturer to avoid any difference of sensitivity and should be returned to the appropriate dosimetry laboratory where films are processed under controlled conditions. These are inexpensive and can record a wide range of exposures. Thermoluminescent dosimeters (TLDs) are used to measure patient dose during radiologic procedures. These consist of a small chip that can be used in the form of rings for staff finger dosimetry. Electronic dosimeters are 50 to 200 times as sensitive as TLDs. These are highly appropriate in cases where low-dose measurement is important, such as in pregnancy. They also provide direct reading so that the wearer will know when radiation exposure occurs and can take appropriate steps to avoid it. Electronic dosimeters have a high initial cost but last up to 10 years. Annual calibration is required for accurate reading and is legally required.

Radiation Exposure in Pregnancy

In females of childbearing age, an attempt should be made to determine who is or who could be pregnant, before the examination involving radiation. A missed period in a regularly menstruating woman should be considered as pregnancy until proved otherwise. Notices should be posted in patient waiting areas instructing women to inform staff or clinicians if they are or may be pregnant. The "28 days rule" states that for all women of child bearing age, non-urgent x-rays should only be performed if the patient is sure that she is not pregnant and that she has had her last period sometime during the previous 28 days. In cases where exposure to the abdomen and pelvis is involved, the 28 days rule should be applied. CT of the abdomen or pelvis and abdominal fluoroscopy, in which the radiation dose to the uterus is high, should only be performed in the first 10 days of the menstrual cycle.

Thousands of women are exposed to ionic radiation each year. Medical exposure is appropriate most of the time, and radiation risk to the fetus is minimal. Although there are radiation risks throughout the pregnancy, this is most significant during organogenesis in the early pregnancy, and risk to the fetus reduces as pregnancy progresses. The central nervous system is most commonly affected, and this occurs after a threshold of 100 mGy, which is roughly equivalent to three pelvic CTs and 20 conventional x-ray examinations. However, this level can be reached with fluoroscopically guided interventional procedures of the pelvis and radiotherapy. Weeks 8 to 25 of pregnancy are the most important for central nervous system development. Exposures greater than 100 mGY may lead to reduced intelligence quotient (IQ), and exposures of 1000 mGY may cause mental retardation. Risk for leukemia and other types of cancer also increases after excessive radiation exposure. In pregnancy, medical and occupational exposure should be justified for benefit versus risk and should be calculated for each individual. Once the decision is made about radiation exposure, every attempt should be made to reduce the fetal exposure during the medical examination.[13] In fluoroscopically guided interventional procedures, exposure may be quite high (10 to 100 mGY) depending on the procedure. After such a procedure, fetal dose and potential risk should be calculated by a knowledgeable person.[14] Most radionuclide procedures are performed with short–half-life radiopharmaceuticals (e.g., technetium-99m) and there is minimal fetal dose, which could be further reduced by oral hydration and frequent voiding. Some radionuclides (e.g., iodine-131) cross the placenta and can pose fetal risk. The fetal thyroid begins accumulating iodine after 10 weeks of gestational age. A high fetal thyroid dose may lead to permanent hypothyroidism. A number of radionuclides are excreted in breast milk, and breastfeeding should be suspended completely after iodine-131 therapy and for 3 weeks after iodine-125 and gallium-67.[15]

In a radiation occupational worker, once pregnancy has been declared, the mother should not receive more than 10 mSv of radiation averaged over her abdomen for the remainder of the pregnancy. Pregnant medical radiation workers may continue to work in the radiation environment as long as there is reasonable assurance that fetal dose can be kept below 1 mSv during the pregnancy.

Conventional radiology examinations generally have a low radiation dose. However, more complex CT examinations and fluoroscopically guided interventional procedures are being performed that involve high radiation exposure. Protocols should be in place in the department and staff should be regularly trained to keep radiation-related morbidity to a minimum.

References

Full references for this chapter can be found on www.expertconsult.com.

Chapter **13**

Magnetic Resonance Imaging

Hifz Aniq and Robert Campbell

Description of Modality

Magnetic resonance imaging (MRI) is based on the principles of nuclear magnetic resonance (NMR), a spectroscopic technique used to obtain microscopic chemical and physical information about molecules. MRI is based on the absorption and emission of energy in the radiofrequency (RF) range of the electromagnetic spectrum. It produces images based on spatial variations in the phase and frequency of the RF energy being absorbed and emitted by the imaged object. A number of biologically relevant elements, such as hydrogen, oxygen-16, oxygen-17, fluorine-19, sodium-23, and phosphorus-31 are potential candidates for producing magnetic resonance (MR) images. The human body is primarily fat and water, both of which have many hydrogen atoms, making the human body approximately 63% hydrogen atoms. Hydrogen nuclei have an NMR signal, so for these reasons clinical MRI primarily images the NMR signal from the hydrogen nuclei given its abundance in the human body. Protons behave like small bar magnets, with north and south poles within the magnetic field. The magnetic moment of a single proton is extremely small and not detectable. Without an external magnetic field, a group of protons assumes a random orientation of magnetic moments. Under the influence of an applied external magnetic field, the protons assume a nonrandom alignment, resulting in a measurable magnetic moment in the direction of the external magnetic field. By applying RF pulses, images can then be created based on the differences in signal from hydrogen atoms in different types of tissue. A variety of systems are used in medical imaging, ranging from open MRI units with magnetic field strength of 0.3 Tesla (T) to extremity MRI systems with field strengths up to 1.0 T and whole-body scanners with field strengths up to 3.0 T (in clinical use). Because of its superior soft tissue contrast resolution, MRI is best suited for evaluation of internal derangement of joints, central nervous system abnormalities, and other pathologic processes in the patient with pain.

The advantages of MRI over other imaging modalities include absence of ionizing radiation, superior soft tissue contrast resolution, high-resolution imaging, and multiplanar imaging capabilities. The time to acquire an MRI image has been a major weakness and continues to be so with the advent of faster computed tomography (CT) scanners (with multislice CT). However, newer imaging techniques (e.g., parallel imaging), faster pulse sequences, and higher field strength systems are addressing this issue. A number of pulse sequences have been invented to highlight differences in signal of various soft tissues. The most common and most basic of pulse sequences include T1-weighted and T2-weighted sequences. T1-weighted sequences have traditionally been considered good for evaluation of anatomic structures. Tissues that show a high signal (bright) on T1-weighted images include fat, blood (methemoglobin), proteinaceous fluid, some forms of calcium, melanin, and gadolinium (a contrast agent). T2-weighted sequences have generally been considered fluid-conspicuity pulse sequences, useful for identifying pathologic processes. Tissues that show a high signal on T2-weighted images include fluid-containing structures (i.e., cysts, joint fluid, cerebrospinal fluid) and pathologic states causing increased extracellular fluid (i.e., sources of infection or inflammation).

Advanced imaging techniques used in medical imaging include MR angiography (MRA), diffusion-weighted imaging, chemical shift imaging (fat suppression), functional imaging of the brain, and MR spectroscopy (MRS). Many of these techniques are especially useful in brain imaging. MRA (either time-of-flight or phase contrast) and diffusion-weighted imaging are useful for the detection and characterization of ischemic insults in the brain. MRS uses the differences in chemical composition in tissues to differentiate necrosis or normal brain matter from tumor.

In musculoskeletal imaging, MR arthrography is a technique available to augment the depiction of internal derangements of joints.[1] Arthrography can be either indirect (intravenous gadolinium is administered and allowed to diffuse into the joint) or direct (a dilute gadolinium solution is percutaneously injected into the joint) to provide distention of a joint, assisting in the evaluation of ligaments, cartilage, synovial proliferation, or intra-articular bodies. MR arthrography has been most extensively used in the shoulder to outline labral-ligamentous abnormalities and to distinguish partial-thickness from full-thickness tears in the rotator cuff. It is also helpful in demonstrating labral tears in the hip, partial- and full-thickness tears of the collateral ligament of the elbow, and bands in the elbow. This technique is also useful in patients after meniscectomy in the knee to detect recurrent or residual meniscal tears, to evaluate perforations of the ligaments and triangular fibrocartilage in the wrist, and to assess the stability of osteochondral lesions in the articular surface of joints. T1-weighted images are often employed with MR arthrography to bring out the T1 shortening effects of gadolinium. Fat saturation is also added to help differentiate fat from gadolinium. A T2-weighted sequence in at least one plane is also necessary to detect cysts and edema in other soft tissues and bone marrow.

Patients in whom MRI is contraindicated include those who have the following: cardiac pacemaker, implanted cardiac defibrillator, aneurysm clips, carotid artery vascular clamp, neurostimulator, insulin or infusion pump, implanted drug infusion device, bond growth/fusion stimulator, and a cochlear or ear implant. In addition, patients who have a history of metalworking should have a pre-MRI screening radiograph of the orbits to evaluate for radiopaque foreign bodies near the ocular globe.

Applications

In imaging of pain in the neurologic system, MRI is useful in cases of trauma, evaluation of the posterior fossa, and evaluation of a nonacute headache. MRI is more sensitive than CT in identifying pathologic intracranial changes. In the setting of acute trauma, CT is the modality of choice for the identification of intracranial hemorrhage. However, in the specific setting of suspected diffuse axonal injury (DAI), MRI is the preferred examination (particularly with gradient-echo sequences). Other considerations come into play, including general availability and practicality of CT versus MRI. Of patients proven eventually to have DAI, 50% to 80% demonstrate a normal CT scan on presentation. Delayed CT may be helpful in demonstrating edema or atrophy, but these are later findings. Characteristic CT findings in the acute setting are small petechial hemorrhages that are located at the gray matter/white matter junction, within the corpus callosum, and in the brainstem. The degree of confidence in CT is moderate, because the only finding may be petechial hemorrhage, and fewer than 20% of patients with DAI demonstrate this finding on CT alone. Gradient-echo sequences are particularly useful in demonstrating the paramagnetic effects of petechial hemorrhages. Gradient-echo imaging often can demonstrate signal abnormality in areas that appear normal in T1- and T2-weighted spin-echo sequences. For this reason it has become a mainstay of MRI of patients with suspected shearing-type injuries. The abnormal signal on gradient-echo images can persist for many years after the injury. The most common MRI finding is multifocal areas of abnormal signal (bright on T2-weighted images) at the white matter in the temporal or parietal corticomedullary junction or in the splenium of the corpus callosum. The degree of confidence is high, because

abnormal signal in the characteristic locations in the clinical setting of recent trauma leaves little doubt about the diagnosis of DAI.

Other MRI applications in neuroimaging include the evaluation of the posterior fossa, venous sinus thrombosis, vasculitis, and further soft tissue characterization after CT has been performed. For nonacute headache and migraines, the U.S. Headache Consortium has developed evidence-based guidelines for the use of neuroimaging in patients with nonacute headache (i.e., headache occurring at least 4 weeks during a patient's lifetime).[2] Based on the studies reviewed, MRI appears to be more sensitive in finding white matter lesions and developmental venous anomalies than CT. The greater contrast resolution and discrimination of MRI, however, appears to be of little clinical importance in the evaluation of patients with nonacute headache. Therefore the recommendation was that data were insufficient to make evidence-based recommendations regarding the relative sensitivity of MRI compared with CT in the evaluation of migraine or other nonacute headache.

Spine imaging using MRI can exquisitely provide information regarding various pathologic entities, including degenerative disk disease, zygapophyseal (facet) joint disease, infection, neoplasm, and fracture (**Fig. 13.1**). With respect to degenerative disk disease, MRI often does not define a specific painful clinical syndrome because of the overlap of multiple nociceptors and their nonspecific appearance in painful versus painless degenerative conditions. Many findings may represent senescent changes that are the sequelae of stress applied during the course of a lifetime. Therefore utilization of MRI within a defined clinical context is paramount.

To improve communication and consistency between providers, there is a standard nomenclature for lumbar spine disk disease endorsed by the North American Spine Society (NASS), the American Society of Spine Radiologists (ASSR), and the American Society of Neuroradiologists. It is important to recognize that the definitions of diagnoses should not define or imply external etiologic events such as trauma, should not imply relationship to symptoms, and should not define or imply need for specific treatment.

Degenerative disk disease (DDD) is a term applied specifically to intervertebral disk degeneration. The term *spondylosis* is often used in general as synonymous with *degeneration*, including both nucleus pulposus and anulus fibrosus processes, but such usage is confusing, so it is best that *degeneration* be the general term. *Degeneration* can be subclassified into spondylosis deformans, which is characterized by marginal osteophytosis without substantial disk height loss, reflecting predominantly anulus fibrosus disease. *Intervertebral osteochondrosis* is the term applied to the condition of mainly nucleus pulposus and vertebral body end plate disease, including anular tearing (fissuring). *Osteoarthritis* is a process of synovial joints. In the spine this term is appropriately applied to the zygapophyseal (facet, Z-joint), atlantoaxial, costovertebral, and sacroiliac joints.

Herniation is defined as a localized displacement of disk material beyond the limits of the intervertebral disk space. Disk material may be nucleus, cartilage, fragmented apophyseal bone, anular tissue, or any combination thereof. Normally, the posterior disk margin tends to be concave in the upper lumbar spine and is straight or slightly convex at L4-5 and L5-S1. The normal margin is defined by the vertebral body ring apophysis

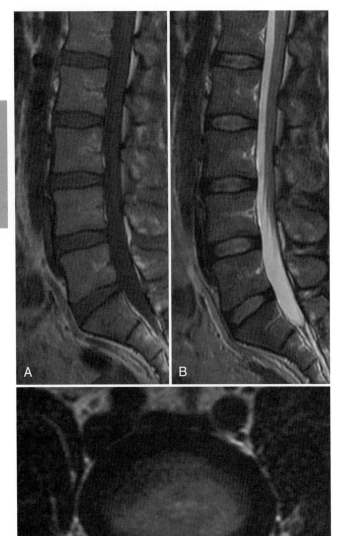

Fig. 13.1 Lumbar spine. Normal MRI appearance of the lumbar inter-vertebral disk: sagittal T1-weighted (A), sagittal T2-weighted without fat suppression (B), and axial T2-weighted through the intervertebral disk level (C). Note that on T1-weighted image the disk is hypointense to the lumbar vertebral body whereas on T2-weighted image it is hyperintense, reflecting normal water content of the nucleus pulposus. On axial imaging, the posterior margin should have a concavity (arrowhead, C,) with the exception of the lumbosacral junction, which may normally have a slight convexity. The disk margins should project no more than 1 or 2 mm beyond the vertebral end plate.

25% (90 degrees) of the disk circumference, or *broad based,* meaning between 25% and 50% (90 to 180 degrees) of the disk circumference. Presence of disk tissue *circumferentially,* meaning 50% to 100% (180 to 360 degrees) beyond the edges of the ring apophyses, may be called *bulging* and is not considered a form of herniation.

Beyond having descriptors of the circumferential extent of the herniation, herniated disks may take the form of protrusion, extrusion, or sequestration (free fragment) based on the shape of the displaced disk material. Protrusion is present if the greatest distance, in any plane, between the edges of the disk material beyond the disk space is less than the distance between the edges of the base in the same plane. In other words, the base against the parent disk margin is broader than any other diameter of the herniation. In the craniocaudal direction, the length of the base cannot exceed, by definition, the height of the intervertebral space. Protrusions may be broad based or focal. Extrusion is present when, in at least one plane, any one distance between the edges of the disk material beyond the disk space is greater than the distance between the edges of the base. In other words, the base against the parent disk margin tends to be narrower than any other diameter of the herniation. Extrusion may be further specified as a "sequestration" if the displaced disk material has lost completely any continuity with the parent disk (**Fig. 13.2**). The term *migration* may be used to signify displacement of disk material away from the site of extrusion, regardless of whether sequestration is present. Herniated disks in the craniocaudal (vertical) direction through a break in the vertebral body end plate are referred to as *intravertebral herniations* (Schmorl's nodes). They often have a round or lobulated appearance and are often incidental and likely to be developmental or post-traumatic rather than purely degenerative.[3]

Anular tears (fissures) are characterized by a focal area of increased signal intensity on T2-weighted images (high-intensity zone) and imply a loss of integrity of the anulus fibrosus, such as radial, transverse, and concentric separations (**Fig. 13.3**). They do not imply that a significant traumatic event has occurred or that the etiology is known. Some tears may have clinical relevance, and others may be asymptomatic and inconsequential components of the aging process. At diskography there is about an 85% concordance of imaging findings with the presence of anular tear. Correlation of the tear with responses to diskography and other clinically relevant observations may enable the clinician to make such distinctions. Another source of diskogenic pain is related to the adjacent vertebral end plate changes. Modic et al[4] proposed a classification of vertebral body end plate marrow changes by MRI. Modic type 1 changes appear as low signal intensity on T1-weighted images and high signal intensity on T2-weighted images (**Fig. 13.4**). Type 2 changes appear high signal on both T1- and T2-weighted images whereas type 3 changes appear of low signal intensity on both T1- and T2-weighted images. The type 1 changes appear similar to edema and may sometimes be mistaken for reactive edema from an adjacent diskitis. Type 2 changes appear similar in signal to fat and represent a reparative phase. Type 3 changes are analogous to diskogenic sclerosis seen on radiographs. Moderate and severe end plate type I and type II abnormalities on MR images may indicate painful disk derangement in patients with low back pain.[5] A grading system for the assessment of lumbar disk degeneration using MRI was described by Pfirrmann et al[6]:

exclusive of osteophytes. Herniations are either *localized* or *generalized,* the latter being defined as greater than 50% (180 degrees) of the periphery of the disk. Localized displacement in the axial (horizontal) plane can be *focal,* signifying less than

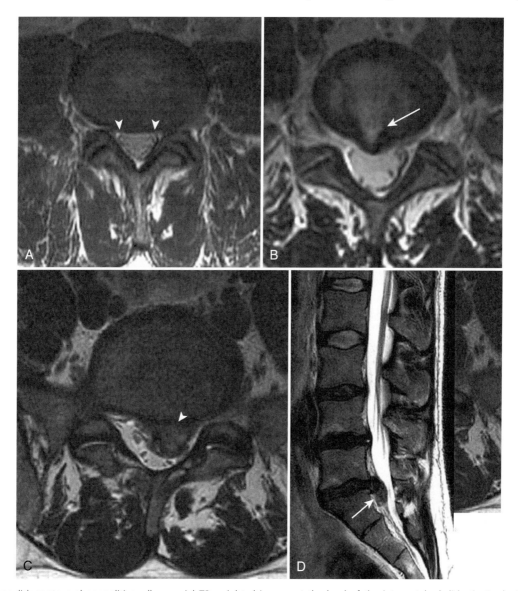

Fig. 13.2 Lumbar disk contour abnormalities: all are axial T2-weighted images at the level of the intervertebral disk. A, Anular bulge. There is generalized displacement of greater than 180 degrees of the disk margin beyond the normal margin of the intervertebral disk space that is the result of disk degeneration with an intact anulus *(arrowheads)*. B, Disk protrusion. The base against the parent disk margin is broader than any other diameter of the herniation. Extension of nucleus pulposus through a partial defect in the anulus is identified *(arrow)* but the herniated disk is contained by some intact anular fibers (may or may not be distinguished at MRI). C and D, L5-S1 disk extrusion: the base against the parent disk margin is narrower than any other diameter of the herniation *(arrowhead),* which migrates inferiorly *(arrow)*. There may be extension of the nucleus pulposus through a complete focal defect in the anulus. Substantial mass effect is present, causing moderate central canal stenosis.

- Grade I: The structure of the disk is homogeneous, with bright hyperintense white signal intensity and a normal disk height.
- Grade II: The structure of the disk is inhomogeneous, with hyperintense white signal. The distinction between nucleus and anulus is clear, and the disk height is normal, with or without horizontal gray bands.
- Grade III: The structure of the disk is inhomogeneous, with intermediate gray signal intensity. The distinction between nucleus and anulus is unclear, and the disk height is normal or slightly decreased.
- Grade IV: The structure of the disk is inhomogeneous, with hypointense dark gray signal intensity. The distinction between nucleus and anulus is lost, and the disk height is normal or moderately decreased.

- Grade V: The structure of the disk is inhomogeneous, with hypointense black signal intensity. The distinction between nucleus and anulus is lost, and the disk space is collapsed.

The following scheme is used to define the degree of canal compromise (stenosis) produced by disk displacement based on the goals of being practical, objective, reasonably precise, and clinically relevant. Canal compromise of less than one third of the canal at a given axial section is "mild," between one and two thirds is "moderate," and over two thirds is "severe" (**Fig. 13.5**). This same scheme may be applied to foraminal narrowing, with the sagittal images playing a primary role in determining the degree of narrowing.

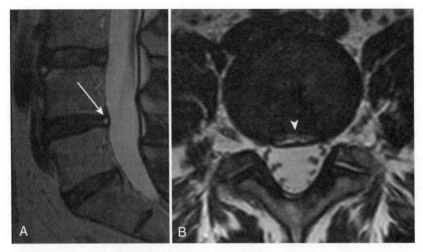

Fig. 13.3 Hyperintense zone (HIZ). **A,** Sagittal T2-weighted image shows a small focus of hyperintensity *(arrow)* within the posterior anulus fibrosus. **B,** Axial T2 at L4-5 disk level shows anular fissure posterocentrally *(arrowhead).*

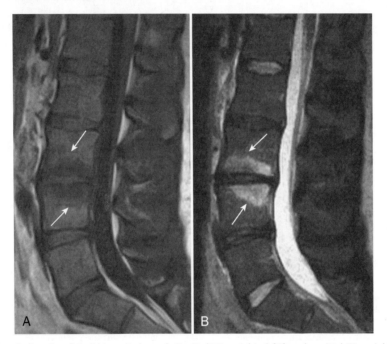

Fig. 13.4 Vertebral marrow signal alteration (Modic type 1 change). Sagittal T1-weighted **(A)** and sagittal T2-weighted **(B)** MR images show disk height loss and desiccation at multiple levels. At the L3-4 level this is associated with rounded areas of signal alteration that abut the end plate and follow fluid-like signal with T1 hypointensity and T2 hypointensity *(arrows).*

Bone Marrow and Bone Marrow Edema–Like (BME) Lesions

Normal bone marrow has three constituents: osseous, myeloid elements, and adipose cells. Hematopoietic (red) marrow has approximately 40% fat content and fatty (yellow) marrow has 80% fat content. The appendicular skeleton tends to have more fatty marrow than hematopoietic marrow. However, normal variations in marrow distribution are important to recognize and should not be confused with pathologic processes. Small differences in the amount and distribution of red marrow from side to side are normal, but marked asymmetry is suggestive of a disease process. An important exception to early and complete red to yellow marrow conversion is seen in the proximal humeral and femoral epiphyses and may

be seen throughout life. This epiphyseal red marrow is curvilinear and located in the subchondral regions of these bones. Heterogeneous marrow signal, in which small focal islands of red marrow occur in predominantly yellow marrow and vice versa, can be seen. Normal marrow on T1-weighted sequences is always isointense or hyperintense to surrounding muscle or intervertebral disk. With BME lesions, they are hypointense on T1-weighted images and have high signal on fluid-sensitive sequences such as T2-weighted or short tan inversion recovery (STIR) imaging.

BME lesions can reflect nonspecific response to injury or excess stress. The pathophysiology is related to increased extracellular fluid, which can be from hypervascularity and hyperperfusion (hyperemia, an inflammatory infiltrate causing resorption, granulation tissue, or a reactive phenomenon

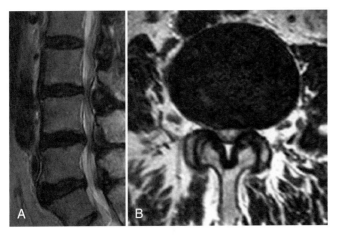

Fig. 13.5 Severe spinal stenosis. Sagittal T2-weighted **(A)** and axial T2-weighted at L3-4 disk level **(B)** MR images show a broad-based disk bulge resulting in greater than two-thirds compromise of the spinal canal.

related to altered biomechanics). Enhancement with gadolinium occurs in BME irrespective of etiology (benign or malignant, infectious or inflammatory). Potential causes include diseases in the following categories: trauma, biomechanical, developmental, vascular, neoplastic, inflammatory, neuropathic, metabolic, degenerative, iatrogenic, and potentially idiopathic conditions (e.g., transient bone marrow edema syndromes).

One of the most common causes of BME is occult injuries. Stress fractures can be subclassified into insufficiency or fatigue fractures. Insufficiency fractures occur with normal stresses in abnormal bone. Fatigue fractures occur in normal bone with excess or superphysiologic stress. MRI is a more sensitive technique for fracture detection and characterization than radiography. Common locations predominate in the lower extremities, including the pelvis (supra-acetabular and parasymphyseal regions), femur (head and neck), tibia (proximal or distal), fibula (distal diaphysis), ankle (posterior calcaneus), and multiple regions in the foot (e.g., metatarsal shaft). Bone contusions (bruises) are considered microtrabecular fractures. On MRI there is no fracture line and the pattern of BME may be a secondary sign of associated ligament or tendon injury. These often occur in a subarticular location from osteochondral impaction injuries. Altered biomechanics can also be an important cause of BME and may reflect bone stress response without fractures and may even be asymptomatic.

Vascular causes of BME may be related to either hyperemic or ischemic causes. Of the hyperemic causes, inflammatory disorders that increase vascularity or disuse may cause subarticular BME patterns. The disuse pattern can be characteristic and parallels the radiographic pattern with multiple rounded areas of fluid-like hyperintensity in a subarticular and metaphyseal distribution. In ischemic lesions, the broad category of osteonecrosis (infarct, avascular necrosis) can have BME early that is associated with the acute painful symptomatology. Pain improvement usually parallels the resolution of the BME signal. The "double line" sign is specific and is characterized by a ring of T1-weighted hypointensity and T2-weighted hyperintensity (**Fig. 13.6**). MR findings may be seen within a few hours after vascular insult. Transient osteoporosis (radiographic) or the MR correlate transient bone marrow edema

syndrome may occur in numerous lower extremity locations, including the hip, knee, talus, tarsals (cuboid, navicular), and metatarsals. It is controversial whether these lesions reflect salvaged avascular necrosis or simply are biomechanical.

In the inflammatory category, infections can cause BME. Often, a difficult differential diagnosis in the clinical setting of diabetic neuropathy is distinguishing osteomyelitis from Charcot arthropathy. MRI may be helpful in differentiating the two. First, the distributions are typically different. Osteomyelitis is more common in the phalanges, distal metatarsals, and calcaneus, whereas neuropathic disease is more common in the Lisfranc and Chopart joints. Second, epicenters can be useful. Neuropathic disease has an articular epicenter and usually multiple joints are involved. Osteomyelitis has a marrow epicenter with focal spread throughout the bone. Third, secondary soft tissue findings such as a subcutaneous ulcer, cellulitis, phlegmon, abscess, and, particularly, a sinus tract strongly support infection.[7] Noninfectious causes in the inflammatory category may also be a source of BME, such as in reflex sympathetic dystrophy (RSD). RSD is a condition characterized by localized or diffuse pain, usually with associated swelling, trophic changes, and vasomotor disturbance. Allodynia, hyperhidrosis, and nail or hair growth changes may also occur. Motor abnormalities have been reported, and contractures may occur in the later stages. Three stages are recognized, with clinical and radiologic features used in the staging. Stage 1 is characterized by the onset of burning type pain, with swelling and edema. Stage 2 reflects more established disease; pain diminishes with the onset of vasoconstriction and subsequent decreased skin temperature. In stage 3, pain is less prominent and the skin can be smooth and/or cyanotic with underlying muscle atrophy. MRI, because of its inherent soft tissue imaging capabilities, has been shown to be useful for the accurate diagnosis of RSD.[8] BME is a nonspecific finding in RSD, but the adjacent soft tissue changes help stage the disease in association with clinical findings. Stage 1 disease is the most accurately demonstrated stage, showing skin thickening, contrast medium enhancement, joint effusion,[9] and, less frequently, soft tissue edema (**Fig. 13.7**). MRI of RSD in stage 2 disease is less accurate. Findings in stage 2 disease include skin thinning and/or thickening and infrequent soft tissue enhancement. In patients with stage 3 RSD, soft tissue enhancement is not seen but muscle atrophy is a common finding (**Fig. 13.8**). Patients with stage 1 or 2 RSD generally do not demonstrate muscle atrophy. Skin changes seen on MRI in stage 3 RSD are variable.

Degenerative conditions can also be associated with BME, such as primary or secondary osteoarthritis. Subchondral cysts are one of the imaging hallmarks of osteoarthritis and can be identified on MRI. Early in the course there are ill-defined areas of BME, and, later, discrete cystic structures form. In the knee, marrow findings are strongly associated with the presence of pain and moderate or larger effusions and synovial thickening are more frequent among those with pain than those without pain adjusted for degree of radiographic osteoarthritis.[10] In addition, focal subchondral BME can be an indicator of focal overlying cartilage defects. A flame-shaped BME lesion in a nonarthritic joint can be a helpful secondary sign of cartilage abnormality. BME lesions can also be seen in a subtendinous location as a response to tendon abnormality from mechanical friction, hyperemia, or biomechanical reasons. This is most common in the foot and ankle.[11]

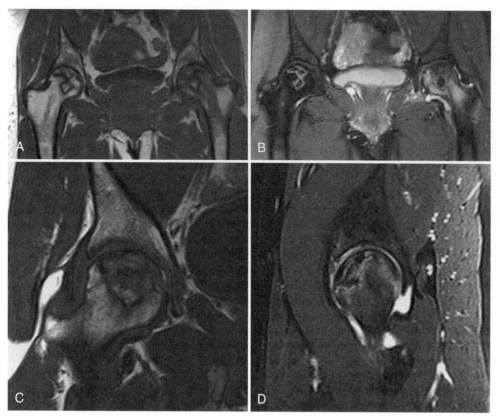

Fig. 13.6 Osteonecrosis. Coronal T1-weighted (A) and coronal short tan inversion recovery (B) images show characteristic serpentine, alternating lines of T1-weighted hypointensity and T2-weighted hyperintensity typical of osteonecrosis. Coronal T1-weighted (C) and sagittal T2-weighted with fat suppression (D) images further show a curvilinear low signal intensity line in the subarticular area of the femoral head suggesting subarticular collapse, a complication of avascular necrosis.

Tendons

Tendons are relatively avascular structures that attach muscles to bones, consisting of dense fascicles of collagen fibers. Because normal tendons (as well as ligaments and cortical bone) have few mobile protons, they are usually of low signal intensity on all pulse sequences. There are a few instances that are exceptions to this rule. The quadriceps tendon at the knee and the distal triceps tendon at the elbow have a striated appearance with alternating areas of linear low- and intermediate-signal intensity. This striated appearance is caused by the fact that several tendons are fusing to form a single conjoined tendon. Similarly, there may be a solitary, vertical high signal intensity line in the midsubstance of many normal Achilles tendons representing the site where the soleus and gastrocnemius tendons are apposed to one another or a vascular channel in the tendon. Another exception may occur when tendons demonstrate slightly increased signal intensity near their osseous insertions. This occurs because the tendon fans out to attach to a bone and fatty material is interposed between tendon fibers. A third reason for a normal tendon to have increased signal intensity is the result of the magic angle phenomenon. The phenomenon results when the tendons are oriented at a 55-degree angle to the direction of the main magnetic field. There will be high signal intensity on short TE sequences (such as T1-weighted, proton-density, and gradient-echo sequences). Differentiation between magic angle phenomena and true pathology can be made by examining long TE sequences (i.e., T2-weighted sequences), where the high signal intensity will disappear if it is due to magic angle phenomenon.

A number of tendon abnormalities may be detected by MRI. The spectrum of tendinopathy encompasses tendinosis, partial tears, complete tears, and tenosynovitis. The term *tendon degeneration* is a broad term synonymous with *tendinopathy.* Degeneration of tendons occurs with aging or from chronic overuse. This is generally painless but weakens the tendon and predisposes to partial or complete tears with minimal trauma. On MRI, a degenerated tendon demonstrates both morphologic and signal alterations. Partial tears represent incomplete disruption of tendon fibers. These can have a variable appearance on MRI. The tendon may be thickened or thinned or remain of normal caliber with abnormal signal being the only evidence of the partial tear. Partial tears can also manifest as longitudinal tears along the length of the tendon (interstitial or split tears) rather than along the transverse plane. Complete tendon tear (rupture) indicates total disruption of fibers so that there are two separate fragments. The resulting fragments may be separated (retracted) for variable distances.

Tenosynovitis is defined as inflammation of the lining of the sheath that surrounds a tendon. Tendon sheaths are present where tendons pass through fascial slings, beneath ligamentous bands, or through fibro-osseous tunnels. A thin layer of fluid exists between the tendon sheath and the tendon itself and allows for smooth gliding of the tendon. Although there are no strict criteria defining the normal amount of tendon sheath fluid, when the diameter of the tendon sheath is greater than the enclosed tendon it is probably pathologic. Tenosynovitis may occur from chronic repetitive motion, inflammatory arthritides, and infection, among other causes. Tendon sheaths that

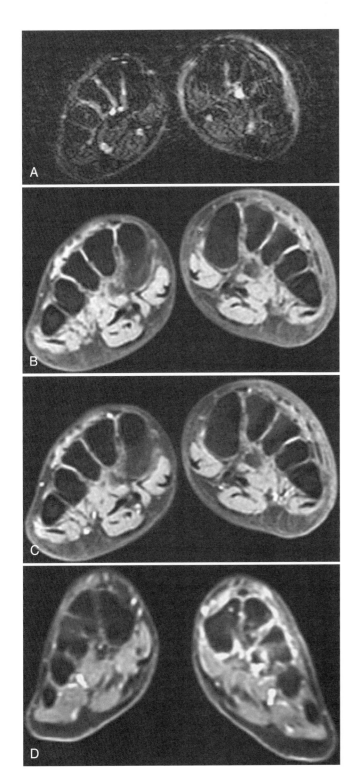

Fig. 13.7 Reflex sympathetic dystrophy stage 1. **A,** Axial T2-weighted fat-suppressed image shows a prominent area of subcutaneous edema over the dorsum of the left midfoot. Axial T1-weighted fat-suppressed **(B)** and axial T1-weighted fat-suppressed post–intravenous gadolinium **(C)** images show skin thickening and enhancement in the area corresponding to subcutaneous edema. **D,** Axial T1-weighted fat-suppressed postcontrast image also shows periarticular enhancement in the left midfoot.

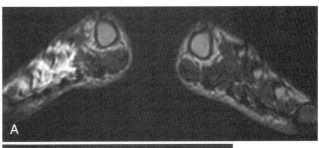

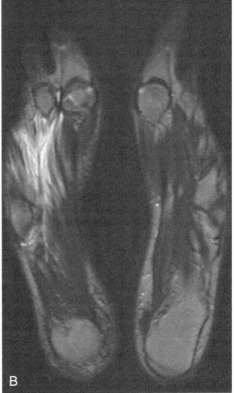

Fig. 13.8 Reflex sympathetic dystrophy stage 3. Coronal T2-weighted **(A)** and axial T2-weighted **(B)** images show prominent T2-weighted hyperintensity in the intrinsic muscles of the right foot reflecting an early stage of muscle atrophy.

can communicate with an adjacent joint, such as the long head of the biceps tendon in the shoulder and the flexor hallucis longus tendon at the ankle, should not be considered to have tenosynovitis simply because of fluid surrounding the tendon. Only if this is disproportionate to the amount of joint fluid do these findings have possible clinical significance.

Ligament Abnormalities

Classification of ligamentous injuries in general is similar to that of tendon abnormalities. Ligament injuries are referred to as *sprains,* whereas muscle injury is correctly referred to as *strain.* Ligaments usually show as low signal intensity on all pulse sequences. Exceptions to this exist in which ligaments such as the anterior cruciate ligament in the knee and deep deltoid fibers in the ankle can have a striated appearance with fatty tissue interspersed between ligament fibers. Grading of ligament injuries (sprain) ranges from microscopic tearing (analogous to tendinosis of tendons) to partial or complete tears. Grade I sprain is when stretching of a ligament occurs or there is microscopic tearing. On MRI these can manifest as either fluid immediately adjacent to or surrounding the ligament or an increase in signal intensity of the ligament. The ligament may be normal or enlarged in thickness. Grade II sprain refers to a partial tear, which indicates disruption of some of the fibers of the ligament. Grade III sprain indicates a complete tear. Partial and complete ligament tears appear on MRI as discontinuity of some or all of the fibers of the ligament with interposed fluid (**Fig. 13.9**).

Cartilage Abnormalities

Over the past decade, MRI of articular cartilage has become a leading area of clinical and research interest. Development of new cartilage-specific sequences has made MRI the optimal imaging modality for the evaluation of cartilage abnormalities and also plays a significant role in determining the appropriate pharmacologic or surgical repair procedures. Articular cartilage lesions may be categorized as degenerative or traumatic.[12] Early degenerative changes may be seen on MRI as abnormality in contour (fibrillation or surface irregularity), changes in cartilage thickness (thinning or thickening), or alterations in cartilage signal intensity. Advanced degenerative changes on MRI manifest as multiple areas of cartilage thinning of varying depth and size. Focal cartilage defects may be associated with corresponding edema-like marrow signal abnormality in the subchondral bone. Subchondral cystic change and sclerosis can also be seen. In contrast, traumatic chondral lesions usually appear on MRI as solitary focal cartilage defects with acutely angled margins. These defects are usually the results

of shearing, rotational, or tangential forces and result in partial- or full-thickness cartilage defects or osteochondral injuries. Linear clefts or fissures may also be seen extending for variable depths within the articular cartilage. These may result in chondral flap lesions or delamination injuries. Associated alterations in subchondral marrow signal may also be seen and should alert the observer to the possibility of overlying articular cartilage abnormality. MRI is reliable for detection and characterization of full-thickness cartilage defects. A number of surgical cartilage repair procedures have been developed to treat cartilage defects. These include local stimulation techniques (abrasion arthroplasty, microfracture, subchondral drilling) and autologous transplantation of cartilage: autologous osteochondral transplantation and autologous chondrocyte implantation.

Muscle and Nerve

Normal skeletal muscles have intermediate signal on all pulse sequences. On T1-weighted sequences, muscles have a mild feathery pattern caused by interposition of fat among the fibers in a muscle and between the adjacent muscles. Individual groups of muscles are identified by fat in the intermuscular fascia. However, in some locations (e.g., the calf) there is a paucity of fat, which makes it difficult to separate the individual muscle groups. On T2-weighted sequences, muscles maintain the intermediate signal and there is no high signal between the muscles apart from normal vascular structures. Muscle abnormalities can be seen as abnormal signals on different sequences, and there may be an increase or a reduction in their size. MRI is extremely sensitive but at the same time it can be quite nonspecific. In the acute phase, high signal on T2-weighted sequences could be due to muscle injury, inflammation, or denervation.[13] In the chronic phase, high signal in

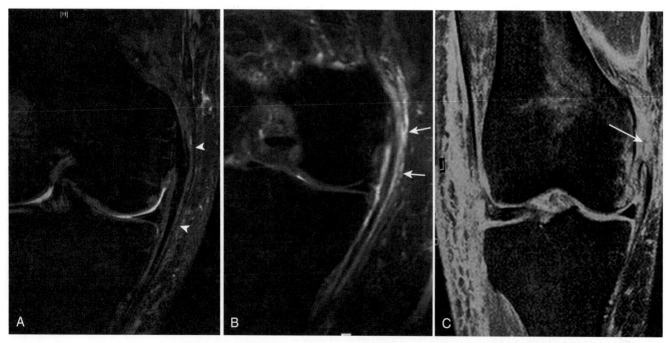

Fig. 13.9 Medial collateral ligament (MCL) tear, coronal T2 fat-saturated sequences of different knees. **A,** MCL sprain as high signal noted around the ligament *(arrowheads)*. The MCL is thickened but its fibers are intact. **B,** Partial-thickness tear as superficial fibers are torn *(black arrow)* but deep fibers are intact. **C,** Full-thickness tear as MCL is completely torn at its femoral attachment *(white arrow)*.

muscle may represent fatty infiltration with reduction in the size of muscle resulting from muscle atrophy. Muscle strains are caused by direct injury to the muscle or caused indirectly by excessive stretching or tension. Muscles that cross two joints are more commonly affected, such as the rectus femoris, gastrocnemius, and biceps femoris. Muscle strains typically occur in the region of myotendinous junction, which is the weakest point of the muscle unit. MRI not only helps in diagnosing muscle strains but is also highly accurate in assessment of severity of muscle injury. In grade I strains, high signal is seen within the muscle because of edema and hemorrhage; however, there is no disruption of fibers. In grade II strains, there is partial tear of the muscle and the gap is filled with edema and hemorrhage. In grade III strains, there is complete tear with muscle retraction[14] (**Fig. 13.10**). Muscle denervation may be multifactorial, but MRI is useful for the assessment of nerve entrapment syndromes and compressive lesions, as well as nerve and nerve sheath tumors. Common nerve entrapment syndromes include suprascapular nerve entrapment in the shoulder (suprascapular nerve), carpal tunnel syndrome in the wrist (median nerve), and cubital tunnel syndrome in the elbow (ulnar nerve).

Other Considerations

Over the past decade dramatic improvements have occurred in MR scanning systems, pulse sequences, and high-resolution coil design. By using a technique called *MR neurography,* imaging of the peripheral nervous system can be performed reliably and quickly. In conjunction with electrophysiologic studies, the specific cause of peripheral nerve disorders can be anatomically localized and diagnosed. MRI has become the technique of choice for the evaluation of patients with malignancy or peripheral nerve masses (e.g., brachial and lumbosacral plexus tumors), nerve sheath tumors, and soft tissue tumors secondarily involving peripheral nerves. This technique is also used to evaluate previously mentioned nerve root compression and entrapment syndromes.

Vertebral compression fractures have a prevalence of 26% in women older than 50 years, and more than 84% of these injuries are associated with pain. Although many patients recover with conservative therapy, a significant number continue to have pain that is refractory to such measures. Traditional immobilization techniques, such as bed rest and bracing, may lead to a vicious cycle in which decreased activity leads to worsened bone density, with resultant fracture formation and more pain. Long-term consequences are physically and psychologically devastating and include physical deconditioning, difficulty breathing and sleeping, depression, and fear of further fracture. Imaging studies are used to guide performance of vertebral augmentation whether patients have acute or chronic fractures. Conventional radiography is helpful but not definitive, because many patients will have with multiple compression deformities. Therefore determining appropriate level(s) to treat on the basis of conventional radiography alone can be problematic. Positive results on scintigraphy are a strong predictor of clinical outcome after vertebroplasty to treat acute fractures, but up to 59% of untreated vertebral fractures are scintigraphically negative at 12 months. One of the strengths of MRI is its high sensitivity for bone marrow edema and the greater anatomic detail it demonstrates compared with conventional radiography or scintigraphy. Therefore MRI has become an important tool in the evaluation of patients before vertebral augmentation because of the combination of its sensitivity in detecting bone marrow edema and its multiplanar capabilities. Acute end plate changes demonstrate increased signal on T2-weighted/STIR images and low signal on T1-weighted images (**Fig. 13.11**). Chronic fractures are often isointense to fatty marrow on both sequences. Information obtained from MRI before vertebral augmentation also is valuable for the evaluation of canal compromise, vertebral body shape, determination of the residual height of the affected vertebral body

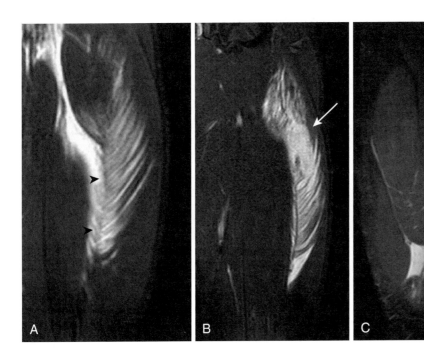

Fig. 13.10 Muscle strain. A, Grade I strain. "Feathery pattern" around the myofascial *plane (black arrowheads)* caused by tracking of fluid and hemorrhage around the muscle fibers. B, Grade II strain. Partial-thickness tear of vastus lateralis muscle. Gap in the muscle is filled with hemorrhage and fluid. C, Grade III strain. Rectus femoris muscle is completely torn with proximal retraction.

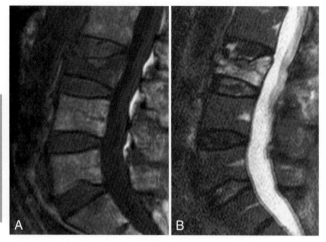

Fig. 13.11 Vertebral compression fracture. Sagittal T1-weighted (A) and sagittal STIR-weighted sequences (B) MR images. A vertebral wedge deformity is present in the L3 vertebra. The marrow signal shows diffuse edema reflecting a subacute unhealed painful fracture.

and identification of other vertebrae that are in the early stages of fracture or collapse.

Conclusion

MRI is the key imaging modality in diagnosis of multiple pathologic entities in the neurologic and musculoskeletal systems relating to pain. With its unparalleled soft tissue contrast, high-resolution imaging, and multiplanar capabilities, MRI is the optimal technique for evaluating structures in the brain and spine, as well as evaluating internal derangement of joints. With newer technologies, including higher field strength magnets and faster pulse sequences, previous limitations of the modality will undoubtedly be overcome and further augment the utility of MRI for the health care provider.

References

Full references for this chapter can be found on www.expertconsult.com.

Intervertebral Disk Stimulation Provocation Diskography

Milton H. Landers

The doctor enters a covenant with the patient; he penetrates his life, affecting his mode of living, often deciding his fate.

Abraham J. Heschel[1]

The diagnostic procedure often referred to as diskography in actuality consists of two separate and distinct components. The first part, diskography (i.e., a picture of the intervertebral disk), involves the injection of contrast medium into the nucleus pulposus of the intervertebral disk to study its internal morphology. This is a static test in which contrast is injected and radiographic images, fluoroscopic and computed tomography (CT), are obtained and evaluated. The second dynamic element of the procedure, the disk stimulation aspect, entails distention of the nucleus pulposus by the pressure produced by the injectate to determine whether a specific disk is involved in generating the patient's pain symptoms. In the most basic description, needles are placed within the intervertebral disks at multiple levels, and contrast material is injected into each disk to place a mechanical load on the disks. The response from the patient is then correlated with the index pain, low back, neck, or thoracic, as previously detailed by the patient and documented.

In the United States, low back pain is a serious individual and societal problem. Approximately 15% to 20% of the population suffers from low back pain each year and 80% over their lifetime. This entity is the second most common cause of lost work and physician visits. Although 90% of low back pain resolves after 6 weeks and another 5% after 12 weeks, approximately 5% will advance from an acute to a chronic condition. One percent of the U.S. population is chronically disabled by low back pain. Although chronic versus acute low back pain accounts for only 5% of cases, it is responsible for greater than 60% of the costs. Approximately $24 billion in medical and $50 billion in total societal costs are directly attributable to this condition.

Chronic neck pain, although somewhat less common than pain of the low back region, is frequently seen in clinical practice. A history of neck pain was noted in 35% to 80% of a population, depending on the group studied.[2-6] The prevalence of thoracic diskogenic pain has not been addressed in the literature.

Although two separate entities, axial pain of the low back or neck is often confused with radiculopathy or radicular pain. By definition, *radiculopathy* is a neurologic condition in which a conduction block of the motor or sensory axons is noted during physical examination. Radicular pain refers to pain originating from spinal nerves or their roots and is described as electrical, shooting, lancinating, and "band-like," with distal, rather than proximal, extremity pain.[7] In contrast, mechanical low back, or cervical, pain (i.e., referred somatic pain) is described as deep, dull, achy, and diffuse and is usually hard to localize. Lumbar radicular pain is associated with a herniated intervertebral disk about 98% of the time,[8] and cervical herniated intervertebral disks also account for cervical radicular pain in the great majority of cases.[9] However, low back pain is rarely associated with herniated disks,[10–13] although their supposed association is a common misconception.

The distinction between radicular and referred somatic pain having been made, we will now focus on the latter for the remainder of this chapter.

Chronic pain involving the cervical, thoracic, or lumbar regions is not a diagnosis; rather, it is a symptom usually attributable to pathology of the spine. It has been well documented that the three structures involved in the majority of chronic low back pain are the sacroiliac joint, the zygapophysial (facet) joints, and the intervertebral disk. Dismissing the sacroiliac joint, the cervical and thoracic segments of the spine are analogous. All of these structures are known to be innervated, have been shown to cause pain, are susceptible to injury or disease, known to be painful, and have been demonstrated to be the source of pain in the clinical setting. All are accompanied by deep, dull, achy low back pain often referred to the hips or buttocks, and physical examination is usually unable to differentiate between the three. The sacroiliac joint accounts for approximately 15% of cases of chronic low back pain,[14,15] and the zygapophysial joint is identified as the "pain generator" in approximately 15% of injured workers[16] and approximately 40% of older persons.[17] Diskogenic pain is known to be highly correlated with internal disk disruption involving extension of radial anular fissures into the outer third of the anulus fibrosus.[18]

Low back pain is a common and often debilitating condition that is frequently caused by pathology involving the intervertebral disk. As noted by Dr. Bogduk[19] in his classic text, "amongst patients with chronic low back pain, the prevalence of internal disc disruption is at least 39%."[20] This makes internal disk disruption the most common cause of chronic low back pain that can be objectively demonstrated, and provocation diskography is the only means of making the diagnosis.

Anatomy of the Intervertebral Disk

The juncture between adjacent vertebrae consists of a three-joint interface: two posterior synovial zygapophysial joints and an anterior intervertebral body joint. Teleologically, the intervertebral body joint requires a soft tissue spacer that allows for anterior-posterior rocking and rotational movement; in addition, this spacer must be deformable and strong enough to allow movement without injury and weight bearing without collapse.

The lumbar intervertebral disk consists of three components: the outer anulus fibrosus, the inner nucleus pulposus, and two cartilaginous vertebral end plates (**Fig. 14.1**). The two vertebral end plates of each intervertebral disk are situated within the ring apophysis of each vertebral body and are in contact with the entire nucleus pulposus but only the inner aspect of the anulus fibrosus. This structure is 0.6 to 1 mm thick and consists of hyaline cartilage and fibrocartilage. The end plates derive collagen fibers from the inner anulus fibrosus. These fibers provide a strong bond between the end plates and the anulus fibrosus, whereas the attachment of the end plates to the vertebral bodies is relatively weak.[21,22] The collagen fibers shared between the anulus fibrosus and the end plates form a capsule around the entire nucleus pulposus.

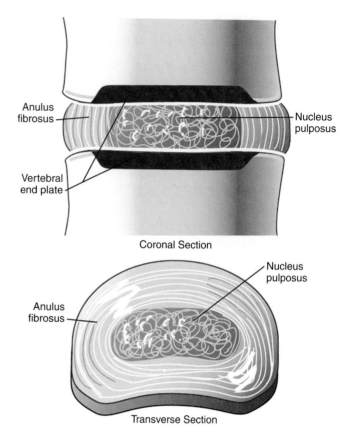

Fig. 14.1 Structure of the lumbar intervertebral disk.

The nucleus pulposus of the lumbar intervertebral disk is a viscous structure. Chemically, it is composed of 70% to 90% water, depending on age,[23–27] along with proteoglycans,[23,24] collagen,[23,28] elastic fibers, and noncollagenous proteins.[23,26,29–31] Being a viscous semifluid, the nucleus pulposus is freely deformable and noncompressible, with biomechanical pressure being transferred to the adjacent anulus fibrosus evenly in all directions.

The lumbar anulus fibrosus is composed of collagen fibers arranged in concentric rings of 10 to 20 lamellae (i.e., sheets), which results in an exceedingly strong ligamentous structure. Within each lamella the collagen fibers are parallel to each other, at approximately 65 degrees from the vertical, and extend between adjacent vertebral bodies. Neighboring lamellae alternate in the obliquity of the fibers between right and left. Although water is the major component of the anulus fibrosus,[23,24,26,27] with regard to dry weight, approximately 50% to 60% of the anulus fibrosus is composed of collagen,[23,26,29,32] with proteoglycans,[23] elastic fibers,[33–36] chondrocytes, and fibroblasts being represented in lesser amounts. Even though both the nucleus pulposus and anulus fibrosus are composed of the same biochemical components, water, collagen, proteoglycans, and other constituents, the proportions vary; specifically, the nucleus pulposus is proteoglycan rich, whereas the anulus fibrosus includes collagen as its major component.

The interface of the lumbar nucleus pulposus and anulus fibrosus is not a clearly delineated boundary. A transition zone, which increases with age, is present in which the inner anulus fibrosus and outer nucleus pulposus merge and take on the biochemical milieu and attributes of each other.[37]

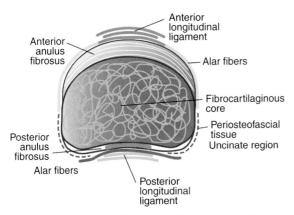

Fig. 14.2 Structure of the cervical intervertebral disk.

The cervical intervertebral disk is known to be distinct from its lumbar counterpart, although there is a relative paucity of literature regarding its unique qualities. At birth, the nucleus pulposus of the cervical intervertebral disk occupies less than 25% of the disk volume, as opposed to 50% in the lumbar levels.[38] After the third decade of life, marked fibrosis of the nucleus pulposus is seen,[39] and unlike the semifluid nucleus pulposus of the lumbar intervertebral disk, the cervical nucleus has a semisolid consistency resembling bar soap. To allow for and in response to cervical movement, fissures are seen originating at the uncovertebral joints and progressing medially into the nucleus pulposus. These clefts have been described as joints of Luschka, or uncovertebral recesses, and should be considered normal in mature individuals.[40–42]

An excellent study by Mercer and Bogduk[43] has documented the gross and microscopic morphology of the cervical intervertebral disk. In the cervical disk, the collagen fibers of the anulus fibrosus do not circumscribe the entire structure as in the lumbar spine. Rather, the anulus fibrosus is an anterior crescent-shaped structure, thick ventrally and tapering toward each uncinate and a small, discrete dorsal paramedian element. The fibers of the cervical anulus fibrosus do not form multiple distinct layers. The transitional fibers of the thin anterior superficial layer and the small posterior component are vertically oriented, whereas deeper fibers form an obliquely interwoven structure that becomes progressively embedded in the proteoglycan matrix of the nucleus pulposus. The posterior lateral aspect of the cervical intervertebral disk is unbounded by an anulus fibrosus and is contained only by fibers of the posterior longitudinal ligament (**Fig. 14.2**). In that the inner cervical intervertebral disk does not form a discrete nucleus as seen in the lumbar and thoracic levels, it might be more accurately referred to as the disk "core."

The thoracic intervertebral disk has been little studied. It is now known that the anatomy of the thoracic disk is somewhat reminiscent of the cervical rather than lumbar model down to the T9-10 level, at which point it adopts the morphology of the lumbar disk.[44]

The blood supply to the intervertebral disk is limited to small branches of the metaphyseal arteries, which penetrate only into the outer aspect of the anulus, and the capillary plexuses beneath the vertebral end plates.[45–48] Diffusion of nutrients through the vertebral end plates and anulus fibrosus allows only a low level of metabolic activity.

Although Roofe had reported the innervation of the anulus fibrosus and posterior longitudinal ligament in 1940,[49] other histologic studies indicated that the intervertebral disk was devoid of nerve endings[50–52] and was reported to lack innervation.[53–55] It is now known that the outer third of the anulus fibrosus is not only innervated but contains a wide variety of simple and complex neural structures[56–60] derived from branches of the sinuvertebral nerves, gray rami communicantes, and lumbar ventral rami.[56,58,59,61] Histochemical studies have shown that the neural tissue present in the intervertebral disk contains peptides specific to nociceptive neural elements.[62,63] Physiologic changes are known to occur in a painful intervertebral disk, including nerve ingrowth into the usually aneural inner anulus,[64] and an increase in nerve growth factor has been demonstrated in painful versus asymptomatic intervertebral disks.[65,66]

Several possible physiologic mechanisms for the production of pain in the intervertebral disk have been postulated. Although mechanical stress across the anulus has been proposed,[61] an inflammatory mechanism appears likely.[67] The nucleus of the intervertebral disk is known to have a low pH[68] and contains a multitude of inflammatory enzymes.[56,69–71] These chemicals, when released secondary to injury or disk degradation, are thought to sensitize neural structures within and in close proximity to the disk.

Therefore the intervertebral disk is innervated, subject to pathology, and known to contain chemicals that produce painful inflammatory responses. Can diskography pinpoint pathology and lead to a diagnosis of pain arising from a suspect intervertebral disk?

Historical Considerations

Diskography has a history that can be more completely appreciated by an understanding of its introduction, and subsequent development, in the context of the prevailing concept of co-evolving knowledge, techniques, and other aspects of medical science in a number of other fields, including pain anatomy and physiology of the intervertebral disk in terms of disk pathology and nociception, the development of myelographic contrast material, and the introduction of advanced imaging techniques, including CT and magnetic resonance imaging (MRI).

During its development, diskography has achieved some notoriety as a "controversial" technique but has subsequently become a standard for the evaluation of certain conditions of the spinal intervertebral disks that cannot otherwise be diagnosed by any other contemporary approach.

Schmorl and Junghans,[72] as referenced in their later work, laid the basis for clinical diskography in their voluminous and pioneering work on the pathology of the intervertebral disk, published in monograph form in 1932. They reported their examination of 10,000 cadaveric spines in which the partially dissected spines were radiographed en bloc; they subsequently completed the dissection and noted the radiographic/pathologic correlations. In many of these specimens they injected red lead into the disk before radiographs, which allowed the first analysis of diskographic morphology. This study led to the terms *protrusion* and *rupture* of the intervertebral disk and introduced diskography as an anatomic study to evaluate the internal structure of the cadaveric disk. Their work also described the progression from radial tear to rupture.

Mixter and Barr's landmark paper in 1934,[73] in which a surgical cure for radiculopathy secondary to a herniated nucleus pulposus was reported, heralded a new era in spinal surgery and led to renewed interest in techniques for diagnosis.

In the late 1930s and early 1940s, lumbar spine diagnostics consisted almost solely of plain film radiographs and myelography. During that period, myelography, which involves placement of contrast within the intrathecal space, was an extremely painful procedure that required general anesthesia. Technical limitations of myelography continue to this day, and are many, including visualization of only the effect of a lesion (i.e., compression of the dura) rather than direct visualization, and imaging limited to the central portion of the spinal canal.

Even though Lindgren reported injection of a normal disk with parabrodil in 1941,[74] fear of injuring disks in a report by Pease[75] in 1935 held up the first clinical trials in humans. It was not until Hirsch[76] showed that the disk was not damaged when injected that clinical studies of diskography became more widespread.

In an attempt to provide diagnostic clarity to the analysis of patients with back and leg pain and to directly visualize the pathology of the intervertebral disk, Dr. Kirk Lindblom[77] was influenced to develop a technique to directly visualize the lumbar intervertebral disks as a clinical examination for investigation of patients with suspected disk pathology. He published a series of papers describing his technique and results and provided the first clinical correlation to the observations.[78-81]

Among other innovations that Lindblom described was a dual-needle approach to the lower disks, albeit this was a transarachnoid (i.e., interpedicular), direct radiographic analysis of both degeneration and herniation, along with the demonstration of fissures directly communicating with the epidural and perineural spaces.[78] Even in the earliest papers, he described disk stimulation and the correlation of pain provocation during disk injection and the patient's symptomatology as a valuable aspect of diskography. This was corroborated by Hirsch,[76] who reported provocation of pain in 16 patients by injection of saline into the disk. Lindblom also advanced the concept that herniations could become asymptomatic with conservative care and the new concept that posterolateral herniations are important to the clinical syndrome of leg pain,[82] although myelography is often insensitive to this pathology.

Further work documenting that disk puncture was not damaging in animals[83] or human cadavers[84,85] was followed by the first report of diskography in the United States by Wise and Weiford in 1951.[86] However, in a recent paper, Carragee et al[87] provide evidence that diskography may not be as benign as has been previously believed.

In 1952, Erlacher performed cadaveric studies to document the accuracy with which the contrast dispersal pattern defined the nuclear space and found complete agreement between the radiographic and the gross dispersal patterns in 200 disks.[88] Cloward, also in 1952, reported on the technique and indications for lumbar diskography.[89]

In his 1960 monograph, Fernstrom[90] reviewed the then current literature. He noted that back and leg pain can occur regardless of whether nerve root compression is present. He also advanced the concept that there are both neurogenic (mechanical compressive) and diskogenic (biochemical irritative) causes for the symptoms.

Early authorities embraced diskography, both lumbar and cervical, as a technique in the diagnosis of disk herniation,[88,89,91-103] including reports of enhanced surgical results when using diskography as a preoperative assessment tool.[104,105]

Hartjes et al[106] compared diskography and myelography and concluded that indications for diskography included specific radiculopathy and a normal myelogram or symptoms with multiple myelographic defects. Some found it superior to oil-contrast myelography,[93,96,107] but others disagreed and thought that lumbar diskography should be reserved for the investigation of unusual or atypical cases.[108]

Although the development and deployment of minimally toxic contrast agents made myelography much safer,[109,110] this technique continued to have the inherent weakness of assessing the effect of lesions in the spine on the dural sac rather than direct visualization of the lesion. In addition, it did not provide the information regarding the reproduction of concordant pain as initiated by disk stimulation that diskography provides.

The development of high-quality CT scanning[111] permitted not only direct visualization of the anatomy in cross section[112] and direct diagnosis of disk herniation,[113] but also supplementary information when myelographic contrast was used.[114-117] The development of CT also enhanced the diagnostic capabilities of diskography. In 1987, Videman et al[118] reported the valuable additional information gained by performing postdiskography CT in 103 cadaveric disks.

The emergence of MRI[119] in 1984 provided noninvasive characterization of a variety of disk lesions[120] and extradural[121] pathology, and it has become the primary modality for diagnosing pathology of the spine. Although MRI provides high spatial and contrast resolution, biochemical diagnostic information has led to further knowledge regarding the pathophysiology of disk disorders,[122,123] and MRI (although quite effective in the detection of disk degeneration)[124-126] does not provide evidence of pain with mechanical stress.

Despite this major advance in the ability to visualize anatomy and tissue characteristics, MRI was still found to be less sensitive than diskography in detecting tears and fissures,[127] although gadolinium enhancement may be of assistance.[128] There was also the problem of normal MRI and abnormal diskography findings.[129,130] Even though these new imaging technologies (i.e., CT and MRI) have helped,[131] they do not tell us whether the pathoanatomy is symptomatic.

The relationship of pain to disk rupture and nerve compression began with Mixter and Barr in 1934.[73] However, as a pathophysiologic lesion, the concept of compression of neural structures has never been sufficient to explain the majority of back pain.[132-134]

A number of authors have described lesions associated with severe pain without neural compression, including painful posterior fissures,[135] acute traumatic interosseous herniation,[136] isolated intervertebral disk resorption,[137] and painful lumbar end plate disruption.[138]

During the ensuing years, the technique used for diskography has undergone certain additional refinements, such as provocation-analgesic diskography[139] and manometry, as introduced by Derby in 1993, that have led to the refinement of the obtained data.[140,141]

The use of cervical diskography for the evaluation of patients with neck, head, and shoulder pain was reported almost simultaneously in the late 1950s by Smith and Nichols[142] and Cloward.[143] Both reports emphasized that stimulation of the disk was a vital aspect of the procedure and used cervical diskography to help in choosing the correct level for surgical procedures.[144,145] The similarities in their work included the basic concept that abnormal disks could exactly reproduce the patient's symptoms, that there was a high incidence of abnormal disks, and that diskography had specific value in differentiating neurogenic from somatic diskogenic pain.[146] The literature has continued to provide evidence of the usefulness of cervical diskography for diagnosis and planning of surgical procedures.[101,102,104,147]

Analgesic diskography, in which local anesthetic is injected into the disk to relieve pain at the level thought to be positive by provocation diskography, has been shown to be of value for diagnosis and staging for cervical procedures.[148] Kofoed[149] used this technique to differentiate thoracic disk pain from thoracic outlet syndrome.

Lumbar and cervical diskography has a long history of providing accurate information about whether the intervertebral disk is a source of pain. By extrapolation it is thought that in a like manner, the thoracic disk can be a significant pain generator. Schellhas et al[150] described a safe technique to access the thoracic intervertebral disk, as well as its role in patient evaluation.[151]

Diskography has become the "gold standard" for the diagnosis of cervical, thoracic, and lumbar diskogenic pain and has established an important position within the diagnostic armamentarium of the spine physician.

Validation of Diskography

Mechanical stimulation of the intervertebral disk has long been known to produce low back pain.[152] However, the use of diskography for detection of clinically painful disks has not been without a certain degree of controversy, which continues to the present day. The enthusiasm of certain early proponents waned,[153] and others questioned its value.[154–157]

Because all interventional procedures are associated with a certain rate of morbidity, if pain secondary to intrinsic intervertebral disk pathology (i.e., diskogenic pain) could be diagnosed by physical examination or imaging studies, invasive provocation diskography would not be indicated. Physical examination has been shown to be unreliable in differentiating low back pain generated from intervertebral disks as distinct from other pain generators.[158,159] Except for a "high-intensity zone" in the area of the posterior anulus on T2-weighted MRI images, which appears to have low sensitivity (28%) but high specificity (86%),[160] there are no specific findings on imaging studies that can be used to differentiate diskogenic from other mechanical sources of pain.[161] Carragee et al[162] have questioned the diagnostic value of the "high-intensity zone," and its prevalence in the asymptomatic population has yet to be determined with accuracy.

For any diagnostic test to be of value, the false-positive rate must be low. In that diskography is a test in which provocation of symptoms is assessed, asymptomatic volunteers should have close to zero positive responders. Unfortunately, some reports, though often based on suspect methodology, have led to questions involving the specificity of diskography in diagnosing diskogenic pain.

The most infamous opposition opinion to the validity of lumbar diskography was by Holt.[163] This 1968 study of inmates at an Illinois state prison reported a high false-positive rate

in a group of asymptomatic volunteers. Multiple flaws are to be found in Holt's methods, including a suspect population of asymptomatic "volunteers," technical competence of the author, and the use of a highly irritating contrast agent. Although criticized immediately, this report was ultimately answered by Simmons et al,[164] who provided a compelling argument why it should not be used as scientific or authoritative evidence against the use of diskography. Walsh et al[165] reproduced Holt's experimental design, with the exception of (1) using nonsuspect subjects; (2) having a single, technically skilled diskographer; (3) utilizing a lateral, "modern," extrapedicular approach; and (4) using nonirritating contrast medium. No positive painful disks were found in the asymptomatic group of volunteers, in contrast to the symptomatic group, in whom high correlation was evident between pain reproduction and pathologic disk morphology.

In an excellent series of papers,[166–168] Eugene Carragee and colleagues indicated that lumbar diskography is associated with a high false-positive rate, up to 75%. However, in a reanalysis of the data as presented by Nikolai Bogduk[169] that took into account the psychiatric history of the volunteers, manometric data, and other criteria as published by the International Association for the Study of Pain (IASP),[170] and the International Spine Intervention Society (ISIS),[1] the false-positive rate dropped to a very low, acceptable level. Because diskography is dependent on a subjective patient response, it is no surprise that questionable Minnesota Multiphasic Personality Inventory (MMPI) scores and any psychological overlay, such as somatization, hypochondriasis, hysteria, and depression, are correlated with overreporting of pain during diskography.[171]

One possible measure of the validity of diskography lies in its predictive value with regard to surgical outcomes. Over the years, when stringent criteria are met, lumbar diskography has been shown to be a good predictor of surgical outcome.[141,172] Colhoun et al[173] used very rigid criteria for evaluating clinical benefit from surgery and noted that in patients with abnormal-appearing disks, 89% of those with a positive diskogram had a positive surgical outcome whereas only 52% of those with a negative diskogram benefited in a significant manner. However, any treatment modality, including surgery, cannot be held to be the "gold standard" for evaluation of any diagnostic procedure unless the specific surgical procedure has been shown to be 100% effective.

In the cervical spine, pathology, as detected by imaging studies, should be considered the norm and cannot predict neck pain. Gore et al[174] used plain film radiography and noted abnormal studies in 70% at age 60, whereas Boden et al[175] performed MRI and reported major or minor abnormalities that could produce pain in 97% of asymptomatic individuals. Although morphologically normal disks on MRI were never painful with diskography, significant anular disruptions were often missed and MRI cannot reliably indicate the source of cervical diskogenic pain.[176] Injuries to the cervical spine were often found at autopsy when previous imaging was normal,[177] thus indicating low sensitivity with routine testing. In numerous papers going back to the late 1960s,[102,104,139,147,178–183] preoperative cervical diskography has been shown to be an excellent predictor of successful outcomes (70% to 90%), as opposed to cervical fusions performed without the benefit of this diagnostic procedure (39% to 50%).

Wood et al[151] performed thoracic diskography on 10 symptomatic and 10 asymptomatic volunteers. In the asymptomatic group, although 3 of the 40 disks stimulated produced significant pain, this discomfort was unfamiliar and nonconcordant and would be classified as a negative response during diagnostic diskography. In contrast, in the symptomatic group, 24 of the 48 disks injected produced marked concordant pain reminiscent of the patient's usual symptoms.

Although the rate of false-positive results with diskography continues to be a legitimate concern, most well-designed studies have substantiated the procedure's diagnostic credibility. The ISIS,[3] the North American Spine Society (NASS),[184] and the Physiatric Association of Spine, Sports, and Occupational Rehabilitation (PASSOR)[185] have all indicated that diskography is an appropriate diagnostic procedure that has value in clinical situations, if performed correctly and interpreted in the context of the totality of the patient's pertinent clinical information.

Physician Training

It is imperative that all physicians performing all other fluoroscopically guided spinal injections, including diskography, have training in the interpretation of real-time fluoroscopic imaging whether cervical, thoracic, lumbar, or sacral. This training must be beyond the level of any residency and most current so-called pain fellowships. Expertise in radiologic interpretation is far beyond the training and proficiency of certified registered nurse anesthetists (CRNAs), physician assistants (PAs), and other so-called midlevel nonphysician providers. Performance of interventional pain procedures constitutes the practice of medicine as noted by at least one judicial body within the United States,[186] and numerous medical specialty societies including the American Medical Association,[187] the ISIS,[188] the American Society of Interventional Pain Physicians,[189] and the American Society of Anesthesiologists.[190] It is the responsibility of the referring physician, whether surgeon or primary care, and the medical facility where the procedure is performed to ensure that that the patient is receiving competent care by a physician who is trained in nonsurgical spine procedures and practicing the specialty of interventional pain using standard-of-care procedural techniques.

Patient Selection

Indications

"Indications for a diagnostic disk puncture [are] long standing sciatica, which was not improved by conservative treatment and which was myelographed by abrodil without definite localization of the disk protrusion."[78]

Much has changed in regard to the diagnosis and treatment of spinal pain since Lindblum proposed the above passé indication for injection into the intervertebral disk. With the advent of CT and MRI, diskography is no longer indicated for diagnosis of radicular pain, sciatica, and elucidation of the external disk morphology. MRI and CT imaging will rule out the so-called red flag conditions of tumor, infection, and fracture, but cannot diagnose the cause of low back pain in the majority of patients. Images, no matter how sophisticated, are just pictures and although they can provide clues as to the origin of the pain, they do not pinpoint a specific pain generator.

Diskography is indicated to diagnose somatic, chronic low back pain with or without referral, and will determine whether one or more specific disks are painful in regard to the patient's pain complaint. In that for the majority of patients the natural history of low back pain evidences improvement and resolution within 3 months, diskography before this time period should be rarely considered and only for specific extraordinary cases. In the past, diskography has been thought of as a preliminary tool to verify that surgery is indicated, but nothing can be farther from the truth. Although many in the United States who are shown to have a positive diskogram do undergo surgical procedures, this is a consequence of social norms, unrealistic patient expectations and insistence, economic variables, medical referral patterns, and the proclivity of some surgeons toward highly invasive procedures. Much as a diagnosis of a malignant carcinoma is sought if suspected whether or not surgery will be indicated, so diskography provides a diagnosis, not the presumption and expectation that any specific treatment modality must follow. At the present time treatments for diskogenic pain are limited, but new technologies including minimally invasive procedures and injectable therapies are being given a high priority, and hopefully will see fruition in the coming years.

Diskography must not be performed for capricious, unjustifiable reasons. For idiopathic low back pain, a well-thought-out algorithm must be used. ISIS has published such an algorithm based on the best evidence available.[191] If a surgeon has planned a surgical procedure at a specific level and there is a question as to whether adjacent intervertebral disks are contributing to the pain complaint, consideration of diskography would be appropriate to determine the condition of these disks.

Although significant objective information can be derived from diskography, the procedure is not only operator dependent, but also requires input from the subject. To proceed with any expectation of accurate data, the patient must understand the basic tenets of the procedure, be able to comply with instructions, and cooperate in order to provide meaningful responses to the ongoing disk stimulation.

Contraindications

Absolute contraindications to the performance of diskography at any level include the following: (1) the patient being unable or unwilling to consent to the procedure; (2) inability to assess the patient's response to the procedure, including sedation, significant analgesic use, or psychiatric overlay; (3) significant localized or systemic infection; and (4) pregnancy. Relative contraindications include (1) anticoagulant therapy or bleeding diathesis; (2) allergy to radiographic contrast, local anesthetic, or antibiotic; and (3) anatomic derangements that would compromise the safe and successful conduct of the procedure.

In regard to cervical diskography, further contraindications exist. Because of the possibility of iatrogenic quadriplegia, an anteroposterior (AP) spinal canal diameter of less than 10 mm is an absolute contraindication, and an AP diameter of less than 11 mm constitutes a relative contraindication, to the performance of cervical diskography at the specific or adjacent levels. In a male patient, a beard, depending on style, can make sterile preparation of the skin and injection field difficult, if not impossible; therefore facial hair is a possible contraindication to cervical diskography.

The Technique of Diskography

Preprocedure and Periprocedure Considerations

Before disk puncture, cervical, thoracic, or lumbar, a medical history and physical examination must be performed to ensure that there are no contraindications to performing diskography and the patient is an appropriate candidate for the procedure. If intravenous sedation is to be used, nothing-by-mouth (NPO) status is verified to conform to institutional guidelines. In females of childbearing age, pregnancy must be ruled out.

Any allergies to non-ionic water-soluble contrast media (iohexol or iopamidol) or other drugs used must be ascertained. If allergies are present, the risks versus benefits of the procedure must be weighed and discussed with the patient. Pretreatment regimens for allergies can be considered, including the use of corticosteroids and H_1 and H_2 blockers. If the risk for an allergic reaction to contrast is significant, the use of saline for the provocation aspect of the procedure can be considered. The use of gadolinium in place of iodinated contrast has been discussed in the literature.[192,193]

Informed consent is obtained with regard to the purpose of, risks and complications inherent in, and alternatives to the procedure. A discussion with the patient concerning the nature of diskography, specifically, the pain provocation aspect, is of the utmost importance. It is imperative that the patient be made aware that the procedure is potentially painful and that during stimulation of the disk, a description of this discomfort in terms of concordance and intensity as compared with the patient's ongoing complaint will be required.

Intravenous access is obtained before the procedure. Because diskitis (i.e., intradiskal infection) is the most common though rare complication, prophylactic antibiotic (cefazolin, 1 g; gentamicin, 80 mg; clindamycin, 900 mg; or ciprofloxacin, 400 mg) is administered intravenously within 30 minutes of needle insertion. Aminoglycosides are not indicated for preprocedure prophylaxis.[194] In sheep studies, Fraser et al[195] noted antibiotic levels in the anulus 30 minutes after intravenous administration, but none was demonstrated at 60 minutes. In addition to intravenous antibiotics, it has long been advocated that antibiotics be mixed with the contrast injected into the disk.[2,196–198] Klessig et al[198] note that cefazolin and gentamicin, 1 mg/mL, and clindamycin, 7.5 mg/mL, exceed the minimum inhibitory concentrations for the three most common organisms implicated in diskitis, *Escherichia coli*, *Staphylococcus aureus*, and *Staphylococcus epidermidis*.

Many patients experience varying degrees of anxiety and discomfort before and during diskography. Intravenous sedation enables the patient to tolerate the procedure and allows the physician to work on a physically quiet subject. For the vast majority of patients, intravenous midazolam has been shown to be quite effective in providing sedation during diskography in doses between 2.0 and 4.0 mg. In addition, this versatile medication often renders the patient amnestic of the procedure. The ultrashort-acting hypnotic propofol is used by some injectionists who have an anesthesia background. This medication enables the practitioner to render the patient unconscious during the needle insertion portion of the study but awaken the patient rapidly for the provocation part of the procedure. However, this author questions the safety of performing any spinal injection on an unconscious, nonresponsive subject as rendered by propofol. All medications used for sedation must be titrated to effect as per patient response. The ability of the patient to tolerate the procedure, while being oriented and conversant, is mandatory. The possibility of oversedation and respiratory depression must be considered. Adequate monitoring, in addition to competence by the physician in airway management and resuscitation, is a minimum requirement.

Although controversial, the author feels that analgesic medications should not be administered routinely before or during diskography. Provocation diskography is a study in which a mechanical load is placed on individual intervertebral disks, and any pain produced must be analyzed by the patient with regard to whether it reproduces the patient's index (i.e., familiar and accustomed) pain. In addition, the intensity of the pain produced needs to be quantified in terms of the patient's usual pain level in regard to a visual or oral analog scale. The validity of the test is based on the patient's response to disk pressurization (i.e., pain provocation). Therefore analgesics, which by definition attenuate the pain response, are contraindicated because their use precludes accurate assessment of the provoked pain by the patient. When analgesics are used, a higher percent of false-negative outcomes would be expected.

Diskography can be performed in any procedure room appropriate for aseptic procedures. Safety concerns require imaging equipment that provides good visualization of the relevant spinal anatomy. This aspect is critically important when performing cervical or thoracic procedures. The ability to view the spine in anteroposterior (AP), lateral, and oblique views is mandatory. Although biplane fluoroscopy has been used, this must be considered as passé. Today, C-arm fluoroscopic units are the imaging tool of choice. The ability to obtain many fluoroscopic views without repositioning the patient makes the use of a quality C-arm safe and efficient. C-arms, which can be rotated into the contralateral oblique view to greater than 50 degrees, allow disk entry from either side. Also required is a radiolucent procedure table, without metal side rails, that can be raised and lowered as needed. Monitoring equipment should include pulse oximetry, a noninvasive blood pressure device, and electrocardiography. Oxygen, airway supplies, drugs, and suction and other resuscitation equipment and supplies should be immediately available. Adequate personnel to monitor the patient and operate the fluoroscope are required.

Sterile technique requires preparation of the skin and draping analogous to that used for surgery. Ten percent povidone-iodine (Betadine solution) or DuraPrep (0.7% iodophor and 74% isopropyl alcohol), or both, is the preparation of choice. If the patient indicates allergies to these preparations, chlorhexidine and alcohol can be safely substituted. Standard draping is used to provide a sterile field and may include the use of sterile towels and fenestrated drapes as per the injectionist's preference. The procedure room staff should be dressed in clean clothes (scrub suits). Masks and surgical caps are mandated for anyone coming in close proximity to the sterile field. The vast majority of injectionists elect to scrub, gown, and glove as for an open surgical procedure. The C-arm image intensifier requires a sterile cover to prevent detritus from falling on the sterile field.

Before commencing with the diskography procedure, the levels to be injected, be they lumbar, thoracic, or cervical, must be selected. This selection is based on the results of physical examination, imaging studies, and the history (pain referral pattern). At the least, the most likely level and the two adjoining levels should be included. Rarely is it necessary to inject more than four segments. When simulating the disks, the patient is blinded regarding the onset and level being stimulated.

Lumbar Diskography Technique

As with all spinal injections, positioning of the patient facilitates the procedure in that it allows good visualization of the target structure, thereby providing easy, precise, and safe access. As noted earlier, most injectionists use a C-arm because of the ability to move the C-arm to obtain various views rather than repositioning the patient. Although the following description assumes C-arm use, modifications in patient positioning can be made by the operator to facilitate performance of the procedure using the less appropriate biplanar fluoroscope.

Historically, before the late 1960s, disk puncture was performed via a posterior (i.e., interpedicular or transdural) approach. This technique is little used today because of the complications that are inevitable with any puncture of the dura. A lateral, or extrapedicular, approach[199,200] is now used, except in rare situations.

The patient is placed in a prone position on the radiolucent procedure table with a pillow or other material under the abdomen to slightly flex the spine and decrease the normal lumbar lordotic curve. Monitoring is initiated and prophylactic antibiotic and light sedation provided. The lower thoracic, lumbar, and sacral regions are prepared and draped as discussed previously.

The target disk is identified with an AP view. The image intensifier of the C-arm is then tilted in a cephalocaudad direction until the subchondral end plate of the vertebral body, caudad to the target disk, is parallel to the x-ray beam. The subchondral plate will be seen as a line rather than an oval. To ensure against the patient mistaking the discomfort from needle placement for provoked pain secondary to disk stimulation, the disk is preferentially approached from the opposite side of the patient's usual pain. In cases in which the pain is central or bilaterally equal, anatomic variation is present, or equipment limitations prevent disk puncture from the contralateral side of the pain, needle insertion from either side is appropriate.

After squaring of the end plate, the C-arm is rotated toward the side of needle insertion into an oblique view until the tip of the superior articular process of the level below appears to lie under the midpoint of the subchondral plate of the inferior end plate of the disk above (**Figs. 14.3A and 14.4A**). Such positioning of the fluoroscope allows needles to be passed via "tunnel vision" (i.e., parallel to the beam of the fluoroscope when the skin puncture site is aligned with the target structure), just lateral to the superior articular process (see Figs. 14.3A and 14.4A). The needle will travel under the segmental nerve (see Figs. 14.3B and 14.4B), which courses medial to lateral and dorsal to ventral, and will puncture the anulus fibrosus of the disk at the midpoint of the disk when seen in lateral and AP views.

Once the oblique view as just described is obtained, the skin overlying the target is marked (see Figs. 14.3A and 14.4A). A skin wheal is made with a 25-gauge, 1.5-inch needle using 1% lidocaine (1 to 2 mL). A 25- or 22-gauge, 3.5-inch needle is then advanced, via "tunnel vision" (i.e., parallel to the x-ray beam), to the level of the superior articular process, and lidocaine (~5 mL) is injected while withdrawing the needle to create an anesthetized tract. Care must be taken with slender individuals to ensure that local anesthetic is not placed within the foramen. If a foraminal injection were to occur, the segmental nerve might be anesthetized to such an extent that the forthcoming disk puncture needle might impale the nerve and cause lasting dysesthesia after the procedure. In addition, local anesthetic within the foramen might anesthetize the innervation of the disk (i.e., the sinuvertebral and ramus communicans nerves), which would alter the discomfort perceived during disk stimulation and possibly result in a false-negative response.

At this juncture, the injectionist can choose either a one- or two-needle technique. Before the routine administration of prophylactic antibiotics,[201] the rate of diskitis with the use of single needles without stylets was reported to be 2.7%, as opposed to 0.7% when a double-needle technique with stylets was used. In a technique involving the use of a single styletted

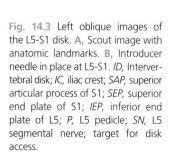

Fig. 14.3 Left oblique images of the L5-S1 disk. A, Scout image with anatomic landmarks. B, Introducer needle in place at L5-S1. *ID*, Intervertebral disk; *IC*, iliac crest; *SAP*, superior articular process of S1; *SEP*, superior end plate of S1; *IEP*, inferior end plate of L5; *P*, L5 pedicle; *SN*, L5 segmental nerve; target for disk access.

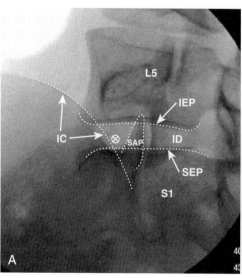

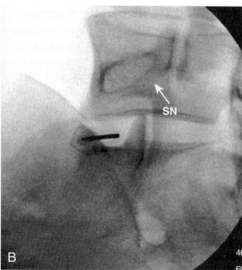

needle, Aprill[197] has reported one case of diskitis in approximately 2000 patients (≈0.05% per patient). Both NASS[184] and ISIS[2] recommend a two-needle approach.

The two-needle technique involves the use of a shorter, larger-gauge introducer needle through which a longer, smaller-gauge needle is advanced past the tip of the introducer needle into the targeted intervertebral disk. The introducer needles are 18 or 22 gauge, 3.5 or 5 inches long, whereas complementary disk puncture needles are 22 or 25 gauge and 6 or 8 inches long. The body habitus of the patient dictates the combination of needles used at each level. Both the introducer and the disk puncture needles should have stylets to prevent skin from being picked up and introduced into, or in close proximity to, the disk. The author advocates that a slight bend, opposite the bevel, be placed at the tip of the disk puncture needle to enable the operator to control the course of (i.e., "steer") the needle during advancement.[202–205]

The introducer needle is passed through the skin wheal at the skin puncture point via a down-the-beam, "tunnel vision"

technique toward the disk entry site. Forward advancement is stopped at the approximate level of the superior articular process, although placement within, or slightly dorsal to, the foramen is acceptable. An AP view with the fluoroscope will indicate the needle tip lying at the lateral extent of the intervertebral disk (**Fig. 14.5A**), whereas a lateral view is used to check needle depth (**Fig. 14.5B**). The stylet is removed from the introducer, and the longer, smaller-gauge disk puncture needle is advanced slowly under active lateral fluoroscopy. The needle will be seen to traverse the intervertebral foramen, and firm resistance will be noted as the needle touches and enters the anulus fibrosus.

Because the ventral ramus crosses the posterolateral aspect of the disk in close proximity to the disk entry site, if radicular pain or dysesthesia is noted by the patient at any point during advancement of the needles, insertion of the needle is stopped, the needle is partially withdrawn, and the course is altered and redirected toward the disk. As discussed, a slight bend on the tip of the disk puncture needle facilitates this change in direction. If more aggressive direction changes are required, the introducer needle can be withdrawn and redirected as well. Contact with the segmental nerve occurs rarely, and if the operator notes this with any frequency, the technique used for disk access and anatomic knowledge needs be questioned.

After contacting the anulus, the disk puncture needle should be advanced under active lateral fluoroscopy into the center of the disk (i.e., into the nucleus pulposus). Because the outer third of the anulus is abundantly supplied with nerve endings, some axial discomfort, with referral into the thigh or buttock, may be felt by the patient. AP and lateral projections are used to ensure good needle placement, with spot images saved for documentation before injection of contrast (**Fig. 14.6**).

Although the technique just presented can be used for disk puncture in more than 95% of lumbar disk levels, occasionally, because of anatomic variations (i.e., overriding iliac crest, osteophytes) or postsurgical changes (i.e., a posterior intertransverse fusion mass or fusion hardware), variations in the procedure must be implemented. A detailed description of the myriad modifications with which an injectionist might

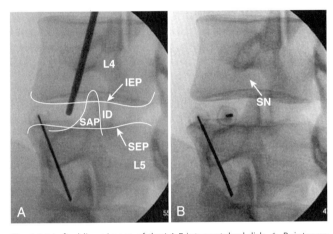

Fig. 14.4 Left oblique image of the L4-5 intervertebral disk. **A,** Pointer on skin over target. **B,** Introducer needle in place at L4-5. Note the insertion angle of the L5-S1 needle as compared to that of L4-5. *ID,* Intervertebral disk; *SAP,* superior articular process of L5; *IEP,* inferior end plate of L4; *SEP,* superior end plate of L5; *SN,* L4 segmental nerve.

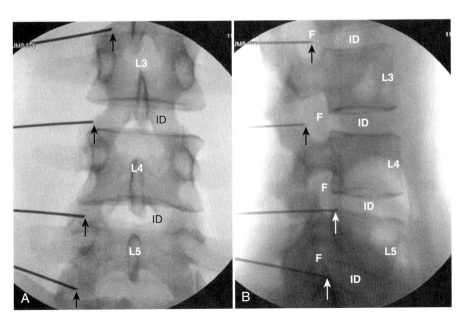

Fig. 14.5 Anterior-posterior (**A**) and lateral (**B**) images of the lumbar spine with introducer needles in place at L2-3, L3-4, L4-5 and L5-S1. *ID,* Intervertebral disk; *F,* foramina. *Arrows* indicate the tips of introducer needles dorsal and lateral to the disks.

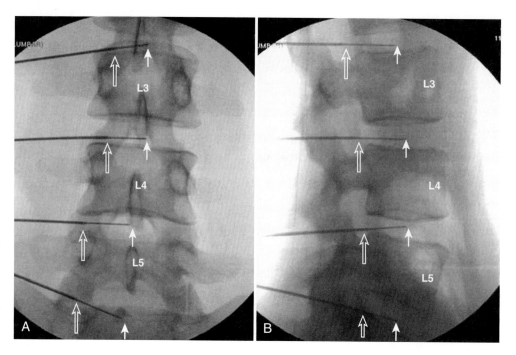

Fig. 14.6 Images of the lumbar spine with introducer needles in place. **A,** Anteroposterior (AP) image. **B,** Lateral image. *Black arrows* indicate tips of the disk puncture needles in the center of the disks; *open arrows* indicate tips of introducer needles dorsal and lateral to disks.

be faced is beyond the scope of this chapter; however, most involve either a more lateral or more medial needle insertion with the disk puncture needle bent or curved to varying degrees (**Fig. 14.7**).

Rarely, the posterior interpedicular, transdural approach must be used to gain access to the disk. This approach increases the chance of morbidity because the dura is twice punctured. The risks and benefits of this technique must be weighed. At levels above the L2-3 intervertebral disk, the posterior approach should not be used because the chance of impaling the spinal cord is high.

Once all needles are positioned within the nucleus pulposus of the disks to be stimulated, injection can proceed. The patient should be blinded with regard to the disk level and initiation of the injection. At this point, the patient must be conversant in order to describe any sensations produced by stimulation of the disk.

Only non-ionic contrast agents safe for myelography (iohexol or iopamidol), and added antibiotic should be used.[198] Under active fluoroscopy, as the injectate is slowly instilled into the disk opening pressure of the disk is exceeded and contrast is seen to flow into the disk nucleus. As the nucleus is filled, the height of the disk space is known to increase rather than the axial cross-sectional area.[206] Pressure is applied slowly, in 0.5 aliquots, until one of four end points is noted: a 3.5 mL volume has been attained, significant pain is noted by the patient, an epidural or vascular pattern is evident, or a maximum pressure of 75 to 100 psi has been reached.[165,207]

During pressurization of the disk, parameters of the injection are recorded on a standardized form by procedure room personnel. The disk level, volume injected, pressure generated, pain description (none, nonconcordant, concordant), vocal or physical patient pain responses, and pain intensity are the minimum required. Images, AP and lateral, of all disks injected must be saved for a permanent record of the study. These images should include AP and lateral both before (see Fig. 14.6) and after (**Fig. 14.8**) contrast administration.

Although a 3 mL syringe has provided good results in the past, most experienced, well-versed diskographers now advocate the use of a manometer to accurately quantify the opening pressure and the pressure generated during disk injection. Derby et al[141] have shown a correlation between surgical outcome and the pressure at which concordant pain is noted by the patient during disk stimulation. The opening pressure in supine patients, at levels known to be without anular disruption, is 20 to 25 psi, whereas disks with anular disruption often have opening pressures of less than 15 psi.[140] Disks that when injected elicit positive concordant pain at less than 15 psi above opening pressure (30 to 40 psi end pressure) are said to be chemically sensitive and have a better prognosis after combined interbody/intertransverse fusion than after intertransverse fusion alone. Pauza et al[208] supported this concept in their study of intradiskal anular thermal lesioning. Patients who experience concordant pain with disk pressures between 15 and 50 psi above opening pressure (30 to 75 psi end pressure) are said to have an intermediate response, whereas a positive response above 50 psi (65 to 75 psi) is not considered clinically significant.[1] With a 3 mL syringe it is difficult to maintain digital (thumb) pressure of greater than 60 to 75 psi.[197] Therefore, with the 3 mL syringe technique (i.e., nonmanometric), pressures can be described as low or high with some degree of accuracy, and pressures that are considered "not clinically significant" are possibly excluded by the confines of the technique. Although exact quantification of pressure by manometry during provocation diskography should be considered the most appropriate technique, nonmanometric studies should be questioned, but not automatically assumed to be invalid, especially when performed by experienced, well-trained diskographers.

Once all disks included in the study have been injected, if the stimulation part of the procedure produces concordant pain at one or more levels, a CT scan of the lumbar spine is appropriate to ascertain the degree of internal architectural disruption within each level. Scout sagittal and axial views, including both bone and soft tissue windows of the levels studied, should be obtained. Axial images need to include 3 to 5 mm contiguous slices, parallel to the subchondral endplates, through each disk injected.

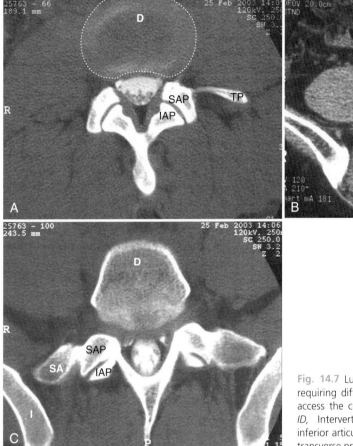

Fig. 14.7 Lumbar axial CT images indicating needle path requiring differing curves on the disk puncture needles to access the center of the disk. **A,** L3-4. **B,** L4-5. **C,** L5-S1. *ID,* Intervertebral disk; *F,* intervertebral foramen; *IAP,* inferior articular process; *SAP,* superior articular process; *TP,* transverse process; *I,* ilium; *SA,* sacral ala.

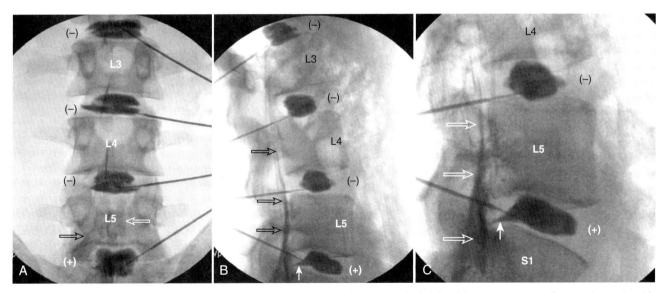

Fig. 14.8 AP and lateral images of the lumbar spine with contrast within the intervertebral disks. *(–),* No provocation of concordant pain with injection; *(+),* positive provocation of concordant pain with injection. *Open arrows,* epidural spread of contrast; *closed arrow,* anular disruption.

Interpretation of Disk Stimulation and Imaging Studies

Diskography is based on the premise that placing a mechanical load on a symptomatic intervertebral disk will reproduce the patient's index pain (i.e., reproduction of the pain is concordant with the ongoing complaint). The pain response must therefore be classified with respect to its location. In most cases, one of three descriptions can be used to characterize the discomfort provoked: (1) "no pain," (2) "nonconcordant" (i.e., dissimilar) pain or pressure, or (3) "concordant" with the patient's familiar pain.

In addition to concordance of the pain, the severity of the response provoked must be of at least moderate to severe intensity (>6on a 10-point visual analog, numerical rating, or other pain scale) to be considered a positive provocation. Acceptance of minimal to moderate pain, or "pressure," as positive would increase the false-positive rate significantly. A recent meta-analysis of the diskography literature by Wolfer et al[209] has shown that when the criteria for diskogenic pain, as detailed in the ISIS Practice Guidelines[2] are used, there is an acceptably low false-positive probability.

IASP,[170] ISIS,[1] and PASSOR[185] stipulate that to be a valid study and make a diagnosis of diskogenic pain, an anatomic, internal control must be present. Therefore provocation diskography cannot be considered valid if all disks stimulated are shown to be concordantly painful, be it one or several. Valid diskography cannot be performed by stimulation of a single level. If all levels are found to be positive to stimulation, the study is described as "indeterminate." By the aforementioned criteria, the diagnosis of diskogenic pain is most ensured when a painful disk on stimulation is shown to have two adjacent asymptomatic levels.

The gross morphology of the internal disk architecture can be studied by examination of the nucleogram in lateral and AP fluoroscopic spot images. Pattern variations indicating abnormalities with regard to nuclear filling, degeneration of the disk substance, and radial fissures have been described.[11,88,210] Pain is often not associated with disk pathology. Full-thickness anular disruption, with contrast flow into the epidural space, is often encountered without a positive pain response. Because pain on injection is thought to be partially due to the mechanical load placed on the disk during pressurization, nonpainful disks with large rents may not be capable of this pressurization, and therefore no painful response is forthcoming. Even disks with large protrusions or extrusions may evidence no pain with high-pressure stimulation. Pathology does not equal pain.

Evaluation by axial CT imaging is integral to the diagnostic diskography study. At a minimum, CT axial images of each disk that shows evidence of concordant pain with stimulation is appropriate. Axial images validate the procedure in that contrast is seen to fill the nucleus and reveals anular fissures.[211–214] Historically, postdiskography CT scans have been performed to make the diagnosis of disk herniation,[215–218] although today MRI is the "gold standard" for this diagnosis. Because CT imaging is an inherent part of diskography and not a separate imaging study per se, correlation between the two components of the test is mandatory, and separate interpretation of the CT scan by a physician radiologist not involved in the actual diskography is not appropriate. Injectionists, no matter what the primary specialty, who are not "comfortable" interpreting the preprocedure MRI, or the postprocedure CT images, should forgo undertaking this, or any other interventional pain/nonsurgical spine procedure, until competence as a spinal diagnostician is ensured.

As noted earlier, the outer third of the anulus, in contrast to the inner third, is known to have a high concentration of nerve endings.[58,59,219] One would expect a correlation between anular disruptions radiating into this area and pain. Because anular tears radiating into the outer third of the disk have been shown to be the primary indicator

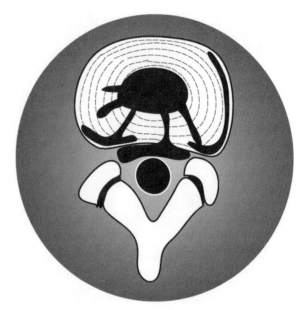

Fig. 14.9 Grades of internal disk disruption. Grade "0," contrast confined to the nucleus pulposus, no anular disruption; grade I, disruption involving the medial third of the anulus fibrosus; grade II, disruption extending to the outer third of the anulus fibrosus; grade III, disruption extending into the outer third of the anulus fibrosus with circumferential spread of contrast of less than 30 degrees; grade IV, disruption extending into the outer third of the anulus fibrosus with circumferential spread of contrast of greater than 30 degrees; grade V, disruption through the outer third of the anulus fibrosus with contrast outside the bounds of the intervertebral disk.

of diskogenic pain,[18,160,220] a grading scale of anular disruption has been developed[221] and modified.[160] The Modified Dallas Diskogram Scale is widely used in reporting findings on the axial post-diskogram CT scan images, and it describes five grades of anular fissures (**Fig. 14.9**).[222] Grade "0" indicates no anular disruption (**Fig. 14.10A**). Grade I describes radial disruption into the inner third of the annulus (**Fig. 14.10B**), whereas in grade II, contrast has spread into the middle third of the annulus (**Fig. 14.10C**). Grade III and grade IV lesions both denote an anular fissure that involves the outer third of the anulus; they are differentiated by a grade IV lesion extending into a circumferential tear involving more than 30 degrees of the disk perimeter (**Fig. 14.10D, E**). A Grade V anular disruption describes a full-thickness tear through the anulus with spread of contrast outside the confines of the disk (**Fig. 14.10F, G**), although some think that this should not be designated as a separate grade of disruption.

Once the procedure has been completed and all images examined, a diagnosis of diskogenic pain may be made if the following requirements are met: (1) stimulation of the disk in question produces concordant pain; (2) the concordant pain is greater than 6 on a visual analog or equivalent scale; (3) the pain is produced at less than 50 psi above opening pressure when a manometer is used; and (4) a negative control disk produces no pain when stimulated.[2]

Though not widely used at present, a numeric scoring system in which points are awarded for the various criteria just presented has been devised[2] and, if used, should markedly decrease the frequency of false-positive studies.

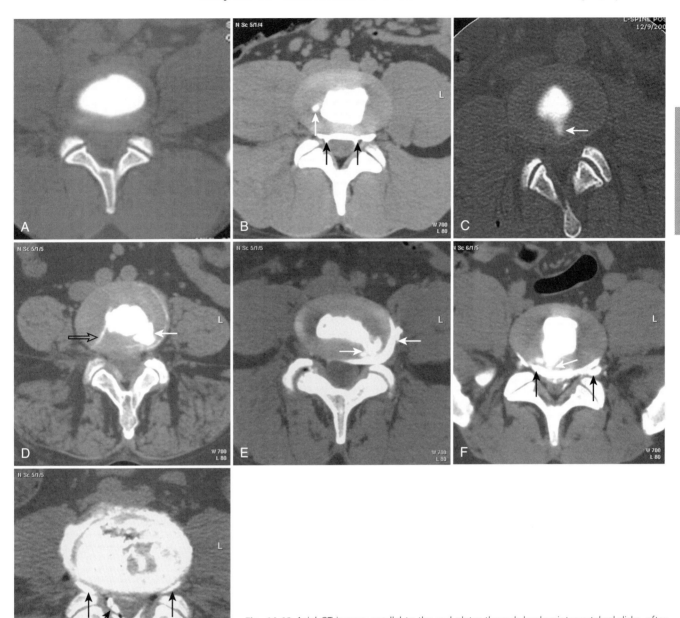

Fig. 14.10 Axial CT images parallel to the end plates through lumbar intervertebral disks, after contrast injection. A, Grade 0. B, Grade I. L4-5 from Figure 14.8. Epidural contrast secondary to a grade V disruption at the infrasegmental level. C, Grade II. D, Grade III. Note needle track, *open arrow*. E, Grade IV. F, Grade V. L5-S1 from Figure 14.8. G, Grade V with grade III degenerative pattern (>50% anular disruption). *Black arrows* indicate epidural spread. *White arrows* indicate anular disruption.

Thoracic Diskography Technique

In the past, surgical procedures for the treatment of painful thoracic intervertebral disks were limited and diskography of the dorsal spine rarely indicated or requested. With newer, less invasive percutaneous disk procedures now at least an option (intradiskal anular thermal lesioning, percutaneous thoracic diskectomy, and chemical modulation), thoracic disk stimulation is gaining in indications.

Because of the close proximity of the lung, which creates the real possibility of iatrogenic pneumothorax, and the relatively small target, thoracic disk stimulation is technically demanding and, as with cervical diskography, should be attempted only by expert spinal injectionists whose skills have been well honed by significant experience in performing fluoroscopically guided procedures. The procedural technique as first described by Schellhas et al[150] and recently codified[223] provides safe access to the thoracic intervertebral disk when the pertinent anatomy is mastered and due diligence afforded.

On a radiolucent procedure table, the patient is placed in the prone position. A thin pillow may be used under the chest or upper part of the abdomen to accentuate the normal kyphotic curve. The posterior thoracic and upper lumbar region is prepared and draped in a sterile manner. At each level to be studied the target disk is identified, and with a cephalocaudad tilt of the C-arm fluoroscope, the end plates are aligned so that they are parallel to the x-ray beam. The end plates will be seen as linear rather than ovoid structures.

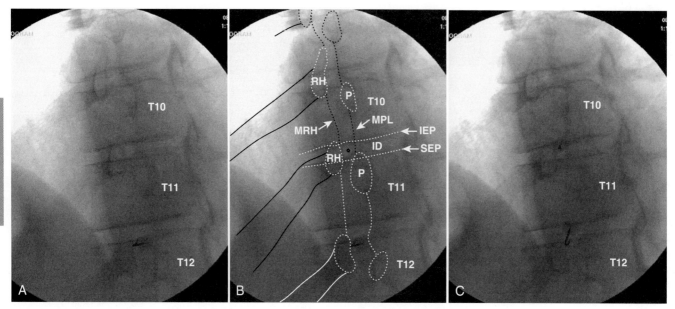

Fig. 14.11 Left oblique view of the thoracic spine at T10-11. **A,** Scout image. **B,** Anatomic landmarks labeled. **C,** Needle at target in anulus of T10-11 disk. Note needle at disk margin, T11-12. *ID,* T10-11 intervertebral disk; *IEP,* inferior end plate T10; *SEP,* superior end plate T11; *MPL,* projected midpedicular line (superior articular process and lamina); *MRH,* projected medial rib head line; *P,* pedicles; *RH,* rib head; *open circle,* target.

In most instances, needle placement will be from the side opposite the usual pain. If pain is in the midline, there is no preference with respect to the side of needle insertion. The C-arm is then rotated obliquely to the side where needle insertion will take place. The spinous processes will appear to move laterally toward the contralateral side, followed by the pedicle and rib head. When the pedicle is positioned approximately 40% of the distance across the vertebral body, rotation of the C-arm should cease. A rectangle or square hyperlucent area, or "box," will be evident and be bounded in the sagittal plane medially by the mid-interpedicular line (lateral superior articular process and lamina) and laterally by a line connecting the medial aspect of the rib heads and costovertebral joints. In the axial plane, the rectangular hyperlucent area is delineated by the superior end plate of the vertebral body caudal to the targeted disk and the inferior end plate of the vertebral body cephalad to the targeted disk (**Fig. 14.11A, B**).

The skin is marked over the hyperlucent box (**Fig. 14.11B**), local anesthetic is injected, and a 25- or 22-gauge, 3.5-inch needle with a slightly bent tip is inserted. Depending on target level and body habitus, a longer, 5-inch needle might be required. The needle is advanced toward the target in small increments with the frequent use of spot fluoroscopy. It is important to stay medial to the medial aspect of the rib heads or the pleura may be penetrated (**Fig. 14.12**). Often, as the needle is advanced, os will be contacted. By withdrawing the needle 1 to 2 mm to disengage the needle tip from the boney contact, and rotating the needle, the bent needle tip will alter direction, and continued advancement of the needle between the rib head and superior articular process should be accomplished without significant difficulty. The unique feel of resistance will be met as the needle tip contacts the disk anulus (**Fig. 14.11C**). After contacting the anulus, the disk is entered under active lateral fluoroscopic guidance and the needle positioned in the center of the disk.

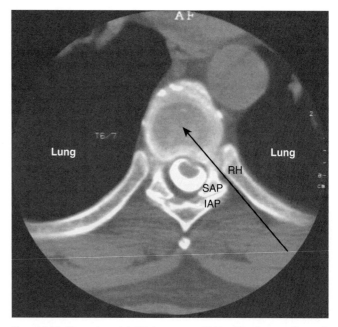

Fig. 14.12 Thoracic axial CT image at T6-7 with the needle path indicated. *IAP,* Inferior articular process; *RH,* rib head; *SAP,* superior articular process.

Once needle position in the center of each disk is verified and documented by AP and lateral imaging (**Fig. 14.13**), contrast is injected under active lateral fluoroscopy. The capacity of injectate in a thoracic intervertebral disk with a competent anulus will range from 0.5 to 2.5 mL, depending on the level, with capacity decreasing as one proceeds cephalad from the lumbothoracic junction. The author prefers to use a manometer for thoracic disk stimulation in that additional objective data can be obtained. During injection of contrast, the volume injected, the patient's pain response, the concordance of pain, the pressure generated or characteristic of the end point (none, soft, or firm), and the pattern of contrast within

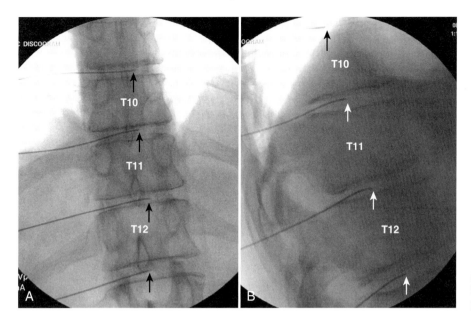

Fig. 14.13 Anteroposterior (A) and lateral (B) images of the thoracic spine with needles in position within the intervertebral disks.

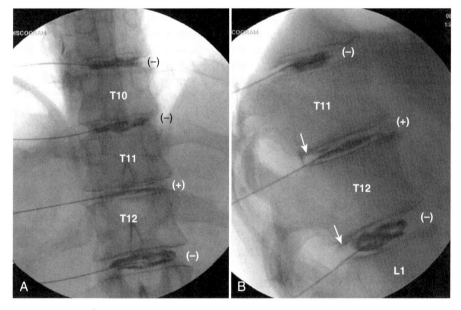

Fig. 14.14 Anteroposterior (A) and lateral (B) images of the thoracic spine after disk stimulation. Contrast is seen within the intervertebral disks at T9-10 through T12-L1. (–), No provocation of concordant pain with injection; (+), positive provocation of concordant pain with injection; *arrows* indicate anular disruption with contrast seen extending into the outer annulus.

the disk, including anular competence, should be recorded. Spot AP and lateral images are saved after disk injection (**Fig. 14.14**).

If desired, following the procedure a CT scan will provide information on pathology involving the internal architecture of each injected intervertebral disk (**Fig. 14.15**) but provides little new information if an anular tear was noted on the fluoroscopic images.

Cervical Diskography Technique

The cervical region is a compact area with a high concentration of vulnerable structures; if these structures are violated, significant morbidity or mortality can occur. Cervical diskography is a technically demanding and unforgiving procedure that requires a precision gained only after much experience with fluoroscopically guided procedures. Although some well-trained diskographers recommend diskography only if positive results will be acted on (i.e., a surgical or a percutaneous

disk procedure is contemplated), this author is adamant that the obtaining of a diagnosis is of paramount importance.

Cervical diskography traces its history back to techniques described by Smith and Nichols[142] and Cloward.[224] Both reports discussed indications for the procedure[144,145] and surgical approaches to treatment.[224,225]

Cord compression or symptoms of myelopathy are absolute contraindications to the performance of cervical diskography. Iatrogenic disk herniation[226] during disk stimulation, and the severe untoward consequences, can result from spinal cord compression.[227] Therefore, before initiation of cervical diskography, high-quality CT or MRI scans, or both, must be examined by the physician performing the procedure to ensure that adequate reserve space within the spinal canal is present at the target level, or levels, to accommodate disk material possibly being forced into the canal during the procedure, with the resulting possible cord compression and morbidity. Axial views must be examined to ensure a sagittal (i.e., AP) diameter of 10 mm or greater.[228] Patients with congenitally narrow

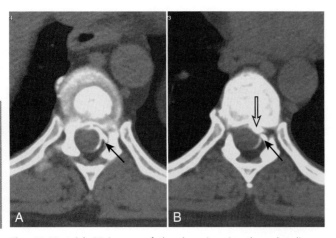

Fig. 14.15 Axial CT images of the thoracic spine through adjacent intervertebral disks after diskography. **A,** Contrast is confined to the nucleus pulposus without anular disruption. **B,** Marked disruption of the internal intervertebral disk architecture. Epidural spread, *dark arrow*, is noted in association with a significant disk protrusion, *open arrow*.

spinal canals may not be candidates for this procedure. If a physician does not possess the competence to interpret the preprocedure CT or MRI scans, he or she is not competent to perform any disk procedure. Review of a report by a radiologist, or assurances by a surgeon, who may or may not be a competent diskographer, are not an adequate substitute for personal interpretation of the imaging studies by the physician actually performing the procedure, and who is solely responsible to ensure that the patient is a safe candidate for the procedure. Physicians who do not "feel comfortable" interpreting MRI and CT images should not be performing cervical diskography under any circumstance.

A high-quality C-arm fluoroscopy unit is required. The patient is placed on a radiolucent procedure table in a supine position. A pillow or triangular sponge is positioned under the upper part of the thorax and shoulders to extend the neck. Before preparation and draping of the skin, verification by preprocedure fluoroscopic screening guarantees adequate visualization in the AP, lateral, and oblique views. Disk puncture should not be attempted at any level if accurate evaluation of needle tip position within the disk cannot be obtained. Depending on the procedural technique used (see later discussion), the body of the C-arm will be either perpendicular to the patient on the left or at the head of the table.

The neck, mandible, clavicular regions, and shoulders are prepared and draped in sterile fashion. Inclusion of the shoulders is necessary so that they may be depressed by the physician to improve lateral visualization of the C6-7 and C7-T1 disks as needed. Beards prevent adequate preparation of the skin and must be removed before the procedure. Prophylactic antibiotic and light sedative medications are administered as previously discussed.

Because the esophagus lies toward the left at the lower cervical levels, a right-sided approach is used for cervical disk access. The skin entry point will be along the medial margin of the sternocleidomastoid muscle with the needle track running lateral to the trachea and esophagus and medial to the carotid artery. Depending on the targeted disk level, other structures may come into play. The hypopharynx can be distended at C2-3, and therefore a slightly more lateral approach is

indicated. Thyroid cartilage is present at C5-6. A more medial approach is necessitated at C7-T1 to avoid the apex of the lung and the common carotid and thyroid arteries.

Although a double-needle technique has been described and advocated,[229] most experienced cervical diskographers today use 25-gauge, 3.5-inch needles with stylet.[228,230] As noted in the lumbar technique, a slight bend in the needle tip facilitates directional control. Local anesthetic, if used, should be limited to the skin because deeper infiltration may track along the cervical sympathetic chain and cause an alteration in the pain response.

Two alternative techniques are used by practitioners to gain access to the cervical disk. The traditional approach involves the use of the fluoroscope in an AP or slightly oblique view, whereas the alternative calls for a foraminal (i.e., anterior oblique) image. The actual needle insertion site and needle tract to the disk are virtually identical with both techniques, as demonstrated in cadaver studies by Dr. Charles Aprill[231] and this author.

With the traditional, less precise, more experience intensive, approach to the cervical intervertebral disk, the C-arm in an AP or slight right oblique view is used to identify the target disk. Cephalocaudad tilt of the image intensifier is used to align the vertebral body end plates. Two hands are used, with the nondominant middle and index fingers advanced toward the anterior aspect of the spine at the skin entry point. This significant digital pressure displaces the laryngeal structures medially, whereas the carotid artery is distracted laterally and can be palpated under the fingers. The spine is felt under the finger tips. With the dominant hand, the needle is then inserted between, directly over, or under the fingers and, with active fluoroscopic guidance, advanced swiftly toward the right anterior-lateral aspect of the spine. Aprill[228] advocates directing the needle so that it touches the superior aspect of the vertebral body caudad to the disk in order to ascertain the depth of the disk. Slight manipulation of the needle, including rotation to make use of bevel control, is then performed to direct the needle into the disk anulus just medial to the uncinate process. With the use of a lateral view and active fluoroscopy, the needle is then advanced into the center of the disk core. AP and lateral images are saved to document needle placement.

The alternative technique for cervical disk access has advantages that include ease of use, excellent visualization of the target disk, ability to use a down-the-beam (i.e., tunnel vision) approach, and somewhat less x-ray exposure to the hands. This approach is adapted for the use of a C-arm and is favored by the author. The fluoroscope is positioned at the head of the table to provide ease of imaging in all planes. A right anterior oblique projection, or foraminal view, is used to visualize the intervertebral foramina at their greatest diameter (**Fig. 14.16A**). The target disk is identified by counting down from C2-3, and the end plates of the chosen disk are aligned by using cephalocaudad tilt of the image intensifier. A target on the disk is chosen that is approximately one third to one half the distance between the uncinate process and the anterior aspect of the disk (**Fig. 14.16B**). The skin entry site is marked with a sterile skin marker and should lie just medial to the sternocleidomastoid muscle and carotid artery (**Fig. 14.17**). If desired, a local anesthetic skin wheal can be made, although if 25-gauge needles are used, this is not necessary. A blunt sterile metal instrument is then pressed firmly against the skin, over the skin entry point, until resistance by the underlying tissues and spine is felt. This decreases the distance between the skin and

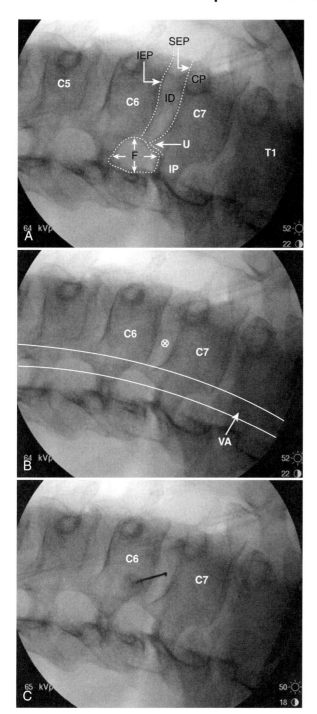

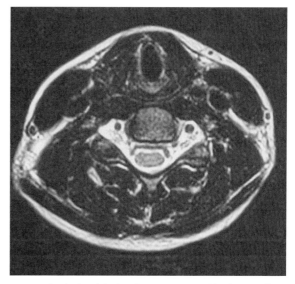

Fig. 14.17 Cervical axial CT view at C5-6 with the needle path. *CA,* Carotid artery; *E,* esophagus; *JV,* internal jugular vein; *T,* trachea; *TH,* thyroid; *VA,* vertebral artery.

Fig. 14.16 Oblique-anterior, "foraminal," views of the cervical spine. **A,** Anatomic landmarks labeled. **B,** Target for safe disk access. **C,** Needle in outer anulus. *ID,* Intervertebral disk; *F,* C6-7 foramen; *IP,* ipsilateral pedicle; *CP,* contralateral pedicle; *IEP,* inferior end plate of C6; *SEP,* superior end plate of C7; *U,* uncinate process.

disk and distracts any vulnerable soft tissue structures away from the needle track. The position over the disk target is verified, and a 25-gauge needle is inserted at the tip of the instrument. With the assistance of active fluoroscopy the needle is quickly maneuvered toward the disk in one movement using rotation to control the needle direction. The patient is asked to refrain from vocalization, coughing, or swallowing during this portion of the procedure in that movement of the soft tissue

and larynx makes needle control difficult. Resistance to needle insertion is felt as the anulus is contacted and entered (**Fig. 14.16C**). Further insertion is halted until depth can be ascertained using a lateral view. Active lateral and AP fluoroscopy is then used to advance the needle to the approximate center of the disk core. Care must be taken to ensure that the needle will not be unintentionally advanced through the posterior aspect of the disk and into the spinal canal and cord. Once all needles are in place, AP, oblique, and lateral images are saved to document needle placement (**Fig. 14.18**).

Whether the traditional or alternative technique is used, once needle position at all disks to be studied is verified, the stylets are removed. The needle hubs are filled with contrast, and a contrast-filled, 3 mL Luer-Lok syringe with small-bore, minimal-volume, Luer-Lok extension tubing attached and connected to each needle. Care must be taken to ensure that the needles are not advanced or withdrawn during connection of the extension tubing. At the present time, manometry is used by few cervical diskographers in that the literature on its benefit has not yet been advanced.

Active, lateral fluoroscopy is used during contrast injection (i.e., disk stimulation). The patient is blinded with respect to initiation of stimulation and the disk level. Injection into the disk proceeds by slowly increasing the pressure on the syringe until the intrinsic, opening, pressure of the disk is overcome and contrast is seen to flow into the disk core. If injection of contrast into the disk is not forthcoming, slight rotation, advancement, or withdrawal of the needle frequently allows flow of contrast to be seen within the disk. Firm resistance is often noted with injection of as little as 0.2 mL, and separation of the disk end plates during injection is expected. Injection into a normal cervical intervertebral disk will be limited to less than 0.5 mL of solution[232] at a sustained high pressure.[233] Intervertebral disks that accept more than 0.5 mL of injectate will be seen to have evidence of abnormalities on imaging studies.

During disk stimulation, parameters of the injection are recorded on a standardized form by procedure room personnel. At a minimum, volume of injectate, the presence

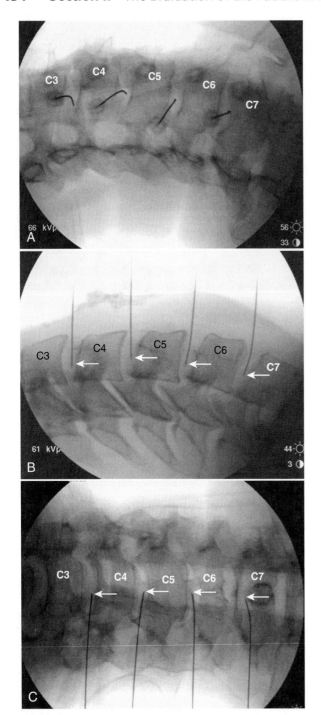

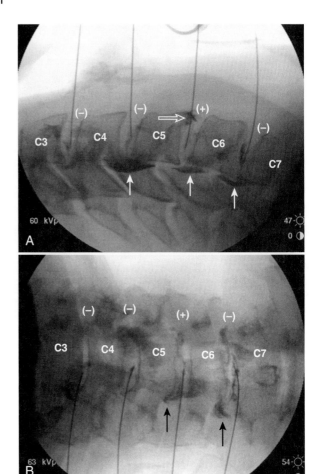

Fig. 14.19 Lateral **(A)** and AP **(B)** images of the cervical spine after disk stimulation. *(–),* No provocation of concordant pain with injection; *(+),* positive provocation of concordant pain with injection; *closed arrow,* filling of the uncovertebral recess (joints of Luschka); *open arrow,* anterior anular disruption.

Fig. 14.18 A, Oblique; B, lateral; and C, AP images of the cervical spine with needles in position within the core of the intervertebral disks C3-4 through C6-7. *Arrows* indicated needle tips in the approximate center of each disk.

or absence of pain, the severity of pain, pain location and description, and concordance must be assessed at each level stimulated.[230] In addition, the pressure generated (soft versus a firm end point) and vocal or physical pain responses are often recorded. Because even at nonpathologic levels cervical disk stimulation is uncomfortable, evaluation of the patient's response requires experience beyond that demanded by the technical aspects of the procedure. Individuals vary in their

pain tolerance, and thus some degree of subjectivity is required by the diskographer.

As per the ISIS *Practice Guidelines,*[230] the injection end points include any of the following: concordant pain greater than 6/10, neurologic symptoms reported by the patient, contrast solution escaping from the disk, displacement of the vertebral body end plates, firm resistance to injection, and the disk accepting no further volume at a reasonable pressure. To be considered a valid study, a negative control level, without pain on stimulation, must be present.

Analgesic diskography,[148] or the injection of local anesthetic and corticosteroid into a painful, pathologic disk, has been advocated by some authors.[228,234] Although there is little consensus among diskographers concerning this practice, and no convincing data validating its use, anecdotal experience has led some to promote this practice.

AP and lateral images of all disks injected, both before and after injection of contrast, must be saved for a permanent record of the study (**Fig. 14.19**). These images confirm injection of contrast into the disk core. However, because changes in the internal architecture of the disk are widespread in mature asymptomatic individuals, little in the way of diagnostic credibility is gained by images alone. Contrast seen to fill one or both of the uncovertebral recesses, or the joints of

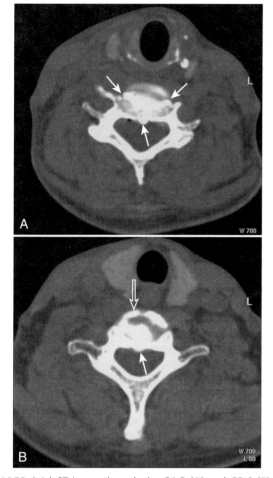

Fig. 14.20 Axial CT image through the C4-5 (A) and C5-6 (B) disks from Figure 14.19. Although significant disruption of the internal disk anatomy is present in both disks, only C5-6 was painful with stimulation. *Closed black arrow,* filling of the uncovertebral recess (joint of Luschka); *open arrow,* anterior anular disruption.

Luschka, is not a sign of abnormal degenerative changes but rather reflects the normal maturation of the cervical intervertebral disk.[228,235] A postprocedure CT scan provides little additional information and should not be considered routine (**Fig. 14.20**). Because of the high frequency of internal disk disruption in nonsymptomatic individuals, the criteria for a diagnosis of diskogenic pain in the cervical region is based solely on the provocation of concordant pain rather than a combination of pain provocation and pathology by imaging studies as in the lumbar and thoracic spine.

Postprocedure Considerations

After completion of the diskogram, independent of the level, sterile self-adhesive dressings are applied to the puncture wounds and the patient is taken to a recovery room with nurses trained to care for patients recovering from spinal injections. Periodic evaluation of the patient, including vital signs, level of comfort, level of consciousness, and visualization of the injection sites, is recommended. Analgesic medications, oral, intramuscular, or intravenous, are provided as needed. Following the recovery period, once stable, the patient can be taken for a postdiskogram CT to provide axial images of the injected disks if deemed appropriate.

Patients are observed for a minimum of 1 hour after the procedure and discharged home with a responsible adult. Discharge instructions include no driving the day of the procedure. The patient is told to expect some increase in discomfort for a few days after the procedure, and a limited prescription of oral analgesics can be provided. Patients are encouraged to call if they feel any unusual or severe pain not relieved by the oral analgesics. Pneumothorax is discussed with all patients who have undergone diskography of the lower cervical and thoracic regions.

Documentation

A detailed record of the procedure must be completed. It is mandatory that this medical-legal document be a true and exact record of the specific procedure. If a template is used, it must be significantly modified to reflect the procedure it purports to detail. This procedure note must included the following information: name of patient; name of injectionist; date of procedure; indication for procedure, history; preinjection diagnosis; postinjection diagnosis; procedures performed; consent; and a detailed narrative of the procedure. See Appendix A.

Complications

A myriad of complications after diskography have been well documented.[195,227,236,237] Complications can be inherent to disk penetration, the medications used, or unintentional misadventures involving needle placement. They range in severity from minor inconveniences, such as nausea and headache, to death.

Historically, diskitis is the most common complication of diskography, with a rate of less than 0.08% per disk injected.[184] Fraser et al[238] provided evidence that all cases of diskitis are due to an infectious process, with the most common organisms being *S. aureus,* *S. epidermidis,* and *E. coli* from the skin, hypopharynx, esophagus, or bowel. In that the intervertebral disk is an essentially avascular structure, it provides an excellent growth medium for bacteria. However, with the use of preprocedure screening for chronic or acute infections, strict aseptic preparation of the skin, styletted needles, meticulous sterile technique, and intravenous and intradiskal antibiotics, diskitis should be an exceedingly rare occurrence today.[196,228]

Whether occurring after diskography or a surgical procedure, diskitis is manifested in similar fashion.[201,239] A patient with diskitis usually has severe, intractable, debilitating pain of the cervical, thoracic, or lumbar spine days to weeks after the procedure; however, mild self-limited cases have been described.[219] Diskitis needs to be ruled out in any postdiskogram patient who notes a marked change in the severity or quality of the pain after the procedure. The workup consists of obtaining laboratory and imaging studies. C-reactive protein levels will increase within days of the onset, whereas the sedimentation rate may remain in the normal range for over a month. Blood cultures will be negative and a complete blood count normal until the end plates are breached. MRI is the imaging study of choice,[240–242] with hyperemia of the end plates and marrow space changes noted on T2-weighted images 3 to 4 days after the onset of symptoms. Radionuclide bone scanning has been shown to be inferior to MRI in specificity and sensitivity.[243] If an adequate sample of tissue can be obtained, disk aspiration or biopsy, or both, will be positive in the acute phase of diskitis, but once the end plates are violated, a sterile environment within the disk is soon noted in response to the patient's immune system.[228]

Once diskitis is suspected, consultations with a spine surgeon and infectious disease specialist are appropriate. Treatment of infections within the disk and sepsis often requires antibiotic therapy. Though rare, abscess or empyema[244-246] may necessitate surgical intervention.

The cervical region has many vulnerable structures packed in a small area. Although vascular structures are plentiful, penetration of a vein or artery will rarely cause any significant problems. Poor technique can result in penetration of the cord either during insertion of the needle or when connecting the syringe to the needle. Good visualization and verification of needle position are mandatory during all parts of the procedure.

Pneumothorax must be considered if marked shortness of breath occurs in a patient who has undergone diskography at levels between C5-6 and T12-L1.

Boswell and Wolfe[247] described a case in which intractable seizures, coma, and death developed in a woman after diskography. Their conclusion was that unintentional intrathecal administration of cefazolin (12.5 mg/mL), which had been included in the contrast agent for prophylaxis of infection, precipitated this catastrophic event. However, misadventure into the spinal canal is nearly impossible if proper technique is used; the operator understands the anatomy and has received appropriate fluoroscopic training; and AP, lateral, and oblique images are obtained and interpreted before injection of contrast as is standard of care.

Conclusion

As with any diagnostic spinal injection procedure, diskography, be it cervical, thoracic, or lumbar, can be performed in a safe manner with the appropriate knowledge, training, and vigilance. However, diskography is more than a technique. Analysis of data obtained from the procedure, along with knowledge of the patient's history, clinical features, and psychologic condition, must be considered before a final diagnosis is determined. A highly invasive procedure, anterior-posterior spinal fusion at multiple levels, may be performed on the basis of your findings. Therefore meticulous technique and awareness of the procedure's limitations are of utmost importance.

Mark Twain once said, "The reports of my death are greatly exaggerated"; this statement could apply to diskography as well. Throughout its history, provocation diskography has been controversial and more than once pronounced "dead." But, like the Phoenix of legend rising from the ashes, or the zombie rising from the grave, diskography is reborn after each notice of its demise. Today diskography lives, and is well recognized as the only diagnostic modality that can be used to determine whether an intervertebral disk is painful to mechanical forces. Provocation disk stimulation is, without a doubt, the "gold standard" for diagnosing diskogenic pain secondary to internal disk disruption.[2,248,249] The technique has been endorsed by the majority of professional organizations whose objectives lie in advancing knowledge of the spine and its myriad pathologies. In the future, although refinements in our use and interpretation of diskography are certain to occur, the procedure will continue to provide information about our patients' afflictions and guide the treatment those modalities offer.

Dedication

This chapter is dedicated to my mentor, friend, and diskographer extraordinaire, Professor Charles N. Aprill.

Acknowledgment

I wish to acknowledge the contribution of John D. Fisk, MD, to the Historical Considerations section.

References

Full references for this chapter can be found on www.expertconsult.com.

Appendix A

Lumbar Diskogram: Sample Procedure Note

Patient name: John Pain
Injectionist: Dr. Needle
History: See previously dictated consultation. Mr. Pain suffers from low back pain with radiation into the left buttock for 2 years.
Preoperative diagnosis: (1) Low back pain etiology unknown. (2) L4-5 disk degeneration with a high-intensity zone. (3) Probable diskogenic pain.
Postoperative diagnosis: (1) L4-5 internal disk disruption, with intermediate pressure diskogenic pain.
Procedures: (1) Injection into lumbar intervertebral disks ×3 levels. (2) Lumbar diskography supervision and interpretation ×3 levels. (3) Sedation ×45 minutes. (4) Interpretation of lumbar CT scan after diskography.

Procedure

Informed consent was obtained from the patient with regard to risks and complications were discussed. Diskitis and the provocative nature of the study were discussed at length. Mr. Pain elected to proceed. He was taken to an operating room with an intravenous drip in place. He was placed in prone position with a pillow under the abdomen to decrease the lordotic curve. Physiologic monitors were attached. Prophylactic cefazolin was give. Sedation with midazolam only was afforded for the duration of the procedure. The patient was conversant throughout the procedure.

The lower thoracic, lumbar, and sacral regions were "prepped" and draped in a sterile manner. A C-arm was used to examine the lumbar spine. Five lumbar, non–rib bearing vertebral bodies were noted. The intervertebral disks at L3-4, L4-5, and L5-S1 were identified sequentially. At each level the superior endplate of the level below the targeted disk was aligned parallel to the beam. A right oblique view was then obtained so that the superior articular process of the level below appeared to lie as closely as possible under the approximate midpoint of the endplate above. At each level sequentially, a skin weal was made with local anesthetic and carried down to the level of the superior articular process. A puncture was made with a 15-gauge needle, through which an 18-gauge introducer needle was passed using "tunnel vision" toward the lateral aspect of the superior articular process at each level. Once all three introducer needles were in place, a lateral view evidenced all introducer needles as lying ventral to the posterior elements and dorsal to the intervertebral disk. Using active lateral fluoroscopy, the 22-gauge disk puncture needles were advanced through the introducer needles and seen and felt to enter the intervertebral disks. The needles were advanced into the center of each disk. No dysesthetic radicular type pain was noted during insertion of any needle. An anteroposterior (AP) view indicated excellent needle position at all levels.

Injection was then made into each disk using an injectate of iopamidol containing gentamycin 2 mg/mL. A manometer was used. During injection, volume injected, opening pressure, final pressure, pain response, and contrast pattern were recorded.

L3-4:
Volume: 1.5 mL
Opening pressure: 22 psi
Final pressure: 90 psi
Pain: None
Remarks: Contrast is noted within the nucleus pulposis in both AP and lateral views. No anular disruption is present.

L4-5:
Volume: 1.25 mL
Opening pressure: 8 psi
Final pressure: 31 psi
Pain: Concordant, 9/10 with vocal and physical pain response. Patient stated, "Oh shucky darn."
Remarks: Contrast is noted within the nucleus pulposus. In lateral view, a posterior anular tear is noted.

L5-S1:
Volume: 2.75 mL
Opening pressure: 14 psi
Final pressure: 90 psi
Pain: Nonconcordant, dissimilar pain, to right, 4/10
Remarks: Contrast is noted within the intervertebral disk. An anular tear to the left is noted.

Mr. Pain tolerated the procedure well, was taken to recovery, and then taken for a postprocedure CT scan. He will follow up with Dr. Surgeon in the near future. He knows to follow up with his physician if any problems were to develop.

Interpretation of Lumbar CT after Diskography

This interpretation should be considered the functional report for the record. It should take precedence over all other reports, past and future, in that correlation with the provocation diskography is an essential part of the interpretation and can only be afforded by the physician actually injecting the intervertebral disks.

Scout sagittal and 3 mm axial views through the lumbar cistern were examined this date. Axial views included bone and soft tissue windows and included contiguous slices, parallel to the end plates, through the intervertebral disks at L3-4, L4-5, and L5-S1. Contrast is noted within the intervertebral disks at all levels noted above.

L3-4:
Contrast is noted within the nucleus pulposus. No anular disruption is present. A grade 0 nuclear pattern is evident.
L4-5:
Contrast is noted within the nucleus pulposus. A grade III posterior left anular disruption is noted.

L5-S1:
Contrast is noted within the intervertebral disk. A wide, left lateral grade IV anular disruption is present with circumferential spread of contrast ~180 degrees.

Interpretation

L3-4

This is a negative level for diskogenic pain. No pain was noted with disk stimulation up to 90 psi. No disruption of the normal internal disk architecture is evident. This is a negative level for diskogenic pain without internal disk disruption, and provides a negative control level.

L4-5

This is a positive level for diskogenic pain. Marked concordant pain was noted at 23 psi above an opening pressure of 8 psi This is a positive level for diskogenic pain at intermediate pressure stimulation, with internal disk disruption.

L5-S1

This is a negative level for diskogenic pain. Although some discomfort was noted at 90 psi, that is, 76 psi above an opening pressure of 14 psi, this pain was nonconcordant, at high pressure, and only at an intensity of 4/10. This is a negative level for diskogenic pain, with disruption of the normal internal disk architecture.

Myelography

Hifz Aniq and Robert Campbell

The correct diagnosis of spinal stenosis and nerve root impingement depends on the precise correlation between a neurologic finding and radiologic imaging studies. Several imaging diagnostic tests exist for spinal disorders. For many years, myelography, computed tomography (CT), and a combination of CT and myelography have been the modalities of choice for evaluation of spinal diseases. The introduction of magnetic resonance imaging (MRI) has revolutionized the way we diagnose and treat these conditions. It is superior to CT because it has better soft tissue contrast, spinal structures can be seen in multiple planes, it allows direct visualization of subligamentous disk prolapse, and it provides the ability to evaluate the spinal cord directly. Like any other diagnostic modality, MRI has its own strengths and weaknesses.

Myelography is a simple and economical modality, but it is an invasive procedure, as contrast is injected into the thecal sac, and it involves radiation. In most cases, lumbar puncture is usually performed at the L3-4 or L4-5 level and non-ionic contrast (iopamidol-300) is injected into the subarachnoid space under fluoroscopic guidance. During injection the foot end of the table is kept slightly down. Erect anteroposterior (AP), lateral, and oblique radiographs are taken. The thecal sac is assessed on AP and lateral views whereas nerve roots are best seen on oblique views. With the use of non-ionic contrast after myelography, morbidity has been significantly reduced. However, patients should be informed of the possibility of nausea, vomiting, headache, and meningitis. Approximately 10% to 15% of patients have postmyelography headache, which usually starts 24 hours after the procedure, attributed to low cerebrospinal fluid (CSF) pressure syndrome. A remote possibility of nerve damage exists during the procedure. For cervical spine myelograms, the lumbar approach for contrast injection can be used in which the patient lies in prone or in decubitus position after the injection for contrast to flow toward the cervical region. Direct cervical puncture can also be performed at the C1-2 level through a lateral approach under fluoroscopy. This approach should be reserved for patients with complete spinal block, severe degenerative change, scoliosis, or infection preventing lumbar puncture. Cervical cord and vertebral artery puncture are potential complications. This approach should be used with caution in cases of suspected Chiari malformation. A standard volume of 10 mL is injected for lumbar regions, 20 mL for ascending lumbo-cervical myelograms, and 10 mL for cervical myelograms after C1-2 lateral puncture.[1] CT examination of the cervical spine is usually performed immediately after the injection, and the lumbar spine CT is performed after an interval of 2 to 3 hours to reduce high contrast between the thecal sac and soft tissues. Multislice CT is performed with coronal and sagittal reformats. Spinal stenosis is assessed by encroachment of the spinal canal secondary to osteophyte formation and vertebral degeneration along with a degree of displacement of the contrast-filled thecal sac (**Fig. 15.1**). Asymmetries of displacement of nerve roots can also be easily accessed using CT myelogram. However, asymmetries caused by disk herniation should be differentiated from normal physiologic variances such as conjoined nerve root spinal ganglia and perineural cysts.

Magnetic resonance myelogram is performed by choosing a particular set of sequences in which the main signal contribution comes from CSF in the thecal sac. In these heavily T2-weighted sequences, signal from tissue other than fluid is almost completely canceled. Magnetic resonance myelography demonstrates the thecal sac and nerve root sleeves similar to conventional myelography and postmyelographic CT. The major advantages of this modality include its noninvasive nature, its lack of ionizing radiation, and no requirement for intrathecal contrast injection.

Many studies have been performed that compared the efficiency of MRI and postmyelography CT scan.[2] Bartlett et al[3] demonstrated that MRI could be quite insensitive for small lateral disk herniation in the cervical exiting foramen. It is difficult to differentiate between soft disk herniation and osteophyte in the neural exiting foramen on MRI. Reul et al[4] proved in their study that MRI overestimates the degree of canal stenosis in the cervical spine compared with postmyelogram CT. However, MRI produced correct measurements in a normal-sized spinal canal. Several reasons for this overestimation were given, including truncation, chemical shift, and CSF pulsation artifacts. The artifacts can alter the shape, anatomic details, and structure of the spine. Truncation and chemical shift artifacts can be avoided by selecting a large data acquisition matrix and by changing the frequency and phase encoding directions, respectively. However, CSF motion artifacts appear to be the most important factor in incorrect measurements. Pulsation of CSF is strongest in the cervical spinal canal. In degenerative spinal narrowing, CSF motions become turbulent and accelerated leading to a reduction in the signal strength, which can look like advanced spinal stenosis, but this will not change the therapeutic management. Overestimation in mild to moderate spinal stenosis could be misleading and dangerous, leading to unnecessary intervention. CT myelogram was found to be highly sensitive and accurate in the diagnosis of spinal stenosis and lateral lumbar recess syndrome.[5] Osteophytes with subperiosteal new bone formation in the vertebral body and its articulations are directed toward the center of the spinal canal and produce spinal stenosis. The extent of this bony involvement is best assessed on CT myelogram (**Fig. 15.2**). CT myelography has a

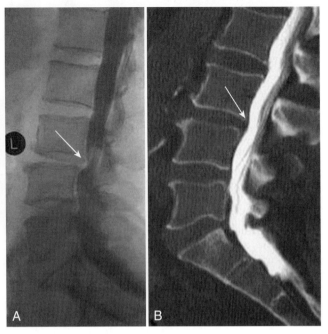

Fig. 15.1 A, Myelogram, lateral view, anterior indentation of contrast-filled thecal scan at the L3-4 level. **B,** Postmyelogram CT, sagittal multiplanar reformation (MPR), anterior indentation at the L3-4 level is due to posterior slip of L3 over L4.

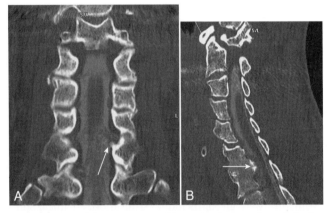

Fig. 15.2 Cervical fusion: osseous ridge. With the use of cervical spine multi-detector computed tomography (MDCT) myelography in a patient after anterior cervical fusion, coronal **(A)** and sagittal **(B)** Multiplanar reformations show an osseous ridge compressing the nerve roots *(arrows).*

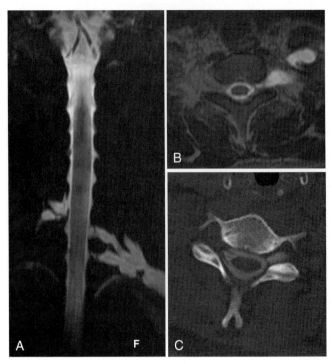

Fig. 15.3 Brachial plexus injury. **A,** Magnetic resonance myelogram, bilateral traumatic meningocele caused by avulsion of the right C6 and left C7-8 nerve roots. **B,** Axial T2 three-dimensional drive sequence shows left C7 root avulsion and traumatic meningocele. **C,** Axial CT myelogram (different patient) shows avulsion of ventral and dorsal roots of left C5 with traumatic meningocele.

significant role in postoperative spine imaging. On MRI, distortion of images may be caused by screws, plates, and pieces of metal. On CT, the contrast-filled thecal sac is less affected by the postoperative metalwork and is also able to demonstrate arachnoid adhesions and CSF leaks.

MR myelography can be used in cases of multisegmental or severe spinal stenosis in which the intrathecal contrast injection may not pass distal to the area of stenosis. On the other hand, this technique overestimates the degree of spinal stenosis compared to conventional MRI. Magnetic resonance and CT myelography are routinely used in brachial plexus injuries. The most common cause of brachial plexus injury is motorcycle accidents involving young adults. In this injury, nerve root avulsion takes place at the preganglionic or postganglionic

segment or a combination of both. The C5 and C6 nerve roots are most commonly involved. Treatment varies in these different types of nerve root avulsions. Conventional MRI may show cord edema and enhancement around the affected nerve root. CT myelography is superior to magnetic resonance myelography as it allows separate evaluation of both the ventral and dorsal nerve roots and detection of intradural nerve defects (**Fig. 15.3**). Magnetic resonance myelogram can show traumatic meningocele and nerve root avulsion but there may be degradation of images because of respiration and swallowing movements. There may be further loss of information on images because of pulsation artifacts from the cervical vessels.[6]

As compared to magnetic resonance scanning, CT myelogram is an invasive procedure and involves significant radiation. New high-resolution magnetic resonance scanning is the investigation of choice for all spinal conditions. It is noninvasive, has better soft tissue contrast, is able to visualize the spinal cord directly, and is free of radiation hazards.[7] However, small percentages of the population have contraindications for MRI scan or are claustrophobic. In these cases CT myelogram can be the alternative modality for diagnosing spine-related problems. Many studies have proved that MRI is the most cost-effective modality for spinal imaging.[8] CT myelogram should be reserved for elective presurgical patients when MRI fails to answer the clinical question or symptoms are not explained by the MRI findings.[9]

References

Full references for this chapter can be found on www.expertconsult.com.

Epidurography

Jeffrey P. Meyer, Miles R. Day, and Gabor B. Racz

Historical Considerations

Epidurography is one of the most commonly performed interventional pain procedures, yet is likely taken for granted by most pain practitioners. The accurate interpretation of epidural contrast patterns is key to the success of many interventional pain procedures, and remains a vital skill in the interventional pain arena.

First described in 1921 by the accidental injection of lipiodol into the epidural space by Sicard and Forestier,[1] epidurography has been performed with many different agents including air,[2] perobrodil,[3] and metrizamide.[4] The use of ionic contrast agents such as diatrizoate (Renografin, Hypaque) led to complications related to both anaphylactic and contrast-induced seizures, and the use of non-ionic contrast agent has now become widely accepted. The use of radiopaque contrast agents to identify correct needle positioning in epidural steroid injections was described by White et al in 1980,[5] and has since become widespread practice.[6–8] Epidural contrast patterns and their interpretation are central to caudal neuroplasty,[7] and have been described in the management of indwelling epidural catheters.[9]

The current practice of epidurography has evolved with necessity. It is currently performed whenever confirmation of epidural localization of needle placement is desired. When performed via the caudal approach, it is useful in delineating the presence of epidural fibrosis, with concomitant nerve root entrapment. In the cervical, thoracic, and lumbar transforaminal approaches, correct needle positioning is confirmed, as well as delineating the extent of spread. Interlaminar epidurography not only confirms correct positioning but defines "safe" runoff patterns that ensure that loculation (and subsequent intrathecal space compression) is not occurring.

Indications

Epidurography is indicated in any instance in which correct needle positioning within the epidural space is desired. Previous reports have identified false-positive rates as high as 25% in the identification of the caudal epidural space,[10] and confirmation of correct needle positioning is necessary for both therapeutic effect and safety. In the presence of failed back/neck surgery syndrome, the pattern of contrast distribution and runoff ensure that loculation is not occurring, and that further volumes may be instilled safely. This is especially important in cervical epidural injections as there is little room within the epidural space for loculation.

In the presence of epidural fibrosis, epidurography is useful in delineating the extent and pattern of fibrosis, along with identifying the affected nerve roots. It provides a baseline from which to gauge the extent of adhesiolysis during cervical, thoracic, and caudal epidural neuroplasty, and guides therapeutic decisions as to the necessity for further interventions.

Epidurography is essential in the performance of cervical interlaminar and transforaminal epidural steroid injections. The possibility of loculation with concomitant cord compression is ever present, and only epidurography is able to adequately identify runoff. In the case of cervical transforaminal injections, the presence of radicular feeder vessels to the spinal cord necessitates that epidurography be performed to ensure that intravascular injection is not occurring.[11] Several reports in the literature detail spinal cord damage following the transforaminal delivery of epidural steroids to the cervical space, and a proposed mechanism for this complication is the delivery of local anesthetic and particulate steroid into these radicular feeder vessels.[12,13]

Clinically Relevant Anatomy

The dorsal epidural space is bounded superiorly by the foramen magnum, inferiorly by the sacral notch, ventrally by the dura mater, and dorsally by the laminar periosteum and ligamentum flavum. It extends to envelop the exiting nerve roots in the foraminal sheath. The space is largest in the sacral canal, and most limited in the midcervical spine. Plica mediana dorsalis are dorsal-median bands that may separate the epidural space into left and right compartments. They are usually incomplete, but may be continuous, limiting contrast spread to the ipsilateral epidural space.[14] The ventral epidural space is bounded superiorly by the foramen magnum, inferiorly by the sacral notch, ventrally by the posterior longitudinal ligament, and dorsally by the dura mater.

The epidural space contains fat, loose connective tissue, and veins. It may also contain radicular arterial feeder vessels for the spinal cord,[14] which are of particular concern when performing cervical transforaminal epidural steroid injections.[13,15]

Materials

Epidurography may safely be performed in non–iodine-allergic patients by the injection of non-ionic, water-soluble contrast material into the epidural space. Because the possibility of intrathecal administration is always present, the choice of contrast agent is based on the intrathecal application of contrast. The only agent currently approved for use is iohexol (Omnipaque). Although available in concentrations of 140 to 360 mg of organic iodine per milliliter, only the 180, 240, and 300 mL of iodine per milliliter are indicated for intrathecal administration. In children, only the 180 mL of iodine per milliliter concentration is indicated. Iopamidol (Isovue) is another water-soluble, non-ionic contrast agent that is available; however, it is not currently approved for intrathecal injection. Gadolinium has been described as an alternative in iodine-allergic patients.[16]

The use of ionic or non–water-soluble contrast agents in epidurography is contraindicated. The possibility of inadvertent intrathecal injection is ever present, and the application of these agents to the intrathecal space may lead to life-threatening seizures. Confirmation of the agent to be injected into the epidural space is mandatory before injection because the consequences of inadvertent injection of agents not approved for epidural use may be life threatening.

Technique

Epidurography may be performed from any of the commonly used approaches to the epidural space. Following confirmation of epidural needle tip positioning by loss-of-resistance, hanging drop technique, or fluoroscopy, a syringe containing 5 mL of contrast agent is attached to the needle. Careful aspiration to assess possible intrathecal or intravascular needle positioning is carried out. The initial injection of contrast is carried out under continuous fluoroscopy to assess the flow of contrast in an epidural pattern. It is advisable to limit the volume of initial contrast injection to the smallest amount possible to ascertain distal spread of contrast in the epidural space. In the presence of suspected epidural fibrosis, loculation surrounding the access point is an ever-present possibility, and injection of even small (1 to 2 mL) volumes of contrast may compress surrounding structures. This is especially important in the cervical and thoracic epidural space.

After confirming that loculation is not occurring, additional volumes of contrast may be injected as necessary to assess the pattern of contrast spread. Contrast injection should always be carried out under continuous fluoroscopy to identify possible vascular runoff patterns, and to assess the continued runoff of contrast material. Contrast will flow to the areas of least resistance, and filling defects may be identified, indicating areas of epidural scarring. Fluoroscopy should be carried out in both the anteroposterior (AP) and lateral projections to confirm spread in an epidural pattern.

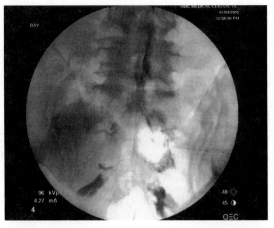

Fig. 16.1 Normal caudal epidurogram.

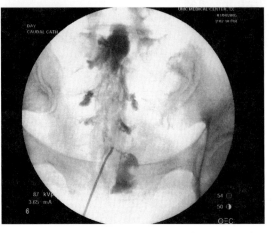

Fig. 16.2 Normal epidurogram—note filling of S1-S3 nerve roots.

Three general patterns of contrast filling may be identified: epidural, subdural, and intrathecal. The epidural pattern is characterized by a reticular pattern limited to the midline epidural space, and flowing in a "Christmas-tree" pattern to fill the exiting nerve roots (**Fig. 16.1**). When obtained, this contrast pattern responds by further filling of ever higher nerve root levels with the administration of additional contrast. In the presence of plica mediana dorsalis, it is not uncommon for this pattern to fill only one half of the epidural space and exiting nerve roots. Contrast should spread both superiorly and inferiorly in a free-flowing pattern (**Fig. 16.2**).

Subdural injection of contrast results in a patchy, fine pattern in the AP projection (**Fig. 16.3**). Lateral fluoroscopy will reveal a solid "line" of contrast extending several levels higher than expected given the volume of contrast injected (**Fig. 16.4**). Subdural therapeutic injections are not recommended, and repositioning of the access needle should be carried out. It is important to note that subdural contrast patterns are very difficult to identify in the AP fluoroscopic projection, emphasizing the necessity for both AP and lateral views to confirm proper needle positioning.

Intrathecal contrast injection reveals a myelographic spread, with outlining of the nerve roots/cauda equina when carried out in the lumbar spine. The injected contrast will not spread to outline the exiting nerve roots, and will be limited to the midline spinal space. In the cervical and thoracic regions, intrathecal

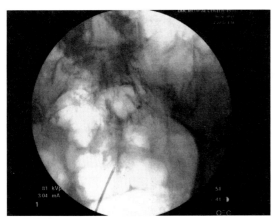

Fig. 16.3 Subdural injection of contrast—note reticular filling pattern.

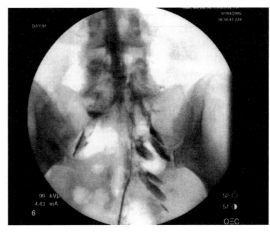

Fig. 16.5 Epidurogram—note filling defect of left S2 level.

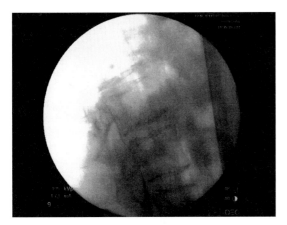

Fig. 16.4 Subdural contrast (2 mL in sacral space)—note extension to L1 level with 2 mL injection.

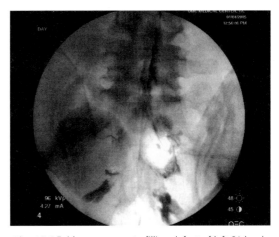

Fig. 16.6 Epidurogram—note filling defect of left S1 level.

injection of contrast will flow laterally, and appear as a "double bar" outlining the spinal cord laterally within the spinal canal.

When performed in the sacral space, epidurography is very effective in identifying areas of epidural scarring that may be targeted via caudal neuroplasty. These areas appear as "filling" defects within the dye spread. It is uncommon for these filling defects to appear below the S2 level, but they are common above S1 (**Figs. 16.5** and **16.6**). Areas of filling defect may be accessed via caudal catheter and the degree of neuroplasty may be assessed by repeat epidurography following injection of hyaluronidase. When performed properly, these filling defects resolve with neuroplasty.

Side Effects and Complications

Epidurography can be safely performed in the cervical, thoracic, lumbar, and sacral spinal canals. Loculation with concomitant spinal cord compression and myelopathy is a real concern in the cervical and thoracic epidural spaces, and the need for visualization of distal runoff cannot be overemphasized. Injection into radicular feeder vessels of the spinal cord is a concern at all levels of the spinal cord, and careful observation for vascular patterns must be maintained.

Injection into the intrathecal space is occasionally observed. Iohexol (Omnipaque) is the only contrast agent approved for intrathecal use, and is therefore the only agent used at our institution. Tonic-clonic seizures with the intrathecal administration of iohexol have been reported,[17] but are a rare complication.

Anaphylactic reactions to injected contrast material may occur. Patients who are allergic to iodine or radiographic contrast material should not be subjected to epidurography until sensitivity testing by appropriate specialists has been performed. Currently, no iodine-free contrast agents are approved for epidural use.

Contrast-induced nephropathy is possible with large volumes of contrast injected, but is rare in epidurography because of the slow reabsorption of contrast and limited concentrations delivered to the kidneys. Total doses of contrast should be limited to the least effective dose in patients with preexisting renal insufficiency.

Conclusion

Epidurography is a commonly performed procedure in interventional pain management. The correct interpretation of epidurograms is essential to the safe practice of epidural access procedures, and helps guide appropriate interventions in the future. All interventional pain management physicians should become proficient at the performance and interpretation of epidurograms to enhance the safety of their practice.

References

Full references for this chapter can be found on www.expertconsult.com.

Chapter **17**

Neural Blockade for the Diagnosis of Pain

Steven D. Waldman

As emphasized in previous chapters, the cornerstone of successful treatment of the patient suffering from pain is a correct diagnosis. As straightforward as this statement is in theory, it may become difficult to achieve in the individual patient. The reason for this difficulty is due to four disparate but interrelated issues: (1) pain is a subjective response that is difficult, if not impossible, to quantify; (2) pain response in humans is made up of a variety of obvious and not so obvious factors that may modulate the patient's clinical expression of pain either upward or downward (**Table 17.1**); (3) our current understanding of neurophysiologic, neuroanatomic, and behavioral components of pain is incomplete and imprecise; and (4) there is ongoing debate by the specialty of pain management of whether pain is best treated as a symptom or as a disease. The uncertainly introduced by these factors can often make accurate diagnosis problematic.

Given the difficulty in establishing a correct diagnosis of a patient's pain, the clinician often is forced to look for external means to quantify or confirm a dubious clinical impression. Laboratory and radiologic testing are often the next procedures the clinician seeks for reassurance. If such testing is inconclusive or the results are discordant with the clinical impression, diagnostic nerve block may be the next logical step. Done properly, diagnostic nerve block can provide the clinician with useful information to aid in increasing the comfort level with a tentative diagnosis. It cannot be emphasized enough, however, that overreliance on the results of even a properly performed diagnostic nerve block can set in motion a series of events that will, at the very least, provide the patient little or no pain relief and, at the very worst, result in permanent complications from invasive surgeries or neurodestructive procedures that were justified solely on the basis of diagnostic nerve block.

The Historical Imperative and Clinical Rationale for Use of Diagnostic Nerve Blocks

Our view of pain has changed over the centuries as our understanding of this universal condition has improved. Early humans viewed pain as a punishment from the deities for a variety of sins as exemplified by the legend of Prometheus. Prometheus was sentenced by Zeus to eternal torture for giving the fire reserved for the gods to mortals (**Fig. 17.1**). The seventeenth-century scientist and philosopher, Descartes (**Fig. 17.2**), changed this view in a single instant by his drawing of a fire burning the foot of a man. Descartes postulated a rational basis for pain premised on the then radical notion that pain was sensed in the periphery and then carried via the nerves and spinal cord to the brain (**Fig. 17.3**).

It is not surprising that concurrent advances in the understanding of the anatomy of the peripheral and central nervous system led scientists and clinicians to seek new ways to stop pain. In 1774 English surgeon James Moore described the use of a "C" clamp to compress the peripheral nerves of the upper and lower extremity to induce anesthesia to decrease the pain of amputation and other surgeries of the extremities.[1] The development and refinement of the syringe and hollow needle led to the idea of injecting substances such as morphine in proximity to the peripheral nerves to relieve pain. Rynd, in 1845, postulated the utility of delivering morphine directly onto a nerve via a hollow trocar.[2] This was a radical departure from the then current practice of surgically exposing the nerve and then topically applying pain relieving agents. It is not surprising that many patients thought that the "cure was worse than the disease." However, it was the landmark clinical discovery of the utility of cocaine as a surgical anesthetic by Carl Koller in 1884

Table 17.1 Factors That Influence Pain

Age
Gender
Socioeconomic status
Ethnicity
Pregnancy
Stress
Chronicity

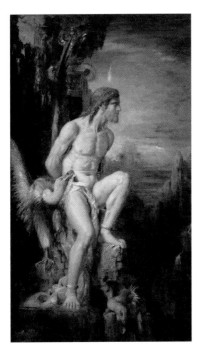

Fig. 17.1 Artist's depiction of Prometheus.

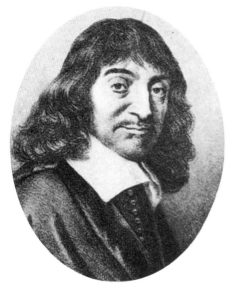

Fig. 17.2 A portrait of Descartes.

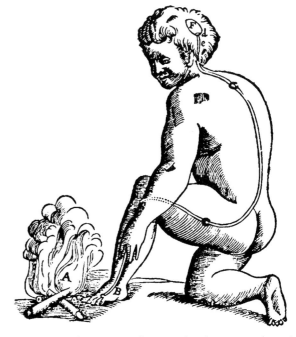

Fig. 17.3 Drawing by Descartes demonstrating the concept that pain is carried via nerves from the periphery to the brain.

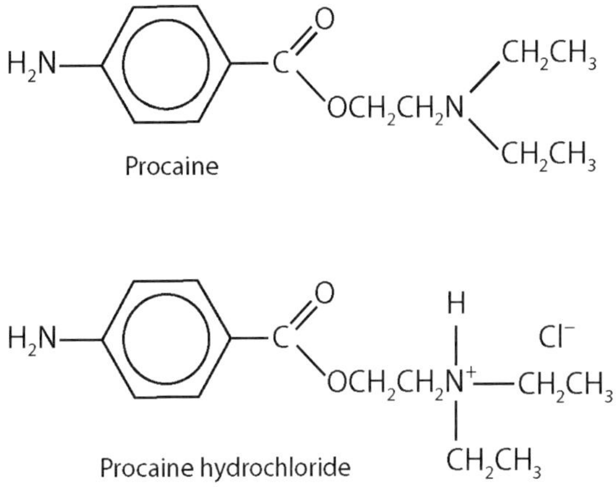

Fig. 17.4 Diagram of chemical structures of procaine and procaine hydrochloride.

that ushered in the era of regional anesthesia.[3] Corning's first spinal anesthetic in 1885 further solidified the concept that blocking nerves could alleviate human suffering, albeit not without complications—as it was Corning himself who may have suffered the first spinal headache following induction of an anesthetic.

As the specialty of regional anesthesia matured, the technical ability to easily and consistently render nerves incapable of transmitting pain increased. The early work of Halstead and Hall, Corning, and others helped refine the "how-to-do-it" aspects of blocking a nerve. However, the relative toxicity of cocaine, which was the only local anesthetic readily available at the time, significantly limited the clinical utility of otherwise technically satisfactory nerve block techniques.

It was not until the synthesis in 1909 by Einhorn of the local anesthetic ester procaine that regional anesthesia was truly safe enough for widespread use (**Fig. 17.4**). Unfortunately, procaine's short duration of action made its use impractical for longer operations; this limitation led to the development of the longer-acting ester class of local anesthetics, such as tetracaine and dibucaine, albeit with increased systemic toxicity. It was the development of the safer amide class of local

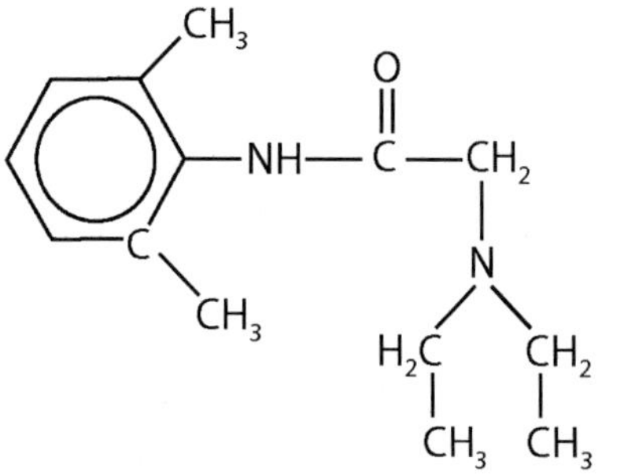

Fig. 17.5 Diagram of chemical structure of lidocaine.

Table 17.2 The Do's and Dont's of Diagnostic Nerve Blocks

Do analyze the information obtained from diagnostic nerve blocks in the context of the patient's history, physical, laboratory, neurophysiologic, and radiographic testing.

Don't overrely on information obtained from diagnostic nerve blocks.

Do view with skepticism discordant or contradictory information obtained from diagnostic nerve blocks.

Don't rely on information obtained from diagnostic nerve block as the sole justification to proceed with invasive treatments.

Do consider the possibility of technical limitations that limit the ability to perform an accurate diagnostic nerve block.

Do consider the possibility of patient anatomic variations that may influence the results of diagnostic nerve blocks.

Do consider the presence of incidents pain when analyzing the results of diagnostic nerve blocks.

Don't perform diagnostic nerve blocks when patients are not currently having the pain you are trying to diagnose.

Do consider behavioral factors that may influence the results of diagnostic nerve blocks.

Do consider that the patient may premedicate before undergoing diagnostic nerve blocks.

anesthetics, such as lidocaine by Löfgren and Lundquist in 1943, that began the most recent chapter in the quest for the ability to block human pain (**Fig. 17.5**).

Just as it seemed that science had finally given doctors the ability to block pain, other scientific advances began to question the construct that Descartes has given us—that pain is a simple function of a stimulus being carried over an anatomically distinct neural pathway. As clinicians were puzzled that patients who had otherwise seemingly perfect nerve blocks continued to have pain during surgical procedures, research scientists were beginning to unravel the mystery of peripheral and central modulation of pain—as well as the role that the sympathetic nervous system plays in the pain response. The quest for answers as to how these disparate neuroanatomic structures affect, modulate, and subserve a patient's pain continues today. It is this quest for answers that brings us to an evaluation of the role that diagnostic nerve blocks play in contemporary pain management.

A Road Map for the Appropriate Use of Diagnostic Nerve Block

It must be said at the outset of this discussion that even the perfectly performed diagnostic nerve block is not without limitations. **Table 17.2** provides the reader with a list of do's and dont's when performing and interpreting diagnostic nerve blocks. First and foremost, the clinician should use with caution the information gleaned from diagnostic nerve blocks and use it only as one piece of the overall diagnostic workup of the patient in pain. Results of a diagnostic nerve block that contradicts the clinical impression that the pain management specialist has formed as a result of the performance of a targeted history and physical examination and consideration of confirmatory laboratory, neurophysiologic, and radiographic testing should be viewed with great skepticism. Such disparate results should never serve as the sole basis for moving ahead with neurodestructive or invasive surgical procedures that, in this setting, have little or no hope of actually helping alleviate a patient's pain.

In addition to the admonitions just mentioned, it must be recognized that the clinical utility of the diagnostic nerve block can be affected by technical limitations. In general, the reliability of data gleaned from a diagnostic nerve block is in direct proportion to the clinician's familiarity with the functional anatomy of the area in which the nerve resides and the clinician's experience in performing the block being attempted. Even in the best of hands, some nerve blocks are technically more demanding than others, which increases the likelihood of a less than perfect result. Proximity of other neural structures

to the nerve, ganglion, or plexus being blocked may lead to the inadvertent and often unrecognized block of adjacent nerves, thereby invalidating the results that the clinician sees (e.g., the proximity of the lower cervical nerve roots, phrenic nerve, and brachial plexus to the stellate ganglion).

Some of these technical obstacles can be decreased, although by no means completely eliminated, by the use of fluoroscopic or computerized tomographic guidance during needle placement. The addition of small amounts of radiopaque contrast medium to the local anesthetic may also increase the accuracy of the block. However, the clinician must be aware that the overreliance on either of these aids may lead to erroneous conclusions. It should also be remembered that the possibility of undetected anatomic abnormality always exists, which may further confuse the results of the diagnostic nerve block (e.g., conjoined nerve roots, the Martin Gruber anastomosis [a median to ulnar nerve connection]).[4]

Because each pain experience is unique to the individual patient and the clinician really has no way to quantify it, special care must be taken to ensure that everybody is in agreement insofar as what pain the diagnostic block is intended to diagnose. Many patients have more than one type of pain. A patient may have both radicular pain and the pain of alcoholic neuropathy. A given diagnostic block may relieve one source of the patient's pain while leaving the other untouched.

If the patient is having incident pain (e.g., pain when walking or sitting), the performance of a diagnostic block in a setting other than one that will provoke the incident pain is of little or no value. This often means that the clinician must tailor the type of nerve block that is to be performed to allow the patient to be able to safely perform the activity that incites the pain. A diagnostic nerve block should never be performed if the patient is not having or is unable to provoke the pain that the pain management specialist is trying to diagnose because there is nothing to quantify.

The accuracy of diagnostic nerve block can be enhanced by assessing the duration of nerve relief relative to the expected pharmacologic duration of the agent being used to block the pain. If there is discordance between the duration of pain relief relative to duration of the local anesthetic or opioid being used, extreme caution should be exercised before relying solely on the results of that diagnostic nerve block. Such discordance can be due to technical shortcomings in the performance of the block, anatomic variations, and, most commonly, behavioral components of the patient's pain.

It must be remembered that the pain and anxiety caused by the diagnostic nerve block itself may confuse the results of an otherwise technically perfect block. The clinician should be alert to the fact that many pain patients may premedicate themselves because of the fear of procedural pain. This also has the potential to confuse the observed results. Obviously, the use of sedation or anxiolytic agents before the performance of diagnostic nerve block will further cloud the very issues the nerve block is, in fact, supposed to clarify.

Specific Diagnostic Nerve Blocks

Early proponents of regional anesthesia, such as Labat and Pitkin, believed it was possible to block just about any nerve in the body.[5] Despite the many technical limitations these pioneers faced, these clinicians persevered. They did so not only because they believed in the clinical utility and safety of regional nerve block but because the currently available alternatives to render a patient insensible to surgical pain were much less attractive. The introduction of the muscle relaxant, curare, in 1942 by Dr. Harold Griffith changed this construct, and in a relatively short time, regional anesthesia was relegated to the history of medicine with its remaining proponents viewed as eccentric at best.[6] Just as the Egyptian embalming techniques were lost to modern man, many regional anesthesia techniques that were in common use were lost to today's pain management specialists. What we are left with today are those procedures that stood the test of time for surgical anesthesia. For the most part, these were the nerve blocks that were not overly demanding from a technical viewpoint and were reasonably safe to perform. Many of these techniques also have clinical utility as diagnostic nerve blocks. These techniques are summarized in **Table 17.3**. A discussion of the more commonly used diagnostic nerve blocks follows.

Neuroaxial Diagnostic Nerve Blocks

Discussed in detail in Chapter 14, differential spinal and epidural blocks have gained popularity as an aid in the diagnosis of pain. Popularized by Winnie, differential spinal and epidural blocks have as their basis the varying sensitivity of sympathetic and somatic sensory and motor fibers to blockade by local anesthetics.[7] Although sound in principle, these techniques are subject to serious technical difficulties that limit the reliability of the information obtained. These difficulties include the following:

1. The inability to precisely measure the extent to which each type of nerve fiber is blocked.
2. The possibility that more than one nerve fiber type is simultaneously blocked, leading the clinician to attribute the patient's pain to the wrong neuroanatomic structure.

Table 17.3 **Common Diagnostic Nerve Blocks**
NEUROAXIAL BLOCKS
Epidural block
Subarachnoid block
PERIPHERAL NERVE BLOCKS
Greater and lesser occipital nerve blocks
Third occipital nerve blocks
Trigeminal nerve block
Brachial plexus block
Median, radial, and ulnar nerve blocks
Intercostal nerve block
Selective nerve root block
Sciatic nerve block
INTRA-ARTICULAR NERVE BLOCKS
Facet block
SYMPATHETIC NERVE BLOCKS
Stellate ganglion block
Celiac plexus block
Lumbar sympathetic block
Hypogastric plexus and ganglion impar blocks

3. The impossibility of "blinding" the patient to the sensation of warmth associated with sympathetic blockade, as well as the numbness and weakness that accompany blockade of the somatic sensory and motor fibers.
4. The breakdown of the construct of temporal linearity, which holds that the more "sensitive" sympathetic fibers will become blocked first, followed by the less sensitive somatic sensory fibers, and last by the more resistant motor fibers. As a practical matter, it is not uncommon for the patient to experience some sensory block before noticing the warmth associated with block of the sympathetic fibers, rendering the test results suspect.
5. Afferent nociceptive input can still be demonstrated in the brain, even in the presence of a neuroaxial block that is dense enough to allow a major surgical procedure.
6. Neurophysiologic changes associated with pain may increase or decrease the firing threshold of the nerve, suggesting that even in the present of sub-blocking concentrations, there is the possibility that the sensitized afferent nerves will stop firing.
7. Modulation of pain transmission at the spinal cord, brainstem, and higher levels is known to exist and may alter the results of even the most carefully performed differential neural blockade.
8. Significant behavioral components to a patient's pain may influence the subjective response the patient reports to the clinician who is performing differential neuroaxial blockade.

In spite of these shortcomings, neuroaxial differential block remains a clinically useful tool to aid in the diagnosis of unexplained pain. The clinician can increase the sensitivity of this technique by (1) use of reverse differential spinal or epidural block, in which the patient is given a high concentration of local anesthetic that results in a dense motor, sensory, and sympathetic block and then observing the patient as the block regresses; (2) use of opioids instead of local anesthetics that remove the sensory clues that may influence patient responses; and (3) repeating the block on more than one occasion using local anesthetics or opioids of varying durations (e.g., lidocaine versus bupivacaine or morphine versus fentanyl) and comparing the results for consistency. Whether or not this technique stands the test of time, Winnie's admonition to clinicians that sympathetically mediated pain is often underdiagnosed most certainly will.

Greater, Lesser, and Third Occipital Nerve Block

The greater occipital nerve arises from fibers of the dorsal primary ramus of the second cervical nerve and to a lesser extent from fibers of the third cervical nerve.[8] The greater occipital nerve pierces the fascia just below the superior nuchal ridge along with the occipital artery. It supplies the medial portion of the posterior scalp as far anterior as the vertex. The lesser occipital nerve arises from the ventral primary rami of the second and third cervical nerves. The lesser occipital nerve passes superiorly along the posterior border of the sternocleidomastoid muscle, dividing into cutaneous branches that innervate the lateral portion of the posterior scalp and the cranial surface of the pinna of the ear. The C2-3 facet joint is exclusively innervated by the third occipital nerve, which is the superficial medial branch of the C3 dorsal ramus.[9] The third occipital nerve also supplies a small patch of skin immediately below the occipital region.

Selective blockade of the greater, lesser, and third occipital nerves can provide the pain management specialist with useful information when trying to determine the cause of cervicogenic headache. By blocking the atlantoaxial, atlanto-occipital, cervical epidural, cervical facet, and greater, lesser, and third occipital nerves on successive visits, the pain management specialist may be able to differentiate the nerves subserving the patient's headache.

Stellate Ganglion Block

The stellate ganglion is located on the anterior surface of the longus colli muscle. This muscle lies just anterior to the transverse processes of the seventh cervical and first thoracic vertebrae.[10] The stellate ganglion is made up of the fused portion of the seventh cervical and first thoracic sympathetic ganglia. The stellate ganglion lies anteromedial to the vertebral artery and is medial to the common carotid artery and jugular vein. It is lateral to the trachea and esophagus.[11] The proximity of the exiting cervical nerve roots and brachial plexus to the stellate ganglion make it easy to inadvertently block these structures when performing stellate ganglion block, making interpretation of the results of the block difficult.

Selective blockade of stellate ganglion can provide the pain management specialist with useful information when trying to determine the cause of upper extremity or facial pain without clear diagnosis. By blocking the brachial plexus (preferably by the axillary approach) and stellate ganglion on successive visits, the pain management specialist may be able to differentiate the nerves subserving the patient's upper extremity pain. Selective differential blockade of the stellate ganglion, trigeminal nerve, and sphenopalatine ganglion on

successive visits may elucidate the nerves subserving facial pain that is often difficult to diagnose.

Cervical Facet Block

The cervical facet joints are formed by the articulations of the superior and inferior articular facets of adjacent vertebrae.[12] Except for the atlanto-occipital and atlantoaxial joints, the remaining cervical facet joints are true joints in that they are lined with synovium and possess a true joint capsule. This capsule is richly innervated and supports the notion of the facet joint as a pain generator. The cervical facet joint is susceptible to arthritic changes and trauma caused by acceleration-deceleration injuries. Such damage to the joint results in pain secondary to synovial joint inflammation and adhesions.

Each facet joint receives innervation from two spinal levels.[13] Each joint receives fibers from the dorsal ramus at the same level as the vertebra, as well as fibers from the dorsal ramus of the vertebra above. This fact explains the ill-defined nature of facet-mediated pain and explains why the branch of the dorsal ramus arising above the offending level must often also be blocked to provide complete pain relief. At each level, the dorsal ramus provides a medial branch that wraps around the convexity of the articular pillar of its respective vertebra and provides innervation to the facet joint.

Selective blockade of cervical facet joints can provide the pain management specialist with useful information when trying to determine the cause of cervicogenic headache and/or neck pain. By blocking the atlantoaxial, atlanto-occipital, cervical epidural, and greater and lesser occipital nerves on successive visits, the clinician may be able to differentiate the nerves subserving the patient's headache and/or neck pain.

Intercostal Nerve Block

The intercostal nerves arise from the anterior division of the thoracic paravertebral nerve.[14] A typical intercostal nerve has four major branches. The first branch is the unmyelinated postganglionic fibers of the gray rami communicantes, which interface with the sympathetic chain. The second branch is the posterior cutaneous branch, which innervates the muscles and skin of the paraspinal area. The third branch is the lateral cutaneous division, which arises in the anterior axillary line. The lateral cutaneous division provides the majority of the cutaneous innervation of the chest and abdominal wall. The fourth branch is the anterior cutaneous branch supplying innervation to the midline of the chest and abdominal wall. Occasionally, the terminal branches of a given intercostal nerve may actually cross the midline to provide sensory innervation to the contralateral chest and abdominal wall.[15] This fact has specific import when utilizing intercostal block as part of a diagnostic workup for the patient with chest wall and/or abdominal pain. The twelfth thoracic nerve is called the subcostal nerve and is unique in that it gives off a branch to the first lumbar nerve, thus contributing to the lumbar plexus.

Selective blockade of intercostal and/or subcostal nerves thought to be subserving a patient's pain can provide the pain management specialist with useful information when trying to determine the cause of chest wall and/or abdominal pain. By blocking the intercostal nerves and celiac plexus on successive visits, the pain management specialist may be able to differentiate which nerves are subserving the patient's chest wall and/or abdominal pain.

Celiac Plexus Block

The sympathetic innervation of the abdominal viscera originates in the anterolateral horn of the spinal cord. Preganglionic fibers from T5-12 exit the spinal cord in conjunction with the ventral roots to join the white communicating rami on their way to the sympathetic chain. Rather than synapsing with the sympathetic chain, these preganglionic fibers pass through it to ultimately synapse on the celiac ganglia.[16] The greater, lesser, and least splanchnic nerves provide the major preganglionic contribution to the celiac plexus. The greater splanchnic nerve has its origin from the T5-10 spinal roots. The nerve travels along the thoracic paravertebral border through the crus of the diaphragm into the abdominal cavity, ending on the celiac ganglion of its respective side. The lesser splanchnic nerve arises from the T10-11 roots and passes with the greater nerve to end at the celiac ganglion. The least splanchnic nerve arises from the T11-12 spinal roots and passes through the diaphragm to the celiac ganglion.

Interpatient anatomic variability of the celiac ganglia is significant, but the following generalizations can be drawn from anatomic studies of the celiac ganglia. The number of ganglia varies from one to five, and ganglia range in diameter from 0.5 to 4.5 cm. The ganglia lie anterior and anterolateral to the aorta. The ganglia located on the left are uniformly more inferior than their right-sided counterparts by as much as a vertebral level, but both groups of ganglia lie below the level of the celiac artery. The ganglia usually lie approximately at the level of the first lumbar vertebra.

Postganglionic fibers radiate from the celiac ganglia to follow the course of the blood vessels to innervate the abdominal viscera. These organs include much of the distal esophagus, stomach, duodenum, small intestine, ascending and proximal transverse colon, adrenal glands, pancreas, spleen, liver, and biliary system. It is these postganglionic fibers, the fibers arising from the preganglionic splanchnic nerves, and the celiac ganglion that make up the celiac plexus. The diaphragm separates the thorax from the abdominal cavity while still permitting the passage of the thoracoabdominal structures, including the aorta, vena cava, and splanchnic nerves. The diaphragmatic crura are bilateral structures that arise from the anterolateral surfaces of the upper two or three lumbar vertebrae and disks. The crura of the diaphragm serve as a barrier to effectively separate the splanchnic nerves from the celiac ganglia and plexus below.

The celiac plexus is anterior to the crus of the diaphragm. The plexus extends in front of and around the aorta, with the greatest concentration of fibers anterior to the aorta.[17] With the single-needle transaortic approach to celiac plexus block, the needle is placed close to this concentration of plexus fibers. The relationship of the celiac plexus to the surrounding structures is as follows: The aorta lies anterior and slightly to the left of the anterior margin of the vertebral body. The inferior vena cava lies to the right, with the kidneys posterolateral to the great vessels. The pancreas lies anterior to the celiac plexus. All of these structures lie within the retroperitoneal space.

Selective blockade of the celiac plexus can provide the pain management specialist with useful information when trying to determine the cause of chest wall, flank, and/or abdominal pain. By blocking the intercostal nerves and celiac plexus on successive visits, the pain management specialist may be able to differentiate which nerves are subserving the patient's pain.

Selective Nerve Root Block

Improvements in fluoroscopy and needle technology have led to increased interest in selective nerve root block in the diagnosis of cervical and lumbar radicular pain. Although technically demanding and not without complications, selective nerve root block is often used in conjunction with provocative diskography to help identify the nidus of the patient's pain complaint. The use of selective nerve root block as a diagnostic maneuver must be approached with caution. Because of the proximity of the epidural, subdural, and subarachnoid spaces, it is easy to inadvertently place local anesthetic into these spaces when intending to block a single cervical or lumbar nerve root. This error is not always readily apparent on fluoroscopy, given the small amounts of local anesthetic and contrast medium used.

Conclusion

The use of nerve blocks as part of the evaluation of the patient in pain represents a reasonable next step if a careful targeted history and physical examination and rational radiographic, neurophysiologic, and laboratory testing fail to provide a clear diagnosis. The overreliance on diagnostic nerve block as the sole justification to perform an invasive or neurodestructive procedure can lead to significant patient morbidity and dissatisfaction.

References

Full references for this chapter can be found on www.expertconsult.com.

Chapter 18

Differential Neural Blockade for the Diagnosis of Pain

Alon P. Winnie and Kenneth D. Candido

Clinically, differential neural blockade is the selective blockade of one type of nerve fiber without blocking other types of nerve fibers. It is an extremely useful diagnostic tool that allows the clinician to observe the effect of a sympathetic block, a sensory block, and, for that matter, a block of all nerve fibers by local anesthetic agents on a patient's pain, and to compare that effect with the effect of an injection of an inactive agent (placebo). Two clinical approaches to the production of differential neural blockade exist: an *anatomic approach* and a *pharmacologic approach*. The anatomic approach is based on sufficient anatomic separation of sympathetic and somatic fibers to allow injection of local anesthetic to block one type only (see discussion later in this chapter). The pharmacologic approach is based on the presumed difference in the sensitivity of the various types of nerve fibers to local anesthetics, so that the injection of local anesthetics in different concentrations selectively blocks different types of fibers.

Because pain is a totally *subjective* phenomenon, what is needed to identify the neural pathway that subserves it is some sort of *objective* diagnostic test, and differential neural blockade is just such a test. Although differential neural blockade is not intended to replace a detailed history, a complete physical examination, and appropriate laboratory, radiographic, and psychologic studies, in our practice it has been a rewarding diagnostic maneuver that has been effective in delineating the neural mechanisms subserving many puzzling pain problems,

and it has been particularly useful in patients who have intractable pain with no apparent cause.

The Pharmacologic Approach

A differential spinal is the simplest pharmacologic approach with the most discrete end points. The first clinical application of this technique[1] was based on the seminal work of Gasser and Erlanger,[2,3] and, although these investigators were wrong about the site of conduction (they believed it took place within the axoplasm), they established forever the relationship between fiber size, conduction velocity, and fiber function. Their classification of nerve fibers based on size is still used today (**Table 18.1**). In a simple but elegant experiment, these researchers showed that when a nerve is stimulated and the response is recorded only a few millimeters away, the record shows a single action potential. Then they demonstrated that, as the recording electrode is moved progressively farther away from the stimulating electrode, the action potential can be shown to consist of several smaller spikes, each representing an impulse traveling at a different rate along a nerve fiber of a different size. The action potentials might be compared to runners in a race who become separated along the course as the faster contestants outstrip the slower. Thus, in a record obtained by a recording electrode 82 mm from the point of stimulation, three waves can be seen; whereas at 12 mm, the potentials are fused, and only one large wave appears (**Fig. 18.1**). It may be seen in **Table 18.1** that the

Table 18.1 Classification of Nerve Fibers by Fiber Size and the Relation of Fiber Size to Function and Sensitivity to Local Anesthetics*

Group/Subgroup	Diameter (μm)	Conduction Velocity (m/sec)	Modalities Subserved	Sensitivity to Local Anesthetics (%)[†]
A (myelinated)				
_A-alpha	15–20	8–120	Large motor, proprioception	1.0
_A-beta	8–15	30–70	Small motor, touch, pressure	↓
_A-gamma	4–8	30–70	Muscle spindle, reflex	↓
_				↓
_A-delta	3–4	10–30	Temperature, sharp pain, nociception	0.5
B (myelinated)	3–4	10–15	Preganglionic autonomic	0.25
C (unmyelinated)	1–2	1–2	Dull pain, temperature, nociception	0.5

*Subarachnoid procaine.
†Vertical arrows indicate intermediate values, in descending order.

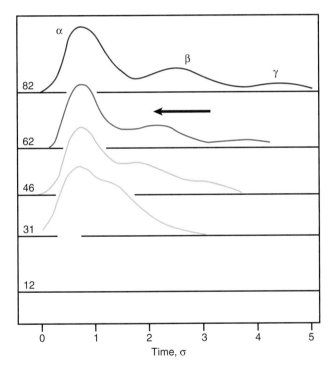

α

β

γ

82

62

46

31

12

0 1 2 3 4 5

Time, σ

Fig. 18.1 Cathode ray oscillographs of the action current in a sciatic nerve of a bullfrog after conduction from the point of stimulation through the distances (mm) shown at the left. The delta wave is not shown. *(Modified from Gasser HS, Erlanger J: Role of fiber size in establishment of nerve block by pressure or cocaine,* Am J Physiol *88:587, 1929.)*

diameter of a nerve fiber is its most important physical dimension, so it is on that basis that they have been subdivided into three classes, A, B, and C fibers, with A fibers being subdivided into four subclasses, alpha, beta, gamma, and delta. It may also be seen that the fiber diameter is an important determinant of conduction velocity—the conduction velocity of A fibers (in meters per second) being approximately 6 times the fiber diameter (in micrometers).[4] In addition, the diameter and myelination of a nerve fiber also determine to some degree the modality or modalities subserved by that fiber[5]: A-alpha fibers subserve motor function and proprioception; A-beta fibers subserve the transmission of touch and pressure; and A-gamma fibers subserve muscle tone. The thinnest A fibers, the A-delta group, convey sharp pain and temperature sensation and signal nociception (tissue damage). The myelinated B fibers are thin, preganglionic, autonomic fibers, and the non-myelinated C fibers, like the myelinated A-delta fibers, subserve dull pain, temperature transmission, and nociception. C fibers are thinner than the myelinated fibers and have a much slower conduction velocity than even A-delta fibers.

Although the relationship between fiber size and sensitivity to local anesthetics originally proposed by Gasser and Erlanger was challenged recently, the "bathed length principle" proposed by Fink[6,7] has restored the functional relationship between fiber size and sensitivity to local anesthetics because the larger the nerve fiber, the greater the internodal distance. It has been postulated that the density of the distribution of sodium channels at the nodes of Ranvier increases with fiber size, so that the "denser channel packing at the nodes" may also result in increased minimum blocking concentration (C_m), so this may be another reason larger fibers require a higher concentration of local anesthetic for blockade than do smaller fibers.[8]

Conventional Sequential Differential Spinal Block

The conventional sequential technique of differential subarachnoid block[9,10] is a refinement of the techniques first used by Arrowood and Sarnoff[1] and later by McCollum and Stephen.[11] The technique has certain inherent shortcomings (see later discussion), which have caused it to be replaced in our practice by the modified technique, but, because this is the prototype of differential neural blockade, understanding the technique and the problems it presents provides insight into the usefulness and the limitations of diagnostic differential spinal blockade using the pharmacologic approach.

Procedure

After detailed informed consent is obtained from the patient, an intravenous infusion is started and prehydration with

Table 18.2 Preparation of Solutions for Conventional Sequential Differential Spinal Blockade

Solution	Preparation of Solution	Yield	Blockade
D	To 2 mL of 10% procaine add 2 mL of normal saline	4 mL of 5% procaine	Motor
C	To 1 mL of 5% procaine add 9 mL of normal saline	10 mL of 0.5% procaine	Sensory
B	To 5 mL of 0.5% procaine add 5 mL of normal saline	10 mL of 0.25% procaine	Sympathetic
A	Draw up 10 mL of normal saline	10 mL of normal saline	Placebo

Table 18.3 Observations After Each Injection

Sequence	Observation
1	Blood pressure and pulse rate
2	Patient's subjective evaluation of the pain at rest
3	Reproduction of patient's pain by movement
4	Signs of sympathetic block (temperature change, psychogalvanic reflex)
5	Signs of sensory block (no response to pinprick)
6	Signs of motor block (inability to move toes, feet, legs)

crystalloid is begun, as for any spinal anesthetic. Similarly, all of the monitors routinely used for spinal anesthesia are applied, including blood pressure, electrocardiography (ECG), and pulse oximetry, and baseline values are recorded. Four solutions are prepared (**Table 18.2**), and the patient is placed into the lateral decubitus position with the painful side down, if possible. After the usual sterile preparation and draping of the back, a 25- to 27-gauge pencil-point spinal needle is introduced into the lumbar subarachnoid space at the L2-3 or L3-4 interspace. The patient is shown the four prepared syringes, all of which appear identical, and is told that each of the solutions will be injected sequentially at 10- to 15-minute intervals. The patient is instructed to tell the physician which, if any, of the solutions relieves the pain. The solutions are referred to as *A* through *D,* so that the physicians can discuss the solutions freely in front of the patient without using the word *placebo.*

Solution A, which contains no local anesthetic, is the placebo. Solution B contains 0.25% procaine, which is the mean sympatholytic concentration of procaine in the subarachnoid space.[1] That is, it is the concentration that is sufficient to block B fibers but is *usually* insufficient to block A-delta and C fibers. Solution C contains 0.5% procaine, the mean sensory blocking concentration of procaine. That is, it is the concentration *usually* sufficient to block, in addition to B fibers, A-delta and C fibers but is insufficient to block A-alpha, A-beta, and A-gamma fibers. Solution D contains 5.0% procaine, which provides complete blockade of all fibers, including sympathetic, sensory, and motor fibers.

To prevent bias, it is extremely important that all of the injections be carried out in exactly the same manner, so that to the patient they are identical to and indistinguishable from one another. It is equally important that the physician make exactly the same observations after each injection (**Table 18.3**). The observations must be carried out in an identical manner after each injection so that the observations themselves do not influence the patient's response. Obviously, an inexperienced clinician who checks only the blood pressure after the sympatholytic injection, or who checks only the response to pinprick after the sensory-blocking injection, and who checks only the motor function after the motor-blocking injection

would clearly reveal the expectation that each sequential injection will produce progressively increasing effects. This would clearly compromise the validity of the information obtained from the procedure.

Interpretation

The conventional sequential differential spinal is interpreted as follows: If the patient's pain is relieved after subarachnoid injection of solution A (the placebo), the patient's pain is classified as "psychogenic." It is well known that some 30% to 35% of all patients with true, organic pain obtain relief from an inactive agent.[12] Therefore relief in response to the normal saline may represent a placebo reaction, but it may also indicate that an entirely psychogenic mechanism is subserving the patient's pain. Clinically, these two can usually be differentiated, because a placebo reaction is usually short-lived and self-limiting, whereas pain relief provided by a placebo to a patient suffering from true, psychogenic pain is usually long-lasting, if not permanent. If the difference between the two is not clinically evident, evaluation by a clinical psychologist or psychiatrist may be deemed to be necessary.

If the patient does not obtain relief from the placebo but does obtain relief from the subarachnoid injection of 0.25% procaine, the mechanism subserving the patient's pain is tentatively classified as sympathetic, provided that concurrent with the onset of pain relief, signs of sympathetic blockade are observed *without* signs of sensory block. Obviously, although 0.25% procaine is the *usual* sympatholytic concentration in most patients, in some patients (who may have a reduced C_m for A-delta and C fibers) relief may be due to the production of analgesia and/or anesthesia. The finding that a sympathetic mechanism is subserving a patient's pain is extremely fortuitous for the patient, because if the pain is truly sympathetically mediated, if treated early enough, it may be completely and permanently relieved by a series of sympathetic nerve blocks.

If 0.25% procaine does not provide pain relief but the subarachnoid injection of the 0.5% concentration does, this usually indicates that the patient's pain is subserved by A-delta and/or C fibers and is classified as somatic pain, *provided that* the patient did exhibit signs of sympathetic blockade after the previous injection of 0.25% procaine and that the onset of pain relief is accompanied by the onset of analgesia and/or anesthesia. This is important because if a patient has an elevated C_m for B fibers, the pain relief from 0.5% procaine could be due to sympathetic block rather than to sensory block.

Table 18.4 Diagnostic Possibilities of "Central Mechanism"

Diagnosis	Explanation/Basis of Diagnosis
Central lesion	The patient may have a lesion in the central nervous system that is above the level of the subarachnoid sensory block. For example, we have seen two patients who had a metastatic lesion in the precentral gyrus, which was the origin of the patient's peripheral pain and was clearly above the level of the block.
Psychogenic pain	The patient may have true "psychogenic pain," which obviously is not going to respond to a block at any level. This is an even more uncommon response in patients with psychogenic pain than a positive response to placebo.
Encephalization	The patient's pain may have undergone "encephalization"—that poorly understood phenomenon whereby persistent, severe, agonizing pain, originally of peripheral origin, becomes self-sustaining at a central level. This usually does not occur until severe pain has been endured for a long time, but once it has occurred, removal or blockade of the original peripheral mechanism fails to provide relief.
Malingering	The patient may be malingering. One cannot prove or disprove this with differential blocks, but if a patient is involved in litigation concerning the cause of his pain and anticipates financial benefit, it is unlikely that any therapeutic modality will relieve the pain. However, empirically, it is our belief that a previous placebo reaction from solution A followed by no relief from solution D strongly suggests that the patient whose pain ultimately appears to have a "central mechanism" is not malingering, since the placebo reaction, depending as it does on a positive motivation to obtain relief, is unlikely in a malingerer. Clearly, there is no way to document the validity of this theory, but it certainly suggests greater motivation to obtain pain relief than to obtain financial gain.

If pain relief is not obtained by any of the first three spinal injections, 5% procaine is injected into the subarachnoid space to block all modalities. If the 5% concentration *does* relieve the patient's pain, the mechanism is still considered somatic, the presumption being that the patient has an elevated C_m for A-delta and C fibers. If, however, the patient obtains no relief in spite of complete sympathetic, sensory, and motor blockade, the pain is classified as "central" in origin, although this is not a specific diagnosis and may indicate any one of the four possibilities in **Table 18.4**.

Disadvantages

The conventional sequential differential spinal technique just described was used by the authors for many years and was effective in pinpointing the neural mechanisms subserving pain syndromes in a multitude of patients. It was particularly effective in establishing a diagnosis in patients with pain syndromes of questionable or unknown etiology. However, the technique has several obvious drawbacks. First of all, it is quite time consuming, because the physician must wait long enough after each injection for the response to become evident, and then to wane, allowing a subsequent solution to be injected. Second, occasionally a patient is encountered whose C_m for sympathetic blockade is greater than 0.25, so when relief is produced by 0.5% procaine, one *might* erroneously conclude that this is somatic pain rather than sympathetic pain. Similarly, a patient may occasionally be encountered who has a lower C_m for sensory blockade than 0.5%, and when 0.25% procaine produces relief, one *might* erroneously conclude that the mechanism is sympathetic rather than somatic. Third, each successive injection with this technique deposits more procaine into the subarachnoid space, so that after the final injection, when all modalities are blocked, it takes quite a while for full function to return. Full recovery is absolutely essential, at least in our pain center, because the vast majority of the patients are outpatients and must be fully able to ambulate before being discharged. This technique demands that the needle remain in place throughout the entire procedure, so the patient must remain in the lateral position throughout the test. Occasionally this is a serious problem, especially when the

Table 18.5 Preparation of Solutions for Modified Differential Spinal Blockade

Solution	Preparation and Solution	Yield
D	To 1 mL of 10% procaine add 1 mL of saline	2 mL of 5% procaine (hyperbaric)
A	Draw up 2 mL of normal saline	2 mL of normal saline

patient's pain is associated with a particular position that cannot be assumed with the needle in situ.

The "Modified Differential Spinal"

In an effort to overcome the disadvantages just described, the conventional technique has been modified in a way that simplifies it and increases its utility.[13–16] For the modified technique, only two solutions need to be prepared, as summarized in **Table 18.5**, namely, normal saline (solution A) and 5% procaine (solution D).

Procedure

As in the conventional technique, after informed consent has been obtained, an infusion started, and the monitors applied, the back is prepared and draped, and a small-bore blunt-tipped spinal needle is used to enter the subarachnoid space. At this point 2 mL of normal saline is injected, and observations are made as in the conventional technique described previously (see **Table 18.3**). If the patient obtains no relief or only partial relief from the placebo injection, 2 mL of 5% procaine is injected, the needle is removed, and the patient is returned to the supine position. Because the injected 5% procaine is hyperbaric, the position of the table may have to be adjusted to obtain the desired level of anesthesia. Once this is accomplished, the same observations are made as after the previous injection (see **Table 18.3**).

Interpretation

If the patient's pain is relieved after the injection of normal saline, the interpretation is the same as if it were relieved by placebo in the conventional differential spinal—that is, the pain is considered to be of psychogenic origin. Again, when the pain relief is prolonged or permanent, the pain is probably truly psychogenic, whereas if relief is transient and self-limited, the response probably represents a placebo reaction.

When the patient does not obtain pain relief after the subarachnoid injection of 5% procaine, the diagnosis is considered to be the same as that when the patient obtains no relief after injection of all of the solutions with the conventional technique—that is, the mechanism is considered to be "central." As in the conventional technique, this diagnosis is not specific; rather, it indicates one of four possibilities (see **Table 18.4**).

Alternatively, when the patient does obtain complete pain relief after the injection of 5% procaine, the cause of the pain is considered to be organic. The mechanism is considered to be somatic (to be subserved by A-delta and/or C fibers) if the pain returns when the patient again perceives pinprick as sharp (recovery from analgesia); whereas it is considered sympathetic if the pain relief persists long after recovery from analgesia.

Fundamental Differences Between the Conventional Technique and the Modified Technique of Differential Spinal

The conventional sequential differential spinal sought to block specific types of nerve fibers with specific concentrations of local anesthetics. At the time when we modified the conventional technique, evidence was accumulating that the exact concentrations of local anesthetics required to block different fiber types are unpredictable, to say the least. Thus we abandoned the practice of injecting predetermined concentrations of local anesthetics in an attempt to selectively block one fiber type at a time and adopted a technique not unlike that used to produce surgical spinal anesthesia—a technique that was much better understood. With that technique, after a placebo injection, a concentration of a short-acting local anesthetic sufficient to produce surgical anesthesia is injected into the subarachnoid space to block all types of fibers, and the patient is observed as the concentration of local anesthetic in the cerebrospinal fluid decreases and the fibers recover sequentially, motor fibers first, followed by sensory fibers, and then sympathetic fibers. Whereas the conventional sequential technique attempted to correlate the *onset* of pain relief with the *onset* of blockade of the various fiber types, the modified technique attempts to correlate the *return* of pain with the *recovery* of the various blocked fibers.

It readily becomes apparent that this modified technique of differential spinal block simplifies the differentiation of sympathetic from somatic mechanisms considerably. With the conventional technique, occasionally the concentration required to produce sympathetic blockade is somewhat greater or somewhat less than the usual mean of 0.25%, and the concentration of procaine required to produce a sensory block is greater or less than the usual mean of 0.5%. Significant diagnostic confusion can result. With the modified technique,

when a patient recovers sensation, the only fibers that remain blocked are the sympathetic fibers; thus pain relief that persists beyond the recovery of sensation clearly indicates a sympathetic mechanism.

Advantages over the Conventional Technique

The major advantage of the modified differential spinal block over the conventional technique is that it takes less time. The modified technique has consistently provided diagnostic information identical to that provided by the conventional technique, but in approximately one third of the time. The conventional differential technique requires a series of injections into the subarachnoid space of progressively increasing concentrations of local anesthetic, so that when the study is complete, the patient has a high level of anesthesia that takes a long time to dissipate. The modified technique requires only a single injection of active drug; so in addition to the test's taking less time, the time for recovery is likewise reduced—a fact of great importance in a busy pain center. The modified technique also minimizes the extent and duration of discomfort for the patient, who does not have to lie so long in the lateral position with the needle in place. In addition, the modified technique allows a better evaluation of the subjective nature of a patient's pain. Because there is no need to keep the needle in the back throughout the procedure, the patient can lie supine, and positional changes or passive movement of the legs that may be necessary to reproduce the pain are much easier. The advantage of the modified approach over the traditional one in differentiating sympathetic from somatic pain has already been described.

Differential Epidural Block

More than 30 years ago, Raj[17] suggested using sequential differential epidural block instead of the conventional sequential differential spinal to avoid spinal headaches after the procedure. With his proposed technique, solution A was still to be the placebo, but solution B was 0.5% lidocaine, which was presumed to be the mean sympatholytic concentration of lidocaine in the epidural space; solution C was 1% lidocaine, the presumed mean sensory blocking concentration in the epidural space; and solution D was 2% lidocaine, a concentration sufficient to block all modalities, sympathetic as well as sensory and motor. In short, the technique Raj proposed for differential epidural block was virtually identical to that used for the conventional differential spinal block, except that the local anesthetic doses were injected sequentially into the epidural space and the concentrations were modified as described earlier.

There were two problems with the technique proposed by Raj. First, because of the slower onset of blockade after each injection of local anesthetic into the epidural space, more time would be required between injections before the usual observations could be made. So a differential epidural block, as proposed by Raj, would take even longer for complete recovery than the conventional differential spinal technique. An even more serious drawback of this approach, however, relates to the fact that, if local anesthetics *occasionally* fail to give discrete end points when injected into the subarachnoid space, the end points are even less discrete with injections into the epidural space. For example, 0.5% lidocaine provides sympathetic blockade when injected epidurally, but it commonly causes sensory block as well. Similarly, whereas 1% lidocaine injected epidurally almost always produces sensory block, it frequently also produces paresis, if not paralysis. As a matter of fact, it was the failure of this technique to provide definitive end points that led Raj to decide not to publish it.

Nonetheless, *conceptually*, a differential epidural approach is inherently appealing because it avoids lumbar puncture and the possibility of post–lumbar puncture headache in a predominantly outpatient population. The major problem with the technique Raj proposed, the lack of discrete end points, was due to the attempt to inject a different concentration of local anesthetic to block each type of nerve fiber, something we had attempted with our conventional differential spinal. Because our modified differential spinal eliminated the occasional confusing end points of the conventional technique, we decided to modify Raj's proposed differential epidural as we had modified our differential spinal. This technique as we perform it is as follows[14–16]:

Informed consent is obtained, an infusion is started, and the various monitors are applied. The patient is placed in the lateral (or sitting) position, and the back is prepared and draped in the usual manner. After a 20-gauge Tuohy-type epidural needle has been placed in the epidural space by the modified loss-of-resistance technique, equal volumes of normal saline and 2% chloroprocaine (or lidocaine) are injected sequentially 15 to 20 minutes apart, and the needle is removed. The volume of each is that required to produce the desired level of anesthesia. After each injection, exactly the same observations are made as for a differential spinal (see **Table 18.3**).

The interpretation is virtually identical to that of a modified differential spinal. If the patient experiences pain relief after the injection of saline, the presumptive diagnosis is "psychogenic pain," a designation that indicates the possibility of either a placebo reaction or true psychogenic pain. If the patient does not experience pain relief after the injection of 2% chloroprocaine (or lidocaine) into the epidural space *in spite of complete anesthesia of the painful area*, the diagnosis is considered to be "central pain," that diagnosis again including the four possibilities described earlier (see **Table 18.4**). When the patient does experience pain relief after the injection of 2% chloroprocaine (or lidocaine), however, the pain is considered organic. It is presumed to be somatic (subserved by A-delta and C fibers) when the pain returns with the return of sensation, and sympathetic when the pain persists long after sensation has been recovered. This approach to differential epidural blockade has been used extensively at our institution and has provided the same valuable information obtained from the modified differential spinal technique without the usual risk of post–dural puncture headache. In addition, differential epidural is a useful alternative to differential spinal when a patient refuses spinal anesthesia or when spinal anesthesia is contraindicated, although both of these situations are rare. A catheter can be placed through a larger epidural needle if it is anticipated that supplemental injections may be necessary to achieve the proper level, but in our experience this has rarely been necessary.

Differential Brachial Plexus Block

Performed in a manner analogous to that of differential epidural block, a differential brachial plexus block can be extremely useful in evaluating upper extremity pain.[18] Two successive injections are made into the perivascular compartment using an approach appropriate to the site of the patient's pain, one injection consisting of normal saline and the other 2% chloroprocaine. Again, the same observations are made after each injection (see **Table 18.3**). If the patient is somewhat naive with respect to the injections carried out at a pain center, it may be sufficient for the placebo injection to consist of local infiltration over the anticipated site of injection of the active agent, as long as all of the appropriate observations are made after the injection. If this does not provide relief, the brachial plexus block is carried out with local anesthetic, inserting the needle through the anesthetized skin. If the patient obtains pain relief from the placebo injection, as with a differential spinal or epidural, the pain is considered psychogenic, whereas if the pain disappears after injection of chloroprocaine into the brachial plexus sheath, it is labeled organic. If the pain returns as soon as the sensory block is dissipated, the mechanism is somatic (i.e., it is subserved by A-delta and C fibers); if the relief persists long after recovery from the sensory block, the mechanism is presumed to be sympathetic. Finally, of course, if the pain does not disappear, even when the arm is fully anesthetized, the diagnosis is central pain, and the same four possibilities are again associated with that response (see **Table 18.4**).

It is significant to note that Durrani and Winnie[19] reported on 25 patients referred to our pain control center with a clinical diagnosis of "classic" reflex sympathetic dystrophy (Complex Regional Pain Syndrome Type I [CRPS Type I]) of the upper extremity—all of whom obtained no relief from a series of three stellate ganglion blocks, even though each patient developed Horner's syndrome after each block. The significance of this report is that, when these patients were subjected to differential brachial plexus block by one of the perivascular techniques, 16 of the 25 patients (who had not obtained relief from three stellate ganglion blocks) exhibited a typical sympathetic response to the brachial plexus block. Perhaps more important, 12 of the 19 patients so treated obtained complete and permanent relief from a series of therapeutic brachial plexus blocks, even though they had failed to do so after a series of stellate ganglion blocks. Thus it would appear that perivascular brachial plexus blocks provide more complete sympathetic denervation of the upper extremity than do stellate ganglion blocks. The success of brachial plexus block and the failure of stellate ganglion blocks in this report might be explained by the fact that the local anesthetic injected at the stellate ganglion failed to reach the nerve of Kuntz, the nerve by which ascending sympathetic fibers may bypass the stellate ganglion.[20,21] Because all of the stellate ganglion blocks at our institution are carried out using a minimum of 8 mL of local anesthetic as well as with fluoroscopic guidance or using ultrasound, however, this is unlikely. A more likely explanation is that stellate ganglion block interrupts only those sympathetic fibers that travel with the peripheral nerves, whereas perivascular brachial plexus block interrupts the sympathetic fibers traveling by both neural and perivascular pathways.[22]

Summary

Controversial aspects aside, the pharmacologic approach to differential neural blockade remains a simple but useful technique—whether carried out at a subarachnoid, epidural, or plexus level—because it provides reproducible, objective, and definitive diagnostic information on the neural mechanisms subserving a patient's pain. Obviously, the results of this test must be interpreted in the light of other diagnostic tests (including psychologic tests) and the results must be integrated with the information obtained from the patient's history and the findings on physical examination. Not infrequently, the results of a differential spinal, a differential epidural, or a differential plexus block provide the missing piece in the complex puzzle of pain.

The Anatomic Approach

To obviate the problems inherent in high spinal (or epidural) anesthesia, particularly in an outpatient or a patient whose pain is in the upper part of the body, it is occasionally safer and more appropriate to use an anatomic approach to differential neural blockade. In this approach, after the injection of a placebo, the sympathetic and then the sensory and/or motor fibers are blocked sequentially by injecting local anesthetic at points where one modality can be blocked without blocking the other. The procedural sequences by which differential nerve blocks are carried out in this approach for pain in the various parts of the body are presented in **Table 18.6**.

Procedure

For pain in the head, neck, and upper extremity, if a placebo injection fails to provide relief, a stellate ganglion block is carried out with any short-acting, dilute local anesthetic. If the sympathetic block cannot be carried out without spillover onto somatic nerves innervating the painful area, the sequential blocks should be carried out on two separate occasions, allowing the sympathetic block to wear off before proceeding with the somatic block. In any case, if the patient does not obtain relief from the stellate ganglion block, a block of the somatic nerves to the painful area should be carried out.

For pain in the thorax, after a placebo injection, the safest procedure (and the one that causes the least discomfort to the patient) is a differential segmental epidural block, as described previously. It must be remembered, however, that, with thoracic pain, relief after an extensive sympathetic block, in addition to suggesting a possible sympathetic mechanism, may indicate visceral rather than somatic pain, because visceral pain is mediated by sympathetic fibers. If it is unwise to carry out a differential thoracic epidural block in a particular

patient because of cachexia, hypovolemia, or dehydration, an alternative is the anatomic approach, using paravertebral or intercostal blocks of the appropriate dermatomes. Failure of these somatic blocks to provide relief implies (but does not prove) a visceral origin for the pain; however, if the blocks provide complete relief and if the pain returns immediately after recovery, a peripheral somatic mechanism is indicated. If the relief provided by the blocks persists long after recovery of sensation, this may indicate a sympathetic mechanism.

When a placebo injection fails to provide relief for abdominal pain, before a celiac block is considered, paravertebral or intercostal blocks of the appropriate dermatomes should be done to make certain that the pain is not somatic (body wall). Patients have a great deal of difficulty localizing "abdominal pain," and therefore they usually cannot differentiate pain that is due to body wall extension of a lesion from pain that is due to true visceral involvement. If the paravertebral or intercostal blocks produce complete anesthesia of the body wall overlying the patient's pain but fail to provide relief, a splanchnic or celiac plexus block should be carried out to confirm that the pain is truly visceral in origin.

If a placebo injection fails to provide relief for pelvic pain, before a superior hypogastric plexus block is attempted, paravertebral or appropriate sacral blocks should be carried out to make certain that the pain is not somatic. If these blocks produce appropriate anesthesia but fail to provide relief, a superior hypogastric block is carried out to establish that the pain is visceral.

For pain in the lower extremities, the pharmacologic approach (differential spinal or epidural) is preferable because it is more precise and less painful than peripheral nerve blocks. Differential peripheral blocks, however, can be used if the pharmacologic approach is contraindicated or undesirable or if subsequent neurolytic blocks are anticipated. After a placebo block, lumbar paravertebral sympathetic blocks are performed at the levels L2-4, and if these fail to provide relief, lumbosacral plexus block (or any appropriate specific peripheral nerve block) is carried out.

Interpretation

Interpretation of the results achieved with differential nerve blocks for head, neck, arm, and leg pain is self-evident. Relief after a placebo injection indicates a psychogenic mechanism,

Table 18.6 **Anatomic Approach: Procedural Sequence for Differential Diagnostic Nerve Blocks**			
Site of Pain		**Technique**	
Head	Placebo block	Stellate ganglion block	Block of C_2; block of trigeminal I, II, III (or specific nerve block)
Neck	Placebo block	Stellate ganglion block	Cervical plexus block (or specific nerve block)
Arm	Placebo block	Stellate ganglion block	Brachial plexus block (or specific nerve block)
Thorax*	Placebo block	Thoracic paravertebral sympathetic block	Lumbar paravertebral somatic block
Abdomen†	Placebo block	Celiac plexus block	Paravertebral somatic or intercostal block
Pelvis†	Placebo block	Superior hypogastric plexus block	Paravertebral somatic or intercostal block
Leg	Placebo block	Lumbar paravertebral sympathetic block	Lumbosacral plexus block (or specific nerve block)

*In our opinion, thoracic paravertebral sympathetic blocks carry such a high risk of pneumothorax that a pharmacologic approach should be used.
†Because of the simplicity of intercostal blocks, as compared with celiac plexus and superior hypogastric plexus blocks, the procedural sequence is altered for abdominal pain (i.e., somatic before sympathetic).

but, as with the pharmacologic approaches, it could indicate either a placebo reaction or true psychogenic pain. Relief after sympathetic blocks indicates a sympathetic mechanism, usually reflex sympathetic dystrophy (CRPS Type I), and relief after blockade of somatic nerves indicates an organic, somatic mechanism. Failure to obtain relief in spite of the establishment of complete anesthesia in the appropriate area would tend to indicate a central mechanism, which could be any of the four possibilities listed in Table 18.4. Interpretation of the results of differential blocks for thoracic and abdominal pain has already been discussed.

Discussion

In spite of the clinical success of the various techniques of differential neural blockade in many centers over the last 35 years, the validity of the results has become controversial. There are two reasons for this: (1) the changes in our understanding of the factors that determine the process of nerve conduction and blockade are believed by some to invalidate the concept of differential neural blockade; and (2) the even greater changes in our understanding of the complexities of chronic pain and the physiologic, anatomic, and psychosocial factors involved are believed to limit the diagnostic utility of neural blockade. To establish both the validity and utility of differential neural blockade in the diagnosis of pain mechanisms, it is essential to understand the bases of this controversy by answering two questions: (1) do the factors recently found to determine nerve conduction and blockade invalidate the concept of differential neural blockade, and (2) do the complexities of chronic pain and the physiolgic, anatomic, and psychosocial factors involved limit the diagnostic utility of differential neural blockade?

Do the Factors Recently Found to Determine Nerve Conduction and Blockade Invalidate the Concept of Differential Neural Blockade?

The pharmacologic approach to differential neural blockade is based on the assumption that local anesthetic agents can selectively produce conduction block of one type of fiber in a nerve while sparing the other types in that nerve.[23] Although the concept of differential block was introduced almost 90 years ago by Gasser and Erlanger,[24] in vitro and in vivo studies carried out over the past 35 years have indicated that the basis of Gasser and Erlanger's explanation of this commonly observed clinical phenomenon was totally erroneous, as was their explanation of the process of nerve conduction itself. From the classic studies Gasser and Erlanger carried out on the peripheral nerves of dogs they concluded that, in general, small-diameter fibers were more readily blocked by cocaine than were larger-diameter fibers. At that time, however, it was believed that the site of action of conduction was the axonal protoplasm. Thus the higher ratio of surface to volume in small-diameter fibers was supposed to make them more "sensitive" (easier to enter and render unexcitable) than large ones. Since that theory was articulated in one form or another this "size principle" has influenced the concept of differential block, has led to clinical use of differential spinal block,[1] and has provided an explanation for the persistent differential losses of function observed during subarachnoid[25] and epidural[26] anesthesia.

It was over 50 years before the concept of Gasser and Erlanger was challenged. Studies by Franz and Perry in vivo[27] and by Fink and Cairns in vitro[28] indicated that all mammalian axons require about the same blocking concentration of local anesthetic, regardless of their diameter, and the issue was rendered even more confusing when Gissen et al[29] demonstrated that the larger the diameter of an axon, the more susceptible it was to conduction block by local anesthetics, a finding diametrically opposed to Gasser and Erlanger's traditional concept. However, as de Jong[30] pointed out, a major flaw in Gissen's study was that the experiments were carried out at room temperature. Because conduction in large fibers is more affected by cold than is conduction in small fibers, relatively little anesthetic may be needed to block large fibers in conditions cooler than body temperature. Subsequently, Palmer et al,[31] using a preparation maintained at body temperature, showed that C fibers were, in fact, more susceptible to conduction block by bupivacaine than were A fibers, but they were unable to demonstrate such differential effects with lidocaine.

This study introduced a new complexity: different anesthetics may affect various axon types differently. In two sequential in vitro studies, Wildsmith et al[32,33] compared the differential nerve-blocking activity of a series of amide-linked local anesthetics with that of a series of ester-linked agents. These studies confirmed Gissen's finding that, in general, A fibers are the most sensitive and C fibers the least sensitive to blockade by local anesthetics but that the absolute and relative rates of development of A fiber blockade were directly related to lipid solubility and inversely related to pK_a. On the basis of the findings of these two in vitro studies, Wildsmith postulated that, in vivo, C fibers could be blocked differentially by an agent of low lipid solubility and high pK_a, because a compound with these properties (such as procaine) might produce blockade of C fibers relatively quickly, but before it could penetrate the great diffusion barriers around A fibers, it would be removed by the circulation. Ford et al[34] tested this hypothesis, studying several local anesthetics in a cat model in vivo and found that, regardless of the local anesthetic, A-alpha fibers were consistently less sensitive to blockade than either A-delta or C fibers, thus reaffirming the original scheme of Gasser and Erlanger.

It remained for Fink[6] to elucidate the importance of two other factors subserving differential neural blockade. First, he pointed out the importance of the nodes of Ranvier, the internodal distance, and the number of nodes bathed by a local anesthetic to differential neural blockade. It has long been known that to block conduction, an adequate concentration of local anesthetic (C_m) applied to a myelinated axon must bathe at least three consecutive nodes.[35] Because the internodal distance increases as the thickness of the axon increases, the probability of three successive nodes of Ranvier being bathed quickly by an injected local anesthetic solution decreases as the internodal distance increases, that is, as the size of the fiber increases (**Fig. 18.2**). In other words, the chance of a local anesthetic solution blocking a given nerve fiber decreases with increasing fiber size. For example, the internodal distance of small A-delta fibers ranges from 0.3 to 0.7 mm, so that a "puddle" of local anesthetic solution only 2 mm long will fully cover three successive nodes. In contrast, large A-alpha fibers have an internodal distance of 0.8 to 1.4 mm, so their *critical blocking length* is at least 5 mm.[27] Thus, because the internodal distance increases with thickness of the axon, the minimal blocking length ranges from 2 to 5 mm.

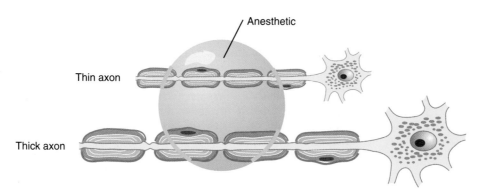

Fig. 18.2   Differential nerve block based on different internodal intervals. Two axons, one thin and one thick, are depicted lying side by side in a puddle of local anesthetic at or above the minimum blocking concentration (C_m). The internodal interval of the thick fiber is twice that of the thin one, so whereas the local anesthetic solution covers three successive nodes of the thin axon, it covers only one node of the thick one. Nerve impulses can skip easily over one node, and even over two, rendered inexcitable by the local anesthetic,[35] so conduction along the thick axon will continue uninterrupted. In the thin axon, however, because three nodes are covered by the local anesthetic solution, impulse conduction is halted. Thus conduction appears to proceed normally in the thick (motor) fiber but is blocked in the thin (sensory) fiber. Such a differential block of thin versus thick nerve fibers occurs in spinal roots during spinal anesthesia (see discussion in text). *(Modified from de Jong RH: Local anesthetics, St Louis, 1994, Mosby, p 89.)*

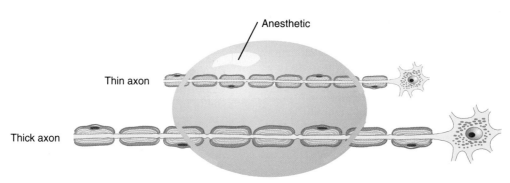

Fig. 18.3   Differential decremental nerve block and frequency-dependent block. When both thick and thin axons have more than three nodes covered by a local anesthetic solution, if the solution is at or above the minimum blocking concentration (C_m) all of the sodium channels are occupied and conduction is blocked in both fibers. However, if the concentration of local anesthetic is below C_m, a significant portion (but not all) of the sodium channels are blocked, so that at each node the action potential undergoes a progressive reduction in amplitude, with resultant decremental slowing of impulse conduction. Such decremental conduction will ultimately extinguish the impulse in the nine exposed nodes of the thin fiber (decremental block); but, although the impulse is slowed in its passage along the five incompletely blocked nodes of the thick fiber, it will resume at full speed when normally conducting membrane is reached again. The lower the concentration of the local anesthetic, the longer must be the exposure length (the number of nodes of Ranvier exposed) to yield complete impulse blockade. Conversely, the more concentrated the local anesthetic solution, the shorter is the exposure length required for complete blockade, up to the point of C_m, when the "three-node principle" again applies. In other words, below C_m, the blocking concentration of local anesthetic is inversely proportional to the length of the nerve it bathes. The greater the frequency of nerve stimulation, the shorter is the exposure length (the number of incompletely blocked nodes) required to yield complete impulse blockade. Such a frequency-dependent block superimposed on decremental block is operant clinically in the zone cephalad to the level of somatic block in a spinal anesthesia (see discussion in text). *(Modified from de Jong RH: Local anesthetics, St Louis, 1994, Mosby, p 91.)*

Next, Fink demonstrated that the differential blockade of the sympathetic nerves observed clinically with spinal anesthesia is probably due, at least in part, to decremental block with a superimposed frequency-dependent effect.[36] Decremental block occurs when a nerve is bathed by a weak concentration of local anesthetic ($<C_m$): Both thick and thin axons have more than three nodes covered by local anesthetic (**Fig. 18.3**); because of the difference in the internodal distance, fewer nodes are bathed by local anesthetic in the thick fiber than in the thin one. Thus, when an impulse arrives at the incompletely blocked thick fiber, although there is a progressive reduction in conduction velocity and elevation of firing threshold as it traverses the incompletely blocked segment,

it resumes full speed when it reaches a segment of normally conducting membrane. Put simply, too few nodes were partially blocked to completely halt conduction. However, in the thin axon, a sufficient number of nodes are partially blocked so that the progressive reduction in the action current at each node ultimately causes the impulse to be blocked. Because the action current decreases in decrements, the phenomenon is referred to as *decremental conduction block*. Because the block is complete in the small axon and incomplete in the large one, this represents a differential (decremental) block.

In this example, decremental block of single impulses has been described, and single impulses allow enough time for membrane recovery. In reality, impulses occur in rapid sequential bursts that allow little time for recovery, and it has been demonstrated repeatedly that, as the rate of stimulation increases, so does the intensity of the block. Presumably, this phenomenon, called *frequency-dependent block,* is due to the fact that, at rapid rates of stimulation, the time between impulses is insufficient for the local anesthetic to unbind, so a fraction of the sodium channels is still blocked when the next impulse arrives. Obviously, frequency-dependent block superimposed on decremental block enhances conduction block by local anesthetics in concentrations considerably below C_m. While frequency-dependent block is clearly a viable mechanism at work in describing how local anesthetics function when injected into the subarachnoid space, this concept must be differentiated from the somewhat related, but distinct, phenomenon associated with local anesthetic peripheral plexus blocks used for extremity anesthesia wherein an individual performs muscular exercise to enhance the onset or spread of an injected local anesthetic.[37,38] In fact, Langen et al[37] at Loyola University were unable to determine any clinical benefit whatsoever from employing frequency-dependent block concepts when instituting vigorous physical exercise following the interscalene injections of bupivacaine in patients undergoing arthroscopic surgery under regional block anesthesia.

Because the conditions necessary for frequency-dependent block in the subarachnoid space include a weak concentration of local anesthetic ($<C_m$) and a train of repetitive stimuli,[39] both conditions are present in the zone cephalad to the level of somatic block in spinal anesthesia: The cerebrospinal fluid concentration of local anesthetic is too low to block somatic axons, but the preganglionic sympathetic fibers carry a normal tonic flow of rapid vasoconstrictor impulses. As a result, frequency-dependent block of the sympathetic fibers is superimposed on decremental block. Another observation of clinical importance is that highly lipid-soluble local anesthetics require more repetitive stimuli to reach maximal frequency-dependent blocking than less lipid-soluble agents,[40] so differential blockade of the sympathetic fibers without blockade of somatic fibers is easier to accomplish with agents of low lipid solubility such as procaine.

Applying these two concepts, Fink pointed out that the anatomy of the spinal roots in the spinal canal of an adult varies considerably at different levels because the spinal cord is substantially shorter than the dural sac that surrounds it. Thus, proceeding cephalocaudad, the length of the spinal roots from the point where they leave the cord to the point where they exit the dura increases from 0.5 cm for the C1 root to 15 cm for the S4 root. With spinal anesthesia, the densest concentration of local anesthetic is nearest the lumbar puncture site. Here the length of the lumbosacral nerve roots allows many nodes of Ranvier of all sizes of fibers to be exposed to the local anesthetic, so a solid block of the lumbosacral roots is rapidly achieved.

Progressively farther craniad, the local anesthetic solution is increasingly diluted by spinal fluid until the cephalad salient is "watered down" to C_m. At that point, fibers with a short internodal distance may still fall within the blocking zone, whereas the distal nodes of thicker fibers with a longer internodal distance may fall well outside the blocking potency range. In other words, small autonomic and nociceptive fibers are still blocked, but the thicker touch and motor fibers no longer are.[41] As fibers cephalad to the C_m zone are exposed to subthreshold local anesthetic concentrations, decremental block and/or frequency-dependent block begins to play a role. The

short-to-long internode-blocking gradient still holds, but now a longer string of nodes must be bathed before an impulse is halted (see **Fig. 18.3**). Because of the shorter internodal intervals of thin fibers, the segment of a thin nerve that needs to be bathed to block conduction is shorter than the segment required to block thick nerves. Thus differential spinal block is observed at threshold-blocking concentrations.[7] The other contribution of Fink, based on the same "bathed length" concept, is seen during epidural anesthesia. The length of the nerve segments from dural sac to intervertebral foramen is both shorter and less variable than that of the intrathecal roots. In fact, the few millimeters of root exposed in the cervical and thoracic epidural space barely span the three-node length of thin nerves, let alone that of thicker nerves. Differential block with epidural analgesia thus can be quite pronounced, a property used to great advantage in providing "pure" postoperative analgesia with epidural infusions of a weak local anesthetic solution.

In an editorial accompanying Fink's article, Raymond and Strichartz[42] summarized the impact of Fink's "innovative" observations on the concept of differential block as follows:

> They link clinical observations to anatomical findings in both humans and animals and to measurements made in vitro on isolated nerves, thereby generating interesting predictions and possibilities. They lead the discussion of differential block away from a broad susceptibility to LA [local anesthetic] according to fiber size to focus on the number of nodes per unit length, which is correlated with fiber size. Clinically, this permits retention of familiar interpretations (based on the size principle) of phenomena consistently seen during epidural and spinal anesthesia; and it does not deny the single fiber data showing similar LA susceptibility across the fiber spectrum (for long exposed segments). The ideas are, in this sense, an extension of the size principle, not a renunciation of it.

From this summary, it is clear that differential neural blockade is a reality. Although the size principle (the thicker the fiber, the harder it is to block) has been replaced by the length principle (the fewer nodes bathed, the harder it is to block), as indicated by de Jong,[43] the clinical outcome remains functionally the same. The thicker the nerve fiber, the broader the internode and the fewer nodes per exposure length. Thus blocking a thick nerve fiber requires a supra-C_m local anesthetic solution because there are too few nodes accessible for decremental block to come into play. In other words, for a given local anesthetic concentration, there will be an interim transition phase in which nociception (pain) conducted by thin fibers is blocked, but touch and motor function conducted by thick fibers remain virtually intact.

Although inconsistencies and contraindications about the mechanisms of differential neural blockade persist, it is conceptually valid, and in our hands, it has proved an invaluable clinical tool for identifying the mechanism subserving a patient's pain.

Do the Complexities of Chronic Pain and the Physiologic, Anatomic, and Psychosocial Factors Involved Limit the Diagnostic Utility of Differential Neural Blockade?

No one could deny that over the last 35 years basic research in the field of pain has produced important insights into the pathophysiology of chronic pain, the anatomic pathways involved in the processing and conduction of pain, and the important psychosocial issues that affect a patient's perception of pain. It is not readily apparent, however, why increases in our understanding of the complexities of pain should invalidate the diagnostic information provided by differential neural blockade. Better understanding of the mechanisms involved in the pain process should actually enhance our ability to interpret the information gained from diagnostic nerve blocks. Yet, just 10 years ago in a review of neural blockade for diagnosis and prognosis,[44] the authors state categorically that "complex physiologic events may confound the simple interpretation of diagnostic blocks"; that "compelling evidence with regard to placebo responses leads to the conclusion that the ambiguity created by these responses is a major impediment to the valid use of neural blockade for diagnosis"; and that "anatomic uncertainties with regard to neuroconnections and structural variability degrade the accuracy of diagnostic information obtained by neural blockade."

Furthermore, the author of an editorial supporting these views states that "several factors, such as the improper use of pain measurement scales, observer errors, problems of placebo effects, and bias introduced by patient expectations, confound the interpretation of studies on the usefulness of neural blockade in the diagnosis of chronic pain," and that "because the treatment [of pain] and prognosis often depend on accurate diagnosis, the incorrect interpretation of the results of a nerve block may result in inappropriate therapy."[45] These platitudes and attitudes do not denigrate differential neural blockade, but the intelligence, knowledge, and clinical judgment of anesthesiologists who are in the practice of pain management. There are few (if any) diagnostic techniques in all of medicine that are infallibly positive or negative or, when taken by themselves, are invariably indicative of a specific etiology. All such tests give false-positive and false-negative results, and knowing this, the experienced clinician integrates the result of any one test with the results of others, with the information gained from a careful history, and with the findings of the physical examination. Of course, caution must be exercised when interpreting any tests, but, interpreted intelligently, the results of differential neural blockade not infrequently provide the missing piece of the puzzle of pain, and the reward for the patient (and the concerned physician) is pain relief.

To abandon differential nerve blocks for the diagnosis of pain until the precise mechanisms subserving pain and its relief are understood would be as foolish as to abandon general anesthesia until the precise mechanism by which general anesthetics work is understood. Even those who decry diagnostic blocks admit that "experienced and observant clinicians have found that these procedures may, on certain occasions, provide information that is helpful in guiding subsequent therapy, so we should not be in haste to dismiss the accumulated judgment of [the] practitioner," and that "the confusion and complexity that typify the diagnosis of chronic pain may justify the selective use of diagnostic blocks that make anatomic and physiologic sense, even if their validity is incompletely proved."[44] It goes without saying that the clinician who employs diagnostic nerve blocks must exercise great care in carrying out the technique, in confirming observed effects in interpreting the results, and in applying them to clinical decisions.

Role of Differential Neural Blockade

Many patients seeking pain relief at a pain control center present no diagnostic problem whatsoever; however, anyone experienced in the diagnosis and management of chronic pain problems has seen many apparently clear-cut diagnoses completely and unexpectedly refuted when one of the techniques of differential neural blockade was used to "confirm" the diagnosis. The concern in such cases is that *if this diagnostic approach had not been used* because the clinician felt that with his or her "experience and expertise in pain management" such supportive evidence was unnecessary, *the true diagnosis would have been missed,* and the patient's therapy, based on the clinical diagnosis, would have been unsuccessful. Human limitations being what they are and pain being the complex process that it is, no one ever develops enough experience or expertise to make the correct diagnosis 100% of the time. Differential neural blockade provides an objective means of *confirming* a diagnosis when the cause of pain appears obvious, and, perhaps more important, a means of *establishing* a diagnosis when there appears to be no demonstrable cause.

Forty years ago we retrospectively reviewed a series of 100 patients referred to our pain control center "because all diagnostic attempts had failed to discover a cause for the patient's pain."[9] Reviewing these difficult cases, we were impressed by the fact that differential neural blockade was effective in identifying the mechanism as sympathetic, somatic, or central in all of these patients (**Table 18.7**). Even more impressive and surprising was the fact that in 74% of the patients, differential neural blockade indicated the mechanism to be sympathetic. A somatic mechanism was implicated in only 18% and a central (including psychogenic) mechanism in only 8%. These findings were important because in the vast majority of these patients, patients in whom a sympathetic mechanism was *unexpectedly* identified, the diagnosis was established early enough that complete and permanent relief could be provided by a series of sympathetic blocks.

These data provide convincing evidence that, at least in patients suffering from pain syndromes of questionable cause, sympathetically maintained pain (sympathetically maintained or mediated pain, reflex sympathetic dystrophy, and complex regional pain syndrome) is not uncommon. All of these patients were referred by specialists who could find no cause for the pain, and indeed, in most of the cases the signs and symptoms were either so bizarre or so seemingly unrelated to any precipitating factor that, had differential blocks not been carried out, we (like the referring physicians) would probably

Table 18.7 Results of Differential Neural Blockade in 100 Patients Referred Because of "No Demonstrable Cause for Pain"

Diagnosis	Incidence (%)
Psychogenic mechanism	5
Sympathetic mechanism	74
Somatic mechanism	18
Central mechanism	3

From Winnie AP, Collins VJ: The pain clinic. I. Differential neural blockade in pain syndromes of questionable etiology, *Med Clin North Am* 52:123, 1968.

have considered the pain to be psychogenic. The importance of establishing a diagnosis in this group of patients was emphasized over 60 years ago by de Takats[46] and 10 years later by Bonica,[47] both of whom pointed out that if such patients are not properly diagnosed and treated in time, they often become addicted to narcotics or become psychotic or even suicidal.

In view of the difficulty of establishing a precise diagnosis in many patients suffering intractable chronic pain and in view of the efficacy of differential neural blockade in doing so in carefully selected patients, it has been and continues to be our practice to use differential neural blockade to confirm the diagnosis in many cases, even when the mechanism appears to be obvious on clinical grounds, and even more frequently to establish a diagnosis when the mechanism is in question or is not known.

References

Full references for this chapter can be found on www.expertconsult.com.

Chapter 19

Spinal Canal Endoscopy

Takashi Igarashi and Lloyd R. Saberski

Historical Considerations

Endoscopy plays a role in the diagnosis and treatment of many different conditions. Endoscopy platforms continue to grow into areas amenable to endoscopic visualization, particularly the epidural space, spinal cord, and contiguous structures. A review of the medical literature shows that clinicians have been working with various types of endoscopes for more than 60 years, with varying degrees of success. Today, fiberoptic technology has been integrated with computer-enhanced imaging to provide a new medium for viewing the central nervous system (CNS). The initial results are promising and will probably pave the way for newer, less invasive means of diagnosis and treatment of CNS pathology.

Direct visualization of the spinal canal and its contents was born in 1931 from the pioneering work of Michael Burman.[1] With each decade since then, myeloscopists and epiduroscopists have attempted to develop a means of fiberoptic visualization that would be easy and safe for application in medical practice. Burman[1] removed 11 cadaver vertebral columns and examined them with rigid arthroscopic equipment and an incandescent light source. As might be expected, the diameter of the trocar in which the lamp was mounted was greater than the average width of the spinal canal—approximately ⅜ inch, or 9.5 mm. Thus the viewing lens was not completely within the spinal canal. In a few locations, the spinal canal was wide enough to accommodate insertion of the endoscope, thereby permitting visualization of the spinal canal contents: the dura mater, blood vessels, and cauda equina. The endoscope's field of view was limited because of its large size to only 1 inch (2.54 cm). In 1931, Burman[1] concluded that myeloscopy was limited by the technology available. With higher-quality instrumentation, a better postmortem examination of the cauda equina could be performed in situ. He believed that visualization of the contents of cadaveric spinal canals would be especially important in establishing the diagnosis of tumor or inflammation. He did not anticipate that an improved device might allow in situ/in vivo, minimally invasive therapy. This was not to be achieved until the 1980s, when both flexible fiberoptic light sources and optics became available.[2]

In 1936, Elias Stern[3] of Columbia University's Department of Anatomy was among the first to describe a spinascope. A working model was built by American Cystoscopes Makers, Inc. The spinascope was designed for in vivo examination of the spinal canal contents in the presence of a spinal anesthetic. The instrument was never actually used, but Stern[3] did envision direct observation of the posterior roots for rhizotomies in patients with intractable pain, as well as sectioning of the anterior roots for incurable spastic conditions. He predicted that technologic improvements might allow the endoscopic platform to replace exploratory laminotomy.

In March 1937 the first anesthetized subject was examined with a myeloscope by J. Lawrence Pool[4,5] of New York (**Fig. 19.1**). Unfortunately, hemorrhage obscured the field of vision and permitted only a fleeting glimpse of the lumbosacral nerve roots. Subsequently, seven patients were examined without complication. The cauda equina and blood flow through epidural vessels were observed. In 1942, Pool published in the journal *Surgery* a summation of 400 cases.[6] In the era before computed tomography (CT) and magnetic resonance imaging (MRI), he reconstructed graphics that established or confirmed the diagnosis via the myeloscope. With images in hand, he approached operations with expectation and avoided extensive explorations. He identified neuritis, herniated nucleus pulposus, hypertrophied ligamentum flavum, primary and metastatic neoplasms, varicose vessels, and arachnoid adhesions.

Despite these successes and the relative ease of performing such examinations, no further reports of similar technique are found in the literature until 1967 because of the widespread acceptance and simplicity of myelography and the need to

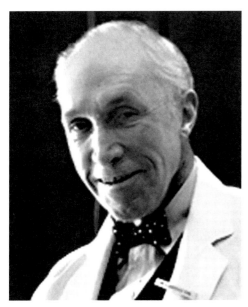

Fig. 19.1 J. Lawrence Pool (1906–2004), one of the pioneers of spinal endoscopy.

sketch observations if performing spinal endoscopy. There was no automatic graphic capture, and photographic equipment of the era did not provide sufficient light for image formation. Dr. Pool, a talented artist, documented his observations with hand-drawn sketches.

In the late 1960s and early 1970s, Yoshio Ooi et al,[7–11] working without knowledge of the American experience, developed an endoscope for intradural and extradural examination. Then available for use in the 1970s was fiberoptic light source technology, which allowed miniaturization and more lumens of light without added heat. The fiberoptic light source technology protected tissues from heat injury because fiberoptic fibers absorb infrared rays and reflect visible rays. The myeloscope could now be miniaturized because a large size was unnecessary for carrying sufficient light. The smaller size allowed the myeloscope to be inserted between lumbar spinous processes in the same manner as a needle for percutaneous lumbar puncture.[12] The procedure was now greatly simplified and no serious complications were reported from their initial 86 patients. Postspinal cephalgia was a common, albeit temporary, complication in 70% of the study patients. Ooi et al[13] recorded detailed descriptions of normal and abnormal anatomy, as well as blurry black-and-white photographic images of the ligamentum flavum, epidural adipose tissue, the surface of the dural sac, and the cauda equina.

From 1967 to 1977, Ooi et al[13] and Satoh et al[14] performed 208 myeloscopic procedures with various types of equipment. Their progress was reported in several publications, culminating in 1981 with their publication on myeloscopy and blood flow changes in the cauda equina during Lasegue's test.[15] The intrathecal space was regularly entered with a 1.8 mm rigid scope. The fiberoptics used were only for the light source; fiberoptic myeloscopes with fiberoptic light sources for direct visualization were still a decade away. The authors noted changes in blood flow in vessels accompanying the cauda equina during straight-leg raising tests. During this maneuver, caudad anterior displacement of the cauda equina leading to

temporary cessation of blood flow was observed. Presumably, this is clinically associated with pain in susceptible patients. Abdominal straining, coughing, and sneezing did not alter blood flow but did cause slight up-and-down movement of the cauda equina in the lateral position. Unfortunately, with the decrease in diameter of the scope, the amount of light available for good-quality pictures was reduced; a larger myeloscope (2.5 mm) was needed for visualization in the epidural space. Myeloscopy epiduroscopy therefore continued to be regarded as having limited value for the diagnosis of spinal stenosis but was thought to be an important aid in the diagnosis of pathology associated with spinal pain syndromes such as arachnoiditis, tumors, and vascular abnormalities. Procedures such as removal of a herniated nucleus pulposus were considered, but because of limitations in flexibility of the rigid scope, insufficient light, and difficulty distinguishing normal from abnormal tissue, the surgical use of spinal endoscopic equipment remained limited. A flexible myeloscope was theorized to have many advantages, but another decade passed before arrival of the micromyeloscope.

Blomberg[16] was the next to describe a method of epiduroscopy and spinaloscopy. It was his interest to study anatomic variation of the epidural space so that a better understanding of epidural anesthesia could be obtained. Using a fiberoptic light source with a small rigid endoscope, he determined that the contents of the epidural space varied widely, especially in regard to the amount of fat and connective tissue. In 12 of 30 postmortem examinations, the epidural contents limited visibility of the epidural space. Adhesions between the dura mater and ligamentum flavum restricted opening the epidural space despite flushing with normal saline. Blomberg was able to position the epiduroscope, which was still similar to the Stern spinascope, to visualize entry of a Tuohy needle through the ligamentum flavum into the epidural space. Dural tenting was seen when an epidural catheter was threaded through the Tuohy needle into the epidural space. Once in the epidural space, the orientation of the catheter varied greatly and was ultimately determined by local anatomy. Blomberg surmised that it was "too early to decide to what extent clinical application is possible with epiduroscopy. Under all circumstances it would be necessary to improve lighting conditions, and to shorten shutter speeds in order to make the method more easily handled."[16]

In 1989, Blomberg and Olsson[17] performed 10 epiduroscopic procedures on patients scheduled for partial laminectomy for herniated lumbar disks. They believed that the conclusions drawn from previous autopsy work were not necessarily transferable to the clinical setting. Their concerns pertained to the absence of circulation in cadavers and to the possible impact of low or completely absent cerebrospinal fluid (CSF) pressure on appearance of the epidural space.[17] They determined that the epidural space was indeed only a potential space that remained open for brief periods when fluid or air was injected. Blomberg and Olsson[17] confirmed the presence of a dorsomedian connective tissue band that divided the epidural space into compartments. They determined that a midline approach to the epidural space was often associated with bleeding and that a paramedian approach was less likely to cause this complication.[18] Blomberg recorded his internal images with videocassette recorder (VCR) tape. The fiberoptic light source combined with computer-assisted exposure allowed adequate video capture.

Shimoji et al[2] were the first group to publish endoscopic experience with both a fiberoptic light source and a flexible fiberoptic catheter instead of the traditional rigid metal endoscopes for myeloscopy. Their experience with small (0.5 to 1.4 mm) flexible fiberoptic scopes was published in 1991. The continued availability of camcorders and VCRs made it possible to have simultaneous video images and a recording of all aspects of the internal procedure. In 10 patients with chronic, intractable spinal pain syndromes, they placed flexible fiberoptic myeloscopes/epiduroscopes into either the subarachnoid space, epidural space, or both via a lumbar paramedian approach through a Tuohy needle. The epidural space was able to be visualized only after withdrawal of the myeloscope from the subarachnoid position because of passage of CSF into the potential epidural space, which gently distended the space, permitted tissues to be less adherent, and allowed the lens to achieve its focal length of 3 to 5 mm. With the tissues adherent to the lens, view of the tissue bed was obliterated. The procedures were performed without sedatives or local anesthetics to allow assessment of patient discomfort. There was an interest in seeing whether chronic pain sources could be identified with a mechanical stimulus. Accurate identification of the spinal level was determined by the simultaneous use of radiographs. In four of the study patients, subarachnoid fiberoptic scopes were advanced to the cisterna magna. In patients with a diagnosis of adhesive arachnoiditis, nerve roots were observed to be matted or clumped by filamentous tissue without evidence of other structural lesions. The excessive connective tissue made observation of the subarachnoid space difficult. Three of the five patients in whom adhesive arachnoiditis was diagnosed before the procedure had either a reduction or complete remission of their pain after the procedure. Although the myeloscopic examinations did not establish the anatomic cause of pain, the authors believed that further study was warranted. There were minimal complications consisting mainly of transient post–dural puncture headaches and fever; the few cases of dysesthesia during the procedure were rectified by slowly withdrawing the scope from the nerve root in question.

In 1991 Saberski and Kitahata[19] began evaluation of several fiberoptic endoscopes for epiduroscopy. The technology had improved, but appropriate indications for epiduroscopy were still not clear. Uncertainty remained about whether epiduroscopy provided a diagnostic advantage over noninvasive imaging procedures—CT and MRI.[19] A number of technologic problems needed to be surmounted before clinical use of such devices could seriously be considered. The fiberoptic endoscopes could visualize tissue immediately in front of the lens when the 2 mm focal length was maintained. This focal distance was difficult to achieve in a potential space such as the epidural space. There was also difficulty getting the endoscopes into the epidural space without damage, even with simultaneous fluoroscopy. The original fiberoptic endoscopes did not have working channels for tissue sampling or delivery of medication. The ideal device needed to be maneuverable, have a working lumen, have a lens with a short focal length, and incorporate a mechanism that prevented tissue from obstructing the lens. By using the caudal approach, Saberski and Kitahata[20] were able to steer a fiberoptic with great difficulty to specific sites and deliver steroid medication to nerve roots via the introducer after removing the fiberoptic. To achieve steering, they curved the naked fiberoptic by wrapping it gently over a finger. When inside the epidural space, they then rotated the proximal end of the fiberoptic, which caused an exaggerated rotation inside the epidural canal. This allowed visualization of more epidural space.

These early therapeutic successes indicated that spinal canal endoscopy was not only possible but also had the advantage of placing medications directly onto structures of concern. This contrasted sharply with the widely accepted technique for epidural steroid injection in which an injection took the pathway of least resistance. Saberski and Kitahata[20] found that normal saline irrigation easily distended the epidural space and allowed the fiberoptic to assume its needed focal length. Once the initial 15 to 20 mL of normal saline was injected, maintenance of only slight positive pressure on the syringe was necessary to keep the epidural space distended.

Saberski and Kitahata[20] also observed that nerves intended for visualization, on the basis of symptoms, electrodiagnostic studies, response to local anesthetic root blockade, and imaging studies, often appeared by spinal canal endoscopy to have fluffy connective tissue over them. The presence of this tissue was not appreciated before the development of spinal canal endoscopy because previous methods of entering the spine were always at the level of interest and were associated with local bleeding. The spinal canal endoscope was floated from the caudal epidural space into position to observe the lumbar epidural anatomy. Any bleeding was far removed from the sites of observation. The "cottony" tissue at times seemed to float in the saline. Some of this material could be irrigated aside to reveal denser connective tissue attached to nerves and contiguous structures. On occasion, an erythematous hue of the perineural tissue was seen after the fluffier tissues were irrigated away. These changes are probably an inflammatory reaction that represents the immune system's response to change.

Concurrent with the work done at Yale, in 1991 Heavner et al[21] reported on endoscopic evaluation of the epidural and subarachnoid spaces in rabbits or dogs and in human cadavers with the aid of a flexible endoscope; the technique used flexible endoscopes with outside diameters of 2.1 and 1.4 mm, respectively. In 1992 Mollmann et al[22] published details of spinaloscopy with a rigid 4 mm endoscope on nonfixed preparations from human cadavers. At the Seventh World Congress of Pain in 1993, Heavner et al[23] reported that in anesthetized dogs, endoscopes could be passed freely from their lumbar epidural insertion sites to the cervical epidural space without producing motor or cardiovascular responses. Significant difficulty with orientation was encountered, thus suggesting that further modifications would be necessary before the vast potential of epiduroscopy could be exploited.[22] In 1994, Rosenberg et al[24] performed epiduroscopy in anesthetized dogs with a thin flexible and deflectable steerable fiberscope. The same year, Schutze and Kurtze[25] published their experience with epiduroscopy in 12 patients with various pain syndromes. They were able to visualize normal and abnormal anatomy. Pronounced adhesions and fibrosis were observed in two patients after failed back surgery. Three permanent epidural catheters were implanted under epiduroscopic control.[25]

Though representing multiple breakthroughs in technology, these devices had limitations that needed to be addressed before further human clinical trials could begin in earnest. A channel for instrumentation and refinements in steering was necessary. An easy-to-steer system with multiple lumens for instrumentation, irrigation, and fiberoptics needed to be developed. In response to these needs, Catheter Imaging

Systems, Inc., Myelotec, Inc., Clarus, K. Storz, and EBI manufactured or supplied various devices that were used for spinal canal endoscopy throughout the 1990s.

By 1996, epidural spinal canal endoscopy was used frequently for the delivery of epidural steroid medication. Many providers throughout the world modified the Saberski/Kitahata techniques to include lysis of adhesions with blunt dissection, volumetric injection, and the use of lasers and balloons. There was a sense that these techniques provided an advantage over other percutaneous blind techniques, but there were few studies to support such use. By 1998, various versions of the technique were common. Insurance carriers began to review whether the literature supported continued reimbursement for such services despite strong advocacy from patients and physicians. Many concluded that there was insufficient peer-reviewed literature or randomized controlled studies and stated that these technologies were experimental and denied reimbursement of services to physicians and hospital/surgery centers.

Despite considerable interest to continue research, a number of factors impeded progress. First of all, the first company to manufacture and distribute a commercial flexible fiberoptic endoscope system for spinal canal endoscopy (Myelotec, Inc.) had limited resources for funding research. Though aware of the need to fund research, Myelotec hoped that commercial sales and widespread use of the technology would be enough to generate revenue for future research. Unfortunately, simultaneous growth within the United States of managed care slowed expansion of the endoscopy field and limited funds for research. It was also extremely difficult to develop randomized controlled studies, even with funding. Most patients were not interested in randomization, and patients opted for surgery or endoscopy, depending on patient preference and clinical circumstance. The demands of insurance review boards for randomized controlled studies seemed particularly harsh with regard to endoscopy because other surgical and minimally interventional procedures were performed in the United Sates with a dearth of outcome data. Although the platform for endoscopy was easy to use and relatively safe and made perfect sense as an option before consideration of surgical procedures involving disks, inflammation, and pain, it was a paradigm shift that required reeducation of physicians, surgeons, insurance companies, and the public. Before the work of McCarron, Saberski, the Saals, and others, disk-related spine disease was usually conceptualized in terms of compression of nerves. The awareness that disk disease and spine pain could be partially or completely a medical inflammatory condition controlled by the immune system was not even a consideration. The focus was on detection of anatomic causes of pain by MRI, with the size of the herniated disk expected to determine the degree of pain. In fact, this specificity theory that size determines pain has been debunked for more than 30 years, yet it is still subscribed to. It is now known that chemical and cell signal change at the tissue bed level in conjunction with changes in receptivity of the CNS determine the quantity of pain. Thus a patient with a small injury can be debilitated and in pain. The pain is every bit real and organic.

The late 1990s concluded with several studies that took advantage of the spinal endoscopic platform, including examination of living anatomy by Igarashi et al[26] in Japan, the risk of dural puncture during combined anesthetic techniques,[27] the effect of epidural fat on epidural catheter placement,[28] the relative effects of age on epidural fat content and local anesthetic dose requirements,[28] and changes in epidural anatomy after epidural anesthesia.[29–31] Kurtze and Schutze[32] from Germany reported on the Internet observations of the epidural space in 139 patients and placed epidural catheters and electrodes under spinal endoscopic guidance. There were numerous case reports showcasing the potential of the endoscopic platform.[19,20,33–35] A distinction was made between management of acute pain and chronic pain syndromes, and it was recognized that a multitude of different pathophysiologies constitute the spinal pain syndrome. Thus the platform was used in many different ways for many different pathologic conditions. Saberski et al[36] indicated that immunoinflammation secondary to acute disk irritation was observed regularly. It appears to be independent of disk compression and may be representative of leaky disk syndromes and an autoimmune response.[36] This raises the likelihood of developing specific chemotherapies to interfere with the immunochemical events in epidural tissue beds. There is discussion but no substantiation that environmental factors and infectious disease may influence the immune system's response to disk antigen/chemical. Animal work has begun in which cell signals and immune responses are being analyzed. When mature, this work could define many common spine afflictions as medical diseases and not surgical disorders.[36]

Since the start of the new century there has been a steady trickle of new publications that have highlighted the potential of epiduroscopy. Richardson[37] published a review of spinal canal endoscopy in the *British Journal of Anaesthesia* during the autumn of 1999. Saberski[38] reported at the World Foundation for Pain Conference, New York, that medical management of patients with spinal canal endoscopy is less expensive and more likely to return a patient to work than similar acute herniated disk patients treated by laminectomy/diskectomy. In 2000, Manchikanti et al[39] showed that the overall safety of spinal canal endoscopy is good and with such a low risk that the gamble on benefit seemingly worthwhile. Richardson et al[40] reported on the association of adhesions and chronic spinal pain in 34 patients and that 1 year after manipulation there was less pain and epidural adhesion, supporting the concept that scarring/adhesion in the epidural space contributes to pain. Manchikanti et al[41] demonstrated that endoscopic adhesiolysis performed in 60 postlaminectomy patients was 100% effective in reducing pain for 30 days but thereafter effectiveness reduced until only 22% at 1 year and then even less at 7%. Saberski,[42] in a pilot study comparing outcome of laminectomy to spinal canal epiduroscopy, showed better long-term outcome with 72% of the epiduroscopy group returning to work and 32% requiring continued opioid medication compared to the postlaminectomy group with only 28% returning to work and 92% continued on opioid. Krasuski et al[43] reported initial improvements in 64%, considerably less than Manchikanti, and relief declined to 50% after 1 month and 32% after 3 months. Hammer et al[44] modified the technique in 2001 and reported on the transforaminal approach to a ventral epidural adhesiolysis. Many considered this to be higher risk given the variability of the major radicular artery feeding the anterior spinal cord, but the procedure had appeal since the ventral-lateral epidural space (the principle areas of spinal canal pathology) were hard to reach from the typical sacral canal entry point. In 2001, Richardson et al[40] performed a prospective case series and concluded that spinal endoscopy may be the diagnostic method of choice for epidural fibrosis.

It has substantial therapeutic and research potential. However, prospective randomized studies are required. Geurts et al[45] in 2002 concluded that epiduroscopy is of value in the diagnosis of spinal root pathology. In sciatica, adhesions unreported by MRI can be identified. Targeted epidural medication, administered near the compromised spinal nerve, results in substantial and prolonged pain relief. Ruetten et al[46] reported that application of laser in epiduroscopy extended possibilities in the treatment of chronic back pain syndrome and showed a potential future option for epiduroscopy. When findings were appropriate, mechanical instruments and the holmium:YAG laser were applied therapeutically; 45.9% of 93 patients presented with positive results in postoperative examination. Pathomorphologic processes corresponding to the multifactorial pain processes, which escape detection in modern imaging procedures, can be diagnosed in the epidural space using epiduroscopy. Therapeutic intervention is possible. However, use is limited because of technical difficulties. Navigation of the endoscope is especially limited with access through the sacral hiatus. Manchikanti et al[47] in 2003 showed spinal endoscopic adhesiolysis in management of chronic low back pain in a preliminary report of a randomized, double-blind trial. The results showed significant improvement in patients undergoing spinal endoscopic adhesiolysis at 1 month, 3 months, and 6 months, compared to baseline measurements, as well as compared to the control group without adhesiolysis. It was concluded that spinal endoscopic adhesiolysis with targeted injection of local anesthetic and steroid is an effective treatment in a significant number of patients without major adverse effects at 6-month follow-up. Igarashi et al's[48] landmark publication in the *British Journal of Anesthesia* in 2004 showed considerable improvement in lumbar spinal stenosis symptoms in the elderly. This article started considerable discussion in the literature from Richardson[49] and Nash[50] debating findings with epiduroscopy. Dashfield et al[51] in 2005 showed that targeted placement of epidural steroid onto the affected nerve root causing sciatica demonstrated no significant reduction in pain intensity, anxiety, or depression compared with untargeted caudal nonendoscopic epidural steroid injection. When analyzed individually, both techniques benefited patients. Mizuno et al[52] in 2007 further reported on adverse events by reporting encephalopathy and rhabdomyolysis induced by iotrolan contrast agent during epiduroscopy. Dural tear during epiduroscopy may have allowed access of contrast media into CSF with neurotoxicity secondary to iotrolan within the CSF contributing to the encephalopathy and subsequent rhabdomyolysis. Avellanal[53] in 2008 reported on the interlaminar approach for epiduroscopy in patients with failed back surgery syndrome and described a 50% reduced outer diameter catheter, which allowed for the interlaminar approach. Komiya et al[54] in 2008 warned of a potential risk of cumulative x-ray dosages in epiduroscopic procedures. Sairyo et al[55] in 2008 showed long-term radiculopathy caused by epidural lipomatosis at the L3-4 intervertebral disk level. The fatty tissue was located on the dorsal side of the dural sac in the spinal canal and compressed the dural sac. The fatty tissue was removed endoscopically. After surgery, the symptoms disappeared, and neurologic deficits normalized. Ruetten et al[56] also in 2008 demonstrated that endoscopic techniques are equal to microsurgical techniques with the benefit of reduced traumatization. The majority of epiduroscopy performed worldwide to date has been done with a disposable steering handle with lumens for fiberoptics and instrumentation. However, Schutze[57] pioneered advances in spinal canal endoscopy using a completely reusable scope made by Karl Storz and has described many novel uses, including placement of epidural electrode arrays, in his recently published book *Epiduroscopy.* In 2008 the second European Consensus Statement regarding epiduroscopy, published in *The Pain Clinic,* laid further groundwork for study and clinical care.[58,59] The World Society of Pain Clinicians' (WSPC's) 2008 meeting in Seoul, South Korea, highlighted presentations from Hanaoka et al[60] on use of spinal canal endoscopy in Japan and Van Seventer[61] from the Netherlands.

Terminology

The original term for endoscopic evaluation of the epidural space was *epiduroscopy.* Coining of the term is credited to Rune Blomberg. In the United States there was considerable reluctance by insurance carriers to reimburse for epiduroscopy because they were not familiar with the term and it did not appear in insurance coding books. The term *spinal canal endoscopy* was adopted because of familiarity in the American insurance market with endoscopy in other body cavities. Spinal canal endoscopy today refers to either epiduroscopy, fiberoptic evaluation in the peridural position, or myeloscopy for subarachnoid visualization.

Epiduroscopy and Spinal Canal Endoscopy Consensus

On September 17, 1998, in Iserlohn and on October 3, 1998, in Bad Durkheim, Germany, an international group of experts drew up a consensus paper titled "Standards for Epiduroscopy."[62] The participants in the working group agreed on the following general principles governing the clinical application of spinal canal endoscopy. The scientific basis for the recommendations for the use of spinal canal endoscopy was provided from publications and the clinical experience of Drs. Groll, Heavner, Kurtze, Leu, Mollmann, Rawal, Saberski, and Schutze.

Spinal canal endoscopy epiduroscopy was defined as percutaneous, minimally invasive endoscopic investigation of the epidural space to enable color visualization of anatomic structures inside the spinal canal: the dura mater, blood vessels, connective tissue, nerves, fat, and pathologic structures, including adhesion fibrosis, inflammation, and stenotic change. The general indications established for spinal canal endoscopy in the diagnosis and treatment of spinal pain syndromes included (1) observation of pathology and anatomy; (2) direct drug application; (3) direct lysis of scarring with medication, blunt dissection, laser, and other instruments; (4) placement of catheter and electrode systems (epidural, subarachnoid); and (5) as an adjunct to minimally invasive surgery.

Indications for Spinal Canal Endoscopy

In selecting patients for spinal canal endoscopy, the provider must realize that there are symptoms pertaining to the chief complaint and the anatomic diagnosis. Both symptom and anatomic variables need to be taken into consideration before selection of the technique. Symptoms thought to be representative of nerve irritation from a variety of causes may be responsive to directed irrigation and placement of anti-inflammatory steroid medications. The chemical mediators responsible for the immuno-inflammation may come from herniated nucleus pulposus, synovium, and other sources. Such irritants can be associated with radiculopathy, canal stenosis, fibrous adhesions, and cysts. Typical symptoms amenable to spinal canal endoscopy include those related to lumbar and sacral radiculopathy: neuralgia and plexopathy from nerve root irritation without significant compressive lesions. The presence of a compressive lesion with signs of progressive neurologic impairment is a contraindication to further placement of fluid into the epidural space. Patient selection based on case reports suggests that better results are achieved in the subgroup of patients with an acute or subacute disk-related spinal pain syndrome who have not undergone back surgery and have no associated pain behavior.[19,20,33–35] This subgroup of patients may be more likely to be responsive to "washout" of chemical irritants and the anti-inflammatory effects of corticosteroids. In addition, changes in CNS plasticity/secondary hyperalgesia may not have developed in this subgroup and thus they may be responsive to peripheral treatment with washout alone. Spinal canal endoscopy is not indicated in patients suffering from biomechanical pain syndromes such as lumbar facet syndrome, sacroiliac joint dysfunction, or myofascial pain syndromes. **Table 19.1** summarizes the indications and contraindications for spinal canal endoscopy.

Rationale for the Caudal Approach

The caudal approach to the epidural space seemed to offer advantage over the paramedian approach. The straight entry into the epidural space contrasted sharply with the approximately 45-degree bend required to pass a catheter into the lumbar epidural space. Thus there was less of a chance of fracturing the fiberoptic. The straight caudal canal placement also made it easier to add additional channels for future surgical procedures and to steer.

The previous work of Odendaal and Van Aswegen[63] supported the caudal approach on an entirely different basis, the kinetics of injected fluids. They injected a radionuclide admixture into the lumbar epidural space of patients with and without previous laminectomy. By monitoring the distribution of the radioactive tracer, these researchers were able to demonstrate poor caudal spread of injectate in patients who had previously undergone laminectomy. In the nonoperated control group, however, there was an even spread of fluid throughout the lumbar and sacral nerve roots. Thus an injection into the lumbar epidural space took the pathway of least resistance and would not necessarily deliver intended steroids to the sacral nerve roots. For these reasons, Cyriax and Cyriax[64] intuitively advocated volumetric caudal injections during the 1960s to 1980s. With such epidural injections the injectate (normal saline, local anesthetic, and steroid) was more likely to go cephalad. Some injectate did escape through the sacral foramen. Using volumes of 25 to 50 mL containing local anesthetic, normal saline, and steroid, Cyriax and Cyriax[64] claimed lasting results in more than 40% of patients. These results were secondary to better spread of the steroid, improved irrigation of the epidural tissue bed, and mobilization of adherent tissues via hydrostatic pressure gradients. It is presumed that the dramatic response was seen in patients with relatively acute disk inflammatory processes, not failed surgical back syndromes. The effect of Cyriax and Cyriax's personal choice for local anesthetic, procaine, on long-term outcome is unknown, but its role cannot be excluded.

The work of Racz et al[65] in Lubbock, Texas, suggested that lysis of epidural adhesions was of significant benefit to many patients with refractory lumbar radiculopathy. Their pioneering work indicated that scar adhesions formed in the epidural space of patients with many chronic spine pain syndromes, after surgery or perhaps as a result of inflammation, and were responsible for pulling and tugging nerve roots and the dural sac. Their innovative technique involved placement of a catheter through the sacral hiatus into the epidural space in close approximation to the root or adhesion in question, which was indicated by an epidurogram. A total volume of 30 to 40 mL of a local anesthetic, steroid, and non-ionic contrast agent was

---

Table 19.1 Indications and Contraindications for Spinal Canal Endoscopy

IDEAL CANDIDATE

Healthy, working, no litigation, minimal medication, no dependent behavior

Indications

Widely accepted indications	Irritative neuralgias: new-onset radiculopathy, radiculopathy associated with postlaminectomy pain syndrome
Probable indications	Adhesion related: postlaminectomy epidural adhesion, low back pain, Tarlov cyst

Contraindications

Strong contraindications	No consent, cauda equina syndrome, urinary dynamic problem, sphincter dysfunction, footdrop, pilonidal cyst, osteomyelitis, anal fissure, raised intracranial pressure, pseudotumor cerebri, CNS tumor, coagulopathy, no sacral hiatus, unable to place a thin needle into the sacral canal, untreated addictive behavior, unstable angina, severe COPD, meningocele/meningomyelocele, inability to lie prone, COPD, CHF, angina, back pain, etc., inadequate facilities, allergy to proposed medications
Relative contraindications	Multiple different complaints of pain, active untreated psychiatric disorders, somatoform process, unrealistic expectations, retinal disease, partial blindness

CHF, Congestive heart failure; *CNS,* central nervous system; *COPD,* chronic obstructive pulmonary disease.

then injected. The results showed significant variability between study groups, probably a consequence of the heterogeneous nature of persistent lumbar radiculopathy. Nonetheless, approximately 50% of the patients had marked improvement, as measured by decreased medication, enhanced function, and reduced visual analog scale scores for 1 to 6 months. Racz et al[65] and Arthur et al[66] concluded that the overlooked epidural adhesions could cause pain, perhaps from compression and irritation of nerves. With spinal canal endoscopy, it is envisioned that a three-dimensional color view of the adhesions and adjacent anatomy will afford the operator an advantage over two-dimensional, black-and-white fluoroscopic projection epidurograms. Thus spinal canal endoscopy will have potential as a platform for the management of chronic spinal canal–based diseases, in addition to its place in the management of acute inflammatory canal diseases.

Work by Serpell et al[67] showed that sustained pressure applied epidurally is transmitted intrathecally and could compromise perfusion or cause barotrauma at remote locations. They noted an initial escape of fluid via leakage into the large sacral root foramina and sheaths. After capacity around 20 mL in ewes was achieved, there was an abrupt increase in CSF pressure with each injection. The range was variable and was reflective of each study animal and of CNS compliance. The researchers concluded that instillation of saline into the epidural space results in an eventual significant increase in CSF pressure. CNS compliance was variable and seemed to deteriorate after instrumentation surgery. Thus scarring associated with surgery predisposed animals to neurologically dangerous pressure. Serpell et al[67] recommend continuous monitoring of CSF pressure in humans. However, Cyriax and Cyriax[64] reported no major long-term complications after 50,000 volumetric caudal injections. Certainly with these injections, even if performed slowly, there were increases in CSF pressure without apparent ill effect. At higher volumes greater than 100 mL, Cyriax and Cyriax did note the potential for retinal hemorrhage with the single-shot caudal injection technique completed in minutes. Cyriax and Cyriax indicated that the retinal hemorrhages resolved without consequence. There are other reports indicating that retinal hemorrhage can occur with routine epidural injections.[68] A few reports have now been made of retinal and macular hemorrhage with varying degrees of blindness after spinal canal endoscopy. In the cases that the authors are aware of, the patients were deeply anesthetized, thus disconnecting the most sensitive monitor for elevated pressure—the patient's own complaint of pain. Patients who have a noncompliant spinal canal will have resistance to injection and will complain of significant pain, both local and remote. The pain will often begin in the lumbar region and migrate cephalad. As a precaution, all injections into the spinal canal for both endoscopic and routine epidural injections should be given incrementally with constant dialog with the patient. When the patient's complaint of pain or discomfort has moved cephalad, the managing physician must take appropriate action determined by the clinical circumstance: alter the technique, infuse less volume, stop the procedure, drain/decompress the epidural space, or other measures. It is noted that the total volume that can be injected into a spinal canal with a series of injections or endoscopies often increases with each subsequent injection, presumably from stretching out the more compliant spinal canals. An injection rate of 1 mL/sec is recommended. Previous work at Yale has determined that rapid injection of fluid greater than 1 mL/sec is more likely to be associated with high peak epidural pressure, measured at times in excess of 300 mm Hg. The rapidity of injection, the size of the syringe, the volume of injection, compliance of the spinal canal epidural space, and turbulence of the injection are all determinants of peak pressure. Peak pressure falls off to preinjection levels abruptly with disconnection of the syringe, as a rule when the total volume is less than 30 to 40 mL.[46,69]

Clinically Relevant Anatomy

The spinal canal extends from the foramen magnum to the sacrum. It is bounded posteriorly by the ligamentum flavum and periosteum and anteriorly by the posterior longitudinal ligament, which lies over the dorsal aspect of the vertebral bodies and disks.

The size of the canal is approximately twice the size of the cord. It is largest in the cervical and lumbar regions, corresponding to enlargements of the spinal cord. At C4 to C6, it measures 18 mm in an anteroposterior direction. The transverse diameter at C4 to C6 measures 30 mm. The thoracic canal is 17 mm in both anteroposterior and transverse measurements. The lumbar canal is 23 and 18 mm, respectively.[70] The canal in cross section appears triangular at the cervical and lumbar levels and is more cylindrical at the thoracic level.

The spinal cord is continuous with the brain and ends with the conus medullaris at the lower border of the L1 vertebra. The dural sac containing the spinal cord and conus, however, runs down to the level of S2. The cauda equina consists of the terminal fibers of the conus, which extend inside the dural sac from L1 to S2. In the fetus, the spinal cord extends down to the coccyx, but as development proceeds, it is drawn upward because of greater growth of the vertebral column; at birth, the spinal cord extends only to L3. Flexing the column draws the cord temporarily higher.[71] In nerves that are not freely movable, such as in arachnoiditis, flexion can cause lancinating pain.

The epidural space surrounds the dural sac. It is bordered posteriorly by the ligamentum flavum and periosteum and anteriorly by the posterior longitudinal ligament. Laterally, the pedicles and the 48 intervertebral foramina bound it. The epidural space extends from the foramen magnum to the end of the dural sac at S2. The sacral canal is technically not part of the epidural space because it has no dural sac.

The posterior epidural space varies greatly. It averages 2 mm at the cervical level, 3 to 5 mm at the thoracic level, and 4 to 6 mm at the lumbar level.[70] The epidural space narrows considerably at L4 through S2. The epidural space anterior to the dura is uniformly narrow, less than 1 mm cephalad through caudad.

The epidural space is rich in content. At the midline connecting the dura to the periosteum posteriorly, there is usually a dorsal median connective tissue band, which can be complete or weblike.[2] Through the epidural space run the internal vertebral venous plexus, the spinal branches of the segmental arteries, the lymphatics, and the dura-arachnoid projections that surround the spinal nerve roots.[70] In addition, fat is abundant, but the amount present seems to bear no relationship to the patient's body fat percentage.[72]

The dura mater covering the spinal cord is a tough elastic tube that forms a loose sheath around the spinal cord. It is composed principally of longitudinal connective tissue fibers, with a proportionately small amount of circular yellow elastic tissue fibers. The spinal dura mater extends from the foramen magnum, to which it is closely adherent by its outer surface, to the S2 vertebra, where it ends in a cul-de-sac. Below this level the dura mater forms the filum terminale and descends to the coccyx, where it fuses with the periosteum.[73]

The paramedian approach for lumbar epidural injections has been advocated by anatomists and spinal endoscopists because vessels concentrate at the midline. It is remarkable to note the success of the epidural anesthetic technique despite the plethora of fat and connective tissue. Even catheters thread better than one might predict. As demonstrated by Blomberg and Olsson,[17] the dura is fairly tough and deflects catheters away, usually cephalad or caudad, depending on the direction of the bevel of the needle and local anatomy.

Technique

Before spinal canal endoscopy, all patients must undergo a thorough and complete history and physical examination. Care should be taken to document this examination carefully with special attention to a complete neurologic examination. Imaging studies should be reviewed, as well as special testing such as electromyography and nerve conduction studies. Lumbosacral, flexion, extension, and oblique plain x-ray views should be reviewed to assess for pathology not amenable to epidural procedures. MRI of the lumbar and sacral spine should be considered to assess the contents of the spinal canal and the presence of spinal stenosis. If a clinical decision is made to offer spinal canal endoscopy, all contraindications and relative contraindications must be addressed and documented in the medical record.

Preparation

Nonsteroidal anti-inflammatory drugs, aspirin, and anticoagulants should be discontinued before spinal canal endoscopy.[74] Appropriate laboratory studies should be considered. As a rule, bleeding associated with spinal canal endoscopy is limited and occurs distally at the introducer's entrance into the sacral hiatus. The patient should use an antibacterial scrub while showering the evening before and carefully cleanse the lumbar spine and sacral areas. The patient is directed to maintain nothing-by-mouth (NPO) status after midnight.

Equipment should be inspected, including disposables, several days in advance to ensure that all needed equipment is available. The procedure must be scheduled for a time when fluoroscopy and a postanesthetic care unit are available. Preprocedure discussion with the anesthesiologist should include patient positioning prone and the need for an awake, responsive patient. It is recommended that voice contact be maintained with the patient throughout the procedure to be able to assess the patient's response to manipulations. Informed consent must be obtained. It is preferable to obtain informed consent before the day of the procedure.

Procedure

1. Preprocedure prophylactic antibiotic coverage is considered. The patient is placed prone with a pillow under the abdomen and the feet internally rotated. Such positioning provides better exposure of the sacral hiatus. The sacral hiatus is identified anatomically by palpating for the sacral cornua (**Fig. 19.2A**). The cornua lie on either side of the midline, just above the natal crease. In instances in which the cornua are not palpable, firm midline palpation just above the natal crease should reveal the spinal canal. A midline position is confirmed with posteroanterior (PA) fluoroscopy.

2. With a 25-gauge or smaller needle, 3 to 5 mL of local anesthetic with epinephrine is placed onto the floor of the sacral canal. The small needle is passed cephalad and should easily slide into the sacral canal.

3. A 17-gauge Tuohy needle is inserted into the sacral hiatus and advanced cephalad. The loss-of-resistance technique can be used to confirm entry into the canal. A lateral fluoroscopic projection will show the needle in the canal (**Fig. 19.2B**). If the needle is noted to be dorsal to the canal false passageway, it should be removed and repositioned.

4. An injection of non-ionic contrast, 5 to 15 mL, followed by PA fluoroscopy will provide an epidurogram. The epidurogram will outline the nerve roots, scar adhesions, and other spinal canal structures (**Fig. 19.2C** and **D**).

5. The flexible end of the guidewire is threaded through the Tuohy needle. The guidewire should thread cephalad. This step should be followed by PA fluoroscopy. Repositioning and flushing the Tuohy needle with normal saline might be necessary to facilitate passage of the guidewire toward the nerve root or roots in question. After confirmation of the position of the wire with PA and lateral fluoroscopy, the Tuohy needle is removed.

6. The dilator and sheath are carefully introduced over the wire (**Fig. 19.2E** and **F**). With a no. 11 scalpel, the wire's aperture is widened to allow easier passage of the introducer. A similar technique is used for central line placement. If significant bleeding occurs, firm pressure is applied with gauze, and additional local anesthetic with epinephrine can be given. Rotary movement as the dilator goes through the soft tissues facilitates passage. As the dilator and sheath are passed cephalad, the wire should be frequently tested to see whether it moves freely. If the guidewire cannot be moved easily, there could be a kink in the wire. PA and lateral fluoroscopy can help check whether there is a kink or loop. If a kink present, it is best to remove dilator and sheath and slide the Tuohy needle back over the guidewire so that the wire can be removed and inspected. If the wire is kinked, a new wire should be used. A kinked wire could misdirect passage of the dilator and introducer catheter.

7. After the dilator and sheath are inserted, the dilator is removed with the introducer sheath left in place (**Fig. 19.2G** and **H**).

8. The side arm of the introducer sheath is flushed with 5 to 10 mL of preservative-free normal saline. The fiberoptic cable is then placed through one of the two lumens in the steering handle. Tubing containing normal saline for irrigation of the spinal canal/epidural space is attached to the second steering handle lumen. The clinician should next orient himself or herself to the steering direction and focus the fiberoptic on a sterile ruler or other recognizable structure.

9. The steering handle containing the fiberoptic scope and tubing for irrigation with preservative-free normal saline is inserted through the introducer. The camera and the video recorder are activated. The steering handle with the fiberoptic is advanced cephalad through the

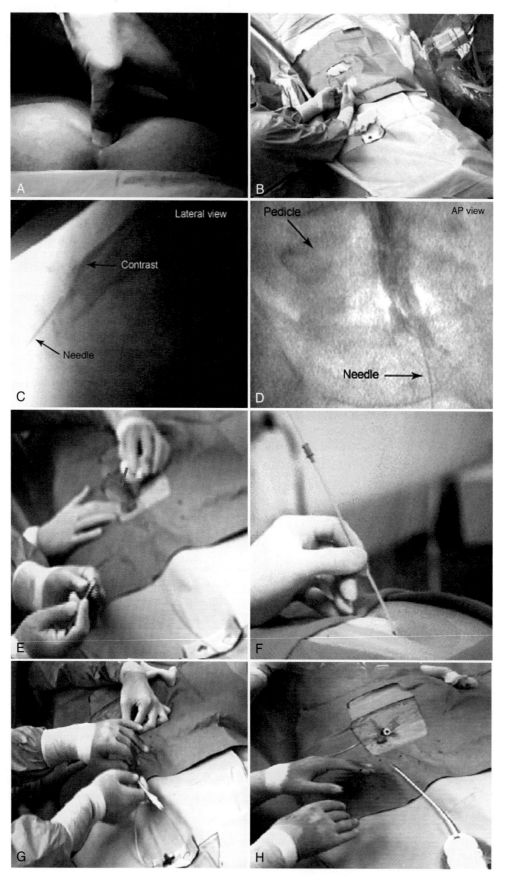

Fig. 19.2 Spinal endoscopy, step-by-step procedure.

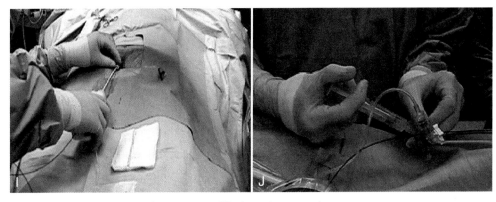

Fig. 19.2–cont'd For legend see opposite page.

sacral canal into the epidural space (**Fig. 19.2I**). To keep the epidural space distended and achieve the correct focal length for fiberoptic visualization, gentle pressure is applied to the normal saline syringe (**Fig. 19.2J**). To complement gentle pressure on the syringe, preservative-free normal saline bags (100 mL pressurized to less than systole for brief periods of 1 to 2 minutes) can be used. This technique often frees the hands for steering. Care should always be taken to ensure that the infusion of normal saline is not excessive. For this reason, small bags of normal saline are chosen. High pressure in the epidural space may be safe for brief periods in some patients with compliant spinal canals. The pressure generated by a bolus from a 10 mL syringe injected at 1 mL/sec can be greater than 300 mm Hg. When using a pressurized bag, the pressure is sustained for 1 to 2 minutes and then reduced to resting pressure to prevent any compromise in perfusion. The amount of fluid injected must be accurately monitored. The amount of preservative-free normal line used is approximately 60 mL per procedure. Most procedures last 30 to 45 minutes after the fiberoptic scope has been placed. Insertion of the introducer can at times be prolonged, depending on patient anatomy and skill of the provider.

Postprocedure Management

After the procedure is completed, a dressing is applied and the patient is taken to the recovery area. In the recovery suite a postprocedure neurologic examination is performed. Any new deficits should be detailed and monitored serially. MRI and neurosurgical consultation should be considered. Patients are instructed to not bathe for 5 days, but showers are acceptable after day 2. Hygiene instructions are important: perineal cleaning after bowel movements should be directed away from the procedural site. The patient should be discharged with a driver and should be observed by a friend or family member for the immediate postprocedure period. A 2- or 3-day supply of postprocedural short-acting opioid such as hydrocodone or oxycodone is appropriate.

Epidural Images

To follow the internal spinal canal anatomy (epidural anatomy), it is critical to maintain one's orientation. Simultaneous use of

fluoroscopy allows the operator to distinguish one level of epidural anatomy from the next. At times when confused about the location/orientation, needles can be inserted into the posterior epidural space. Blomberg's photographs of epidural catheters passing into the spinal canal epidural space illustrate this nicely. It is best to proceed with each spinal canal endoscopy with the objective of examining specific areas as opposed to a general exploration of the canal, epidural space, and contents. In this way the time that a spinal canal is subjected to insufflation with normal saline and potentially hazardous hydrostatic pressure is reduced.

The epidural space consists of fatty tissue, fibrous connective tissue, blood vessels, and nerve roots, and it is referred to as a potential space because the infusion of solution may change the morphology.[17,75] During epiduroscopy, saline is infused into the epidural space to create the endoscopic visual field and to release adhesions simultaneously. Therefore it should be kept in mind that the patency of the visualized epidural space may be different from that of the actual epidural space. To establish the orientation of the epidural space, it is important to rotate and fix the endoscope to the guide catheter or to the cable for the image guide, so as to achieve consistency of orientation while observing movement of the catheter via the endoscopic monitor and the fluoroscopy monitor. When the direction of the image movement on the monitor is opposite to the direction of endoscope movement, the vertical and horizontal directions of the image on the monitor are reversed, which may lead to mishandling of the endoscope. Therefore the orientation should be carefully established before and after insertion of the endoscope. Since the manual control of endoscopy consists of a combination of three techniques—lateral movement, axial rotation, and insertion/withdrawal—the obtained images may be seen in a slightly rotated state depending on the rotation of the endoscope. Various epidural spaces constructed by the dura, fatty tissue, nerve root, and yellow ligament can be observed depending on the site of observation, such as dorsal and ventral sides.

Normal Findings of the Spinal Endoscopy

In the sacral epidural space, the visual field of epiduroscopy entirely comprises fatty tissue in many cases, since abundant fatty tissue is present in the sacral epidural compared to the lumbar epidural space. Saline infusion creates a space among the fatty tissue, which ensures the visual field and facilitates endoscopic advancement to the lumbar region.

In the lumbar epidural space, the dura, fatty tissue, fibrous connective tissue, blood vessels, and nerve roots (**Fig. 19.3A**) can be clearly observed. Thin blood vessels are present on the surfaces of the dura and fatty tissue (**Fig. 19.3B**). The yellow ligament shows a slightly more whitish color than fat, and the surface blood vessels are unclear (**Fig. 19.3C**). Fibrous connective tissue shows a varying morphology, such as a filamentous shape (**Fig. 19.3D**) or an adherent form (**Fig. 19.3E**), and macroscopically appears very soft. Saline infusion generally creates a cavity between the dura and fatty tissue in the lumbar epidural space. The patency of this space varies depending on the volume of saline infused, the amount of fibrous connective tissue, the strength of adhesion between the dura and the surrounding tissues, and the cross-sectional area of the spinal canal. When the endoscope is advanced toward the cranial side in the epidural space, regions with and without fatty tissue alternately appear because the fatty tissue of the epidural space is present in a ladder arrangement at the thoracic to lumbar level.[26,76,77]

When air bubbles with saline are introduced into the epidural space, the original epidural space construction may be obscured, and assessment of the endoscopic image may be difficult. When some air bubbles are seen in the visual field, an image reflected by the bubbles may be seen as an unidentifiable structure, to which particular attention should be paid.

Abnormal Findings of the Spinal Endoscopy

In patients who have undergone spinal surgery, adhesions between the dura and surrounding tissue (**Fig. 19.3F**), scar tissue, and irregularly growing connective tissue are often present in the surgical vertebral levels in the epidural space. Scar tissue is harder than normal connective tissue, contains reduced blood flow in many cases, and appears pale. In contrast, connective tissue that has grown irregularly involving congestion, redness, and vascularization may be seen. The lysis of adhesions and scar tissue is possible on epiduroscopy (**Fig. 19.3F-G**),[78] but ensuring an appropriate endoscopic visual field and simultaneous lysis of adhesions may be difficult depending on the degree of adhesions and the scar tissue properties. In patients with no medical history of spinal surgery, connective and fatty tissues accompanied by congestion and redness may be also noted. In patients with a herniated intervertebral disk, the relationship between the prolapsed herniated mass, nerve root, and congestion and redness of the tissue around the herniated disk can be observed (**Fig. 19.3H**).[78] In many lumbar spinal stenosis patients with monosegmental symptoms, congestion and redness are seen in the tissue around the affected nerve root (**Fig. 19.3I**).[48] In lumbar spinal stenosis patients with multisegmental symptoms, connective tissue with impaired blood flow is present at affected vertebral levels in many cases (**Fig. 19.3J**).[48]

The epiduroscopic findings, combined with the information provided by the patient's disease history, physical examination, x-ray radiography, and MRI, may facilitate a close assessment of the pathology of low back and leg pain.

Side Effects and Complications

For spinal canal endoscopy to be performed, the epidural space must be distended with preservative-free normal saline. This allows the fiberoptic scope to achieve its required focal length and reveals intricate epidural structure that would not otherwise be possible. A possible complication of this technique is the generation of significant epidural pressure that could affect local perfusion. The epidural pressure generated can be transmitted cephalad through CSF and affect perfusion at more remote levels.[67] For these reasons it is essential that the procedure be performed on lightly sedated, well-informed, cooperative patients who can inform the provider of pain at remote areas. If such a complaint is articulated, the provider should consider adjusting the technique or terminating the procedure. An example is the spontaneous development of a headache or altered vision during endoscopy.

Complications of spinal canal endoscopy generally pertain to improper needle placement and generation of excessive epidural hydrostatic pressure.[67] Excessive pressure can potentially affect both local and distant perfusion. A new onset of scapular or neck pain during the procedure suggests elevated pressure and may portend retinal hemorrhage. Patient complaints of pain from small-volume distention of the epidural space usually signify a noncompliant epidural space and may permit transmission of pressure far from the site of fluid administration via CSF. Be very careful to keep the epidural fluid volume low and maintain contact with the patient throughout the procedure. Alert patients can inform the operator of sensations and changes inside their body as they occur. The operator uses clinical judgment during the procedure to determine whether an adjustment or termination of the procedure is necessary.

Potential complications include pain at and remote from the surgical site, transient dysesthesias, paresis, paralysis, blindness, other visual changes, post–dural puncture headache, local surgical site bleeding, infection, and allergic reactions.

Pain at the surgical site is generally self-limited. Pain at sites other than the surgical site, such as severe headache, dysesthesia, and extreme back pain, require evaluation and documentation in the medical record. Such pain may be caused by epidural hematoma, cord ischemia, or elevated hydrostatic pressure. Paresis, paralysis, and pain can be complications of needle trauma, epidural hematoma, elevated hydrostatic pressure, ischemia and nerve injury (avulsion and traction transection). Visual changes and blindness have been reported. The incidence is very low, and such complications have previously been reported with routine epidural injections. They presumably result from transmission of spinal canal pressure cephalad into the brain via CSF and cause retinal perfusion or macular hemorrhage. Local surgical site bleeding is unlikely to cause neurologic complications because the site is just above the coccyx. Bleeding may predispose to infection. However, infection is rare. A soapy scrub by the patient is suggested before the procedure, prophylactic antibiotics should be administered, sterile preparation and draping should be performed, the wound should be kept dry for 3 days, and after a bowel movement the anus should be wiped away from the surgical site posterior to anterior.

Conclusion

The technology of spinal canal endoscopy has developed slowly over the twentieth century. Contributions have been made by many innovators; however, only recently has this technique been developed and refined sufficiently to be used clinically. Further study is needed to determine whether this technique has advantages over alternative, currently used techniques of delivery of medication into the epidural space.

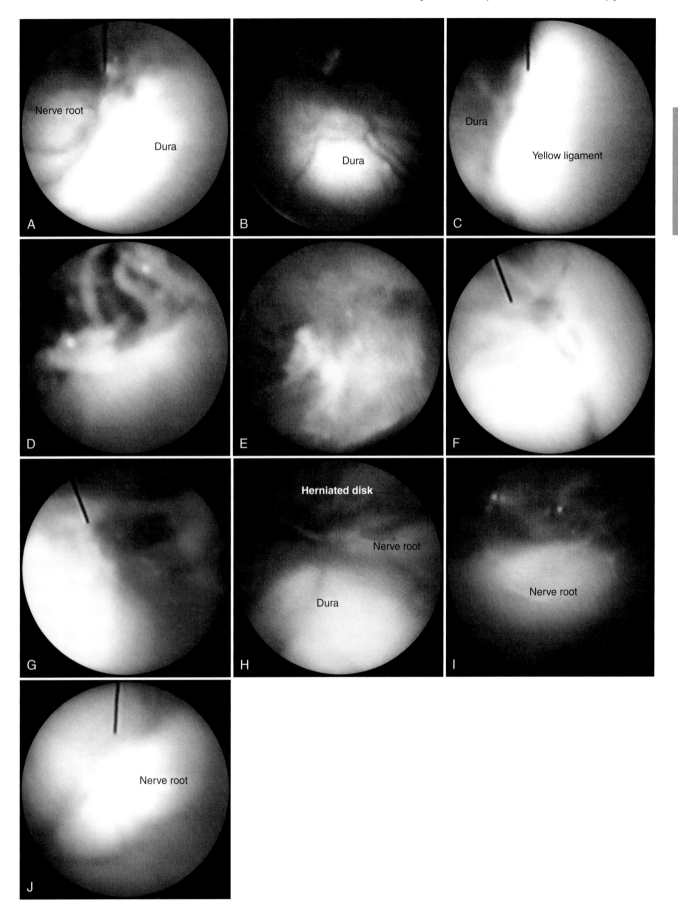

Fig. 19.3 Spinal endoscopy, findings. *(A-H, Reprinted courtesy of Igarashi T, Hirabayashi Y, Seo N: Epiduroscopic findings,* Pain Clinic *19:171–177, 2007; I-J, Reprinted courtesy of Igarashi T, Hirabayashi Y, Seo N, et al: Lysis of adhesions and epidural injection of steroid/local anaesthetic during epiduroscopy potentially alleviate low back and leg pain in elderly patients with lumbar spinal stenosis,* Br J Anaesth *93:181–187, 2004).*

Real-time direct visual examination of the epidural anatomy currently enables the identification of epidural pathology and localization of pain generators there. This ability to examine epidural pathology apart from operative trauma and to direct the delivery of medication is not duplicated by any other technique available at present. The future may hold the promise of minimally invasive and effective therapy for both radicular and perhaps other forms of disabling back pain. Other exciting possibilities for this technology may include removal of extradural or intradural scar tissue, cyst drainage, biopsy, study of cell biology and inflammatory mediators, and retrieval of foreign bodies. The authors believe that the possibility of modifying the inflammatory process by blocking mediators of inflammation holds the greatest promise. Today, the technique can be used safely and effectively to deliver medication to pathology under direct vision. It opens new doors for the diagnosis and treatment of pathology accessible through the epidural space.

References

Full references for this chapter can be found on www.expertconsult.com.

Electromyography and Nerve Conduction Velocity

Bernard M. Abrams

Electromyography (EMG) is usually performed by neurologists or physiatrists; it enters the realm of the anesthesiologist and pain specialist for several reasons: (1) it can be a valuable asset in localization of areas involved in peripheral pain problems; (2) it can provide evidence that the painful area or mechanism is a more central one by ruling out peripheral problems; and (3) it may provide documentation as to cause, location, timing, and prognosis for nerve injuries that occur in the anesthetic and perianesthetic time frame. In addition, EMG is a procedure performed on physician referral; a working knowledge of how it is performed, of the indications, and of reasonable expectations for information derived from the results helps the nonelectromyographer to order appropriate testing, advise the patient about the testing, and better assess the adequacy of the testing and the physician performing the test.

EMG is a useful extension of the clinical neurologic examination and, therefore, is an adjunct in the diagnosis and management of pain. Conditions in which EMG may be of use include painful peripheral neuropathies, entrapment neuropathies, traumatic nerve injuries, radicular and multiradicular problems,

lumbar or cervical spinal stenosis, arachnoiditis, and painful myopathies. The problems inherent in applying electrodiagnostic techniques to pain diagnosis and management are similar to those encountered in history taking, physical examination, radiologic and other imaging procedures, and therapeutic diagnostic testing. Pain is a subjective experience, and the final diagnosis of the etiology and presumptive treatment of a pain syndrome is a clinical diagnosis that can only be supported with relevant data, including EMG. No "litmus test" exists to objectify symptoms of pain, and the final diagnosis of a pain syndrome is a clinical one that can be supported only by relevant data, such as EMG. In this regard, EMG is no different from radiology, other forms of imaging, or laboratory tests.

History

The existence of electrical activity resulting from muscular contractions was first described by Galvani.[1] The first experimental work with EMG was performed by Lord Adrian in 1925. In 1928, Proebster first described the presence of "spontaneous irregular action potentials in denervated muscle."[1] In its progression to clinical application, EMG made a major step forward with the use of the cathode ray oscilloscope by Erlanger and Gasser, and the concentric needle electrode and loud speaker.[2] Vast numbers of nerve injuries in World War II and later conflicts added impetus to the study of nerve and muscle with electrodiagnostic techniques.

A few definitions are in order before proceeding. The term *electromyography* previously caused considerable confusion because, strictly speaking, it referred to the evaluation of muscle function (and indirectly nerve, nerve root, and anterior horn cell) via needle insertion into the muscle. In time, the term became a more inclusive one, embracing nerve conduction velocity testing and other less frequently performed tests, such as the H⁻ and F⁻ reflexes, cranial nerve reflexes, and studies of the neuromuscular junction. The all-inclusive term *EMG* is used here to include these tests. *Electrodiagnosis* originally referred to muscle testing in the form of chronaxie and threshold determinations but now embraces all electrical testing of the nervous system and includes evoked potentials. The national organization was originally called the American Association of Electromyography and Electrodiagnosis (AAEE) and is now known as the American Association of Neuromuscular and Electrodiagnostic Medicine (AANEM), which reflects the modernization of terminology and the vast expansion of the scope of electrodiagnostic testing.

EMG is a method of testing both the physiologic state and the anatomic integrity of lower motor neuron structures, their sensory components, and some spinal and brainstem reflex pathways.[3] The lower motor neuron is composed of the anterior horn cells, nerve root, plexus, peripheral nerves, neuromuscular junction, and muscles. Longmire[4] pointed out the puzzling dichotomy in the medical literature on pain and electrodiagnostic testing. In standard textbooks on electrodiagnostic testing,[5–9] little mention is found of painful syndromes. On the other hand, perusal of standard pain textbooks[1,10,11] reveals cogent attempts to correlate neurophysiologic studies in pain diagnosis and management. The reason for the paucity of references in standard textbooks appears to be, at least in part, the attitudes of some pain specialists themselves who point out "nevertheless, it should be emphasized that large caliber afferent fibers are physiologically unrelated to pain, a submodality mediated by small caliber fibers. Additionally, the test is unable to explore the bases for positive sensory phenomenon, generated by dysfunction of large caliber afferent channels."[12]

EMG and nerve conduction are extremely useful investigative techniques in evaluating the patient in pain because they satisfy two fundamental steps[12] in the assessment of a neuropathic pain syndrome before any attempt at therapy. First, they rigorously establish the presence or absence of a peripheral nervous system lesion, and second, they determine the relevance of an established peripheral lesion to the subjective clinical symptom. In brief, electrodiagnostic techniques may occasionally be helpful in diagnosing central nervous system disorders[10] but are more often useful in disorders of the nerve roots, plexus lesions, neuropathies, and disorders of the peripheral nerves, and less frequently in painful myopathies. Neuromuscular junction disorders, amyotrophic lateral sclerosis, and other anterior horn cell disorders (except poliomyelitis in its acute stage) rarely produce pain. After the discussion of test procedures and their interpretation, a full discussion of the clinical correlates of electrodiagnostic testing is made.

The Electrodiagnostic Method

The four essential components of any electrodiagnostic measurement system are: (1) electrodes; (2) a stimulator; (3) a high-gain differential amplifier; and (4) a recording display or central processing device.[4] Computer-assisted analysis systems may be added.

The EMG apparatus amplifies and displays biological information derived from either surface or needle electrodes. Electrical information may be recorded from muscles, nerves, or other nervous system structures and is generally displayed on an oscilloscope. In addition to the visual display, a permanent recording may be made; audio amplification may allow it to be heard over a loud speaker, and analog or digital signals may also be used. Electrical nerve stimulation is used to simulate nerves to measure nerve conduction and latencies of the evoked responses. Modern EMG equipment ranges from simple to complex with even "notebook"-type devices coupled with electrodes and stimulators for maximum portability. A representative EMG machine is shown in **Figure 20.1**.

For nerve conduction studies, surface skin electrodes (**Fig. 20.2**) are used to record a compound muscle or nerve action potential; in needle electromyography, needle electrodes are used with a strong trend toward disposable needles (**Fig. 20.3**). For sensory testing, ring electrodes are used for measurement (**Fig. 20.4**). Modern EMG equipment is manufactured by numerous companies and is generally standardized to allow reliable and reproducible testing by different laboratories,[10] but normative data should be established by each individual laboratory.[8,13,14] Extra precautions

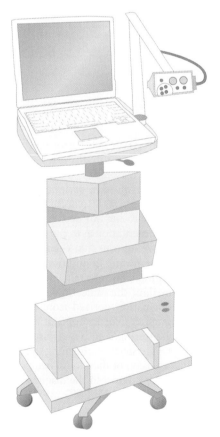

Fig. 20.1 **A typical electromyography machine.**

must be taken with patients on warfarin or other antico-agulant therapy, patients with hemophilia or other blood dyscrasias, patients who are HIV positive, and patients with a cardiac pacemaker, neuromodulatory implant, or transcutaneous stimulator.[3] Beyond placement of a needle through an infected site, there are probably no absolute, but only relative contraindications for EMG. Extremely anxious adults and some children occasionally need seda-tion. Aftereffects of EMG are negligible, with rare bruising, although occasionally a highly suggestible or litigious patient may complain vehemently of increased pain or disability. Conversely, occasionally a patient may proclaim extravagant therapeutic effects from electromyography.

Physiologic Mechanisms

Production of Muscle Potentials

When an impulse arrives at the region of the junction between nerve and muscle, the muscle fiber is thrown into an almost simultaneous contraction, assuming that the threshold for activation is exceeded. This is brought about by a wave of exci-tation that moves rapidly along the fiber surface and stimulates

the contractile substance as it moves (excitation-contraction coupling). The stimulus is transmitted along the fiber by an excitable membrane that surrounds the muscle fiber. The action potential results from the breakdown of the surface membrane potential, which is associated with critical changes in ionic permeability. In the resting muscle fiber, the poten-tial difference across the surface membrane is 90 mV, with a negative charge on the inside surface. During excitation, the resting potential temporarily reverses to a potential of approx-imately 40-mV negativity on the outside surface. This action potential travels along the muscle fiber at velocities from 3.5 to 5 m/sec in different fibers. Conduction along the fine intra-muscular branches of the anterior horn cell occurs so rapidly that all the muscle fibers in a motor unit are activated almost simultaneously.[15]

In extracellular recording, as in EMG, the electrode picks up the action potential as it is conducted by volume conduc-tion through the medium surrounding the active fiber. The impedance of the external medium is small compared with the impedance of the interior of the fiber; therefore, the volt-age of the extracellularly recorded potential is maximally only 2% to 10% of the intracellularly recorded potential. The functional unit for reflex or voluntary motor activity is the motor unit. The motor unit (**Fig. 20.5A**) is the group of muscle fibers innervated by a single anterior horn cell. The number of fibers per motor unit varies considerably from muscle to muscle. Generally, the finer the control exerted by a muscle, the fewer fibers per motor unit. Eye muscles may have as few as 5 to 7 muscle fibers per motor unit, whereas the gastrocnemius may have as many as 3500 muscle fibers per motor unit. Antigravity muscles, such as the back extensors or gastrocnemius, have much larger numbers of fibers per motor unit because they require less fine control and greater endur-ance. The motor units in various muscles cover different areas of muscle cross section (e.g, 55 mm in the biceps brachii and

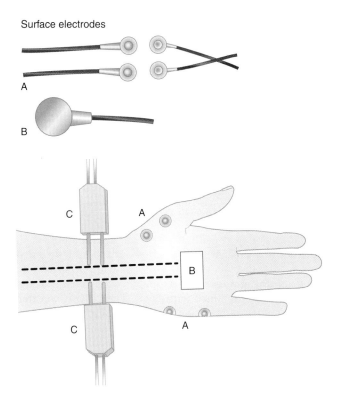

Fig. 20.2 **Typical setup for nerve conduction studies with repre-sentative surface electrodes and stimulating electrodes.** A, Surface electrodes. B, Ground electrodes. C, Stimulating electrodes.

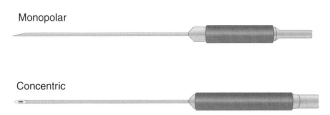

Fig. 20.3 **Needle electrodes for electromyography.**

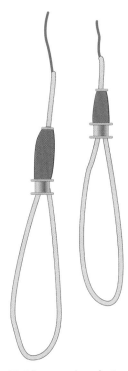

Fig. 20.4 **Sensory ring electrodes.**

8 to 9 mm in the rectus femoris, anterior tibial, and opponens pollicis muscles). The distribution of fibers is such that fibers from several different motor units are intermingled (see **Fig. 20.5B**), which is why four to six motor units can be identified with EMG from the same intramuscular recording point. In normal muscle, single motor unit potentials can be differentiated only during weak, voluntary contraction.[13,16] The potentials from different motor units are recognized by their frequency of discharge, amplitude, and morphology, which vary for each motor unit (some being more or less excitable). The different potentials often differ in appearance because of the differential distance of the recording electrode from the individual fibers of the activated motor units and the differential distribution of the motor end plates in the

several units within "range" of a concentric or single needle electrode in one position in the muscle. An upward deflection on the oscilloscope is considered electrically negative, whereas a downward deflection is considered electrically positive. In the immediate vicinity of a potential, there is an upward or negative deflection.

Nerve Conduction

The cell membrane (axolemma) of a nerve axon separates the intracellular axoplasm from the extracellular fluid.[8] The unequal distribution of ions between these fluids produces a potential difference across the cell membrane, with a resting potential of about 70 mV, negative inside with respect to the outside of the cell membrane. When a nerve fiber is stimulated, it causes a change in the membrane potential, and a rapid but brief flow of sodium ions occurs through ionic channels inward across the cell membrane, giving rise to an action potential. The way an action potential is conducted along an axon depends on whether the axon is myelinated or unmyelinated.[17] In a myelinated fiber, the action potential is regenerated only at the nodes of Ranvier, so that the resulting action potentials "jump" from node to node (salutatory conduction). The velocity of nerve conduction depends on the diameter of a myelinated fiber. Small myelinated fibers may conduct as slowly as 12 m/sec, whereas large motor and sensory fibers conduct at a rate of 50 to 70 m/sec in humans. In an unmyelinated fiber in a human, the conduction rate is about 2 m/sec.

Several factors influence nerve conduction velocity, other than whether or not the axon is myelinated. Among these factors are the temperature of the limb,[18] the age of the patient (with infants having slowed conduction velocities and older adults having increasingly slowed conduction with age), and the height of an individual, which may increase the internodal distances of the nodes of Ranvier.[8]

The Basic Examination

must be combined with the clinical examination of the patient by the electromyographer and should include a grading of muscle strength. Of prime importance is for the electromyographer to personally correlate clinical data with those data obtained with EMG. The EMG is an extension of the neurologic examination, and each examination must be planned individually. No "cookbook formula" can be followed. Because EMG is an extension of the clinical examination, the patient must be evaluated fully, and the problem tentatively assigned to the portion of the affected anterior horn cell unit. The electromyographer determines the segment or segments of the peripheral nervous system suspected to be involved, and the examination is planned to either substantiate or invalidate the presumptive clinical diagnosis.

Conducting the Examination

The needle examination is designed to determine: (1) the integrity of muscle and its nerve supply; (2) the location of any abnormality, and (3) any abnormalities in the muscle itself. The electrodes may be monopolar or concentric (see **Fig. 20.3**). The examination proceeds through the following steps: (1) determination of

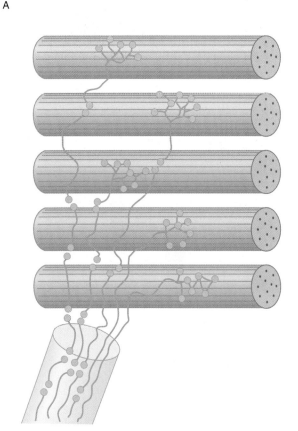

Motor Unit

A

B

Fig. 20.5 **A,** Anatomy of the motor unit. **B,** Intermingling of fibers.

the activity of the muscle in a relaxed state[9,13]; (2) evaluation of any insertional activity that arises; (3) assessment of the activity seen on weak voluntary effort; (4) recruitment (i.e., the more or less orderly addition of motor units as effort increases); and (5) determination of the pattern seen on maximal voluntary effort (known as the *interference pattern,* a term that derives its name from interference with the discernment of the initial muscle action potentials from the resting baseline).

Needle Electrode Findings in Normal Muscle

Insertional Activity

When a needle is inserted into a normal muscle, it evokes a brief burst of electrical activity that lasts no more than 2 to 3 sec, a little longer than the actual movement of the needle.[10] This activity is described as insertional activity and is generally 50 to 250 mV in amplitude (**Fig. 20.6A**). These insertional potentials are believed to represent discharges from muscle fibers produced by injury, mechanical stimulation, or irritation of the muscle fibers.

Spontaneous Activity (at Rest)

When the needle is stationary and the muscle is relaxed, no electrical activity should be present in normal muscle, except when the needle is in the area of the motor end plate (see **Fig. 20.6B**). Two types of end plate "noise" are normal: (1) low amplitude and undulating (see **Fig. 20.6C**), which probably represents extracellular miniature end plate potentials (MEPP); and (2) higher amplitude intermittent spike discharges, which probably represent discharges of a single muscle fiber excited by intramuscular nerve terminals irritated by the needle. Any other spontaneous activity at rest is abnormal. An increase in duration of insertional activity may be seen in loss of innervation or primary muscle fiber disease.[10]

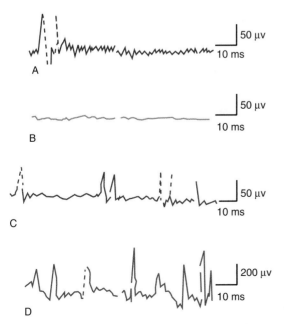

Fig. 20.6 **Potentials recorded from muscle.** A, Needle insertion. B, Resting muscle. C, End plate potentials. D, Voluntary contraction.

Reduction may occur in myopathies or in more advanced degeneration, in which muscle tissue has been replaced by fat or fibrous connective tissue.[19]

Voluntary Activity

Voluntary activity of the muscle is analyzed after the muscle is studied at rest. The motor unit action potential is analyzed. As previously mentioned in the discussion of physiology, the term *motor unit* refers to the number of muscle fibers supplied by one motor neuron and its axon. This unit varies from muscle to muscle and may be as few as 5 to 10 fibers to more than 1000 muscle fibers. When a motor neuron discharges, it activates all the muscle fibers in the motor unit. The force of contraction determines the number of motor units brought into play.[14,16] This begins with a single motor unit (see **Fig. 20.6D**) that fires and can be identified on the screen by its distinctive morphology. As the effort is increased, other motor units come into play, which still can be individually discerned and have their own individual morphology and audio representation on the loud speaker. As the contraction increases, the firing rate of each individual motor unit action potential increases and is subsequently joined by other motor unit action potentials whose firing rates also increase. In many ways, this action resembles an orchestra with different instruments being "recruited" to join in the musical number. This phenomenon is known as the *principle of orderly recruitment* (**Fig. 20.7**). In normal muscle, the strength of a voluntary muscle contraction is directly related to the number of individual motor units that have been recruited and their firing rate.[16,20] Analysis of motor units includes waveform, amplitude, and interference patterns.

Waveform

Most units are biphasic or triphasic. The number of phases is determined by the number of baseline crossings of the wave. Motor units that cross the baseline more than five times are termed *polyphasic.* Although occasionally seen in healthy muscles, they do not exceed 15% of the total number of motor units. In some muscles, polyphasic motor units are more prevalent. Polyphasic potentials are a measure of fiber synchrony.

Amplitude

The amplitude of a motor unit depends on the number of fibers in the motor unit and the type of EMG needle used. Monopolar needles are associated with larger amplitude normal values than bipolar or coaxial needles. Normal amplitude ranges from 1 to 5 mV. Because the motor units are the sum of the action potentials of each muscle fiber of the unit, a larger motor unit has a larger amplitude, and a smaller motor unit has a smaller amplitude.

Interference Pattern

With maximum voluntary effort, a large number of motor units are brought into play and their firing rate increases. They tend to "interfere with each other," and thus, they cannot be recognized further as individual motor units (see **Fig. 20.7**), which gives rise to the interference pattern. In a normal muscle, a "full" interference pattern is seen.

Various abnormalities may occur that indicate the presence of total denervation: neurogenic paresis, peripheral type; or neurogenic paresis, anterior horn cell type. In addition, myogenic paresis may be detected.

Generally, on the basis of abnormal findings with a well-planned examination, the presence of a radiculopathy, generalized neuropathy, or focal mononeuropathy or plexopathy can be determined. The following are needle abnormalities in abnormal muscles: (1) insertional activity (increased or decreased); (2) spontaneous activity (fibrillations, positive sharp waves, or fasciculations; **Fig. 20.8**); (3) abnormalities of voluntary motor unit activity, especially recruitment (**Fig. 20.9**); and (4) abnormal motor unit morphology (e.g., excessive or extreme polyphasia).

Nerve Conduction Studies

Nerve conduction studies are of value in determination of whether a disease of nerve is present and in determination of the distribution of a neuropathy (e.g., mononeuritis, polyneuropathy,

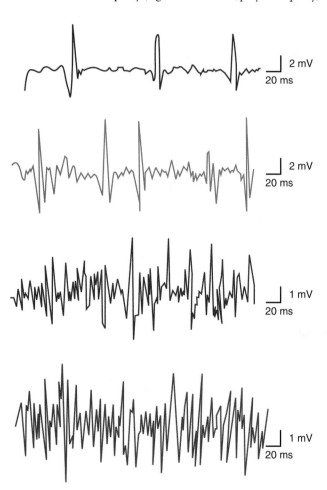

Fig. 20.7 **Increasing levels of firing associated with increased muscular force.**

or mononeuritis multiplex). These studies may provide valuable information in the differential diagnosis of the etiology of a neuropathy, determining the point in a nerve where there is conduction block, locating an entrapment site, and studying the progress of a disease of a peripheral nerve (e.g., whether the condition is improving or staying the same; whether there is reinnervation of a previously sectioned nerve; whether conduction along the nerve is adequate or normal, which is important in diseases of the neuromuscular junction such as myasthenia gravis or the myasthenic syndrome).

Motor nerve conduction velocity studies may be carried out with the insertion of a needle electrode in a muscle innervated by the nerve under study or with the use of surface electrode over that muscle (**Fig. 20.10**). For example, the first dorsal interosseus muscle may be examined to determine the function of the ulnar nerve (**Fig. 20.11**). The nerve is stimulated (in the case of the ulnar nerve, at the elbow), and the latency (length of time for an impulse to arrive and make a "spike" on the oscilloscope screen) of the response is determined. The response is generally a spike-like large motor unit action potential. The ulnar nerve is then stimulated at the wrist or axillary region. The difference in latencies between the two points of stimulation and the distance between the two points of stimulation provide the basis for the calculation of the conduction velocity. The conduction velocity is measured by the formula:

$$ncv \text{ (m/sec)} = dmm \div pml \text{ (msec)} - dml \text{ (msec)}$$

where *dmm* is the distance between the two stimulus points in millimeters; *pml* and *dml* are the proximal and distal motor latencies, respectively, in milliseconds; and *ncv* is the nerve conduction velocity in meters/second.[3]

Textbooks of stimulation points and pick-up points are readily available.[7,8] Normal values are usually established for each nerve in individual laboratories, whereas normal valuest for commonly tested sensory and motor nerves are generally available. Median nerve stimulation is comparable with ulnar nerve stimulation (**Fig. 20.12**).

The F Wave
Definition of the F Wave

Motor conduction velocity along the whole axon, including proximal portions, can be studied by eliciting the F-wave response, a small late muscle response that occurs from backfiring of anterior horn cells.[21–23] F waves may be obtained from almost any mixed nerve that can be stimulated, but the median, ulnar, peroneal, and posterior tibial nerves are the most commonly used. If the standard distal motor conduction velocities are normal but the F-wave value is prolonged, then slowing must be occurring somewhere more proximal to the distal normal segment. The method used to determine F-wave

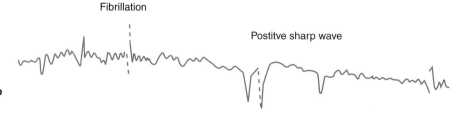

Fig. 20.8 **Fibrillations and positive sharp waves (denervation potentials).**

Normal

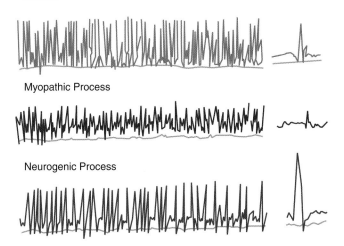

Myopathic Process

Neurogenic Process

Fig. 20.9 **Patterns of abnormal motor unit recruitment.**

latency varies from laboratory to laboratory; the F-wave value with each successive stimulus shows variability of several milliseconds, with some examiners averaging 10, 30, or 50 responses, and some taking the shortest of 10 or 20 responses. Limb temperature and arm or leg length may influence the results. Comparison with the opposite limb may be helpful if that limb is asymptomatic.

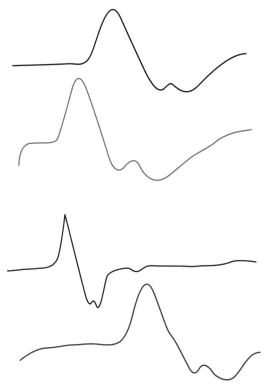

Fig. 20.11 **Responses from the abductor digiti minimi from stimulation at various sites of the ulnar nerve.** A, Below elbow. B, Wrist. C, Axilla. D, Above elbow.

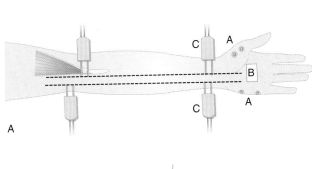

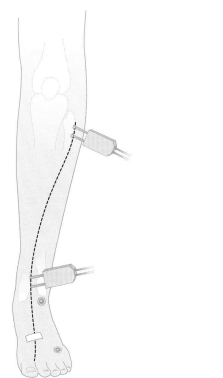

Fig. 20.10 A, Setup for typical upper extremity nerve conduction study. B, Setup for typical lower extremity nerve conduction study.

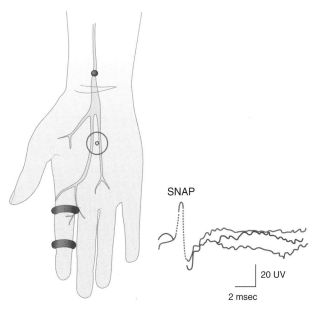

Fig. 20.12 **Typical setup for median nerve stimulation.** *Inset*: Evoked sensory nerve action potential from median nerve stimulation at the wrist.

Complications and Pitfalls

In addition to variability in F waves and how they are obtained in different laboratories, many electromyographers overuse (or at least overperform) the F-wave study in cases in which proximal slowing in a nerve or nerve root is not even in the differential diagnosis. The most accepted use of the study is in suspected early Guillain-Barré syndrome when usual distal nerve conduction studies are still normal, usually in the first 10 days of the illness. Use of F waves is highly controversial in the workup of radiculopathies.[24,25]

H-Reflex

Definition of the H-Reflex

The H-reflex, or Hoffmann reflex, is obtained with electrode stimulation of the posterior tibial nerve in the popliteal space—at a slow rate with long duration—with submaximal electrical shock and recorded with surface electrodes over the gastrocnemius-soleus complex. The impulse travels up the sensory fibers to the spinal cord, synapses with the alpha motor neuron, and returns down the motor fibers to the calf muscle. H-reflex latencies are long, in the 40-msec to 45-msec range. They are mostly carried out in the S1 root distribution and cannot be recorded consistently from other muscles. For determination of a delay or an asymmetry, the opposite leg should always be studied for comparison.[26-29]

The H-reflex is somewhat more useful than the F wave, but the main reason for this study is in the workup of a suspected S1 radiculopathy, in which the history or physical examination results are suggestive but the EMG results are normal.[30] In most cases, when an absent H-reflex is found, which suggests a problem with S1 conduction, an absent or depressed ankle reflex has already been seen in the physical examination, so the study is, for many, redundant.

Pitfalls occur when the opposite leg is not studied to show a normal H-reflex as a contrast. If the H-reflex is bilaterally absent, it may reflect a generalized disease (e.g., peripheral neuropathy). Older patients do not have good H-reflexes as a rule; this finding may be normal. In addition, a unilaterally absent H-reflex with normal needle EMG examination results does not indicate when the injury occurred. It could be the result of a previous remote injury.

Quantitative Sensory Testing

Quantitative Sudomotor Axon Reflex Test

Quantitative sensory testing takes various forms, including the quantitative somatosensory thermotest, with a controlled ramp of ascending or descending temperature through a Peltier device.[31] Measurement of threshold for cold sensation reflects function of small-caliber A-delta myelinated afferents. Threshold for warm sensation reflects function of warm-specific small unmyelinated afferent channels. Cold pain and heat pain thresholds test the function of unmyelinated C-fiber polymodal nociceptors and, to a lesser extent, A-delta fiber nociceptors. Certain abnormal patterns are characteristic of dysfunction of small-caliber peripheral afferents.[32] To obtain maximum information from a quantitative somatosensory thermotest, testing of both hot and cold sensations is necessary.[33] Quantitative sensory testing performed at different sites along an extremity in cases of polyneuropathy yields useful information about progression of the pathologic process along the extremity, provides an estimate of the progression of the disease, and serves as a baseline for evaluation of treatment and further progression or improvement of the disease.

Quantitative sudomotor axon reflex test (Q-SART) is a quantitative thermoregulatory sweat test that has been used to detect postganglionic sudomotor failure in neuropathies[34,35] and preganglionic neuropathies with presumed transsynaptic degeneration.[36] In patients with distal small fiber neuropathy, it is the most sensitive diagnostic test.[37] Various commercial devices have been used in an attempt to differentiate axonal and demyelinating polyneuropathies.[38]

Clinical Correlations

Clinical correlations can be based on careful history, clinical examination, and electrodiagnostic studies. Electrodiagnostic studies are best for separating neuropathy from myopathy and determining whether a neuropathy is generalized mixed or focal, axonal or demyelinating, thereby giving important clues as to etiology. Nerve trauma can be followed serially to determine recovery. With careful attention to anatomic detail, the diagnosis of radiculopathy or plexopathy can often be made.

Nerve Trauma

After injury, such as a laceration, the nerve is often completely severed. At rest, denervation potentials are recorded in the muscles supplied by that nerve in the form of positive sharp waves or fibrillation potentials, and on electromyography, no motor unit action potentials are seen. However, sometimes an injury is incomplete and the type of nerve lesion and its extent are uncertain.

Neurapraxia is the mildest form of nerve injury and consists of conduction loss without associated axonal structural changes. This form of conduction block often occurs with compressive or ischemic nerve injuries, such as mild entrapment neuropathy or compression (e.g., radial nerve palsy or "Saturday night palsy"). In neurapraxic injuries, focal demyelination occurs. Serial nerve conduction determinations along the course of the nerve enable one to locate the site of the conduction block. The prognosis for complete recovery is generally good, and healing occurs within days or weeks, barring further injury.

In axonotmesis, disruption of the axon in its myelin sheath occurs, for a more severe form of nerve injury. The neural tube, which consists of the endoperineurium and the epineurium, remains intact. The nerve undergoes wallerian degeneration with fragmentation of the axon distal to the site of injury. Motor and sensory loss occur with associated atrophy of supplied muscles and loss of reflexes. After about 4 to 5 days, the distal segments of the nerve become inexcitable. In 1 to 2 weeks, positive sharp waves are seen in the EMG on needle examination. In 2 to 3 weeks, fibrillation potentials are seen in the involved muscle segments. The intact neural tube forms "lattice" for the regenerating axon, and the prognosis for recovery is generally good, but not as favorable as in neurapraxia.

Neurotmesis is the most severe form of nerve injury and consists of severe disruption or transection of the nerve. Nerve regeneration and recovery are often incomplete or nonexistent and may necessitate surgical reanastomosis to attempt recovery of nerve integrity. Neuromas may form and are commonly associated with pain. Only serial EMG and nerve conduction studies over time can determine the difference between axonotmesis and neurotmesis in some cases, and in almost all cases, electrical signs of recovery precede clinical ones.

Nontraumatic Neuropathies

In nontraumatic neuropathies, segmental demyelination is generally associated with slowing of nerve conduction velocities and temporal dispersion of evoked responses. With axonal degeneration, however, reduction of the evoked response amplitudes with mild terminal slowing of nerve conduction velocities is typical. An EMG provides early information regarding reinnervation before clinical recovery is evident. The earliest positive evidence of reinnervation is the appearance during voluntary effort of motor units that are of low amplitude in the beginning but are highly polyphasic ("nascent units"). They may be present several weeks before clinical evidence of functional recovery.

Polyneuropathy

EMG and nerve conduction determinations are useful in diagnosis of polyneuropathy and in determination of whether a pathologic process is axonal, or demyelinating, or mixed. A diagnosis of polyneuropathy is made when abnormal nerve conduction and EMG findings are bilateral and relatively symmetrical. Generalized peripheral neuropathies often associated with pain are noted in **Table 20.1**.[39-44]

Electrodiagnostic findings characteristic of axonal neuropathy are:

- Abnormally low or absent sensory nerve action potential amplitude
- Abnormally low or absent compound muscle action potential amplitude

Table 20.1 Generalized Peripheral Neuropathies

Diabetes mellitus
Polyneuropathy associated with insulinoma
Polyneuropathy associated with nutritional deficiency
Alcohol–nutritional deficiency polyneuropathy
Vasculitis-associated neuropathy
Amyloidosis neuropathy
Toxic neuropathy (e.g., arsenic and thallium)
HIV-related distal symmetrical polyneuropathy
Fabry's disease
Guillain-Barré syndrome (acute inflammatory demyelinating polyneuropathy)
Chronic inflammatory demyelinating polyneuropathy
Cryptogenic sensory, or (much less commonly) sensorimotor, polyneuropathy
Polyneuropathy as a result of neoplasms, including those that are paraneoplastic

HIV, human immunodeficiency virus.

- Normal distal latencies for sensory and motor potentials
- Normal or near normal sensory and motor conduction velocities

If a disease process affects the large-diameter axons, some slowing of conduction velocity occurs; the velocity is seldom reduced by more than 20% to 30% of normal value. However, fibrillations and positive sharp waves are present in muscles innervated by affected nerves and are generally worse distally. The feet muscles are more involved than the hand muscles, and the leg muscles are more involved than the arm muscles. Motor unit potentials are decreased in number with deficient recruitment and an incomplete interference pattern. Some motor units are of increased amplitude and duration.

In contrast, diffuse demyelinating neuropathy is characterized by reduction of conduction velocities, usually more than 40% of the normal range. Distal latencies are also prolonged. The sensory nerve action potentials and compound muscle action potentials usually have low amplitudes and temporal dispersion. A needle EMG shows no fibrillations or positive sharp waves unless secondary axonal degeneration is present. In a pure demyelinating neuropathy, no denervation of muscle fibers occurs. Motor units are decreased in number. Decreased recruitment is attributable to conduction block in some fibers. Usually no significant change is seen in the duration, amplitude, or morphology of motor units, but the number of polyphasic units may be increased if demyelination of terminal axons is present.

Once electromyographic determination is made of whether or not a neuropathy is primarily axonal or demyelinating, one can then consider clinically which neuropathies are diffusely axonal and which are demyelinating. Subacute and chronic diffuse axonal types include most toxic and nutritional neuropathies as from uremia, diabetes, hypothyroidism, HIV disease, paraneoplastic disease, dysproteinemias, and amyloidosis. Patients with diabetes usually begin with slow conduction velocities, in the 32-m/sec to 38-m/sec range in the lower extremities. Fibrillations and positive waves in the intrinsic foot muscles are a later finding.

Demyelinating polyneuropathies include hereditary motor and sensory neuropathies types 1 and 3, Refsum's disease, multifocal leukodystrophy, and Krabbe's disease. Acute nonuniform demyelinating diseases include Guillain-Barré syndrome, diphtheria, and acute arsenic intoxication, whereas chronic demyelinating diseases include chronic inflammatory demyelinating polyneuropathy (CIDP), idiopathic disease, and neuropathies that accompany HIV disease, and various paraproteinemias, dysproteinemias, and osteosclerotic myeloma.[45]

Mononeuropathies, Compression Neuropathies, and Entrapment Neuropathies

A mononeuropathy is obviously one that affects only a single nerve. Its clinical implications generally are different from a polyneuropathy, and a far higher percentage of affected patients have traumatic or microtraumatic etiologies. Subtypes include compression neuropathy, in which acute or chronic compression of a nerve results in varying degrees of nerve impairment, and entrapment neuropathy, in which a nerve is subjected to an anatomic situation with either inadequate space for transit of the nerve or an unyielding anatomic structure that compresses the nerve.

In entrapment neuropathies and compression neuropathies, the most commonly involved nerves are the median, ulnar, radial, common peroneal, and tibial. Entities such as trauma, vasculitis, diabetes mellitus, leprosy, and sarcoidosis can affect any nerve in the body. Electrophysiologic studies are of great assistance in localizing the pathologic process to the individual nerve and in differentiating mononeuropathy from diffuse polyneuropathy, plexopathy, or radiculopathy.

Median Nerve

The median nerve is most commonly entrapped at the wrist as it passes through the carpal tunnel but may also be injured at the elbow where it passes between the two heads of the pronator teres or, less frequently, is compressed by a dense band of connective tissue (the ligament of Struthers immediately above the elbow).[46,47]

The median nerve is derived from C6 through T1 nerve roots (lateral and medial cords of the brachial plexus). The diagnosis of carpal tunnel syndrome is made with demonstration of localized slowing of sensory and motor conductions across the wrist as evidenced by prolonged sensory and motor distal latencies.[1] In addition, with advanced changes, denervation may be found in the form of fibrillations, positive sharp waves, and reduced motor units with polyphasia in median nerve–innervated hand muscles.

Pronator Teres and Anterior Interosseous Syndromes

The pronator teres and anterior interosseous syndromes are proximal compression or entrapment neuropathies of the median nerve. The pronator teres syndrome may show normal distal latency of sensory and motor determinations at the wrist and no evidence of denervation in median nerve–innervated hand and forearm muscles except for the pronator teres.[47] The anterior interosseous nerve is a motor nerve that is a branch of the median nerve with its origin just distal to the pronator teres.[47] Denervation may be seen in the flexors of the thumb and index finger.

Ulnar Nerve

The ulnar nerve is derived from the C8 and T1cervical and thoracic nerve roots (medial cord of the brachial plexus) and is usually compressed, entrapped, or injured at the elbow but occasionally at the wrist in the canal of Guyon or deep in the palm ("silver beater's palsy"). EMG studies help to differentiate C8-T1 radiculopathy from plexopathy or more distal ulnar neuropathy.[48,49]

When the lesion is at the wrist at the canal of Guyon, usually both motor and sensory fibers are involved and the amplitude of the sensory and motor action potentials is reduced. Distal sensory and motor latencies across the wrist are prolonged, and no focal slowing of motor conduction velocity or decrement of the compound motor action potential across the elbow is found. With a deep palmar branch lesion, no sensory abnormality is seen, and all of the changes are in a motor distribution distal to the lesion.[50] When the lesion is at the elbow, slowing of nerve conduction across the elbow may be found, often as reduced as 25% to 40% below normal value. Normal values depend on the method of determination (i.e., arm straight versus arm bent). The sensory potential at the wrist may be delayed or absent, and EMG may show denervation in intrinsic hand muscles and in the flexor carpi ulnaris, a muscle innervated just below the elbow by the ulnar nerve in some cases.

Radial Nerve

The radial nerve is a continuation of the posterior cord of the brachial plexus and receives fibers from the C5 through C8 cervical nerve roots. It is usually involved at the spiral groove of the humerus, often as the result of a humeral fracture. With a lesion at the spiral groove, the triceps muscle is often spared on EMG, but all of the extensor muscles in the forearm are involved. An isolated superficial radial nerve lesion sometimes occurs at the wrist ("handcuff neuropathy"), with the only electrophysiologic abnormality a diminution or absence of the radial sensory potential elicited over the radial aspect of the wrist.

Posterior Interosseous Syndrome

The posterior interosseous syndrome (sometimes referred to as complicated or resistant lateral epicondylitis or tennis elbow) occurs from entrapment of the radial nerve branch in the region of the elbow at the arcade of Fröhse between the two heads of the supinator muscle. The EMG shows involvement of the extensor carpi ulnaris, extensor digitorum longus, extensor pollicis longus, and extensor indicis with sparing of the more proximal supinator and extensor carpi radialis and brevis.[51] Sensation is unaffected.

Common Peroneal Nerve

The common peroneal nerve is derived from L4 through S1 lumbar and sacral nerve roots but is usually primarily from the L5 lumbar nerve root. It may be compressed at the head of the fibula. Peroneal nerve conduction studies show reduced compound motor action potentials as recorded from the extensor digitorum brevis at the ankle with stimulation above the fibular head and normal below the fibular head and at the ankle.

Posterior Tibial Nerve at the Ankle

The posterior tibial nerve is derived from the L4 through S2 lumbar and sacral nerve roots and may be compressed in the tarsal tunnel. Nerve conduction studies show prolongation of the distal motor and sensory latencies of the tibial nerve.[52–54] This syndrome is relatively uncommon.

Sciatic Nerve

The sciatic nerve arises from the L4, L5, S1, S2, and S3 lumbar and sacral nerve roots. A controversial syndrome is entrapment by the piriformis muscle as it passes through the sciatic notch. A lesion of the sciatic nerve is defined and localized with detailed needle examination of muscles in the lower extremity.

Other Uncommon Neuropathies

The numerous potential mononeuropathies include those that involve the long thoracic nerve; the dorsal scapular, suprascapular, and musculocutaneous nerves; and the axillary nerves in the shoulder girdle and upper extremity. In the pelvic girdle, the femoral, obturator, saphenous, and lateral femoral cutaneous nerves, and the genitofemoral, ilioinguinal, superior gluteal, and inferior gluteal nerves, are potentially involved.

Needle EMG reveals denervation changes in muscles supplied by the affected nerves. Cutaneous nerve conduction may reveal abnormalities in pure sensory neuropathies, such as the lateral femoral cutaneous nerve (meralgia paresthetica), and careful EMG differentiates it from a high (L1, L2) radiculopathy. Nerve conduction studies are rarely of assistance in the other conditions delineated previously.[55]

Radiculopathies

Radiculopathies are diseases of the nerve roots and must be differentiated from plexopathies and from complex individual nerve root and nerve lesions. Roots are commonly involved by compression, especially in the cervical and lumbar regions, but may also be involved by diseases such as diabetes mellitus, herpes zoster, carcinomatous infiltration, lymphomatous infiltration, sarcoidosis, and infectious processes. Motor and sensory nerve conduction velocities are rarely useful because the lesion in a radiculopathy is proximal to the dorsal root ganglion and motor and sensory nerve conductions are usually normal, although potentials may be reduced in amplitude if the lesion is severe enough to cause axonal loss. The H-reflex is absent or delayed when the S1 nerve root is involved. Typically, nerve root lesions are diagnosed with abnormal needle examination results in the appropriate paraspinal and limb muscles.[56]

Because most limb muscles are supplied by more than one nerve root, a normal study does not exclude the diagnosis of radiculopathy; however, abnormal EMG results provide objective evidence of impairment of physiologic function in the nerve root and localize the lesion to one or more nerve roots in addition to giving information about the severity of the involvement in the pathologic process.[1]

Plexopathies

In plexopathies, motor conduction studies are useful in excluding a peripheral nerve lesion; otherwise, results are generally normal except that the amplitudes of compound muscle action potentials may be reduced. Sensory nerve conductions are usually helpful only in excluding other lesion sites, such as peripheral nerves. Again, the needle examination is the most helpful element of the examination and requires knowledge of plexus anatomy and innervation of muscles by specific portions of the plexus under investigation.[57]

Anterior Horn Cell Disorders

Disorders of the anterior horn cell usually do not manifest with prominent pain except in the acute febrile stage of poliomyelitis.

Disorders of the Central Nervous System

EMG and nerve conduction study results are almost always normal in diseases of the central nervous system not complicated by peripheral nerve disease.

Primary Muscle Disorders

Many primary disorders of muscle are painless. These disorders include the congenital muscular dystrophies. However, many acquired myopathies (e.g., polymyositis) are painful, and

Table 20.2 Painful Myopathies

Dermatomyositis

Polymyositis

Necrotizing myopathies

Toxic and drug-induced myopathies

  Cholesterol-lowering agents: Cyclosporine, Labetalol, Propofol

  Alcohol

  Amphilic: Chloroquine, Hydrochloroquine, Amiodarone

  Antimicrotubular: Colchicine, Vincristine

  Mitochondrial: Zidovudine and other anti–HIV-AIDS drugs

  Inflammatory: L-tryptophan, D-penicillamine, cimetidine, L-dopa, phenytoin, lamotrigine, interferon-alpha, hydroxyurea, imatinib

  Hypokalemic: Diuretics, laxatives, amphotericin, toluene abuse, licorice, corticosteroids, alcohol abuse

  Critical care myopathy

  Unknown mechanism: corticosteroids

  Nondepolarizing neuromuscular agents: Omeprazole, Isotretinoin, Finasteride, Emetine

Sepsis

HIV-AIDS, human immunodeficiency virus–acquired immunodeficiency syndrome

metabolic muscle disorders, (e.g., glycogen and lipid storage diseases) may include pain and muscle cramps in their symptomatology. Most manifest as myalgias. **Table 20.2** lists some of the painful myopathies. A large number are toxic in origin.[58] One of the clearest uses of EMG is in differentiating myopathies from neuropathic processes. Needle examination should clearly differentiate neuropathy from myopathy. In myopathy, the motor potentials are reduced in amplitude and may be polyphasic. In addition, the potentials show paradoxical recruitment, with more potentials seen on the oscilloscope screen than normally seen for that degree of muscular effort. In inflammatory myopathies, such as polymyositis, marked signs of muscle irritability may be found in the form of fibrillations and positive sharp waves. In polymyositis and metabolic and congenital muscle disorders, nerve conduction study results are generally normal. EMG study results are usually normal in myofascial pain syndromes, fibromyalgia, and polymyalgia rheumatica.[59–61]

Conclusion

EMG and nerve conduction studies are useful in localizing neuromuscular disease sites and in providing information about the nature of the process (demyelinating, axonal, primary muscle disease, radiculopathy, plexopathy, and so on) but cannot directly determine the etiology (e.g., diabetes, Guillain-Barré syndrome, polymyositis, tumor, ruptured disc, and so on). The etiology must be inferred from anatomic location, symptoms, and the examination bolstered by the EMG in certain instances. That process is discussed in detail in Chapter 5.

Figure 20.13 presents a summary of EMG findings in various conditions. In addition, normal study results do not mean the patient has no pain. Electrodiagnostic studies in the

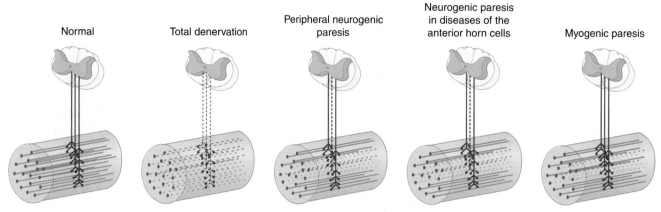

Normal   Total denervation   Peripheral neurogenic paresis   Neurogenic paresis in diseases of the anterior horn cells   Myogenic paresis

Fig. 20.13 **Summary of normal and abnormal findings in needle EMG for various conditions.**

EMG laboratory as usually performed measure only activity related to the motor fibers, the larger sensory fibers, and the muscles. Sympathetic and small unmyelinated (C) fibers are not evaluated except with quantitative sensory testing.

In addition, the timing of the EMG in relation to injury or onset of symptoms may be quite important. Early after nerve injury (0 to 14 days), the EMG may show only electrical silence, which may not be helpful. If any motor units are seen at that time, the nerve to that muscle is at least partially intact. Fibrillation potentials in denervated muscles appear only after 2 to 3 weeks. If reinnervation is occurring, small, polyphasic recovery or "nascent" units are noted. Serial studies after nerve injury are more helpful in determining recovery than a single study.

Cost-containment issues have become extremely important, and Medicare and other insurers have developed guidelines for appropriate testing for various conditions. In response, the American Association of Neuromuscular and Electrodiagnostic Medicine has also issued its own practice testing guidelines.[62]

In conclusion, EMG and nerve conduction studies may find, confirm, and localize disease processes, but the relevance of the findings to the patient's pain must remain a clinical determination.

References

Full references for this chapter can be found on www.expertconsult.com.

Evoked Potential Testing

Howard J. Waldman and Steven D. Waldman

Although they are underused by many pain management specialists, evoked potentials (EPs) are a useful diagnostic test to help in identification of abnormalities of the peripheral and central nervous system that may help explain why the patient is having pain or functional disability. EP testing is also useful in helping prove the absence of neural pathway abnormalities in the patient with otherwise unexplained visual or hearing loss or unexplained numbness. Such information is extremely useful with a clinical impression of behavioral issues influencing a patient's pain response.

What Are Evoked Potentials?

EPs are electrophysiologic responses of the nervous system to externally applied sensory stimuli. EP testing can provide information on the peripheral and the central sensory nervous system pathways that is unobtainable with electromyelography (EMG) and magnetic stimulation evaluations. EP testing provides objective and reproducible data to delineate sensory system lesions that are unsuspected or are clinically ambiguous on the basis of history and physical examination findings alone. EP testing can provide information on the anatomic location of nervous system lesions and help to monitor progression or regression.[1-4]

EP responses are of very low amplitude (0.1 to 20 µV) and are obscured by random electrical "noise," such as muscle artifact, electroencephalographic activity, and interference from surrounding electrical devices. Extraction of the EP response is accomplished with computer averaging. This technique summates the EP response, which is "time-locked" to the applied sensory stimuli, and minimizes unwanted noise interference.[1,3]

A variety of stimuli may elicit evoked potentials, but the most commonly used are visual, auditory, and somatosensory. These three stimuli give rise to visual evoked potentials (VEPs), brainstem auditory evoked potentials (BAEPs), and somatosensory evoked potentials (SEPs), which evaluate functions of their respective sensory systems.[3,5]

EP responses consist of a sequence of peaks and waves characterized by latency, amplitude, configuration, and interval between individual peaks (interpeak latency). In this manner, EP responses are similar to conventional nerve conduction study (NCS) responses and magnetically stimulated motor EPs.

A standardized nomenclature exists for the individual peaks and waves of the various EP responses.[6-9] The peaks and waves may be identified by polarity (positive or negative), by latency (e.g., the positive wave that occurs at 100 msec in VEP testing is designated P100), by the anatomic site where the response was recorded (e.g., Erb's point), or by simple numbering in sequence (e.g., waves I through V in the BAEP). Normal values for EP responses are generally established by each electrophysiology laboratory, with use of 2.5 or 3.0 standard deviations from mean values as the upper limits of normal.[1,3,10]

Instrumentation

The EP equipment, like that for EMG, is a biological amplifier. In its most basic form, EP equipment consists of recording electrodes attached to specific areas over the scalp, spine, and extremities. Input from the electrodes is routed to an amplifier, which filters, averages, displays, and records data.[3] Electrodes are placed on the scalp much as for conventional electroencephalography, following the international 10-20 system according to which electrodes are located at distances 10% or 20% of the total distance between bony landmarks of the skull.[11] The configuration of electrode placement for a specific test is referred to as a montage.

Specific Evoked Potential Tests

The three most commonly used EP tests are the VEP, BAEP, and SEP. For most patients who consult a pain specialist, SEPs have the most clinical utility. A fourth test, cognitive evoked potentials, also is discussed briefly.

Visual Evoked Potentials

VEPs are used in evaluation of pathology that affects the visual pathways. They are primarily generated in the visual cortex and, therefore, may be affected by pathology anywhere along the visual pathways, from the corneas to the visual cortex.[6,12] A reversing checkerboard pattern projected through a video monitor is most often used to stimulate the visual pathways (pattern-reversal VEP). Each eye is tested individually to localize abnormalities to the affected side. Generally, 100 pattern reversals (trials) are needed to obtain a clearly defined response. The test is repeated to confirm reproducibility of responses. The resultant VEP consists of three peaks. The primary peak of interest occurs at approximately 100 msec, has positive polarity, and is thus referred to as the P100 peak. The remaining two peaks have negative polarities and latencies of approximately 75 and 145 msec, respectively.[1,10] The upper limits of normal for the P100 response are about 117 to 120 msec, with a differential latency between eyes of no more than 6 to 7 msec.[3]

VEP testing is useful in the diagnosis of many conditions that affect the visual pathways but is most often used in the diagnosis of multiple sclerosis (MS; **Fig. 21.1**). The demyelination of the optic nerve that occurs in MS has the same effect as demyelination in peripheral nerves (i.e., slowing of conduction velocity), which results in increased response latency. If axonal loss also occurs, response amplitude is also reduced.[1,13–15] These abnormalities correspond to the changes seen in demyelination and axonopathy found in conventional NCS. In patients with MS, the most common abnormalities are increased P100 latency and increased interocular latencies. Reduction of P100 amplitude may also occur, although this is generally associated with compressive or ischemic lesions.[1] In patients suspected to have MS, VEP abnormality rates are approximately 63%, and they approach 85% in patients with confirmed MS.[1] VEP abnormalities may antedate typical changes of MS seen on magnetic resonance imaging (MRI).[1] MS may also produce abnormalities of BAEP and SEP; therefore, testing of all three may improve the diagnostic yield over that of VEP alone.[16,17]

Ocular disorders, tumors, inflammatory conditions, and ischemia of the optic pathways may be associated with VEP abnormalities.[18–20] VEP abnormalities have also been reported in a variety of cerebral degenerative disorders and neuropathies with central nervous system (CNS) involvement.[1–20] A few reports are found of VEP abnormalities in patients with migraine headaches.[21–25] VEP testing has been used for visual screening of infants and persons who are suspected of having visual pathway disease but are unable to respond to or comply with conventional ophthalmologic or optometric testing.[10,22]

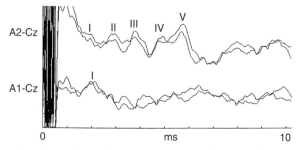

Fig. 21.1 *Upper trace,* Normal brainstem auditory evoked potential response shows waves I through V. *Lower trace,* Abnormal brainstem auditory evoked potential response obtained from a patient with a left acoustic neuroma. Wave I is present, but waves II through V are absent. *(From Waldman SD, editor:* Interventional pain management, *ed 2, Philadelphia, 2001, Saunders, p 185, Fig. 14.11, with permission.)*

Brainstem Auditory Evoked Potentials

In the manner that visual stimuli are used to evaluate visual pathways, auditory stimuli are used to assess the auditory pathways. The auditory pathway extends from the middle ear structures through the eighth cranial nerve (CN VIII) and brainstem to the auditory cortex.[1,3,10] Auditory stimuli presented to each ear individually produce the BAEPs, which consist of a series of waves that correspond closely to these auditory pathway structures. BAEP evaluation, therefore, allows relatively specific localization of auditory pathway pathology. BAEP responses are recorded from electrodes placed on the scalp, near or on each ear. The most commonly used auditory stimulus is brief electrical pulses, referred to as clicks, which are presented to each ear through audiologic earphones. (Earphones that fit *into* the auditory canal can also be used.) These click stimuli may be varied in frequency, intensity, and rate. A well-defined BAEP response generally requires 1000 to 2000 stimuli.

The typical BAEP response consists of a sequence of seven positive waves, of which the first five are used clinically. They are numbered sequentially with Roman numerals I through V and occur within the first 10 msec after presentation of auditory stimuli. Each wave closely corresponds to structures along the auditory pathway that are believed to generate it. Wave I is thought to be generated by CN VIII, wave II by CN VIII and the cochlear nucleus, wave III by the lower pons, and waves IV and V by the upper pons and lower midbrain.[1,2,10,26] Diagnosis of the anatomic site of pathology is based on which wave or waves show increased latency or are absent (see Fig. 21.1). Determination of interpeak latency is important because disorders such as peripheral hearing loss may increase the latency of the entire BAEP response but do not change the interpeak latency relationships. Severe hearing loss may render recording of the BAEP impossible because of degradation of the response.[1,26] BAEP response amplitudes vary considerably among healthy subjects. To reduce intersubject variability, the ratio of wave I and wave V amplitudes is calculated. If the wave V amplitude is reduced in comparison with wave I, an intrinsic brainstem impairment is implied. A reduction of wave I to wave V amplitude ratio suggests possible hearing impairment.[4,27]

BAEP testing may aid in the diagnosis of a variety of diseases that affect the auditory pathways. The BAEP may be abnormal in 32% to 64% of persons with MS,[26,28] although it is less sensitive than either VEP or SEP testing.[15,29,30] BAEPs are particularly useful in the diagnosis of cerebellopontine angle tumors, such as acoustic neuromas (see Fig. 21.1). BAEP testing has been found to be superior to routine audiometry and computed tomography in the diagnosis of cerebellopontine angle tumors[31,32] and appears to be at least as sensitive as, and less expensive than, MRI for this diagnosis.[1] BAEPs are also useful in: (1) the evaluation of strokes and tumors that involve the auditory pathways[10,12,29,33]; (2) the evaluation of, and as a predictor of outcome for, persons with comas and head injuries[34–36]; and (3) the diagnosis of a variety of neurodegenerative disorders, such as Friedreich's ataxia, in which the responses are abnormal.[37] BAEP abnormalities have been reported in association with Arnold-Chiari malformations, postconcussion syndrome, vertebrobasilar transient ischemic attacks, basilar migraines, and spasmodic torticollis.[38,39] These responses are used in audiometric screening of infants and of patients with mental deficiency who are unable to undergo routine audiometric testing.[26,40]

Somatosensory Evoked Potentials

SEPs assess the function of somatosensory pathways via stimulation of sensory nerves. SEPs may be recorded with stimulation of mixed or pure sensory nerves in the upper and lower extremities, in dermatomal areas of the skin, and from some cranial nerves with sensory function. The somatosensory pathway consists of the peripheral nerve, dorsal columns of the spinal cord, medial lemniscus, ventroposterior lateral thalamus, and primary sensory cortex.[1,10,41] SEPs appear to be related to the senses of joint position, touch, vibration, and stereognosis but are not related to pain and temperature sensation.[1,6]

Typically, SEPs are obtained through electrical stimulation of a peripheral nerve after recording electrodes are placed at sites along the somatosensory pathway. In upper and lower extremity SEPs, stimulation is generally applied at the more distal portion of major nerves, with recording sites along the extremity, over certain spinous processes, and on the scalp over regions that correspond to the somatosensory cortex. In SEP evaluation of dermatomal sensory areas, stimulation is performed over an area of skin that is innervated by a given dermatome (e.g., lateral foot for the S1 dermatome), and recording is usually limited to the scalp.[1,3,42]

SEP responses consist of a group of waveforms, each corresponding to the anatomic site of the recording electrode (**Figs. 21.2** and **21.3**). Abnormalities are manifested as increased latency, reduced amplitude, or absence of a given wave. The anatomic site of the lesion is determined by the point at which the abnormality is seen in a wave corresponding to recording

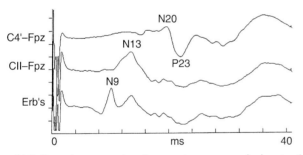

Fig. 21.2 Normal upper extremity somatosensory evoked potential response obtained with stimulation of the median nerve at the wrist shows responses recorded from Erb's point (N9), the second cervical vertebra (N13), and the cortex (N20-P23). *(From Waldman SD, editor:* Interventional pain management, *ed 2, Philadelphia, 2001, Saunders, p 186, Fig. 14.12, with permission.)*

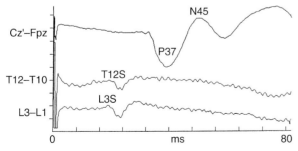

Fig. 21.3 Normal lower extremity somatosensory evoked potential response obtained with stimulation of the tibial nerve at the ankle shows responses recorded from the third lumbar vertebra (L3S), the 12th thoracic vertebra (T12S), and the cortex (P37-N45). *(From Waldman SD, editor:* Interventional pain management, *ed 2, Philadelphia, 2001, Saunders, p 186, Fig. 14.13, with permission.)*

electrode sites along the somatosensory pathway.[1,10,41] The SEP is analogous to conventional nerve conduction testing, in which the site of the NCS abnormality corresponds to the site of disease. Because peripheral nerve disorders may prolong response latencies along the entire length of the somatosensory pathway, interpeak latency determinations are important.[41,43] In addition, conventional nerve conduction testing of the peripheral portions of the nerve can help to exclude peripheral neuropathy.

SEPs are often abnormal in persons with MS. SEP testing is frequently performed in conjunction with VEP and BAEP testing to enhance diagnostic sensitivity—SEP being the most sensitive of the three modalities.[1,10,45] SEP abnormalities are more often seen in patients with MS with sensory symptoms and are more common in the lower extremities.[44,45] Generally, conventional NCS are used in evaluation of sensory disturbances of the peripheral nerve, although SEP may be recordable from the scalp (because of amplification effects of the cerebral cortex) when sensory never action potentials (SNAPs) are unrecordable. This amplification effect may be particularly useful in evaluation of some entrapment neuropathies, such as meralgia paresthetica, in which recording of the response from the peripheral nerve is technically difficult or impossible.[41,46,47] SEPs are useful in the diagnosis of brachial plexus lesions and may be complementary to conventional EMG. SEP may help to confirm axonal continuity and to determine whether lesions are preganglionic or postganglionic.[25,26] Ulnar nerve SEP may be useful in the diagnosis of thoracic outlet syndrome and appear to be complementary to EMG testing.[48-53]

The use of SEPs in the diagnosis of radiculopathy has been controversial.[3,46,54-64] Many studies that use SEP of peripheral nerves in the diagnosis of radiculopathy have found the test to be of limited utility. This limitation was attributed to "overshadowing" of abnormalities in a single nerve root by contributions from uninvolved nerve roots that supply the same peripheral nerve. Recording of SEP from a dermatomal area supplied by a single nerve root (e.g., the webbed space between the great and first toes innervated by the L5 nerve root) represents an attempt to circumvent this problem.[55-59] Dermatomal SEPs have been generally found to improve diagnostic yield; however, EMG testing remains the most sensitive electrodiagnostic test for radiculopathy.[1,3,46,55,58,65]

Somatosensory EPs are frequently abnormal in patients with myelopathy, and they may be abnormal in the presence of normal EMG evaluation results.[50,66-69] Serial SEPs have been found useful in determination of the extent of spinal cord trauma and may help in determination of prognosis for recovery.[45,70]

SEPs recorded from the trigeminal nerve have been reported to be abnormal in persons with MS-related trigeminal neuralgia and with parasellar and cerebellopontine angle tumors that affect the trigeminal nerve. Alterations of trigeminal SEP also relate well to successful treatment of trigeminal neuralgia with retrogasserian injection of glycerol and thermocoagulation-induced lesions. Trigeminal SEPs generally have not been found to be useful in the diagnosis of "idiopathic" trigeminal neuralgia.[71-74]

Other uses of SEPs are evaluation of spinal cord syndromes, such as transverse myelitis, syringomyelia, and spinal cord ischemia; and of tumors, infarctions, and hemorrhages that involve the somatosensory pathways of the brainstem and cortex.[1,10,45] Some neurodegenerative disorders, such as

Huntington's chorea, and some neuropathies that involve the central somatosensory pathways may also be associated with SEP abnormalities.[1,10]

Cognitive Evoked Potentials

Cognitive EPs, or endogenous event-related potentials, are long-latency EPs related to cognitive processing. Testing consists of random presentations of infrequent stimuli (rare stimuli) interspersed with different, more frequently occurring stimuli (common stimuli). The subject is instructed to attend to the infrequent stimuli only. Normal persons produce a P300 response with a latency of approximately 300 msec and positive polarity. The P300 response latency may be abnormally prolonged or reduced in amplitude in disorders that impair cognition, such as dementias, autism, schizophrenia, and Huntington's chorea.[1,3,10,75–77]

Conclusion

EMG and EP testing are essential tools in the diagnosis of neuromuscular disorders. They provide reliable and reproducible information on function of the nervous system that would not be obtainable through other means. They provide an extension of the clinical examination and are complementary to laboratory, radiologic, and other evaluations. Development of new techniques and improvements in old ones continue to expand the clinical utility of these tests. For example, the addition of transcranial magnetic stimulation has allowed evaluation of central motor pathways that had not been possible with EMG or other EP testing. Further refinements in cognitive EP testing may allow greater understanding of the nature and complexity of cognitive processing. The clinical neurophysiology laboratory is an increasingly important part of the total clinical milieu. With this thought in mind, the prudent practitioner will find greater utility and put more reliance on these tests for evaluation of patients, now and in the future.

References

Full references for this chapter can be found on www.expertconsult.com.

The Measurement of Pain: Objectifying the Subjective

Darin J. Correll

The International Association for the Study of Pain defines pain as "an unpleasant sensory and emotional experience associated with actual or potential tissue damage, or described in terms of such damage."[1] The idea that pain is an emotion is not new. During the fifth and sixth centuries BC, Siddharta Gautama (the Buddha) taught that pain is a part of life, is the result of desire, and could be ended only with the mind; in the fourth century BC, Aristotle wrote, "pain is the passion of the soul."

Pain has been suggested to be composed of the following three levels: sensory-discriminative (e.g., location, intensity), motivational-affective (e.g., depression, anxiety), and cognitive-evaluative (e.g., thoughts of the cause and significance).[2] Others have described pain as "a complex, subjective, perceptual phenomenon with a number of dimensions—intensity, quality, time course, impact, and personal meaning—that are uniquely experienced by each individual and, thus can only be assessed indirectly. Pain is a subjective experience and there is no way to objectively quantify it."[3] Still others have said that "emotion is not simply a consequence of pain sensation that occurs after a noxious sensory message arrives at the somatosensory cortex; rather, it is a fundamental part of the pain experience."[4]

It may seem obvious that pain is a subjective experience because people have unique, individual responses to the same stimulus (e.g., same surgery); however, different responses could result from some physiologic differences in the nociceptive pathways and not related to affective interpretation at all. So, do we know that pain is a subjective experience?

Is Pain a Subjective Experience?

Several brain areas are activated by nociceptive stimulation, including the anterior cingulate cortex, frontal and prefrontal cortices, primary and secondary somatosensory cortices, thalamus, basal ganglia, cerebellum, amygdala, and hippocampus.[5] These areas form a cerebral signature for the pain experience.[6] The primary and secondary somatosensory cortices have a role in the location and intensity of a painful stimulus.[7] The anterior cingulate cortex is involved in the affective aspects of pain (i.e., the subjective experience of unpleasantness).[8,9] The insula seems to serve as an integrator between the two and encodes intensity and location and also affect.[10] The amygdala appears to link sensory experiences to emotional arousal and negative emotional associations.[11]

Evidence that pain is indeed a subjective experience comes from psychophysical studies in which pain sensation and pain unpleasantness were shown to represent two distinct dimensions of pain.[12] Studies were performed on subjects who had a painful stimulus applied and then had hypnotic suggestions of either enhancing or decreasing the pain unpleasantness or intensity.[13] When the hypnotic suggestion related to unpleasantness was given, only the subjective pain rating changed, whereas when the hypnotic suggestion related to intensity was given, both the subjective rating and the pain intensity rating changed. These results suggest that pain sensation is a cause of pain unpleasantness.

Humans have been equipped with the capability of negative emotion for a purpose. In terms of pain, it allows people to be aware of and adjust to tissue trauma. Therefore, pain is instrumental in guiding behavior needed for self preservation and preservation of the species.[4] Unlike the somatosensory cortex, the limbic system is complexly interconnected, and processing of the affective quality of pain may outlast the sensory processing.[4] Thus, the emotional aspect of pain may be more important for the clinical manifestation of pain and its control than the sensory component because patients do not suffer from the sensory intensity but rather from the negative emotional quality.[4] This has been shown by the fact that patients who have cingulotomies,[14] insular cortex lesions,[15] or prefrontal lobotomies[16] can appreciate the sensory characteristics of pain but do not have emotional responses to it nor properly appreciate its meaning.

Another line of evidence that pain is indeed a subjective experience and not just the result of differences in nociceptive pathways comes from functional brain imaging studies. One functional magnetic resonance imaging (fMRI) study showed that as the magnitude of expected pain increased, activation increased in the thalamus, insula, prefrontal cortex, and anterior cingulate cortex; when the expected pain was manipulated, expectations of decreased pain reduced both the subjective experience of pain and the activity in the primary somatosensory cortex and the affective areas of the brain (insula, prefrontal cortex, and anterior cingulate cortex).[17] Another fMRI study showed that both suggestion-induced pain and nociceptive pain activate the secondary somatosensory cortex and the anterior cingulate cortex.[18] Other imaging studies performed in patients that have pain in the absence of known nociceptive input show the physiologic reality of these experiences by the extensive neural activation that occurs.[6]

Another major line of evidence that pain is subjective comes from study of the placebo effect. Patients who are given a positive placebo suggestion of analgesia tolerate pain better than do those given a neutral suggestion, and those given a negative placebo suggestion tolerate pain less well than do those given a neutral suggestion.[19] A patient's understanding of the therapeutic intervention seems to be crucial to the placebo analgesic effect.[20] Verbally induced expectations affect pain, thus suggesting that placebo responses are mediated by expectation.[21] An open injection of a painkiller in full view of a patient who knows what is going on and what to expect is more effective than a hidden injection in which the patient does not know to expect any effect.[22–25] Different verbal instructions about certain and uncertain expectations of analgesia produce different placebo analgesic effects.[26] The study of placebo effects shows that "subjective" constructs such as expectation and value have physiologic bases that are powerful modulators of perceptual processes.[27] The use of fMRI has shown that placebo administration with expectation of analgesia is associated with a reduction in the activity of pain-responsive regions (anterior cingulate, insular cortex, and thalamus) during a painful experience.[28] Positron emission tomography has shown that the same regions of the brain affected by opioids are affected by placebo, specifically, the anterior cingulate cortex, orbitofrontal cortex, and anterior insula.[29] In other studies, expectations of pain relief have been shown to reduce perceived pain as much as an analgesic dose of morphine.[30]

The use of examples of placebo in this discussion is solely to show the subjective nature of pain and is not meant to endorse the use of placebo for pain management without the patient's consent and certainly never to discredit the patient's report of pain or punish the patient. The American Pain Society opposes the inadequate treatment of pain with any therapeutic modality, including the use of placebo. An analgesic effect from a placebo does not provide any useful information about the genesis or severity of the pain. The deceptive use of placebo and misinterpretation of the placebo response to discredit the patient's pain report are unethical and should be avoided.[31]

Another line of evidence that pain is a subjective experience comes from studies of the effects of emotional states on the pain experience. The relationship between reported pain intensity and the peripheral stimulus that evokes pain depends on many factors, such as the level of arousal, anxiety, depression, attention, and expectation or anticipation.[32] In general, acute pain has more associated anxiety, and chronic pain states have more associated depression.

Anxiety directed toward a painful stimulus increases attention to the stimulus, and anxiety directed away from the stimulus to an external event decreases pain sensitivity.[33] Moderate levels of fear and anxiety enhance attention to salient events such as pain, thereby augmenting its perceived intensity, whereas high levels of fear may become more salient than pain, in which case fear and anxiety attenuate the pain.[34] Patients with higher trait anxiety (a greater disposition to experience anxiety) tend to exacerbate perceived pain stimulation.[35]

Depression has also been associated with the experience of heightened pain and emotional distress in response to pain.[36,37] The mechanism by which depression exerts its effect on pain-related emotional distress may be through response expectancy, as seen by the fact that patients who are prone to catastrophize have a heightened pain and emotional response to painful stimulation.[38]

Can We Objectify Pain?

That we will ever be able to evaluate pain without reliance on the individual's perceptions is highly unlikely.[3] Noninvasive functional brain imaging has allowed an objective window to the mind, but we are still a long way from objective measures of consciousness.[39] As our understanding of the brain increases, we may develop better tools, but we will also need to rely on patients to express their experience in some fashion.

In the meantime, we do need standardized measures to have some consistency and an ability to communicate with patients and between providers. However, individual differences in the accuracy of pain reports are considerable.[40] The reporting consistency of pain has also been shown to be weak within patients.[41] Therefore the idea that patients in pain examine their consciousness to come up with a number to match a discrete internal stimulus before making a report of the sensory and affective qualities of the experience seems false. Rather, it is an attempt to construct meaning, influenced by and with reference to a range of internal and external factors and private meanings.[41] This is a function of the fact that numerous brain structures involved not only in sensation but also cognition, emotion, and memory are activated with each pain experience.

However, other studies have supported the notion that patients can capture their conscious experience and accurately report on a painful experience. The use of fMRI has shown more frequent and robust activation of the somatosensory cortex, anterior cingulate cortex, and prefrontal cortex in individuals who were highly sensitive to pain versus those who were insensitive to pain, whereas activation in the thalamic relay centers showed no difference.[42] This may point to the mechanisms involved in the central nervous system that are responsible for between-individual differences in pain sensitivity. This difference is unlikely to come from peripheral or spinal differences, because the thalamic activation was the same, but rather from factors within the cognitive domain of the cortex. These findings do not, however, differentiate whether these cortical structures are the effectors or the targets of modulation of the individual pain experience. Even if unique patterns of cortical activation can be characterized in large numbers of patients for a given pain state, the subjective report will probably remain the most reliable index of the experience.[42] The most important finding was that individuals with similar patterns of activation in the primary somatosensory cortex, anterior cingulate cortex, and prefrontal cortex provide similar subjective reports of pain, thus suggesting that people can accurately capture their conscious experience via introspection.[42]

Pain Assessment

The Joint Commission in the United States has set standards for the assessment of pain in hospitalized patients, as outlined in **Table 22.1**.[43] Pain assessment should be ongoing, individualized, and documented. Patients should be asked to describe their pain in terms of the following characteristics: location, radiation, mode of onset, character, temporal pattern, exacerbating and relieving factors, and intensity.

Pain has been suggested to be considered the "fifth vital sign."[44] Although pain cannot be considered vital, nor is it a sign, the suggestion that it be routinely measured along with temperature, pulse, blood pressure, and respiratory rate is a powerful reminder to health care providers to attend to their patients' suffering.[45] Unfortunately, simple routine documentation of pain levels has not been shown in and of itself to lead to any improvement in the quality of pain management.[46] However, proper assessment is still a desirable goal before appropriate treatment.

The ideal pain measure should be sensitive, accurate, reliable, valid, and useful for both clinical and experimental conditions and able to separate the sensory aspects of pain from the emotional aspects.[47] The greatest difficulty in measurement of pain is that, because it is subjective, its measurement relies on patients to give an accurate assessment of their state. For a test to be valid, it needs to have a strong correlation with its underlying variable. Because this is not possible with subjective experiences such as pain, any measurement or number obtained is only an estimation of pain.[48] Medicine has always been strongly attracted to diagnostic methods that promise to objectify what is inherently subjective, such as a patient's report of pain.[49] It would be ideal if pain could be measured like other variables in medicine, such as weight, blood pressure, and electrolyte levels, but as yet it cannot, so surrogate measures of the experience are needed.

The measures presently available fall into two general categories: single-dimension scales and multidimensional scales. The numbers obtained from these instruments must be viewed as guides and not absolutes. Care must be taken not to solely rely on the results of the measurement but instead to wholly evaluate patients clinically so that their experience is not misinterpreted. "It remains a clinical art to combine patients' reports, behavioral observation, and physiologic measurement with the history, physical exam, laboratory information, and overall clinical context in guiding clinical judgments and therapeutic interventions."[50] The following sections describe only some of the available scales.

Single-Dimension Scales
Visual Analog Scale

The Visual Analog Scale (VAS; **Fig. 22.1**) is most commonly a straight 100-mm line, without demarcation, that has the words "no pain" at the left-most end and "worst pain imaginable" (or something similar) at the right-most end.[51] Patients are instructed to place a mark on the line that indicates the amount of pain that they feel at the time of the evaluation. The distance of this mark from the left end is then measured, and this number is used as a numeric representation of the severity of the patient's pain.

The benefit of the VAS is that it has been validated and shown to be sensitive to changes in a patient's pain experience.[52–54] It is quick to use and relatively easy to understand for most patients.[52,55] It avoids the imprecise use of descriptive words to describe pain and allows a meaningful comparison of measurements over time. The latter is possible because

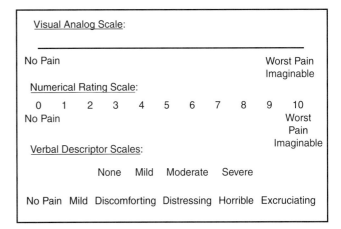

Fig. 22.1 **Single-dimension pain scales.**

Table 22.1 The Joint Commission Pain Assessment and Management Standards for Hospitals

1. The hospital respects the patient's right to pain management.
2. The hospital educates all licensed independent practitioners on assessing and managing pain.
3. The hospital assesses and manages the patient's pain. The hospital conducts a comprehensive pain assessment that is consistent with its scope of care, treatment, and services and the patient's condition.
4. The hospital uses methods to assess pain that are consistent with the patient's age, condition, and ability to understand.
5. The hospital assesses and reassesses its patients. The hospital defines, in writing, criteria that identify when additional, specialized, or more in-depth assessments are performed for pain.
6. Based on the patient's condition and assessed needs, the education and training provided to the patient by the hospital include any of the following: discussion of pain, the risk for pain, the importance of effective pain management, the pain assessment process, and methods for pain management.

the VAS has been shown to have ratio scale properties, which means that changes in VAS measurements represent actual percent differences between the measures.[56,57]

One disadvantage of the VAS is that it attempts to assign a single value to a complex, multidimensional experience. Some patients have trouble deciding how to choose a single number to represent their pain sensation. In addition, they often have no real concept of what "worst pain imaginable" actually means because every experience of pain is different and one can never know whether the present experience is the "worst." Thus, although the VAS is looked at as linear, it actually has a false ceiling at the upper-most end. If a patient marks the pain at the 100-mm end and then at a later time decides that it has become worse, the patient has no way to document this change.

Another disadvantage of the VAS is that because it offers a value for the patient's pain intensity, care providers assume that this represents a specific "amount" of pain and base treatment decisions on it. It is commonly accepted that a value of 30 mm or less represents an acceptable treatment goal. One study showed that for most patients, a VAS score greater than 30 mm (with a mean of 49 mm) represents "moderate pain" and a score greater than 54 mm (with a mean of 79 mm) represents "severe pain."[58] However, another study has shown that the number generated from the VAS is actually meaningless because the value for "moderate pain" ranged from 22 to 65 mm.[59] Disagreement also exists about what amount of change in the VAS is necessary for it to be considered an acceptable improvement in pain from the patient's perspective. Some suggest a 30% reduction in the VAS,[60] whereas others claim that at least a 50% reduction is needed to be considered meaningful relief to patients.[61,62]

Numeric Rating Scale

The numeric rating scale (NRS; see Fig. 22.1) is similar to the VAS in that it is bounded at the left-most end with "no pain" and at the right-most end with "worst pain imaginable" (or something similar). The difference is that instead of a line without marks, numbers from 0 to 10 are spaced evenly across the page. Patients are instructed to circle the number that represents the amount of pain that they are experiencing at the time of the evaluation. A variation of this scale is the verbal numeric scale (VNS), in which patients are asked to verbally state a number between 0 and 10 that corresponds to their present pain intensity.[63,64]

The benefits of the NRS and VNS are that they are validated[52,63,64] and quick and easy to use. The VNS is especially straightforward to use clinically, particularly in the acute setting, when speed of evaluation is of importance.

Disadvantages of the NRS and VNS are similar to those of the VAS in that they attempt to assign a single number to the pain experience. They also have the same ceiling effect in that if a value of "10" is chosen and the pain worsens, the patient officially has no way to express this change. In practice, at least with the VNS, patients often rate their pain as some number higher than 10 (e.g., "15 out of 10") in an attempt to express their extreme level of pain intensity.

Also similar to studies of the VAS, attempts have been made to define what is considered a meaningful change in the NRS. At least a 30% reduction or an absolute reduction in the value of at least 2 has been suggested as representing meaningful pain relief to patients.[65,66] However, that these scales are actually linear is

unlikely; the numbers and the changes between them represent different things to different individuals.

Verbal Descriptor Scale

A verbal descriptor scale (VDS; see Fig. 22.1) is a list of words, ordered in terms of severity from least to most, that describe the amount of pain that a patient may be experiencing. Patients are asked to either circle or state the word that best describes their pain intensity at that moment in time.

The benefits of VDS instruments are that they have been validated and are simple for patients to understand and quick to use.[52,67] The disadvantage of all single-dimensional scales—assigning a single value (in this case one adjective) to the pain experience—is also seen with the VDS. Another disadvantage is that a VDS forces patients to select words that are not of their own choosing to describe their pain. In addition, like the VAS and NRS, changes in pain over time are difficult to interpret and probably have different meanings to each individual. This may especially be a problem with the VDS when only a limited number of possible choices are offered to the patient (i.e. only four to six words).

Multidimensional Scales
McGill Pain Questionnaire

The McGill Pain Questionnaire (MPQ; **Fig. 22.2**) is a form that contains three different parts for assessment of a patient's pain experience.[68] One part consists of line drawings of the back and front of a human body that patients use to mark where they are experiencing pain. The second part is a six-word VDS that patients use to record their present pain intensity. The third part of the form is composed of 78 adjectives divided into 20 sets that describe the sensory, affective, and evaluative qualities of the patient's pain.

The benefits of the MPQ are that it is valid, reliable, and consistent in its ability to assign seemingly appropriate descriptions to a given pain experience.[55,69–73] The MPQ may be able to discriminate between different types of pain syndromes.[74,75] Moreover, it has been shown to be sensitive to changes in the amount of pain experienced by patients in response to receiving various analgesic therapies in both the acute and chronic setting.[76–79]

One disadvantage of the MPQ is its length. The MPQ should take from 5 to 15 minutes to complete, which for some patients may be seen as more trouble than it is worth. In addition, this amount of time is prohibitive for use on a repeated basis over a short period (e.g., in a clinical acute pain setting). Another potential disadvantage of the MPQ is that it may not be able to adequately assess the specific multidimensional aspects of pain (sensory, affective, and evaluative) because of a lack of validity in the scoring or the consistency of the test.[80,81]

Short-Form McGill Pain Questionnaires

The short-form McGill Pain Questionnaire (SF-MPQ; **Fig. 22.3**) contains three different parts for assessment of a patient's pain experience.[82] In addition to a six-word VDS and a VAS that patients use to record their present pain intensity are 15 adjectives that describe the sensory (11 words) and affective (4 words) qualities of the patient's pain.

The SF-MPQ has been validated and appears to correlate well with the original long-form MPQ.[83] Like the long form, the

McGill Pain Questionnaire

Patient's Name _____   Date _____   Time _____ am/pm

PRI: S _____   A _____   E _____   M _____   PRI(T) _____   PPI _____
      (1-10)   (11-15)   (16)   (17-20)   (1-20)

BRIEF	RHYTHMIC	CONTINUOUS
MOMENTARY	PERIODIC	STEADY
TRANSIENT	INTERMITTENT	CONSTANT

1 FLICKERING ___
QUIVERING ___
PULSING ___
THROBBING ___
BEATING ___
POUNDING ___

2 JUMPING ___
FLASHING ___
SHOOTING ___

3 PRICKING ___
BORING ___
DRILLING ___
STABBING ___
LANCINATING ___

4 SHARP ___
CUTTING ___
LACERATING ___

5 PINCHING ___
PRESSING ___
GNAWING ___
CRAMPING ___
CRUSHING ___

6 TUGGING ___
PULLING ___
WRENCHING ___

7 HOT ___
BURNING ___
SCALDING ___
SEARING ___

8 TINGLING ___
ITCHY ___
SMARTING ___
STINGING ___

9 DULL ___
SORE ___
HURTING ___
ACHING ___
HEAVY ___

10 TENDER ___
TAUT ___
RASPING ___
SPLITTING ___

11 TIRING ___
EXHAUSTING ___

12 SICKENING ___
SUFFOCATING ___

13 FEARFUL ___
FRIGHTFUL ___
TERRIFYING ___

14 PUNISHING ___
GRUELLING ___
CRUEL ___
VICIOUS ___
KILLING ___

15 WRETCHED ___
BLINDING ___

16 ANNOYING ___
TROUBLESOME ___
MISERABLE ___
INTENSE ___
UNBEARABLE ___

17 SPREADING ___
RADIATING ___
PENETRATING ___
PIERCING ___

18 TIGHT ___
NUMB ___
DRAWING ___
SQUEEZING ___
TEARING ___

19 COOL ___
COLD ___
FREEZING ___

20 NAGGING ___
NAUSEATING ___
AGONIZING ___
DREADFUL ___
TORTURING ___

PPI
0 NO PAIN ___
1 MILD ___
2 DISCOMFORTING ___
3 DISTRESSING ___
4 HORRIBLE ___
5 EXCRUCIATING ___

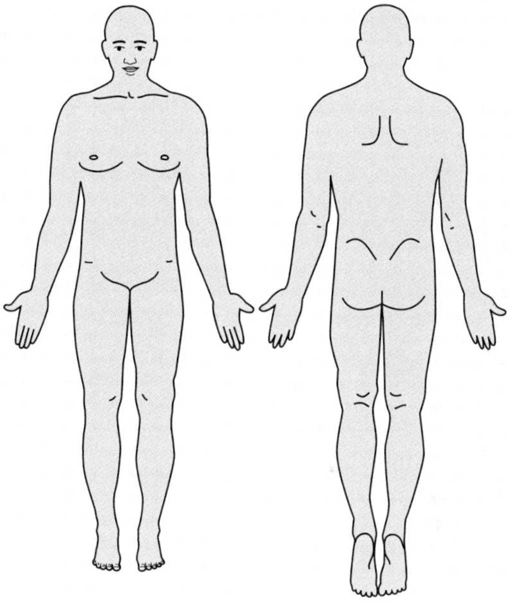

E = EXTERNAL
I = INTERNAL

COMMENTS:

Fig. 22.2 **McGill Pain Questionnaire.** *(From Melzack R: The McGill Pain Questionnaire: major properties and scoring methods, Pain 1:277, 1975.)*

SHORT-FORM McGILL PAIN QUESTIONNAIRE
RONALD MELZACK

PATIENT'S NAME: _____   DATE: _____

	NONE	MILD	MODERATE	SEVERE
THROBBING	0) _____	1) _____	2) _____	3) _____
SHOOTING	0) _____	1) _____	2) _____	3) _____
STABBING	0) _____	1) _____	2) _____	3) _____
SHARP	0) _____	1) _____	2) _____	3) _____
CRAMPING	0) _____	1) _____	2) _____	3) _____
GNAWING	0) _____	1) _____	2) _____	3) _____
HOT-BURNING	0) _____	1) _____	2) _____	3) _____
ACHING	0) _____	1) _____	2) _____	3) _____
HEAVY	0) _____	1) _____	2) _____	3) _____
TENDER	0) _____	1) _____	2) _____	3) _____
SPLITTING	0) _____	1) _____	2) _____	3) _____
TIRING-EXHAUSTING	0) _____	1) _____	2) _____	3) _____
SICKENING	0) _____	1) _____	2) _____	3) _____
FEARFUL	0) _____	1) _____	2) _____	3) _____
PUNISHING-CRUEL	0) _____	1) _____	2) _____	3) _____

PPI

NO PAIN |————————————————————————| WORST POSSIBLE PAIN

0 NO PAIN   _____
1 MILD   _____
2 DISCOMFORTING   _____
3 DISTRESSING   _____
4 HORRIBLE   _____
5 EXCRUCIATING   _____

Fig. 22.3 **McGill Pain Questionnaire-Short Form.** *(From Melzack R: The Short-Form McGill Pain Questionnaire, Pain 30:191, 1987.)*

SF-MPQ may be used to discriminate between different types of pain syndromes.[82] Also like the long form, it has been shown to be sensitive to changes in pain brought about by various analgesic therapies in both the acute and chronic setting.[84–86]

The SF-MPQ was not designed specifically for assessment of symptoms of neuropathic pain and does not contain questions to address the mechanisms of this type of pain. To deal with this, a revised version of the short-form McGill Pain Questionnaire (SF-MPQ-2; **Fig. 22.4**) was developed.[87] Seven questions were added to the SF-MPQ, and the scale for each was changed to an 11-point NRS. The dimensions of pain that are measured are continuous, intermittent, neuropathic, and affective.

Although the SF-MPQ and SF-MPQ-2 may take only around 5 minutes to complete, they are still too cumbersome for repeated use in an acute pain setting. The other disadvantages mentioned previously for the long-form MPQ may also apply to these short-form versions.

Brief Pain Inventory

The Brief Pain Inventory (BPI; **Fig. 22.5**) is used to evaluate a patient's pain experience through a number of different scales.[88] Line drawings of the front and back of a human body are included for patients to mark the location of their pain. Patients are asked to list the treatments or medications

Short-Form McGill Pain Questionnaire-2 (SF-MPQ-2)

This questionnaire provides you with a list of words that describe some of the different qualities of pain and related symptoms. Please put an X through the numbers that best describe the intensity of each of the pain and related symptoms you felt during the past week. Use 0 if the word does not describe your pain or related symptoms.

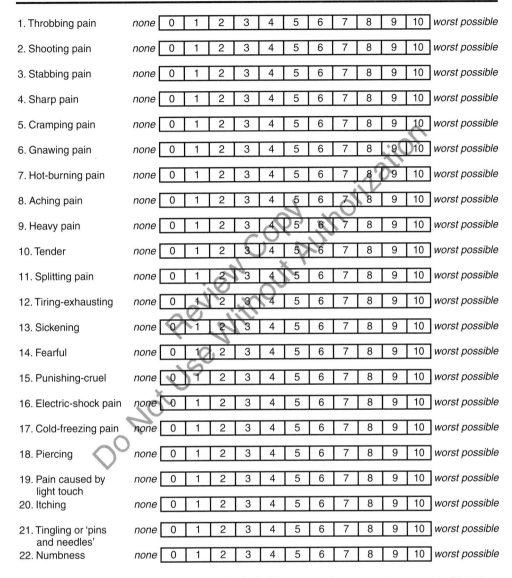

Fig. 22.4 **McGill Pain Questionnaire-Short Form 2.** *(From Dworkin RH, Turk DC, Revicki DA, et al: Development and initial validation of an expanded and revised version of the Short-form McGill Pain Questionnaire (SF-MPQ-2), Pain 144:35, 2009.)*

that they are using and how much relief they have provided in the past 24 hours. In addition, patients fill out 11 different NRS questions that ask about pain intensity (present and least, most, and average for the past 24 hours) and the effect of the pain on the ability to function during various activities of daily living.

The benefits of the BPI are that it has been validated and shown to be reliable in a number of different pain states.[89–92] It is an excellent tool to use for monitoring the effect of pain or treatment of pain, or both, in terms of a patient's functional ability or disability over time.[93] Its major disadvantage is that it takes

5 to 15 minutes to complete (depending on which form is used), thus making it less desirable for repeated use in an acute setting.

Scales for Neuropathic Pain

In addition to the previously mentioned SF-MPQ-2, other scales are available for assessment of neuropathic pain. The Neuropathic Pain Scale (NPS) was designed specifically for assessment of the qualities seen in patients with neuropathic pain.[94] The scale consists of 10 questions, five of which ask about the specific sensations sharp, dull, hot, cold, and itchy. Three of the questions ask patients to rate the intensity of their pain: overall, on the surface, and deep. One question has patients rate how unpleasant the pain is for them, and the final one asks patients to describe the time quality of the pain experience (i.e., "all the time" or "sometimes").

The benefits of the scale are that it is validated and can be used to help determine the underlying physiologic mechanism of the neuropathic pain.[94] It is also used to determine the effects of different analgesic therapies on the various qualities of the neuropathic pain.[95] Length is again one of

---

Brief Pain Inventory (Short Form)

Study ID#_____ Hospital#_____
Do not write above this line.

Date: _____

Time: _____

Name: _____
          Last   First   Middle initial

1) Throughout our lives, most of us have had pain from time to time (such as minor headaches, sprains, and toothaches). Have you had pain other than these everyday kinds of pain today?

        1. yes   2. no

2) On the diagram, shade in the areas where you feel pain. Put an X on the area that hurts the most.

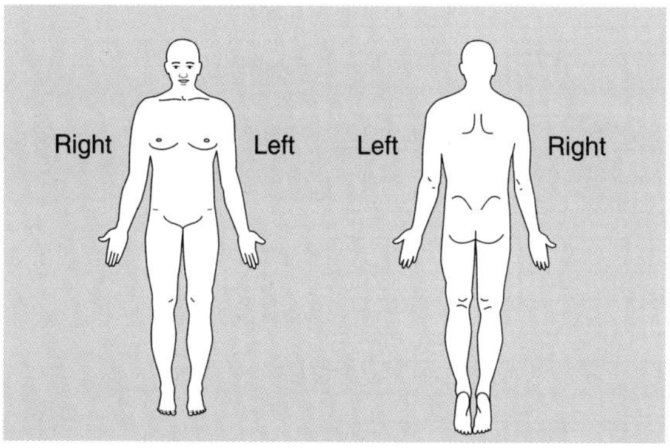

Right   Left   Left   Right

3) Please rate your pain by circling the one number that best describes your pain at its **WORST** in the past 24 hours.

0	1	2	3	4	5	6	7	8	9	10

No Pain   Pain as bad as you can imagine

4) Please rate your pain by circling the one number that best describes your pain at its **LEAST** in the past 24 hours.

0	1	2	3	4	5	6	7	8	9	10

No Pain   Pain as bad as you can imagine

5) Please rate your pain by circling the one number that best describes your pain on the **AVERAGE.**

0	1	2	3	4	5	6	7	8	9	10

No Pain   Pain as bad as you can imagine

6) Please rate your pain by circling the one number that tells how much pain you have **RIGHT NOW.**

0	1	2	3	4	5	6	7	8	9	10

No Pain   Pain as bad as you can imagine

---

7) What treatments or medications are you receiveing for your pain?

_____

8) In the past 24 hours, how much **RELIEF** have pain treatments or medications provided? Please circle the one percentage that most shows how much relief you have received.

0% 10% 20% 30% 40% 50% 60% 70% 80% 90% 100%
No Relief   Complete Relief

9) Circle the one number that describes how, during the past 24 hours **PAIN HAS INTERFERED** with your:

A. General Activity:

0	1	2	3	4	5	6	7	8	9	10

Does not interfere   Completely interferes

B. Mood

0	1	2	3	4	5	6	7	8	9	10

Does not interfere   Completely interferes

C. Walking Ability

0	1	2	3	4	5	6	7	8	9	10

Does not interfere   Completely interferes

D. Normal work (includes both work outside the home and housework)

0	1	2	3	4	5	6	7	8	9	10

Does not interfere   Completely interferes

E. Relation with other people

0	1	2	3	4	5	6	7	8	9	10

Does not interfere   Completely interferes

F. Sleep

0	1	2	3	4	5	6	7	8	9	10

Does not interfere   Completely interferes

G. Enjoyment of life

0	1	2	3	4	5	6	7	8	9	10

Does not interfere   Completely interferes

Fig. 22.5 Brief Pain Inventory. *(From Cleeland CS, Ryan KM: Pain assessment: global use of the Brief Pain Inventory,* Ann Acad Med Singapore *23:129, 1994.)*

its disadvantages, especially in the acute setting. It is thought to possibly be best suited for research as opposed to clinical settings.[96] The major disadvantage is that it cannot differentiate neuropathic from nonneuropathic pain.

The Leeds Assessment of Neuropathic Symptoms and Signs (LANSS; **Fig. 22.6**) is a seven-item scale that consists of a five-part pain questionnaire answered by the patient and a two-part sensory test performed on the patient by a provider.[97] The patient answers questions, using "yes" or "no", about specific qualities of how the pain has felt over the prior week and the skin's appearance and sensitivity. The sensory tests assess for the presence of allodynia and an altered pinprick threshold. Each of the items has a specific numeric value that when scored produces a final number from 0 to 24. A score greater than or equal to 12 suggests that some neuropathic mechanism is likely contributing to the patient's pain.

The benefits of the scale are that it has been validated and tested in a number of clinical settings.[98–100] The scale also has been used to monitor treatment effects from analgesics.[101] Unlike the NPS, it is used to establish the prevalence of neuropathic pain in a patient with pain of both neuropathic and nonneuropathic origins or with symptoms that are not obviously of a specific origin. A disadvantage, again, is length of time, especially in an acute setting. In addition, as with any scale, it is not 100% sensitive or specific and thus cannot be expected to be used to fully replace a comprehensive clinical evaluation because 10% to 20% of patients with a diagnosis of neuropathic pain are missed.[102] Also, patients could score as if they have neuropathic pain when in fact they do not.

Which Scale Is Best?

In an outpatient chronic pain setting, use of one of the general multidimensional scales or neuropathic pain scales is probably best. Assessment of all aspects of the patient's pain experience is important, and the length of these surveys is less prohibitive when they are used only occasionally. If the functionality of the patient is also of importance, use of the BPI is probably best. With a definite or even questionable neuropathic component to the patient's pain, a scale that can assess this is needed (e.g., SF-MPQ-2, LANSS).

In the acute inpatient setting, the multidimensional forms are generally too long for repeated use. If the pain

---

THE LANSS PAIN SCALE
Leeds Assessment of Neuropathic Symptoms and Signs

NAME _____   DATE _____

This pain scale can help to determine whether the nerves that are carrying your pain signals are working normally or not. It is important to find this out in case different treatments are needed to control your pain.

A. PAIN QUESTIONNAIRE

• Think about how your pain has felt over the last week.
• Please say whether any of the descriptions match your pain exactly.

1) Does your pain feel like strange, unpleasant sensations in your skin? Words like pricking, tingling, pins and needles might describe these sensations.

   a)   NO - My pain doesn't really feel like this .... (0)
   b)   YES - I get these sensations quite a lot .... (5)

2) Does your pain make the skin in the painful area look different from normal? Words like mottled or looking more red or pink might describe the appearance.

   a)   NO - My pain doesn't affect the color of my skin .... (0)
   b)   YES - I've noticed that the pain does make my skin look different from normal .... (5)

3) Does your pain make the affected skin abnormally sensitive to touch? Getting unpleasant sensations when lightly stroking the skin, or getting pain when wearing tight clothes might describe the abnormal sensitivity.

   a)   NO - My pain doesn't make my skin abnormally sensitive in that area .... (0)
   b)   YES - My skin seems abnormally sensitive to touch in that area .... (3)

4) Does your pain come on suddenly and in bursts for no apparent reason when you're still? Words like electric shocks, jumping and bursting describe these sensations.

   a)   NO - My pain doesn't really feel like this .... (0)
   b)   YES - I get these sensations quite a lot .... (2)

5) Does your pain feel as if the skin temperature in the painful area has changed abnormally? Words like hot and burning describe these sensations.

   a)   NO - I don't really get these sensations .... (0)
   b)   YES - I get these sensations quite a lot .... (1)

Fig. 22.6 Leeds Assessment of Neuropathic Symptoms and Signs. *(From Bennett M: The LANSS pain scale: the Leeds Assessment of Neuropathic Symptoms and Signs,* Pain *92:147, 2001.)*

(Continued)

B. SENSORY TESTING

Skin sensitivity can be examined by comparing the painful area with a contralateral or adjacent non-painful area for the presence of allodynia and an altered pin-prick threshold (PPT).

1) ALLODYNIA

Examine the response to lightly stroking cotton wool across the non-painful area and then the painful area. If normal sensations are experienced in the non-painful site, but pain or unpleasant sensations (tingling, nausea) are experienced in the painful area when stroking, allodynia is present.

   a)   NO - normal sensation in both areas .... (0)

   b)   YES - allodynia in painful area only .... (5)

2) ALTERED PIN-PRICK THRESHOLD

Determine the pin-prick threshold by comparing the response to a 23 gauge (blue) needle mounted inside a 2 ml syringe barrel placed gently on to the skin in a non-painful and then painful areas.

If a sharp pin prick is felt in the non-painful area, but a different sensation is experienced in the painful area e.g. none/blunt only (raised PPT) or a very painful sensation (lowered PPT), an altered PPT is present

If a pin-prick is not felt in either area, mount the syringe onto the needle to increase the weight and repeat.

   a)   NO - equal sensation in both areas .... (0)

   b)   YES - altered PPT in painful area .... (3)

SCORING:

Add values in parentheses for sensory description and examination findings to obtain overall score.

TOTAL SCORE (maximum 24) ....

If score <12, neuropathic mechanisms are **unlikely** to be contribution to the patient's pain
If score ≥12, neuropathic mechanisms are **likely** to be contributing to the patient's pain

Fig. 22.6–Cont'd

Fig. 22.7 Faces Pain Scale. *(From Bieri D, Reeve R, Champion G, et al: The FACES pain scale for the self-assessment of the severity of pain experienced by children: development, initial validation and preliminary investigation for ratio scale properties, Pain 41:139, 1990.)*

Table 22.2 Pain Assessment in Advanced Dementia Scale

	0	1	2	Score
Breathing Independent of vocalization	Normal	Occasional labored breathing. Short period of hyperventilation.	Noisy labored breathing. Long period of hyperventilation. Cheyne-Stokes respirations.	
Negative vocalization	None	Occasional moan or groan. Low-level speech with a negative or disapproving quality.	Repeated troubled calling out. Loud moaning and groaning. Crying.	
Facial expression	Smiling, or inexpressive	Sad. Frightened. Frown.	Facial grimacing.	
Body language	Relaxed	Tense. Distressed pacing. Fidgeting.	Rigid. Fists clenched. Knees pulled up. Pulling or pushing away. Striking out.	
Consolability	No need to console	Distracted or reassured by voice or touch.	Unable to console, distract, or reassure.	
				TOTAL

(From Warden V, Hurley AC, Volicer L: Development and psychometric evaluation of the Pain Assessment in Advanced Dementia (PAINAD) scale, *J Am Med Dir Assoc* 4:9, 2003.)

state of interest is acute postoperative pain and the patient was not in a chronic pain state previously, the somatic portion of the experience is probably a major component and use of the single-dimension scales (e.g., VAS, NRS, VNS, VDS) probably gives adequate information for treatment. However, if the patient has chronic pain or underwent surgery for an emotionally charged condition (e.g., cancer), the affective qualities of pain are likely major determinants of the experience, so attempts to address, at least in a limited fashion, the multidimensional aspect, may be helpful. Multiple VAS, NRS, or VNS instruments are possible to use to address the various issues that appear to be important to patients. The exact questions for best assessment of patients in the acute setting are still to be determined, but one set of questions that has been suggested is to ask patients specifically about the following aspects of their experience: pain, anxiety, depression, anger, fear, and interference with physical activity.[103] These recommendations come from a study of patients in the postoperative period who were evaluated with the Multidimensional Affect and Pain Survey, a form that consists of 101 descriptors of pain and emotion. The study showed no correlation between a single pain intensity NRS and any somatosensory pain descriptors. Rather, four of the descriptors from the emotional pain supercluster (depressed mood, anger, anxiety, and fear) were highly predictive of the pain NRS.[104] These findings also add more evidence that pain is indeed subjective.

Use of the single-dimension scales to track the change in a patient's pain rating over time or after an intervention is often more helpful than trying to use them to measure an absolute level of pain at a given point in time. In addition, measurement of pain is best not only at rest but also with activity because patients must be able to do certain things, such as get out of bed, cough, and breathe deeply, to limit possible complications like venous thrombosis and pneumonia.[105]

Assessment of the Elderly or Cognitively Impaired

If an elderly patient is cognitively intact, it appears that a VAS or an NRS can be used effectively. However, the VAS has been suggested as the least preferred method by the elderly.[106] If any question exists about the cognitive abilities of the patient, one may choose to use a VDS or the Faces Pain Scale, both of which have been shown to be easy to understand and use in this population.[107,108] The Faces Pain Scale (**Fig. 22.7**) is a visual scale with six somewhat

Table 22.3 Functional Pain Scale

0 = No pain

1 = Tolerable (and does not prevent any activities)

2 = Tolerable (but does prevent some activities)

3 = Intolerable (but can use telephone, watch TV, or read)

4 = Intolerable (but cannot use telephone, watch TV, or read)

5 = Intolerable (and unable to verbally communicate because of pain)

Ideally, all patients should reach a 0 to 2 level, preferably 0 to 1. It should be made clear to the respondent that limitations in function only apply if limitations are a result of the pain being evaluated.
(From Gloth FM, Scheve AA, Stober CV, et al: The Functional Pain Scale: reliability, validity, and responsiveness in an elderly population, *J Am Med Dir Assoc* 2:110, 2001.)

realistically drawn faces that range from a content-looking smiling face to a distressed-looking face.[109]

Other examples of instruments that have been developed and validated specifically for pain assessment in the elderly, who cannot self report, and the cognitively impaired are the Pain Assessment in Advanced Dementia (PAINAD) scale (**Table 22.2**)[110] and the Functional Pain Scale (FPS; **Table 22.3**).[111] The PAINAD is a simple observer-based tool that generates a pain score between 0 and 10 based on an assessment of five different patient behaviors. The FPS is a six-point scale that includes both patient-based subjective components and observer-based objective measures of seeming tolerability of pain and interference with normal daily activities.

Conclusion

Multiple lines of evidence support the fact that pain is subjective. No truly objective measure of pain is available, nor might any be appropriate. Instruments exist that can yield useful information, and patients can effectively relate what is needed to treat pain, even if the experience cannot be fully objectified. One just needs to understand the limitations of the measures, use sound clinical judgment, and always listen to the patient.

References

Full references for this chapter can be found on www.expertconsult.com.

Chapter 23

Neuropathic Pain: Neuropsychiatric, Diagnostic, and Management Considerations

Brian Hainline

Introduction

Neuropathic pain is associated with multidimensional suffering: physical, emotional, cognitive, and social. Although general consensus exists among pain medicine physicians and clinicians that neuropathic pain differs from nociceptive pain, controversy is found regarding the definition and pathophysiology of neuropathic pain. This chapter explores the physiology, diagnosis, and management of neuropathic pain, with the premise that neuropathic pain is a neuropsychiatric condition that is best managed in a multidisciplinary treatment facility.

Definitions

The International Association for the Study of Pain (IASP) defines neuropathic pain as pain initiated or caused by a primary lesion or dysfunction in the nervous system.[1] This commonly accepted view of neuropathic pain has been challenged by a group of neurologists, neuroscientists, clinical neurophysiologists, and neurosurgeons who established a task force in collaboration with the IASP's special interest group on neuropathic pain. This group has redefined neuropathic pain as pain that arises as a direct consequence of a lesion or disease that affects the somatosensory system.[2] Whereas this revised definition follows classical nosology for neurologic disorders, it does not allow for a broader classification of neuropathic pain that is in keeping with emerging mind-body science.[3–5]

This chapter uses the standard definition from the IASP, which indicates that neuropathic pain is initiated or caused by a primary lesion or dysfunction in the nervous system. Although the term dysfunction may be considered by some to be a nebulous term without delineated boundaries,[6] it is in keeping with neurophysiologic data from functional brain imaging studies that show perturbed neurophysiologic function in patients with neuropathic pain. The perturbed function is widespread in the limbic brain and is not limited to the somatosensory system.

When emerging data challenge our traditionally held views, we must decide, personally and as a society, if we will allow our view to be reconsidered. The practice and study of medicine is an ever-evolving phenomenon that is determined by both society and science.[7] Pain medicine is a perfect example of how society and science have merged to create a new discipline of medicine, one that must take into account social and scientific evidence that may push the boundaries of classical neurological nosology.[3] Pain medicine physicians and clinicians must understand how science is influenced by philosophy, psychology, sociology, religion, and other attributes that determine what doctors look for and what they seek to cure.[7] This influence may seem arbitrary because the driving force may not be science itself.[8] The current boundary between psychiatry and neurology is an example of how disparate forces and decisions created an arbitrary chasm in a previously unified field of study; some have argued that at its very foundation this boundary has led to a baseless cleavage of brain-based disorders into two separate medical specialties.[9] If we consider neuropathic pain as a neuropsychiatric condition, then we are arguing that there is an indelible inseparability of brain and thought, mind and body, and mental and physical.[9–13]

Even defining neuropathic pain as a neuropsychiatric condition may lead to limitations in terms of management. Because of the myriad manifestations of neuropathic pain, the belief that a single physician trained in the combined fields of neurology and psychiatry could adequately manage the multidimensional suffering of a patient with neuropathic pain is naive.[3] Neuropathic pain is a complex neurophysiologic condition with neurologic, behavioral and physical manifestations. The multitude of treatment failures in patients with neuropathic pain by physicians and clinicians with a single focus of management should lead to a reassessment of the best way to manage this condition.[3,14] As discussed in this chapter, the myriad of clinical manifestations of a neuropathic pain patient require a multidimensional, team-oriented management approach.[3,15]

Pain Processing and Perception

The IASP defines pain as "an unpleasant sensory and emotional experience which we primarily associate with tissue damage or describe in terms of such damage, or both."[1] Pain is often defined as either acute pain or chronic pain, but such definitions are clinical and do not necessarily correlate with neurophysiologic counterparts. A more useful consideration, both clinically and scientifically, is of pain as either nociceptive pain or neuropathic pain, which is in keeping with emerging clinical and neuroscientific models of pain.[14]

The normal processing of nociceptive pain begins in the peripheral nervous system in primary afferent neurons. These neurons, known as nociceptors, distinguish noxious from innocuous events. The transmitting nerves may be lightly myelinated or unmyelinated and are specialized to respond to mechanical, heat, thermal, and chemical stimuli. Threshold activation of nociceptive afferent neurons leads to afferent transmission of signals to the spinal cord. Most afferent input occurs by way of the dorsal root (**Fig. 23.1**), although some fibers traverse the ventral root. Nociceptive input can be modified within the spinal cord.[16] Both nociceptive-specific neurons and more nonspecific, wide–dynamic range cells can be activated from these afferent sensory pathways.

In the most simplistic view of pain processing, nociceptive-specific cells in the spinal cord ascend to the contralateral thalamus by way of the neocortical spinothalamic tract. From the thalamus, afferent pathways then activate both primary and secondary somatosensory cortices, which mediate sensory-discriminative perception (see Fig. 23.1). However, pain processing pathways are more complex. Wide–dynamic range cells, which are activated by innocuous and noxious stimuli, can amplify afferent stimuli.[16] In addition, more widespread ascending pathways from the spinal cord to the brain activate multiple brainstem and subcortical regions, limbic pathways, and both ipsilateral and contralateral cortical brain regions, which mediate affective-motivational and cognitive perception (see Fig. 23.1). These pathways intermingle with regions of the brain that mediate emotions, autonomic activity, attention and localization, motor planning, and cognition.[17]

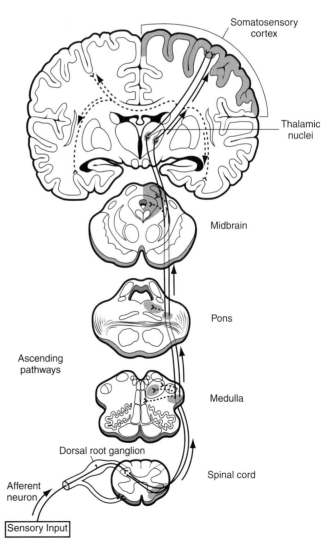

Fig. 23.1 **Ascending pain pathways.** *Solid lines:* Sensory-discriminative pathways. *Broken lines:* Affective-motivational and cognitive pathways.

Descending pain pathways also influence the perception of pain (**Fig. 23.2**). The midbrain periaqueductal gray matter subserves the endogenous opiate system.[18] The endogenous opioids consist of endorphins and enkephalins, which regulate the pain response, homeostasis, immune function, and the normal stress response. Activation of the periaqueductal gray matter leads to inhibition of dorsal horn neurons and subsequent analgesia, primarily through an excitatory conduction with the dorsal raphe nucleus. The dorsal raphe nucleus (serotonergic) and locus ceruleus (noradrenergic) are two other brainstem centers that relay key descending pain-inhibitory pathways (see Fig. 23.2). These brainstem centers are modified by cortical, subcortical, and limbic pathways.[17]

Additional brain regions are intimately involved in pain modulation through the activation of endogenous neurotransmitters, including acetylcholine, γ-aminobutyric acid (GABA), vasoactive intestinal polypeptide, oxytocin, somatostatin, cholecystokinin, vasopressin, histamine, prolactin, and cannabinoids.[19–21] A host of endogenous neurotransmitters either inhibit or augment pain perception in a complex interplay that is mediated from cortical, limbic, and brainstem centers (see Fig. 23.2). These pain-modulating pathways and their neurochemical substrate are one basis for the pharmacologic management of pain.[22]

Whereas nociceptive pain and acute pain are sometimes considered interchangeable terms, acute pain—pain that has arisen within a short period of time after perceived injury to the individual—may possibly transform into neuropathic pain within hours or days.[14] Thus, acute pain is not necessarily interchangeable with nociceptive pain. The transition from nociceptive pain to neuropathic pain is not seamless or clear cut. Patient descriptions of pain help to shed some light on this transition. For example, activation of thermal or chemical nociceptors may lead to an immediate experience of a burning, freezing, or tingling sensation. The experience, generally speaking, is not complex, and an immediate behavioral response of limb or body withdrawal occurs. Similarly, activation of a mechanical nociceptor may lead to an immediate withdrawal of the affected limb, with the perception of a pressure-like discomfort.

Contrast this with the subsequent descriptions that were offered by patients with neuropathic pain.

> *"I feel as though someone has pulled the skin off my left arm and is then constantly rubbing salt into the wound."*
> *"I feel as though my leg is on fire. My skin feels burnt, and it is as though someone is taking a claw and tearing into my skin 24 hours a day."*
> *"I feel as though someone has taken a hot poker knife and is jabbing it deep into my right eye. If I could pull my eye out, only to remove the sensation, I would gladly do so."*

These descriptions suggest the complex conscious experience of neuropathic pain.

Pain and Functional Brain Imaging

Functional brain imaging has revolutionized our understanding of pain processing and has become a cornerstone of defining and understanding neuropathic pain.[4,5,23,24] Functional brain imaging studies provide a window into neurophysiology and neuroanatomy that is not possible with traditional anatomic brain imaging studies (magnetic resonance imaging [MRI] and computerized axial tomography) or postmortem neuropathologic studies.[24] Functional brain imaging studies challenge the manner in which we view traditional concepts of injury, lesion, nosology, and neuroanatomic correlates. For example, axotomized hind limb cortical spinal neurons are incorporated into the sensory motor circuits of the unaffected forelimbs of adult rats that have been rendered a thoracic spinal cord injury. Mapping of these novel, nonclassical neural pathways is possible through voltage-sensitive dye imaging and blood-oxygen level–dependent functional MRI.[25] Such ongoing advances in neuroscience lead us to probe further into the plasticity and reorganization potentials of the brain, a cornerstone of neuropathic pain transformation.

The two main techniques used in functional brain imaging are positron emission tomography (PET) and functional MRI (fMRI), which measure energy consumption in activated brain regions.[5] Functional brain imaging has mapped out the pain neuromatrix, which is the area of the brain that processes the pain response. The pain neuromatrix includes: the primary and secondary somatosensory cortices, which mediate sensory-discriminative features of pain;

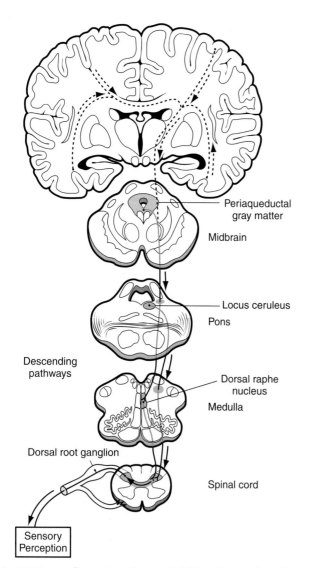

Fig. 23.2 Descending pain pathways. *Solid lines:* Sensory-discriminative pathways. *Broken lines:* Affective-motivational and cognitive pathways.

Periaqueductal gray matter

Midbrain

Locus ceruleus

Pons

Descending pathways

Dorsal raphe nucleus

Medulla

Dorsal root ganglion

Spinal cord

Sensory Perception

the anterior cingulate cortex and insula, which mediate affective-motivational components of pain; and the prefrontal cortex, which mediates cognitive aspects of pain. The thalamus serves as the gateway between the cortex and the brainstem and spinal cord pathways.[3,24]

Functional brain imaging studies have shown that neuropathic pain is associated with an increase in regional blood flow in the primary and secondary somatosensory cortices, or areas that mediate sensory-discriminative pain.[5,26] This response may be bilateral.[5] On the other hand, patients with neuropathic pain have a decrease in brain metabolism in the orbitofrontal and insular cortices.[24] In addition, pain perception in patients with neuropathic pain is mediated primarily by the anterior cingulate gyrus as opposed to the primary somatosensory cortex.[5,24] Patients with neuropathic pain reveal a reduction in metabolism in the contralateral thalamus in body regions affected by the neuropathic pain.[24] Functional brain imaging studies reveal clearly that the limbic brain is intimately involved in the perception and manifestation of neuropathic pain.

Functional brain imaging studies shed some light as to how a neuropathic pain syndrome develops. The six main mechanisms involved in the transformation from nociceptive pain to neuropathic pain are: (1) activity increased scenarios of the pain neural matrix; (2) recruitment of cortical areas beyond the classical pain neural matrix; (3) cortical reorganization and maladaptive neural plasticity; (4) alterations in neural chemistry; (5) structural brain changes; and (6) disruption of the brain default mode network.[24] Such changes cannot be predicted from peripheral or central nervous system lesions alone and reflect a dynamic interplay between the nervous system and the environment that is the hallmark of brain plasticity and reorganization.

Functional brain imaging studies help us understand why neuropathic pain may not manifest clinically along classically defined pain dermatomes. For example, patients with complex regional pain syndrome have a substantial reorganization of the somatotopic map within the primary somatosensory cortex: the cortical hand representation shrinks contralateral to the affected arm in patients with this condition, and the head position shifts toward the mouth.[23,24] These studies help us understand the clinical manifestation of complex regional pain syndrome along a broad regional area of an affected limb,[23] as opposed to along a strict dermatome.[6] Similar changes have been identified in patients with carpal tunnel syndrome, phantom limb pain, and herpes simplex virus infections with secondary neuropathic pain.[23,24] When patient conditions improve, whether through behavioral or pharmacologic strategies, the somatotopic reorganization reverses.[27,28]

Such studies take us to the forefront of emerging mind-body medicine, which teaches us that the brain and environment communicate interactively and bidirectionally.[11,13,29,30] Thus, as we increasingly understand brain function, especially through the window of functional brain imaging, we understand that we can affect changes in the brain by any combination of psychologic intervention, environment manipulation, psychopharmacology, molecular biology, cell transplantation, or neurosurgical procedures.[12,31–33] This evolving view of the mind-brain does not allow for a split of mind function and brain function and encourages an investigation into the meaning of dysfunction.

Functional brain imaging studies reveal that the brain may reorganize after injury or perception of injury.[23,24] Thus, plasticity, which is the ability of the central nervous system to adapt or to reorganize in response to new internal or external environmental requirements,[34] may underlie the basis of neuropathic pain. The cause of such reorganization is becoming increasingly revealed through functional brain imaging studies and application of clinical observation. These exciting data challenge and encourage pain medicine to move beyond a simplistic lesion-oriented and single pain pathway model. Functional brain imaging studies show unequivocally that the pathways that mediate both emotional and physical pain comingle, which begs for a more integrative neuropsychiatric explanation of neuropathic pain phenomena.

Genetic Predisposition to Pain

Emerging neuroscience has revealed that genetic factors may increase the risk of psychiatric morbidity, while not necessarily coding for a specific psychiatric disorder. Such genetic alterations are sometimes referred to as endophenotypic traits.[35] Endophenotypic factors affect circuitry essential for affective function, cognition, stress, and immune activity—all functions that are also altered in neuropathic pain. Some studies have shown specific vulnerabilities to the development of neuropathic pain.

The "s" allele of the 5-HTTLPR gene is associated with numerous alterations in brain function and morphology, including the processing and experience of pain.[36,37] Distinct clinical correlations with such genetic changes are not yet available, but other emerging genetic psychiatric work shows a possible link with neuropathic pain conditions. For example, individuals who carry both the "s" allele of the 5-HTTLPR gene with the met-BDNF allele show a protective effect with regard to loss of gray matter volume in the anterior cingulate cortex and the risk of development of depression in the context of environmental adversity early in life.[35] This finding is significant because the anterior cingulate cortex plays a crucial role in pain signaling and even predicts treatment response to antidepressants.[38]

A number of genes have been identified that modulate human nociception, and alterations in these genes may be a risk factor for impaired pain processing and subsequent neuropathic pain development.[39] These include, but are not limited to, genes coding for opioid receptors; transient receptor potential cation channels; fatty acid, amino hydrolase, and GTP cyclohydrolase; and spinal cord N-methyl-d-aspartate (NMDA) acid receptors.[40,41] An association has been shown between a polymorphism of catechol-O-methyl-transferase—an enzyme involved in catecholamine metabolism—and sensory and affective patient pain ratings. Methionine homozygous carriers show a diminished mu-opioid receptor response to pain and a stronger subjective experience of pain when compared with heterozygous subjects.[42] Other studies have shown a connection between a gene coding for the D4 dopamine receptor and vulnerability toward fibromyalgia. Such emerging genetic studies show an intriguing possible relationship between genetic predisposition and the manner in which the individual responds to external threat, perceived tissue damage, emotional processing, and the experience of pain.[35]

The gene encoding the sodium channel Nav1.7 may be a target for modulating pain disorders. A mutation in this gene can result in the inability to perceive pain,[43] and a gain of function mutations in this gene leads to enhanced pain perception, potentially causing erythromelalgia, a neuropathic pain condition in which patients experience burning pain after warm stimuli or exercise.[44]

Psychological Comorbidity and Predisposition

Division of vulnerabilities to neuropathic pain into psychologic, genetic, and physical factors is simplistic. However, our common clinical experience is often compartmentalized, and thus, it is useful to define matters in such compartments, so long as it is also understood that such compartmentalization does not present the more fluid reality of pain perception. Psychologic factors associated with neuropathic pain can be considered in terms of both comorbid conditions with neuropathic pain and predispositions to the development of neuropathic pain.

Depression is the most common comorbidity associated with neuropathic pain. Some studies reveal a depression prevalence rate approaching 100% in patients with neuropathic pain.[45] The relationship between pain and depression is complex. Although depression is not an independent risk factor for the development of neuropathic pain, patient with depression report higher levels of pain than patients without depression.[46,47] Depression augments the impairment associated with neuropathic pain, and the likelihood of successful treatment of neuropathic pain is very low if depression is not treated successfully.[45]

Anxiety also has a high comorbid association with neuropathic pain. Some postulate that neuropathic pain may be an expression of chronic post-traumatic stress disorder.[48–51] Functional and metabolic similarities exist between neuropathic pain and post-traumatic stress disorder.[52,53] Clinical data tell us that some patients adapt to prior traumatic stress with chronic behavioral strategies and then have neuropathic pain develop years later in a response to a perceived injury. The hypothesis is that the perceived injury—the inciting event—becomes associated with the prior traumatic experience, resulting in an alteration in pain pathways and the perception of pain.[54] This point is important because some patients may avoid discussing prior trauma because of fearfulness or lack of trust. Other patients may be unaware of prior trauma.[54]

Post-traumatic stress disorder is diagnosed in about 10% of patients with chronic neuropathic pain.[55] However, patients referred for psychologic treatment of neuropathic pain report rates of post-traumatic stress disorder approaching 50% or higher.[56,57]

Clinical studies have shown that unresolved post-traumatic stress can help maintain neuropathic pain for years and can activate physical pain many years later as well.[54] This has important clinical implications. For example, in a study of 100 patients for spinal surgery, 95% of patients had a successful outcome if they had no history of physical, sexual, or emotional trauma; only 15% of patients had a successful outcome if they recalled three or more prior traumatic events.[58] Thus, patients with significant history of trauma may do poorly when surgery is performed in an attempt to relieve pain. Surgery may be perceived by the individual (consciously or unconsciously) as yet another traumatic event.[54] Such literature shows that psychologic factors can predict treatment success and must be an integral part of pain management.

Psychologic maladaptations may be a significant factor for some individuals who have development of chronic pain. Studies have shown that patients with neuropathic pain have a statistically significant increased incidence rate of childhood abuse.[59–62] Such statistics, however, do not lay a foundation for a causal relationship between childhood abuse and neuropathic pain and should not lead to an assumption that patients with neuropathic pain have an underlying psychologic or psychosomatic illness. Ultimately, the dysfunction and misprocessing that occurs in individuals with neuropathic pain needs to be understood in terms of biologic predisposition and the individual's processing of internal and external perception.[17]

Sleep deprivation is common in patients with neuropathic pain, and sleep deprivation alone causes a hyperexcitable state that amplifies the pain response.[63] Other comorbid conditions can exist at the social support level. If social support is inadequate, the patient with neuropathic pain has a lower likelihood of effectively managing pain. Dysfunction may also exist at a spiritual level in that some patients believe they deserve to have pain and they place such reasoning within a religious or metaphysical context.[14]

Examples of Neuropathic Pain Syndromes

An exhaustive discussion of neuropathic pain syndromes is beyond the scope of this chapter. A brief discussion of some common neuropathic pain syndromes follows.

Chronic Low Back Pain

Although chronic low back pain is ubiquitous, no single satisfactory treatment regimen exists for this problem. Too often, chronic back pain is viewed as a biomechanical problem that can be fixed by way of either local injections or surgical therapy. However, it is more useful to view chronic low back pain as neuropathic pain that may also manifest with superimposed, nociceptive-mediated, biomechanical features.[14]

Patients with chronic low back pain, without active nociceptive symptomatology, have essentially constant pain that is position independent. Pain may be across the lower back and may be radiating into one or both legs. Pain is often described as having a burning quality to it but may also be described as stabbing, cramp-like, or deep pressure. Patients may describe position-dependent pain superimposed on chronic, position-independent pain. For example, patients with chronic back pain with associated segmental lumbar instability have acute, severe pain with sudden positional changes. Patients with lumbar stenosis have development of progressively severe low back pain, with or without leg pain, on walking or standing. Patients with active facet syndrome have sudden pain with back extension. Distinguishing between these variations is important when obtaining a history and performing an examination. Treatment may combine interventions targeted at the nociceptive-mediated, biomechanical pain while addressing the overall neuropathic pain syndrome.[14]

The multitude of failed back surgeries is a testament to the fact that low back surgery, including laminectomy and diskectomy, spinal fusion, and disc replacement, are not the answers to patients with chronic low back pain.[64] However, the converse position that chronic low back pain is simply "myofasciitis"[65] does not advance the scientific and clinical understanding of chronic low back pain as a neuropathic pain condition. As with all neuropathic pain syndromes, chronic low back pain represents a transformation from nociceptive pain into neuropathic pain that must take into account the patient's underlying perception.[66,67] The clinician's management should shift so that the chronic nature of the pain becomes the guiding principle for multidisciplinary management.

Postherpetic Neuralgia

Postherpetic neuralgia is one of the better-studied neuropathic pain syndromes and exemplifies how a peripheral nerve insult can lead to dysfunction of the central nervous system. Postherpetic neuralgia is caused by reactivation of the varicella zoster virus along a single dermatome related to either a spinal dorsal root ganglion or a brainstem cranial nerve ganglion. Pain develops along the same dermatome as the rash. The initial pain of postherpetic neuralgia is an appropriate, nociceptive response to irritation of the peripheral nerve. However, postherpetic neuralgia becomes transformed into neuropathic pain in a substantial number of individuals.[68] Such pain, as with other neuropathic pain syndromes, affects multiple aspects of life, including affect, physical activities, social interactions, self esteem, and sleep.

The transition from nociceptive pain to neuropathic pain may be from deafferentation of the second order neurons of the spinothalamic tract as a result of primary sensory neuronal death. However, this has not been conclusively shown, and pain transformation may involve other aspects of sensory processing, including an alteration in descending inhibitory signals. This is the key point in all neuropathic pain syndromes. The transition from nociceptive pain to neuropathic pain is likely multifactorial and differs from individual to individual. Whether the transforming event is a "lesion" with subsequent deafferentation in the classic lesion-oriented model of traditional neurology or whether the transforming event is more one of processing, thus raising the possibility that the transformation is physiologically based, is irrelevant in terms of the clinical manifestation. Ultimately, the central nervous system expression of neuropathic pain involves similar pathways, and the overlap between physiologic dysfunction and physical dysfunction becomes blurred, both causally and from a management viewpoint.

Patients who suffer with postherpetic neuralgia typically describe a burning, stabbing, or lancinating pain along the affected dermatome. Pain is unremitting and hypersensitive to touch, and this leads to considerable behavioral changes to protect this region of the body. As with all neuropathic pain states, treatment directed to the peripheral nerve alone is unrewarding; successful management involves a multidisciplinary approach. Future research efforts are directed at a preventative vaccine in the elderly and other at-risk individuals.[69]

Diabetic Peripheral Neuropathy

Peripheral neuropathy develops in up to 60% to 70% of patients with diabetes.[70] A substantial number of such patients present with neuropathic pain, but no clear distinguishing peripheral nerve feature is found between patients with diabetic neuropathic pain and those who have a nonpainful peripheral neuropathy.[71] Diabetic peripheral neuropathy is another example of how peripheral nociceptive pain transforms into neuropathic pain through dysfunction of the nervous system.

Patients with painful diabetic neuropathy typically have pain in a stocking distribution. Pain is often burning and may be sharp or lancinating. Often, pain is worse in a recumbent position and is somewhat better with weight bearing. There may be associated allodynia (hypersensitivity to touch), thus leading to avoidance type behavior. Patients often have severe interruption of sleep because the pain is typically worse at nighttime. Other aspects of the patient's life, as with all neuropathic pain syndromes, are often affected, with a breakdown of affect, social support, and self esteem.[72] Treatment directed simply at the peripheral nerves is not successful.

Complex Regional Pain Syndrome

Complex regional pain syndrome, formerly known as reflex sympathetic dystrophy, is a controversial neuropathic pain condition.[2,3,6,14] Unlike postherpetic neuralgia and diabetic neuropathy, the inciting event of complex regional pain syndrome may not be so evident. Very often, the inciting event is a seemingly innocuous injury to the soft tissue, and the perceived injury then becomes transformed into an unrelenting, debilitating pain syndrome. The term reflex sympathetic dystrophy, although still commonly in use, was changed in favor of complex regional pain syndrome because the pain of complex regional pain syndrome is not simply related to dysfunction of the sympathetic nervous system; in addition, dystrophic changes are not universal, and the transformation from an inciting event into chronic pain is not reflexive. Complex regional pain syndrome is divided into type I, no evidence of peripheral nerve injury, and type II, documented peripheral nerve injury.[73]

Complex regional pain syndrome illustrates the enormous complexity of neuropathic pain. Often, the inciting event is a seemingly trivial trauma. Indeed, the inciting event can be so trivial that patients are often led to believe they are fabricating the pain. In addition, because no clear cut, satisfactory pathophysiologic explanation exists for the severe transformed pain, some authors have even doubted the neuropathic nature of this syndrome and have concluded that complex regional pain syndrome is a somatoform disorder.[74]

Complex regional pain syndrome is diagnosed with the following four diagnostic criteria: (1) the presence of an initiating noxious event for a cause of immobilization; (2) continuing pain, allodynia, or hyperalgesia with which the pain is disproportionate to any inciting event; (3) evidence at some time of edema, changes in skin blood flow, or abnormal sudomotor activity in the region of the pain; and (4) the condition is excluded by the existence of a condition that otherwise would account for the degree of pain and dysfunction.[75] Thus, the diagnosis is made on clinical grounds, taking into account objective, autonomic nervous system pathophysiology; complex regional pain syndrome is not simply a diagnosis of exclusion.

Augmented autonomic (sympathetic) activity early in the course of complex regional pain syndrome led to sympathetic blockade becoming one of the hallmarks of treatment. Although pain relief from sympathetic blockade helps to support the diagnosis of complex regional pain syndrome, sympathetically independent neuropathic pain develops early in the course of this condition and is unresponsive to peripheral sympathetic blockade.[76,77]

Some authors have argued that complex regional pain syndrome has nothing to do with the sympathetic nervous system, confusing the difference between transient sympathetic nervous system dysfunction and transformed neuropathic pain.[78,79] The sometimes seemingly trivial inciting event of complex regional pain syndrome has led some to speculate that this is an emotionally based condition. However, no identifiable psychologic predisposition to the development of complex regional pain syndrome has been identified.[80,81]

Pain From Central Nervous System Injury

A variety of chronic pain states have been described after well-documented central nervous system injury, including trauma, multiple sclerosis, cerebrovascular accidents, infections, spinal cord syrinx, and neoplasms.[82–86] All have in common a well-documented lesion of the central nervous system. However, what is not clear is why some patients with such lesions have development of a transformed pain syndrome, whereas others with the same lesion have development of a neurologic deficit without neuropathic pain. The clinical manifestations of neuropathic pain can become the overwhelming presentation in such patients, with development of the same comorbidities as individuals with other neuropathic pain syndromes.[87,88]

Diagnosis

History

Clinicians can confidently diagnose neuropathic pain by taking a careful history, performing a focused physical examination, and judiciously using ancillary diagnostic studies.[22] When obtaining a history, understanding the presenting characteristic of pain is important. The five most important characteristics are: (1) temporal qualities, including: acute, recurrent, or chronic; daily variation; onset and duration; (2) intensity, including: average pain; pain at its worst; pain at its least; pain at the time of history taking; (3) topography, including: localized versus regional pain, superficial versus deep pain, and focal versus radiating pain; (4) quality, including: burning; aching; freezing; stabbing; electric shock-like; tooth achy; cramping; knifelike; and (5) palliative and precipitating factors, including: physical activities; emotional stressors; nutritional triggers; and circadian rhythms.

Use of a rapid rating scale, such as the Brief Pain Inventory or the Visual Analog Scale, is beneficial for patients.[89] Patients rate temporal aspects of pain from 0 (no pain) to 10 (the worst imaginable pain). Such rating scales are not only helpful in following patients but also aid in understanding the relationship between the patient and pain. Some patients rate their pain as a constant "10," yet they appear in no acute distress, which suggests a disassociation between their perception of pain and their physical manifestations.

Clinicians should spend considerable time trying to understand the inciting event of pain. This may provide insight into a disease state or injury that has otherwise been underdiagnosed. In addition, understanding the patient's perception of the inciting event is critical and takes into account life experiences.[14,54] Daily activities need to be considered, including physical limitations of pain and the amount of daily exercise. Some patients are so debilitated that they are essentially homebound, performing little in the way of even sedentary activities. The support system must be explored, including the immediate family and the patient's work environment, if appropriate. Often, patients with neuropathic pain feel alone and abandoned and essentially become imprisoned with pain. Many patients have discontinued all sexual activity as a manifestation of depression, rejection, or fear that such activity will further exacerbate pain.

In addition to a general medical history, careful attention must be paid to any prior psychiatric conditions or prior episodes of prolonged pain-related conditions. This history may provide important insight into the patient's adaptive responses over time. Childhood trauma must be considered, although probing into childhood trauma must be done in a delicate and noninvasive manner. Although a high incidence rate of childhood trauma and abuse is found in patients with chronic pain, one cannot suggest or assume that a patient with neuropathic pain has experienced such trauma. The role of stress in the exacerbation and maintenance of pain should be explored. Alcohol and drug histories are critical because one facet of chronic neuropathic pain treatment may be the use of opioid analgesics.[54]

A careful search for comorbid medical conditions is important. The three most common comorbid conditions include depression, anxiety, and sleep deprivation. If these conditions are not managed properly, successful pain management is unlikely. Simple questions may suffice. For example, asking patients if they have felt depressed or hopeless, or if they have lost pleasure, may uncover an otherwise undiagnosed depression. Pain centers often use more formal depression scales as part of an initial assessment.[3,15] Family history may provide a clue to possible genetic predispositions to psychiatric disease, pain syndromes, or both.

The patient's expectations of treatment must be assessed.[63] Expectation that a simple procedure or medication will lead to a complete alleviation of pain is unrealistic. Realistic goals must be set. Too often, patients arrive with an expectation of obtaining a concise anatomic explanation of pain coupled with a quick-fix, simplistic treatment. Once the clinician begins to discuss neuropathic pain, patients may fail to understand the mind-body implications of this condition. This may lead patients to feel a lack of validation, which can undermine future treatments.

Once neuropathic pain is diagnosed, multidisciplinary management should begin. Patients need to appreciate that the ultimate goal of treatment is to reduce pain, increase function, and improve quality of life. The focus on complete cessation of pain alone may lead to treatment failure. Patients should feel that they are in an integral component of treatment and they are ideally participating in the process and not simply focused on a cure of their pain.[14]

Physical Examination

Careful physical examination should include vital signs, a focused musculoskeletal and extremity examination, and a neurologic examination. Patients with neuropathic pain generally do not present in acute distress, and vital signs should be stable. The musculoskeletal examination may show evidence of chronic maladaptation as a result of prolonged muscle spasm and avoidance-type behavior or may reveal evidence of active mechanical signs of an entrapped nerve or of an irritated spinal segment.

The extremity examination may show altered autonomic activity, for example, a change in hair growth or nail bed pattern, a change in extremity color or temperature, or extremity swelling out of proportion to injury. Such changes are the hallmark of complex regional pain syndrome. Patients with diabetes may present with diminution in peripheral blood flow, which can aggravate peripheral neuropathic pain.

The sensory aspect of a neurologic examination is exceedingly important. In addition to testing for the presence or absence of primary sensory modality perception (vibration, proprioception, light touch, and pinprick), the examiner should test for alterations in sensory experience that are consistent with neuropathic pain. Allodynia is hypersensitive pain in response to a normally non-noxious mild stimulus. Hyperalgesia indicates an increased sensation of pain in response to a normally painful stimulus, such as a pinprick. Hyperpathia is a prolonged painful experience after pinprick assessment.

Other aspects of the neurologic examination may be abnormal, either as a result of a documented lesion or as a functional aberration from central nervous system dysfunction. For example, dystonia has been well described in complex regional pain syndrome or in patients with a basal ganglia lesion.[90] Tremor may develop with peripheral neuropathy or may manifest as a physiologic aberration in chronic pain.

Ancillary Studies

Ancillary studies should be used to help diagnose medical conditions that can mimic or comingle with the patient's clinical condition. For example, deep venous thrombosis presents as extremity swelling and abnormal temperature sensation and can sometimes mimic complex regional pain syndrome or coexist with this condition. MRI of the lumbar spine can sometimes uncover a lesion in the cauda equina that can mimic the clinical manifestations of chronic low back without an identifiable nociceptive cause. Electromyography (EMG) and nerve conduction studies can differentiate active denervation along a nerve dermatome that may manifest concomitantly with chronic postlaminectomy neuropathic pain. Ultimately, all ancillary diagnostic tests are taken in conjunction with the history and examination to secure a diagnosis that then becomes the springboard for effective management.

Management

Treatment for neuropathic pain should be multidisciplinary.[91] Although many pain centers focus on anesthesiology-based procedures, such procedures are but one aspect of an important component of successful pain management. A general discussion of the principles of multidisciplinary treatment follows; such principles can be applied to any neuropathic pain state. Treatment must be individualized for the physical manifestation of pain and the patient's psychosocial adaptation.

Psychologic Therapies

Because of the high prevalence rate of depression and anxiety with neuropathic pain, psychologic therapies are an important component of successful neuropathic pain management.[92,93] Although patients may be resistant to psychologic therapies, fearing that their pain is viewed as "psychosomatic," clinicians must stress the importance of psychologic intervention because this not only helps manage depression and coping skills but may also uncover a previously undiagnosed repressed trauma or other significant life event.[54]

Cognitive-behavioral therapy helps patients understand the interplay of pain perception, affect, and daily thought patterns. The focus is to develop positive thoughts in patients.[94] This type of therapy also implements specific cognitive-behavioral techniques such as relaxation training and biofeedback, which enable positive pain coping skills. Patients with neuropathic pain may resist insight-oriented therapy. The author's experience is that many patients with neuropathic pain are sufficiently disassociated from their emotions that such therapy is not possible. Insight-oriented therapy should only be recommended once a trusting bond forms between the patient and the clinician and a solid clinical foundation exists to explore a relationship between emotions and neuropathic pain. Group therapy is extremely beneficial, especially for patients who feel they are uniquely alone in their neuropathic pain experience. Family therapy becomes important in helping other family members understand that neuropathic pain is a real medical condition. Patients need to be validated within the family, and they also need to understand that at times they isolate themselves from their family because of pain.

In some cases, acute psychiatric intervention becomes necessary in chronic pain management. Long-term treatment is sometimes associated with a sudden insight or flashback into previously unrecognized trauma, severe depression, or poorly managed anxiety,[54] and a skilled psychiatrist may be needed to help manage such conditions.

Pharmacologic Therapy

Several pharmacologic strategies are used in treatment of chronic pain.[95] A general discussion follows of various classes of drugs frequently used in neuropathic pain management. The best-studied conditions for use of pharmacologic management are diabetic neuropathic pain and postherpetic neuralgia. Other neuropathic pain syndromes are less well studied regarding efficacy of pharmacologic therapy. Nonetheless, several generalizable treatment strategies exist.

Anticonvulsants

Anticonvulsants are first-line pharmacologic treatment for neuropathic pain syndromes.[96–98] Carbamazepine, phenytoin, valproate, and clonazepam were the first anticonvulsants to be well studied in treatment of neuropathic pain, especially with such conditions as trigeminal neuralgia and diabetic peripheral neuropathy.[97] Gabapentin has been well documented in many well-controlled studies as an effective medication for treatment of postherpetic neuralgia and other neuropathic pain conditions.[97–99] The list has extended to several other anticonvulsants, including pregabalin, topiramate, oxcarbazepine, lamotrigene, zonisamide, valproate, and levetiracetam.[22,100–106]

Anticonvulsants reduce neuronal hyperexcitability. Their effectiveness in treatment of neuropathic pain is through several different primary mechanisms, including reduction of neuronal influx of sodium and calcium; indirect or direct enhancement of the inhibitory effects of γ-aminobutyric acid; and reduction in activity of the excitatory neurotransmitter glutamate through depletion of its storage sites or through blockade of NMDA receptors.[107]

The initial choice of drugs should be based on clinician comfort and relative indications. One can take advantage of the side-effect profile of some medications, for example, topiramate for weight loss and zonisamide for sedative side effects. Anticonvulsants are administered with the dosing schedules commonly used for treatment of epilepsy. Generally speaking, only one anticonvulsant should be prescribed at a time, and upward titration should be based on efficacy and tolerability.[105] Anticonvulsants may be used in conjunction with other medications described subsequently. Only gabapentin and pregabalin are approved by the US Food and Drug Administration (FDA) for treatment of neuropathic pain, specifically postherpetic neuralgia and diabetic neuropathic pain.

Antidepressants

Antidepressants, like anticonvulsants, are first-line pharmacologic treatment for neuropathic pain. Numerous studies have established the efficacy of tricyclic antidepressants (TCAs) in treatment of a variety of neuropathic pain disorders.[22,105,107–110] Indeed, tricyclic antidepressants may be more efficacious in treatment of diabetic neuropathic pain than pregabalin, gabapentin, serotonin selective reuptake inhibitors (SSRIs), and serotonin-norepinephrine reuptake inhibitors (SNRIs).[111] In addition, a combination of a tricyclic antidepressant with gabapentin may be more effective than use of either drug alone in treatment of diabetic neuropathic pain.[112] The sedative side effects of TCAs often provide a useful adjunct in treatment of patients with comorbid sleep deprivation. Because of potential anticholinergic and cardiac side effects, TCAs are typically begun in low dosage (10 mg nightly) and titrated upward as tolerated and needed.

Serotonin selective reuptake inhibitors, serotonin-norepinephrine reuptake inhibitors, and norepinephrine-dopamine reuptake inhibitors are also effective in treatment of neuropathic pain.[22,105,107,111,113–117] These agents become particularly useful when patients present with comorbid depression, anxiety, or both. Antidepressants alleviate neuropathic pain primarily through their ability to modulate descending pain pathways by blocking the reuptake of norepinephrine and serotonin.[118] Antidepressants may also reduce hyperexcitability by blocking sodium and calcium channels and by binding to adenosine and NMDA receptors.[107] In addition, antidepressants may improve neuropathic pain by improving comorbid conditions of depression and anxiety.[119–121]

Opioid Analgesics

Opioid analgesics are the most potent prescription analgesics. Although wide acceptance is seen for prescribing opioid analgesics in cancer patients, acceptance is not so universal in treatment of patients without cancer.[14] Problems arise because of a lack of acceptance in using such medication long term in patients without cancer, combined with a fear of causing drug addiction.[15,122]

Common practice in pain medicine clinics is for patients to sign a controlled substance agreement if they are to begin chronic opioid analgesic treatment. Such agreements help provide clarity with regard to intent of opioid usage and the manner in which medications will be used. The controlled substance agreement usually stipulates that patients may only obtain opioid analgesics from one physician, may only use one pharmacy, and may only take medication in the manner prescribed. Patients must return for monthly visits, and they are subject to random drug screening. Although a contract may seem harsh, the medical literature supports the usage of such contracts, which help to minimize opioid analgesic abuse by drug-seeking patients.[94]

Initially, short-acting opioid analgesics should be prescribed. When a patient's daily opioid need is discerned, clinicians should switch to a long-acting medication, which enables patients to obtain a steady state of pain relief. Short-acting opioids taken on an as-needed basis can reinforce pain and may lead to addiction.[123] Once a long-acting medication has been prescribed, short-acting medications should be used for breakthrough pain only. When patients with neuropathic pain take opiate analgesics for legitimate medical reasons (i.e., for pain control), there is little risk that patients will become addicted to these medications.[124,125] Addiction is a broader behavioral phenomenon in which individuals plan their lives in an obsessive manner around obtaining and taking a particular substance (opioids, alcohol) or around participating in a certain activity (gambling, sex). Patients may develop tolerance to opiate analgesics, necessitating an increased dosage, or they may become dependent on the medication after long-term use, meaning that sudden medication discontinuation would cause drug withdrawal.

Tramadol hydrochloride is a unique opioid-like medication. Tramadol does have weak mu-opioid receptor agonism and also enhances the inhibitory affect of descending serotonergic and adrenergic systems. Tramadol is efficacious in a variety of neuropathic pain conditions and can be used as a first-line medication before a more traditional opioid analgesic is prescribed.[105]

Topical Analgesics

The most well-studied topical analgesic is a 5% lidocaine patch,[126] which may be especially useful in well-localized pain syndromes such as postherpetic neuralgia. Capsaicin may also be effective in relatively localized neuropathic pain conditions. High-concentration (8%) capsaicin dermal patch, applied locally for 1 hour, may provide sustained pain relief in patients with postherpetic neuralgia and painful HIV neuropathy.[127,128]

Other Adjunctive Medications

Tizanidine is a centrally acting alpha₂-adrenergic agonist with prominent antispasticity effects. This medication may be an important adjunct in patients who present with chronic muscle spasm or tension-type headache.[107] Baclofen, a GABA agonist, may benefit patients with chronic muscle spasm or paroxysmal pain.[129] In addition, intrathecal baclofen is effective in reducing both spasticity and pain in patients with spinal cord injury and other central pain syndromes with spasticity.[130,131] Mexiletine is an antiarrhythmic drug with demonstrable efficacy in treatment of some neuropathic pain conditions. Clonidine, another central alpha₂-adrenergic agonist, may be helpful in treatment of complex regional pain syndrome and related conditions when taken orally or transdermally.[107] Neuroleptics and benzodiazapines are sometimes useful in and of themselves or in treatment of comorbid conditions.[132]

Pulse therapy with corticosteroids or nonsteroidal antiinflammatory drugs should be considered when patients have development of acute musculoskeletal pain superimposed on chronic neuropathic pain. For example, some patients with chronic low back pain have acute radicular pain develop with active, mechanical stretch signs on examination. In such patients, a 1-week to 2-week course of nonsteroidal antiinflammatory drugs or oral corticosteroids can help break the cycle of acute or chronic pain. Long-term corticosteroid and nonsteroidal antiinflammatory drug usage has little role in the treatment of chronic, neuropathic pain.[14]

Some evidence shows that NMDA receptor antagonists ameliorate chronic neuropathic pain. Ketamine infusions have been studied, but the high toxicity rate of hallucinations and anorexia limit this medication's usefulness. Smaller doses of ketamine may be useful in select circumstances.[133,134] Oral NMDA receptor antagonist drugs have shown little efficacy in treatment of chronic, neuropathic pain.

Interventional Strategies

Several anesthesiology-based interventions are appropriate as one aspect of multidisciplinary pain management. A mistaken notion in some pain practices is that management should be primarily intervention based. Indeed, in some practices, the failure of one intervention leads to an escalation in intervention strategies, often to the detriment of the patient.[135]

Therapeutic injections may be helpful for diagnostic purposes and may sometimes provide an important break in the chronic cycle of pain.[136] Once a successful therapeutic injection is obtained, physical therapy and other strategies should be used immediately to help the patient overcome maladaptive postures. Sympathetic blockade, which by definition does not include primary sensory or somatic block, has been used both diagnostically and therapeutically in complex regional pain syndrome and related conditions.[137] However, the lack of benefit from sympathetic blockade does not preclude the diagnosis of complex regional pain syndrome. As with other therapeutic injections, a successful sympathetic blockade should be followed immediately by progressive physical therapy.[138,139]

Epidural and transforaminal corticosteroid injections may benefit patients with back conditions that have a demonstrable mechanical component, such as lumbar disc herniation and lumbar stenosis.[140] Similarly, facet blocks may facilitate breaking the cycle of chronic facet locking or provide transient relief in patients with segmental lumbar instability.[141] Such relief allows the patient to begin more progressive physical therapy strategies.[14]

Spinal cord stimulation relies on the principle that a stimulator, placed in the dorsal spinal cord, blocks central pain processing from a peripheral pain generator. Spinal cord stimulators should be considered only in patients who have relatively well-localized extremity or axial pain and who have exhausted all other treatment strategies.[142] Too often, spinal cord stimulators are placed as part of a rapid escalation in interventional techniques, when other multidisciplinary strategies have been neglected.[14]

Intrathecal administration of opioid analgesics takes advantage of very low–dose opioid coupled with strong binding to spinal cord receptors, with minimal systemic side effects. Such strategies are particularly useful in patients who have shown a positive effect to opioid analgesics but who cannot tolerate systemic side effects.[143] These medications may be combined with intrathecal clonidine, which also has independent pain-alleviating effects, and baclofen, which may be useful in alleviating spasticity.

Other surgical interventions must be approached with caution, including spinal surgery. Other than for trigeminal neuralgia, placing a lesion in the nervous system or performing decompressive surgery in an attempt to alleviate chronic, neuropathic pain pathway has yielded equivocal results.[135]

Physical Therapy

Most patients with neuropathic pain have developed several maladaptive physical manifestations. This is especially so in patients with chronic low back pain, but it also holds true for patients with severe extremity neuropathic pain. Physical therapy should be an important consideration in treatment of chronic neuropathic pain.[14]

Some physical therapy, such as craniosacral technique and myofascial release, is more intuitive and may help patients understand the link between physiology and physical pain perception.[14] In these therapies, patients lie on a table and are extremely quiet, and the therapy is quite subtle. More conventional physical therapy includes the use of a transcutaneous electrical nerve stimulation (TENS) unit, which may alleviate localized pain, and the use of other modalities. In addition, range-of-motion strengthening exercises and spine stabilization exercises help overcome chronic maladaptations.

Complementary Strategies

Acupuncture is recognized by the World Health Organization as an effective treatment for pain. Several evidenced-based studies show the efficacy of acupuncture in treatment of pain, although the difficulty of employing sham acupuncture leads to methodologic flaws.[144] Acupuncture is not a stand-alone treatment but should be considered as part of a multidisciplinary approach, especially in patients who wish to explore nonpharmacologic strategies.

Nutritional counseling should be considered in patients with chronic neuropathic pain. Some patients have poor eating habits, often as a result of chronic nausea or depression. Other patients have a diet that consists primarily of high-carbohydrate and high-fat or junk food intake; we can never underestimate the immediate gratifying effects of such foods, and poor eating habits often become part of a cycle of self treating underlying anxiety and depression.[145]

Massage therapy can be used both to desensitize areas of hyperalgesia and to help alleviate muscular and emotional stress. In some cases, massage therapy becomes a transition into developing greater insight into the interplay between physiology and physical pain perception.[146]

Mirror Therapy

Mirror therapy has proven efficacious for neuropathic pain treatment, notably phantom limb pain and complex regional pain syndrome. Mirror therapy consists of putting a patient in a rectangular box with a mirror placed vertically and sagittally. Patients place their affected limb (the limb with neuropathic pain) in the nonreflecting side of the mirror, and the normal limb is placed on the reflecting side. When the patient is told to move the normal limb, they receive the visual impression that the painful limb is moving normally and without pain; thus, the illusion is that the neuropathic limb has been restored.

Mirror therapy can lead to remarkable improvement in limb function and pain perception. Authors postulate that mirror therapy is efficacious because visual stimuli override tactile and proprioceptive stimuli.[147,148] This postulation furthers the argument that pain pathways are not simple hierarchic, autonomous modules, but are rather in a state of dynamic mind-body equilibrium with connections that adapt according to changes in the environment and perception.

Conclusion

Neuropathic pain is a neuropsychiatric condition in which pain is initiated or caused by a primary lesion or dysfunction in the nervous system. Understanding the complexity of neuropathic pain becomes the cornerstone for appropriate diagnosis and management. Successful management depends on realistic patient-physician expectations and an individualized, multidisciplinary approach that takes advantage of the ever-evolving armamentarium of evidenced-based treatments.

References

Full references for this chapter can be found on www.expertconsult.com.

Section III

Generalized Pain Syndromes Encountered in Clinical Practice

Part A

Acute Pain Syndromes

Chapter 24

Management of Acute and Postoperative Pain

Steven D. Waldman

Pain is the most common medical symptom among civilized populations. The National Pain Survey[1] estimated that more than 76 million Americans have pain that is severe enough to need medical care. In this survey of individuals with pain severe enough to seek medical attention, 25 million had acute pain as a result of surgery or trauma, with other causes of acute pain further increasing this number. Societal costs of pain in terms of medical bills, reduced productivity, and absenteeism are staggering. Although much of the medical and lay literature focuses on chronic pain, acute pain is also a major problem. About 8% of the US population experiences acute or postoperative pain each year; this figure is relatively constant throughout the industrialized nations of the world.

Despite the high prevalence worldwide, acute and postoperative pain is poorly managed, as studies have repeatedly shown.[2,3] The following factors are noted in discussions of the reasons for inadequate pain management:

- Appropriate adjuvant drugs, such as simple analgesics and nonsteroidal anti-inflammatory drugs (NSAIDs), are often overlooked.
- Patients receive significantly fewer opioids than are ordered by their physicians.
- Nursing staff and physicians are overly concerned about drug addiction.

- Selection of analgesics is often irrational and confined to a limited number of the available options.
- Physicians' knowledge of the nature and properties of the analgesics selected is often inadequate.

Physicians can do many things to help minimize and alleviate needless suffering from acute or postoperative pain.[2] This chapter provides an overview of strategies that are useful in management of acute pain syndromes commonly encountered in clinical practice. Each approach has advantages and disadvantages. Armed with an understanding of the individual patient's needs, physicians can provide optimal pain relief that results in a high degree of patient satisfaction.

Prophylactic Measures Useful in Management of Acute and Postoperative Pain

An explanation of the cause and the expected course of acute or postoperative pain in detail can do much to alleviate patient stress and anxiety. In addition, the use of relaxation techniques (e.g., breathing and body maneuvers) may help relieve pain. In surgery, subsequent postoperative pain can be decreased with gentle intubation, careful positioning and transfer of the patient, adequate muscle relaxation, and minimization of surgical trauma.

Pharmacologic Measures

Nonsteroidal Anti-Inflammatory Drugs

NSAIDs are a chemically heterogeneous class of drugs that can reduce fever, pain, and inflammation without producing chemical dependence.[4] Regardless of their diverse structures, all NSAIDs decrease inflammation by their inhibitory effect on prostaglandin synthesis (**Fig. 24.1**).[5] NSAIDs also inhibit platelet function, decrease white blood cell chemotaxis, and impede production of the byproducts of inflammation and the chemical messengers of pain. All of these actions may explain in part the efficacy of this class of drugs in the management of many of the acute pain syndromes frequently seen in clinical practice.

Selection of Nonsteroidal Anti-Inflammatory Drugs

Many NSAIDs are available. Busy clinicians need not be familiar with each drug, but they should have a working knowledge of one or two agents in each of the pharmacologic groups, as follows:

- Proprionic acid derivatives: ibuprofen and naproxen
- Salicylates: aspirin and choline salicylate
- Anthranilic acid derivatives: indomethacin and ketorolac
- Oxicams: piroxicam
- Cyclooxygenase-2 inhibitors: celecoxib

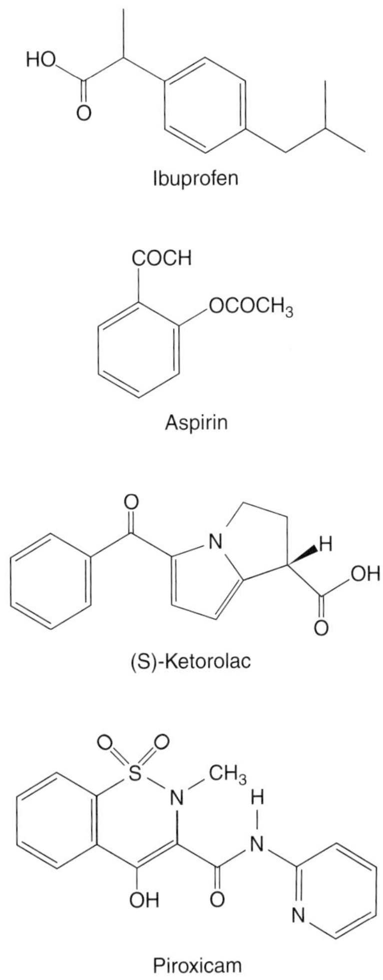

For each drug, physicians should be aware of the need for a loading dose, time from onset of activity to peak effect, routes of administration, cost, and side-effect profile. Also, efficacy may be enhanced by choosing a drug that can be given via a nonoral route (e.g., rectal administration of indomethacin, intramuscular administration of ketorolac tromethamine). By capitalizing on the unique properties of each drug, physicians can tailor a treatment plan to meet each individual patient's needs. **Table 24.1** lists practical suggestions for choosing an NSAID.

Because of the great variation in dosage ranges and frequency of administration of NSAIDs, physicians should review carefully the properties of the agent chosen. In general, dosing should be started at the low end of the recommended range and titrated upward as therapeutic response and side effects dictate. A loading dose should be used if indicated, especially for abortive treatment of headache. Under no circumstances should the recommended ceiling dose be exceeded. **Table 24.2** lists practical suggestions for administering NSAIDs.

Side Effects of Nonsteroidal Anti-Inflammatory Drugs

Considering their diversity in chemical structure, NSAIDs are extremely well tolerated. In addition, compared with all of the other drugs currently used in treatment of acute pain, NSAIDs have among the most favorable risk-to-benefit ratios.[6] As with all medications, NSAIDs can cause side effects, ranging from minor annoyances (e.g., dyspepsia, diarrhea, constipation) to life-threatening conditions (e.g., gastrointestinal hemorrhage, hepatic dysfunction, renal insufficiency).[7] Consequently, physicians need to anticipate the potential for side effects and choose and use NSAIDs appropriately.

Fig. 24.1 The heterogeneous structures of some common nonsteroidal anti-inflammatory drugs.

Table 24.1 Guidelines for Choosing a Nonsteroidal Anti-Inflammatory Drug

Assess patient's renal, cardiac, and gastrointestinal status before starting drug treatment.

Determine best route of administration.

Identify drugs that are appropriate for route of administration desired.

Select familiar agent among the drugs whose time between onset of activity and peak effect is appropriate for pain syndrome being treated.

Table 24.2 Guidelines for Administering Nonsteroidal Anti-Inflammatory Drugs

Review properties of agent selected.

Start at low end of dosing range.

Use loading dose when appropriate.

Do not exceed ceiling dose.

Ensure that equianalgesic doses are given if route of administration is changed.

NSAIDs can cause a decline in renal function in patients at high risk, such as patients with hypertensive or diabetic nephropathy, or with overuse or misuse. Because identification of patients with borderline renal function purely on clinical grounds is often impossible, the clinician faced with a patient who has acute or postoperative pain should strongly consider obtaining a baseline measurement of the serum creatinine level before beginning NSAID therapy. This measurement alerts physicians to preexisting renal problems that may be exacerbated by NSAID use and enables them to attribute to the drug any changes in renal function that occur during therapy in patients who had normal function at baseline.[8]

NSAIDs generally should be taken with food to minimize gastrointestinal side effects. A history of dyspepsia and gastrointestinal upset may indicate the need for the concurrent use of gastric cytoprotective agents. A history of gastric ulceration or hemorrhage necessitates that NSAIDs be used only after medications that are free of gastrointestinal side effects have failed to control the pain adequately. In this event, histamine blocking and cytoprotective agents should be given concurrently with NSAIDs and patients should be monitored carefully for occult gastrointestinal blood loss. NSAID therapy should be discontinued at the first sign of gastrointestinal difficulties.

The concurrent use of two or more NSAIDs increases the risk of side effects, as may the concurrent use of an NSAID and a simple analgesic (e.g., acetaminophen). Patients with acute pain must be questioned carefully about their use of over-the-counter agents because patients may fail to mention such use during the initial pain evaluation.

Opioid Analgesics

Effective use of opioids for acute pain requires a working knowledge of their potency, opioid class, side effects or toxicity, and duration of effect and the principles of dosing. Regardless of the route of administration, failure to take these factors into account can result in suboptimal pain relief.

Potency

"Weak" opioids are those typically administered orally to patients with mild to moderate pain. These include preparations that contain codeine, propoxyphene, oxycodone hydrochloride, meperidine hydrochloride, pentazocine hydrochloride, or hydrocodone bitartrate. None of these drugs has a ceiling dose, but at high doses, their use may be limited by side effects or toxicity (e.g., seizures from meperidine or propoxyphene, psychotomimetic effects from pentazocine, gastrointestinal intolerance from codeine).[9] "Strong" opioids include morphine sulfate, methadone hydrochloride, levorphanol tartrate, hydromorphone hydrochloride, and fentanyl citrate. These drugs also seem to have no ceiling dose in terms of analgesia, but side effects (e.g., respiratory and central nervous system depression) may limit upward titration of doses to obtain pain relief.

Class

Opioids can be divided into pure agonists (i.e., morphine, hydromorphone, methadone, levorphanol, meperidine, codeine, propoxyphene, fentanyl, hydrocodone, and oxycodone) and agonist-antagonists (i.e., pentazocine, nalbuphine hydrochloride, butorphanol tartrate, buprenorphine hydrochloride, and dezocine; **Fig. 24.2**).[10] The agonist-antagonist class is characterized by a balance of agonism and competitive antagonism at

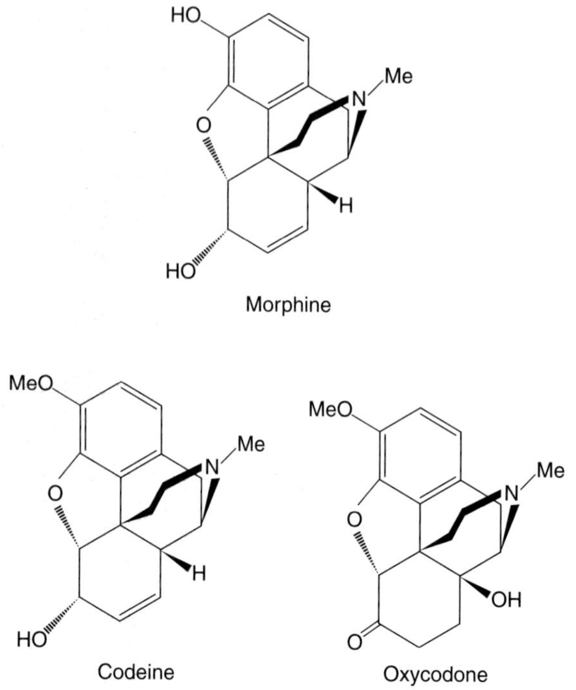

Fig. 24.2 Some common opioid agonists.

one or more of the opiate receptors.[9,11] All agonist-antagonist agents have a ceiling effect above which respiratory depression occurs and analgesic effect reaches its capacity. These agents have the potential to reverse such agonist effects as analgesia and a lesser propensity than pure opioid agonists to produce physical dependence. Administration of an agonist-antagonist agent to a patient who is physically dependent on an agonist agent may cause an acute opioid abstinence syndrome, which may be confused with uncontrolled pain. Agonist-antagonists, particularly pentazocine, also have prominent psychotomimetic effects.[9,11] The lack of an oral form of most of these agents may limit their clinical utility in the acute pain setting; however, dezocine may have a special place in the management of postoperative pain and warrants further evaluation.[10]

Toxicity

Because meperidine is commonly used, special mention should be made of its potential toxicity when taken long term or in high doses, as may occur with patient-controlled analgesia. Meperidine is metabolized to normeperidine.[11] This compound has a half-life about four times that of the parent drug, and its accumulation in plasma may result in signs of central nervous system excitation (e.g., myoclonus, tremor, seizures). The risk of toxicity precludes the long-term or high-dose use of meperidine in the management of acute or postoperative pain.

Duration of Effect and Dosing

These factors are an important consideration in opioid selection. Opioids with a short half-life (e.g., hydrocodone, oxycodone, morphine, hydromorphone) must be administered at least every 4 hours, whereas methadone, the opioid with the longest half-life, usually can be given every 6 hours.[9,11] If around-the-clock dosing in a frequency appropriate to the chosen opioid is not provided, periods of inadequate pain control result.

In patients with moderate pain that is not relieved with simple analgesics and NSAIDs, a reasonable next step is the addition of a weak opioid analgesic (e.g., 30 to 60 mg of codeine or 5 mg of oxycodone plus 325 mg of acetaminophen, aspirin, or another NSAID). The dose of the opioid can be increased until side effects or toxicity preclude further increases. If a weak opioid does not provide adequate pain relief, therapy with a strong opioid alone or in combination with simple analgesics or NSAIDs is indicated. Morphine elixir, 5 to 10 mg every 4 hours, is a reasonable choice. In elderly patients and patients with compromised hepatic or renal function, the starting dose should be low to avoid side effects.

If pain remains severe after the initial dose of a strong opioid, the dose can be doubled. If partial analgesia occurs, daily dose titration is usually appropriate. An effective approach involves the concurrent use of a fixed around-the-clock dose, usually every 4 hours, together with a "rescue dose," which is usually equal to 5% to 10% of the total daily dose and is administered every 1 to 2 hours as needed for "breakthrough" pain. This approach provides patients with some control over analgesic dosing and can be used to estimate the amount of opioid patients need.

Route of Administration of Opioid Analgesics

Oral administration of opioids is preferred whenever patients with acute pain can tolerate it. Other routes are available, however, and each has specific advantages and disadvantages.

INTRAMUSCULAR ADMINISTRATION

In patients who are unable to take medication orally, opioids can be administered intramuscularly.[12] Disadvantages of this route include pain on administration, variable and sometimes slow onset of effect, and peaks and valleys of analgesic effect.[12]

INTRAVENOUS BOLUS

Delivery of opioids via intravenous bolus has the advantages of a rapid onset of effect and a high level of efficacy in terms of pain relief.[9,11,12] Compared with the use of pumps and patient-controlled analgesia devices, this method of drug administration is relatively inexpensive. Disadvantages include more pronounced peaks and valleys of analgesic effect and side effects and a relatively short duration of analgesic.[12]

CONTINUOUS INFUSION

Continuous infusion of opioids achieves a high level of pain relief when the minimal effective analgesic concentration has been reached.[11,12] Peaks and valleys of effect are decreased with this route of administration, which results in fewer side effects than are seen with intravenous bolus or intramuscular administration of opioids. Generally, the level of patient satisfaction is high.

One disadvantage of continuous infusions of opioids is the significant delay in onset of analgesic activity if a bolus dose is not given with the infusion. Another is that the cost, in terms of infusions and the labor needed during setup and monitoring, is considerable. Also, the nursing staff may express some resistance to this method because of a perceived possibility of an increased risk of respiratory depression and other side effects.[13]

PATIENT-CONTROLLED ANALGESIA

Many of the objections to continuous infusion of opioids have been overcome with the advent of patient-controlled analgesia devices. Instead of medical personnel determining an appropriate infusion regimen and administering it, the patient is given an element of control.[14] The drug administration rate is titrated against the desired end point—analgesia.

Advantages of patient-controlled analgesia include a high level of efficacy after the minimal effective analgesic concentration has been reached, lower rates of side effects than are seen with other methods, and high patient satisfaction.[12] These advantages have led to the rapid acceptance of patient-controlled analgesia in the treatment of acute and postoperative pain. Labor and cost savings also are positive factors. Disadvantages include the cost of the device and the drugs used with it, the significant delay in implementation in some institutions that do not use this method routinely, the need for special pumps and supplies that may not be readily available, and significant nursing staff resistance at some institutions.[13]

Neural Blockade in the Management of Acute and Postoperative Pain

Neural blockade with a local anesthetic may be used to identify specific pain pathways and to aid in diagnosis of the origin and site of the pain. Therapeutic neural blockade with a local anesthetic plus a corticosteroid, an opioid, or, rarely, a neurolytic agent can be useful in relieving a variety of acute pain syndromes. Neural blockade should not be viewed as stand-alone therapy for most acute pain syndromes; rather, it should be intelligently integrated into a comprehensive treatment plan.[15]

Sympathetic Neural Blockade
Sphenopalatine Ganglion
ANATOMY

Located in the pterygopalatine fossa, posterior to the middle turbinate, the sphenopalatine (i.e., pterygopalatine, nasal, or Meckel's) ganglion comprises the largest group of neurons in the head outside the brain. The ganglion, a triangular structure 5 mm in diameter, is covered by a layer of connective tissue and mucous membrane that is 1 to 5 mm thick. It gives rise to major branches of the trigeminal nerve, carotid plexus, facial nerve, and superior cervical ganglion.[16]

INDICATIONS

Blockade of the sphenopalatine ganglion with a local anesthetic is useful in the management of acute migraine, acute cluster headache, and a variety of facial neuralgias. It also may relieve status migrainosus and chronic cluster headache.[17–19]

TECHNIQUE

Blockade of the sphenopalatine ganglion is accomplished with application of a local anesthetic to the mucous membrane overlying the ganglion.[16] With the patient in the supine position, the cervical spine is extended, and the anterior nares space is inspected for polyps, tumors, and foreign bodies. A small amount of 2% lidocaine viscous solution, 4% lidocaine hydrochloride topical solution, or 10% cocaine hydrochloride solution is instilled into each

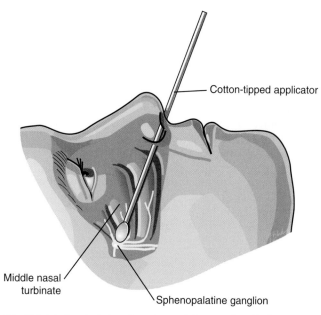

Fig. 24.3 Injection technique for sphenopalatine ganglion block. *(From Waldman SD: Sphenopalatine ganglion block. In Atlas of interventional pain management, ed 3, Philadelphia, 2009, Saunders, p 13.)*

nostril. The patient is asked to inhale briskly through the nose. This inhalation draws the local anesthetic into the posterior nasal pharynx, serving the double function of lubricating the nasal mucosa and providing topical anesthesia to allow easier passage of a 35-inch cotton-tipped applicator into each nostril.

These applicators are saturated with a local anesthetic and advanced along the superior border of the middle turbinate until the tip contacts the mucosa overlying the ganglion (**Fig. 24.3**). Local anesthetic (1.2 mL) is placed alongside each applicator, which acts as a tampon, keeping the anesthetic in contact with the mucosa overlying the ganglion and allowing it to diffuse through the mucosa to the ganglion. The applicators are removed after 20 minutes. The patient's pulse rate, blood pressure, and respiration rate must be monitored for untoward effects as a result of blockade.

PRACTICAL CONSIDERATIONS

Clinical experience has shown that sphenopalatine ganglion blockade can be useful in aborting acute attacks of migraine or cluster headache.[16–20] Because of its simplicity, sphenopalatine ganglion blockade lends itself to use at the bedside, in the emergency department, and in the headache or pain clinic. For patients with acute headache, this procedure can be combined with oxygen inhalation through the mouth (via mask) while the applicators are in place.[18,19] It may be used on a once-daily basis for chronic headache and facial pain, with the endpoint being total pain relief. The author's clinical experience indicates that five successive treatments usually bring pain relief.

COMPLICATIONS

Epistaxis is the major complication of blockade of the sphenopalatine ganglion, and it occurs more often during winter months, when forced-air heating may cause drying of the nasal mucosa. Given the highly vascular nature of the nasal mucosa,

attention must be paid to the total dose of local anesthetic used if toxic effects are to be avoided.[16] Occasionally, patients experience significant orthostatic hypotension after the procedure. For this reason, they should be moved to a sitting position after the procedure, monitored carefully, and allowed to walk only with assistance.

Stellate Ganglion Block
ANATOMY

Located between the anterior lateral surface of the seventh cervical vertebral body and the neck of the first rib, the stellate ganglion lies central to the vertebral artery and the transverse process. It is separated from the transverse process by the longus colli muscle and is medial to the common carotid artery and jugular vein and lateral to the trachea and esophagus.[21]

INDICATIONS

Blockade of the stellate ganglion is used to treat acute vascular insufficiency of the upper extremities, frostbite of the face and upper extremities, and acute herpes zoster.[21–23] Other indications are early treatment of reflex sympathetic dystrophy of the face, neck, upper extremities, and upper thorax and sympathetically mediated pain caused by malignant disease. It also may provide short-term palliation of some atypical vascular headaches.

TECHNIQUE

The medial edge of the sternocleidomastoid muscle is identified at the level of the cricothyroid notch (C6), and the muscle is displaced laterally with two fingers. Pulsations of the carotid artery should be identified. The skin medial to the carotid pulsation is prepared with alcohol, and an 11/2-inch 22-gauge needle is advanced until contact is made with the transverse process of C6 (**Fig. 24.4**). The needle is withdrawn about 2 mm, careful aspiration is performed, and 7 mL of 0.5% preservative-free bupivacaine hydrochloride is injected. Pulse rate, blood pressure, and respiration rate should be carefully monitored.

PRACTICAL CONSIDERATIONS

Daily stellate ganglion blockade with a local anesthetic is beneficial for the previously mentioned pain syndromes. To avoid undue anxiety, the unique side effect of Horner's syndrome should be explained to patients before the block is administered. The local anesthetic should never be injected if the transverse process of C6 cannot be identified with the needle because doing so leads to an unacceptably high rate of potentially life-threatening complications.

COMPLICATIONS

Hematoma, hoarseness caused by blockade of the laryngeal nerves, difficulty in swallowing, and pneumothorax can occur.[21] Because of the proximity of the great vessels of the neck, intravascular injection—with almost immediate toxic effects from the anesthetic—is a distinct possibility unless aspiration and needle placement are carefully carried out. Epidural and subarachnoid anesthesia can occur if the needle is allowed to pass between the transverse process of C5 and C6 and impinge on the cervical root.

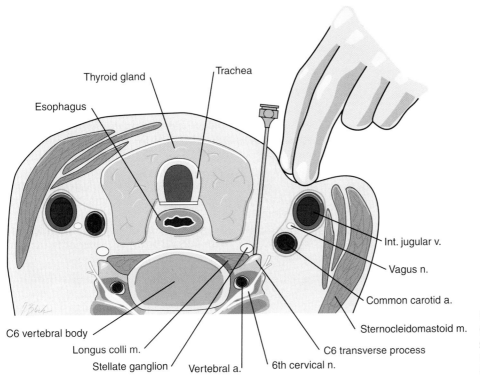

Fig. 24.4 Injection technique for stellate ganglion block. *(From Waldman SD: Stellate ganglion block. In Atlas of interventional pain management, ed 3, Philadelphia, 2009, Saunders, p 132.)*

Celiac Plexus Block
ANATOMY

Situated in the prevertebral area at the level of the T12-L1 vertebral body, the celiac plexus is composed of the right and left celiac, superior mesenteric, and aorticorenal ganglia and the dense network of connecting sympathetic nerve fibers (**Fig. 24.5**).[24]

INDICATIONS

Blockade of the celiac plexus with a local anesthetic is indicated to determine whether flank, retroperitoneal, or upper abdominal pain is sympathetically mediated via the celiac plexus.[24,25] Daily blockade with a local anesthetic palliates pain from acute pancreatitis.[26] According to clinical reports, celiac plexus blockade with a local anesthetic or corticosteroid or both carried out early in the course of acute pancreatitis may reduce markedly the associated morbidity and mortality.

TECHNIQUE

Diagnostic blockade of the celiac plexus with a local anesthetic may be performed without radiographic guidance. Many pain management specialists believe, however, that neurolytic blockade can be performed most safely with the guidance of computed tomographic (CT) scan, or fluoroscopy if CT scan is unavailable. Radiographic guidance should improve not only the safety but also the efficacy of the following technique.

The patient is well hydrated with intravenous fluids and placed prone on the CT scan table. A scout film is obtained to identify the T12-L1 interspace. A CT scan is taken through this area and reviewed for the position of the aorta relative to the vertebral body; the position of the intraabdominal and

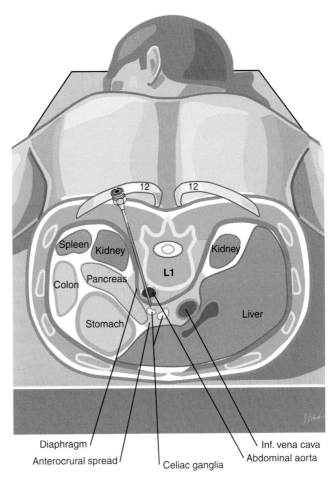

Fig. 24.5 Injection technique for celiac plexus block. *(From Waldman SD: Celiac plexus block. In Atlas of interventional pain management, ed 3, Philadelphia, 2009, Saunders, p 345.)*

retroperitoneal organs; and distortion of normal anatomy caused by tumor, previous surgery, or adenopathy.

The level at which the scan was taken is marked with gentian violet on the patient's skin, which is prepared with antiseptic solution. At about 10 cm left of the midline, the skin and subcutaneous tissue are anesthetized with 1% lidocaine using an 11/2-inch 22-gauge needle. A 13-cm 22-gauge styleted Hinck needle is inserted through the anesthetized area and advanced until the posterior wall of the aorta is encountered. The needle is advanced into the aorta, and the stylet is removed. Free flow of arterial blood should be present. After a well-lubricated 5-mL glass syringe filled with preservative-free saline solution is attached to the Hinck needle, the needle is advanced through the anterior wall of the aorta with use of the loss-of-resistance technique (see Fig. 24.5).[27] The glass syringe is removed, and a small amount of 0.5% lidocaine in solution with water-soluble contrast medium is injected through the needle. Another CT scan is taken at the same level. The scan is reviewed for needle placement and, most importantly, for contrast medium spread. Contrast medium should be seen in the area surrounding the aorta but not in the retrocrural area. When satisfactory needle placement and spread of contrast medium have been confirmed, 12 to 15 mL of absolute alcohol or 6% aqueous phenol is injected through the needle. The needle is flushed with a small amount of saline solution and removed. The patient should be monitored carefully for hemodynamic changes, including hypotension and tachycardia, as a result of the profound sympathetic blockade induced.

PRACTICAL CONSIDERATIONS

CT scan–guided celiac plexus neurolysis with the loss-of-resistance technique has been shown to be safe and efficacious in the treatment of the pain syndromes mentioned.[25] This procedure may be performed with patients in the lateral position if they are unable to lie prone because of such factors as intractable abdominal pain or the presence of colostomy or ileostomy appliances.

Celiac plexus blockade avoids spread of the neurolytic substance onto the lumbar plexus. Posterior retrocrural spread of the local anesthetic and contrast medium, which are injected before the neurolytic substance, alerts the physician to the possibility of this complication and provides the opportunity to reposition the needle.

COMPLICATIONS

The most feared complications of celiac plexus blockade arise from inadvertent injection of neurolytic substance onto the lumbar plexus or from epidural, subarachnoid, or intravascular injection. Inappropriate needle placement can result in damage to the kidneys.[24] If the needle is placed too far anteriorly, injection into the pancreas, peritoneal cavity, or liver can occur. As mentioned, the incidence of these complications can be reduced markedly with CT scan guidance.

When properly performed, this technique results in profound sympathetic neural blockade. In cancer patients with compromised cardiac reserve, resultant hypotension can be life threatening. Patients should be well hydrated before the procedure, and blood pressure should be monitored closely after the procedure. Because orthostatic hypotension

may persist for several days, patients should be cautioned not to stand up without assistance until compensation has occurred.

Lumbar Sympathetic Ganglion
ANATOMY

The lumbar sympathetic nerve lies along the anterolateral surface of the lumbar vertebral bodies and anteromedial to the psoas muscle. The anterior vena cava lies just anterior to the right sympathetic chain, and the aorta lies anterior and slightly medial to the right sympathetic chain (**Fig. 24.6**).[28] Sympathetic innervation of the lower extremities arises from preganglionic fibers that originate from the cell bodies located in the T10-L2 level of the spinal cord. Nearly all postganglionic fibers that lead to the lower extremities leave the sympathetic chain interval below L2. Anterior to the chain are the visceral peritoneum and the great vessels.

INDICATIONS

Blockade of the lumbar sympathetic nerve with a local anesthetic is indicated to determine whether lower extremity pain is sympathetically mediated via this chain and to detect sympathetic dystrophy of the lower extremity. The lumbar sympathetic chain may be blocked with a local anesthetic to ascertain whether blood flow to the lower extremities and greater pain relief would be achieved by destroying the chain with

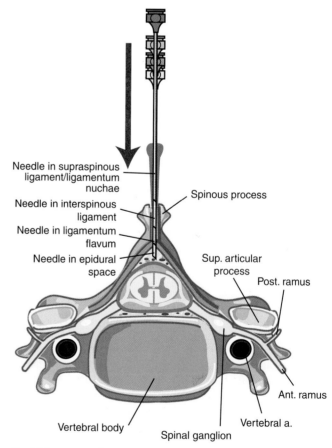

Needle in supraspinous ligament/ligamentum nuchae

Spinous process

Needle in interspinous ligament

Needle in ligamentum flavum

Needle in epidural space

Sup. articular process

Post. ramus

Ant. ramus

Vertebral body

Vertebral a.

Spinal ganglion

Fig. 24.6 Anatomy of the lumbar epidural space. *(From Waldman SD: Lumbar sympathetic block. In Atlas of interventional pain management, ed 3, Philadelphia, 2009, Saunders, p 404.)*

a neurolytic substance (e.g., phenol, alcohol, radiofrequency lesioning) or surgically excising a portion of the chain. This procedure is used therapeutically for acute peripheral vascular insufficiency, ischemia from frostbite, acute herpes zoster of the lower extremities, and a variety of peripheral neuropathic pains of the lower extremities.[29]

TECHNIQUE

The technique used for lumbar sympathetic blockade and neurolysis is similar to that for celiac plexus neurolysis. The patient is placed in the prone position on the CT scan table with a pillow under the abdomen to allow flexion of the thoracolumbar spine and opening of the space between adjacent transverse processes. A scout film is taken to identify the L2 vertebral body. The skin overlying the transverse process of L2 is marked with gentian violet and prepared with povidone-iodine. The skin and subcutaneous tissue are anesthetized with 1% lidocaine with use of an 11/2-inch 22-gauge needle. A 13-cm 22-gauge styleted needle is advanced through the anesthetized area until the tip rests against the vertebral body. The needle is redirected in a trajectory to pass just lateral to the vertebral body. A well-lubricated glass syringe filled with preservative-free saline solution is attached, and the loss-of-resistance technique is used to advance the needle through the body of the psoas muscle. As soon as the needle tip passes through the fascia of the muscle, a loss of resistance is felt, indicating that the needle is adjacent to the sympathetic chain (see Fig. 24.6). A small amount of local anesthetic and water-soluble contrast medium is injected to ensure appropriate spread of the contrast material in the prevertebral region, and 12 mL of 0.5% preservative-free lidocaine or absolute alcohol is injected through the needle. The needle is flushed with preservative-free saline solution and removed. The patient should be observed carefully for hypotension and tachycardia from sympathetic blockade.

PRACTICAL CONSIDERATIONS

CT scan guidance during lumbar sympathetic neurolysis can decrease markedly the risk of complications. Patients should be told that some backache is likely because of trauma to the muscles of posture by the needle. They also should be advised that after lumbar sympathetic blockade, the affected lower extremity may feel hot and be swollen as compared with the unaffected extremity. This side effect is normal and resolves with time.

COMPLICATIONS

Complications of lumbar sympathetic blockade are similar to those of celiac plexus neurolysis. Because the needle tip is more medial in its trajectory, damage to lumbar nerve roots at their exit from the spinal column is possible.[28]

Somatic Neural Blockade

Similar to sympathetic neural blockade, somatic neural blockade should be only one part of a comprehensive diagnostic and treatment plan for patients who have pain syndromes. The failure to use rational pharmacologic therapy as a first step or in conjunction with somatic neural blockade results in less than optimal results for patients with acute and postoperative pain.

Epidural Nerve Block
ANATOMY

The epidural space extends from the foramen magnum, where the periosteal and spinal layers of dura fuse with the sacrococcygeal membrane (**Figs. 24.7** and **24.8**). Its anterior portion is bounded by the posterior longitudinal ligament, which covers the posterior aspect of the vertebral body and the intravertebral disk. The epidural space is posteriorly bounded by the anterior lateral surface of the vertebral lamina and the ligamentum flavum and laterally bounded by the pedicles of the vertebra and the intravertebral foramen. From a technical viewpoint, the ligamentum flavum is the key landmark for identification of the epidural space. It is composed of dense fibroelastic tissue and is thinnest in the

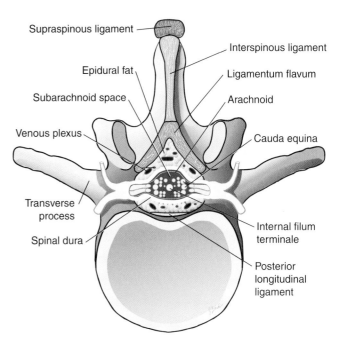

Fig. 24.7 Injection technique for cervical epidural block. *(From Waldman SD: Cervical epidural block. In* Atlas of interventional pain management, *ed 3, Philadelphia, 2009, Saunders, p 171.)*

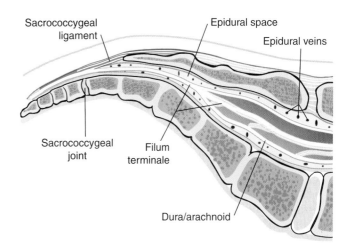

Fig. 24.8 Anatomy of the triangular sacrum. *(From Waldman SD: Caudal epidural block. In* Atlas of interventional pain management, *ed 3, Philadelphia, 2009, Saunders, p 442.)*

cervical region. In men, the epidural space is narrowest in the cervical region (anteroposterior diameter 2 to 3 mm when the neck is flexed).

INDICATIONS

Epidural nerve blockade with a local anesthetic or corticosteroid or both can be used to diagnose and treat a variety of acute pain syndromes. It relieves pain from acute cervical, thoracic, and lumbar strain and radiculopathy; tension-type headache; bilateral sympathetically mediated pain (e.g., reflex sympathetic dystrophy); pain caused by peripheral vascular insufficiency; and ischemic pain from frostbite.[30-32] In addition, this procedure is valuable in the management of acute herpes zoster and postherpetic neuralgia of the extremities or trunk.[33]

TECHNIQUE

Epidural nerve blockade is carried out most easily with the patient in the sitting position and the cervical spine flexed and the forehead resting on a padded bedside table. The arms should rest comfortably in the patient's lap or at his or her sides. After the skin overlying the appropriate intervertebral space is prepared with antiseptic solution, a sterile fenestrated drape is placed over the area.

The spinous process and intervertebral space are carefully palpated to identify the exact midline position. The skin and subcutaneous tissue at the midline are anesthetized with 1% preservative-free lidocaine or 0.25% preservative-free bupivacaine. An 18-gauge or 20-gauge Hustead or Tuohy needle is inserted into the anesthetized area in a midline, slightly cephalad trajectory. On removal of the stylet, a well-lubricated 5-mL glass syringe filled with preservative-free saline solution is attached to the epidural needle. With continuous pressure applied on the plunger of the syringe, the epidural needle is carefully advanced until the tip impinges on the dense ligamentum flavum. A sudden loss of resistance is felt as the tip of the needle passes through the ligamentum flavum into the epidural space; 0.5 mL of air is injected through the needle to confirm epidural placement (**Fig. 24.9**).

After careful aspiration, 0.5% preservative-free lidocaine or 0.25% preservative-free bupivacaine combined with a depot corticosteroid preparation or preservative-free opioid, such as morphine or fentanyl, is injected, and the epidural needle is removed. A 4 × 4–inch gauze pad is placed over the injection site, and pressure is applied. The patient is returned to the supine position, and blood pressure, pulse rate, and respiration rate are monitored closely until recovery is complete.

Thoracic and lumbar epidural block can be performed in the sitting, lateral, or prone position with use of the loss-of-resistance technique described previously. In addition, the caudal approach to the epidural space offers numerous theoretical advantages over the lumbar approach to the epidural space, including the markedly decreased incidence of postdural puncture headaches and the fact that caudal epidural block can be performed with a 25-gauge needle in the presence of anticoagulation. This latter advantage is useful in patients who are fully anticoagulated after lower extremity salvage procedures and in patients anticoagulated for deep venous thrombosis. The caudal approach to the epidural space is amenable to the administration of opioids via single injection or continuous infusion.

PRACTICAL CONSIDERATIONS

Epidural nerve blockade with a corticosteroid may be used early in the course of treatment of the pain syndromes described until other methods (e.g., use of antidepressants, physical therapy) become effective. Experience suggests that epidural neural blockade is most efficacious when it is performed in the following manner:

- The initial block is achieved with 80 mg of methylprednisolone and 7 mL of 0.25% preservative-free bupivacaine in the cervical region, 10 mL in the lower thoracic region, or 12 mL in the lumbar region or in the alternative 0.5 mg of preservative-free morphine in the cervical and upper thoracic region, 10 mg of preservative-free morphine in the lower thoracic and upper lumbar region, and 12 mg of preservative-free morphine via the caudal approach to the epidural space.[33]

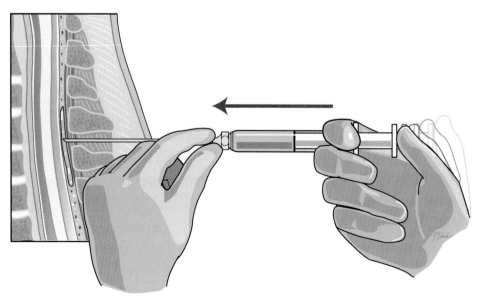

Fig. 24.9 Correct needle placement for epidural nerve block. *(From Waldman SD: Cervical epidural block. In Atlas of interventional pain management, ed 3, Philadelphia, 2009, Saunders, p 134.)*

- Subsequent blocks are administered every other day with 40 mg of methylprednisolone being substituted for the initial 80-mg dose and the appropriate amount of preservative-free bupivacaine or morphine. Six blocks may be given in this manner, with the endpoint being complete pain relief.
- The amount of methylprednisolone should be decreased in patients who have diabetes or who have received systemic corticosteroid therapy.[34,35]

COMPLICATIONS

Because epidural nerve blockade interrupts somatic and sympathetic nerve conduction, cardiovascular changes (e.g., hypotension, tachycardia) may occur and can produce devastating complications if they are not identified and treated promptly.[36] Respiratory compromise or failure may result from blockade of the phrenic nerve or respiratory centers of the brainstem. For this reason, epidural nerve blockade should be performed only by personnel trained in airway management and resuscitation. Appropriate monitoring of vital signs is imperative, and resuscitation equipment must be readily available.

Other major complications include damage to neural structures, epidural hematoma, and epidural abscess. These complications occur rarely but can be life threatening.[37] Minor untoward effects and complications of epidural nerve blockade include pain at the injection site, inadvertent dural puncture, and vasovagal syncope.

Trigeminal Nerve Block
ANATOMY

The trigeminal nerve is the largest of the cranial nerves and contains sensory and motor fibers. It can be approached extraorally via the coronoid notch into the pterygopalatine fossa.[38] The fossa is a triangular space between the pterygoid process of the sphenoid bone and the maxilla of the upper part of the infratemporal fossa.

INDICATIONS

Trigeminal nerve blockade with a local anesthetic and corticosteroid is an excellent adjunct to drug treatment of trigeminal neuralgia.[38,39] This procedure affords rapid palliation of pain while doses of oral medications are being titrated to effective levels. It also may be valuable in alleviation of atypical facial pain. Other indications include pain in maxillary neoplasms, cluster headache uncontrolled with sphenopalatine ganglion blockade, and acute herpes zoster in the area of the trigeminal nerve that is not controlled with stellate ganglion blockade.

TECHNIQUE

Palpation of the coronoid notch is facilitated by opening and closing the patient's mouth. The notch should be encountered about 4 cm anterior to the acoustic auditory meatus. The skin is anesthetized with antiseptic solution, and an 11/2-inch 22-gauge needle is directed through the middle of the coronoid notch. The tip of the needle may encounter the lateral lamina of the pterygoid process (**Fig. 24.10**). If blockade of the maxillary nerve is desired, the needle is withdrawn into the subcutaneous tissue and the tip is redirected 1 cm more anterior and 1 cm more superior to the first bony contact. Paresthesias may be elicited in the area of the maxillary nerve. If blockade of the mandibular nerve is desired, the needle is withdrawn into the subcutaneous tissue and the tip is redirected 1 cm more posterior and 1 cm more inferior to the first bony contact. Paresthesias may be elicited in the area of the mandibular nerve. After careful aspiration, 5 to 7 mL of 0.5% preservative-free bupivacaine with 80 mg of methylprednisolone is injected. Subsequent daily nerve blockade is carried out in a similar manner, with the dose of methylprednisolone lowered to 40 mg.

PRACTICAL CONSIDERATIONS

This procedure is an excellent emergency treatment of uncontrolled pain of trigeminal neuralgia. It can be used while doses of carbamazepine, baclofen, phenytoin sodium, or other medications are being titrated.[39] In patients with atypical facial pain from temporomandibular joint dysfunction, trigeminal nerve blockade makes physical therapy and range-of-motion exercises of the joint possible.

COMPLICATIONS

The major complication of trigeminal nerve blockade is inadvertent vascular injection.[38] The pterygopalatine fossa is traversed by many arteries and veins. Careful and frequent aspiration should be carried out during injection of the local anesthetic. Needle damage to this vasculature can result in significant hematoma formation. Patients should be advised of the potential for this untoward effect and informed of its self-limiting nature so that they are not unduly alarmed if it occurs.

Intercostal Nerve Block
ANATOMY

The thoracic spinal nerves give off the white and gray rami communicantes of the sympathetic system, which communicate with particular ganglia of the sympathetic chain. Distal to the rami communicantes, the nerve trunk divides into the dorsal and ventral branches. The dorsal branch innervates

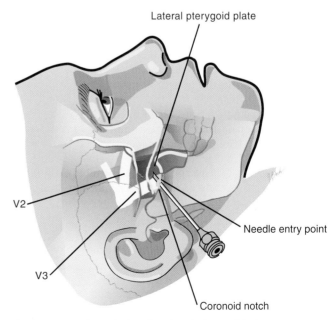

Fig. 24.10 Injection technique for trigeminal nerve block. *(From Waldman SD: Trigeminal nerve block. In Atlas of interventional pain management, ed 3, Philadelphia, 2009, Saunders, p 48.)*

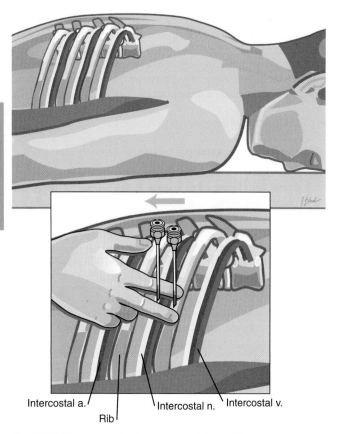

Intercostal a.
Rib
Intercostal n.
Intercostal v.

Fig. 24.11 Correct needle placement for intercostal nerve block. *(From Waldman SD: Intercostal nerve block. In Atlas of interventional pain management, ed 3, Philadelphia, 2009, Saunders, p 296.)*

Table 24.3 Useful Somatic Nerve Blocks in the Management of Acute and Postoperative Pain

Nerve Block	Indication
Occipital nerve block	Postcraniotomy pain
Auriculotemporal nerve block	Postcraniotomy pain
Glossopharyngeal nerve block	Glossopharyngeal neuralgia
Phrenic nerve block	Intractable hiccups
Cervical plexus block	Carotid artery and neck surgery
Cervical epidural block	Acute herpes zoster and upper extremity pain
Brachial plexus block	Shoulder and upper extremity surgery
Median, radial, and ulnar nerve blocks	Upper extremity and hand surgery
Intercostal nerve blocks	Fractured ribs, chest wall pain, metastatic lesions to chest wall, liver pain, postoperative pain
Thoracic epidural block	Vertebral compression fractures, postoperative pain
Ilioinguinal, iliohypogastric, and genitofemoral nerve blocks	Groin and pelvic pain
Obturator nerve block	Hip fracture pain
Femoral nerve block	Femoral fractures
Lumbar epidural block	Vertebral compression fractures, postoperative pain
Lumbar plexus and sciatic nerve blocks	Lower extremity pain
Ankle block	Foot and ankle pain

the skin and muscles of the back and the periosteum of the vertebra. The ventral branch follows the rib via the costal sulcus, traveling into the dorsal thoracic region between the two laminae of the intercostal muscles and into the lateral and ventral portions of the thorax. This intercostal nerve travels in tandem with the intercostal artery and vein.[40]

INDICATIONS

Intercostal nerve blockade with a local anesthetic or corticosteroid or both can be performed at the bedside or in the outpatient setting. This procedure may palliate pain from acute traumatic or pathologic rib fractures, chest wall metastasis, intercostal neuralgia, or thoracotomy and is useful for right upper quadrant pain from hepatic metastasis.[41–43] Intercostal nerve blockade also may reduce pain caused by percutaneous drainage devices (e.g., chest or nephrostomy tubes). Clinically significant improvement in pulmonary function has been shown in patients treated with this procedure.

TECHNIQUE

Intercostal nerve blockade can be performed with the patient in the sitting, lateral decubitus, or prone position. The rib in the anatomic region to be blocked is identified with palpation, and the skin in the posterior axillary line is prepared with antiseptic solution. An 11/2-inch 22-gauge needle attached to a 5-mL syringe is advanced vertically until contact with the rib is made. The needle is withdrawn into the subcutaneous tissue and "walked off" the inferior margin of the rib (**Fig. 24.11**).

Care must be taken not to advance the needle more than 0.5 cm. After careful aspiration, 3 to 5 mL of 0.5% or 0.75% preservative-free bupivacaine is injected, and the needle is removed. This procedure may be repeated at each level subserving the pain.

PRACTICAL CONSIDERATIONS

Therapeutic intercostal nerve blockade is an excellent adjunct in the treatment of a variety of acute pain syndromes. Its simplicity allows its use in the emergency department or at the bedside, provided that appropriate resuscitation equipment and drugs are readily available. The highly vascular nature of the intercostal region mandates careful monitoring of the total amount of local anesthetic used. With the use of a long-acting protein-bound local anesthetic (e.g., 0.75% bupivacaine), intercostal nerve blockade can be performed daily to provide long-lasting relief from pain caused by trauma or surgical incision.

COMPLICATIONS

The major complication of intercostal nerve blockade is inadvertent and unrecognized pneumothorax. The incidence rate of this complication is about 0.5% to 1%.[41] If the patient is being maintained on positive-pressure ventilatory support, tension pneumothorax can occur. As mentioned, systemic toxic effects from vascular uptake of the local anesthetic may occur if dosing guidelines are not carefully observed.

Other Somatic Nerve Blocks

As can be seen from the discussion of some of the nerve blocks commonly used in the management of acute and postoperative pain, these techniques are a reasonable next step if pharmacologic modalities fail to control the patient's pain adequately. Many somatic nerve blocks are useful as anesthesia-sparing adjuncts to general anesthesia and as adjuncts to analgesia in the postoperative period. **Table 24.3** provides an overview of other somatic nerve blocks that have utility in the management of acute and postoperative pain.

Conclusion

Most pain is controllable. Patient education and careful intraoperative technique are useful prophylactic measures. Simple analgesics and NSAIDs reduce pain, fever, and inflammation and are well tolerated when dosing guidelines are followed carefully. In patients with pain that is not controlled with these measures, the addition of a weak opioid analgesic is reasonable. If relief is still inadequate, a stronger opioid alone or in combination with another analgesic may be needed. The advent of patient-controlled analgesia has diminished some of the objections to continuous intravenous infusion of opioids. Various acute pain syndromes respond to blockade of the sympathetic or somatic neural pathways. Knowledge of the appropriate anatomic structures and careful technique are mandatory with this method. It should be considered only one part of a comprehensive treatment plan.

References

Full references for this chapter can be found on www.expertconsult.com.

Chapter 25

Burn Pain

Shelley A. Wiechman, Sam R. Sharar, and David R. Patterson

Historical Considerations

Burn injuries are a widespread medical hazard and a frequent cause of human suffering in the contemporary world. Burn injuries often gain more attention through tragic and mass casualty events, such as the 1942 Cocoanut Grove nightclub fire in Boston (491 deaths), the 1981 Stardust Nightclub fire in Dublin (48 deaths), and the 2003 Station Concert Club fire in Warwick, RI (96 deaths). However, often neglected in the public eye are common, survivable injuries that can force survivors to experience recurrent and often intense pain associated with both the injury itself and its days to months–long treatment. Because death rates for burn injuries have declined (e.g., 33% between 1985 and 1995[1]), primarily because of improved surgical care, more people with large burns are surviving and facing unique physical and psychologic rehabilitation challenges, such as scarring (disfigurement), contractures, amputations, pain, and psychologic adjustment. An estimated 1.25 million burn injuries occur annually in the United States, resulting in more than 51,000 acute hospitalizations.[2] Each survivor has a number of potential important medical challenges, including burn wound management, prevention of infectious complications, pulmonary function (in cases of smoke inhalation), nutritional demands, physical and rehabilitation therapy requirements, and, particularly in the case of large or aesthetically disfiguring burns, long-term issues of psychosocial adjustment. Central to most of these issues is the pain associated not only with the burn injury itself but also with the ongoing, therapeutic medical care (e.g., wound debridement, aggressive physical therapy, and occupational therapy).

Media publicity surrounding fires or explosions with casualties has resulted in increased attention to, and improved medical care of, various aspects of patient care. This is particularly true for issues of fire safety, inhalation injury, and wound care management but has not necessarily been the case for pain management, which until recently has been underprioritized in this population. As an example, a national survey of US burn centers in 1982 reported that 17% of centers used no analgesics or anesthesia for hospitalized children during burn wound debridement and that 8% recommended no analgesic medications at all.[3] In addition, burn pain treatment techniques have historically been applied more liberally in adults than in children, as demonstrated by Schechter[4] who reported in 1985 that in a large teaching hospital, children hospitalized for burns of up to 20% body surface area (BSA) received an average of 1.3 opioid doses per day, compared with 3.6 opioid doses per day for adults with similar BSA injuries. In the ensuing 30 years since these reports, the active participation of clinical behavioral scientists, anesthesiologists, nurses, some burn surgeons, and other burn team members in improving burn pain assessment and management has led to both a broader application of conventional analgesic techniques and the introduction of newer analgesic techniques in burn patients. These advances aside, recent observations are reported that inadequate burn pain management still exists during both the acute and the rehabilitation phases of care and can directly influence long-term functional outcome.[5] With encouragement from The Joint Commission's declaration that pain should be regarded as a fifth vital sign,[6] however, an increased emphasis on pain assessment and management has occurred more recently in all medical settings, including burns. Additionally encouraging is that a review of research presented at the American Burn Association annual meeting reported that the research category of "pain/anxiety/patient comfort" was the third most popular of 10 burn-related clinical and laboratory research areas.[7] Hopefully, then, continued clinical improvements in the acute and long-term analgesic management of burn survivors will be a trend in the years to come.

The Clinical Syndrome Signs, Symptoms, and Physical Findings

Acute burn injury pain results from the combination of thermal tissue injury of the dermal sensory organs and acute inflammatory response[8] that is, at least in the early postburn period, related to the depth of tissue injury (**Figs. 25.1** and **25.2**). Superficial, or first-degree, burns (e.g., sunburn) are characterized by tissue injury that is limited to the epidermal skin layer and an inflammatory response in the superficial dermal layers that results in hyperemia (manifest as erythema), an intact epidermis (no skin blistering), and sensitization of dermal sensory organelles that results in hyperalgesia and mild to moderate pain. Partial-thickness (i.e., second-degree) burns involve tissue injury that extends to variable depths into the dermis. Superficial second-degree burns involve only the upper, papillary dermis and are more likely to heal spontaneously; deep second-degree burns involve the deeper, collagen-dense reticular dermis and are more likely to need surgical treatment. Because second-degree burns consistently injure or inflame sensory receptors in the dermis, these burns are associated with marked hyperalgesia and produce moderate to severe pain. Full-thickness, or third-degree, burns are characterized by complete destruction of the dermis, including its sensory and vascular structures, so that although pain may still be a presenting symptom, hypalgesia to cutaneous stimulation is common, as is a leathery skin texture and lack of capillary refill. Acute pain symptoms with third-degree burns are typically minimal, but can be variable, and are universally present with respect to the transition zone between burned and unburned skin. All burn injuries that involve the dermis (i.e., second-degree and third-degree) result in sensitized and reorganized states of both peripheral mechanoheat receptors and dorsal horn neurons. Models of these cellular alterations provide a conceptual framework for understanding how such peripheral neuronal injuries that are present after a burn can cause acute and subacute pain, hyperalgesia, and chronic pain and are described elsewhere.[8]

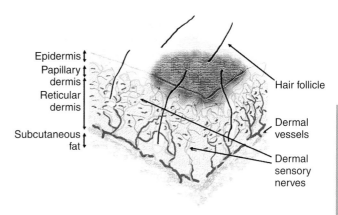

Fig. 25.1 **Anatomic layers of the skin.**

Discussions on definition and measurement of burn pain typically focus on the variable of pain intensity, with less emphasis on variables of pain quality. In one of the earlier studies in this area, Perry and Heidrich[3] reported that burn patients typically report their pain as severe or excruciating, despite administration of opioid analgesics. However, an important note is that burn pain varies greatly from patient to patient, shows substantial fluctuation over the time course of hospitalization, and can be unpredictable because of the complex interaction of anatomic, physiologic, psychosocial, and premorbid behavior issues.[9] In contrast to the approximate relationship between burn depth and pain described previously for the acute postinjury period, burn pain that is reported after the initial injury is not reliably correlated with the size or depth of a burn. Specifically, a patient with a superficial (second-degree) burn may show substantially more pain than one with a full-thickness (third-degree) burn as a result of both physical factors (e.g., location and mechanism of the injury, individual differences in pain threshold and tolerance, response to analgesics) and psychologic factors (e.g., previous pain experiences, anxiety, depression). Emotional distress, including traumatic memories, guilt or loss of loved ones or family members, anticipatory fears about treatment and recovery, and unexpected confinement in the hospital environment all may contribute to, and complicate, the postburn pain experience.

Indirect assessments of pain and nociception with measures of sympathetic nervous system activation (e.g., hypertension, tachycardia, and tachypnea) that may be of value in other acute pain settings are notoriously inaccurate in the acute burn victim. One reason for this is that a generalized increase in sympathetic tone often occurs, particularly in seriously injured burn patients, in response to the combination of immediate postburn intravascular hypovolemia and as much as a 100% increase in resting metabolic rate. Accordingly, a critical realization is that predicting the amount of nociception or suffering a patient will experience based on the nature of, or the physiologic response to, the burn injury is not possible; furthermore, the patient's pain experience can change dramatically—for better or for worse—over the course of both inpatient and outpatient care.

As a result of this unpredictability, a more useful paradigm for describing acute and subacute burn pain is to base it on the clinical settings in which it commonly occurs. This approach is also useful because analgesic treatment decisions can also be based on such a classification. It follows that acute burn pain is generally classified into four clinical settings (**Fig. 25.3**)[10]:

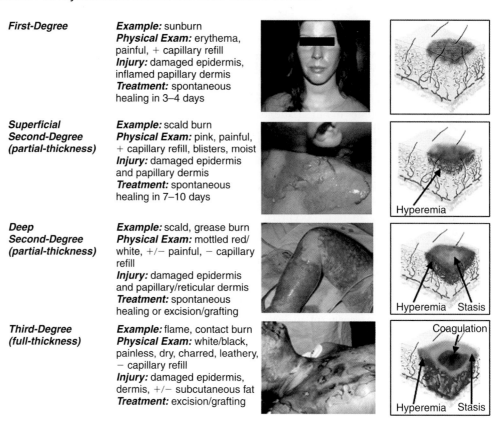

First-Degree

Example: sunburn
Physical Exam: erythema, painful, + capillary refill
Injury: damaged epidermis, inflamed papillary dermis
Treatment: spontaneous healing in 3–4 days

Superficial Second-Degree (partial-thickness)

Example: scald burn
Physical Exam: pink, painful, + capillary refill, blisters, moist
Injury: damaged epidermis and papillary dermis
Treatment: spontaneous healing in 7–10 days

Hyperemia

Deep Second-Degree (partial-thickness)

Example: scald, grease burn
Physical Exam: mottled red/white, +/− painful, − capillary refill
Injury: damaged epidermis and papillary/reticular dermis
Treatment: spontaneous healing or excision/grafting

Hyperemia   Stasis

Third-Degree (full-thickness)

Example: flame, contact burn
Physical Exam: white/black, painless, dry, charred, leathery, − capillary refill
Injury: damaged epidermis, dermis, +/− subcutaneous fat
Treatment: excision/grafting

Coagulation

Hyperemia   Stasis

Fig. 25.2 Definitions and examples of partial-thickness and full-thickness burn injuries. *(Images and illustrations courtesy of Nicole Gibram, MD, University of Washington Burn Center)*

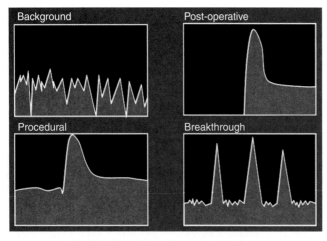

Background   Post-operative

Procedural   Breakthrough

Fig. 25.3 Four clinical burn pain settings.

(1) background: pain that is present while the patient is at rest, results from the thermal tissue injury itself, and is typically of low-moderate intensity and long duration; (2) procedural: brief but intense pain generated by wound care (e.g., debridement and dressing change) or rehabilitation activities (physical and occupational therapies); (3) breakthrough: unexpected spiking of pain levels that occurs when current analgesic efforts are exceeded, either at rest or during procedures; and (4) postoperative: a predictable and temporary (2 to 5 days) increase in pain symptoms after burn excision and grafting, in large part as a result of the creation of new wounds in the process of skin graft harvesting and autografting.

Burn pain that lasts longer than 6 months or remains after all burn wounds and skin graft donor sites have healed is viewed as chronic and is thus a challenge primarily in the outpatient setting. The mechanisms and treatment of chronic burn pain are inadequately studied and poorly understood. Although most acute burn pain results from tissue damage, one must be aware that pain from nerve damage may also be present, particularly in severe injuries associated with extremity amputations, and represent an anatomic source for chronic burn pain symptoms. Acute and chronic pain, arising from such nerve damage, is often treated differently than conventional burn pain and is addressed elsewhere in this text.

Testing

The history and physical examination that should be a mandatory part of initial burn care negate the need for specialized testing for diagnosis of acute burn pain. The assessment of chronic pain conditions (e.g., complex regional pain syndromes [CRPS]) and associated psychologic disorders that can accompany some burn injuries (e.g., depression from disfigurement or functional impairment issues) is not unlike that in other pain settings and is described in more detail elsewhere in this text. However, because of the high incidence rate (25% to 74%) of psychiatric diagnoses in patients admitted for burn care (e.g., depression, character disorder, and substance abuse),[11] one should maintain a high index of suspicion for these diagnoses, and a low threshold for collaborative patient management with clinical psychologists or psychiatric professionals throughout the management period. Burn injuries often occur because something has gone wrong in a patient's life, be it an Axis I psychiatric disorder, domestic abuse, homelessness, substance abuse, or suicidal (and parasuicidal) behavior.

Differential Diagnosis

A history and physical examination usually leave little doubt as to the etiology of burn pain, whether acute or chronic (although with an increasing admission rate of burn admission through illegal methamphetamine laboratory explosions, the clinician must be forever vigilant for suspicious causes). In addition, however, other pain findings may be consistent with associated trauma (e.g., blunt trauma associated with a motor vehicle crash and subsequent car fire) or premorbid medical issues (e.g., substance abuse histories that may alter the management picture). Although these associated findings rarely affect the diagnosis of acute burn pain, they certainly may complicate its treatment.

Treatment

General Treatment Philosophy

The highly variable nature of burn pain makes reliable prediction through clinical assessment of either the patient or the burn wound difficult, and universally agreed-on burn pain management protocols simply do not exist. What's more, the state of the science is not at a point where types of opioid analgesics and other pain interventions have been clearly shown to be superior to one another. Further, not only is opioid analgesic dosing variable based on patient weight, factors such as drug tolerance and the extreme nociception associated with burn injuries make specific dosing suggestions a challenge. As a result, the analgesic approaches to burn pain are variable and often institution-specific. In a recent survey of pediatric pain control practices in 82 North American burn centers,[12] for example, opioid analgesic use for procedural wound care and background pain control was ubiquitous, and a large fraction of responders (77%) also reported the adjunctive use of nonpharmacologic analgesic techniques (mostly limited to distraction). However, only a limited number of responders reported the routine use of general anesthesia for exceptionally challenging wound care procedures (21%), the regular consultation of pain specialists (17%), or the use of an established protocol for the critically important first inpatient wound care procedure (33%).

Many burn centers advocate a structured approach to burn analgesia that incorporates both pharmacologic and non-pharmacologic therapies, targets the specific clinical pain settings unique to the burn patient (see Fig. 25.3), and yet can be individualized to meet specific patient needs and institutional capabilities. Such structured protocols help to avoid the undertreatment of burn pain that has been reported all too frequently[3] despite education regarding the importance of adequate analgesia and the low risks for addictive and other side effects. The source of such undertreatment has been conceptualized in psychodynamic terms by Perry, Heidrich, and Ramos.[13] Specifically, some staff members required to perform repeated and painful procedures on burn patients have a subconscious need for patients to demonstrate pain as a means to create a psychologic distance between themselves and the realities of burn care. Alternatively, the unfounded fear of creating psychologic dependence on opioid analgesics in patients may also explain the reluctance of some burn care staff to aggressively treat burn pain. However, currently no evidence shows that opioid addiction occurs more commonly in burn patients without premorbid substance abuse issues than in other patients populations that need such analgesics for acute pain.[14]

Development of succinct, yet detailed, institutional guidelines has been advocated to assist physicians and nurses who do not specialize in pain control avoid extremes of dosing with the choice of pharmacologic analgesics that target specific analgesic needs.[15,16] For maximal simplicity and utility, such guidelines are recommended to be safe and effective over a broad range of ages, to be explicit in dosing parameters, to have a limited formulary to maximize staff familiarity, and to allow the bedside nurse flexibility to respond quickly to the changing needs of the patient.[16] An example of such pharmacologic dosing guidelines from the author's institution is shown in **Table 25.1**. In addition, the regular use of a weight-based pediatric medication worksheet (placed at the bedside and in the patient record) that contains all analgesic and resuscitation drugs likely to be administered for each particularly pediatric patient provides a supplemental safeguard against accidental overdose. This safeguard is particularly needed in the young pediatric age group where analgesic risks and clinical unfamiliarity may both be elevated.[17]

The generalized burn pain management paradigm should involve both pharmacologic and nonpharmacologic analgesic techniques, selected on the basis of institutional availability and experience and patient factors.[11,18] In general, selection of an analgesic regimen is first based on the answers to two general questions: (1) what is the clinical setting or challenge for which analgesia is needed (i.e., treatment of background versus procedural versus breakthrough versus postoperative pain); and (2) what specific treatment limitations are imposed by the patient (presence of intravenous [IV] access, endotracheal intubation/mechanical ventilation, or opioid tolerance) or by clinical facilities (available monitoring capabilities, training and skills of burn care staff)? For example, the presence or absence of IV access (particularly in children, in whom IV access may be challenging to obtain) directly influences pharmacologic analgesic options. Similarly, patients who are mechanically ventilated are largely "protected" from the risk of opioid-induced respiratory depression and thus can be administered larger doses of opioids. Tolerance may be a relevant issue in patients who need prolonged opioid analgesic therapy or in those with substance abuse histories. Because of the development of drug tolerance with prolonged medical use (>2 weeks) or recreational abuse of opioids (both commonly seen in burn patients), doses needed for burn analgesia may significantly exceed those recommended in standard guidelines. One clinically important consequence of drug tolerance is the potential for opioid withdrawal to occur during inpatient burn treatment. Thus, the period of inpatient burn care is not an appropriate time to institute deliberate opioid withdrawal or detoxification measures in patients who have a premorbid history of opioid abuse because a strategy such as this ignores the very real, acute pain analgesic needs of these patients. Such practices might also lead to illegal drug seeking in hospitalized patients, with associated health risks and hospital system problems. Similarly, when reductions in analgesic therapy are considered as burn wounds heal, reductions should occur via careful taper to prevent acute opioid withdrawal syndrome. Patients with substance abuse histories should be provided with the proper counseling and referral sources and weaned off of opioid medications at discharge or soon after. However, weaning during acute care can potentially be construed as a form of punishment that may serve to exacerbate their addiction problem.

Table 25-1 Example of Institutional Burn Pain Medication Guidelines

	ICU (No PO Intake)	ICU (Taking PO)	Ward (Large Open Areas)	Ward (Small Open Areas/Predischage)
Background pain	Continuous morphine sulfate (IV) drip	Scheduled methadone or MS Contin	Scheduled methadone or MS Contin	Scheduled NSAIDs/acetaminophen or scheduled oxycodone or none
Procedural pain	Morphine sulfate (IV) or fentanyl (IV)	Oxycodone, fentanyl IV, or fentanyl (Actiq)	Oxycodone, fentanyl (IV), Nitrox (IH), or fentanyl (Actiq)	Oxycodone
Breakthrough pain (prn dosing)	Morphine sulfate (IV) or fentanyl (IV)	Oxycodone	Oxycodone	NSAIDs/acetaminophen or oxycodone
Background anxiolysis	Scheduled lorazepam (IV) or continuous lorazepam (IV) drip	Scheduled lorazepam	None or scheduled lorazepam	None
Procedural anxiolysis	Lorazepam or midazolam (IV)	Lorazepam	None or lorazepam	None
Discharge or transfer pain medications	N/A	For transfer to ward: wean drips, establish PO pain medication early; anticipate dose tapering as needs decrease	Oxycodone for procedural pain; methadone taper or MS Contin; taper if applicable	Oxycodone or NSAIDs for procedural pain

ICU, intensive care unit; IH, by inhalation; IV, intravenously; N/A, not applicable; NSAIDs, nonsteroidal anti-inflammatory drugs; PO, by mouth, prn, as needed. Representative pain and sedation management guideline for adult (nonpediatric, nongeriatric) burn patients from the University of Washington Burn Center. General medication recommendations are provided for specific pain and anxiolysis needs encountered in various intensive care units and ward care settings. Medication options are intentionally limited (for simplicity) and do not include specific dose recommendations (to allow for individual patient variability). Complex or refractory cases are managed through special consultation with the burn care team or pain specialists.

Because nociception at the wound site is the predominant mechanism of pain and suffering in patients with acute burn injuries, pharmacologic treatment with potent opioids analgesics, anxiolytics, or other anesthetics is the first line and cornerstone of therapy. In addition, nonpharmacologic methods of treatment of burn pain are also extremely useful but are best applied only after optimal pharmacologic therapy has been established (although abiding by nonpharmacologic *principles* for pain control in all cases is important, such as minimizing the adversity of wound care and making the environment as patient friendly as possible). Brief descriptions of the analgesic goals and potential general therapeutic options for each of the four clinical settings of burn pain are presented subsequently (see also Fig. 25.3).

Background Pain Management

Background pain is relatively constant and is mild to moderate in severity and is consequently best treated pharmacologically with mild-to-moderately potent analgesics administered so that plasma drug concentrations remain relatively constant throughout the day. Examples include continuous IV opioid infusions (with or without patient-controlled analgesia [PCA]), oral administration of long-acting opioids with prolonged elimination (methadone) or prolonged enteral absorption (sustained-release morphine, sustained release oxycodone), or oral administration on a regular schedule of short-acting oral opioid analgesics or nonsteroidal anti-inflammatory agents (NSAIDs). Background pain decreases with time as the burn wound (and associated donor sites) heals, so that analgesics can be slowly tapered. Nonpharmacologic techniques applicable to background pain might include approaches to enhance coping, relaxation, information provision, and participation (see subsequent discussion).

Procedural Pain Management

Pain associated with burn wound care presents a unique and significant challenge for the medical staff in that potent sedation or analgesia is often needed on a daily basis, yet general anesthesia is either too dangerous, expensive, or logistically challenging to use on an ongoing basis. Thus, the provision of moderate sedation (formerly conscious sedation) or deep sedation (as defined by the American Society of Anesthesiologists [ASA][19]) is frequently needed and should conform to the sedation guidelines set by the ASA[19] and adopted by The Joint Commission. For example, the institutional capability to provide adequate monitoring (pulse oximetry, independent patient observer) for moderate sedation by nonanesthesiologists may also dictate which specific agents are used for procedural analgesia, as some of the more potent opioids (e.g., remifentanil) or anesthetics (e.g., ketamine) may result in depths of sedation that far exceed the intended target of moderate sedation. Careful individual and institutional interpretation of sedation levels is necessary to ensure safety and practicality in meeting the appropriate sedation guidelines. The use of potent opioid analgesics and anxiolytics should only occur in settings with adequate monitoring, personnel, and resuscitation equipment appropriate for the degree of sedation anticipated. For most wound debridement procedures, opioid analgesia, with or without the concurrent use of anxiolytic sedatives (e.g., benzodiazepines), typically produces a clinical response consistent with moderate sedation.

In contrast to background pain, procedural pain is significantly more intense but shorter in duration; therefore, pharmacologic analgesic regimens for procedural pain are best comprised of moderately-to-highly potent opioids that have a short duration of action, often in combination with benzodiazepine class anxiolytics. Intravenous access is helpful in this setting because opioid analgesics with a rapid onset of action and short duration (e.g., fentanyl, remifentanil) may be used, as can other IV anesthetic agents such as ketamine and dexmedetomidine. In the absence of IV access, orally administered opioid analgesics are commonly used, although their relatively long durations of action (2 to 6 hours) may potentially limit postprocedure treatments such as rehabilitative or nutritional therapies. Oral ketamine,[20] oral transmucosal fentanyl,[21,22] and inhaled nitrous oxide[23] are agents of particular use when IV access is not present because of their rapid onsets and short durations of action. Finally, when a particularly painful dressing change or one that requires extreme cooperation in a noncompliant patient (e.g., face debridement in a young child) is anticipated, the provision of brief general anesthesia[24,25] or regional anesthesia in the burn unit setting may be indicated.

Anticipatory anxiety is an important issue that can develop with the repeated (usually daily) performance of such wound care. When adequate analgesia is not provided for an initial, painful procedure, the effectiveness of analgesia for subsequent procedures is reduced, in large part from anticipatory anxiety and heightened arousal.[26,27] Thus, efforts to provide effective procedural burn sedation should begin as early in the hospitalization as possible, preferably with the first (and often most painful) wound care procedure. In addition, nonpharmacologic analgesic techniques are of particular value in the clinical setting of procedural pain and are discussed subsequently in detail.

Breakthrough Pain Management

Breakthrough pain occurs when the comfort provided by background pain therapies is exceeded and can be the result of inadequate analgesic support (e.g., undertreatment, development of opioid tolerance) or predictable changes in the burn wound itself that may produce increased pain (e.g., proliferation of epidermal skin buds during the spontaneous burn healing process). Recognition of the correct cause of the breakthrough pain is paramount so that the appropriate change in pharmacologic or nonpharmacologic management can rapidly take place.

Postoperative Pain Management

Postoperative pain is an anticipated and temporary (2 to 5 days) increase in background pain that occurs after burn excision or grafting procedures and is most commonly the result of increased pain from newly created wounds at the skin graft harvesting site. Pharmacologic management of postoperative pain includes a temporary increase in background opioid analgesic support but can also include the use of continuous regional block techniques in the immediate postoperative period.[28] One of the most useful nonpharmacologic analgesic techniques in this setting is information provision, so that patients also anticipate both the increase and the temporary nature of the postoperative pain.

Pharmacologic Approaches to the Management of Burn Pain

Three consistent observations can be made in describing pharmacologic approaches for burn analgesia. First, for patients with injuries extensive enough to need hospitalization, potent opioid analgesics form the cornerstones of pharmacologic pain control, whereas the mild to moderate analgesia provided by NSAIDs or acetaminophen may provide some degree of opioid-sparing effect but have limited use until the later rehabilitative or outpatient phases of treatment. Second, because burn pain is largely influenced by the parameters of care (background, procedural, and postoperative pain), pharmacologic choices for analgesia should target each of the four clinical pain settings individually. Finally, because burn pain varies somewhat unpredictably throughout hospitalization, analgesic regimens should be continuously evaluated and reassessed to avoid problems of undermedication or overmedication. Pain assessment is facilitated by the regular use of standardized, self-report scales for adults and older children and observational scoring systems for the very young, as described elsewhere in this text. Of special note is that the reliance on nurse assessment of patient burn pain can be problematic; it is well documented that nurse and patient assessments of burn pain and analgesic effects are not always comparable.[29–31] Unfortunately, nursing staff assessments frequently underestimate the need for analgesic therapy in the burn setting (a problem that is echoed in the evaluations of physicians and other health care professionals). Thus, whenever possible, patient reports of pain should be elicited and should be the basis for analgesic decisions, rather than observations of the staff.

Opioid Analgesics

The most commonly used analgesics in the treatment of burn pain are opioid agonists, in part because: (1) they are potent; (2) the benefits and risks of their use are familiar to most care providers; and (3) they provide some dose-dependent degree of sedation that can be advantageous to both burn patients and staff, particularly during burn wound care procedures. The wide spectrum of opioid analgesics available for clinical use provides dosing flexibility (i.e., variable routes of administration, variable durations of action) that is ideal for the targeted treatment of burn pain. The pharmacokinetics of opioid analgesics in burn patients are not consistently different from nonburn patients,[32,33] although decreased volume of distribution and clearance and increased elimination half-life have been reported for morphine.[34] Similarly, pharmacodynamic potency of opioids has inconsistently been reported as increased[35] and decreased[34] in burn patients.

The route of opioid administration is an important issue in burn patients, with the principal choice between IV or oral administration dictated by the severity of burn (critically ill patients need IV access and may have abnormal gut function) and the high risk of burn patients for development of intravascular catheter-related sepsis (hence, physician reluctance to maintain long-term IV access).[36] Intramuscular opioid administration is avoided because of the need for repeated, painful injections and because of variable vascular absorption from unpredictable compartmental fluid shifts and muscle perfusion in burn patients, particularly those undergoing burn shock resuscitation immediately after the burn injury. PCA with IV opioids offers the burn patient a safe and efficient method of achieving more flexible analgesia. PCA also offers patients the nonpharmacologic benefit of control coping by allowing some degree of control over their medical care, which often is a major issue for burn patients whose waking hours are often completely scheduled with care activities ranging from wound care to physical and rehabilitation therapy, all within the foreign confines of the hospital. Studies that compare PCA opioid use with other routes of administration in the burn population have shown positive, but limited, benefits of PCA.[37] Finally, oral transmucosal administration of opioids is reported in burn patients[21,22] and appears to be particularly advantageous in those patients without IV access and in children.

Nonopioid Analgesics

The list of nonopioid analgesics in widespread use for the treatment of burn pain is currently limited, although not without potential benefit. Oral NSAIDs and acetaminophen, as outlined previously, are only mild analgesics that exhibit a ceiling effect in their dose-response relationship, rendering them unsuitable for the treatment of typical, severe burn pain, except to the degree that they provide a limited opioid-sparing effect. However, they are of benefit in treatment of minor burns, particularly in the outpatient setting. The opioid agonist-antagonist drugs (e.g., nalbuphine, butorphanol) produce "mixed" actions at the opiate receptor level, theoretically providing analgesia (agonist property) with lesser side effects (antagonist properties), but also exhibit ceiling effects. Although studies have shown this class of drugs to be effective in treatment of burn pain,[38] experience with them is both limited and suggestive of efficacy in patients with only relatively mild burn pain.

Centrally acting alpha$_2$ agonists have been proposed as potential analgesic agents for burn pain based on their known mechanisms of action in other acute pain states. In case reports, clonidine has shown analgesic efficacy in burned children[39,40]; the efficacy of dexmedetomidine is limited to anecdotal reports to date.

Anxiolytics

Aggressive surgical treatment and debridement of burn wounds, together with the persistent and repetitive qualities of background and procedural burn pain, make burn care an experience that creates significant anxiety in most patients of all ages. The recognition that anxiety can exacerbate acute pain has led to the common practice in US burn centers of use of anxiolytic drugs in combination with opioid analgesics, a practice that has become more widespread in the past two decades.[3,12] Intuitively, this practice is particularly useful in premedicating patients for wound care because of the anticipatory anxiety experienced by these patients before and during such procedures. However, benzodiazepine therapy has also been shown to improve postoperative pain scores in nonburn[41] and burn[42] settings. Specific to burns, patients who appear most likely to benefit from this therapy are not necessarily those with high trait (premorbid) anxiety but rather those with either high state (at the time of the procedure) anxiety or high baseline pain scores.[42]

Anesthetics

Given the brief, but intense pain associated with many burn wound procedures, the provision of a limited duration general anesthetic may at first glance seem a reasonable analgesic approach. However, the repeated (often daily) need for such procedures poses economic and logistic obstacles that makes general anesthesia not feasible. Nonetheless, the provision of deep sedation with carefully titrated inhaled or IV anesthetic agents, brief general anesthetics, and regional analgesic techniques have a large role in procedural burn pain settings.

Inhaled nitrous oxide is an analgesic agent safe for administration by nonanesthesia personnel and provides safe and effective analgesia without loss of consciousness for moderately painful procedures in other health care settings. It is also used for the treatment of burn pain,[23,43] typically as a 50% mixture in 50% oxygen and self administered by an awake, cooperative, spontaneously breathing patient via a mouthpiece or mask. Although the level of sedation achieved with such inhalation is typically light (minimal or moderate by ASA definitions), the analgesic effect of the drug can be very good. Furthermore, the technique allows patients some degree of control in their medical care (i.e., deciding when to breathe and when not to breathe the agent during the procedure) and can consequently benefit patients psychologically. On the negative side, nitrous oxide has also been implicated in a small but measurable incidence of toxicity issues (e.g., spontaneous abortion, bone marrow suppression) to patients or staff exposed for prolonged periods,[44,45] although not in the setting of burn pain treatment.

Certain aggressive wound care procedures are, in terms of invasiveness, on a scale well below that of surgical burn care (and associated general anesthesia) yet are nonetheless difficult to perform on a conscious patient (e.g., the removal of hundreds of skin staples from recently grafted wounds, meticulous wound care of recently grafted and often tenuous skin on the face or neck, or wound care procedures in variably cooperative children). For such cases, deep sedation or general anesthesia with intravenous agents may be indicated, in spite of the logistic or economic challenges they present. Historically, IV or intramuscular ketamine has been used for these procedures[46,47]; more recently, oral ketamine use is described for pediatric burn patients.[20] However, ketamine use is limited by the potential risk of associated emergence delirium reactions (5% to 30% incidence rate), particularly in the elderly. Alternatively, propofol has been reported safe and effective when administered by appropriately trained physicians (anesthesiologists) in the burn setting[48] and has even been suggested to be a potential drug for PCA delivery for less aggressive wound care procedures.[49] Propofol is particularly advantageous because it can be titrated to effect in terms of both level of consciousness and duration of action with continuous IV infusion techniques and carries the benefit of a rapid awakening with a minimal risk of nausea.

The extension of full anesthetic care capabilities outside of the operating room and into the burn ward has been implemented in high-volume, specialized burn centers.[24,25] This has been facilitated by the recent introduction into clinical anesthetic practice of a variety of drugs with a rapid onset and short duration of action, a more rapid awakening and recovery, and fewer associated side effects— ideal qualities for agents to be used for procedural burn wound care—that include IV propofol, IV remifentanil, and inhaled sevoflurane. The provision of brief, dense analgesia or anesthesia in a comprehensively monitored setting by individuals specifically trained to provide the service appears safe and efficient, both in terms of allowing wound care to proceed rapidly under ideal conditions for patient and nursing staff and in terms of cost-effective use of the operating room only for true surgical burn care procedures.

Regional anesthetic blockades in various forms may also be considered for inpatient burn pain management. Neuraxial administration of local anesthetics (or opioid analgesics) via an epidural catheter seem to be of benefit in patients with lower extremity burns, resulting in both background and procedural analgesia and autonomic sympathectomy and peripheral vasodilation (of theoretical benefit to wound healing). However, such use has only been reported anecdotally.[50] A major drawback of this technique is that the accompanying indwelling catheter can become densely colonized with infectious organisms at the wound site, thus increasing the risk for the serious complication of epidural abscess formation[51] Targeted non-neuraxial regional blockade, in contrast, is relatively easy to perform, carries minimal risks, and has been reported primarily for lower extremity analgesia after skin graft harvesting (fascia iliaca block). This technique can be used both for immediate postoperative analgesia (one-shot injection[52]) and for prolonged postoperative analgesia (continuous local anesthetic infusion via indwelling catheter[28]).

Local anesthetics are of obvious use in regional blockade for wound care procedures but may also be considered for burn pain analgesia in the form of a topical gel. The use of topical local anesthetics on burn wounds is controversial. The commonly available prilocaine (2.5%)–lidocaine (2.5%) cream (eutetic mixture of local anesthetics [EMLA]), when administered at a total dose of 2g, had no effect in a study on burn pain in volunteers.[53] Topical 5% lidocaine applied at 1 mg/cm^2 offered analgesic benefit in one study without associated side effects[54]; however, enthusiasm for its use is significantly tempered by reports of local anesthetic-induced seizures from enhanced systemic absorption at open wound sites.[55]

Nonpharmacologic Approaches to the Management of Burn Pain

Pharmacologic and nonpharmacologic treatments should be complementary in treatment of pain and anxiety in the burn patient. Considerable empirical evidence for the efficacy of nonpharmacologic treatments has been reported with burn pain, particularly when used as an adjunct to opioid analgesics. Beginning nonpharmacologic treatments as early as possible in the patient's hospital course is important to prevent anticipatory anxiety and the subsequent anxiety-pain cycle. Before the various nonpharmacologic techniques are explained in detail, the psychologic factors that come into play during burn care that can exacerbate pain should be understood. Perhaps the most important example of such a process is the potential loss of control that burn patients experience and its relation to coping.

Coping with Decreased Control

The experience of sustaining a burn injury, and enduring the many subsequent treatments, taxes a person's coping resources by reducing the sense of control. Most patients describe feelings of having less control in the hospital setting because of a number of factors, including high pain levels, the unfamiliar environment, a forced dependency on caregivers, the lack of input into daily schedules and routines, and the uncertainty about the future (e.g., appearance, wound status, work, or even survival). Such uncertainty about the nature and outcome of treatment often leads to feelings of helplessness in both adults and children. Patients and staff need effective strategies to maximize a patient's sense of control.[27]

For selection of appropriate strategies, one should understand the types of coping mechanisms that patients might be actively using and also ones of which they are not aware and may be of potential use.[27] The two-process model of control is applicable in this respect to both adults and children.[56] This model distinguishes between primary, secondary, and relinquished control strategies. Primary control is when persons manipulate the situation or environment to fit their needs; secondary control is when persons modify themselves to better fit the situation. Relinquished control describes the coping style of

"giving up" and often involves a process of emoting or withdrawal and depression. Research has shown that flexible coping, using both primary and secondary control strategies, is most adaptive.[57] Selection of a coping style that suits the particular situation works better than strict adherence to one approach. Patients who assertively request more medication in response to pain are demonstrating adaptive primary coping, and those who mediate or pray while having a particularly bad day are likely illustrating secondary coping strategies; both can be useful under some circumstances. On the other hand, adults and children who rely too much on a relinquished control style show greater psychologic distress.[58,59] This type of coping often leads to learned helplessness and is characterized by negative catastrophic thoughts, more pain behaviors, higher pain levels, and slower physical recovery.[27,60] The nonpharmacologic pain management techniques listed in the remainder of this chapter ideally help patients regain some control over their environment through primary or secondary control coping techniques.

A number of nonpharmacologic treatments are available for use with burn pain. In choosing the most effective approach, the team should be guided by the manner in which patients have typically responded to stressful medical procedures. Such responses lie on a continuum that ranges from giving up control to the health care professional and desiring little information to seeking out as much information as possible and actively participating in care. Those patients who wish to give up control to the health care professional have a tendency toward cognitive avoidance and likely use various types of distraction techniques to avoid the painful stimuli. These patients are said to have more of an avoidant coping style. Those who seek out information about the procedure and like to participate as much as they can often find distraction techniques distressing; for them, trying to ignore a procedure may serve to relinquish too much control. Such patients are thought to have more of an approach coping style.[61] One should note that both coping styles can be adaptive and it is best for the care team to support an individual's coping style rather than try to change the natural response. Also important to note is that patients may change their coping style depending on the procedure. For example, patients may find it is easier to use distraction techniques for short procedures such as receiving injections, whereas they are more comfortable attending to details of their long wound care sessions and participating when possible. Patients may also change their coping style as they become more familiar and comfortable with the environment. The approach avoidance coping continuum and the interventions that can be considered along it are illustrated in **Table 25.2**. Techniques (e.g., imagery or hypnosis) may fall into various places on the continuum, and depending on the outcome goals and script, the continuum can be a useful heuristic to guide clinicians in choosing an appropriate technique for a specific patient. The remainder of this section describes the nature of various nonpharmacologic interventions for burn pain management and how they fall on the continuum.

Avoidance
DISTRACTION

The types of distraction techniques available to reduce burn pain are limited only by the creativity of patients and health care professionals. Common distraction techniques used with children include bubble blowing, singing songs, reading a story, and counting. Generating strategies for adults may

Table 25-2 Control Coping Continuum and Nonpharmacologic Techniques	
Avoidance Coping style	1. Avoidance
|	Distraction
|	Imagery
|	Hypnotic analgesia
|	Virtual reality
|	2. Relaxation
|	Deep breathing
|	Progressive relaxation
|	3. Operant Techniques
|	Regular medication schedule
|	Quota system
|	Positive reinforcement
|	4. Information
|	Medication effects
|	Procedures
|	Timelines
|	5. Cognitive Restructuring
|	Thought stopping
|	Cognitive reappraisal
Approach Coping Style	6. Participation
	Setting schedules
	Wound care

require a bit more creativity, but adults can do a number of things, including engaging in enjoyable conversation during the procedure, listening to music, playing a video game, or immersing themselves in interactive virtual reality (see subsequent discussion) during the procedure.

IMAGERY

Patients who use imagery simply create or recreate an image in their mind, presumably one that they find pleasant and engaging. Types of imagery can be infinite and depend on the desired goals. For example, many people use healing imagery to facilitate recovery from overcoming disease or injury. In the case of burn injuries, they might imagine processes such as increased blood flow to the injured area in an effort to carry away damaged tissue and rebuild new tissue or decreased inflammation in the injured area. Although healing imagery can be an effective means of helping the burn patient feel more in control of the situation, it forces a person to focus on their injury and is consequently not a distraction technique when used in this way. In contrast, relaxation imagery tends to work best for pain control and is a better example of use of imagery for distraction. Before a painful procedure, the patient elicits a "safe" or "favorite" place to go. This can be a place where they have been before (e.g., a favorite vacation spot) or simply a place that they imagine to be relaxing and safe. Some common examples include the beach, a spot for camping or hiking or fishing, a grandmother's kitchen, or a childhood bedroom. The clinician then collects as many details as possible about what this place looks like (the colors, the sounds, the smells, objects in this place), and the patient practices the imagery; before the procedure, patients are encouraged to relax through deep breathing, closing their eyes, and imagining this favorite place. The clinician simply cues the patient with the details that they have provided before beginning relaxation. Next, the patient is encouraged to imagine this place during subsequent wound care, and if necessary, the clinician is present during the wound care to facilitate "taking them" to this place. Children often enjoy more active forms of imagery that relate to fantasy, such as taking a magic carpet ride or jumping on a broomstick with Harry Potter and flying through the woods at Hogwarts.[62]

Numerous imagery scripts have been published and can be used when a person is unable to think of a safe or favorite place.[63] These scripts often entail a person "flying" or "floating on a cloud" through beautiful places. An important note is that a patient should be asked about any fears such as heights, flying, or water so that use of these images does not actually create more anxiety.

Imagery is usually most effective when all of the senses are incorporated to make it as realistic and absorbing as possible. Most people need practice to be able to create vivid images, and some people are unable to visualize much at all, particularly when they are in significant pain and are too distracted. Virtual reality may be a better option for these patients (see subsequent discussion).

HYPNOTIC ANALGESIA

Although hypnosis involves much more than just avoidance or distraction, the end result is often similar in that this technique takes a person's focus off of the painful procedure. Hypnosis is an altered state of consciousness characterized by an increased receptivity to suggestion, ability to alter perceptions and sensations, and an increased capacity for dissociation.[64] Several features make it a unique method of pain control that differs markedly from imagery or relaxation. In fact, hypnosis may or may not lead to relaxation depending on the nature of the suggestions. In turn, it is not necessary for a patient to be relaxed or even in a deep hypnotic state for suggestions to be useful.[65] The belief is that the dramatic shift in consciousness that occurs with hypnosis is the cornerstone of an individual's ability to change awareness of pain.[66] Hypnosis involves several stages, including building clinician-patient rapport, enhancing relaxation through deep breathing, suggestions for deepening the hypnotic state and narrowing attention, providing posthypnotic suggestions, and alerting.[67] A full hypnotic induction for burn care is published in Patterson's[64] *Clinical Hypnosis for Pain*, as are inductions for the patient in the intensive care unit (ICU) or a crisis situation. In addition, the rapid induction analgesia format was described by Patterson[67] and originally published by Barber.[68] Hypnosis should only be used by trained clinicians who can assess the risks and benefits of this powerful technique. As an example, patients with a history of sexual abuse may have a tendency to dissociate too easily and are not served by hypnosis in some instances.

Hypnotic analgesia has increased in popularity with recent reports that it can reduce medical costs[64,69] or possibly even facilitate wound healing.[70,71] Although the mechanism for how hypnosis works is not fully understood, hypnotic analgesia has shown demonstrable brain function changes in neuroimaging studies.[72] A metaanalysis by Montgomery, DuHamel, and Redd[73] reported analgesic effects in most studies that used hypnosis for clinical and experimental pain. A more recent review by Patterson and Jensen[74] indicated that anecdotal reports of hypnotic pain relief have been published for decades on virtually every type of pain imaginable. They found 17 randomized controlled studies on the use of hypnosis for acute pain and concluded that the evidence for hypnotic analgesia was strong and seems to be related to the trait of hypnotizability. Several studies have shown the efficacy of hypnosis for patients with burn injuries.[75-77] Patterson, Adcock, and Bombardier[78] have

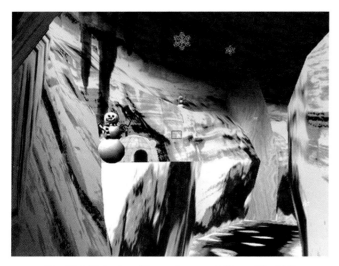

Fig. 25.4 **Virtual reality environment "SnowWorld."**

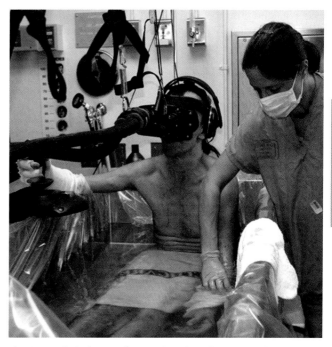

Fig. 25.5 **Clinical use of virtual reality distraction during burn wound care.**

proposed several reasons why patients with burn injuries may make good candidates for hypnotic analgesia. First, the intense nature of burn pain motivates patients to engage in this technique that they might normally disregard. This is supported by research findings that show that patients with higher baseline pain levels have a greater drop in pain after hypnosis than patients with lower baseline pain levels.[75,79] Second, the behavioral regression that often occurs after a traumatic injury makes patients more willing to be taken care of by others. Third, patients with burn injuries often experience a dissociative response as a means of coping that may moderate hypnotizability. Finally, although burn pain associated with procedures is the most intense, it is also the most amenable to hypnotic analgesia; because these procedures are often planned in advance, patients can be adequately prepared for these aversive events with hypnosis.

Despite occasional dramatic responses to hypnosis in burn patients, not every patient benefits from this technique, and resources for a trained clinician may not be available on every burn unit. Research into ways of making hypnosis more available to patients and more effective for those with low hypnotizability scores would be valuable.[80] These goals could be accomplished by eliminating the need for a live hypnotist with either audiotaped or computer-assisted hypnosis and by making hypnosis less effortful for those with low hypnotizability scores or whose cognitive effort is compromised from pain. Patterson[64] discusses every element of this and the following section (virtual reality) in much more detail in a recent book.

VIRTUAL REALITY

Immersive virtual reality (VR) is a technology that isolates patients from the outside world, including any threatening stimuli associated with health care. Immersive VR uses a helmet or goggles that block the user's view of the real world and gives the patient the illusion of going into the three-dimensional computer-generated environment, a condition known as presence.[64] This quality makes immersive VR particularly effective in capturing participants' attention.[81] In the burn pain setting, a virtual environment called "SnowWorld" is used (**Fig. 25.4**)[82] in which patients float through an icy canyon and are able to direct snowballs at virtual snowmen and igloos as they appear. The image of snow was specifically

chosen because its connotation of cooling is in direct contrast to the sensations often associated with burn pain.

VR is effective in theory because attention involves the limited selection of relevant information from a variety of inputs or tasks, and each human has a finite amount of it available.[83,84] The strength of the illusion, or presence, is thought to reflect the amount of attention drawn into the virtual world.[85] Because it is designed to be a highly attention-grabbing experience, VR is thereby thought to reduce the amount of conscious attention available to process pain (**Fig. 25.5**). Less attention to pain can reduce perceived pain intensity and unpleasantness and can also reduce the amount of time patients spend thinking about pain. VR has been shown to be effective in reducing pain in a number of clinical studies that used it for pain distraction.[82,86-88] Virtual reality technology can also be used to administer hypnotic analgesia and is particularly effective with patients who have difficulty imagining a scene.[64,81]

Relaxation
DEEP BREATHING
Deep breathing, or diaphragmatic breathing, is one of the least time-consuming techniques to use and is easiest for adults and children to learn. When a person becomes anxious or experiences pain, breathing can become shallow and irregular because of the increased muscle tension in the chest wall. Such shallow breathing, known as thoracic breathing,[89] leads to an increase in muscle tension and subsequent heightened pain. Teaching patients to become aware of this cycle, and teaching deep breathing techniques that allow them to break it, usually leads to a relaxation response that can alleviate some pain. Bubble blowing and blowing on a pinwheel are helpful tools to use with children to encourage deep breathing. Adults can be taught to place a hand on their stomach and take a breath deep enough to passes through their chest and fills their stomach (shallow breathing is more in the chest and does not cause

as much hand movement on the stomach). Their hand should rise and fall with the stomach. The exhalation is the most important part of the deep breath and should not be rushed. Diaphragmatic breathing is central to all forms of relaxation and is simple and time efficient.[89]

PROGRESSIVE MUSCLE RELAXATION

Patients tend to use muscles inefficiently[89] when they experience stress such as pain, which results in muscle bracing that can lead to an increase in pain. Progressive muscle relaxation is a technique developed by a physician, Edmund Jacobson, after he observed increased muscle tension in hospitalized patients and discovered that those with more tension took longer to recuperate and had poorer outcomes.[90] He taught patients to systematically focus on a muscle group, tense and relax it, and then progress to a different group. This progression usually starts with the distal muscle groups and moves to the proximal ones until total body relaxation is achieved. Most patients are able to learn this technique with practice, facilitated by scripts or audiotapes. If a person is unable to actively tense a muscle group because of pain or injury, he or she can still imagine each muscle becoming progressively "warm, heaving and relaxed," a process known as autogenic training.[64] Patients repeat each statement to themselves as they hear in on a tape (e.g., "My right hand is heavy, my right hand is relaxed, my right hand is becoming warm…").

Operant Techniques

Operant techniques rely on the principles of reinforcement learning and are based on the assumption that patients repeat behaviors that have positive consequences and avoid those that lead to punishment.[64] These principles can be applied in various ways to alleviate burn pain.

REGULAR MEDICATION SCHEDULING

Many inpatient acute care settings administer pain medication on a *pro re nata* (prn) or "as needed" basis (i.e., waiting for patients to report they are in pain before providing analgesic medications). From a behavioral perspective, waiting to medicate patients until they report pain reinforces them for pain behaviors; this can later become problematic.[10] The reinforcing properties of this process come from the euphorigenic properties of short-acting opioid analgesics and the attention received from caregivers and family for displaying pain behaviors. In contrast, providing opioid analgesics on a regular schedule minimizes the potential for these reinforcing properties of drugs and attention to worsen the pain problem. The superiority of regularly scheduled medications over prn dosing has been shown with nonburn pain[91] and has also been confirmed in background pain management for burn-injured children.[92] Simply put, treating pain before it occurs with regularly scheduled medication is a superior approach based on psychologic, and neurophysiologic and pharmacologic, principles.

Although research has shown that there is little chance of creating a chronic drug problem when opioid analgesics are given for acute pain in patients with no substance abuse histories, there is a risk of exacerbating a preexisting substance abuse problem.[93] Therefore, adherence to a regular opioid schedule is even more important for patients with substance abuse histories. Patients with drug histories often have frequent pain reports or drug-seeking behaviors and typically have lower tolerance for pain. They may also approach multiple caregivers for medications that create staff splitting and caregiver resentment toward the patient. Adhering to a regular medication schedule and having only one caregiver responsible for discussing or changing medications and doses can help alleviate some of these problems. As noted previously, patients who present with premorbid opioid abuse issues, or who are on methadone maintenance programs, still need to receive adequate levels of opioid analgesics to manage the acute burn pain. The consequences of patients self administering street narcotics for pain control can be extremely disruptive, if not fatal for the patient.

QUOTA SYSTEM

Patients can become easily overwhelmed through the multiple invasive therapies involved in burn care. They can also lose a sense of control and develop a type of learned helplessness. The quota system is one of the more effective techniques to address this. The quota system is an operant technique often used by burn providers to promote a sense of mastery among patients undergoing painful wound care procedures and difficult physical therapies.[94] Caregivers are encouraged to pace their procedural demands in a manner that is consistent with what is within the individual's level of tolerance by taking baseline measurements for each task that needs to be performed and gradually (10% per day) increasing the demands of each task. Rest is used as the reinforcement for successfully reaching a quota or, in other words, meeting a predetermined level of exercise (task). Goals for each task are determined based on what was done the previous day, and patients are expected to work until the goal is accomplished, rather than work until they feel pain or fatigue. This technique puts more control in the hands of the patient and consequently offsets the syndrome of learned helplessness discussed previously. It also avoids reinforcement of pain behaviors. The quota system is based on the notion that although physical therapies after a burn injury are painful, this pain itself is not damaging and does not negatively impact outcome. As discussed subsequently, patients are taught the difference between hurt and harm.

POSITIVE REINFORCEMENT

Positive reinforcement is another operant principle that is often successful with patients with burn injuries, particularly children. There is no intrinsically rewarding aspect of sustaining a burn injury or going through the care necessary for recovery. In fact, children often see the treatment for a burn injury as a punishment. Explaining to children that they are not undergoing painful procedures because they have done anything wrong, particularly if they see themselves as responsible for their injury, is often important. Children need to be rewarded for participation in the recovery process and for displaying appropriate behavior. For example, a common practice on a burn unit is use of a sticker board and prize box in each child's room. Behavioral expectations are established in advance and define what responsibilities the child has for that day, such as wound care, physical and occupational therapy, eating meals, etc. Children receive a reward (sticker) for each responsibility that they accomplish. Once they have a set amount of stickers, they are able to pick a prize from the prize box. This practice is known in the behavioral literature as establishing a token economy. Other creative means of positive reinforcement can also be effective, such as reading stories, watching movies or television, or offering adult attention. When children are frequently reinforced for good behavior or for completing a therapeutic goal, it lessens the need for punishment for bad behavior and makes the hospital environment more tolerable. In essence, the positive consequence after the adverse care on the burn unit is designed to be more prominent for the child; when reinforcement is not working, it is often because the magnitude of the reward is not sufficient.

With use of positive reinforcement, caregivers should also be careful not to reward (i.e., ignore) inappropriate behaviors such as tantrums or escape or avoidance behavior. For example, children often have a tantrum during wound care to try and get the nurse to cease what he or she is doing. If the nurse complies and stops wound care, the child has just been reinforced for the tantrum and learns to scream and cry to avoid a critical component of care. Once reinforced, this tactic then is likely to be tried in situations outside of wound care and in the next day's wound care. In contrast, once a behavioral expectation has been established (i.e., "we need to do our wound care now"), staff and parents need to commit to following through on the task, regardless of the child's response. Some of these responses can be avoided by allowing children to determine when their wound care will be, or to assist in the wound care, and by giving them positive reinforcement throughout wound care.

However, although minimizing attention to acting out in response to pain is often important, it is also important that reinforcement contingencies for children not be based on bravery or stoic pain. It is a subtle form of punishment to withhold rewards in wound care except when the child reacts calmly. Rather, acting out is ignored and the child is rewarded for successfully completing a therapy or wound care session. Ignoring pain behavior during wound care should only be considered after the burn team has done everything possible to minimize pain, in terms of both pharmacology and decreasing adversity of wound care (e.g., less caustic cleaning agents, longer water soaks).

Information

Patients differ in how much information they wish to receive about medical care. Most patients, however, find that the unknown is anxiety provoking and that receiving general information is helpful in reducing some anxiety. It is important to ask a patient how much detail they desire to know and follow their individual proclivities in providing information. Patients may benefit from information in several elements of burn care. First, side effects from medication can be worrisome, particularly for those who have no experience with potent opioid analgesics. Letting patients know that weird dreams, itching, and constipation are normal effects of pain medications and that long-term opioid dependency or addiction is unlikely can help alleviate these concerns. Second, some patients may not want to know details of procedures or tests but nevertheless should be warned that they will occur and told why and when they will occur. This information then allows patients to garner their coping skills and appropriately prepare for the situation. Finally, patients often report that not knowing the medical plan or timeline for upcoming surgeries, treatments, etc, is one of the biggest stressors in burn care. The nature of wound healing is such that the medical team

cannot predict whether the burn will need surgery or will heal on its own. Once this determination is made, however, it is important to sit down with patients and lay out a timeline for upcoming surgeries, dressing removals, therapies, rehabilitation, estimated discharge dates, and long-term care plans.

Cognitive Restructuring

Patients' thoughts about burn pain can be can be modified to reduce their perceptions of pain. Such cognitive restructuring is frequently used as a coping technique for patients with chronic pain.[95,96] Studies have identified the maladaptive thought pattern of catastrophizing as being particularly influential in how patients perceive pain. Teaching patients to recognize when they are engaging in catastrophic thoughts and to learn how to change that style will likely lead to a positive change in how they experience pain. A few reports in the literature have used this technique for various type of acute pain, including that from dental work and surgical procedures.[97] A handful of studies have investigated this approach with burn pain.[27,98] These techniques are likely to only be successful with patients who want to use more of an approach coping style because it forces them to be aware and tend to their thoughts of pain.

THOUGHT STOPPING

The first step in cognitive restructuring is to identify and stop negative catastrophizing thoughts. Thoughts such as "this is really going to hurt" and "I can't handle this pain" only lead to an increase in anxiety and a subsequent increase in pain. Patients can learn to recognize such negative thoughts and stop them, perhaps by picturing a stop sign or red light in their mind. They can also distract themselves by turning their attention to another topic. Children as young as 7 years of age have been taught to use this technique successfully.[27,99]

REAPPRAISAL

Ideally, patients should transform their catastrophic thoughts into positive, or at least neutral, statements. This is known as reappraisal, or reframing. For example, a patient may change the thoughts in the previous example to "I have been through this wound care procedure before, and it did not hurt as much as I thought it would" or "however much this hurts, it will go away." Patients may also benefit from being taught the difference between hurt and harm when interpreting pain sensations.[100] Specifically, an increase in pain is often a good sign with respect to burn wound healing. As discussed previously in the chapter, deep (third-degree) burns often destroy nerve endings and limit the capacity for nociception. In deep burns that begin to heal, or in more shallow burns, skin buds develop that are highly innervated and sensitive to pain and temperature.[10] An explanation of this healing process to patients can help them to understand the nature of their pain and to reframe negative thoughts into reassuring, positive ones.

The treatment for burn wounds, including daily removal of bandages and the aggressive washing of the open wounds, is counterintuitive to what most adults and children instinctively believe should be the appropriate treatment for open wounds. Most of us are taught to believe that we do not touch open wounds, and we certainly should not rub them aggressively. An explanation that this type of treatment, and the subsequent pain, is necessary to heal the wound can help patients to reframe any negative beliefs they may have toward wound care. Given the counterintuitive nature of the information, patients often must be given this information repeatedly; they have to have trust in the staff member (particularly children), and combining the information with relaxation or hypnosis is often useful.

Participation

Allowing patients who have more of an approach coping style to participate in their own burn care and recovery is one of the simplest and most effective ways to increase their sense of control and reduce anxiety. We often use the technique of forced choice for children to create more of a sense of control over their environment without overwhelming them with choices. When a child needs to accomplish an unpleasant task, parents and caregivers can often create a situation where the child is given two choices in how to proceed with the task. For example, children who have difficulty in wound care may be given the choice of having the nurse wash their arm or of washing the arm themselves. Or if children need to get out of bed to walk, they can be given the choice of either doing it before lunch or after lunch. They must choose one of the two options, and if they cannot decide within a certain time frame, they are told that the nurse or parent will decide for them. This method is likely to fail if more than two choices are given or if a child is presented with an option that caregivers or parents have no intention of allowing. Although patient participation may not be feasible in all aspects of burn care, several areas lend themselves to giving patients more control (e.g., uncomplicated wound care, physical therapy, nutritional intake).

SETTING SCHEDULES

Adults and children may benefit from having input into when certain tasks are done, such as wound care or physical therapy. Although open-ended choices in this matter are not feasible, a choice of two or three options may be reasonable. For example, patients can be given the choice of having wound care before lunch or after lunch, or physical therapy immediately after wound care in the morning or in the later afternoon. If a scheduling choice is not possible, sufficient notice of when the event will occur can help patients to adequately prepare themselves.

WOUND CARE

Patients who use more of an approach coping style can participate in their own wound care in a variety of different ways. One simple way is to allow the patient to choose if and what type of music is played during wound care. Patients are often encouraged to create a repeatable routine for each wound care procedure, in which they mentally prepare and do certain things the same way every day in an effort to help reduce anxiety. Because patients have different nurses from day to day, the patient must let the nurses know what works best and the details of the routine. Patients should be encouraged to take responsibility for communicating these plans to their nurse or therapist. Patients can also regulate the pace of wound care by asking for periodic breaks or by telling a nurse to wash slower or faster. One useful approach is to give children a set number of "timeout cards" (around five) that allow them a short (30-second) break during wound care. They can use them at any time until they are gone. Often, patients progress to the point of wanting to assist the nurses in their own wound care, particularly after they have

been in the hospital for some time. Easy ways to assist are to have them unwrap their bandages or wash areas that are easily reachable or particularly painful. Finally, patients preparing for hospital discharge may even want to perform their entire wound care independently if possible.

Side Effects and Complications
Analgesic Management Based on Valid Pain Assessment

As with any type of pain management paradigm, therapeutic burn pain decisions are related to what analgesic techniques to use, what drugs to use, and what drug doses to use, all of which hinge dramatically on the valid assessment of the patient's pain. Pain assessment is no less challenging in burn patients and may be further complicated by the multiple premorbid or comorbid psychologic issues that frequently accompany the burn injury.[11] As already noted, patient reports of pain are preferred because they differ from (and are typically greater than) those reported by burn caregivers.[29–31] However, patient reports are not always possible, as in cases of severely injured, noncommunicative (intubated and mechanically ventilated) adults or young children who cannot provide meaningful pain reports. Pain assessment in burns has been extensively reviewed, with details on appropriate tools for various clinical settings described elsewhere in adults[31] and children.[18]

Although pain assessment in the clinical and research setting has traditionally relied on patient reports (0 to 10 verbal scales, 0 to 10 visual analog scales [VAS], or 0 to 10 graphic rating scales [GRS]), increasing interest is found in assessment of patient satisfaction with pain control as an alternative measure of analgesic success. For example, asking a patient for a "treatment or analgesic goal" with the same measurement scale as for pain intensity can be useful. This concept has been recommended for clinical use by The Joint Commission[6] but is not in widespread use. However, in limited studies in the burn population,[101] those patients who experience the least amount of pain (by standard pain ratings) appear to have greater analgesic satisfaction than do those who report pain ratings that most closely match their stated analgesic treatment goals. Thus, the ideal choice and interpretation of pain assessment tools in burn pain settings is yet to be defined.

Complications From Excessive Analgesic Medications

The wide spectrum of untoward side effects associated with potent benzodiazepines, opioid analgesics, and anesthetics is well known and ranges from the relatively benign (e.g., transient nausea) to life threatening (e.g., respiratory depression). The prevention and treatment of these various analgesic side effects is detailed elsewhere in this text. However, general recommendations should include that all analgesia and sedation procedures be carried out under the guidelines published by the American Society of Anesthesiologists[19] and supported by The Joint Commission.[6] These guidelines include requirements for appropriate physiologic and consciousness monitoring and for appropriate training of all caregivers who administer pharmacologic sedation. Specifically, because the desired level of sedation (typically a moderate level) cannot be guaranteed in a given patient with a given pharmacologic regimen, providers must be trained and skilled at managing the next greater depth of sedation (deep sedation), including airway, respiratory, and cardiovascular support, in the event this level of sedation unexpectedly occurs.

Overlooking Anxiety

One of the biggest mistakes made in burn pain management is not recognizing anxiety and treating it accordingly. As mentioned previously, anxiety exacerbates, and often precedes, pain. Poorly managed pain, particularly early in the hospitalization, leads to anticipatory anxiety for any future procedures. An effective pain management program needs to target anxiety and pain, with use of both pharmacologic and nonpharmacologic techniques. For assessment of anxiety, one can ask patients to rate both their pain and their anxiety on separate 0 to 10 scales. In both adults and children who are unable to distinguish between pain and anxiety, staff should watch for behavioral signs, such as the display of pain behaviors before a procedure even begins. Taal and Faber[102,103] have published the *Burn Specific Anxiety Scale*, which is a measure validated with burn patients that focuses on anxiety during burn care procedures.

Staff Changeover

Patients have many caregivers during their hospitalization. Inconsistencies in the care that patients receive from various staff members can frustrate them and make pain and anxiety harder to manage. The familiarity and training that staff has had in nonpharmacologic pain management techniques also vary significantly. Inpatient units often have a shortage of nurses, and nursing time may be stretched between multiple patients. Thus, even when health care providers are well trained in nonpharmacologic techniques, they may not have adequate time to apply them effectively. Most burn centers recognize the importance of having psychologists and other specialists trained in these techniques as part of the burn team. These individuals may be available to assist in applying the techniques in many cases; however, it is not reasonable to assume that they will be available to meet every patient's daily needs. Therefore, they should continue to train nurses and patients in these techniques to the extent possible. Differences in how nurses perform wound care and lack of training in nonpharmacologic techniques can cause patients to lose confidence in the medical team and make pain even harder to manage. Thus, empowering patients to direct their own care by sharing with caregivers their care needs and preferences is even more necessary.

Mismatch of Techniques and Coping Style

As mentioned previously, matching various nonpharmacologic techniques to patient coping style is crucial. For example, one can see the problem in using a distraction technique with patients who have a high need for control and desire to participate in their wound care. Further, providing a patient who is closer to the avoidance end of the control continuum with too much information on a medical procedure may actually increase anxiety. Again, periodic assessment of a person's preference is important because patients often shift where they are on the continuum of control during hospitalization.

Inadequate Planning "Surprises"

Even with the most vigilant preparation, unplanned procedures, quick changes in schedules, and other "surprises" are bound to occur. These unplanned procedures can cause significant anxiety for patients and may increase pain levels. Teaching patients distress tolerance and to "expect the unexpected" and providing them with quick strategies to use when the unexpected occurs can go a long way toward decreasing anxiety and pain. Patients may even get to the point of being able to anticipate the chaos often associated with acute inpatient hospitalization. Although seemingly counterintuitive to the clinician, this is an example of the patient adopting a secondary coping mechanism as described previously.

Premorbid Psychologic Problems

Patients with preexisting problems, including anxiety disorders, substance abuse, and chronic pain, have even more difficulty with the management of acute pain and anxiety. As noted previously, preinjury psychologic problems are common in burn patients and are much higher than in the general population.[11] A burn injury and its subsequent treatment can often exacerbate depression in patients with this premorbid diagnosis. Treatment for depression should not only continue on the burn unit but should be pursued even more aggressively. Patients with DSM-IV revised (American Psychiatric Association) Axis II personality disorders often cause great difficulty for the staff. Caregivers need to be educated about such personality disorder and understand that a person with a burn injury will not be "cured" of such while on the burn unit. Psychologists or psychiatrists should be consulted to devise appropriate behavior plans and to train staff in managing such patients. Often patients with substance abuse problems have a strong reliance on the pharmacologic management of pain. Depending on the drug of choice, they may have a lower pain tolerance or display more pain behaviors. Specialists, such as anesthesiologists, may need to be consulted. Patients with substance abuse problems should still be offered nonpharmacologic approaches and should be encouraged to use them. Sufficient medication for acute pain through a regular medication schedule (versus prn) is particularly important for these patients. In the instance of premorbid anxiety and chronic pain problems, patients should be encouraged to use whatever coping techniques they have used in the past to manage these problems. Burn hospitalization and care may be an ideal time for such patients to learn new such techniques.

Wound Care Environment

Nurses can help make wound care procedures more relaxing by having the dressings and necessary supplies prepared in advance and laid out before the patient arrives in the tank room, by keeping the room warm, by having relaxing music playing low in the background, by dimming bright lights, by reducing clutter in the tank room, by keeping their voices low, and by speaking in relaxed tones. When a patient comes into a tank room that is not prepared and is cold and uninviting and encounters nurses who are rushed, an atmosphere of tension and anxiety for both the nurses and the patient is created. When a patient expresses significant anxiety and pain, the nurses must remain calm because patients often pick up on the anxiety or discomfort of the staff. Also, any painful procedure, including wound care, should be done in a location outside of the patient's room, particularly with children. A pediatric patient must feel that his or her room is a relaxing place that can be viewed as a safe retreat after painful procedures or therapies. Keeping the patient's room as a safe area also leads to more restful sleep.

Conclusion

The control of burn pain continues to be a challenge that demands creativity and continued staff training on pain assessment, traditional pharmacologic analgesic approaches, and adjunctive nonpharmacologic techniques. Pharmacologic analgesics need to be administered by appropriately trained and experienced staff, under appropriate monitoring conditions. Likewise, assessment of a patient's coping style and matching of nonpharmacologic techniques accordingly are crucial. Assessment is necessarily ongoing because patient coping styles and preferences may change throughout the hospitalization.

Future directions in burn pain management include improvements in the diagnostic and prognostic assessment of burn wounds and prediction of which analgesic techniques are best suited for individual patients. With regard to burn wound diagnosis, improved early and accurate definition of burns that will heal only with surgical excision and grafting helps minimize the number of patients who currently undergo days to weeks of hopeful watching of the burn wound, waiting for the wound to declare itself as self healing or not. There is a subpopulation of these patients who undergo days and weeks of painful wound care and significant background pain, only to discover that the burn could have been treated initially with excision and grafting, thus avoiding the prolonged period burn pain. With regard to predicting the most effective analgesic techniques in an individual burn patient, advances in both pharmacologic and nonpharmacologic techniques are anticipated. Pharmacologic analgesia potential for specific drugs may be more accurately predicted as genetic screening for opioid metabolic enzymes comes into common clinical practice, thus enabling caregivers to choose the most appropriate drug and dose for a given metabolic genotype.[104] Similarly, tools that predict the success of non-pharmacologic analgesic interventions will undoubtedly be developed. One such example is the assessment of hypnotizability (Stanford Hypnotic Clinical Scale[105]) that predicts the potential success of hypnotic analgesia in individual patients. With numerous such genetic and behavioral screening tools available for clinical use, one can imagine the power and clinical benefit of identifying and implementing, early in the clinical course of the burn patient, the most effective pharmacologic and nonpharmacologic analgesic techniques for a particular patient, thereby maximizing analgesic benefit and minimizing analgesic side effects.

References

Full references for this chapter can be found on www.expertconsult.com.

Sickle Cell Pain

Samir K. Ballas

Acknowledgements

Supported in part by the Sickle Cell program of the Commonwealth of Pennsylvania for the Philadelphia Region.

Introduction

The healthy adult hemoglobin (Hb A) is a tetramer of 2 alpha-globin chains and 2 beta-globin chains $(\alpha_2\beta_2)$.[1,2] Each chain contains a heme moiety that carries oxygen. Thus, the major function of hemoglobin is to transport oxygen from the lungs to all organs and tissues throughout the body. Hemoglobinopathies are disorders of the structure or function of Hb A. They are broadly divided into two major groups: structural variants and thalassemias. Structural variants are, most commonly, the result of single base mutation in the globin genes. Thalassemias are characterized by decreased synthesis of globin chains. Thus beta-thalassemia major or Cooley's anemia is the result of lack of or decreased synthesis of the beta-globin chains of hemoglobin.[1,2]

The sickle hemoglobin (Hb S) is the most common structural variant of normal hemoglobin, followed by hemoglobin C (Hb C). Both of these hemoglobins are the result of single base mutation in the 6th codon of exon I of the beta-globin gene responsible for the synthesis of the beta-globin chain hemoglobin. In the case of Hb S, glutamic acid is replaced by valine; in Hb C, glutamic acid is replaced by lysine. These mutations change the net charge of the variant hemoglobin, thus allowing their separation via electrophoresis.[3,4]

Sickle cell syndromes, also collectively referred to as sickle cell disease (SCD), are generic terms for a group of chronic inherited disorders of hemoglobin structure in which the affected individual inherits two mutant globin genes (one from each parent), at least one of which is always the sickle mutation. Sickle cell anemia (SS) is the homozygous state in which the sickle gene is inherited from both parents. Other sickle cell syndromes result from the coinheritance of the sickle gene and a nonsickle gene, such as Hb C, Hb O^{Arab}, Hb D, beta$^+$-thalassemia, beta^0-thalassemia, etc. **Table 26.1** lists the common sickle cell syndromes among Africans and African-Americans. Structural variants of hemoglobin are inherited in an autosomal codominant manner according to Mendelian principles. Thus, if one parent is healthy and the other has sickle cell anemia, then all children have sickle cell trait.

Pathophysiology

Sickle cell anemia is almost synonymous with pain, and the acute painful crisis is its hallmark. The most important pathophysiologic event in SS that explains most of its clinical manifestations is vasoocclusion.[5-8] The primary process that leads to vascular occlusion is the polymerization of Hb S on deoxygenation, which, in turn, results in distortion of the shape of red blood cells (RBCs), cellular dehydration, and decreased deformability and stickiness of RBCs that

Table 26.1 Major Types of Sickle Cell Syndromes and Their Typical Hematologic Parameters

Disease	Abbreviation	Genotype	Hb (g/dL)	Retic (%)	MCV (fl)	Hemoglobin Composition			
						Hb A %	Hb A$_2$* %	Hb S %	Hb F %
Sickle cell anemia									
1. No alpha-gene deletion	SS	β^S/β^S; $\alpha\alpha/\alpha\alpha$	7.0-8.0	10-20	85-110	0	2.5-3.5	75-96	1-20
2. Deletion of 2 alpha-genes	SS, α-Thal	β^S/β^S; $-\alpha/-\alpha$	9.0-10.0	6-12	70-80	0	3.0-4.5	75-94	1-20
Sickle-beta°-thalassemia	S-β°-Thal	$\beta^S/\beta°$ thal	7.0-10.0	6-15	60-70	0	4.0-6.0	70-90	1-20
Sickle-beta$^+$-thalassemia	S-β$^+$-Thal	β^S/β^+ thal	>10.0	5-10	60-70	10-20	4.0-6.0	65-85	1-15
Hb SCD	SC	β^S/β^C	>10.0	5-10	75-85	0	45-50	50	1-6
Sickle cell trait	AS	β^A/β^S	12-16	1.0-2.0	>82	55-57	2.5-3.5	40	<1.0

Note that all disorders may be associated with variable degrees of alpha gene deletions.
HbSCD, hemoglobin sickle-cell disease; MCV, mean corpuscular volume; Retic, reticuloyte count.
*Hb A$_2$ and Hb C have the same electrophoretic mobility at alkaline pH and are not separable on routine analysis; they can be separated, however, with high-pressure liquid chromatography (HPLC).

promotes their adhesion to vascular endothelium (**Fig. 26.1**). Vascular occlusion causes damage of the tissues supplied by the occluded vessel and is also responsible for creating a state of chronic vascular inflammation that explains many features of SCD.[9–11] Tissue damage and vascular inflammation generate a number of inflammatory mediators that initiate an electrical impulse of pain transmitted along peripheral nerves (Aδ and C fibers) to the dorsal horn of the spinal cord. The impulse ascends along the spinothalamic tract to the thalamus, which is a major relay station of the central nervous system (CNS). The thalamus interconnects reversibly with other centers, most notably with the limbic system and reticular formation (mediators of emotion and memory). At the same time, the CNS inhibits the transmission of the painful stimulus at the level of the dorsal horn via a descending pathway that begins in the periaqueductal gray matter of the midbrain. Eventually, the modified electrochemical impulse that started at the site of vasoocclusion is sent to the cerebral cortex, where it is perceived as pain by the patient. Pain perception is thus a subjective phenomenon and is the result of a complex interplay among enhancing and inhibiting factors at the level of the CNS.

Types of Sickle Pain

Sickle cell pain can be classified in a number of ways.[12–14] Pathophysiologically, sickle cell pain could be nociceptive or neuropathic; temporally, it could be acute or chronic; anatomically, it could be somatic, visceral, unilateral, bilateral, localized, or diffuse; pathologically, it could be mild, moderate, or severe; and etiologically, it could be the result of the disease itself, of therapy, or of comorbid conditions. The etiologic classification of sickle pain is listed in **Table 26.2** and includes pain syndromes that are unique to SCD. These include acute pain syndromes, chronic pain syndromes, and neuropathic pain. Other types of pain that are not unique to SCD, such as postoperative pain and pain from comorbid conditions, are described elsewhere in this book and are not addressed here.

Acute Sickle Cell Pain Syndromes
Acute Painful Episodes (Painful Crises)

The acute painful sickle cell crisis is the hallmark of SCD and is the most common symptom among patients with this disease. It is defined as new onset of pain that lasts at least 4 hours for which there is no explanation other than vasoocclusion and that requires therapy with parenteral opioids or ketorolac in a medical facility.[15] Most painful episodes, however, are mild in nature or of moderate severity and are usually treated at home with oral analgesics, bed rest, adequate oral hydration, and the application of local measures, such as a heating pad to the painful area.[12,16] Severe painful episodes necessitate treatment in the emergency room or hospital. About 95% of hospital admissions of adult patients with sickle cell disease are for the treatment of acute painful episodes.[17] The frequency and severity of these painful episodes vary considerably among patients and in the same patient from time to time.[12] Infection, stress of any kind, and emotional upheaval may precipitate a painful crisis.[12,18] In most patients, however, no obvious factor precedes the crisis.[12,19] Objective signs of a painful crisis, such as fever, leukocytosis, joint effusions, and tenderness, occur in about 50% of patients at initial presentation.[12,19] The acute painful episode (painful crisis) evolves through four phases: prodromal, initial, established, and resolving.[12,20,21] Objective laboratory signs do occur during these phases in most patients provided the tests are done serially and compared with established steady-state values.[12,20,21] Moreover, recent studies have suggested a vasoocclusive "phenotype" that consists of patients with relatively higher hemoglobin levels who clinically display increased frequency of pain, acute chest syndrome, and avascular necrosis.[22] About 10% to 15% of patients with SS have very frequent severe crises (10 to 20/y). This subset of patients is almost always hospital or emergency room bound and evokes considerable resentment among some health care providers who, in turn, develop stereotyped misconceptions about SCD in general. Pain usually involves the low back, legs, knees, arms, chest, and abdomen in decreasing order of

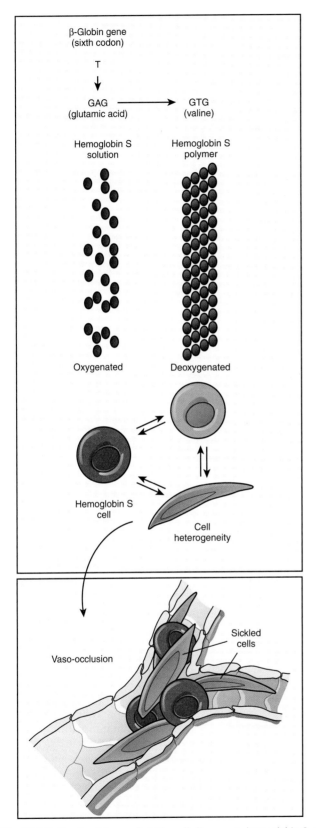

Fig. 26.1 Pathophysiology of sickle cell disease. In hemoglobin S, a substitution of T for A in the sixth codon of the beta-globin gene leads to the replacement of a glutamic acid residue by a valine residue. On deoxygenation, hemoglobin S polymers form, causing cell sickling and damage to the membrane. Some sickle cells adhere to endothelial cells, leading to vasoocclusion. *(Reproduced from Steinberg MH: Management of sickle cell disease, N Engl J Med 340:1022, 1999, with permission.)*

Table 26.2 Etiologic Classification of Pain Syndromes Unique to Sickle Cell Disease

ACUTE PAIN SYNDROMES
Acute painful sickle cell crises
Acute chest syndrome
Right upper quadrant syndrome
Left upper quadrant syndrome
Hand-foot syndrome (dactylitis)
Priapism
CHRONIC PAIN SYNDROME
With objective signs
Avascular (aseptic) necrosis
Leg ulcers
Without objective signs
Intractable chronic pain
NEUROPATHIC PAIN SYNDROMES UNIQUE/COMMON IN SICKLE CELL DISEASE
Mental nerve neuropathy
Ischemic optic neuropathy
Spinal cord infarction
Other neuropathies

frequency.[12,23] Pain may be throbbing, sharp, dull, or stabbing in nature. Bone marrow infarcts are associated with the most severe pain that is pounding-stabbing in nature and forces the patient to assume certain postures (crouching, raising legs, etc) in an effort to mitigate the intensity of the pain.[12,23]

Acute Chest Syndrome

This is an acute illness characterized by fever or respiratory symptoms, accompanied by a new pulmonary infiltrate on a chest x-ray.[15] The full-blown clinical picture of acute chest syndrome includes chest pain, fever, dyspnea, hypoxia, pulmonary infiltrates on chest x-ray, and a decreasing Hb level. These signs and symptoms vary from the very mild, to the very severe, which may be life threatening. The syndrome may be caused by pneumonia, pulmonary infarcts from in situ sickling, fat embolism, or pulmonary embolism. Diagnostic workup should include chest x-ray, sputum and blood cultures, monitoring of arterial blood gases, monitoring of Hb levels, ventilation and perfusion (V/Q) scans, monitoring for fat bodies in sputum and urine, and ruling out thrombophlebitis in the pelvis or lower extremities as possible sources of emboli. Treatment includes antibiotic therapy, oxygen, and, in severe cases, transfusion or exchange transfusion to bring the percentage of Hb S to less than 30% and keep the Hb level 9 to 10 g/dL. Caution should be exercised in giving opioids (especially the slow-release preparations) or nonsteroidal anti-inflammatory drugs (NSAIDs) to the hypoxic patient to avoid possible respiratory depression or bronchospasm, respectively,. Heparin is usually reserved for the patient with a proven pulmonary embolism. Repeated attacks of acute chest syndrome with pulmonary infarcts predict the onset of pulmonary failure with cor pulmonale and terminal adult respiratory distress syndrome.[24–28]

Right Upper Quadrant Syndrome

Chronic hyperbilirubinaemia, cholelithiasis, and gall bladder disease are common in patients with sickle cell disease. At least two thirds of patients with sickle cell anemia have hepatomegaly, and 75% have cholelithiasis. About 90% of patients with cholelithiasis undergo cholecystectomy either prophylactically or after an episode of acute calculus cholecystitis. Most cholecystectomies are currently performed via laparoscopy, a much simpler procedure than laparotomy, and are associated with less morbidity.[29–31]

Hepatic crisis (also called sickle cell intraheptic cholestasis) is the sudden onset of right upper quadrant pain, progressive hepatomegaly, increasing bilirubin levels (mostly indirect), and prolongation of prothrombin and partial thromboplastin times. The levels of liver enzymes (γ-glutamyl transpeptidase [γGT] and alanine amino transferase [ALT]) are also increased, but not to those levels seen in acute viral hepatitis. Liver biopsy shows engorgement of hepatic sinusoids with sickled erythrocytes. Hepatic crises vary in severity from minor episodes to severe life-threatening situations. Total blood exchange is a recommended for the severe variety. Blood exchange is indicated if the total bilirubin level increases progressively to values greater than 50 g/L. At that level, the prothrombin time values are usually prolonged. Blood exchange should be total in nature; that is, whole blood is removed and replaced with red cells and fresh frozen plasma to correct the coagulation abnormality.[29,32–35]

Left Upper Quadrant Syndrome
ACUTE SPLENIC SEQUESTRATION CRISIS

This rapid intrasplenic trapping of cellular elements of the blood causes a precipitous fall in hemoglobin level and is often associated with a relative or absolute thrombocytopenia and hypovolemia.[15] In its full blown picture, acute splenic sequestration is characterized by a pentad of: (1) rapid fall in hemoglobin level; (2) rise in reticulocyte count; (3) fall in platelet count; (4) sudden increase in spleen size associated with acute pain and tenderness in the left upper quadrant; and (5) signs and symptoms of hypovolemia. Minor episodes may resolve spontaneously, but severe episodes can be fatal and may be mistaken for the sudden infant death syndrome. Treatment of acute splenic sequestration consists of rapid restoration of intravascular volume and oxygen-carrying capacity. This goal is achieved with the transfusion of sickle-negative RBCs at a rate of 15 to 20 mL/kg with careful monitoring to avoid sudden overexpansion of blood volume that may precipitate pulmonary edema. After successful treatment, the spleen usually shrinks within a few days and gradually regains its baseline size. Splenectomy has been recommended for patients who survive the initial severe episode and for patients who have recurrent episodes of acute sequestration.[36–38]

Acute Splenic Infarction

This acute ischemic necrosis of the spleen is a result of venous or arterial compromise. In patients with sickle cell, this is due to the inability of the rigid sickle red cell to negotiate the splenic circulation. In SS, multiple infarcts during childhood commonly result in a scarred, contracted, autoinfarcted spleen by adulthood. Clinically, it is characterized by acute left upper quadrant pain that may be referred to the left shoulder; imaging studies show evidence of necrotic or ischemic splenic parenchyma.[15,39]

Hand-Foot Syndrome (Dactylitis)

This acute pain syndrome occurs most commonly in infants and young children between the ages of 6 months and 2 years, with a few case reports up to 7 years, The clinical picture is characterized by acute painful swelling with limited range of motion of one or more extremities. It is caused by inflammation from ischemic infarction of the bone of the affected extremity, resulting in swelling, redness, and pain in affected areas. Fever and leukocytosis may be present. The episode is usually self limiting and resolves within 1 week, but recurrent attacks are common. Treatment is symptomatic, and if the attack persists, acute osteomyelitis should be ruled out.[40,41]

Priapism

Priapism is a painful, persistent, unwanted erection of the penis. Diagnosis is based on patient self report. During an episode, priapism can be confirmed with physical examination findings of a fully erect tender penis and symptom of pain in the penis or scrotum. Priapism could be stuttering, with episodes (lasting up to 4 hours) that are often recurrent, or prolonged, with episodes lasting 4 hours or longer and carrying the risk of ischemia, fibrosis, and impotence. Stuttering priapism responds well to diazepam or pseudoephedrine. Patients who become impotent may benefit from psychologic counseling and the insertion of penile implants. A practical and relatively simple approach to manage outpatients with priapism includes aspiration of the corpora cavernosa followed by irrigation with a dilute epinephrine solution. Patients who do not respond to this approach are potential candidates for exchange transfusion or surgery.[15,42,43]

Chronic Sickle Cell Pain Syndromes

The two types of chronic sickle cell pain are: chronic pain from obvious pathology (leg ulcers and avascular necrosis) and intractable chronic pain with no obvious objective signs.

Leg Ulcers

Leg ulcers are ulcerations of the skin and underlying tissues of the lower extremities, especially the medial or lateral surfaces of the ankles. Trauma, infection, and severe anemia may predispose patients to ulcer formation. They could be mid or large and severe. Severity may be based on depth or duration. Depth is usually used most often in describing the severity of leg ulcers; the deeper the ulcer, the worst the prognosis.[15,44–46]

Leg ulcers tend to be indolent and intractable and heal slowly over months to years. The pain may be severe, excruciating, penetrating, sharp, and stinging in nature. In most patients, oral or parenteral opioid analgesics are needed to achieve some pain relief. The prevalence rate is about 5% to 10% in adult patients. Leg ulcers are more common in males and older patients and less common in patients with alpha-gene deletion, relatively high Hb level, or high levels of Hb F. They seem to be associated with the severity of hemolysis, priapism and pulmonary hypertension. Moreover, leg ulcers have been reported to be more common in carriers of the Central African republic beta-gene cluster haplotype and associated with single nucleotide polymorphism in Klotho, tyrosine kinase (endothelial), and genes of the transforming growth factor–beta/bone morphogenetic protein pathway.[44–48]

Principles of management of leg ulcers include prevention, education, infection control, débridement, and compression bandages. Débridement could be surgical or medical. Osteomyelitis may complicate chronic leg ulcers, especially those with deep wounds, and it is advisable to rule out this complication with a bone scan or magnetic resonance imaging (MRI) and bone biopsy if needed. Recent advances in the management of leg ulcers include topical applications of analgesics, including opioids for pain, and topical application of a platelet-derived growth factor prepared autologously.

Avascular Necrosis

Avascular necrosis (AVN) is a condition that results in dead bone tissue because of an interruption in blood supply, most likely as a result of vasoocclusion. Bones near a joint, especially the hip, are primarily affected. AVN is also referred to as aseptic necrosis, osteonecrosis, or ischemic necrosis of the bone. Necrosis and subsequent bone changes in bones are evident radiographically. Plain films may be normal early in disease, whereas MRI techniques show early changes and provide more detail on the degree of bony involvement. Early plain film findings of AVN of the femoral head include femoral head lucency and sclerosis. As disease advances, subchondral collapse, flattening of the femoral head, narrowing of the joint space, and femoral head collapse occur. Early MRI findings include increased low-intensity signals on T1 and high-intensity signals on T2 images, indicating bony necrosis.

Severity is assessed with a combination of clinical features, pain, and limitation of movement, and radiologic findings with plain films or MRI. Often, the need for surgical intervention is based on clinical and radiographic findings and subsequently, the classification or staging with radiographic techniques. Ficat and Steinberg are two of the more popular staging systems for osteonecrosis in patients with SCD.[15,49–52]

Intractable Chronic Pain Without Obvious Objective Signs

This type of pain is not associated with obvious signs. The only symptom is the patient's self report of pain that does not go away. Often, distinguishing a persistent acute painful episode from a chronic pain syndrome is difficult. Worse still is a patient with chronic pain maintained on high-dose oral opioids who has an acute painful episode develop over and above the chronic pain syndrome: a situation in which the dose of opioids could be increased to phenomenal levels to achieve pain relief. The pathophysiology of intractable chronic pain is unknown. It appears to result from "central sensitization," a situation where repeated and frequent pain stimuli lower the pain threshold to a degree that ambient innocuous events cause severe pain. It is unknown at which point this occurs or what the factors are that may transform an acute painful episode into a chronic pain syndrome. Surgery, severe acute painful episodes, and severe emotional stresses are some of the proposed causes.[12,13,53]

Neuropathic Pain

Neuropathic pain is characterized by sensations of burning, tingling, shooting, lancination, and numbness. These symptoms may occur in the presence or absence of obvious central or peripheral nerve injury. The mechanism of neuropathic pain presumably involves aberrant somatosensory processing in the central or peripheral nervous system. Sickle cell pain could have a neuropathic component, but this aspect of sickle cell pain has not been well characterized. A thorough history and physical examination are essential to determination of whether sickle cell pain is associated with a neuropathic component. Mental nerve necropathy,[54,55] trigeminal neuralgia,[56] acute proximal median mononeuropathy,[57] entrapment neuropathy,[58] acute demyelinating polyneuropathy,[58] ischemic optic neuropathy,[59] orbital infarction,[60] orbital apex syndrome,[61] and spinal cord infarction[62] have been described in SCD anecdotally. Management of neuropathic pain involves the use of anticonvulsants among other medications. Gabapentin appears to be the anticonvulsant that is used for this complication most often.

Management of Sickle Cell Pain
Nonpharmacologic Management of Pain

Nonpharmacologic management of pain includes the use of heat or cold packs, distraction, relaxation, massage, music, guided imagery, self hypnosis, self motivation, and acupuncture. Although no controlled clinical trials report the efficacy of these methods in the management of sickle cell pain, many anecdotal reports of their efficacy in pain management, both by patients and providers, are found.[12]

Pharmacologic Management of Pain

Pharmacologic management of sickle cell pain includes three major classes of compounds: nonopioids, opioids, and adjuvants.[12,13,63] Nonopioids include acetaminophen, NSAIDs, topical agents, and corticosteroids. Most commonly used opioid analgesics include the mu-agonists, although the mixed agonist/antagonist buprenorphine and the partial agonist pentazocine have achieved some popularity, especially in Europe. Adjuvants commonly used in the management of sickle cell pain include antihistamines, benzodiazepines, antidepressants, anticonvulsants, and phenothiazines. Details of these pharmacologic agents are well described in other chapters of this book. Suffice to say here is that the short-acting opioids are usually used to treat acute pain, whereas controlled-release opioids and long-acting opioids are used in the management of chronic pain.

Pain Management of Outpatients

Acute painful episodes of mild or moderate severity are usually treated at home with a combination of nonpharmacologic and pharmacologic modalities.[12,13,63] Home treatment of pain usually follows the three-step analgesic ladder proposed by the World Health Organization.[64] Mild pain is treated with nonpharmacologic agents alone or in combination with a nonopioid. More severe pain entails the addition of an opioid with or without an adjuvant. Oxycodone and acetaminophen formulations are most often used for the home treatment of pain.[12,65]

Pain Management in the Day Unit

Severe acute sickle cell painful episodes are usually treated in a medical facility with parenteral analgesics. Progress in this area has been the advent of day hospitals (or day units) where patients are promptly evaluated by a team of experts in the management of sickle cell pain, without the delay that is common in hospital emergency rooms.[66] Available data in the literature show that management of patients with severe acute painful episodes in such facilities, especially those that operate on a 24-hour basis, reduces the frequency of hospital admissions significantly.

Pain Management in the Emergency Department

Treatment of acute sickle cell painful episodes in the emergency department (ED) follows the principles of thorough assessment, treatment with analgesics or adjuvants, coordination of cure, monitoring, outcome, and disposition. The major problem in the ED is the length of waiting time to initial analgesia, which could be up to several hours. Specific treatment in the ED should be based on the history or the computerized version of the treatment plan if available. Usually analgesics are given individually every 2 hours for a total of three doses. Adjuvants may also be given intravenously or orally as needed. If the pain is resolved or reduced to a level with which the patient is comfortable, the patient is discharged with instructions for follow up by the primary care physician. Otherwise, the patient is admitted to the hospital.[12,62,63]

Management of Sickle Cell Pain in the Hospital

Successful management of the acute painful crisis in the hospital should include the following steps:[12,13,63,67]

1. Multidimensional assessment to determine the location of pain, its intensity, its quality, precipitating factors, modifying factors, and triggers and to determine mood, relief, and sedation

2. Choice of analgesics (opioids or nonopioids), adjuvants, and hydration, if needed; such choices are individualized based on the medical history and the assessment of the patient in question. If the acute painful episode is superimposed on chronic pain for which the patient is taking long-acting or controlled-release opioids with short-acting opioids for breakthrough pain, keep the long-acting or controlled-release opioids the same and discontinue the short-acting ones.

3. Determination of the route and method of administration of analgesics. These, again, should be individualized; parenteral analgesics are usually administered either on a fixed schedule or via a patient-controlled analgesia (PCA) pump.

4. Titration of the dose of analgesics to achieve relief with which the patient is comfortable

5. Maintenance of the dose that achieves adequate relief. Consider opioid rotation (i.e. change the opioid chosen initially to an equianalgesic opioid if its usage does not achieve or maintain relief).

6. Plan to treat breakthrough pain, neuropathic pain if present, and side effects of the crisis or the analgesics if present.

7. Taper the dose of analgesics once the patient uses the PCA pump less frequently or the intensity of pain decreases by 2 or more points.

8. Gradually switch to oral analgesics using tables of equianalgesic doses as an initial guide. One example is to decrease the parenteral dose by 25% and replace it with an equianalgesic oral dose. The latter should be adjusted according to its effect to achieve pain relief with which the patient is comfortable.

9. Prevent withdrawal with either clonidine patch or methadone.

10. Plan for discharge and follow-up.

Preventative Therapy

Measures to reduce the morbidity and mortality of SS include prophylactic penicillin therapy (or other antibiotic when there is sensitivity to penicillin) in infants and children[68] and hydroxyurea in adults.[69,70] Patients who responded to hydroxyurea experienced significant reduction in the incidence of acute painful episodes, acute chest syndrome, transfusion requirement, and mortality.[69–71] The beneficial effects of hydroxyurea are thought to be from its induction of Hb F production.

Conclusion

The clinical manifestations of SCD fall into four major categories: (1) pain; (2) anemia and its sequelae; (3) organ failure, including infection; and (4) comorbid conditions. Acute painful episodes are the hallmark of SCD and the most common cause of hospitalization. Advances in the pathogenesis of SCD focused on the sequence of events that occur between polymerization of deoxyhemoglobin S and vasoocclusion. Management of SCD continues to be primarily palliative in nature, including supportive, symptomatic, and preventive approaches to therapy. Pain management entails the use of nonpharmacologic and pharmacologic modalities. Pain management should follow certain principles that include an assessment stage, treatment stage, reassessment stage, and adjustment stage. Chronic sickle cell pain may be the result of certain complications of the disease, such as leg ulcers and avascular necrosis; intractable chronic pain may be the result of central sensitization. Management of chronic pain should take a multidisciplinary approach. The ultimate goals of management of sickle cell pain should be pain relief, improved physical functioning, reduced psychosocial distress, and improved quality of life.

References

Full references for this chapter can be found on www.expertconsult.com.

Acute Headache

Seymour Diamond and George R. Nissan

Acute headache is often a presenting symptom in the emergency department setting. One study noted the occurrence rate of headache as the chief symptom on admission to range from 0.36% to as high as 2.5% of patients.[1] The incidence of headache with significant mortal or fatal outcome is not frequent.[2] However, it is of the utmost importance to rule out organic disease in the patient with an acute headache. After the appropriate diagnosis has been established, a treatment plan can be implemented.

When a patient with acute headache is encountered in an emergency department setting, the physician must be familiar with the various categories of headaches. In an acute setting, a helpful approach is to divide headaches into three categories: organic, vascular, and tension-type.[3] Multiple disease processes are included in the category of organic headaches (**Table 27.1**) and are only rarely seen in an emergency department setting; the physician is more likely to see vascular headaches in up to 20% of patients with an acute headache.[4] Tension-type headache is, by far, the most prevalent diagnosis among patients with acute headache. Both migraine and tension-type headaches are discussed in other chapters of this textbook.

Signs and Symptoms

All patients with acute headache should be interviewed extensively regarding headache history, including location, severity, character, associated symptoms, and any precipitating factors (**Table 27.2**). Any recent-onset headaches or changes in headache pattern should be thoroughly investigated to rule out organic disease and possible life-threatening illness. A detailed headache history should also include risk factors for vascular disease, family history, and medication history.

Patients must be encouraged to describe the headache pain as accurately as possible because the clinical details may suggest the location and pathogenesis of the pain. The timing of the headache, particularly if the headache appears suddenly or on awakening in the early morning, often has diagnostic value in secondary headache disorders. A sentinel headache, which is a sudden-onset severe headache that disappears, may be a precursor to impending hemorrhage and can occur days or weeks before subarachnoid hemorrhage.

The site of pain can be an important consideration in the headache history because pathologic lesions are more likely than others to produce headache.[5] Lesions in the posterior cerebral and vertebral arteries are most likely to be accompanied by headache, whereas lesions in the anterior cerebral artery are least likely. Lesions in the carotid, middle cerebral, and basilar arteries commonly produce headache. Posterior circulation strokes are more likely to cause headache than are anterior circulation strokes.

The age of the patient is important in the consideration of primary headache disorders versus secondary headache disorders, which can include intracranial masses such as abscesses and brain tumors, and intracranial and extracranial vascular disorders. Patients with primary headache disorders such as migraine, tension-type, and cluster headaches are likely to have onset of symptoms before the age of 25 years. The typical presentation is unilateral or bilateral head pain. No associated neurologic dysfunction is usually observed, with the exception of aura preceding or associated with migraine. In contrast, patients with intracranial pathology are often older than age 45 years and have some neurologic symptoms. Only rarely do the symptoms caused by intracranial lesions overlap with those of primary headache disorders.[6]

Table 27.1[3] Organic Causes of Headache

STROKE
Hemorrhagic
Thrombotic
Embolic
INFECTION
Meningitis
Brain abscess
Encephalitis
Sinusitis
INFLAMMATION
Temporal arteritis
Vasculitis
BRAIN TUMOR
Primary
Metastatic
HYPERTENSION
Hypertensive headache
Malignant (accelerated) hypertension
Hypertensive encephalopathy

From Solomon GD: Classification and mechanism of headache. In Diamond ML, Solomon GD, editors: *Diamond and Dalessio's the practicing physician's approach to headache,* ed 6, Philadelphia, 1999, Saunders, p 8.

Table 27.2 Components of Headache History

Onset
Frequency
Location
Duration
Severity and character
Prodromata
Associated symptoms
Precipitating factors
Sleep pattern
Emotional factors
Family history
Medical, surgical, or obstetric history
Allergies
Current medications
Previous medications and therapies

Adapted from Diamond S: *Diagnosing and managing headaches,* ed 4, Caddo, OK, 204, Professional Communications.

Physical and Neurologic Examination

Physical examination of the patient with acute headache should include the following:

- Measurement of vital signs, including blood pressure in both arms
- Palpation of the carotid and superficial temporal arteries
- Auscultation of the carotid arteries for bruits
- Evaluation of the neck for signs of meningismus
- Evaluation of the cranium for any evidence of trauma

- A thorough funduscopic examination to rule out:
  - Arteriovenous nicking
  - Blurring of the optic disks
  - Papilledema

Neurologic examination should include the following:

- Complete mental status examination
- Assessment of
  - Cranial nerves
  - Muscle strength and motor tone
  - Upper and lower extremity reflexes
- Sensory examination
- Tests for coordination and gait

Any abnormalities uncovered during the neurologic examination should warrant an immediate further investigation.

Testing

The physical examination and headache history usually facilitate the choice of diagnostic tests to be ordered in the evaluation of the acute headache. A complete blood count (CBC) should be obtained if infection or anemia is suspected, which can be a precursor of a hypoxia-associated vascular headache. Evaluation of electrolytes and renal function should be undertaken in patients who have been vomiting, appear dehydrated, or have been taking excessive amounts of analgesics, either prescribed or over-the-counter. An erythrocyte sedimentation rate (ESR) according to the Westergen method should be obtained on all patients older than the age of 50 years who present with acute headache or a change in the character of the headache to rule out temporal arteritis. If the ESR is elevated, a temporal artery biopsy should be scheduled as soon as possible and treatment with corticosteroids should be initiated immediately to avoid irreversible blindness.

After the complete history and physical examination, the next step in diagnosis of a secondary headache disorder usually requires a computed tomographic (CT) scan of the head. The CT scan is generally preferable to magnetic resonance imaging (MRI) for the evaluation of acute subarachnoid hemorrhage, acute head trauma, and bony abnormalities. In an emergency department setting, the CT scan affords easier monitoring of the patient and is less time consuming to obtain. It detects most, but not all, abnormalities that cause headache and is usually sufficient to exclude conditions that necessitate immediate treatment. A CT scan is also indicated for patients with hypertension and a change in sensorium with focal neurologic symptoms to rule out intracerebral bleeding or hydrocephalus. Although sensitivity of a CT scan decreases as time from onset of symptoms elapses, in nearly 90% of patients with subarachnoid hemorrhage, the abnormality is seen on CT scan. Obstructive hydrocephalus can often be diagnosed with CT scan and may appear as a mass obstructing the ventricular system.

When the findings on CT scan are inconclusive or when significant physical signs or symptoms are observed, an MRI is indicated to narrow the list of differential diagnoses. In contrast to CT scanning, which uses the attenuation of an x-ray beam by the body, MRI measures the response of the body to a strong magnetic field. Fat, subacute blood, and highly paramagnetic substances such as gadolinium are highlighted on T1-weighted images. T2-weighted images highlight tissues with protons that remain in phase with each other for a long

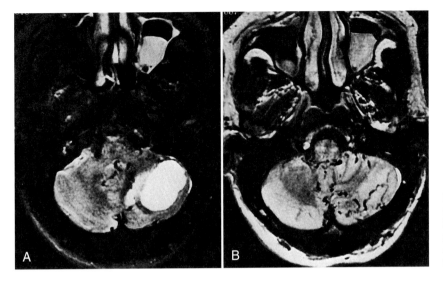

Fig. 27.1 **Cerebellar hemorrhage in the subacute stage.** A, On the axial T2-weighted spin-echo image, the hemorrhage appears bright. B, The proton density-weighted spin-echo image of an adjacent slice shows multiple flow voids, consistent with an arteriovenous malformation.

time after the radiofrequency pulse is turned off; the prototypical bright signal is *water*. The addition of gadolinium to T1-weighted magnetic resonance images causes enhancing structures to appear bright and is analogous to the enhancement seen on contrast-enhanced CT scan in which breakdown of the blood-brain barrier has occurred. Gadolinium enhancement is useful in imaging tumor, acute infarctions, infectious and inflammatory conditions, and vascular abnormalities.

An MRI of the brain usually follows the CT scan for further definition of the anatomic position of the lesion before surgery. MRI is more sensitive than CT scan for detection of posterior fossa and cervicomedullary lesions, ischemia, white matter abnormalities, cerebral venous thrombosis, subdural and epidural hematoma, neoplasms, meningeal disease, cerebritis, and brain abscess.[7]

Magnetic resonance angiography (MRA) is usually indicated for suspicion of aneurysm, either by unusual headache presentation or by family history of aneurysm. Small aneurysms, less than 5 mm in size, are less reliably imaged than larger ones, and considerable debate exists surrounding the use of MRA for the detection of aneurysms.[8] When aneurysm is strongly suspected because of symptoms and physical findings, catheter angiography remains the standard. If findings on MRI suggest vasculitis, catheter angiography is also indicated.

If subarachnoid hemorrhage, meningitis, or both are suspected in the patient with acute headache, a lumbar puncture should be performed. If a focal lesion is suspected, a CT scan must be obtained before a lumbar puncture. In patients with subarachnoid hemorrhage, xanthochromia—a yellow-tinged supernatant caused by the enzymatic breakdown of in vivo red blood cells—is always present in the cerebrospinal fluid (CSF) within 7 to 12 hours. In bacterial meningitis, white blood cells with decreased glucose and elevated protein levels are present in the spinal fluid. The CSF opening pressure should always be measured in these cases, and the spinal fluid should be sent immediately for culture. For patients with fever, neck stiffness, and vomiting, treatment with appropriate intravenous antibiotics should be initiated immediately.

An electroencephalogram (EEG) is usually not indicated for the patient with acute headache because it has minimal diagnostic significance in these cases. If symptoms suggest possible seizure disorder, such as an atypical migrainous aura or episodic loss of consciousness, then an EEG is appropriate. If a structural lesion such as a neoplasm is suspected, CT scan or MRI of the brain is preferred.

Differential Diagnosis

As stated earlier in this chapter, we will focus on the approximately 10% of patients who present with an acute headache and are found to have a secondary cause rather than a primary headache disorder such as migraine, tension-type, and cluster headaches. Organic causes of headache are primarily divided into five categories:

- Strokes
- Infections
- Inflammatory disorders
- Tumors
- Hypertension

Stroke and Subarachnoid Hemorrhage

Cerebrovascular disorders and stroke are included in the differential diagnosis for patients with acute headache older than the age of 35 years and with a history of cardiac or peripheral vascular disease. In evaluation of a patient with acute headache, modifiable risk factors for stroke are important to consider, including hypertension, coronary artery disease, diabetes mellitus, hyperlipidemia, history of stroke, cigarette smoking, and obesity. Overall, headache occurs in about one fourth of patients with acute stroke.[9] This figure includes up to 16% of patients who experience an acute headache with a transient ischemic attack (TIA). In patients with cerebellar hemorrhage, up to 65% to 80% experience an acute headache (**Fig. 27.1**).[10] Headache is less likely to occur in a lacunar infarct and in a deep basal ganglia stroke, most likely because of the lack of innervation of small intracerebral arterioles.

Approximately 10% of all cerebrovascular accidents are related to the presence of a subarachnoid hemorrhage (SAH), which has a nearly 50% mortality rate.[11] The most common causes of subarachnoid hemorrhage are ruptured berry aneurysms, arteriovenous malformations, and trauma.

These patients present with an acute headache that is usually described as "the worst ever." The headache associated with aneurysmal rupture usually is bilateral, and the intensity becomes severe in a very brief interval. A transient loss of consciousness associated with the onset of bleeding is sometimes noted. Other associated symptoms include nausea, vomiting, meningismus, and focal neurologic symptoms. Up to 15% of patients experience seizures. Papilledema and meningeal signs may not be evident for approximately 7 hours after SAH. CT scan of the head without contrast is imperative as early as possible because subarachnoid blood can be found in up to 85% of cases if the CT scan is performed immediately after the event.[12] The sensitivity of the CT scan decreases to 74% after 3 days.

Infections
Bacterial Meningitis

One of the most life-threatening conditions that can manifest as an acute headache is bacterial meningitis. Meningitis should be suspected in all patients who present with headache, fever, and stiff neck, regardless of age or season. Headache is often the first symptom and rapidly increases in severity over several minutes. Patients typically describe a generalized or frontal headache that can radiate into the occipital region and the neck and spine. Associated symptoms include severe pain, fever, photophobia, phonophobia, nausea, vomiting, altered consciousness, nuchal rigidity, and rarely, seizures. In examination of the patient with suspected meningitis, an inability to completely extend the legs (Kernig's sign) and forward flexion of the neck may result in flexion at the hips and knees (Brudzinski's sign).

The age of the patient can often determine which bacterial organism is most likely responsible for the meningitis. In children aged 2 to 5 years, *Haemophilus influenzae* is the most prevalent cause of bacterial meningitis. *Neisseria meningitidis* is more frequently the causative organism in older children and adolescents, and *Streptococcus pneumoniae* is more frequent in adults older than the age of 40 years. Patients with immunosuppression or who are undergoing immunosuppressive therapy are particularly susceptible to bacterial meningitis.

If no contraindications exist, including increased intracranial pressure, mass lesions, or coagulopathy, then lumbar puncture should be performed immediately without neuroimaging. The CSF should be sent for Gram stain and bacterial cultures, and determination of CSF glucose, protein, and cell counts should be performed.

Brain Abscess

The incidence rate of brain abscess in the United States is approximately 1 per 100,000; the condition is predominantly found in children and in those older than 60 years.[13] Headache is the most common initial symptom of brain abscess. Associated signs and symptoms include drowsiness, confusion, seizures, and focal neurologic deficits. The primary site of the abscess determines the accompanying signs and symptoms. Papilledema is present in less than half of all patients at presentation.[14] Most abscesses are the result of an infection elsewhere in the body (i.e., paranasal sinuses, middle ear, mastoid, pulmonary sites, and infective endocarditis). In up to 20% of patients, no source of infection is identified.[15]

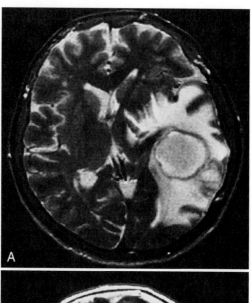
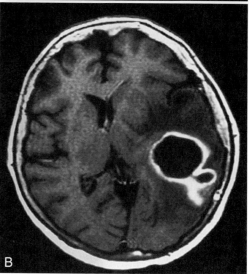

Fig. 27.2 Nocadia abscess. A, Axial T2-weighted (spin-echo [SE], 2500/70) image illustrates the abscess capsule as a hypointense ring, highlighted by areas of increased signal intensity both centrally (necrotic core) and peripherally (edema). Note that the hypointense ring is thinner and less hypointense toward the deep white matter. **B,** Axial post-contrast T1-weighted (SE, 600/20, gadolinium diethylenetriaminepentaacetic acid [Gd-DTPA]) image at the same level shows a ring-enhancing lesion, surrounded by low-signal-intensity vasogenic edema. A satellite lesion (daughter abscess) is seen at the periphery of the abscess.

Early in the course of infection, fever and leukocytosis may occur and resolve as the abscess becomes encapsulated. Approximately 1 week after the onset of headache, nausea and vomiting usually begins, perhaps from increased intracranial pressure.[15] Neuroimaging with either CT scan or MRI of the brain confirms the diagnosis of brain abscess (**Fig. 27.2**).

Other Infectious Disorders

Other infectious disorders that may be associated with acute headache include viral and bacterial encephalitis, human immunodeficiency virus, Lyme disease, fungal infections, and protozoan infections.

Inflammatory Disorders

Early diagnosis and management of temporal (giant cell) arteritis is essential in a patient with acute headache who is over the age of 50 years and who had been asymptomatic before headache onset. Headache is the most common presenting symptom of temporal arteritis in elderly patients and can be associated with weight loss, night sweats, low-grade fever, jaw claudication, and aching of joints.[16] When this cluster of symptoms is present, the term polymyalgia rheumatica is used. A 2:1 female-to-male preponderance is found.

The headache associated with temporal arteritis usually is throbbing and continuous, focally worse in the temporal region and localized to the affected scalp vessels. Pain that occurs with chewing is also a characteristic symptom. On examination, many patients have painful, swollen, and erythematous superficial temporal arteries. The involved arteries generally dictate which physical signs manifest. Temporal arteritis is often associated with an elevated ESR or an elevated C-reactive protein (CRP) value. An ESR of greater than 40 mm/hr in the presence of correlating symptoms indicates the need for a temporal artery biopsy. Initiation of early treatment is critical because of the possibility of irreversible blindness in one or both eyes in up to 50% of untreated cases.

Other less common systemic vasculitides include polyarteritis nodosa and Kawasaki disease, which are both of the medium vessel vasculitis class, and several small vessel vasculitides. These include Wegener's granulomatosis, microscopic polyarteritis, and Churg-Strauss syndrome, which are all affiliated with the presence of antineutrophil cytoplasmic antibodies (ANCA). Henoch-Schönlein purpura, cryoglobulinemic vasculitis, Goodpasture's syndrome, and leukocytoclastic vasculitis are not associated with the presence of ANCA.

Brain Neoplasms

One of the most common fears in patients with acute headache is the possibility of a brain tumor. Headache is an initial symptom in 20% of patients with brain tumor and can occur in up to 60% during the disease (**Fig. 27.3**).[17] It is a common symptom in patients with infratentorial tumors and uncommon in patients with pituitary tumors, craniopharyngiomas, or cerebellopontine angle tumors.[18] Headache is a frequent manifestation of increased intracranial pressure (ICP), although elevation of ICP is not required for its production. The headache associated with brain tumors is usually bilateral and described as dull, aching, and rarely throbbing, similar to the presentation of a tension-type headache. The pain is usually worse on the side ipsilateral to the tumor, and increases in ICP resulting from Valsalva's maneuvers or exertion may exacerbate the pain. Headaches that are worse in the morning occur in approximately one third of patients.

In patients with a history of headaches, suspicion should arise when headaches become more severe or are accompanied by neurologic signs or symptoms. Nausea and vomiting accompany the headache in up to one half of patients. Focal signs may occur depending on the area of the brain involved. Increased blood pressure may also be present. CT scanning, or preferably MRI, of the brain is indicated with suspicion of an intracranial neoplasm.

A clinical disorder that is not a neoplasm but is worth mentioning in this section is idiopathic intracranial hypertension, which is also called pseudotumor cerebri or benign intracranial hypertension. The disorder is one of elevated CSF pressure and occurs predominantly in women in the childbearing years. More than 90% of patients are obese, and more than 90% are women. The mean age at the time of diagnosis is 32 years. The primary manifesting symptom is headache; associated signs and symptoms can include transient episodes of visual loss, diplopia from sixth cranial nerve paresis, papilledema, and pulse-synchronous tinnitus.

The headache associated with idiopathic intracranial hypertension is usually a severe daily headache that is described as a pulsatile pain that increases in intensity. Most of the patients describe the headache as the most severe head pain ever (91%) and different from previous headaches (85%). Nausea and neck stiffness are commonly seen. The headache can awaken the patient from sleep in more than 60% of cases.[19] In the absence of papilledema, a lumbar puncture is indicated to confirm the diagnosis in patients with suspicious symptoms. The resting spinal pressures vary from 220 to 600 mm of water. The CSF is always clear and colorless with an unusually low protein count. The remaining cellular constituents are normal.

Hypertensive Headache

Essential hypertension is generally not a cause of acute headache. Headaches can develop when the diastolic blood pressure is greater than or equal to 110 mm Hg. The elevation in blood pressure is usually a manifestation of a secondary disorder, such as acute nephritis or acute pressor reactions. The degree of elevation of blood pressure may not necessarily correlate with the severity of the acute headache. The headache is usually bilateral, although it can occur at the occiput and can also be global. Patients usually describe the pain as severe, throbbing or bursting in nature. The headache is usually most severe in the early morning on awakening and gradually improves throughout the day. Symptoms of catecholamine release, such as tremors or palpitations, can occur.

If intracerebral bleeding is suspected, then neuroimaging with CT scan or MRI of the brain should be undertaken. If a secondary cause of the hypertensive headache, including acute nephritis, is suspected, then a complete renal workup and follow-up is essential after the blood pressure has been adequately controlled and palliative measures for the headache are initiated.

Treatment

Stroke and Subarachnoid Hemorrhage

Treatment of ischemic stroke now includes thrombolytic therapy with recombinant tissue-type plasminogen activator (rt-PA) if given within 3 hours of symptom onset, which can improve long-term outcomes. A small but significant risk of symptomatic intracranial hemorrhage is found with rt-PA use. Because most patients present outside the 3-hour window period, most patients with stroke are treated with aspirin or antiplatelet agents to reduce the risk of recurrent stroke. Heparin and low–molecular-weight heparin sometimes are used in the treatment of ischemic stroke in patients with comorbid atrial fibrillation, basilar artery thrombosis, or

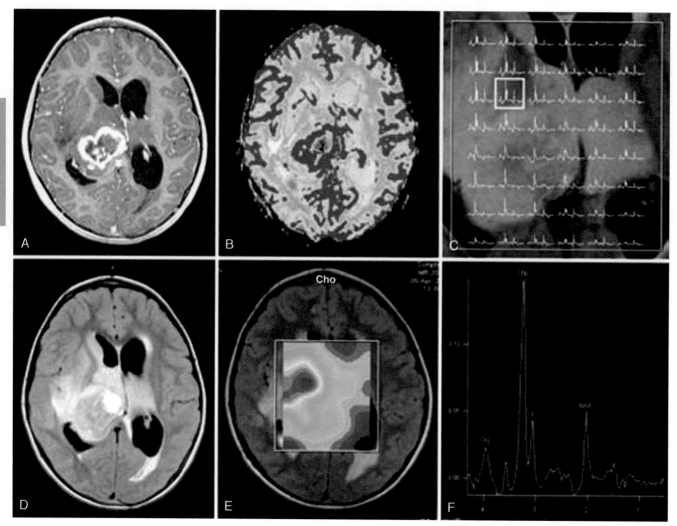

Fig. 27.3 A 70-year-old woman with a histologically confirmed grade III/IV glioma. A, Axial T1-weighted image after gadolinium shows a lesion in the right thalamic region with heterogeneous peripheral contrast enhancement with a central cystic/necrotic region. **B,** Axial fluid-attenuated infusion recovery image shows increase in T2 signal within the lesion with moderate surrounding edema. The patient also has hydrocephalus and transependymal edema around the ventricles. **C,** Gradient-echo axial digital still camera magnetic resonance imaging (DSC) MRI with relative cerebral blood volume (rCBV) color overlay map shows a high rCBV of 3.70 in keeping with a high-grade glioma. A thick rind of markedly increased perfusion is seen (see also cine-movie on www.clinicalmri.com). **D,** Choline (Cho) color overlay metabolite map showing the region of increased Cho which again does not correspond exactly to the region of highest rCBV seen on the DSC MRI study in **C. E,** Spectral map shows regions of Cho elevation within the region of abnormal signal and tumor infiltration beyond the region of enhancement, particularly anteriorly and potentially across the midline into the left thalamus. The central areas do not show substantial amount of lipids/lactate as compared with a grade IV lesion. **F,** Spectrum (TE 144 ms) from the peritumoral region showing marked Cho elevation with respect to creatine (Cr) and *N*-acetyl aspartate (NAA), indicating tumor infiltration.

progressive infarction. However, no long-term neurologic benefit is associated with the use of heparin, and the increased risks of intracranial and extracranial bleeding often negate its use in the treatment of acute ischemic stroke. During and after hospitalization, physical and occupational therapy are part of the overall treatment plan.

Subarachnoid hemorrhage treatment involves surgical obliteration of the aneurysm responsible for the SAH (**Fig. 27.4**). Multiple aneurysms are present in up to 20% of patients, and four-vessel cerebral angiography is preferred because both ruptured and unruptured aneurysms may be revealed. Several randomized controlled trials have shown that oral nimodipine reduces the vasospasm that is associated with poor outcomes in SAH. Catheter-based deployment of detachable coils or balloons prevents rebleeding and affords the opportunity to treat complications appropriately should they arise. The most

serious early complications of SAH include rebleeding, vasospasm with delayed ischemic deficit, obstructive hydrocephalus, seizures, hyponatremia and volume depletion from a central salt-wasting syndrome, pulmonary edema, and cardiac arrhythmias. Despite considerable diagnostic and therapeutic advances, the mortality rate of SAH is still 25%.

Infections

Bacterial meningitis is a life-threatening emergency and should be treated immediately with intravenous antibiotics after lumbar puncture is performed. The antibiotics should be administered before receiving CSF Gram stain and culture results. Analgesics and antipyretics may also be given to treat the associated headache. In addition, intravenous fluid hydration should accompany the antibiotics. The choice of antibiotics should be

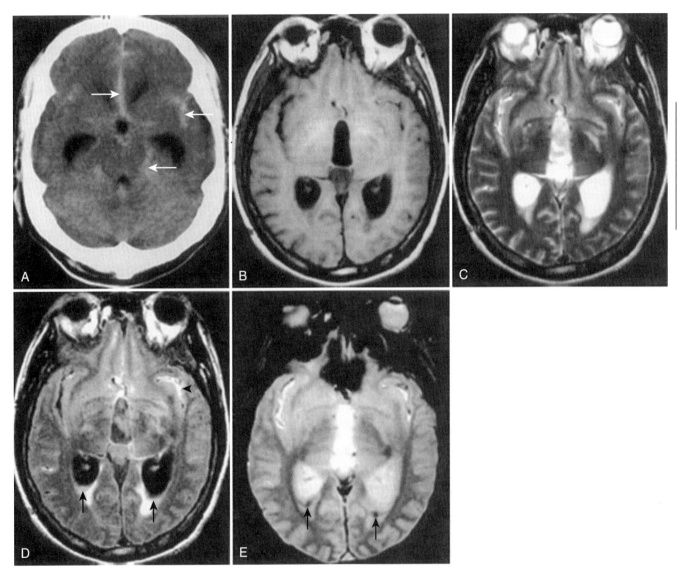

Fig. 27.4 Acute SAH from a ruptured aneurysm of the anterior communicating artery in a 40-year-old man. CT and MRI scans were performed 2 days after hemorrhage. The images shown are at the level of the sylvian fissures and lateral ventricles. A, A CT scan shows SAH as areas of high attenuation in the interhemispheric fissure, left ambient cistern, and left sylvian fissure *(arrows)*. B, A T1-weighted MRI scan (433/ 14/2) shows no high signal-intensity areas. C, A T2-weighted MRI scan (4000/100/2) shows no low signal-intensity areas. D, A fluid-attenuated inversion recovery image (9002/2200/133) shows SAH as an area of high signal intensity in the left sylvian fissure *(arrowhead)* and blood in bilateral occipital horns of the lateral ventricles *(arrows)*. E, A gradient-echo T2-weighted image (567/20/25) shows blood as a low signal-intensity area in bilateral occipital horns of the lateral ventricles *(arrows)*.

made based on the most likely organisms involved and the age of the patient. If pneumococcal meningitis is suspected, then intravenous vancomycin and ceftriaxone should be administered until Gram stain and culture results are available, secondary to the high level of *S. pneumoniae* resistance to penicillin in the United States. If the patient has immunosuppression, then *Listeria* meningitis is also a consideration, and treatment with intravenous ampicillin should also be included.

The treatment of a brain abscess may necessitate needle aspiration or excision of the abscess, ideally before antibiotics are initiated. Intravenous antibiotics are administered for a minimum of 6 weeks and are used to cover the possibility of polymicrobial infection. In nontraumatic brain abscesses, anaerobic streptococci are most commonly implicated. In surgical and posttraumatic cases, staphylococci

and Enterobacteriaceae are most commonly involved, which necessitates the addition of intravenous vancomycin in place of penicillin.[20] Steroids are indicated only when the intracranial pressure is markedly elevated because the antibiotic penetration is compromised with concomitant steroid use. Fungal abscesses are more common in patients with HIV and immunocompromise, and appropriate antifungal agents should be administered in these cases.

Temporal Arteritis

If temporal arteritis is suspected, treatment should be started immediately with steroids; most patients need a starting dose of prednisone 40 to 60 mg daily. A temporal artery biopsy should be performed as soon as possible after steroid initiation to avoid histologic suppression or alteration of vasculitis in the biopsy specimen. Despite steroid treatment, continued histologic evidence of vasculitis may be found up to 6 weeks after initiation of treatment, even with clinical resolution of symptoms.[21] The dose of prednisone is then tapered by 2.5-mg to 5-mg decrements every 1 to 3 weeks as tolerated. The headache associated with temporal arteritis usually resolves within days after the initiation of steroid treatment. The ESR or CRP values may improve within a few days and may become normal within 1 or 2 weeks.

Patients treated with long-term steroids should be instructed regarding possible complications, including diabetes mellitus, steroid myopathy, vertebral compression fractures, psychosis, and infections from immunosuppression. Data are limited regarding the use of steroid-sparing agents, including dapsone, azathioprine, and cyclophosphamide, and the toxicity of these agents should be considered before their incorporation into the treatment regimen.

Brain Neoplasms and Pseudotumor Cerebri

The prognosis of a brain neoplasm is determined by tumor grade and anatomic location. Tumor resectability, which greatly influences prognosis, is determined by the proximity of the tumor to essential neuroanatomic structures. Resectability is also affected by the degree of demarcation between tumor and normal brain tissue. For example, astrocytomas frequently extend beyond the gross tumor margin, whereas meningiomas have a well-defined demarcation between tumor and normal tissue. Once the diagnosis of a malignant intracranial tumor is established, whether the tumor is a metastatic or a primary lesion is important to distinguish. The presence of multiple lesions on contrast-enhanced MRI or CT scan of the brain favors a metastatic process, although metastases can manifest as a single lesion in up to 50% of patients.

Patients with vasogenic edema from an intracranial neoplasm should be treated with steroids. Intracranial hypertension is usually accompanied by a headache and vomiting, papilledema, decreased level of consciousness, and MRI or CT scan evidence of significant mass effect or impending hydrocephalus (**Fig. 27.5**). The typical loading dose of dexamethasone is 10 mg intravenously followed by a maintenance dose of 4 mg four times daily. A neurosurgeon should be consulted emergently because deterioration from intracranial hypertension can occur rapidly.

Management of pseudotumor cerebri includes a structured weight reduction program for all obese patients and may involve gastric surgery when medications and diet fail. The most commonly used oral agents to reduce intracranial pressure include furosemide and acetazolamide, which are usually started at a dose of 250 mg twice daily.[22] The headache associated with pseudotumor cerebri usually responds to nonsteroidal anti-inflammatory agents (NSAIDs) and non-narcotic analgesics. Chronic headaches may respond to migraine prophylactic agents, including tricyclic antidepressants, beta blockers, anticonvulsants, and so on. Repeated lumbar punctures have unproven efficacy and are not currently recommended in the treatment regimen. Neurosurgical procedures, including lumboperitoneal shunting (LPS) and optic nerve

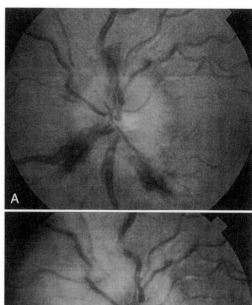
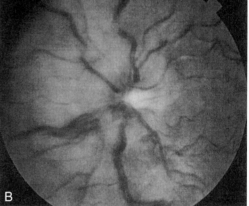

Fig. 27.5 Asymmetric, moderate papilledema with nerve fiber layer hemorrhages. A, Right eye; **B,** left eye. *(From Friedman DI: Pseudotumor cerebri, Neurosurg Clin North Am 1999;10:609–621.)*

sheath fenestration, should be reserved for patients with progressive visual loss on medical therapy. Optic nerve sheath fenestration rarely improves headache, so if headache accompanies visual loss, LPS should be considered the procedure of choice.

Hypertensive Headache

Control of blood pressure is most important in a patient with a hypertensive headache because end-organ damage may occur from the hypertensive state. The general goal is to reduce the mean arterial pressure by approximately 20% to 25% or to reduce the diastolic blood pressure to 100 to 110 mm Hg. If central nervous system, cardiovascular, or renal damage is occurring, prompt treatment with intravenous medication is indicated. If hypertensive encephalopathy is evident, preferred intravenous agents include nitroprusside, labetalol, or diazoxide infusion. The blood pressure should return to normal levels within 24 hours of treatment. No available studies have proven that intravenous treatment should be initiated in patients with severe hypertension but no end-organ damage.

After treatment is initiated to control blood pressure levels, the headache may be treated with analgesics. The headache usually resolves within 2 days after the reduction of blood pressure. If hypertensive encephalopathy is present, the headache may persist for up to 7 days.

Conclusion

Although the incidence of headache with significant morbid or fatal outcome is not frequent, it is essential to recognize organic causes as part of the differential diagnosis. The headache history and physical examination provide important clues to facilitate the choice of diagnostic tests and subsequent treatment regimen. For the clinical practitioner, it is preferable to divide organic causes of headache into the five categories discussed in this chapter: stroke, infection, inflammatory disorders, tumor, and hypertension. The physician should be aggressive in diagnosing the acute headache to rule out life-threatening illness and should be reassured that organic causes of headache occur rarely.

References

Full references for this chapter can be found on www.expertconsult.com.

Part B

Neuropathic Pain Syndromes

Chapter **28**

Evaluation and Treatment of Peripheral Neuropathies

Steven D. Waldman, Corey W. Waldman, and Katherine A. Kidder

The peripheral neuropathies are one of the most common, yet most misunderstood, causes of pain, numbness, and functional disability encountered in clinical practice. Although the exact incidence of peripheral neuropathy is unknown because of a lack of standardized diagnostic criteria, failure to include this heterogeneous group of diseases in the differential diagnosis of pain would lead to much frustration for the clinician and unnecessary suffering for the patient. This chapter provides the physician with a concise roadmap to aid in the diagnosis and treatment of peripheral neuropathies.

History and Physical Examination

Anatomic Classification System

Although peripheral neuropathy has many causes, the relatively consistent signs and symptoms associated with this group of diseases make it easy to consider in the differential diagnosis of patients with pain. Similar to the sympathetically maintained pain syndromes, a universal classification system for the peripheral neuropathies is unavailable. A useful method, however, is the grouping of patients suspected to have peripheral neuropathy based on clinical presentation with the anatomic distribution of symptoms as a starting point in the evaluation process (**Table 28.1**). To accomplish this first step, the clinician must obtain a careful history from the patient

and perform a careful physical examination with an eye to identifying neurologic findings that show the isolated or more diffuse nature of the disease process. The clinician must direct efforts at determining whether the patient's symptoms stem from an isolated mononeuropathy, such as carpal tunnel syndrome, or a symmetric polyneuropathy, such as diabetic polyneuropathy.[1] Such efforts are crucial if the clinician is to bring order to this myriad group of diseases that manifest in such a clinically similar manner.

Verbal Descriptors of Peripheral Neuropathy

A patient with peripheral neuropathy often presents with a constellation of symptoms that may contain reports of pain, numbness, weakness, and lack of coordination (**Table 28.2**).[2] The adjectives used to describe the pain component of the neuropathy often include burning, tingling, hot, stabbing, and shock-like. The adjectives used to describe the numbness component of the neuropathy often include dead, cold, and wooden. Weakness often is described in terms of what the patient could do in the past and is now unable to do (e.g., I am unable to stand on my tiptoes, my little finger catches on the side of my pocket when I try to retrieve my keys, my foot slaps the ground when I walk; **Fig. 28.1**). Incoordination is often described by the patient as clumsiness, inability to button a shirt, or inability to pick up small items.

Table 28.1 Classification of Common Peripheral Neuropathies Based on Anatomic Distribution

SYMMETRIC POLYNEUROPATHIES

Diabetic polyneuropathy

Toxic neuropathies

Alcohol-induced

Drug-induced (e.g., chemotherapy, nitrofurantoins)

Heavy metal poisoning

Inflammatory neuropathies

Guillain-Barré syndrome

Vasculitic neuropathy

Chronic inflammatory demyelinating polyradiculopathy

Nutrition-related neuropathies

Thiamine-deficiency neuropathy

Cobalamin-deficiency neuropathy

Vitamin E–deficiency neuropathy

Cancer-related neuropathies

Paraneoplastic syndromes

Plexopathies from tumor infiltration

Peripheral nerve compromise from tumor infiltration

Infectious neuropathies

Leprosy

HIV-related neuropathy

Lyme disease

Organ failure–related neuropathies

Renal failure

Hepatic failure

Pulmonary failure

Organ transplant–related neuropathy

MONONEUROPATHIES

Entrapment neuropathies (e.g., carpal tunnel syndrome)

Trauma to a specific nerve (e.g., post–inguinal hernia ilioinguinal neuropathy)

MULTIPLE MONONEUROPATHIES*

Leprosy

Diabetic multiple mononeuropathies

HIV-related neuropathies

Sarcoidosis-related neuropathy

*All multiple mononeuropathies can manifest initially as a simple mononeuropathy and progress in a nonsymmetric pattern to involve other nerves.

Table 28.2 Verbal Descriptors of Peripheral Neuropathy

PAIN

Burning

Tingling

Raw

Searing

Hot

Stabbing

Shock-like

NUMBNESS

Dead

Asleep

Cold

Wooden

Walking on sand

Novocaine wearing off

WEAKNESS

I am unable to stand on my tiptoes.

My little finger catches on the side of my pocket when I try to retrieve my keys.

My foot slaps the ground when I walk.

LACK OF COORDINATION

Clumsiness

Inability to button a shirt

Inability to pick up small items

Temporal Classification of Peripheral Neuropathy

In additional to the aforementioned clinical descriptors that help point the clinician toward a diagnosis of peripheral neuropathy, classification of the patient's clinical symptoms in terms of a timeframe is useful. **Table 28.3** provides an arbitrary but useful framework for the temporal classification of peripheral neuropathies. Acute peripheral neuropathies have presented and evolved in 4 weeks or less.[3] Subacute peripheral neuropathies have evolved in 4 to 8 weeks. Chronic peripheral neuropathies have evolved in greater than 8 weeks to years. Much overlap is found in this temporal classification system, but the clinician may find this approach especially useful in classifying patients who present with more than one type of neural compromise (e.g., double-crush syndrome).

Targeted Medical and Surgical History

Table 28.4 provides the clinician with a framework of salient points of the medical history when questioning a patient with suspected peripheral neuropathy.[4] As a starting point, the clinician should ascertain whether the patient has a history of any systemic illness known to be associated with peripheral neuropathy. Specific questions as to the presence of diabetes, collagen-vascular disease, or hepatic, renal, or endocrine abnormalities need to be asked.[5] Also, a careful inquiry into potential causes of acute electrolyte disturbances should be undertaken. In addition, a careful surgical history should be obtained with special attention to surgeries that suggest previous neurologic compromise (e.g., carpal tunnel surgery, ulnar entrapment at the elbow release, laminectomy). Perhaps most important in a patient with a suspected peripheral neuropathy is obtaining a detailed medication history. As summarized in **Table 28.5**, numerous drugs are implicated in peripheral neuropathy. Some of these drugs are obvious to the clinician

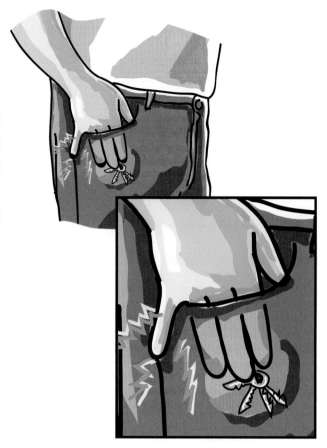

Fig. 28.1 **Functional disability associated with ulnar nerve entrapment.**

Table 28.4 Medical and Surgical History

SYSTEMIC ILLNESSES ASSOCIATED WITH PERIPHERAL NEUROPATHIES
Diabetes
Acute electrolyte disturbances
Collagen-vascular diseases
Hepatic disease
Renal disease
Thyroid disease
Other endocrine diseases
Amyloidosis
Sarcoidosis
NUTRITIONAL STATUS EVALUATION
Vitamin deficiencies
Anorexia
Malabsorption syndrome
HEREDITARY DISEASES
Charcot-Marie-Tooth disease
Fabry's disease
Refsum's disease
SURGICAL HISTORY
Carpal tunnel syndrome and other entrapment neuropathies
Laminectomies
Cancer surgeries

Table 28.3 Classification of Peripheral Neuropathies Based on Time of Onset

Acute peripheral neuropathies	Manifest and evolve in ≤4 wk	Example: Guillian-Barré syndrome
Subacute peripheral neuropathies	Manifest and evolve in 4 to 8 wk	Example: Leprosy
Chronic peripheral neuropathies	Manifest and evolve in >8 wk to years	Example: Diabetes

Table 28.5 Common Drugs Associated with Peripheral Neuropathy

Antiretrovirals
Chloroquine
Cisplatin
Colchicine
Dapsone
Disulfiram
Gold salts
Isoniazid
Metronidazole
Nitrous oxide
Nitrofurantoins
Paclitaxel
Phenytoin
Pyridoxine overuse
Thalidomide
Vinca alkaloids

(e.g., chemotherapeutic agents), and some less so, such as vitamin overuse, which occurs with increasing frequency as patients become more concerned about a healthy diet.[6]

Targeted Family History

Perhaps nowhere in the specialty of pain medicine is the family history more helpful than in the diagnosis of peripheral neuropathy. Although a comprehensive discussion of the heritable diseases associated with peripheral neuropathies is beyond the scope of this chapter, several generalizations can be made:

(1) A significant number of heritable peripheral neuropathies exists (the most common being Charcot-Marie-Tooth disease, with an incidence rate of 1:2500 patients).

(2) Failure to diagnose these disorders early on can lead to significant problems for the patient in the future.

(3) The history of both parents, siblings, and children relative to signs and symptoms that suggest a peripheral neuropathy is important.

Table 28.6 Occupations and Behaviors Associated with Peripheral Neuropathies

Occupation or Behavior	Offending Agent
Agriculture	Organophosphates
Alcohol overuse	Nutritional or vitamin deficiencies
Anesthesia delivery (anesthesiologists, nurse anesthetists, dentists)	Nitrous oxide
Dry cleaning	Trichloroethylene solvent
Homosexuality	HIV
Intravenous drug abuse	HIV
Painters	Hexacarbon solvents
Plastics manufacturing	Acrylamide residue
Rayon manufacturing	Carbon disulfide
Plumbers or building demolition crews	Lead
Tobacco abuse	Paraneoplastic syndromes
Tree sprayers, copper smelters, or jewelers	Arsenic
Vegetarian diet	Cobalamin deficiency

HIV, human immunodeficiency virus.

Table 28.7 Components of the Physical Examination in a Patient with Suspected Peripheral Neuropathy

Examination of the feet

Neurologic examination

Deep tendon reflexes

Pathologic reflexes

Manual muscle testing

Sensory examination

Autonomic nervous system evaluation

Eye examination

Skin, hair, and nail examination

Organ system examination

(4) All family members should be asked whether they have any difficulty walking.

(5) All family members should be asked whether they or any other family members need canes, walkers, or wheelchairs.

(6) All family members should be asked whether they or any family members have "funny-looking feet" or have foot problems. Many patients with peripheral neuropathy have pain and functional disability that they and their physicians have attributed erroneously to arthritis or aging.[7]

Social History

From a statistical perspective, with the exception of alcohol exposure, the incidence of patients with a toxic neuropathy is extremely small. Because removal or limiting of the patient's ongoing exposure to nerve-damaging substances is possible, however, careful inquiry about high-risk occupations and behaviors is important. As summarized in **Table 28.6**, certain occupations and behaviors put the patient at greater risk for the development of peripheral neuropathies, some of which are reversible if the cause is identified and removed in a timely manner. As the number of patients with HIV increases and the mean survival time grows, the number of patients presenting to the pain center with HIV as the underlying cause of peripheral neuropathy will increase. Remember that the increasing use of often neurotoxic retroviral drugs in the treatment of HIV can also be responsible for the development of peripheral neuropathy.

Review of Systems

A targeted review of systems aids the clinician in identification of systemic diseases that are often a factor in the evolution of a patient's peripheral neuropathy. To maximize the useful information received from the review of systems, the questions asked should be tailored to ferret out underlying diseases. Polyuria and polydipsia might point the clinician toward a diagnosis of diabetes mellitus.[8] Temperature intolerance might suggest possible thyroid disease. Arthralgias and musculoskeletal symptoms might suggest a diagnosis of collagen-vascular disorders. Previous lung cancer might point the clinician toward a paraneoplastic syndrome. Although uncommon, conversion disorders may mimic the signs and symptoms of peripheral neuropathy. A carefully performed review of symptoms may be time consuming, but it often helps identify the underlying cause of a previously undiagnosed peripheral neuropathy and allows the clinician to implement treatment.

Physical Examination

The targeted physical examination can often provide the clinician with important clues to aid in diagnosis of peripheral neuropathy (**Table 28.7**). Although the patient may encourage the clinician to focus the examination on a numb hand or numb feet, many of the physical findings associated with peripheral neuropathy are identified in locations far removed from the anatomic region the patient is concerned about.

Foot Examination

Perhaps the best single piece of advice that can be given regarding the non-neurologic portion of the physical examination is to have patients take off their shoes. Many heritable peripheral neuropathies are associated with abnormal-looking feet. Often, such physical findings are overlooked because patients are embarrassed about the way their feet appear and go to great lengths to avoid exposing their feet. Embarrassment coupled with the functional disability the peripheral neuropathy imposes can cause patients with peripheral neuropathy to avoid activities such as running or swimming. Many patients with feet affected by peripheral neuropathy relate that the first time they realized that their feet "weren't right" was when they saw their footprints in the dirt or sand when playing barefoot as a child. These abnormal footprints are often the result of pes cavus or pes planus deformities, which are easily identified on physical examination. In addition to these structural abnormalities of the foot, patients with peripheral neuropathy often have additional physical findings develop as a result of distal denervation of the joints of the phalanges and tarsal and metatarsal bones, such as claw toes, hammer toes, and the like. If the peripheral neuropathy remains undiagnosed and untreated, the clinician may observe Charcot neuropathic joint destruction, characteristic plantar foot ulcers called mals perforans, and ultimately necrotic acropathy as repeatedly traumatized phalanges become ischemic and autoamputate (**Figs. 28.2** and **28.3**).

Neurologic Examination

The neurologic examination of a patient suspected to have peripheral neuropathy can yield important information to aid the clinician in diagnosis and treatment. Most peripheral neuropathies have in common the following findings on physical examination: (1) reflex changes; (2) weakness; and (3) sensory deficit (**Table 28.8**). In addition to this classic triad of physical findings, many patients with peripheral neuropathy have significant autonomic dysfunction, especially patients with diabetic polyneuropathy.

The next step in the neurologic examination of suspected peripheral neuropathy is careful manual motor testing. Similar to deep tendon reflex evaluation, this provides more objective information than the sensory examination, which largely depends on the patient's subjective response. As in the deep tendon reflex evaluation, when testing the muscle groups, the clinician should assess not only the presence or absence of muscle weakness but also the pattern in which any abnormality occurs. Muscle weakness associated

with the polyneuropathies tends to be symmetric, although the length-dependent polyneuropathies tend to affect the distal motor groups preferentially. Asymmetric weakness is seen most commonly in the entrapment neuropathies, such as

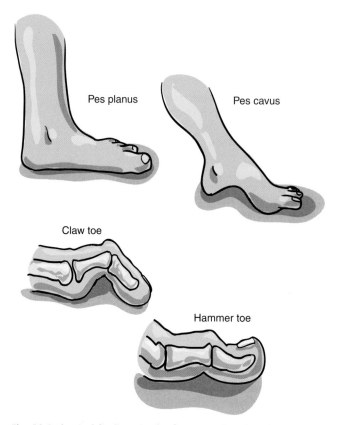

Fig. 28.2 Physical findings in the foot associated with peripheral neuropathy.

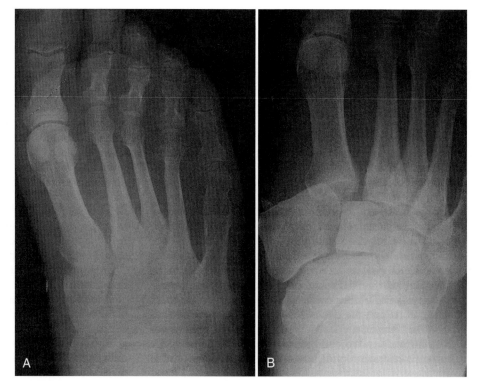

Fig. 28.3 **A** and **B,** Magnetic resonance imaging of Charcot joint. *(From Resnick D: Diagnosis of bone and joint disorders, ed 4, Philadelphia, 2002, Saunders, p 2123.)*

carpal tunnel syndrome, although serious systemic diseases, such as amyloidosis, may manifest as an isolated mononeuropathy that may be misdiagnosed as a simple entrapment neuropathy. Plexopathies may manifest with a confusing pattern of muscle weakness and pain that may seem out of proportion to the patient's physical findings. Electromyography (EMG) combined with magnetic resonance imaging (MRI) helps with correct diagnosis.

Finally, the sensory examination is performed. As mentioned previously, obtaining clinically useful information from the sensory examination is more difficult than gleaning information from the deep tendon reflex and motor examination because the clinician must rely on the patient's subjective responses. For this reason, the clinician must confirm findings of abnormal pain sensation with side-to-side temperature sensation evaluation in the affected areas. The clinician should not ignore sensory and temperature testing of the thoracoabdominal regions; more subtle neuropathic changes are often missed. Testing of vibration sense and proprioception also helps confirm the pattern of the neural compromise: symmetric versus asymmetric, diffuse versus localized. All of this information can be used to confirm the clinical diagnosis.

Eye Examination

Although beyond the scope of expertise of most clinicians who care for patients in pain, eye symptoms in the presence of peripheral neuropathy should raise the index of suspicion that a peripheral neuropathy exists. The report of dry eyes is often associated with Sjögren's syndrome. Uveitis is often associated with the inflammatory systemic diseases associated with peripheral neuropathies, such as Behçet's disease, inflammatory bowel disease, and sarcoidosis. Optic atrophy has long been known to be associated with Charcot-Marie-Tooth disease, and scleritis is commonly seen in patients with vasculitis and connective tissue disease. Any of these symptoms warrants immediate referral to an ophthalmologist.

Skin, Hair, and Nail Examination

As in the ophthalmologic examination, the clinician who cares for the patient in pain may not have adequate clinical expertise to diagnosis the myriad abnormalities of the skin, hair, and nails associated with peripheral neuropathies. The presence of such abnormalities should strengthen the clinical impression that peripheral neuropathy is the correct diagnosis, however, and prompt referral to a qualified dermatologist to help sort things out. Obvious findings on the skin, nail, and hair examination are summarized in **Table 28.9**.

Finding of Organomegaly

The finding of organomegaly, although nonspecific, is often associated with peripheral neuropathies. Hepatomegaly and splenomegaly are often seen in patients with amyloidosis,

Table 28.8 Triad of Physical Findings in Peripheral Neuropathy

Loss of deep tendon reflexes

Weakness

Loss of sensation

sarcoidosis, AIDS, and collagen-vascular diseases. Chronic alcohol abuse also can lead to hepatosplenomegaly, as can a variety of heritable causes of peripheral neuropathy, such as Tangier disease. An enlarged tongue is thought to be pathognomonic for amyloidosis. Whether or not ultimately associated with peripheral neuropathy, the finding of organomegaly should alert the clinician to search diligently for the systemic disease responsible for this physical finding.

Neurophysiologic Testing

Neurophysiologic testing, including the rational use of nerve conduction testing, EMG, and in selected patients quantitative sensory testing, is invaluable in the evaluation of a patient suspected to have peripheral neuropathy.[9] Neurophysiologic testing is an extension of the targeted history and physical examination, rather than a replacement for it. In most instances, the results of neurophysiologic testing are used to confirm or fine tune a diagnosis of peripheral neuropathy, rather than make the diagnosis. For the purposes of this chapter, the following generalizations may break down in the individual patient, given the highly complex subject matter, but may serve to improve the basic understanding of the clinician faced with the presumptive diagnosis of peripheral neuropathy. Neurophysiologic testing is discussed in detail in Chapter 20.

Sensory Nerve Conduction Testing

Sensory nerve conduction testing is usually the starting point for neurophysiologic testing of suspected peripheral neuropathy for confirming or excluding sensory nerve involvement.[10] For the purposes of this discussion, assume that normal sensory nerve action potentials mean that the cells of the dorsal root ganglion and the large myelinated axons are healthy and that if the patient is having numbness, the pathologic process lies proximal to the dorsal root ganglion, or the patient has common small fiber or nociceptive neuropathy. This

Table 28.9 Common Skin, Nail, and Hair Changes Associated with Peripheral Neuropathies

Abnormal Physical Finding	Cause
Foot ulcers	Diabetes
Angiokeratomas	Fabry's disease
Pruritus	Renal and liver failure
Hair loss	Hypothyroidism, thallium poisoning
Mees' lines	Heavy metal poisoning, especially arsenic
Clubbing of digits	Pulmonary failure, lung cancer
Livedo reticularis	Cryoglobulinemia
Tight curly hair	Giant axonal neuropathy
Hypopigmentation	Leprosy, sarcoid
Hyperpigmentation	Cobalamin deficiency
Vesicles and bullae	Porphyria

information can lead the clinician to look to diagnoses other than peripheral neuropathy to explain the patient's symptoms (e.g., myelopathy).

Motor Nerve Conduction Testing

Motor nerve conduction studies represent another piece of the neurodiagnostic puzzle in the diagnosis of peripheral neuropathy. The motor nerve conduction test is performed by stimulating a nerve and recording a response for the corresponding muscle. The motor nerve conduction study is useful in the identification and localization of lesions of the motor neuron, root, plexus, and peripheral nerve. As with sensory nerve conduction studies, side-by-side comparisons are useful.

Needle Electromyography

Needle EMG is most useful in helping the clinician determine whether loss of motor unit fibers innervating the muscle has occurred.[11] EMG needle examination shows the presence of muscle denervation by identifying: (1) the presence of muscle fibrillation and positive sharp waves; (2) the presence of increased amplitude of motor unit potentials; (3) the presence of an increased recruitment pattern; (4) the presence of an increased firing rate to offset the loss of motor nerve fibers; and (5) the presence of reduced recruitment of motor units as the muscle contracts. Although the information obtained from EMG needle examination is extremely useful in helping diagnose the myriad causes of muscle weakness and pain, EMG generally provides less specific information in and of itself regarding the presence of peripheral neuropathy relative to the nerve conduction testing.

Quantitative Sensory Testing

Quantitative sensory testing is gaining acceptance as a useful adjunct in the evaluation of peripheral neuropathies.[12] Although its widespread use has been limited by the lack of third-party reimbursement, quantitative sensory testing is extremely helpful in diagnosis of a relatively large subset of patients who clinically have peripheral neuropathy but in whom conventional nerve conduction testing and EMG are nondiagnostic. This subset of patients have in common damage to small nociceptive fibers that may not be identified on nerve conduction testing, which focuses primarily on large fiber function. Diseases that have a propensity to cause such damage include idiopathic distal painful neuropathy, HIV-related neuropathy, and some subsets of painful diabetic polyneuropathy. Because quantitative sensory testing still requires patient participation, it cannot be considered a true "objective" neurophysiologic test, and in patients with suspected small fiber neuropathy, a confirmatory skin biopsy for analysis of intraepidermal small nerve fibers and peripheral nerve biopsy (e.g., sural nerve) may be helpful.

Autonomic Reflex Testing

As mentioned previously, the autonomic nervous system is often profoundly affected by peripheral neuropathies. Despite the frequency of autonomic dysfunction in patients with peripheral neuropathies, given the lack of easy and readily available testing of autonomic dysfunction, this component of the patient's disease often may go overlooked and be undertreated. If the patient is experiencing significant abnormalities of sweating, orthostatic hypotension, hypertension,

Table 28.10 Treatment Strategies for Most Common Causes of Peripheral Neuropathy

Disease	Treatment
Diabetes	Control hyperglycemia
Nutritional and vitamin deficiencies	Add missing nutrients or vitamins or both
Alcohol overuse	Abstain from alcohol
HIV-induced neuropathy	Improve nutrition and symptomatic treatment
Amyloidosis	Liver transplantation
Toxic substances	Removal of toxic substances
Uremia	Vigorous dialysis and renal transplantation
Cryoglobulinemias	Plasmapheresis and immunosuppression
Guillain-Barré syndrome	Plasmapheresis
Porphyria-induced neuropathy	Glucose infusions and hematin
Entrapment neuropathies	Surgery, splinting

HIV, human immunodeficiency virus.

tachycardia or bradycardia, gastrointestinal hypomotility, or urinary retention, referral to a center skilled in diagnosis of autonomic dysfunction is indicated.

Magnetic Resonance Imaging and Computed Tomography

Although not specific tests for the diagnosis of peripheral neuropathy per se, MRI and computed tomographic (CT) scan are useful adjuncts in the evaluation of a patient thought to have peripheral neuropathy because of their ability to help diagnose accurately many of the underlying pathologies associated with peripheral neuropathy. MRI and CT scan are of particular clinical use in evaluation of the central nervous system, axial skeleton, brachial and lumbar plexus, and anatomic area of suspected entrapment neuropathy (e.g., the tarsal tunnel). The clinician should use these methods early on in the diagnostic workup of patients who present with pain, numbness, weakness, and functional disability because they often may provide a specific diagnosis without the need for more invasive testing.

Treatment of Common Peripheral Neuropathies

The goal of the evaluation of the patient suspected of having peripheral neuropathy is the identification of the specific cause of the patient's pain, numbness, weakness, and functional disability. Such identification allows a treatment plan to be designed specifically to treat the underlying pathologic process and avoid further nerve damage. **Tables 28.10** and **28.11** provide the clinician with treatment strategies that have been shown to be useful in the treatment of specific types of peripheral neuropathy. Although use of the diagnostic approach as outlined previously allows the clinician to make such a specific diagnosis in many instances, a relatively large subset of

Table 28.11 Treatment Strategies for Painful Peripheral Neuropathies

Treat any underlying disease or diseases thought to contribute to the patient's problem (e.g., better control of hyperglycemia in diabetes).

Remove any toxic substance that may cause ongoing damage to the nerve (e.g., removal of thallium or lead exposure).

Use simple analgesics, nonsteroidal anti-inflammatory drugs, and opioids to provide acute symptomatic relief.

Use adjuvant analgesics, such as tricyclic antidepressants and anticonvulsants (e.g., amitriptyline and gabapentin).

Use topical pharmacologic treatments, such as topical lidocaine patches, capsaicin, and analgesic balms.

Use somatic and sympathetic nerve blocks and neuroaugmentation techniques, such as spinal cord stimulation, in carefully selected patients.

Use occupational and physical therapy to instruct the patient how to protect insensate areas and joints and to restore and maintain function.

Use nonpharmacologic pain relief techniques (e.g., hypnosis, guided imagery, coping strategies, acupuncture, contrast baths).

Table 28.12 Adjuvant Analgesics in Pharmacologic Management of Painful Peripheral Neuropathies

Drug	Starting Dose	Maximum Daily Dose
ANTIDEPRESSANTS		
Amitriptyline	25-50 mg at bedtime	200 mg
Nortriptyline	25 mg at bedtime	200 mg
Desipramine	25 mg at bedtime	200 mg
Trazodone	50 mg at bedtime	300 mg
ANTICONVULSANTS		
Gabapentin	100 mg at bedtime	3600 mg in divided doses
Pregabalin	50 mg three times daily	200 mg three times daily
Phenytoin	100 mg at bedtime	400 mg in divided doses
Topiramate	25 mg daily	300 mg twice daily
Carbamazepine	100 mg at bedtime	1200 mg in divided doses
ANTIARRHYTHMICS		
Mexiletine	150 mg at bedtime	200 mg three times daily

Table 28.13 Use of Gabapentin for Management of Painful Peripheral Neuropathies

Start with 100 mg at bedtime for 2 nights.

Increase to 100 mg twice daily for 2 days.

Increase to 100 mg three times daily for 2 days.

Increase to 300 mg four times daily.

Increase to 400 mg at bedtime and 300 mg three times daily.

Increase to 400 mg four times daily.

patients remains in whom a specific cause of the neuropathy cannot be identified. Most of these patients seem to have some form of idiopathic small fiber nociceptive neuropathy. Treatment for these patients centers primarily on symptom management and restoration of function.

After ensuring that all that can be done to make a specific diagnosis has been done, and any specific treatments have been implemented (e.g., better control of hyperglycemia), the clinician should determine what symptoms cause the patient the most distress. Frequently, the numbness, functional disability, or sleep disturbance associated with the peripheral neuropathy bothers the patient more than pain. By focusing on the most troublesome aspects of the disease first, the clinician can maximize success and avoid making the cure worse than the disease by doing too much too soon.

In general, the clinician is strongly recommended to avoid the temptation to treat everything at once with polypharmacy and to begin treatment with monotherapy targeted at the most problematic symptoms. For pain alone, treatment should begin with simple analgesics or nonsteroidal anti-inflammatory drugs with an eye to end-organ side effects (**Table 28.12**). Topical lidocaine patches or capsaicin also may be considered. If dysesthesia or numbness is present, a good starting point is gabapentin, or pregabalin, which should be started slowly as outlined in **Table 28.13**. If sleep disturbance is a prominent feature of the patient's pain report, the use of amitriptyline in a starting nighttime dose of 35 to 50 mg is indicated. Given the relative resistance of neuropathic pain to treatment with opioids, and given the increasingly obvious downside to the use of long-term opioid therapy in this setting, the routine use of opioids as a primary treatment of the symptoms of peripheral neuropathy should be discouraged.

Conclusion

Peripheral neuropathies are a common problem encountered in clinical practice. The conditions are often misdiagnosed, so a patient with peripheral neuropathy may present to the pain specialist feeling frustrated, discouraged, sleep deprived, and often iatrogenically addicted to narcotic analgesics. The goal of evaluation of peripheral neuropathies is identification of specific types of peripheral neuropathies with an eye to implementation of specific successful treatment strategies. When this is not possible, the goal is to rule out other treatable causes of the patient's symptoms and to begin a rational course of treatment that maximizes results and minimizes iatrogenic complications.

References

Full references for this chapter can be found on www.expertconsult.com.

Chapter **29**

Acute Herpes Zoster and Postherpetic Neuralgia

Steven D. Waldman

Herpes zoster is an infectious disease that is caused by the varicella-zoster virus (VZV), which also is the causative agent of chickenpox (varicella). Primary infection in the nonimmune host manifests itself clinically as the childhood disease chickenpox. During the course of primary infection with VZV, the virus is postulated to migrate to the dorsal root or cranial ganglia. The virus then remains dormant in the ganglia, producing no clinically evident disease. In some individuals, the virus may reactivate and travel along peripheral or cranial sensory pathways to the nerve endings, producing the pain and skin lesions characteristic of shingles. The reason for reactivation in only some individuals is not fully understood, but a theory is that a decrease in cell-mediated immunity allows the virus to multiply in the ganglia and spread to the corresponding sensory nerves, producing clinical disease.[1]

Patients with malignant disease (particularly lymphoma) undergoing immunosuppressive therapy (chemotherapy, steroids, radiation) or with chronic diseases generally have debilitated conditions and are more likely than the healthy population to have acute herpes zoster develop.[2] These patients all have in common a decreased cell-mediated immune response, which may be the reason for the propensity for shingles. This may also explain why the incidence rate of shingles increases dramatically in patients older than 60 years and is relatively uncommon in persons younger than age 20 years.

Signs and Symptoms

As viral reactivation occurs, ganglionitis and peripheral neuritis cause pain, which is generally localized to the segmental distribution of the posterior spinal or cranial ganglia affected. Approximately 52% of cases involve the thoracic dermatomes, 20% the cervical region, 17% the trigeminal nerve, and 11% the lumbosacral region.[2] Rarely, the virus may attack the geniculate ganglion, resulting in facial paralysis, hearing loss,

vesicles in the ear, and pain. This combination of symptoms is called the Ramsay Hunt syndrome.[3]

Herpetic pain may be accompanied by flu-like symptoms and generally progresses from a dull, aching sensation to unilateral, segmental, band-like dysesthesias and hyperpathia. Because the pain of herpes zoster usually precedes the eruption of skin lesions by 5 to 7 days, erroneous diagnosis of other painful conditions (e.g., myocardial infarction, cholecystitis, appendicitis, or glaucoma) may be made. Some pain specialists believe that in some immunocompetent hosts, when reactivation of virus occurs, a rapid immune response may attenuate the natural course of the disease and the rash may not appear. This segmental pain without rash is called zoster sine herpete and is, by necessity, a diagnosis of exclusion. In most patients, however, clinical diagnosis of shingles is readily made when the rash appears. Like chickenpox, the rash of herpes zoster appears in crops of macular lesions, which progress to papules and then to vesicles. At this point, should the diagnosis of herpes zoster be in doubt, it can be confirmed with isolation of the virus from vesicular fluid (differentiating it from localized herpes simplex infection) or with Tzanck smear of the base of the vesicle, which reveals multinucleated giant cells and eosinophilic intranuclear inclusions.

As the disease progresses, the vesicles coalesce and crusting occurs. The area affected by the disease can be extremely painful, and the pain tends to be exacerbated by any movement or contact (e.g., with clothing or sheets). As healing takes place, the crusts fall away, leaving pink scars in the distribution of the rash that gradually become hypopigmented and atrophic. As a general rule, the quicker all the vesicles in a given patient appear, the quicker the rash heals.

The clinical severity of the skin lesions of herpes zoster varies widely from patient to patient, although the severity of skin lesions and scarring tends to increase with age as does the duration of pain (**Fig. 29.1**). In most patients, the hyperesthesia and

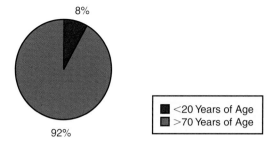

Fig. 29.1 **Postherpetic neuralgia: pain 1 year after attack.**

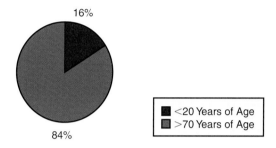

Fig. 29.2 **Postherpetic neuralgia: pain beyond lesion healing.**

pain generally resolve as the skin lesions heal; in some, however, pain may persist beyond lesion healing. This most common and feared complication of herpes zoster is called postherpetic neuralgia; the elderly are affected at a higher rate than the general population with acute herpes zoster (**Fig. 29.2**).

The symptoms of postherpetic neuralgia can vary from a mild self-limited problem to a debilitating, constantly burning pain that is exacerbated by light touch, movement, anxiety, and temperature change. This unremitting pain may be so severe that it often completely devastates the patient's life and can lead to suicide. The desire to avoid this disastrous sequela to a usually benign self-limited disease dictates all therapeutic efforts for the patient with acute herpes zoster.

Treatment

Basic Considerations

The therapeutic challenge of the patient with acute herpes zoster is twofold: the relief of acute pain and symptoms, and the prevention of complications, including postherpetic neuralgia. The consensus of most pain specialists is that the earlier in the natural course of the disease that treatment is initiated, the less likely the development of postherpetic neuralgia.[4] Because the older patient is at highest risk for postherpetic neuralgia, early and aggressive treatment for this group of patients is mandatory.

Careful initial evaluation, including a thorough history and physical examination, is indicated to rule out occult malignant or systemic disease that may be responsible for the patient's immunocompromised state and to allow early recognition of changes in clinical status that may presage the development of complications, including myelitis or dissemination of the disease.

Treatment Options

There are as many therapeutic approaches to the treatment of acute herpes zoster as there are clinicians treating the disease.

Inherent problems in assessment of the efficacy of a specific treatment are that the disease has many different clinical expressions and the natural history of the disease, and the incidence of complications, including postherpetic neuralgia, cannot be predicted reliably in any single patient. Most studies of the efficacy of a proposed treatment have failed to take these problems into account; therefore, only the most general conclusions may be reached.

Nerve Blocks

Sympathetic neural blockade appears to be the treatment of choice to relieve the symptoms of acute herpes zoster and to prevent the occurrence of postherpetic neuralgia.[5] Sympathetic nerve block appears to achieve these goals by blocking the profound sympathetic stimulation that is a result of the viral inflammation of the nerve and ganglion. If untreated, this sympathetic hyperactivity can cause ischemia from decreased blood flow of the intraneural capillary bed. If this ischemia is allowed to persist, endoneural edema forms, increasing endoneural pressure and causing a further reduction of endoneural blood flow with irreversible nerve damage. This damage appears to preferentially destroy large myelinated nerve fibers, which are metabolically more active, and to spare small fibers. Skin biopsy studies in patients with acute herpes zoster reveals a striking loss of epidermal-free nerve endings, which in all likelihood further contributes to the patient's pain.[6]

Noordenbos was first to report this phenomenon and correlate it with the pain symptomatology of herpes zoster. He postulated that large neural fibers modulate or inhibit entry of pain impulses into the central nervous system (CNS), whereas small fibers enhance entry of pain impulses into the CNS. Therefore, enhanced transmission of painful stimuli, and misinterpretation of the non-noxious stimuli of the small fibers as pain by the CNS, results if large fibers are preferentially destroyed. Interestingly, the theory of Noordenbos' "fiber dissociation" predated Melzack and Wall's gate control theory by 6 years. His theory may also explain the clinical finding of Winnie and others that sympathetic neural blockade is more efficacious when used early in the course of the disease by presumably interrupting the neural ischemia before irreversible large fiber changes occur.[7]

For patients with acute herpes zoster that involves the trigeminal nerve (**Fig. 29.3**) and the geniculate, cervical, and high thoracic regions, blockade of the stellate ganglion with a local anesthetic on a daily basis should be implemented immediately. For patients with acute herpes zoster that involves the thoracic, lumbar, and sacral regions, daily epidural neural blockade with local anesthetic should be implemented immediately (**Fig. 29.4**). As vesicular crusting occurs, the addition of steroids to the local anesthetic may decrease neural scarring and further decrease the incidence of postherpetic neuralgia. These sympathetic blocks should be continued aggressively until the patient is pain free and should be reimplemented at the return of pain. Failure to use sympathetic neural blockade immediately and aggressively, especially in the elderly, may sentence the patient to a lifetime of suffering.

Drug Therapy

Opioid analgesics may be useful in relieving the aching pain that is often present during the acute stages of herpes zoster as

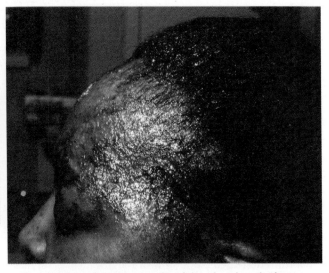

Fig. 29.3 **Acute herpes zoster involving the trigeminal nerve.**

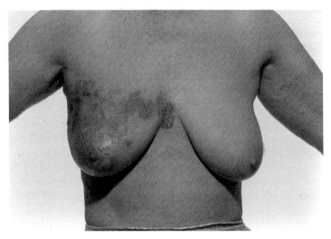

Fig. 29.4 **Acute herpes zoster involving the thoracic dermatome.**

sympathetic nerve blocks are being implemented. These drugs are less effective in the relief of the neuritic pain that is often present. Careful administration of potent, long-acting narcotic analgesics (e.g., oral morphine elixir or methadone) on a time-contingent rather than an as-needed (prn) basis may represent a beneficial adjunct to the pain relief provided with sympathetic neural blockade. Because many patients with acute herpes zoster are elderly or have severe multisystem disease, close monitoring for the potential side effects of potent narcotic analgesics (e.g., confusion or dizziness, which may cause a patient to fall) is warranted. Daily dietary fiber supplementation and milk of magnesia should be started along with narcotic analgesics to prevent the side effect of constipation.

Antidepressants may be useful adjuncts in the initial treatment of the patient with acute herpes zoster.[8] On an acute basis, these drugs help alleviate the significant sleep disturbance that is commonly seen in this setting. In addition, the antidepressants may be valuable in helping ameliorate the neuritic component of the pain, which is treated less effectively with narcotic analgesics. After several weeks of treatment, the antidepressants may exert a mood-elevating effect that may be desirable in some patients. Care must be taken to observe closely for CNS side effects in this patient population. These

drugs may cause urinary retention and constipation that may be mistakenly attributed to herpes zoster myelitis.

Anticonvulsants may also be of value as an adjunct to sympathetic neural blockade in the management of pain from acute herpes zoster. They may be particularly useful in relieving persistent paresthetic or dysesthetic pain. As with the narcotic analgesics and antidepressants, careful monitoring for CNS side effects is mandatory. Gabapentin at a bedtime dose of 300 mg is a reasonable starting place, with the dosage of this drug increased by 300 mg in divided doses every 48 to 72 hours as side effects allow. If carbamazepine is used, rigid monitoring for hematologic parameters, especially in patients undergoing chemotherapy or radiation therapy, is indicated. Phenytoin should not be used in patients with lymphoma because the drug may induce a pseudolymphoma-like state that is difficult to distinguish from the actual disease. Pregablin has also been shown to be efficacious in decreasing allodynia.[9]

Minor tranquilizers (e.g., diazepam) have a limited place in the adjunctive therapy of pain of acute herpes zoster. Although anxiety is often present in this setting, these drugs may actually increase pain perception. In addition, the addiction potential and CNS side effects limit their usefulness. Anxiety may be treated pharmacologically with hydroxyzine or, perhaps more appropriately, with behavioral interventions (e.g., monitored relaxation training and hypnosis).

A limited number of antiviral agents, including famcyclovir, acyclovir, and perhaps interferon, have been shown to shorten the course of acute herpes zoster.[10] Of these drugs, famciclovir and acyclovir appear to have fewer side effects. A difference of opinion exists as to whether these drugs prevent the occurrence of postherpetic neuralgia. They are probably useful in attenuating the disease in patients with immunosuppression and may provide symptomatic relief. Careful monitoring for side effects is mandatory with the use of these relatively toxic drugs.

In the past, corticosteroids have been advocated as an adjunct in the treatment of acute herpes zoster. Proponents of this approach cite more rapid healing and a decreased incidence of postherpetic neuralgia. Other studies have been unable to confirm these findings. Local infiltration of affected skin areas with corticosteroid with or without local anesthetic may be of value as an adjunct to sympathetic neural blockade in decreasing localized areas of pain not amenable to other treatment modalities. Some authors believe that corticosteroids may increase the risk of dissemination in patients with immunosuppression if used before vesicular crusting. Our experience has not confirmed this to be the case.

Adjunctive Treatments

Local application of ice packs to the lesions of acute herpes zoster may provide relief in some patients. Application of heat increases pain in most patients, presumably because of increased conduction of small fibers, but is beneficial in an occasional patient and may be worth trying if application of cold is ineffective. Transcutaneous electrical nerve stimulation and vibration may also be effective in a limited number of patients. The favorable risk-to-benefit ratio of all these methods makes them reasonable alternatives for patients who cannot or will not undergo sympathetic neural blockade. As a last resort, spinal cord stimulation may be considered in those patients in whom no other treatment methods have provided pain relief.

Topical application of aluminum sulfate as a tepid soak provides excellent drying of the crusting and weeping lesions of acute herpes zoster, and most patients find these soaks soothing. Zinc oxide ointment may also be used as a protective agent, especially during the healing phase, when temperature sensitivity is a problem. Topical lidocaine patches provide some patients with postherpetic neuralgia symptomatic relief, but this method should not be used on broken or inflamed skin or skin with active lesions.[11] Topical capsaicin has also been advocated as a treatment for postherpetic neuralgia; however, experience has shown that this treatment is poorly tolerated by many patients.[12,13] Disposable diapers can be used as an absorbent padding to protect healing lesions from contact with clothing and sheets.

Complications

In most patients, acute herpes zoster is a self-limited disease. In the elderly and in patients with immunosuppression, however, complications may occur.[2] Cutaneous and visceral dissemination may range from a mild rash that resembles chickenpox to an overwhelming, life-threatening infection in those who already have severe multisystem disease. Myelitis may cause bowel, bladder, and lower-extremity paresis. Ocular complications from trigeminal-nerve involvement range from severe photophobia to keratitis with loss of vision.

Conclusion

In view of the devastating effects of inadequately treated acute herpes zoster on the patient, the family, and society in terms of cost and lost productivity, healthcare professionals must initiate immediate and aggressive treatment for all patients with acute herpes zoster.

References

Full references for this chapter can be found on www.expertconsult.com.

Complex Regional Pain Syndrome Type I (Reflex Sympathetic Dystrophy)

Andreas Binder, Jörn Schattschneider, and Ralf Baron

Complex regional pain syndrome types I and II (CRPS I and CRPS II) share most of the same pathophysiologic, clinical, and therapeutic features. Therefore, all main information regarding CRPS in general is included in this chapter dealing with CRPS I. Specific information on CRPS II is added in Chapter 31.

Until the 1990s, CRPSs were recognized as poorly defined pain disorders that mostly confused basic researchers, clinicians, and epidemiologists, rather than stimulating their scientific activities. The reasons for this confusion were that diagnostic criteria were defined vaguely, underlying pathophysiologic mechanisms were unknown, and therapeutic

options were limited. No data on incidence, prognosis, and prevention were available, and research on mechanisms focused primarily on pain and controlled treatment studies were absent. However, insight into pathophysiologic mechanisms has progressed dramatically since the 1990s. Researchers became aware that CRPS I and II are not just neuropathic pain syndromes. Based on this notion, it has become obvious that multiple different pathophysiologic mechanisms may occur in different individual patterns.[1] These consist of somatosensory changes (including pain) that interact with changes related to the sympathetic nervous system, peripheral inflammatory changes, and changes in the somatomotor system.[2]

Definition

The International Association for the Study of Pain (IASP) *Classification of Chronic Pain* redefined pain syndromes formerly known as *reflex sympathetic dystrophy* and *causalgia*. The term *complex regional pain syndrome* describes "a variety of painful conditions following injury which appears regionally having a distal predominance of abnormal findings, exceeding in both magnitude and duration the expected clinical course of the inciting event often resulting in significant impairment of motor function, and showing variable progression over time."[3]

These chronic pain syndromes contain different additional clinical features including spontaneous pain, allodynia, hyperalgesia, edema, autonomic abnormalities, and trophic signs. In CRPS I (reflex sympathetic dystrophy), minor injuries or fractures of a limb precede the onset of symptoms. CRPS II (causalgia) develops after injury to a major peripheral nerve.

History

The American Civil War physician Weir Mitchell observed that approximately 10% of patients with traumatic partial peripheral nerve injuries in the distal extremity had a dramatic clinical syndrome that consisted of prominent, distal, spontaneous burning pain. In addition, patients reported exquisite hypersensitivity of the skin to light mechanical stimulation. Furthermore, movement, loud noises, or strong emotions could trigger their pain. The distal extremity showed considerable swelling, smoothness and mottling of the skin, and, in some cases, acute arthritis. In most cases, the limb was cold and sweaty. Weir Mitchell named this syndrome "causalgia." He was emphatic that the sensory and trophic abnormalities spread beyond the innervation territory of the injured peripheral nerve and often were remote from the site of injury. The nerve lesions giving rise to this syndrome were always partial; complete transection did not cause it. Because of this and the peripheral signs of the disease, Weir Mitchell concluded that, in addition to disease of the nerve, some process in the skin or other peripheral tissue was responsible for the pain.

After World War II, Leriche for the first time reported that sympathectomy dramatically relieved causalgia. This notion was supported by several large clinical series, primarily in wounded soldiers. Richards described the clinical features of causalgia and the effect of sympatholytic interventions in hundreds of cases. He repeatedly stressed the dramatic response of causalgia to sympathetic blockade: "One of the outstanding surgical lessons that was learned during World War II was that interruption of the appropriate sympathetic nerve fibres is almost invariably effective in the treatment of causalgia. When the sympathetic chain is blocked by a local anaesthetic, complete relief occurs almost immediately." The finding that sympatholysis relieves causalgic pain gave rise to the concept of *sympathetically maintained pain.*

In the years between World Wars I and II, the concept that sympathetic outflow could influence pain was extended to a group of patients without detectable nerve injury. These patients developed asymmetrical distal extremity pain and swelling (**Fig. 30.1**). The disorder had first been described by Sudeck early in the century. Precipitating events include fracture or minor soft tissue trauma, low-grade infection, frostbite,

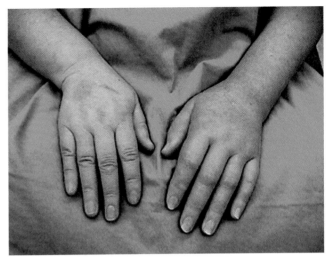

Fig. 30.1 Clinical picture of patient with complex regional pain syndrome type I of the upper left extremity after distortion of the left wrist. *(From Baron R: Complex regional pain syndromes. In McMahon SB, Koltzenburg M, editors: Wall and Melzack's textbook of pain, ed 5, London, 2006, Elsevier, pp 1011–1027.)*

and burns, as well as stroke and myocardial infarction. The swelling and pain often develop at a site remote from the inciting injury, without any obvious local tissue-damaging process at the site of pain and swelling. This syndrome was named *reflex sympathetic dystrophy* because vasomotor (altered skin color and temperature) and sudomotor abnormalities (altered sweat production) are common, the pain and swelling are often spatially remote from the inciting injury, and patients typically obtain dramatic relief with sympathetic block.

Epidemiology

Incidence and Prevalence

A population-based study on CRPS I calculated an incidence of approximately 5.5 per 100,000 person-years at risk and a prevalence of approximately 21 per 100,000.[4] In contrast, a European population-based study using a different diagnostic approach calculated a much higher incidence of 26.2 per 100,000 for CRPS in general.[5] CRPS I develops more often than does CRPS II. Retrospective analyses revealed CRPS prevalences following fractures of between 0.03% and 37%.[6,7] Estimations suggested an overall incidence of CRPS I of 1% to 2% after fractures, 12% after brain lesions, and 5% after myocardial infarction. However, the data for brain lesions and myocardial infarctions are relatively high and must be interpreted with some care because of the lack of uniform diagnostic criteria in the past. Preceding trauma such as fracture or surgery is the most common (≈40%) inciting event in CRPS I. However, in approximately 10% of the patients, CRPS develops after minor trauma, and in 5% to 10% of patients it develops spontaneously. No correlation exists between the severity of trauma and CRPS presentation.[8] Female patients are more often affected than male patients, and the female-to-male ratio ranges from 2:1 to 4:1. CRPS shows a distribution over all ages, with a mean age peak of 37 to 50 years and highest incidence rates at 61 to 70 years. The epidemiologic differences may reflect ethnicity, socioeconomic factors, and diagnostic criteria.

Clinical Presentation

The most common precipitating event is trauma affecting the distal part of an extremity (65%), especially fracture, a post-surgical condition, contusion, and strain or sprain. Less common incidents are central nervous system (CNS) lesions such as spinal cord injuries and cerebrovascular accidents, as well as cardiac ischemia.

Patients with CRPS I develop asymmetrical distal extremity pain and swelling without an overt nerve lesion (**Table 30.1**; see also Fig. 30.1). These patients often report a burning spontaneous pain felt in the distal part of the affected extremity. Characteristically, the pain is disproportionate in intensity to the inciting event. The pain usually increases when the extremity is in a dependent position. Stimulus-evoked pain is a striking clinical feature; these pains in clude mechanical and thermal allodynia or hyperalgesia. These sensory abnormalities often appear early, are most pronounced distally, and have no consistent spatial relationship with individual nerve territories or to the site of the inciting lesion. Typically, pain can be elicited by movement of and pressure on the joints (deep somatic hyperalgesia), even if these joints are not directly affected by the inciting lesion. Autonomic abnormalities include swelling and changes of sweating and skin blood flow. In the acute stages of CRPS I, the affected limb is often warmer than the contralateral limb. Patients with initially cold skin temperature ("cold" CRPS type) are thought to have an unfavorable course of the disease (see the later discussion of prognosis) and have been found to present with different clinical findings, such as increased incidence of dystonia, sensory loss, and cold-induced pain.[9] Sweating abnormalities—either hypohidrosis or, more frequently, hyperhidrosis—are present in many patients with CRPS I. The acute distal swelling of the affected limb depends on aggravating stimuli. Because the swelling may diminish after sympathetic blocks, it is probably maintained by sympathetic activity.

Trophic changes such as abnormal nail growth, increased or decreased hair growth, fibrosis, thin glossy skin, and osteoporosis may be present, particularly in chronic stages. Restrictions of passive movement are often present in patients with long-standing cases and may be related to both functional motor disturbances and trophic changes of joints and tendons.

Weakness of all muscles of the affected distal extremity is often present. Small, accurate movements are characteristically impaired. Results of nerve conduction and electromyography studies are normal, except in patients in very chronic and advanced stages of the disorder. Approximately half of the patients have a postural or action tremor, which represents an increased physiologic tremor. In approximately 10% of cases, dystonia of the affected hand or foot develops.[10]

Table 30.1 Signs and Symptoms of Complex Regional Pain Syndrome

Sign or Symptom	Duration		
	2–6 mo (%)	>12 mo (%)	Total from 0–12 mo (%)
Pain	88	97	93
Increase of complaints after exercise	95	97	96
NEUROLOGIC			
Hyperesthesia/allodynia	75	85	76
Coordination deficits	47	61	54
Tremor	44	50	49
Muscle spasm	13	42	25
Paresis	93	97	95
SYMPATHETIC			
Hyperhidrosis	56	40	47
Color difference	96	84	92
Temperature difference	91	91	92
Changed growth of hair	71	35	55
Changed growth of nails	60	52	60
Edema	80	55	69
ATROPHY			
Skin	37	44	40
Nails	23	36	27
Muscle	50	67	55
Bone (diffuse/spotty osteoporosis on radiograph)	41	52	38

Modified from Veldman PH, Reynen HM, Arntz IE, et al: Signs and symptoms of reflex sympathetic dystrophy: prospective study of 829 patients, *Lancet* 342:1012, 1993.

Spatial Distribution

Predominantly, CRPS occurs in one extremity. Retrospective studies in large cohorts showed a distribution in the upper and lower extremity from 1:1 to 2:1. In 113 retrospectively reviewed cases, symptoms occurred in 47% of patients on the right side, in 51% on the left side, and in 2% bilaterally. Multiple extremities were affected in up to 7%.[4,11–13]

Time Course

For therapeutic reasons, every effort should be undertaken to diagnose CRPS as early as possible. CRPS mostly starts acutely; that is, the cardinal symptoms may appear within hours or days. At the onset, the main symptoms of CRPS are spontaneous pain, generalized swelling, and difference in skin temperature on the symptomatic side. These early symptoms already develop in areas and tissues that are not affected by the preceding lesion. Thus, swelling and pain provide valuable information for an early diagnosis of CRPS. Before the onset of CRPS, pain is felt inside the area of the preceding lesion. After the onset of CRPS, however, the pain becomes diffuse and felt deep inside the distal extremity and the swelling generalizes, yet the initial pain may already have disappeared.

To some extent, the tendency of symptoms to generalize may be a physiologic phenomenon in post-traumatic states that will disappear without any treatment. Exact differentiation between these physiologic diffuse post-traumatic reactions and the development of "real" CRPS is not possible at present.

Stages

A sequential progression of untreated CRPS has been repeatedly described. Each stage of CRPS (usually three are proposed) differs in patterns of signs and symptoms. Nevertheless, this concept has come into question. In 2002, the clinical validity of this concept was tested in 113 patients by Bruehl et al.[12] Using a cluster analysis, the investigators identified 3 subgroups that could be differentiated by their symptoms and signs regardless of disease duration. The sequential concept relies on the course of untreated CRPS; however, so far all studies performed to test the clinical validity of this concept investigated patients already under treatment. Furthermore, vascular disturbances and skin temperature measurements indicated different thermoregulatory types, depending on time.

In conclusion, it is questionable whether staging of CRPS is appropriate. A much more practical approach, one with direct therapeutic implications, is to grade CRPS according to the intensity of the sensory, autonomic, motor, and trophic changes as being mild, moderate, or severe (see later).

Psychology

Most patients with CRPS exhibit significant psychological distress, most commonly depression and anxiety. Many patients become overwhelmed by the pain and associated symptoms and, without adequate psychosocial support, may develop maladaptive coping skills. Based on these symptoms, the tendency is to ascribe the origin of CRPS to emotional causes, and investigators have proposed that CRPS is a psychiatric illness. In fact, sometimes it is difficult to recognize the organic nature of the symptoms. However, when describing the clinical picture in the 1940s, Livingston was convinced: "The ultimate source of this dysfunction is not known but its organic nature is obvious and no one seems to doubt that these classical pain syndromes are real." Covington[14] drew the following conclusions about psychological factors in CRPS:

1. No evidence was found to support the theory that CRPS is a psychogenic condition.
2. Because anxiety and stress increase nociception, relaxation and antidepressive treatment are helpful.
3. The pain in CRPS is the cause of psychiatric problems and not the converse.
4. Maladaptive behavior by patients, such as volitional or inadvertent actions, is mostly the result of fear, regression, or misinformation and does not indicate a psychopathologic condition.
5. Some patients with conversion disorders and factitious diseases have been diagnosed incorrectly with CRPS.

In summary, Covington concluded that the widely proposed "CRPS personality" is clearly unsubstantiated. This assumption was further strengthened when no differences in psychological patterns were found in patients with radius fracture who developed CRPS I in comparison with patients who recovered without developing CRPS I.[15]

In a study supporting this view, an even distribution of childhood trauma, of pain intensity, and of psychological distress was confirmed in patients with CRPS in comparison with patients with other neuropathic pain and chronic back pain.[16] Further studies demonstrated a high rate of psychiatric comorbidity, especially depression, anxiety, and personality disorders, in patients with CRPS. These findings are also present in other patients with chronic pain and are more likely a result of the long and severe pain disease.[17] Compared with patients with low back pain, patients with CRPS showed a higher tendency to somatization but did not show any other psychological differences.[18] In 145 patients, 42% reported stressful life events in close relation to the onset of CRPS, and 41% had a previous history of chronic pain.[19] Thus, stressful life events could be risk factors for the development of CRPS.

Genetics

One of the unsolved features in human pain diseases is that a minority of patients develop chronic pain after seemingly identical inciting events. Similarly, in certain nerve lesion animal models, differences in pain susceptibility were found to result from genetic factors. The clinical importance of genetic factors in CRPS is not clear. A mendelian law does not seem to affect the incidence and prevalence, but familial occurrence has been described.[20] Evidence indicates that certain genotypes are predisposing risk factors for the development of CRPS. A single nucleotide polymorphism of the alpha$_1$-adrenoreceptor was identified as a risk factor for the development of CRPS I.[21] Human leukocyte antigen (HLA) associations with different phenotypes showed an increase in A3, B7, and DR(2) major histocompatibility complex (MHC) antigens in a small group of patients with CRPS in whom resistance to treatment was associated with positivity of DR(2). In a cohort of 52 patients with CRPS, class I or II MHC antigens were typed. The frequency of HLA-DQ1 was found to be significantly increased compared with control frequencies.[22] In patients with CRPS who progressed toward multifocal or generalized tonic dystonia, an association with HLA-DR13 was noted, and an association of fixed dystonia with HLA-B62 and HLA-DQ8 was reported.[23,24] Furthermore, a different locus, centromeric in HLA class I, was found to be associated with the spontaneous development of CRPS, a finding suggesting an interaction between trauma severity and genetic factors that describe CRPS susceptibility.[25] No associations have been identified for different cytokines, inflammatory neuropeptides, neutral endopeptidase, the SCNA9 sodium Na1.7 channel, and mutations of different dystonia predicting genes (DYT genes).

Pathophysiologic Mechanisms

Sensory Abnormalities and Pain

Based on numerous animal experimental findings, spontaneous pain and various forms of hyperalgesia at the distal extremity are thought to be generated by processes of peripheral and central sensitization. In patients with acute CRPS I, somatosensory profiling revealed heat and cold hyperalgesia in combination with warm and cold hypoesthesia, whereas in chronic CRPS I, thermal hyperalgesia declined and thermal hypoesthesia increased.[26] Similar but minor deficits were found at the contralateral nonaffected extremity. In addition, up to 50% of patients with chronic CRPS I develop hypoesthesia and hypoalgesia in the entire half of the body or in the upper quadrant ipsilateral to the affected extremity. Systematic quantitative sensory testing has shown that patients with these generalized hypoesthesias have increased thresholds to mechanical, cold, warmth, and heat stimuli compared with the responses generated from the corresponding contralateral healthy body side. Patients with these extended sensory deficits have longer disease duration, greater pain intensity, a higher frequency of mechanical allodynia, and a greater tendency to develop changes in the somatomotor system than do patients with spatially restricted sensory deficits.

These changed somatosensory perceptions are likely the result of changes in the central representation of somatosensory sensations in the thalamus and cortex. Accordingly, positron emission tomography (PET) studies demonstrated adaptive changes in the thalamus during the course of the disease.[27] The magnetoencephalographic (MEG) first somatosensory (SI) responses were increased on the affected side, a finding indicating processes of central sensitization. Psychophysical and transcranial magnetic stimulation (TMS) studies suggested sensory and motor hyperexcitability within the CNS.[28] Furthermore, MEG and **functional magnetic resonance imaging (fMRI)** studies uncovered networks of hyperalgesia and allodynia involving nociceptive, motor, and attention processing and demonstrated a shortened distance between little finger and thumb representations in the SI cortex on the painful side (**Fig. 30.2**).[29–32] This latter cortical reorganization was reversible and correlated with pain reduction and improvement of tactile impairment.[33–35] This cortical reorganization may not be CRPS specific, however, but may give a suitable hypothesis for the observed sensory features in CRPS.[29] Using fMRI, Lebel et al[36] demonstrated that patients who had recovered from CRPS still had significant differences in CNS reactivity to sensory stimuli.

The dependency of these phenomena on structural or functional changes in the peripheral nerve system is not known. However, skin preparations from patients with CRPS I showed diminished axonal density[37] and mixed decreased and increased innervation of epidermal and vascular structures and sweat glands.[38] The relevance of these findings to distinct pathophysiologic mechanisms remains unclear.[39]

Autonomic Abnormalities
Denervation Supersensitivity

A partial nerve lesion is the important preceding event in CRPS II. Therefore, investigators have generally assumed that abnormalities in skin blood flow within the territory of the lesioned

nerve are the result of peripheral impairment of sympathetic function and sympathetic denervation. During the first weeks after transection of vasoconstrictor fibers, vasodilatation is present within the denervated area. Later, the vasculature may develop increased sensitivity to circulating catecholamines, probably because of up-regulation of adrenoceptors.

Central Autonomic Dysregulation

Sympathetic denervation and denervation hypersensitivity cannot completely account for vasomotor and sudomotor abnormalities in CRPS. First, patients with CRPS I have no overt nerve lesion, and, second, in CRPS II, the autonomic symptoms spread beyond the territory of the lesioned nerve. In fact, direct evidence indicates a reorganization of central autonomic control in these syndromes.[2,40]

Hyperhidrosis, for example, is found in many patients with CRPS. Resting sweat output and thermoregulatory and axon reflex sweating are increased in patients with CRPS I.[41] Increased sweat production cannot be explained by a peripheral mechanism because, unlike blood vessels, sweat glands do not develop denervation supersensitivity. Moreover, exaggerated CGRP levels may enhance sweat gland activation.[42]

To study cutaneous sympathetic vasoconstrictor innervation in patients with CRPS I, Baron and Wasner et al[43–45] analyzed central sympathetic reflexes induced by thermoregulatory (whole-body warming, cooling) and respiratory stimuli. Sympathetic effector organ function (i.e., skin temperature and skin blood flow) was measured bilaterally at the extremities by infrared thermometry and laser Doppler flowmetry. Under normal conditions, these reflexes do not show interside differences. In patients with CRPS, three distinct vascular regulation patterns were identified related to the duration of the disorder:

1. In the warm regulation type (acute stage, <6 months), the affected limb was warmer and skin perfusion values were higher than contralaterally during the entire spectrum of sympathetic activity. Even massive body cooling failed to activate sympathetic vasoconstrictor neurons.[44] Consistently, direct measurements of norepinephrine levels from the venous effluent above the area of pain showed a reduction in the affected extremity.[44,46]

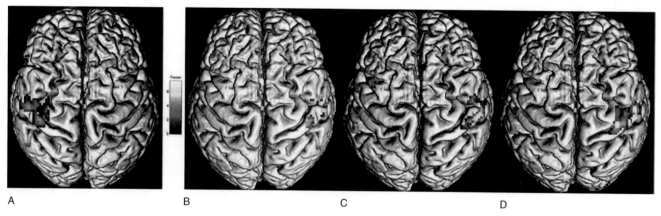

Fig. 30.2 Central reorganization of the somatosensory cortex in a patient with complex regional pain syndrome type I on the right hand. **Functional magnetic resonance imaging (fMRI)** after mechanical stimulation of digits 1 and 5 on both sides. Shrinkage of the hand representation that recovers after successful treatment. A, Acute stage: nearly complete absence of the fMRI signal on the left hemisphere; normal representation on the contralateral side. B to D, Normalization of the representation after 3 (B), 6 (C), and 12 (D) months of the course. *(From Pleger B, Tegenthoff M, Ragert P, et al: Sensorimotor retuning in complex regional pain syndrome parallels pain reduction, Ann Neurol 57:425, 2005.)*

2. In the intermediate type, temperature and perfusion were either elevated or reduced depending on the degree of sympathetic activity.
3. In the cold type (chronic stage), temperature and perfusion were lower on the affected side during the entire spectrum of sympathetic activity. Norepinephrine levels, however, were still lower on the affected side.[45]

These data support the idea that CRPS I is associated with pathologic unilateral inhibition of cutaneous sympathetic vasoconstrictor neurons that leads to a warmer affected limb in the acute stage.[43,45] The locus of pathophysiologic changes underlying such disturbed reflex activity must be in the CNS. Secondary changes in neurovascular transmission may induce severe vasoconstriction and cold skin in chronic CRPS.[47,48] Accordingly, alpha-adrenoceptor density has been reported to be increased in skin biopsies of patients with CRPS I.[49] Furthermore, skin lactate was increased in patients with CRPS, a finding indicating an enhanced anaerobic glycolysis, probably as a result of vasoconstriction and chronic tissue hypoxia.[19,50]

The few microneurographic studies of small sympathetic nerve fascicles that have been performed so far in patients with CRPS, however, have not confirmed the presence of reflex abnormalities.[51] The average skin sympathetic activity (i.e., a combination of vasoconstrictor and sudomotor activity) was not different on the two sides.[51]

In one study performed in patients suffering from the cold type of CRPS, iontophoresis of acetylcholine into the skin of the affected and unaffected extremity revealed a decrease of the vasodilatory response in the CRPS extremity.[52] Additionally, expression of endothelial nitric oxide synthase and endothelin-1 was observed to be increased in skin tissue of amputated CRPS limbs.[53] The pathophysiology of the hereby proven endothelial dysfunction in cold-type CRPS is not known so far. However, it can be assumed that production of free radicals is triggered by tissue hypoxia and tissue acidosis as a result of peripheral vasoconstriction. Thus, the production of free radicals is responsible for the observed endothelial function. The vasoconstrictor- and nociceptor-sensitizing agent endothelin-1 seems not to be involved in the pathophysiology of CRPS.[54]

Neurogenic Inflammation

Some of the clinical features of CRPS, particularly in its early phase, could be explained by an inflammatory process.[55] Consistent with this idea, corticosteroids are often successfully used in acute CRPS.[56]

Increasing evidence indicates that a localized neurogenic inflammation may be involved in the generation of acute edema, vasodilatation, and increased sweating. Scintigraphic investigations with radiolabeled immunoglobulins show extensive plasma extravasation in patients with acute CRPS I.[57] Analysis of joint fluid and synovial biopsies in patients with CRPS have shown an increase in protein concentration and synovial hypervascularity. Furthermore, synovial effusion is enhanced in affected joints, as measured with MRI. In patients with acute untreated CRPS I, neurogenic inflammation was elicited by strong transcutaneous electrical stimulation through intradermal microdialysis capillaries. Protein extravasation that was simultaneously assessed by the microdialysis system was provoked only on the affected extremity as compared

with the normal side. Furthermore, axon reflex vasodilatation was increased significantly. The time course of electrically induced protein extravasation in these patients resembled that observed[58] after application of exogenous substance P or showed no differences from healthy controls. Additionally, high substance P levels may be caused by impaired substance P inactivation in acute stages of CRPS.[59] As further support of a neurogenic inflammatory process, systemic calcitonin gene-related peptide (CGRP) levels were found to be increased in acute CRPS but not in chronic stages.[60,61] In the fluid of artificially produced skin blisters and venous blood, significantly higher levels of interleukin-6 (IL-6) and tumor necrosis factor-α (TNFα), and IL-2 were observed in the involved extremity as compared with the uninvolved extremity and patients with CRPS I, respectively.[62] Because these findings persisted although pain and signs of CRPS I improved, the direct relationship between clinical signs and symptoms and proinflammatory cytokines was questioned.[63] However, proinflammatory cytokine levels were also significantly elevated, first in patients with CRPS who complained of mechanical hyperalgesia more than in patients with CRPS who did not have hyperalgesia[64] and, second, in the venous blood of the affected limb compared with the unaffected contralateral extremity.[61] Moreover, analysis of the cerebrospinal fluid in CRPS I and II revealed higher levels of proinflammatory IL-1β and IL-6, whereas TNF levels did not differ from levels in patients with painful conditions of other origin.[65,66]

Moreover, in suction blisters of patients with cold-type CRPS, the vasoconstrictive neuropeptide endothelin-1 was found to be significantly increased.[67] Thus, in summary, these data indicate that up-regulation of neuropeptides causing neurogenic inflammation and impaired inactivation of those substances contribute to symptom diversity in CRPS.[68]

As an indicator of an exogenous infection, a significantly higher seroprevalence of erythrovirus (formerly parvovirus) B19 was observed in patients with CRPS I.[69,70] Other studies investigated whether an exogenous *Campylobacter* infection may trigger autoimmune activation.[70,71] However, the importance of antecedent infections, as well as detected autoantibodies against autonomic nervous system structures,[72,73] in the pathophysiology of CRPS (e.g., in the generation of facilitated chronic inflammation) is yet not known.

Thus, evidence indicates that inflammatory processes are involved in the pathogenesis of early CRPS. However, the exact mechanisms of the initiation and maintenance of these inflammatory reactions are unclear.[74] One central issue is whether the sympathetic nervous system may contribute to the early inflammatory state. De novo expression of adreno-receptors on macrophages after an experimental nerve lesion supports this idea. However, this concept has yet to be proven in patients with CRPS. **Figure 30.3** illustrates the possible interactions among sympathetic fibers, afferent fibers, blood vessels, and non-neural cells related to the immune system (e.g., macrophages), interactions that theoretically lead to the inflammatory changes observed in patients with CRPS.

Motor Abnormalities

Approximately 50% of the patients with CRPS show decreased active range of motion, increased amplitude of physiologic tremor, and reduced active motor force of the affected extremity. In approximately 10% of cases, dystonia of the affected

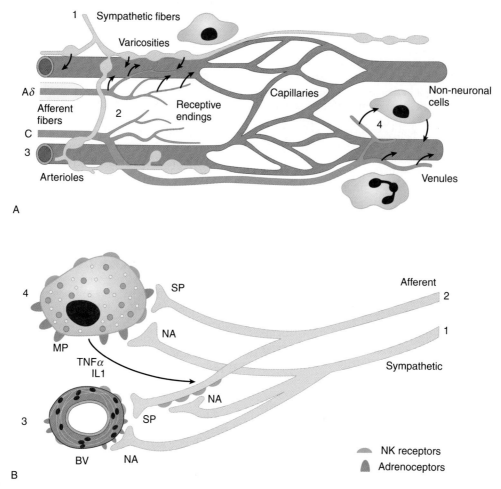

Fig. 30.3 A, The micromilieu of nociceptors. The microenvironment of primary afferents is thought to affect the properties of the receptive endings of myelinated (A) and unmyelinated (C) afferent fibers. This has been particularly documented for inflammatory processes, but one may speculate that pathologic changes in the direct surroundings of primary afferents may contribute to other pain states as well. The vascular bed consists of arterioles (directly innervated by sympathetic and afferent fibers), capillaries (not innervated and not influenced by nerve fibers), and venules (not directly innervated but influenced by nerve fibers). The micromilieu depends on several interacting components: neural activity in postganglionic noradrenergic fibers (1) supplying blood vessels (3) causes release of norepinephrine and possibly other substances and vasoconstriction. Excitation of primary afferents (A-delta [Aδ] and C fibers) (2) causes vasodilatation in precapillary arterioles and plasma extravasation in postcapillary venules (C fibers only) by the release of substance P (SP) and other vasoactive compounds (e.g., calcitonin gene–related peptide [CGRP]). Some of these effects may be mediated by non-neuronal cells such as mast cells and macrophages (4). Other factors that affect the control of the microcirculation are the myogenic properties of arterioles (3) and more global environmental influences such as a change of temperature and metabolic state of the tissue. **B,** Hypothetical relationships among sympathetic noradrenergic nerve fibers (1), peptidergic afferent nerve fibers (2), blood vessels (3), and macrophages (4). The activated and sensitized afferent nerve fibers activate macrophages (MP) possibly by SP release. The immune cells start to release cytokines, such as tumor necrosis factor-α (TNFα) and interleukin-1 (IL1), which further activate afferent fibers. SP (and CGRP) released from the afferent nerve fibers reacts with neurokinin-1 (NK1) receptors in the blood vessels (arteriolar vasodilatation, venular plasma extravasation, neurogenic inflammation). The sympathetic nerve fibers interact with this system on three levels: (1) through adrenoceptors (mainly α) on the blood vessels (vasoconstriction); (2) through adrenoceptors (mainly β) on macrophages (further release of cytokines), and (3) through adrenoceptors (mainly α) on afferents (further sensitization of these fibers). BV, blood vessels; NA, norepinephrine. *(A, Modified from Jänig W, Koltzenburg M: What is the interaction between the sympathetic terminal and the primary afferent fiber? In Basbaum AI, Besson J-M, editors:* Towards a new pharmacotherapy of pain, *Chichester, 1991, Wiley, 1991, pp 331–352; B, Modified from Jänig W, Baron R: Complex regional pain syndrome: mystery explained?* Lancet Neurol *2:687, 2003.)*

hand or foot develops with delayed onset.[75] It is unlikely that these motor changes are related to a peripheral process (e.g., influence of the sympathetic nervous system on neuromuscular transmission or contractility of skeletal muscle). These somatomotor changes are more likely generated by changes of activity in the motoneurons (i.e., they have a central origin). Maihofner et al[76] used kinematic analysis of target reaching and grip force analysis to assess motor deficits quantitatively in patients with CRPS. These results pointed to abnormalities in cerebral motor processing and were confirmed in an fMRI study. A pathologic sensorimotor integration located in

the parietal cortex was found that may induce abnormal central programming and processing of motor tasks. Larger brain activation during the movement of the affected limb may indicate impaired inhibitory mechanisms within the motor areas. The motor performance was also slightly impaired on the contralateral unaffected side.[76,77] Furthermore, sustained disinhibition of the motor cortex was found in patients with CRPS on the contralateral as well as the ipsilateral hemisphere.[78,79] Repetitive TMS applied to the motor cortex contralateral to the affected extremity in CRPS I showed the potential to modulate (i.e., decrease) pain.[80,81]

According to this view, a neglect-like syndrome was clinically described as being responsible for the disuse of the extremity.[82,83] Delayed recognition of hand laterality that is related to the duration and pain intensity[84] in CRPS I and impairment of body perception[85] and self-perception of the affected extremity that is related to pain intensity, illness duration, and extent of sensory deficits[86] may contribute to disuse, impaired motor planning, and function. A controlled study also supported incongruence between central motor output and sensory input as an underlying mechanism in CRPS. Using the method of mirror visual feedback, the visual input from a moving unaffected limb to the brain was able to reestablish the pain-free relationship between sensory feedback and motor execution. After 6 weeks of therapy, pain and function were improved as compared with the control group.[87,88] A study extension comparing the combined therapy regimen of hand laterality recognition training, imagination of movements, and mirror movements demonstrated the efficacy of this approach to reduce pain and disability.[89]

Sympathetically Maintained Pain
Definition

On the basis of experience and clinical studies, the term *sympathetically maintained pain* (SMP) was redefined. Patients with neuropathic pain who presenting with similar clinical signs and symptoms can clearly be divided into two groups by the negative or positive effect of selective sympathetic blockade or antagonism of alpha-adrenoceptor mechanisms. The pain component that is relieved by specific sympatholytic procedures is considered SMP. Thus, SMP is now defined as a symptom or the underlying mechanism in a subset of patients with neuropathic disorders and not as a clinical entity. The positive effect of sympathetic blockade is not essential for the diagnosis. Conversely, the only way to differentiate between SMP and sympathetically independent pain (SIP) is the efficacy of a correctly applied sympatholytic intervention.[8]

Studies on Patients

Clinical studies in CRPS support the idea that nociceptors develop catecholamine sensitivity.[90] Intra-operative stimulation of the sympathetic chain induces an increase of spontaneous pain in patients with causalgia (CRPS II) but not in patients with hyperhidrosis. In CRPS II and post-traumatic neuralgias, intracutaneous application of norepinephrine into a symptomatic area rekindled spontaneous pain and dynamic mechanical hyperalgesia that had been relieved by sympathetic blockade. This finding supports the idea that noradrenergic sensitivity of human nociceptors is present after partial nerve lesion. In addition, intradermal norepinephrine, in physiologically relevant doses, was demonstrated to evoke greater pain in the affected regions of patients with SMP than in the contralateral unaffected limb and in control subjects.[91]

Baron et al[92] performed a study in patients with CRPS I by using physiologic stimuli of the sympathetic nervous system. Cutaneous sympathetic vasoconstrictor outflow to the painful extremity was experimentally activated to the highest possible physiologic degree by whole-body cooling. During the thermal challenge, the affected extremity was clamped to 35°C (95°F) to avoid thermal effects at the nociceptor level. The intensity as well as the area of spontaneous pain and mechanical hyperalgesia (dynamic and punctate) increased significantly in patients who had been classified as having SMP by positive sympathetic blocks but not in patients with SIP (**Fig. 30.4**). The experimental setup

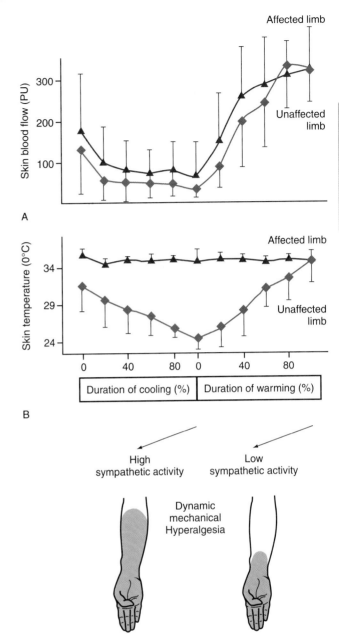

Fig. 30.4 Experimental modulation of cutaneous sympathetic vasoconstrictor neurons by physiologic thermoregulatory reflex stimuli in 13 patients with complex regional pain syndrome (CRPS). With the help of a thermal suit, whole-body cooling and warming were performed to alter sympathetic skin nerve activity. The subjects were lying in a suit supplied by tubes in which running water of 12°C (54°F) and 50°C (122°F), respectively (inflow temperature), was used to cool or warm the whole body. By these means, sympathetic activity can be switched on and off. **A,** High sympathetic vasoconstrictor activity during cooling induces a considerable drop in skin blood flow on the affected and unaffected extremity (laser Doppler flowmetry). Measurements were taken at 5-minute intervals at the fingertips (mean + SD). **B,** On the unaffected side, a secondary decrease of skin temperature was documented. On the affected side, the forearm temperature was clamped at 35°C (95°F) by a feedback-controlled heat lamp to exclude temperature effects on the sensory receptor level. Measurements were taken at 5-minute intervals (mean + SD). **C,** Effect of cutaneous sympathetic vasoconstrictor activity on dynamic mechanical hyperalgesia in one patient with CRPS who had sympathetically maintained pain. Activation of sympathetic neurons (during cooling) leads to a considerable increase of the area of dynamic mechanical hyperalgesia. SD, standard deviation. *(From Baron R, Schattschneider J, Binder A, et al: Relation between sympathetic vasoconstrictor activity and pain and hyperalgesia in complex regional pain syndromes: a case-control study, Lancet 359:1655, 2002.)*

used in the latter study selectively altered sympathetic cutaneous vasoconstrictor activity without influencing other sympathetic systems innervating the extremities (i.e., piloerector, sudomotor, and muscle vasoconstrictor neurons). Therefore, the interaction of sympathetic and afferent neurons measured here was likely to be located within the skin as predicted by the pain-enhancing effect of intracutaneous norepinephrine injections.[91] The relief of spontaneous pain after sympathetic blockade was more pronounced than changes in spontaneous pain that could be induced experimentally by sympathetic activation. One explanation for this discrepancy may be that complete sympathetic block affects all sympathetic outflow channels projecting to the affected extremity.

In addition to a coupling in the skin, a sympathetic-afferent interaction is also likely to occur in other tissues, in particular in deep somatic domains such as bone, muscle, and joints. Supporting this view, these structures in particular are extremely painful in some patients with CRPS.[93] Furthermore, some patients may have CRPS characterized by a selective or predominant sympathetic-afferent interaction in deep somatic tissues sparing the skin.[44] Additionally, nonresponsiveness to sympathetic blockades or modulation of sympathetic activity may be explained by the observation that the SMP component is not a constant phenomenon over time and decreases during the course of the disease.[93]

Summary of Pathophysiologic Mechanisms

In light of the numerous studies on pathophysiologic mechanisms in CRPS, investigators are currently at a turning point in recognizing that important elements of CRPS pathophysiology are obviously located within the CNS. Therefore, CRPS can be described as a neurologic disease (**Fig. 30.5**), including the autonomic, sensory, and motor systems as well as cortical areas involved in the processing of cognitive and affective information. In addition to these neural abnormalities, the inflammatory component appears to be particularly important in the acute phase of the disease.

Diagnosis

The diagnosis of CRPS I and II follows the IASP clinical criteria established in 1994.[8] If two clinical signs are joined by "or" and if either sign is present or both are, the condition of the statement is satisfied. For CRPS I (formerly known as reflex sympathetic dystrophy), the criteria are as follows:

1. Type I is a syndrome that develops after an initiating noxious event.
2. Spontaneous pain or allodynia/hyperalgesia occurs, is not limited to the territory of a single peripheral nerve, and is disproportionate to the inciting event.

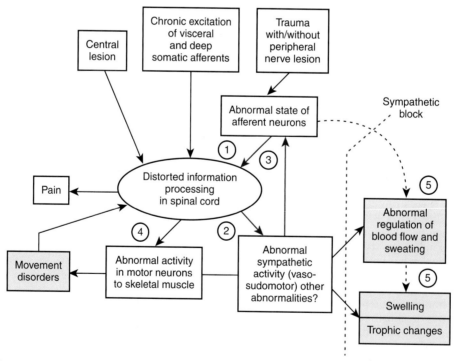

Fig. 30.5 General explanatory hypothesis about the neural mechanisms of generation of complex regional pain syndrome (CRPS) types I and II after peripheral trauma with and without nerve lesions, long-term stimulation of visceral afferents (e.g., myocardial infarction) and of deep somatic afferents, and, rarely, central trauma. The clinical observations are *shaded*. Note the vicious circle *(solid arrows)*. An important component of this circle is the excitatory influence of postganglionic sympathetic axons on primary afferent fibers in the periphery. The numbers indicate changes of activity in peripheral neurons that have not been measured directly in patients with CRPS but that have been postulated on the basis of measurements of effector responses of somatic sensations (including pain): 1, afferent traumatized neurons; 2, sympathetic neurons; 3, sympathetic-afferent coupling; 4, motoneurons; 5 *(interrupted arrow;* hypothetical mechanism), antidromically conducted activity in peptidergic afferent C fibers that leads to increased blood flow (arteriolar vasodilatation) and venular plasma extravasation, both of which hypothetically contribute to increased blood flow and to swelling. The *dotted line* represents the effect of sympathectomy or sympathetic blocks on the positive vicious feedback circuit. *(From Baron R: Complex regional pain syndromes. In McMahon SB, Koltzenburg M, editors:* Wall and Melzack's textbook of pain, *ed 5, London, 2006, Elsevier, pp 1011–1027.)*

3. The patient has or has had evidence of edema, skin blood flow abnormality, or abnormal sudomotor activity in the region of the pain since the inciting event.

4. This diagnosis is excluded by the existence of conditions that would otherwise account for the degree of pain and dysfunction.

Pain is essential for the diagnosis, and "spontaneous" indicates pain without external cause. Motor symptoms and findings are not included in this classification, although they are common and can include tremor, dystonia, and weakness.

In 2007, revised diagnostic criteria ("Budapest criteria") were proposed, segregated by clinical and research indications (**Table 30.2**).[94] For fulfilling the diagnostic criteria in the clinical use, at least one symptom in at least three categories and at least one sign in at least two categories must be present. A validation study indicated improved specificity in comparison with the 1994 IASP criteria (see later).[95]

Diagnostic Tests

The diagnosis of CRPS is based on the clinical criteria described earlier. However, several tests and procedures are valuable diagnostic tools that can add information to confirm

Table 30.2 Revised Diagnostic Criteria for Complex Regional Pain Syndrome: Budapest Criteria

CATEGORIES OF CLINICAL SIGNS OR SYMPTOMS

1. Positive sensory abnormalities
Spontaneous pain
Mechanical hyperalgesia
Thermal hyperalgesia
Deep somatic hyperalgesia

2. Vascular abnormalities
Vasodilatation
Vasoconstriction
Skin temperature asymmetries
Skin color changes

3. Edema, sweating abnormalities
Swelling
Hyperhidrosis
Hypohidrosis

4. Motor, trophic changes
Motor weakness
Tremor
Dystonia
Coordination deficits
Nail, hair changes
Skin atrophy
Joint stiffness
Soft tissue changes

INTERPRETATION FOR CLINICAL USE

≥1 symptom of ≥3 categories each
AND ≥1 sign of ≥2 categories each
Sensitivity, 0.85; specificity, 0.60

INTERPRETATION FOR RESEARCH USE

≥1 symptom of 4 categories each
AND ≥1 sign of ≥2 categories each
Sensitivity, 0.70; specificity, 0.96

Adapted from Harden RN, Bruehl S, Stanton-Hicks M, et al: Proposed new diagnostic criteria for complex regional pain syndrome, *Pain Med* 8:326, 2007.

the diagnostic impression about autonomic, sensory, and motor function and dysfunction.

Osseous changes are common in CRPS. Thus, three-phase bone scintigraphy can provide valuable information. Homogeneous unilateral hyperperfusion in the perfusion (30 seconds after injection) and blood-pool phases (2 minutes after injection) are characteristic and help to exclude differential diagnoses (e.g., osteoporosis resulting from inactivity). At 3 hours after injection, the mineralization phase shows increased unilateral periarticular tracer uptake (**Fig. 30.6**). Pathologic uptake in the metacarpophalangeal or metacarpal bones is thought to be highly sensitive and specific for CRPS. Although a gold standard for comparison is as yet unknown, it is useful to rule out pain syndromes of other origin. Bone scintigraphy shows significant changes only during the subacute period (≤1 year). A negative finding does not exclude the presence of CRPS. Bone scintigraphy has high specificity (75% to 100%) but low sensitivity (31% to 69%) for CRPS, with moderate interrater reliability. Endosteal and intracortical excavation, subperiosteal and trabecular bone resorption, spotty and localized bone demineralization, and osteoporosis have been thought to be specific signs of CRPS, but these signs are positive only in chronic stages. A comparison of radiography and three-phase scintigraphy in early postfracture CRPS showed lower sensitivity and specificity of radiography. MRI is suggested as being more reliable than radiographic examination and probably also than scintigraphy, but its value remains to be confirmed in further studies.

Quantitative sensory testing can provide information about the sensory symptom profile (function or dysfunction of unmyelinated and myelinated afferent fibers) by using psychophysical testing of thermal pain and vibratory thresholds. However, no sensory profile is characteristic for CRPS.

Autonomic testing with the quantitative sudomotor axon reflex test (QSART) can provide information about the function of sudomotor reflex loops. Swelling can be quantified by measuring water displacement. Autonomic vascular function can be tested by laser Doppler flowmetry[44,45,96] and infrared thermography.

Skin temperature measurements are an easy way to determine vascular function and may be particularly helpful for the diagnosis of CRPS. Wasner et al[97] performed a study using controlled thermoregulation (whole-body warming, cooling) to change cutaneous sympathetic vasoconstrictor activity. Skin temperature at the affected and unaffected limbs (infrared thermometry) was measured under resting conditions (before temperature challenge in the office at room temperature) and was continuously monitored during controlled modulation of sympathetic activity. Only minor skin temperature asymmetries were present between both limbs under resting conditions in most patients. However, during controlled thermoregulation, temperature differences between both sides increased dynamically and were most prominent at a high to medium level of vasoconstrictor activity. In patients suffering from painful limbs of other origin and in healthy volunteers (control groups), only minor side differences were noted in temperature both at rest and during thermoregulatory changes of sympathetic activity. When comparing the diagnostic value of skin temperature asymmetries in CRPS, sensitivity was only 32% under resting conditions but increased up to 76% during controlled alteration of sympathetic activity.

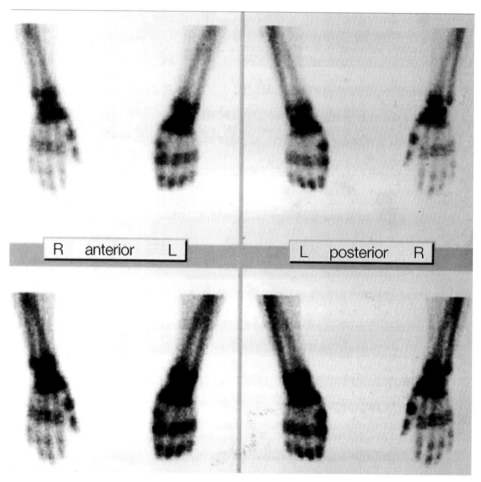

Fig. 30.6 Three-phase bone scintigraphy in a patient with complex regional pain syndrome type I of the upper left extremity: characteristic increased unilateral periarticular tracer uptake. *(From Baron R: Complex regional pain syndromes. In McMahon SB, Koltzenburg M, editors: Wall and Melzack's textbook of pain, ed 5, London, 2006, Elsevier, pp 1011–1027.)*

Specificity was 100% at rest and 93% at controlled thermo-regulation (**Fig. 30.7**). A sum score built from long-term skin temperature measurements, including temperature dynamics, reached a sensitivity of 73% and specificity of 67% compared with patients with other pain syndromes, regardless of clinical symptoms and signs.[98]

In conclusion, the degree of unilateral vascular disturbances in CRPS and the temperature side differences depend critically on environmental temperature and spontaneous sympathetic activity. However, the maximal skin temperature difference that occurs during the thermoregulatory cycle distinguishes, with high sensitivity and specificity, CRPS from other extremity pain syndromes.

Validation of Clinical Diagnostic Criteria

The definition of standardized diagnostic criteria for CRPS in 1994 was a major advance in the classification of regional pain disorders associated with vasomotor or sudomotor abnormalities.[8] Based on these criteria, clinical research on mechanisms was performed on a much more homogeneous group of patients and was therefore comparable for the first time. Validation of these CRPS diagnostic criteria showed adequate sensitivity (i.e., cases of actual CRPS rarely missed). The inclusion of motor and trophic signs and symptoms, for example, improved specificity to 85% without losing sensitivity.[12] However, both internal and external validation research suggested that these criteria led to overdiagnosis of CRPS.[99,100]

Possibly because of this drawback, the newer terminology did not replace the former denominations immediately.

The newer diagnostic criteria have been validated.[95] In this study, the 1994 IASP criteria showed high sensitivity (1.00) and low specificity (0.41), but the Budapest criteria for clinical use improved specificity to 0.68, whereas sensitivity of 0.99 was reached. Meeting the criteria for the diagnosis of CRPS varies according to the diagnostic criteria used.[101]

Differential Diagnosis

Because of the lack of a gold standard for the diagnosis of CRPS, the risk of overdiagnosing must be taken into account. To differentiate CRPS from other neuropathic and other pain syndromes, a detailed history and physical examination are mandatory and must be performed according to the specifications outlined earlier.

Post-Traumatic Neuralgia

Many patients with post-traumatic neuropathy have pain but do not have the full clinical picture of causalgia (CRPS II). In these cases, in contrast to patients with causalgia, the pain is located largely within the innervation territory of the injured nerve. Although the patients with post-traumatic neuropathy often describe their pain as burning, they exhibit a less complex clinical picture than do patients with causalgia, and they do not have marked swelling or progressive spread of symptoms. The cardinal symptoms are spontaneous burning pain,

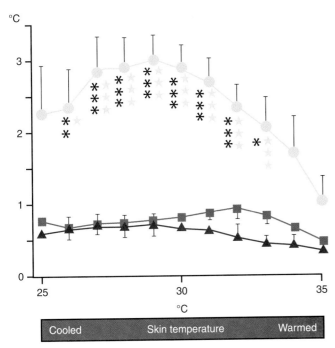

Fig. 30.7 Average absolute side differences in skin temperature of the fingers (toes) of both hands (feet) in 25 patients with complex regional pain syndrome (CRPS) *(circles)*, in 20 healthy controls *(triangles)*, and in 15 control patients with extremity pain of other origin *(squares)* during a controlled thermoregulatory cycle (controlled alteration in cutaneous sympathetic activity). The level of the overall cutaneous sympathetic vasoconstrictor activity was estimated indirectly by using the skin temperature on the unaffected side (or the right side in healthy controls) as a reference value. A skin temperature on the healthy side of 25°C (77°F) indicates a high level, a temperature of 30°C (86°F) indicates an intermediate level, and a temperature of 35°C (95°F) indicates a complete inhibition of sympathetic vasoconstrictor activity to the skin (mean ± SEM). CRPS compared with healthy controls *(asterisks)*; CRPS compared with control patients with extremity pain of other origin *(stars)*: one symbol, *P* <.05; two symbols, *P* < .01; three symbols, *P* < .001. *(From Wasner G, Schattschneider J, Heckmann K, et al: Vascular abnormalities in reflex sympathetic dystrophy [CRPS I]: mechanisms and diagnostic value, Brain 124:587, 2001.)*

hyperalgesia, and mechanical and especially cold allodynia. These sensory symptoms are confined to the territory of the affected peripheral nerve, although allodynia may extend beyond the border of nerve territories for some centimeters. Spontaneous pain and evoked pain are felt superficially and not deep inside the extremity, and the intensity of both types of pain does not depend on the position of the extremity. Patients with post-traumatic neuropathy occasionally obtain relief with sympatholytic procedures, although much less often than do patients with CRPS.

Following the IASP classification, it is possible to use the term *neuralgia* for this type of neuropathic pain (pain within the innervation territory of a lesioned nerve, e.g., post-traumatic neuralgia). However, the definition of CRPS II includes the statement that symptoms may also be limited to the territory of a single peripheral nerve. Therefore, the term *complex regional pain syndrome type II* provides a window to include these localized post-traumatic neuropathies. An inherent weakness of this definition of CRPS II is that different syndromes with different underlying mechanisms are obviously included.

Neuropathies (e.g., diabetic polyneuropathy) may also manifest with spontaneous pain, skin color changes, and motor deficits, but they are distinguished by their symmetrical distribution and the patient's history. Furthermore, all kinds of inflammations or infections (e.g., rheumatism, phlegmon) may induce intense unilateral skin warming. Unilateral arterial or venous occlusive diseases can cause unilateral pain and vascular abnormalities and must be excluded. Repetitive artificial occlusion of the blood supply to one limb (as in the psychiatric factitious disorders, artifact syndrome) may induce secondary structural changes of the blood vessels with consecutive abnormalities in perfusion and may therefore mimic the symptoms and signs of CRPS.

Treatment

A lack of understanding of the underlying pathophysiologic abnormalities and the absence of objective diagnostic criteria result in inherent difficulties in conducting clinical trials with therapeutic modalities. Therefore, only few evidence-based treatment regimens for CRPS are available so far; these are summarized in **Table 30.3**. In fact, six literature reviews of outcome studies found discouragingly little consistent information regarding the pharmacologic agents and methods for treatment of CRPS.[102–107] Moreover, the methodology was often of low quality within the 50 randomized controlled trials available. In the absence of more specific information about pathophysiologic mechanisms and treatment of CRPS, one must rely additionally on outcomes from treatment studies for other neuropathic pain syndromes. Furthermore, the still hypothetical mechanism-based treatment concept must be transferred from ideas derived from animal experiments on peripheral nerve lesions to the situation in patients with CRPS. However, functional imaging and neurophysiologic studies indicate that a reduction of pain does not reduce the burden of illness only. Moreover, it can contribute to the reversibility of cortical reorganization and thereby lead to an improvement of functional (i.e., motor function) and sensory capacity.

Pharmacologic Therapy
Nonsteroidal Anti-Inflammatory Drugs

Nonsteroidal anti-inflammatory drugs (NSAIDs) have not been investigated in the treatment of CRPS to date. However, from clinical experience, these drugs can control mild to moderate pain.

Opioids

Opioids are clearly effective in postoperative, inflammatory, and cancer pain. The use of opioids in CRPS has not been studied. In other neuropathic pain syndromes, compounds such as tramadol, morphine, oxycodone, and levorphanol are clearly analgesic when compared with placebo. However, no long-term studies have been conducted on oral opioid use for treatment of neuropathic pain, CRPS included. Even without solid scientific evidence, the expert opinion of pain clinicians is that opioid use could be and should be part of a comprehensive pain treatment program. Given that some patients with neuropathic pain may obtain considerable pain relief, opioids should be prescribed immediately if other agents do not achieve sufficient analgesia.

Table 30.3 Pharmacologic Treatment of Complex Regional Pain Syndromes (Randomized Controlled Trials)

Agent	Result	No. Patients	Reference, year
ANTICONVULSANTS			
Gabapentin	Positive	85 (of 305)	Mellick and Mellick, 1995[110]
Gabapentin	Weak effect on pain	46	van de Vusse et al, 2004[111]
SODIUM CHANNEL BLOCKERS			
Lidocaine (IV)	Positive	16	Wallace et al, 2000
CORTICOSTEROIDS			
Prednisone (oral)	Positive	23	Christensen et al, 1982[56]
Prednisone (oral)	Positive	34	Braus et al, 1994[112]
Prednisone (oral)	Positive	60	Kalita et al, 2006[113]
Methylprednisolone	Negative	21	Munts et al, 2010[114]
CALCIUM-REGULATING DRUGS			
Clodronate (IV)	Positive	31	Varenna et al, 2000[122]
Alendronate (IV)	Positive	20	Adami et al, 1997[121]
Alendronate (oral)	Positive	39	Manicourt et al, 2004[123]
Pamidronate (IV)	Positive	27	Robinson et al, 2004[124]
Calcitonin (intranasal)	Positive	66	Gobelet et al, 1992[119]
Calcitonin (intranasal)	Negative	38	Bickerstaff and Kanis, 1991
Calcitonin (subcutaneous)	Negative	24	Gobelet et al, 1986
Calcitonin (intranasal/oral)	Negative	35	Sahin et al, 2006
FREE RADICAL SCAVENGERS			
DMSO (topical)	Positive	26	Geertzen et al, 1994[127]
DMSO (topical)	Equal to N-Acetylcysteine	112	Perez et al, 2003[125]
DMSO (topical)	Negative	31	Zuurmond et al, 1996[126]
N-Acetylcysteine (oral)	Equal to DMSO	112	Perez et al, 2003[125]
Mannitol (IV)	Negative	41	Perez et al, 2008
NMDA ANTAGONIST			
Ketamine (IV)	Positive	19	Schwartzman et al, 2009[117]
Ketamine (IV)	Positive	30	Sigtermans et al, 2009[118]
Ketamine (topical)	Positive	20	Finch et al, 2009[116]
VASODILATOR			
Tadalafil (oral)	Positive (cold-type CRPS)	24	Groeneweg et al, 2008[67]
SEROTONIN (5-HT₂) ANTAGONIST			
Sarpogrelate hydrochloride (oral)	Negative	30	Ogawa et al, 1998[129]

CRPs, complex regional pain syndrome; DMSO, dimethylsulfoxide; IV, intravenous; NMDA, N-methyl-D-aspartate.
Adapted from Baron R: Complex regional pain syndromes. In McMahon SB, Koltzenburg M, editors: *Wall and Melzack's textbook of pain*, ed 5, London, 2006, Elsevier, 2006, pp 1011-1027; Bickerstaff DR, Kanis JA: The use of nasal calcitonin in the treatment of post-traumatic algodystrophy, *Br J Rheumatol* 30:291, 1991. Gobelet C, Meier JL, Schaffner W, et al: Calcitonin and reflex sympathetic dystrophy syndrome. *Clin Rheumatol* 5:382, 1986. Perez RS, Pragt E, Geurts J, et al: Treatment of patients with complex regional pain syndrome type I with mannitol: a prospective, randomized, placebo-controlled, double-blinded study. *J Pain* 9:678, 2008. Sahin F, Yilmaz F, Kotevoglu N, et al: Efficacy of salmon calcitonin in complex regional pain syndrome (type 1) in addition to physical therapy. *Clin Rheumatol* 25:143, 2006. Wallace MS, Ridgeway BM, Leung AY et al: Concentration-effect relationship of intravenous lidocaine on the allodynia of complex regional pain syndrome types I and II, *Anesthesiology* 92:75, 2000.

Antidepressants

Tricyclic antidepressants (TCAs) have been intensely studied in different neuropathic pain conditions but not in CRPS. Solid evidence indicates that (selective) reuptake inhibitors of serotonin and norepinephrine (e.g., amitriptyline, duloxetine) and selective norepinephrine blockers (e.g., desipramine) produce pain relief in diabetic or postherpetic neuropathy. No studies have been performed on patients with CRPS.

Sodium Channel Blocking Agents

Lidocaine administered intravenously was effective in a small trial conducted in CRPS I and II regarding spontaneous and evoked pain.[81] Carbamazepine has not been tested in CRPS.

γ-Aminobutyric Acid Agonists

Intrathecally administered baclofen is effective in the treatment of dystonia in CRPS.[108] Oral baclofen has been effective in the treatment of trigeminal neuralgia. No further trials in CRPS are available, and no evidence indicates an analgesic effect of baclofen, valproic acid, vigabatrin, and benzodiazepines in CRPS.

Gabapentin

Promising preliminary evidence was revealed by two studies on patients with CRPS that showed an analgesic effect of gabapentin.[109,110] A randomized, double-blind, placebo-controlled trial demonstrated a mild effect of gabapentin on pain only and a good effect on sensory deficit symptoms in CRPS I.[111] Gabapentin is effective in conditions such as painful diabetic neuropathy and postherpetic neuralgia.

Corticosteroids

Orally administered prednisone, 30 to 40 mg daily, has demonstrated efficacy in the improvement of the entire clinical status (≤75%) of patients with acute CRPS (< 13 weeks)[56] and in CRPS of patients with stroke.[112,113] No evidence has been obtained for a single 60-mg intrathecal bolus of methylprednisolone.[114] A small trial of intravenous immunoglobulin treatment in 12 patients indicated positive effects, but further confirmation[115] with other immune-modulating therapies, such as immunoglobulins or immunosuppressive drugs, is needed.

N-Methyl-D-Aspartate Receptor Blockers

Clinically available compounds that are demonstrated to have N-methyl-D-aspartate (NMDA) receptor–blocking properties include ketamine, dextromethorphan, and memantine. Three randomized controlled trials on topical and intravenous ketamine proved significant reductions of spontaneous pain and evoked pain, respectively.[116–118]

Calcium-Regulating Drugs

Calcitonin, administered three times daily intranasally, demonstrated significant pain reduction in patients with CRPS.[119] However, three other trials showed negative results, and different meta-analyses showed conflicting evidence of the efficacy of calcitonin.[102,103,106,120] Clodronate (300 mg daily intravenously), alendronate (7.5 mg daily intravenously or 40 mg orally daily), and pamidronate (60 mg intravenously in a single dose) produced significant improvements in pain and movement range in acute CRPS.[121–124] The mode of action of all these compounds in CRPS is unknown and may rely on the interaction with CRPS-related bone resorption and a direct analgesic effect.

Free Radical Scavengers

A placebo-controlled trial was performed using the free radical scavengers dimethylsulfoxide (DMSO) 50% topically and N-acetylcysteine (NAC) orally for the treatment of CRPS I.[125] Both drugs were found to be equally effective; however, DMSO seemed more favorable for warm-type CRPS I and NAC more effective for cold-type CRPS I. The results were negatively influenced by longer disease duration. A previous trial with DMSO failed to show a positive result in CRPS[126]; however, DMSO was shown to be more effective than regional blocks with guanethidine in a small population of patients with CRPS.[127]

Transdermal application of the alpha$_2$-adrenoceptor agonist clonidine, which is thought to prevent the release of catecholamines by a presynaptic action, may be helpful when small areas of hyperalgesia are present.[128]

Miscellaneous Agents

The phosphodiesterase inhibitor tadalafil was investigated in 24 patients suffering from cold-type CRPS of the lower limb. In addition to physical therapy, oral intake of 10 mg daily for 4 weeks and 20 mg daily for the following 8 weeks led to a significant reduction in pain intensity compared with placebo.[67] Sarpogrelate hydrochloride, a selective serotonin (5-HT$_2$) receptor blocker, as an add-on medication was ineffective to reduce pain additionally.[129]

Interventional Therapy at the Sympathetic Nervous System Level

Currently, two therapeutic techniques to block sympathetic activity are used:

1. Injections of a local anesthetic around sympathetic paravertebral ganglia that project to the affected body part (sympathetic ganglion blocks)
2. Regional intravenous application of guanethidine, bretylium, or reserpine (which all deplete norepinephrine in the postganglionic axon) to an isolated extremity blocked with a tourniquet (intravenous regional sympatholysis [IVRS])

Many uncontrolled surveys published in the literature review the effect of sympathetic interventions in CRPS. In CRPS, approximately 70% of the patients report full or partial response.[130] The efficacy of these procedures is, however, still controversial and was questioned in the past.[104,106,131] In fact, the specificity and long-term results as well as the techniques used have rarely been adequately evaluated.

Sympathetic Ganglion Blocks

One controlled study in patients with CRPS I showed that sympathetic ganglion blocks with local anesthetic had the same immediate effect on pain as a control injection with saline.[132] However, after 24 hours, patients in the local anesthetic group were much better, a finding indicating that nonspecific effects are important initially and that evaluating the efficacy of sympatholytic interventions is best done after 24 hours. With these data in mind, the uncontrolled studies mentioned earlier must be interpreted cautiously. Only 10 of 24 studies reviewed assessed long-term effects. A meta-analysis of studies assessing the effect of local anesthetic sympathetic blockade for CRPS failed to draw conclusions concerning the effectiveness of this procedure, mainly as a result of small sample sizes.[133]

Intravenous Regional Sympatholysis: Open Studies

No improvement compared with baseline was found for IVRS with reserpine and guanethidine,[134] nor were differences in IVRS results reported between guanethidine and lidocaine.[135]

Guanethidine and pilocarpine versus placebo showed no differences after application of four blocks.[136] However, stellate blocks with bupivacaine and regional blocks with guanethidine demonstrated a significant improvement of pain compared with baseline but no differences between these two therapies.[137] One study demonstrated that IVRS with bretylium and lidocaine produced significantly longer pain relief than did lidocaine alone.[138] No effect was obtained by IVRS with droperidol.[139] Hanna and Peat[140] demonstrated a significant improvement of pain after a single IVRS bolus of ketanserin. Bounameaux and associates[141] failed to show any significant effect with the same procedure. Bier's block with methylprednisolone and lidocaine in CRPS I did not provide a short-term or long-lasting benefit compared with placebo.[142]

A desperate need exists for controlled studies that assess the acute as well as the long-term effects of sympathetic blockade and IVRS on pain and other CRPS symptoms, in particular motor function. Well-performed sympathetic ganglion blocks should be performed, rather than IVRS.[143]

Surgical Sympathectomy

Only limited evidence is available regarding the efficacy of thoracoscopic or surgical sympathectomy, and meta-analysis again did not permit a conclusion to be drawn about the efficacy of this method.[144] Four open studies reported partly long-lasting benefits of sympathectomy in CRPS I and II.[145–148] The most important independent factor in determining a positive outcome of sympathectomy is a time interval of less than 12 months, best within 3 months after CRPS onset, between the inciting event and sympathectomy.[145,147] Videoscopic lumbar sympathectomy is as effective as is open surgical intervention.[149]

Baron and Maier[43] investigated skin blood flow, sympathetic vasoconstrictor reflexes, and pain after surgical sympathectomy in a small cohort of patients with CRPS. Postoperatively, no vasoconstriction resulting from deep inspiration (vasoconstrictor reflex) could be elicited at the affected extremity, a finding indicating complete sympathetic denervation. Additionally, the skin temperature at the affected hand increased. After 4 weeks, skin temperature decreased without signs of reinnervation. This denervation supersensitivity was associated with the recurrence of pain and is thought to rely on vascular supersensitivity to cold and circulating catecholamines. Only 2 of 12 patients experienced long-term pain relief.

Irreversible sympathectomy may be effective in selected cases. Because of the risk of development of adaptive supersensitivity, even on nociceptive neurons and consecutive pain increase and prolongation, these procedures should not be broadly recommended.

Stimulation Techniques and Spinal Drug Application

Transcutaneous electrical nerve stimulation (TENS) may be effective in some cases and has minimal side effects.

Epidural spinal cord stimulation (SCS) showed efficacy in one randomized study in selected patients with chronic CRPS.[150] These patients had previously undergone unsuccessful surgical sympathectomy. The pain-relieving effect was not associated with peripheral vasodilatation, a finding suggesting that central disinhibition processes are involved. Sensory detection threshold was not affected by the stimulation, but one trial identified brush-evoked allodynia as a negative predictor of treatment outcome, whereas age, disease duration, pain intensity and localization, and mechanical hypoesthesia did not predict SCS efficacy.[151,152] At 5-year follow-up, pain intensity, global perceived effect, treatment satisfaction, and health-related quality of life did not differ between those receiving physical therapy and SCS and patients receiving physical therapy alone.[153] A meta-analysis showed that in selected patients, SCS can relieve pain and allodynia and can improve quality of life.[154] Other stimulation techniques (i.e., peripheral nerve stimulation with implanted electrodes, repetitive TMS, and deep brain stimulation [sensory thalamus and medial lemniscus, motor cortex]) have been reported to be effective in selected cases of CRPS.[80,155,156]

In selected patients with severe refractory CRPS, the epidural application of clonidine showed pain reduction in high doses (700 µg) and in lower doses (300 µg).[157] However, the drug was associated with marked side effects (e.g., sedation and hypotension).

Intrathecally administered baclofen (50/75 µg daily) showed preliminary efficacy in the treatment of dystonia in CRPS.[108] The effect was more pronounced at the upper extremity and showed a high-variability on the long-term. An open-label study reported 89 adverse events during the treatment with intrathecally administered baclofen, and the investigators advocated an improvement of patient selection and application technique.[158] Intrathecally administered glycine showed no significant effect on CRPS-related dystonia in a randomized placebo-controlled cross-over trial in 19 patients.[159]

Physical Therapy and Occupational Therapy

The use of physical and occupational therapy in CRPS is recommended.[160] Clinical experience clearly indicates that physical therapy is of utmost importance to achieve recovery of function and rehabilitation. Standardized physical therapy has produced long-term relief of pain and of physical dysfunction in children.[161]

Physical therapy and, to a lesser extent, occupational therapy are able to reduce pain and improve active mobility in CRPS I.[162] Lymph drainage provides no benefit when applied together with physical therapy in comparison with physical therapy alone.[163] Patients with initially less pain and better motor function are predicted to benefit to a greater degree than are others.[164] Physical therapy of CRPS is both more effective and less costly than either occupational therapy or control treatment.[165]

Mirror visual feedback treatment in CRPS I has been shown to reduce pain and improve function. Studies have demonstrated that the combination of hand laterality recognition training, imagination of movements, and mirror movements reduces pain and disability in patients with CRPS.[87–89,166,167] Using a mirror image of the unaffected limb also enhances the recovery of tactile acuity.[168] The order of training—laterality recognition, movement imagination, mirror movements—is important for treatment success.

Thus, physical and occupational therapy and attentional training have become important parts of a successful therapeutic approach to CRPS.

Psychological Therapy

Although evidence indicates a psychological impact on patients with CRPS, only one study addressed the efficacy of psychological treatment. A prospective, randomized, single-blind trial of cognitive-behavioral treatment was conducted together with physical therapy of different intensities in children and adults and showed a long-lasting reduction of all symptoms in both arms of the trial.[169] Fear of injury or reinjury by moving the affected limb is thought to be a possible predictor of chronic disability. Thus, in a small group of patients, graded exposure therapy was successful for decreasing pain-related fear, pain intensity, and disability.[170]

Treatment Guidelines

Given the limited data available, the treatment of CRPS still remains largely empirical.[105] Treatment should be immediate and most importantly directed toward restoration of full function of the extremity. This objective is best attained in a comprehensive interdisciplinary setting with particular emphasis on pain management and functional restoration.[171,172] A treatment algorithm is proposed in **Figure 30.8**. Pain specialists should include neurologists, anesthesiologists, orthopedic surgeons, physical therapists, psychologists, and the general practitioner.

The severity of the disease determines the therapeutic regimen. Pain reduction is the precondition with which all other interventions must comply. All therapeutic approaches must not hurt. During the acute stage of CRPS when the patient still suffers from severe pain at rest and during movements, it is usually impossible to carry out intensive active therapy. Painful interventions and, in particular, aggressive physical therapy at this stage often lead to deterioration. Therefore, immobilization and careful contralateral physical therapy should be the acute treatments of choice, and intense pain treatment should be initiated immediately. First-line analgesics and co-analgesics are opioids, antidepressants, and calcium channel–modulating anticonvulsants. Additionally, corticosteroids should be considered if inflammatory signs and symptoms are predominant. Sympatholytic procedures, preferably sympathetic ganglion blocks, should identify the component of the pain that is maintained by the sympathetic nervous system.

For efficacy, a stepwise treatment protocol should be followed. Calcium-regulating agents should be used in cases of refractory pain. If resting pain subsides, first passive physical therapy, mirror therapy, and then later active isometric therapy, followed by active isotonic training should be performed in combination with sensory desensitization and lateralization programs until restitution of complete motor function. Psychological treatment must flank the regimen, to strengthen coping strategies and to discover contributing factors. In refractory cases, spinal cord stimulation and epidural clonidine could be considered. If refractory dystonia develops, intrathecal baclofen application is worth considering.

Children

CRPS I and CRPS II also occur in children. The diagnosis seems to be delayed more often than in adults. The incidence increases with puberty, and girls are predominantly affected, with a ratio of 4:1. In contrast to adults, children with CRPS more often have lower limb involvement (5.3:1). The mean age was 12.5 years in a cohort of 396 children. Children may present with primarily colder affected extremities and less pronounced neurologic and sympathetic symptoms.[173] Significant emotional dysfunction was demonstrated in a small number of children with CRPS. A possible association of intensive, parentally forced sports and leisure activities with the occurrence of the inciting trauma was discussed. A sign of escape from parents' excessive demands was hypothesized.

Diagnostic bone scintigraphy in children seems to be of minor value compared with adults because images show higher variability and often decreased diffuse uptake. To minimize exposure to radiation, scintigraphy should not be performed in children on a routine basis.

Limited attention has been paid to differences in the response to therapy in children. So far, conservative strategies, such as analgesics, TENS, and cognitive and behavioral pain management techniques, as well as physical therapy, have been empirically effective in treating childhood CRPS and in preventing symptom prolongation. Between 50% and 90% of children with CRPS I in one study showed good long-term resolution of all symptoms.[124] However, a retrospective follow-up study with a median follow-up period of 12 years showed a disease course comparable to that in adults, and this finding calls into question the previous results.[173]

Prevention Studies

Only three reliable randomized placebo-controlled prevention studies have been conducted to date. Zollinger et al[174] proved a significantly reduced incidence of CRPS after Colles' fracture after vitamin C (500 mg/day) treatment. This result was confirmed in a second trial.[175] Preoperatively administered guanethidine did not prevent CRPS in patients undergoing fasciotomy for Dupuytren's disease.[176]

The recurrence rate of CRPS in patients with a history of CRPS undergoing surgery of the formerly affected extremity was significantly reduced by a perioperative stellate ganglion block.[177]

Prognosis

The disease duration is variable, and CRPS may persist over decades. In rare cases, causally directed therapy (e.g., decompression of an entrapment syndrome) may lead to complete recovery.

A 5.5-year follow-up study showed that 62% of patients were still limited in their activities of daily living; pain and motor impairment were the most important factors.[127] Over a period of 8 years, no significant changes in symptom severity in patients with CRPS I were observed irrespective of an initial warm or cold CRPS type.[178] In more than 60% of patients with CRPS II, the complaints remained unchanged even after 1 year of intensive therapy.[179] In contrast, a retrospective population-based study reported a resolution of symptoms in 74% of patients with CRPS I.[4] In a 13-month follow-up study in a small cohort and a follow-up study at 2 to 11 years, most patients still suffered from impairments of the affected extremity, although other clinical features of CRPS had resolved.[180,181]

The severity, rather than the origin, seems to determine the disease course. Age, sex, and affected side are not associated with the outcome.[4] Fractures may be associated with a higher

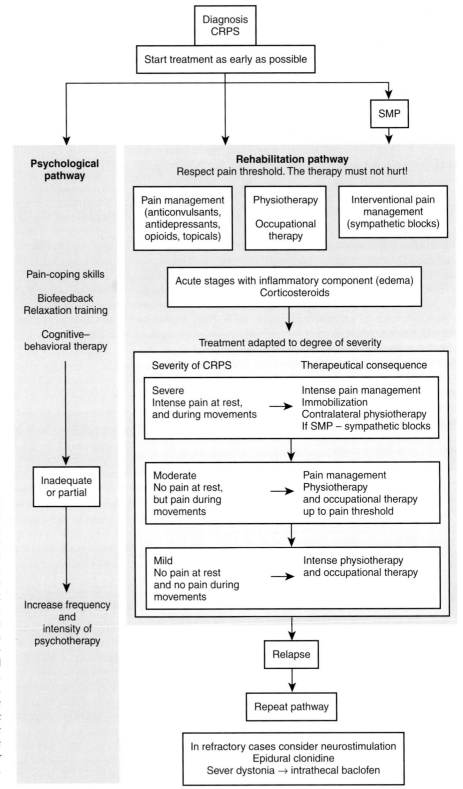

Fig. 30.8 Treatment algorithm: During the acute stage of complex regional pain syndrome (CRPS) with severe pain at rest, immobilization and careful contralateral physical therapy are the treatments of choice. Sympatholytic procedures, preferably sympathetic ganglion blocks, should identify the component of the pain that is maintained by the sympathetic nervous system. If resting pain subsides, physical therapy should be performed in combination with sensory desensitization programs and pain therapy. If movement-induced pain subsides, physical therapy and occupational therapy should be intensified. SMP, sympathetically maintained pain. *(Modified from Baron R, Binder A, Ulrich W, et al: Complex regional pain syndrome: reflex sympathetic dystrophy and causalgia, Nervenarzt 73:305, 2002; and Stanton-Hicks M, Burton A W, Bruehl SP, et al: An updated interdisciplinary clinical pathway for CRPS: report of an expert panel, Pain Pract 2:1, 2002.)*

resolution rate (91%) than are sprains (78%) or other inciting events (55%).[4] In one study, spontaneous-onset CRPS had a longer disease duration than did trauma-induced CRPS.[182] In 1183 patients, the incidence of recurrence was 1.8% per year.[183] Patients with recurrent CRPS were significantly younger but did not differ in gender or primary localization. Recurrence of CRPS manifests more often with few symptoms and signs and

spontaneous onset. A low skin temperature at the onset of the disease may predict an unfavorable course and outcome.[13,178] A retrospective analysis of 1006 cases of CRPS showed an incidence of severe complications in approximately 7%. These complications included infection, ulceration, chronic edema, dystonia, and myoclonus. Mostly female and younger patients with CRPS of the lower limb were affected.[184]

Conclusion

CRPS is clinically characterized by pain, abnormal regulation of blood flow and sweating, edema of skin and subcutaneous tissues, active and passive movement disorders, and trophic changes of skin, appendages of skin, and subcutaneous tissues. It is classified into type I (reflex sympathetic dystrophy) and type II (causalgia).

Patients with CRPS exhibit changes that occur in somatosensory systems that process noxious, tactile and thermal information, in sympathetic systems innervating skin (blood vessels, sweat glands), and in the somatomotor system. These observations indicate that the central representations of these systems are changed and that CRPS, in particular type I, is a systemic disease involving these neuronal systems. Patients with CRPS also demonstrate peripheral changes, such as edema, signs of inflammation, sympathetic-afferent coupling (as a basis for SMP), and trophic changes, which cannot be explained by the central changes but also cannot be considered independently of those central changes. Therefore, CRPS cannot be reduced to one system or to one mechanism only. This view is based on clinical observations, experimentation on humans, and experimentation on animals.

So far, very few evidence-based treatment regimens for CRPS have become available. Treatment of the individual patient is empirical and uses evidence-based techniques that have been proven effective in other neuropathic conditions. Treatment should be immediate and most importantly directed toward restoration of full function of the extremity. This objective is best attained in a comprehensive interdisciplinary setting with particular emphasis on pain management and functional restoration.

The key future question to be asked in research is this: What is the organizing principle leading to this complex syndrome? The changing views of pathophysiologic interactions will shift the focus of research efforts, will bring about diagnostic reclassification and redefinition of CRPS, and finally will lead to novel therapeutic approaches.

The essential task to be addressed in therapy is to perform controlled, multicenter studies that assess the short-term and long-term effects of drug and interventional therapies, as well as the effects of physical therapy and psychotherapy.

Acknowledgments

This work was supported by the German Ministry of Research and Education, German Research Network on Neuropathic Pain (BMBF, 01EM05/04). Thanks are given to Professor Dr. C. Maier for his support and contribution of Figure 30.2. This chapter was adapted from Baron R: Complex regional pain syndromes. In McMahon SB, Koltzenburg M, editors: *Wall and Melzack's textbook of pain,* ed 5, London, 2006, Elsevier, 2z006, pp 1011-1027, with permission.

References

Full references for this chapter can be found on www.expertconsult.com.

Chapter **31**

Complex Regional Pain Syndrome Type II (Causalgia)

Andreas Binder and Ralf Baron

Definition

The International Association for the Study of Pain (IASP) *Classification of Chronic Pain* redefined pain syndromes formerly known as *reflex sympathetic dystrophy* and *causalgia*.[1] The term *complex regional pain syndrome* (CRPS) describes "a variety of painful conditions following injury which appears regionally having a distal predominance of abnormal findings, exceeding in both magnitude and duration the expected clinical course of the inciting event often resulting in significant impairment of motor function, and showing variable progression over time."

These chronic pain syndromes comprise different additional clinical features, including spontaneous pain, allodynia, hyperalgesia, edema, autonomic abnormalities, and trophic signs. In contrast to CRPS type I (CRPS I, reflex sympathetic dystrophy), CRPS type II (CRPS II, causalgia) develops after injury to a major peripheral nerve.

Epidemiology

Incidence and Prevalence

A population-based study on CRPS I calculated an incidence of approximately 5.5 per 100,000 person-years at risk and a prevalence of approximately 21 per 100,000. An incidence of 0.8 per 100,000 person-years at risk and a prevalence of approximately 4 per 100,000 were reported for CRPS II.[2] Thus, CRPS II develops less often than does CRPS I. The incidence of CRPS II in peripheral nerve injury varies from 2% to 14% in different series, with a mean of approximately 4%.[3] In contrast, a European population-based study using a different diagnostic approach calculated a higher incidence of 26.2 per 100.000 for CRPS in general.[4] Female patients are predominantly affected,

with a ratio of approximately 2:1 to 4:1. The upper extremity without side preference is affected in approximately 60% of patients.[4]

Clinical Presentation

The symptoms of CRPS II are similar to those of CRPS I, the only exception being that a lesion of peripheral nerve structures and subsequent focal deficits are mandatory for the diagnosis. The symptoms and signs spread beyond the innervation territory of the injured peripheral nerve and often occur remote from the site of injury, but a restriction to the territory is not in conflict with the current definition.

Pathophysiologic Mechanisms

Pathophysiologic Concepts in Complex Regional Pain Syndrome After Stroke and Spinal Cord Injury

CRPS may occasionally develop after lesions of the central nervous system.[5] In patients with stroke, risk factors for recurrent initiating events (e.g., trauma of the affected extremity) that may self-perpetuate a vicious cycle of CRPS include visual deficits, neglect, paresis of the shoulder girdle, and somatosensory deficits. Accordingly, affected extremities after brain injury are associated with a higher risk of CRPS than are unaffected extremities.

CRPS after spinal cord injury is relatively rare, ranging from 5% to 12% in selected cohorts. It develops within a few months, more often unilaterally at the upper extremity in tetraplegic patients. Medullary gunshot wounds seem to predispose to the development of CRPS. As in patients with stroke, the association of paresis with limb trauma may initiate a vicious pathophysiologic cycle. Additionally, CRPS may contribute to contractures in the course of spinal cord injury.

Diagnosis

The diagnosis of CRPS I and CRPS II follows the IASP clinical criteria established in 1994.[6] If two clinical signs are joined by "or," if either sign is present, or if both occur, the condition of the statement is satisfied.

Complex Regional Pain Syndrome Type II (Formerly Causalgia)

1. Type II is a syndrome that develops after nerve injury. Spontaneous pain or allodynia/hyperalgesia occurs and is not necessarily limited to the territory of the injured nerve.
2. Evidence of edema, skin blood flow abnormality, or abnormal sudomotor activity in the region of the pain is present or has been present since the inciting event.
3. This diagnosis is excluded by the existence of conditions that would otherwise account for the degree of pain and dysfunction.

Pain is essential for the diagnosis, and "spontaneous" indicates pain without an external cause. Motor symptoms and findings are not included in this classification, although they are common and can include tremor, dystonia, and weakness.

In 2007, the IASP published revised diagnostic CRPS criteria (the "Budapest criteria") that have been validated (see Table 30.2 in Chapter 30).[7,8] These clinical criteria show a sensitivity of 0.99 and a specificity 0.68.

However, the diagnostic situation became more complicated after publication of a proposed redefinition of neuropathic pain as "pain arising as a direct consequence of a lesion or disease affecting the somatosensory system."[9] Because pain is generalized distally in CRPS II, the criterion of a distinct, neuroanatomically plausible distribution is not fulfilled, thus making it impossible to reach the grade of "definite neuropathic pain" within the additionally proposed grading system. These issues become even more problematic in CRPS I (see Chapter 30).

Differential Diagnosis

Because of the lack of a gold standard for the diagnosis of CRPS, the risk of overdiagnosis must be taken into account. To differentiate CRPS from other neuropathic and pain syndromes, a detailed history and physical examination must be performed according to the specifications just outlined.

Post-Traumatic Neuralgia

Many patients with post-traumatic neuropathy have pain but do not have the full clinical picture of CRPS II. In these cases, in contrast to patients with CRPS II, the pain is located largely within the innervation territory of the injured nerve. Although these patients often describe their pain as burning,

they exhibit a less complex clinical picture than do patients with CRPS II and do not have marked swelling or progressive spread of symptoms. The cardinal symptoms are spontaneous burning pain, hyperalgesia, and mechanical and especially cold allodynia. These sensory symptoms are confined to the territory of the affected peripheral nerve, although allodynia may extend beyond the border of nerve territories for some centimeters. Spontaneous pain and evoked pain are felt superficially and not deep inside the extremity, and the intensity of both types of pain does not depend on the position of the extremity. Patients occasionally obtain relief with sympatholytic procedures, although much less often than do patients with CRPS.

Following the IASP classification, it is possible to use the term *neuralgia* for this type of neuropathic pain (pain within the innervation territory of a lesioned nerve, e.g., post-traumatic neuralgia). However, the 1994 IASP definition of CRPS II includes the statement that symptoms may also be limited to the territory of a single peripheral nerve. Therefore, the term *CRPS II* provides a window to include these localized post-traumatic neuropathies. An inherent weakness of this definition of CRPS II is that different syndromes with different underlying mechanisms are obviously included.

Neuropathies (e.g., diabetic polyneuropathy) may also manifest as spontaneous pain, skin color changes, and motor deficits, but neuropathies are distinguished by their symmetrical distribution and the patient's history. Furthermore, all kinds of inflammations or infections (e.g., rheumatism, phlegmon) may induce intense unilateral skin warming. Unilateral arterial or venous occlusive diseases can cause unilateral pain and vascular abnormalities and must be excluded. Repetitive artificial occlusion of the blood supply to one limb (as in the psychiatric factitious disorders, artifact syndrome) may induce secondary structural changes of the blood vessels with consecutive abnormalities in perfusion and may therefore mimic CRPS symptoms and signs.

Prognosis

The disease duration is variable, and CRPS II may persist over decades. In rare cases, causally directed therapy (e.g., decompression of an entrapment syndrome) may lead to complete recovery.

A 5.5-year follow-up study showed that 62% of patients were still limited in their activities of daily living; pain and motor impairment were the most important factors.[10] In more than 60% of patients with CRPS II, the complaints remained unchanged even after 1 year of intensive therapy.[11] In contrast, a retrospective population-based study reported resolution of symptoms in 74% of the patients with CRPS I.[2] In a 13-month follow-up study in a small cohort, nearly all patients still suffered from functional impairment of the affected extremity, although most of the other clinical features of CRPS had resolved.[12]

References

Full references for this chapter can be found on www.expertconsult.com.

Chapter 32

Phantom Pain Syndromes

Laxmaiah Manchikanti, Vijay Singh, and Mark V. Boswell

Historical Considerations

Phantom sensation or pain is the persistent perception that a body part exists or is painful after it has been removed by amputation or trauma. The first medical description of postamputation phenomena was reported by Ambrose Paré, a French military surgeon, in 1551 (**Fig. 32.1**).[1,2] He noticed that amputees complained of severe pain in the missing limb long after amputation. Civil War surgeon Silas Weir Mitchell[3] popularized the concept of phantom limb pain and coined the term *phantom limb* with publication in 1871 of a long-term study on the fate of Civil War amputees (**Fig. 32.2**). Herman Melville immortalized phantom limb pain in American literature, with graphic descriptions of Captain Ahab's phantom limb in *Moby Dick* (**Fig. 32.3**).

The three most commonly used terms are *phantom sensation, phantom pain*, and *stump pain*. Phantom sensation refers to any sensation of the missing limb or organ except pain. In contrast, phantom pain refers to painful sensations referred to the missing organ or limb. Stump pain refers to pain in the stump.

Phantom sensations may occur in any part of the body but are most often described in the extremities. Phantom sensation of the tongue, nose, breast, bladder, uterus, rectum, penis, and other organs have been described in the literature.[4–11]

The Clinical Syndrome

Epidemiology

Phantom limb sensation is an almost universal occurrence at some time during the first month following surgery. Patients generally describe the limb in terms of definite volume and length and may try to reach out with or stand on the phantom limb.[4] Phantom limb sensation is strongest in amputations above the elbow and weakest in amputations below the knee.[12] It is more frequent in the dominant limb of double amputees.[13] The incidence of phantom limb sensation increases with the amputee's age.[4] Phantom limb sensation in 85% to 98% of the amputees is seen in the first 3 weeks after amputation,[14] whereas in a small proportion of patients (approximately 8%), phantom limb sensation may not occur until 1 to 12 months following amputation.[15] Most phantom sensations generally resolve after 2 to 3 years without treatment, except when phantom pain develops.

The incidence of phantom limb pain has been reported to vary from 0% to 88%.[16–36] Prospective evaluations[31,37] suggest that in the year after amputation, 60% to 70% of amputees experience phantom limb pain, but it diminishes with time.[14,31] Sherman and Sherman,[26] in a survey of 590 war veteran amputees, reported that 85% of these veterans had phantom pain. These investigators also studied 2694 amputees and showed that 51% experienced severe phantom limb pain.[27]

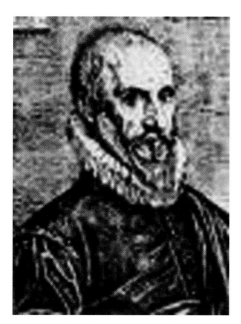

Fig. 32.1 **Ambrose Paré.**

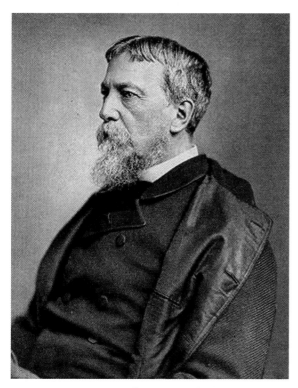

Fig. 32.2 **Silas Weir Mitchell.**

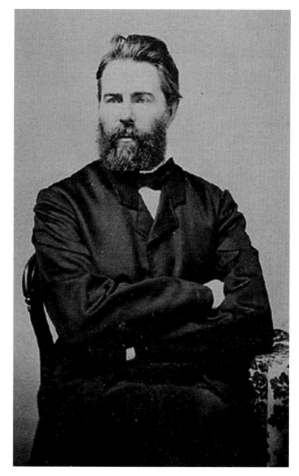

Fig. 32.3 **Herman Melville.**

Phantom limb pain has been reported to occur as early as 1 week and as late as 40 years after amputation.[4,33,34] Although phantom pain may diminish with time and eventually fade away, some prospective studies indicate that even 2 years after amputation, the incidence is almost the same as at onset.[31,37] Investigators have reported that nearly 60% of patients continue to have phantom limb pain[24,31] after 1 year, whereas in the first month following amputation, 85% to 97% of patients experience phantom limb pain.[24,29,30] Although phantom limb pain may begin months to years after an amputation, pain starting after 1 year following amputation occurs in fewer than 10% of patients.[4]

Stump pain is reported with a prevalence of up to 50% of amputees.[16,18,21–23,35,36] Stump pain results in disuse of the limb prosthesis in approximately 50% of patients.[16,18,21–23,35,36] The stump pain usually coincides with the development of phantom limb pain.[37] In one study, investigators showed that 88% of patients with phantom pain also reported stump pain.[23] In another study, stump pain was reported in only 50% of patients.[30]

Phantom limb pain is also associated with multiple pain problems in other areas of the body. Reports have indicated headache or pain in joints in 35% of patients, sore throat in 28% of patients, abdominal pain in 18%, and back pain in 13%.[38]

Disability and Risk Factors

Sherman et al[27] reported that of all amputees, 51% experienced phantom limb pain severe enough to hinder lifestyle on more than 6 days per month, 21% reported daily pain over a 10- to

The incidence of phantom limb pain increases with more proximal amputations. The reports of phantom limb pain after hemipelvectomy ranged from 68% to 88%; and following hip disarticulation, the incidence was 40% to 88%.[28,30] However, wide variations exist with reports of phantom limb pain after lower extremity amputation; reported rates are as high as 72%[21] and as low as 51% after upper limb amputation.[22] Further, a 0% prevalence was reported in below-knee amputations compared with a 19% prevalence in above-knee amputations.[30]

14-hour period, and 27% had pain for more than 15 hours per day. Multiple risk factors identified for phantom pain include phantom sensations, stump pain, pain before the amputation, cause of amputation, prosthesis use, and years elapsed since the amputation.[39] The most important risk factors for phantom pain were "bilateral amputation and lower limb amputation." The risk for phantom pain ranged from 0.33 for a 10-year-old patient with a distal upper limb amputation to 0.99 for an 80-year-old patient with a bilateral lower limb amputation, of which one side was an above-knee amputation. Van der Schans et al[40] showed that amputees with phantom pain had a poorer health-related quality of life than amputees without phantom pain. Sunderland,[41] based on the frequency and severity of pain and the degree to which pain interferes with the patient's lifestyle, proposed a classification to divide patients into four groups:

- Group I patients have mild, intermittent paresthesias that do not interfere with normal activity, work, or sleep.
- Group II patients have paresthesias that are uncomfortable and annoying but do not interfere with activities or sleep.
- Group III patients may have pain that is of sufficient intensity, frequency, or duration to be distressful; however, some patients in group III have pain that is bearable, that intermittently interferes with their lifestyle, and that may respond to conservative treatment.
- Group IV patients complain of nearly constant severe pain that interferes with normal activity and sleep.

The usual course of phantom limb pain is to remain unchanged or to improve.[4,27,31] Up to 56% of patients report improvement or complete resolution.[27]

Ehde and coworkers[21] evaluated not only the characteristics of phantom limb sensation, phantom limb pain, and residual limb pain, but also pain-related disability associated with phantom limb pain, in a retrospective, cross-sectional survey of 255 participants after lower limb amputation. Seventy-two percent of patients with phantom limb pain were classified into two low pain-related disability categories: grade I, low disability/low pain intensity, 47%, or grade II, low disability/ high pain intensity, 28%.

Etiology

Of the three conditions, namely, phantom sensations, phantom pain, and stump pain, phantom sensations are the easiest to explain. It is believed that, throughout life, an individual's body image develops from proprioceptive, tactile, and visual inputs.[42] Once a cortical representation of the body image is established, it is unchanged following limb amputation.[4,7]

The etiology and pathophysiologic mechanisms of phantom pain are not clearly defined. However, both peripheral and central neuronal mechanisms are likely. In addition, psychological mechanisms have also been proposed. Independently, none of the theories fully explain the clinical characteristics of this condition.

Nikolajsen and Jensen[43] described several clinical observations suggesting that mechanisms in the periphery, either in the stump or in the central parts of sectioned primary afferents, may play a role in the phantom limb percept. These observations are as follows:

- Phantom limb sensations can be modulated by various stump manipulations.

- Phantom limb sensations are temporarily abolished after local stump anesthesia.
- Stump revisions and removal of tender neuromas often reduce pain, at least transiently.
- Phantom pain is significantly more frequent in those amputees with long-term stump pain than in those without persistent pain.
- Although obvious stump disease is rare, altered cutaneous sensibility in the stump is a common, if not universal, feature.
- Changes in stump blood flow alter phantom limb perception.

Experimental support for these clinical observations may exist. First, peripherally, spontaneous and abnormal evoked activity following mechanical or neurochemical stimulation is observed in nerve-end neuromas.[44,45] This increased activity is assumed to be the result of a novel expression or up-regulation of sodium channels.[46,47] Thus, the increased sensitivity of neuroma to norepinephrine may, in part, explain the exacerbation of phantom pain by stress and other emotional states associated with increased catecholamine release from sympathetic efferent terminals that are in proximity to afferent sensory nerves and sprouts.[43] Investigators have also shown that cell bodies in the dorsal root ganglion have similar abnormal spontaneous activity and increased sensitivity to mechanical and neurochemical stimulation.[48] Thus, abnormal activity from neuromas and dorsal root ganglion cell bodies may contribute to the phantom limb percept, including pain.

The second mechanism is considered at the spinal cord level. The increased barrage from neuromas and from dorsal root ganglia cells is thought to induce long-term changes in central projecting neurons in the dorsal horn, including spontaneous neuronal activity, induction of immediate early genes, increases in spinal cord metabolic activity, and expansion of receptive fields.[49,50] Nikolajsen and Jensen[43] noted that the pharmacology of spinal sensitization involves an increased activity in N-methyl-D-aspartate (NMDA) receptor–operated systems,[51] and many aspects of the central sensitization can be reduced by NMDA receptor antagonists. This finding was further confirmed in human amputees with one aspect of such central sensitization: the evoked stump or phantom pain produced by repetitive stimulation of the stump by non-noxious pinprick can be reduced by the NMDA receptor antagonist ketamine.[52] Besides the functional changes in the dorsal horn, an anatomic reorganization also has been described.[53] Investigators have shown that peripheral nerve transection results in a substantial degeneration of afferent C-fiber terminals in lamina II, thus reducing the number of synaptic contacts with second-order neurons in lamina II, which normally respond best to noxious stimulation. Consequently, central terminals of Aβ mechanoreceptive afferents, which normally terminate in deeper laminae, sprout into lamina II and may form synaptic contacts with vacant nociceptive second-order neurons. As a result of this organization, evocation of pain is seen with simple touch, by Aβ-fiber input.

The third element is the supraspinal or central mechanism. Based on peripheral and spinal cord mechanisms, it is reasonable to assume that amputation produces a cascade of events in the periphery and in the spinal cord, and these changes eventually sweep more centrally and alter neuronal activity in cortical and subcortical structures. Investigators have shown that thalamic stimulation results in phantom sensation and pain in amputees.[54] This finding suggests that plastic changes in the thalamus are involved in the generation of chronic pain because normally such stimulation does not evoke pain. Other studies in humans have documented a cortical reorganization after amputation using multiple cerebral imaging techniques.[55–70]

Psychological theories have also been put forth to explain the cause of phantom pain. Whereas a biopsychosocial mechanism may be involved in development and persistence of phantom pain, no consistent personality disorders or clinical syndromes have shown to be increased in incidence in patients with phantom limb pain. However, psychological disturbances related to the loss of a limb or feelings of dependence, as well as chronic pain and disability, may lead to a host of psychological problems in these patients.[36,71–76] Patients reporting phantom limb pain have been shown to be more rigid, compulsive, and self-reliant than their cohorts.[14]

The cause of stump pain is often associated with definite pathologic findings that may account for the pain in the stump or the phantom, such as skin disease, circulatory disturbances, infection of the skin or underlying tissue, bone spurs, or neuromas. However, stump pain and phantom pain may occur without obvious stump disorders.

Symptoms and Signs

Phantom sensations are painless. Patients generally describe the sensations in their phantom limb either as normal or as pleasant warmth and tingling.[4] The strongest sensations come from body parts with the highest brain cortical representation, such as fingers and toes.[4,7,77] The phantom limb may undergo "telescoping," in which the patient loses sensations from the midportion of the limb, with subsequent shortening of the phantom.[25] During telescoping, the last body parts to disappear are those with the highest representation in the cortex, such as the thumb, index finger, and big toe. Telescoping occurs only with painless phantoms, and it is most common in the upper extremity. Lengthening of the phantom may occur if pain returns. **Figure 32.4** illustrates telescoping of the phantom limb sensation in the upper extremity.

Phantom pain is primarily localized in distal parts of the missing limb.[14,22,25–27,31,78–82] Phantom pain is usually intermittent.

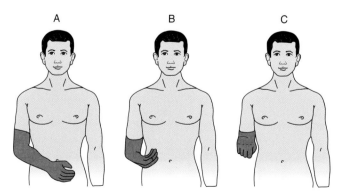

Fig. 32.4 **Illustration of telescoping of the phantom limb.** The highly innervated areas (hands) remain, whereas the midportion of the phantom limb shortens in length.

Only a few patients are in constant pain. Episodes of pain are reported to occur at daily or weekly intervals, with only a few patients reporting monthly, yearly, or rare episodes. The duration of individual attacks may last from seconds to hours, but rarely days or longer.

The pain is usually described as burning, aching, or cramping.[30,83] However, pain may also be described as crushing, twisting, grinding, tingling, drawing, stabbing with needles, knifelike, sticking, burning, squeezing, sharp, shocklike, excruciating, and so on.[27,30,31,35,83] Phantom pain may mimic preamputation pain—not only in location, but also in character.[27,79] The frequency with which preamputation pain persists as phantom pain is highly variable, from 12.5% to 80%.[14,28,31,37,79,84] Several investigators have considered preamputation pain as a risk factor for phantom pain,[24,43,80,85] even though other investigators have not agreed.[22,28,86]

Phantom pain may be modulated by multiple factors, both internal and external. Exacerbations of pain may be produced by trivial, physical, or emotional stimuli. Anxiety, depression, urination, cough, defecation, sexual activity, cold environment, or changes in the weather may worsen phantom limb pain.[25,26,28,30,31,42,83,87] Investigators have also reported that general, spinal, or regional anesthesia in amputees may cause the appearance of phantom pain in otherwise pain-free subjects.[77,88–92]

In contrast to phantom pain, stump pain is often located in the stump itself and is frequently described as pressing, throbbing, burning, or squeezing.[87] Other descriptions have included a stabbing sensation or an electrical current. An additional variant involves complaints of spontaneous movements of the stump ranging from painful, hardly visible myoclonic jerks to severe clonic contractions lasting as long as 2 days.

Physical Examination

Physical examination is not very useful except for the trigger points in the stump to reproduce the phantom limb pain. Physical examination may reveal altered sensitivity in the stump. Neuromas are also found in only 20% of patients. The stump may be cold, and thermography may be a useful diagnostic test if symptoms consistent with reflex sympathetic dystrophy are present. Sherman and coworkers[51] demonstrated an inverse relationship between pain intensity and skin temperature in patients who described burning, throbbing, or tingling in the phantom limb or stump.

Diagnostic Testing

At present, no proven diagnostic test exists for evaluating phantom pain or stump pain except for the physical abnormalities noted on physical examination. However, the patient's response to sympathetic blocks may be assessed by the use of diagnostic sympathetic blocks to assist in therapeutic management.

Differential Diagnosis

The usual course of phantom limb pain is to remain unchanged or to improve gradually. Investigators have shown that up to 56% of patients report improvement or even complete resolution.[27] Thus, if symptoms of phantom limb pain increase in severity or if they start after long periods of time after amputation, a differential diagnosis must be entertained. Multiple causes, which may increase phantom limb pain other than changes in the weather, autonomic stimulation, and so on, to be entertained in the differential diagnosis include radicular pain, angina, postherpetic neuralgia, and metastatic cancer.

■ Radicular pain in the phantom limb may be associated with disk herniation.[93]
■ Increased levels of pain in the phantom limb may be triggered by new-onset herpes zoster or reactivation of herpes zoster by suppressed immunologic mechanisms.[94,95]
■ Angina may manifest as exacerbated phantom limb pain.[96,97]
■ In patients undergoing amputation secondary to malignant disease, if phantom limb pain increases significantly, metastatic disease should be evaluated.

Treatment

Phantom limb pain often requires a multimodal approach to treatment. Treatment options include behavioral techniques, antidepressants, anticonvulsants, opioid and nonopioid analgesics, neural blockade, spinal cord stimulation (SCS), and motor cortex stimulation (MCS). However, no data are available from large randomized controlled trials to guide treatment options. As a general rule, initial treatment should be low risk, low cost, and noninvasive, with more expensive and invasive treatments reserved for patients in whom conservative care fails. However, treatment of phantom limb pain or stump pain continues to be difficult and has generally not been very successful.

Halbert et al[98] conducted a systematic review to evaluate evidence for the optimal management of acute and chronic phantom pain. These investigators concluded that a gap exists between research and practice in the area of phantom limb pain. Nevertheless, since 2000, clinical trials have examined treatments for phantom limb pain. Surveys suggest that although physicians believe that treatments are effective,[99] fewer than 10% of patients with phantom limb pain receive lasting relief from prescribed medical treatments.[27] Even then, clinicians have been restricted by the lack of clinical trials that would aid in treatment decisions and by the absence of evidence-based treatment guidelines. In a literature review in 1980, 43 methods for treating phantom limb pain were identified; however, it was concluded that few of these methods produced relief, and that placebo responses were common.[100] Multiple investigators also have recommended treatment for phantom limb pain in line with the management of neuropathic pain states.[101–103] The literature review suggests, however, that trials of treatments for neuropathic pain rarely include patients with phantom limb pain.

Early trials concentrated on the reduction of established postoperative phantom limb pain, but newer approaches have used analgesic agents administered before amputation.[104] Treatment approaches continue to be based on the assumption that long-term phantom limb pain is the result of functional or structural changes in the central nervous system in response to noxious somatosensory input.[105] Thus, therapies are directed at early reduction of pain.

Halbert et al[98] summarized that their review was limited by the poor quality of the included trials. Although these investigators identified 186 articles, they were able to use only 12 trials. Of the 12 trials, only 3 randomized, controlled studies with parallel groups and 3 randomized cross-over trials were identified. These investigators also mentioned the following challenges associated with examining phantom limb pain: extremely low numbers of amputees, a high mortality rate among the amputees, and interventions designed to examine operative and perioperative treatments that were ethically unacceptable.

Prevention

Increasing knowledge of the mechanisms involved in the development and perpetuation of neuropathic pain theoretically should allow a rational approach to its prevention. However, initially hopeful attempts such as the use of presurgical and postsurgical epidural blockade have been questioned, and the utility of this approach is controversial.[106] Advances in neuroimaging techniques are unveiling some keys to the problem. The current emphasis is on the adaptive processes taking place in the central nervous system following deafferentation. In this sense, it seems that the ability to prevent postamputation pain will depend on a capability to modulate the plasticity of the central nervous system. Feria[106] stated that the problem needs a broad-based approach, including control of perioperative pain and inflammation, adequate information and follow-up of the patients, correct surgical technique and long-term rehabilitation, and the use of pharmacologic and behavioral approaches reflecting current knowledge.

Multiple investigators have attempted psychological preparation, drug therapy, epidural anesthesia, and regional nerve blocks, among other approaches, to reduce the occurrence of phantom limb pain and to delay or stop the process of progression from acute to chronic pain. At least some postamputation pain may be prevented by appropriate psychological preparation of patients.

Epidural Anesthesia

Gehling and Tryba[107] showed that preoperative, intraoperative, and postoperative epidural anesthesia was associated with a significant reduction of phantom limb pain 12 months after amputation. These investigators concluded, however, that a reduction of phantom limb pain by postoperative epidural anesthesia alone could not be confirmed on the basis of the analyzed data. They also concluded that perioperative epidural anesthesia has been shown to be effective for the prophylaxis of phantom limb pain. This technique does not completely abolish phantom limb pain, but rather increases the number of patients with a milder form of phantom pain.

Investigators in 4 trials[108–111] assessed preoperative epidural pain relief and were unable to provide definitive evidence to support its routine use. The results of 2 studies involving a small number of patients suggested that epidural analgesia may help, but findings were inconsistent. The first study showed relief at 7 days, 6 months, and 1 year postoperatively.[109] The second study,[108] however, showed less phantom limb pain in the intervention group at 1 week, 6 months, and 1 year, and the difference reached significance only at 6 months. The largest of the studies[110] showed no difference in phantom pain at 7 days, 3 months, 6 months, and 12 months. In a randomized prospective study by Lambert et al,[111] 30 patients scheduled for lower limb amputation were randomly assigned epidural bupivacaine or an intraoperatively placed perineural catheter for intraoperative and postoperative administration of bupivacaine. All patients had general anesthesia. The results showed no significant difference between perioperative epidural block and perineural infusion of local anesthetic. However, phantom pain after 3 days in the epidural group was 29%, at 6 months it was 63%, and at 12 months it was 38%. Thus, it is not known whether epidural anesthesia reduces the prevalence of phantom limb pain.

Regional Anesthesia

Multiple trials assessed perineural,[111–113] and intraneural[114] bupivacaine blocks, either at the time of surgery or immediately postoperatively. Despite some early benefits, no difference in pain was reported between the intervention and control groups in the postoperative period.[112,113] Perineural block was similar to infusion of local anesthetic through epidural catheter.[111] Evaluation of continuous brachial plexus analgesia showed prevention of the establishment of phantom limb pain, which did not reappear during follow-up of 1 year.[115] Nerve sheath catheter analgesia also showed reduced prevalence.[116]

Other Interventions

Other treatments assessed for prevention of phantom limb pain included administration of calcitonin, ketamine, intravenous lidocaine, and transcutaneous electrical nerve stimulation (TENS).[117–121] A study of intravenous calcitonin,[121] in which 8 patients were evaluated, showed that only 2 patients developed phantom limb pain after 10 days of intravenous treatment with salmon calcitonin; the prevalence of phantom limb pain remained at 25% in systematic follow-up examinations after 3, 6, and 12 months. However, in another study,[117] intravenous calcitonin reduced phantom limb pain in the early postoperative period, but phantom limb pain on longer-term follow-up was not adequately controlled. The effectiveness of ketamine was studied in a prospective, observational study with historical controls with 14 patients in each group.[120] The results showed that phantom limb pain remained high at 72%, even though only 9% of the patients after ketamine, compared with 71% of the patients in the control group, complained of severe phantom limb pain. TENS was assessed in the 2-week postoperative period, and the treated group reported less pain at 4 weeks.[118] However, by 12 months, no difference was noted between the groups.

Management of Established Phantom Pain Syndrome

Drug Therapy

Medical therapy is the most common modality of treatment for phantom pain syndromes. The most frequently used classes of medications are antidepressants and anticonvulsants.

Antidepressants

Many randomized, controlled clinical trials have shown a beneficial effect of tricyclic antidepressants and sodium channel blockers in different neuropathic pain conditions. Even though no controlled trials in phantom pain have been performed, the drugs are generally considered to be effective, at least in some patients.[122–125] Tricyclic antidepressants have been thoroughly studied in other denervation syndromes, such as postherpetic neuralgia and diabetic neuropathy.[125]

Wilder-Smith et al[123] studied 94 treatment-naïve post-traumatic limb amputees with phantom pain who were randomly assigned to receive individually titrated doses of tramadol, placebo double-blind comparison, or amitriptyline open comparison for 1 month. These investigators concluded that in the treatment-naïve patients, both amitriptyline and tramadol provided excellent and stable phantom limb and stump pain control with no major adverse events. In contrast, another study conducted by Robinson et al[124] evaluated 39 persons with amputation-related pain lasting more than 6 months in a 6-week randomized controlled trial of amitriptyline (titrated up to 125 mg per day) or an active placebo. These investigators concluded that no differences existed between the treatment group and outcome variables. This finding did not support the use of amitriptyline in the treatment of postamputation pain.[124]

Canovas et al[122] assessed the analgesic effectiveness and tolerance of amitriptyline versus nefazodone for the management of neuropathic pain. Of the 120 patients included in this study, fewer than 10 patients suffered with phantom limb pain. The quality of pain was burning and cutting in 62.3% of the cases, lancinating in 40%, and sharp in 25%. The results demonstrated that after 3 months of therapy, the amitriptyline-treated group showed a pain severity of 2 ± 0.9, and in the nefazodone-treated group, pain severity was 3 ± 1.1. Pain relief was greater than 75% (excellent) in 42 patients treated with amitriptyline and in 36 patients treated with nefazodone; it was between 50% and 75% (good) in 18 patients treated with amitriptyline and in 12 patients treated with nefazodone; and pain relief was less than 50% (poor) in 3 patients treated with amitriptyline and 3 patients treated with nefazodone. These investigators concluded that both drugs were effective for the management of neuropathic pain. The group of patients treated with nefazodone showed a lower incidence of side effects, except for nausea and vomiting. The amitriptyline-treated group showed a significant incidence of orthostatic hypotension, dry mouth, nausea, and vomiting.

Anticonvulsants

Among the anticonvulsants, carbamazepine is the most commonly used.[126,127] Elliott et al[126] and Patterson[127] reported cases of lancinating phantom limb pains that improved with oral carbamazepine. Logan[128] reported incomplete relief with carbamazepine but complete relief with chlorpromazine in long-standing phantom limb pain. No evidence indicates that carbamazepine is effective for pains that are not of the intense, brief, lancinating type.

Currently, gabapentin is the most common anticonvulsant used for phantom limb pain. Other than sedation, side effects are rare, and patients become tolerant to sedation with time. Because gabapentin has no known long-term toxicity, monitoring of blood levels, as with other anticonvulsants, is not necessary. The effectiveness of gabapentin in postamputation phantom limb pain was studied in a randomized, double-blind, placebo-controlled, cross-over study by Bone and coworkers.[129] These investigators evaluated analgesic efficacy of gabapentin in phantom limb pain in patients attending a multidisciplinary pain clinic. Each treatment lasted 6 weeks, separated by a 1-week washout. The daily dose of gabapentin was titrated in increments of 300 to 2400 mg of the maximum tolerated dose. Nineteen eligible patients were randomized, of whom 14 completed both arms of the study. Both placebo and gabapentin treatments resulted in reduced Visual Analog Scale (VAS) scores compared with baseline. However, pain intensity difference was significantly greater than placebo for gabapentin therapy at the end of the treatment. These investigators concluded that after 6 weeks, gabapentin monotherapy was better than placebo in relieving postamputation phantom limb pain. No significant were reported differences in mood, sleep interference, or activities of daily living.

Serpell et al[130] evaluated the use of gabapentin in neuropathic pain in a randomized, double-blind, placebo-controlled trial of 305 patients in a wide range of neuropathic pain syndromes, including phantom limb pain in 2% of patients. These investigators concluded that at an average dose of 900 to 2400 mg per day, gabapentin was well tolerated and was associated with significant pain control with few secondary effects (dizziness and somnolence), most of which were transient and occurred during the titration phase. Nikolajsen et al[131] also examined whether postoperative treatment with gabapentin could reduce postamputation residual phantom pain and concluded that gabapentin administered in the first 30 postoperative days after amputation did not reduce the incidence or intensity of postamputation pain.

Local Anesthetics

Analgesic effects of intravenous lidocaine and morphine on postamputation pain were evaluated in a randomized double-blind, active placebo-controlled, cross-over trial by Wu and coworkers.[119] An intravenous bolus followed by an intravenous infusion of morphine, lidocaine, and the active placebo (diphenhydramine) were performed on 3 consecutive days. The results showed that 31 of 32 subjects enrolled completed the study. Eleven subjects had both stump and phantom pains, and 11 and 9 subjects had stump and phantom pain alone, respectively. These investigators concluded that stump pain was diminished by both morphine and lidocaine, whereas phantom pain was diminished only by morphine. This finding suggested that the mechanisms and pharmacologic sensitivity of stump pain and phantom pain are different. Mexiletine (the oral congener of lidocaine) also has been reported to be effective.[132]

N-Methyl-D-Aspartate Receptor Antagonists

The effects of an NMDA receptor antagonist have been examined in different studies.[51,133–135] In a double-blind, placebo-controlled study, intravenous ketamine reduced pain, hyperalgesia, and "wind-up"–like pain in 11 amputees with stump and phantom pain.[52] In another controlled trial by the same investigators,[133] 19 patients received memantine, an NMDA receptor antagonist available for oral use, in a blinded, placebo-controlled, cross-over fashion. Memantine failed to have any effect on spontaneous pain, allodynia, or hyperalgesia. In another randomized, double-blinded, placebo-controlled trial,[135] memantine failed to demonstrate a significant clinical benefit of the NMDA receptor antagonist in chronic phantom limb pain.

Experimental and clinical literature supports the effectiveness of ketamine in blocking central sensitization by its effects on NMDA receptor.[136–138] Studies have reported low-dose ketamine infusion to be effective in the treatment of complex regional pain syndrome (CRPS).[136,138] No studies are available in managing phantom limb pain.

In a double-blind cross-over trial,[139] dextromethorphan was studied for attenuation of phantom pain in 3 patients with cancer-related amputations. Results showed that oral dextromethorphan effectively reduced postamputation phantom limb pain, and it bestowed improvement in feeling and minimized sedation in comparison with the pretreatment or placebo conditions, with no side effects. Capsaicin also was tried in phantom limb pain.[140,141] In this study of 24 patients, which was conducted in double-blind fashion, the investigators concluded that capsaicin may be used as an alternative treatment for phantom limb pain.

Beta-Adrenergic Blockers

Beta-adrenergic blockers have also been suggested for treatment of phantom limb pain, based on three cases.[142] However, in a double-blind cross-over trial of propranolol up to 240 mg daily, the investigators were unable to show significant improvement in post-traumatic neuralgias.[143]

Benzodiazepines

Some investigators have reported a beneficial effect of benzodiazepines.[144] The general impression is that benzodiazepines do not produce substantial pain relief, however.

Opioids

Opioid analgesics with or without other drugs are considered the mainstay of treatment in modern medicine. Generally, it is stated in textbooks that opioid analgesics are not effective in producing long-term pain relief in patients with phantom limb pain.[27] However, evidence suggests that opioids can be used safely for years with a limited risk of drug dependence.[4,27,43,66,102,145–147] Further, patients undergoing amputation related to systemic medical diseases have only a 42% 5-year survival rate; thus, the risk of opioid addiction may be weighed against quality-of-life issues.[36] In a review of five patients who were taking methadone, 10 to 20 mg daily, a 50% to 90% reduction in pain at 12 to 26 months' follow-up was reported.[147]

Wilder-Smith et al[123] studied the treatment of 94 treatment-naïve post-traumatic limb amputees with phantom pain who were randomly assigned to receive individually titrated doses of tramadol (mean dose, 448 mg) or placebo (double-blind comparison for 1 month). These investigators found that tramadol provided excellent and stable phantom limb and residual limb pain control, with no major adverse events.

In a placebo-controlled trial, Huse et al[66] studied the efficacy of oral long-acting morphine sulfate in a double-blind cross-over design in 12 patients after unilateral leg or arm amputation. The dose of morphine sulfate was titrated up to at least 70 mg per day, and at its highest, 300 mg per day. Pain, reorganization of somatosensory cortex, and pain thresholds were assessed before and after treatment. Significant pain reduction was found with morphine sulfate therapy but not with placebo. A clinically relevant response to morphine sulfate (pain reduction of more than 50%) was evident in 42%, and partial response (pain reduction of 25% to 50%) was noted in 8% of the patients. In addition, neuromagnetic imaging using magnetographic and cephalographic recordings of 3 patients showed initial evidence of reduced cortical reorganization with morphine sulfate treatment concurrent with the reduction of pain intensity. These investigators concluded that opioids show efficacy in the treatment of phantom pain and may also potentially influence cortical reorganization.

Wu et al,[146] in a randomized double-blind trial, compared the analgesic effects of intravenous morphine and lidocaine on postamputation stump and phantom pains. A bolus of morphine, lidocaine, and an active placebo (diphenhydramine) were used over a span of 3 consecutive days. The results showed that 31 of 32 subjects enrolled completed the study. Eleven subjects had both stump and phantom pains, and 11 and 9 subjects had stump and phantom pain alone, respectively. Compared with placebo, morphine reduced both residual limb and phantom pain significantly. In contrast, lidocaine decreased residual limb pain but not phantom pain. Consequently, the investigators concluded that the mechanisms of residual limb pain and phantom pain are different.

Neural Blockade

Nerve blocks are commonly used in the treatment of phantom limb pain, and although physicians performing these blocks report a high success rate, it has not been substantiated.[99] These blocks range from trigger point injections to neurolytic sympathetic blocks with stump injections, sympathetic blocks, peripheral nerve blocks, and epidural or subarachnoid blocks. However, investigators have shown that only 14% of patients with phantom limb pain report even a significant temporary change, whereas less than 5% report a large permanent change or cure.[27] The use of neural blockade in the treatment of phantom limb pain is largely based on anecdotal reports in the literature.[148–150]

Blankenbaker[148] reported that sympathetic blocks are successful if amputees are treated soon after the onset of phantom limb pain. Halbert et al,[98] in a systematic review to evaluate evidence of the optimal management of acute and chronic phantom pain, were unable to find any trials to meet the criteria for inclusion.

Lesions of the dorsal root entry zone have been reported to provide long-term pain relief in patients with phantom limb pain following avulsion of nerve roots or amputation.[83,151,152] Investigators have reported that 36% of patients had pain relief on follow-up at 6 months to 4 years following dorsal root entry zone lesions.[83,152] However, they reported very poor relief in patients with stump pain alone.

Botulinum toxin A injections in phantom limb pain have also been used for residual limb pain control. It is conceivable that muscle tension, perhaps resulting from cortical reorganization, may contribute to phantom pain as a trigger of spinal reflexes, and botulinum toxin A, by muscle relaxation in the stump or through inhibition of the release of various neurotransmitters, may lead to analgesia.[153] In a small pilot trial, researchers injected 100 IU of botulinum toxin A in four muscle trigger points of an amputation stump and reported that the injection reduced phantom pain approximately 60% to 80%.[154] Further, Kern et al,[155] in a study using 2500 IU of botulinum toxin type B to the arm of amputation stumps,

5000 IU for one amputation of a lower leg, and 2500 IU to the other leg amputation of a patient with a low baseline body weight, reported that all patients experienced a reduction in stump pain that lasted for many weeks.

Other reports included a reduction in the frequency of pain at attacks, cessation of "balloon feelings," improvement in stump allodynia, and decreased occurrence of involuntary stump movements.[155] In addition, quality of sleep at night significantly improved at least in one patient. Kern et al[156] suggested that by diminishing muscle tone, pain, and hyperhidrosis, botulinum toxin may facilitate prosthetic use. Dahl and Cohen[157] treated six soldiers with residual limb and phantom pain with a series of perineural etanercept injections. These investigators reported that five of the six patients were significantly improved with respect to residual limb pain at rest and with activity, functional capacity, and psychological well-being 3 months after injections.

Neuromodulation

TENS has been used with some success in the treatment of phantom pain. However, the results are inconclusive and not encouraging. SCS, deep brain stimulation (DBS) of the thalamic nucleus ventralis chordalis, and MCS are all used in managing phantom limb pain, with variable success.

Some investigators have reported excellent relief with TENS. One investigator reported success in five of six patients with phantom pain following TENS treatment.[158] Another reported a 66% reduction in pain lasting less than 10 hours.[159] Yet other investigators reported good to excellent results in only 25% of patients treated with TENS.[160] Stimulation of the contralateral extremity with TENS also has been shown to have favorable response in some patients.[161,162]

Evaluations of SCS have shown encouraging results in neuropathic pain, including reflex sympathetic dystrophy.[163,164] Thus, spinal cord posterior column stimulation is the most common neurosurgical technique used for the treatment of phantom limb pain. The selection process is very crucial. Response to TENS or percutaneous electrical stimulation may predict a response to dorsal column stimulation.[165] Even with appropriate patient selection, investigators have reported that only 65% of patients receive a greater than 25% reduction in pain immediately after surgical implantation.[166] Further, the success rate of dorsal column stimulation steadily declines over time, and a greater than 50% long-term pain reduction is present in only one third of patients who originally showed improvement.[167,168]

SCS may not cause any improvement in patients with severe pain and phantom limb sensations. In one case report, investigators showed that good to excellent results were observed in five patients, as judged by decreased pain and increased functional status with decrease in medication.[169] However, in another report, dorsal column stimulation provided minimal relief in patients with phantom limb pain.[170] Yet another report showed that dorsal column stimulation showed improvement in only 25% of patients.[171] Thus, one should weigh the risk-to-benefit ratio with caution and diligence. However, Siegfried et al[172] reported that 51% of patients with SCS had a 50% or more decrease in pain, but without long-term follow-up.

Intracranial neurostimulation caused initial pain relief in 80% of patients with sensory thalamic stimulation,[173] and 86% of patients had significant relief with DBS.[174] Thalamic stimulation, in contrast to SCS, may block spontaneous neuronal activity, which has been proposed to mediate phantom sensation in some models.[54] Thus, some investigators believe that it may be more effective than SCS. In addition, Bittar et al[175] concluded that DBS has been used successfully for the treatment of phantom limb pain, with resultant decreased pain, decreased opiate intake, and improved quality of life. Bittar et al[176] also published a meta-analysis supporting this pain improvement, especially in patients with burning pain. Sol et al[177] used long-term MCS in three patients with intractable pain after upper limb amputation. Functional magnetic resonance imaging (MRI) correlated with anatomic MRI permitted frameless image guidance for electrode placement. Pain control was obtained for all patients initially, and relief was stable for two of the three patients at 2-year follow-up. However, it has not thus far been proven. Percutaneous stimulation of the periosteum has been used, even though it has not been well studied.[178]

Neurosurgical Techniques

Some investigators have reported multiple neurosurgical techniques apart from electrical stimulation, including intrathecal implantable devices, stereotactic thermocoagulation lesions, and cordotomy. Some of these treatments may have more serious complications than benefits.[26,179] Sporadic success has been reported with many physical therapy modalities, including ultrasound or vibration, heat or cold, massage therapy, and stump percussion.[99] Investigators noted that neither surgeons nor patients reported good success rates with currently recommended surgical procedures.[27,99]

Stump Revision

Patients with continued phantom limb pain as well as issues related to the stump with vascular insufficiency, infection, or extensive neuromas may undergo stump revision. This approach may provide benefit in 50% of patients.[30]

Physical Therapy

Physical therapy has been shown to be useful, especially the educational aspect with attention to stump and preparation for prosthesis. The reason is that phantom limb pain is most commonly seen in patients who are unable to use a prosthesis within the first 6 months following amputation.

Acupuncture

Electroacupuncture has been shown to provide relief from phantom limb pain of the arm.[180] Short-term relief has been reported with the first few acupuncture treatments; no long-term improvement in patients with a history of nerve damage, including phantom limb pain, has been reported.[181]

Electroconvulsive Therapy

A case report of electroconvulsive therapy (ECT) with study of regional cerebral blood flow[182] suggested that total resolution of pain in this particular patient and the regional cerebral blood flow of the anterior cingulate cortex and insula were related to the analgesic effectiveness of the ECT. In another case report,[183] the investigators reported that two patients with severe phantom limb pain refractory to multiple therapies, without concurrent psychiatric disorder, enjoyed substantial pain relief of phantom pain on long-term follow-up at 3.5 years.

Psychological Therapies

Multiple psychological modalities have been attempted in managing phantom limb pain.[68,184–190] Psychotherapy was reported to yield good results.[68] Relaxation training with or without biofeedback or hypnosis has been studied.[184–190] Investigators reported that in 12 of 14 patients with chronic phantom limb pain, significant improvement was noted with muscular relaxation training to disrupt the pain-anxiety-tension cycle.[184] In this study, patients required an average of 6 treatments to produce therapeutic effect. This approach was also associated with decreased anxiety levels and increased pain relief. In a case report, a combination of electromyography and thermal biofeedback was shown to be effective in a patient with extreme phantom limb pain at 12-month follow-up.

Hypnotic suggestion of stocking-glove anesthesia may lead to a reduction in phantom limb pain.[186,187] Investigators showed that 45% of patients were successfully hypnotized, and 35% had successful improvement in phantom limb pain.[187] Relapses occurred soon after the discontinuation of the treatment in 34% of the patients. In a case report describing 2 patients who used hypnotic imagery as a treatment for phantom limb pain,[188] the investigators concluded that hypnotic procedures appear to be a useful adjunct to established strategies for treating phantom limb pain.

Side Effects and Complications

Most complications result from problems related to the stump, prosthesis, and management techniques. An improper prosthesis may cause a multitude of problems, including psychological problems, as well as local irritation and neuroma formation. Physical therapy may increase or exacerbate pain levels. Acupuncture and neural blockade therapy may cause complications related to needle insertion, drugs, and physiologic and pharmacologic effects of various drugs. Neuroablation techniques may cause serious complications ranging from minor persistent neurologic deficits to hemiplegia and incontinence. Neuroablation techniques may also increase pain by loss of inhibitory control. Neurosurgical techniques may be associated with significant complications.

Conclusion

Phantom pain syndromes are a common consequence of the removal of a limb or organ. Approximately two thirds of patients complain of phantom pain following limb removal. However, in fewer than 10% of patients, this pain manifests as a severe, incapacitating condition. The understanding of phantom limb pain has improved substantially since the 1990s as a result of experimental studies that showed a series of morphologic, physiologic, and biologic changes resulting in hyperexcitability in the nervous system. Prevention of phantom pain by various modalities has shown to be ineffective. Similarly, most treatment modalities of chronic phantom pain syndrome are in their infancy and are not well studied. At present, no evidence-based approach to managing phantom pain syndromes is available.

References

Full references for this chapter can be found on www.expertconsult.com.

Part C

Pain of Malignant Origin

Chapter 33

Identification and Treatment of Cancer Pain Syndromes

Steven D. Waldman

Pain is extremely prevalent in cancer patients. It is a major impediment to an adequate quality of life and may undermine efforts to assess and treat the underlying disease.[1] Pain severe enough to require treatment with opioids occurs in about one third of patients undergoing active treatment and in more than two thirds of those with advanced disease.[2] Although extensive clinical experience indicates that most cancer patients can attain acceptable pain relief, compelling evidence indicates that treatment often is inadequate.[2,3] In a small portion of patients, this inadequacy results from the refractoriness of pain or the patient's reluctance to comply with effective therapy; far more often, however, uncontrolled cancer pain reflects a failure of clinical management. Physicians and nurses often seem unaware of the problem of cancer pain and frequently compromise treatment with inappropriate concerns about the risks of therapy (particularly addiction) and ignorance about the assessment and treatment of pain.[2,4]

A comprehensive approach to managing cancer pain can have a gratifying outcome and should be reviewed as a fundamental element in the treatment of the cancer patient. Simple pharmacologic approaches alone can provide relief in more than 70% of cancer patients with pain, and other treatment modalities, which include nerve blocks and neurodestructive procedures, can help many others.[3] This review describes the basic principles of pain evaluations and treatment in cancer patients and discusses advances that may further improve the results of therapy.

Pain

Pain assessment in the cancer patient requires understanding of the relationships among pain, nociceptive, and suffering.[5] *Nociception* refers to the activity in the afferent nervous system induced by potentially tissue-damaging stimuli. A comprehensive assessment will identify a nociceptive lesion in most patients with cancer pain. *Pain* is the perception of nociception. It is strongly influenced by affective and cognitive processes unique to the individual. These processes may result in an intensity of pain that is either greater or less than that anticipated by the degree of tissue damage. *Suffering* is a construct that refers to a more global response, which is related to unrelieved symptoms (including pain) and many perceived losses, including those related to evolving physical disability, social isolation, financial concerns, loss of role in the family, and fear of death. It is important for the clinician to recognize that suffering may occur in the absence of active nociception.

Clinical interventions targeted solely at the complaint of pain, particularly at the nociceptive component, are unlikely to offer measurable benefit to patients whose complaints are an expression of a more global degree of suffering. Indeed, such treatment plans often are perceived by patient and family as lacking in compassion.

Establishing a Pain Diagnosis

The goals of pain assessment in the cancer patient are to identify the underlying nociceptive lesion, clarify the various non-nociceptive contributions to the pain, and determine the degree and causes of suffering. From this information a "pain diagnosis" can be elaborated; practically, this is a problem list that can be used to target specific problems for treatment and organize a multimodal therapeutic approach.

The first step in establishing the diagnosis is to characterize the pain complaint fully. Specific inquiries should evaluate onset, duration, severity, quality, location, radiation, temporal characteristics, provocative and palliative factors, and course. A medical history should access both previous and current use of analgesic and other drugs. The physicians should elicit any history of chronic nonmalignant pain, long-term opioid use, or substance abuse. The extent of disease at the time of evaluation and the patient's general medical condition also should be assessed. An integral part of this initial evaluation is the assessment of the affective, behavioral, and social disturbances related to the pain. Patients with cancer pain commonly experience anxiety and vegetative signs, such as sleep disturbances, lassitude, and anorexia.

After taking an adequate history, the physician should perform a general medical and neurologic examination. The physical examination, like the history, should attempt to clarify the specific pain syndrome, determine the extent of the disease, clarify the nature of the specific nociceptive lesions underlying the pain, and assess the degree of physical impairment (**Table 33.1**).[6]

After obtaining a working clinical diagnosis from the history and physical examination, the physician should consider appropriate laboratory, electrodiagnostic, or radiographic procedures; these evaluations further clarify the nature of the nociceptive lesion presumed to underlie the pain. The primary clinician must carefully review all test results, including radiographs, to obtain clinicopathologic correlation for the pain. It is important that the clinician avoid overreliance on past test results when the patient's clinical status has changed, if incorrect diagnosis is to be avoided. When in doubt, this is one clinical setting in which repeating tests will often yield important clinical information. Effective analgesic treatment should be provided to the patient throughout the evaluation, particularly during procedures; the psychological impact of the evaluation will be far less adverse and the quality of tests enhanced if the patient's cooperation is not compromised by pain.

The pain diagnosis can be clarified in most patients after this comprehensive assessment is completed. The problem list may include the following: the pain itself; the physical and psychological disturbances contributing to the pain; associated symptoms; physical impairments; and the psychological, social, or familial problems that independently augment the patient's suffering. These problems can be prioritized according to their impact on the patient's quality of life, and therapeutic interventions can be staged appropriately.

Therapeutic Approach to Cancer Pain Management

Antineoplastic therapies should be considered a first step in the analgesic management of patients whose pain is a direct effect of the neoplasm. Radiation therapy provides adequate analgesia in more than one half of patients treated, and pain is a common primary indication for this modality.[7] Although toxicity and unpredictable pain relief limit the utility of chemotherapy as

an analgesic intervention, some patients obtain symptomatic relief by the administration of chemotherapeutic drugs.[8] The variable analgesic response and risks associated with surgical extirpation of a neoplasm limit surgery as a primary analgesic therapy. However, tumor resection performed for other indications, such as vertebral body resection for epidural spinal

Table 33.1 Cancer Pain Syndromes

PAIN SYNDROMES ASSOCIATED WITH DIRECT TUMOR INVOLVEMENT

Bone

Base of skull
  Orbital
  Parasellar
  Sphenoidal sinus
  Middle cranial fossa
  Clivus
  Jugular foramen
  Occipital condyle

Vertebral body
  Atlantoaxial
  C7-T1
  L1
  Sacral
  Generalized bone pain

Nerves

Peripheral nerve syndromes
  Paraspinal tumor
  Chest wall tumor
  Retroperitoneal tumor

Leptomeningeal metastases

Painful polyneuropathy

Brachial, lumbar, and sacral plexopathies

Epidural spinal cord compression

Viscera

Blood Vessels

Mucous Membranes

PAIN ASSOCIATED WITH CANCER THERAPY

Postoperative

Thoracotomy

Mastectomy

Radical surgery of the neck

Amputation

Postchemotherapy

Painful polyneuropathy

Aseptic necrosis of bone

Pseudorheumatism caused by steroids

Postradiation

Fibrosis of brachial or lumbosacral plexus

Myelopathy

Radiation-induced peripheral nerve tumors

Mucositis

PAIN INDIRECTLY RELATED OR UNRELATED TO CANCER

Myofascial Pain

Postherpetic Neuralgia

Chronic Headache Syndromes

cord compression, may provide analgesia.[9] Although all patients with cancer pain should be considered for antineoplastic therapy, most pain management depends on the expert application of one or more primary analgesic modalities. Pharmacotherapy is the most important of these.

Pharmacologic Approaches

Three categories of analgesic medications—nonsteroidal anti-inflammatory drugs (NSAIDs), opioid analgesics, and the so-called adjuvant analgesics—are used in the pharmacotherapy of cancer pain. The Cancer Pain Relief Program of the World Health Organization developed guidelines for the selection of drugs from these categories.[10] The approach, known as the analgesic ladder, can be summarized as follows: For mild pain, an NSAID is administered, and an adjuvant is added if a specific indication for one exists. If the regimen fails to control pain or if the patient presents with moderate to serve pain, a so-called weak oral opioid is administered in combination with an NSAID; again, adjuvants are added if indicated. If maximal doses of this opioid do not control the pain or if the patient's pain is severe, a so-called strong opioid is administered, with or without an NSAID or adjuvant drugs. Considerable expertise is required to select and administer specific drugs appropriately within this general framework. Guidelines are described subsequently.

Nonsteroidal Anti-Inflammatory Drugs and the Cyclooxygenase-2 Inhibitors

All NSAIDs including the cyclooxygenase-2 (COX-2) inhibitors inhibit cyclooxygenase and thereby reduce tissue levels of prostaglidins.[11] This anti-inflammatory effect probably contributes to the analgesic efficacy of NSAIDs and is the basis for the traditional view that these drugs are peripherally acting, although a central mechanism may also underlie the analgesic effects of this class. Even though the COX-2 inhibitors have a more favorable gastrointestinal side effect profile relative to the nonselective NSAIDs, concerns about their causative role in cardiac side effects makes the use of these drugs in cancer pain management less clear.[12] The analgesia provided by NSAIDs is characterized by a ceiling dose, beyond which additional dosage increments produce no further analgesic effect. Although published dosing guidelines exist for each NSAID, individual differences in both the ceiling dose and dose-related toxicity vary widely. Consequently, the standard recommended dose may be inappropriate for any given patient. This consideration is especially salient in cancer patients, who may have altered NSAID pharmacokinetics or a predisposition to adverse effects on the basis of multisystem disease or the coadministration of other drugs. This observation suggests the value of dose titration in this population. The analgesia provided by NSAIDs also is characterized by a lack of demonstrable tolerance or physical dependence.

Drug Selection and Administration

The NSAIDs (**Table 33.2**) are useful alone for mild to moderate pain and, in combination with opioids, provide additive analgesia to patients with more severe pain. Anecdotally, patients with bone pain or pain associated with grossly inflammatory lesions appear most likely to benefit from NSAIDs.

NSAIDs must be used cautiously in older patients and should be considered relatively contraindicated in cancer patients with renal insufficiency, congestive heart failure, hypertension, or a remote history of peptic ulcer disease. In patients with mild bleeding or ulcer diatheses, including some patients with thrombocytopenia or coagulopathy, a history of peptic ulcer disease, or concurrent use of acrogenic medications such as steroids, the preferred drugs are those with the least potential to damage the gastric mucosa and to impair platelet aggregation. These drugs are acetaminophen and two salicylates, choline magnesium trisalicylate and salsalate.[13] Acetaminophen traditionally has been considered the safest drug for patients with significantly impaired renal function; however, evidence of renal toxicity from long-term acetaminophen use suggests caution in the use of this drug.[14] Acetaminophen should also be used cautiously in patients with significant hepatic disease. Of the various subclasses, the toxicity of the pyrazoles—of which only phenylbutazone is available in the United States—is greatest; however, the use of the drug has been supplanted by newer NSAIDs.

It is reasonable to explore the dose-response relationship when NSAIDs are administered to cancer patients. Because the clinician cannot know whether the optimal NSAID dose for a given patient is higher or lower than the standard recommended dose, therapy should be initiated with a relatively low dose, and the dose should then be increased to identify the ceiling dose or the most efficacious dose that yields tolerable side effects. Using ibuprofen as an example, the clinician should consider that the ceiling dose has been reached if an increase in the dose from 400 mg four times daily to 600 mg four times daily produces no additional analgesia. If the 400-mg dose is effective, dosing should continue at this level; if it is inadequate, the drug should be discontinued, and the trial of another drug should begin. If the higher dose produces additional analgesia but relief is still inadequate and no significant side effects are noted, the dose can be increased further.

Dose titration, however, cannot proceed without limit because of the potential for dose-related toxicity. In the absence of studies establishing the safety of very high NSAID doses in the cancer population, the physician must base selection for the maximum NSAID dose on clinical experience and customary use. A reasonable maximum is 1.5 to 2 times the standard recommended dose. If relatively high doses (higher than the standard recommended dose) are used, patients should be monitored every 1 to 2 months for occult gastrointestinal bleeding or changes in renal or hepatic function.

The administration of an NSAID must continue for a duration adequate to judge clinical effects. The efficacy of a drug can usually be determined in 2 to 3 weeks. Clinical experience suggests that 1 week is typically long enough to clarify the need for further dose titration during the initial trial of a drug.

If an NSAID proves to be ineffective, consideration should be given to a trial of another. Because patients may respond poorly to one NSAID but very well to another, switching to a different drug is reasonable if the target symptom continues to be mild pain (or mild residual pain during opioid therapy).

Opioid Analgesics

Effective administration of opioids requires a working knowledge of pharmacology and dosing principles in cancer pain. The most important points of these dosing guidelines are summarized in the next subsection.[15]

Opioid Selection and Administration

Opioid selection is based on a variety of pharmacologic factors and patient variables. Important considerations

Table 33.2 Simple Analgesics and Nonsteroidal Anti-Inflammatory Drugs

Chemical Class	Generic Name	Time Between Doses (hr)	Recommended Starting Doses (mg/day)*	Maximum Recommended Doses (mg/day)
p-Aminophenol	Acetaminophen	4–6	1,400	6,000
	Comments: Overdosage produces hepatic toxicity; not anti-inflammatory and thus not preferred as first-line analgesic or coanalgesic in patients with bone pain or pain from grossly inflammatory lesions; lack of GI or platelet toxicity may be important in some cancer patients			
Salicylates	Aspirin	4–6	1,600	6,000
	Comments: Standard for comparison; may be tolerated as well as some of the newer NSAIDs			
	Diflunisal	12	1,000 ×1, then 500 q12h	1,500
	Comment: Less GI toxicity than aspirin			
	Salsalate	12	1,500 × 1 then 1,000 q12h	4,000
	Choline magnesium trisalicylate	12	1,500 × 1 then 1,000 q12h 4,000	4,000
	Comments: Unlike other NSAIDs, these have minimal GI toxicity and no platelet aggregation, despite potent anti-inflammatory effects; may be particularly useful in some patients			
Propionic acids	Ibuprofen	4–8	1,200	4,200
	Comment: Available over the counter			
	Naproxen	12	500	1,000
	Naproxen sodium	12	550	1,100
	Fenoprofen	6	800	3,200
	Ketoprofen	6–8	150	300
Acetic acids	Indomethacin	8–12	75	200
	Comments: Available in sustained-release and rectal formulations; higher incidence of side effects, particularly GI and central nervous system, than propionic acids			
	Tolmetin	6–8	600	2,000
	Sulindac	12	300	400
	Comment: Some reports suggest less renal toxicity than other NSAIDs			
	Diclofenac sodium	6	75	200
Oxicams	Piroxicam	24	20	40
	Comment: Administration of 40 mg for more than 3 weeks associated with high incidence of peptic ulcer, particularly in older patients			
Fenamates	Mefenamic acid	6	500 × 1, then 250 q6h	1,000
	Comment: Not recommended for use longer than 1 week and therefore not indicated in cancer pain therapy			
	Meclofenamic	6–8	150	400
Pyrazoles	Phenylbutazone	6–8	300	400
	Comments: Not a first-line drug because of risk of serious bone marrow toxicity; not preferred for cancer pain therapy; if used, frequent monitoring of blood count needed in early therapy, in addition to other tests			

*Starting dose should be one half to two thirds of recommended dose in the older patients, those taking multiple drugs, and those with renal insufficiency. Doses must be individualized. Low initial doses should be titrated upward if tolerated and clinical effect is inadequate. Doses can be incrementally increased weekly. Studies of NSAIDs in the cancer population are meager; dosing guidelines are thus empirical.

GI, gastrointestinal; NSAID, nonsteroidal anti-inflammatory drug.

include the division of opioids into "weak" and "strong" opioid classes, differential toxicities, pharmacokinetic distinctions, and duration of effect (**Table 33.3**). The so-called weak opioids are those typically administered orally to patients with mild to moderate pain; they include preparations containing codeine, propoxyphene, oxycodone, hydrocodone, or dihydrocodeine. Meperidine and pentazocine are sometimes used but are not recommended for reasons discussed subsequently.

With the exception of pentazocine, none of these drugs has a ceiling dose, the property that would be the pharmacologic basis for their designation as weak. Rather, their customary use at relatively low doses, which are adequate to treat only moderate pain in nontolerant patients, is based on other considerations, such as toxicity at high doses (e.g., seizures from meperidine, psychotomimetic effects of pentazocine, and possible gastrointestinal intolerance from codeine).

Recognition that these drugs are not inherently weak provides added therapeutic flexibility because if the patient's pain is not controlled at the usual doses, and the drug is well tolerated, consideration can be given to increasing the dose, rather than switching to another drug.

In the United States, the reasonable weak opioid for the second rung of the analgesic ladder is typically a combination product containing an NSAID and an opioid, such as 30 to 60 mg of codeine or 5 mg of oxycodone combined with 325 mg of aspirin or acetaminophen. The dose of this drug can be increased until the risks associated with the NSAID become prohibitive. With an acetaminophen- or aspirin-containing product, three tablets every 4 hours is a prudent maximum dose.

The opioids can be divided into the pure agonist class (e.g., morphine, hydromorphone, methadone, meperidine, and oxycodone) and the agonist-antagonist class (pentazocine, nalbuphine, dezocine, butorphanol, and buprenorphine). The

Table 33.3 Agonist Opioid Analgesics

Drug	Dose (mg) Equianalgesic to Morphine Sulfate 10 mg*	Peak Effect (hr)	Duration (hr)	Toxicity
Morphine	10 mg IM	0.5–1	3–6	Constipation, nausea, sedation most common; respiratory depression most serious; itch and urinary retention uncommon
Controlled-release morphine	20–60 PO	3–4	8–12	Same as morphine
Hydromorphone	1.5 IM 7.5 PO Comment: Used for multiple routes	0.5–1 1–2	3–4 3–4	Same as morphine
Oxymorphone	1 IM 10 rectally Comment: No oral formulation	0.5–1 1.5–3	3–6 4–6	Same as morphine
Meperidine hydrochloride	75 IM Comment: Not preferred for cancer pain because of potential toxicity	0.5–1	3–4	Same as morphine, plus CNS excitation; contraindicated in those taking monoamine oxidase inhibitors
Heroin	5 IM	0.5–1	4–5	Same as morphine
Methadone hydrochloride	10 IM Comments: Risk of delayed toxicity caused by accumulation is a significant problem; dosing should start on prn basis, with close monitoring	0.5–1.5	4–6	Same as morphine
Codeine	130 IM 200 PO Comments: Usually combined with NSAID	1.5–2	3–6	Same as morphine
Propoxyphene hydrochloride	200 mg	1.5–2	3–6	Same as morphine, cardiac arrhythmias
Hydrocodone bitartrate	30 mg	0.5–1	3–4	Same as morphine

*Dose that provides analgesia equivalent to 10 mg intramuscular morphine.
CNS, central nervous system; IM, intramuscularly; NSAID, nonsteroidal anti-inflammatory drug; PO, by mouth; prn, as needed.

agonist-antagonist class is characterized by a balance between agonists and competitive antagonists at one or more of the opioid receptors; based on receptor interactions, these drugs can be additionally categorized into partial agonists and the mixed agonist-antagonists, which include pentazocine, nalbuphine, dezocine, and butorphanol.[16]

Agonist-antagonist drugs are characterized by a lesser propensity to produce physical dependence and by a ceiling effect for respiratory depression and, probably, for analgesia. These drugs have the potential to reverse effects in patients receiving agonist opioids. Administration to patients physically dependent on an agonist drug may cause an abstinence syndrome. The mixed agonist-antagonist subclass, particularly pentazocine, also has prominent psychotomimetic effects. These characteristics, combined with the lack of oral formulations, justify the conclusions that agonist-antagonist drugs are not preferred for cancer pain management. The only exception to this generalization may be sublingual buprenorphine, which has achieved some acceptance because of the potential value of the route of administration and its relatively long duration of action.

Thus, the management of severe cancer pain in the tolerant patient generally relies on the pure agonist drugs—morphine, hydromorphone, and methadone. Oxycodone as a single entity is sometimes used as well. Meperidine is not preferred because

it is metabolized to normeperidine, a compound with significant central nervous system toxicity, including myoclonus, tremulousness, and seizures.

In most countries, morphine is the first-line drug for cancer pain. Newer information about morphine metabolites may influence this use, however. Morphine is metabolized to an active compound, morphine 6-glucuronide, which is cleared by the kidney. The metabolite may contribute to the clinical effects of the parent compound, particularly in patients with relatively high concentrations as a result of renal insufficiency. Patients with renal failure were reported to develop respiratory compromise during morphine treatment and were found to have high levels of the metabolite in the plasma, with no measurable morphine.[17] Given the available data, it is reasonable to administer morphine cautiously to patients with stable renal insufficiency and to consider an alternative opioid in those with unstable renal function, in whom the amount of morphine 6-glucuronide may change and unpredictably influence drug effects.

The most important pharmacokinetic parameter in drug selection is its half-life. Regardless of the drug, dose, or route of administration, four to five half-lives are required to approach steady-state plasma levels. This becomes a clinical issue only in the case of methadone, the half-life of which may be so long that drug accumulation can continue for a week or longer when dosing is instituted or the dose is increased. Failure to recognize this potential for accumulation has resulted in serious delayed toxicity. Methadone should be used as a second-line agent in patients with the potential for significantly prolonged drug metabolism and in those who are at particular risk of adverse drug effects. Such patients include older persons, patients with organ failure (lungs, kidneys, liver, or brain), and those whose compliance or communication with the physician is in question.

Another important consideration in opioid selection is duration of analgesic effect. The opiates with short half-lives, such as morphine and hydromorphone, must be administered at least every 4 hours, whereas methadone—the opioid with the longest half-life—can often be administered every 6 hours and sometimes even less frequently. Controlled-release formulations of morphine and other opioid agonists can be given every 8 to 12 hours.

In summary, morphine, oxycodone, and hydromorphone are the preferred first-line drugs for severe cancer pain in older patients and in patients with major organ dysfunction. However, morphine should be used cautiously, if at all, in the patient with changing renal function. In the younger, compliant patient without organ failure, therapy can begin with morphine or with any other drug on the third rung of the analgesic ladder. A favorable previous experience with one of these drugs may be considered in this decision. Patients who may benefit from less frequent dosing should be considered for a trial of controlled-release morphine, usually after titration with an immediate-release morphine formulation.

The physician should start with the lowest dose that produces analgesia. Relatively nontolerant patients with severe pain, including those in whom a trial with a weak opioid has failed, are generally administered an opioid intramuscularly at a dose equivalent to 5 to 10 mg of morphine. Patients who are switched from a higher dose of an opioid to an alternative drug should begin at a dose that is one half to two thirds the equianalgesic dose of their current medication. This reduction is recommended in the expectation that a new drug will have relatively greater effects, as a result of incomplete cross-tolerance between opioids. To avoid side effects, older patients and those with compromised hepatic or renal function should receive even lower starting doses. Clinical experience also suggests that a switch to methadone should be accompanied by a greater decrement, perhaps to one third the equianalgesic dose.

Dose titration is the most important principle in opioid therapy. The dose should be gradually increased until favorable effects occur or intolerable and unmanageable side effects supervene. If pain remains severe after the initial dose, the subsequent dose can be doubled. If partial analgesia occurs, dose titration can usually follow on a daily basis. A useful approach involves concurrently administering a fixed, around-the-clock dose together with a "rescue dose," which is usually equal to 5% to 10% of the total daily dose and is offered as needed every 1 to 2 hours for breakthrough pain. This approach provides the patient with some personal control over analgesic dosing and can be used to estimate the increment in the fixed dose. For example, a patient receiving 100 mg of morphine every 4 hours, who required six rescue doses of 60 mg during the previous 24 hours, has demonstrated the need for at least an additional 360 mg/day; hence, it is reasonable to increase the fixed dose to 160 mg every 4 hours and simultaneously to increase the rescue dose to 90 mg, thereby maintaining it at 10% of the total daily dose.

For all agonist drugs except methadone, the rescue dose medication should be the same as the drug administered on a fixed basis. When methadone is administered around the clock, concurrently administering an opioid with a short half-life, such as morphine or hydromorphone, will avoid unanticipated toxicity from drug accumulation.

Scheduled around-the-clock dosing should be used in all patients who endure relatively constant pain. However, as needed dosing may be valuable in selected circumstances. The use of the rescue dose is described previously. In addition, as needed dosing without a concurrent fixed dosing regimen may have advantages in some settings, including the following: (1) defining the analgesic requirement in a nontolerant patient who is beginning opioid therapy; (2) titrating methadone at less risk of drug accumulation; and (3) facilitating dose changes during rapidly changing nociception, such as that occurring with radiation therapy to a painful bony lesion.

The physician should always choose an appropriate route of administration. If the patient can swallow and absorb the drug, the oral route is always preferable. Many other routes of opioid administration are available, however, and clinicians who manage patients with cancer pain should have knowledge of those routes used more frequently (**Table 33.4**). The usual starting place for the implementation of opioid therapy in the management of cancer pain is with immediate-release oral formulations, rather than sustained-release formulations and novel routes of administration (e.g., transdermal fentanyl).

The clinician must also be aware of equianalgesic doses. As noted, awareness of equianalgesic doses is necessary to change drugs or routes of administration safely. These ratios, which were developed from controlled single-dose studies of relative potency, are available for parenteral and oral dosing. The relative potency of drug administration by other routes (e.g., epidural or sublingual) is not known and complicates the management of patients treated with these approaches.

Published equianalgesic doses should be viewed as broad guidelines. The dose of a new drug must be reduced in all patients because of anticipated incomplete cross-tolerance, and this reduction should be greater in patients predisposed to adverse effects by advanced age or organ failure. Dose titration is almost always required after a switch to a new drug or route of administration.

Side Effects

Opioid side effects vary greatly among patients. The pattern and severity of side effects vary from drug to drug in the same patient. This observation suggests that a trial with an alternative opioid should be undertaken if tolerable side effects occur during dose titration. Early and appropriate management of side effects may enhance patient comfort and permit dose escalation to proceed.

Common side effects include constipation, sedation, and nausea. Opioid-induced constipation is so common that many practitioners believe that laxatives should always be administered concurrently with the opioid. This probably is the best course in older patients and in others with predisposing factors for constipation (e.g., use of other drugs with

Table 33.4 Routes of Administration

Route	Comment
Oral	Preferred in cancer pain management
Buccal	Variable absorption limits clinical utility
Sublingual	Efficacy of morphine controversial
Rectal	Available for morphine, oxymorphone, and hydromorphone Customarily used as if dose is equianalgesic to oral dose
Transdermal	Kinetics that mimic continuous infusion
Intranasal	May be efficacious with some drugs
Subcutaneous Repetitive bolus Continuous infusion Continuous infusion with PCA	Advent of ambulatory infusion pumps permits outpatient continuous infusion Can be accomplished with any drug with a parenteral formulation
Intravenous Repetitive bolus Continuous infusion PCA (with or without infusion)	This route indicated if other routes unavailable or not tolerated Infusion most useful in obviating bolus effect (i.e., peak concentration toxicity or pain breakthrough at the trough)
Epidural	Epidural catheter can be percutaneous portal, depending on life expectancy Intrathecal usually administered by subcutaneous pump
Intracerebroventricular	Rarely indicated but efficacious

PCA, patient-controlled analgesia.

constipating effects or intra-abdominal neoplasm); younger patients without these factors can be observed for the development of constipation and treated only if needed. Constipation can usually be managed by an increase in fiber consumption and the use of one of the following therapies[18]: (1) an osmotic laxative, such as magnesium citrate, milk of magnesia, or sodium citrate, administered every 2 or 3 days; (2) long-term administration of a stool softener and a contact laxative (senna, bisacodyl, or phenolphthalein); or (3) long-term administration of lactulose, beginning at a dose of 15 to 30 mL twice daily, and titrated upward as needed.

The choice of therapy should be based on the specific needs and desires of the patient.

Sedation, if not transitory, can usually be reversed with a small dose of a psychostimulant, with dextroamphetamine or methlyphenidate.[19] The starting dose is 2.5 to 5 mg once or twice daily and is gradually increased if needed. Some patients also benefit from a change in the dosing interval or opioid administered.

Nausea usually can be managed by an antiemetic, such as metoclopramide, prochlorperazine, haloperidol, or ondansetron. Because tolerance to this effect often develops within 1 or 2 weeks, it is often useful to administer one of these drugs on a fixed schedule for a brief time after nausea begins and then discontinue it to determine whether treatment is still needed. If movement-induced nausea or vertigo is prominent, an antivertiginous medication, such a meclizine, cyclizine, or scopolamine, may be helpful. Finally, if epigastric fullness or early satiety is a significant complaint, a trial of metoclopramide, a drug that enhances gastric emptying, is appropriate.

Opioid drugs can cause psychotomimetic effects (ranging from nightmares to frank psychosis), dry mouth, itch, or urinary retention (usually in men with prostatism or patients with pelvic cancer). Management includes discontinuation of other nonessential drugs with additive side effects, a change to an alternative opioid, and symptomatic treatment, if available (e.g., antihistamines for those with uncomfortable itch).

Tolerance

The physician should be aware of tolerance, a poorly understood phenomenon defined as a need for increasing doses to maintain opioid effects. The need for escalating doses may not reflect the primary effect of tolerance, however, and most patients who require rapidly increasing doses have progression of painful lesions or an increase in the level of psychological distress. Indeed, if progressive disease is not clinically overt, the need for increasing opioid doses should be considered a possible indication for reevaluation of the neoplasm.

When pharmacologic tolerance does occur, it typically manifests as a reduction in the duration of analgesia after a dose. This can usually be managed by dose escalation or an increase in dosing frequency. Tolerance has no limit, and, in an effort to maintain analgesia, doses can become extremely high; for example, a dose higher than that equivalent to 35,000 mg of morphine has been reported.[20]

Tolerance to respiratory depression usually develops rapidly, and drug-induced respiratory compromise is rare in patients receiving long-term opioid therapy. Should respiratory symptoms occur, they almost always have another cause, such as pneumonia or pulmonary embolism. Patients who are receiving high opioid doses may show great sensitivity to the antagonist drugs; therefore, naloxone (0.4 mg in 10 mL of saline) should be given slowly until the respiratory rate improves. A return to consciousness, which is often accompanied by a severe narcotic abstinence syndrome and the return of pain, should not be viewed as the goal of this intervention. Repeated doses of naloxone are usually required because of its relatively short half-life.

Distinction Between Physical Dependence and Addiction

Physical dependence is a pharmacologic property of opioid drugs defined by an abstinence syndrome that occurs after abrupt discontinuation of the drug or administration of an antagonist. Presumably, all patients administered high enough doses for a long enough period of time will become physically dependent. This situation presents no difficulties in management if the opioid dose is tapered before discontinuation and if antagonist drugs, including the agonist-antagonist analgesics, are avoided.

In contrast, addiction is a psychological and behavioral syndrome characterized by psychological dependence (drug craving and overwhelming concern with drug acquisition) and aberrant drug-related behaviors, including drug selling or hoarding, acquisition of drugs from nonmedical sources, and unsanctioned dose escalation. Unlike with physical dependence, little evidence supports the conclusion that otherwise normal patients with painful medical diseases are at substantial risk of developing addiction from the administration of opioids in a medical context.[21] It is uncommon for addiction to develop in a patient with no drug abuse history who is administered opioids for the treatment of cancer pain. Concern about addiction should never inhibit the aggressive management of this symptom.

Adjuvant Analgesics

Adjuvant analgesics are drugs with other specific indications that may be effective in the management of selected types of pain. They include the tricyclic antidepressants, anticonvulsants, neuroleptics, corticosteroids, and other miscellaneous drugs.

Tricyclic Antidepressants

Extensive literature supports the use of tricyclic antidepressants as analgesics in a wide variety of chronic pain syndromes.[22] In cancer patients, these drugs generally are administered for neuropathic pain (usually related to nerve infiltration or compression) or pain associated with prominent sleep disturbance or depression. To reduce the risk of side effects, it is usually prudent to titrate the opioid first and then add the adjuvant.

The initial dose of a tricyclic antidepressant should be low (e.g., 10 to 25 mg of amitriptyline). If the initial dose is tolerated, doses should be titrated upward gradually. The analgesic dose is usually 50 to 150 mg/day, typically administered as a single nighttime dose. Higher doses should be administered if the drug is ineffective and has produced no significant side effects. Depression is a prominent component of the pain syndrome.

Anticonvulsants

Anticonvulsants can be useful in the management of paroxysmal lancinating neuropathic pains,[23] such as those accompanying nerve infiltration by tumor. Gabapentin, carbamazepine, phenytoin, clonazepam, and valproate are used for this indication. Baclofen is a non-anticonvulsant drug that also may be efficacious in managing paroxysmal lancinating neuropathic pains. These drugs can have significant hematologic or hepatic adverse effects, and cancer patients should be monitored carefully during treatment.

Oral Local Anesthetics

Mexiletine has demonstrated efficacy in painful diabetic polyneuropathy,[24] and it has been used to treat diverse neuropathic pain.[25] This drug is available only in parenteral formulation and has a side effect profile, including its limited applicability to bedridden patients with advanced disease; in this setting, the sedative and anxiolytic properties of the drug can be salutary. Given the lack of evidence of analgesic effects and potential for side effects, other neuroleptics should be considered as second-line agents for continuous neuropathic pain that is refractory to other measures. These drugs remain primary therapy for pain patients with delirium or nausea.

Corticosteroids

Methylprednisolone is efficacious as an analgesic in patients with advanced cancer.[26] Clinical experience suggests that any of the corticosteroids may be useful in patients with pain from diffuse bony metastasis or tumor infiltration of neural structures. Dexamethasone is often chosen because of its modest mineralocorticoid effect. Dosing is empirical, and the duration of effect is undetermined.

Miscellaneous Drugs

Although hydroxyzine has been reported to be analgesic,[27] clinical responses at the usual oral doses have been disappointing. The drug may be a reasonable adjuvant in patients with pain complicated by nausea or anxiety.

In addition to corticosteroids, refractory bone pain has been treated with calcitonin, diphosphonates, and L-dopa.[28,29] Although experience with these agents is limited, trials are indicated in select patients with bone pain that is unresponsive to radiation therapy and drug treatment with opioids, NSAIDs, and corticosteroids.

Nonpharmacologic Approaches

A majority of cancer patients can achieve adequate pain relief through the expert application of pharmacologic therapies alone. Some patients attain a better quality of relief or balance between analgesia and side effects through the complementary use of adjunctive nonpharmacologic approaches. One or more of these approaches may become the primary analgesic therapy for the relatively small number of patients who fail to gain any meaningful relief from systemic drugs. The following review describes the most important of the nonpharmacologic therapies used in the management of cancer pain (**Table 33.5**).

Anesthetic Approaches

Neural Blockade

Neural blockade should be intelligently integrated into the multimodal approach, which includes an optimal trial of opioid therapy (see earlier). For some patients, the early use of neural blockade is indicated to provide immediate relief of uncontrolled pain and thereby allow time for opioid titration. Transient blockade also can be useful for patients with positional pain who must undergo procedures. Neural blockade of longer duration may be appropriate in patients who fail to obtain relief with routine noninvasive procedures.

Intercostal Nerve Block

Intercostal nerve block with a local anesthetic or corticosteroid can be performed at the bedside or in the outpatient setting. This procedure may palliate pain secondary to pathologic rib fractures or chest wall metastasis, post-thoracotomy pain, or right upper quadrant pain secondary to hepatic metastasis.[30] Intercostal blocks also may reduce pain caused by percutaneous drainage devices, such as chest or nephrostomy tubes. Studies have demonstrated a clinically significant improvement in pulmonary function in patients treated with this procedure.[31] The major complication is pneumothorax, which occurs in 0.5% to 1.0% of patients.

Table 33.5 Nonpharmacologic Approaches to Cancer Pain
Anesthetic approaches
Neural blockade
Intercostal nerve block
Interpleural catheters
Epidural nerve block
Sympathetic nerve block
Celiac plexus block
Neurostimulatory approaches
Physiatric approaches
Neurolytic anesthetic and neurodestructive approaches

Interpleural Catheters

Studies have demonstrated that local anesthetic instillation into the pleural space through a catheter may be effective in the management of some acute and chronic cancer pains.[32] This simple technique may be performed at the bedside or on an outpatient basis. Although the primary indications are essentially the same as those for intercostal nerve blocks, several reports suggest that this technique also can reduce pain below the diaphragm.[33] Complications of interpleural catheters are similar to those of intercostal nerve block. If the patient has significant pleural disease or pleural effusion, the dose of local anesthetic must be decreased to avoid toxic blood levels. If long-term use is anticipated, the catheter should be tunneled to avoid the risk of subcutaneous infection and empyema.

Epidural Nerve Block

Epidural nerve block with local anesthetic infusion or repeated local anesthetic injections with or without steroid has been demonstrated to provide pain relief in a variety of cancer pain syndromes.[34] These techniques can be safely performed at the bedside or on an outpatient basis, provided appropriate monitoring and resuscitation equipment are readily available. Epidural nerve blocks can be used to gain rapid control of pain while other approaches are implemented, to facilitate lengthy diagnostic or therapeutic procedures, or to provide primary analgesic therapy for specific syndromes (e.g., steroid-induced spinal compression fractures or acute herpes zoster).

Epidural blockade interrupts both somatic and sympathetic nerve conduction; cardiovascular complications, including hypotension and tachycardia, may occur. Respiratory compromise is possible if inadvertent blockade of the phrenic nerve or brainstem respiratory centers occurs. These procedures should be performed only by personnel trained in airway management and resuscitation.

Other major complications of epidural blockade include damage to neural structures, epidural hematoma, and epidural abscess. Although these complications are rare, they may occur more frequently in cancer patients who are immunocompromised and who may have coagulopathy. In spite of these potential complications, epidural block with local anesthetic or steroids has a positive risk-to-benefit ratio in the treatment of cancer pain, and this technique is probably underused.

Sympathetic Nerve Block

Many cancer pain syndromes are mediated, at least in part, by sympathetic efferent activity (known as sympathetically maintained pain). Syndromes that may benefit from interruption of the sympathetic nervous system by stellate ganglion or lumbar sympathetic nerve block with local anesthetics include postmastectomy pain and acute herpes zoster. Complications of these procedures are uncommon and include bleeding at the injection site, infection, inadvertent dural puncture, and trauma to neural structures. Because sympathetic neural blockade may induce profound cardiovascular changes, the practitioner must be ready to treat hypotension and tachycardia during the procedure.

Celiac Plexus Block

Celiac plexus block, in which a neurolytic solution is injected into the region of the celiac plexus, is useful in the management of pain caused by upper abdominal and retroperitoneal tumors, including the pain of pancreatic malignancy. Extensive clinical experience suggests a very favorable risk-to-benefit ratio with this procedure, and it is appropriate to consider it in selected patients early in the course of pain management.[35] Complications include bleeding, infection, and damage to neural structures or intra-abdominal organs. The incidence of these serious complications is substantially decreased by performing the procedure under the guidance of computed tomography. Because the celiac plexus is a major sympathetic ganglion, profound hypotension and orthostatic changes should be expected and treated aggressively.

Spinal Opioids

Spinal opioid administration, like neural blockade, must be integrated into a comprehensive pain treatment plan. In contrast to local anesthetics, spinal opioids produce effects through activation of opioid receptors in the spinal cord; sympathetic or motor function is not compromised.[36]

The short-term use of spinal opioids may be appropriate in patients receiving primary antineoplastic treatments that are expected to provide long-term relief of pain, patients with severe movement-related pain who are unable to undergo diagnostic or therapeutic procedures, and patients with very severe pain (pain emergencies) that cannot be controlled quickly by other cancer pain treatment modalities. Long-term administration of spinal opioids should not be implemented until more conservative approaches—specifically, trials of systemic opioids—have failed to control the pain without also causing intolerable side effects. Other factors to be considered before implementing a long-term trial include physiologic and behavioral abnormalities that may interfere with the ability of the patient to assess his or her pain relief, the presence of coagulopathy or infection, and the adequacy of the support system necessary to institute this therapy.[37]

Many techniques have been developed to deliver spinal opioids. An implanted pump can be used to administer drugs continuously into the subarachnoid space, and epidural administration can be implemented by using any of a variety of approaches, including a percutaneous catheter, a subcutaneous tunneled catheter connected to an implanted portal, or a tunneled catheter connected to a pump. Epidural opioids can be administered by continuous infusion or repetitive bolus. Although morphine continues to be the agent used most frequently, other opioids, such as hydromorphone, have been delivered successfully, and combinations of opioids and local anesthetics are innovations that may improve the outcome in some patients who fail to attain adequate relief with spinal opioids alone. The selection of a specific drug, site of delivery, and technique is based on many factors, including the clinical status (e.g., life expectancy) of the patient, characteristics of the drug, and patient preference.[37–39]

Side effects of spinal opioids may or may not be systemically mediated. Because the epidural space is highly vascular, any drug administered by this route will rapidly enter the systemic circulation. If systemic redistribution is sufficiently great, the patient may experience the same side effects that would occur with oral or parenteral administration of the drug. The degree of systemic redistribution is determined by numerous factors, including the lipid solubility of the drug and the dose. The most dreaded side effect of spinal opioids—respiratory depression—is exceedingly rare in the cancer population, presumably as a result of the opioid tolerance induced by previous intake of opioid drugs. Aggressive treatment of side effects may permit continuation of the therapy at analgesic doses.

Physiatric Approaches

The use of orthotics and prostheses and the techniques applied in physical and occupational therapy are intended to prevent impairment of function. In addition, however, these approaches may have value as analgesic techniques. For example, a patient with malignant vertebral collapse may obtain considerable relief from back pain with a brace, and an arm splint may benefit a patient whose pain is caused by neoplastic infiltration of the brachial plexus. Aggressive physical therapy may prevent the development of painful contractures or joint ankylosis, and myofascial pains, which are common in the cancer population, may improve with local massage, application of heat and cold, or passive muscle stretching.

Physical and occupational therapy may also enhance the cancer patient's sense of personal control over pain and encourage the maintenance of independent function, with potentially great psychological benefits. The use of physiatric techniques in the management of patients with cancer pain should be expanded.

Neurostimulatory Approaches

It is well known that stimulation of afferent neural pathways may relieve pain. The most widely applied of such techniques is transcutaneous nerve stimulation. The safety of this approach suggests that a trial can be recommended for patients with localized pain, particularly neuropathic pain. Beneficial effects, if any, usually are transitory, and other analgesic approaches are almost always necessary. The invasive neurostimulatory procedures, including percutaneous electrical nerve stimulation, dorsal column stimulation, and deep brain stimulation, are rarely used in cancer patients and should be considered only by practitioners experienced in cancer pain therapy. These procedures require an invasive technique to implant the apparatus. Given the immunocompromise, fragile medical

status, and limited experiences with these approaches in cancer patients, these techniques have a very limited role in this setting.

Neurolytic Anesthetic and Neurosurgical Approaches

The use of neurolytic celiac plexus block is discussed previously. Other neurolytic procedures have been developed to interrupt somatosensory transmission at various levels of the nervous system, from peripheral nerves to the cerebrum. Other neurolytic techniques are not intended to block afferent information. These include lobotomy and cingulotomy—which are now rarely performed and purportedly relieve suffering without necessarily altering pain—and chemical or surgical hypophysectomy.[40] Studies of hypophysectomy, which can be performed by injecting alcohol into the pituitary gland, indicate that the procedure can reduce pain from disseminated cancer in a majority of patients for several months. The tumor need not be hormone dependent for the procedure to be successful.[41] The use of neurolytic procedures, most of which are intended to isolate the painful site from the central nervous system, is best limited to patients with localized nociceptive pain. These procedures should be considered only when more conservative approaches have failed to control the pain adequately.

Psychological Approaches

Some patients with cancer pain have psychiatric disorders, such as major depression or anxiety disorder, and require formal psychological assessment and treatment.[42] All patients, including those with no psychiatric disease, benefit from supportive interaction with staff, during which disease-related issues can be addressed openly. Some patients also may be candidates for specific cognitive approaches to pain control, including hypnosis, relaxation training, and distraction techniques.[42] Although these cognitive interventions have not been studied adequately in cancer patients, experience suggests that they may be particularly useful in patients with predictable pain (e.g., pain that accompanies dressing changes) and in those with pain associated with high levels of anxiety.

Conclusion

Pain management is a compelling issue in the care of patients with cancer. Adequate pain relief allows the patient the greatest opportunity to live normally during the early stages of disease and to have an optimal quality of life if the cancer progresses. Effective symptom control also eases the burden on the family, who otherwise may experience helplessness as uncontrolled pain occurs in a loved one. Ongoing and careful assessment, a systematic approach to pharmacotherapy, and the judicious use of other approaches are fundamental elements of the successful management of cancer pain.

References

Full references for this chapter can be found on www.expertconsult.com.

Chapter 34

Radiation Therapy in the Management of Cancer Pain

Scott C. Cozad

History

Ionizing radiation was coincidentally discovered by Frederic Röntgen, while experimenting with Crooke's tubes. He presented his finding to the Physical Society at Würzburg, Germany on December 28, 1895. The discovery of radium by the Curies followed in 1898. Therapeutic applications, including palliation of pain, ensued almost immediately.[1]

In spite of more than a century of use, the mechanism of action of radiation is still unsettled. Some cytotoxic effect is likely, as shown by Hillman et al.[2] In experimental prostate cancer cell lines grown in bone, irradiation with photon or neutron beams was evaluated, with or without interleukin-2 (IL-2). A dose-dependent inhibition of tumor growth was found. Additional delay was noted with the addition of IL-2 to photon irradiation, but IL-2 alone had no effect. Histologic sections confirmed areas of tumor destruction with fibrosis and inflammatory changes. Compared with controls, viable tumor cells were noted in 10% to 40% of the specimens, depending on radiation dose.

The early response for radiation implies other mechanisms as well. Hoskin et al[3] found an association between urinary markers of bone resorption before and after radiation and subsequent pain relief. These findings suggested that bone, not tumor effects, determines response. Osteoclastic production of cytokines, which stimulate pain receptors, may also play a role.

This theory fits well with emerging concepts of bone metastases. Normal bone homeostasis is maintained by a balance between osteoclasts and osteoblasts. Both are necessary for the development and propagation of metastases.[4] Products of normal bone turnover such as type I collagen have been shown to attract cancer cells in vitro.[5-7] Once the nonmineralized surface is broken down by collagenase, which is produced by osteoblasts, bone matrix resorption by osteoclasts can proceed, with resultant release of cytokines that can further attract and promote the growth of bone cancer cells and lead to the recruitment of additional osteoclasts.[8] Once the process has proceeded sufficiently, direct destruction of bone by tumor cells can occur.[8,9] Further clarification of the relative contributions of these different mechanisms will be important in defining the role and timing of radiation in the treatment of osseous metastases.

Indications for Radiation in Pain Management

Metastatic disease to bone is the most common cause of pain in oncology practice.[10] Approximately 100,000 new cases are diagnosed annually in the United States,[11] with an overall incidence of twice this number. Pain may be caused by any of the following several mechanisms, more than one of which could be present in any given case[10]:

- Stimulation of endosteal nerve by humoral or cytokine agents
- Stretching of the periosteum by tumor mass
- Fractures with disruption of the periosteum
- Tumor growth into neural structures

Special cases of this last mechanism would include spinal cord compression with resultant myelopathy, cauda equina syndrome with bowel and bladder dysfunction and lower motor neuron leg weakness, and brachial plexopathy from tumors in the lung apex or celiac plexopathy, usually from pancreatic carcinoma. Other indications for radiation therapy are pain secondary to central nervous system (CNS) metastases, visceral organ involvement, and trigeminal neuralgia.

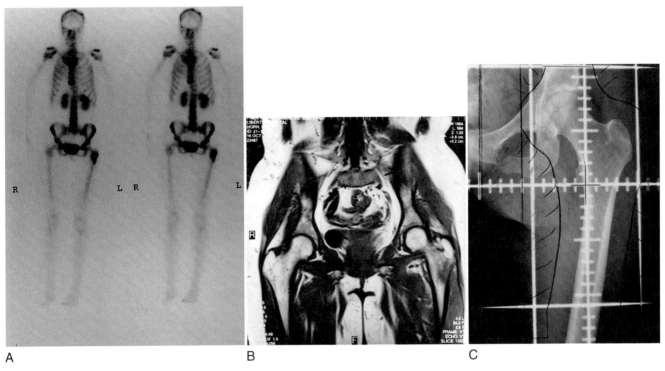

A   B   C

Fig. 34.1 A, Bone scan showing marked uptake in the left greater trochanter. B, T1-weighted magnetic resonance imaging scan showing marrow replacement. C, Simulation film showing treatment field for the patient in A and B. Note the essentially normal appearance of bone in the trochanteric area.

Testing

Treatment with radiation depends on accurate diagnosis and precise localization of the lesion or lesions. Signs or symptoms of pain and neurologic deficits are helpful in locating the general site of involvement and in guiding effective use of imaging studies. Plain films are very specific but lack sensitivity; they require more than 50% trabecular bone destruction or a 1.0-cm lesion for detection (**Fig. 34.1**).[12] Bone scans are much more sensitive. They have a false-negative rate of approximately 8% but may have a false-positive rate as high of 40% to 50%, depending on the number of lesions. Computed tomography (CT) scan or magnetic resonance imaging (MRI) may be necessary to confirm the diagnosis of metastases and to define the extent of the lesion and associated soft tissue mass, if present. These studies are also helpful in identifying the position of normal structures in the area as the radiation oncologist begins to conceptualize techniques for treatment.

Treatment Technique

After a diagnosis is established, the process of simulation follows to localize the treatment area. Depending on the area to be treated, history of prior radiation, and presence of sensitive normal structures, the simulation treatment planning process may be either simple or complex (**Fig. 34.2**). After this step is completed, a set of physical data relating to both the patient and the treatment delivery system will have been generated for use in calculating "beam on" time to deliver the prescription dose.

The optimal prescription dose has been the subject of numerous randomized trials (**Table 34.1**).[13–27] These trials can be

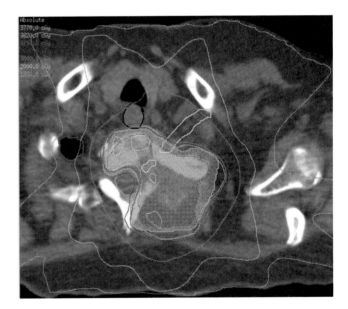

Fig. 34.2 Computed tomography–generated setup and isodose lines a patient with prostate carcinoma metastatic to the left sacral iliac area with a soft tissue mass. The *solid orange area* is the area of soft tissue mass and gross bone involvement. The *heavy orange lines* are the 100% isodose line. Note the oblique field angles to avoid the bowel in this patient who had previously received radiation to the pelvic area.

divided into those evaluating different multifraction schedules, those evaluating multifraction versus single-fraction schedules, and those evaluating single fraction of higher versus lower dose. These trials had various entry criteria and methodologies for response of evaluation and thus cannot be directly compared.

Table 34.1 Optimal Prescription Dose Trials

Reference	Fractionation Schedule (No. Patients in Trial)	Pain Relief (%) (Partial or Complete)	Duration	Retreatment	Reossification	Fracture	Toxicity
Kirkbride et al[13]	4.0 Gy × 5	40 (P = .03)	—	—	—	—	—
	8.0 Gy × 1	32					
	(N = 398)						
Bone Pain Trial Working Party[14]	3.0 Gy × 10	78	—	10%	—	2/378	No change 61% with symptoms
	4.0 Gy × 5						
	8.0 Gy × 1	78	—	23%	—	7/383	
	(N = 761)						
Steenland et al[15]	4.0 Gy × 6	71	24 wk	7%	—	2%	No change
	8.0 Gy × 1	71	20 wk (time to progression)	25%		4%	
	(N = 1,171)						
Nielsen et al[16]	5.0 Gy × 4	60	60% control (for groups as a whole at 6 mo)	14/119	—	5%	35%
	8.0 Gy × 1	60		25/120		5%	35%
	(N = 239)						
Gaze et al[17]	4.5 Gy × 5	89	25 wk (mean)	—	—	—	37%
	10.0 Gy × 1	84	22.5 wk (mean)				37%
	(N = 265)						
Cole[18]	4.0 Gy × 6	~80	—	0%	—	1/13	33%/22%
	8.0 Gy × 1	~85		25%		0/16	77%/30% (upper/lower GI)
	(N = 29)						
Price et al[19]	3.0 Gy × 10	~85	57%	4/148 (3%)	—	1/148	No change
	8.0 Gy × 1	~85	59% (at 1 year)	15/140 (11%)		0/140	
	(N = 288)						
Hartsell et al: RTOG 97-14[20]	3.0 Gy × 10	66	10% (for group as a whole: progression 3 mo)	—	—	—	17%
	8.0 Gy × 1	65					10% Grade 2–4 acute toxicity
	(N = 949)						
Niewald et al[21]	3.0 Gy × 10	68	245 days	1	20%	4%	—
	4.0 Gy × 5	83	247 days (mean duration)	1	28%	6%	
	(N = 100)						

Study	Dose						
Rasmusson et al[22]	3.0 Gy × 10	69	12 mo	—	~70%	—	Minimal
	5.0 Gy × 3	66	12 mo	—	~76%	—	Minimal
	(N = 217)						
Okawa et al[23]	2.0 Gy × 15	76	—	—	—	—	—
	4.5 Gy × 5	75					
	2.0 Gy bid × 5 (900)	78					
	(N = 80)						
Madsen[24]	4.0 Gy × 6 (2 fractions/wk)	47	—	—	—	—	8/30
	10.0 Gy × 2 (over 3 wk)	48					10/27 Slight/severe nausea
	(N = 57)						
Tong: RTOG[25]	Solitary metastases						
	2.7 Gy × 15	85	29 wk	—	—	18%	—
	4.0 Gy × 5	82	20 wk			4%	
	(N = 266)						
	Multiple metastases						
	3.0 Gy × 10	82	23 wk	—	—	8%	—
	3.0 Gy × 5	85	20 wk			5%	
	4.0 Gy × 5	83	17 wk			7%	
	5.0 Gy × 5	78	15 wk			9%	
	(N = 750)						
Jeremic et al[26]	4.0 Gy × 1	57	42 wk	42%	—	6%	19%/13%
	6.0 Gy × 1	72	50 wk	44%		7%	18%/11%
	8.0 Gy × 1	78	47 wk (mean time to progression)	38%		7%	22%/15% Grade 1–2 upper/lower GI toxicity
	(N = 327)						
Hoskin et al[27]	8.0 Gy × 1	76	No change at 12 wk	20%	—	—	—
	4.0 Gy × 1	53		9%			
	(N = 270)						

bid, twice daily; GI, gastrointestinal; RTOG, Radiation Therapy Oncology Group.

In general, approximately one third of patients will have a complete pain response, and an additional one third will have a partial response. With the exception of single-fraction treatment of 4.0 Gray (Gy), little, if any, apparent difference is noted in pain response by dose or fractionation. This conclusion is still challenged based on the following:

- Uncontrolled or unreported use of analgesics in most of the studies
- Differences in retreatment rates in favor of higher dose
- Improvement in remineralization rates at higher dose
- Differences in durability of response
- Lack of toxicity and quality-of-life data

To address these shortcomings in future trials, a consensus conference agreed on entry criteria, treatment technique, end points, reporting of analgesic use, and statistical analysis.[28]

In light of the uncertainties, especially of various secondary end points, the specific radiation prescription requires consideration of the anticipated toxicities and life expectancy of the patient. A decision should also take into account the patient's preference because many patients may prefer a short multifraction schedule over single fraction if the risk of pathologic fracture or retreatment is lower.[29] The cited studies suggest more favorable responses in patients with breast or prostate cancer and in those with less intense pain at the time of treatment.

Hemibody Radiation and Radiopharmaceuticals

In an effort to increase pain responses and avoid progression at new sites, wide-field radiation to the upper, middle, or lower body was piloted by the Radiation Therapy Oncology Group (RTOG).[30] Doses of 6.0 to 8.0 Gy in a single fraction led to pain relief in 73%; however, severe or life-threatening gastrointestinal (GI) or hemologic toxicity was seen in 10%. A phase III fractionation trial was subsequently performed. Poor response was seen for a dose of 8.0 Gy at 4.0 Gy twice daily compared with 15.0 Gy in five fractions or 12.0 Gy at 3.0 Gy twice daily for 2 days. Overall response was 91%, with 12% severe acute toxicity.[31]

An alternative approach is the use of bone-seeking radionuclides including strontium-89 (^{89}Sr), samarium-153, and rhenium-188. ^{89}Sr is the most extensively studied. Its use requires blastic lesions, and the overwhelming experience has been in patients with prostate and breast cancer. Initial therapy with these agents requires adequate blood counts, usually a white blood cell count greater than 3000 and a platelet count greater than 100,000. Repeated treatment can lead to significant cytopenia. Treatment has not consistently led to measurable tumor response, decreased bone turnover markers, or remineralization.[32] Therefore, these agents are unsuitable for lytic lesions, bone fracture, spinal cord compression, or neuropathic syndromes.

In a small trial from Germany, no difference in pain relief was noted in patients treated with ^{89}Sr compared with placebo.[33] A similar study of only 32 patients reached a contradictory conclusion, with significant pain response in metastatic prostate carcinoma.[34] Differences in result may be explained by the higher doses of ^{89}Sr and control of hormonal manipulation in the latter trial.

Strontium has also been directly compared with external beam radiation or as an adjunct. Either treatment by itself led to pain relief in 61% to 65% of patients, with no significant differences. Fewer patients receiving ^{89}Sr required treatment to new sites, 36% versus 58%.[35]

Porter et al[36] found that the addition of ^{89}Sr to external beam radiation did not improve pain responses but did decrease new sites of pain. A similar trial from Norway found no significant benefit from ^{89}Sr, although the investigators noted a 10% difference in the number of new sites, with fewer seen in the ^{89}Sr arm of the trial.[37] Time to development of new sites of disease was 4 months.

The application of wide-field or systemic radiation does not improve on pain responses compared with focal radiation alone. Although a reduction or delay for new sites occurs, this is at the cost of significant acute GI or hemologic toxicity, especially in pretreated patients.

Bisphosphonates

Bisphosphonates are preferentially delivered to sites of bone resorption or formation, where they are incorporated into osteoclasts, on which they have an inhibitory effect. Ongoing studies suggest that these agents may also cause apoptosis of tumor cell lines and inhibit adhesion of tumor cells to bone matrix elements.[38,39] Bisphosphonates have been recommended in patients with lytic disease, based on the ability of these drugs to limit complications such as pathologic fracture, spinal cord compression, and need for radiation.[40,41] Time to progression for metastatic complications was 10 to 13 months, comparatively longer than the 4 months achieved with ^{89}Sr. Initial studies primarily focused on osseous metastases secondary to breast cancer, but newer, more potent agents, have demonstrated similar outcomes for a wide range of solid tumors.[42]

Given the mechanism of action, the lack of hematologic or GI side effects, and the applicability to a wide range of tumor systems, the use of combinations of bisphosphonates and radiation is an attractive therapeutic approach. Animal studies suggest that administration of bisphosphonates preceding radiation may lead to greater bone remineralization.[43] Early studies in human subjects suggest improved pain relief and remineralization as well.[44–46] Trials evaluating newer agents, timing, and duration of bisphosphonates are investigating these promising areas of research.

Neuropathic Pain

Neuropathic pain is caused by pressure on or direct invasion of neural structures and is characterized by symptoms in a dermatome distribution. It is often described as a burning sensation but may manifest as an area of hypoesthesia or dysesthesia. This pain is often thought of as being intractable to common analgesics and is more resistant to relief from radiation.

The Trans-Tasman Radiation Oncology Group specifically studied this group of patients.[47] Entry into the study required neuropathic pain; most patients had spine involvement but without spinal cord compression. An interim analysis of the first 90 patients randomized to either a single fraction of 8.0 Gy or five fractions of 4.0 Gy revealed an overall pain response of 59%. This response rate is similar, albeit at the lower end of the range, to responses reported for uncomplicated bone pain.

Spinal Cord Compression

Although most patients entering the Trans-Tasman trial had spine lesions, spinal cord compression was an exclusion. In this population, radiation is also a well-established therapy. Although numerous studies have been conducted, information on pain relief is scarce because the usual end point is neurologic function. In general, for a given functional level, radiation has been considered equivalent to surgical decompression followed by radiation.[48–51] This paradigm was challenged by Patchell et al.[52] In this randomized trial, patients undergoing anterior decompression and stabilization followed by radiation had improved neurologic outcomes and ability to ambulate compared with patients managed with radiation alone. Narcotic use was significantly less as well. The surgical approach used in this trial was more aggressive than that commonly employed, and perhaps more importantly, surgery was initiated within 24 hours.

Plexopathy

Involvement of the brachial plexus by superior sulcus tumors or the celiac plexus by retroperitoneal tumors, most commonly pancreatic carcinoma, can cause severe pain. The natural history of these conditions is markedly different because the former can be treated curatively, whereas the latter signifies advanced disease and is only palliated by currently available therapy.

Superior sulcus tumors often manifest with pain in the upper chest, neck, shoulder, and arm. The distribution corresponds to the trunk of the brachial plexus involved and indicates the position of the tumor in the upper portion of the lung (**Fig. 34.3**).

Approaches to superior sulcus tumors without evidence of metastases have historically included surgery or a short course of radiation followed by surgery. This approach was extensively reported by Paulson[53] and leads to approximately 25% long-term survival. Local failure was the dominant recurrence pattern; approximately 40% of patients had treatment failure at the primary site. Many of these patients experienced local symptoms, including pain subsequent to the relapse.

Current treatment consists of preoperative radiation and chemotherapy. The Southwest Oncology Group (Intergroup 0160) reported the results of this approach in a phase II trial.[54] Radiation was delivered to a dose of 45.0 Gy in 25 fractions concurrent with cisplatin and VP-16 (etoposide). Seventy-five percent of patients entered had Eastern Cooperative Oncology Group performance status 1 resulting from pain. Although no specific data on pain relief were given, 92% of patients had a complete resection. Equal proportions had a pathologic complete response, microscopic residual tumor, or gross residual tumor. The plateau for survival curves was 55% for all patients. The pattern of recurrence was altered as well with marked improvement in control at the primary site.

In contrast, patients with locally advanced pancreatic cancer treated with combined chemoradiation have a 2-year survival of approximately 10%.[55–58] Fifty percent to 60% of these patients can, however, have clinical regression of their disease

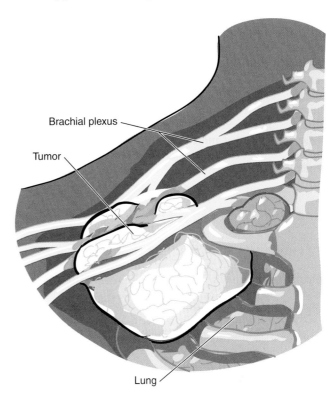

Fig. 34.3 Brachial plexus and nerve distribution in relation to the upper chest. Superior sulcus tumors often manifest with pain in the upper chest, neck, shoulder, and arm. The distribution corresponds to the trunk of the brachial plexus involved and indicates the position of the tumor in the upper portion of the lung.

and accompanying pain relief. This finding compares favorably with chemotherapy alone, in which 5% treated with 5-fluorouracil and 24% treated with gemcitabine achieved a clinical benefit, primarily pain relief.[59]

Visceral Pain

Neoplastic involvement of organs can lead to pain, primarily by capsular distention. Pain is usually diffuse and dull because it is transmitted by visceral nerve fibers. The liver is commonly involved in advanced metastatic disease, with accompanying pain. Although liver pain is often thought of as too sensitive to radiation for treatment, numerous reports of palliative radiation exist. Phillips and Karnofsky et al[60] reported complete relief in 26 of 30 patients with various primary carcinomas involving the liver who were treated at Memorial Sloan-Kettering Cancer Center in New York. The RTOG reported various fractionation schedules.[61,62] Pain relief was achieved in 55%. Mass effect, fever, and nausea were also improved in approximately one half of the patients. No cases of radiation hepatitis occurred at doses lower than 30.0 Gy. Median survival overall is 3 to 4 months and is highly dependent on performance status and extent of extrahepatic disease. Because many patients have extensive metastases and corresponding poor performance status, radiation is rarely employed in this setting.

Brain Metastases

Involvement of the CNS by metastatic disease is usually a late event. Manifestations depend on the area of involvement, and headache is a component of presentation in 52% to 55%.[63–65] Radiation treatment is usually delivered over 2 to 3 weeks to the whole brain, although resection or stereotactic radiation for selected patients is increasingly used. Headaches improve in 85% to 95%, with one half to two thirds of patients having complete resolution. Benefits in neurologic and cognitive function and decreased seizure activity are also common. Median survival rates are highly dependent on performance or neurologic status and can be as limited as a few weeks for those presenting with severe deficits or neurologic class IV but generally are 4 to 6 months.

Trigeminal Neuralgia

Trigeminal neuralgia can be a debilitating disease occurring as a consequence of tumors of the gasserian ganglion, associated with multiple sclerosis, or idiopathically. The pain is lancinating and often repetitive in the distribution of one or more divisions of cranial nerve V. It may be bilateral and can have an accompanying sensory component. When conservative management fails or is not tolerated, more invasive procedures are indicated. One potential option is stereotactic radiosurgery.

The first system used in this setting was the Gamma Knife, developed by Leksell in 1951.[66] Current models consist of a spherical shell housing 201 cobalt-60 sources that can be differentially unshielded to produce a highly conformal radiation dose distribution around a target. An important characteristic of this is the steep dose gradient outside of the target area that allows for sparing of normal structures.

The root of the affected nerve is identified as it exits the pons by MRI. Treatment is delivered in one fraction, with the patient immobilized in a rigid ring fixed to the skull with pins placed under local anesthesia. Pain relief with radiosurgery has been reported in 75% to 89% of those treated,[67–69] although with further follow-up this rate may decrease to 50% to 60%.[70,71] Higher response rates are seen in patients with shorter symptom duration who have not undergone surgical intervention. Toxicity primarily consists of new sensory deficits, seen in 7.3% in the University of Maryland series. Toxicity is increased with dose escalation higher than the standard 70.0 Gy, or longer length of nerve treated, without a concomitant improvement in pain relief.[72]

Controlled trials comparing radiosurgery with surgical approaches have not been performed. Pain relief in series of microvascular decompression tends to be in the range of 70% to 90%, although typically younger patients with better prognoses are selected for this approach.[73]

In a retrospective review of patients matched for prior surgical procedures and Barrow Neurologic Index, radiosurgery led to excellent or good outcomes (Barrow Neurologic Index 1 or 2) in 29% and 10% compared with 33% and 0% in those treated with glycerol rhizotomy. Complications, primarily facial numbness, were higher in the glycerol rhizotomy group (53%) compared with the radiosurgery group (33%).[74]

Cost Effectiveness

In clinical practice, the cost of intervention is usually considered last. However, it is an important consideration from the viewpoint of public policy. The agency for Healthcare Policy and Research of the Department of Health and Human Services published clinical practice guidelines on pain management. As discussed in the *New England Journal of Medicine*,[75] these guidelines called for certain measures, including the following:

- A collaborative, interdisciplinary approach
- An individualized plan agreed on by patients, families, and caregivers
- Ongoing assessment
- Both drug and nondrug therapies
- Institutional policies on pain management and monitoring

Given the prevalence of pain in cancer patients, effective management will carry a high aggregate cost. This is balanced against the cost of uncontrolled pain, which can lead to complications and hospitalizations, as well as the indirect losses from decreased quality of life.

In a pilot study from the Cleveland Clinic in Ohio that evaluated cost effectiveness, 66 patients treated by radiation for bone metastasis were evaluated.[76] Entry required a Karnofsky performance status of 70% and an estimated survival of 6 months. Radiation fractionation was chosen by the physician; the most common prescription was 30.0 Gy in 10 fractions in 75% of patients. On a 10-point scale, pain scores at rest improved by 4 points, and with movement they improved by 5 points. Cost was based on Medicare-allowable charges and ranged from $1,200 to $2,500 for radiation compared with an estimated $9,000 to $36,000 for 9 months of oral narcotics. These costs are in close agreement with other estimates of $1,000 to $4,000 monthly for oral narcotics.[77]

The radiation costs are similar to those seen in a national survey of Swedish practices. This study found the cost of a palliative course of radiation to be $2,000. The investigators concluded that radiation therapy was underused in the palliative setting.[78]

Conclusion

- Radiation palliates pain in a large proportion of patients with bone metastases.
- Preservation of osseous and neural function is beneficial.
- Pain from other types of metastases such as visceral and CNS metastases can also be improved.
- A rapidly increasing indication is stereotactic radiosurgery for trigeminal neuralgia.
- Radiation is cost effective in the palliative care setting.

References

Full references for this chapter can be found on www.expertconsult.com.

Neural Blockade with Local Anesthetics and Steroids in the Management of Cancer Pain

P. Prithvi Raj

Pain is one of the most prevalent symptoms among patients with advanced cancer. Numerous studies have shown that 30% to 50% of all cancer patients undergoing chemotherapy or other antitumor treatments and 50% to 80% of those with advanced cancer suffer severe pain.[1]

Drug therapy remains the foundation of cancer pain management. Numerous studies have demonstrated that the World Health Organization (WHO) three-step hierarchy for pain management is effective in controlling pain for 70% to 90% of patients with cancer.[2] However, for the 10% to 30% of cancer patients whose pain is not being controlled by the WHO three-step ladder or for patients who are experiencing severe side effects of the treatments, regional anesthetic techniques can be valuable. This chapter focuses on the role of regional anesthetic techniques in the treatment of cancer pain.

Role of Regional Anesthetic Techniques for the Treatment of Cancer Pain

No clear consensus exists on when more invasive therapies should be used in cancer patients, but as a general rule of thumb, therapies should start with more conservative, low-risk procedures and progress to more invasive, high-risk procedures that are justified by the presence of severe refractory pain. The United States Agency for Health Care Policy and Research (AHCPR) has published guidelines for the management of cancer pain.[3,4] Although the report focuses more on the pharmacologic management of cancer pain, the agency endorses the use of regional anesthetic techniques for the treatment of severe cancer pain. However, the report is critical of the lack of well-controlled studies on the outcome of interventional techniques for cancer pain.

In 1996, the American Society of Anesthesiologists published guidelines for the treatment of cancer pain that focused more on regional anesthetic techniques.[5] The take-home message from these published guidelines is "first do no harm." If more conservative noninvasive measures have not been tried in the patient with cancer pain, the clinician should not forge ahead to more invasive, high-risk procedures. Although 70% to 90% of patients can be successfully treated with conservative measures outlined in the WHO three-step ladder, cancer patients who are suffering from severe, unrelieved pain or who are experiencing debilitating side effects of systemic therapy should not be denied the benefits of regional anesthetic techniques that can turn a major pain crisis into a manageable situation.[6] **Table 35.1** summarizes the indications for regional anesthetic techniques in cancer pain.

Local Anesthetic Injections

Although temporary, local anesthetic regional anesthesia is a valuable tool in the management of cancer pain.[7,8] Because the effects are temporary, the role of regional anesthesia must be clearly outlined to the patient, family, and health care providers. It can be distressing to the patient to experience significant pain relief with regional anesthesia only to have the severe

Table 35.1 Indications for Regional Anesthesia Techniques in Cancer Pain Management

Pain unrelieved by the World Health Organization three-step hierarchy of pain management

Unacceptable side effects with systemic therapies

Pain crisis

Patient's desire to avoid systemic therapy

From Wallace MS, Leung AY, McBeth MD: Malignant pain. In Raj PP, editor: *Textbook of regional anesthesia*, Philadelphia, 2002, Churchill Livingstone, p 562.

Table 35.2 Diagnostic Blocks in Cancer Pain Management

ANATOMIC SOURCE OF PAIN

Intra-articular injection

Trigger point injection

Peripheral nerve block

VISCERAL VERSUS SOMATIC PAIN

Intercostal nerve block: differentiates thoracoabdominal wall pain from thoracic and abdominal visceral pain

Celiac plexus block: differentiates abdominal wall pain from abdominal visceral pain

Hypogastric plexus block: differentiates pelvic wall pain from pelvic visceral pain

Cervicothoracic ganglion (stellate-T4) block: differentiates thoracic wall pain from thoracic visceral pain

SYMPATHETIC VERSUS SOMATIC PAIN

Stellate ganglion block: differentiates sympathetically mediated pain from somatic pain of the head, neck, and upper extremity

Lumbar sympathetic block: differentiates sympathetically mediated pain from somatic pain of the lower extremity

Differential spinal block: differentiates sympathetically mediated pain from somatic spinal pain

From Wallace MS, Leung AY, McBeth MD: Malignant pain. In Raj PP, editor: *Textbook of regional anesthesia*, Philadelphia, 2002, Churchill Livingstone, p 562.

pain return after a few hours. Local anesthetic neural blockade regional anesthesia serves several purposes: (1) diagnosis, (2) prognosis, and (3) therapy.

Diagnosis

For diagnostic purposes, regional anesthesia can be valuable in determining the pathway or mechanism of the pain. **Table 35.2** gives examples of useful diagnostic blocks. The anatomic source of the pain can be diagnosed with a variety of regional anesthesia techniques. Joint pain resulting from cancer (i.e., osteonecrosis, sacroiliac joint metastasis) can be diagnosed with intra-articular injections. Muscle spasms as a result of tumor invasion of bony structures can be diagnosed with trigger point injections, and peripheral nerve blocks can identify the peripheral neural pathway of the pain.

Although thoracoabdominal pain is often described as more localized and sharp as compared with thoracic and visceral pain, which is described as diffuse and dull, it can sometimes be difficult to differentiate visceral pain from thoracoabdominal wall pain, especially as the pain becomes more severe. For thoracic pain, intercostal blocks can differentiate between thoracic wall and visceral pain. With the exception of the cardiac structures, most of the sensory innervation of the thoracic viscera travels through the T1-T4 sympathetic ganglion. Therefore, cervicothoracic sympathetic blocks can be used to diagnose thoracic visceral pain. For abdominal pain, intercostal, celiac plexus, and hypogastric plexus blocks can differentiate between abdominal wall pain and visceral pain.

Sympathetic blocks can be used to diagnose sympathetically mediated pain and to guide treatment. Because somatic peripheral nerves contain both sympathetic and somatic fibers, it is necessary to block the sympathetic nervous system at locations that are free of somatic nerves. This can be accomplished at the stellate ganglion for diagnosis of head, neck, and upper extremity pain and at the lumbar ganglion for diagnosis of lower extremity pain.

The technique of differential blockade may be useful in cancer pain diagnosis. Since the description of this technique by Winnie and Collins,[9] this technique has generated much controversy. Both in vitro and in vivo studies have cast doubt on the existence of a differential effect of local anesthetics on varying sizes of nerve fibers. Although zones of differential sensory block after neuraxial local anesthetics have been demonstrated in humans,[10–13] both in vivo and in vitro studies have produced conflicting results.[14,15] Differential blockade can be achieved with the following different techniques: (1) spinal, (2) epidural, and (3) peripheral somatic blocks. All three techniques commonly use 2% lidocaine, which results in motor, sensory, and sympathetic block. The block is then evaluated as it regresses to determine whether the pain correlates with the return of somatic sensory function or sympathetic function.

The use of placebo injections (i.e., saline) is controversial, and these injections should be used with caution in cancer patients. As many as one third of the patients will respond to placebo, and that does not necessarily mean that they do not have pain.[16] In addition, saline injected into trigger points has been reported to be as effective as local anesthetic injection.[17]

Prognosis

Before any permanent neurolytic procedure, it is recommended that a prognostic local anesthetic block of the nerve to be ablated be performed. An exception is for the terminally ill patient who incurs extreme inconvenience during performance of the block. An example is a patient with terminal pancreatic cancer and severe pain who may experience severe discomfort from positioning during the block. Many practitioners would proceed with the neurolytic block in this setting. If numbness and motor blockade are unlikely to result from the block (i.e., celiac plexus block), it is more acceptable to proceed with the permanent neurolytic block without a diagnostic block.

The purpose of prognostic blocks is to allow the patient to experience not only the pain relief that may result from the block but also the numbness and motor blockade that may be produced. The numbness and motor blockade may be more distressing to the patient than the pain itself.[18] Unfortunately, the prognostic value for long-term pain relief from a positive regional anesthesia result is not guaranteed.[19] However, a negative regional anesthesia result almost certainly predicts failure, a finding that supports the use of prognostic regional anesthesia before an ablative procedure is undertaken.

Therapy

Regional anesthesia is useful in the management of myofascial pain, sympathetically mediated pain, long-term treatments using catheter techniques and continuous delivery, and in crisis management of severe pain.

Reflex muscle spasms caused by tumor invasion of deep tissues can be debilitating. Some patients receive long-term benefit from trigger point injections of local anesthetics. If long-lasting benefit results, trigger point injections can be repeated at intervals of 1 to several weeks.[20] As tumors encroach on the nervous system, neural damage can result.[21] This neural damage can lead to complex regional pain syndromes that may be responsive to sympathetic blockade. It is known that the pain relief from such blockade can far outlast the duration of the local anesthetic.[22,23] In these cases, the sympathetic blockade can be repeated at intervals of 1 to several weeks. Whereas the use of sympathetic blockade in chronic benign pain is focused more to improve function, the use of this technique in cancer pain is focused more on pain control.

Continuous regional anesthesia can be achieved by placement of catheters at peripheral nerve sites, epidurally or intrathecally. The brachial plexus and lumbar plexus are the most common sites for placement of peripheral nerve catheters. A case report on long-term continuous axillary plexus blockade demonstrated no adverse effects for up to 16 days.[24] Other sites that can be cannulated include the intercostal nerve, celiac plexus, hypogastric plexus, stellate ganglion, and lumbar sympathetic ganglion.[25] The ease and low complication rate of epidural catheters favor this technique over peripheral nerve catheters for long-term management of localized pain (i.e., lower extremity, sacrum, upper extremity).[26] Even the long-term delivery of cervical epidural local anesthetics is safe, and studies have shown that high concentrations of local anesthetic do not result in phrenic nerve block.[27] Several studies have been conducted on the use of intrathecal local anesthetics in combination with opioids for the treatment of cancer pain,[28–32] with bupivacaine doses as high as 100 mg/day. It can be concluded from these studies that a sensory motor block does not occur at doses lower than 30 to 40 mg/day. In one case report on severe refractory cancer pain, the patient received daily intrathecal bupivacaine doses as high as 800 mg/day.[33]

Some cancer patients develop severe pain refractory to opioid analgesics, even at high doses. These patients can benefit from continuous techniques to give them respite from the debilitating pain and allow a drug holiday from the opioids. This approach may also provide pain control until palliative techniques such as chemotherapy, radiation therapy, and radionuclide therapy take effect.

Treatments of Cancer Pain with Glucocorticoid

Opioids are widely used in the management of cancer pain, but sufficient pain relief without side effects is sometimes difficult to obtain. Although intrathecal or epidural opioid injections may be a good option for cancer pain treatment, patients develop side effects similar to those seen with oral opioids, and a catheter must be implanted for continuous opioid injection.[34] Oral glucocorticoids are used palliatively for cancer pain treatment, especially in patients with bone metastases.[35] Small-dose betamethasone has been used intrathecally once a week. Sufficient pain relief was achieved in about a half of the patients, and no clinical complications were seen. Therefore, certain types of uncontrollable cancer pain can be better treated with intrathecal betamethasone, especially in patients with vertebral metastases whose pain is frequently difficult to control. In contrast to epidural procedures, the intrathecal technique is easy and safe to perform in the lumbar region. Therefore, the intrathecal injection of betamethasone has a technical advantage over other anesthetic procedures for the management of cancer pain.

Indications for Intraspinal Steroid Injections

When conventional treatments for cancer pain are not successful, intrathecal injection of small-dose betamethasone may be a useful approach, especially in patients with vertebral bone metastases. Intrathecal betamethasone may induce long-lasting analgesia without adverse effects. As a result, intrathecal betamethasone may be able to improve activities of daily living and quality of life in patients with cancer pain.

Invasion or compression of nerves by growing tumors is a common source of pain. It is thought that inflammation plays a major role in the production of pain.[36,37] However, other pain mechanisms responsive to the local application of steroids that have been postulated include weak local anesthetic action,[38] change in activity in dorsal horn cells,[39] and reduced ectopic discharge from neuromas.[40,41] The local instillation of steroid in the compartment of the affected neural structure (i.e., brachial plexus, lumbar plexus, intercostal nerve) can result in significant and prolonged pain relief. If the tumor invades the vertebral column and compresses nerve roots, epidural steroid injection (ESI) can be very helpful. Steroids that may be used locally or epidurally include methylprednisolone, triamcinolone, betamethasone, and dexamethasone.[42,43] Although not performed routinely, the intrathecal delivery of steroids has been used for lumbar radiculopathy. Concern exists about inducing arachnoiditis with this technique, but many reports failed to show any serious adverse events.[43–45] A comprehensive review by Abram and O'Connor[46] concluded that most cases of arachnoiditis following subarachnoid steroid injections occurred with multiple injections over a prolonged time period.

The list of indications is quite extensive and includes several well-described conditions such as lumbar or cervical radiculopathy, spinal stenosis, postlaminectomy syndrome, failed back syndrome, postherpetic neuralgia, complex regional pain syndrome, pelvic pain syndromes, phantom limb pain, and periaxial malignant disease and tumor invasion.[47] Conversely, the list of contraindications is relatively short and includes sepsis, local infection, anticoagulation or coagulopathy, and hypovolemia (relative contraindication).

White et al,[48] in a study of 304 patients, found that the response to ESI was most closely related to onset of symptoms, the presence of nerve root compression, and the lack of any associated psychological issues. Others investigators[49–53] identified some of the primary positive and negative predictive factors of the response to ESI. Factors associated with the patient's history that correlated with a favorable response to the procedure include the presence of radicular pain and radicular numbness, relatively short duration of symptoms (<6 months), advanced educational background, absence of previous back surgery, and young age. Findings on the physical examination or in diagnostic studies that correlated well with a positive response to ESI include the presence of dermatomal sensory loss, motor loss correlating with the involved nerve root, positive straight leg raise test, positive findings on electromyography involving the affected nerve root, and radiographic confirmation of a herniated disk affecting the suspected nerve root. Negative predictive factors that have been identified include pain duration of greater than 6 to 24 months, occupational injuries, previous back surgery, primarily axial pain, injury-related litigation, history and examination consistent with myofascial pain syndrome, and the so-called nonorganic physical signs (Waddell's signs).

The mechanism of action of epidural steroids also remains somewhat controversial. It is known, however, that the enzyme phospholipase A_2 is contained in relatively high concentrations within the nucleus pulposus of intervertebral disks.[54] This enzyme initiates the release of arachidonic acid from cell membranes and thus starts an enzymatic cascade that—in the presence of annular tears or severe degenerative disk disease—can cause chemical irritation (or radiculitis) of an adjacent nerve root. Steroids induce the synthesis of a phospholipase A_2 inhibitor that inhibits arachidonic acid metabolism one step earlier in the pathway when compared with nonsteroidal anti-inflammatory drugs. In addition, steroids have been shown to have an effect on local membrane depolarization. Johansson et al[55] demonstrated that local administration of methylprednisolone blocks the transmission of C fibers but not A-beta fibers. The effect was noted to be reversible, a finding that suggests a direct membrane action of the steroid.

The efficacy of ESI for back pain, neck pain, and radicular pain remains fairly controversial. This is partly because most of the literature has been hindered by poor study design or inconclusive data. Kepes and Duncalf[56] concluded, in 1985, that the role of steroids in this subgroup of patients was not warranted. However, their study included patients who were treated with both epidural and systemic steroids. Benzon[57] concluded, in a study of patients with lumbosacral radiculopathy who were treated only with ESI, that epidural steroids were effective in the treatment of patients with acute radiculopathy.

More recently, Koes et al[58] concluded that epidural steroids were not effective in patients with chronic back pain without evidence of ongoing radiculopathy; however, 50% of the patients in this review who had ongoing radiculopathy showed a positive response. These investigators reviewed all available randomized controlled trials published up to 1994 and determined that only four studies adhered to acceptable standards of quality, and only two of those studies supported the use of epidural steroids in the treatment of radicular pain.

In 1995, Watts and Silagy[59] performed a meta-analysis of the same data using odd ratios, with the goal of answering the question: "Do epidural steroids work?" In this meta-analysis, these investigators defined efficacy as at least 75% improvement for short-term (60 days) and long-term (1 year) outcomes. With an odds ratio greater than 1 suggestive of efficacy and greater than 2 suggestive of significant efficacy, these investigators determined that ESI had an odds ratio of 2.61 for short-term outcomes and 1.87 for long-term outcomes. This meta-analysis provided quantitative evidence of the efficacy of epidural steroids in the management of radicular pain.

In 1998, McQuay and Moore[60] sought the answer to the question: "How well do epidural steroids work?" These investigators used the same data as Watts and Silagy, in addition to the work of Carette et al,[61] and they used the used the number needed to treat (NNT) as the measure of clinical benefit. In the short-term outcomes group, the NNT was 7. In other words, to achieve a goal of 75% improvement in pain in 1 patient, the clinician would have to treat 7 patients with ESI. However, when a more reasonable goal of 50% improvement in pain was the standard, the NNT was slightly less than 3. In the long-term group, the NNT corresponding to 50% improvement at 12 months was 13. The investigators also noted no difference in the functional level or the need for subsequent surgery in these patients after receiving the injections. These data seem to indicate a significant short-term improvement in leg pain, but minimal improvement in back pain or function, after ESI for radiculopathy.

Relatively few long-term follow-up studies are available in the literature with regard to ESIs. Most patients report a diminished effect after 120 days. However, Dilke et al[62] reported 36% with complete relief and 55% with partial relief at 3 months. Ridley et al[63] noted that 65% of their patients reported sustained relief at 6 months. At 1 year, Green et al[64] reported that 41% of their patients experienced sustained relief, whereas White et al[48] reported persistent improvement after 6 months in 34% of patients with acute pain, but in only 12% of patients with chronic pain. In this study, White et al also concluded that ESIs are most appropriately used in the presence of root compression, root irritation, or annular tears. ESIs are least effective when given for chronic degenerative disk disease, herniated disks without neurologic deficit, spinal stenosis, and functional low back pain.

The response time to epidural steroids is between 4 and 6 days in most patients (59%), but many other patients (37%) experience an earlier effect, and a few patients (4%) respond after 6 day.[23] Therefore, it is advisable to allow at least 7 days between each injection. The decision to proceed with another ESI after the initial one is usually based on the results of the first injection. A positive response to the initial injection—usually measured by a subjective claim by the patient of 50% reduction in pain—is considered a good indication that the patient will receive further benefit from additional injections. Brown[65] demonstrated that no further benefit to the patient generally occurs after three injections. Duration of pain or onset of symptoms has also been positively correlated with the response to ES1s.[66-68] Patients with symptoms lasting than 3 months have response rates of 83% to 100%. Those with symptoms lasting up to 6 months have a response rate of 67% to 81%, and the response rate is 44% to 69% in patients with symptoms for more than 6 months.

The preponderance of the literature supports the use of ESIs as another treatment modality in the comprehensive management of patients with chronic back and neck pain. Some controversy exists over the mandatory use of fluoroscopy, mainly because of the less than 100% certainty of epidural steroid placement as a result of intravascular or other extraepidural location of the needle or catheter tip.[69,70] The absolute efficacy depends on the diagnosis and amount of pain relief deemed "successful." ESIs are particularly beneficial in patients with signs of acute or ongoing radiculopathy. These injections play a vital role in the armamentarium of the pain management specialist.

Use of Betamethasone as an Intrathecal Glucocorticoid

Betamethasone was injected in the intrathecal space one to four times in one study during the 4-week study period, depending on the patient's physical and mental condition. In four patients with bone metastasis in the lumbar vertebrae, the intrathecal approach was chosen to avoid the metastatic region.[71]

The intrathecal use of glucocorticoid may be effective for the treatment of inflammatory or neurologic injury associated pain in the spinal cord and roots because this technique has an inhibitory action on prostaglandins and other algogenic substances. However, adverse effects related to neurotoxicity of intrathecal glucocorticoid have been reported.[72] In a previous study, investigators reported that intrathecal betamethasone produced long-lasting analgesia without any adverse effects in patients with advanced pelvic and perineal cancer.[73] Intrathecal injection of glucocorticoid may alleviate intractable pain caused by inflammation and sensitization without the development of neurotoxicity in the spinal cord and nerve roots, when the injection consists of a small dose of glucocorticoid that includes relatively safe preservatives.

One can choose betamethasone as the glucocorticoid for intrathecal injection because of its water solubility, the presence of small-dose additives in the solution, its safety in animal studies, and the fact that the intrathecal use of betamethasone is recommended by the drug manufacturer for meningeal leukemia, cerebrospinal meningitis, and malignant lymphoma.

Safety of Intrathecal Glucocorticoid

Several arguments have been put forth concerning the safety of intrathecal injection of steroids. Complications such as arachnoiditis and meningitis have been reported.[74] Nelson and Landau[75] argued that the intrathecal administration of glucocorticoids is unsafe and indicated that intrathecal glucocorticoids could lead to the development of neurotoxicity in the spinal cord and meninges. However, the safety of intrathecal glucocorticoids has been advocated in some clinical and experimental studies. In the clinical study by Kotani et al,[76] no complications were reported in 89 patients with postherpetic neuralgia who received four doses of intrathecal methylprednisolone acetate (60 mg) containing propylene glycol. Langmayr et al[77] indicated that, after lumbar disk surgery, intrathecal betamethasone provided significant pain reduction without any disadvantageous effects.

Latham et al[78] showed in sheep that repeated intrathecal administration of 5.7 mg (1 mL) betamethasone containing benzalkonium chloride did not result in pathologic changes. However, large doses of betamethasone, such as 11.4 mg (2 mL) and more, were associated with dose-dependent neurotoxicity. Furthermore, investigators found that intrathecal triamcinolone diacetate containing polyethylene glycol did not induce spinal neurotoxicity in a rat model.[79] It is believed that the chemicals responsible for neurotoxicity when glucocorticoids are administered intrathecally are not the glucocorticoids themselves, but the additives such as antioxidants, preservatives, and excipients that are present in the injected solution.[80]

Analgesic Effects of Intrathecal Glucocorticoid

Glucocorticoids have multipurpose use and offer symptomatic relief in the management of patients with cancer pain. Principally, the analgesic effect of glucocorticoids is assumed to occur in inflammatory conditions. The analgesic effects of intrathecal steroids have been observed in both human and animal studies.[77,78,81] In patients with postherpetic neuralgia, the intrathecal injection of methylprednisolone with lidocaine induced excellent and long-lasting analgesia for burning pain, lancinating pain, and allodynia.

It is thought that the long-lasting analgesia that results from the intrathecal injection of betamethasone is achieved through a decrease in the inflammatory reactions in the injured nerves and a reduction in algogenic substances such as prostaglandins, glutamate, and substance P in the spinal cord. The suppression of spinal glial activation and the inhibition of inflammatory cells and cytokines may accelerate the analgesic effects.[82,83] Almost all of 10 patients studied showed an immediate analgesic effect within 30 minutes, which was followed by long-lasting analgesia; this finding was similar to the first observation in the previous 3 patients reported. The effects of steroids are not expected to be immediate because the changes in gene expression and synthesis of proteins take several hours.[84]

In the traditional theory of steroid action, steroids bind to intracellular receptors and modulate nuclear transcription. Anti-inflammatory effects of glucocorticoids are induced by the inhibition of phospholipase A_2 resulting from lipocortin production through fundamental steroid pharmacology. However, this mechanism for the analgesic effect of intrathecal glucocorticoid does not explain the immediate analgesia that was seen in patients studied. This rapid effect may be transmitted by specific membrane-bound receptors.[85,86] Although a relationship between immediate and long-lasting analgesia is unknown, all the patients with long-lasting analgesia had immediate analgesia after the first intrathecal betamethasone treatment. Given these findings, the mechanism of the analgesic effects of intrathecal glucocorticoid should be studied in greater depth in the future.

Acknowledgment

Portions of this chapter were adapted from Wallace MS, Leung AY, McBeth MD: Malignant pain; and Bender JB, Lord EAR, Burton AW: Outcomes using procedures for nociceptive pain. In Raj PP, editor: *Textbook of regional anesthesia*, Philadelphia, 2002, Churchill Livingstone, 2002, with permission; and from Taguchi H, Oishi K, Sakamoto S, et al: Intrathecal betamethasone for cancer pain in the lower half of the body: a study of its analgesic efficacy and safety, *Br J Anaesth* 98(3):385–389, 2007.

References

Full references for this chapter can be found on www.expertconsult.com.

Chapter **36**

Neural Blockade with Neurolytic Agents in the Management of Cancer Pain

Erin F. Lawson and Mark S. Wallace

Background and History

Neural blockade with neurolytic agents has been documented for the treatment of pain for more than a century. In 1904, Schloesser was the first to report alcohol neurolysis for the treatment of trigeminal neuralgia.[1,2] White, in 1935, applied alcohol neurolysis to the upper thoracic ganglia for the treatment of angina pain.[3] Doppler used phenol neurolysis to destroy presacral sympathetic nerves for treatment of pelvic pain in 1926.[3] In 1947, Mandl also studied phenol, for cervical ganglion neurolysis.[3] Today, the role of neurolytic agents is well established in the approach to cancer pain. Blocking neuronal transmission has the potential to relieve otherwise refractory cancer pain. However, because all currently available neurolytic agents have the potential for adverse outcomes, the use of these agents is controversial in nonmalignant or nonterminal pain.

Patient Selection

Neurolytic agents are employed to produce long-lasting pain relief through disabling or destroying nerves. Because of the potential for morbidity, neurolytic agents are selected after noninvasive and less invasive therapies have failed. Classically, these agents are used in the setting of malignant pain when life expectancy is short. This indication is the focus of this chapter. Pain is frequently inadequately controlled in cancer patients,[4] a situation leading to unnecessary suffering, physical debilitation, psychological deterioration, and avoidance of treatment. Cancer pain management has been identified as an international priority focus for improvement by the World Health Organization (WHO).[5] The WHO analgesic ladder usually establishes effective pain management for cancer patients with a less invasive approach, but neurolytic procedures are required in 29% of patients.[6] Although the approach may be more controversial, patients without cancer but with certain chronic pain conditions are also potential candidates for neurolysis. For example, some pain physicians advocate for sympathetic neurolysis for patients with complex regional pain syndrome.[7]

Newer approaches such as pulsed radiofrequency ablation have widened the potential pool of candidates for denervation because of the decreased risk of permanent neurologic sequelae. For use of traditional nonselective neurolytic agents, however, a conservative approach continues to prevail. The use of chemical neurolytic blocks for chronic nonmalignant pain is controversial and is not recommended. Furthermore, it is critical that only experienced and skilled persons who are equipped to treat immediate effects perform these blocks.[8] Finally, radiographic guidance is recommended when appropriate.

Locations and Applications

Neurolysis is used to provide pain relief by interrupting pain transmission. It can therefore theoretically be applied anywhere along the sensory pathway. Peripheral nerves, sympathetic ganglia, and dorsal roots are all examples of potential targets for neurolysis. Peripheral nerve neurolysis is effective for painful symptoms limited to a single nerve distribution. Because most peripheral nerves are mixed, peripheral neurolysis carries a high risk of motor block as well.[7] It is important to perform a prognostic block with local anesthetic first, to assess efficacy.

Table 36.1 An Overview of Neurolytic Agents

Agent	Strength (%)	Unique Property	Negative Properties	Systemic Toxicity
Alcohol	50–100	Hypobaric, fast onset	Painful on injection, risk of neuritis (peripheral nerves)	Disulfiram-like reaction
Phenol	4–15	Hyperbaric, painless, slow onset	Shorter-lived, affinity for vasculature	Convulsions, cardiovascular collapse
Glycerol	50	Historically applied to gasserian ganglion for treatment of trigeminal neuralgia	Inability to control the spread	Severe headache or local dysesthesia
Capsaicin	8	Nociceptor selective, topical	Painful application, used only for localized neuropathic pain	
Ammonium salts	10	Sensory fiber selective, motor intact, lack of postblock neuritis	Nausea and vomiting, headache, and paresthesia	Nausea and vomiting, headache, and paresthesia

The local anesthetic block determines the appropriateness of the location of the block and also provides the patient with an opportunity to evaluate the effect with a short term block. If the patient is uncomfortable with the numb sensation or motor weakness, a neurolytic block is not indicated.

Sympathetic blocks are generally indicated for treatment of painful symptoms that are not confined to a dermatomal distribution, pain resulting from damage of peripheral nerve branches, pain caused or maintained by increased sympathetic tone, or pain produced by circulatory disturbances. Stellate ganglion neurolysis is appropriate for upper extremity and possibly facial pain. Celiac plexus neurolysis is indicated for pain of the upper abdominal viscera. Lumbar plexus neurolysis targets pain in the lower extremity. Superior hypogastric plexus neurolysis targets lower abdominal or pelvic visceral pain. Finally, ganglion impar neurolysis treats sympathetically maintained perineal pain.

Intrathecal neurolysis or rhizolysis of the dorsal root provides a sensory block without a motor block. Positioning is of the utmost importance. Thus, selection of neurolytic agent (hypobaric versus hyperbaric) and patient cooperation are critical. Epidural neurolysis may also be chosen to treat pain in the upper abdominal wall, thorax, or upper extremity. Because positioning is less critical, this approach may be an option when positioning for subarachnoid neurolysis is difficult.

Neurolytic Agents

Table 36.1 provides an overview of the neurolytic agents commonly used in clinical practice, and **Table 36.2** summarizes the clinical indications for each agent. An understanding of the unique properties of each agent is crucial to optimize success and minimize complications.

Phenol
Mechanism of Action

Phenol causes nonselective tissue destruction by coagulating proteins.[9] Phenol denatures axonal proteins and initiates wallerian degeneration. Intrathecal administration of phenol causes degeneration of large and small nerve fibers within the nerve roots but not the ganglia or spinal cord.[10] Regeneration following phenol neurolysis is faster than regeneration following alcohol and is complete in approximately 14 weeks.[11]

Dosing

Concentrations lower than 1% to 2% act as a local anesthetic. Concentrations higher than 5% are required for neurolysis.[12] The highest concentration possible in water or saline is approximately 6.67%. Higher concentrations require a mixture in glycerin. Phenol may also be mixed with radiopaque dye for injection.

Application and Clinical Pearls

Phenol is toxic to vasculature, to which it has an affinity.[9] Therefore, this agent is controversial for celiac plexus neurolysis or use in other highly vascular locations. Phenol is not painful on injection and produces a milder blockade compared with alcohol. Phenol neurolysis generally lasts for several months.[12] Because phenol is hyperbaric compared with cerebrospinal fluid (especially when mixed with glycerol), patients must be positioned with the painful side down during intrathecal injection, to coat the dorsal roots. Phenol diffuses out of glycerin slowly and allows for patient positioning following injection. In addition, because of the high viscosity of glycerin, at least a 20-gauge needle is required.

Alcohol
Mechanism of Action

Alcohol destroys nerve function by inducing local wallerian degeneration when the agent is applied to peripheral nerves.[13] Subarachnoid application causes wallerian degeneration and demyelination and degeneration in the dorsal roots, posterior columns, and dorsolateral tract of Lissauer secondary to direct contact.[14] Attempts at neuronal regeneration in peripheral nerves and spinal cord are observed 1 to 3 months following neurolysis.[14]

Dosing

Alcohol is available in the United States in a 95% concentration in 5-mL vials. At concentrations of up to 33% applied to peripheral nerves, alcohol destroys sensory nerves without injury to motor nerves and provides analgesia without paralysis.[11] At doses higher than 33% applied to peripheral nerves, alcohol may cause paralysis. For intrathecal neurolysis, concentrations between 50% and 100% are typically used. Forty percent alcohol is equipotent to 3% to 5% phenol.[11]

Table 36.2 Use of Neurolytic Agents for Neural Blockade*

Procedure	Indication	Agent/Strength/Volume	Unique Issues	Side Effect and Complications
Sphenopalatine ganglion block	Trigeminal neuralgia, posttraumatic headache, cluster headache, migraine headache, sphenopalatine neuralgia, atypical facial pain	Phenol 6% <1 mL	Various techniques described	Hematoma if the maxillary artery punctured, hypesthesia and numbness of the palate, maxilla, or posterior pharynx
Stellate ganglion block	Cancer pain, upper extremity CRPS, postherpetic neuralgia, phantom pain, cluster headache	Phenol 6% 1–2 mL; absolute alcohol <1.5 mL		Erosion, thrombosis, or spasm of major blood vessels; cerebral infarction, prolonged hoarseness, brachial plexus injury
Thoracic sympathetic blocks	Cancer pain, CRPS upper extremity, peripheral neuropathy, brachial plexalgia, vascular disorders	Phenol 6%–10% 2–5 mL		Neuraxial injection, intravascular injection, nerve injury, PTX
Celiac plexus block	Pain of upper abdominal viscera	Alcohol 50% 10 mL each side for retrocrural, transcrural, or splanchnic approach		Diarrhea, hypotension, sexual dysfunction, paraplegia, PTX, bowel injury, bleeding
Lumbar sympathetic block	Lower extremity CRPS, peripheral neuropathy	Phenol 6%–10% 5 mL each side		Bleeding, nerve root injury, genitofemoral neuritis, paralysis, neuraxial injection, renal puncture or trauma
Superior hypogastric plexus block	Pelvic visceral pain	Phenol 10% 8–10 mL		Intravascular injection, neuraxial injection, discitis, urinary injury, bladder/bowel incontinence
Ganglion impar block	Vulvar cancer pain, chronic perineal pain, sacral postherpetic neuralgia	Phenol 10% 2–6 mL		Rectal trauma
Subarachnoid block	Well-localized unilateral pain limited to a few dermatomes	Absolute alcohol or phenol 6% in glycerin ≤1 mL	Alcohol is hypobaric; phenol is hyperbaric; positioning less critical	Painful setup, coagulum with CSF (do not aspirate CSF before injection), bowel/bladder incontinence, lower extremity weakness
Epidural block	Well-localized bilateral pain limited to a few dermatomes	Absolute alcohol, injected in 0.1–0.2 mL increments; phenol 10% in glycerol volume 1.5 mL/dermatome, up to 10mL	Less predictable spread than with intrathecal route	Motor block, numbness, neuritis, deafferentation pain
Peripheral nerves	Well-localized somatic pain	Absolute alcohol 1–2 mL; phenol 6%–12% aqueous 1–2 mL		Neuritis, motor weakness
Cranial nerves		Phenol 6%–12%; aqueous 1 mL	CT guidance or use of digital subtraction fluoroscopy recommended	Neuritis

*The strengths and volumes of the neurolytic agents shown here are not supported by scientific literature but are based only on clinical experience. This table is intended for example only and should be interpreted for use by experienced clinicians.
CRPS, complex regional pain syndrome; CSF, cerebrospinal fluid; CT, computed tomography; PTX, pneumothorax.
Data from Day M: Sympathetic blocks: the evidence, *Pain Pract* 8:98–109, 2008; Finch PM: Sympathetic neurolysis. In Raj PP, editor, *Textbook of regional anesthesia*. Philadelphia, 2002, Chruchill Livingstone; Patt RB: *Cancer pain*, Philadelphia, 1993, Lippincott; Wong GY, Carns PE: Neurolytic celiac plexus block. In deLeon-Casasola O, editor, *Cancer pain: pharmacological, interventional and palliative care approaches*, Philadelphia, 2006, Saunders.

Application and Clinical Pearls

Alcohol rapidly spreads from the injection site and thus requires larger volumes. Moreover, because alcohol is also easily absorbed into the bloodstream, blood alcohol levels increase following injection.[15] Peak blood alcohol levels are usually lower than the legal limit for driving unless accidental intravascular injection has occurred. Alcohol is hypobaric compared with cerebrospinal fluid. During intrathecal neurolysis, the patient must be positioned with the painful side up, to coat the appropriate dorsal roots. Because alcohol is painful on injection, local anesthetic injection is needed before peripheral nerve blocks are performed. However, intrathecal neurolysis with alcohol is generally well tolerated, with transient mild burning. Alcohol is toxic to vasculature and connective tissue, and it causes vasospasm and necrosis, respectively. Accidental intravascular injection may cause thrombosis.[9] Therefore, small volumes should be used, and the needle should be flushed with sterile saline before it is withdrawn.[11]

Glycerol

The mechanism of action of glycerol is unclear, but the agent appears to cause wallerian degeneration following intraneuronal injection.[11] Glycerol is most commonly used to treat trigeminal neuralgia and is rarely used to treat cancer pain. However, radiofrequency lesioning for this syndrome is gaining favor over the use of glycerol. A concentration of 100% is typically used for neurolysis.

Ammonium Compounds

Ammonium sulfate 10% has been used successfully to treat intercostal neuralgia without causing painful postprocedure neuritis.[16] Intrafascicular injection was shown to be less neurotoxic than phenol 5% and to spare motor function in animal models.[17,18] Complications such as nausea and vomiting, headache, and paresthesia led to the abandonment of the clinical use of ammonium salts.[19]

Hypertonic Solutions

Hypertonic saline (10% sodium chloride) has been used in percutaneous epidural neuroplasty for the treatment of radiculopathy and low back pain. Intrathecal hypertonic saline (10% to 15%) has been shown to decrease pain by 50% in cancer patients for up to 3 months.[20] However, serious complications have been reported from the use of hypertonic saline, including death.[21]

Vanilloids

Capsaicin, the active ingredient in hot chili peppers, and resiniferatoxin (RTX) are vanilloids that ultimately desensitize certain pain fibers. These vanilloids activate the transient receptor potential vanilloid 1 (TRPV1) receptor on unmyelinated C-fiber nociceptors and cause it to open. The following influx of calcium and sodium ions depolarizes the nociceptive afferent terminals and leads to pain signaling and subsequent desensitization.[22] After C-fiber depolarization by capsaicin or RTX, these nociceptors release stored neuropeptides and are then desensitized. Capsaicin and RTX cause early desensitization of nociceptors by inducing a conduction block and delayed desensitization by down-regulating TRPV1 receptors.[23] TRPV1 receptors have been identified in visceral organs, spinal cord, and dorsal root ganglion.[23] Because this agent is selective for nociceptors, its application in chronic nonmalignant pain is widely accepted.

Speed of onset and duration of analgesia depend on dose, duration, and frequency of exposure.[24] The topical application of low-dose capsaicin (<1%) as an adjunct to the treatment of postherpetic neuralgia, postmastectomy pain, and diabetic neuropathy is well established.[25] However, this technique provides only temporary relief. NGX-4010, a high-concentration (8%) capsaicin patch, is a new approach that has proven effective in the treatment of distal sensory polyneuropathy associated with human immunodeficiency virus infection[26,27]

and postherpetic neuralgia.[28] This treatment involves one 60-minute application of high-dose capsaicin and requires topical and or oral analgesics for tolerance; it provides pain relief for up to 12 weeks.[28] Intrathecal RTX has been shown to reduce pain in a canine model of bone cancer.[29] Phase I clinical trials in cancer patients will start soon.

Clostridial Neurotoxin

Botulinum toxin is neurotoxic to cholinergic nerves by inhibiting striated and smooth muscle contraction. Botulinum toxin (BTX) has seven serotypes (A to G) that consist of a heavy chain bound to a light chain by a disulfide bond.[30] The toxin heavy chain first binds to the nerve terminal and facilitates internalization of the light chain, which then internally interferes with neurotransmitter vesicle docking on the plasma membrane required for release.[30] The vesicular docking is mediated by the soluble N-ethylmaleimide–sensitive factor attachment protein receptor (SNARE) complex, which is the target for the BTX light chain. Normal nerve terminal function that eventually recovers following BTX occurs by restoration of the SNARE complex.[31] BTX is too large to penetrate the blood-brain barrier and is inactivated by retrograde axonal transport; therefore, it has no direct central nervous system effect.[31]

BTX effectively inhibits muscle contraction by blocking presynaptic acetylcholine release from nerve terminals. By the same effect, BTX may be used on the autonomic nervous system to alleviate hyperhidrosis, hypersalivation, or hyperlacrimation.[31] Botulinum toxin A has also been shown to have analgesic properties by inhibiting release of calcitonin gene–related peptide from afferent nerve terminals,[32] substance P from dorsal root ganglia, and glutamate in the dorsal horn.[31] BTX treatment is effective in the treatment of painful muscle spasticity and myofascial pain. In cancer patients, BTX has been shown to improve symptoms of radiation fibrosis syndrome.[33] Its effect on neuropathic pain is also potentially useful for painful cancer conditions.[34]

Clinical Approach

Currently, three BTX products are approved for use in the United States: onabotulinumtoxinA (Botox/Botox Cosmetic), abobotulinumtoxinA (Dysport), and rimabotulinumtoxinB (Myobloc). Dosage units differ among the BTX products and are not comparable or convertible.[35] BTX may be diluted in local anesthetic or sterile saline, and optimal dilutions have not been established for treatment of pain. BTX is injected into striated muscle in increments of units. Paresis develops within 5 days and lasts several months. Therapy failure occurs secondary to the development of antibodies against BTX and is characterized by a spectrum from smaller effect and shorter duration to no effect.[31]

Complications include local effects such as muscle atrophy, dysphagia, dysphonia, and ptosis, depending on the site of injection. Systemic adverse reactions to BTX-A and BTX-B including dyspnea, respiratory compromise, weakness, and death have mostly occurred in children treated for spasticity associated with cerebral palsy. Serious systemic complications have been reported between 1 day and several weeks following treatment.[36]

Limitations

Following neurolysis, the nerves typically regenerate over time, with return of pain. Nerves may regrow unpredictably and may form neuromas. In such cases, not only does pain return, but also it is often worse than the initial pain experience. However, with terminal cancer pain, onset of this complication often exceeds the life expectancy of the patient. Therefore, the life expectancy of the patient should be considered when neurolytic procedures are performed for pain management. Furthermore, neurolysis does not necessarily provide complete neuronal blockade. The neurolytic block often clinically provides less analgesia than the local anesthetic block.[9]

Complications

Complications arise from all aspects of the procedure. Complications at the needle entry site include infection, bleeding, perforation of a viscus or organ, pneumothorax, unintentional subarachnoid or epidural injection, vascular laceration or injection, and peripheral nerve trauma. Complications of sympathectomy, especially with celiac plexus block, include hypotension, which may be severe and prolonged, diarrhea, and sexual dysfunction. Because these agents are nonselective, potentially catastrophic complications are possible.

Complications of the neurolytic agent include motor block, paraplegia, neuropathic pain and dysesthesias, skin ulceration, soft tissue and muscle injury, phlebitis, thrombosis, and tissue ischemia.[9] Motor block is common and even expected with peripheral or neuraxial neurolysis because of the nonselective nature of most neurolytic agents. However, weakness and paraplegia may also occur during sympathetic blocks secondary to vascular injury. Bowel or urinary incontinence is possible following intrathecal neurolysis.[14] Although less devastating, neuralgias, hypesthesia, and anesthesia following neurolysis may be very distressing to patients expecting relief of suffering. These complications are more common following traditional neurolytic agents such as alcohol.

Future Considerations

Neurolysis for the treatment of refractory cancer pain continues to be an effective option. However, given the nonspecificity and complications associated with currently available agents, further research in the area is needed. Intrathecal RTX holds the greatest promise because of the high specificity for the unmyelinated C fibers that transmit pain. However, a side effect of this therapy may be an inability to detect thermal pain that could lead to thermal injuries. Therefore, patients require close observation and counseling on this risk.

References

Full references for this chapter can be found on www.expertconsult.com.

The Role of Spinal Opioids in the Management of Cancer Pain

Steven D. Waldman

Spinal opioids were first administered in humans in the late 1970s to palliate cancer pain that was unrelieved by all traditional treatments.[1] The choice of cancer pain as a first proving ground for this exciting new treatment derived from the favorable risk-to-benefit ratio in these terminally ill patients who had intractable cancer pain, as well as from the frustration born of the inability to control cancer pain in such patients without the use of invasive neurodestructive procedures.

The initial positive results of these early clinical trials led to rapid and widespread acceptance of spinal opioids as a treatment for cancer pain. As a result, spinal opioids have dramatically influenced the way intractable pain of malignant origin is managed. The continued decline in the number of neurodestructive procedures performed to palliate cancer pain attests to this fact.[2]

Etiology of Cancer Pain

To evaluate and treat the cancer pain patient adequately, it is helpful to delineate the specific pathophysiologic processes responsible for the pain. Precise evaluation allows the development of a rational treatment plan.

More than two thirds of cases of cancer pain result from direct tumor involvement of pain-sensitive structures.[3] Bone pain, which is probably related to disruption of the sensitive periosteum, is most common, followed by neuropathic pain caused by invasion of neural structures and visceral pain caused by obstruction of hollow viscus. Pain also may be a side effect of cancer treatment, including surgery, chemotherapy, and radiation therapy; 10% of patients have pain that is unrelated to the cancer or its treatment.[4] Failure to recognize this last group can lead to the use of inappropriate treatment modalities.

Designing a Treatment Plan for Cancer Pain

Primary Cancer Treatments

When the pathophysiologic mechanism of the patient's pain is determined, an appropriate pain treatment plan can be designed. One should first determine whether any primary antineoplastic therapies are available and are likely to provide long-lasting pain relief.[5] Hormonal treatments for prostate and breast cancer and radiation therapy for bony metastatic disease fall into this category, as does surgical decompression of a bowel obstruction or laminectomy for spinal tumor. If the possibility of primary antineoplastic therapy exists, pain treatment should be approached as in the patient with acute pain. Analgesic therapy in this setting should be flexible and easily withdrawn, to allow the opportunity for rapid adjustment should the primary antineoplastic therapy prove to have analgesic consequences. If palliation of cancer pain by primary treatment modalities is impossible or if these efforts are ineffective, the implementation of analgesic treatments need not be constrained by the requirement of easy reversibility.

Pharmacologic Treatments

The World Health Organization (WHO) estimates that every day at least 3.5 million people worldwide have cancer pain.[6] Numerous reports have indicated that cancer pain is inadequately treated in many of these patients.[7] In an effort to provide a systematic approach to the pharmacologic treatment of cancer pain, the WHO Cancer Pain Relief Program developed an "analgesic ladder" to guide the selection of pharmacotherapy for cancer pain (**Fig. 37.1**).[6]

According to this approach, cancer patients with mild pain should first be administered simple nonopioid analgesics, such as aspirin, acetaminophen, or other nonsteroidal anti-inflammatory agents. Adjuvant drugs, such as tricyclic antidepressants and antiemetics, are added to provide additional analgesic effects or palliation of other symptoms. Patients who fail to achieve adequate relief with these drugs or who present with moderate cancer pain should be treated with a "weak" narcotic analgesic, such as codeine and tramadol, with or without adjuvant analgesics. A nonopioid analgesic also should be given, and adjuvants are added as needed. Virtually all patients require a laxative. Finally, patients who fail to attain pain relief with these drugs or who present with severe pain should be administered a "strong" narcotic agonist, such as morphine, with or without adjuvant analgesics. Opioids have no ceiling effect, and doses should be titrated upward until analgesia occurs or intolerable and unmanageable side effects are noted.[5]

Studies have suggested that if the first three steps of the therapeutic ladder are used appropriately, pain relief can be expected in at least 70% of patients with cancer pain.[8] Pitfalls in the use of the therapeutic ladder involve failure to individualize treatment, failure to use appropriate routes of administration, failure to anticipate side effects, and failure to progress rapidly up the pain ladder to control acute pain breakthrough aggressively.

Neural Blockade

For the 30% of patients who do not obtain relief with the routine implementation of the analgesic ladder, a trial of neural blockade with local anesthetics alone or combined with long-acting steroids (corticosteroids such as methylprednisolone)

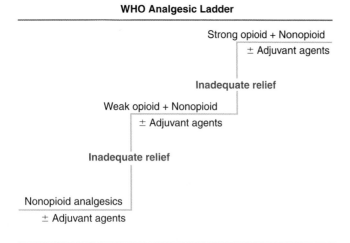

WHO Analgesic Ladder

Strong opioid + Nonopioid
± Adjuvant agents

Inadequate relief

Weak opioid + Nonopioid
± Adjuvant agents

Inadequate relief

Nonopioid analgesics
± Adjuvant agents

Fig. 37.1 **World Health Organization analgesic ladder.** *(From Zech DF, Grond S, Lynch J, et al: Validation of World Health Organization guidelines for cancer pain relief: a 10-year prospective study, Pain 63:65, 1995.)*

may be indicated.[9] Neural blockade should not be viewed as a stand-alone treatment for cancer pain, but it should be intelligently integrated into the therapeutic ladder. Patients with acute pain from a pathologic rib fracture may undergo intercostal nerve block simultaneously with implementation of opioid therapy.[10] Other acute pain problems amenable to neural blockade include acute vertebral compression fractures, post-thoracotomy or postlaparotomy pain, painful chest and nephrostomy tubes, painful biliary drainage catheters, and acute herpes zoster.[11] Neural blockade also may provide pain relief during painful procedures, such as biopsies and interventional radiology procedures.

Many cancer pain syndromes are mediated at least in part by the sympathetic nervous system.[9] Acute cancer pain syndromes that may benefit from interruption of the sympathetic nervous system by neural blockade with local anesthetics include postmastectomy upper extremity pain, biliary and ureteral colic, pancreatitis, acute herpes zoster, and vascular insufficiency.[11,12]

Spinal Opioids
Indications

Similar to neural blockade, spinal opioid administration must be integrated into a comprehensive pain treatment plan. In contrast to local anesthetics, spinal opioids produce effects through activation of opioid receptors in the spinal cord[13] and do not compromise sympathetic or motor function. Spinal opioids may be useful in many situations not otherwise amenable to neural blockade.[14]

Spinal opioids may be useful acutely as a palliative measure in patients receiving primary antineoplastic treatments expected to provide long-term relief of pain. They may be used transiently to allow patients with severe movement-related pain to undergo diagnostic or therapeutic procedures.[2] Finally, short-term administration of spinal opioids may be useful for aggressive treatment of "pain emergencies" that cannot be quickly controlled with other cancer pain treatment modalities.

Long-term administration of spinal opioid should not be implemented until the approach outlined in the analgesic ladder proves unable to control the pain. This recommendation recognizes that these more traditional treatments have a more favorable risk-to-benefit ratio than do spinal opioids.

Patient Selection

Proper patient selection is crucial if spinal opioids are to be used successfully to treat cancer pain.[15] Factors to be considered include the following: physiologic and behavioral abnormalities that may interfere with the patient's ability to assess pain relief; the presence of coagulopathy or infection, which may preclude the injection of spinal opioids; and the adequacy of the support system necessary to obtain, prepare, and administer spinal opioids.[2,15]

Choice of Drug

The choice of the specific opioid to be administered is based on an analysis of three variables: (1) onset of action, (2) duration of action, and (3) side effect profile. Although onset of action may be of paramount importance in the patient with acute pain, it is of little importance when choosing a spinal opioid for the treatment of chronic cancer pain. In general, the onset of analgesia correlates with the lipophilicity of the opioid.[16] Duration of action has a direct bearing on the mode of administration (bolus versus continuous infusion) required to obtain around-the-clock pain relief. Factors that may determine the duration of action of spinal opioids include lipophilicity, receptor affinity, intrinsic agonist activity of the opioid, rate of disassociation from spinal cord binding sites, and removal of the opioid through the circulation of the spinal cord.[17] Although generalizations can be made regarding the side effect profile of each spinal opioid, significant patient-to-patient variability exists. To use spinal opioids successfully, the clinician must anticipate and treat side effects aggressively (see later).

Route of Administration

Epidural and subarachnoid routes for administration of spinal opioids to cancer patients have advantages and disadvantages.[2] An important factor in selecting the route of administration is the technical expertise of the anesthesiologist in identifying the epidural space. When technical expertise is lacking, the subarachnoid route is preferred.

SUBARACHNOID ROUTE

The subarachnoid route bypasses the dura and deposits the opioid in close proximity to receptors in the spinal cord.[18] This deposition results in a faster onset and a longer duration of action, but also a higher incidence of centrally mediated side effects. Because the dura must be punctured to inject the opioid, the risk of post–dural puncture headache exists. If infection occurs, meningitis rather than epidural abscess will result.

EPIDURAL ROUTE

The major advantage of the epidural route of administration is the ability to place the opioid at any dermatomal level.[2,15] This ability has proved especially useful in the treatment of upper body pain, such as that caused by superior sulcus lung tumors.[19] The epidural route is not associated with post–dural puncture headache, and if infection occurs, epidural abscess rather than meningitis will result. Because higher doses of opioid are necessary to obtain analgesia, a slightly greater incidence of systemic side effects, such as hives and bronchospasm, may be seen with epidural administration.[2,14]

Dosage

As a general rule, the dosage of epidurally administered opioid equianalgesic to the subarachnoid dosage approximates a ratio of 10:1.[16] The initial epidural dose of morphine administered in the lumbar region is approximately 5 mg, whereas the subarachnoid dose is approximately 0.5 mg. **Table 37.1** provides recommended starting doses of commonly used spinally administered opioids for the relatively nontolerant patient. Because most patients with cancer pain have a variable degree of opioid tolerance (related to the dose and duration of prior opioid intake), these doses may be too low to initiate therapy in an individual patient. The increase in the starting dose is empirical, based on the judgment of the clinician that the patient is tolerant to the agent. The development of guidelines for the selection of the dose has been hampered by the lack of studies to determine the relative potency of spinal opioids compared with opioids administered by other routes.

Intermittent Bolus versus Continuous Infusion

The duration of action of spinally administered opioids should be the major determinant of the mode of administration.[16] Drugs with a longer duration of action, such as morphine (18 to 20 hours), are more suitable for intermittent injection. Drugs with a short duration of action, such as fentanyl, must be administered by continuous infusion to provide around-the-clock pain relief.[2,15]

Side Effects

Side effects can be systemic or centrally mediated.[14,16,17] Because the epidural space is highly vascular, any drug administered by this route enters the systemic circulation.[18] If the epidural dose is high enough, the patient may experience the same systemic side effects that would occur with intravenous administration of the drug. These side effects include the release of histamine that may result in urticaria or wheezing and occasionally gastrointestinal side effects.

Centrally mediated side effects of spinal opioids include pruritus, nausea and vomiting, urinary retention, sedation, and late respiratory depression.[14,16,20] Although potentially life-threatening, the actual occurrence of late respiratory depression in a patient with cancer pain is exceedingly rare, presumably because of opioid tolerance induced by prior intake of these drugs. An opioid-naïve patient is at higher risk for this potentially serious problem.[20]

Treatment of the side effects of spinal opioids, with the exception of respiratory depression, should be directed at symptomatic relief.[16,21] The clinician and patient must be aware of the potential side effects to anticipate and recognize the need for treatment. For milder symptoms, reassurance is often all that is required. Adjuvant drugs to treat pruritus, nausea and vomiting, or other symptoms can be given if necessary. A standing order for bladder catheterization as needed should be considered for the first few doses of spinal opioids in nontolerant patients. If symptoms persist, or if respiratory depression occurs, minute doses of narcotic antagonists, such as naloxone, or administration of small amounts of agonist-antagonist drugs, such as nalbuphine, also can be used.[16,20] These drugs should be titrated carefully to avoid reversal of the analgesic properties of systemic or spinally administered opioids because patients in this setting may experience increased sensitivity to narcotic antagonists. **Table 37.2** provides an example of standing post–spinal opioid orders that have worked well in a variety of clinical settings for cancer patients.

Table 37.1 Recommended Starting Doses of Commonly Used Spinally Administered Opioids

Drug	Epidural Dose (mg)	Volume/ Diluent (mL)	Duration (hr)
Meperidine	50 Lumbar	5 Lumbar	7
	5 Cervical	1 Cervical	7
Morphine	5 Lumbar	0.5 Lumbar	18
	0.5 Cervical	0.1 Cervical	18
Fentanyl	0.1 Lumbar	5 Lumbar	4
	0.01 Cervical	0.1 Cervical	4

Table 37.2 Post–Spinal Opioid Injection Standing Orders

1. Measure vital signs every 15 min × 1 hr, every 30 min × 1 hr, then every hour × 4 hr, then every 4 hr × 24 hr.

2. Check and record respiratory rate every hour × 24 hr.

3. Maintain patient supine with head of bed up 30 degrees for 30 min after injection.

4. Administer naloxone (Narcan) intravenous push for respirations <6/min as follows: Dilute 1 ampule of naloxone (0.4 mg) with 8 mL of normal saline, and give 3 mL every 5 min until respirations >10/min. Notify pain management physician if this is done.

5. Administer diphenhydramine (Benadryl) 50 mg intramuscularly every 4–6 hr as needed for severe itching.

6. Give droperidol (Inapsine) 2.5 mg intramuscularly every 4 hr as needed for nausea in the absence of any other standing antiemetic order.

7. If patient develops hypotension, administer ephedrine intravenous push in 10-mg increments every 3–5 min to a total of 50 mg. Notify pain management physician if ephedrine is given. *Note:* To effect an accurate dose of ephedrine, mix 1 mL of ephedrine (50 mg/mL) with 4 mL of sterile normal saline to equal 50 mg in 5mL or 10 mg in 1mL.

8. If not sedated, patient may be up with assistance 30 min after injection of spinal opioids.

9. Document pain complaints carefully (i.e., onset, intensity, location, duration, precipitating and alleviating factors).

10. If any problems or questions arise, contact pain management physician.

11. Monitor for urinary retention, and insert straight catheter as needed for urinary retention. Notify pain management physician if this is done.

Conclusion

Spinal opioids represent a great advance in cancer pain management. Proper selection of patients is crucial if optimal results are to be achieved. The long-term administration of opioids and other drugs into the epidural or subarachnoid space is in its infancy. Advances in the pharmacology of spinal drugs and the development of new delivery system technology in time no doubt will expand the options available for the relief of cancer pain.

References

Full references for this chapter can be found on www.expertconsult.com.

Neurosurgery in the Management of Cancer Pain

Nicholas Kormylo and Mark S. Wallace

About one third of all cancer patients experience disease-related pain. In patients with advanced disease, the number increases to 80%.[1] In early stages, pain is most likely to be nociceptive. However, neuropathic pain can occur as the cancer spreads and damages distal peripheral nerves, nerve plexuses, dorsal roots, or the central nervous system. When pain is not sufficiently treated with basic analgesics, opioid and adjuvant medications provide acceptable relief for most patients. In more refractory cases, intrathecal delivery is a good alternative for patients, especially those experiencing dose-limiting side effects of oral pain medications.

Neuropathic pain has historically been the more difficult pain to treat because it sometimes is unresponsive to neuropathic pain medications, opioids, and even intrathecal medications. However, neuropathic pain generators can occur at numerous locations in the nervous system, both peripherally and centrally. Therefore, neuroablative procedures distal to the pain generator will have no effect and can possibly worsen the pain. Ablative neurosurgical procedures may be considered in end-stage refractory cancer pain; however, the risks should be considered seriously. In addition, neuroablative procedures can induce neuropathic pain and therefore should be reserved for patients with a short life expectancy. Patient selection is critical because the procedures can be associated with significant potential morbidity. When successful, however, the procedures can offer the patient with refractory cancer pain dramatic relief of symptoms and a substantially improved quality of life.

Patient Selection

Overall health status and life expectancy must be taken into consideration when selecting patients for neuroablative surgical procedures. Patients with poorly controlled pain often cannot tolerate even simple procedures and may require general anesthesia. Suitability for general anesthesia therefore must also be considered. Cancer patients with advanced disease may have large pleural or pericardial effusions, significant ascites, coagulopathies that are difficult to correct, or anterior mediastinal tumors. These comorbidities present an especially elevated risk. Another consideration is the patient's life expectancy. Although patients with a short life expectancy have a lower risk of developing neuropathic pain from the neuroablative procedure, they may have a higher risk of morbidity and mortality.[2] Therefore, the risks and benefits of performing the neuroablative procedure must be assessed carefully before proceeding.

The patient's psychological status should also be taken into account before the procedure. Patients with dementia, severe confusion, agitation, or otherwise altered mental status usually do not respond well to any pain intervention, whether conservative or invasive. However, the needs of these patients should not be ignored, and more conservative measures are usually just as effective.

Dorsal Root Entry Zone Lesioning

The dorsal root entry zone (DREZ) consists of the central portion of the dorsal roots, Lissauer's tract, and the outer layers of the dorsal horn.[3] DREZ lesioning is intended to destroy preferentially the more lateral nociceptive fibers in the dorsal rootlets as well as the excitatory medial portion of Lissauer's tract (**Fig. 38.1**). Ideally, medial fibers in the dorsal rootlets are spared to avoid loss of proprioception. The target structures can be accessed through the dorsal lateral sulcus. Ablative techniques include microbipolar cautery, radiofrequency thermocoagulation, carbon dioxide laser, and ultrasound lesioning.[4]

The procedure is most valuable in patients with well-defined, localized pain and should be limited to thoracic dermatomes or functionless extremities. DREZ lesioning has been used most often for brachial plexus avulsion, but it has also been successful in patients with other peripheral nerve injuries, postherpetic neuralgia (especially with a strong allodynic

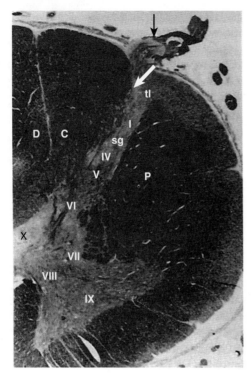

Fig. 38.1 **Rexed laminae (I to IX).** Rexed's lamination of the dorsal horn (I to VI). Transverse hemisection of the spinal cord (at the lower cervical level) with myelin stained by luxol-fuchsin and showing the myelinated rootlet afferents that reach the dorsal column. The *black arrow* designates the pial ring of the dorsal rootlet (diameter, 1 mm). The *white arrow* shows the MDT target. (DC, dorsal column; P, pyramidal tract; sg, substantia gelatinosa; tl, tract of Lissauer; MDT, microsurgical DREZotomy). *(From Sindou MP: Dorsal root entry zone legions. In Burchiel KJ, editor,* Surgical management of pain, *New York, 2002, Thieme Medical Publishers, pp 701-713.)*

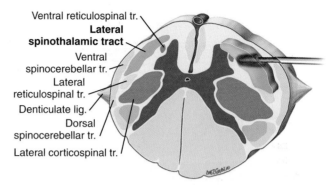

Fig. 38.2 **Schematic drawing of the target-electrode relation and main anatomic structures in percutaneous cordotomy.** *(From Kanpolat Y, Ugur HC, Ayten M, et al:* Computed tomography-guided percutaneous cordotomy for intractable pain in malignancy, *Neurosurg 64[Suppl 1]:178, 2009.)*

component), painful localized spasticity, and segmental spinal cord injuries. DREZ lesioning does not improve pain originating below the spinal cord segment treated. In cancer patients, DREZ lesioning has been effective for Pancoast's syndrome, invasive tumors of the abdominal wall or trunk involving few dermatomes, or tumors involving peripheral nerves, nerve plexuses, or dorsal roots. In one series, 87% of 46 patients with cervicothoracic level lesioning and 78% of 35 patients with lumbosacral level lesioning had a good result, defined as withdrawal of narcotics.[4]

Anterolateral Cordotomy

The purpose of anterolateral cordotomy is to interrupt the spinothalamic tract. The spinothalamic tract transmits pain and temperature sensations from the contralateral side of the body to the thalamus. Anterolateral cordotomy is useful to treat unilateral, nociceptive pain, usually below the C5 dermatome. Cordotomy can relieve the evoked component of neuropathic pains, including allodynia and intermittent shooting pains, but it is ineffective for constant painful dysesthesias.[5] The procedure is used almost exclusively for cancer pain because the level of analgesia diminishes over time. Results are initially excellent, with success rated at 95% at the time of discharge. Satisfactory analgesia decreases over time. Rosomoff et al[6] reported satisfactory analgesia 84% at 3 months, 43% at 1 to 5 years, and then 37% at 5 to 10 years.

Anterolateral cordotomy can be performed open or percutaneously. Percutaneous procedures can be performed under local anesthesia with light sedation, and allow functional mapping prior to lesioning (**Fig. 38.2**). Percutaneous procedures require no incision and can be much more easily repeated in cases of inadequate pain relief.[7]

Complications are frequently attributed to inadvertent lesioning of the corticospinal and reticulospinal tracts, which are both also located in the anterolateral quadrant. High cordotomies can therefore impair both voluntary and involuntary breathing. Fortunately, this complication is rare with unilateral cordotomies and is often mild or transient.[8] Bowel and bladder incontinence and significant ipsilateral weakness occur in 2% to 10% of patients. Postprocedure dysesthetic syndrome, a burning sensation throughout the analgesic area, can occur in 1% to 10% of patients.[6]

Myelotomy

Commissural myelotomy is designed to interrupt the decussating fibers of the spinothalamic tract as they cross the midline. A longitudinal incision is made extending over several spinal cord segments. The expected responses would be bilateral pain relief and sensory changes restricted to the spinal segments treated. Although pinprick analgesia does occur in the expected distribution, pain relief often extends well beyond these limits. Pain relief can extend much farther caudal or rostral to the levels of spinothalamic neurons interrupted during the surgical procedure.[6]

Small midline posterior lesions at C1 and T10 were also reported to provide unexpectedly large distributions of relief from visceral pain, even though in some cases the lesions were probably too shallow to reach the decussating spinothalamic fibers.[9] Evidence exists for an important visceral pain pathway in the posterior columns that is a possible anatomic explanation for the success of these procedures, referred to as punctate midline myelotomies. Punctate midline myelotomies are much less extensive procedures and can be performed percutaneously.

Myelotomies are an option for bilateral visceral cancer pain, especially in the pelvic and perineal distributions. This option may be superior to the only other surgical alternative, bilateral cordotomy, which is associated with a significant risk

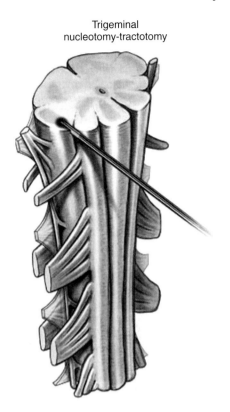

Trigeminal
nucleotomy-tractotomy

Fig. 38.3 Diagrammatic representation of trigeminal nucleotomy-tractotomy procedure. *(From Raslan AM, Burchiel KJ: Neurosurgical advances in cancer pain management, Curr Pain Headache Rep 14:477, 2010.)*

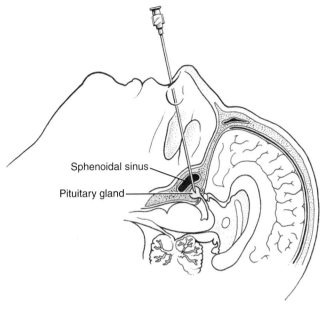

Sphenoidal sinus

Pituitary gland

Fig. 38.4 Pituitary ablation. *(From Cousins MJ, Bridenbaugh PO, Carr DB, et al, editors:* Cousins and Bridenbaugh's neural blockade in clinical anesthesia and pain medicine, *ed 4, New York, 2009, Lippincott Williams & Wilkins.)*

of bladder dysfunction. Published results for commissural myelotomy from 1927 to 1997 showed initial complete relief of pain in 92% (161 of 175 patients). By the time of last follow-up or death, this rate decreased to 59% (103 of 175 patients).[6] Results published for punctate midline myelotomy in patients with advanced disease cancer from 1997 to 2004 showed relief of pain for the duration of life span in 19 of 23 patients. Postoperative survival times ranged from 2 weeks to 31 months. All patients were reported to have used lower opiate dosages, and 5 patients did not use any opiates for the remainder of life.[10]

Dorsal Rhizotomy

Dorsal rhizotomy involves surgical sectioning of the dorsal roots or ablation with radiofrequency lesions. The technique has been used for cancer pain, but long-term results have not been encouraging. Pain tends to recur over time as the area of anesthesia decreases because of peripheral and central collateral sprouting.[11,12] Because proprioceptive fibers are destroyed along with the target pain fibers, dorsal rhizotomy is usually not appropriate for extremity pain. Deafferentation pain is a

frequent complication. Pagni et al[13] reported anesthesia dolorosa in 8 of 15 patients after long-term follow-up.

Single dorsal root involvement in the thoracic region, confirmed by local anesthetic blocks, may be the best indication for dorsal rhizotomy. For pelvic and perineal pain, the S2 and S3 roots usually need to be ablated bilaterally, and this procedure will result in bowel and bladder incontinence if it is not already present.[14] Because of poor long-term outcomes and high complication rates, dorsal rhizotomy has largely been supplanted by intrathecal medication delivery and spinal or peripheral nerve stimulation (**Fig. 38.3**).

Hypophysectomy

Hypophysectomy can be effective for widespread bone pain resulting from endocrine-sensitive cancers such as breast and prostate. Hypopituitarism can occur, as well as diabetes insipidus on occasion. The mechanism of pain relief is still unknown. In a series of nine patients reported by Hayashi et al,[15] all patients became completely pain free within a few days after the procedure. This absence of pain persisted for the duration of follow-up or end of life, ranging 1 to 24 months.[15] Earlier series published efficacy rates ranging from 76% to 90% (**Fig. 38.4**).[16–18]

References

Full references for this chapter can be found on www.expertconsult.com.

Palliative Care in the Management of Cancer Pain

Fadi Braiteh and Eduardo Bruera

Worldwide, most cancer patients still present with advanced-stage disease. For many patients, the only sensible treatment options remain pain relief and palliative care. Effective approaches to palliative care are available to improve the quality of life for cancer patients.

Palliative Care

Palliative care is a discipline that has changed its names frequently and encountered multiple definitions. One can find different nomenclature varying from palliative medicine to supportive care to hospice care.[1]

In 2002, the World Health Organization (WHO) provided a newer, more appropriate definition of palliative medicine.[2] According to this definition, palliative care:

- Provides relief from pain and other distressing symptoms
- Affirms life and regards dying as a normal process
- Intends neither to hasten nor to postpone death
- Integrates the psychological and spiritual aspects of patient care
- Offers a support system to help patients live as actively as possible until death
- Offers a support system to help the family cope during the patient's illness and in their own bereavement
- Uses a team approach to address the needs of patients and their families, including bereavement counseling, if indicated

- Will enhance quality of life and may also positively influence the course of illness
- Is applicable *early* in the course of illness, in conjunction with other therapies that are intended to prolong life, such as chemotherapy or radiation therapy, and includes those investigations needed to understand and manage distressing clinical complications better

The WHO broadened its approach to palliative care. The 2002 definition clearly emphasizes the superior outcome of the early delivery of palliative care. It extends the spectrum of care to the family because the health and wellbeing of family members is also important.[3] It stresses the relevance of palliative care to all life-threatening conditions and recognizes the preventive component of the discipline by understanding that end-of-life problems have their origins at an earlier time in the trajectory of disease. This definition reinforces the unquestionable focus of palliative care on quality of life.[1,3]

Because traditions, cultural attitudes, health systems, and resources vary widely among countries, the framework into which palliative care service must fit varies accordingly. The WHO designed three sets of general recommendations for countries according to the level of resources available (**Table 39.1**).[4] Palliative medicine is an emerging medical specialty recognized in the United States, Canada, Australia, and the United Kingdom and is rapidly being established in most of the world. The term *palliative care* is most frequently used for interdisciplinary care delivered by a team including physicians, nurses, counselors, chaplains, and rehabilitation professionals.[5]

Table 39.1 Priority Actions for National Cancer Control Programs According to Level of Resources

Component	All Countries	Scenario A: Low Level of Resources	Scenario B: Moderate Level of Resources	Scenario C: High Level of Resources
Pain relief and palliative care	Implement comprehensive palliative care that provides pain relief, other symptom control, and psychosocial and spiritual support Promote national minimum standards for management Ensure availability and accessibility of opioids Provide education and training for caregivers and public	Ensure that minimum standards for pain relief and palliative care are progressively adopted by all levels of care in targeted areas and that there is a high coverage of patients through services provided mainly by home-based care	Ensure that minimum standards for pain relief and palliative care are progressively adopted by all levels of care and nationwide there is rising coverage of patients through services provided by primary health care clinics and home-based care	Ensure that national pain relief and palliative care guidelines are adopted by all levels of care and nationwide there is high coverage of patients through a variety of options, including home-based care

World Health Organization: *National cancer control programmes: policies and managerial guidelines,* ed 2, Geneva, 2002, World Health Organization, p 164.

Cancer Pain Epidemiology

Three percent of the population of the United States is living with cancer. Many of these patients have pain that is caused by the disease or by the treatment they are receiving for the disease. Annually, more than 500,000 persons have terminal cancer, and 60% to 80% of them have severe pain. The prevalence of pain complaints ranges from 20% to 50% of all cancer patients in early stages, and it may rise to between 55% and 95% in patients with advanced disease.[6] Although 75% will have moderate to severe pain, more than 80% of patients with cancer can find relief when their pain is managed with simple noninvasive procedures.

Many guidelines for the management of cancer pain have been revised,[7–9] and major efforts are being made to broaden their application worldwide.[10] However, poor assessment techniques and misconceptions of pain management remain major barriers to adequate pain relief in cancer patients.[11]

Considerable variability exists in the treatment of cancer pain. Surveyed oncologists recognized that 86% of patients with cancer pain were undertreated, and 31% of the physicians waited until the patient's prognosis for death was 6 months or less before they would initiate maximal analgesia.[12] Several studies documented disparities in cancer pain treatment among cancer patients. The Eastern Cooperative Oncology Group physicians demonstrated that most cancer pain is undertreated, and particularly at risk for poor pain management, as identified in earlier studies, are women, minorities, and older persons.[11,13–16]

Pain occurs within the context of complex syndromes. Some of these affect the expression of pain, such as depression, anxiety, constipation, and dyspnea. Pain treatment itself can also inflict multiple different symptoms causing distress, including nausea, constipation, cognitive impairment, neurotoxicity, sedation, and hallucinations.

Clinical Assessment of the Palliative Care Patient

Pain is one of the most feared consequences of cancer.[17] Successful control of pain in a cancer patient depends on adequate broad assessment of the patient's satellite comorbidities and symptoms. The unidimensional pain assessment can lead to pharmacologic overtreatment and toxicities.[18]

A thorough history and physical examination are required. In the cancer patient, an organic process responsible for the patient's complaints of pain can usually be identified. A new onset of pain in an established patient is, by principle, caused by recurrent or metastatic disease until otherwise proven.

The purposes of assessment are multiple. Assessment of symptoms for intervention in the terminally ill patient has the ultimate goal of improving the quality of life, but it also influences the course of the disease. Pain can kill.[19] Laboratory data showed that pain can inhibit immune function and enhance tumor growth.[20,21] Therefore, appropriate cancer pain management can enhance life expectancy. Uncontrolled pain was found to be a major factor in suicidal deaths in cancer patients.[22,23] Depression can also kill. A high level of depressive symptoms is an independent risk factor for mortality in community-residing older adults,[24] independent of suicide incidence. Cachexia up-regulates cytokine production and enhances tumor progression.[25] In one report, the degree of interference with activity and enjoyment of life was greater when the pain was caused by cancer than when it had another cause.[26]

Assessment of Cancer Pain: The Edmonton Symptom Assessment System

In one study, pain occurred in 67% of patients with metastatic cancer.[11] When asked about barriers to good pain management in their own practice setting, 76% of surveyed oncologists[11] cited poor assessment of pain as the major problem. This finding is consistent with the strong predictive role of the discrepancy between patients' and physicians' assessments of the patients' pain and inadequate analgesia. Many diagnostic tools are available for assessment of pain intensity. The most common tools used in clinical practice are the Edmonton Symptom Assessment System (ESAS)[27,28] and the Verbal or Visual Analog Pain Scales. In addition, the Memorial Pain Assessment Card allows us to distinguish pain intensity from both pain relief and global suffering.[29]

Pain assessment scores should not be interpreted blindly by a rigid therapeutic intervention. One should carefully consider the wide spectrum of the underlying pain and suffering mechanisms. Unidimensional pain rating scales can miss the affective dimensions on pain expression and their impact. Multidimensional rating scales that include the various pain-related symptoms identify those affective dimensions and allow optimal palliation. The affective dimensions such as delirium, catastrophizing, somatization, depression, and anxiety are components of suffering, and they can have considerable impact on the expression of pain.

Besides the usual assessment tools of pain such as numeric rating scales or visual analog scales, valid tools have been developed to help in daily assessment: the ESAS, the Memorial Delirium Assessment Scale (MDAS), and the CAGE questionnaire.[30–32]

The ESAS consists of 10 visual analog scales (0 = best, 10 = worst) for pain, fatigue, drowsiness, nausea, anxiety, depression, appetite, dyspnea, insomnia, and sense of well-being.[27] The ESAS is a simple, validated tool that is completed by the patient and allows for screening and monitoring for the most common symptoms in patients with advanced incurable illness.[28,33] The information is displayed as a graph, to allow for fast interpretation of the relative intensity of different symptoms and over time. The MDAS is a validated tool that that allows for screening, assessment of severity, and follow-up of delirium. It is superior to traditional cognitive assessment tools such as the Mini-Mental State Examination (MMSE) because it assesses not only cognition but also perceptual, thought, and psychomotor abnormalities. This tool can be administered accurately by different health care professionals after one single training session of less than 1 hour.[34] The CAGE questionnaire consists of four simple questions used to screen for alcoholism (cutting down, annoyance, guilty feeling, and eye-opener). An abnormal CAGE score (defined as a positive answer to at least two of the four questions) has been shown to have prognostic value in the opioid management of cancer pain.[35]

Types of Pain

The key step in pain assessment is characterization of the pain complaint, which can be somatic, visceral, or neuropathic.

Somatic nociceptive pain is usually described as a well-localized, sharp aching in the complaint area, with or without throbbing or pressure sensation. It is caused by the activation of nociceptors in the affected tissue secondary to damage of peripheral and deep tissues. The causes of somatic pain are usually related to bone disease and postsurgical pain.

Visceral pain is poorly localized and diffuse. It can be crampy, squeezing, colicky, or gnawing because it is usually associated with distention of a hollow viscus, stretching of the capsule of a solid organ, or invasion of an internal organ by a tumor. Sometimes, it is referred to other anatomic areas beyond the area of the pathologic process. Visceral pain is also frequently associated with autonomic activation manifested by nausea, vomiting, perspiration, and peripheral vasospasm.

Neuropathic pain is commonly described as burning, sharp, shooting, or tingling. A pain that a patient "cannot describe" is probably neuropathic pain. It can be caused either by direct injury to nervous tissue by the cancer itself (e.g., tumor infiltration of a nerve, plexus, or the spinal cord) or by antineoplastic therapy (e.g., peripheral neuropathy caused by cisplatinum, paclitaxel, vincristine or postradiation neuritis or fibrosis). It is sometimes associated with motor neurologic deficits. Neuropathic pain is difficult to control and is associated with a high incidence of suffering.[36]

Edmonton Classification System for Cancer Pain

Pain is a subjective sensation and therefore more difficult to assess, but research has identified certain features to influence its response to different treatments. The Edmonton Staging System (ESS) (**Fig. 39.1**) provides a clinical staging system for cancer pain and includes known prognostic factors for the response to treatment. The system is accurate in predicting the outcome of patients with cancer pain. Three stages are identified:

Stage 1: Indicates good prognosis for pain control
Stage 2: Indicates intermediate prognosis
Stage 3: Indicates poor prognosis

Patients with visceral, bone, or soft tissue pain, who are receiving low doses of opioids, whose cognitive status is intact, and who have no severe psychological distress are classified in stage I and are more likely to respond well to analgesic treatment. Patients with features such as incidental pain, neuropathic pain, tolerance to the present opioid, a past history of alcoholism, severe psychosocial distress, and cognitive impairment are classified in stage 3 and have a diminished likelihood of good response to analgesic treatment. In patients with stage 3 pain, assessment of the complex pain will guide a multiaxial intervention to reduce suffering.

The effectiveness of a staging system in predicting the outcome of patients with cancer pain was found to be limited when 55% of patients with a poor prognosis were able to achieve pain control during a 3-week assessment period.[37] However, the system is highly accurate in predicting patients with good prognosis.[37] This lack of specificity makes this staging system impractical in certain situations. "A new onset of pain or change in character or intensity of an established pain raises the strongest possibility of metastatic disease or a tumor growth of the original site." A more recent version of the ESS is the Edmonton Classification System for Cancer Pain. This staging system has confirmed the prognostic value of some critical findings such as neuropathic or incidental mechanism, psychosocial distress, or chemical coping.[37]

Multidimensional Assessment: Pain in Palliative Care

The multidimensional nature of pain and the overall expressions of suffering fall under the label of pain. In palliative care, a complex spectrum of various symptoms has been reported by patients: pain in 41% to 76%, depression in 33% to 40%, anxiety in 57% to 68%, nausea in 24% to 68%, constipation in 65%, sedation or confusion in 46% to 60%, dyspnea in 12% to 58%, anorexia in 85%, and asthenia in 90%.[11,15,28,38]

Instruments for the Measurement of Multiple Symptoms

Results from palliative studies are often difficult to compare because many different evaluation tools are used. No consensus has been reached about which instruments are most appropriate. Many different questionnaires are used in palliative care, but no selection of questionnaires can cover all the palliative needs of all patients. Examples include the European Organization for Research and Treatment of Cancer Quality of Life-Core 30 (EORTC QLQ-C30), the Palliative Care Outcome

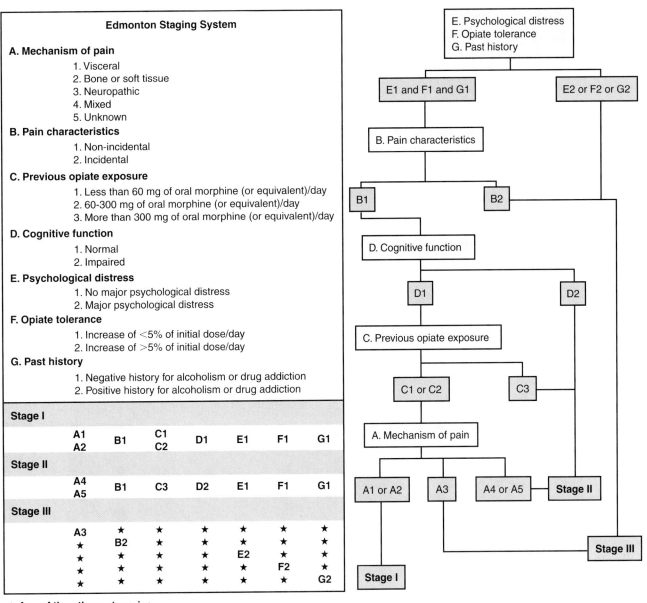

Fig. 39.1 **Edmonton Staging System.**

Scale (POS), and the McGill Quality of Life Questionnaire (MQOL),[39-41] the Functional Assessment of Chronic Illness Therapy (FACIT), the Brief Pain Inventory (BPI), the Memorial Symptom Assessment Scale (MSAS), the Hospital Anxiety and Depression Scale (HADS), the Edinburgh Depression Scale (EDS), the ESS, and the ESAS. Few of those tools are practical for the daily clinical setting.

To minimize the burden on patients, questionnaires should be brief and manageable, and they should be validated.[42] The ESAS is a 10-item patient-rated symptom visual analog scale developed for use in symptom assessment of patients in palliative care.[27] It has been validated[28] when compared with other multidimensional symptom assessment instruments—the MSAS,[43] a multidimensional quality-of-life instrument; the FACIT; and the self-administered BPI.[44]

Measurement of Specific Symptoms and Its Instruments

FATIGUE

Fatigue, the most common symptom in advanced cancer, affects 60% to 90% of patients, as identified by diverse criteria.[45] Cancer-related fatigue is characterized by an unusual, persistent, subjective sense of tiredness that interferes with usual functioning.[46]

The modes of expression are physical (e.g., decreased energy), cognitive (e.g., decreased concentration), and affective (e.g., decreased motivation) modes of expression.[47] Fatigue is a multidimensional syndrome with major contributing factors, including cancer cachexia, depression, pain, opioid medications, radiation therapy, and chemotherapy agents.

Deconditioning and anemia are common among cancer patients as well.[48] Unlike fatigue in healthy individuals, cancer-related fatigue occurs despite adequate amounts of rest or sleep. It occurs early, often before the diagnosis of cancer, and increases during the course of cancer treatment and progression. Fatigue persists long after cancer treatment is completed and can be reported in 17% of cancer survivors more than 1 year after treatment.[49]

Several fatigue assessment tools exist and include functional capacity tests, subjective assessments during function, and objective and subjective assessments of function. A multidimensional fatigue assessment incorporating multiple characteristics of fatigue and their impact on function, such as the Functional Assessment of Cancer Therapy-Anemia Scale[50] and the Piper Fatigue Self-Report Scale,[51] can be more informative but also more time-consuming to administer. Simpler unidimensional scales, such as a numeric scale (0 to 10), can be used, especially for screening because patients are often reluctant to discuss fatigue with their physicians, who, in turn, do not frequently assess this symptom. When screening reveals moderate (4 to 6) or severe (7 to 10) fatigue, then a more focused history and physical examination should be performed with attention to possible etiologic factors.[48]

The goal of treatment can be to reduce fatigue intensity, to help patients function at a stable fatigue level, or both. Fatigue management involves specific (targeting potentially reversible causes of fatigue such as anemia or hypothyroidism) and symptomatic (targeting symptoms because no obvious or reversible cause of fatigue can be identified) intervention and treatment measures. Specific interventions include treating other endocrine abnormalities such as hypogonadism—evidence of opioid-induced hypothalamic hypogonadism is strong[52]—as well as managing pain, insomnia, depression, and anxiety. Treatment of anemia with red blood cell transfusion and epoetin alpha has been shown to improve quality-of-life outcomes, including fatigue.[53] Symptomatic interventions such as education, counseling, and pharmacologic and nonpharmacologic measures may be used. Sleep hygiene measures can be initiated for insomnia, and thyroid hormone replacement may be initiated for hypothyroidism. Patients with mood disorders should be referred for counseling and possible pharmacologic therapy. Medications that contribute to fatigue should be discontinued, if possible. Prednisone, 20 to 40 mg/day for a limited period of 2 to 4 weeks, has been shown to decrease fatigue, although the mechanism of action is unknown. Prolonged regimens can potentially induce myopathy and worsen fatigue.

Psychostimulants, such as methylphenidate, have been used to treat opioid-induced somnolence, reduce pain intensity, treat depression, and improve cognition.[54] Preliminary results show that patient-controlled methylphenidate administration rapidly improved fatigue and quality of life. Patients were able to appropriately titrate their methylphenidate to their symptom distress.[55] Modafinil has been studied in cancer fatigue; it is a psychostimulant with potentially fewer side effects than methylphenidate. Progestational agents, traditionally used to improve appetite, were shown to have a beneficial effect on activity levels in patients after a 10-day treatment course.[56] Thalidomide, which is thought to act through inhibiting tumor necrosis factor-α and modulating interleukins, has been shown to improve the sensation of well-being in patients with cancer cachexia, and it may also be beneficial for

cancer-related fatigue.[57] Monoclonal anti-interleukin antibodies, pentoxifylline and bradykinin antagonists, and alpha-melanocyte–stimulating hormone offer fields for future investigation in the treatment of cancer-related fatigue.[58] Donepezil appears to improve sedation and fatigue in patients receiving opioids for cancer pain.[59] Alternative approaches such as acupuncture, healing touch, and massage therapy are promising.[60] Adding massage therapy and healing touch to standard care improves pain scores, mood disturbance, and fatigue in patients receiving cancer chemotherapy.[61]

NAUSEA

Chronic nausea is a common symptom in patients with advanced cancer, with a frequency of 32% to 98%.[62] It is mandatory to screen for nausea in the palliative care setting and to distinguish it from chemotherapy-induced nausea. Ondansetron and the newer selective 5-hydroxytryptamine (anti–5-HT$_3$) granisetron and palonosetron, along with the neurokinin-1 (NK-1) receptor antagonist aprepitant, reduce chemotherapy-induced nausea significantly, but these agents have less promising effects on chronic nausea.[63,64] The reason is the difference in the pathophysiology of nausea. Causes of nausea and vomiting include gastrointestinal motility disorders, metabolic derangement, raised intracranial pressure, chemotherapy and radiation therapy, psychosomatic factors, and opioids (**Table 39.2**).

Gastroparesis caused by autonomic dysfunction is one of the most frequent problems in patients with cancer.[65] More than 80% of terminal cancer patients receive opioid analgesics for pain and dyspnea. Opioids induce nausea and

Table 39.2 Etiology of Nausea in the Palliative Care Setting

Preexisting comorbidities	Congestive heart failure, hypothyroidism, or neurologic disorders
Cancer	Paraneoplastic neurologic syndromes
Cancer treatment	Chemotherapy, radiotherapy, immunotherapy, or surgery
Endocrine abnormalities	Hypothyroidism or hypogonadism
Cancer/treatment complications	Anemia, sepsis, pulmonary and cardiac disorders, renal and hepatic failure, metabolic complications, dehydration, hypoxia, autonomic failure, or neuromuscular disorders
Psychological factors	Anxiety, depression, or stress
Medications	Opioids, hypnotics, anxiolytics, antihistamines, antiemetics, or antihypertensives
Cachexia/malnutrition	
Deconditioning	
Sleep disorders	
Interrelationship with other physical symptoms	

vomiting by direct stimulation of the chemoreceptor trigger zone,[66] decrease gastric emptying and gastrointestinal motility, and induce constipation.

Opioids stimulate nausea and vomiting by an action on the chemoreceptor trigger zone in the area postrema by increasing vestibular sensitivity and delaying gastric emptying.[67] In most patients, nausea can be well controlled using safe and simple antiemetic regimens such as metoclopramide, haloperidol, and phenothiazines.[67] Different drugs have been proposed to treat nausea and vomiting induced by opioids. Opioid rotation and change of route of administration may widen the therapeutic window of opioids in some circumstances.

Management of nausea in the palliative care setting includes assessment for constipation. The patient undergoes a rectal examination, and abdominal radiographs are reviewed and assessed for constipation. Appropriate management of constipation with laxatives, stool softeners, and enemas is fundamental.

Haloperidol, a potent narrow-spectrum drug with antidopaminergic activity, is frequently used before broad-spectrum drugs such as methotrimeprazine.[67] **Figure 39.2** summarizes management options including metoclopramide and steroids.

Metoclopramide is a benzamide derivative with gastrointestinal motility and antiemetic activity.[68] Efficient treatment requires frequent administration around the clock of short-acting formulations of metoclopramide to ensure a sustained plasma concentration to suppress nausea, vomiting, and other gastrointestinal symptoms associated with cancer. Controlled-release metoclopramide reduces gastrointestinal symptoms in patients with advanced cancer and has an easier administration regimen.[69] Metoclopramide should be maximized in the form of continuous infusion with the added steroids. In the postoperative period, it is important to discuss with the surgeon whether any procedure has been performed on the intestinal lumen because prokinetic agents are associated with a risk of perforation or dehiscence of sutures.

Ondansetron, in doses of 4 to 16 mg, may be effective in preventing opioid-induced emesis when the opioids are administered by the intravenous or intraspinal route.[70,71] Once the antiemetic measures are exhausted and the obstruction cannot be reversed (approximately 50% of obstructions reverse spontaneously), then the approach is palliative desiccation of the secretions with octreotide or glycopyrrolate.

DYSPNEA

Dyspnea, the uncomfortable awareness of breathing, is a frequent and distressing symptom in patients with advanced cancer and is often difficult to control. Studies have shown that the incidence of dyspnea in terminally ill patients with cancer ranges from 20% to 80%.[72,73] Evidence indicates that good

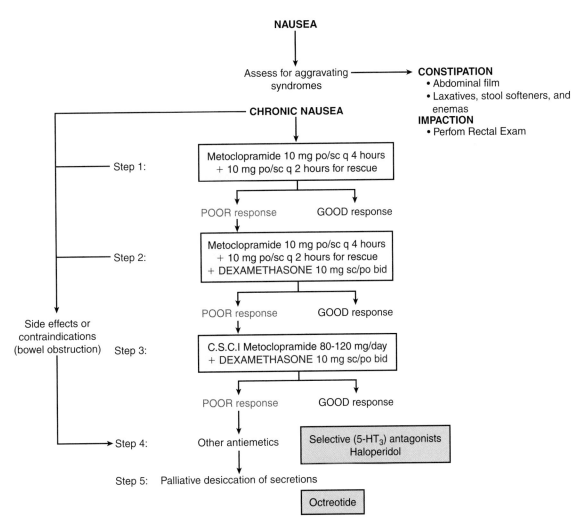

Fig. 39.2 **Algorithm for management of chronic nausea.** po, orally; sc, subcutaneously.

symptom control, even by experienced palliative care teams, is achieved less frequently for dyspnea than for other symptoms such as pain or nausea.[74]

Very limited research has been conducted on the frequency and correlates of dyspnea in patients with advanced cancer.[75] Bruera et al[73] conducted several prospective and randomized control trials investigating the dimensions of this problem and the outcomes of oxygen supplementation. Lung involvement, anxiety, and maximum inspiratory pressure all influence the intensity of dyspnea in patients with advanced cancer.[73] Supplemental oxygen is proven to be beneficial to patients with hypoxia and dyspnea at rest,[76,77] but it did not improve the physical function or performance in patients with nonhypoxic dyspnea associated with cancer.[78] Intermittent injections of subcutaneous morphine are safe and effective for the management of dyspnea in terminal cancer.[79] These injections decrease the intensity of dyspnea without statistically modifying oxygen saturation, respiratory rate, or the end-tidal arterial partial pressure of carbon dioxide.[80] Controversy exists regarding the superiority of aerosolized opiates in relieving dyspnea.[81]

DROWSINESS

Opioid-induced sedation is a major complication in patients with cancer pain.[82] Several approaches have been attempted for improvement of sedation—opioid dose reduction, opioid rotation, neuraxial analgesia, and the use of psychostimulants.[83]

Methylphenidate has been found to reduce opioid-induced sedation and to increase cognitive function and analgesia in patients with cancer pain. Clinical applications are limited by the development of tolerance, potential aggravation of agitation or anxiety, and concerns about cardiovascular safety and addiction.[54] Donepezil is a long-acting selective acetyl-cholinesterase inhibitor that Bruera et al[59] studied for its effectiveness in opioid-induced sedation and related symptoms in patients with cancer pain. Significant improvements in sedation, fatigue, anxiety, well-being, depression, anorexia, and problems with sleep were observed.[59]

SLEEP DISTURBANCES

Sleep problems are commonly inadequately assessed in routine clinical care. Insomnia is more frequent in cancer patients than in the general population.[84] Prevalence of cancer-related sleep disturbance is estimated between 24% and 95% and persists even years after treatment and cure of cancer.[85,86] The prevalence of sleep disturbances tends to be higher in women and in older persons.[86] This heterogeneous complaint may involve difficulties in falling asleep, trouble staying asleep, early-morning awakening, or complaints of nonrestorative sleep with corresponding sleep efficiency of less than 85%.[86]

Sleep disorders may generate a further burden of distress to patients and families, and symptoms such as depression, anxiety, pain, and fatigue tend to be exacerbated. Sleep disturbance scores of cancer patients and community subjects were significantly correlated with fatigue severity.[87] Inadequate pain control can be considered a risk factor for sleep disturbances in patients with advanced cancer.[88] Anxiety, falling asleep, waking, early awakening, getting back to sleep, and nightmares were significantly associated with fewer hours slept.[89] Sleep disturbances coexisted with psychiatric conditions such as depressive and anxiety disorders, which can be consequences of this disturbance.

Depression may influence sleep, but persistent insomnia can precipitate depression.[90] In patients with advanced cancer, medications contribute to insomnia. Insomnia is a well-known side effect of dexamethasone, and other antiemetic medications have also been found to disturb sleep.

Research suggests that stress-reduction programs tailored to the cancer setting help patients cope with the effects of treatment and improve their quality of life. Tibetan yoga, which incorporates controlled breathing and visualization, mindfulness techniques, and low-impact postures, had a positive effect on improving the subjective sleep quality, fastening the sleep latency, prolonging sleep duration, and reducing the use of sleep medications among cancer patients.[91]

APPETITE DISTURBANCES

Poor appetite in patients with advanced cancer is part of both cachexia and gastroparesis syndromes. Anorexia, early satiety, nausea, vomiting, bloating, and postprandial fullness may all be, at least partially, the result of gastroparesis caused by autonomic dysfunction.[92] Investigators conducted a prospective randomized, placebo-controlled trial using fish oil in patients with advanced cancer and loss of weight and appetite. Fish oil did not significantly influence appetite, tiredness, nausea, well-being, caloric intake, nutritional status, or function after 2 weeks compared with placebo.

Limited evidence exists for effectiveness of cannabinoids on appetite stimulation, and cannabinoids have minor or no overall nutritional advantages in acquired immunodeficiency syndrome (AIDS) or cancer cachexia. The remaining indications are largely supported by anecdotal case reports and by small, uncontrolled case series.[93] The main active compound present in marijuana is tetrahydrocannabinol (THC). Nabilone, levonantradol, and dronabinol are potent synthetic cannabinoids.

The two proven indications for the use of the synthetic cannabinoid dronabinol are chemotherapy-induced nausea and vomiting and AIDS-related anorexia. This drug is superior to low doses of metoclopramide in patients receiving moderately emetogenic chemotherapy but inferior to high-dose metoclopramide in patients receiving cisplatin-based chemotherapy.[93-95] With the newer antiemetics available, dronabinol remains a fourth-line agent for this indication after high-dose metoclopramide plus dexamethasone, 5-HT$_3$ antagonists, and NK-1 antagonists.[96] Other possible uses that may prove beneficial in the oncology population include analgesia, muscle relaxation, mood elevation, and relief of insomnia.

The main limitation of cannabinoids has been the high frequency of adverse effects on the central nervous system.[97] These consist mostly of perceptual abnormalities, including occasional hallucinations, dysphoria, abnormal thinking, depersonalization, and somnolence.[98]

DEPRESSION

Psychological distress of terminally ill cancer patients has major impact on their clinical care. One half of cancer patients in one study were diagnosed with a psychiatric disorder, and most of them had an adjustment disorder or major depression.[99] In published data, 3% to 35% of cancer patients experience full-syndrome post-traumatic stress disorder (PTSD), but little is known about this incidence in the terminally ill patients with advanced cancer.[100] Psychological distress can have a severe negative impact on patients with advanced or terminal cancer, including reduced quality of life,[101] significant suffering,[102] a request for physician-assisted suicide or euthanasia,[103] and suicide,[104] as well as psychological distress in family members.[105] In one study, the incidences at baseline among terminally ill patients diagnosed with adjustment disorders, major depression, and PTSD were 16.3%, 6.7%, and 0%, respectively—those patients experienced lower performance status, concern about being a burden to others, and lower satisfaction with social support. On follow-up, only 10.6% were diagnosed with adjustment disorders, and the rate of major depression increased to 11.8%.[106]

Depression is a significant symptom for approximately 25% of patients in palliative care, but it is frequently unrecognized and untreated.[107] Factors include failure of patients to disclose complaints[108] and attribution by physicians of somatic symptoms of depression to the cancer illness.[109] Consequently, nearly 80% of the psychological and psychiatric morbidity in patients with cancer is unrecognized and untreated in general oncologic practice.[110]

Most palliative medicine physicians surveyed in the United Kingdom assessed patients for depression routinely in 73% of cases; 27% used the HADS, and 10% asking the patient "Are you depressed?" The most frequently prescribed medications were selective serotonin reuptake inhibitors (80%). Fewer than 6% of practitioners prescribed psychostimulants.[111]

One study illustrated that effective tools for depression do not have to be complex. The single question "Are you depressed?" proved to be the tool with the highest sensitivity, specificity, and positive predictive value when compared with HADS and the EDS. It is crucial to have a psychiatric counselor on the palliative care team or access to an oncologist-psychiatrist familiar with the common syndromes that affect the terminally ill and their families in the inpatient or outpatient setting. The counselor should be experienced with special treatment delivery framed. In the literature, the focus is on depression risk factors such as younger age, female gender, physical symptoms (pain) and functioning, cancer site (pancreatic cancer), cancer therapy (chemotherapy, radiation therapy), brain metastasis, hypercalcemia, and use of steroids, several types of concerns (existential concerns), past history of major depression, and lack of social support.[112] Systemic screening, with a low threshold for referral for professional assessment by psychiatrist or psychologist experienced in palliative care, is highly beneficial.

ANXIETY

Despite a wide variability across studies, prevalence rates of anxiety and depressive disorders in cancer patients have been found to be as high as 49% and 53%, respectively.[113] Meta-analysis confirmed that relaxation training had a significant effect on the emotional adjustment variables of depression, anxiety, and hostility of cancer patients in acute medical treatment.[114]

WELL-BEING

Patients with advanced cancer often experience physical, psychological, social, and existential distress associated with the disease or its treatment. Subjective health-related quality of life is thought to characterize the interaction between the circumstance or experiences associated with illness and the patient's

personal values and expectations.[115,116] Many tools attempt further evaluation and scoring of the subjective quality of life and service effectiveness in the form of patient reported outcomes such as the Self-Perception and Relationship Tool, the Ferrans and Powers Quality of Life Index, the Functional Living Index-Cancer Scale, the Functional Assessment of Cancer Therapy Scale, the Short Form-36 Health Survey, and the General Well-Being Scale.[117-119] The "well-being" scoring between 0 and 10 in the ESAS could be a valid summary of subjective quality of life that integrates all the symptoms of distress.

Assessment of Cognitive Impairment

The symptom of distress resulting from pain and delirium will further increase suffering among patients with advanced cancer. One of the main reasons for inadequate pain treatment is poor assessment of cognitive function. Delirium occurs in 26% to 44% of cancer patients admitted to hospital or hospice. Approximately 90% of patients experience delirium in the hours to days before death. *Delirium* is defined as a disturbance of consciousness and attention with a change in cognition or perception (**Fig. 39.3**). In addition, it develops suddenly and follows a fluctuating course related to the cancer, metabolic disorders, or the effects of drugs (**Table 39.3**).

Frail older patients are at high risk for delirium. The presence of delirium causes extreme distress for the patient and the patient's family. The treatment proposes a clinical challenge for the physician (**Fig. 39.4**). Terminally ill older patients also have distinct needs because of the coalescence of symptoms, accumulation of debility, and increasing dependence on the caregiver.

STEP 1: Team training in recognition and management of delirium in general

- Regular use of the term "delirium" and no others
- Train the team in key concepts
- Inclusion of MMSE (or other screening tests) as a routine tool in the evaluation of the patient

STEP 2: Systematic screening of risk factors for delirium and prevention of opioid-induced neurotoxicity

- Psychological distress (examination)
- Previous abuse of substances
- Renal failure or dehydration
- Pre-existing progressive cognitive failure
- Incidental or neuropathic pain
- Abundance of drugs

STEP 3: Evaluation of delirium

- Recognize changes in the mental state of the patient
- Identify cognitive decline and attention disturbances through clinical examination, MMSE or other tests
- Rule out other causes of cognitive changes: dementia, depression or psychosis
- Verification of DSM-IV criteria
- Maintain evaluation of delirium; use specific tests to follow-up with the patient

Fig. 39.3 **Three-step approach to detect delirium in cancer patients.** MMSE, Mini-Mental Status Examination. *(From American Psychiatric Association: Diagnostic and Statistical Manual of Mental Disorders, Fourth Edition, Text Revision, Washington, DC, 2000, American Psychiatric Association.)*

Managing delirium is of major importance in end-of-life care and frequently gives rise to controversies and to clinical and ethical dilemmas. Excluding terminal delirium, delirium is reversible in 50% of cases.[120] These dilemmas are rooted in the poor recognition or even misdiagnosis of delirium, despite its frequent occurrence. Delirium generates major distress to the patient, the family, and even the health care providers. It opens the field to misinterpretation of symptoms and creates behavioral management challenges for health care professionals. The challenge is to recognize when delirium is potentially reversible, all the while knowing that most patients die after a nonreversible, terminal episode that can be qualified as end-stage delirium.

Greater educational efforts are required to improve the recognition of delirium and lead to a better understanding of its impact on end-of-life care. Awaiting the development of low-burden instruments for assessment, communication strategies, and family education regarding the manifestations of delirium should be further integrated into the management of delirium. The challenge is to identify the reversibility components of delirium and to target precipitating factors superimposed onto baseline vulnerability.[121]

The MDAS is a simple and validated tool for the screening and follow-up of delirium. Scores of 7 out of 30 or higher are the most sensitive (98%) and specific (96%) for the diagnosis of delirium in cancer patients.[120] Delirium is associated with changes in the circadian distribution of breakthrough analgesia, which is possibly related to reversal of the normal circadian rhythm.[122] Delirium precipitated by opioids and other psychoactive medications and dehydration is frequently reversible with change of opioid or dose reduction, discontinuation of unnecessary psychoactive medication, opioid rotation, or hydration, respectively.[123] Haloperidol is the

Table 39.3 Etiology of Delirium in the Palliative Care Setting

Intracranial disease	Systemic disease
Brain neoplasm	Organ failure
Leptomeningeal disease	Cardiac
Postictal disorder	Hepatic
Medications	Renal
Psychoactive agents	Respiratory
Opioids	Infection
Benzodiazepines	Pulmonary
Anticholinergics	Urinary tract
Selective serotonin	Decubitus ulcer
reuptake inhibitors	Hematologic
Tricyclic antidepressants	Anemia
Antihistamines	Dissemination intravascular
Others	coagulation
Steroids	Metabolic
Ciprofloxacin	Dehydration
Histamine H_2-blockers	Hypercalcemia
	Hyponatremia, hyperkalemia
	Hypoglycemia

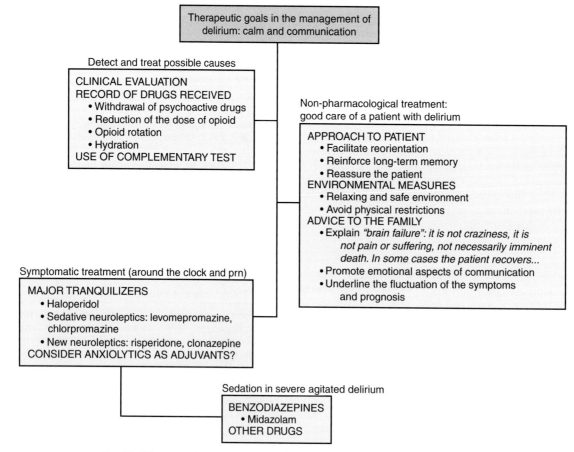

Fig. 39.4 **Therapeutic approach to delirium in patients with advanced cancer.**

most frequently used drug, and newer neuroleptics such as risperidone or olanzapine are being tested with good results. Methylphenidate has been used for hypoactive delirium. A crucial step in the management is withdrawal of benzodiazepine compounds. These drugs are major contributors or precipitators of delirium and should be reserved for sedation in patients with severe agitated delirium after failure of the foregoing measures.

Community Issues and Adjunct Treatments

Psychological Support

To make a positive impact on the overall quality of life, one needs to address suffering in addition to managing nociception and pain. Pain is usually only one of the components of suffering, which can be defined as a more global aversive experience. Other contributors to suffering can be depression, anxiety, fatigue, and social isolation.

The Angry Patient

When the clinician is faced with an angry patient, expressive supportive counseling may be counterproductive. The required steps in assessing an angry patient start with ruling out an agitated delirium syndrome. Once delirium diagnosis is excluded, mood status is assessed, mainly for depression, because 25% of cancer patients may develop depression. Anxiety is another mood disorder that may affect cancer patients as part of the delirium syndrome or as a component of their depression. In fact 15% to 20% of depressive episodes manifest with agitation.

The third step is use of the CAGE questionnaire to identify a missed diagnosis of chemical coping mechanism; anger may be a patient's conscious strategy to obtain opioids. Anger can be merely adaptive, and the possibility that a patient's anger is a personality trait should be further explored.

Communication and Family Involvement

Good communication is the foundation of an atmosphere of sensitivity and compassion; it can elicit honesty and openness. Better communication and better interpersonal care can translate into improvements in patient satisfaction,[124] compliance with medical recommendations, and health outcomes.[125]

Ong et al[126] found that doctor-patient communication during oncologic consultation is related to patients' quality of life and satisfaction. The affective quality of the consultation seems to be the most important factor in determining these outcomes. Communication with patients and with their families is crucial. The word "family" is used in the broad spectrum to designate the relatives and other people important to the patient and involved in the patient's care. Research revealed that relatives are intensely attuned to the conditions and reactions of their loved ones. They perceive discomfort the way caregivers would but have a tendency to associate

more pain as a reason for discomfort in nonverbal patients.[127] Communication facilitates development of relationships, allows exchange of information, and assists in medical decision making.[128]

In one study, medical decision-making preferences were assessed in a palliative care setting where physicians were trained in communication skills.[129] Approximately 63% of patients chose a shared approach with physicians, when physicians predicted the shared decision making only in 38% of the cases.[130] Agreement on decision-making preferences occurs in 38%[131] to 42%.[2] Physicians, even those highly trained in communication skills, are not good at predicting decision-making preferences. Asking the patient directly, rather than assuming a prediction of the level of involvement, should be the foundation of a decision-making preference.

Families may have little knowledge of the disease and its prognosis and may have low expectations of pain relief or unrealistically high expectations of curative treatment. Patients with narrowed disparities between expectations and reality have a better quality of life. Older cancer patients, those living with others, those enrolled in managed care organizations, and those who report better than expected experience are more likely to have a higher overall health-related quality of life.[132] Communication empowers the family and the patient by involving them in decision making with regard to treatment. The clinician should explain treatment in detail so patients can give informed consent or refusal and should create an environment in which patients are in control.[133]

Communication strategies and education of the family regarding the manifestations of delirium are paramount in managing delirium, which is a major cause of distress for the family and a risk factor for iatrogenic harm when it is misdiagnosed. Delirium-related symptoms can cause great distress in both patients and family members.[134] Most patients with delirium recall their delirium as highly distressing. Delirium is also upsetting for spouses, caregivers, and nurses who are caring for delirious patients.[134]

The degree of emotional distress of family members concerning terminal delirium was studied. More than two thirds of bereaved family members perceived all delirium-related symptoms, other than somnolence, as distressing or very distressing when these symptoms occurred frequently.[135] It is crucial to counsel families about terminal delirium and to explain the potential causes, course, possible interventions, and outcomes. The key point is to prepare families for potential future delirium episodes and the high likelihood of recurrence. Communication is crucial in the setting of delirium requiring terminal sedation. In fact, the percentage of patients who were terminally sedated varied from 4% in the hospice setting to 10% in the tertiary palliative care unit. Uncontrolled delirium is only one of the indications for sedation.

Other centers reported terminal sedation indications to be dyspnea, pain, general malaise, agitation, and nausea.[136] Terminal sedation should be restricted to patients with uncontrollable symptoms such as delirium, dyspnea, suffocation, and dramatic hemorrhage. Midazolam seems to be the agent most commonly used. Before its induction, a thorough assessment of the underlying reversible factors, such as medications, should be undertaken.

Treatment

Principles of Management

Besides a physician and a nurse, members of various disciplines, such as psychology, social work, nutrition, rehabilitation, pastoral care, pharmacology, speech therapy, and respiratory care, can be efficiently involved in patient care to address the complex needs of these patients.[137]

The treatment of nociceptive cancer pain, once fully assessed, is mainly achieved with pharmacologic analgesics but can involve multiple treatment modalities. These include antitumor therapy, nonanalgesic adjuvant pharmacologic management, psychosocial therapy, and, occasionally, invasive therapy including nerve blocks and neuroablative procedures and various nonpharmacologic treatments (**Table 39.4**).

Effective pain management is best achieved by a broad-based assessment platform of the pain and other symptoms, an interdisciplinary interventional approach, and an extensive plan of action involving patients, their families, and health care providers. Barriers to effective pain management (**Fig. 39.5**) include a sense of fatalism, denial, the desire to be "the good patient," geographic barriers, and financial limitations. The physician should do the following:

- Initiate prophylactic anticonstipation intervention in every patient treated with opiates. Unlike nausea, complete tolerance to the constipation does not generally develop.
- Discuss pain and its management with patients and their families.
- Encourage patients to report their pain, and explain to them that many safe and effective ways to relieve pain are available.
- Understand that some patients may be reluctant to report pain because of "opiophobia" or because of a spiritual belief in the meaning of pain and suffering as part of the healing process.
- Explain the reality of risks of addiction and the spectrum of the side effects, their prevention, and interventions to control them.
- Consider the cost of proposed drugs and interventions.
- Communicate the pain assessment and its management with other clinicians treating the patient.
- Know state and local regulations regarding controlled substances.

The WHO introduced a simple and effective method for cancer pain management (**Fig. 39.6**) based on titration of therapy.[138] This approach should allow adequate pain control in most (90%) cancer patients[139] and in most (75%) terminally ill patients.[140] The WHO guides cancer pain treatment through a five-concept approach. Oral administration of medications is the preferred route. Medications should be administered on an around-the-clock basis rather than on an as-needed basis. The dosages should be individualized for each patient. Vigilance and consideration of details and side effects when administering or prescribing the various drugs are crucial.

Interventional Procedures for Intractable Pain in Palliative Care

In the setting of failure to control a pain syndrome, the clinician should consider interventional pain management such as

Table 39.4 Cancer Pain Management Modalities

A. Systemic analgesic therapy
1. Nonopioid analgesics
2. Opioid analgesics
3. Adjuvant agents
   Antidepressants
   Anticonvulsants
   Local anesthetics
   Corticosteroids
   Other
4. Side effect management

B. Invasive therapy
1. Peripheral nerve blocks
2. Plexus blocks
3. Neuraxial therapy
4. Neuroablative techniques

C. Antitumor therapy

D. Psychosocial therapy

E. Nonpharmacologic therapy
1. Heat or cold application
2. Exercise
3. Counterstimulation (TENS)
4. Relaxation/imagery
5. Distraction/reframing
6. Hypnosis
7. Peer group support
8. Pastoral counseling
9. Occupational therapy aids
10. Physical therapy appliances

intrathecal catheter or pump opioid infusion. It is crucial to consider a safe road map toward such an intervention with the following five safety checkpoints (**Table 39.5**): (1) Is the pain refractory? (2) Does the pain have non-nociceptive components (somatization, delirium, and chemical coping)? (3) Is the pain mainly nociceptive? (4) What is the likelihood of response to the intervention? (5) What are the logistics of postintervention pain service and its availability to the patient?

Conclusion

Multidisciplinary acute care is the most successful approach in the management of complex symptoms in patients with advanced cancer. Multidimensional approaches to cancer pain allow a comprehensive assessment of the nonorganic components of pain, such as psychosocial distress, which do not respond to escalating doses of opioid medication. Additionally, nociceptive pain is just one component of the suffering, and improving the patient's quality of life requires targeting all variables when possible. Not recognizing these complex interactive syndromes will lead to misdiagnosis and mismanagement, with tremendous harm to the patient, caregivers, and family. The health care provider's frustration can be reduced by better management of the patient. The following five interventions are needed during consultation in the palliative care pain management setting for optimal service to dying patients: (1) a digital rectal examination, (2) the CAGE score test, (3) the MMSE, (4) evaluation for supportive counseling, and (5) the do not

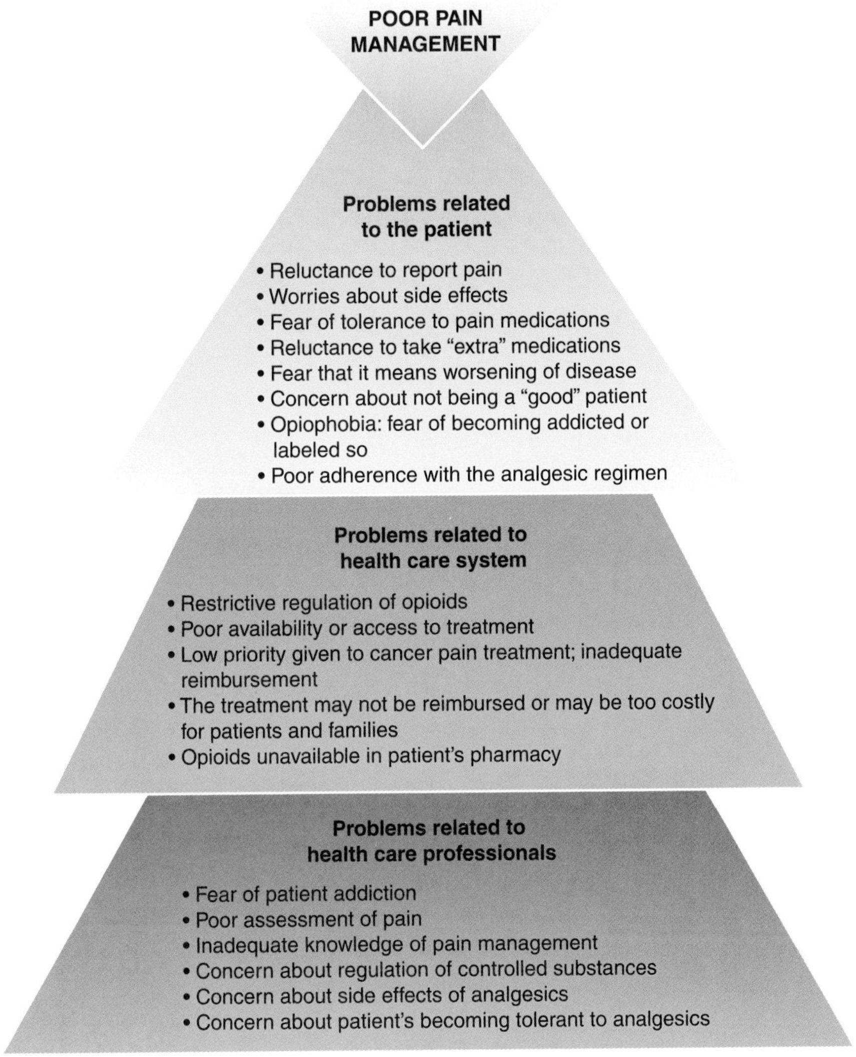

POOR PAIN MANAGEMENT

Problems related to the patient

- Reluctance to report pain
- Worries about side effects
- Fear of tolerance to pain medications
- Reluctance to take "extra" medications
- Fear that it means worsening of disease
- Concern about not being a "good" patient
- Opiophobia: fear of becoming addicted or labeled so
- Poor adherence with the analgesic regimen

Problems related to health care system

- Restrictive regulation of opioids
- Poor availability or access to treatment
- Low priority given to cancer pain treatment; inadequate reimbursement
- The treatment may not be reimbursed or may be too costly for patients and families
- Opioids unavailable in patient's pharmacy

Problems related to health care professionals

- Fear of patient addiction
- Poor assessment of pain
- Inadequate knowledge of pain management
- Concern about regulation of controlled substances
- Concern about side effects of analgesics
- Concern about patient's becoming tolerant to analgesics

Fig. 39.5 **Barriers to effective pain management.**

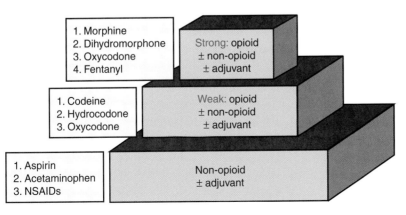

1. Aspirin
2. Acetaminophen
3. NSAIDs

Non-opioid ± adjuvant

1. Codeine
2. Hydrocodone
3. Oxycodone

Weak: opioid ± non-opioid ± adjuvant

1. Morphine
2. Dihydromorphone
3. Oxycodone
4. Fentanyl

Strong: opioid ± non-opioid ± adjuvant

Fig. 39.6 **World Health Organization analgesic ladder for cancer pain management.** NSAIDs, nonsteroidal anti-inflammatory drugs.

Table 39.5 Checklist for Administration of Interventional Opioids

Is the pain refractory?
 Are the opioids adequately titrated?
 Is rotation of opioids done?
 Are adjuvants used?
 Are other side effects treated?

Is the pain mainly nociceptive?

Have non-nociceptive components of pain expression been taken into consideration?
 Somatization
 Delirium
 Chemical coping

Likelihood of response
 Will the pain syndrome respond to intrathecal opioids (consider components of deafferentation pain and anatomic location)?

Have logistics of postintervention pain care in the community been considered and resolved?

resuscitate (DNR) status determination. These interventions should be administered early, sometimes even repeatedly. The patient will not benefit from a palliative care service consultation unless these five protocols have been followed.

References

Full references for this chapter can be found on www.expertconsult.com.

Part D

Pain of Dermatologic and Musculoskeletal Origin

Common Sports Injuries

Steven D. Waldman

Injuries incurred during recreational sports activities are becoming increasingly common with the new emphasis in recent years on physical and cardiovascular fitness. For the purposes of this chapter, the clinician can classify sports injuries into two broad classes: (1) accidental traumatic injuries and (2) overuse injuries (**Table 40.1**). On one hand, accidental traumatic injuries are, for the most part, readily apparent and do not present significant diagnostic challenges. Overuse injuries, on the other hand, can manifest in a more subtle manner

and may elude easy diagnosis. The following discussion will center on some of the most common sports injuries and will provide the clinician with a concise approach to diagnosis and treatment. Some of the syndromes discussed here can also result from activities not related to sports. Several of these conditions, such as carpal tunnel syndrome, DeQuervain tenosynovitis, and biceps tendinitis, are important pain syndromes that are described in greater detail in separate chapters; this chapter discusses them from the sports injury perspective.

Supraspinatus Tendinitis

Supraspinatus tendinitis can manifest as either an acute or a chronic painful condition of the shoulder. Acute supraspinatus tendinitis will usually occur in a younger group of patients following overuse or misuse of the shoulder joint. Inciting factors may include carrying heavy loads in front and away from the body, throwing injuries, or the vigorous use of exercise equipment. Chronic supraspinatus tendinitis tends to occur in an older group of patients and manifests in a more gradual or insidious manner without a single specific event of antecedent trauma. The pain of supraspinatus tendinitis will be constant and severe with sleep disturbance often reported. The pain of supraspinatus tendinitis is felt primarily in the deltoid region.[1] It is moderate to severe in intensity and may be associated with a gradual loss of range of motion of the affected shoulder. The patient will often awaken at night when he or she rolls over onto the affected shoulder.

Signs and Symptoms

The patient suffering from supraspinatus tendinitis may attempt to splint the inflamed tendon by elevating the scapula to remove tension from the ligament, giving the patient

Table 40.1 Types of Overuse and Traumatic Sports Injuries

Overuse Sports Injuries	Traumatic Sports Injuries
Tendinitis	Torn ligaments
Bursitis	Torn and ruptured tendons
Muscle strains	Fractures
Entrapment neuropathies	Dislocations Meniscal tears Muscle sprains Lacerations

a "shrugging" appearance (**Fig. 40.1**). There is usually point tenderness over the greater tuberosity. The patient will exhibit a painful arc of abduction and complain of a catch or sudden onset of pain in the midrange of the arc caused by impingement of the humeral head onto the supraspinatus tendon. Patients with supraspinatus tendinitis will exhibit a positive Dawbarn sign, which is pain to palpation over the greater tuberosity of the humerus when the arm is hanging down that disappears when the arm is fully abducted.[2] Early in the course of the disease, passive range of motion is full and without pain. As the disease progresses, patients suffering from supraspinatus tendinitis will often experience a gradual decrease in functional ability with decreasing shoulder range of motion making simple everyday tasks such as hair combing, fastening a brassiere, or reaching overhead quite difficult. With continued disuse, muscle wasting may occur and a frozen shoulder may develop.

Testing

Plain radiographs are indicated in all patients with shoulder pain. Based on the patient's clinical presentation, additional testing including complete blood count, erythrocyte sedimentation rate, and antinuclear antibody testing may be indicated. Magnetic resonance imaging (MRI) scan of the shoulder is indicated if rotator cuff tear is suspected and to help confirm the diagnosis (**Fig. 40.2**). The injection technique mentioned subsequently will serve as both a diagnostic and therapeutic maneuver.

Differential Diagnosis

Because supraspinatus tendinitis may occur after seemingly minor trauma or develop gradually over time, the diagnosis will often be delayed. Tendinitis of the musculotendinous unit of the shoulder frequently coexists with bursitis of the associated bursae of the shoulder joint, creating additional pain and functional disability. This ongoing pain and functional

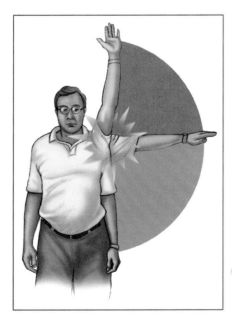
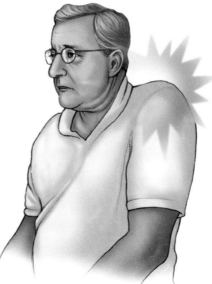
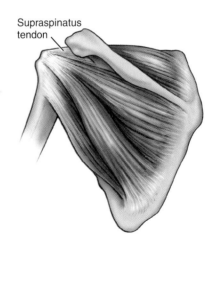

Supraspinatus tendon

Fig. 40.1 Patients with supraspinatus tendinitis exhibit point tenderness of the greater tuberosity and a painful arc of abduction. *(From Waldman SD:* Atlas of uncommon pain syndromes, *ed 2, Philadelphia, 2008, Saunders, p 58.)*

disability can cause the patient to splint the shoulder group with resultant abnormal movement of the shoulder, which puts additional stress on the rotator cuff. This can lead to further trauma to the entire rotator cuff. It should be remembered that with rotator cuff tears, passive range of motion is normal, but active range of motion is limited in contradistinction to frozen shoulder in which both passive and active ranges of motion are limited. Rotator cuff tear rarely occurs before age 40 except in cases of severe acute trauma to the shoulder. Cervical radiculopathy may rarely cause pain limited to the shoulder, although in most instances, there is associated neck and upper extremity pain and numbness.

Treatment

Initial treatment of the pain and functional disability associated with supraspinatus tendinitis should include a combination of nonsteroidal anti-inflammatory drugs (NSAIDs) or COX-2 inhibitors and physical therapy. The local application of heat and cold may also be beneficial. For patients who do not respond to these treatment modalities, the following injection technique may be a reasonable next step. The use of physical therapy including gentle range-of-motion exercises should be introduced several days after the patient undergoes this injection technique for shoulder pain. Vigorous exercises should be avoided because they will exacerbate the patient's symptoms.

To inject the supraspinatus tendon, the patient is placed in the supine position with the forearm medially rotated behind the back. This positioning of the upper extremity will place the lateral epicondyle of the elbow in an anterior position and make its identification easier. After identifying the lateral epicondyle of the elbow, the humerus is traced superiorly to the anterior edge of the acromion. A slight indentation just below the anterior edge of the acromion marks the point of insertion of the supraspinatus tendon into the upper facet of the greater tuberosity of the humerus. The point is marked with a sterile marker.

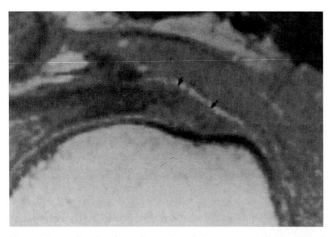

Fig. 40.2 Tendinosis of tendinopathy of the rotator cuff. A coronal oblique protein density-weighted (TR/TE, 2000/25) spin-echo magnetic resonance image (MRI) reveals increased signal intensity in the distal part of the supraspinatus tendon (*arrows*). There was no further increase in signal intensity in T2-weighted spin-echo MRIs. The peribursal fat plane is intact. (*From Kjellin I, Ho CP, Cervilla V, et al: Alterations in the supraspinatus tendon at MR imaging: correlation with histopathologic findings in cadavers, Radiology 181:837, 1991.*)

Proper preparation with antiseptic solution of the skin overlying the shoulder, subacromial region, and joint space is then carried out. A sterile syringe containing 1.0 mL of 0.25% preservative-free bupivacaine and 40 mg of methylprednisolone is attached to a 1½-inch 25-gauge needle using strict aseptic technique. With strict aseptic technique, the previously marked point is palpated and the indentation indicating the insertion of the supraspinatus tendon is reidentified with the gloved finger. The needle is then carefully advanced perpendicularly at this point through the skin and subcutaneous tissues through the joint capsule until it impinges on bone.[3] The needle is then withdrawn 1 to 2 mm out of the periosteum of the humerus and the contents of the syringe are gently injected. Slight resistance to injection should be felt. If no resistance is encountered, either the needle tip is in the joint space itself or the supraspinatus tendon is ruptured. If significant resistance to injection occurs, the needle tip is probably in the substance of a ligament or tendon and should be advanced or withdrawn slightly until the injection proceeds without significant resistance. The needle is then removed and a sterile pressure dressing and ice pack are placed at the injection site.

The major complication of this injection technique is infection. This complication should be exceedingly rare if strict aseptic technique is followed. The possibility of trauma to the supraspinatus tendon from the injection itself remains an ever-present possibility. Tendons that are highly inflamed or previously damaged are subject to rupture if they are directly injected. This complication can be greatly decreased if the clinician uses gentle technique and stops injecting immediately if significant resistance to injection is encountered. Approximately 25% of patients will complain of a transient increase in pain following this injection technique and should be warned of this possibility.

Rotator Cuff Tendinopathy and Tear

Rotator cuff tendinopathy and tears represent a common cause of shoulder pain and dysfunction encountered in clinical practice. A rotator cuff tear will frequently occur after seemingly minor trauma to the musculotendinous unit of the shoulder. However, in most cases, the pathology responsible for the tear is usually a long time in the making and is most often the result of ongoing tendinitis. The rotator cuff is made up of the subscapularis, supraspinatus, infraspinatus, and teres minor muscles and associated tendons (**Fig. 40.3**).[4] The function of the rotator cuff is to rotate the arm to help provide shoulder joint stability along the other muscles, tendons, and ligaments of the shoulder.

The supraspinatus and infraspinatus muscle tendons are particularly susceptible to the development of tendinitis for several reasons.[5] First, the joint is subjected to wide ranges of motion that are often repetitive in nature. Second, the space in which the musculotendinous unit functions is restricted by the coracoacromial arch, making impingement a likely possibility with extreme movements of the joint. Third, the blood supply to the musculotendinous unit is poor, making healing of microtrauma more difficult. All these factors can contribute to tendinitis of one or more of the tendons of the shoulder joint. Calcium deposition around the tendon may occur if the inflammation continues, making subsequent treatment more difficult.

Bursitis often accompanies rotator cuff tears and may require specific treatment. In addition to the previously mentioned pain, patients suffering from rotator cuff tear will often experience a gradual decrease in functional ability with decreasing shoulder range of motion, making simple everyday tasks such as hair combing, fastening a brassiere, or reaching over head quite difficult. With continued disuse, muscle wasting may occur and a frozen shoulder may develop.

Signs and Symptoms

Patients with rotator cuff tear will frequently complain that they cannot lift the arm above the level of the shoulder without using the other arm to lift it (**Fig. 40.4**). On physical examination, the patient will have weakness on external rotation if the infraspinatus is involved and weakness in abduction above the level of the shoulder if the supraspinatus is involved. Tenderness to palpation in the subacromial region is often present. Patients with partial rotator cuff tears will exhibit loss

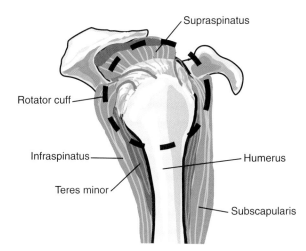

Fig. 40.3 The rotator cuff is a functional musculotendinous unit composed of four muscles, their fascia, and tendons. *(From Waldman SD: Physical diagnosis of pain: an atlas of signs and symptoms, ed 2, Philadelphia, 2010, Saunders, p 82.)*

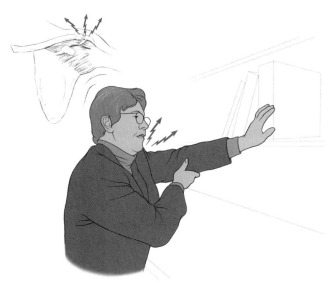

Fig. 40.4 Inability to elevate the arm above the level of the shoulder is the hallmark of rotator cuff disturbance. *(From Waldman SD: Atlas of common pain syndromes, ed 2, Philadelphia, 2008, Saunders, p 89.)*

of the ability to smoothly reach overhead. Patients with complete tears will exhibit anterior migration of the humeral head, as well as a complete inability to reach above the level of the shoulder. A positive drop arm test, which is the inability to hold the arm abducted at the level of the shoulder after the supported arm is released, will often be present with complete tears of the rotator cuff (**Figs. 40.5 and 40.6**).[6] The Moseley

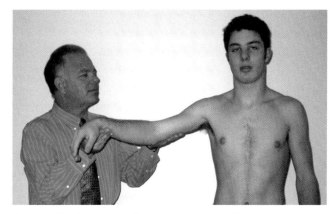

Fig. 40.5 The drop arm test for complete rotator cuff tear. *(From Waldman SD: Physical diagnosis of pain: an atlas of signs and symptoms, ed 2, Philadelphia, 2010, Saunders, p 86.)*

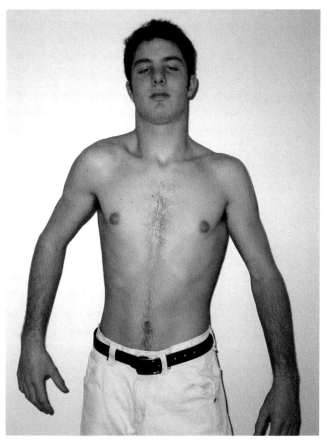

Fig. 40.6 A patient with a complete rotator cuff tear will be unable to hold the arm in the abducted position, and it will fall to the patient's side. The patient will often shrug or hitch the shoulder forward to use the intact muscles of the rotator cuff and the deltoid to keep the arm in the abducted position. *(From Waldman SD: Physical diagnosis of pain: an atlas of signs and symptoms, ed 2, Philadelphia, 2010, Saunders, p 86.)*

test for rotator cuff tear—performed by having the patient actively abduct the arm to 80° and then adding gentle resistance, which will force the arm to drop if complete rotator cuff tear is present—will also be positive. Passive range of motion of the shoulder is normal, but active range of motion is limited.

The pain of rotator cuff tear is constant and severe and is made worse with abduction and external rotation of the shoulder. Significant sleep disturbance is often reported. The patient may attempt to splint the inflamed subscapularis tendon by limiting medial rotation of the humerus.

Testing

Plain radiographs are indicated in all patients with shoulder pain. Based on the patient's clinical presentation, additional testing including complete blood count, erythrocyte sedimentation rate, and antinuclear antibody testing may be indicated. MRI scan of the shoulder is indicated if rotator cuff tear is suspected.

Differential Diagnosis

Because rotator cuff tears may occur after seemingly minor trauma, the diagnosis will often be delayed. The tear may be either partial or complete, further confusing the diagnosis, although careful physical examination can help distinguish the two. Tendinitis of the musculotendinous unit of the shoulder frequently coexists with bursitis of the associated bursae of the shoulder joint, creating additional pain and functional disability. This ongoing pain and functional disability can cause the patient to splint the shoulder group with resultant abnormal movement of the shoulder, which puts additional stress on the rotator cuff. This can lead to further trauma to the rotator cuff. It should be remembered that with rotator cuff tears, passive range of motion is normal but active range of motion is limited, in contradistinction to frozen shoulder in which both passive and active ranges of motion are limited. Rotator cuff tear rarely occurs before age 40 except in cases of severe acute trauma to the shoulder.

Treatment

Initial treatment of the pain and functional disability associated with rotator cuff tear should include a combination of the nonsteroidal anti-inflammatory agents or COX-2 inhibitors and physical therapy. The local application of heat and cold may also be beneficial. For patients who do not respond to these treatment modalities, injection of the rotator cuff may be a reasonable next step before surgical intervention.

Bicipital Tendinitis

The tendons of the long and short heads of the biceps, either alone or together, are particularly prone to the development of tendinitis, which is known as *bicipital tendinitis*.[7] The etiology of this syndrome is usually, at least in part, due to impingement on the tendons of the biceps at the coracoacromial arch. The onset of bicipital tendinitis is usually acute, occurring after overuse or misuse of the shoulder joint. Inciting factors may include activities such as trying to start a recalcitrant lawn mower, practicing an overhead tennis serve, or overaggressive

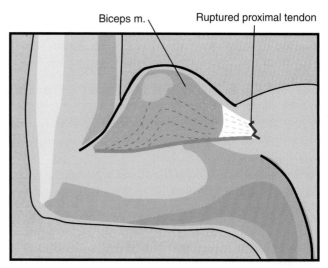

Fig. 40.7 "Popeye" deformity associated with ruptured long tendon of the biceps. *(From Waldman SD: Physical diagnosis of pain: an atlas of signs and symptoms, ed 2, Philadelphia, 2010, Saunders, p 78.)*

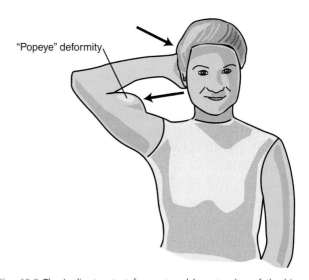

Fig. 40.8 The Ludington test for ruptured long tendon of the biceps. *(From Waldman SD: Physical diagnosis of pain: an atlas of signs and symptoms, ed 2, Philadelphia, 2010, Saunders, p 79.)*

follow-through when driving golf balls. The biceps muscle and tendons are susceptible to trauma and to wear and tear from overuse and misuse as mentioned earlier. If the damage becomes severe enough, the tendon of the long head of the biceps can rupture, leaving the patient with a telltale "Popeye" biceps (**Fig. 40.7**). This deformity can be accentuated by having the patient perform the Ludington maneuver, which is having the patient place his or her hands behind the head and flex the biceps muscle (**Fig. 40.8**).[8]

Signs and Symptoms

The pain of bicipital tendinitis is constant and severe and is localized in the anterior shoulder over the bicipital groove (**Fig. 40.9**). A catching sensation may also accompany the pain. Significant sleep disturbance is often reported. The patient may attempt to splint the inflamed tendons by internal rotation of the humerus, which moves the biceps tendon from

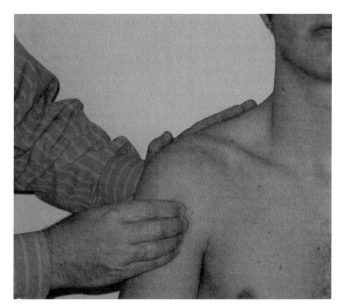

Fig. 40.9 Palpation of the long tendon of the biceps. *(From Waldman SD: Physical diagnosis of pain: an atlas of signs and symptoms, ed 2, Philadelphia, 2010, Saunders, p 78.)*

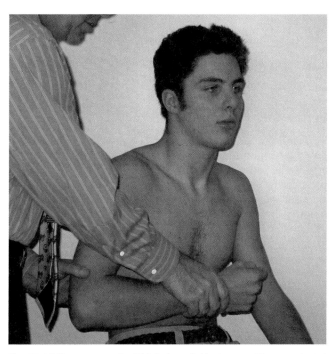

Fig. 40.10 Yergason test for bicipital tendinitis. *(From Waldman SD: Physical diagnosis of pain: an atlas of signs and symptoms, ed 2, Philadelphia, 2010, Saunders, p 70.)*

beneath the coracoacromial arch. Patients with bicipital tendinitis will exhibit a positive Yergason sign, which is production of pain on active supination of the forearm against resistance with the elbow flexed at a right angle (**Fig. 40.10**).[9] Bursitis often accompanies bicipital tendinitis.

In addition to this pain, patients suffering from bicipital tendinitis will often experience a gradual decrease in functional ability with decreasing shoulder range of motion, making simple everyday tasks such as hair combing, fastening a brassiere, or reaching over head quite difficult. With continued disuse, muscle wasting may occur and a frozen shoulder may develop.

Testing

Plain radiographs are indicated in all patients with shoulder pain. Based on the patient's clinical presentation, additional testing including complete blood count, erythrocyte sedimentation rate, and antinuclear antibody testing may be indicated. MRI scan of the shoulder is indicated if rotator cuff tear is suspected. The injection technique described later will serve as both a diagnostic and therapeutic maneuver.

Differential Diagnosis

Bicipital tendinitis is usually a straightforward clinical diagnosis. However, coexisting bursitis or tendinitis of the shoulder from overuse or misuse may confuse the diagnosis. Occasionally, partial rotator cuff tear can be mistaken for bicipital tendinitis. If the clinical situation dictates, consideration should be given to primary or secondary tumors involving the shoulder, superior sulcus of the lung, or proximal humerus. The pain of acute herpes zoster, which occurs before the eruption of vesicular rash, can also mimic bicipital tendinitis.

Treatment

Initial treatment of the pain and functional disability associated with bicipital tendinitis should include a combination of NSAIDs or COX-2 inhibitors and physical therapy. The local application of heat and cold may also be beneficial. For patients who do not respond to these treatment modalities, the following injection technique with local anesthetic and steroid may be a reasonable next step.

Injection for bicipital tendinitis is carried out by placing the patient in the supine position. The arm is then externally rotated approximately 45 degrees. The coracoid process is then identified anteriorly. Just lateral to the coracoid process is the lesser tuberosity. The lesser tuberosity will be more easily palpated as the arm is passively rotated. The point overlying the tuberosity is marked with a sterile marker.

Proper preparation with antiseptic solution of the skin overlying the anterior shoulder is carried out. A sterile syringe containing 1.0 mL of 0.25% preservative-free bupivacaine and 40 mg of methylprednisolone is attached to a 1½-inch 25-gauge needle using strict aseptic technique. With strict aseptic technique, the previously marked point is palpated and the insertion of the bicipital tendon is reidentified with the gloved finger. The needle is then carefully advanced at this point through the skin and subcutaneous tissues and underlying tendon until it impinges on bone (**Figs. 40.11 and 40.12**).[10] The needle is then withdrawn 1 to 2 mm out of the periosteum of the humerus and the contents of the syringe are gently injected. There should be slight resistance to injection. If no resistance is encountered, either the needle tip is in the joint space itself or the tendon is ruptured. If significant resistance to injection occurs, the needle tip is probably in the substance of a ligament or tendon and should be advanced or withdrawn slightly until the injection proceeds without significant resistance. The needle is then removed and a sterile pressure dressing and ice pack are placed at the injection site.

The major complication of this injection technique is infection. This complication should be exceedingly rare if strict aseptic technique is followed. The possibility of trauma to the bicipital tendon from the injection itself remains an ever-present possibility. Tendons that are highly inflamed or previously

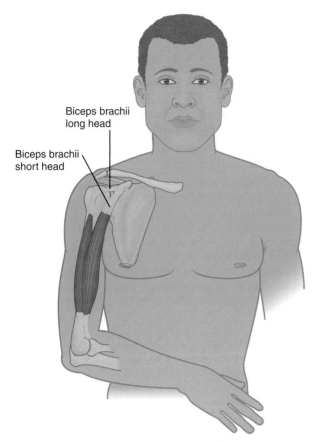

Fig. 40.11 Drawing of clinically relevant anatomy for injection for bicipital tendinitis. *(From Waldman SD: Atlas of pain management injection techniques, ed 2, Philadelphia, 2007, Saunders, p 54.)*

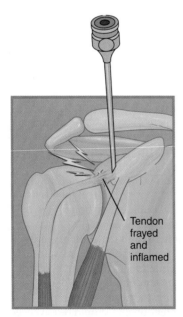

Fig. 40.12 Injection technique for bicipital tendinitis. *(From Waldman SD: Atlas of pain management injection techniques, ed 2, Philadelphia, 2007, Saunders, p 95.)*

damaged are subject to rupture if they are directly injected. This complication can be greatly decreased if the clinician uses gentle technique and stops injecting immediately if significant resistance to injection is encountered. Approximately 25% of patients will complain of a transient increase in pain following

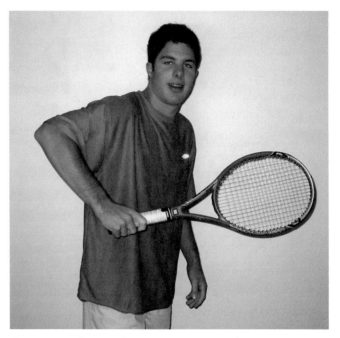

Fig. 40.13 Mechanism of elbow injury in tennis players. *(From Waldman SD: Physical diagnosis of pain: an atlas of signs and symptoms, ed 2, Philadelphia, 2010, Saunders, p 130.)*

intra-articular injection of the shoulder joint and should be warned of this possibility.

Lateral Epicondylitis

Tennis elbow (also known as lateral epicondylitis) is caused by repetitive microtrauma to the extensor tendons of the forearm.[11] The pathophysiology of tennis elbow is initially caused by microtearing at the origin of the extensor carpi radialis and extensor carpi ulnaris. Secondary inflammation, which can become chronic as the result of continued overuse or misuse of the extensors of the forearm, may occur. Coexistent bursitis, arthritis, and gout may also perpetuate the pain and disability of tennis elbow.

Tennis elbow occurs in patients engaged in repetitive activities that include hand grasping (e.g., politicians shaking hands) or high-torque wrist turning (e.g., scooping ice cream at an ice cream parlor). Tennis players develop tennis elbow by two separate mechanisms: first, increased pressure grip strain as a result of playing with too heavy a racquet; and second, making backhand shots with a leading shoulder and elbow rather than keeping the shoulder and elbow parallel to the net (**Fig. 40.13**). Other racquet sport players are also susceptible to the development of tennis elbow.

Signs and Symptoms

The pain of tennis elbow is localized to the region of the lateral epicondyle. It is constant and is made worse with active contraction of the wrist. Patients will note the inability to hold a coffee cup or hammer. Sleep disturbance is common. On physical examination, there will be tenderness along the extensor tendons at, or just below, the lateral epicondyle. Many patients with tennis elbow will exhibit a bandlike thickening within the affected extensor tendons.[11] Elbow range of motion will be

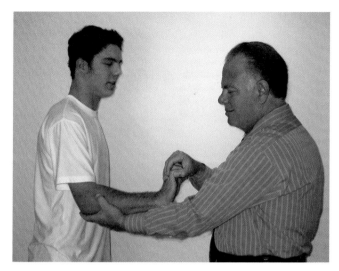

Fig. 40.14 Test for tennis elbow. *(From Waldman SD: Physical diagnosis of pain: an atlas of signs and symptoms, ed 2, Philadelphia, 2010, Saunders, p 130.)*

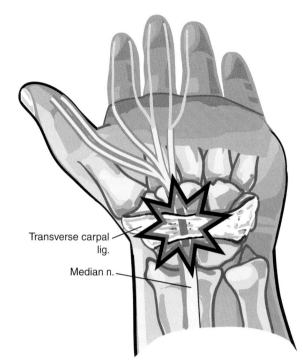

Transverse carpal lig.

Median n.

Fig. 40.15 Carpal tunnel syndrome: relevant anatomy. *(From Waldman SD: Physical diagnosis of pain: an atlas of signs and symptoms, ed 2, Philadelphia, 2010, Saunders, p 162.)*

normal. Grip strength on the affected side will be diminished. Patients with tennis elbow will demonstrate a positive tennis elbow test.[12] The test is performed by stabilizing the patient's forearm and then having the patient clench his or her fist and actively extend the wrist. The examiner then attempts to force the wrist into flexion (**Fig. 40.14**). Sudden severe pain is highly suggestive of tennis elbow.

Testing

Electromyography will help distinguish cervical radiculopathy and radial tunnel syndrome from tennis elbow. Plain radiographs are indicated in all patients with tennis elbow to rule out joint mice and other occult bony pathology. Based on the patient's clinical presentation, additional testing including complete blood count, uric acid, erythrocyte sedimentation rate, and antinuclear antibody testing may be indicated. MRI scan of the elbow is indicated if joint instability is suspected. The injection technique described later will serve as both a diagnostic and therapeutic maneuver.

Differential Diagnosis

Radial tunnel syndrome and occasionally C6-7 radiculopathy can mimic tennis elbow. Radial tunnel syndrome is an entrapment neuropathy that is the result of entrapment of the radial nerve below the elbow. Radial tunnel syndrome can be distinguished from tennis elbow in that with radial tunnel syndrome, the maximal tenderness to palpation is distal to the lateral epicondyle over the radial nerve, whereas with tennis elbow, the maximal tenderness to palpation is over the lateral epicondyle.

The most common nidus of pain from tennis elbow is the bony origin of the extensor tendon of extensor carpi radialis brevis at the anterior facet of the lateral epicondyle. Less commonly, tennis elbow pain can originate from the extensor carpi radialis longus at the supracondylar crest, or, rarely, more distally at the point where the extensor carpi radialis brevis overlies the radial head. As mentioned earlier, bursitis may accompany tennis elbow. The olecranon bursa lies in the posterior aspect of the elbow joint and may also become inflamed as a result of direct trauma or overuse of the joint. Other bursae susceptible to the development of bursitis exist between the insertion of the biceps and the head of the radius, as well as in the antecubital and cubital areas.

Treatment

Initial treatment of the pain and functional disability associated with tennis elbow should include a combination of NSAIDs or COX-2 inhibitors and physical therapy. The local application of heat and cold may also be beneficial. Any repetitive activity that may exacerbate the patient's symptoms should be avoided. A Velcro band placed around the extensor tendons may also help relieve the symptoms of tennis elbow. For patients who do not respond to these treatment modalities, injection of the lateral epicondyle may be a reasonable next step.

Carpal Tunnel Syndrome

Carpal tunnel syndrome is the most common entrapment neuropathy encountered in clinical practice. It is caused by compression of the median nerve as it passes through the carpal canal at the wrist. The more common causes of compression of the median nerve at this anatomic location include flexor tenosynovitis, rheumatoid arthritis, pregnancy, amyloidosis, and other space-occupying lesions that compromise the median nerve as it passes though this closed space.[13] This entrapment neuropathy manifests as pain, numbness, paresthesias, and associated weakness in the hand and wrist; these symptoms radiate to the thumb, index, middle, and radial half of the ring fingers (**Fig. 40.15**), and may also radiate proximal to the entrapment into the forearm. Untreated, progressive motor

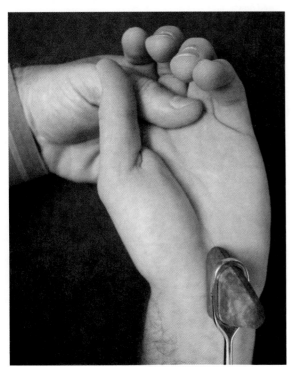

Fig. 40.16   The Tinel sign for carpal tunnel syndrome. *(From Waldman SD: Physical diagnosis of pain: an atlas of signs and symptoms, ed 2, Philadelphia, 2010, Saunders, p 164.)*

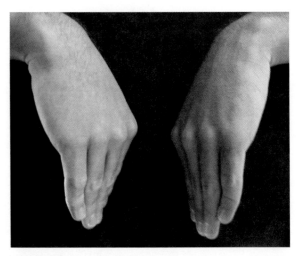

Fig. 40.17 The Phalen test for carpal tunnel syndrome. *(From Waldman SD: Physical diagnosis of pain: an atlas of signs and symptoms, ed 2, Philadelphia, 2010, Saunders, p 165.)*

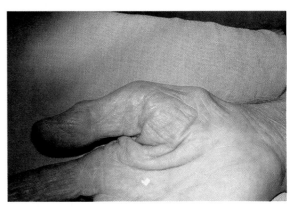

Fig. 40.18 Thenar muscle atrophy. Chronic entrapment of the median nerve in the carpal tunnel or more proximally can produce thenar atrophy as seen in this patient. *(From Nathan DJ: Soft tissue. In Klippel JH, Dieppe PA, editors:* Rheumatology, *ed 2, London, 1998, Mosby, p 4.)*

deficit and, ultimately, flexion contracture of the affected fingers can result. The onset of symptoms is usually after repetitive wrist motions or from repeated pressure on the wrist, such as resting the wrists on the edge of a computer keyboard. Direct trauma to the median nerve as it enters the carpal tunnel may also result in a similar clinical presentation.

Signs and Symptoms

Physical findings include tenderness over the median nerve at the wrist. A positive Tinel sign over the median nerve as it passes beneath the flexor retinaculum is usually present (**Fig. 40.16**).[14] A positive Phalen test is highly suggestive of carpal tunnel syndrome. The Phalen test is performed by having the patient place his or her wrists in complete, unforced flexion for at least 30 seconds (**Fig. 40.17**).[15] If the median nerve is entrapped at the wrist, this maneuver will reproduce the symptoms of carpal tunnel syndrome. Weakness of thumb opposition and wasting of the thenar eminence are often seen in advanced carpal tunnel syndrome, although because of the complex motion of the thumb, subtle motor deficits may be easily missed (**Fig. 40.18**). Early in the course of the evolution of carpal tunnel syndrome, the only physical finding, other than tenderness over the nerve, may be the loss of sensation on the thumb, index, middle, and radial half of the ring fingers.

Testing

Electromyography will help distinguish cervical radiculopathy and diabetic polyneuropathy from carpal tunnel syndrome. Plain radiographs are indicated in all patients with carpal tunnel syndrome to rule out occult bony pathology. Based on the patient's clinical presentation, additional testing

including complete blood count, uric acid, erythrocyte sedimentation rate, and antinuclear antibody testing may be indicated. MRI scan of the wrist is indicated if joint instability or a space-occupying lesion is suspected. The injection technique described later will serve as both a diagnostic and therapeutic maneuver.

Differential Diagnosis

Carpal tunnel syndrome is often misdiagnosed as arthritis of the carpometacarpal joint of the thumb, cervical radiculopathy, or diabetic polyneuropathy. Patients with arthritis of the carpometacarpal joint of the thumb will have a positive Watson's test and radiographic evidence of arthritis (**Fig. 40.19**). Most patients suffering from a cervical radiculopathy will have reflex, motor, and sensory changes associated with neck pain, whereas patients with carpal tunnel syndrome will have no reflex changes and motor and sensory changes will be limited to the distal median nerve. Diabetic polyneuropathy will generally manifest as symmetric sensory deficit involving the entire hand rather than limited to the distribution of the median nerve. It should be remembered that cervical radiculopathy and median nerve entrapment may coexist as the so-called double crush

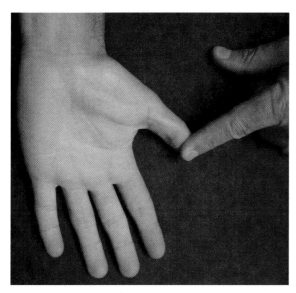

Fig. 40.19 The Watson stress test for arthritis of the carpometacarpal joint of the thumb. *(From Waldman SD: Physical diagnosis of pain: an atlas of signs and symptoms, ed 2, Philadelphia, 2010, Saunders, p 160.)*

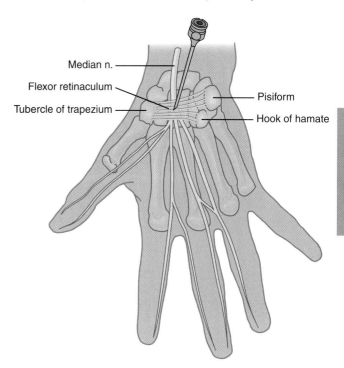

Fig. 40.20 Injection technique for carpal tunnel syndrome. *(From Waldman SD: Atlas of pain management injection techniques, ed 2, Philadelphia, 2007, Saunders, p 256.)*

syndrome. Because carpal tunnel syndrome is commonly seen in patients with diabetes, it is not surprising that diabetic polyneuropathy is usually present in diabetic patients with carpal tunnel syndrome.

Treatment

Mild cases of carpal tunnel syndrome will usually respond to conservative therapy; surgery should be reserved for more severe cases. Initial treatment of carpal tunnel syndrome should consist of treatment with simple analgesics, NSAIDs or COX-2 inhibitors, and splinting of the wrist. At a minimum, the splint should be worn at night, but ideally it should be worn 24 hours a day. Avoidance of repetitive activities thought to be responsible for the evolution of carpal tunnel syndrome (e.g., keyboarding, hammering) will also help ameliorate the patient's symptoms. If the patient fails to respond to these conservative measures, a next reasonable step is injection of the carpal tunnel with local anesthetic and steroid.

Carpal tunnel injection is performed by placing the patient in a supine position with the arm fully abducted at the patient's side and the elbow slightly flexed, with the dorsum of the hand resting on a folded towel. A total of 3 mL of local anesthetic and 40 mg of methylprednisolone is drawn up in a 5 mL sterile syringe. The clinician then has the patient make a fist and at the same time flex his or her wrist to aid in identification of the palmaris longus tendon. After preparation of the skin with antiseptic solution, a ⅝-inch 25-gauge needle is inserted just medial to the tendon and just proximal to the crease of the wrist at a 30-degree angle (**Fig. 40.20**). The needle is slowly advanced until the tip is just beyond the tendon.[16] A paresthesia in the distribution of the median nerve is often elicited and the patient should be warned of this. The patient should be instructed that should a paresthesia occur, he or she is to say "There!" as soon as the paresthesia is felt. If a paresthesia is elicited, the needle is withdrawn slightly away from the median nerve. Gentle aspiration is then carried out to identify blood. If the aspiration test is negative and no persistent paresthesia into the distribution of the median nerve remains, 3 mL of solution is slowly injected, with

the patient being monitored closely for signs of local anesthetic toxicity. If no paresthesia is elicited and the needle tip hits bone, the needle is withdrawn out of the periosteum and after careful aspiration, 3 mL of solution is slowly injected.

For patients who fail these treatment modalities, surgical release of the median nerve at the carpal tunnel is indicated. Endoscopic techniques are showing promise and appear to result in less postoperative pain and dysfunction.

De Quervain Tenosynovitis

De Quervain tenosynovitis is caused by an inflammation and swelling of the tendons of the abductor pollicis longus and extensor pollicis brevis at the level of the radial styloid process.[17] This inflammation and swelling is usually the result of trauma to the tendon from repetitive twisting motions. If the inflammation and swelling becomes chronic, a thickening of the tendon sheath occurs with a resulting constriction of the sheath (**Fig. 40.21**). A triggering phenomenon may result with the tendon catching within the sheath, causing the thumb to lock or "trigger." Arthritis and gout of the first metacarpal joint may also coexist and exacerbate the pain and disability of de Quervain tenosynovitis.

De Quervain tenosynovitis occurs in patients engaged in repetitive activities that include hand grasping (e.g., politicians shaking hands) or high-torque wrist turning (e.g., scooping ice cream at an ice cream parlor). It may also develop without obvious antecedent trauma in the parturient.

The pain of de Quervain tenosynovitis is localized to the region of the radial styloid. It is constant and is made worse with active pinching activities of the thumb or ulnar deviation of the wrist. Patients will note the inability to hold a coffee cup or turn a screwdriver. Sleep disturbance is common.

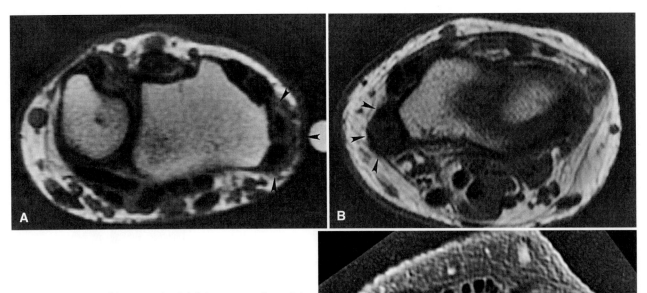

Fig. 40.21 A, T1 axial image, wrist. Painful mass over the radial styloid process in the postpartum woman proved to be fibrosis surrounding the extensor pollicis brevis and abductor pollicis longus tendons *(arrowheads),* causing obliteration of the subcutaneous fat that normally surrounds these tendons. **B,** T1 axial image, wrist (different patient than in **A**). The tendons of the first dorsal compartment are not discrete, low-signal structures like other wrist tendons and appear enlarged *(arrowheads).* The subcutaneous fat surrounding the tendons remains normal in this patient. **C,** T1 fat-saturation image with contrast, axial wrist (different patient than in **A** and **B**). There is increased signal and size of the tendons of the first dorsal compartment and contrast enhancement surrounding the tendons *(arrowheads)* from extensive tenosynovitis. *(From Kaplan PA, Helms CA, Dussault R, et al, editors:* Musculoskeletal MRI, *Philadelphia, 2001, Saunders, p 259.)*

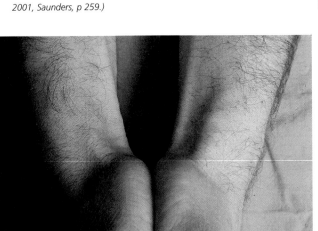

Fig. 40.22 De Quervain tenosynovitis. *(From Fam AG: The wrist and hand. In Klippel JH, Dieppe PA, editors:* Rheumatology, *ed 2, London, 1998, Mosby, p 4.)*

Signs and Symptoms

On physical examination, there will be tenderness and swelling over the tendons and tendon sheaths along the distal radius with point tenderness over the radial styloid (**Fig. 40.22**). Many patients with de Quervain tenosynovitis will exhibit a creaking sensation with flexion and extension of the thumb. Range of motion of the thumb may be decreased because of the pain and a trigger thumb phenomenon may be noted. Patients with de Quervain tenosynovitis will demonstrate a positive Finkelstein

test (**Fig. 40.23**).[18] The Finkelstein test is performed by stabilizing the patient's forearm and then having the patient fully flex his or her thumb into the palm and actively force the wrist toward the ulna. Sudden, severe pain is highly suggestive of de Quervain tenosynovitis.

Testing

There is no specific test to diagnose de Quervain tenosynovitis. The diagnosis is generally made on clinical grounds. Electromyography will help distinguish de Quervain tenosynovitis from neuropathic processes such as cervical radiculopathy and cheiralgia paresthetica. Plain radiographs are indicated in all patients with de Quervain tenosynovitis to rule out occult bony pathology. Based on the patient's clinical presentation, additional testing including complete blood count, uric acid, erythrocyte sedimentation rate, and antinuclear antibody testing may be indicated. MRI scan of the wrist is indicated if joint instability is suspected. The injection technique described subsequently will serve as both a diagnostic and therapeutic maneuver.

Differential Diagnosis

Entrapment of the lateral antebrachial cutaneous nerve, arthritis of the first metacarpal joint, gout, cheiralgia paresthetica, and occasionally C6-7 radiculopathy can mimic de Quervain tenosynovitis. Cheiralgia paresthetica is an entrapment neuropathy that is the result of entrapment of the superficial

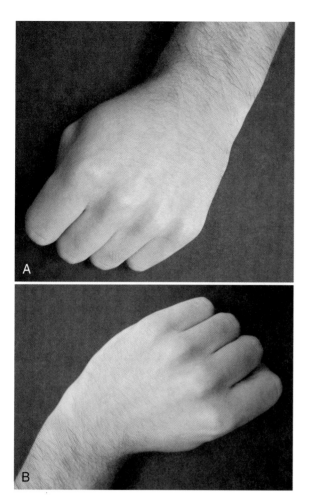

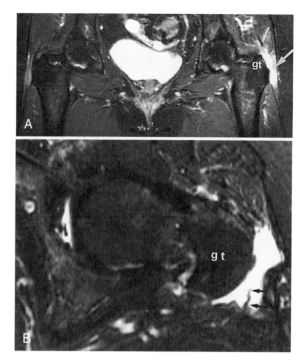

Fig. 40.24 Greater trochanteric bursitis and torn gluteus medius tendon. **A,** Coronal STIR image shows focal high signal around the greater trochanter *(gt; arrow)*. The torn and retracted gluteus medius tendon also is seen *(small arrow)*. **B,** Axial image shows the well-defined fluid collection that is compatible with greater trochanteric bursitis. The gluteus medius bursitis often is seen in association with gluteus medius tendon tears. *(From Kaplan PA, Helms CA, Dussault R, et al, editors:* Musculoskeletal MRI, *Philadelphia, 2001, Saunders, p 351.)*

Fig. 40.23 **A** and **B,** the Finkelstein test for de Quervain tenosynovitis. *(From Waldman SD: Physical diagnosis of pain: an atlas of signs and symptoms, ed 2, Philadelphia, 2010, Saunders, p 157.)*

branch of the radial nerve at the wrist. All these painful conditions can coexist with de Quervain tenosynovitis.

Treatment

Initial treatment of the pain and functional disability associated with de Quervain tenosynovitis should include a combination of NSAIDs or COX-2 inhibitors and physical therapy. The local application of heat and cold may also be beneficial. Any repetitive activity that may exacerbate the patient's symptoms should be avoided. Nighttime splinting of the affected thumb may also help avoid the trigger finger phenomenon that can occur on awakening in many patients suffering from this condition. For patients who do not respond to these treatment modalities, injection of the inflamed tendons may be a reasonable next step.

Trochanteric Bursitis

Trochanteric bursitis is a commonly encountered pain complaint in clinical practice. The patient suffering from trochanteric bursitis will frequently complain of pain in the lateral hip that can radiate down the leg, thereby mimicking sciatica.[19] The pain is localized to the area over the trochanter. Often, the patient will be unable to sleep on the affected hip and may

complain of a sharp, catching sensation with range of motion of the hip, especially on first arising. The patient may note that walking upstairs becomes increasingly more difficult. Trochanteric bursitis often coexists with arthritis of the hip joint, back and sacroiliac joint disease, and gait disturbance.

The trochanteric bursa lies between the greater trochanter and the tendon of the gluteus medius and the iliotibial tract (**Fig. 40.24**). This bursa may exist as a single bursal sac or in some patients may exist as a multisegmented series of sacs that may be loculated in nature. The trochanteric bursa is vulnerable to injury from both acute trauma and repeated microtrauma. Acute injuries frequently take the form of direct trauma to the bursa via falls directly onto the greater trochanter or previous hip surgery, as well as from overuse injuries, including running on soft or uneven surfaces. If the inflammation of the trochanteric bursa becomes chronic, calcification of the bursa may occur.

Signs and Symptoms

Physical examination of the patient suffering from trochanteric bursitis will reveal point tenderness in the lateral thigh just over the greater trochanter. Passive adduction and abduction, as well as active resisted abduction of the affected lower extremity, will reproduce the pain. Sudden release of resistance during this maneuver will markedly increase the pain (**Fig. 40.25**).[20] There should be no sensory deficit in the distribution of the lateral femoral cutaneous nerve as seen with meralgia paresthetica, which is often confused with trochanteric bursitis.

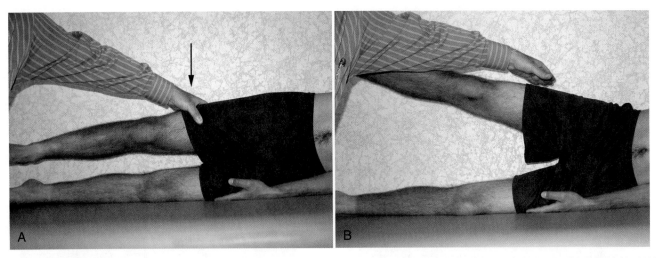

Fig. 40.25 **A** and **B,** The resisted abduction release test. *(From Waldman SD: Physical diagnosis of pain: an atlas of signs and symptoms, ed 2, Philadelphia, 2010, Saunders, p 271.)*

Testing

Plain radiographs of the hip may reveal calcification of the bursa and associated structures consistent with chronic inflammation. MRI scan is indicated if occult mass or tumor of the hip or groin is suspected. Complete blood count and erythrocyte sedimentation rate are useful if infection is suspected. Electromyography will help distinguish trochanteric bursitis from meralgia paresthetica and sciatica. The injection technique described later will serve as both a diagnostic and therapeutic maneuver.

Differential Diagnosis

Trochanteric bursitis frequently coexists with arthritis of the hip, which may require specific treatment to provide palliation of pain and return of function. Occasionally, trochanteric bursitis can be confused with meralgia paresthetica because both manifest with pain in the lateral thigh. The two syndromes can be distinguished in that patients suffering from meralgia paresthetica will not have pain on palpation over the greater trochanter. Electromyography will help sort out confusing clinical presentations. The clinician must consider the potential for primary or secondary tumors of the hip in the differential diagnosis of trochanteric bursitis.

Treatment

A short course of conservative therapy consisting of simple analgesics, NSAIDs, or COX-2 inhibitors is a reasonable first step in the treatment of patients suffering from trochanteric bursitis. The patient should be instructed to avoid repetitive activities that may be responsible for the development of trochanteric bursitis (e.g., running on sand). If the patient does not experience rapid improvement, the following injection technique is a reasonable next step.

Injection of the trochanteric bursa can be carried out by placing the patient in the lateral decubitus position with the affected side up. The midpoint of the greater trochanter is identified. Proper preparation with antiseptic solution of the skin overlying this point is then carried out (**Figs. 40.26** and **40.27**). A syringe containing 2.0 mL of 0.25% preservative-free bupivacaine and 40 mg of methylprednisolone is attached to a 1½-inch 25-gauge needle.

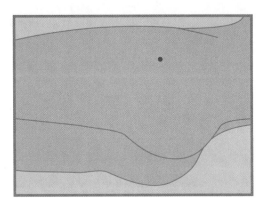

Fig. 40.26 Patient positioning for trochanteric bursa injection. *(From Waldman SD: Atlas of pain management injection techniques, ed 2, Philadelphia, 2007, Saunders, p 361.)*

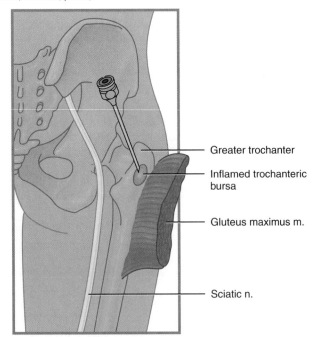

Greater trochanter

Inflamed trochanteric bursa

Gluteus maximus m.

Sciatic n.

Fig. 40.27 Injection technique for trochanteric bursitis. *(From Waldman SD: Atlas of pain management injection techniques, ed 2, Philadelphia, 2007, Saunders, p 221.)*

The pain of adductor tendinitis is sharp, constant, and severe with sleep disturbance often reported. The patient may attempt to splint the inflamed tendons by adopting an adductor lurch type of gait, that is, shifting the trunk of the body over the affected extremity when walking. In addition to this pain, patients suffering from adductor tendinitis will often experience a gradual decrease in functional ability with decreasing hip range of motion, making simple everyday tasks such as getting in or out of a car quite difficult. With continued disuse, muscle wasting may occur and an adhesive capsulitis of the hip may develop.

Signs and Symptoms

On physical examination, the patient suffering from adductor tendinitis will report pain on palpation of the origins of the adductor tendons and will exhibit a positive Waldman knee squeeze test (**Fig. 40.29**). Active resisted adduction will reproduce the pain as will passive abduction.[23] Tendinitis of the musculotendinous unit of the hip frequently coexists with bursitis of the associated bursae of the hip joint, creating additional pain and functional disability. Neurologic examination of the hip and lower extremity will be within normal limits unless there has been concomitant stretch injury to the plexus or obturator nerve.

Testing

Plain radiographs are indicated in all patients with hip, thigh, and groin pain. Based on the patient's clinical presentation, additional testing including complete blood count, erythrocyte sedimentation rate, and antinuclear antibody testing may be indicated. MRI scan of the hip is indicated if aseptic necrosis or occult mass is suspected. Radionuclide bone scanning should be considered if the possibility of occult fracture of the pelvis is being considered. Electromyography can help rule out compression neuropathy or trauma of the obturator nerve, as well as plexopathy and radiculopathy. Injection of the insertion of the adductor tendons will serve as both a diagnostic and therapeutic maneuver.

Differential Diagnosis

Internal derangement of the hip may mimic the clinical presentation of adductor tendinitis. Occasionally, indirect inguinal hernia can produce pain that can be confused with adductor tendinitis. If trauma has occurred, consideration of the possibility of occult pelvic fracture, especially in those individuals with osteopenia or osteoporosis, should be entertained and radionuclide bone scanning should be obtained. Avascular necrosis of the hip may also produce hip pain, which can mimic the clinical presentation of adductor tendinitis. Entrapment neuropathy and/or stretch injury to the ilioinguinal, genitofemoral, and obturator nerves, as well as plexopathy and radiculopathy, should be considered if there is the physical finding of neurologic deficit in patients thought to suffer from adductor tendinitis because all of these clinical entities may coexist.

Treatment

Initial treatment of the pain and functional disability associated with adductor tendinitis should include a combination of NSAIDs or COX-2 inhibitors and physical therapy.

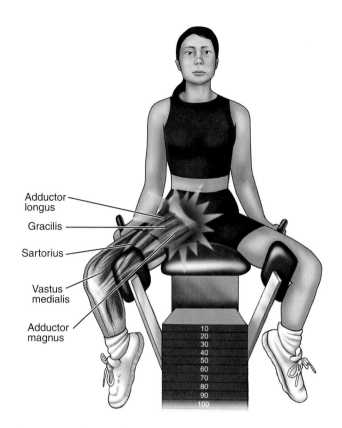

Fig. 40.28 Mechanism of injury in adductor tendinitis. *(From Waldman SD: Atlas of uncommon pain syndromes, ed 2, Philadelphia, 2008, Saunders, p 252.)*

Before needle placement, the patient should be advised to say "There!" immediately if he or she feels a paresthesia into the lower extremity, indicating that the needle has impinged on the sciatic nerve. Should a paresthesia occur, the needle should be immediately withdrawn and repositioned more laterally. The needle is then carefully advanced through the previously identified point at a right angle to the skin directly toward the center of the greater trochanter.[21] The needle is advanced very slowly to avoid trauma to the sciatic nerve until it hits the bone. The needle is then withdrawn back out of the periosteum and, after careful aspiration for blood and if no paresthesia is present, the solution is then gently injected into the bursa. There should be minimal resistance to injection.

Adductor Tendinitis

The increased use of exercise equipment for lower extremity strengthening has resulted in an increased incidence of adductor tendinitis. The adductor muscles of the hip include the gracilis, adductor longus, adductor brevis, and adductor magnus muscles.[22] The adductor function of these muscles is innervated by the obturator nerve, which is susceptible to trauma from pelvic fractures and compression by tumor. The tendons of the adductor muscles of the hip have their origin along the pubis and ischial ramus and it is at this point that tendinitis frequently occurs (**Fig. 40.28**). These tendons and their associated muscles are susceptible to the development of tendinitis because of overuse or trauma caused by stretch injuries. Inciting factors may include the vigorous use of exercise equipment for lower extremity strengthening and acute stretching of the musculotendinous units as a result of sports injuries (e.g., sliding into bases when playing baseball).

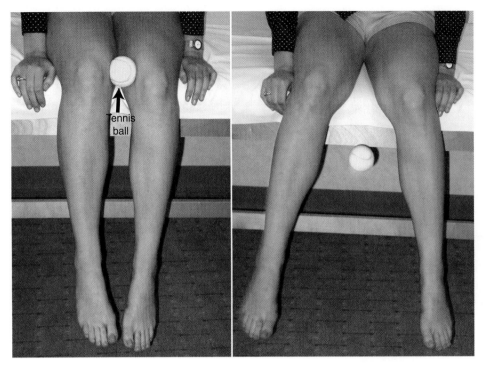

Fig. 40.29 The Waldman knee squeeze test for adductor tendinitis. *(From Waldman SD: Physical diagnosis of pain: an atlas of signs and symptoms, ed 2, Philadelphia, 2010, Saunders, p 307.)*

The local application of heat and cold may also be beneficial. For patients who do not respond to these treatment modalities, the injection of the insertion of the adductor tendons of the hip with local anesthetic and steroid may be a reasonable next step.

Medial Collateral Ligament Syndrome

Patients with medial collateral ligament syndrome will have pain over the medial knee joint and increased pain on passive valgus and external rotation of the knee.[24] Activity, especially involving flexion and external rotation of the knee, will make the pain worse, with rest and heat providing some relief. The pain is constant and characterized as aching in nature. The patient with injury to the medial collateral ligament may complain of locking or popping with flexion of the affected knee. The pain may interfere with sleep. Coexistent bursitis, tendinitis, arthritis, and/or internal derangement of the knee may confuse the clinical picture following trauma to the knee joint.

The medial collateral ligament syndrome is characterized by pain at the medial aspect of the knee joint. It is usually the result of trauma to the medial collateral ligament from falls with the leg in valgus and externally rotated, typically during snow skiing accidents or football clipping injuries (**Fig. 40.30**). The medial collateral ligament is a broad, flat, band-like ligament that runs from the medial condyle of the femur to the medial aspect of the shaft of the tibia where it attaches just above the groove of the semimembranosus muscle. It also attaches to the edge of the medial semilunar cartilage. The ligament is susceptible to strain at the joint line or avulsion at its origin or insertion.

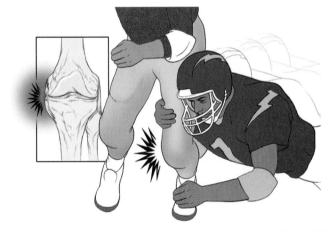

Fig. 40.30 Medial collateral ligament syndrome is characterized by medial joint pain that is made worse with flexion or external rotation of the knee. *(From Waldman SD: Atlas of common pain syndromes, ed 2, Philadelphia, 2008, Saunders, p 253.)*

Signs and Symptoms

Patients with injury of the medial collateral ligament will exhibit tenderness along the course of the ligament from the medial femoral condyle to its tibial insertion. If the ligament is avulsed from its bony insertions, tenderness may be localized to the proximal or distal ligaments, whereas patients suffering from strain of the ligament will exhibit more diffuse tenderness. Patients with severe injury to the ligament may exhibit laxity of the joint when valgus and varus stress is placed on the affected knee (**Fig. 40.31**).[25] Because pain may produce muscle guarding, MRI scanning of the knee may be necessary to confirm the clinician's clinical impression.

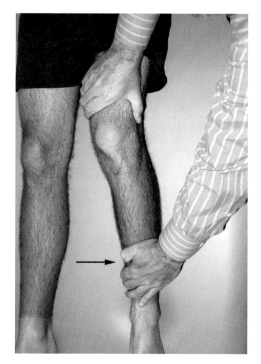

Fig. 40.31 The valgus stress test for medial collateral ligament integrity. *(From Waldman SD: Physical diagnosis of pain: an atlas of signs and symptoms, ed 2, Philadelphia, 2010, Saunders, p 334.)*

Joint effusion and swelling may be present with injury to the medial collateral ligament, but it is also suggestive of intra-articular damage.

Testing

Plain radiographs are indicated in all patients with medial collateral ligament syndrome pain. Based on the patient's clinical presentation, additional testing including complete blood count, erythrocyte sedimentation rate, and antinuclear antibody testing may be indicated. MRI scan of the knee is indicated if internal derangement or occult mass or tumor is suspected. Bone scan may be useful to identify occult stress fractures involving the joint, especially if trauma has occurred.

Treatment

Initial treatment of the pain and functional disability associated with injury to the medial collateral ligament should include a combination of NSAIDs or COX-2 inhibitors and physical therapy. The local application of heat and cold may also be beneficial. Avoidance of any repetitive activity that may exacerbate the patient's symptoms should be avoided. For patients who do not respond to these treatment modalities and who do not have a lesion that will require surgical repair, injection of the medial collateral ligament may be a reasonable next step.

Prepatellar Bursitis

The prepatellar bursa is vulnerable to injury from both acute trauma and repeated microtrauma. The prepatellar bursa lies between the subcutaneous tissues and the patella.[26] This

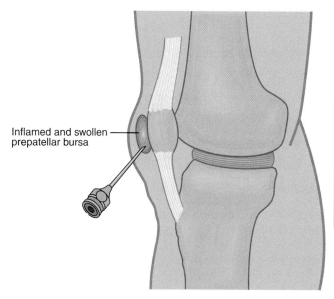

Fig. 40.32 Correct needle placement for injection of the prepatellar bursa. *(From Waldman SD: Atlas of pain management injection techniques, ed 2, Philadelphia, 2007, Saunders, p 272.)*

bursa may exist as a single bursal sac or in some patients may exist as a multisegmented series of sacs that may be loculated in nature. Acute injuries frequently take the form of direct trauma to the bursa via falls onto the knee or from patellar fractures, as well as from overuse injuries, including running on soft or uneven surfaces (**Fig. 40.32**). Prepatellar bursitis may also result from jobs requiring crawling or kneeling such as in carpet laying or scrubbing floors; hence the other name for prepatellar bursitis is *housemaid's knee*. If the inflammation of the prepatellar bursa becomes chronic, calcification of the bursa may occur.

Signs and Symptoms

The patient suffering from prepatellar bursitis will frequently complain of pain and swelling in the anterior knee over the patella that can radiate superiorly and inferiorly into the area surrounding the knee.[27] Often, the patient will be unable to kneel or walk down stairs. The patient may also complain of a sharp, catching sensation with range of motion of the knee, especially on first arising. Prepatellar bursitis often coexists with arthritis and tendinitis of the knee joint and these other pathologic processes may confuse the clinical picture.

Testing

Plain radiographs of the knee may reveal calcification of the bursa and associated structures including the quadriceps tendon, which is consistent with chronic inflammation. MRI scan is indicated if internal derangement, occult mass, or tumor of the knee is suspected. Electromyography will help distinguish prepatellar bursitis from femoral neuropathy, lumbar radiculopathy, and plexopathy. The following injection technique will serve as a diagnostic and therapeutic maneuver. Antinuclear antibody testing is indicated if collagen vascular disease is suspected. If infection is considered, aspiration, Gram stain, and culture of bursal fluid are indicated on an emergent basis.

Differential Diagnosis

Because of the unique anatomy of the region, not only the prepatellar bursa but the associated tendons and other bursae of the knee can become inflamed and confuse the diagnosis. The prepatellar bursa lies between the subcutaneous tissues and the patella. The bursa is held in place by ligamentum patellae. Both the quadriceps tendon and the prepatellar bursa are subject to the development of inflammation following overuse, misuse, or direct trauma. The quadriceps tendon is made up of fibers from the four muscles that compose the quadriceps muscle: the vastus lateralis, the vastus intermedius, the vastus medialis, and the rectus femoris. These muscles are the primary extensors of the lower extremity at the knee. The tendons of these muscles converge and unite to form a single, exceedingly strong tendon. The patella functions as a sesamoid bone within the quadriceps tendon with fibers of the tendon expanding around the patella thereby forming the medial and lateral patellar retinacula, which help strengthen the knee joint. These fibers are called expansions and are subject to strain, and the tendon proper is subject to the development of tendinitis. The suprapatellar, infrapatellar, and prepatellar bursae may also concurrently become inflamed with dysfunction of the quadriceps tendon. It should be remembered that anything that alters the normal biomechanics of the knee can result in inflammation of the prepatellar bursa.

Treatment

A short course of conservative therapy consisting of simple analgesics, NSAIDs or COX-2 inhibitors, and a knee brace to prevent further trauma is a reasonable first step in the treatment of patients suffering from prepatellar bursitis. If the patient does not experience rapid improvement, injection of the prepatellar bursa is a reasonable next step. The use of local heat and gentle range-of-motion exercises should be introduced after the acute inflammation begins to subside.

Deltoid Ligament Strain

The deltoid ligament is susceptible to strain from acute injury from sudden overpronation of the ankle or from repetitive microtrama to the ligament from overuse or misuse, such as long distance running on soft or uneven surfaces. The deltoid ligament is exceptionally strong and is not as subject to strain as the anterior talofibular ligament.[28] The deltoid ligament has two layers (**Fig. 40.33**). Both attach above to the medial malleolus. A deep layer attaches below to the medial body of the talus with the superficial fibers attaching to the medial talus and the sustentaculum tali of the calcaneus and the navicular tuberosity.

Signs and Symptoms

Patients with strain of the deltoid ligament will complain of pain just below the medial malleolus. Plantar flexion and eversion of the ankle joint will exacerbate the pain (**Fig. 40.34**). Often patients with injury to the deltoid ligament will note a "pop" followed by significant swelling and inability to walk.

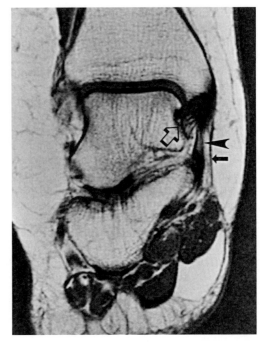

Fig. 40.33 Medial ankle ligaments: normal. T1 coronal image, ankle. Two layers of the deltoid (medial) ligament are seen on routine MRI. The deep tibiotalar ligament is striated *(open arrow)*. The more superficial tibiocalcaneal ligament *(arrowhead)* may have vertical striations also. The thin, vertical, low-signal structure superficial to the tibiocalcaneal ligament is the flexor retinaculum *(solid arrow)*. *(From Kaplan PA, Helms CA, Dussault R, et al, editors:* Musculoskeletal MRI, *Philadelphia, 2001, Saunders, p 835.)*

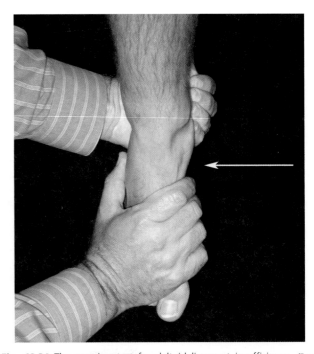

Fig. 40.34 The eversion test for deltoid ligament insufficiency. *(From Waldman SD: Physical diagnosis of pain: an atlas of signs and symptoms, ed 2, Philadelphia, 2010, Saunders, p 409.)*

On physical examination, there will be point tenderness over the medial malleolus. With acute trauma, ecchymosis over the ligament may be noted. Passive eversion and plantar flexion of the ankle joint will exacerbate the pain.[29] Coexistent bursitis and arthritis of the ankle and subtalar joints may also be present and confuse the clinical picture.

Testing

Plain radiographs are indicated in all patients with ankle pain. Based on the patient's clinical presentation, additional testing including complete blood count, erythrocyte sedimentation rate, and antinuclear antibody testing may be indicated. MRI scan of the ankle is indicated if disruption of the deltoid ligament, joint instability, or occult mass or tumor is suspected. Radionuclide bone scanning should be used if occult fracture is suspected.

Differential Diagnosis

Avulsion fractures of the calcaneus, talus, medial malleolus, and the base of the fifth metatarsal can mimic the pain of injury to the deltoid ligament. Bursitis and tendinitis, as well as gout of the midtarsal joints, may coexist with deltoid ligament strain and may confuse the diagnosis. Tarsal tunnel syndrome may occur following ankle trauma and may further confuse the clinical picture.

Treatment

Initial treatment of the pain and functional disability associated with deltoid ligament strain should include a combination of NSAIDs or COX-2 inhibitors and physical therapy. The local application of heat and cold may also be beneficial. Avoidance of repetitive activities that aggravate the patient's symptoms, as well as short-term immobilization of the ankle joint, may also provide relief. For patients who do not respond to these treatment modalities, injection of the deltoid ligament may be a reasonable next step.

Achilles Bursitis

Achilles bursitis is being seen with increasing frequency in clinical practice as jogging has increased in popularity. The Achilles tendon is susceptible to the development of bursitis both at its insertion on the calcaneus and at its narrowest part at a point approximately 5 cm above its insertion. Additionally, the Achilles tendon is subject to repetitive motion injury, which may result in microtrauma that heals poorly as a result of the tendon's avascular nature.[30] Running is often implicated as the inciting factor of acute Achilles bursitis. Bursitis of the Achilles tendon frequently coexists with Achilles tendinitis, creating additional pain and functional disability. Calcium deposition around the Achilles bursa may occur if the inflammation continues, making subsequent treatment more difficult.

Signs and Symptoms

The onset of Achilles bursitis is usually acute occurring after overuse or misuse of the ankle joint. Inciting factors may include activities such as running and sudden stopping and starting as when playing tennis. Improper stretching of the gastrocnemius and Achilles tendon before exercise has also been implicated in the development of Achilles bursitis, as well as acute tendinitis and tendon rupture. The pain of Achilles bursitis is constant and severe and is localized in the posterior ankle. Significant sleep disturbance is often reported. The patient may attempt to splint the inflamed Achilles bursa by adopting a flat-footed gait to avoid plantar flexing the affected foot. Patients with Achilles bursitis will exhibit pain with resisted plantar flexion of the foot. A creaking or grating sensation may be palpated when passively plantar flexing the foot because of coexisting tendinitis.[31] As mentioned earlier, the chronically inflamed Achilles tendon may suddenly rupture with stress or during vigorous injection procedures to treat Achilles bursitis.

Testing

Plain radiographs are indicated in all patients with posterior ankle pain. Based on the patient's clinical presentation, additional testing including complete blood count, erythrocyte sedimentation rate, and antinuclear antibody testing may be indicated. MRI scan of the ankle is indicated if joint instability is suspected. Radionuclide bone scanning is useful to identify stress fractures of the tibia not seen on plain radiographs. The injection technique described later will serve as both a diagnostic and therapeutic maneuver.

Differential Diagnosis

Achilles bursitis is generally easily identified on clinical grounds. Because tendinitis frequently accompanies Achilles bursitis, the specific diagnosis may be unclear. Stress fractures of the ankle may also mimic Achilles bursitis and may be identified on plain radiographs or radionuclide bone scanning.

Treatment

Initial treatment of the pain and functional disability associated with Achilles bursitis should include a combination of NSAIDs or COX-2 inhibitors and physical therapy. The local application of heat and cold may also be beneficial. Avoidance of repetitive activities responsible for the evolution of the bursitis (e.g., jogging) should be encouraged. For patients who do not respond to these treatment modalities, the following injection technique with local anesthetic and steroid may be a reasonable next step.

Injection for Achilles bursitis is carried out by placing the patient in the prone position with the affected foot hanging off the end of the table. The foot is gently dorsiflexed to facilitate identification of the margin of the tendon to aid in avoiding injection directly into the tendon.[32] The tender points at the tendinous insertion and/or at its most narrow part—approximately 5 cm above the insertion—are identified and marked with a sterile marker (**Fig. 40.35**).

Proper preparation with antiseptic solution of the skin overlying these points is then carried out. A sterile syringe containing 2.0 mL of 0.25% preservative-free bupivacaine and 40 mg of methylprednisolone is attached to a 1½-inch 25-gauge needle using strict aseptic technique. With strict aseptic technique, the previously marked points are palpated. The needle is then carefully advanced at this point alongside the tendon through the skin and subcutaneous tissues with care being taken not to enter the substance of the tendon (**Fig. 40.36**). The contents of the syringe are then gently injected while slowly withdrawing the needle. There should be minimal

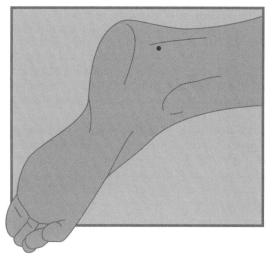

Fig. 40.35 Foot positioning for injection for Achilles bursitis. *(From Waldman SD: Atlas of pain management injection techniques, ed 2, Philadelphia, 2007, Saunders, p 329.)*

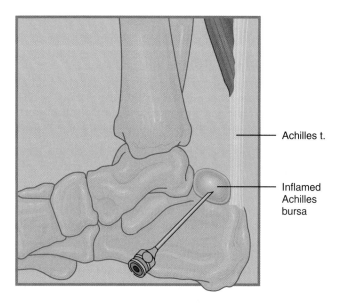

Achilles t.

Inflamed Achilles bursa

Fig. 40.36 Injection technique for Achilles bursitis. *(From Waldman SD: Atlas of pain management injection techniques, ed 2, Philadelphia, 2007, Saunders, p 329.)*

resistance to injection. If there is significant resistance to injection, the needle tip is probably in the substance of the Achilles tendon and should be withdrawn slightly until the injection proceeds without significant resistance. The needle is then removed and a sterile pressure dressing and ice pack are placed at the injection site.

Sesamoiditis

Sesamoiditis is being seen with increased frequency in clinical practice because of the increased interest in jogging and long-distance running. The sesamoid bones are small rounded structures that are embedded in the flexor tendons of the foot and are usually in close proximity to the joints.[33] These sesamoid bones decrease friction and pressure of the flexor tendon as it passes in proximity to a joint. Sesamoid

bones of the first metatarsal occur in almost all patients, with sesamoid bones being present in the flexor tendons of the second and fifth metatarsals in a significant number of patients.

Although the sesamoid bone associated with the first metatarsal head is affected most commonly, the sesamoid bones of the second and fifth metatarsal heads are also subject to the development of sesamoiditis. Sesamoiditis is characterized by tenderness and pain over the metatarsal heads. The patients often feel that they are walking with a stone in their shoe. The pain of sesamoiditis worsens with prolonged standing or walking for long distances and is exacerbated by improperly fitted or padded shoes. Sesamoiditis is most often associated with pushing off injuries during football or repetitive microtrauma from running or dancing.

Signs and Symptoms

On physical examination, pain can be reproduced by pressure on the affected sesamoid bone. In contradistinction to metatarsalgia, in which the tender area remains over the metatarsal heads, with sesamoiditis, the area of maximum tenderness will move along with the flexor tendon when the patient actively flexes his or her toe (**Fig. 40.37**). The patient with sesamoiditis will often exhibit an antalgic gait in an effort to reduce weight bearing during walking. With acute trauma to the sesamoid, ecchymosis over the plantar surface of the foot may be present.

Testing

Plain radiographs are indicated in all patients with sesamoiditis to rule out fractures and identify sesamoid bones that may have become inflamed. Based on the patient's clinical presentation, additional testing including complete blood count, erythrocyte sedimentation rate, and antinuclear antibody testing may be indicated. MRI scan of the metatarsal bones is indicated if joint instability or occult mass or tumor is suspected. Radionuclide bone scanning may be useful in identifying stress fractures of the metatarsal bones or sesamoid bones that may be missed on plain radiographs of the foot.

Differential Diagnosis

Primary pathology of the foot including gout and occult fractures may mimic the pain and disability associated with sesamoiditis. Entrapment neuropathies such as tarsal tunnel syndrome may also confuse the diagnosis, as may bursitis and plantar fasciitis of the foot, both of which may coexist with sesamoiditis. Metatarsalgia is another common cause of forefoot pain and may be distinguished from sesamoiditis by the fact that the pain of metatarsalgia is over the metatarsal heads and does not move when the patient actively flexes his or her toes, as is the case with sesamoiditis. Primary and metastatic tumors of the foot may also manifest in a manner analogous to arthritis of the midtarsal joints.

Treatment

Initial treatment of the pain and functional disability associated with sesamoiditis should include a combination of NSAIDs or COX-2 inhibitors and physical therapy. The local application of heat and cold may also be beneficial. Avoidance of repetitive activities that aggravate the patient's symptoms, as well

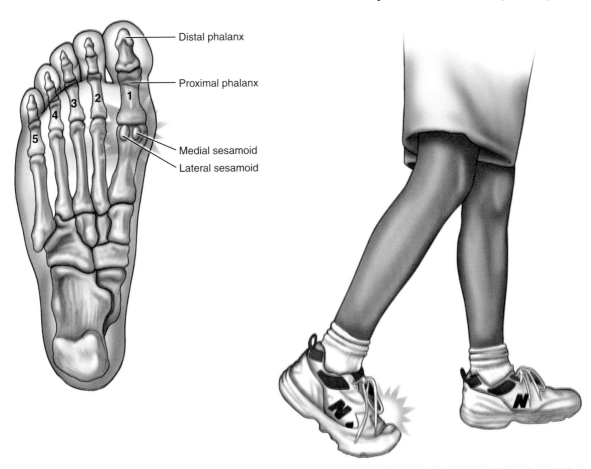

Fig. 40.37 Mechanism of injury in sesamoiditis. *(From Waldman SD:* Atlas of uncommon pain syndromes, *ed 2, Philadelphia, 2008, Saunders, p 318.)*

as short-term immobilization of the midtarsal joint, may also provide relief. For patients who do not respond to these treatment modalities, injection of the affected sesamoid bone with local anesthetic and steroid may be a reasonable next step.

Plantar Fasciitis

Plantar fasciitis is characterized by pain and tenderness over the plantar surface of the calcaneus.[34] Occurring twice as commonly in women, plantar fasciitis is thought to be caused by an inflammation of the plantar fascia. This inflammation can occur alone or can be part of a systemic inflammatory condition such as rheumatoid arthritis, Reyiter's syndrome, or gout. Obesity also seems to predispose to the development of plantar fasciitis, as does going barefoot or wearing house slippers for prolonged periods (**Fig. 40.38**). High-impact aerobic exercise and jogging with excessive heel strike have also been implicated.

Signs and Symptoms

The pain of plantar fasciitis is most severe on first walking after non–weight bearing and is made worse by prolonged standing or walking. Characteristic radiographic changes are lacking in plantar fasciitis, but radionuclide bone scanning may show increased uptake at the point of attachment of the plantar fascia to the medial calcaneal tuberosity.

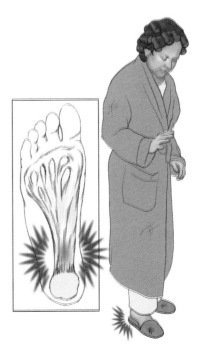

Fig. 40.38 The pain of plantar fasciitis is often localized to the hindfoot and can cause significant functional disability. *(From Waldman SD:* Atlas of common pain syndromes, *ed 2, Philadelphia, 2008, Saunders, p 309.)*

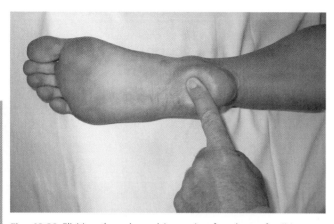

Fig. 40.39 Eliciting the calcaneal jump sign for plantar fasciitis. *(From Waldman SD: Physical diagnosis of pain: an atlas of signs and symptoms, ed 2, Philadelphia, 2010, Saunders, p 379.)*

On physical examination, the patient will exhibit a positive calcaneal jump sign when pressure is applied over the plantar medial calcaneal tuberosity (**Fig. 40.39**).[35] The patient's foot may also be tender along the plantar fascia as it moves anteriorly. Pain will be increased by dorsiflexing the toes, which pulls the plantar fascia taut, and then palpating along the fascia from the heel to the forefoot.

Differential Diagnosis

The pain of plantar fasciitis can often be confused with the pain of Morton's neuroma or sesamoiditis. The characteristic pain on dorsiflexion of the toes associated with plantar fasciitis should help distinguish these painful conditions of the foot. Stress fractures of the metatarsals or sesamoid bones, bursitis, and tendinitis may also confuse the clinical picture.

Testing

Plain radiographs are indicated in all patients with pain thought to be emanating from plantar fasciitis to rule out occult bony pathology and tumor. Based on the patient's clinical presentation, additional testing including complete blood count, prostate-specific antigen, erythrocyte sedimentation rate, and antinuclear antibody testing may be indicated. MRI scan of the foot is indicated if occult mass or tumor is suspected. Radionuclide bone scanning may be useful to rule out stress fractures not seen on plain radiographs. The following injection technique will serve as both a diagnostic and therapeutic maneuver.

Treatment

Initial treatment of the pain and functional disability associated with plantar fasciitis should include a combination of the NSAIDs or COX-2 inhibitors and physical therapy. The local application of heat and cold may also be beneficial. Avoidance of repetitive activities that aggravate the patient's symptoms, as well as avoidance of walking barefoot or with shoes that do not provide good support—combined with short-term immobilization of the affected foot—may also provide relief. For patients who do not respond to these treatment modalities, injection technique with local anesthetic and steroid may be a reasonable next step. Extracorporeal shock wave treatment has recently been shown to be useful in the treatment of recalcitrant cases and may help the patient avoid surgical fasciotomy.[36]

Conclusion

Painful sports injuries are a common problem confronting the clinician given today's ever-increasing interest in physical and cardiovascular fitness. Understanding the problems of misuse and overuse, as well as rapidly identifying potentially dangerous injuries, is the mainstay of the successful diagnosis and treatment of these common afflictions. Often the biggest barrier to successful treatment is the patient's unwillingness to modify his or her exercise routine. The concept of relative rest with the patient resting the affected anatomic area—while continuing to maintain the remainder of the workout routine—can go a long way toward overcoming this obstacle to success. Because the areas most frequently injured during sports injuries often have poor blood supplies (e.g., tendon, cartilage), the risk of further damage if the acute injury is not aggressively treated remains ever present. The use of injectable anti-inflammatory steroids is extremely effective in the treatment of many of the foregoing conditions, but it must be used with care to avoid further injury to already compromised and weakened anatomic structures.

References

Full references for this chapter can be found on www.expertconsult.com.

Fibromyalgia

Steven D. Waldman

Fibromyalgia is one of the most common painful conditions encountered in clinical practice. It is thought to affect approximately 2% of women and 0.5% of men.[1] Fibromyalgia is a chronic pain syndrome that affects a focal or regional portion of the body. The sine qua non of fibromyalgia is the finding of myofascial trigger points on physical examination. Although these trigger points manifest as localized areas of tenderness, the pain of fibromyalgia is often referred to other areas. This referred pain is often misdiagnosed or attributed to other organ systems, leading to extensive evaluations and ineffective treatment. Whether fibromyalgia is a distinct clinical entity or simply a point on the spectrum of a disease called *chronic musculoskeletal pain syndrome* is the subject of much debate.[2]

Although pain is the central symptom of fibromyalgia, it is important for the clinician to recognize that this disease affects many aspects of the patient's clinical well-being. Poor exercise tolerance and easy fatigability with routine activities are present in many patients with fibromyalgia.[3,4] Some investigators believe that chronic fatigue syndrome is simply one variation of fibromyalgia.[5] Part and parcel to fatigue is the frequent presence of sleep disturbance with nonrestorative sleep patterns predominating rather than insomnia.[6] Poor concentration and faulty short-term memory are also common, as is depressive affect.[7] Abnormalities of the hypothalamic-pituitary-adrenal axis and irritable bowel syndrome are also common in patients suffering from fibromyalgia. Treatment of these somatic, psychologic, and behavioral abnormalities must be an integral part of any successful treatment plan for fibromyalgia.[8] Treating only the pain without taking these other difficulties into account will yield less than optimal results.

The trigger point is the pathognomonic lesion of fibromyalgia pain and is thought to be the result of microtrauma to the affected muscles.[9] Stimulation of the myofascial trigger point will reproduce or exacerbate the patient's pain. Often, stiffness and joint pain will coexist with the pain of fibromyalgia, increasing the functional disability associated with this disease and complicating its treatment. Fibromyalgia may occur as a primary disease state or may occur in conjunction with other painful conditions including radiculopathy, the collagen vascular diseases, overuse syndromes, and chronic regional pain syndromes.[10–12]

Although the exact etiology of fibromyalgia remains unknown, tissue trauma seems to be the common denominator. Acute trauma to muscle as a result of overstretching will commonly result in the development of fibromyalgia. More subtle injury to muscle in the form of repetitive microtrauma can also result in the development of fibromyalgia, as can damage to muscle fibers from exposure to extreme heat or cold. Extreme overuse or other coexistent disease processes, such as radiculopathy and the overuse syndromes, may also result in the development of fibromyalgia.

In addition to tissue trauma, a variety of other factors seem to predispose the patient to develop fibromyalgia. The "weekend athlete" who subjects his or her body to unaccustomed physical activity may often develop fibromyalgia. Poor posture while sitting at a computer keyboard or while watching television has also been implicated as a predisposing factor to the development of fibromyalgia. Previous injuries may result in abnormal muscle function and may also predispose to the subsequent development of fibromyalgia. All these predisposing factors may be intensified if the patient also suffers from poor nutritional status or coexisting psychologic or behavioral abnormalities, including depression.

Signs and Symptoms

The sine qua non of fibromyalgia is the identification of myofascial trigger points.[9] The trigger point is the pathologic lesion of fibromyalgia of the cervical spine and is characterized by a local point of exquisite tenderness in the affected muscle. Mechanical stimulation of the trigger point by palpation or stretching will produce not only intense local pain but referred pain as well. In addition to this local and referred pain, there will often be an involuntary withdrawal of the stimulated muscle that is called a *jump sign* (**Fig. 41.1**). This jump sign is characteristic of fibromyalgia and is associated with stiffness of the affected area, pain on range of motion, and pain referred into other anatomic areas in a nondermatomal or peripheral nerve distribution or pattern.

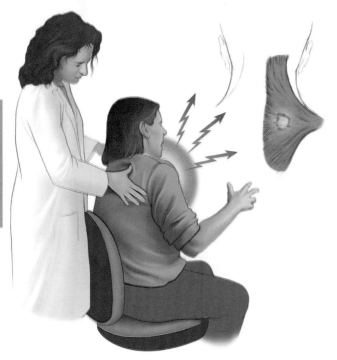

Fig. 41.1 Palpation of a trigger point will result in a positive jump sign. *(From Waldman SD: Atlas of common pain syndromes, ed 2, Philadelphia, 2008, Saunders, p 56.)*

Although the referred pain has been well studied and occurs in a characteristic pattern, it is often misdiagnosed and attributed to diseases of organ systems in the distribution of the referred pain. This often leads to extensive evaluation for nonexistent disease and ineffective treatments. Taut bands of muscle fibers are often identified when myofascial trigger points are palpated. In spite of this consistent physical finding in patients suffering from fibromyalgia, the pathophysiology of the myofascial trigger point remains elusive, although many theories have been advanced. Common to all of these theories is the belief that trigger points are the result of microtrauma to the affected muscle. This microtrauma may occur as a single injury to the affected muscle or as the result of repetitive microtrauma or chronic deconditioning of the agonist and antagonist muscle unit.

Testing

The exact pathophysiologic processes responsible for the development of fibromyalgia remain unknown, and no specific test exists that will positively diagnose the disease.[9] Biopsies of clinically identified trigger points have not revealed consistently abnormal histology. The muscle hosting the trigger points has been alternatively described as "moth eaten" or containing "waxy degeneration." Increased plasma myoglobin has been reported in some patients with fibromyalgia, but this finding has not been reproduced by other investigators. Electrodiagnostic testing of patients suffering from fibromyalgia has revealed an increase in muscle tension in some patients. Again, this finding has not been reproducible. However, whatever the pathophysiology of fibromyalgia, there is little doubt that the clinical findings of trigger points in the affected muscles and associated jump sign exist in combination with a clinically recognizable constellation of symptoms that are consistently diagnosed as fibromyalgia.

Differential Diagnosis

The diagnosis of fibromyalgia of the cervical spine is made on the basis of clinical findings rather than specific diagnostic laboratory, electrodiagnostic, or radiographic testing. For this reason, a targeted history and physical examination with a systematic search for trigger points and identification of a positive jump sign must be carried out on every patient suspected of suffering from fibromyalgia. Because of the lack of objective diagnostic testing, the clinician must also rule out other coexisting disease processes that may mimic fibromyalgia, including primary inflammatory muscle disease and collagen vascular disease.[10,11] The judicious use of electrodiagnostic and radiographic testing will also help identify coexisting pathology such as herniated nucleus pulposus and rotator cuff tears. The clinician must also identify coexisting psychologic and behavioral abnormalities that may mask or exacerbate the symptoms associated with fibromyalgia and other coexisting pathologic processes.[12]

Treatment

The treatment of fibromyalgia involves the use of techniques that will help eliminate the trigger point that may be the source of the perpetuation of this painful condition.[9,13] It is hoped that the interruption of the pain cycle by the elimination of trigger points will allow the patient to experience prolonged relief. The mechanism of action of each of the aforementioned modalities is poorly understood, and trial and error in developing a treatment plan is the expected norm.[14] A multidisciplinary approach is often associated with better long-term results[15] Because underlying sleep disturbance, depression, and a substrate of anxiety are present in many patients suffering from fibromyalgia, the inclusion of antidepressant compounds as an integral part of most treatment plans represents a reasonable choice.[16]

In addition to these treatment modalities, a variety of additional treatments are available for the treatment of fibromyalgia. The therapeutic use of heat and cold is often combined with trigger point injections and antidepressant compounds to effect pain relief and normalize sleep. Some patients will experience decreased pain with the use of transcutaneous nerve stimulation or electrical stimulation to fatigue-affected muscles. Although not currently approved by the Food and Drug Administration, the injection of minute quantities of botulinum toxin A directly into trigger points has recently gained favor in the treatment of persistent fibromyalgia that has not responded to traditional treatment modalities.[17] Pregabalin has also been shown to be useful in the management of fibromyalgia.

Trigger point injections are an extremely safe procedure if careful attention is paid to the clinically relevant anatomy in the areas to be injected.[18] Care must be taken to use sterile technique to avoid infection, as well as the use of universal precautions to avoid risk to the operator. Most side effects of trigger point injection are related to needle-induced trauma to the injection site and underlying tissues. The incidence of ecchymosis and hematoma formation can be decreased if pressure is placed on the injection site immediately following trigger point injection. The avoidance of overly long needles will help decrease the incidence of trauma to underlying structures. Special care must be taken to avoid pneumothorax when injecting trigger points in proximity to the underlying pleural space.

Conclusion

Fibromyalgia is a common disorder that commonly coexists with a variety of somatic and psychologic disorders. Fibromyalgia is often misdiagnosed. In patients suspected of suffering from fibromyalgia, a careful evaluation to identify underlying disease processes is mandatory.

Treatment is focused on blocking the myofascial trigger and achieving prolonged relaxation of the affected muscle. Conservative therapy consisting of treatment with the antidepressant compounds and trigger point injections with local anesthetics or saline is the starting point for the treatment of fibromyalgia of the cervical spine. Adjunct therapies including physical therapy, therapeutic heat and cold, transcutaneous nerve stimulation, and electrical stimulation can be used on a case-by-case basis. For patients who do not respond to these traditional measures, consideration should be given to the use of botulinum toxin A, which has been shown to be a safe and effective treatment for this disorder.

References

Full references for this chapter can be found on www.expertconsult.com.

Chapter 42

Painful Neuropathies Including Entrapment Syndromes

Charles D. Donohoe

Pain management has evolved extremely rapidly as a distinct medical subspecialty. Its meteoric growth aptly reflects medicine's dismal record of inadequate pain treatment. To date, most pain management practitioners are trained anesthesiologists. These physicians are now evaluating patients with pain through direct referral from a primary care physician or, in many cases, as the only treating physician. In essence, they are functioning in a primary diagnostic role similar to a neurologist or rheumatologist. This could easily be a precarious situation without clinical insight into other medical disciplines, including rheumatology, radiology, infectious disease, and clinical neurology.

The cause of neuropathic pain is a vast topic. This chapter focuses on only a few painful neuropathies, including certain entrapment syndromes that highlight the many practical subtleties in clinical diagnosis (**Table 42.1**). The intention is to debunk the concept that any clinician with a coding book, a vial of steroids, and a 22-gauge needle can present himself or herself to patients as a pain expert. Pain is truly a common symptom, but its proper evaluation requires an uncommonly broad knowledge and experience in general medicine.

Anesthesiologists and other non-neurologists have limited experience with laboratory studies, electrodiagnosis, electromyography (EMG), nerve conduction velocity (NCV), and neuroimaging (computed tomography [CT] and magnetic resonance imaging [MRI]). For pain specialists, these are basic tools. Using these modalities properly and realizing their intrinsic limitations will distinguish pain management physicians in their field. In the words of George Bernard Shaw, "Beware of false knowledge, it is more dangerous than ignorance."

This chapter outlines painful neuropathies frequently encountered in a neurologic practice. The chapter provides a few basic concepts on which the pain management physician can build and ultimately develop confidence in the role of a pain specialist.

Clinical Evaluation of Painful Neuropathies

The evaluation of painful neuropathies begins with the history. This is the most important part of the diagnostic process. The nature of the pain, its duration, description, provocative factors, and association with other clinical findings, such as weakness and sensory loss, constitute essential information. The history includes a detailed past medical history for prior conditions, such as cancer, diabetes, thyroid disorders, connective tissue diseases, surgeries, and constitutional symptoms, such as fever or weight loss. The history sets the stage and proper focus for the physical examination and the proper selection of diagnostic studies, including blood work, CT, MRI, magnetic resonance angiography, and electrodiagnosis (NCV and EMG). If the history does not provide any clear direction as to the nature or location of the pathology, the hope that extensive laboratory work, electrodiagnosis, and neuroimaging will provide miraculous clarification is highly remote.

In my experience, laboratory work is frequently overlooked by primary care physicians and specialists alike. A basic panel includes complete blood count, erythrocyte sedimentation rate, thyroid-stimulating hormone, serum vitamin B_{12}, serum protein electrophoresis with immunofixation, and complete chemical profile including lipids and hemoglobin A-1 C. The evaluation of any painful neuropathy should address the possibility of underlying diabetes. This disease is epidemic in the United States and now the type 2 variant is seen commonly in adolescents.[1] The laboratory work should be done in a fasting state. A fasting glucose below 100 mg/dL is considered normal; 100 to 125 mg/dL is considered impaired fasting glucose. A plasma glucose level above 126 mg/dL is consistent with a provisional diagnosis of diabetes. This diagnosis can be confirmed using a 75 g glucose load. If the 2-hour postload glucose

Table 42.1 Painful Neuropathies

Nerves	Vascular/Inflammatory	Compression/Entrapment
CN III (oculomotor)	Pupil reactive—diabetic CN III palsy	CN III palsy with pupil dilated and unreactive Compression due to posterior communicating artery aneurysm
CN V (trigeminal)	—	Trigeminal neuralgia—CN V compression by vascular loop at root entry zone
Combined CNs III, V, and VI (abducens)	Tolosa-Hunt syndrome (cavernous sinus inflammation) (see Fig. 42.5)	—
Upper extremity	Brachial neuritis (neuralgic amyotrophy, Parsonage-Turner syndrome) (see Fig. 42.8)	Carpal tunnel syndrome (median nerve compression at the wrist) Cubital tunnel syndrome (ulnar nerve compression at the elbow)
Lower extremity	Lumbosacral plexus neuropathy (diabetic amyotrophy, Bruns-Garland syndrome, proximal diabetic neuropathy)	Meralgia paresthetica (lateral femoral cutaneous nerve compression below inguinal ligament) Tarsal tunnel syndrome (tibial nerve compression in tarsal tunnel)

CN, cranial nerve.

is below 140 mg/dL, it is considered normal. If glucose is 140 to 199 mg dL, it is designated as impaired glucose tolerance. A level above 200 mg/dL is consistent with diabetes.

Impaired glucose tolerance and impaired fasting glucose represent high-risk states for the ultimate development of diabetes, cardiovascular disease, and metabolic syndrome (abdominal obesity, dyslipidemia, and hypertension). These states can be associated with several of the neuropathic conditions mentioned in this chapter before clear-cut diabetes is manifest. The practical importance of the proper identification of these prediabetic states is supported by early evidence suggesting that they may be positively affected by preventive weight loss and exercise in postponing a wide range of diabetic complications. If testing is limited to a single casual glucose measurement, the opportunity to identify these prediabetic states may be lost. Although the use of hemoglobin A-1 C as a diagnostic criteria for diabetes remains somewhat controversial, it is more convenient and certainly less cumbersome than a glucose tolerance test. It is noteworthy that certain diabetologists believe that the hemoglobin A-1 C with the 6.5% cut off identifies one third fewer cases of undiagnosed diabetes than does a fasting plasma glucose of 126 mg/dl or greater. In short, diabetes is one of the most common and important conditions underlying painful neuropathy, and its identification can be aided by understanding the laboratory criteria.

In contrast to laboratory evaluation, in which there are objective parameters, the other cornerstones of neurologic diagnosis, electrodiagnosis (EMG and NCV) and neuroimaging (CT and MRI), require practical insight and experience into the proper use of these valuable studies. EMG and NCV are extremely helpful in identifying conditions such as carpal tunnel syndrome, brachial neuritis, and lumbosacral plexopathy. These studies depend on the technical expertise, clinical insight, and diligence of the electromyographer. The adage that a bad laboratory is worse than no laboratory at all is true. As in many branches of medicine, electrodiagnosis has its superstars, its average performers, and many players who have no business being on the field. The results of these studies cannot be viewed as truly definitive and always must be correlated with the clinical history and the physical examination. In my experience, many patients have been subjected to unnecessary surgeries, and other clinical mistakes have been made based on sloppy, inaccurate electrodiagnosis.

CT and MRI have revolutionized neurologic diagnosis. It is now more than 30 years since the introduction of CT, and it is almost impossible to consider the field of neurology without these tools. CT and MRI are extremely sensitive. This sensitivity detects pathology, such as disk protrusions, osteophytic spurring, and facet degenerations, in many individuals who are completely asymptomatic.[2] Such pathologic findings increase statistically with advancing age, and neuroimaging results always must be correlated with the history and physical examination.[3]

There is considerable interobserver variability with respect to the interpretation of MRI, and terms such as *disk protrusion, disk extrusion,* and *moderate* and *severe spinal stenosis* are subjective and observer dependent. The pain management physician should review all imaging studies and over time develop his or her own expertise with these modalities. The pain management physician has a tremendous advantage over the radiologist in that he or she has examined the patients as well as the imaging studies. That added insight is crucial in the proper use of these technologies.

Cranial Nerves

Knowledge of the anatomic relationships of the cranial nerves (CNs) is essential in evaluating facial pain and localizing neurologic pathology (**Figs. 42.1** and **42.2**): CN III (oculomotor nerve), CN IV (trochlear nerve), CN V (trigeminal nerve), CN VI (abducens nerve), and CN VII (facial nerve). Acute and chronic cranial neuropathies may be associated with pain and present difficulty for the specialist trained predominantly as an anesthesiologist. The most commonly involved CN is the facial nerve (CN VII) (**Fig. 42.3**). Although there are many causes of facial nerve involvement, the idiopathic variant (Bell's palsy) is more commonly seen (**Table 42.2**).

Disease states of the oculomotor nerves (CNs III, IV, and VI) manifest with diplopia and varying degrees of pain. Dysfunction of CN VI and dysfunction of CN III are the most common oculomotor neuropathies seen in clinical practice.

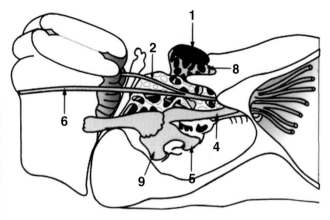

Fig. 42.1 Anatomic diagram of cavernous sinus, showing structure of cavernous sinus. *1 = carotid artery, 2 = oculomotor nerve, 3 = trochlear nerve, 4 = ophthalmic nerve, 5 = maxillary nerve, 6 = abducens nerve, 7 = pituitary gland, 8 = sympathetic nerve, 9 = mandibular nerve.*

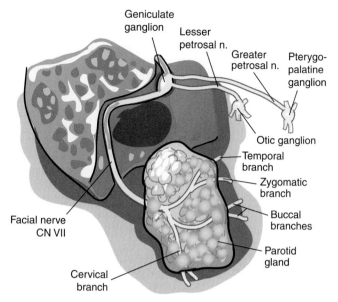

Fig. 42.3 Anatomy of the facial nerve (CN VII).

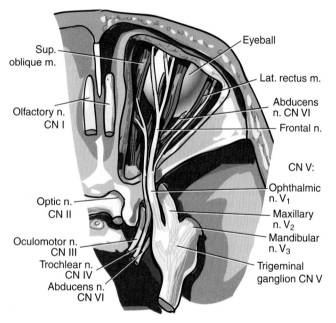

Fig. 42.2 Anatomy of cranial nerves I to VI.

Table 42.2 Differential Diagnosis of Facial Paralysis (Cranial Nerve VII)

Idiopathic	Bell's palsy (diagnosis of exclusion) Melkersson-Rosenthal syndrome (recurrent swelling of face [lip] with facial paralysis)
Infectious	Herpes zoster oticus (Ramsay-Hunt syndrome) Acute and chronic otitis media Lyme disease
Neoplastic Extracranial	Parotid tumors Metastatic Facial nerve neurinomas
Intracranial	Cholesteatoma Glomus tumors Acoustic neuroma Squamous cell carcinoma Metastatic
Trauma and iatrogenic	Newborn paralysis Fractures of petrous pyramid and other temporal bone fracture Penetrating injuries to the parotid gland
Inflammatory	Sarcoidosis Wegener's granulomatosis

The combination of the two, CNs III and VI, is the most commonly observed multiple cranial neuropathy.

Classic oculomotor nerve (CN III) involvement includes ptosis (drooping of the eyelid) and a globe that does not move upward, downward, or medially. If CN VI is intact, lateral movement is preserved. The trochlear nerve (CN IV) is rarely involved as a painful condition, and its action (intorsion of the eye) is best seen when CN III function is interrupted.

In my experience with the oculomotor nerves, an isolated CN VI palsy and CN III palsy are the two most commonly encountered entities. CN VI palsy can be caused by myriad factors (**Table 42.3**), as can CN III palsy (**Table 42.4**). Involvement is frequently secondary to infarction of the nerve trunk associated with diabetes and hypertension (diabetic ophthalmoplegia). In CN III palsy, a droopy eye, with or without pain, that is unable to look upward, downward, or medially should prompt immediate concern. If the pupil is normal

in size and reacts briskly to light, this suggests CN III paresis resulting from microvascular infarction of the central core of CN III, a condition often found in diagnosed or undiagnosed diabetics. It is believed that the more peripheral fibers, those that innervate the pupil, are spared. With this variant of CN III palsy, when pupillary function is preserved, the initial periorbital pain, which may be quite intense, usually resolves in 1 to 2 weeks, and the function of the ocular muscles returns spontaneously in 3 to 4 months.

Table 42.3 Abducens (Cranial Nerve VI) Palsies Associated with Pain

NONLOCALIZING	DIABETES/HYPERTENSION
	Increased intracranial pressure (e.g., pseudotumor cerebri)
	Lumbar puncture or spinal anesthesia
	Basal meningitis
LOCALIZING	
Pontine (ipsilateral facial palsy, horizontal gaze weakness, and contralateral hemiparesis)	Tumor
	Demyelinating disease (multiple sclerosis)
	Infarction
Cavernous sinus (in combination with disorders of CNs III and IV and first division of CN V)	Inflammation (Tolosa-Hunt syndrome)
	Tumor
	Vascular (aneurysm, dural fistula, carotid/cavernous fistula)
Clivus and middle cranial fossa (in combination with facial numbness [CN V], facial weakness [CN VII], and hearing loss [CN VIII])	Tumor (acoustic neuroma, nasopharyngeal carcinoma, perineural spread of head and neck cancer, meningioma, chordoma)
	Infection (meningitis, petrositis, human immunodeficiency virus [HIV], immunocompromised opportunistic infections)

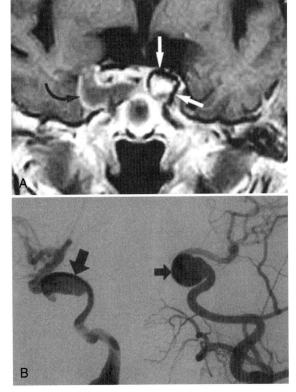

Fig. 42.4 Bilateral saccular aneurysms of internal carotid arteries in cavernous sinuses in a 67-year-old woman with diplopia. A, Axial T2-weighted image shows large signal void *(arrows)* resulting from aneurysm of internal carotid artery in both cavernous sinuses. B, Digital subtraction angiogram of both internal carotid arteries shows partially thrombosed aneurysms of internal carotid artery of right cavernous sinus *(large arrow)* and another aneurysm of internal carotid artery of left cavernous sinus *(small arrow)*.

Table 42.4 Oculomotor (Cranial Nerve III) Palsies Associated with Pain

Aneurysm

Diabetic ophthalmoplegia

Migraine

Inflammation (orbital pseudotumor, cavernous sinus [Tolosa-Hunt syndrome])

Infection (contiguous sinusitis, mucormycosis [other fungi])

Neoplasm (lymphoma, meningioma, nasopharyngeal carcinoma)

Vascular (arteritis, carotid-cavernous fistula, cavernous sinus thrombosis)

With external compression of the nerve resulting from a tumor or the pulsations of a posterior communicating artery aneurysm, the peripheral aspect of the nerve is damaged early and the pupil is found to be dilated and unreactive to light. Assigning a benign etiology to CN III palsy because pupillary function is intact, although having a statistical foundation, is not absolute. It has been found that such pupillary sparing is found in 8% to 15% of patients with isolated CN III palsy resulting from aneurysms.[4] In addition, patients with aneurysmal CN III palsy may have pupillary sparing on initial presentation, but if followed closely, the pupil becomes dilated and ultimately unreactive to light within 3 to 5 days.

Brain and orbital imaging with high-field MRI and magnetic resonance angiography of the circle of Willis is indicated (**Fig. 42.4**). Some insurance-based protocols suggest in a painful CN III palsy with pupillary sparing, neuroimaging is not indicated. However, in the real world of clinical medicine, even delaying imaging carries too much risk. These patients exhibit a high level of concern and rightfully so. Normal imaging studies are psychologically reassuring and medically relevant to the patient and the physician.

Abnormalities of CN VI are more common than abnormalities of CN III. It is the most common CN to exhibit bilateral involvement. Its action innervating the lateral rectus muscle moves the globe laterally. Impaired function of any of the extraocular muscles is not limited to involvement of CNs III, IV, and VI. Eye movements may be impaired as a result of processes directly affecting the muscle rather than the nerve. These include myasthenia gravis, thyroid eye disease, and orbital pseudotumor and may cause pain.

In the setting of involvement of multiple cranial nerves or bilateral involvement, skull-based tumors and neoplastic or

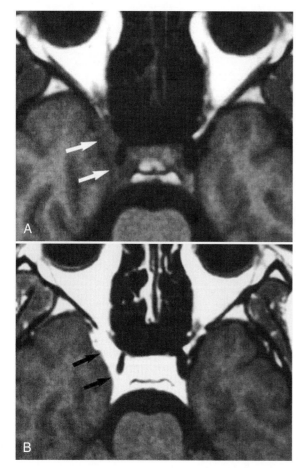

Fig. 42.5 Tolosa-Hunt syndrome in a 21-year-old woman with painful ophthalmoplegia. Unenhanced **(A)** and contrast-enhanced **(B)** axial T1-weighted images reveal homogeneous infiltrating lesion *(arrows)* narrowing carotid artery in orbital apex and in anterior cavernous sinus, which shows homogeneous intense enhancement.

infectious meningeal infiltrates are causes where delayed diagnosis or misdiagnosis frequently occurs. With multiple CN palsies in which initial contrast-enhanced neuroimaging (CT or MRI) is normal, lumbar puncture and cerebrospinal fluid analysis for cells, cytology, protein, glucose, and culture should be considered. Imaging, repeat imaging, lumbar puncture, and referral to physicians in allied specialties, such as otorhinolaryngology (ears, nose, and throat) and neuro-ophthalmology, is an appropriate way to proceed in cases with multiple CN palsies where a specific diagnosis remains elusive (**Fig. 42.5**).

These cases are often difficult ones. Patients are frustrated because they can see that obviously there is something wrong. The physician is frustrated because the initial laboratory studies and imaging examinations can be normal. This situation ultimately results in doctor shopping, loss of continuity, and misplaced trust in the concept that "we've done everything and it's all normal." In evaluating patients in pain with multiple CN palsies, the physician should be willing to start over from the beginning, repeat previously "normal" studies, continue to follow the patient regularly, and enlist the help of allied specialists. Although the locations and causes of multiple CN palsies are diverse, tumor is the underlying diagnosis in more than one quarter of these cases. This fact alone places a premium on rapid and accurate diagnosis.[5]

Neuralgia and Neuropathy of the Trigeminal Nerve (Cranial Nerve V)

Although the sharp, electric, lancinating, unilateral pain of trigeminal neuralgia is quite distinctive, 90% of patients experience paroxysms of pain for over 1 year before receiving an accurate diagnosis and treatment. With an incidence of 4 cases per 100,000 in the United States, many medical practitioners and dentists see very few cases during their careers. It is a diagnosis made predominantly in middle-aged or older individuals and is so characteristic that it can be made over the telephone. Despite its striking pattern, about one third of patients with trigeminal neuralgia undergo unnecessary dental extractions and a variety of expensive treatments for temporomandibular joint disorders.[6]

Most pain specialists are familiar with the sharp, shooting, electric shock–like pain that can last several seconds to minutes with pain-free intervals between attacks. Less well appreciated is when this classic form of trigeminal neuralgia, particularly if left untreated, is transformed into an aching, throbbing, or burning pain that is almost constant in nature and present at least 50% of the time. The persistence of this background pain is its most significant attribute and may signify advancing neural injury. The progression of the lancinating episodic pain into pain with a more constant nature or the combination of both should be noted when evaluating trigeminal neuralgia.

Trigeminal neuralgia should be distinguished from trigeminal neuropathy. In classic trigeminal neuralgia, the basic pathophysiologic feature has been postulated to be compression of the trigeminal nerve root by a blood vessel at or near the root entry zone. In classic trigeminal neuralgia, there is little sensory loss other than hypoesthesia that may be identified at the nasolabial fold. In trigeminal neuropathy, objective sensory loss is more apparent in any or all of the three divisions of the trigeminal nerve. In the case of the mandibular nerve, CN V_3, sensory loss is identified over the skin of the lower face, including the mandibular teeth, the mucosa of the mandibular gingiva, the floor of the mouth, and the anterior two thirds of the tongue. In addition, the mandibular nerve provides motor innervation to the muscles of mastication, the mylohyoid muscle, and the anterior belly of the digastric muscle. Facial pain associated with objective sensory loss in any or all territories of the trigeminal nerve, with or without weakness of the muscles of mastication, signifies involvement of the trigeminal nerve other than trigeminal neuralgia.

In evaluating patients with facial pain, the physician should be aware of perineural spread. Perineural spread is a mechanism whereby a benign or malignant head and neck tumor, an infectious process such as rhinocerebral mucormycosis, or a granulomatous process such as sarcoidosis can spread along the tissues of the neural sheath (**Fig. 42.6**). The most common signs of this process include pain and paresthesias in the second and third divisions of the trigeminal nerve and involvement of the facial nerve often misdiagnosed as Bell's palsy.

The most common malignancies associated with head and neck perineural spread are tumors of the salivary gland, particularly adenoid cystic carcinoma of the parotid, squamous cell carcinoma, and melanoma. These head and neck tumors and other skull-based tumors frequently are missed or have long delays in their proper identification. Facial pain associated with objective facial sensory loss, weakness of chewing, or

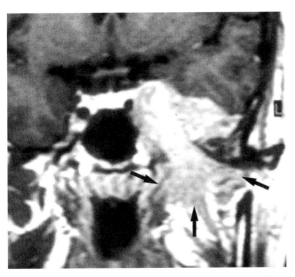

Fig. 42.6 Perineural spread of adenoid cystic carcinoma of parotid gland in a 36-year-old woman with diplopia and left-sided hemifacial pain. Coronal contrast-enhanced T1-weighted image shows strongly enhancing infiltrating mass in left parapharyngeal space *(arrows)* extending into cavernous sinus through widened foramen ovale.

facial weakness should be viewed as an ominous clinical complex. Initial CT and MRI can be normal. A high index of suspicion in these cases with a low threshold for repeat imaging and alerting the radiologist to focus on the skull base is crucial to making these difficult diagnoses. The pain management physician should be suspicious of facial pain associated with multiple cranial nerve palsies. These cases are fraught with misdiagnosis, delayed diagnosis, initial normal neuroimaging, patient dissatisfaction, and ultimately considerable liability.

The use of the term *atypical facial pain* is discouraged. This is a label and not a true medical diagnosis. It says more about the physician's lack of insight than it does about the nature of the facial pain. Although in certain circles *atypical facial pain* is also used as a euphemism for somatoform disorder, any premature tendency to ascribe facial pain to psychogenic mechanisms is also discouraged. Facial pain, particularly when associated with atypical features, is best viewed in a professional and nonjudgmental fashion. In cases that are not clear-cut, the best policy is frequent patient follow-up examinations, repeat neuroimaging, referral to other specialists, and resistance to suggesting stress as the primary mechanism. There already are too many amateur pain specialists competing with countless amateur psychiatrists.

Facial Neuropathy (Cranial Nerve VII)

Acute idiopathic facial neuropathy (Bell's palsy) is the most common cranial neuropathy. The main symptom is usually unilateral facial weakness that begins abruptly and can be preceded by severe pain behind the ipsilateral ear. It has an annual incidence of about 30 per 100,000. The facial weakness usually reaches a maximum within 24 hours after onset. Patients may experience altered taste and hyperacusis in the ipsilateral ear. Although patients often complain of numbness about the face, objective sensory loss is rarely found. Most medical students have seen Bell's palsy, yet it is not unusual to see misdiagnosis in the emergency department, where it is frequently confused

with stroke. Bell's palsy can recur in 5% to 10% of patients, particularly patients with diabetes or a family history.

Bell's palsy is a diagnosis of exclusion (see Table 42.2). Most patients with Bell's palsy do not experience protracted periods of pain, and if painful facial paralysis remains unresolved after 6 to 8 weeks, the patient should undergo contrast-enhanced MRI of the head, internal auditory canals, and parotid gland with and without contrast enhancement. Neoplastic invasion of the facial nerve may mimic signs and symptoms of Bell's palsy. When the clinical picture does not fit, or when a patient with a previously diagnosed Bell's palsy is not experiencing improvement or is developing increasing facial pain, facial numbness, diplopia, or dysarthria, this is a red flag. The pain of Bell's palsy generally improves within 1 to 2 weeks and is usually localized behind the ipsilateral ear.

Perineural spread is a well-described phenomenon in which a head and neck tumor can migrate away from its primary site along the neural sheath.[7] This most commonly occurs in the distribution of the second and third divisions of the trigeminal nerve and the facial nerve. As expected, squamous cell carcinoma would be the most common, followed by many others, including adenoid cystic carcinoma, lymphoma, melanoma, sarcoma, and salivary gland malignancies.

Imaging, and frequently repeat imaging, is essential in these cases. CT is superior for bone detail at the skull base, whereas MRI excels in soft tissue detail. In this subgroup of patients with skull-based malignancies, incredible delays in diagnosis are common. It is not unusual for these patients to have seen several physicians. Each new physician is lulled into a false sense of security by reports of previously normal imaging studies. I have seen a patient with four MRI studies over an 18-month period, interpreted as normal, before a parotid tumor causing protracted facial pain and paralysis (incorrectly identified as Bell's palsy) became sufficiently conspicuous on a fifth MRI study to make a diagnosis of adenoid cystic carcinoma.

Carpal Tunnel Syndrome

Carpal tunnel is the most common focal compression neuropathy. It results from compression of the median nerve at the wrist. This syndrome affects 3% of adult Americans and is about three times more common in women than in men. It is extremely common in diabetic patients with neuropathy, where its prevalence increases to almost 40%. Other medical causes include acromegaly, rheumatoid arthritis, renal failure, hypothyroidism, and amyloidosis. The cause of carpal tunnel syndrome has been linked to work-related repetitive wrist activity, although the validity of this relationship continues to be challenged.[8]

Classic symptoms of carpal tunnel syndrome are pain, numbness, and paresthesias in the distribution of the median nerve, although numbness of the entire hand may be a more common initial clinical complaint. Symptoms usually are worse at night and as the compression becomes more severe can awaken patients from sleep on a nightly basis. These patients often exhibit a tendency to flick their wrist as if they were shaking a thermometer in an attempt to relieve the painful paresthesias ("flick sign"). In my experience, a patient who exhibits the flick sign on a nightly basis or several times a week generally requires carpal tunnel surgical release. Although Tinel's sign and a positive Phalen maneuver are classically described with carpal tunnel syndrome, they are notoriously

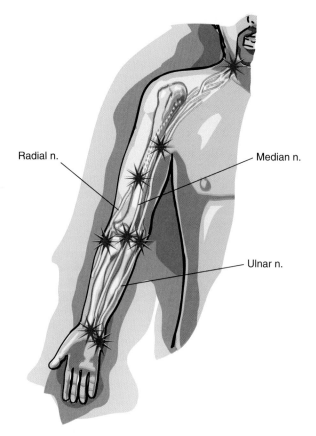

Fig. 42.7 Double-crush syndrome. A proximal nerve lesion makes the distal nerve more vulnerable to injury. It is a concept that remains unproven.

unreliable. Diminished sensation in a median distribution and weak thumb abduction are far more strongly correlated with abnormal NCV studies.[9]

Regarding NCV studies, although they are recognized as a diagnostic gold standard for carpal tunnel syndrome, 25% of patients with positive clinical histories and examinations for carpal tunnel syndrome can have normal NCV studies. These studies essentially assess demyelinization and axonal loss by determining conduction velocities, distal latencies, and response amplitude.[10] The largest diameter axons of the motor or sensory nerve disproportionately contribute to these measurements. The conduction velocity of a nerve is the conduction velocity of the fastest fibers. If in some patients with carpal tunnel syndrome the smaller diameter axons in the median nerve were preferentially compressed, but the larger diameter axons were spared, it is understandable that clinically they may complain of significant entrapment, but have normal median sensory and motor nerve conduction results. In the end, carpal tunnel syndrome remains a clinical diagnosis.

Much has been made of the double-crush syndrome (**Fig. 42.7**), particularly in relationship to carpal tunnel syndrome. The concept of double-crush as postulated by Upton and McComas[11] in 1973 suggests that the presence of a proximal lesion, such as a cervical root compression involving the C6 or C7 roots, renders the distal median nerve more susceptible to mild compression producing carpal tunnel symptoms. The beauty of the double-crush concept lies not in the strength of its scientific foundation, but rather

in the ease with which it can be applied. Carpal tunnel syndrome whose characteristics are atypical or that does not respond to surgery can be explained by a coexistent cervical root lesion. In the lower extremity, peroneal neuropathy that appears after a total knee arthroplasty can be linked with an unsuspected lumbosacral radiculopathy from osteoarthritic involvement.

These are all common situations, and linking them together casually can provide an explanation for almost anything. It can provide an excuse for a suboptimal result or a reason to do additional surgery based on how strongly the practitioner believes in the double, triple, or quadruple sites of crush. In my opinion, there is no scientific evidence to prove that a proximal root lesion, either in the upper or in the lower extremities, results in a magnified susceptibility of a distal nerve to an insult such as compression that would have been otherwise inadequate to cause symptoms.

It is ironic that the hypothesis of Upton and McComas, who were firm advocates of conservative management of entrapment neuropathies and cervical root lesions, ultimately would gain wide acceptance as a universal impetus supporting more surgery, more nerve blocks, and more chiropractic manipulations in treating a variety of symptoms where the initial treatment had failed. The "principle" of double-crush likely has been frequently misapplied in medicolegal settings and worker's compensation cases, and its usage has only added to the vast body of pseudoscience and misinformation that so characterizes these proceedings.[12]

Carpal tunnel syndrome remains a clinical diagnosis that is frequently supported by electrodiagnostic studies. Despite reported advances in ultrasound and MRI evaluation of the carpal tunnel, these modalities remain unproven adjuncts to the clinical examination. Although recognized in some circles as the diagnostic gold standard for carpal tunnel syndrome, electrodiagnostic studies, including NCV, have distinct limitations. Many asymptomatic individuals can have abnormal NCV suggestive of median neuropathy at the wrist. Equally important to note is that surgery may be effective in patients with clinical symptoms who have normal NCV studies.

Although carpal tunnel surgery is effective, it is performed too often and often prematurely. We believe that the decision regarding surgery should be based on significant symptoms that do not respond to conservative measures, including splinting and local combined injections of a corticosteroid and anesthetic into the carpal tunnel. If these patients are followed, many improve with or without treatment. Persistent wrist pain, nocturnal awakening associated with the flick sign, and thenar muscle weakness or atrophy are the best indicators of the need for surgery.

Brachial Neuritis

Brachial neuritis (neuralgic amyotrophy, Parsonage-Turner syndrome) is a rare but exquisitely painful syndrome involving the shoulder girdle.[13] Its incidence is approximately 1.6 cases per 100,000 person-years; Bell's palsy has an incidence of 30 cases per 100,000 person-years. In my practice, we see one such patient about every 2 years. The first symptom is severe sharp, stabbing, throbbing, or aching pain that begins abruptly in the shoulder girdle, scapular area, or hand. The pain is of high intensity and is exacerbated by any movement

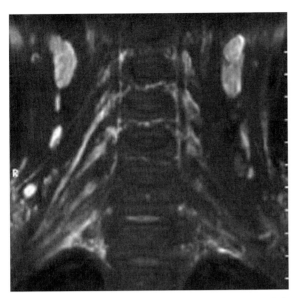

Fig. 42.8 Diffuse plexitis of unclear origin in the right branchial plexus. Note bright signal involving multiple roots of the right brachial plexus (left side of figure).

of the shoulder. The pain may be bilateral in 10% to 20% of cases. There is a distinct male-to-female predominance ranging from 2:1 to 4:1.

This condition initially goes unrecognized, and the patient develops a sense of desperation as he or she travels from physician to physician hoping for a specific diagnosis. The patient typically walks with the affected arm supported by the uninvolved arm. After several weeks, the pain subsides, and the patient becomes aware of weakness followed by atrophy. This weakness usually involves the shoulder girdle muscles, but the hand or forearm also may be involved. A patchy proximal sensory loss in the arm also may be noted.

This condition is most common in young and middle-aged men. Its cause is unknown, but it has been linked to multiple antecedent events, including vaccinations, viral and bacterial infections, surgery, and trauma not involving the shoulder. Biopsy specimens of the involved plexus have shown florid inflammation, and the disorder is believed to have an immune-mediated origin. The clinical findings are predominantly that of a lower motor neuron lesion. Fasciculations and hyperreflexia are not seen. Deep tendon reflexes may be diminished. Involvement of the axillary and suprascapular nerves is the most common combination resulting in weakness and atrophy in descending order of frequency of the deltoid, serratus anterior, biceps, and triceps.

MRI or CT myelography should be considered to rule out cervical radiculopathy, particularly at C5-6, or a neoplasm. MRI neuronography with special sequences to identify the brachial plexus is an evolving technique that may help in ruling out carcinomatous infiltration of the plexus (**Fig. 42.8**). Nerve conductions often reveal loss of sensory or reduction in motor amplitudes with preserved conduction velocities. Needle EMG shows denervation including fibrillations and positive waves in affected muscles 2 to 3 weeks after the onset. These EMG changes may be bilateral, even when only one extremity is involved clinically.[14] Treatment is largely symptomatic, and in the face of such intense pain, opioid analgesics and corticosteroids are often necessary.

The diagnosis, although often delayed, frequently is made based on a history of the sudden onset of neuropathic pain in the shoulder girdle, followed by weakness and atrophy. The prognosis is good, although the period of improvement may be protracted. Approximately 80% of patients recover by 2 years, and almost 90% make a functional recovery by 3 years. In its initial stages, brachial neuritis can be misdiagnosed as cervical radiculopathy, rotator cuff disease, entrapment neuropathy, or drug-seeking behavior.

The diagnosis usually is made by a careful review of the history and a thorough physical examination. In the current climate of clinical medicine, the days of detailed history taking and careful neurologic examination are quickly disappearing. Brachial neuritis is such a condition that when one has seen a case, its clinical characteristics are not forgotten. The patient is in terrible pain and describes the shoulder as being "on fire." The patient typically is a young or middle-aged man whose shoulder pain does not respond to opioids. MRI of the cervical spine may be normal or show moderate age-related degenerative changes that have nothing to do with the current problem.

By keeping this diagnosis in mind, referring to an experienced electromyographer, and offering reassurance that the process is a benign one with a good outcome, the pain management physician's contribution to the patient's well-being is enormous. A pain specialist, who may actually be functioning in a primary diagnostic role, should not underestimate the healing power of face-to-face interaction with the patient. In the end, it is the essence of the physician's role.

Meralgia Paresthetica

Meralgia paresthetica is a painful neuropathy caused by lateral femoral cutaneous nerve compression below the inguinal ligament (**Fig. 42.9**). This entrapment neuropathy was reported more than 100 years ago. The involved nerve is purely sensory, and there is no associated weakness or loss of deep tendon reflexes. The symptoms of meralgia paresthetica consist of varying degrees of pain, paresthesias, and numbness in the upper lateral thigh (see Fig. 42.9). The pain may be worsened by standing, walking, or adduction of the thigh. The most common area of hypoesthesia is frequently described in the trouser pocket area. Touch may evoke an unpleasant sensation when the hand is placed in the pocket. Physical examination reveals sensory loss along the lateral aspect of the upper thigh, but the objective loss of sensation is often in a much smaller area than the subjective area of pain and paresthesias.

This is another diagnosis made predominantly based on history and physical examination. Although electrodiagnostic studies, including NCV and evoked potentials, have been reported useful, these are extremely technically difficult and have not been reliable or helpful in clinical practice. In situations in which the clinical findings are atypical, including a more extensive area of sensory involvement supplied by the lateral femoral cutaneous nerve, or if there is any weakness, CT or MRI of the spine and pelvis is indicated. Imaging studies are indicated for patients who are at risk of neoplastic disease, have bleeding disorders, or those on anticoagulation, who are at added risk of a retroperitoneal hematoma.

The major issue is a proper diagnosis and putting the patient at ease. Meralgia paresthetica usually improves spontaneously.

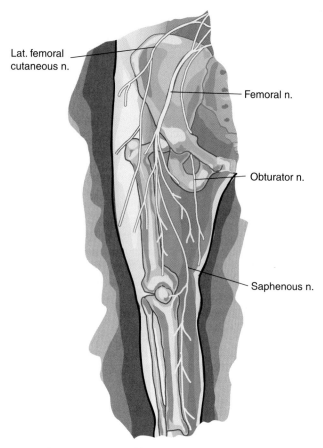

Lat. femoral cutaneous n.

Femoral n.

Obturator n.

Saphenous n.

Fig. 42.9 Anatomy of lateral femoral cutaneous nerve.

The cause is usually idiopathic, although it has been reported in relation to transfemoral angiography, tight bandaging, laparoscopic repair of inguinal hernias, iliac bone crest harvesting, seatbelt injury, weight gain and weight loss, pregnancy, and gymnastic practice in which the uneven parallel bars are used. Diabetics have a higher incidence of this entrapment neuropathy.[15]

Management should be conservative including addressing the causative factors, such as losing weight, wearing looser clothing, or avoiding activities that exacerbate the discomfort. Analgesic patches, such as lidocaine (Lidoderm), and medications used in treating neuropathic pain, such as gabapentin (Neurontin) and pregabalin (Lyrica), have been found to be useful. If conservative treatments fail, local anesthetic injections lateral to the inguinal ligament with hydrocortisone and local anesthetics can provide temporary relief. Rarely, if ever, is surgical decompression necessary. This is a diagnosis that, when recognized, should alleviate the fears of the patient and set the proper stage for spontaneous recovery. It is another example where the history and physical examination are the primary tools.

Lumbosacral Plexus Neuropathy

Lumbosacral plexus neuropathy is a condition that begins with neuropathic pain involving the hip and the thigh. The pain is described as aching and stabbing and exhibits neuropathic qualities of electric-like shocks and burning with

excessive tenderness to touch (allodynia). This anterior thigh and hip pain is followed by proximal lower limb muscle weakness and atrophy. The patient has particular difficulty rising from a squatting position. The knee jerk is usually absent, and sensory loss may be noted over the anterior thigh. Ankle jerks may be reduced, particularly if the patient has an underlying diabetic neuropathy. In diabetics, this condition is known by a variety of names, including diabetic lumbosacral radiculoplexus neuropathy, diabetic amyotrophy, proximal diabetic neuropathy, and Bruns-Garland syndrome. Diabetics and nondiabetics can present in a similar fashion. A significant historical detail is that recent weight loss of 10 to 40 lb is commonly reported predating the onset of symptoms.

Electrodiagnostic testing, including EMG and NCV, is helpful in supporting this diagnosis. The skill of the electromyographer is crucial. It also is important to consider MRI of the lumbar spine and pelvis to rule out an intraspinal process and MRI or CT of the pelvis to exclude malignant invasion of the lumbar plexus, a psoas abscess, or, in patients who are on anticoagulation, a retroperitoneal hematoma. The average age of these patients is 65 to 70 years, and many unrelated asymptomatic findings on MRI of the lumbar spine can confuse the picture. The role of MRI neuronography in detecting signal abnormalities within the lumbosacral plexus is still under development.

This is a condition that presents a characteristic clinical picture requiring recognition. It can remain undiagnosed for months, and over time a substantial percentage of cases can show bilateral hip girdle involvement. Differential diagnosis includes iatrogenic causes of femoral neuropathy, including nerve trauma resulting from abdominal surgery, lithotomy positioning during delivery, or gynecologic procedures and urologic procedures in which sharp flexion of the hip can compress the inguinal ligament. Careful clinical examination, history, and appropriate electrodiagnostic studies can differentiate these conditions from lumbosacral plexus neuropathy.

Diabetic and nondiabetic lumbosacral plexus neuropathies are similar. Both neuropathies are associated with weight loss and often begin focally in the anterior thigh with severe neuropathic pain.[16] Biopsy suggests ischemic damage secondary to microvasculitis. Although unequivocal improvement occurs over time in most patients, total recovery is rare. The role of immunomodulating therapies is currently under evaluation. This diagnosis should be considered in middle-aged to elderly patients with severe anterior thigh pain and muscle weakness with or without diabetes. It is another condition sufficiently rare that misdiagnosis and delayed diagnosis is common. Although seen fairly commonly in neurologic practice, it may present a problem for an anesthesiology-based pain specialist.

Tarsal Tunnel Syndrome

Although tarsal tunnel syndrome is touted to be the lower extremity counterpart to carpal tunnel syndrome, this entity is far less common and of far less clinical significance as a common pain syndrome involving the lower extremity. Tarsal tunnel syndrome is caused by entrapment of the posterior tibial nerve and its tibial branches, the medial or lateral or calcaneal nerves, within the tarsal tunnel. This tunnel is located posterior and inferior to the medial malleolus and is formed by the flexor retinaculum. Causative factors include trauma with post-traumatic fibrosis, tenosynovitis, and ganglion formation affecting the nerves or tendons. The tarsal tunnel is different from the carpal tunnel in the hands in that the flexor retinaculum is thin compared with the thick volar carpal ligament. In addition, the tarsal tunnel is compartmentalized by several deep fibrotic septations that run between the tendons and the neurovascular bundle. In contrast to carpal tunnel syndrome, tarsal tunnel syndrome is less commonly associated with systemic diseases, such as diabetes, inflammatory arthritis, acromegaly, or hypothyroidism.[17]

The onset of tarsal tunnel syndrome is usually unilateral and insidious. The most common symptom is burning, tingling numbness over the territory of the plantar nerve. When symptoms are localized to the plantar surface of the medial two toes, the median plantar nerve is involved. When the lateral plantar nerve is involved, the numbness and paresthesias involve the surface of the lateral two toes. The calcaneal branch of the nerve supplies the plantar and medial surface of the heel. Symptoms classically are aggravated by activities such as prolonged standing or walking and are relieved by rest. In tarsal tunnel syndrome, the nocturnal aggravation of symptoms seen with carpal tunnel syndrome is far less common. Loss of strength in the intrinsic foot muscle has not been reported with tarsal tunnel syndrome. The most common reported objective findings are a positive Tinel sign at the tarsal tunnel and sensory impairment in the territory of any of the terminal branches.

MRI may be helpful in evaluating the tarsal tunnel for space-occupying or compressive lesions. The differential diagnosis includes lumbosacral radiculopathy, interdigital neuroma, plantar fasciitis, or posterior tibial tendonitis. MRI is helpful in evaluating rare cases, including neurilemoma, ganglion cysts, and post-traumatic neuroma.

NCV studies are the test of choice in confirming the diagnosis of tarsal tunnel syndrome. EMG is generally not helpful. With respect to NCV, distal motor latency has a low diagnostic sensitivity; sensory nerve conduction studies are far superior in confirming the diagnosis. There are technical difficulties in performing these studies, however, and the sophistication of the electromyographer is crucial. In most cases, the diagnosis rests on clinical grounds, and treatment should be conservative, including resting the ankle, use of a foot orthosis, nonsteroidal anti-inflammatory agents, or local injection of corticosteroids. My overall impression is that this disorder is frequently considered, but rarely found in clinical neurologic practice. For every case of tarsal tunnel syndrome, we see hundreds of cases of carpal tunnel syndrome.

Conclusion

Pain is the most common symptom that brings a patient to a physician. This pain is evaluated most effectively when an experienced physician spends ample time with the patient obtaining a targeted history and physical examination. The time and thoroughness of the physician's interview is in itself therapeutic in relieving patient anxiety. This is reflected in a euphoric response of relief and hope: "I finally found someone who is listening to me."

Society has currently devalued this essential interpersonal part of medicine. This devaluation is glaringly reflected in the inequities of the insurance system, in which imaging, dangerous invasive procedures, and novel but unproven technologies are favorably reimbursed over basic cognitive consultative services. Self-preservation is inherent in human nature, and physicians have responded accordingly. Office visits are short and frequently conducted by physician "extenders" who often order multiple tests. Follow-up visits are rare, and the patient is ultimately informed of the test results over the telephone by a secretary. Patient and physician dissatisfaction is at an all-time high.

Most painful neuropathies are diagnoses that are almost exclusively made by this devalued history and physical examination. Some are common (Bell's palsy and carpal tunnel syndrome) and some are less common (trigeminal neuralgia and branchial neuritis). Often there are no specific treatments, and the basic therapeutic process is one of making a specific diagnosis, educating the patient, providing symptomatic treatment, and reassuring the patient that he or she will improve over time. Keep learning. We see and can recognize only what we know.

References

Full references for this chapter can be found on www.expertconsult.com.

III

Chapter 43

Osteoarthritis and Related Disorders

Paul Creamer, Bruce L. Kidd, and Philip G. Conaghan

Historical Considerations

Osteoarthritis (OA) is the most common form of disease of synovial joints, and a frequent cause of chronic pain in older people. It is characterized pathologically by focal areas of loss of articular cartilage with overgrowth of subchondral and marginal bone, and clinically by use-related pain and joint stiffness.

OA was first differentiated from other forms of arthritis at the beginning of the twentieth century,[1] when pathologic and radiologic studies indicated that there were two major forms of joint disease: the *atrophic* form, occurring in younger people and characterized by synovial inflammation and bone erosion (this included rheumatoid arthritis and sepsis), and the *hypertrophic* form of arthritis, a condition of older people in which there was overgrowth of bone around affected joints. Hypertrophic arthritis subsequently became known as *osteoarthritis* (because of the prominent involvement of bone) or *degenerative arthritis* because of its relationship to age and the development of a belief that it was a consequence of wear and tear and tissue degeneration.

However, during a period of renewed interest in connective tissue research in the 1970s, along with the development of animal models of OA, it became apparent that there was increased turnover of matrix in both the articular cartilage and subchondral bone in hypertrophic arthritis, challenging the concept of degenerative joint disease. More contemporary studies have reemphasized the involvement of the bone, synovium, and capsule in OA, which is now seen as an active disease process involving the whole joint organ and as the response of a synovial joint to injury or altered biomechanics.

Epidemiologic studies delineating the main risk factors for OA have aided the development of current concepts of the disease.[2] We know that, in addition to age, joint injury and certain forms of activity predispose joints to OA, and that obesity and genetic and hormonal factors are also associated with it. **Figure 43.1** summarizes the contemporary view of the pathogenesis of OA.

The Clinical Syndrome

The science of OA has featured three different approaches to the disease:

1. Epidemiologists have studied the incidence, prevalence, and associations of joint damage in the community, defining OA radiographically.
2. Clinical scientists have concentrated on a minority of those with joint damage or symptoms (i.e., those who present to doctors complaining of joint pain).
3. Basic science has been dominated by biochemical and biomechanical studies of the properties of articular cartilage.

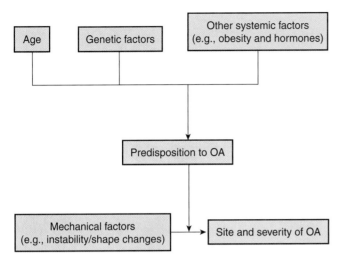

Fig. 43.1 A schematic representation of current views on the pathogenesis of osteoarthritis. OA, osteoarthritis.

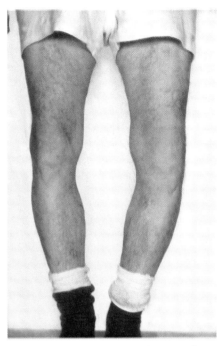

Fig. 43.2 Clinical photograph of a man with osteoarthritis of the knee joint who has the typical medial compartment involvement, resulting in a varus deformity (making him bowlegged); note the marked wasting of the quadriceps muscles but absence of any effusion in the joint.

Unfortunately, there is a paucity of common ground among these three groups.

Health scientists like to believe that they can unravel disease pathways that lead us from genetic and environmental causes of pathology or pathophysiology, directly to the symptoms and signs of a condition. OA does not fit comfortably into this paradigm. John Lawrence made a seminal observation in the 1960s—showing that the relation between radiographic evidence of OA in a joint and the amount of pain was poor, and that severely damaged joints were often asymptomatic.[3] This observation has been substantiated and enhanced by more recent work.[4] The "disconnect" between pathology and pain (the main symptom of OA) can be seen as a problem or an opportunity. It is a problem for the reductionist, who will offer the obvious explanation that we are simply looking at the wrong pathologic features when we take a radiograph of the joint; but it is an opportunity for the physician, who can then ask what the likely causes of pain are in any individual patient, without recourse of having to assess the degree of joint damage. The basic scientist can only sit on the sidelines and wonder if he or she has selected the right tissue to study (possibly not in our view: bone may be a better target than cartilage).

OA can affect any synovial joint in the body. The joints that most often cause clinical problems include the apophyseal joints of the spine (particularly in the midcervical and lower lumbar spine), the interphalangeal joints and first carpometacarpal joint (thumb base) in the hands, the knee (particularly the medial tibiofemoral and lateral patellofemoral compartments), the hip, and the first tarsometatarsal joint. One of the joints least likely to be affected is the ankle; shoulder disease is uncommon, whereas elbow OA is relatively common pathologically, but rarely symptomatic. The greatest burden of disease arises from knee disease, which affects some 25% of those over age 55, and from hip disease requiring joint replacement surgery.

The symptoms and signs of OA, as well as the disease associations, do vary somewhat between the different joint sites affected. However, a number of features are common to all symptomatic OA joints. These include pain, usually use-related; short-lasting *gelling* of the joint after inactivity (difficulty initiating movement after rest); limitation of movement, with pain at the end of the range and often crepitus (creaking of the joint during movement); tenderness over the joint line and palpable bony swelling around it; and, in some cases, signs of mild inflammation.

Spinal OA is a particularly difficult problem to investigate or understand because back pain is particularly poorly associated with any definable pathology. For this reason, and because back pain is dealt with elsewhere in this book (see Section IV, Part H), we will not deal with OA of spinal joints any further. Brief descriptions of the main features of OA of the most common peripheral joint sites are discussed subsequently. We then return to the subject of pain.

The Knee

There are two main groups of people who get knee OA: a younger male group, in whom there is often an antecedent history of joint trauma (such as cruciate ligament rupture or meniscal injury) or a work history that predisposes to the condition (bearing weight while in full-knee flexion); and an older female group in whom there is usually a family history of OA, often apparent from the presence of Heberden nodes on the fingers. Obesity is a strong predisposition in both groups. Overall, there are far more women than men with knee OA. The condition most often affects the medial tibiofemoral and lateral patellofemoral compartments, but as it progresses, more of the knee joint becomes involved.[5]

Knee OA manifests with pain and stiffness. Reduced flexion, as well as weakness of the quadriceps muscles, may contribute to disability. The predominant involvement of the medial tibiofemoral joint often results in varus deformity (**Figs. 43.2** and **43.3**). The natural history is one of slow progression, often punctuated by short-lasting *flares* of increased pain—although only a minority of the total number of people affected (some 25% of all people older than age 55) suffer enough to need a joint replacement, indicating that most cases stabilize at some stage.[5]

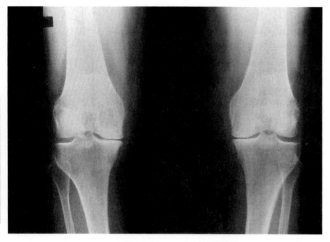

Fig. 43.3 A radiograph of patient with osteoarthritis of similar nature to that illustrated in Figure 43.2. Note the narrowing of the medial joint space in both knees, caused by loss of articular cartilage, and the early osteophyte formation.

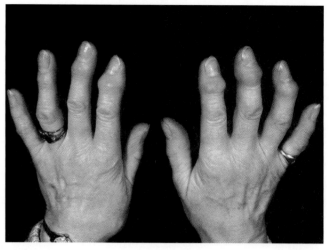

Fig. 43.4 Clinical photograph of someone with interphalangeal osteoarthritis. Note the large swellings of the distal interphalangeal joints (Heberden nodes) associated with some inflammation, and the earlier changes in the proximal interphalangeal joints resulting in Bouchard nodes.

The Hip

Hip OA manifests over a wide age range (twenties to nineties), but most often starts in the fifties or sixties. There is a roughly equal sex incidence. Several different anatomic types have been described, based on the direction of migration of the femoral head (superolateral or medial/concentric) or the degree of osteophyte formation (hypertrophic or atrophic), and these may be genetically distinct.[6] Predisposing factors include anatomic abnormalities of the hip such as dysplasia (the percent that can be attributed to such problems is disputed); certain occupations, particularly farming; a family history; and obesity (although this is much less important for hip OA than it is for knee disease).

The usual manifestation is pain on walking. The pain may be felt in the buttock, groin, thigh, or knee (hip disease manifesting with knee pain is a common source of diagnostic confusion). Stiffness and difficulty with selected activities are common complaints. The natural history is variable: some progress steadily, but others have relatively stable complaints for years, followed by a relatively sudden deterioration with the development of severe pain. A minority of instances resolve spontaneously.

The Hand

The principal joints affected are the interphalangeal joints (distal more than proximal) and the first carpometacarpal joint (thumb base). However, every other joint of the hand can, and often is, affected to some degree. Hand OA is extremely common in women (much less so in men) and strongly related to age, family history, and trauma. The classic features of hand OA are firm swellings of the distal (Heberden nodes) or proximal (Bouchard nodes) joints (**Fig. 43.4**). These swellings consist of chondrophyte or osteophyte and are sometimes associated with hyaluronan-filled cysts.

The presentation of interphalangeal joint OA may be an insidious one in older age, with the gradual and often largely painless development of swellings of the interphalangeal joints. However, in many cases it is more dramatic, with the sequential development of painful, hot, red swellings of these joints, most often in women in their fifties. This has led to the concept of *menopausal arthritis* and is strongly associated with

the idea that there is a form of *generalized osteoarthritis* in which there is a strong genetic predisposition to the development of OA in multiple joint sites.[7] The exact process in this common condition is unclear; it is important to recognize and differentiate OA from systemic forms of inflammatory joint disease, such as psoriatic arthritis. The natural history is one of resolution of pain but not swelling or joint stiffness, leaving most of those affected with knobby fingers that do not move as well as they once did.

Thumb-base OA is somewhat different. It is more clearly related to overuse or injury, and may be precipitated by damage to the ligaments that stabilize the joint in many cases. It causes use-related pain and can be a source of significant discomfort and disability to people who need fine movements of their fingers and the pinch grip in their daily activities (surgeons and those who do needlework, for example).

Why Are Osteoarthritic Joints Sometimes Painful?

The question needs asking because of the poor correlation between structural evidence of joint damage and the presence and severity of joint pain. The data of Creamer et al[8] suggest that OA joint damage predisposes to pain, but that there is little correlation between pain severity and the extent of joint damage thereafter—indicating that there might be a threshold point of predisposition to a painful condition.

Pain mechanisms in OA have received surprisingly little attention in the past, although this is now changing. We know that use-related pain in OA is common, that rest pain and night pain sometimes occur, and that a variety of patterns of pain are described by different patients, varying from a dull ache to stabbing sharp pains.[9] We also know that there are diurnal and other rhythms to pain severity, perhaps related to activity. However, attempts to discriminate between OA and other rheumatologic disorders, such as rheumatoid arthritis, through verbal descriptions of pain have generally proved unsuccessful, and we have not clearly defined the different experiences of pain in patients with OA. Similarly, we know precious little about the likely causes of OA pain.

The abandonment of the Cartesian model of pain in the late nineteenth century, the recognition that the nervous system is not fixed or "hard wired," and the adoption of biopsychosocial models in the mid to latter part of the twentieth century have radically changed our approach to pain. It is now appreciated that the perception of pain arises in response to a complex series of underlying neurophysiologic events involving transduction of stimuli, transmission of encoded information, and subsequent modulation of this activity at both peripheral and more central levels. In all but acute situations, the relation between tissue injury and resultant symptoms becomes less well defined and more susceptible to extraneous influences originating both within and external to the individual. The relevance of this to chronic diseases such as OA is obvious and the model goes a long way toward explaining the heterogeneous symptoms described by individuals with this disorder.

All musculoskeletal structures, with the exception of cartilage, receive an extensive supply of sensory fibers that include rapidly conducting A beta fibers, which are activated by nonnoxious stimuli such as movement and light touch, as well as A delta and C fibers, which, under normal circumstances, only respond to noxious or damaging stimuli. In the presence of persistent injury or inflammation the release of local mediators acts to sensitize the receptors on these latter fibers such that hitherto innocuous events such as walking or simply weight bearing now become painful. Parallel changes occurring at more central levels (central sensitization) lead to augmentation of pain perception and referred pain and tenderness away from the initial site of injury.

Given that many or possibly the majority of OA joints remain pain free, the pivotal question arises as to the nature of underlying mechanisms whereby an asymptomatic but diseased joint becomes symptomatic. It is possible to speculate that OA is essentially a painless disorder rendered symptomatic by additional factors. One noteworthy feature of symptomatic OA is the diffuse nature of the pain and widespread tenderness that accompanies symptomatic disease. Such widespread hypersensitivity argues strongly that tissue factors are not solely responsible for the clinical picture and implies that altered central pain processing is also involved. This, in turn, raises the further question as to whether such altered central processing might persist in the absence of ongoing abnormal peripheral input or whether it serves simply to amplify sensory information from diseased tissues. Support for a dissociation between peripheral input and altered central processing in some circumstances comes from follow-up studies of individuals with OA who go on to have joint replacement surgery. These show that nearly 20% remain unsatisfied with the outcome, with ongoing pain being the strongest predictor of lower levels of satisfaction.[10]

Several lines of evidence point to the importance of mediators released from either synovium or bone. The presence of inflammation has been convincingly demonstrated in OA, and mediator-induced sensitization of articular nociceptors provides a convincing mechanism by which symptoms might occur. Consistent with this, the presence of knee pain has been shown to correlate with magnetic resonance imaging (MRI) findings of moderate or larger effusions, as well as synovial thickening.[11] Periosteum, subchondral, and bone marrow are richly innervated with sensory fibers and are potential sources of OA pain. Bone marrow lesions detected on MRI are more prevalent in individuals with OA who have knee pain than in those who are symptom free.[12] Increased intraosseous pressure arising from impaired venous drainage has long been linked with OA, probably explaining the immediate benefits of surgical procedures such as an osteotomy.[13]

Although there is good evidence that synovial and capsular problems, as well as increased intraosseous pressure, are all associated with pain in OA, it is also clear that periarticular problems, secondary to deformity and mechanical abnormalities, are common; for example, trochanteric bursitis around the hip and anserine bursitis around the knee are common accompaniments of OA of those joints.

An intervention study by Creamer et al[14] lends support to the variable contributions of altered peripheral and central nociceptive mechanisms to pain generation. The authors studied pain in people with bilateral knee OA in response to an injection of local anesthetic or placebo into one knee. Pain was temporarily reduced to almost nothing in the injected knee in some but not all patients; importantly, pain often got better in the contralateral knee.

Psychophysical studies of patients with symptomatic OA have reported diffuse alteration of pain perception in response to various stimuli,[15] with subjects having increased pain intensity and significantly larger referred and radiating pain areas than matched controls. It is highly unlikely that local changes to nociceptive activity account for these findings and point to the presence of enhanced central pain processing in OA. Consistent with this, studies that have combined psychophysical methods with functional brain imaging have reported increased activation in the brainstem of OA patients following punctuate stimulation compared to controls.[16] OA pain has also been shown to be associated with increased activity in areas concerned with the processing of fear and emotions, including the cingulate cortex, the thalamus, and the amygdala.[17] This is in accord with other studies showing an important relationship between psychosocial factors and pain reporting in OA, particularly anxiety, depression, catastrophizing, coping strategies, and social isolation.[18–20]

It seems likely that OA pain reflects a state of altered pain processing such that everyday stimuli are perceived as being painful. These changes are likely to arise in response to a critical interaction with particular joint, bone, and periarticular factors that may well vary among individuals. The resultant sensitization of nociceptive pathways at both peripheral and central levels is then dependent on constitutional factors unique to an individual, such as gender, age, and previous history, as well as environmental factors, including culture and lifestyle. If this is true, the unpredictability of pain responses to different interventions, which we experience in the management of OA, would not be surprising.

Diagnosis and Investigation

Diagnosis of OA may be considered in two ways. First, it may be considered as a *clinical diagnosis* depending entirely on recognition of the patterns described previously and differentiation of true OA joint pain from referred or periarticular problems. For example, the American College of Rheumatology Classification Criteria for knee OA include knee pain and age over 40 years with morning stiffness lasting less than 30 minutes and crepitus on motion.[21] The European League Against Rheumatism (EULAR) recommendations for diagnosis of knee OA confirm from research evidence

Table 43.1 Clinical and Differential Diagnosis of Knee and Hip Osteoarthritis

Typical features suggesting OA	Pain—deep, often poorly localized, worse on use Stiffness—localized to involved joints, rarely exceeds 30 minutes Crepitus on active motion Limited range of movement No systemic features	
Differential Diagnoses to Consider	**Knee**	**Hip**
Other arthritis	Rheumatoid arthritis, gout, CPPD	Rheumatoid arthritis, seronegative spondyloarthropathy
Bone disease	Avascular necrosis Paget's disease	Avascular necrosis Paget's disease
Soft tissue	Meniscal or ligament injuries, bursitis (anserine, prepatella)	Trochanteric bursitis, tendinopathy
Referred pain	From hip	From spine, sacroiliac joint

CPPD, calcium pyrophosphate dihydrate deposition; OA, osteoarthritis.

and expert consensus that clinical assessment alone enables a confident diagnosis to be made.[22] They highlight the symptoms of persistence of pain and reduced function, as well as limited morning stiffness. A reasonable working diagnostic approach to OA is to assume that knee pain in those older than age 50 is due to OA unless another cause can be found, especially if pain is worse on use and is associated with stiffness after inactivity and restricted movement. **Table 43.1** indicates the typical features of OA and some of the alternative diagnoses that should be excluded at the hip and knee.

It should be noted that experts consider examination to be an important part of diagnosis; crepitus, restricted movement, and bony enlargement are the three useful examination findings.[22]

Second, OA can be defined by *pathologic changes*. Histopathology is, in general, unavailable and we rely on radiographs and other imaging modalities such as MRI as surrogates. No other investigations are of value, except perhaps use of synovial fluid analysis to differentiate simple OA from crystal-related disorders (discussed later).

Conventional Radiography

Plain radiographs are useful in confirming that established OA is present and in defining which joints (or parts of joints) are affected. It should be noted that how radiographs are taken will affect the outcome: multiple views (posteroanterior, skyline, and lateral) will detect more OA than a single posteroanterior view.[23] Weight-bearing views are essential if assessing knee cartilage loss. Taken serially, they also allow assessment of the progression of anatomic changes, but care must be taken when comparing serial films to ensure appropriate patient repositioning (this is one of the major problems with clinical trials using radiographs as outcome measures).

They are also of value in excluding other causes of joint pain (e.g., fracture, avascular necrosis, or Paget's disease of bone). Unfortunately radiographs do not accurately represent pathology because early changes (which may be confirmed by arthroscopy or MRI) are not seen on radiographs.[24] A normal radiograph does not exclude OA. Radiographs cannot indicate

Table 43.2 Managing Osteoarthritis

Factors That Influence the Seeking of Medical Care for Osteoarthritis

Disease severity (pain, disability)

Sudden worsening of symptoms

Socioeconomic or occupational factors

Comorbidity

Cultural expectations (such as influences of family or friends)

Coping strategies

Availability of services and ease of access to them

The Aims of Managing Osteoarthritis

Education and empowerment of patient and caregivers

Alleviating pain

Improving disabling effects by encouraging participation in activities

Reducing the risk of progression

the impact of disease on the individual or allow a prognosis to be made. Possible indications for obtaining radiographs in a patient with knee pain might be:

- Knee pain that suddenly gets worse
- Acute inflammation or other signs that suggest a diagnosis other than OA (**Table 43.2**)
- Possible referral of pain from spine to hip or hip to knee
- Investigation before surgery

Typical changes of OA on a plain radiograph include joint space narrowing (generally assumed to reflect articular cartilage loss) and osteophyte, sclerosis, and cyst formation (**Fig. 43.5**). These same features are seen at all sites affected by OA, although the correlation between radiographic features and symptoms may vary (e.g., osteophytes at the distal interphalangeal joint are often asymptomatic, whereas at the hip there is a closer correlation with pain).

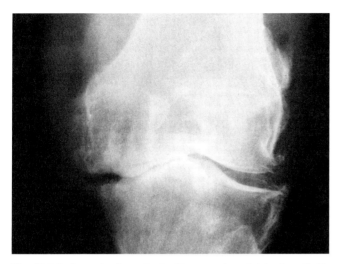

Fig. 43.5 Radiograph of a patient with severe knee joint osteoarthritis and associated chondrocalcinosis. The joint space has disappeared in the medial joint compartment, and there has been major remodeling of the subchondral bone with associated sclerosis and changes in contour. The chondrocalcinosis is seen in the lateral compartment, where there is still some cartilage. Fairly large osteophytes are also present.

In general, there is surprisingly little overlap between the clinical and radiographic diagnosis of OA. Community studies indicate that the risk of knee pain increases with radiographic severity of OA. In the National Health and Nutrion Examination Survey-I study, for example, among subjects ages 65 to 74, knee pain was reported by 8.8% of subjects with normal radiographs, 20.4% with grade 1 OA, 36.9% with grade 2, and 60.4% with grade 3 or 4.[25] However, about 10% of individuals with knee pain have completely normal radiographs, whereas up to 40% of subjects with severe radiographic changes apparently are pain free. If pain severity, rather than presence, is used as an outcome, there is even less association with radiographic change. Several studies now confirm that once an individual with knee pain becomes a patient seeking medical care there is virtually no relationship between radiographic severity and level of reported pain.[4,26] An interesting analysis that used a within-person, knee matched, case control design in OA patients with discordant knee pain demonstrated a strong relationship between radiographic OA and pain, with individual features (especially joint space narrowing) also strongly associated with pain.[27]

A number of other imaging modalities can provide information about OA, although none are currently useful in routine clinical practice.

Isotope Bone Scans

Isotope bone scans appear to predict progression of radiographic OA and the need for surgery at the knee[28] and hand,[29] suggesting that bone responses may be a critical feature in the progression of OA.

Ultrasonography

Ultrasonography has many advantages over conventional radiography (e.g., it can image multiple joints in real time in the clinic and does not involve radiation exposure). In the hands of a trained ultrasonographer, it is a useful tool in both small and large joints. With respect to differential diagnosis

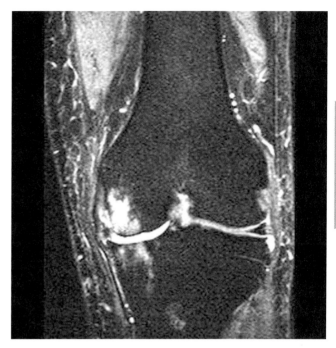

Fig. 43.6 MRI of an osteoarthritic knee: coronal STIR sequence demonstrating high signal (white area) of both medial tibial and medial femoral bones. This is bone marrow edema. Note that the adjacent meniscus is severely degenerated.

of OA, in the small joints of the hands or feet, ultrasound may determine joint space narrowing, synovitis, periarticular erosions, and occasionally crystals.[30] Of course, both inflammatory arthritis and OA joints may have synovitis present. In the knee, ultrasound is able to distinguish both synovial hypertrophy and effusions, although care should be taken because there is little consensus on definitions for these abnormalities. A large study of 625 painful OA knees demonstrated that 34% had effusions and 17% had synovial hypertrophy (14% had both).[31] Although clinically detected effusions correlated modestly with ultrasonographic effusions, no other clinical symptom or sign was predictive of the presence of ultrasonographic synovitis or effusions. Importantly, these imaging-detected effusions were subsequently demonstrated to be a modest independent predictor of later knee replacement surgery.[32]

If treating synovial inflammation is demonstrated to be critical in the management of OA, then ultrasound may well provide a simple and relatively cheap tool for monitoring patients. Ultrasound has the added benefit of providing a tool for guided injection therapy.[33]

Magnetic Resonance Imaging

MRI offers huge potential to the field of OA because it is able to image all the structural components involved in this whole-organ disease. Radiographs image calcified bone, whereas MRI presents a *proton map,* and the amount of information that MRI can provide is very much dependent on the particular sequences used. For example, the use of the intravenous contrast agent gadolinium allows optimal detection of synovitis, whereas fat-suppressed sequences allow for detection of bone marrow edema (**Fig. 43.6**). Unlike conventional radiographs, MRI also has the advantage, like computed tomography, of being tomographic and therefore more sensitive in detecting abnormalities such as osteophytes (**Fig. 43.7**).

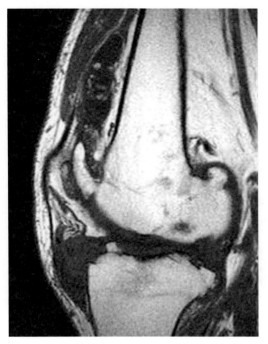

Fig. 43.7 MRI of an osteoarthritic knee: sagittal T1-weighted image demonstrating large patellofemoral osteophyte. A posterior femoral condyle osteophyte is also visible.

Optimal sequence setting will depend on the information to be obtained because clinical trials may require different information from clinical practice.

Preliminary work from large MRI cohorts of OA subjects is emerging; most of this work involves knee OA. Generally, abnormalities of all tissues are present with increased frequency with increasing radiographic Killgren-Lawrence grade.[34] There is no consensus yet on the best ways to quantify or score these multi-abnormal features. However, the ability of MRI to image joint pathology not seen on conventional radiographs has been highlighted. In a preliminary report of 445 knees with minimal radiographic abnormalities, MRI detected abnormal cartilage morphology in more than 75%, whereas abnormalities of bone marrow, menisci, ligaments, and synovium were seen in 30% to 60%.[35] The old belief that "there is no pathology because the radiograph is normal" is clearly wrong. The sensitivity of MRI creates a new conundrum, however: How will OA be defined structurally in the MRI era, when radiographs are normal?

Such information throws important new light on our concepts of structure-pain relationships. Generally, more abnormal features correlate with pain. MRI is now providing us with ideas on candidates for structural associations of pain. One MRI study of 150 OA knees suggested that synovial hypertrophy and effusions were associated with pain.[36] Bone marrow edema, a feature described only with MRI and associated with histologic fibrosis and remodeled trabeculae, has also been associated with knee pain in another large cohort,[37] although this association is not universal and may relate to the size of the lesions. Bone marrow edema has been associated with compartment-specific progression of joint space loss; this risk for progression persisted even after correction for alignment, another known risk factor for structural progression.[38] MRI has also highlighted the relevance of extra-articular features (e.g., bursitis or iliotibial band syndrome) in causing knee pain.[39]

MRI holds the promise of creating subcategories of OA for targeted therapy, but much more work needs to be done to validate these abnormalities against relevant clinical outcomes and then provide methods that reliably quantify the abnormalities.

Differential Diagnosis

Four issues need to be thought about in the differential diagnosis of OA: (1) the differentiation of OA from periarticular problems, referred pain, and generalized musculoskeletal pain (as in fibromyalgia); (2) crystal-associated arthropathies; (3) diffuse idiopathic skeletal hyperostosis (DISH); and (4) the development of complications.

Many aspects of the differentiation of OA from periarticular disorders, referred pain, or generalized musculoskeletal pain have just been discussed. However, it must be stressed that OA often occurs with periarticular or generalized musculoskeletal pain. Thus OA of the hip may be complicated by coexisting trochanteric bursitis, or knee OA by anserine bursitis, and anyone with OA may develop pain amplification, generalized pain, or fibromyalgia as well. The frequent coexistence of OA with other morbidity—including depression (its dominance in older people may complicate the situation, making it difficult for the clinician to be certain what the main causes of pain are)—creates uncertainty about the choice of interventions.

Calcium-containing crystals are often present in the tissues and synovial fluid of joints affected by OA. The two main categories are calcium pyrophosphate dihydrate (CPPD) and basic calcium phosphates (BCPs), principally hydroxyapatite. The presence of CPPD crystals appears to be a marker of more hypertrophic forms of OA (extensive osteophyte formation and subchondral bone sclerosis) and BCP crystals of more atrophic forms (with destruction of bone). Whether these forms of OA should be regarded as distinct entities (such as pyrophosphate arthropathy or apatite-associated destructive arthropathy) or merely ends of the spectrum of OA changes in joints is contentious, although we favor the spectrum approach versus the distinct entity approach. In addition, these crystals, if released in sufficient quantity into the synovial space, can cause attacks of acute arthritis (pseudogout in the case of CPPD crystals). Pseudogout is the most common form of acute arthritis seen in older people and is particularly likely to occur after surgery for another condition or during an intercurrent illness. The synovial fluid may be blood stained; chondrocalcinosis is usually seen on the radiograph (see Fig. 43.5); and CPPD crystals can be seen in synovial fluid using polarized light microscopy. It is sometimes difficult to distinguish OA from chronic gout pain when the two arthritides coexist, commonly in the first metatarsophalangeal joint. The presence of early morning stiffness in the affected joint or other acutely inflamed joints may favor the diagnosis of gout, but sometimes a pragmatic pharmacologic reduction of uric acid may be required to exclude ongoing gout.

DISH is a condition characterized by extensive enthesophyte ossification in the spine leading to bridging of vertebrae, and associated with peripheral enthesophyte ossification. It is a common age-related disorder, with a male-to-female preponderance of 2:1 associated with obesity, diabetes, gout, hypertension, and hyperinsulinemia. It leads to stiffening of the spine and of central peripheral joints such as the shoulder and hip, as well as, in some cases, peripheral joints. The development of peripheral bony enthesopathies may cause pain in some cases, but pain is not nearly as prominent a feature as in OA.

Severe complications of OA are rare, but exacerbations of pain are common, and physicians must be aware of the possibility of a serious complication, particularly if the nature of the pain is different, or if an exacerbation is persistent. The most common complication is acute crystal arthritis (see earlier discussion). Acute increase in pain is associated with a warm effusion and crystals can be found in the synovial fluid. The main differential diagnosis is septic arthritis, which can coexist with an acute crystal-related synovitis. Trauma may also lead to rupture of a tendon or ligament, increasing joint instability. Finally, osteonecrosis can occur, particularly at the hip and knee, resulting in severe exacerbation of pain followed by accelerated joint destruction.

The Management of Osteoarthritis

Currently, there is no good evidence for disease-modifying therapy in OA; treatment is aimed at reducing the consequences of OA, of which pain is the most important. Important principles include the following: avoidance of iatrogenic complications (OA is rarely life threatening and risks of side effects are increased in older persons, the group most at risk of OA); empowerment of patients to improve self-efficacy over pain control and acknowledgment that pain in OA is, like most chronic pain, the result of an interaction between structural factors, host characteristics, and the environment. Implicit in this model is the concept of *individualization:* The development of a treatment strategy for each patient should be based on his or her particular needs and expectations, as well as the evidence base. Management of OA requires a team approach involving health care professionals and the patient to develop a package of care tailored to the individual.[40]

Most data on management of peripheral joint OA focus on the knee, although it seems likely that general management principles will hold for the other common joint sites (hip, hand). There are good reasons for the knee to assume predominance because it is the joint site associated with most morbidity. In a population of 100,000 individuals, some 7500 will have knee pain and disability caused by OA. Clearly, the burden of such a prevalent condition falls mainly on primary care physicians, and management should be focused on the community rather than the hospital.

Not all individuals with knee pain seek medical attention, even those with severely painful and disabling symptoms. Why some individuals elect to seek care whereas others do not is unclear but probably does not simply reflect disease severity (see Table 43.2). Physicians do not see people who are representative of all of those in the community with OA.

Treatments for OA are listed in **Table 43.3**. Several guidelines for the management of lower limb OA have been produced recently,[41–44] usually by consensus statements from expert panels. These provide a good summary of the evidence base underlying nonsurgical interventions, but their use in daily practice is limited by a number of factors:

- Guidelines are designed to be applied to groups of patients, whereas an individualized approach to management is likely to be more effective. Clearly, the need for weight reduction, for example, is greater in some patients than in others.

Table 43.3 Therapeutic Options in the Management of Osteoarthritis

Education	Patient and spouse or family
Weight loss	For the overweight
Social support interventions	Telephone, help lines, support groups, formal cognitive
Exercise	Muscle strengthening, patellar strapping, aerobic exercise (walking, swimming, cycling)
Orthotics/footwear	Aids and appliances, joint protection, insoles
Dietary supplements	Glucosamine, vitamins C and D; ginger, avocado, and soybean extracts, fish oils
Topical drugs	Topical NSAIDs, rubefacients, capsaicin
Oral drugs	Analgesics (paracetamol, codydramol, opiates) NSAIDs Cyclooxygenase-2–selective NSAIDs
Intra-articular treatment	Corticosteroids Hyaluronans
Surgical interventions	Tidal lavage and débridement Osteotomy Total joint arthroplasty
Other	Acupuncture, TENS

NSAIDs, nonsteroidal anti-inflammatory drugs; TENS, transcutaneous electrical nerve stimulation.

- By definition, they can evaluate only available data, which for some (especially physical) interventions is sparse. Most published research has examined drugs (59%) or surgery (27%).[45] Most (94%) report positive results, suggesting a bias against publishing negative findings. The EULAR guidelines reviewed 674 papers of which 564 concerned drug or surgical therapy (of which 365 were nonsteroidal anti-inflammatory drugs (NSAIDs)).[43]
- Recommendations made in guidelines may not be practical because of local constraints or lack of resources.
- Guidelines do not distinguish between provision of primary and secondary care.
- In practice, treatments are rarely applied sequentially: rather, combinations of interventions are applied simultaneously. The effect of such "packages" of care is unknown.
- Despite good evidence for many nonsurgical treatments in OA, most patients remain undermanaged and significant improvement could be made simply by making better use of the therapies currently available.

Table 43.4 indicates the issues that should be considered when planning treatment. The age of the patient is probably the least important but may affect the decision to consider surgery. Exactly how age affects this decision is not clear. Surgeons may prefer to operate on older people, reducing the chances of having to perform difficult revision surgery in the future; patients themselves may feel that younger, more active individuals should have the chance of total joint

Table 43.4 Issues to Be Considered When Planning Management of the Patient with Osteoarthritis

Age

Comorbidities

Risk factors

Impact of osteoarthritis

Individual preference

Availability of services

replacement (TJR). Comorbidity should be considered. Does the patient have contraindications to use of NSAIDs? Does the patient have cardiovascular disease limiting mobility more than the OA? Would the patient have a high operative risk if TJR were to be considered? Risk factors for OA should be assessed: is the patient obese or at risk of occupational overuse? Are there psychosocial factors that may confer a worse prognosis? The impact of OA should be assessed using the International Classification of Function model, including pain severity, impairment of function, and the effect on the individual.

The patient's preference for treatment should be explored and attempts should be made to identify the issues that are of importance to that individual. The treatment plan should be developed through a dynamic partnership between patient and doctor. Finally, management is necessarily affected by local service provision such as length of waiting list, access to physiotherapy, and so on.

Given the variability introduced by the factors described, it is rarely practical to follow the standard sequential approach to managing patients advocated by guidelines. For all individuals with OA electing to seek medical care, a minimum care package should be offered including education, exercise, advice on weight reduction, correction of adverse mechanics, and advice on use of simple analgesics.

Education and Empowerment

Education is particularly important in OA. Much depends on the patient assuming control for his or her own care. It should aim to dispel myths such as the inevitability of OA or that "nothing will help" and provide information on the disease process, likely outcome, available treatments (and how to use them), and help with lifestyle adaptations to the disease. "Medicalization" should be avoided if possible: The concept of gradual joint failure with a variety of outcomes is preferable to a "disease" label. Although it is difficult to prove that education itself affects important outcomes such as pain, it may be that education allows a reduction in perceived helplessness, disability, and impact. Meta-analysis suggests that, overall, both patient education and exercise regimens have a modest, yet clinically important, influence on patients' well-being.[46] More remains to be learned about how and when to deliver education packages.

Exercise

Specific muscle-strengthening exercises (e.g., quadriceps for knee) can significantly reduce pain and disability and can be delivered at home.[47] Graded aerobic exercise programs have

also been shown to be safe and effective for most individuals with knee OA and may be slightly more beneficial than isometric exercises. Importantly, compliance can be maintained at 60% to 70% with appropriate encouragement and support.[48] Hydrotherapy and Tai Chi can also provide sustained improvement in physical function.[49] Participation in regular exercise can be encouraged by giving patients advice and backing this up with written instructions and literature; by making the exercises practical and enjoyable; and by regularly reinforcing the benefits of remaining active. The mechanism by which aerobic exercise reduces knee pain is unclear. In addition to acting to strengthen local muscles (e.g., quadriceps), it may also reduce obesity and has documented psychologic effects, including promoting independence, self-confidence, and self-esteem. Exercise is a good example of a treatment for OA that puts patients very much in control of their own management.

Weight Reduction

Obesity is an important risk factor for knee OA because subjects who lose weight are less likely to progress radiographically or to develop symptoms.[50] Proving that weight loss reduces existing pain levels is difficult, largely because of the difficulty in achieving significant weight reduction. Dieting is often combined with exercise, which itself has an effect on symptoms of OA. More remains to be learned about the best ways of encouraging weight loss, and different approaches may be effective in different individuals. Overall, weight reduction is a powerful, disease-modifying intervention that deserves intensive effort in all obese patients with lower limb OA.

Biomechanical Approaches

OA is primarily a biomechanical condition and therapies directed at realignment, correction of deformity, and improved gait are effective and safe. Comfortable shoes with shock-absorbing insoles can reduce pain in OA. Heel wedges are a method of correcting the abnormal biomechanics seen in knee OA. A laterally elevated (valgus) insole may decrease lateral thrust and reduce pain in subjects with medial compartment OA (**Fig. 43.8**). Knee braces and Neoprene sleeves, combined with muscle-strengthening programs, can reduce pain—probably more by improving proprioception and patellar tracking than by physically realigning the tibiofemoral joint.[51] Provision of a cane or walking stick may reduce pain and improve function by "unloading" the joint. Taping of the patella (**Fig. 43.9**), designed to apply medial glide and medial tilt with unloading of the infrapatellar fat pad or pes anserinus, is an effective treatment that has been shown to improve pain by as much as 40%. This effect is greater than that seen with a control tape and persists for up to 3 weeks after stopping treatment.[52]

Medication

Patients should be informed about drug options but many choose not to use drugs. It should be made clear to patients that drugs are purely for symptom relief and that it is entirely reasonable, if preferred, to "put up with the pain" rather than take medication. The main indication for drug therapy in OA is pain. Pharmacologic therapy should always be added to a program of nonpharmacologic modalities discussed earlier. This is particularly relevant in older persons who are at high risk for adverse reactions to drugs.

Varus knee
(right, viewed from behind)

Correction with
lateral heel wedge

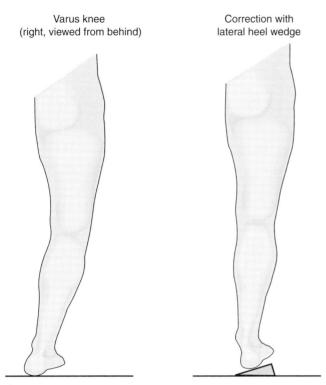

Fig. 43.8 A laterally elevated (valgus) insole within footwear can have the effect of correcting the varus deformity of the knee joint commonly seen in osteoarthritis and correcting much of the biomechanical abnormality. The shoe wedge should be combined with subtalar strapping to maintain the correction. *(Adapted from Toda Y, Segal N: Usefulness of an insole with subtalar strapping for analgesia in patients with medial compartment osteoarthritis of the knee,* Arthritis Rheum *47:468, 2002.)*

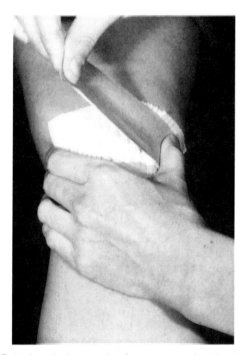

Fig. 43.9 A clinical photograph of someone undergoing taping for patellofemoral osteoarthritis. The operator is shifting the patella medially with her thumb while applying tape to keep it in that position, thus relieving pressure on the diseased lateral facet of the joint.

Analgesics

Non-opioid analgesics remain the drugs of first choice for symptomatic OA; paracetamol should be given at full dose, up to a maximum of 1 g four times a day, for a reasonable time before other drugs are considered. Paracetamol is superior to placebo and comparable in effectiveness to both ibuprofen and naproxen in patients with knee OA. Compound analgesics including codeine are more powerful. Some patients with severe end-stage OA of the hip or knee who are not candidates for total joint arthroplasty because of comorbid medical condition may require chronic treatment with opioid analgesics; in these patients, long-acting preparations of oxycodone or morphine may be used.

Concerns about patient addiction and vulnerability to legal action have led physicians to be reluctant to prescribe these drugs. In fact, addiction rates in otherwise psychologically stable individuals are very low. Reluctance to use powerful opiates is one example of the discrepancy that may exist between patient and doctor in analyzing the risk-benefit trade-off of interventions: Doctors perceive their patients to be suffering less than patients perceive themselves to be; as a result, patients are willing to accept greater risks to achieve pain reduction.

Topical Creams

Topical creams, either capsaicin or NSAIDs, can be helpful as either monotherapy or when added to oral analgesics, especially in patients with OA of the hand or knee if only one or a few joints are involved. In addition, they afford patients a measure of self-control over their therapy, which may in itself be beneficial. Capsaicin cream needs to be applied three or four times per day, and care must be taken to avoid getting the cream into the eyes or on mucous membranes because of severe burning. Most patients tolerate capsaicin cream, but some notice burning and rash that requires discontinuation.

Nonsteroidal Anti-inflammatory Drugs

A variable proportion of patients will not respond to paracetamol, alone or in combination with a topical agent, and derive additional benefit from oral NSAIDs. It is reasonable to try NSAIDs if nonpharmacologic therapy and paracetamol have failed to provide adequate symptomatic relief. There is no clear evidence to suggest superiority of one NSAID over another either in efficacy or toxicity. General principles of NSAID use in OA include the following: use of the minimum effective dose; avoidance of using more than one NSAID simultaneously; assessment of benefit after about a month (and cessation of a particular NSAID if no benefit is seen); and encouragement of "intelligent noncompliance" (i.e., patients should not feel obliged to take the NSAID if they do not have pain). The patient should be reassessed at 1 month and the additional benefit of NSAIDs, over and above that of analgesia, should be assessed.

The introduction of COX-2–selective NSAIDs in the 1990s raised the hope that their unique mode of action would reduce gastrointestinal toxicity. Although this may be the case, this has been tempered by concerns over other toxicities, notable cardiovascular, which have led to the withdrawal of at least one agent (rofecoxib) and recommendations for caution when using others in patients at risk of cardiac disease.[53] Coxibs such as etoricoxib and celecoxib are more effective than placebo in

OA and response at 2 weeks predicts long-term (12-week) response,[54] but as with NSAIDs, use of coxibs should only be considered after a trial of analgesia and nondrug therapy.

Nutriceuticals

Many patients seek alternative or complementary medications. Glucosamine is widely used and appears to be relatively safe. Claims for a disease-modifying effect remain controversial, but there may be a modest reduction in pain and stiffness by mechanisms that currently remain unclear.[55] In the Glucosamine/chondroitin Arthritis Intervention Trial (GAIT),[56] patients with symptomatic knee OA were randomised to five treatment groups: glucosamine, chondroitin sulphate, a combination of glucosamine and chondroitin sulphate, celecoxib, and placebo. Primary outcome was a decrease of at least 20% in pain measured by the Western Ontario and McMasters Universities Osteoarthritis Index (WOMAC) score. This outcome was reached in 64% of the glucosamine group, 65% of the chondroitin sulphate group, 67% of the combination, 70% of the celecoxib, and 60% of the placebo group.

Intra-Articular Steroids

Intra-articular steroids are widely used in patients with OA, particularly knee or thumb-base OA. Hip OA is also amenable to steroid injection, although confirmation that the injection is correctly located (e.g., by ultrasound control) is recommended. There is good evidence supporting steroid efficacy, but only for up to 4 weeks.[57] This contrasts with clinical practice suggesting that some patients have a sustained response to intra-articular steroid. Triamcinolone hexacetonide at a dose of 40 mg with or without anesthetic is suitable for the knee, and postinjection rest of the injected joint may improve response. Efforts to identify clinical predictors of response have proved largely unsuccessful.

Intra-Articular Hyaluronan

Intra-articular hyaluronan (previously hyaluronic acid) has also been shown to be effective in reducing pain in patients with mild-to-moderate knee OA confirmed by radiography; this therapy requires weekly injections for 3 to 5 weeks, and at least one study has suggested greater efficacy than a single injection of intra-articular steroids. However, the magnitude of the effect is small and must be weighed against cost and the invasive nature of the intervention. Several preparations, which differ largely in molecular weight, are available and may be of value in those patients whose symptoms persist despite standard treatment and in whom surgery is contraindicated.

The Placebo Effect in Osteoarthritis

The GAIT study described earlier confirmed previous findings of a high placebo response in OA. A meta-analysis of 198 trials found an effect size of 0.51 (comparing favorably with most active treatments) in placebo arms compared to 0.03 in untreated arms, leading the authors to conclude that "placebo is effective in the treatment of OA, especially for pain, stiffness and self-reported function."[58] Not all OA is equally affected by the placebo response; the effect is twice as high in hand OA as at the hip, for example. Harnessing the placebo response becomes a valid therapeutic goal in OA, though how this can be achieved is less clear.[59]

Surgery
What Operation?

For knee OA, arthroscopic debridement and lavage is a relatively noninvasive option for milder disease, although benefit appears to be short lived.[60] If the medial tibiofemoral joint is mainly affected, hemiarthroplasty can be performed. Osteotomy (division and realignment of the femur or tibia) is effective at relieving pain and correcting biomechanics and does not preclude more extensive surgery at a later date. At the hip, "resurfacing" procedures such as the Birmingham hip may have a role in men under age 50, but the failure rate in women is four to five times greater than full total hip replacement (THR), mainly because of fracture through the femoral head. In general, therefore, surgery in OA means TJR.

Who Currently Gets Total Joint Replacement?

OA is the main disease leading to THR or total knee replacement (TKR), accounting for up to 94% of THRs.[61] Current rates of joint replacement vary greatly between different countries, and within the United Kingdom there are large (threefold) variations in rates of THR between different regions. Rates of TJR are increasing rapidly, especially as revision surgery (currently 10% in the United Kingdom and 16% in the United States). It is predicted that in the United States by 2030 there will be a 175% increase in THR and a 670% increase in TKR, making these the commonest elective surgical procedures.[62]

Women tend to have worse function at the time of surgery than do men. American data suggest that the elderly, obese, and African American populations are less likely to get a TJR than are middle-aged, middle-class whites despite the fact that there is no evidence that older obese patients have worse outcomes. United Kingdom studies confirm that social deprivation reduces the chance of having a TJR.[63] Risk factors for TJR include pain, radiographic evidence of severe OA, obesity, and heavy manual work.[64]

Who Should Be Referred for Total Joint Replacement?

TJR is an effective but expensive intervention.[61] Although results from TJR in OA are generally excellent, outcomes do vary, with measurable perioperative death and morbidity rates and a small number of patients suffering continuing pain and disability in spite of a replacement.

There are currently no evidence-based indications for TJR in OA. Consensus-based criteria for who should get TJR have been produced in, for example, New Zealand.[65] In general, TJR is recommended for moderate-to-severe persistent pain, disability, or both that is not substantially relieved by an extended course of nonsurgical (medical) management.

Individuals undergoing TJR vary widely in preoperative severity of pain and disability. Although all groups show improvement in terms of function at 3 months, greatest benefit is seen in those with lower baseline disability. There is therefore a potential trade-off between operating on more people who have less severe disability because those patients achieve greatest benefit and limiting surgery to those fewer patients with more severe disease, accepting that some of their disability may never improve, even with TJR. Geographic variations suggest that this determinant is already operating: Patients in

Australia having TJR have lower disability than those in the United States; those in the United Kingdom are most disabled at the time of surgery.

Prevention of Osteoarthritis

The risk factors for large-joint OA are becoming well understood. Although some (race, gender, age, genetic predisposition) are unchangeable, others are modifiable, raising the possibility of primary prevention. Individuals at high risk for knee OA include those with obesity, a family history of "generalized OA" as manifested by presence of nodal OA in the hands, a history of injury, and a high-risk occupation.

Obesity is a major risk factor for development and progression of knee OA and, to a lesser extent, hand and hip OA. Weight reduction has been shown to be disease modifying. Although weight reduction is part of all guidelines for the management of lower limb OA, strategies to reduce the community prevalence of obesity might also reduce the incidence of OA; conversely, the rapid rise in obesity in most Western countries has major implications for the community burden of OA in the future. Tackling obesity in the general population requires major public health initiatives and is likely to be achievable only by a combination of reducing intake (changing what we eat—particularly what our children eat) and increasing energy expenditure by promoting aerobic exercise. Again, exercise is beneficial in established OA but may also have a role in primary prevention: quadriceps weakness is a risk factor for development of OA.[66]

Repetitive adverse loading of the knee (during occupation or extreme competitive sports) is another potentially avoidable risk factor.[50] Occupations involving heavy physical work, especially prolonged kneeling and squatting, have approximately twice the risk for knee OA. This risk interacts with that of obesity so that individuals with a body mass index (BMI) greater than 30 who also have occupational risk factors have a greatly increased odds ratio for developing knee OA of about 14.[67] Not only is the risk of OA increased, but once an individual has OA, the combination of intense physical activity at work and a high BMI significantly increases the risk when undergoing TKR.[64] In this high-risk group, it would be possible to aggressively support weight reduction or discourage obese individuals from performing such jobs. Alterations in work practice by avoiding prolonged work in high-risk postures or using supporting knee pads may theoretically reduce OA.

Injury (e.g., meniscal damage at the knee) is a powerful, potentially preventable risk factor for later OA. The role of intervention for problems of alignment, joint laxity, and nutritional status is less clear.

Barriers to the Prevention and Management of Osteoarthritis

Some of the main problems encountered when attempting to make a difference in the huge health burden caused by OA include the following:

- The perception that OA is an inevitable consequence of aging for which little can be done. Something can be done for most people with OA problems, and there is potential for prevention.
- The belief that exercise may worsen the disease. Although there may be a place for rest during acute flares of pain, there is a risk that rest will lead to a cycle of disuse, muscle atrophy, weakness, and increased pain. Therefore appropriate exercise is important.
- The importance of nonpharmacologic therapies tends to be underestimated, even though at least two (weight reduction and quadriceps strengthening) are potentially both disease modifying and preventive.
- Therapies are not exclusive. For example, intra-articular steroid injections may provide only short-term relief, but they can be used to reduce acute pain so that immediate exercise therapies can be instituted in the pain-free window.
- Packages of care, involving a large number of behavioral and other nonpharmacologic interventions, are likely to be the way forward for both prevention and treatment. However, it is difficult to test this hypothesis because it is difficult to obtain funding for complex intervention trials or for the testing of nonpharmacologic treatments.
- There is a need for treatment to be individualized.

Conclusion

Although thought to be one of the major causes of chronic pain in older people, OA remains poorly understood and difficult to treat effectively. There is an urgent need for more research into the causes and treatment of pain in OA, using the biopsychosocial model, in addition to the reductionist research being undertaken on its pathogenesis.

References

Full references for this chapter can be found on www.expertconsult.com.

The Connective Tissue Diseases

Steven D. Waldman

The connective tissue diseases are a heterogeneous group of syndromes that have in common a number of features, including the following: (1) they are multisystem diseases; (2) there is significant overlap of the signs and symptoms associated with these diseases; (3) blood vessels and connective tissue are frequently affected; (4) significant abnormalities of the immune response exist that often account for the tissue damage associated with these diseases; (5) these diseases affect females more commonly than males; and (6) onset occurs more often in winter than in summer in the Northern Hemisphere (**Table 44.1**).[1] Common connective tissue diseases include rheumatoid arthritis, systemic lupus erythematosus, systemic sclerosis (also known as scleroderma), polymyositis and dermatomyositis, polymyalgia rheumatica, temporal arteritis, and polyarteritis nodosa (**Table 44.2**). Previously known as the collagen vascular diseases, the term *connective tissue diseases* is now preferred because it more accurately reflects the fact that collagen is just one type of connective tissue affected in patients suffering from this group of diseases.

Rheumatoid Arthritis

Rheumatoid arthritis (RA) is the most common of the connective tissue diseases with approximately 1.5% of the population affected. The cause of RA is unknown but there appears to be a genetic predisposition to the development of this disease. Environmental factors may trigger the activation of RA and initiate the autoimmune response that ultimately can lead to potentially devastating multisystem disease. The possibility of an infectious etiology has gained new credence as the pathophysiologic processes behind Lyme disease are being elucidated.

The disease can occur at any age with the juvenile variant termed *Still disease*. Patients between 22 and 55 years of age are most often affected with increasing incidence with age.[2] Women are affected 2.5 times more often than men. Although the clinical diagnosis of RA is usually obvious in full-blown cases, the variability of presentation, severity, and progression can make the disease more difficult to diagnose. Because of the nonspecific nature of the signs and symptoms of RA, as well as the significant overlap of symptoms associated with other connective tissue diseases, the American College of Rheumatology has promulgated useful guidelines to assist the clinician in its diagnosis. These guidelines are presented in **Table 44.3**.

Table 44.1 **Common Features of the Connective Tissue Diseases**

They are multisystem diseases.

There is significant overlap of the signs and symptoms associated with these diseases.

Blood vessels and connective tissue are frequently affected.

There are significant abnormalities of the immune response, which often accounts for the tissue damage associated with these diseases.

These diseases affect females more commonly than males.

Onset occurs more commonly in winter than in summer in the Northern Hemisphere.

Table 44.2 **The Connective Tissue Diseases**

Rheumatoid arthritis (RA)

Systemic lupus erythematosus (SLE or lupus)

Polymyositis-dermatomyositis (PM-DM)

Systemic sclerosis (SSc or scleroderma)

Sjögren syndrome (SS)

Various forms of vasculitis

Signs and Symptoms

The onset of the disease may be subtle with nonspecific early signs and symptoms. Easy fatigability, malaise, myalgias, anorexia, and generalized weakness are often the first symptoms the patient with RA may experience. Ill-defined morning stiffness most often will progress to symmetric joint pain with color, tenosynovitis, and fusiform joint effusions (**Fig. 44.1**).[3] The rubor accompanying many of the other inflammatory arthritides (e.g., gout, septic arthritis) is not a predominant

---

Table 44.3 **Clinical Classification Criteria for Rheumatoid Arthritis***

Using history, physical examination, and laboratory and radiographic findings, four of the following symptoms must be present, with the first four symptoms present a minimum of 6 weeks:
- Morning stiffness 1 hour
- Arthritis of three or more of the following joints: right or left PIP, MCP, wrist, elbow, knee, ankle, or MTP
- Arthritis of wrist, MCP, or PIP joint
- Symmetric involvement of joints
- Rheumatoid nodules over bony prominences, or extensor surfaces, or in juxta-articular regions
- Positive serum rheumatoid factor
- Radiographic changes including erosions or bony decalcification localized in or adjacent to the involved joints

*From the American College of Rheumatology Subcommittee on Osteoarthritis Guidelines: Arthritis Rheum 43(9):1905, 2000.
MCP, metacarpophalangeal; MTP, metatarsophalangeal; PIP, proximal interphalangeal.

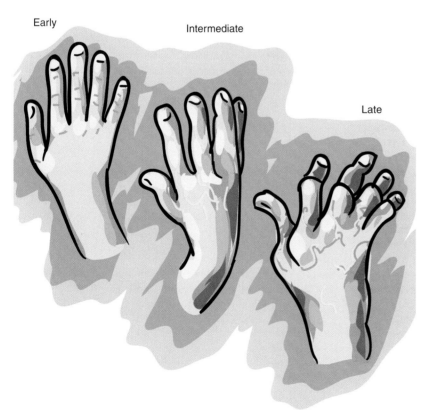

Early   Intermediate

Late

Fig. 44.1 Stages of rheumatoid arthritis.

feature of RA. The wrists, knees, ankles, fingers, and bones of the feet are most often affected, although any joint can be affected. Untreated, the synovitis becomes worse and joint effusions are common (**Fig. 44.2**). Tendons may become inflamed and may spontaneously rupture.[4] Ultimately, the destruction of the cartilage and supportive bone will result in severe disability and pain. Deformities of the affected joints—including flexion contractures and ulnar drift of the fingers and wrist as a result of slippage of the extensor tendons off the metacarpophalangeal joints—will ultimately occur with poorly treated or untreated disease (see Fig. 44.1).

Extra-articular manifestations of RA are common. Carpal tunnel syndrome is frequently associated with RA and, in fact, may point to diagnosis if the clinician thinks about it.[5] Carpal tunnel syndrome and the other entrapment neuropathies such as tardy ulnar palsy are the result of proliferation and thickening of the affected connective tissue. Ruptured Baker cysts are not uncommonly seen in patients with RA and can mimic deep vein thrombosis leading to unnecessary anticoagulation therapy (**Fig. 44.3**).[6] Other extra-articular manifestations of RA include rheumatoid nodules, which are painless masses that appear under the skin and around the extensor tendons. These nodules can also occur in the lung. Ocular manifestations are common, and uveitis and iritis can be severe. Vasculitis and anemia can also occur and if undiagnosed can lead to life-threatening multisystem organ failure. Pericarditis and pleuritis herald significant extra-articular disease and must be treated aggressively.[7]

These signs and symptoms of RA are the result of the autoimmune response associated with the disease. Immunologic abnormalities associated with RA include inflammatory immune complexes in the synovial fluid, as well as antibodies that are produced by the patient's own plasma cells. Among these antibodies is a substance called *RF factor*, which also serves as the basis of the serologic test used in the diagnosis of RA. As RA progresses, the patient's own T-helper cell lymphocytes infiltrate the synovial tissue of the joints. These T-helper cells produce cytokines that facilitate the inflammatory response and contribute to ongoing joint damage. Macrophages and their cytokines (e.g., tumor necrosis factor, granulocyte-macrophage colony-stimulating factor) are also abundant in diseased synovium. Increased adhesion molecules contribute to inflammatory cell migration and retention in the synovial tissue. Increased macrophage-derived lining cells are prominent along with some lymphocytes and vascular changes in early disease.

Prominent immunologic abnormalities that may be important in pathogenesis of RA include immune complexes found in joint fluid cells and in vasculitis. Plasma cells produce antibodies (e.g., rheumatoid factor [RF]) that contribute to these complexes. Lymphocytes that infiltrate the synovial tissue are primarily T-helper cells, which can produce proinflammatory cytokines. Macrophages are also present in the diseased synovium of the patient suffering from RA and produce additional cytokines, which attract other cells involved in the inflammatory response, further perpetuating joint damage, as well as setting the stage for vasculitis. These cells produce a variety of other substances that damage the joint, including fibrin, prostaglandins, collagenase, and interleukin-2. This ongoing inflammatory response leads to thickening of the synovium of the affected joints with pannus formation.

Laboratory Findings

A normochromic normocytic anemia is a common finding in patients suffering from RA with the patient's hemoglobin being mildly decreased with levels greater than 10 g/dL usually

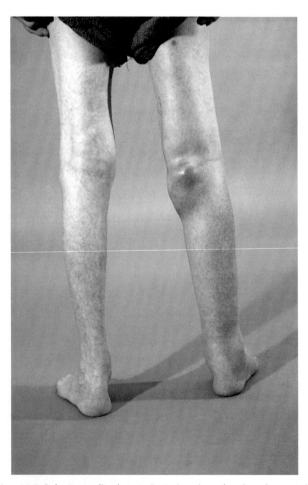

Fig. 44.3 Baker's popliteal cyst. Posterior view showing rheumatoid swelling behind the right knee. Swelling of the lower limb was related to venous compression by popliteal synovitis. *(From Klippel JH, Dieppe PA, editors: Rheumatology, ed 2, Philadelphia, 1997, Mosby, p 5.3.10.)*

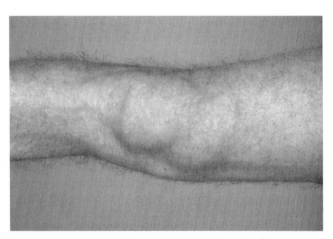

Fig. 44.2 Early rheumatoid arthritis of the knee showing extension of a small effusion into the suprapatellar pouch. *(From Klippel JH, Dieppe PA, editors: Rheumatology, ed 2, Philadelphia, 1997, Mosby, p 5.3.4.)*

seen unless there has been chronic bleeding from vasculitis of the stomach, kidneys, and so on. Neutropenia can occur in a small percentage of patients with RA and is usually associated with splenomegaly, which is termed *Felty syndrome*. Thrombocytosis and mild-to-moderate hypergammaglobulinemia may also be present. The erythrocyte sedimentation rate (ESR) is elevated in more than 90% of patients suffering from RA as is the C-reactive protein.

Antibodies to the aforementioned gamma globulins can be detected by a latex agglutination test and are called *rheumatoid factors* (RFs).[8] Although not 100% diagnostic for RA, RF titers greater than 1:160 dilution are highly suggestive of the disease and their presence makes the diagnosis of RA one of exclusion. The RF titer is indicative of the severity of the disease with higher titers signaling more severe disease. These titers will drop and can be used as a rough measure of the success of the various treatments available for RA.

Synovial fluid analysis of patients suffering from active RA will reveal a leukocytosis consisting of predominantly polymorphonuclear cells with lymphocytes and monocytes also present. The viscosity is decreased and the protein levels are increased. Unlike the crystal arthropathies, no crystals are present.

Radiographic Findings

Early in the course of the disease, the radiographic findings of RA are nonspecific and are often limited to soft tissue swelling and a suggestion of increased synovial fluid. As the disease progresses, osteochondral destruction and pannus formation become more evident. The earliest specific radiographic findings of RA are most often found in the second and third metacarpophalangeal joints and the third proximal interphalangeal joints.[9] Fusiform soft tissue swelling, concentric loss of the joint space, and periarticular loss of bone are also seen, as are marginal erosions of the articular surfaces that have lost their protective articular cartilage (**Fig. 44.4**). Superficial erosions beneath inflamed tendon sheaths may also occur. With further destruction of the joint, complete loss of the articular space can be seen and a variety of deformities and deviations of the joints and bones may occur (e.g., boutonnière and swan-neck deformities of the digits; **Fig. 44.5**). The characteristic ulnar drift or deviation of the metacarpophalangeal joints is pathognomonic of RA; this can be diagnosed by visual inspection of the affected joints and is vividly demonstrated on plain radiographs and magnetic resonance imaging (**Fig. 44.6**).

Differential Diagnosis

As mentioned earlier, the nonspecific nature of many of the signs and symptoms associated with RA, coupled with the significant overlap of symptoms associated with the other causes of arthritis and the connective tissue diseases, may make the diagnosis of RA challenging.[1] The American College of Rheumatology diagnostic guidelines presented in **Table 44.3** may help decrease the confusion, but the clinician should be cautioned that more than one form of arthritis may coexist and synovial fluid analysis, which is often overlooked, may be the quickest way to sort things out.[10]

Osteoarthritis can be difficult to distinguish from early or mild RA because nontraumatic osteoarthritis is often symmetric, with joint swelling and pain. Like RA, rubor is not a prominent feature of osteoarthritis when compared

with the crystal and infectious arthropathies. Osteoarthritis preferentially affects the proximal and distal interphalangeal joints (as characterized by Heberden and Bouchard nodules), first carpometacarpal and first metatarsophalangeal joints, knee, shoulder joints, and spine early in the course of the disease, whereas RA preferentially affects the second and

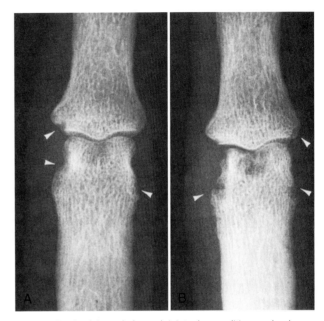

Fig. 44.4 Proximal interphalangeal joint abnormalities: early changes. A, Initial radiographic changes include soft tissue swelling, joint space narrowing, and marginal erosions *(arrowheads)*. B, Subsequently (in another digit), further loss of interosseous space and progressive erosions are evident *(arrowheads)*. Note that the erosive changes are more extensive on the proximal phalanx than on the middle phalanx. *(From Resnick D: Diagnosis of bone and joint disorders, ed 4, Philadelphia, 2002, Saunders, p 897.)*

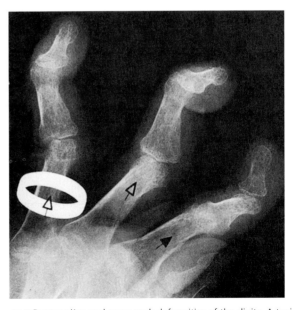

Fig. 44.5 Boutonnière and swan-neck deformities of the digits. A typical swan-neck deformity of the third and fourth digits *(open arrows)* and boutonnière deformity of the second digit *(closed arrow)* are evident in this patient with rheumatoid arthritis. *(From Resnick D: Diagnosis of bone and joint disorders, ed 4, Philadelphia, 2002, Saunders, p 899.)*

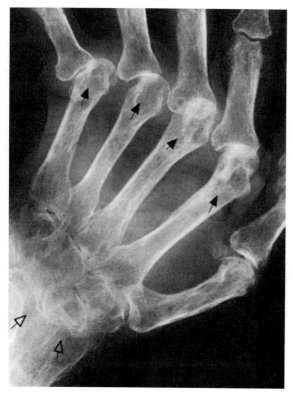

Fig. 44.6 Ulnar deviation of metacarpophalangeal joint. The simultaneous occurrence of ulnar deviation at the metacarpophalangeal joints *(solid arrows)* and radial deviation at the radiocarpal joint of the wrist *(open arrows)* is well shown in this patient. The resulting appearance is termed the *zigzag deformity. (From Resnick D: Diagnosis of bone and joint disorders, ed 4, Philadelphia, 2002, Saunders, p 901.)*

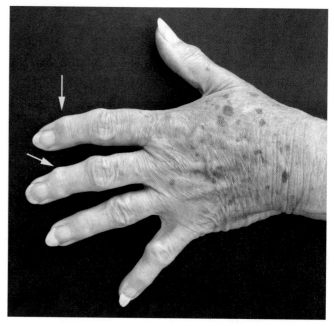

Fig. 44.7 The Heberden node sign for osteoarthritis of the distal interphalangeal joints. *(From Waldman SD: Physical diagnosis of pain, ed 2, Philadelphia, 2010, Saunders, p 184.)*

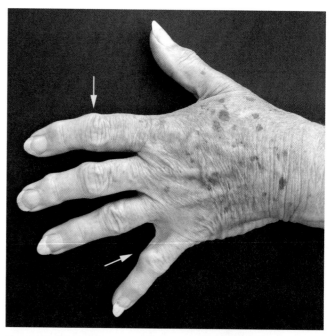

Fig. 44.8 The Bouchard node sign for osteoarthritis of the proximal interphalangeal joints. *(From Waldman SD: Physical diagnosis of pain, ed 2, Philadelphia, 2010, Saunders, p 185.)*

third metacarpophalangeal joints and the third proximal interphalangeal joints (**Figs. 44.7** and **44.8**). The absence of significantly elevated RF and ESR, rheumatoid nodules, and systemic symptomatology can also help distinguish RA from osteoarthritis. Evaluation of the synovial fluid in patients suffering from osteoarthritis will reveal white blood cell counts much lower than those seen in RA.

After osteoarthritis, systemic lupus erythematosus is probably the disease most commonly confused with active RA, although all the other connective tissue diseases can, at times, be difficult to distinguish from RA. These diseases will be discussed in greater detail subsequently, and the diagnostic criteria presented should aid the clinician in the differential diagnosis of confusing clinical presentations of symmetric arthritis.

In addition to the connective tissue diseases and crystal arthropathies (e.g., gout and pseudogout), amyloidosis, celiac disease, and sarcoidosis may also mimic RA, as can acute rheumatic fever secondary to streptococcal infections. Infectious arthritis usually manifests as a monoarticular or asymmetric arthritis, as does Lyme disease and Reiter's syndrome. Ankylosing spondylitis preferentially affects males and involves the sacroiliac joints and axial skeleton to a much greater extent than the peripheral joints.

Treatment

Although no cure for RA exists, most patients will experience good-to-excellent palliation of their symptoms and decrease the potential for severe disability with appropriate treatment

of their disease.[11] Despite optimal treatment, 8% to 10% of patients suffering from RA will experience serious disability that will interfere with the ability to provide self-care and carry out their activities of daily living.

The initial treatment of RA should focus on two factors: (1) rest and protection of affected joints and (2) aggressive treatment of the acute inflammatory process. The failure to rest and splint the joints acutely inflamed by RA can often lead to irreversible joint damage with attendant pain and disability. Splinting may also help slow the progression of hand and foot deformities that can be so distressing and disabling to the patient suffering from RA. Aggressive treatment of the inflammatory response associated with acute RA requires skillful use of the drugs discussed subsequently.

Pharmacologic Treatment with Anti-Inflammatory Agents

Acute inflammation should be treated aggressively with the nonsteroidal anti-inflammatory drugs (NSAIDs), such as aspirin, ibuprofen, and the like. These drugs have significant renal, gastrointestinal, and hepatic side effects and must be used with caution. For patients with gastrointestinal side effects, enteric-coated products or the nonacetylated salicylates, such as salsalate or choline magnesium salicylate, may be considered. The addition of cytoprotective drugs such as misoprostol or the proton pump inhibitors such as ranitidine may also help decrease the incidence of gastrointestinal side effects and allow the RA patient to continue to take these much-needed drugs.[12] For patients who cannot tolerate the NSAIDs, the COX-2 inhibitors may be considered with an eye to their potential cardiac side effects. Fish oil supplementation may also help suppress intra-articular prostaglandins, as well as promote cardiovascular health. Whether these drugs alter the ultimate course of the disease remains an area of intense debate.

Although NSAIDs are generally the first line of treatment for acute RA, it should be remembered that corticosteroids can provide dramatic relief of the pain and disability associated with acute exacerbations of the disease. Unfortunately, two major problems are associated with the use of corticosteroids in the treatment of acute RA: (1) corticosteroids tend to become less effective in suppressing the acute inflammatory response over time, and (2) this class of drugs has significant side effects with chronic use. Like the NSAIDs, it is unclear whether treatment with corticosteroids will alter the ultimate course of RA in the individual patient, although the ability of this class of drugs to palliate the acute symptoms of RA is unsurpassed. In general, daily treatment of RA with corticosteroids should be limited to those patients who are unable to tolerate other treatment options or in those patients with life-threatening extra-articular manifestations of the disease (e.g., pericarditis, pleurisy, nephritis). Injection of acutely inflamed and painful joints with small amounts of anti-inflammatory steroid may be useful to provide symptomatic relief, stop the inflammatory process, and allow the patient to avoid all the side effects associated with the systemic administration of this class of drugs.

Pharmacologic Treatment with Disease-Modifying Drugs

As mentioned, it is unclear whether an NSAID or a corticosteroid as a sole therapeutic agent can effectively modify the course of RA. For this reason, there is a move toward the use of disease-modifying drugs such as methotrexate, hydroxychloroquine, sulfasalazine, penicillamine, and gold salts earlier in the course of the disease. Methotrexate is an immunosuppressive drug that is reasonably well tolerated and is increasingly becoming a first-line drug in the treatment of RA (see later discussion).[13] Gold is available as a parenteral solution that is usually administered via intramuscular injection on a weekly basis; it is also available as an oral formulation. Although

effective in the treatment of RA, gold salts are not without side effects. These side effects include significant renal and hepatic toxicity, as well as potentially life-threatening skin and blood dyscrasias.

If gold therapy is ineffective or causes toxic side effects, oral penicillamine may be considered. Potentially serious side effects associated with penicillamine therapy include bone marrow suppression, renal damage, a lupus-like syndrome (Goodpasture syndrome), and myasthenia gravis. Careful monitoring for these potentially life-threatening side effects is mandatory, and the drug should be used only by those familiar with its potential toxicity.

Hydroxychloroquine can also provide symptomatic relief for the patient suffering from mild to moderately active RA. Reasonably well tolerated, the major serious side effects of this drug include myopathy, which may be irreversible, and ophthalmologic side effects, including reversible corneal opacities and potentially irreversible retinal degeneration. Both of these serious side effects require careful neurologic and ophthalmologic monitoring while the drug is being used.

Sulfasalazine, which is used primarily for treatment of ulcerative colitis, may also be used to treat RA. Less toxic than gold salts and penicillamine, it is slower acting but generally well tolerated. An enteric-coated product has increased its tolerability. Monitoring of basic hematologic and blood chemistries to identify the relatively uncommon hematologic, renal, and hepatic side effects should be carried out in all patients treated with this drug.

Pharmacologic Treatment with Immunosuppressive Drugs

In addition to the aforementioned disease-modifying drugs, the immunosuppressive drugs including methotrexate, azathioprine, and cyclosporine are increasingly being used relatively early in the course of RA. These drugs have in common their ability to suppress active inflammation in RA. Generally well tolerated, these drugs are not without side effects. Careful monitoring for bone marrow suppression, hepatic and renal dysfunction, and pneumonitis is mandatory. The potential of the immunosuppressive drugs to trigger malignancy is of real concern, especially with prolonged use of azathioprine.

As mentioned, the immunosuppressive drug methotrexate is now being used early in the course of active RA. It can be given orally as a once a week dose and is generally well tolerated. Side effects include interference with folic acid metabolism, which requires concomitant folic acid replacement. Methotrexate also has significant hepatotoxicity in some patients, and any elevation of liver function tests and potentially fatal fibrosis of the liver requires immediate attention and liver biopsy. Although rare, fatal pneumonitis has been reported with the use of methotrexate in the treatment of RA.

Etanercept and infliximab are new disease-modifying drugs that have shown promise when given alone or in combination with methotrexate in the management of RA.[14] Both etanercept and infliximab block tumor necrosis factor alpha, a protein that the body produces during the inflammatory response.[15] The increased amounts of tumor necrosis factor alpha seen in patients with acute RA accelerate the inflammatory response and contribute to the pain, swelling, and stiffness associated with the disease. The mechanism of action for these drugs is thought to be via the binding of free tumor necrosis factor alpha, thereby decreasing the amounts available to promote the inflammatory response. Given via subcutaneous injection twice a week, etanercept is well tolerated with rare side effects including neurologic dysfunction, optic neuritis, and occasionally pancytopenia. Infliximab is given via intravenous infusion, and these infusions are often accompanied by chills, fever, blood pressure abnormalities, and rash. These drugs should not be used in patients with active infections because even minor infections may become life threatening as a result of the drug's ability to suppress the inflammatory response. Reactivation of tuberculosis has also been reported following administration of these drugs when treating RA.

Treatment with Physical Modalities, Orthotics, and Physical and Occupational Therapy

As mentioned earlier, the pharmacologic treatment of the pain and disability of RA is only one part of a successful treatment strategy. Just as acute inflammation must be aggressively treated to avoid further joint destruction, the aggressive use of physical modalities, orthotics, and physical and occupational therapy is paramount to modify the relentless progression of inadequately treated RA.[16]

The use of local heat and cold can provide significant symptomatic relief for the pain, swelling, and stiffness of RA. Although conventional wisdom suggests that the application of heat should be avoided in the acutely inflamed joint, many patients suffering from RA find superficial moist heat to provide significant symptomatic relief. Other patients find the use of superficial cold more beneficial. Deep-heating modalities such as ultrasound and diathermy should be avoided during the acute phases of RA, but may be useful as part of a comprehensive rehabilitation program for joints that are no longer acutely inflamed.

The use of orthotic devices to prevent joint deformity is an integral part of the treatment of the patient with RA. The use of night splints to slow the progression of ulnar drift should be considered early in the course of the disease. The use of shoe inserts and careful fitting of shoes can also help preserve function and ease pain. Protection of the elbows and Achilles tendons during periods of bed rest will also decrease the development of rheumatoid nodules at pressure areas. As the acute inflammation is brought under control, a gentle physical therapy program that focuses on reconditioning, joint protection, and restoration of range of motion and function should be undertaken.

Perhaps nowhere else in medicine is the role of patient education and the use of assistive devices more important than in the care of the patient suffering from RA. Instruction in proper lifting techniques and joint protection strategies and training in the use of assistive devices such as jar openers and button hooks are paramount if preservation of joint function is to be achieved.

Surgical Treatment Options

Surgical treatment should be limited to the repair of acute joint injuries (e.g., subluxated joints, torn cartilage, ruptured tendons) and the release of associated entrapment neuropathies. Total joint arthroplasty is indicated in those patients with severely damaged joints that are compromising the patient's ability to

provide self-care and carry out his or her activities of daily living. It should be remembered that patients suffering from RA are at particular risk for C1-2 subluxations and that early surgical treatment may be required to avoid fatal spinal cord injury (**Fig. 44.9**). Any surgical interventions should include a concurrent plan of physical medicine and rehabilitation to avoid further loss of function in the postoperative period.

Systemic Lupus Erythematosus

The second most common connective tissue disease encountered in clinical practice, systemic lupus erythematosus (SLE) is a disease of unknown etiology.[17] Ninety percent of patients suffering from SLE are women. There is an increased incidence of this disease among African Americans and Asians.[18] Affecting the joints, skin, blood vessels, and major organ systems, SLE has the potential to cause much suffering and disability, although a milder, less virulent variant of the disease is less problematic.

Signs and Symptoms

As mentioned, SLE manifests in a wide spectrum. The clinical picture can range from a mild, nonprogressive disease to an aggressive syndrome affecting multiple organ systems and producing life-threatening sequelae.[19] SLE may manifest as an acute febrile illness with arthralgias and rash that are difficult to distinguish from the acute febrile exanthemas with involvement of the central nervous system and other major organ systems; or the onset may be much more subtle and insidious, leading to significant delays in diagnosis. Manifestations referable to any organ system may appear.[20] Either the cutaneous manifestations or the almost universal complaint of polyarthralgias usually lead the clinician to think about the diagnosis of SLE.[21]

Although polyarthritis is present in more than 90% of patients with SLE, in contradistinction to RA, the joint disease

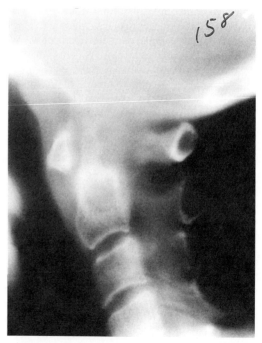

Fig. 44.9 Computed tomography (CT) scan of cervical spine showing erosion of the odontoid. *(From Klippel JH, Dieppe PA, editors: Rheumatology, ed 2, Philadelphia, 1997, Mosby, p 5.4.5.)*

associated with SLE tends to be much less destructive and deforming.[22,23] This form of nonerosive arthritis called *Jaccoud arthritis* is usually seen in SLE patients who present acutely with a constellation of symptoms reminiscent of acute rheumatic fever. In rare patients, significant joint destruction and deformity resembling that seen in RA can be observed.[24]

The characteristic cutaneous lesion associated with SLE is the butterfly rash (**Fig. 44.10**).[21] A variant form of SLE, which is characterized by discoid cutaneous lesions, is known as discoid lupus erythematosus (**Fig. 44.11**). The discoid variant of the disease tends to be milder with less systemic involvement than SLE (**Fig. 44.12**). Recurrent mouth ulcers and focal areas of alopecia are reasonably common, as are purpuric lesions secondary to small vessel vasculitis (**Figs. 44.13** and **44.14**). Photosensitivity is reported by more than 44% of patients suffering from SLE.[25]

In addition to the joint and dermatologic manifestations of SLE, the clinician will do well to remember that this disease can affect virtually any organ system. **Table 44.4** provides some of the common extra-articular manifestations of SLE. These include vasculitis, pleuritis, pneumonitis, myocarditis, endocarditis, pericarditis, glomerulonephritis, hepatitis, splenomegaly, and generalized adenopathy (**Fig. 44.15**).[21,26]

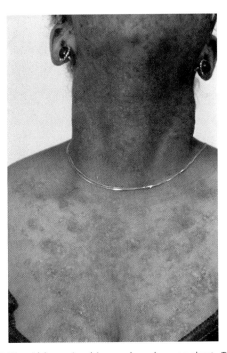

Fig. 44.12 Discoid lupus involving neck and upper chest. The lesions have characteristic central scarring. *(From Klippel JH, Dieppe PA, editors: Rheumatology, ed 2, Philadelphia, 1997, Mosby, p 7.1.3.)*

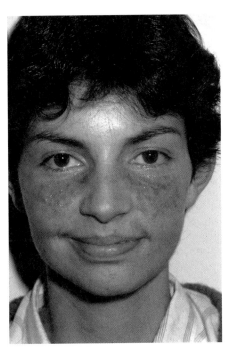

Fig. 44.10 Erythematous malar rash of systemic lupus erythematosus. Note that the rash does not cross the nasolabial fold. *(From Klippel JH, Dieppe PA, editors: Rheumatology, ed 2, Philadelphia, 1997, Mosby, p 7.1.3.)*

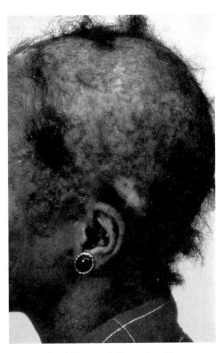

Fig. 44.13 Scarring discoid lupus of the scalp with permanent alopecia. *(From Klippel JH, Dieppe PA, editors: Rheumatology, ed 2, Philadelphia, 1997, Mosby, p 7.1.4.)*

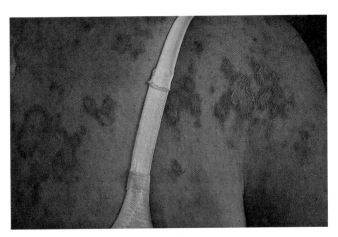

Fig. 44.11 Subacute cutaneous lupus lesions. *(From Klippel JH, Dieppe PA, editors: Rheumatology, ed 2, Philadelphia, 1997, Mosby, p 7.1.3.)*

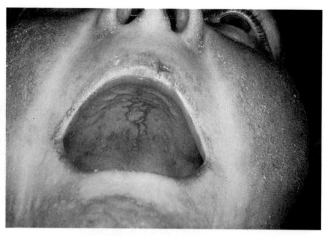

Fig. 44.14 Mouth ulcers in a patient with systemic lupus erythematosus. *(From Klippel JH, Dieppe PA, editors: Rheumatology, ed 2, Philadelphia, 1997, Mosby, p 7.1.4.)*

Table 44.4 Extra-Articular Manifestations of Systemic Lupus Erythematosus

Dermatologic manifestations	Butterfly rash Discoid lesions Focal alopecia Maculopapular lesions
Vascular manifestations	Vasculitis Thrombosis
Pulmonary manifestations	Pleuritis Pleural effusion Pleurisy Pulmonary embolus
Cardiac manifestations	Myocarditis Endocarditis Pericarditis Renal Manifestations Proteinuria Glomerulonephritis
Hepatic manifestations	Hepatitis
Hematologic manifestations	Pancytopenia Leukopenia Thrombocytopenia Hypercoagulable state
Neurologic manifestations	Headaches Seizures Peripheral neuropathy Stroke Confusion Psychosis
Generalized lymphadenopathy	
Splenomegaly	

Hematologic side effects including pancytopenia, thrombocytopenia, leukopenia, and a hypercoagulable state with secondary pulmonary and coronary artery embolic phenomenon and/or thrombosis can occur. Neurologic dysfunction including headaches, seizures, confusion, and occasionally frank psychosis can occur.[27]

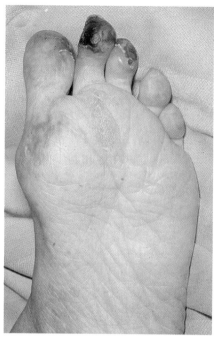

Fig. 44.15 Gangrene of the toe in a patient with systemic lupus erythematosus and vasculitis. *(From Klippel JH, Dieppe PA, editors: Rheumatology, ed 2, Philadelphia, 1997, Mosby, p 7.1.4.)*

Laboratory Findings

The antinuclear antibody (ANA) test is positive in more than 98% of patients suffering from SLE.[28] Occasional false positives occur in those patients with serology that is positive for syphilis, and positive ANA titers can occur from drug-induced lupus-like states. If the clinical diagnosis is in doubt or if a patient's presentation is highly selective for SLE but the ANA is negative, more specific testing for the presence of anti–double-stranded DNA antibody can help clarify the situation because high titers of anti–double-stranded DNA antibody are highly specific for SLE.

The ESR is significantly elevated in most patients suffering from SLE. In contradistinction to RA with consistently elevated C-reactive protein levels, C-reactive protein levels are surprisingly low, even in the face of active disease. As mentioned earlier, a wide range of hematologic abnormalities including pancytopenia, thrombocytopenia, leukopenia, and coagulopathy may be present. The presence of high levels of anticardiolipin antibodies should alert the clinician to the significantly increased possibility of hypercoagulability.

Differential Diagnosis

SLE is obvious when a patient (particularly a young woman) is febrile with an erythematous skin rash, polyarthritis, evidence of renal disease, intermittent pleuritic pain, leukopenia, and hyperglobulinemia with anti–double-stranded DNA antibodies. Early-stage SLE can be difficult to differentiate from other connective tissue disorders and may be mistaken for RA if arthritic symptoms predominate. Mixed connective tissue disease has the clinical features of SLE with overlapping features of systemic sclerosis, rheumatoid-like polyarthritis, and polymyositis or dermatomyositis (see later discussion).[21,26]

As mentioned earlier, several drugs in current clinical use can produce a clinical syndrome that resembles SLE and can also produce a positive ANA test. These drugs include hydralazine, procainamide, and several beta blockers. The lupus-like symptoms and positive ANA generally disappear after discontinuation of the offending drug.

Treatment

In general, if SLE is diagnosed early in the course of the disease and its effects on the joints and other organ systems are appropriately treated, the long-term prognosis of this disease is much better than for many of the other connective tissue diseases. The rational treatment of SLE is driven by the severity and extra-articular manifestations of the disease because long-term studies have shown that much of the morbidity and, in some cases, mortality associated with SLE are iatrogenically introduced complications of treatment. For purposes of treatment, SLE is divided into mild and severe disease classifications.

Mild SLE is manifested by fever, arthralgias, headache, rash, and mild pericarditis. Severe SLE is characterized by the symptoms of pleural effusions, severe pericarditis, myocarditis, renal dysfunction, thrombocytopenic purpura, vasculitis, hemolytic anemia, hypercoagulable state, and significant central nervous system involvement.[29-32] The patient with severe SLE must be viewed as suffering from a potentially life-threatening emergency and treated as such.

Mild SLE is treated symptomatically with an eye toward early identification of renal damage and the development of a hypercoagulable state. The NSAIDs and aspirin (especially if thrombosis is a concern) are an excellent starting point in the treatment of mild SLE. The antimalarial drugs such as chloroquine, hydroxychloroquine, or quinacrine can be added if dermatologic or joint manifestations are a problem. It should remembered that lupus is a disease that, like multiple sclerosis, is characterized by remissions and exacerbations, and also like multiple sclerosis, it has an extremely unpredictable course. Failure to recognize warning signs of increasing renal, cardiac, hematologic, or pulmonary dysfunction can have disastrous results.

The classification of a patient's lupus as severe represents a need for aggressive treatment with corticosteroids and close monitoring for occult system failure. Prednisone at a starting dose of 60 mg/day is indicated at the first sign of trouble although some experienced clinicians will use high-dose intravenous methylprednisolone at a dosage of 1000 mg for 3 to 4 days, especially if florid central nervous system symptoms are present. The addition of immunosuppressive drugs such as azathioprine or cyclophosphamide is also useful if there is significant renal disease. The risk of thrombosis as heralded by high anticardiolipin antibodies may suggest a need for prophylactic anticoagulation.

As severe SLE is controlled, suppression of the autoimmune and inflammatory response is usually required. This is best accomplished with low-dose corticosteroids or low-dose immunosuppressive therapy. The effectiveness of suppressive therapy can be monitored by the subjective clinical response to the therapeutic regimen chosen and objectified by following titers of anti–double-stranded DNA antibody. The clinician should be vigilant for exacerbation of the inflammatory and autoimmune response as the corticosteroids are tapered, and such exacerbations should

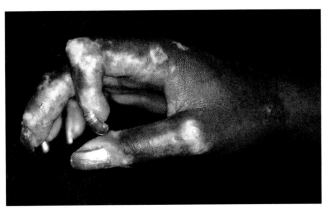

Fig. 44.16 Digital and hand scleroderma. Advanced changes of scleroderma have caused digital contractions and limitation of finger movement. *(From Klippel JH, Dieppe PA, editors:* Rheumatology, *ed 2, Philadelphia, 1997, Mosby, p 7.9.3)*

be treated promptly to avoid sequelae. Intercurrent infections can be problematic for the patient suffering from SLE and should be treated aggressively. The clinician should also be aware that, even in the face of excellent disease control, pregnancy is associated with flaring of symptoms, and spontaneous abortions and late-term fetal demise are common.

Scleroderma and Systemic Sclerosis

Scleroderma is a connective tissue disease of unknown etiology that is characterized by diffuse fibrosis of the skin and connective tissue, vascular damage, arthritis, and abnormalities of the esophagus, gastrointestinal tract, kidneys, heart, and lungs.[33] This fibrosis is the result of abnormal collagen deposition in the affected structures. The disease may be localized to the skin or a single organ system or may cause severe multisystem disease.[34] There is a trend to call the systemic variant of the disease *systemic sclerosis* to more accurately reflect the multisystem nature of the disease. Like SLE, the severity and course of the disease vary widely from patient to patient. Scleroderma is four times more common in women than in men and its onset is rare before age 30 or after age 50. Exposure to contaminated cooking oils, polyvinyl chloride, and silica has also been implicated as risk factors for the development of scleroderma.

Signs and Symptoms

Unlike RA, the onset of scleroderma can be very subtle and insidious. The initial complaints of patients suffering from scleroderma usually reflect the pain or deformity associated with swelling and loss of range of motion of the digits (sclerodactyly) and the associated Raynaud phenomenon.[35] Polyarthralgias and dysphagia can also be prominent initial features of the disease.

Most distressing to the patient are the cutaneous changes associated with scleroderma. Most often, the unsightly changes of sclerodactyly cause the patient to initially seek medical attention (**Fig. 44.16**). The skin changes of scleroderma tend to be symmetric, affecting the distal upper extremities first. Untreated, the skin will become shiny and atrophic looking with a swollen, taut appearance. Hyperpigmentation and telangiectases of the digits, face, chest, and lips may also occur (**Fig. 44.17**). A mask-like facies may appear, which can be quite distressing to the patient and family (**Fig. 44.18**). Subcutaneous calcifications of the fingers and over the elbows, ankles, and knees may cause further pain and deformity (**Fig. 44.19**). Ulcerations of the skin overlying these calcifica-

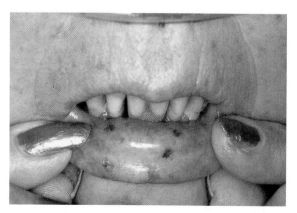

Fig. 44.17 Facial telangiectases. Punctate telangiectases are present on the lips and cheeks of this woman with long-standing limited scleroderma. *(From Klippel JH, Dieppe PA, editors:* Rheumatology, *ed 2, Philadelphia, 1997, Mosby, p 7.9.4)*

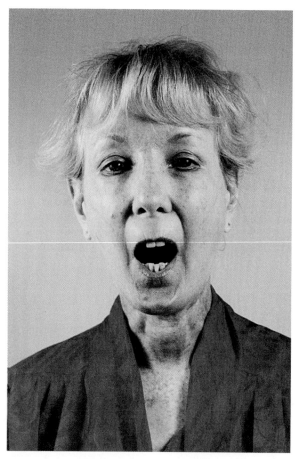

Fig. 44.18 Facial scleroderma. Taut, smooth skin over the face of a woman with long-standing disease. Oral aperture is reduced and radial furrowing is present around the lips. *(From Klippel JH, Dieppe PA, editors:* Rheumatology, *ed 2, Philadelphia, 1997, Mosby, p 7.9.6)*

tions and the fingertips caused by the trophic nature of the skin and vasculitis are common.[36]

Tendinitis and bursitis, especially of the large joints, can contribute to pain and disability and can accelerate loss of range of motion of already compromised joints. Flexion contractures of the fingers, wrists, and elbows caused by fibrosis of the synovium and overlying skin can be particularly problematic and very difficult to treat once they have occurred.

Complicating the cutaneous and musculoskeletal manifestations of the disease is the almost universal complaint of dysphagia caused by impaired esophageal motility.[37] Fibrosis of the esophagus and lower esophageal sphincter can further exacerbate the problem of dysphagia as a result of acid reflux induced distal to esophageal strictures. Hypomotility of the small intestine can result in malabsorption, and diffuse fibrosis of the large intestine can further compromise gastrointestinal function.

Pulmonary fibrosis, pleurisy, and pleural effusions can compromise pulmonary function. Untreated, this fibrosis may affect the small vessels of the lung, and pulmonary hypertension with all of its attendant problems may develop. The fibrosis associated with scleroderma may also affect the muscle and conduction system of the heart. Cardiac arrhythmias may result, and compromised cardiac output secondary to myocardial fibrosis (combined with pulmonary hypertension) may result in treatment-refractory congestive heart failure. The onset of pulmonary and cardiac symptoms early in the course of the disease is a poor prognostic sign.

The kidneys are most often the most severely affected by scleroderma with fibrosis of the small arteries of the kidneys, resulting in the rapid deterioration of renal function and malignant hypertension. This deterioration of renal function

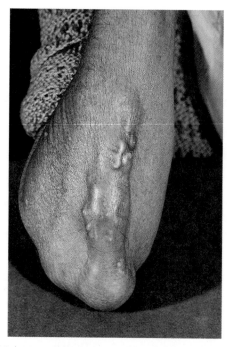

Fig. 44.19 Subcutaneous calcinosis. Extensive calcinosis is present on the exterior surface of the forearm in a patient with limited scleroderma. *(From Klippel JH, Dieppe PA, editors:* Rheumatology, *ed 2, Philadelphia, 1997, Mosby, p 7.9.4)*

may be exacerbated when concomitant heart failure is present. Untreated, it is the unremitting deterioration of renal function that is fatal in patients suffering from scleroderma.[32]

Laboratory Findings

Although the diagnosis of scleroderma is most often made on clinical grounds, confirmatory laboratory testing is sometimes useful when the diagnosis is in question or if a variant of scleroderma (e.g., calcinosis, raynaud phenomenon, esophogeal involvement, sclerodactyly, and telangiectasia [CREST] syndrome) is being considered (see later discussion).[38] ANA titers are elevated in more than 90% of patients suffering from scleroderma. Although not pathognomonic for the disease, the presence of high ANA titers at least points the clinician in the direction of connective tissue disease. If the diagnosis of scleroderma is still in question, the pattern of the ANA testing may be helpful. In patients with scleroderma, specific ANA testing will show an antinucleolar pattern, whereas patients with CREST syndrome will demonstrate an anticentromere pattern. Approximately one third of patients suffering from scleroderma will have a positive rheumatoid factor that may confuse the picture. The ESR will often be elevated in scleroderma, but frequently not to the extent seen in RA and SLE.

Differential Diagnosis

Because of the often subtle and insidious onset of scleroderma, the diagnosis may be delayed or confused with other connective tissue diseases or other systemic diseases of the heart, lungs, joints, skin, and kidneys. Variants of scleroderma can manifest in myriad fashion and confuse the clinical picture. CREST syndrome is one such variant. Its constellation of systems include calcinosis, Raynaud phenomenon, esophageal dysfunction, sclerodactyly, and telangiectasia (**Figs. 44.20** and

44.21).[38] Also known as limited cutaneous scleroderma, this variant of scleroderma has a much more benign course and an infinitely better prognosis.[39] Scleroderma that is limited to the skin and adjacent connective tissue, but without multisystem involvement can also occasionally make the diagnosis of scleroderma more difficult.[40] Like CREST syndrome, the clinical course and prognosis of this localized variant of scleroderma is relatively benign. Mixed connective tissue disease (MCTD), which combines elements of polymyositis, SLE, and scleroderma, can also present a diagnostic dilemma.[41] If MCTD is being considered in the differential diagnosis of scleroderma, testing for the presence of antinuclear ribonucleoprotein antibody will prompt the clinician to suspect that MCTD is the culprit rather than classic scleroderma.

Treatment

The treatment of scleroderma has its basis in the treatment of specific organ system dysfunction related to the disease rather than any treatment that is specifically aimed at the underlying disease itself. Early treatment of organ system dysfunction is critical if the clinician hopes to improve the quality of life and prognosis for the patient suffering from scleroderma. Nowhere is this statement more valid than when dealing with renal dysfunction. The early use of angiotensin-converting enzyme inhibitors and vasodilators such as

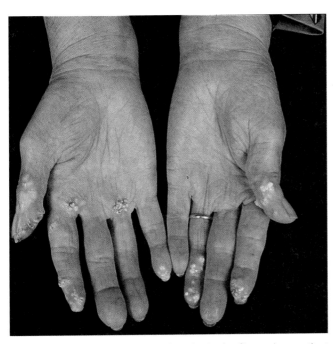

Fig. 44.20 Calcific subcutaneous deposits in the fingers in a patient with limited scleroderma (CREST). *(From Klippel JH, Dieppe PA, editors: Rheumatology, ed 2, Philadelphia, 1997, Mosby, p 7.12.5)*

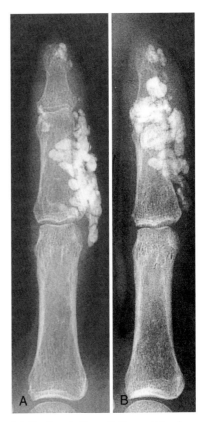

Fig. 44.21 A, Calcifications in the soft tissue of the fingers in a patient with scleroderma. B, Following treatment with low-dose sodium warfarin for 18 months, there is redistribution of the calcifications without a decrease in extent. *(From Klippel JH, Dieppe PA, editors: Rheumatology, ed 2, Philadelphia, 1997, Mosby, p 7.12.5)*

minoxidil is indicated to control hypertension and improve renal blood flow.[42]

The use of NSAIDs and corticosteroids in low doses to treat synovitis, arthritis, and myositis should be considered early in the course of the disease.[43] The calcium channel blockers may help ameliorate the symptomatology associated with Raynaud phenomenon, and there is anecdotal evidence that topical nitroglycerin ointment may also help provide symptomatic relief. Methotrexate and penicillamine may help slow the progression of fibrosis, especially of the skin and digits.[44] Immunosuppressive drugs may be of value in uncontrolled, rapidly progressive disease.[45,46]

Treatment of reflux with histamine blocking agents, bed blocks, and multiple small feedings may also provide symptomatic relief and help prevent lower esophageal erosions and stricture.[47] Oral antibiotics may also be used if malabsorption secondary to bacterial overgrowth in dilated small intestine and bowel is a problem. As with the other connective tissue diseases, the rational use of occupational and physical therapy can help decrease pain and preserve and improve function.

Polymyositis and Dermatomyositis

Less common than RA, SLE, or scleroderma, polymyositis is a connective tissue disease of unknown etiology.[48] The disease is characterized by muscle inflammation that progresses to degenerative muscle disease and atrophy.[49] There are many variants of polymyositis, including dermatomyositis, which is from a clinical viewpoint simply polymyositis with significant cutaneous manifestations.[50] Affecting women twice as frequently as men, polymyositis can overlap with basically all of the connective tissue diseases, making diagnosis on purely clinical grounds somewhat more challenging.[51] Generally not occurring in adults before age 44 or after age 60, there is a childhood variant that carries a poor prognosis. The clinician should aware that there is a strong correlation with the presence of malignancy in patients with polymyositis, and a search for underlying malignancy must be an integral part of any diagnostic workup and treatment plan of patients suspected of having polymyositis.[48] Whether the malignancy serves as a trigger to the autoimmune response to muscle in this disease or is simply a trigger to an unknown cascade of events has yet to be elucidated. There is a greater incidence of malignancy in those patients suffering from dermatomyositis relative to polymyositis. The type and location of tumor are not consistent, making the search for associated occult malignancy all the more difficult.

Signs and Symptoms

The onset of polymyositis is often preceded by an acute infection, often viral in nature. The onset of symptoms may be acute or may come on gradually with the patients thinking that they simply have not shaken the initial febrile illness. Patients generally present with rash and muscle weakness as the initial symptoms with the proximal muscle groups affected initially more commonly than the distal muscle groups. Myalgias and polyarthralgias may be present, as may constitutional symptoms resembling polymyalgia rheumatica (see later discussion).[52] In some patients the onset of profound muscle weakness may be rapid with the patient presenting with the inability to rise

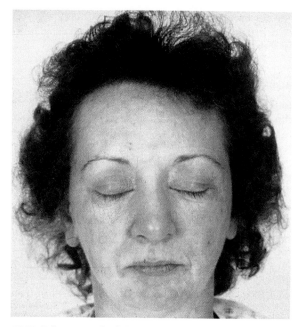

Fig. 44.22 Heliotrope rash of dermatomyositis. The erythematous and/or violaceous rash over the eyelids of this patient with dermatomyositis and breast cancer is a characteristic cutaneous feature. *(From Klippel JH, Dieppe PA, editors:* Rheumatology, *ed 2, Philadelphia, 1997, Mosby, p 7.13.5)*

from a sitting position or the complaint of the inability to raise the arms above the head to comb or curl the hair.

In rare patients, weakness of the muscles controlling the vocal cords may cause dysphagia, which may be mistaken for myasthenia gravis or a stroke. In severe cases, acute respiratory insufficiency may occur and the association of recent febrile illness may yield the mistaken diagnosis of Guillain-Barré disease. Involvement of the gastrointestinal tract may lead to symptoms as described previously in scleroderma. Cardiac arrhythmias and conduction defects are seen in many patients suffering from polymyositis, as is renal failure, due to acute myoglobulinemia from rhabdomyolysis in acute exacerbations of the disease. In general, the small muscles of the hands and feet are spared, as are the muscles of facial expression.

When patients with polymyositis exhibit significant cutaneous manifestations, for clinical purposes the diseases is called dermatomyositis.[53] A heliotrope periorbital blush is pathognomonic for the disease (**Fig. 44.22**). There may be a peeling or splitting of skin over the radial sides of the digits that is highly suggestive of dermatomyositis (**Fig. 44.23**). A generalized maculopapular rash may also appear (**Fig. 44.24**). Subcutaneous calcific nodules may be present in many patients with undiagnosed and untreated disease.

Laboratory Testing

No specific diagnostic test exists for polymyositis or dermatomyositis.[54] The ESR is usually elevated, as are the serum muscle enzyme determinations, especially in acute disease. The monitoring of creatine kinase (CK) levels may serve as a useful guide as to the efficacy of treatment. Approximately 60% of patients with polymyositis have antibodies to thymic nuclear antigen.

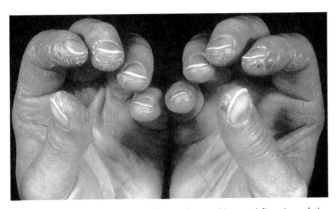

Fig. 44.23 "Machinist's hands." Note the cracking and fissuring of the distal digital skin of the finger pads in this patient with dermatomyositis. *(Courtesy of Dr. Frederick W. Miller. From Klippel JH, Dieppe PA, editors:* Rheumatology, *ed 2, Philadelphia, 1997, Mosby, p 7.13.5)*

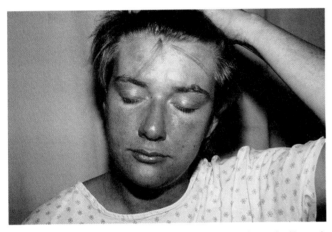

Fig. 44.24 The facial rash of dermatomyositis. Note the malar-like rash of dermatomyositis, which involves the nasolabial area (an area often spared in systemic lupus erythematosus). Patchy involvement of the forehead and chin is also present in this patient. *(From Klippel JH, Dieppe PA, editors:* Rheumatology, *ed 2, Philadelphia, 1997, Mosby, p 7.13.4)*

Differential Diagnosis

As with the other connective tissue diseases, the overlap of symptoms can make the diagnosis of a specific disease difficult on purely clinical grounds. The findings of proximal muscle weakness, characteristic skin rash (in the case of dermatomyositis), positive electromyography, and elevated serum muscle enzymes strongly support the diagnosis of polymyositis or dermatomyositis. If the diagnosis is still in doubt, muscle biopsy may help clarify the situation because in most cases it will be diagnostic.

Treatment

Corticosteroids are the first drug of choice for acute polymyositis.[55,56] A starting dose of 60 mg is usually adequate to control the acute inflammatory response and improve the clinical symptoms. The corticosteroids can be tapered based on both the clinical response to the drug and the decrease in elevated serum CK to normal. The minimum dose of corticosteroid necessary to control symptoms and depress CK should be used to avoid steroid-induced myopathy, which may confuse the clinical management and exacerbate the

patient's disability. A trial of immunosuppressive drugs including methotrexate, cyclosporine, azathioprine, and cyclophosphamide may be considered if corticosteroids fail to control the disease or the side effects associated with the drug preclude its use. It should be remembered that weakness unresponsive to the aforementioned therapies may be secondary to associated malignancies (i.e., paraneoplastic syndrome) and that treatment of the tumor may be required to ameliorate the patient's weakness. The use of physical and occupational therapy to optimize function and to help the patient learn to use assistive devices is indicated early in the course of the disease.

Polymyalgia Rheumatica

Polymyalgia rheumatica (PMR) is a connective tissue disease of unknown etiology that occurs primarily in patients older than 60 years of age.[57] It occurs in females twice as commonly as males and may be associated with temporal arteritis.[58] PMR is characterized by a constellation of musculoskeletal symptoms that includes deep, aching pain of the cervical, pectoral, and pelvic regions; morning stiffness; arthralgias; and stiffness after inactivity.[59] Constitutional symptoms consisting of malaise, fever, anorexia, weight loss, and depression may be so severe as to mimic the cachexia and inanition of malignancy.[60] Unlike polymyositis, there is no significant proximal muscle weakness, but rather the feeling of more generalized weakness and lassitude. In contradistinction to polymyositis, muscle biopsies and electromyography are normal.

Signs and Symptoms

The onset of polymyalgia rheumatica is variable with some patients experiencing a rather acute, fulminant onset of symptoms and with other patients experiencing a more gradual onset of symptoms more like a flu syndrome that "just won't go away." It is often the deep muscle aching and overwhelming feeling of fatigue that will lead the patient to seek medical attention. The astute physician may pick up on the gelling phenomenon (stiffness after periods of inactivity), which is common with PMR, and make the diagnosis on clinical grounds while awaiting confirmatory laboratory results (see next section).

Laboratory and Radiographic Testing

The consistent finding in patients with PMR is the markedly elevated ESR.[59,61] Values are consistently over 100 mm/hour. The C-reactive protein is also consistently elevated in patients with untreated PMR. As mentioned, objective tests for inflammatory muscle disease are negative despite the often dramatic muscle pain that patients report with this disease. In spite of the complaint of arthralgias, plain radiographs of the joints fail to reveal significant effusions or joint destruction that is often seen with RA and some of the other connective tissue diseases.

Differential Diagnosis

PMR is most often confused with other systemic diseases such as hypothyroidism, depression, or malignancy (e.g., multiple myeloma). It is often initially misdiagnosed as polymyositis, but can easily be distinguished from polymyositis by simple electromyography, which is negative in PMR and extremely positive in polymyositis. The relative absence of acutely inflamed joints and lack of evidence of destruction on plain radiographs of the small joints, coupled with the absence of rheumatoid nodules and a negative RF factor, should point the clinician away from the diagnosis of RA.

Treatment

The mainstay of treatment of PMR is the use of prednisone at a starting dose of 15 to 20 mg/day.[61] The symptoms of PMR will usually respond dramatically to the relatively low doses of steroids and the drug should be tapered as the clinical situation dictates. Unlike many of the other connective tissue diseases where the ESR serves as a useful marker as to the effectiveness of treatment, the ESR may remain significantly elevated in otherwise symptom-free patients.[61,62] It should be remembered that temporal arteritis is often seen concomitantly with PMR, and if temporal arteritis is suspected, a much higher dose of prednisone in the range of 60 to 100 mg should be used to decrease the risk of blindness (see later discussion) until temporal artery biopsy can be obtained to confirm the diagnosis.

Temporal Arteritis

Temporal arteritis (TA) is a collagen vascular disease of unknown etiology that occurs almost exclusively in the older patient.[63] It is also referred to in the literature as giant cell and/or cranial arteritis. TA occurs slightly more commonly in females than in males. Etiology and pathogenesis of TA are unknown. Estimated prevalence is about 1 per 1000 in patients more than 50 years of age. TA is often seen concomitantly with polymyalgia rheumatica.[58]

TA is a disease that affects elastin-containing arteries.[64] It has a predilection for the cranial arteries, but the carotid arteries, coronary arteries, aorta, and occasionally peripheral arteries may be involved in the pathogenesis of the disease. The venous system is rarely involved in patients suffering from TA. Arteritis is the main feature of TA with the intima and inner layer of media of the artery being thickened by an inflammatory process (**Fig. 44.25**). The infiltration of lymphocytes

and the presence of giant cells as a result of this inflammation are diagnostic for the disease (**Fig. 44.26**). The arteritis may involve large segments of the affected artery or may manifest as multifocal areas with skin lesions.[65]

Signs and Symptoms

The patient with temporal arteritis is almost always over 50 years of age. As mentioned earlier, there is a slight female preponderance. The patient will often present with the complaint of severe temporal or occipital headache although in some patients the only symptoms are ophthalmologic (e.g., blurred vision, scotomata, amaurosis fugax).[63] Approximately 20% of patients with TA may present with the sudden onset of blindness caused by ischemic optic neuritis, which is often permanent.[66] Scalp tenderness is common. In rare patients, involvement of the peripheral arteries may point the clinician in the direction of atherosclerosis and confuse the diagnosis.

Pain on chewing with jaw claudication is pathognomonic for TA.[67,68] Profound fatigue, lassitude, anorexia, weight loss, and deep muscle aching as seen in polymyalgia rheumatica are common and may initially be attributed to depression or other systemic diseases. Arthritis, fever, and carpal tunnel syndrome occur in many patients with TA. However, it is the finding of a swollen, tortuous, dilated, indurated temporal artery that frequently leads to the diagnosis of TA (**Fig. 44.27**).

Laboratory Testing

As with polymyalgia rheumatica, extreme elevations of the ESR are invariably present in patients suffering from TA with levels frequently greater than 100 mm/hour. A normocytic normochromic anemia is present in the majority of patients with TA. Other serum markers for connective tissue disease (e.g., ANA, RF) are rarely, if ever, present, and no specific blood test is available to diagnose TA.

Although the diagnosis of TA is usually made on clinical grounds, unfortunately sometimes after permanent blindness has occurred, it is the temporal artery biopsy that is needed to confirm the diagnosis. The clinician's tendency to delay or try to

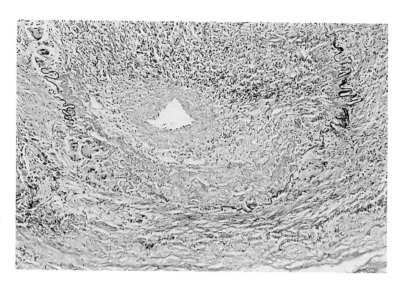

Fig. 44.25 Elastic stain of temporal artery showing disruption of elastic lamina in giant cell arteritis and narrowing of the lumen. *(From Klippel JH, Dieppe PA, editors: Rheumatology, ed 2, Philadelphia, 1997, Mosby, p 7.21.5)*

avoid temporal artery biopsy and the tendency to avoid initiation of treatment with high-dose steroids without a firm diagnosis should be assiduously avoided. If the diagnosis of temporal arteritis is being considered, treatment with at least 60 mg/day of prednisone should be started on an emergent basis while awaiting temporal artery biopsy. Failure to do so could result in permanent blindness. The clinician should remember that the physical examination of the temporal artery may be completely normal even in the presence of florid disease on biopsy, and a normal physical examination should never tempt the clinician to delay treatment. In general, biopsy should be obtained within 3 days of starting high-dose prednisone to avoid false-negative biopsy results.

Differential Diagnosis

The diagnosis of TA is generally straightforward if the clinician thinks about it. The headache associated with TA may be confused with migraine or tension-type headache and the symptom of jaw claudication may be attributed to a toothache given the prevalence of poor dentition in the elderly population. If eye symptoms are the primary presenting complaint, patients may delay treatment, thinking that they "just need new glasses." If there is predominant involvement of the peripheral arteries, the claudication symptoms may be attributed to the much more commonly occurring disease of atherosclerosis. Rarely, this peripheral involvement may lead to the erroneous diagnosis of Takayasu pulseless arteritis.

Treatment

As mentioned, if there is a clinical suspicion that a patient is suffering from temporal arteritis, treatment with high-dose prednisone at a dose of at least 60 mg/day should be instituted on an emergent basis to prevent blindness.[63,68] Temporal artery biopsy should be obtained as soon as possible with a goal of having a tissue diagnosis within 3 days of initiation of therapy to avoid treatment-induced false-negative biopsy results. If the patient continues to experience significant symptomatology on a starting dose of 60 mg of prednisone, hospitalization and administration of 1000 mg doses of methylprednisolone should be implemented immediately. Methotrexate, azathioprine, and dapsone have also been used in those patients who are unable to tolerate treatment with prednisone or experience flaring of ophthalmologic symptoms when high-dose prednisone is tapered.

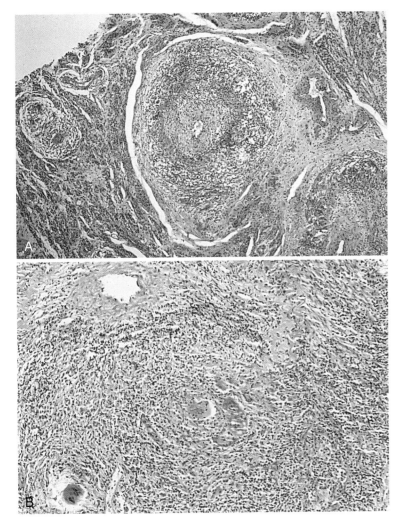

Fig. 44.26 Histology of giant cell arteritis. A, Low-powered view of arterial wall showing infiltration by lymphocytes and plasma cells. B, High-powered view showing giant cells in close relationship to elastic lamina. *(From Klippel JH, Dieppe PA, editors:* Rheumatology, *ed 2, Philadelphia, 1997, Mosby, p 7.21.5)*

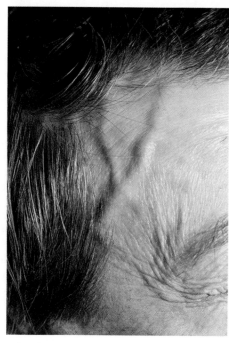

Fig. 44.27 Dilated temporal arteries in a patient with giant cell arteritis. *(From Klippel JH, Dieppe PA, editors:* Rheumatology, *ed 2, Philadelphia, 1997, Mosby, p 7.21.3)*

Conclusion

The connective tissue diseases are a heterogeneous group of disorders that are commonly encountered in clinical practice. The overlap of symptoms associated with these diseases often leads to delayed diagnosis or misdiagnosis. The multisystem nature of these diseases allows the potential for not only much pain and functional disability, but life-threatening sequelae. Early and accurate diagnosis is paramount if these potentially devastating diseases are to be successfully managed.

References

Full references for this chapter can be found on www.expertconsult.com.

Polymyalgia Rheumatica

Brian L. Hazleman

Historical Considerations

The first description of polymyalgia rheumatica (PMR) is believed to have been made in Scotland by Dr. William Bruce in 1884. In 1957, Barber[1] suggested the present name. In 1960, Paulley and Hughes[2] reported on 67 patients, emphasizing the occurrence of "anarthritic rheumatism" in giant cell arteritis (GCA), providing more solid clinical evidence for the relation between PMR and GCA. Histologic support came from the work of Alestig and Barr[3] and Hamrin et al,[4] confirming the coexistence of the two conditions. Both disorders almost always affect patients age 50 years or over. A systemic inflammatory response and a marked response to glucocorticoid therapy are common to both.

Clinical Features

Patients usually locate the source of their pain and stiffness to the muscles. The onset is most common in the shoulder region and neck, with eventual involvement of the shoulder and pelvic girdles and the corresponding proximal muscle groups. Involvement of distal limb muscles is unusual. The symptoms are usually bilateral and symmetric. Stiffness is usually the predominant feature, is particularly severe after rest, and may prevent the patient from getting out of bed in the morning. The muscular pain is often diffuse and movement accentuates the pain; pain at night is common. Muscle strength is usually unimpaired, although the pain makes interpretation of muscle testing difficult. There is tenderness of involved structures, including periarticular structures such as bursae, tendons, and joint capsules, although the muscle tenderness is generally not as severe as that in myositis. In late stages, muscle atrophy may develop, with restriction of shoulder movement. An improvement of shoulder range is rapid with corticosteroid therapy, unlike that seen in frozen shoulder. Occasionally the painful arc sign of subacromial bursitis is present; this is important to recognize because a local injection of corticosteroid will give relief and save the patient from an increase in systemic corticosteroid dosage.

PMR has traditionally been viewed as a condition affecting muscles and many reports have emphasized the rarity of joint involvement.[5] Recent emphasis has been given to a possible association between synovitis and the muscle symptoms in PMR.[6] It has also been suggested that both axial and peripheral synovitis often occur. Inflammatory synovitis and effusions have been noted by several authors; the reported incidence varies from 0% to 100% in different series.[7,8]

Several essential features characterize PMR: (1) the musculoskeletal symptoms are usually bilateral and symmetric, affecting the shoulder and pelvic girdles; (2) stiffness is usually the predominant feature; it is particularly severe after rest and may prevent the patient from getting out of bed in the morning; (3) muscle strength is unimpaired although the pain makes interpretation of muscle testing difficult; and (4) systemic features include low-grade fever, fatigue, weight loss, and an elevated erythrocyte sedimentation rate (ESR).

The variety of symptoms and lack of specificity of signs and symptoms make such studies difficult, and the epidemiology of PMR has been less well defined. It is a common disease, at least in Northern European countries and northern states of the United States. Women are affected twice as often as men. One group, using a questionnaire in 656 patients over a period of 65 years, found a prevalence of arteritis/polymyalgia of 3300 per 100,000.[9] PMR has been found to account for 1.3% to 4.5% of the patients attending rheumatic disease clinics, but clearly these figures are influenced by the type of clinical load.

Familial aggregation of cases of PMR and GCA has been reported by several workers.[10-13] Clustering of cases in time and space suggests that, in addition to a genetic predisposition, environmental factors may be important. One author noted that 9 of 11 cases seen over 6 years in a practice of 3000 lived in one small part of the same village, and of these, 2 lived in the same house, 2 were neighbors, and 2 others were close friends.[14]

Table 45.1 Differential Diagnosis of Polymyalgia Rheumatica

Neoplastic disease
Muscle disease
Joint disease
Polymyositis
Osteoarthritis, particularly cervical spine
Myopathy
Rheumatoid arthritis
Infections (e.g., bacterial endocarditis)
Connective tissue disease
Bone disease, particularly osteomalacia
Multiple myeloma
Hypothyroidism
Fibromyalgia
Parkinsonism
Lymphoma
Shoulder problems (e.g., capsulitis)

Table 45.2 Baseline Clinical Investigations Useful in the Diagnosis of Polymyalgia Rheumatica

Full blood count
Biochemical profile
Protein electrophoresis
Urinary Bence Jones protein
Thyroid function test
Rheumatoid factor
Radiographs of chest and affected joint(s)
Erythrocyte sedimentation rate (ESR) measurement
Acute phase protein (e.g., C-reactive protein) measurement
Muscle enzymes (if indicated)
Specific investigations
Temporal artery biopsy: for suspected giant cell arteritis (GCA), not for polymyalgia rheumatica

Imaging in Polymyalgia Rheumatica

Scintigraphy, magnetic resonance imaging, ultrasonography, and fluorodeoxyglucose–positron emission tomography have all been used to detect synovitis in proximal joints and periarticular studies. Bilateral subacromial bursitis and trochanteric bursitis are the most frequent lesions present in almost all patients who have pain in the shoulder and pelvic girdles. Ultrasound evidence of bilateral shoulder bursitis may support the diagnosis of PMR in patients with a normal ESR. However, bursitis can also be seen in patients with rheumatoid arthritis.[15]

Approximately 12% of PMR patients present with remitting seronegative symmetric synovitis with pitting edema (RS3PE), a condition characterized by extensor tendon synovitis of hands and feet and distal extremity swelling mostly over the dorsum of the hands and wrists.

The presence of erosions in peripheral joints points toward a diagnosis of arthritis rather than PMR.

Differential Diagnosis

Differential diagnosis of PMR is listed in **Table 45.1**.

Testing

Table 45.2 lists baseline clinical investigations that are used to help make the diagnosis of PMR and exclude other conditions. The diagnosis of PMR is initially one of exclusion. There is an extensive differential diagnosis in an older patient with muscle pain, stiffness, and an elevated ESR. No specific diagnostic tests exist, and diagnosis depends on having a high index of suspicion supported by history, examination, and raised inflammatory markers. The differential diagnosis is large because the prodromal phases of several serious conditions can mimic PMR. In practice, nonspecific clinical features and the frequent absence of physical signs make diagnosis difficult.

Despite a typical pattern of musculoskeletal symptoms and the presence in many of significant systemic features, there is often a considerable delay of several months before diagnosis.

Patients and physicians also tend to ascribe the symptoms to degenerative joint disease expected in an older population, or even to psychologic illness. In others, the systemic features of the disease and the laboratory abnormalities can lead to diagnostic confusion and often extensive investigation.

A hidden malignancy can mimic the symptoms of PMR, but these patients do not usually respond to corticosteroids. There is more diffuse pain and absent or minimal morning stiffness. Although there is no evidence to suggest that malignancy is more common in patients with PMR than in other people, deterioration in health or a poor initial response to corticosteroids must always be taken seriously and a search for an occult neoplasm should be undertaken.

The distinction between late-onset rheumatoid arthritis (RA) and PMR can be difficult, especially at onset. Polymyalgic symptoms may be the predominant clinical feature in older-onset RA, whereas a transient symmetric pauciarteritis or polyarteritis is frequently found with PMR. Indeed, many studies of PMR have included patients who eventually were diagnosed with seropositive or seronegative RA.[16] Be aware of the possibility of RA if (1) there are peripheral joint signs such as synovitis, (2) there is failure to respond to an adequate dose of steroids, and (3) the initial dose of steroid cannot be reduced without exacerbating the symptoms.

There has been little evidence to support a concept of primary muscle disease in PMR. Serum aldolase and creatine phosphokinase levels are normal and there is no abnormality on electromyography. Muscle biopsy has shown type II atrophy alone and there is no evidence of inflammatory changes. There have been reports of focal changes in muscle ultrastructure and abnormalities of mitochondrial form and function, similar to those associated with inherited mitochondrial myopathies (MMs).[17,18] These abnormalities are not caused by gene deletions or mutations associated with MMs and persist even after successful treatment. The significance of these changes is unclear. Arteritis in skeletal muscle appears to be uncommon. Liver biopsy can show nonspecific inflammatory changes or focal liver cell necrosis. There are occasional reports of granulomata and hepatic arteritis. Synovial biopsy has shown nonspecific inflammatory changes with lymphocytic infiltration of knees, sternoclavicular joints, and shoulders.

Table 45.3 Diagnostic Criteria for Polymyalgia Rheumatica

1. Age over 65
2. Erythrocyte sedimentation rate (ESR) >40 mm/hr
3. Bilateral upper-arm tenderness
4. Morning stiffness of more than 1 hr
5. Onset of illness less than 2 wk
6. Depression and/or weight loss

Various authors have tried to set out diagnostic criteria for PMR, all of which include a combination of age, clinical features, and an elevated ESR. Bird et al[19] list six diagnostic criteria, three of which are required for the diagnosis of PMR (Table 45.3). The presence of any three of these criteria has a 92% sensitivity and an 80% specificity for the diagnosis of PMR. If an additional criterion of a rapid response to oral steroid therapy is added, the specificity is increased to 99%.[20] Although ESR is usually significantly elevated in PMR, in some patients ESR is normal or only slightly elevated. In these patients and in those presenting with systemic features, other causes of illness should be excluded.

Treatment

Unless there are any contraindications, patients should be started on 15 mg prednisolone per day. This dose should bring rapid relief of symptoms within days. Larger doses are rarely required. If there is no rapid response, reconsider the diagnosis. The dose of prednisolone should be titrated down slowly, according to symptoms rather than the ESR. The dose can often be reduced fairly rapidly to 10 mg per day and then reduced by 1 mg daily every 4 to 6 weeks. Then the dose should be reduced more slowly, aiming to have the patient off steroids by around 2 years, although some patients may require small doses of steroids for longer periods (Table 45.4).

As patients are weaned off steroid therapy, some patients may require a small dose of anti-inflammatory drugs to reduce the muscle pain. Relapses are common and should be diagnosed on clinical grounds. They are usually caused by a too-rapid decrease in dose of corticosteroid and should be treated by increasing the dose again and then decreasing the dose more slowly. Relapses are more common in the first 6 to 12 months of treatment but can occur in the months after stopping corticosteroids. A few patients may need low-dose treatment indefinitely. It should be remembered that steroid therapy has risks and side effects, including the increased risk of osteoporosis. Bone loss is rapid in the early stages of steroid therapy and bone protection therapy should be considered at the time of starting steroid therapy, particularly in those patients 65 years or older or with a history of fragility fracture.

Two randomized control studies[21,22] have investigated the efficacy of methotrexate in polymyalgia rheumatica. The results suggest that methotrexate may be effective in reducing the incidence of flares and the amount of prednisolone needed to maintain a remission when the drug is started at disease onset and given for at least 1 year at a dose of a least 10 mg per week.

A number of studies[23,24] have reported on tumor necrosis factor alpha–blocking agents in PMR; these have proved encouraging in long-standing disease. There is also fairly convincing evidence of a role for interleukin 6 (IL6) in PMR and

Table 45.4 Treatment of Polymyalgia Rheumatica

Initial dose	Prednisolone 10–20 mg daily for 1 month.
Reduce dose	By 2.5 mg every 2–4 weeks until dose is 10 mg, then by 1 mg every 4–6 weeks (or until symptoms return).
Maintenance dose	About 5 mg by 6 months after start of treatment and then further reductions by 1 mg until symptoms return. Most patients require treatment for 3–4 years, but withdrawal after 2 years is worth attempting.
Special points	In patients who cannot reduce prednisolone dosage because of recurring symptoms or who develop serious steroid-related side effects, azathioprine and methotrexate have been shown to have a modest steroid-sparing effect.
Main side effects	Weight gain, skin atrophy, edema, increased intraocular pressure, cataracts, gastrointestinal disturbances, diabetes, osteoporosis.
Risk of side effects	Increased risk with high initial doses (>30 mg) of prednisolone, maintenance doses of 10 mg, and high cumulative doses. Maintenance doses of 5 mg are relatively safe.

therefore IL6 blockade with tocilizumab (a humanized anti–IL6 receptor monoclonal antibody) appears to be a promising new drug for treatment.

Conclusion

The cardinal symptoms of PMR—prolonged morning stiffness in the shoulder and pelvic girdles with an elevated ESR—are generally straightforward. However, PMR is essentially a diagnosis of exclusion. Because the differential diagnosis is extensive, it is important to exclude more sinister conditions at the outset with screening blood investigations. PMR is exceedingly rare in those younger than 50 years of age and occasionally the ESR is misleading, being normal or only slightly raised.

Of particular importance is the link between PMR and GCA. Many believe the two represent opposite ends of the spectrum of the same disease. In any patient who presents with PMR, it is mandatory to ask about headache, scalp tenderness, and jaw claudication because the catastrophic result of untreated GCA is irreversible blindness. In such cases, higher doses of steroids are required with possible referral for temporal artery biopsy.

Diagnosis of PMR can be difficult to make; however, when diagnosed correctly, treatment is highly effective. In prednisolone-resistant cases, response to steroid-sparing agents has been disappointing. Patient education is paramount, and patients should be warned that treatment is typically necessary for at least 2 years, with some patients requiring long-term maintenance therapy.

References

Full references for this chapter can be found on www.expertconsult.com.

Section IV

Regional Pain Syndromes

Part A

Pain in the Head

IV

Chapter 46

Migraine Headache

Seymour Diamond and George J. Urban

Historical Overview

Migraine has been identified, in some form, since ancient times. One of the first (and still questionable) citations about migraine is believed to be at least 6000 years old.[1] More detailed descriptions of headaches, including migraine, are traced to the time of Hippocrates, who first identified headaches as a distinct disorder.[1] Also, Hippocrates first described a few of the well-known clinical features of migraine such as unilateral location of the pain, associated vomiting, and a possible visual aura that appeared as a shining light in one of the eyes followed by severe headache.

More citations about the clinical details have been traced to the first century AD (Greco-Roman period). Medical historians believe that the first accurate description of migraine was provided by Aretaeus of Cappadocia, a Greek physician who wrote a book describing different neurologic disorders including epilepsy, headaches, and hysteria.[2,3] Aretaeus also gained fame by proposing the very first classification of headache disorders, which has affected all future efforts at nomenclature. Aretaeus divided all headache types into three major categories: cephalalgia, cephalea, and heterocrania. This particular system provided the basis for the First International Classification of Headache Disorders.[4] Because Aretaeus was a migraine sufferer himself, he had a unique opportunity to study and describe his own headache, enabling him to detail his visual aura as well as a few associated symptoms, such as photophobia and phonophobia.

Later, in the second century AD, another Greek physician—Galen of Pergamon—added to the headache literature with more clinical and even pathophysiologic information.[5] He subscribed to a connection between the human brain and abdomen because nausea and vomiting were commonly associated with the headache attack. He thus explained the pathogenesis of migraine: yellow bile irritates brain meninges thus causing pain. He attributed the unilateral location of the headache by using information regarding anatomic structures of the human brain and head. He wrote that falx cerebri separates two halves of the brain and protects the unaffected side (side without headache pain) from being affected by the irritating yellow bile. Galen was the first to describe the throbbing pattern of the pain during an acute migraine. He also provided some pathophysiologic explanations of this phenomenon, asserting that the pain originates in blood vessels. Thus he established some basis for the future vascular theories of migraine pathogenesis.

During the sixteenth century, the headache known as *heterocrania* (named by Aretaeus of Cappadocia) or *hemicrania* (named by Galen of Pergamon) was labeled migraine, a term derived form Galen's *hemicrania,* which was first changed to the Latin *hemicranium.* The term was then transformed into *emigranea, migranea, megrim,* and finally *migraine.*[1] In the second half of the seventeenth century, an English physician, Thomas Willis, wrote a textbook of neurophysiology in which he devoted two chapters to a discussion of different headache problems.[6] He expanded the vascular theory first proposed by Galen and identified two actions of the blood vessels during a migraine attack—vasoconstriction and vasodilation. Thomas Willis was not only a remarkable scientist but also a very thorough physician. He attempted to treat migraine using various remedies. Willis was the first to discover the efficacy of *potus cophey*—coffee.

In the eighteenth century, it was discovered that the brain and nervous system, in addition to the blood vessels, are involved in migraine pathogenesis in which weather changes, peculiarities of diet, and stress can play a role as migraine triggers.[7] In the mid–nineteenth century E. Sieveking attempted to find a relation between epilepsy and migraine, because about 60% of his patients with epilepsy were also diagnosed with migraine.[8] He also observed their common physiologic feature (which is still actively discussed in our day)—paroxysmal activity of both epilepsy and migraine.[8,9] Later, the same correlation was applied to status migraine analogous to status epilepticus.[10] These similarities between migraine and epilepsy created the basis of a new migraine treatment with the use of anticonvulsants.[11]

The twentieth century saw multiple achievements in determining the pathophysiology of migraine, as well as the beginning of a new era of specific, highly effective, antimigraine medications. In 1916 pure ergotamine was introduced and in 1928 it was compared to placebo.[11] The classic headache treatise, *Headache and Other Head Pain,* was written by Harold G. Wolff in 1948.[12] Dr. Wolff's book included all clinical and pathophysiologic data available at that time.

Pathogenesis

Further migraine studies identified the specific role serotonin plays in migraine pathogenesis, thus leading to the introduction of a totally new class of preventive medications—serotonin antagonists and abortive agents—serotonin agonists.[11] Also, toward the end of the twentieth century, the first international classification and diagnostic criteria for headache disorders, cranial neuralgias, and facial pain were published.[4]

Although our understanding of migraine has expanded, we are opening new horizons in diagnostic and treatment options—helping us recognize the need for new, more accurate classifications and diagnostic criteria. These requirements were addressed in the second edition of the International Classification of Headache Disorders as proposed by the International Headache Society in September 2003.[13] The study of migraine is still in process and continues to afford us important information that can lead to a better understanding of this disorder and provide us with opportunities in diagnosis and treatment.

Recently, increasing attention has been devoted to the theory of central sensitization. *Central sensitization* is a collective term that reflects the tendency to decreased thresholds to non-painful stimuli, clinically presented as *hyperalgesia* (decreased pain threshold) or *cutaneous allodynia* (pain response to a nonpainful stimuli). Central sensitization is primarily attributed to activation (sensitization) of peripheral C fibers in the trigeminal system. These fibers could be activated by a variety of factors (mechanical, chemical, or thermal). Once activated, C fibers start releasing multiple transmitters (calcitonin gene-related peptide [CGRP], substance P, glutamate) from their central terminals in the nucleus caudalis of the trigeminal system and from their peripheral terminals that produce the sterile neurogenic inflammation described earlier. These events will further activate the C fibers by an increased level of histamine (5-HT) and prostaglandin E_2 elevated synthesis, which is observed in the area of the neurogenic inflammation. Plasma extravasation can be blocked by ergot alkaloids, aspirin, indomethacin, and triptans. The release of C-fiber transmitters could be decreased by activation of m-opiate and 5-HT$_{1D}$ receptors (by using their agonists) or increased by activation of N-methyl-D-aspartate (NMDA) receptors. The release of inflammatory peptides (prostaglandin E_2 and others) could be diminished by using a nonsteroidal anti-inflammatory drug (NSAID). Another important feature of central sensitization is the increase of intracellular calcium in postsynaptic neurons that will activate protein kinase C and nitric oxide synthase (NOS). Activated protein kinase C will phosphorylate membrane-bound proteins changing the activity (activating) NMDA receptors so that these receptors could respond to glutamate—not only during depolarization but also at resting membrane potentials. NOS will cause synthesis of nitric oxide (NO) (vasodilator).

In central modulation of trigeminal pain, functional brain imaging with positron emission tomography (PET) has demonstrated activation of the contralateral dorsal midbrain, including the ventrolateral periaqueductal gray matter and, in the dorsal pons, near the locus ceruleus. This brainstem dysfunction may disinhibit the brain and lower the threshold for developing migraine. In contrast, cortical spreading depression (CSD) may activate the trigeminal system.

Two neurologic events play a major role in the development of migraine: cortical spreading depression and cortical hyperexcitability. CSD is triggered when enhanced cortical activity coincides with other triggering factors. CSD induces the release of a variety of vasoactive and inflammatory substances that could activate and/or sensitize the meningeal trigeminal afferents.

The pain process in migraine is likely to be a combination of activation of the nociceptive pain-producing intracranial structures, and indirectly by facilitation or lack of inhibition of pain signals.

Thus all these steps of reactions will cause the increased excitability of neurons in the trigeminal nuclei or central sensitization. Sensitization of the C fibers occurs in the periphery (meningeal C fibers); peripheral sensitization and sensitization of the neurons of trigeminal nuclei occur in central sensitization. From that point of view, peripheral sensitization explains the intracranial hypersensitivity (aggravation of pain by bending over, coughing, walking, and so on), whereas central sensitization demonstrates the extracranial hypersensitivity (cutaneous allodynia). Prevalence of cutaneous allodynia (CA) in headache sufferers appears to be more common and more severe in patients with migraine and transformed migraine than with other primary headache disorders. Among migraineurs, CA is associated with the female gender, increased headache frequency and body mass index, disability, and depression.[14]

The presence or absence of cutaneous allodynia may be crucial in determining the outcome of triptan treatment.[15]

Patent Foramen Ovale

Patent foramen ovale (PFO) is relatively common in the general population, ranging from 25% to 35% based on autopsy studies.[16] PFO has been associated with number of clinical syndromes including cryptogenic stroke, decompression illness in scuba divers, and migraine. Transesophageal echocardiogram (TEE) has been the preferred diagnostic test. Injection of agitated saline to visualize microbubbles passing from the right to left atrium can augment the findings of the TEE. Transcranial Doppler (TCD) has also been used to detect PFOs. Theoretically, right-to-left shunt may allow different substances, such as platelet factors, atrial natriuretic peptide and other vasoactive amines, and microemboli, to bypass the lungs and reach the brain. The presence of PFO in migraine patients has been documented, especially in patients diagnosed with migraine with aura, reaching a 41% to 48% occurrence.[17,18]

In the NOMAS study of 1101 stroke-free subjects, 13% self-reported migraine with aura.[19] However, no statistical difference was demonstrated between prevalence of PFO in self-reported migraine and the control group (about 15%). PFO was slightly more prevalent in migraine with aura (19%) than in migraine without aura (11%).

Table 46.1 Classification of Migraine

1.1. Migraine without aura

1.2. Migraine with aura
   1.2.1. Typical aura with migraine headache
   1.2.2. Typical aura with nonmigraine headache
   1.2.3. Typical aura without headache
   1.2.4. Familial hemiplegic migraine
   1.2.5. Sporadic hemiplegic migraine
   1.2.6. Basilar-type migraine

1.3. Retinal migraine

1.4. Complications of migraine
   1.4.1. Chronic migraine
   1.4.2. Status migrainosus
   1.4.3. Persistent aura without infarction
   1.4.4. Migrainosus infarction
   1.4.5. Migraine-triggered seizure

1.5. Probable migraine
   1.5.1. Probable migraine without aura
   1.5.2. Probable migraine with aura
   1.5.3. Probable chronic migraine

Table 46.2 Diagnostic Criteria of Migraine Without Aura

At least five headache attacks fulfilling criteria B–D:

A. Headache attack lasting 4–72 hours (untreated or unsuccessfully treated)

B. Headache has at least two of the following characteristics:
   1. Unilateral location of the pain (involves one half of the head)
   2. Throbbing or pulsating quality of the pain
   3. Moderate or severe pain intensity
   4. Aggravation by or causing avoidance of routine physical activity

C. During headache at least one of the following:
   1. Nausea and/or vomiting
   2. Phonophobia and photophobia

D. Not attributed to another disorder

Table 46.3 Most Common Premonitory Symptoms

Fatigue	Irritability
Cognitive change	Elation
Poor concentration	Physical hyperactivity
Difficulty in finding words	Yawning
Muscle pain/stiffness	Photophobia/phonophobia
Food craving	Increased bowel/bladder activity

The closure of septal defect in patients with migraine and paradoxic cerebral embolism resulted in complete resolution of migraine symptoms in 56% and significant reduction in migraine frequency in 14% of patients.[20]

However, the evidence of any benefit on migraine headache following PFO closure is not convincing. The first double-blind randomized trial, MIST I, did not achieve the primary efficacy end point of cessation of migraine attacks at 3 and 6 months after the procedure.[21]

Therefore surgical closure of PFO to reduce frequency of migraine headaches is not recommended.

Clinical Presentation

Migraine is one of the most common primary headache disorders. According to epidemiologic studies, migraine occurs in approximately 18% of females and 5% of males.[22] Migraine occurrence involves the most professionally active age-group in the population with the highest prevalence between ages 25 and 55, with a female-to-male ratio of 3:1.[23] The World Health Organization ranked migraine nineteenth among all diseases that may cause disability.[13]

For diagnostic purposes, we use classification and diagnostic criteria proposed by the International Headache Society in 2003 (**Table 46.1**).[13] Criteria for migraine diagnosis are presented in **Table 46.2**.[13] Typically, patients with migraine will fulfill these criteria although there are some exceptions. First, the duration of an acute migraine attack may be briefer than 4 hours. We have observed in childhood migraine that an attack may last 1 or 2 hours.[24] In many cases of childhood migraine, the symptoms vary from the typical presentation because the headache may be located bilaterally or may involve the entire head.[25] Also, in adults with migraine, the attack may start as a typical unilateral headache but when it reaches its peak, the pain may radiate to the opposite side of the head thus becoming a generalized headache.

A majority of patients with migraine may experience vague or more pronounced warning symptoms. Blau[26] suggested that these symptoms were not simply warnings of migraine but were, in fact, an integral part of the migraine process. He termed this phase of migraine the *prodrome*. Prodromal or premonitory symptoms (**Table 46.3**) are noted in approximately 70% of migraine attacks and may occur as early as 24 to 48 hours before the headache. The neurotransmitters, dopamine and serotonin, are possibly involved in the development of premonitory symptoms.

The pathophysiologic substrate of migraine consists of cerebral blood vessels, venous sinuses, trigeminal nerve, and upper cervical dorsal roots. The acute attack involves activation of the pain-producing structures; release of CGRP, substance P (SP), and NO; and a sterile neurogenic inflammation. The trigeminocervical complex is stimulated by different triggers (neuronal and chemical: prostaglandins, serotonin, histamine) through which the series of reactions will cause the increase of concentrations of such vasoactive peptide as SP and CGRP.[27] Also, concentration of NO (another potent vasodilator) will be elevated.[28] These changes will result in vasodilatation followed by exudation of plasma in to the surrounding tissue, a phenomenon described as a sterile neurogenic inflammation.[29] All these changes will produce a headache.

Clinical Example of Patient with Migraine

A female patient 24 years of age complains of severe, throbbing headache located more frequently (but not always) in the area of the left temple and forehead. The duration of the headache varies but usually lasts 24 hours. The headache is always associated with nausea, occasionally vomiting, and photophobia and phonophobia to the extent that the patient prefers to remain in a dark quiet room and, if possible, to sleep rather than do any physical activity that would exacerbate the headache. The patient's medical history and physical and neurologic examinations are normal.

The two major subgroups of migraine, migraine with aura and migraine without aura, are distinguished by a set of neurologic symptoms—the aura—which is typically visual in nature and precedes the headache by 30 to 60 minutes. Characteristically, the aura is focal, limited in time, and totally and completely reversible. The aura or prodrome manifests the initial vasoconstriction.[30] These neurologic symptoms have a gradual onset, developing over 5 to 20 minutes, and usually continue for less than 60 minutes. In order of frequency, the aura symptoms include scotoma (blind spots); teichopsia or fortification spectra; sensory symptoms (positive—pins and needles; negative—numbness); dysphasia; and visual changes. Approximately 99% of patients with migraine with aura describe visual symptoms.[31] The visual aura itself may consist of photopsia (flashing light) or scotoma (partial loss of sight). One of the most characteristic features of visual auras is the fortification spectrum (the arc of zigzag scintillating lights).[25] About 80% of patients with visual auras indicate that the aura usually precedes the headache itself.[32] Visual aura is rarely observed during or after the headache phase.[33]

The aura phenomenon has been attributed to the spreading depression of Leão, which represents the decrease of cerebral blood flow in cortex that starts posteriorly and spreads anteriorly without crossing the ischemic threshold.[33,34] A few hours later, areas that were exposed to the mentioned oligemia will become hyperemic.

Clinical Example of Patient with Migraine with Aura

The clinical presentation of a patient with headache pain itself might be the same as in the previous example. However, the patient will also mention that occasionally, or possibly with each acute migraine headache, an aura will occur. Approximately 40 to 60 minutes before the headache onset, the patient may start seeing flashing lights or zigzag lines or experience tunnel vision. These visual changes will last for a few minutes (10 to 40 minutes) and then will spontaneously disappear after the severe unilateral, throbbing headache has started.

In some cases, the typical aura may be followed by a headache that does not fulfill diagnostic criteria for migraine. In this case, we may suppose that the patient has typical aura with nonmigraine headache. In this case, other organic causes should be considered that may mimic typical aura (e.g., transient ischemic attack, multiple sclerosis).

In some older patients with a history of migraine with typical aura, the headache alters and the patient may finally lose the migraine headache although the aura persists. In those cases, patients will experience a typical aura that fulfills all the previously cited criteria but will not suffer a headache during the aura or within the 60 minutes following those symptoms. We can describe this situation as typical aura without headache.[35,36]

Other types of migraine with aura may occur, although rarely. Hemiplegic migraine has motor weakness as part of the aura. The diagnostic criteria for hemiplegic aura are provided in **Table 46.4**.[13] Two types of hemiplegic aura have been identified. The first, familial hemiplegic migraine (FHM),[37] has a genetic substrate that has been identified. Patients with FHM type 1 have mutations in the CACNA1A gene on chromosome 19,[13,38] and patients with FHM type 2 have mutations in the

Table 46.4 Diagnostic Criteria of Hemiplegic Migraine

I. At least two attacks fulfilling criteria B and C

  A. Aura consisting of fully reversible motor weakness and at least one of the following:
    1. Fully reversible visual symptoms (visual aura)
    2. Fully reversible sensory symptoms (sensory aura)
    3. Fully reversible dysphasic speech disturbance

  B. At least two of the following:
    1. At least one aura symptom develops gradually over ≥5 minutes and/or different aura symptoms occur in succession over ≥5 minutes
    2. Each aura symptom lasts more than 5 minutes but less than 24 hours

  C. Headache fulfilling criteria B–D for migraine without aura (see Table 46.2) begins during the aura or follows onset of aura within 60 minutes

II. Not attributed to another disorder

ATP1A2 gene on chromosome 1. In addition to the diagnostic criteria listed in **Table 46.4**), we should note that patients with FHM should have at least one first- or second-degree relative with headache attacks that fulfill criteria A through D for hemiplegic migraine (see Table 46.4).[13,39] Also, patients with FHM1 may experience cerebellar symptoms (nystagmus and progressive ataxia) and are frequently diagnosed with chronic progressive cerebellar ataxia—the pathogenesis of which is also linked to the nineteenth chromosome.[40]

The other type of hemiplegic migraine is sporadic, and has the same occurrence and diagnostic criteria but without the genetic substrate described earlier. The patient with the sporadic form of hemiplegic migraine would not necessarily have a first- or second-degree relative with headache attacks fulfilling criteria A through D for hemiplegic migraine (see Table 46.4).[13,41,42] The diagnosis of hemiplegic migraine should be established only after a thorough physical and neurologic examination and with the use of methods of neurovisualization (MRI, MRA).[43]

Clinical Example of Patient with Hemiplegic Migraine

A 36-year-old female patient complains about severe, throbbing unilateral headache, which is always associated with nausea, vomiting, photophobia, and phonophobia, and which has lasted up to 3 days. Occasionally, the patient has also experienced episodes of numbness and pronounced muscle weakness of the right side of the face and right arm and leg. She cannot drive a car or feed herself with her right hand. Her husband advises that during these episodes, her face is asymmetric for up to 1 day. She has continued to experience some numbness and weakness (but not as severe) for another 1 or 2 days. Her medical history, physical and neurologic examinations, and magnetic resonance imaging (MRI) and magnetic resonance angiography (MRA) are negative.

Another form of migraine with neurologic symptoms is basilar artery migraine, which is rare. The nucleus of its clinical presentation are symptoms that originate from the brainstem or both hemispheres (posterior part of the brain that is supplied by the vertebrobasilar artery system). One of the characteristic features of basilar artery migraine is bilateral

Table 46.5 Diagnostic Criteria of Basilar-Type Migraine

At least two attacks fulfilling criteria B–D

A. Aura consists of at least two of the following fully reversible symptoms but no motor weakness:
 1. Dysarthria
 2. Vertigo
 3. Tinnitus
 4. Hypacusia
 5. Diplopia
 6. Visual symptoms simultaneously in both nasal and temporal fields of both eyes
 7. Ataxia
 8. Decreased level of consciousness
 9. Simultaneously bilateral paresthesias

B. At least one of the following:
 1. At least one aura symptom develops gradually over ≥5 minutes and/or different aura symptoms occur in succession over ≥5 minutes
 2. Each aura symptom lasts more then 5 minutes but less than 24 hours

C. Headache fulfilling criteria B–D for migraine without aura (see Table 46.2) begins during the aura or follows onset of aura within 60 minutes

D. Not attributed to another disorder

Table 46.6 Diagnostic Criteria of Retinal Migraine

At least two attacks fulfilling criteria B and C

A. Fully reversible monocular positive and/or negative visual phenomena (scintillations, scotoma, or blindness) confirmed by examination during an attack or (after proper instructions) by the patient's drawing of a monocular field defect during an attack

B. Headache fulfilling criteria B–D for migraine without aura (see Table 46.2) begins during the visual symptoms or follows them within 60 minutes

C. Normal ophthalmologic examination between attacks

D. Not attributed to another disorder

Table 46.7 Diagnostic Criteria of Chronic Migraine

A. Headache fulfilling criteria C and D for migraine without aura (see Table 46.2) on more than 15 days a month for more than 3 months

B. Not attributed to another disorder

Table 46.8 Diagnostic Criteria for Status Migrainosus

A. The present attack in a patient with migraine without aura is typical of previous attack except for its duration

B. Headache has both of the following features:
 1. Unremitting for more than 72 hours
 2. Severe intensity

C. Not attributed to another disorder

neurologic presentation of the aura signs. The diagnostic criteria are presented in **Table 46.5**.[13] During the acute basilar artery migraine attack, the headache itself may not manifest as bilateral pain or as a headache located in the occipital region. Basilar artery migraine is difficult to differentiate from migraine with typical sensory aura (paresthesias) in which the paresthesias are also a part of an aura. In the last case, the sensory phenomenon should be bilateral.[40]

Clinical Example of Patient with Basilar-Type Migraine

A 17-year-old male patient complains of severe, throbbing bilateral headache located in the occipital area, associated with severe nausea and vomiting and paresthesias of both legs and arms, which usually begin in the periphery and gradually radiate to the extremities. During these episodes, the patient also experiences dizziness and vertigo. The duration of these symptoms ranges between 20 and 40 minutes, and symptoms usually occur simultaneously with the headache. The history, physical, and neurologic examinations, as well as MRI and MRA, are negative.

Retinal migraine is associated with monocular visual loss, which is usually preceded by scintillating scotoma. The migraine episode may continue for several hours and occasionally without close association with a headache. This type of migraine is usually a diagnosis of exclusion with other causes being ruled out.[44] The diagnostic criteria are presented in **Table 46.6**.[13]

Some patients may experience more frequent migraine episodes (with or without aura). If the migraine frequency is more than 15 days a month, and the patient experiences such frequency for more than 3 months, we may consider chronic migraine. Diagnostic criteria are presented in **Table 46.7**.[13] Also, it is important that the diagnosis should be established in the absence of medication overuse.[13,45-47] The vast majority of patients with chronic migraine will report a history of episodic migraine in the past.[47,48]

Another complication of migraine is status migrainosus. This condition is characterized by incapacitating severe migraine lasting more than 72 hours. During this episode, patients may experience continuous nausea and/or frequent copious vomiting, which may cause severe dehydration and require urgent hospitalization. During status migrainosus, the standard migraine abortive medications are not effective and the patient may need intravenous drug administration to resolve the headache status (another reason for hospital admission). The diagnostic criteria for status migrainosus are presented in **Table 46.8**.[13]

Persistent aura without infarction should be considered when the migraine aura persists longer than 1 week without any radiographic evidence of infarction.[13] In those cases with prolonged aura associated with ischemic changes located in the areas consistent with aura presentation (considering that these changes had been proved by methods of neuroimaging), the diagnosis of migrainosus infarction can be established.[13]

Migraine-triggered seizure is a rare situation in which migraine aura is followed within 1 hour by a seizure.[13] In those cases when migraine-like headache does not fulfill at least one of the required diagnostic criteria and all other causes of the headache are ruled out, the diagnosis of probable migraine should be made.[13]

It is essential that the patient undergo a thorough examination. For many patients, completing the headache history is a difficult task, especially when little attention has been paid to such features as headache frequency, duration, location, and quality of the pain. Also, the associated symptoms should be evaluated and the physician should determine the type of aura the patient is experiencing because these two factors will affect treatment selections. We should also obtain information regarding previous treatment history and prior pitfalls in therapy. The history is probably the most important factor in establishing the diagnosis. To obtain more accurate information, we ask each of our patients to maintain a daily calendar to record any headache episodes, possible triggers, and medications used. The calendar details the following information: date of headache; time of onset and ending; severity (using a 10-point visual analog scale in which 10 is the most severe); triggers (psychic, physical, emotional); and food and drink excesses. Patients should also indicate their treatment (which medications were taken and the dosage) as well as relief of headache (again using a 10-point visual analog scale in which 0 equals complete relief).[49] This calendar is easy to maintain and does not require a great deal of time to complete. It is also important to use the calendar for treatment evaluation purposes (determining the dynamics of the headache pattern, medication intake, possible triggers, and so on).

In addition to a thorough physical and neurologic examination, neuroimaging may be necessary. For all our primary headache patients, we recommend an MRI of the brain, with and without contrast, if they have never undergone this test or if the last MRI was obtained more than 6 months earlier. Also, if the headache pattern had changed dramatically over the past few months, we also recommend repeating the study. An MRI and MRA of the head and neck should be undertaken in those patients complaining of severe, throbbing headaches associated with aura (especially hemiplegic, basilar, or retinal), or if the headache is exacerbated during or immediately after physical exercise, coughing, sneezing, or bending. The MRI and MRA are used to rule out other possible causes of the headache (brain tumor, aneurysm, intracranial hypertension, and so on). In acute subarachnoid hemorrhage, head trauma, or bone abnormalities, CT scanning should be ordered.[50] Lumbar puncture (LP) should be performed if a patient complains of the worst headache ever or the first ever but very severe headache, or if the headache is associated with fever or other signs of infection.[50] Also, we should be aware of a common complication of LP—low cerebral spinal fluid (CSF) pressure or post-LP headache. This adverse effect from an LP may be reduced by using a smaller needle.[51]

Treatment

Using the information we have obtained during the history and examinations and having established the diagnosis, we may select our treatment options. The goal of treatment is to reduce the patient's disability and improve quality of life. For that purpose, we use abortive, symptomatic, and preventive methods of treatment. At our clinic, we do not limit our treatment options to pharmacologic methods but also engage nonpharmacologic methods of treatment (biofeedback, relaxation techniques, physical therapy, and so on). It is important to educate patients regarding diagnosis and treatment, explaining possible side effects and benefits. We should also inform the patient that we are starting a treatment process that requires the patient's compliance, and if needed, will make corrections and changes in the treatment in the future.

We recommend the following basic rules:

1. Maintain regular sleep pattern (if possible, patients should awaken at the same time every day because oversleeping may trigger a migraine attack).
2. Maintain regular meal pattern (missing meals or fasting may trigger headache).
3. All patients should follow a low-tyramine and low-caffeine diet.[30]
4. Coping strategies (may help to handle stress more efficiently, thus decreasing its ability to trigger migraine).[30,47]

We have also established certain rules regarding abortive therapy:

1. Abortive agents should be taken as soon as possible at the beginning of a migraine attack.
2. Abortive agents should not be taken on a daily basis.

The most potent abortive agents are the triptans (5-HT agonists). Seven triptans are now available: sumatriptan, zolmitriptan, naratriptan, rizatriptan, almotriptan, frovatriptan, and eletriptan. These agents may be prescribed in a variety of administrative routes: oral tablets, nasal sprays, orally disintegrating tablets, and subcutaneous injections. The 5-HT agonists have variable affinity to the different $5\text{-}HT_1$ receptors and inhibit release of 5-HT, norepinephrine, acetylcholine, and substance P. Thus the triptans reduce the sterile neurogenic inflammation, described previously, and cause potent vasoconstriction in the cranial blood vessels.[52]

Because the triptans are potent vasoconstrictors, these medications should never be administered intravenously. The triptans should not be prescribed to patients with a history of ischemic heart disease, hypertension, myocardial infarction, or Prinzmetal angina.[53] Triptans should also be avoided in patients with hemiplegic and basilar-type migraine, and should never be used concomitantly with ergotamine-containing medications and monoamine oxidase inhibitors (MAOIs). The triptans differ in the time of action onset, as well as in the duration of action—factors to be considered when deciding which triptan should be prescribed. If the patient experiences difficulties in identifying an impending migraine (e.g., patient with chronic daily headache) or the headache attack develops within a very brief period of time (a few minutes), we should consider triptans with a fast onset of action (rizatriptan[54]—for oral triptans or parenteral sumatriptan). In those patients experiencing prolonged migraine (longer than 24 hours), we recommend the use of triptans with a longer half-life, such as frovatriptan.

Generally, patients may take another triptan tablet 1 to 2 hours after the first dose if needed. However, triptan intake should be limited to only 2 days a week. We also recommend that a 4-day hiatus be maintained between days of use. The most common side effects are a tingling sensation, chest pain, nausea and vomiting, and tightness of the throat.

Another highly effective group of antimigraine medications are the ergotamine-containing medications, ergotamine and dihydroergotamine (DHE). Because these agents are also potent vasoconstrictors, they should be avoided in patients with unstable hypertension, ischemic heart disease, history of myocardial infarction, impaired renal and hepatic function, infection, and pregnancy. DHE is available as a nasal spray and in parenteral preparation for subcutaneous, intramuscular, or intravenous administration. We also use DHE intravenously for treating patients with status migrainosus and other intractable forms of headaches. In this case, DHE 0.5 to 1.0 mg is administered intravenously over 2 to 3 minutes in combination with metoclopramide (10 mg) every 8 hours for 3 days. The most common side effects are nausea, vomiting, and chest symptoms in the form of tightness, pressure, or pain.[55]

NSAIDs are also effective in migraine management because of their ability to inhibit inflammation. These agents are particularly effective in patients with mild-to-moderately severe migraine episodes. The most common side effects are nausea, abdominal distress, diarrhea, and dyspepsia. Recently, medications from the family of cyclooxygenase-2 (COX2) inhibitors (celecoxib) are being widely used because of their decreased effect on the gastrointestinal system. Phenothiazines (chlorpromazine, prochlorperazine) and new atypical antipsychotic agents (haloperidol, risperidol, ziprasidone) may also be beneficial owing to their dopaminergic and adrenergic effects, as well as their sedative and antinausea actions.[56]

For those patients with contraindications to the aforementioned medications or for those in whom these medications were not effective, we may consider opioid analgesics. In this case, patients should be advised about all possible side effects and complications of these agents, as well as possible addiction problems and rebound phenomenon. We should avoid prescribing opioid analgesics for patients with chronic migraine because of the high risk of abuse.

For those patients who have been diagnosed with chronic migraine or who experience prolonged incapacitating migraines, we recommend prophylactic therapy. Preventive medications may be used singly or in combination with other prophylactic agents.

We recommend starting prophylactic treatment with beta blockers. The drug of choice from this group is the nonselective beta blocker propranolol. Propranolol efficacy in migraine is attributed to its preventive effect resulting from its ability to block beta-adrenergic receptors in the blood vessels, thus preventing their dilation and also possibly reducing platelet aggregation. Propranolol is effective in doses of 80 to 240 mg daily. The long-acting form of the drug enhances patient compliance with a once-daily dosage. The most common side effects are low blood pressure, decreased heart rate, fatigue, and depression.[57] These medications should be avoided in patients with asthma, chronic obstructive lung disease, congestive heart failure, or atrioventricular conduction disturbances. After long-term treatment, a slow tapering is recommended.[30] Other beta blockers used in migraine prevention are timolol, nadolol, and metoprolol. For those patients with asthma, the use of a cardioselective beta blocker such as metoprolol is indicated.

The calcium channel blockers, such as verapamil, have been used effectively in migraine prevention. These medications block calcium influx, which is essential for vasoconstriction, platelet aggregation, and the release of serotonin from the platelets. Verapamil is effective in doses of 120 to 360 mg daily. The most common side effects are constipation, flushing, low blood pressure, and nausea.[58] Gradual reduction of the dosage is also recommended. The potential efficacy of verapamil in migraine prevention is not evidence based. Other calcium channel antagonists (CCAs) such as nimodipine and nifedipine have not demonstrated efficacy in migraine prevention.

The antidepressants are among the most potent preventive agents for chronic migraine and other forms of chronic daily headaches. These agents could be considered in patients with chronic migraine and concomitant depression. The tricyclic antidepressants (TCAs) are especially effective because of their ability to block serotonin reabsorption, and their anticholinergic and antihistaminic activity. All antidepressants require at least 2 to 3 weeks to elicit their effect, and the headache sufferer should be instructed to be patient and not abruptly terminate treatment. For those headache patients who also experience sleeping difficulties, the TCA of choice is amitriptyline (starting at 10 or 25 mg at bedtime slowly, increasing every 5 to 7 days, up to 100 mg if needed).[59] Other sedating TCAs include nortriptyline (starting from 10 or 25 mg at bedtime, increasing every 5 to 7 days up to 100 mg if needed) or doxepin (starting at 25 mg at bedtime slowly, increasing every 5 to 7 days up to 150 mg if needed). For patients who do not require a sedating TCA, protriptyline is indicated. In patients with prolonged chronic migraine and/or prominent psychologic problems (depression, anxiety), a combination of these medications should be used.[30,53] The most common side effects are constipation, blurred vision, dry mouth, decreased libido, orthostatic hypotension, and weight gain. These medications should be avoided in patients with low-angle glaucoma or prostatic hypertrophy. To increase the efficacy of prophylactic treatment, antidepressants may be used in combination with beta blockers or calcium channel blockers.

Another type of antidepressant used in patients with chronic migraine are the MAOIs (phenelzine, isocarboxazid).[60] These medications are not first-line drugs and should be considered only when patients fail all other standard prophylactic methods of treatment. These limitations are due to the extensive interactions between different groups of medications (most TCAs and all selective serotonin reuptake inhibitors [SSRIs] are contraindicated with concomitant use of an MAOI).[60] Diet restrictions are essential for patients on MAOI therapy to avoid hypotensive problems. Generally, we prescribe this type of medication for patients admitted into our hospital unit (Diamond Inpatient Headache Unit). At that facility, we are able to instruct them on the intricacies of this medication, and the dietary and drug restrictions associated with MAOI therapy. We recommend starting phenelzine at 15 mg twice daily, and increasing it by 15 mg every 7 days up to 15 mg four times a day, if needed. Isocarboxazid should be started at 10 mg twice daily, and slowly increased by 10 mg every 7 days up to 10 mg four times a day, if needed. All patients on MAOI therapy should be instructed to wear medical identification to alert emergency personnel that the patient is on MAOI therapy and drug precautions must be followed.

Another class of preventive medications used in migraine prophylaxis are the anticonvulsants. Divalproex sodium may be efficiently used in combination with TCAs and beta blockers. The most common side effects of divalproex therapy are nausea, hepatotoxicity, weight gain, and gastrointestinal distress. This medication should be avoided in patients with a history of hepatitis and abnormal liver function. Liver function tests should be performed before treatment and monitored at regular intervals during therapy.

Another anticonvulsant, topiramate, has demonstrated efficacy in different clinical studies.[61,62] Unlike other centrally acting drugs, topiramate is weight neutral and may be associated with weight loss—another benefit from this medication. We recommend starting treatment with 25 mg once a day, increasing the dose by 25 mg increments every week up to 100 to 200 mg per day if needed. The most common side effects are numbness in the hands, metallic taste when drinking carbonated beverages, cognitive dysfunction, and light-headedness. This medication should not be used in patients with a history of kidney stones. Caution is advised in patients with glaucoma.

A few double-blind, placebo-controlled trials have provided mixed results regarding botulinum toxin type A efficacy as a preventive agent in patients with frequent migraine attacks.[63,64] Until more data are available, we recommend using botulinum toxin type A for patients with intractable headache or in those who cannot tolerate other medications.[65]

For all forms of therapy, we should stress that the most common treatment mistake is its preliminary discontinuation (2 to 3 weeks after treatment was initiated). A brief treatment interval simply does not provide sufficient time to evaluate the efficacy of the preventive medication.

In addition to pharmacologic methods of treatment, we also highly recommend the use of nonpharmacologic interventions: biofeedback, physical therapy, stress management therapy, relaxation training, and psychologic and/or psychiatric consultations. According to our data, patients with chronic migraine and medication-overuse headaches have altered coping strategies that they use to cope with severe pain, chronic pain, and stress.[66] Biofeedback techniques, relaxation exercises, and psychotherapy may help modify the existing (and perhaps not efficient) coping strategies and modify the patient's attitude toward the pain. These interventions may possibly teach new and more effective strategies to be used in the patient's daily life by reducing the severity and, in some cases, the frequency of the headaches. We believe that by using a multidisciplinary approach to headache patients, we may achieve improvement in the treatment of patients with migraine.

References

Full references for this chapter can be found on www.expertconsult.com.

Chapter 47

Tension-Type Headache

Frederick G. Freitag

Historical Considerations

Our concepts of what constitutes tension-type headache have been undergoing revision over the past several years. To a degree, this represents the continuing evolution of our understanding of this disorder. In past decades, tension-type headache was referred to as *muscle contraction* or *muscle tension headache, psychogenic headache, interval headache*, or *depressive headache*. Each of these terms describes components of the headache that individual clinicians thought were the cause of the headache or its association with other disease states. The term *muscle tension headache* was used to describe the musculoskeletal quality of the pain and its distribution in the head and neck area. Although association with musculoskeletal etiologies dates to the nineteenth century, it was Blumenthal and Fuchs[1] who made the direct association with the scalp and neck muscles. The vascular system was believed to contribute to the headache process; this was the reverse from that associated with migraine, and it was vasoconstrictive not vasodilatory. The term *psychogenic headache* and its variants were used by prominent headache physicians such as Ryan[2] and Wolff.[3] Diamond[4] used the term *depressive headache* to characterize headaches relieved by antidepressant medications. The term *interval headache*[5] was used to describe those headaches that patients with migraine headache might experience between their distinct migraine headache attacks. This process of describing tension-type headache began, in great part, with the work of Olesen et al[5] because, at that time, the potential associated symptoms and description of interval headache provided areas of overlap with migraine headache. Frequency of the headaches was the only differentiating element. Interval headache could occur with daily or near-daily frequency. More recently, work by Lipton et al[6] examining the treatment of migraine with sumatriptan led to further differentiation of the true tension-type headache from those tension-type headaches occurring in patients with migraine—and possibly representing a mild or early form of migraine headache. Now, the most recent version of the International Headache Society diagnostic criteria provides a truly clear differentiation between migraine headache and tension-type headache.[7]

The Clinical Syndrome—Signs, Symptoms, and Physical Findings

Tension-type headache is divided into four groups based on the relative frequency of the headaches. In general though these are considered as just two groups, episodic and chronic. The most common headache worldwide is infrequent episodic tension-type headache. It would seem that this is the headache that most people experiences when they have had a stressful day. However, the actual prevalence of tension-type headache is much lower. A study by Schwartz et al[8] estimated the overall prevalence of episodic tension-type headache at 38.3% of the population. Increased prevalence was found in the 30- to 39-year-old age-group, reaching nearly 47% of the women in this age range. Those individuals of African American descent had a substantially lower overall prevalence rate of 22.8%. The prevalence rates also increased with increasing levels of education, being highest in those with graduate school level education where the rate approached half of the population. By contrast, chronic tension-type headache had a far lower prevalence of about 2%. Women were more likely than men to experience the chronic form of the disorder. The prevalence declined with increasing education compared to the increase seen with the episodic form. Although we expect episodic tension-type headache to have little impact on function, Schwartz et al[8] found that 8.3% of individuals lost days from work and nearly half worked at decreased levels of effectiveness. Those with the chronic form were more highly affected with one fifth of patients missing work.

Tension headache is characterized by a number of clinical features (**Table 47.1**). The headache is a dull ache; it may be localized frontally or occipitally or may be more generalized, often in a bandlike distribution about the head. The pain can extend into the neck where it may be associated with stiffness or limitation of motion. Chewing may be affected if there is involvement of the temporalis muscles or the muscles of mastication. Although the pain may be diffuse, it is not severe, except in those patients who have migraine headache that starts as a tension-type headache. It is devoid of other associated physical symptoms, such as nausea, that we traditionally associate with migraine headache. Although symptoms of photophobia and phonophobia are hallmarks of migraine, patients with

Table 47.1 Clinical Characteristics of Tension-Type Headache

Symptoms of Tension-Type Headache

Less than 15 days per month: episodic

15 or more days per month: chronic

Bandlike or localized unilateral or anterior or posterior pain

Mild to moderate; typically may be severe in chronic

Dull aching pain, tightening, pulling

Increased headache with muscle activity (chewing)

With or without pericranial muscle tenderness

No exertional exacerbation

May have photophobia or phonophobia but not both

No nausea

No aura or premonitory symptoms

Coexisting issues and contributors: TMJ syndrome, minimal cervical dystonia, postural mechanical dysfunction of cervical spine, sleep disorder, anxiety, depression

TMJ, temporomandibular joint.

tension-type headache may have one of these symptoms, but not both. Describing tension-type headache, we might say that it is everything that is not found associated with migraine. The pain is self-limited and abates with the use of simple analgesics or removal of oneself from the stressful environment that may have contributed to the headache. As noted, this can be associated with involvement of the pericranial muscles. In most cases, this would be characterized by localized tenderness to palpation of the muscles. If there is involvement of an associated joint, such as in the neck or the temporomandibular joint, there may be limitation of motion. Patients rarely seek medical attention for episodic tension-type headache. Its presentation in the clinical setting should raise the suspicion for the migraine-like headache that fails to meet all the criteria for migraine, such as migrainous headache.

The manifestation of chronic tension-type headaches is very similar to that seen in the episodic versions. The most striking difference in presentation is the persistence of the headaches. Although, by definition, they occur at least 15 days in a month, it is rare to see a patient with the chronic form of headache where the headache is not daily (or near daily) over the course of months, years, and even decades. More variability may be present in the clinical presentation of chronic tension-type headache than in the episodic form. About 16% of patients with episodic headache will have evolution of their headaches to the chronic stage.[9] Although the pain is still most commonly described as a dull, aching sensation, there may be more notation of tightness and pulling sensation, especially with increased involvement of the pericranial muscles. This increased muscle spasm and tenderness is one of the risk factors for the development of chronic tension-type headache from the episodic forms. Other factors that have been suggested as being responsible for this but which continue to lack consistent evidence for serving as responsible etiologies include local inflammations modulated by chemical mediators, and muscle ischemia. What has been demonstrated to be consistently implicated in the development of chronic headache from episodic is the occurrence of allodynia and central sensitization.[10]

This may account for the observation that pain intensity may escalate in patients who have the headache on a long-standing basis. This is also more likely to be seen in patients whose headache is unassociated with the pericranial muscles. In the older terminology this increased pain intensity, which may be rated at maximal levels of severity, would have been associated with psychogenic or depressive headache. Typically when there is an element of depression present in these patients they may describe their pain as being worse in the morning on awakening, yet not waking them from sleep. In those with higher levels of chronic anxiety associated with these headaches, the pattern may be one of increasing severity throughout the day or of a spike in the headache pain in the later afternoon hours.

In patients with these chronic forms of tension-type headache there may also be the development of chronic alterations in their sleep patterns. Most typically, the patient has a concomitant problem with insomnia. Sometimes this is an initiating sleep disorder and occurs more frequently in patients with anxiety versus the frequent nighttime awakenings and difficulty falling back to sleep that occurs more commonly with depressive-type headache. More unusual than the insomnia problem is that of chronic fatigue with patients sleeping in excess of 10 hours per night and requiring a daytime nap as well.

Involvement of the pericranial muscles in these chronic tension-type headaches may be associated with pain or may be found with chronic spasticity of the muscles without associated palpatory tenderness. Diamond and Dalessio[11] postulated a multistep process contributing to the involvement of the pericranial and cervical muscles in tension-type headache. They suggested that local factors in the muscle tissue could provoke a local neural impulse, thereby initiating a reflex response at the spinal cord level, leading to muscle contraction but also to a polysynaptic relay (**Fig. 47.1**) of the stimulus to thalamic and cortical levels. Reflexively, the brain activates the reticulospinal system sending impulses through this efferent tract to the gamma efferent fibers at the spinal cord level causing activation of the muscle spindle. This would lead to a monosynaptic reflex through the ventral cord to efferent peripheral nerves augmenting the muscle contraction. In the absence of blocking factors, the increased muscle tone would lead to inhibition of the muscle spindle. If local factors continue to elicit activation of the afferent paths, or if changes in cortical activity promote reticulospinal efferent transmission, the muscle fibers would experience increasing muscle tone to the point of spasm and associated pain. Similarly, there appears to be changes in both the descending and ascending pain tracts. One study evaluated the sensitivity of the nociceptive reflex in chronic tension-type headache (CTTH) patients and showed a decreased threshold for activation of the reflex in CTTH, suggesting dysfunction of descending inhibition.[12] There is now accumulating evidence from animal studies that analogous facilitatory tracts exist that arise from similar areas in the brainstem.[13] There can be substantial overlap in the patient presenting with temporomandibular joint (TMJ) disorders and the patient presenting with CTTH when the temporalis muscles are involved. Patients may have spasm and pain in these muscles with additional pain being generated from the joint because of compressive effects from the muscle spasm, yet not have a true TMJ syndrome. These patients, if they are experiencing substantial conflict in their life, may exhibit bruxism and clenching—creating muscle pain and joint tenderness as well but without having a TMJ syndrome.

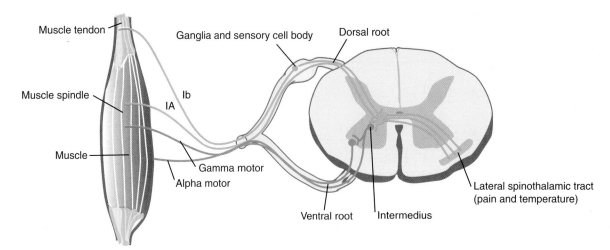

Fig. 47.1 Multisynaptic reflexes involved in regulation of muscle pain and spasm.

Postural mechanical factors involving the cervical spine may also be present in patients with tension-type headache with pericranial muscle involvement. Underlying disk disease or degenerative joint disease of the apophyseal joints of the cervical spine may lead to increased localized muscle spasm and pain. Patterns of altered cervical mechanics may occur chronically, compounding the cervical contribution to the headache process. Although direct neural import from the cervical spine as a cause of headache would be limited to the upper two cervical segments and their interplay with the trigeminal nucleus caudalis, the structure of the neck musculature is such that even distant imitating factors may produce muscle spasm and pain referred to higher cervical levels. Elements of cervical dystonia may also be found in this group of patients with chronic tension-type headache. Typically, the amount of dystonia present is somewhat minimal and may be reflected by a slight tilt of the head toward the side of the dystonia. Involvement of muscles in the anterior and lateral neck is typically associated with this pattern of pericranial muscle involvement.

Physical examination findings are generally absent or minimal in the episodic varieties of tension-type headache. Transient tenderness on palpation or palpatory muscle spasm may be present if there is involvement of distinct muscle groups (**Figs. 47.2, 47.3,** and **47.4**) in the head and neck region. In patients with chronic tension-type headache, where there is no involvement of the pericranial muscles, normal findings on examination is the rule. Despite the pain sometimes being of maximal intensity, there is a paucity of findings on examination. Pericranial muscle involvement patterns, as noted earlier, may be present, especially if the patient is examined in the headache phase.

Diagnostic testing must be considered in patients with tension-type headache (**Table 47.2**). In the primary headache disorder—such as migraine and tension-type headache—the incidence of abnormal radiologic findings in patients with a normal physical and neurologic examination is rare[14] or even nonexistent, as may be the case in tension-type headache. Despite this, neuroimaging (e.g., magnetic resonance imaging [MRI], computed tomography [CT]) should be strongly considered in the patient with a normal neurologic examination if (1) the headaches are rapidly increasing in frequency; (2) the headaches are associated with dizziness or lack of coordination; (3) there is a history of paresthesias associated with the headaches; or (4) the headache awakens the patient from sleep.

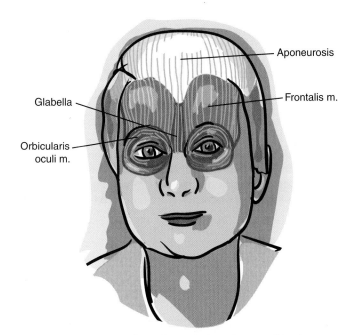

Fig. 47.2 Areas of muscle pain in frontal region of head.

The choice of MRI versus CT scan is determined in part by the clinical suspicions of the physician. If an acute cerebral bleed is suspected or if nasal sinus disease is being investigated, CT scan is most valuable. When other disease entities are being considered, an MRI with contrast enhancement is the test of choice. The resolution available with MRI, lack of interference with braces or fillings, and the ability to visualize the posterior fossa make MRI the preferred diagnostic test. Plain skull radiographs may be helpful in the older patient with a new onset of headache to examine for Paget disease. Plain radiographs of the cervical spine and/or MRI of the cervical spine can be helpful in evaluating for concomitant conditions that might influence or cause tension-type headache.

Baseline chemistries and blood counts should be considered in the evaluation, especially if the patient will be taking daily preventive medications. This should include thyroid evaluation because hypothyroidism can manifest with a headache resembling tension-type headache.

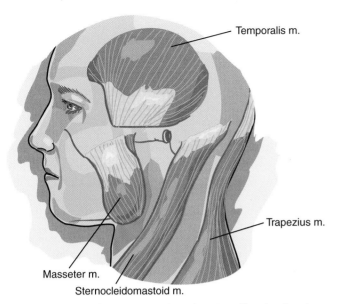

Fig. 47.3 Areas of muscle pain in lateral portion of head and neck.

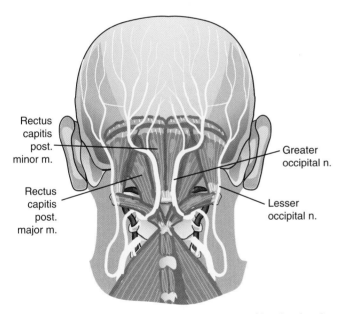

Fig. 47.4 Areas of muscle pain in posterior regions of head and neck.

Table 47.2 Diagnostic Testing in the Tension-Type Headache Patient

Neurologic and head and neck examination

CT scan of sinuses

MRI of brain with and without contrast

Cervical spine radiographs and/or neurodiagnostic scan

Skull radiograph

Thyroid function tests

Baseline laboratory studies if using daily medications

Psychologic testing (MMPI, Beck's Inventory of Depression and Anxiety)

CT, computed tomography; MMPI, Minnesota Multiphasic Personality Inventory; MRI, magnetic resonance imaging.

Table 47.3 Diagnostic Concerns in Tension-Type Headache

Differential Diagnosis

Migraine

Chronic migraine

Medication overuse headache

Hemicrania continua

New daily persistent headache

TMJ syndrome

Naso-sinus disease

Secondary tension-type headache related to coexisting medical disease, disorders of the eyes, and musculoskeletal disorders (e.g., fibromyalgia, arthritis)

TMJ, temporomandibular joint.

In patients in whom psychiatric comorbidity[15] is present, the use of appropriate assessment by a psychologist and a screening psychologic questionnaire should be considered. There are at least two components to the pain that patients may experience. One is the physical component of pain. The other is an emotional component, which is commonly referred to as suffering. One study examined the relationship between pain and scores on specific psychologic testing.[16] This study found that those who were characterized as bearing a heavy emotional burden may increase the affective dimension of pain, which is also called suffering. This personality profile was more significant for its effect on pain than depression, or conversion or a normal profile, independent of sex, age, and baseline pain levels. Additionally, there is evidence for behaviors that result in less assertiveness and increased difficulty expressing emotions.[17] We use the Minnesota Multiphasic Personality Inventory (MMPI). Beck's Inventory of Depression and Anxiety may prove helpful for comprehensive treatment of the patient with chronic tension-type headache. On the MMPI, patients with a significant physical response to stress have elevation of the first three scales. These are the Hy, D, and Hs scales, short for hypochondriac, depression, and hysteria. Typically the Hy and Hs scales are higher than the D scale. If the D scale is the most elevated of the three, further assessment for depression should be undertaken. Elevation of the scores on the Beck's Inventory of Depression and Anxiety may serve as guides to the intensity of behavioral intervention that may be required.

Differential Diagnosis

Perhaps the area that is most challenging in the tension-type headache patient may be differentiating tension-type headache (**Table 47.3**) from migraine headache. This becomes more problematic with daily and near-daily headache, which is more likely to have similarities to chronic migraine.

Chronic migraine is a newer term for those patients who have a history of typical episodic migraine but have developed a now near-daily pattern of headache. In the past, this phenomenon has been known as *migraine with tension-type headache, mixed headache, combined headache, migraine with interval headache, transformed migraine,* and *chronic daily headache.*

Migraine, by definition, is typically a moderate or severe headache attack that may be unilateral and may be exacerbated by physical activity, with the pain having a throbbing or pulsatile component. Normally the attacks have well-defined beginning and ending points with duration of headache between 4 and 72 hours. During the attack, patients have nausea and/or vomiting and/or photophobia and phonophobia. These symptoms will occur if the attack is permitted to go to maximal intensity of pain without successful treatment. Intervention by the patient even with medication that is not capable of fully alleviating the migraine may blunt the intensity of the associated symptoms and characteristics of the headache or alleviate entire components. This intervention and the failure to obtain this information in the headache history is perhaps the most common reason for migraine and tension-type headache to be misdiagnosed. The alleviation or blunting of the migraine symptoms can readily make the migraine attack appear to be a tension-type headache. Because migraine may associated with events that trigger the attacks, if these are of a psychologic nature such as stress, the physician may be even more likely to attribute the headache as a tension-type headache rather than migraine. Biologically, tension-type headache differs from migraine with factors such as biologic peptides. Several studies have examined calcitonin gene-related peptide,[18] substance P,[19] neuropeptide Y, and vasoactive intestinal peptide. These peptides do not change during pain versus pain-free times, nor do they differ from a control nonheadache population.

Migraine may evolve over time to a daily or near-daily headache. Although it may maintain the typical migraine characteristics for many of the headaches, patients may experience a blunting of the migraine characteristics as part of the evolutionary process. Chronic migraine terminology has been developed to aid in the clinical diagnosis of patients as part of the revised International Headache Society guidelines. The headache occurs on 15 or more days per month for at least 3 months, and has two of the following four characteristics as would occur for migraine without aura: (1) unilaterality; (2) throbbing or pulsatile pain; (3) moderate or severe intensity; or (4) exacerbation by physical activity. Additionally, the patient must still experience nausea and/or vomiting or photophobia and phonophobia with the headaches. Again the effects of acute treatment intervention are important to appreciate. In the patient with frequent use of acute medication, overuse headache may occur and further cloud the diagnosis.

The older, other terms for this type of headache should be briefly reviewed for understanding. In the previous version of the International Headache Society criteria, the term *chronic migraine* was not used; rather, this type of headache pattern had to be classified as migraine headache and tension-type headache in one form or another based on the exact migraine and tension-type headache that was occurring and based on which headache was the more frequent. Combined headache and mixed headaches also reflected this dual diagnosis in abbreviated form. *Transformed migraine* was used to reflect the evolution of migraine from an episodic pattern with well-defined pain-free intervals to the daily or near-daily headache pattern. *Chronic daily headache* has been used to describe this type of headache and as a collective term for all of the daily or near-daily headaches, including *transformed migraine, chronic tension-type headache, chronic cluster headaches, new daily persistent headache,* and *hemicrania continua.*

Therefore, in the evaluation of the patient with possible tension-type headache, it is important to assess for several key factors. First, does the patient have a history of migraine headaches? If the patient has this in his or her history, tracking any changes in the migraine pattern may lead to a diagnosis of chronic migraine rather than chronic tension-type headache. Second, it is necessary to know if the attacks of headache that the patient is describing are treated or untreated headaches. If they are untreated and fail to meet criteria for migraine, the diagnosis of tension-type headache is likely. If the attacks the patient describes are treated attacks, it is best to obtain information on any attacks the patient may have had, but that went untreated. This second query is of importance in the patient whose headaches remain episodic because the partially treated episodic migraine without aura may appear to be a tension-type headache. A third factor to consider, more in differentiating episodic tension-type headache from the chronic variety, relates to the overuse of medications for acute treatment. Just as may occur in the migraine patient, so too in the tension-type headache, the overuse of acute medications may cloud the true diagnosis because only after the patient has been free of medication overuse for at least 3 months can the diagnosis be established with certainty.

Patients with chronic significant accommodation disorders of the eyes may develop headache that is referred to the forehead and vertex and may resemble tension-type headache. If accommodation disorders are suspected, a simple examination of the vision by an ophthalmologist or optometrist may provide needed information.

The nasal sinus regions may lead to headache with episodic infection, as well as with chronic disorders of the sinuses. Overlap syndromes with migraine and tension-type headache may occur in these patients and require an appropriate examination of the nasal passages and, if necessary, a CT scan without contrast using coronal sections to establish the diagnosis. The absence of abnormal findings on examination or on scanning helps to eliminate the nasal sinus areas as a cause of the pain. On examination of the nasal passage, the patient with headache from this origin would be expected to have mucopurulent discharge and evidence of contact between the nasal septum and the turbinates. CT scan findings would reflect acute infection with significant air-fluid levels or complete obliteration of the sinus cavities by fluid. In an interesting experiment, Wolff[20] demonstrated that it required 200 mm Hg raised steadily over time to elicit pain from the maxillary sinuses and that sustained pressure over several hours of 50 to 80 mm Hg was needed to elicit even the sensation of pressure from the maxillary sinus cavity. Similarly, pain from engorgement of the nasal turbinates did not occur until these pressures had been achieved and maintained for several hours.

Pain in the temporalis muscle, which extends over the TMJ to attach to the mandible, may be a source of pain in tension-type headache. Because of the effects of sustained contraction of this muscle on the TMJ, there may be pain specifically elicited from this joint associated with tension-type headache. Differentiation from TMJ syndrome is necessary. In patients with TMJ syndrome, the jaw will have limitation in opening. This can be simply assessed in the office by having the patient insert the approximated first and second fingers jointly into the mouth. The ability to do so is a simple screening procedure for assessing the adequacy of the range of motion of this joint. Additionally, there is an audible click or pop of the joint on opening. Not only must audible noise be elicited from the joint but also this should be associated with acute pain in the joint region. Oral examination should reveal malocclusion of the teeth. If this is not obvious to the medical practitioner, appropriate referral to a dental professional should be made for the patient.

Treatment Considerations

Treatment of tension-type headache may involve both pharmacotherapeutic agents and other approaches (**Table 47.4**). The pharmacotherapy of tension-type headache includes medications for acute treatment and medications for the chronic form of tension-type headache for preventive treatment. The other approaches to tension-type headache may include behavioral approaches, such as counseling and biofeedback, and physical methods, including physical therapy, manipulative treatments, and injection treatments. The acute medications for tension-type headache are primarily directed for use as analgesic relief of the pain. Muscle-relaxant agents are used both as episodic acute treatments and as part of preventive treatment.

Because the pain of tension-type headache is mild to moderate in intensity for the majority of patients, the use of opioids should be avoided in this headache disorder, except for isolated headaches in patients who are well known to the treating clinician. Patients with chronic tension-type headache with daily or near-daily headaches are susceptible to becoming dependent on opioids if they are a primary pain medication.

Simple analgesics are the starting point for treating tension-type headache acutely. Acetaminophen, aspirin, and the over-the-counter nonsteroidal anti-inflammatory drugs (NSAIDs) provide effective relief clinically. Because daily, excessive use of these agents may be linked to medication overuse headache, patients should be counseled in their appropriate use to avoid these sequelae. Combination analgesic agents with caffeine have been proven effective in clinical trials.[21,22] From a study by Kubitzek et al,[23] caffeine may not serve as an adjunct in pain relief but may confer a portion of the analgesic activity.

The NSAIDs, both at over-the-counter and at prescription strengths, have been demonstrated to be useful in tension-type headache (**Table 47.5**). Diclofenac potassium at both the

12.5 and 25 mg strengths, ibuprofen at 400 mg,[24] and ketorolac at 60 mg[25] by intramuscular administration have all been demonstrated to be effective. These results, along with clinical experience, suggest that the range of NSAIDs is effective in patients with tension-type headache. Similar results might

Table 47.5 Guidelines for Use of Selected Abortive Therapies in the Treatment of Tension-Type Headache

Medication	Dose/Route/Clarification
NSAIDS (MAJOR SIDE EFFECTS ARE GI RELATED)	
Acetylsalicylic acid	650 mg (2 regular-strength tablets) stat (PO)
Celecoxib	200–400 mg
Diclofenac	12.5–100 mg (PO)
Diflunisal	500 mg q8–12hr
Etodolac	200–400 mg q6–8hr
Fenoprofen	300–600 mg tid–qid
Flurbiprofen	100 mg stat, repeat in 1 hr (PO)
Ibuprofen	400–600mg q6hr (PO)
Ketoprofen	100 mg stat, then 50 mg if needed in 1 hr
Ketorolac	60 mg (IM); limit use to one dose
Meclofenamate	200 mg stat, repeat 1× after 1 hr (PO)
Mefenamic acid	50 mg q4–6hr prn
Naproxen sodium	550 mg stat, then 275 mg in 1 hr (PO)
Tolmetin	400–600 mg tid prn
MUSCLE RELAXANTS WITH/WITHOUT ANALGESICS	
Baclofen	5–20 mg tid–qid (PO); do not abruptly discontinue drug
Carisoprodol	350mg tid (PO); short-term use only—habit-forming; subject to abuse by users of illicit drugs
Carisoprodol 200 mg and aspirin 325 mg	1 tablet tid (PO); short-term use only—habit-forming; subject to abuse by users of illicit drugs
Chlorzoxazone	500 mg qid
Cyclobenzaprine	10 mg tid (PO)
Metaxalone	800 mg (2 tablets) tid–qid (PO)
Methocarbamol	1000 mg qid (PO)
Orphenadrine citrate	100 mg bid (PO)
Orphenadrine citrate 50 mg, aspirin 770 mg, and caffeine 60 mg	1 tablet bid–tid (PO)
Tizanidine	2 mg qid
OTHER	
Isometheptene mucate 65 mg, dichloralphenazone 100 mg, and acetaminophen 325 mg	2 capsules stat, then 1qhr to maximum of 5 capsules/24 hr or 2 capsules stat, then repeat 2 capsules in 1 hr (PO)

Table 47.4 Treatment of Tension-Type Headache

Acute: simple and combination analgesics, skeletal muscle relaxants

Preventive medications: anxiolytics, SSRIs and novel antidepressants, tricyclic antidepressants, MAOIs, botulinum toxin type A

Behavioral approaches: biofeedback, cognitive-behavioral treatment

Physical modalities: TENS, physical therapy, manual manipulative treatment, trigger point injection, neuroaxial and facet injection

MAOIs, monoamine oxidase inhibitor(s); SSRIs, selective serotonin reuptake inhibitor(s); TENS, transcutaneous electrical nerve stimulation.

GI, gastrointestinal; IM, intramuscular(ly); NSAIDs, nonsteroidal anti-inflammatory drugs; PO, by mouth.

Table 47.6 **Antidepressants and Receptor Affinity**

Drug	Serotonin Inhibition	Norepinephrine Inhibition	Dopamine Inhibition	Sedative Effects	Anticholinergic Effects	Histamine Inhibition
Amitriptyline	Moderate	Weak	Inactive	Strong	Strong	Moderate
Doxepin	Moderate	Moderate	Inactive	Strong	Strong	Strong
Nortriptyline	Weak	Fairly potent	Inactive	Mild	Moderate	Mild
Imipramine	Fairly potent	Moderate	Inactive	Moderate	Strong	Mild
Protriptyline	Weak	Fairly potent	Inactive	None	Strong	None
Desipramine	Weak	Potent	Inactive	Mild	Moderate	Mild or none
Trimipramine	Weak	Weak	Inactive	Moderate	Moderate	Moderate
Amoxapine	Weak	Potent	Moderate	Mild	Mild	Mild
Maprotiline	Weak	Moderate	Inactive	Moderate	Moderate	Moderate

also occur with the newer COX-2 inhibitors, which may offer improvement in gastrointestinal safety for patients. Which of these analgesic agents and the strength of the preparation are issues of individual patient response and clinician preference?

A variety of skeletal muscle relaxants and antispasticity agents find their way into treatment of tension-type headache. Unfortunately, the use of these agents is merely anecdotal because there are no well-defined controlled trials relating to tension-type headache. There have been studies with tizanidine in the treatment of chronic daily headache, but most of these patients had medication overuse headache in addition to migraine.

For patients with chronic tension-type headache the use of episodic treatments may not be appropriate. The daily use of analgesics may have health consequences, potentiate the occurrence of medication overuse headache, or lose efficacy over time. The same scenario commonly occurs with the muscle-relaxant agents. The relatively brief half-lives of many of these medications are likely responsible for the overuse phenomenon, as well as their diminished efficacy over time.

To minimize these issues and attempt to induce a remission of these headaches, the use of daily preventive medications may be in order. Although several of the long-duration antispasticity agents such as baclofen or tizanidine may be of benefit, the mainstay of preventive treatment in tension-type headache is the antidepressant medications.[26] Again there is a paucity of well-controlled trials with these agents to support their use; much of the literature is intermixed with chronic daily headache, which includes patients with chronic migraine among other diagnoses. Practically, antidepressants are most likely to afford relief from the chronic recurrent headaches regardless of the etiologic issues underlying their cause. The antidepressants fall into three major groups: the tricyclic antidepressants (TCAs), the monoamine oxidase inhibitors (MAOIs), and the selective serotonin reuptake inhibitors, as well as other novel antidepressants. The TCAs have the best clinical efficacy for tension-type headache, perhaps because of their breadth of pharmacologic activity, which may produce a direct analgesic effect.

The range of pharmacologic effects of TCAs (**Table 47.6**) needs to be appreciated for optimal selection of an agent based on the patient's tolerance of medications, coexisting illnesses, associated mood disorders, and sleep habits. Typically, it is wise to inquire whether a patient has a concomitant sleep disorder. Patients with insomnia usually fare best with a sedating TCA with or without a mild benzodiazepine to initiate sleep. Patients with chronic fatigue and daytime tiredness tolerate a TCA such as protriptyline quite well. The anticholinergic effects contribute to the dry mouth, constipation, and blurred vision that patients may experience as adverse events. The sedative effects are linked in part to the antihistaminic effects of these drugs. This antihistaminic effect may also contribute to carbohydrate cravings and weight gain, as well as coupling with the anticholinergic activity to adversely affect cognitive issues.

The MAOIs are not commonly used outside of specialty clinics because of the issues related to drug interactions, dietary restrictions, and the potential for serious adverse events to occur with these interactions. However, in refractive patients who have failed to achieve benefit with more traditional therapies, they have proven efficacy.[27]

The newer antidepressants have been used in treating chronic daily headache but, again, much of this use has been in patients with chronic migraine or combination headache disorders. In general, in the absence of coexisting psychiatric disease, the efficacy of these compounds in headache tends to be limited. However, they possess comparatively exceptional tolerability compared to the TCAs. Novel agents that have activity at both norepinephrine and serotonin reuptake sites[28, 29] may have potentially better efficacy in the patient with headache without regard for coexisting psychiatric disease. Other types of agents have been used as well, including the Alzheimer's medication memantine, which has proven modestly effective.[30]

Of the nonpharmacologic techniques for tension-type headache, the preferred approach based on efficacy would be the combination of biofeedback along with cognitive-behavioral counseling.[31] These techniques focus not only on the stress issues, which may contribute to the headaches, but on muscle relaxation training in biofeedback to offer a specific method to help reduce the pain of associated headaches. In the training for biofeedback, the patient has surface electrodes attached to the scalp, face, and/or neck region of pain to register the amount of muscle activity. Through guided exercises, patients learn to control the underlying muscle tension and help to alleviate the headache. The technique requires a combination of hands-on training with a therapist experienced in its use along with regular at-home practice sessions. Aggressive multidisciplinary treatment programs of about 100 hours' duration prove to be highly effective and significantly more effective than brief programs of 20 hours' duration.[32]

Massage and physical therapy have been examined in the treatment of tension-type headache. Although specific patients who have postural mechanical factors at play in their headaches may benefit from these treatments, the techniques, in general, produce little in the way of positive benefits. Manual therapies performed by a chiropractor or osteopathic physician have also been studied in the treatment of tension-type headache. The results have been mixed. Some studies report significant benefit, but others report little, if any. Combining manipulative therapy with traditional medical therapies for prevention of tension-type headaches may be more effective than either one alone.[33] Many issues have clouded these results, including diagnosis of the headaches being treated, the techniques used, and the choice of blinding or alternative active controls for assessment of outcome of these studies. Proper assessment of the patient for alterations in muscle tone, postural, and mechanical effects—coupled with appropriate and comprehensive diagnosis—may lead to successful treatment with these techniques.

The use of injections such as trigger pointing, epidural, and cervical facet injection is covered elsewhere in this text. They remain useful adjuncts in the management of tension-type headache. For patients with localized areas of muscle pain and tenderness, injections may be useful as part of a comprehensive treatment program. Specific techniques to address tension-type headache have been examined with the use of botulinum toxin type A (BttA). The trials have been small and lacking in solid control groups but have suggested that some patients will benefit from the injections.[34,35] The mechanism by which BttA exerts its effects in tension-type headache may be by direct effects at the neuromuscular junction, as well as by potential central effects that may modulate the pain tracks centrally. The choice of injection sites (**Table 47.7**) is typically guided by the patient's areas of pain and associated muscle spasm. It is important to assess the mechanics that may contribute to the pain. For example, minimal cervical dystonia may occur involving the sternocleidomastoid muscle. The chronic shortening of the muscle may not be painful but the pull exerted on the posterior muscles on the opposite side of the neck may be the source of the pain. Injecting into the area of pain fails to alleviate the problem and may intensify the situation in some patients, whereas injection into the affected sternocleidomastoid muscle produces relaxation of the spasticity and relief of the pain on the posterior opposite side of the neck. Repetitive injections with BttA may be required to demonstrate an adequate response. There may be a high rate of placebo response with the initial series of injections, or the results may be minimal or brief. Repeating the injections

Table 47.7 Botulinum Toxin Type A Treatment for Tension-Type Headache

BOTULINUM TOXIN TYPE A

Dose: 25 to 200 units

Injection locations: frontalis (bilateral even if unilateral headache), glabellar, temporalis, mastoid, sternocleidomastoid, rectus capitis, cervical paraspinal, trapezius

Repeat treatment in 2 to 3 months based on headache pain recurrence

will minimize placebo effects and may demonstrate more robust relief of the headaches, as well as expand the duration of relief from the headaches and neck pain. Side effects tend to be negligible for most patients beyond the initial discomfort of the injections. Cost may be prohibitive for many patients because its use in headache has not been approved by the Food and Drug Administration and many insurance companies have elected to consider the treatment experimental pending further studies and approval processes. Another approach that has been used in chronic headache, including tension-type headache, is the use of neurostimulators such as occipital nerve stimulators. These are still considered experimental and should be reserved for those who have a long history of refractive headaches to other medical and behavioral therapies. There is evidence that their use may modulate central brain pain pathways.[36]

Although tension-type headache is ubiquitous, only a relatively small percentage of the population has these headaches occurring with sufficient frequency and severity to cause them to seek medical attention. This small group may experience substantial impact from their disease on productivity and quality of life. Assessment of the headaches includes assessment for other headache disorders, which may overlap it, such as a chronic migraine. Coexisting diseases that may contribute to the process, such as mood disorders and mechanical disorders of the spine and neck, require investigation.

Treatment is optimized by appropriate use of acute medications and preventive treatments that may include drugs in the antidepressant classes, along with nonpharmacologic modalities and other alternative treatments ranging from biofeedback to manual therapy to the use of BttA injections.

References

Full references for this chapter can be found on www.expertconsult.com.

Cluster Headache

George J. Urban and Seymour Diamond

Cluster headache, a distinctive and extremely painful primary headache disorder, is called by some sufferers a "killer" or "suicide" headache. The International Headache Society (IHS)[1] defines *cluster headache* as

> a severe unilateral, orbital, supraorbital, and/or temporal pain lasting 15 to 180 minutes untreated and associated with at least one of the several signs [**Table 48.1**] ipsilateral with the pain, occurring in frequency of attacks from one every other day to eight times a day.

History and Terminology

The earliest description of cluster headache occurred in the eighteenth century, when Gerhard van Swienten, a founder of the Vienna School of Medicine and the personal physician to the Empress Maria Theresa, presented an illustrative case of episodic cluster headache that was published (in Latin) in 1745 in his textbook of clinical medicine.[2] His description, which follows, actually fulfills the criteria established by the IHS in 1988 for episodic cluster headache[3]:

> A healthy robust man of middle age [was suffering from] troublesome pain which came on every day at the same hour at the same spot above the orbit to the left eye, where the nerve emerges from the opening of frontal bone: after a short time the left eye began to redden, and to overflow with tears; then he felt as if his eye was slowly forced out of his orbit with so much pain, that he nearly went mad. After a few hours all these evils ceased, and nothing in the eye appeared at all changed.

Other incomplete accounts can be found in European medical literature in the eighteenth and nineteenth centuries. The first recorded account of cluster headache in the English medical literature has been traced to Wilfred Harris in 1926, in which he elaborated on the topic of *migrainous neuralgia*—a term used for cluster headache.[4] Harris identified differential features among migrainous neuralgia, trigeminal neuralgia, and migraine. He noted typical unilaterality in short duration of excruciating headache attacks, frequency, autonomic features, and periodic occurrence of headaches and remission between cycles. His treatment recommendation consisted of

Table 48.1 Signs Associated with Cluster Headache Attack

Ipsilateral conjunctival injection and/or lacrimation
Ipsilateral nasal congestion and/or rhinorrhea
Ipsilateral eyelid edema
Ipsilateral forehead and facial sweating
Ipsilateral miosis and/or ptosis
A sense of restlessness or agitation

barbiturate, ergotamine, and, in intractable cases, an injection of alcohol into the gasserian ganglion.

Bayard Taylor Horton is considered the father of cluster headache treatment. His precise description of headache referred to "erythromelalgia of the head"[5] or "histaminic cephalalgia."[5] His devotion to the study of cluster headache forever linked his name to cluster headache—*Horton's headache*. Horton introduced the use of histamine desensitization in the treatment of chronic cluster headaches following an observation that an injection of histamine would provoke a brief, unilateral, intense headache with symptoms similar to those of cluster headache in susceptible individuals.[6]

The term *cluster headache* was established in 1952 by Kunkle et al[7] to describe a typical periodic pain pattern. This term has been accepted worldwide under the English name or under a translated name in particular languages.

A variety of other titles are associated with cluster headache, although many refer to cluster-like headache. These other terms used in the past include *histaminic cephalalgia; Horton's headache; migrainous neuralgia; sphenopalatine neuralgia; petrosal neuralgia; red migraine; Raeder's syndrome; erythromelalgia; Bing's erythroprosopalgia; Bing's headache; Bing's syndrome; Sluder's syndrome; periodic migrainous neuralgia; ciliary neuralgia; hemicrania intermittent;* and *neuralgia spasmodica.*

Prevalence and Epidemiology

Cluster headache is a relatively uncommon headache disorder. A limited number of studies address the prevalence of cluster headache in the United States and worldwide. Results of these studies vary greatly in range and are inconclusive.

In Sweden, Ekbom et al[8] studied the prevalence of migraine and cluster headache in a homogeneous population of 9803 18-year-old men. They found a prevalence of 0.09% for cluster headache, which is approximately 19 times less than the prevalence of migraine headache in the same age group of men. The flaw of the study is that the sample group is not representative across the population, not even for the mean age of the onset of this disorder.

A population-based study in Olmsted County, Minnesota,[9] has drawn its results from the screening of 6476 patient records over a 3-year period. The overall age- and gender-adjusted incidence was 9.8 per 100,000 (0.01%) for males. In the same group, migraine occurrence was about 25 times higher. Included among the few weaknesses in this screening is that subjects were already experiencing headaches and did not represent the general population. Olmsted County is racially and socioeconomically homogeneous and the study is based on a small number of cluster cases.

Most recently, 1838 individuals from the Vågå study[10] were examined and 7 were found to fulfill the IHS criteria for cluster headache, corresponding to a prevalence of 381 per 100,000 (0.38%). In the small European country of San Marino with an entire population of 21,792, D'Alessandro et al[11] derived a cluster headache prevalence of 0.13% for males and 0.009% for females. The overall prevalence was 69 per 100,000 (0.07%). Kudrow[12] estimated the prevalence of cluster headache at 0.24%. His higher estimate may be attributed to a larger cohort of cluster headache patients consulting him.

Familial Occurrence and Genetics

The involvement of genetic factors in cluster headache is unclear and highly controversial. Some diseases with genetically determined predisposition have been associated with the presence of the human leukocyte antigen (HLA) antigen. However, Cuypers and Altenkirch[13] have failed to find any significant deviations in HLA antigen frequencies in patients with episodic cluster headache. All of their five patients with chronic cluster headaches carried the HLA-A$_1$ antigen—a finding that is nonetheless inconclusive because of the small number of subjects. Similarly, the genetic importance of CACNAA1A gene mutation that has been found in some neurologic disorders, including familial hemiplegic migraine, is doubtful.[14]

Recently, some evidence has emerged suggesting familial occurrence and inheritance of cluster headache. El Amrani et al[15] studied 186 probands (144 men and 42 women) with documented cluster headache diagnosis. A positive family history of cluster headache was found in 12 men and 8 women (a total of 10.75%), with 22 affected first-degree relatives (3.4%). No statistical difference was determined between probands with acute and chronic cluster headaches, although patients with the chronic type had a higher prevalence of familial occurrence. The authors could not demonstrate any mode of inheritance from this study. Likewise, Kudrow[12] noted the occurrence of cluster headache in first-degree relatives in about 3% of patients.

In another study, Russell et al[16] found a positive family history of cluster headache in 7% of 366 families—representing a fourteenfold increased risk of cluster headache in first-degree relatives of probands and twofold in second-degree relatives. It has been suggested that the inheritance in some families may be through an autosomal dominant gene.

Clinical Picture

Cluster headache is characterized by recurrent bouts of extremely painful, unilateral headache attacks, of relatively short duration, and associated with symptoms and signs of autonomic dysfunction. The attacks are clustered over a period of several weeks and separated from another cycle by totally asymptomatic remission. Cluster headache is part of trigeminal autonomic cephalalgia and is divided into episodic and chronic types (**Table 48.2**).

Demographics

Traditionally, cluster headache has been considered a "male" headache disorder. The gender ratio varies from 3.5:1 to 6.7:1 in favor of males. A higher female occurrence has been reported by some investigators at larger, specialized headache clinics. This discrepancy can be explained by the tendency of headache clinics to attract patients with cluster headache and better recognition of the disease.

Table 48.2 International Headache Society Classification of Cluster Headache

3.1. Cluster headache
    3.1.1. Episodic cluster headache
    3.1.2. Chronic cluster headache

3.2. Paroxysmal hemicrania
    3.2.1. Episodic paroxysmal hemicrania
    3.2.2. Chronic paroxysmal hemicrania (CPH)

3.3. Short-lasting unilateral neuralgiform headache attacks with conjunctival injection and tearing (SUNCT)

3.4. Probable trigeminal autonomic cephalalgia
    3.4.1. Probable cluster headache
    3.4.2. Probable paroxysmal hemicrania
    3.4.3. Probable SUNCT

From The International Classification of Headache Disorders, ed 2, *Cephalalgia* 24(suppl 1), 2004.

In a large case series, Horton[17] reported male-to-female ratio in 1176 patients to be 6.7:1 and Kudrow[12] found male-to-female preponderance among 425 patients to be 5:1. Manzoni[18] noted a decreasing trend of male-to-female ratio to 3.5:1 in the Italian population over several years. Similar findings were observed in the Swedish population[19] with a decline of male predominance comparing years before and after 1970. This study also showed a significant shift in proportion of females with respect to age at onset. The highest male-to-female ratio is in persons ages 40 to 49 and 30 to 39 years at onset (8.4:1 and 6.5:1, respectively), and lowest in the 40- to 69- and 10- to 19-year age-groups, at onset (2.3 to 2.5:1 and 3.2:1, respectively). In a review of 225 charts of cluster patients, Urban et al[20] reported 4:1 male preponderance.

No racial or ethnic prevalence has been documented. In the study by Rozen et al,[21] 25% of 32 women were African American, and 17.4% of 69 male patients were African American, which is consistent with Kudrow's findings.[22] These racial differences, however, should not be generalized.

Age of Onset

Cluster headache can begin at any age, including childhood and in the elderly. Onset at both extremes warrants detailed investigations to rule out secondary headache. The average mean age of onset in the various series is 31.5 years.[23] It is noteworthy that the diagnosis is commonly delayed by several years either because of unrecognized clinical symptoms or misdiagnosis as migraine, trigeminal neuralgia, or a sinus or dental problem. A slightly lower mean age of onset was noted in women (27.1%) as compared with 29.7% in men was found in several studies.[21–24]

Childhood onset is relatively rare and therefore not always recognizable. Three of nine cluster headache sufferers in a Swedish population of almost 10,000 18-year-old men had onset of symptoms before age 8 years.[8] In the study by Maytal et al,[25] 35 patients were identified with onset of cluster at or before 18 years of age. Seven of these subjects were 5 to 12 years old at the onset of the headaches. Other authors[11,19,25] also reported early onset before age 6 years. During childhood, the clinical features of cluster headaches are similar to those starting in adulthood. Treatment, however, is limited.

Periodicity

The main distinguishing feature of cluster headache is its periodicity. The term *cluster* derives from attacks tending to occur repeatedly within a relatively limited time span (called *period, cycle, bout,* or *cluster*). On average, a cluster period lasts 6 to 12 weeks and by definition cannot last longer than 12 months. The length of the cycle may vary considerably interindividually and intraindividually. In the study by Manzoni et al[26] of 189 cluster headache patients, 78% of the cycles lasted 1 to 2 months. In another study of 225 patients with cluster headache, Urban et al[20] reported 69% of patients reporting headache cycles with durations of up to 4 months. With treatment, the number of patients in this category increased to 75%. Frequency of cycle also varies, but more than one half of patients' cycles occur one or fewer time per year.

Some investigators suggested that cluster cycles occur annually, and in spring and fall seem to be slightly more prevalent.[16,27–29] However, Kudrow[30] found that an increased number of cluster cycles occur in February and June—coinciding with an increased number of daylight hours. It appears that cluster onset occurs 7 to 10 days before the longest and shortest days of the year. However, in some patients, the number of cycles decreases following the 1-hour resetting of clocks for daylight-saving and standard times in April and October, respectively. This observation with the fact that cycles start in most patients at the same time each year—circannual occurrence—suggests involvement of the biologic clock located in the suprachiasmatic nucleus of the hypothalamus.

Another typical cluster headache feature is a circadian periodicity and predictability of acute cluster headache attacks. The majority of patients experience attacks almost exclusively nocturnally, awakening the individual usually 2 to 3 hours after falling asleep, between midnight and 2 AM. This timing corresponds with the rapid eye movement phase of sleep when rapid fluctuation in autonomic functions occurs. The nocturnal episodes make patients anxious and apprehensive to fall asleep and many will remain awake to avoid an attack. Some patients report that daytime attacks are associated with napping or relaxation. Similarly, biofeedback relaxation during the cluster cycle may induce an acute episode in many patients. The clockwork regularity of daily attacks is also indicative of dysfunction of the modulatory role of the suprachiasmatic nucleus.

Attacks

The attacks are characterized by severe pain and associated symptoms. The pain is distinguishable by its localization, unilaterality, character, severity, and duration. The localization of pain is usually uniform. Typically, pain starts retro-orbitally, periorbitally, supraorbitally, or temporally. The pain area extends over a relatively small region that is easily identified by the patient with the finger or as the intersection of two lines in an area behind the eye. The ocular region is affected in 90% of cluster headache patients. When the pain is confined to the maxillary or mandibular region, it is described as lower-half syndrome.

In some patients, the pain may start in other parts of the head in extratrigeminal territory, including the occipital and cervical regions. The prevalence of neck pain and neck-related symptoms is not unusual. Solomon et al[31] found that in 10%

of their patients the neck was the initial site of pain in addition to the orbital distribution. In 37% of the subjects, the pain radiated to the nuchal area. Their patients also reported neck stiffness (40%) and tenderness (29%), and precipitation, aggravation, or amelioration by head movement. The nuchal symptoms in patients with cluster headache are probably related to the convergence of pain fibers from the first division of the trigeminal nerve and from upper cervical nerve roots.[31]

The pain is strictly unilateral and autonomic symptoms occur ipsilateral to the pain. In most cases, the attacks occur on the same side with every attack and every cycle. A slight predominance has been observed in right-sided headache attacks with 49% right side, 38% left side, and 13% that may shift sides or be bilateral.[22] It is atypical that the side of the pain would change during the attack, although some patients report a shift in sides between attacks or from cycle to cycle. Meyer et al[32] documented similar findings. Among 328 cluster patients, 14% experienced pain side shift. On the remaining 328 individuals without the side shift, no statistical significant difference was demonstrated between the occurrence of right-sided and left-sided pain (54% vs. 46%). The prevalence of side shift was similar for episodic and chronic cluster headache.

The pain may be preceded by prodromal symptoms heralding an oncoming attack of excruciating pain. This may manifest as a vague discomfort or poorly describable feeling in the region of one eye, temple, forehead, or neck. Fatigue, euphoria, depression or mood changes, apathy, irritability, and photophobia and phonophobia may be experienced.

Symptoms that occur minutes or a few hours before the cluster attack are reported by up to 61%. In 8% of the patients, premonitory symptoms occur days or weeks before the cluster cycle.[33] Usually the patient does not spontaneously report this information because the prodrome may precede the attack by hours and the intensity of the pain may cause the patient to ignore warning signs. Therefore the clinician should actively inquire about those symptoms. Although cluster patients do not typically describe an aura, some patients have identified its presence.[29,34,35] Silberstein et al[36] described five patients with visual symptoms and one with olfactory aura, lasting 5 to 120 minutes, and always occurring before headache onset.

The character of the pain is also distinguishable from migraine and other headaches. Adjectives given to the degree of pain vary largely and the pain may change character during the attack. The pain is commonly described as boring, pressing, or burning, but also as piercing, stabbing, screwing, tearing, or sharp, knife-like, "a hot poker in the eye," and occasionally as pulsating, throbbing, tightening, squeezing, or aching. A lingering dull pain, the soreness may persist in the painful area for some time, perhaps for hours, and may resemble a tension-type headache or mild migraine attack. In some cases, the pain continues until the next attack. Cutaneous allodynia-hypersensitivity of the scalp in the affected area may also be present. Ashkenazi and Young[37] studied brush allodynia (BA) in 10 patients (all male, mean age 39.3). Seven had episodic cluster headache (ECH) and three had chronic cluster headache (CCH). Two patients were experiencing an acute attack when tested for BA. In total, 4 (40%) of the 10 patients had BA (2 [28.6%] of the 7 with ECH and 2 [66.7%] of the 3 with CCH). Median disease duration was 22 years for patients with BA and 12 years for patients without BA. Of the two patients suffering an acute attack, one had BA ipsilateral to the headache, which was reduced 20 minutes after treatment in addition to reduced headache severity. The presence of BA in cluster headache may be related to cluster headache type (episodic vs. chronic) and to the duration of the disease. These results also support the concept that allodynia in cluster headache may result from a time-dependent process of neuronal sensitization.

The severity of cluster attacks is notorious for its excruciating level of pain. Cluster headache is nicknamed as the "killer" or "suicide" headache, indicating the mental status of a sufferer during the unbearable attack. The headache has been described as the most severe form of pain a human can endure. It is not unusual for women who experience cluster headache to describe the pain as much worse than that associated with labor and delivery. The intensity of pain is the only feature of an attack that prompts a patient to visit a medical facility. The onset is usually sudden, with rapid crescendo, or peaks within a short time of 10 to 20 minutes. The intensity of pain is milder at the beginning and the end of the cluster period and more severe in the middle. Application of ice or heat may sometimes alleviate the pain.

The posturing and behavior during the painful attack are also typical and differ from an attack of migraine. Usually, patients cannot remain still and may rock back and forth while in a standing, kneeling, or sitting position. These patients hold their head in both hands, pace the floor, or leave the house for colder, outside air. They are restless and may even become violent during the attack. Facial expressions show grimacing and the horror of pain. In a futile attempt to alleviate the excruciating pain, the patient may vigorously rub the affected temple with the thumb, knuckles, fist, or a dull or sharp object such as a pen or screwdriver. Patients may bang their head against the wall or hit hard objects with their fists. Such violent and self-destructive behavior leads to injuries and sometimes to suicide.

Duration of the cluster attack averages between 40 and 90 minutes. Briefer and more prolonged attacks occur less frequently with the exception of the chronic form. At the onset and end of a cluster period, attacks are generally briefer. In the series by Manzoni et al,[27] 73% reported attacks with durations ranging from 30 to 120 minutes. Some reports have noted that females tend to experience longer attacks on average by 30 minutes.[11] Also, nocturnal attacks seem to be more severe and longer.

Associated symptoms (**Table 48.3**) are another pathognomonic feature of cluster headache. These symptoms typically accompany the attack but on occasion may precede it. By definition, these symptoms are ipsilateral to the affected side. The most common accompanying sign is lacrimation, which is reported by more than 80% of cluster headache patients. On occasion, lacrimation may manifest bilaterally. Conjunctival injection occurs slightly less frequently than lacrimation, described probably by 60% of these patients, is usually of a moderate degree, and may persist beyond the attack. Nasal congestion, with or without rhinorrhea, occurs in about 70% of cluster sufferers. Initially, the nasal mucosa swells to varying degrees causing stuffiness or congestion and may lead to nasal secretion of a clear and thin mucus. Nasal discharge often accompanies lacrimation, which may indicate that the discharge is indeed tears directed through the lacrimal duct to the nose. It is believed, though, that those two phenomena exist separately. The nasal stuffiness, lacrimation, and conjunctival injection are called the classic triad of cluster headache.

Table 48.3 Associated Symptoms (More Than 5%)

Ocular
Lacrimation
Conjunctival injection
Partial Horner syndrome
Photophobia
Blurred vision

Vascular
Facial flushing
Prominence and/or tenderness of temporal artery
Eye puffiness

Neurologic
Cutaneous allodynia
Visual aura
Vertigo
Neck muscle stiffness or tenderness

Nasal
Congestion/stuffiness
Rhinorrhea

Gastrointestinal
Nausea
Vomiting

Cardiac
Tachycardia/bradycardia
Blood pressure fluctuation
Arrhythmia

Photophobia also occurs frequently in around 60% to 70% of these patients. Some cluster headache sufferers may also experience phonophobia, nausea, and vomiting. Other symptoms and signs may include facial flushing, increased forehead or generalized sweating, prominence or bulging of the frontal or temporal blood vessels, and blurred vision. The term *partial Horner syndrome* accompanying cluster headache indicates that only two components of a Horner syndrome are present—miosis and ptosis, but without anhidrosis. This syndrome is observed on the ipsilateral side and occurs throughout the cluster period with a great variation—between 16% and 84%.[22] In some cases, these symptoms may persist indefinitely. The pathophysiology of the cluster headache–related Horner-like syndrome is unclear. It is speculated that patients with the partial Horner syndrome may represent a subgroup of cluster headache sufferers.

Other systemic findings may accompany the cluster attack. Cardiovascular changes are sometimes present in the form of blood pressure fluctuation, tachycardia during the onset of the attack, bradycardia after the attack, and occasional various types of arrhythmia (including transient episodes of atrial fibrillation, premature ventricular beats, and first-degree atrioventricular [AV] block or sinoatrial [SA] block).[38] Cluster sufferers do not, for the most part, report autonomic symptoms—only 3% are affected.[39]

Trigger Factors

During the cluster cycle, acute attacks can be induced by alcohol, nitroglycerin, or histamine. The provoked attack occurs usually after the latency of 30 to 50 minutes. All three substances are vasodilators, which may suggest that vasodilatation is part of the mechanism of cluster headache. Alcohol has been known to provoke the cluster attack—but only during the cycle. Many patients will voluntarily abstain from alcohol during the cycle until the headaches are in remission. It is interesting that some patients report that alcohol in a large amount may postpone attacks by a few days. In the chronic form, alcohol consumption may reduce the number of attacks.

Nitroglycerin (1 to 3 mg) can induce an acute attack in a cluster sufferer that is identical to a spontaneous attack. This action—drug-induced headache—can occur only during an active period, and after a latency of 30 to 50 minutes. The provoked attack delays the next expected spontaneous attack. To provoke the bout, the patient should be outside of the refractory period—within 8 hours of a previous spontaneous attack.[23]

Histamine administration induces an acute cluster attack in 75% of patients.[40] Both cluster and noncluster headache patients respond within 5 minutes to histamine infusion with a bilateral, throbbing, moderate-to-severe headache of transitory nature that lasts for 5 to 10 minutes. This headache is not accompanied by typical cluster autonomic symptoms. Again, after the latency of 20 to 50 minutes, a unilateral headache similar to a spontaneous cluster attack will occur.[41]

The mechanism underlying the provocation of attacks by these vasodilatory agents is not entirely clear. Fanciullacci et al[42] suggest that histamine and nitroglycerine activates the trigeminal vascular system. Calcitonin gene-related peptide (CGRP), one of the most potent endogenous vasodilators, is present in the trigeminal sensory neurons that supply the cephalic blood vessels. CGRP basal plasma levels were significantly higher during a cluster period than in remission, and an increase in CGRP was directly related to the peak of a nitroglycerin-induced attack and reversed after sumatriptan-induced alleviation. This activation is possible only during the phase of trigeminal vascular hyperactivity.

Kudrow and Kudrow[43] found that nitroglycerine causes oxygen desaturation at a larger magnitude and is longer in duration in active cluster patients. These researchers indicate that hypoxia may play a role in the mechanism of cluster attack as suggested by higher occurrence of attacks at night during sleep and at high altitudes.

Cluster Headache, Personality, and Psychologic Factors

Traditionally, certain personality traits have been assigned to different headache sufferers. This situation has been supported by observations of clinicians, researchers, and/ or patients' acquaintances, as well as psychologic profiling. More than 30 years ago, Graham[35] observed and described the physical appearance of male cluster patients and ascribed to them particular behavioral characteristics. He observed the preponderance of masculine or sometimes hypermasculine males with leonine facial features that were often associated with paradoxically gentle—even meek—personalities. Graham described the "leonine-mouse" syndrome depicting these patients as "mice living inside of lions." Such patients appear to be dependent and helpless, but also ambitious and diligent, heavy smoking, heavy drinking, executive-type men.

In many instances, in our own clinical experience and that of other headache specialists, this portrayal is fairly accurate. However, some researchers have not been able to document those discrepancies and their results are controversial. Cuypers et al[44] compared the personalities of 40 cluster headache patients to those of 49 migraineurs. This study revealed a slightly elevated score for nervousness and a slightly diminished score for masculinity—but no significant difference between migraine and cluster patients. Similarly, Kudrow and

Sutkus[45] did not find a discrepancy in personality in those two headache groups. Levi et al[46] analyzed the results of a Swedish personality inventory and obtained outcomes indicating higher levels of anxiety, socializing difficulties, and more hostile attitudes toward others. The study of Pfaffenrath et al[47] is more controversial, as no statistically significant differences were noted between the various types of primary headaches. However, patients with cluster headache showed the highest number of abnormalities but also the highest percentage of completely normal results.

In classic works, cluster headache patients have been described as heavy drinkers and smokers. Kudrow[22] found that 78% of 280 cluster patients smoked an average of 33 cigarettes per day. A higher percentage (84%) of smokers were described by Manzoni et al[27] in their study of 180 patients. The higher smoking rate is present in both male and female patients. Alcohol has been consumed in higher prevalence in cluster patients than in non–cluster headache controls. Manzoni et al[27] reported alcohol drinking in more than 90% of 180 patients with cluster headache and significant proportions drank heavily. Similarly, Levi et al[48] found heavy social drinking or alcoholism in 67%. However, 79% of their subjects decreased their alcohol consumption during the active cluster cycles.

The significance of tobacco and alcohol overuse is unclear. Smokers have been found to have low monoamine oxidase (MAO) activities in platelets—a factor that has also been documented in cluster patients who do not smoke.[49] Thus smoking may increase the risk for cluster headache in predisposed individuals with reduced MAO activity.

Women and Cluster Headache

Cluster headache is predominantly a male headache disorder with a male-to-female ratio ranging from 3.5:1 up to 7:1. The gender ratio appears to be declining,[17] which can be attributed to new social and habitual activities of women, hormonal changes, or unknown causes. Many similarities and some peculiarities have been observed in the clinical presentation of women with cluster headache as compared to men. A higher coexistence of cluster and migraine headache in women has been recognized, and many female cluster headache sufferers are misdiagnosed with migraine. In women, cluster headache seems to start earlier in life, at a mean age of 27, as compared to 30 years of age in men.[19,20,23] Women may have bimodal distribution of the age of onset. Typically, the female sufferer will report the initial onset of cluster headaches at age 20 and the second peak around age 50 years or later.[20,50] Furthermore, females show a significantly higher mean age of onset of the primary chronic form as compared to the episodic type.[18] The frequency of attacks per day, character of pain, location, and duration of cycles and remission seem to be equivalent to those of male sufferers. Rozen et al[21] noted a briefer duration of individual attacks in women that was approaching, but not reaching, statistical significance. Their finding was in contrast to Kudrow's study[22] that reported a longer duration of cluster attacks in women.

The associated symptoms are also similar in character and frequency in female and male cluster headache sufferers. However, women less commonly experience Horner syndrome, but complain of an equal frequency of lacrimation, rhinorrhea, and nasal congestion—suggesting less sympathetic dysfunction than found in men. However, the parasympathetic activation is similar to

male cluster sufferers.[20] Women usually have more migrainous symptoms, such as nausea and vomiting.

It has been known that migraine in women is commonly influenced by hormonal changes. Migraine is affected by the natural fluctuations of female hormones at menarche, menstruation, pregnancy, perimenopause, or menopause. Also, the administration of hormone supplement therapy (oral contraceptives, hormone replacement therapy) has a direct or indirect role in migraine development and course. The role of hormonal factors in female cluster patients is less recognized. In reviewing the literature, only a limited number of anecdotal reports identified cases in which the menstrual cycle directly coincided with cluster attacks. Rozen[51] described a woman who experienced one attack of typical cluster headache during each menstrual period. Ekbom and Waldenlind[52] analyzed 34 females with cluster headache. No relation between cluster headaches and menstruation was demonstrated in 25 of 26 women of childbearing age. Eight reported 13 pregnancies since the initial onset of cluster headache. During pregnancy, six women experienced remission of their cluster cycles. The researchers observed a significantly lower number of childbirths in cluster patients, when compared to a general population, as well as a lower parity rate. An infertility rate and premature menopause was noted in 11% of cases. Those results may be interpreted as possible hypofertility suggesting impairment in the hypothalamic-pituitary axis.

Chronic Form

The term *chronic cluster headache* describes attacks occurring for more than 1 year without remission or with a remission lasting less than 1 month.[1] Primary chronic cluster headache starts de novo, and secondary chronic cluster headache evolves from the episodic type. Some patients may alternate between chronic and episodic spontaneously or as a result of treatment.

About 4% to 26% of cluster headache patients experience the chronic form. In a series of 554 patients with cluster headache, Ekbom et al[19] identified 12% of patients with the chronic form and male-to-female ratio of 4.5:1, which is approximately the same proportion as the episodic form. In some studies conducted by headache centers and larger neurologic groups,[28,53] the higher occurrence of the chronic form can be explained by the difficult or complex patient population at those centers. The chronic form usually starts between age 30 and 35 years, with greatly reduced occurrence of onset in men after age 50. Women show a significantly higher mean age of onset of the primary chronic form as compared to the episodic type.[18] Manzoni et al[26] found that, over a 10-year follow-up period, 80% of the patients maintained the primary episodic form and 12% evolved to a secondary chronic type. Only 53% maintained the primary chronic form de novo. A small percentage may acquire the combined forms. From this study, the encouraging observation is that almost one third of their patients who started with chronic cluster headaches transitioned into the episodic form. The clinical presentation is similar to the episodic form, although the attack frequency may be higher. However, the lower limit of the attacks can be as few as once weekly, and there may be a tendency toward higher rates of diurnal attacks.

Possible predictive factors in the evolution of chronic cluster headaches appear to be late onset, occurrence of more than one cluster cycle per year, brief remission periods, and possibly heavy smoking. Head injury, increased alcohol consumption, caffeine consumption of more than six servings per day, and prolonged duration of cluster periods (more than 8 weeks) may be additional risk factors.[54]

Mechanism and Pathophysiology

The pathogenesis of cluster headache is unknown. Many methodologic problems affect the study of cluster headache patients, including differences between active cycles and remission, as well as during and between the attacks. All of these factors may play a decisive role in understanding the mechanism of cluster headache. The intensity, brevity, and behavior of patients during the cluster attack may be prohibitive to conducting investigational studies. To establish any unifying explanation for cluster headache, three major aspects of this disorder must be considered: (1) the trigeminal distribution of the pain; (2) the ipsilateral autonomic features; and (3) the periodicity of attacks.

The Source of the Pain

The location of pain is very consistent anatomically as well as laterality. Typically, the pain is located in trigeminal distribution, and in most cases, in the periocular or retro-ocular area. The fact that cluster headache developed in a patient following the ipsilateral orbital exenteration suggests the involvement of the retro-orbital structures.[55] The pain may emerge from pain fibers in the cranial nerves—anywhere along their course from the peripheral nerve endings to neurons of central endings in the brainstem or upper cervical cord. Anatomically, the intracavernous segment of the internal carotid artery and/or surrounding cavernous sinus has been suggested as a likely site of involvement. Positron emission tomography (PET) studies, conducted during the induced cluster attacks, demonstrated activation in the region of the cavernous sinus.[56] On magnetic resonance imaging (MRI), Sjaastad and Rinck,[57] however, did not find any definitive pathology in, or in the vicinity of, the cavernous sinus in 14 patients diagnosed with cluster headache. However, none of their patients were studied during the cluster attack; therefore the negative study does not exclude any changes occurring during an acute attack of cluster headache.

The cavernous sinus region is packed with various structures that are implicated in the mechanism of a cluster attack. The cavernous sinus is occupied by the sympathetic fibers to the internal carotid artery, the dural sinuses and veins, and the eye, as well as the internal carotid artery itself and the branches of its nerves. This is the site where the trigeminal, parasympathetic, and sympathetic fibers converge. An inflammatory process in the cavernous sinus and branching veins (venous vasculitis) has been suggested as causing vascular congestion and damage to local sympathetic fibers.[58] An inflammatory process as a causative factor may explain why corticosteroids are effective in aborting the cluster cycle.

Vascular and Hemodynamic Changes

In cluster headache patients, studies of cerebral blood flow (CBF) during and between cluster attacks have not demonstrated consistent results. Cluster headache is associated with the dilation of proximal tributaries of the internal carotid artery but without consistent changes in CBF. Transcranial

Doppler and CBF studies have shown, in both spontaneous and nitroglycerin-induced attacks, a bilateral decrease in middle cerebral artery blood flow velocities—with more pronounced decrease on the symptomatic side, suggesting vasodilation during the cluster attack.[59]

Waldenlind et al[60] were able to capture two spontaneous cluster attacks in one patient with magnetic resonance angiography (MRA). Imaging showed a markedly dilated, ipsilateral ophthalmic artery during both attacks with subsequent decrease of the vessel lumen after the attack. No other change in the internal carotid artery or other intracerebral arteries on either side was demonstrated. This patient had normal MRA findings during the clinical remission.

It is known that vasodilators such as alcohol, nitroglycerin, and histamine can induce an acute attack in individuals during the cluster cycle. The induced attack, however, starts after latency of at least 30 minutes. It is unclear if the vasodilatory effect of these drugs is responsible for the attack, or if it results from the activation of the trigeminal vascular system.[42]

In recent years, the discovery of the increased incidence of patent foramen ovale (PFO) with right-to-left shunt (RLS) in patients with migraine both with and without aura has created much debate. Finocchi et al[61] evaluated 40 subjects with cluster headache to identify the presence of PFO. These patients were compared to 40 subjects without headache. Seventeen cluster headache patients (42.5%) had a PFO compared to only seven control subjects (17.5%). Right-to-left shunt in PFO is a possible additional mechanism through which lower brain oxygenation may be a trigger factor. In another study, Morelli et al[62] reported on 30 patients with cluster headaches, of whom 37% documented positive transcranial Doppler contrast monitoring for evaluation of RLS. Low-grade RLS was present in 72% of the patients with positive results and 28% showed high-grade RLS. Transesophageal echocardiography confirmed the presence of PFO in all cases.

Autonomic Changes

The autonomic symptoms that accompany cluster attack are an integral part of the cluster headache. These symptoms are described in not only an anatomic vicinity of cluster headache but also are more systemic as presented by cardiovascular changes. Clinical and experimental observation demonstrates dysfunction of the autonomic nervous system. Both parasympathetic and sympathetic nerves innervate cerebral blood vessels. The cranial parasympathetic innervation is provided via the seventh cranial nerve and supplies both lacrimal and nasal mucosal glands. The activation of the cranial parasympathetic system explains lacrimation, nasal congestion, and rhinorrhea as well as vasodilation either directly or indirectly through vasoactive neuropeptides such as vasoactive intestinal polypeptide and nitric oxide synthase.

Transient or incomplete paralysis—dysfunction of the ocular sympathetic nerve supply producing a partial Horner syndrome—is most likely localized in the cavernous sinus. The impairment of sympathetic activity during the cluster periods was corroborated by the pupillometric study done by Fanciullacci et al.[63] The most likely explanation for autonomic symptoms is a combination of parasympathetic hyperactivity and sympathetic hypofunction as the result of central dysregulation.

Biochemical and Hormonal Changes

Activation of the trigeminal vascular system occurring during attacks of migraine, cluster, or chronic paroxysmal hemicrania triggers the release of vasoactive neuropeptides such as substance P, CGRP, and neurokinin A. Histamine, a potent vasoactive substance, has been considered by Horton[64] to be a major "player" in cluster headache. Anthony and Lance[65] studied serum histamine levels from 20 patients with cluster headache during 22 attacks. They found histamine levels during the headache periods in 19 of 22 attacks to be significantly higher than during the preheadache phase by a mean increase of 20.5%. Appenzeller et al,[66] from temporal skin biopsies in cluster headache patients, found evidence of mast cell degranulation and histamine release in proximity to cutaneous nerves. The clinical importance of histamine in cluster headache is still unclear because the H_1 and H_2 receptors antagonists fail to abort or reduce the cluster attack under controlled trial settings,[67] as well as in real-life clinical conditions.

As documented by D'Andrea et al,[68] dopamine platelet levels were significantly higher in cluster headache patients, in both the active period and remission phase, as compared to control subjects. During cluster headache, increased activity in the dopaminergic system results in reduced 24-prolactin production, which was found in all phases of the disease, as well as the blunted prolactin response to thyrotropin-releasing hormone that stimulates prolactin release. Dopamine also represents the main inhibiting factor of prolactin release, thus it seems that the increased dopaminergic activity in cluster headache is part of a hypothalamic derangement.

Because the majority of cluster headache patients are males, particular attention has been directed toward sex hormone level changes. Surprisingly, low plasma testosterone levels were found in a population with cluster headache suggesting hypothalamic-pituitary axis involvement. The reduced plasma levels of testosterone, however, have been found during the active cluster periods, as well as in patients diagnosed with migraine with aura,[69] and those suffering from trigeminal neuralgia and radicular pain.[70] This finding indicates that a low plasma level of testosterone is a reaction to pain rather than a causative factor. Other alterations in secretion and responses in production of luteinizing hormone, cortisol, prolactin, growth hormone, follicle-stimulating hormone, and thyroid-stimulating hormone have been observed in cluster headache.

Recently, melatonin and its rhythmic secretion have received marked attention. Melatonin release from the pineal gland is regulated from the suprachiasmatic nucleus and is closely synchronized with the hours of sleep and wakefulness. Normally, melatonin levels are low during the day. The secretion is inhibited by light via retinal-hypophyseal pathway and increases during darkness and sleep. During cluster headache cycles, 24-hour production of melatonin is reduced and the nocturnal peak in melatonin concentration is blunted.[71] These observations prompted Leone et al[72] to use melatonin in the prophylaxis of cluster headaches.

Chronobiologic Changes

The cyclic occurrence of cluster headache periods and attacks and their circannual and circadian periodicity suggest pathology or dysfunction of the biologic clock or pacemaker. In mammals, the biologic clock is located in the suprachiasmatic nucleus and its lesion leads to abnormal circadian activities.

The alterations in circadian secretion of testosterone, prolactin, melatonin, and cortisol occur simultaneously with cluster attacks. The hypothalamic activation in the area of the suprachiasmatic nucleus has been documented by PET during both spontaneous and nitroglycerin-induced cluster attacks.[56] Voxel-based morphometric analysis of MRI has documented an increase in hypothalamic volume in the inferior posterior hypothalamus,[73] which is almost identical to the area of activation seen on PET. This structural difference was seen only in cluster headache patients.

Carotid Chemoreceptor

Cluster headache attacks commonly occur at higher altitudes,[74] during sleep, and in association with sleep apnea.[75] Oxygen inhalation is highly effective in aborting attacks, which may suggest a role of hypoxemia in the pathogenesis of cluster headache. On the basis of these observations, Kudrow[74] proposed a hypothesis of a possible role of the carotid body in cluster headache. During the cluster headache attack, the disinhibition of the parasympathetic and inhibition of sympathetic systems affect the carotid body, which is the most sensitive chemoreceptor, resulting in it reacting to hypoxemia by diminished activity.

Synthesis of Pathophysiology

Cluster headache has been well defined clinically for several decades. However, its pathophysiology has been poorly understood. To understand and explain the mechanism of cluster headache, several unique features have to be considered. The following cannot be explained on the basis of only peripheral or central theory: circannual and circadian rhythm; male preponderance; strict unilaterality and the first division of trigeminal nerve distribution; extreme intensity of pain; and characteristic autonomic symptoms. Traditionally, cluster headache and migraine headache have been described as vascular headache disorders. Recent studies of the trigeminal system, brainstem, and vascular changes in the cavernous sinus support the theory that cluster headache disorders are of neurovascular origin with both peripheral and central involvement.

Cluster headache has been attributed to a structural lesion in the cavernous sinus caused by episodic local inflammation with resulting venous congestion and injury to the traversing sympathetic fibers of the intracranial internal carotid artery and its tributaries. This peripheral hypothesis is supported by findings of regional orbital vasodilatation on MRA[60] and activation in the region of the cavernous sinus by PET studies.[56] Studies of transcranial Doppler and CBF in both spontaneous and nitroglycerin-induced attacks suggest vasodilation during the cluster attack.[59] Furthermore, peripheral vascular involvement is suggested by (1) induction of cluster attacks with vasodilators such as nitroglycerin, alcohol, and histamine; (2) finding of increased levels of vasoactive neuropeptides such as CGRP and VIP during the attacks; and (3) the therapeutic effect of vasoconstrictors, including ergotamine and sumatriptan. The pain is transmitted by activation of the ophthalmic division of the trigeminal nerve and autonomic symptoms are mediated by parasympathetic activation of the seventh cranial nerve.

These peripheral changes, however, cannot explain rhythmicity, nocturnal occurrence, and hormonal irregularities in cluster patients. PET studies[56] demonstrated activation in the ipsilateral anteroventral hypothalamus, which is the area involved in the control of circadian rhythm, sleep-wake cycling, and circadian secretion of hormones. It is also the area where morphometric analysis of MRI documented an increase in hypothalamic volume.[73] On the basis of localization of morphologic and functional changes, it has been suggested that the anatomic location for the central origin of cluster headache is the dysfunctional biologic clock (pacemaker) in the hypothalamic gray area, which is also known as the suprachiasmatic nucleus. Thus vascular changes are secondary to activation of the trigeminal vascular system.

Cluster Variants

Cluster variants are a group of uncommon headache disorders that differ from cluster headache in certain features of clinical presentation and treatment response. However, these disorders share the autonomic symptoms. The International Classification of Headache Disorders[1] divides the cluster variant group into paroxysmal hemicrania with its episodic and chronic variant, and the short-lasting unilateral neuralgiform headache attacks with conjunctival injection and tearing (SUNCT).

Paroxysmal Hemicrania

Paroxysmal hemicrania is defined as a headache with at least 20 attacks of severe unilateral orbital, supraorbital, or temporal pain lasting 2 to 30 minutes accompanied by at least one of the autonomic signs and symptoms typical of cluster headache. The attacks should have a frequency of no less than five per day for more than one half of the time and are completely preventable by therapeutic doses of indomethacin. Episodic variants occur in periods with durations ranging from 7 days to 1 year, separated by pain-free periods lasting at least 1 month.

Chronic paroxysmal hemicrania (CPH) is defined as a series of attacks that occur for more than 1 year without remission or with remission lasting less than 1 month. CPH was first described in 1974 by Sjaastad and Dale.[76] CPH is a rare headache disorder and since 1974, approximately 120 cases have been described in the English-language literature. Compared to cluster headache, CPH is more prevalent in females, ranging from 62%[77] to 80% to 90%.[22] The mean age of onset is usually 30 to 40 years, with the range from 6 to 75 years of age.[77] Occasionally, head trauma may precede the onset of CPH.

The pain is strictly unilateral, mostly felt in the temporal, orbital, or maxillary regions. The quality of pain is usually described as sharp, throbbing, boring, piercing, or stabbing, and typically is rated as severe to excruciating. During the attacks, patients attempt to remain still in contrast to the erratic, sometimes bizarre, behavior of cluster patients. Alcohol or certain neck movements may precipitate attacks. Most patients experience a brief attack duration—between 10 and 15 minutes—with the maximum duration about 60 minutes. The mean attack frequency is between 3 to 13 in 24 hours, but there are reports of up to 40 attacks per day. No pronounced circadian or circannual periodicity has been observed.

By operational diagnostic criteria, the attacks should be accompanied by at least one of the following ipsilateral autonomic features: conjunctival injection, lacrimation, nasal congestion, or rhinorrhea. Other symptoms such as ptosis, photophobia, nausea, and facial flushing are not unusual. Seventy-five percent of patients do not report any coexisting primary headaches and there are no reports of familial occurrence of CPH.

The pathophysiology of CPH is unknown, but there are many similarities in biochemical, electrophysiologic, and blood flow studies with cluster headache. Increased levels of CGRP and VIP were observed in patients with CPH, with a return to normal levels after use of indomethacin.[78] Blood-flow studies and MRI studies demonstrated in some patients are identical to those with cluster headache. The autonomic symptoms are attributed to cranial parasympathetic activation. No distinct rhythmicity or hormonal changes have been observed, in contrast to cluster headache, and no findings show the activation of the hypothalamus. CPH appears to lack the central part of pathogenesis, but there is a definite peripheral neurovascular element present.

The responsiveness to indomethacin is a condition sine qua non for establishing the diagnosis. Some patients with a convincing clinical picture fail to respond to indomethacin but will be successful with other therapy. The standard treatment for CPH is indomethacin at doses of 25 to 50 mg, three times per day. Occasionally, a lower dose is sufficient for maintenance therapy. The beneficial effect usually occurs within 1 to 5 days after initiation of treatment. Anecdotal reports of successful treatment of CPH with other nonsteroidal anti-inflammatory agents, such as naproxen,[79] have been published, as have reports of other drugs such as acetazolamide[80] and verapamil.[81] Oxygen was found to be beneficial in the acute treatment of some patients.[77] Combination treatment has been recommended with gastroprotective agents to reduce the risk of gastrointestinal side effects. It should be noted that indomethacin can cause a diffuse, low-grade headache. Another adverse reaction may include pseudotumor cerebri. Instances of symptomatic or secondary CPH have also been reported. Underlying causes include vascular pathologies such as aneurysm, intracranial and extracranial space-occupying processes, inflammatory or infectious diseases, and other disorders.[82]

Short-Lasting Unilateral Neuralgiform Headache Attacks with Conjunctival Injection and Tearing

Described initially by Sjaastad et al[83] in 1989, SUNCT is a very rare primary headache syndrome characterized by short-lasting attacks of unilateral headache often accompanied by prominent lacrimation and conjunctival injection of the ipsilateral eye. To fulfill the diagnostic criteria, at least 20 attacks of periorbital or temporal headache lasting 5 to 240 seconds must be reported. Attacks occur with a frequency from 3 to 200 per day and are not attributed to another disorder. This debilitating headache disorder is noteworthy for its resistance to treatment, including indomethacin. Originally, this disorder had been observed only in males. Recently, a few SUNCT cases have been described in females, with a ratio of 3:8.[84]

Characteristically, SUNCT is described as a short-lasting episode, typically lasting less than 120 seconds, with paroxysms with a rather abrupt onset and end. The pain is severe, stabbing or burning in quality, and is associated with ipsilateral massive conjunctival injection and lacrimation. The autonomic phenomena disappear on conclusion of the attack. Patients may experience up to 30 episodes per hour with a mean frequency of 28 attacks per day.[84]

The pathogenesis of this syndrome is unknown, but SUNCT has also been reported in a few patients with posterior structure lesions such as cerebellopontine angle arteriovenous malformations and a cavernous hemangioma of the brainstem that is demonstrated on MRI.[85,86] Therefore all patients with SUNCT syndrome should undergo MRI investigation of the posterior fossa.

SUNCT syndrome is remarkably refractory to treatment. Most drugs that are effective in other short-lasting headaches are not useful. Two female patients responded to gabapentin[87,88] in doses of 800 to 900 mg per day. One male patient responded to topiramate,[89] and two other patients to lamotrigene.[90]

Testing

As with other primary headache disorders, no biologic marker or diagnostic procedure has been identified that could confirm the diagnosis of cluster headache. Diagnosis is established on the basis of a headache history. With the exception of a possible ipsilateral, partial Horner syndrome, the physical and neurologic examinations are essentially normal. In the majority of patients, the history of cluster headache is not ambiguous and once the temporal pattern has been identified, establishing the diagnosis should not be difficult.

MRI of the brain is essential in the investigation of cluster headache. An MRI should be ordered when the level of suspicion is increased as in any new case (especially when the temporal pattern is not as yet clearly defined) or in patients presenting with atypical features such as (1) atypical location; (2) prolonged duration of attacks; (3) age of onset above 50; (4) cluster headache in females; (5) migraine symptoms; (6) chronic form de novo; (7) atypical neurologic signs; and (8) an abnormal neurologic examination. Established patients with a history of typical cluster headaches should undergo scanning when manifesting new symptoms or signs, unusual pattern, globalization of headache, new onset of coexisting headache, and new neurologic or mental changes.

Conventional electrophysiologic techniques, such as electroencephalography and evoked potentials, have demonstrated nonspecific changes. Some studies of trigeminal somatosensory evoked potentials have shown abnormalities of the trigeminal pathway present in patients with cluster headache—more on the symptomatic side and during the cluster period. Cerebrospinal fluid studies in cluster headache are nonrevealing; therefore lumbar puncture is not essential in routine investigations of cluster headache.

Differential Diagnosis

The diagnosis of cluster headache is not difficult in its typical form. When a patient presents with the initial attack or a fairly new history (with the periodicity of attack still undetermined), the diagnosis may be more confusing. Similarly, the physician may be confronting a diagnostic dilemma with an elderly patient, a patient with an atypical presentation, or cluster headache in combination with migraine or rebound headache. Despite a typical clinical presentation, many patients are commonly misdiagnosed as atypical migraine, sinusitis, trigeminal neuralgia, or temporal arteritis.

The significant differences between cluster headache and migraine are presented in **Table 48.4**. Sinusitis is usually bilateral and follows rhinitis, common cold, or influenza. Pain is rarely as intense as during the cluster attack, and no periodicity or nocturnal occurrence is noted. The pain of sinusitis is rather continuous, dull, pressure-like, or pulsating and is accompanied by purulent nasal secretion. Sinusitis usually resolves with antibiotic treatment.

Trigeminal neuralgia is more common in middle-aged and older women, and is characterized by very brief attacks that last only seconds and are described as lancinating, shocklike, unilateral pain, mainly localized in the second and third divisions of the trigeminal nerve. The attacks occur several times a day without a nocturnal preponderance, and no autonomic symptoms accompany the pain. The acute attack of trigeminal neuralgia can be triggered by touching the face, brushing the teeth, or eating. However, the histamine or nitroglycerin-provocative tests are negative.

The diagnosis of temporal arteritis should be considered in any recent onset of unilateral headache in individuals older than age 50. In this disorder, a higher prevalence has been noted in females and the pain is less severe than in cluster attacks. The headache is accompanied by systemic symptoms such as night sweating, fever, malaise, polymyalgia, muscle stiffness and ache, anorexia and weight loss, and claudication pain on chewing. The diagnosis is confirmed by an elevated sedimentation rate by Westergren method and a biopsy of the temporal artery.

Tolosa-Hunt syndrome (recurrent painful ophthalmoplegia) is a rare disorder similar in certain features to cluster headache. The clinical presentation includes a headache that (1) is usually unilateral and periorbital; (2) is of lesser intensity, intermittent, or more continuous; (3) does not cycle in

Table 48.4 Characteristics of Cluster Headache versus Migraine

	Cluster Headache	Migraine
Male to female ratio	5:1	1:3
Onset of disease (mean)	25 to 30	10 to 15
Hereditary factors	Rarely	70%
Duration of cycle	2 to 3 months	No cycle
Seasonal occurrence	Spring and fall	No
Frequency of attack	1 to 2 a day and daily	Sporadic
Duration of attack	1 to 2 hours	Several hours
Onset of attack	Any time; typically 12 AM to 3 AM	Any time; typically AM or early PM
Localization of pain	Very localized, periorbital	Temporal, hemicranial, global
Rapidity of onset	Abrupt	Evolves over several hours
Unilateral headache	Almost 100%	70%
Character of pain	Boring, burning	Pulsating
Associated symptoms	Ipsilateral lacrimation, rhinorrhea, congestion, Horner syndrome	Nausea, vomiting, photophobia/ phonophobia
Aura	No	Yes
Affected by menstruation	No	Yes

clusters; and (4) has no associated autonomic symptoms. Tolosa-Hunt syndrome is caused by granulomatous infiltration of the superior ophthalmic vein and cavernous sinus.

Secondary Cluster Headaches

Primary cluster headache has no known cause. Occasionally, cluster headache results from an underlying intracranial or, less often, extracranial pathology. It may occur in 3% to 5% of cluster patients. Cluster-like or symptomatic cluster headaches should be suspected when the clinical presentation is atypical. A detailed neurologic examination and brain scanning, preferably MRI and MRA of both intracranial and extracranial carotid arteries, is essential. The level of suspicion should be increased with any deviation from typical cluster symptomatology such as (1) an absence of typical periodicity or unexplained progression to a chronic stage despite adequate treatment; (2) new onset of cluster headache after age 50; (3) change in character or location of pain; (4) prolonged attacks; (5) unresponsiveness to abortive therapy; (6) background headache; (7) new symptoms; (8) presence of neurologic signs other than Horner syndrome; and (9) onset of a new type of headache during the cluster cycle.

The origin of secondary cluster headache can be divided into three categories:

1. Intracranial
   - Tumors and other mass lesions
   - Vascular abnormalities
   - Inflammatory
2. Extracranial
3. Post-traumatic cluster headaches

Several reports have been published of pituitary adenoma, meningioma, metastatic lesion, and other intracranial space-occupying lesions associated with onset of cluster headache or change in the pattern and clinical presentation. Milos et al[91] described a 37-year-old man with a history of episodic cluster headache for 4 years when the frequency of attacks gradually increased and, incidentally, acromegaly was observed during evaluation. After resection of growth hormone–producing adenoma his cluster attacks abated. Similarly, other patients cited by Milos et al[91] experienced cluster headache associated with prolactinoma. The site of an intracranial mass can be located anywhere in relation to the midline or cavernous sinus. Tentorial meningioma in the posterior fossa,[92] parasellar meningioma, trigeminal neurinoma, sphenoidal sinus aspergilloma, and brain metastasis of lung cancer have all been reported in association with cluster headache with subsequent remission after surgical treatment of the mass.

Similarly, AV malformations, intracranial aneurysm or pseudoaneurysm, and carotid artery dissection or aneurysmal thrombosis at different locations may account for new onset or worsening of preexisting cluster headache. It is important to note that those patients usually have a normal neurologic examination.

Gentile et al[93] presented a case report of a male patient with typical cluster headache attacks who was diagnosed with multiple sclerosis. Demyelinating lesions involving the trigeminal nerve root inlet area were identified on the ipsilateral side.

Extracranial lesions, such as an upper cervical meningioma[94] and nasopharyngeal carcinoma without intracranial infiltration,[95] causing cluster symptoms cannot be explained by direct influence on the central factor of cluster headache mechanism.

Disturbance in and around the cavernous portion of the carotid artery does not account for cluster headache in patients with vertebral artery aneurysm or cervical meningioma. An explanation for such phenomena remains to be suggested.

Post-traumatic headaches manifesting with typical or atypical cluster headaches have a relatively low incidence.[96] The onset of pain is usually rapid, with a relatively brief duration. The majority of those patients have incurred only minor head injury, with or without neck trauma.

Therapy

As with management of other primary headaches, the right balance of value and risk should be found. The patient should understand the pathophysiology of cluster headache and that it is not a result of a catastrophic intracranial organic disorder. The treating physician must establish definable expectations of management with each patient, so they will understand the natural process and progress of the disease. The patient needs to responsibly participate in his or her own care. The treatment goal is relief of cluster attack and the shortening of cluster cycle. An established patient should be instructed to contact the physician's office as soon as possible at the start of the next cycle to initiate treatment within the first stage of the cluster period. Successful treatment requires symptomatic or abortive treatment and prophylactic medication (**Tables 48.5 and 48.6**). Lifestyle adjustment may help avoid precipitating attacks during the vulnerable periods. Alcohol consumption should be discouraged, although many patients will preemptively abstain because of fear of provoking the attacks. Daytime napping is not recommended. It is important to not discontinue prophylactic treatment prematurely.

Abortive Treatment

The rapid onset and brief duration of excruciating headache attacks limits the use of conventional analgesics. Therefore oral opioid-analgesics are inappropriate in the management of acute cluster attacks.

Oxygen

Oxygen was introduced as an effective treatment of acute cluster attacks by Horton[17] and has since been the standard of care for symptomatic relief. Inhaled 100% oxygen should be delivered via a nonrebreathing facial mask and inhaled slowly at a

Table 48.5 Therapy of Acute Attack

Oxygen
Sumatriptan SQ or NS
Zolmitriptan NS
DHE IM/SQ/IV
Ergotamine tartrate
Ketorolac IM
Chlorpromazine
Lidocaine viscous solution—intranasal
Cocaine—intranasal
Capsaicin—intranasal

DHE, dihydroergotamine; IM, intramuscularly; IV, intravenously; NS, nasal spray; SQ, subcutaneously.

flow rate of 7 to 8 L/min for 15 minutes, providing relief to about 70% of patients within 15 minutes.[97] The oxygen tank, reduction valve, and mask can be rented for home use and used at the beginning of an attack. The patient should be prohibited from smoking in proximity of the oxygen tank.

Sumatriptan

With the entry of the triptans to the migraine therapeutic armamentarium, new therapeutic options have been introduced in the abortive treatment of cluster attacks. In particular, subcutaneous sumatriptan with very short T_{max}, and rapid onset of action, has been effective in the symptomatic relief of cluster attacks. Complete relief within 15 minutes was achieved by 74% of patients in a placebo-controlled study and was well tolerated as reported by the Sumatriptan Cluster Headache Study Group.[98] No evidence has been reported that repetitive daily use of sumatriptan for several weeks or months would cause tachyphylaxis or rebound phenomenon. Chronic cluster patients appear to respond to sumatriptan at a lower rate. Oral sumatriptan is not recommended because of the longer time to onset of action. Sumatriptan nasal spray (20 mg) is less effective than the injectable form.

The common adverse reactions are local injection-site reaction, nausea and vomiting, chest and throat pressure sensation, and flushing. These side effects are usually temporary and short-lasting. Sumatriptan use should be limited to patients who suffer no more than one attack per day to avoid overuse. Another limiting factor to this therapy is the cost of the drug. Sumatriptan is contraindicated in patients with ischemic heart disease and uncontrolled hypertension.

Dihydroergotamine

Dihydroergotamine (DHE) is available in injectable and intranasal formulations. The intravenous administration of DHE (1 mg) rapidly aborts cluster attack within 15 minutes, but it

Table 48.6 Prophylactic Therapy

Corticosteroids
Verapamil
Lithium
Ergotamine
Topiramate
Valproic acid
Gabapentin
Doxepin
Indomethacin
Clonidine
Naratriptan
Frovatriptan
Methysergide
Baclofen
Melatonin
Occipital nerve injection
Histamine desensitization
Civamide-intranasal

is not practicable because of difficulties in intravenous self-administration. In 54 hospitalized patients with cluster headache, intravenous DHE provided complete relief in all patients during treatment.[99] The intramuscular and subcutaneous administration is slower in obtaining relief because of the time to maximal concentration, but it remains an option. Intranasal formulation is a more convenient route of treatment in ambulatory patients. However, no efficacy data are available from larger studies. DHE is contraindicated in patients with coronary or peripheral ischemic disease.

Zolmitriptan

Zolmitriptan has been used as an effective agent for acute treatment of migraine attacks. In a double-blind study,[100] 124 patients with episodic and chronic cluster headaches required at least one dose of zolmitriptan (10 mg, 5 mg, or placebo). Mild or no pain at 30 minutes was reported by 60%, 57%, and 42%, respectively. It is important to note that these rates do not approach those of oxygen or injectable sumatriptan.

Cittadini et al[101] evaluated the efficacy of intranasal zolmitriptan (ZNS) in 92 patients with acute cluster headache. Zolmitriptan intranasal 5 and 10 mg doses were effective within 30 minutes, and well tolerated in the treatment of acute cluster headache. At 30-minutes after treatment, headache relief rates were placebo (21%), ZNS 5 mg (40%), and ZNS 10 mg (62%).

Eletriptan

Zebenholzer et al[102] reported 16 patients with acute cluster headaches who were treated with eletriptan. In eight of these cases, the use of eletriptan 40 mg twice daily for 6 days significantly reduced the frequency of the cluster attacks. However, this treatment was not markedly effective in aborting the cluster headache cycle.

Lidocaine

Anesthetic action of lidocaine on the sphenopalatine ganglion was studied by Kittrelle et al[103] and showed favorable responses in aborting cluster attacks. Lidocaine 4% viscous solution is instilled in the nostril ipsilateral to the pain in a carefully positioned patient with the body supine and the head extended over the head of a bed, inclined to the side of pain. The positioning is cumbersome, especially during a painful attack, but topical effect may be effective in some patients.

Cocaine

Barre[104] reported 80% or better reduction in intensity of cluster attacks induced by nitroglycerin within 2.5 minutes in 10 of 11 patients treated with cocaine 10% solution. Cocaine was instilled by nasal dropper to the sphenopalatine foramen region. Cocaine may be a valuable adjunctive abortive therapy in a cohort of patients who are refractory to oxygen or sumatriptan or patients with cardiac ischemic disease. The risk for addiction is slight when used for a limited interval of 4 to 12 weeks.

Other Agents

Anecdotal reports indicate marginal effectiveness of other drugs in aborting cluster attacks. Ketorolac intramuscularly or intravenously, chlorpromazine intramuscularly or intravenously, diphenhydramine HCl, and valproate sodium intravenously may help reduce or abate the cluster attacks in some patients.

In an open-label trial, Rozen[105] investigated the use of olanzapine as an abortive agent in five patients with cluster headache. Olanzapine reduced the acute pain of the cluster attack by at least 80% in four of five patients, and two patients became headache free after taking the drug. Olanzapine typically alleviated pain within 20 minutes after oral dosing and treatment response was consistent across multiple-treated attacks. The only reported adverse event was sleepiness.

Subcutaneous administration of octreotide, a somatostatin analog, was studied in two small, randomized, double-blind trials and was demonstrated to be moderately effective in the treatment of acute cluster headache attacks. A significant difference was noted when comparing octreotide to placebo. Fifty-two percent of the study subjects were able to totally abort or reduce the cluster attack to mild within 30 minutes of treatment with octreotide (100 mcg).[106]

Prophylactic Treatment

The purpose of prophylactic therapy is to reduce the frequency, duration, and severity of attacks, and interrupt the cycle of cluster headache. The prophylactic treatment should be initiated at the onset of a new cycle simultaneously with symptomatic therapy. The patient should remain on the prophylactic regimen for at least 2 to 4 weeks after the last cluster attack to ensure that treatment is not discontinued prematurely within the cycle. Discontinuation of treatment should be gradual. Continuation of therapy beyond the cycle will not guarantee prevention of future cluster cycles. The next new cycle should be treated at the beginning, preferably within the first week.

Corticosteroids

Corticosteroids are effective inductive agents in suppressing attacks at the beginning of a cluster cycle during the interval when the standard prophylactic therapy is taking effect. This method of treatment was introduced by Horton[64] in 1952. The mechanism of action is not known. In appropriate doses, the corticosteroids usually provide relief within 1 to 2 days. Kudrow[12] reported significant relief in 77% of 77 patients with episodic cluster headache and partial relief in another 12% who initiated treatment with prednisone 40 mg, gradually tapering the dose over the course of 3 weeks. Treatment with prednisone is usually initiated with 60 to 80 mg doses per day for 2 to 3 days followed by 10 mg decrements every 2 to 3 days.

Dexamethasone 8 mg per day for 2 weeks, followed by 4 mg a day for 1 week, may be used as an alternative. During the tapering of the corticosteroids, some cluster attacks may recur. Therefore simultaneously with inductive therapy, other prophylactic agents should be initiated. Steroids are less effective in chronic cluster headache. Long-term use of these drugs should be avoided because of the potential for frequent, well-known adverse reactions.

Verapamil

The mechanism of action of the calcium channel blockers in preventing cluster headache is not clear. Possible modes of action of verapamil in the hypothalamus are most likely caused by an effect on the low- or high-voltage-activated Ca^{2+} channels.[107] Verapamil is the most commonly used of these agents and is the most effective. However, at least 1 week of treatment is required before the drug demonstrates efficacy. Verapamil was first reported to be effective in cluster headaches in 1983.[108] The initial dose ranges from 240 to 360 mg, but some patients may require up to 600 mg/day. Up to 80% of patients with episodic cluster headache report a significant reduction in the number of the acute attacks, as well as the consumption of analgesics within 2 weeks of treatment.[109] In a subsequent larger study involving 48 patients,[110] 69% of the patients improved by more than 75%. The average dose for episodic cluster was 354 mg/day and 572 mg/day for the chronic form.

Verapamil is usually well tolerated although constipation is a frequent and unpleasant side effect. A high dose of the agent may cause hypotension, bradycardia, or other cardiac abnormalities; therefore patients should be monitored carefully. The prescribing physician should be aware of any potential drug-drug interaction.

Several other calcium channel blockers have been tried in cluster headache prophylaxis, including nifedipine and nimodipine. In small trials,[108] both nifedipine (at doses of 30 to 180 mg/day) and nimodipine (at doses of 120 mg/day) proved to be useful in the episodic and the chronic forms of cluster headache.

Lithium Carbonate

The first line of treatment of chronic cluster headache is lithium carbonate. The reason for introducing lithium to cluster treatment during the 1970s was that cyclic features of cluster headache somewhat reminded an observer of manic-depressive disorder. Multiple trials have been undertaken that studied the effectiveness of lithium in both episodic and especially chronic forms of cluster headache.

In 1977, Kudrow[111] reported a marked and sustained improvement in 27 of 28 patients with unresponsive chronic cluster headache. The treatment was started at doses of 300 to 600 mg/day and increased by the end of the fourth week to 600 to 900 mg/day. A dramatic response was seen in many patients during the first week of treatment. Ekbom[112] described immediate partial remission in eight patients with chronic cluster headache. The average headache index improved within 2 weeks by 85.3%. In contrast, only 4 of 11 patients with episodic cluster responded with almost complete suppression of the cluster cycle.

A larger series evaluating 90 patients with episodic and chronic cluster headache (68 and 22, respectively) showed similar results.[113] One half of patients with the chronic type showed a definite, constant improvement both short- and long-term. Of the 68 patients with episodic cluster, 26 proved highly responsive, 26 were partially responsive, and 16 were refractory to treatment. However, a double-blind crossover study compared verapamil 360 mg/day with lithium 900 mg/day in 30 chronic cluster patients and failed to show a superiority for lithium.[114]

The mechanism of action of lithium in cluster headache is unknown. Lithium has no measurable effect on cerebral hemodynamics.[115] It is conceivable that lithium has a central neurogenic effect influencing the biologic clock in the area of the suprachiasmatic nucleus.

The initial starting dose of lithium carbonate is 300 mg three times per day, or 450 mg of the sustained-release form once or twice per day. Lithium has a narrow therapeutic window and the serum concentration ranges between 0.4 and 0.8 mEq/L, which is effective for cluster headache and is usually lower than that required for treatment of bipolar disorder. The serum concentration should be measured at least 6 hours after the last dose and should not exceed 1.0 mEq/L.

Side effects include fatigue, tremor and other cerebellar symptoms, thirst, edema, weight gain, polyuria, and abdominal discomfort. Renal and thyroid function should be monitored on a regular basis. The concomitant use of diuretics and NSAIDs is not recommended because it may increase the serum concentration of lithium to toxic levels.

Ergotamine Derivates

Ergotamine has lost its popularity with the introduction of sumatriptan. Ergotamine is useful in recurrent and predictable attacks, when it can be used as a targeted prophylaxis. Nocturnal attacks can be prevented by use of ergotamine tartrate 2 mg at bedtime. However, triptans as abortive therapy must be avoided. Ergotamine can be used in a combination preparation with caffeine or belladonna and phenobarbital. in approximately 80% of cluster headaches. Kudrow[12] documented benefit from ergotamine administered by various routes. Adding ergotamine to the regimen of lithium and/or verapamil increases the response to this combination. The vasoconstrictive effect of ergotamine is believed to be one of the mechanisms of action.

Adverse reactions are fairly common and include nausea and vomiting, numbness, itching, and pain in the extremities. Contraindications to ergotamine include peripheral vascular disease, coronary artery disease, uncontrolled hypertension, fever, sepsis, pregnancy, and within 24 hours of using triptans.

Methysergide

Methysergide, a semisynthetic ergot derivative, is no longer available in the United States. In the pretriptan era, methysergide was a staple in the management of cluster headache. Methysergide is a serotonin antagonist with antihistaminic and anticholinergic actions. The efficacy of methysergide in cluster treatment has been reported in a larger series by Friedman and Elkind,[116] who treated 54 patients with cluster headache. The beneficial effect of 6 to 8 mg/day ranged from 50% to 70%, comparable to that of verapamil or lithium.

Methysergide was used extensively after its introduction as a prophylactic agent until the discovery of its tendency to cause retroperitoneal fibrosis. We do not know if the fibrotic reaction is dose-related or idiosyncratic. Patients with lung or connective-tissue diseases are more likely to develop this complication. Other side effects include leg pain, nausea, peripheral edema, paresthesias, and chest pain. To reduce the incidence of fibrotic reaction, a therapeutic window for 2 or more months is recommended after 5 to 6 months of continuous therapy. Periodic imaging of the chest and abdominal cavity and monitoring renal function are recommended.

Valproic Acid

Valproic acid, a gamma-aminobutyric acid (GABA) agonist successfully used in migraine headache, has been also proved to be efficacious in cluster headache prophylaxis. An open-label study in 15 patients confirmed a 73% favorable response rate to valproic acid at doses of 600 to 2000 mg/day.[117]

In another open-label trial,[118] 26 patients with episodic or chronic cluster headache were treated with divalproex sodium (equal proportions of valproic acid and valproate sodium) at a mean daily dose of 850 mg. The mean decrease of headache frequency in chronic cluster for a 28-day period was 53.9%, and 58.6% in the episodic type. Common side effects may include hand tremor, nausea, weight gain, and hair loss.

Topiramate

Anecdotal reports have described the effectiveness of topiramate in both episodic and chronic cluster headache.[119] Topiramate, an antiepileptic drug extensively used in migraine prophylaxis, at doses of 50 to 125 mg/day produced rapid improvement with remission occurring 1 to 3 weeks into the treatment. A larger prospective trial involving 26 patients with episodic or chronic cluster headache confirmed the beneficial effect of topiramate in prophylactic treatment of cluster headache.[120] In 15 patients, the remission was induced at a mean time of 14 days, but in 7 patients, remission was obtained within the first week of treatment.

The mechanism of action is not known, but may include enhancement of GABA antinociceptive property and blockage of voltage-dependent Na^+ channels. Adverse reactions of topiramate include appetite suppression, weight loss, cognitive impairment, paresthesias, taste distortion, and increased risk for renal calculi. These last three side effects are explained by the action of topiramate as a carbonic anhydrase inhibitor.

Gabapentin

In an open study,[121] eight patients with intractable cluster headache received gabapentin at the daily dose of 900 mg. All patients were headache-free at a maximum of 8 days after starting the treatment. Patients with the episodic type remained headache-free at 3 months after discontinuation of therapy. Patients with chronic cluster were headache-free during the 4 months after initiation of treatment while receiving this medication.

The mechanism of action of gabapentin, an anticonvulsant, is not known. However, it is speculated that gabapentin reduces pain messages by suppressing glutamate activity and enhancing GABA within the central nervous system. Side effects may include fatigue and light-headedness.

Indomethacin

Although some trigeminal-autonomic headaches respond in an absolute manner to indomethacin, no large studies are available for evaluating this medication for prophylactic treatment of cluster headache. Only anecdotal evidence has been reported to suggest that indomethacin may reduce the frequency and intensity of cluster attacks.

Other Drugs
CLONIDINE

Clonidine, an alpha$_2$-adrenergic presynaptic agonist, regulates the sympathetic tone in the central nervous system. The efficacy of clonidine at doses of 5 to 7.5 mg delivered transdermally over 1 week was evaluated in a study involving 13 patients with both episodic and chronic forms of cluster headache.[122] The mean weekly frequency of attacks decreased from 17.7 to 8.7; the pain intensity measured on a visual scale (from 0 to 100) decreased from 98 to 41. The duration decreased from 59 to 34 minutes. In many patients, the beneficial effect of clonidine started during the first 24 hours of treatment. Possible explanation of action is central sympathetic inhibition. High doses of clonidine may cause hypotension, dizziness, fatigue, drowsiness, dry mouth, and constipation.

BACLOFEN

Baclofen, a GABA$_B$ analog, has been shown to possess antinociceptive activity and is used primarily as an antispasmodic agent in multiple sclerosis, as well as in some cases of painful neuralgias and neuropathy. Hering-Hanit and Gadoth[123] reported baclofen, at the daily dose of 15 to 30 mg in three divided doses, to be safe and effective in prevention of cluster headaches. Within 1 week of treatment, 12 of 16 patients reported the cessation of attacks.

TIZANIDINE

Tizanidine, a central muscle relaxant, is structurally related to clonidine and has a similar mechanism of action. D'Alessandro[124] used tizanidine as concomitant therapy in five patients refractory to treatment. The medication, administered daily at 12 to 24 mg in divided doses, proved to be effective in abating attacks in three patients. One patient reported marked improvement, and only one patient failed to respond. Tizanidine is generally well tolerated, but sleepiness, fatigue, vivid dreams, and dry mouth may be unpleasant side effects for some patients.

CHLORPROMAZINE

Occasionally, use of chlorpromazine (a phenothiazine) has been tried to reduce and prevent cluster attacks. Caviness and O'Brien[125] used chlorpromazine at doses ranging from 75 to 700 mg/day. Twelve of thirteen patients with cluster headache reported complete relief within 2 weeks of treatment. However, the authors suspected that some improved patients underwent spontaneous remission. Side effects may be common and include tiredness, drowsiness, stupor, restlessness, agitation, dystonia, tardive dyskinesia, and jaundice.

DOXEPIN

Doxepin, a tricyclic antidepressant with high affinity to H$_1$ receptors, has occasionally been used as adjunctive therapy in chronic cluster headache. The usual dose is 25 to 100 mg at night. Drowsiness, dry mouth, urinary retention, and weight gain may affect patient compliance.

NARATRIPTAN

Naratriptan, a 5-HT$_{1B,1D}$ agonist, is an effective and well-tolerated antimigraine agent with a relatively long half-life (6 hours). Several authors reported on the effectiveness of naratriptan in cluster headache prophylaxis.[126–128] Naratriptan was used as adjunctive treatment in 11 refractory cluster patients at doses of 2.5 mg at bedtime or twice a day. Complete cessation or marked improvement has been reported in seven of these patients. Patients tolerated daily use of naratriptan over longer intervals without clinically significant side effects. While a patient is on naratriptan, other triptan or ergotamine preparations including DHE are contraindicated.

CYPROHEPTADINE

Anecdotally, cyproheptadine, an antihistamine, has been used in doses of 4 mg three times a day to prevent cluster headaches. Drowsiness, increased appetite, and weight gain are common side effects.

CLOMIPHENE

Clomiphene citrate is a synthetic nonsteroidal, ovulatory stimulant, which alters hypothalamic estrogen receptors, thus producing an increase in luteinizing hormone and follicle-stimulating hormone levels with subsequent increase in testosterone production. Rozen[129] reported a case of a refractory chronic cluster patient who noted significant improvement resulting from treatment with clomiphene 50 mg per day.

PRAMIPEXOLE

Pramipexole is a nonergoline dopamine agonist with selective activity at dopamine receptors at D2, D3, and D4 receptor subtypes. In a case report by Palmieri,[130] a patient with a 20-year history of chronic cluster headaches became headache-free following therapy with pramipexole.

GREATER OCCIPITAL NERVE BLOCKADE

Injection of 1% lidocaine (3 mL) and triamcinolone (40 mg) to the greater occipital nerve (GON) ipsilateral to the side of cluster headache in 14 patients provided moderate-to-good response in 9 patients, and 5 had no response.[131] GON blockade may offer an alternative in transitional cluster therapy for some patients.

CAPSAICIN

Capsaicin, a derivate of homovanillic acid found in hot peppers, has been shown to cause the release of substance P (SP) and other neuropeptides from primary sensory nociceptive neurons. The first exposure to capsaicin activates these neurons that antidromically generate neurogenic inflammation, clinically causing an intense burning-pain sensation, local flushing, and edema. Desensitization occurs after the first exposure, with the neurons becoming less sensitive to stimulation including capsaicin itself. Repeated application of capsaicin depletes the nerve terminals of SP. Capsaicin cream applied topically in the nostril ipsilateral to the pain twice daily for 7 days significantly reduces headache intensity.[132] A drawback to this treatment is the unpleasant, burning, and painful sensation produced at the beginning of the application. Not every patient is willing to endure the initial pain, and therefore this agent has never gained widespread acceptance in the treatment of cluster headache.

CIVAMIDE

Civamide, a synthetic isomer of capsaicin, has been found to be significantly more potent at depleting SP and CGRP than capsaicin, and is less irritating. The release of CGRP and SP results in dilation of intracranial arteries and an increase of vascular permeability and perivascular inflammatory response. The effect of intranasal civamide has been examined in the double-blind study conducted by the Intranasal Civamide Study Group in multiple centers in the United States.[133] Eighteen cluster headache subjects who received civamide and 10 who received placebo over a 7-day treatment period and a 20-day post-treatment period showed a significantly greater percent decrease in the number of headaches from baseline to post-treatment during days 1 through 7.

MELATONIN

Some authors have found melatonin to be moderately effective as a preventive treatment in both episodic and chronic cluster headache.[72,134] The treatment is based on circadian rhythmicity and observation of reduced serum melatonin levels in patients during a cluster period.[71] Another group did not find any benefit in adding melatonin as adjunctive therapy in patients with cluster headache who had incomplete relief of their headaches on standard therapy.[135]

HISTAMINE DESENSITIZATION

Some patients with chronic cluster headaches do not respond to standard treatment and require a course of intravenous histamine desensitization. Histamine desensitization was introduced by Horton[6] in 1941, who recommended it as the treatment of choice for chronic cluster headache. He noted: "Histamine treatment is as specific for this syndrome as insulin is in treatment of diabetes mellitus."

The idea behind this treatment was a speculative pathogenesis of cluster symptoms, to be an "anaphylactoid reaction at the cellular level" toward histamine. To increase tolerance against endogenous histamine, Horton desensitized his patients by giving increasing doses of histamine subcutaneously. This suggestion was based on similar desensitization treatment for allergies. The intravenous route of histamine desensitization has also been found to be beneficial in the treatment of intractable chronic cluster headache.[136] However, enthusiasm for this treatment has gradually diminished. It requires hospitalization for several days and, in our current atmosphere of restricted use of inpatient resources, the treatment has been abandoned almost totally. At the Diamond Headache Clinic, the only center in the United States where this treatment is still provided, the report from 1986 indicates at least a 75% reduction in cluster attacks in 25 of 64 patients. All but 9 patients demonstrated a partial reduction in their cluster attacks.[137] On the initial day of treatment, histamine is administered intravenously (2.75 mg histamine phosphate diluted in 250 mL of normal saline) followed by 5.5 mg of histamine phosphate in each consecutive dose. The infusion rate starts at 10 mL/hr and the rate is increased hourly up to 120 mL/hr. The rate of infusion is based on the patient's tolerability. Two to three doses are administered daily to a total dose of 110 mg. Side effects include flushing, nausea, cough, abdominal discomfort, and headache. These reactions can be limited by reducing the rate of infusion.

Surgical Management of Cluster Headache

A small percentage of patients with chronic cluster headache do not respond to pharmacologic therapy and may benefit from surgical treatment. This form of intervention should be reserved for patients refractory to both outpatient and inpatient therapy, when a combination of different effective medications has failed, or in patients with a contraindication to pharmacologic treatment. Surgical management should be considered only in patients with chronic cluster headache who suffer from strictly unilateral headaches. This selection should

be absolute to avoid recurrence on the contralateral side after surgery in those whose attacks alternate sides. Patients with atypical cluster features should be excluded. Surgical candidates should have a stable psychologic profile so as not to aggravate or trigger major depressive episodes with suicidal ideation in case of treatment failure.

Although a variety of surgical procedures have been used (**Table 48.7**) in the treatment of chronic cluster headache, these options have yielded only mixed results. Among neurosurgeons,[138] the consensus is that no one procedure provides consistent long-lasting relief; radiofrequency lesion and nerve avulsion are reasonable first-stage procedures. Procedures that carry the least risk should be implemented before more complicated surgeries. Most surgical techniques have been directed toward the sensory trigeminal system or parasympathetic fibers of the nervus intermedius, the greater superficial petrosal nerve, or the sphenopalatine ganglion.

The temporary benefit of lidocaine instillation anesthesia or cocainization of sphenopalatine ganglion has produced a more permanent procedure to provide long-lasting relief than has sphenopalatine ganglion nerve block. However, sphenopalatine gangliectomy or chemical or physical destruction of the ganglion failed to have enduring results. Because of their high unpredictability, these procedures are rarely performed.

Surgical intervention directly involving the trigeminal nerve such as nerve sectioning of the first branch, chemical denervation (using local anesthetic, alcohol, glycerol, or phenol), peripheral nerve avulsion, and trigeminal root section via the posterior fossa have not shown adequate and prolonged relief than has sphenopalatine ganglion nerve block. Partial or complete retrogasserian sensory root lesion seems to be more effective. Nervus intermedius rhizotomy seems to be another approach that may benefit some cluster sufferers. The nervus intermedius relays parasympathetic impulses that mediate most of the autonomic features accompanying the cluster attack and the vasodilation of the external carotid arterial tree.[139] Seven of Sachs'[140,141] nine patients obtained relief from resection of the nerve for several months to years. Complications related to this surgery include hearing and taste loss, vertigo, and facial palsy.

Resection of the greater superficial petrosal nerve on the symptomatic side, performed by Gardner et al[142] in 26 patients with unilateral headache, offered fair to excellent relief in 75%. However, only one half of these patients had cluster headaches. Watson et al[138] were unsuccessful in only one of four

Table 48.7 Surgical Management of Chronic Cluster Headache

INVOLVING SENSORY TRIGEMINAL NERVE

Chemical denervation of the supraorbital and infraorbital nerves
Avulsion of supraorbital, infraorbital, supratrochlear nerve
Chemical denervation of the Gasserian ganglion
Retrogasserian glycerol injection
Radiofrequency ganglio-rhizolysis
Trigeminal root section
Gamma knife radiosurgery

INVOLVING THE AUTONOMIC PATHWAYS

Lesion of the greater superficial petrosal nerve
Lesion of the nervus intermedius
Sphenopalatine ganglion blockade

cases using this procedure. An effort to improve the rate of success in surgical intervention led to different combined procedures such as section of the greater superficial petrosal nerve or nervus intermedius and neurolysis of the sensory root of the trigeminal nerve.

Microvascular decompression of the trigeminal nerve, with or without section of the nervus intermedius, was reported to be effective in chronic cluster headache by Lovely et al.[143] The purpose of the procedure is to remove a vascular loop that is compressing the nerve. In 50% of 30 initial procedures, greater than 90% pain relief was achieved and 50% or greater relief was reported in 73.3% of patients.

Gamma knife is a noninvasive stereotactic radiosurgery that applies gamma radiation at the trigeminal root entry zone. The technique has been used somewhat anecdotally and has a low complication rate. The procedure appears to be effective initially but has a high recurrence rate.

More recent surgical methods seem to be more encouraging and safer. The radiofrequency wave thermocoagulation of the gasserian ganglion performed via percutaneous access to selectively destruct poorly myelinated pain fibers has low morbidity and mortality rates and can be repeated if pain returns. Onofrio and Campbell[144] reported excellent results using this technique in 54% of their 26 patients during a 10-month to 5-year follow-up period. Similar results were shown by Mathew and Hurt[145] over 6 to 63 months of observation in 27 patients. The procedure is relatively safe, has a low recurrence rate, and a low mortality rate. A small percentage of patients undergoing percutaneous radiofrequency ganglio-rhizolysis may experience mild complications such as infection, damage to adjacent structures, temporary trigeminal motor weakness, anesthesia dolorosa, keratitis, and postoperative herpes simplex in the denervated area. However, these effects do not outweigh the benefit from the surgery. Corneal and cutaneous anesthesia within the first and second branch of the trigeminal nerve is essential if relief of the pain of cluster attack is to be achieved.

Hypothalamic Stimulation

The observation of increased activity of the posterior hypothalamic region during spontaneous and nitroglycerin-induced cluster headaches prompted some investigators to stimulate that region to alleviate the pain or to terminate chronic cluster headache. Several studies performing deep brain stimulation (DBS) of the posterior hypothalamus have demonstrated promising results. Leone et al[146] reported long-term cessation of cluster attacks in more than 12 patients with chronic, drug-refractory cluster headache. Continuous hypothalamic DBS achieved by stereotactically implanted electrodes-stimulators was demonstrated to be effective, safe, and tolerable alternative therapy in treatment of intractable, refractory, chronic cluster headache. Other investigators documented similar results.[147]

Conclusion

Cluster headache, although a relatively rare headache disorder, has a special place in headache pathophysiology and management. Establishing the diagnosis is facilitated if the physician is cognizant about the disorder. Most patients respond to treatment and if therapy is initiated within the first week of the cycle, the prognosis is excellent. Education, especially for a newly diagnosed patient, is important for the patient to understand the origin and natural course of the disorder. For the individual experiencing a first-ever cluster cycle, imaging provides significant reassurance. Appropriate management of patients with cluster headache should include flexible availability for a return visit in case of a new cycle. Treatment should be undertaken without waiting for more than a few days.

In the last decade, major steps have been reached in research and treatment of migraine headache, particularly with the introduction of triptans. Unfortunately, lack of interest and especially funding in cluster research—on both a basic level and within the pharmaceutical industry—has had a negative impact on the genesis of cluster headache treatment.

References

Full references for this chapter can be found on www.expertconsult.com.

Medication Overuse Headache

Roger Cady, Curtis P. Schreiber, and Kathleen Farmer

Most intriguing, yet often frustrating, are patients with daily or near-daily headaches who insist they need daily analgesic in order to function. The quantity of analgesic they require is often staggering, and they frequently are seeking medical advice in hopes of being prescribed an even more potent analgesic medication. There is often a history spanning years to decades of increasingly frequent severe, disabling headaches and a concomitant history of escalating analgesic use. Confounding this clinical scenario is that patients assure the medical provider that they only seek medication in order to function effectively and that they have had experiences where the medication was unavailable and have endured severe, unrelenting headaches that often result in repeated visits to the emergency department. Reviewing these patients' histories, one frequently finds that they have multiple medical providers.

The clinical dilemmas are obvious. Are these patients overtly seeking drugs? Are they accurately conveying to us that without their daily use of medications, headache would prevent them from functioning? Or is the medication itself maintaining the headache? What are the therapeutic and management options for these chronic headache patients?

Definition of Medication Overuse

The underlying premise of medication overuse headache is that acute medication used to treat migraine or tension-type headache can over time in susceptible individuals escalate and maintain the frequency and disability of the headache pattern. Essentially, episodic primary headache is transformed into a chronic headache pattern with acute medication being the primary catalyst for this process. The science supporting this phenomenon is weak at best, but the clinical observation that frequent use of acute medication associates with frequent episodes of headache is obvious. Further, numerous clinical studies have observed that withdrawal of the offending medication results in improvement of the underlying headache pattern. Rarely, however, is medication withdrawal the only intervention provided to these patients.

In 2004 the International Headache Society (IHS) defined *medication overuse headache* as a pattern of greater than or equal to 15 days of primary headache per month for at least 3 months associated with predefined quantities of specific acute medication usage. In the IHS taxonomy, overuse of acute medications was divided into medication usages of greater than 15 days a month for 3 months for simple analgesics and caffeine-containing combination analgesics. For opioids, butalbital, and triptans, the threshold was placed at 10 days per month. These quantities were determined by expert consensus.

In its original construct of medication overuse headache the concept of improvement after withdrawal of medication was a critical component of diagnosis. However, this criterion has been dropped in favor of the clinical observation that the underlying headache pattern has worsened since the use of the offending medication was initiated. Thus the term *probable medication overuse headache*, which was used until improvement was documented, has been dropped and quantity limits of various medications imposed in its place.

Section IV—Regional Pain Syndromes

Complicating matters has been the evolving definition of chronic migraine and the newer concept of intractable migraine. At the heart of this debate is the fact that there is not clear agreement on what constitutes either of these diagnostic constructs. Thus it is difficult to quantity which IHS-defined headache is worsening and whether or not this is related to medication or the disease of headache itself or both.

Classification of Chronic Headache

The 2004 edition of The International Classification of Headache Disorders of the IHS for the first time acknowledged chronic migraine.[1] Chronic forms of tension-type headache and cluster had been included in the 1988 classification system. *Chronic migraine* was defined as headaches fulfilling IHS criteria for episodic migraine on 15 or more days per month over a period of at least 3 months and without evidence of medication overuse. Since 2004 several attempts have been made to refine the diagnostic criteria since it was quickly realized that the original definition was overly restrictive and would preclude research of chronic migraine.

In 2006 an appendix definition of chronic migraine was introduced suggesting a headache frequency of 15 or greater days of "headache"[2] but only 8 or more needed to fulfill IHS criteria for migraine. In addition, response to migraine-specific medication (triptan or ergotamine) used by the patient before development of all necessary IHS diagnostic symptoms was considered evidence of the treated headache being a migraine. Zeeberg et al[3] recently published a study comparing these two diagnostic definitions with a third requiring only 4 days of IHS-defined migraine and concluded that the 2006 appendix diagnosis was the most applicable to clinic populations.

Chronic tension-type headache was defined as headaches fulfilling criteria for tension-type headache occurring more than 15 days per month for greater than 3 months without evidence of analgesic overuse. This diagnosis is complicated, and the Spectrum study demonstrated that tension-type headache responded to triptan medication, at least in migraine patients, and suggested that common biologic mechanisms were shared in both primary headache types.

Arguably, the most significant advancement in the latest IHS revision was the inclusion of chronic migraine and medication overuse headache in the diagnostic taxonomy (**Table 49.1**). In acknowledging chronic migraine, the IHS indirectly supported clinical observations that episodic migraine can evolve into chronic headache, thus lending credibility to a potential transformational process for migraine. Further, symptomatic medications were considered a possible factor in maintaining chronic primary headache patterns. The IHS taxonomy expanded the association of chronic headache and medication overuse by providing a diagnosis for each headache syndrome that is related to a specific medication that is being overused (**Table 49.2**). However, because many patients overuse multiple medications and different quantities each month, it makes this aspect of the classification cumbersome in clinical practice. Even more confusing, the classification system also continued to recommend independent diagnosis of each episode of headache a patient experiences—thus necessitating the use of multiple diagnoses when more than one type of primary headache can be defined in an individual patient. Patients are the source of historical information, and their belief (often fostered by past misunderstandings of primary headaches) in

Table 49.1 International Headache Society Diagnostic Criteria for Chronic Migraine and Medication Overuse Headache

MIGRAINE

1. Migraine headache occurring on 15 or more days per month for more than 3 months in the absence of medication overuse and not attributable to other disorder

   2. Headache has at least two of the following four characteristics:
   Unilateral location
   Pulsating quality
   Moderate-to-severe intensity
   Aggravated with activity

3. During the headache, at least one of the following:
   Nausea and/or vomiting
   Photophobia and phonophobia

MEDICATION OVERUSE HEADACHE

1. Headache greater than 15 days per month that has developed or markedly worsened during medication overuse

2. Headache resolves or reverts to its previous pattern with 2 months of discontinuing the overused medication

Table 49.2 Quantities of Selected Medications Associated with Medication Overuse Headaches

Ergotamine intake 10 or more days a month for >3 months

Triptan intake on 10 or more days a month for >3 months

Simple analgesic intake on 15 or greater days per month for >3 months

Opioid intake on 10 or more days a month for >3 months

Combination medications on 10 or more days a month for >3 months

Headache Classification Committee of the International Headache Society: The international classification of headache disorders, *Cephalalgia* 24(suppl 1):8, 2004.

unique etiologies to different clinical presentations of primary headache clearly influences symptom description provided to clinicians and consequently the diagnostic labels medical providers give to patients. This diagnostic confusion often made clinical application of the IHS criteria burdensome in clinical practice. Further, the IHS taxonomy continued to state that clinicians should use the criteria to diagnose each attack of headache and not use the diagnostic labels provided by the IHS to define patients.

In 2006 diagnostic criteria provided as an appendix to the 2004 classification defined *chronic migraine* as 15 or greater days of headache per month with at last 8 fulfilling IHS criteria for migraine 1.1 or 1.2 or responding to migraine-specific therapies used before all IHS symptoms have developed.[2] The other days of headache can fulfill diagnostic criteria for probable migraine or tension-type headache. This represents a clear departure from the operational rules of earlier taxonomy schemes as it defines patients with a pattern of headache rather than dissecting out individual headache diagnoses. This was necessitated by the restrictive nature of the original criteria and concern that research could not be conducted on chronic migraine unless the criteria were more clinically relevant. The need for medication overuse headache to be excluded continues to be required, although recent studies suggest that some preventive medications may be effective without discontinuation of overused acute medications.[4]

Complicating diagnostic issues is the developing concept of intractable migraine. This diagnostic concept is not a formal part of the IHS criteria, but considerable interest has recently developed in an attempt to define a group of patients refractory to pharmacologic treatment. Thus when evaluating a patient with chronic migraine, physicians are confronted with several operational dilemmas. Medication overuse headache is defined based on frequent headaches associated with defined quantities of medication use per month, such as 10 days of triptan use or 15 days of combination analgesics. These quantities were established by consensus criteria, and there is no scientific basis for the quantities that the IHS determined to define medication overuse. Nor is there any recognition of biologic differences in patient populations. This is akin to defining alcoholism solely on the basis of quantity of alcohol consumed and holding the entire population to this definition; there is no requirement for improvement with medication withdrawal. This makes it nearly impossible to differentiate a patient with intractable primary headache from medication overuse headache if that patient has a history of "overusing" acute medication in the past. It is hoped that these diagnostic inconsistencies will be corrected as sound science emerges.

The Debate Over the Role of Analgesics in Patients with Analgesic Overuse

The idea that substances or withdrawal of substances may complicate or provoke headaches has been suggested for many years. In 1940 Dreisbach[5] reported caffeine withdrawal headache; in 1949 Wolfson and Graham[6] reported ergotamine tolerance and withdrawal headache; and in 1951 Peters and Horton[7] coined the term *rebound headache* referring to the severe headache that occurred when "vasoactive substances" were withdrawn from patients with underlying headache disorders. However, it was not until 1982 that Kudrow[8] and concurrently Isler[9] published studies implicating overuse of commonly employed analgesics used in treating primary headache disorders as a factor in maintaining primary headache patterns. Further, withdrawal of the offending analgesic resulted in rebound headache and, with time, a reduction in headache frequency after the offending medications were discontinued.

In Kudrow's study, a population of 200 patients with daily headaches was divided into two groups. Group 1 was prescribed amitriptyline in addition to daily symptomatic medication; group 2 discontinued daily symptomatic medication before using amitriptyline for prophylaxis. The mean improvement of group 1 was 20% as compared with a mean improvement of 72% for group 2. This study noted that it could take up to 3 months for improvement to occur. Isler's study of 235 patients, many of whom were overusing ergotamine, reported that those using more than 30 tablets a month suffered twice as many headaches as those using less than 30 tablets a month.

Mathew et al,[10] in a retrospective analysis, expanded the concept of chronic headache significantly by characterizing a clinical transformation or "evolutive" process by which patients with primary headaches transitioned from an episodic to a chronic headache condition. This landmark study noted the frequently associated analgesics overused by the chronic headache

population and it described several important comorbid conditions observed to be associated with this patient population. In addition, the different medications and the quantities of use of these various analgesics were reported. Thus an important paradigm shift occurred: from the current IHS approach of clinical analysis of each episode of headache to an approach of making diagnoses based on the evolution of the headache pattern over time. This transition, although intuitive to many clinicians, remains an enigma to the academic community that was sought to provide to regulatory agencies worldwide a diagnostic classification system for use in clinical trials of medications.

Later, Mathew et al[11] observed that patients with analgesic-dependent headache patterns were less responsive to both preventive medications and other abortive medications unless the offending medications were first discontinued. He used the terms *evolutive* and *transformational migraine* to describe the observed changes in the headache pattern in this patient population.

In 1985 Rapoport et al[12] published findings on 70 patients with daily headaches using 14 or more analgesics per week. They reported that with discontinuation of the offending analgesic, 66% had improved significantly within 1 month and that 81% had improved within 2 months. The use of either amitriptyline or cyproheptadine significantly added to the success reported in this patient population. These studies demonstrated that successful patient responses were attained by withdrawing frequently used analgesics. This research expanded the concept that symptomatic medications were mechanistically an important component in the etiology of chronic headaches.

Despite these important studies, the fact that few effective nonanalgesic options were available for treating migraine until the advent of the triptans in the early 1990s prevented the concept of analgesic rebound headache from being widely disseminated outside the headache community. With the advent of triptan medications, it was hoped that these migraine-specific medications would provide an option for reducing and perhaps preventing analgesic-maintained headaches. However, reports of triptan overuse headaches began to appear in the literature soon after the regulatory approval of sumatriptan, being formally reported in 1996 by Gobel et al.[13] Today, triptan rebound is considered a potential consequence of all triptans. Thus it appears that a diverse group of symptomatic medications are implicated in maintaining chronic primary headache disorders. This prompted the IHS nomenclature committee to include the diagnosis of medication overuse headache and it cites analgesics, ergotamines, caffeine, and triptans as all being associated with this phenomenon.[1]

Medication Overuse: Cause or Consequence of Headache?

Chronic primary headaches are common, affecting an estimated 2% to 4% of the American population.[14] Although several headache specialists report near-epidemic proportions of analgesic-maintained headache patients in their specialty-based practices, not all patients with chronic headache appear to overuse symptomatic medications. Several large epidemiologic studies conducted outside the United States where over-the-counter analgesics are not commonly available suggest that factors other than medication overuse may be involved in initiating and maintaining chronic headaches. Ravishankar[15] reported that less than 5% of a population of 1000 patients in India with chronic migraine had concomitant medication overuse. Although many studies report that discontinuation of overused symptomatic medications resulted in the chronic headache reverting to an episodic headache pattern, rarely did any of these studies assess the discontinuation of symptomatic medication isolated from other interventions, such as education and the use of preventive medications. For example, the study by Mathew et al[16] of 200 patients found that 20% improved over 2 months by discontinuing overused symptomatic medications only. However, 80% improved over 2 months by discontinuing medication and using preventive medications. Further, the benefits of analgesic withdrawal appear in many studies to be short-lived. Pini et al[17] reported that, after 4 years, only one third of treated patients still refrained from daily analgesics. In addition, those who returned to daily analgesic use had better quality-of-life scores than those who no longer used daily analgesics.

Given the significant rate of analgesic relapse of nearly 60%, the debate has become whether analgesics are a cause or consequence of chronic daily headaches. Dodick[18] has suggested that, whereas symptomatic medication can be associated with rebound headache, chronic migraine itself may be a progressive brain disorder that leads to overuse of symptomatic medication and that this may be a more common reason for chronic headache than overuse of medication. This debate has crystallized given research by Welch et al[19] documenting iron deposition in the periaqueductal gray area (PAG) in migraineurs with histories of long-standing, frequent migraine. The authors hypothesized that this may reflect oxidative damage in this important pain inhibitory nucleus secondary to long-standing uncontrolled migraine. More recently, Kruit et al[20] reported that subclinical cerebellar white matter lesions are noted on magnetic resonance imaging (MRI) scans of individuals with long-standing histories of frequent migraine. These results suggest that for some patients, migraine may indeed be a progressive neurologic disease.[21]

Proposed Mechanisms of Chronic Headache and Analgesic Rebound Headache

Over the preceding three decades, the pathophysiology of migraine has changed significantly and has evolved from a stress to a vascular and now into a neurologic disorder. In addition, the notion that tension-type headache is a disorder of muscular etiology has been largely dispelled and a more unified model of primary headache appears to be emerging. The once-popular notion that migraine and tension-type headache are distinct pathophysiologic diseases has little scientific support—at least in the portion of the population capable of having migraine.[22] (The Spectrum Study found that migraine sufferers have various presentations of headaches that respond equally to migraine-specific medication.)

In 1980 Raskin and Appenzeller[23] proposed a continuum model of migraine with *migraine with aura* on one end of the spectrum of headache activity and *chronic tension-type headache* on the other. Between these two extremes fell the different clinical phenotypes of primary headache disorders observed in clinical practice. This model also suggested that, as migraine became more chronic, the threshold for the next migraine was lowered and that analgesics and ergotamine expedited this change in the threshold to migraine. Mathew[24] observed that,

when migraine was an episodic condition, patients complained of associated neurovascular and gastrointestinal symptoms but as it transformed into a more chronic condition, there was a greater association of myogenic and psychological symptoms. This original observation may have found recent support in the American Migraine II study, with the population screening positive for migraine reporting the greatest frequency of primary headaches also reporting the greatest number of physician diagnoses of primary headaches.[25]

In 2002 Cady et al[26] expanded this concept by proposing the "convergence hypothesis," which suggested that primary headaches, at least in the migraine population, evolved from a single pathophysiologic mechanism. This model correlated the clinical phases of migraine with presumed underlying pathophysiologic mechanisms of the evolving process of migraine (**Fig. 49.1**). Different clinical diagnoses common to the migraine population were explained by the level of pathophysiologic disruption associated with a specific migraine attack.[26] Later, expanding this model to explain the evolution of episodic into chronic headache, it was suggested that the threshold to activating the migraine process was influenced by several factors beyond analgesics including genetics, biology, trauma (both physical and psychologic), and uncontrolled headaches, and that uncontrolled migraine can become a progressive neurologic disease in a subset of primary headache sufferers (**Fig. 49.2**).[27]

Mechanisms of Medication Overuse Headache

The mechanism of analgesic rebound or medication overuse headache is unknown, but data suggest that this phenomenon is more common and perhaps unique to those individuals with migraine. Lance et al[28] reported that analgesic overuse did not increase the frequency of headaches in those without a history of migraine. Based on a study of individuals taking daily analgesics for arthritis, the authors postulated suppression or down-regulation of already suppressed nociceptive mechanisms caused by excessive use of symptomatic medications as a possible explanation for analgesic rebound headaches. Later, Hering et al[29] reported a reduction of serotonin in the blood of patients with chronic headaches and that these levels increased significantly when the offending symptomatic medication was discontinued.

Fields and Heinricher[30] proposed increased nociception resulting in activation of "on cells" in the ventromedial medulla as a possible mechanism of analgesic rebound. Mathew[31] reported that stimulation of 5-HT-1 receptors was abortive for acute episodes of migraine but that activation of 5-HT-2 receptors increased pain transmission. Srikiatkochorn[32] found an increase of 5-HT-2A receptors on platelets in patients with chronic migraine and analgesic overuse that decreased once the offending medication was withdrawn. Current theories suggest that, with medication overuse, there is a decrease in central serotonin and up-regulation of 5-HT-2A receptors leading to central hyperalgesia. Recent work by Ossipov et al[33] and Mao et al[34] has suggested that prolonged used of opioids can produce a state of hyperalgesia.

Thus, the debate continues as to whether escalating headache attacks lead to more frequent medication use or whether escalating medication use leads to increases in headache

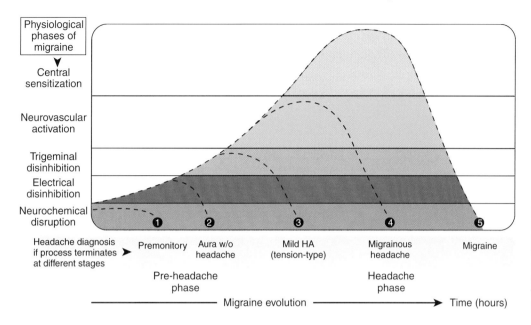

Fig. 49.1 Model of convergence hypothesis, which suggests that primary migraine headaches evolve from a single pathophysiologic mechanism. In this model, the clinical phases of migraine correlate with presumed underlying pathophysiologic mechanisms.

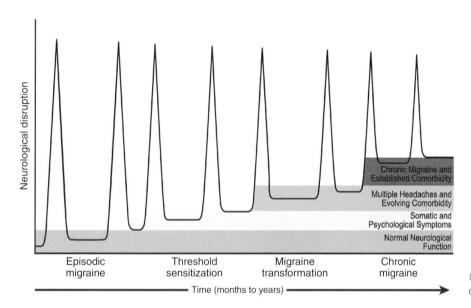

Fig. 49.2 Evolution of migraine from attacks to disease.

frequency. Suffice it to say that once patients are caught in a web of chronic primary headaches and using acute medications frequently, they have significant treatment needs and will undoubtedly find greater benefit from discontinuing the offending medication than continuing a pattern of failure.

Clinical Features of Medication Overuse Headache

Medication overuse headache or analgesic-rebound headache is characterized by a sustained pattern of headaches—medication—headaches—and more medication. Typically, headaches occur on a daily or near-daily basis and the offending medication often appears to be the only medication capable of bringing relief, albeit temporary. The primary headache is low grade, waxing and waning, with pain varying in intensity,

location, and severity. Superimposed on this headache pattern are periods of more intense headache activity. These headaches generally occur with characteristics suggestive of migraine. Often even mild physical and mental perturbations in daily activities trigger severe headaches.

Complicating this clinical scenario is the fact that this population of patients also exhibit psychologic disruptions such as depression and symptoms such as irritability and memory difficulties. Commonly, the patient complains of sleep disturbance and predictable early morning headaches that often necessitate pharmacologic intervention. A detailed history often reveals the need for dose escalation of the medication(s) being overused. In addition, patients will frequently use medication in anticipation of headaches. Patients caught in the web of medication overuse generally believe that their medication is not as effective as it once was but also believe it is a lifeline for preventing severe disabling headaches. Further, they frequently have experienced severe withdrawal headaches when they have been without medication or medication use has been delayed. Consequently, the stage is set for a strong belief in their need for symptomatic medications.

Clinical Evaluation of the Headache Patient with Suspected Medication Overuse

It is paramount that clinicians have a high index of suspicion when evaluating chronic or transforming headache disorders associated with frequent use of symptomatic medications.

Several factors in a patient's history are suggestive of medication overuse headache. Patients caught in this web often begin treatment efforts early in the morning because presumably overnight the blood levels of the offending analgesic may have decreased to the point of causing a mini–withdrawal syndrome, including the symptom of headache. Thus a history of early morning headache is common. Further, the history of having stopped the potentially offending analgesics at some point for several days resulted in a severe "rebound" headache. Patients often interpret this as evidence that they "need" their medication but, in fact, it may be evidence that withdrawal of medication caused the headache and that medication overuse is maintaining the headache condition.

Several investigators have attempted to ascertain the threshold quantity of different analgesics that can result in chronic medication-induced headache patterns. Others have suggested that the time period of exposure is also critical. These studies, although interesting, are retrospective evaluations of patients from tertiary headache centers. Consequently, therapeutic efforts to manage these patients are frequently beyond simply discontinuing an offending medication. Given these limitations, the IHS has proposed a list of substances, including several symptomatic medications, that by consensus appear to relate to chronic headache disorders.

Recently, Limmroth et al[35] looked at duration of exposure to various therapeutic acute agents and the development of chronic daily headache. In their study, they suggest that duration of triptan therapy of 1.7 years using 18 doses per month could result in medication overuse headache. Using ergots for 2.7 years with an average of 37 doses per month or analgesics 4.8 years using 114 doses per month was also considered to result in medication overuse headaches. Combination analgesics were not evaluated in this study. The limitations of this study reside in the different study populations in that those patients selected by medical providers for triptan therapy may have had more severe migraine or have been suffering migraine for a longer duration than those using analgesics.

Taking a Headache History of a Patient with Medication Overuse

When patients have frequent headaches it is critical to determine the frequency and quantity of symptomatic medications the patient is using. Determining how many days a week the patient requires acute treatment is often challenging because patients often provide answers that are vague or reveal that

the amount of medication being used is difficult to determine because its use varies depending on therapeutic need. It is critical that providers press for accurate, quantifiable answers about all symptomatic medications being used by the patient including over-the-counter medications.

Medication overuse headaches should be suspected when there is a daily or near-daily pattern of headache and the patient uses any symptomatic medication on an average of more than 2 days a week. In addition, medication overuse should be suspected whenever patients report that their usual symptomatic medication is less effective than it had been in the past. Frequently, patients will convey the fact that medication controls their headache reasonably well unless there is a delay in administration. It is vital to determine the use of both prescription and nonprescription medications because many patients fail to realize that over-the-counter preparations are, in fact, medications.

The following questions may assist the provider in determining if medication overuse is a likely component of a chronic headache pattern:

1. Is the patient using analgesics to treat other types of pain or medical conditions?
2. How does the patient determine when to treat?
3. Is medication used in anticipation of headache?
4. Is there fear of developing a severe disabling headache if medications are not taken?
5. Are the medications used for headache treatment effective (i.e., do they get a pain-free response or only partial relief)?
6. What is the duration of effective relief that a dose of medication provides?
7. How long does a specific quantity of symptomatic medication typically last?

These questions provide a framework for assessing the role of medication as a contributing factor for chronic headache. In addition, they allow the patient and the provider to communicate about the relationship of chronic primary headaches and symptomatic medications. It is essential that these questions are explored in a nonjudgmental manner and that the provider is in alliance with the patient to solve this vexing clinical situation.

Psychologic Evaluation of the Patient with Medication Overuse Headache

The evolution of episodic headaches into daily ones usually occurs over time, perhaps more than a decade.[36] During this evolutionary time period, individuals have maintained their ability to function through self-management and by following the advice of well-meaning friends, relatives, and medical providers. Today more than ever patients have access to a myriad of treatment ideas. They find advice on the Internet and from talk shows, books, and many different health care practitioners. Often the message for headache sufferers is that their headaches should be something they are able to control on their own through lifestyle and adequate stress management.

Often, by the time headache sufferers seek medical consultation, they have failed with multiple self-treatment attempts. They are fearful that headaches will continue to worsen to the point of ultimately taking away their ability to function. Specifically, they may fear the loss of a scholarship, job, or marriage. At this juncture, patients often feel psychologically and physically vulnerable, worrying that headaches are an expression of physical and mental inadequacy. A recent study found that, before symptoms of depression or anxiety appear, there is an increase in somatic pain complaints. As the impact of headaches reaches severe (60+ on the Headache Impact Test [HIT-6] or 21+ on the Migraine Disability Assessment [MIDAS]), the number of somatic complaints increases to a significant degree, from an average of 5.0 at no or mild headache impact to 7.5 at severe headache impact. In fact, in this study of 93 individuals with disabling headaches, 71% complained of back pain and 54% were bothered by pain in arms, legs, joints, or lower abdomen.[37] From the patient's perspective, headache is but one of several medical conditions that is affecting the patient's life.

Another study measured the link between 391 pain patients and their analgesic medication using the Leeds Dependence Questionnaire. The researchers found that those with migraine (both episodic and chronic) were more profoundly linked to analgesics than were those with rheumatic disease.[38] Clearly, the fear of an attack of migraine intensifies the importance of analgesics. This finding was confirmed in another study utilizing the Severity of Dependence Scale among 405 Norwegians with chronic migraine.[39] A third study found that 66.8% of medication overuse headache patients were considered dependent on acute treatments of headaches according to the DSM-IV criteria, the majority of whom overused opioid analgesics. Interestingly, affective symptoms did not appear to predict dependence. The authors concluded that medication overuse among headache patients appears to belong to the spectrum of addictive behaviors. For this reason, behavioral management should augment pharmacologic intervention.[40] Another group of researchers found a significantly increased familial risk for chronic headache, drug overuse, and substance abuse, suggesting that a genetic factor may be involved.[41]

Psychologic Assessment Tools

Several objective measurements have been devised to help clinicians to assess and define the headache sufferer with chronic primary headaches. These tools, although not specifically designed to define the population overusing medication, are valuable in defining the psychologic and medical needs of this population. Headache impact tools are simple to use even in a busy clinical setting and should be considered an invaluable way to document therapeutic efficacy of management efforts in this population of patients:

1. HIT-6[42] or MIDAS[43] to assess the impact of the headaches on the individual's life. These tests can also be used to follow the progress of patients over time.
2. Visual analog scale (VAS) of pain severity to measure pain levels before and after interventions. It is presented graphically with a 10 cm line and end point adjective descriptors ("the worst imaginable pain" on one end and "no pain" on the other). The patient is asked to place a mark along the line to indicate the current pain level. A difference of 13 mm between consecutive ratings of pain is the minimum change in a pain rating that is clinically significant.[44]
3. Symptom index to record somatic symptoms associated with headaches. As mentioned, chronic daily headache is often one of several pain complaints.
4. Zung Depression Inventory[45,46] to measure the level of depression and suicide potential of the patient, which is a measure of the psychologic effect that headaches are having on the individual.
5. State Trait Anxiety Scale[47] to indicate the level of anxiety both at the present time and throughout the person's life. High anxiety generally implies that the individual is using medication to anticipate headaches and lessen the anxiety over not being able to perform in a certain setting because of headaches.
6. Minnesota Multiphasic Personality Inventory-2 (MMPI-2)[48] to appraise an individual's behavioral adaptation to the current life situation. It consists of 567 true/false statements, which usually takes a patient 1½ to 2 hours to complete. It is an objective, valid, and reliable instrument that uncovers significant psychopathology that may complicate management and serve as a basis for referral.

Psychologic testing of patients with chronic headache reflects a greater incidence of behavioral abnormalities. The MMPI-2 profile may be a 3-1 or 1-3, often called "Conversion V," that may also be interpreted as a call for help. After treatment, when headaches return to episodic, the MMPI-2 usually normalizes.

Using the MMPI-2, researchers compared the personality profiles of patients with medication overuse headaches and episodic headaches. They found that both groups exhibited very similar patterns. Scale 1 (Hypochondriasis) and Health Concerns were the only significantly differing scales. There were no significant differences in the scores of the scales measuring dependence-related behavior. The authors concluded that "pseudo-addiction" may better explain their findings, that is, headache patients use medications to relieve pain that enables them to function and maintain a normal lifestyle.[49]

In addition, a history of substance abuse, especially alcoholism, or physical and/or mental abuse appears more frequently in the chronic headache population, particularly among those who are refractory to treatment.

Management of Medication Overuse Headache

Perhaps the most critical aspect of managing a patient who is suffering from medication overuse headache is for the clinician to avoid being overly judgmental. In many instances, medication overuse begins subtly and symptomatic medications are prescribed to the patient without knowledge of the risks. At times, patients may present for evaluation unsuspecting that medications are actually maintaining their headache pattern. Others may be aware of their reliance on medication but see no alternative. They fear discontinuing the medication instead of understanding the potential benefits of freeing themselves from medication dependency. Still other patients may view their reliance on medication as addiction and feel angry and guilty. Rarely, patients approach the clinician with the intent of using the complaint of headache to surreptitiously acquire specific medications. Thus managing medication-maintained headache requires time, clinical skills, and clear communication between the medical provider and the patient. It is important to approach the patient with medication overuse headache confidently and with compassion.

Education

Education is the cornerstone of effective management for patients caught in the trap of medication overuse headache. From patients' perspective, it is often difficult to understand that discontinuing the only medication that provides relief, albeit temporary, will be beneficial. Clinicians are often met with considerable skepticism and fear when they recommend to their patients that the medication must be stopped. Likewise, clinicians can offer no guarantee that discontinuing medication will improve the underlying headache pattern. However, they can convey that there is good evidence suggesting that most patients do, in fact, improve after stopping overused abortive migraine medications and that not stopping the medication will likely perpetuate and worsen the cycle of daily headaches.

The key component of education includes a clear explanation of medication overuse headache and the spiral of ever-escalating headache that occurs with this medical condition. It is also valuable to explain that uncontrolled migraine may evolve into a progressive neurologic disease that can impair the patient's ability to perform in all aspects of life.

Designing a Treatment Plan

Historically, analgesic withdrawal was often performed in the hospital setting. This is still a reasonable and preferred treatment approach for the more complicated spectrum of this patient population. However, in an era of managed care, most often patients will be managed in an outpatient setting. If patients agree to detoxification, it is critical to be frank and honest about the benefit of discontinuing an overused medication whether detoxification is done on an inpatient or outpatient basis. This education includes the fact that improvement might not be realized for 2 to 3 months (or not at all) and that in all likelihood there will be a period of increased headache, a fact that many patients already know. Regardless, it is critical that clinicians establish a clear rationale for medication withdrawal and provide a plan for its implementation.

The Initial Visit

During the initial visit, many clinicians choose to provide education and do not discontinue the offending medication at that time. Instead the patient is instructed to change the use of the offending medication from symptom-based to time-based administration. This has the advantage of allaying a patient's fear and permits the patient to be open about the quantities of medication being consumed. During that same visit the patient is advised to withdraw from dietary caffeine and other potential dietary factors that may exacerbate the underlying headache pattern, such as tyramine and nitrates. The patient is given a date for discontinuing the medication that is generally not more than 2 weeks away from the first visit. This provides an opportunity for the patient to arrange a short leave of absence from work or family commitments when the withdrawal is commenced. A prophylactic medication can be provided, although it is unlikely to provide its full pharmacologic

benefit until the acute medication withdrawal has been completed. Finally, the patient is provided a headache diary in which headaches and all medication usage are recorded. Many clinicians insist that the patient sign a medication contract with the "rules" clearly defined. Finally, whenever possible, behavioral therapy with a psychologist skilled in pain and headache management should be strongly recommended.

During the initial visit, a strategy for medication withdrawal should be improvised. Several factors should be considered in determining which approach is most appropriate for a specific patient. If patients are using significant quantities of opioid or butalbital combination products, the risk of withdrawal seizure should be assessed. Phenobarbital with its longer half-life can be substituted for butalbital as a convenient and effective withdrawal strategy. Generally, patients are started on 90 mg and the dose is adjusted up or down based on the presence of agitation or sedation. Each week the phenobarbital dose can be reduced by 30 mg. A similar strategy can be employed with opioids, as a short-acting medication is converted to a long-acting formulation and then slowly withdrawn over several weeks. When these strategies are employed, it is critical to communicate to the patient that this medication is not being used as an acute treatment for headache and that the patient is provided with an appropriate abortive for acute intervention. In addition, a clonidine patch can be prescribed to diminish the intensity of some of the withdrawal symptoms. Typically the 0.1 mg patch is used. Dose is patient dependent, but a typical regimen is to apply two patches for 1 week followed by one patch for 1 week, then discontinued.

In general, the authors recommend that withdrawal of overused symptomatic medications be done rapidly rather than using a slow taper. It is valuable to include the patient in these decisions and provide a realistic structure wherein both provider and patient have clear input into the decision-making process. Abrupt withdrawal may result in an intense rebound headache of shorter duration, whereas tapering may buffer withdrawal headache but may prolong the symptomatic time period. If withdrawal is done too slowly, undoubtedly migraine triggering events will ensue and a severe breakthrough headache will occur. This may result in a desperate patient using more medication than the withdrawal schedule permits. Although a temporary worsening of headache often occurs with rapid withdrawal, many patients are able to discontinue medications and have improvement in the headache pattern without an escalation in headaches. It is difficult to predict which patient will have a difficult time. Regardless of the method employed, patients need to be assured that they will not be abandoned and that several bridge therapies exist that can attenuate, although not necessarily prevent, all headaches.

Bridge or Transition Therapies

The concept of bridge therapy is to provide a short-term treatment that will attenuate the rebound headache and other symptoms of medication withdrawal through the time period when the nervous system is most vulnerable. Although commonly employed by headache specialists, these therapies have not been rigorously evaluated in large, placebo-controlled, randomized studies. The first of these was described by Tfelt-Hansen[50] in 1981. Patients were hospitalized and treated with sedatives for an average of 9 days and three fourths were

Table 49.3 Bridge (Transition) Therapies for Medication Withdrawal Headache

Dihydroergotamine (DHE): 0.5–1 mg IV, IM, or SC q8hr for 1 day, then q12hr for 2 days, then qd for 2 days. Metoclopramide 10 mg can be given 30 min before DHE for prevention of nausea. Common adverse events include nausea, vomiting, muscle cramps. Avoid in patient with coronary disease or significant risk factors, peripheral vascular disease, gastric ulcer, sepsis.

Naratriptan: 1–1.25 mg bid for 5 days with an additional 2.5 mg within any 24-hour time period provided for breakthrough headache. Adverse events are uncommon but may include triptan sensations. Avoid in patients with coronary heart disease or significant coronary risk factors, hypertension, hemiplegic or basilar migraine.

Diphenhydramine: 25–50 mg IM or IV tid.

Various neuroleptics (e.g., chlorpromazine): 6.25–12.5 mg IV q 8–12hr.

Magnesium sulfate: 1–2 g IV qd for 3–5 days or 1 g bid for 3–5 days.

Steroids: rapid tapering dose of oral or parenteral steroids such as prednisone 60 mg q am for 3 days then 40 mg q am for 2 days; 30 mg q am for 2 days; 20 mg q am for 2 days; 10 mg q am for 2 days; 5 mg q am for 2 days; then discontinue.

Occipital and cervical epidural nerve blocks with local anesthetics (such as 0.25% bupivacaine). Some physicians add long-acting steroids to the bupivacaine.

bid, twice a day; IM, intramuscularly; IV, intravenously; qd, every day; SC, subcutaneously; tid, three times a day.

reported improved. In 1986 Raskin[51] reported on the use of repetitive doses of intravenous dihydroergotamine (DHE) in hospitalized patients. Patients received nine doses of DHE 0.5 to 1 mg over a 5-day period in a tapering schedule. This protocol has been occasionally modified by several other headache specialists but still remains the standard for detoxification of patients in analgesic rebound. Generally, antidopaminergic medications such as metoclopramide are given with the DHE as an antiemetic agent. Subcutaneous sumatriptan has also been used in management of analgesic rebound with 6 mg given twice daily for 5 days.

More recently, oral triptans have been used as bridge therapies and are especially attractive in an outpatient setting. Triptans with longer half-lives, such as naratriptan and frovatriptan, appear particularly suited for this role. Typically, naratriptan 1 mg (or half of a 2.5 mg tablet) twice daily for 5 to 7 days with 2.5 mg as a rescue dose for breakthrough headaches, with a total daily dose not to exceed 5 mg, is commonly used by headache specialists. Frovatriptan 2.5 mg daily with an additional 2.5 mg for breakthrough migraine, with a daily dose not exceeding 5 mg, is an alternative. Many specialists also have recommended a burst of prednisone 60 to 80 mg tapered over 7 to 14 days as adjunctive therapy or a short tapering course of dexamethasone (12 mg, 8 mg, 4 mg) for three consecutive mornings[52] (**Table 49.3**).

Psychologic Support

In today's health care environment it is often difficult to convince third-party payers or patients that effective management of chronic medical conditions requires more than a prescription and 10 minutes of time. However, successfully managing patients with chronic debilitating headaches and associated medication overuse is one clinical situation in which psychologic support is critical. There are several levels of support to consider, including individual psychotherapy, biofeedback, group therapy, and patient support organizations. Integrating psychologic therapy into a medical treatment plan early on improves treatment response. A group of researchers[53] studied the effects of short-term psychotherapy on the therapeutic response of 26 patients with medication overuse headaches. At 12 months into the study, the group with psychotherapy had a

significantly greater decrease in headache frequency and medication intake. The relapse rate was also significantly lower in the group with psychotherapy (15.3%) compared to the group without psychotherapy (23%).

The biopsychosocial treatment model integrates medical, physical, psychological, and spiritual therapy into the treatment plan (**Fig. 49.3**). In other words, medication overuse headache is more than an acute episode of headache that has become chronic. During this transformational process, it becomes a health problem that affects the patient's entire life and, likewise, factors other than analgesics may be affecting the patient's chronic headache, such as biologic, behavioral, and social factors. Physical problems, such as the diagnosis of a medical disease other than headaches, may short-circuit the system that is expressed by chronic headaches.

Trauma, whether psychologic or physical, such as an automobile accident or a burglary of one's home, can be fodder for chronic headaches. Social factors, such as divorce, separation, loss of job, or relocation, are high-impact events that affect the chronic headache condition, as well as responsiveness to treatment.

These individuals desire the opportunity to discuss these issues in a supportive environment, either with a therapist or within a support group. Once they realize they are not alone, that others may be attempting to cope with as many problems as they are, they are encouraged to follow the treatment plan and venture into the realm of being a doer rather than a victim. For chronic problems, there is no linear relationship between cause and effect. By recognizing that the chronic headache has progressed over time, even years, patients see therapy as a process of healing the nervous system by several avenues, not just medication. This realization is at times essential for patients to respond to a treatment strategy.

What if Medication Withdrawal Does Not Result in Patient Improvement?

As previously discussed, withdrawal from medication does not always result in an improvement in the underlying daily headache pattern. If a patient persists in a debilitating chronic

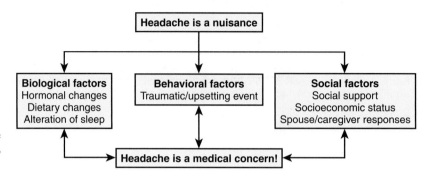

Fig. 49.3 Biopsychosocial model of chronic pain. *(Adapted from Keefe FJ, Bonk V: Psychosocial assessment of pain in patients having rheumatic diseases, Rheum Dis Clin North Am, 25:81, 1999.)*

headache pattern, decisions about chronic maintenance with symptomatic medications should be discussed. Few data are available, but in a study by Saper et al,[54] the clinical outcome of a population of patients with chronic headache using maintenance opioids found that only 25% responded. The obvious difficulty is predicting which patients will respond to a stable dose of opioids without escalation and concomitant reduction in efficacy over time. If analgesic maintenance is recommended, it is critical that patients be followed regularly and that providers document objective improvement in functional status.

Far more difficult is the patient frequently using non-opioid abortive medications such as triptans and presumably controlling disabling headaches but requiring medication more than three times a week. In this scenario, clinicians are often triangulated between the needs of their patient and the restrictions of the payer of the pharmaceutical benefits. Managed care concerns often revert to tactics that imply clinicians are outside of normative prescription behavior standards, although the reality is that this patient population has never been studied by the stringent regulatory standards used to establish accepted evidence. Ironically, patients in this clinical scenario may have daily headaches but report that if they use a triptan early in the headache process, they can abort the impending headache and maintain normal function. For this reason, patients do not want to alter this management strategy. In truth, we do not know the long-term consequences of using abortive medications, such as triptans, on a chronic basis. But once the medications have been appropriately withdrawn without benefit and there has been documented deterioration in the patient's functional status, the question then becomes, Should symptomatic medications be used on a chronic basis? Without scientific proof to guide decisions, one can decide this based only on individual assessment with risks and benefits fully discussed with the patient. Hopefully, over time, as more migraine sufferers develop the need for frequent abortive medication, pharmaceutical and regulatory agencies will see the need to evaluate this question more completely.

Long-Term Care Needs

Patients in medication overuse headache patterns almost always require long-term, ongoing headache management that will span decades of their lives. Through the lifetime of episodic migraine there is a significant chance that patients will, at some point, develop chronic headache. It is important for providers and patients to realize that, although it is convenient to blame medication overuse, there is a significant chance of developing chronic headache even after medication withdrawal has been successful.

The evolution from episodic to chronic primary headache is clearly about more than the headaches patients experience. Often, disruptions of sleep or mood are the first signal that a migraine patient is transitioning to a chronic daily headache pattern. Physiologic and neurologic function between headaches becomes abnormal in that symptoms such as irritability, fatigue, lethargy, and a sense of feeling "blue" or hypervigilant occur. These characteristics may become the basis for diagnosis of several disorders considered comorbid with migraine. Ironically, medication overuse can be a catalyst that signals the transformation of episodic migraine into a chronic headache pattern. Therefore it is essential that patients understand the risks of migraine transformation, which may become a progressive neurobiologic disorder that leads to a chronic pain syndrome. Because overly zealous pharmacologic interventions can be a catalyst for this process, it is critical to set limits on the use of symptomatic medications early in the management of headache patients.

Maintaining medical care that optimizes treatment response can also potentially circumvent daily headache patterns associated with medication overuse. This often appears as a paradox because treatment failure or partial treatment responses often encourages use of additional medication. A treatment diary is invaluable in assessing response to treatment and medication use. The hallmark of quality headache care is to provide these tools for episodic headaches, thereby preventing the development of chronic headaches and the subsequent need to rescue patients from them.

Conclusion

Medication overuse headache can be a challenging clinical syndrome to manage. It is far easier to prevent than to treat. Clinicians should be mindful of medication overuse headache in all headache patients they manage. Central to preventing this medical condition is to provide clear guidelines on frequencies and quantities of medication used as abortive. Further, clear goals defining treatment success should be provided to all patients when prescribed migraine therapies. Patients should be advised to seek reevaluation whenever the goals of treatment are not being met, which includes reviewing the effectiveness of acute therapy, as well as the institution of preventive measures.

Once patients are having chronic headaches associated with medication overuse it is paramount to discontinue the potentially offending medication for at least 2 months. Providing effective education, psychologic support, preventive medications, and a bridge therapy for acute care are invaluable components of successful management of this condition. With a cogent approach to medication overuse headache, most patients can be successfully managed and clinicians often find the condition of analgesic rebound headache rewarding to manage.

References

Full references for this chapter can be found on www.expertconsult.com.

Chapter 50

Trigeminal Neuralgia

M. Alan Stiles and James J. Evans

Historical Considerations

Trigeminal neuralgia has been identified in the medical literature for centuries. Trigeminal neuralgia is the classic neuropathic pain syndrome and is thought first to have been described by Aretaeus in the first century AD. Many physicians have penned descriptions of this affliction; the first to describe it comprehensively was John Locke in 1677. He described a patient as having

> ...such violent and exquisite torment, that it forced her to such cries and shrieks as you would expect from one upon the rack, to which I believe hers was an equal torment, which extended itself all over the right side of her face and mouth. When the fit came there was, to My Lady's own expression of it, as it were a flash of fire all of a sudden shot into all of those parts, and at every one of those twitches which made her shriek out, her mouth was constantly drawn to the right side towards the right ear by repeated convulsive motions, which were constantly accompanied by her cries... These violent fits terminated of a sudden and then My Lady seemed to be perfectly well.[1,2]

John Hunter (1728–1793), an English physiologist and surgeon, described trigeminal neuralgia in his *Treatise on the Natural History of the Human Teeth* in 1778 as follows:

> This pain is seated in some one part of the Jaws. As simple pain demonstrates nothing; a Tooth is often suspected, and is perhaps drawn out; but still the pain continues, with this difference however, that it now seems to be in the root of the next Tooth: it is then supposed either by the patient or the operator, that the wrong Tooth was extracted; wherefore, that in which the pain now seems to be, is drawn, but with as little benefit. I have known cases of this kind, where all the Teeth of the affected side of the Jaw, have been drawn out, and the pain has continued in the Jaw; in others, it has had a different effect, the sensation of pain has become more diffused, and has at last, attacked the corresponding side of the tongue. In the first case, I have known it recommended to cut down upon the Jaw, and even to perforate and cauterize it, but all without effect. Hence it should appear, that the pain in question, does not arise from any disease in the part, but entirely a nervous affection.

In 1912, Osler captured the essence of the clinical description of trigeminal neuralgia as it was understood in his time:

> In advanced cases the paroxysms follow one another rapidly and without assignable cause, and in the intervals the patient may never be quite free from pain. They are inaugurated by almost any form of external stimulus, by a draught of air, by movement of the facial muscles or of the tongue in speaking, by touching the skin, particularly over those points from which the pain seems to take its origin, by the act of swallowing, especially when the pain involves the mucous membrane field of distribution of the nerve. It is not a self-limited disease. In some instances the neuralgia reaches such a frightful intensity that it renders the patient's life insupportable. In former years suicide was not an uncommon consequence.[3]

Clinical Syndrome

Trigeminal neuralgia is a severe, almost exclusively unilateral, neuropathic pain located within the distribution of the trigeminal nerve and manifesting as paroxysmal, high-intensity, stabbing pain lasting seconds. Each attack may be followed by a refractory period, a period of relief that lasts seconds, minutes, or even hours. The burst of pain can occur spontaneously or can be triggered by stimulating a specific area of the face known as a *trigger zone.* Trigger zones can be difficult to locate; they exist anywhere within the trigeminal distribution, including intraorally. The trigger zone is located in the same division of the trigeminal nerve as the pain. For this reason, patients characteristically avoid touching the face, washing, shaving, biting or chewing, or any other maneuver that stimulates the trigger zones and produces the pain.[4] This avoidance is an invaluable clue to the diagnosis. With almost every other facial pain syndrome, patients massage, abrade, or apply heat and cold to the painful area; in trigeminal neuralgia, however, exactly the opposite occurs: patients avoid any stimulation of the face or mouth. The pain is often characterized as an "electric shock" and is typically accompanied by a unilateral grimace, hence the designation *tic douloureux.* The pain may occur daily for weeks or months and then cease, sometimes for years, before returning; these are known as periods of remission.

Although this disorder has been described clinically for centuries, the etiology of trigeminal neuralgia and the other cranial neuralgias is not fully understood. The integrity of the myelin sheath has been the focal point of investigation for years; however, the only agreement is that a dysfunction of the trigeminal sensory system exists.[5] Trigeminal neuralgia is classified as primary (idiopathic or type 1), or secondary (type 2), which results from compression or irritation, tumor, or disease, such as multiple sclerosis.

Intermittent trigeminal neuralgia is uncommon in multiple sclerosis, with an incidence between 1% and 2%.[6,7] Conversely, the incidence of multiple sclerosis among patients with trigeminal neuralgia is approximately 3%. Patients with multiple sclerosis and trigeminal neuralgia typically have a classic trigeminal neuralgia history, except that the trigeminal neuralgia appears at a younger age when patients have multiple sclerosis than when the disease occurs in its idiopathic form. Some patients with multiple sclerosis have recurrent episodes of face pain that are generally long-lasting, not stabbing or lancinating, and without associated trigger zones. These patients are assumed not to have true trigeminal neuralgia, but rather a form of atypical facial pain. Trigeminal neuralgia can occur as the first manifestation of multiple sclerosis, but this is rare. Most patients who have trigeminal neuralgia in association with multiple sclerosis have significant physical signs of multiple sclerosis for many years before the facial pain begins. Most patients, for example, have paraparesis or paraplegia, which are disorders of sensory function. Bilateral trigeminal neuralgia occurs more often than expected in patients with multiple sclerosis.

On rare occasions, trigeminal neuralgia may be a manifestation of brainstem disease and has been reported to result from pontine infarction.[8] Neoplasms involving the trigeminal nerve generally produce constant neuropathic pain associated with sensory loss. Animal models have not been able to reproduce the pain of trigeminal neuralgia, and this limits the ability to study the condition on a basic science level.

Testing

The diagnosis of trigeminal neuralgia is made from the clinical history. No medical testing is available to confirm the diagnosis; however, some investigators have mentioned a response to carbamazepine as being diagnostic. When the condition is found, magnetic resonance imaging (MRI) and evoked potential testing are strongly recommended to rule out secondary causes. Typically, the neurologic examination is normal. Clinically, the onset of trigeminal neuralgia is generally after the age of 50 years, although it can occur at any age. Women are affected twice as often as men. Patients usually have no sensory loss in idiopathic trigeminal neuralgia as measured by ordinary sensory testing, although some investigators refer to occasional sensory findings.[9–12] In contrast, sensory disturbances in the distribution of the trigeminal nerve are relatively common when patients have multiple sclerosis or a structural lesion involving the trigeminal nerve or roots. Such sensory loss may even involve the inside of the mouth. Some investigators postulate that if left untreated, trigeminal neuralgia may become more atypical, accompanied by sensory disturbances and constant pain.[13]

Fromm et al[14] described 18 patients whose initial trigeminal pain was not characteristic of neuralgia, but rather suggested a toothache or sinus pain, and frequently lasted several hours. Often this pain was set off by jaw movements or by drinking hot or cold liquids. Then, at some later time, ranging from several days to 12 years, more typical trigeminal neuralgia developed in the same general area as the initial pain. Six of these patients became pain free while they were taking carbamazepine or baclofen. These investigators designated the problem *pretrigeminal neuralgia.* This neuralgia must be differentiated from trigeminal tumors, atypical facial pain, atypical odontalgia, and facial migraine, among other entities. An MRI scan emphasizing the middle and posterior fossa is recommended as a diagnostic study in this situation.

In rare instances, trigeminal neuralgia is accompanied by hemifacial spasm. The combination has been designated *tic convulsif.*[15] Tic convulsif is characterized by periodic contractions of one side of the face, accompanied by great pain. It may be confused with the facial contortions on the involved side that can accompany the paroxysms of true trigeminal neuralgia.[15] Painful tic convulsif is reported to be more severe in women than in men. It may begin in or about the orbicularis oculi as fine intermittent myokymia, with some spread thereafter into the muscles of the lower part of the face. Occasionally, strong spasms involve all the facial muscles on one side almost continuously. Rarely, the face becomes weak, and some of the facial muscles atrophy. Tic convulsif is usually indicative of a tumor, ectatic dilation of the basilar artery, or a vascular malformation compressing the trigeminal and facial nerves.[16]

Differential Diagnosis

Cluster-Tic

Trigeminal neuralgia in combination with cluster headache has been termed *cluster-tic syndrome.*[17,18]

Glossopharyngeal Neuralgia

Glossopharyngeal neuralgia is an uncommon craniofacial pain syndrome characterized by severe, transient, stabbing, or burning pain felt in the ear, base of the tongue, tonsillar fossa, or area beneath the angle of the jaw. Occasionally, pain spreads to other areas of the face, including the external auditory canal (otic variety) or neck (cervical variety). The distribution is in the sensory areas of the glossopharyngeal nerve, as well as the auricular and pharyngeal branches of the vagus nerve. It can be mistaken for trigeminal neuralgia with a mandibular nerve distribution.

The pain is frequently triggered by chewing, swallowing, talking, yawning, or coughing. Generally, the attacks of pain come in paroxysms and are lightning-like, but some patients have a more constant aching, burning, or pressure sensation. Glossopharyngeal neuralgia may be associated with severe bradycardia, hypotension, or transient asystole, resulting in syncope or convulsions.[19,20] The diagnosis can be confirmed if pain relief results from either topical anesthesia to the pharynx or glossopharyngeal block at the jugular foramen. As with trigeminal neuralgia, MRI and evoked potential testing are strongly recommended to rule out secondary causes.

Geniculate Neuralgia

Geniculate neuralgia is an unusual condition caused by impairment of the sensory part of the seventh cranial nerve. In general, it is related to a herpes zoster infection of the geniculate ganglion. It is characterized by severe pain in the tympanic membrane, the walls of the auditory canal, the external auditory meatus, and the external structure of the ear. The pain is typically deep and may radiate toward other regions of the face. A herpetic rash in the auricle or in the external auditory canal may accompany the pain. The disease may be associated with peripheral facial palsy (Ramsay Hunt syndrome), difficulty with hearing, vertigo, and tinnitus. The pain may persist for more than 6 months and produce chronic postherpetic neuralgia. The pain is usually constant and has a burning, dysesthetic quality.

Tic-like Neuritides of the Fifth Cranial Nerve Associated with Tumors and Other Pathologic Processes

These relatively uncommon and painful states resemble trigeminal neuralgia, but they can usually be differentiated because each painful paroxysm is commonly a sustained high-intensity ache of several minutes' duration, whereas true trigeminal neuralgia is characterized by recurrent, brief, painful jabs lasting usually seconds. Cushing divided these neuralgias resulting from tumor involvement of the trigeminal sensory root, the trigeminal ganglion, or the fifth nerve into four groups on the basis of the site of the tumor.[15]

Herpetic and Postherpetic Neuralgia of the Trigeminal Nerve

Herpetic involvement of the trigeminal nerve is more common in older patients and in immunosuppressed patients. These patients are also at higher risk to develop postherpetic neuralgia.[21] The pain of herpes zoster, in contrast to tic, is steady and sustained. Although the pain often spontaneously regresses within 2 or 3 weeks, it may persist for several months. When the pain occurs in persons more than 70 years of age, as it frequently does, its duration may be a year or more. Rarely, it persists indefinitely. The pain is unilateral. The quality of the pain is usually both burning and aching (gnawing). It is non-throbbing and relatively uniform, and it usually diminishes gradually in intensity. It may be accompanied by a paroxysmal shooting, jabbing pain or by sharp, radiating pain produced by light mechanical stimuli. It may be experienced in any part of the distribution of the fifth cranial nerve, although involvement of the forehead is most common. Examination soon after onset reveals erythema and the typical herpetiform lesions of the skin associated with hyperalgesia and paresthesia. Examination later reveals hypesthesia and paresthesia of the involved areas, and sometimes scarring and pigmentation of the skin. The patient may have weakness of the masseter and pterygoid muscles on the ipsilateral side.

Herpetic and Postherpetic Neuralgia of Cervical Dorsal Root Ganglia

Steady pain in the face and ear, the back of the head, and the neck, associated with vertigo and palsy of the ipsilateral side of the face, results from widespread inflammation involving the gasserian and glossopharyngeal and the first two or three dorsal root ganglia, as well as the dorsal horns of the cervical portion of the cord. The pain has the qualities and duration described earlier. As with all herpes, the patient may have slight or moderate palsy. Herpetiform lesions may or may not be present.

Occipital Neuralgia

Occipital neuralgia remains a controversial subject, presumably because many physicians use the term broadly and non-specifically for any pain in the occipital area. The term should be reserved for paroxysmal or continuous, unilateral, burning, jabbing, or stabbing occipital pain in the distribution of the greater occipital nerve.[22,23] The pain frequently radiates to the frontal region. It is usually accompanied by hypoalgesia, hyperalgesia, or dysesthesia in the affected area and circumscribed tenderness over the nerve as it crosses the superior nuchal line.

Occipital neuralgia can be caused by trauma, injury, inflammation, or compression of the greater occipital nerve somewhere along its course from the C2 dorsal root to the periphery.[24] Although postherpetic occipital neuralgias have been described, most cases are caused by trauma or focal irritation of the nerve or its parent dorsal ramus.[25] In most cases, however, a clear-cut pathophysiologic relationship between the C2 root and the symptom complex is lacking. Myofascial trigger points in the suboccipital muscles (particularly the splenius capitis, splenius cervicis, multifidus, semispinalis capitis, and semispinalis cervicis) cause referred occipital pain that may prove difficult to distinguish from occipital neuralgia. Blockade of the occipital nerves with local anesthetic and steroid can be extremely effective in the management of the pain of occipital neuralgia.

Raeder's Syndrome

Raeder's paratrigeminal syndrome is a rare problem characterized by oculosympathetic paralysis, with ptosis, miosis, and the sudden onset of severe frontotemporal burning, aching pain, often in a periorbital or trigeminal distribution.[26–28] Normal sweating is present in the supraorbital area of the ipsilateral forehead. In essence, Raeder's syndrome consists of ordinary Horner's syndrome without the anhidrosis seen in the usual cases. This combination of signs may have many different causes, but the nature of the deficits points to a process involving the region of the carotid siphon.

Raeder's original cases all had evidence of involvement of one or more cranial nerves (e.g., optic, oculomotor, trochlear, trigeminal, abducens) caused by various parasellar lesions (e.g., infiltrating tumors, head injury).[26] In most subsequent reports, cranial nerve involvement has not been a prominent feature. The eponym has become a source of confusion because it has been applied indiscriminately to all types of cases in which oculosympathetic paralysis is associated with head pain.

Patients with Raeder's syndrome may be divided into two groups: (1) patients with episodic pains that are clearly cluster headaches and (2) patients with more constant pain and definite lesions (aneurysms, tumors, trauma, infections, dissections) involving the internal carotid artery and impinging on the first division of the trigeminal nerve.[29]

Raeder's syndrome has some value in localizing the site of disease in cases of oculosympathetic paralysis and head pain, but it has no value in distinguishing the cause of the process.

Atypical Facial Pain

Atypical facial pain or facial pain of unknown cause is characterized by a deep burning or aching pain that is continuous and poorly localized. The pain may be unilateral or bilateral and does not necessarily follow the distribution of the peripheral nerves. It may be accompanied by sensory changes, such as allodynia, dysesthesia, and paresthesia.[30] The usual sufferers are middle-aged women. Sleep and facial functions, such as eating and talking, are rarely affected, except when pain is located intraorally. Some patients have a history of trauma or a dental or surgical procedure before the onset of pain.

In 1993, Pfaffenrath et al[31] suggested modifying the International Headache Society diagnostic criteria for atypical facial pain (**Box 50.1**). Because Pfaffenrath's criteria could apply to pain symptoms of separate causes, clinicians further categorized these pains according to their specialty in hopes

---

Box 50.1 Criteria for Atypical Facial Pain: Suggested Modifications

- Pain is present daily and persists for most or all of the day, but it may also appear in attacks and with remissions.
- Pain is confined at onset to a limited area on one or both sides of the face. It may spread to the upper and lower jaws or to a wider area of the face or neck. The pain can have different qualities and be perceived as superficial or deep, but it is altogether poorly localized.
- Pain is not associated with sensory loss or other physical signs, but it is often associated with dysesthesia.
- Laboratory investigations including radiographs of face and jaws do not demonstrate relevant abnormalities.
- Pain may be initiated by operation or injury to the face, teeth, or gums, but it persists without any demonstrable cause.

Adapted from Pfaffenrath V, Rath M, Pollmann W, et al: Atypical facial pain: application of the IHS criteria in a clinical sample, *Cephalalgia* 13(Suppl 12):84, 1993.

---

of a better understanding of the condition and of directing treatment toward correcting the cause of the pain. Facial pain of unknown origin was also categorized by Graff-Radford,[32] who proposed an outline to help clinicians compartmentalize their clinical findings and to create a more uniform approach to treating these disorders with limited knowledge of the cause (**Box 50.2**).

Treatment

Medical Management

Initial management of trigeminal neuralgia is medical, and surgical therapy should be considered if medical treatment fails or cannot be tolerated and if secondary causes are found during the initial workup of the patient.[33,34] It is important to discuss all treatment options with the patient early in the treatment process. A neurosurgical consultation early in the medical management of the patient allows the patient time to assimilate the multiple treatment options. It is impossible to predict which patients may become refractory to medications, so patients must understand treatment options before they desperately seek surgery after months of failed medication trials. The patient's preference for either medical or surgical treatment as first-line therapy must be a part of decision making as well, and this can be facilitated by having an early consultation with a neurosurgeon.

The medical treatment of trigeminal and other cranial neuralgias is based on the capacity of the drugs employed to decrease nerve hyperexcitability, either peripherally or centrally. Clinically, pharmacologic therapies are aimed at providing rapid and sustainable pain relief with the least number of side effects. Unfortunately, the clinical trials in trigeminal neuralgia are not adequate for a full understanding of each medication's impact on this disease. Each patient is evaluated individually, by taking into account age, other systemic illnesses, and previous medications tried, and then medication choices are made.

Generally, treatment is begun with an antiepileptic medication that has proven antineuralgic properties. Initial doses should be low and titrated upward gradually, with close clinical monitoring, until either the maximum tolerated dose or the pain-free dose is attained. For years, the standard has been carbamazepine, 100 to 200 mg two or three times daily, which provides benefit in more than 75% of patients. Today, clinicians can choose from multiple medications, but a response to carbamazepine has been described as being almost diagnostic.

Box 50.2 Facial Pain of Unknown Origin (Atypical Facial Pain)

I. Neuropathic pain
  A. Intermittent
    1. Trigeminal neuralgia
    2. Glossopharyngeal neuralgia
    3. Occipital neuralgia
    4. Nervus intermedius neuralgia, etc.
  B. Continuous
    1. Trigeminal dysesthesia
    2. Trigeminal dysesthesia, sympathetically maintained
II. Myofascial pain

If the initial medication is not tolerated because of side effects, then an alternative medication is used. For example, if carbamazepine is not tolerated, other medications, including baclofen,[35–41] sodium valproate,[42] gabapentin,[43–47] lamotrigine,[44,45,48–52] oxcarbazepine,[53–57] topiramate,[53,58,59] felbamate,[60] zonisamide, vigabatrin, pregabalin, and clonazepam,[61,62] are sometimes effective, but adequate formal studies of the therapeutic efficacy of most of these agents have not been performed. A continuing need exists for new antineuralgic medications because of the limited tolerance and limited efficacy of those agents already available.[63] Blockade of the trigeminal nerve and its branches with local anesthetic and steroid can be extremely effective in the management of the acute pain of trigeminal neuralgia while the patient waits for pharmacologic interventions to become effective.

Those clinicians who have followed patients with trigeminal neuralgia for more than a few years realize that the disease often goes into remission, and a patient may enter remission during a treatment course. If the patient has been without an attack for several months, slow tapering of the current medication can be beneficial, and if the patient has entered a remission period, no medication will be necessary until the remission period ends. Patient compliance with medication regimens is essential to determining what benefit, if any, is being obtained. Patients with trigeminal neuralgia often taper the medication themselves as pain relief is sustained, only to have the pain start again. Patients must be counseled to be extremely compliant to achieve maximum benefit from the medications.

If only limited benefit is realized with one medication and side effects prohibit higher doses, a second medication may be used. Often a combination of antiepileptic medications is needed to relieve pain completely. Surgical options may be considered after multiple medication failures, the patient's intolerance of side effects, or pain escalation. When a patient has consulted with a surgeon early in the treatment phase, this transition is easier for both the patient and the treating physicians and is achieved in a more timely manner, thereby limiting the patient's suffering.

Surgical Management

Surgical treatment of trigeminal neuralgia is considered for patients in whom medical treatment has failed or who are unable to tolerate medical treatment because of side effects. *Failure* of medical therapy is a relative term that takes into account the number, duration, maximum dosage, and intolerable side effects of medications used to attempt to control the pain of trigeminal neuralgia. On occasion, patients who are so significantly impaired by pain that they are rendered unable to chew or drink may be offered surgery before medical treatment has failed, or has even begun, to avoid the delay that may be associated with titrating medications to therapeutic doses.

Burchiel[64] separated the diagnosis of idiopathic trigeminal neuralgia into type 1 and type 2. Type 1 (or typical) trigeminal neuralgia is characterized by unilateral, lancinating, very brief attacks of pain in one or more of the trigeminal nerve distributions. Between attacks, the patient has no intervening pain. The neurologic examination is normal, and the patient often has a history of at least a temporary or prolonged initial good response to carbamazepine. Type 2 (or atypical) trigeminal neuralgia is similar to type 1, yet it has a component of more constant, aching facial pain between the bouts of severe lancinating, paroxysmal pain. In addition, patients with type 2 trigeminal neuralgia may have some facial sensory loss and a history of poor response to medications. It is possible that type 2 trigeminal neuralgia represents an advanced stage of type 1.

Both type 1 and type 2 cases are believed to be caused by arterial or venous compression of the trigeminal nerve in the area of transition from central to peripheral myelin (Obersteiner-Redlich zone) near the root entry zone of the nerve to the brainstem. Operations such as microvascular decompression (MVD) directly address the underlying disorder. This procedure requires a general anesthetic and retrosigmoid craniotomy or craniectomy and therefore has historically been reserved for young, healthy patients. The remainder of surgical interventions for trigeminal neuralgia are directed at other areas along the course of the trigeminal pathway, such as the trigeminal tracts in the brainstem, the retrogasserian nerve root, the trigeminal (gasserian) ganglion, or the peripheral trigeminal nerve distributions (V1 to V3).

In addition to MVD, the most common surgical interventions for trigeminal neuralgia used today include percutaneous procedures directed at the gasserian ganglion or retrogasserian trigeminal nerve root and Gamma Knife radiosurgery (GKRS) treatment of the cisternal portion of the trigeminal nerve. The percutaneous techniques include glycerol (retro) gasserian rhizotomy, radiofrequency (RF) rhizotomy, and balloon compression of the trigeminal nerve. These percutaneous procedures produce a chemical, thermal, and physical injury, respectively, to the trigeminal nerve and ganglion. GKRS produces a radiation-induced injury of the trigeminal nerve. The percutaneous procedures, GKRS, and MVD are addressed subsequently.

Percutaneous Procedures

Percutaneous glycerol retrogasserian rhizotomy, otherwise known as a glycerol rhizotomy, is widely used for patients with type 1, type 2, or multiple sclerosis–related trigeminal neuralgia. Historically, this procedure was performed using absolute alcohol[64,65] or phenol and subsequently with a phenol/glycerol mixture injected into the trigeminal cistern. Later, Hakanson[64,66] reported that glycerol alone (without phenol) could relieve facial pain with less facial sensory loss.

Investigators reported that approximately 90% of patients achieved complete or immediate pain relief following glycerol injection, and 77% had good or excellent pain control over approximately a 10-year follow-up.[67,68] Facial sensory loss may occur following glycerol rhizotomy as follows: 32% to 48%, mild; 13%, moderate; 6%, dense.[68,69] Facial dysesthesia has been reported in approximately 2% to 22% of patients,[68] and anesthesia dolorosa has been noted in less than 1%.[69] Transient perioral herpes outbreak is seen in up to 3.8% to 37% of patients up to 1 week postoperatively.[68,69] Aseptic meningitis has been reported in 0.6% to 1.5% of patients.[68,69] An intraoperative vasovagal response can occur in 15% to 20% of cases and does not usually require aborting the procedure.[68,69]

Percutaneous balloon compression of the trigeminal nerve is based on the concept of squeezing, manipulating, or compressing the trigeminal nerve. Surgeons in the 1950s and 1960s reported that patients who had the trigeminal nerve traumatized during surgery seemed to have a better outcome with respect to pain relief. In 1983, Mullan and Lichtor[70] reported a percutaneous technique for compression of the gasserian ganglion using a Fogarty catheter. Currently, percutaneous balloon compression is mainly indicated for patients with type 1 or 2 (classic, idiopathic) trigeminal neuralgia and multiple sclerosis–related trigeminal neuralgia.

As with the other percutaneous techniques, pain relief following percutaneous balloon compression of the trigeminal nerve is usually immediate, but it can be delayed and may occur as long as 1 week after the procedure. Numbness in the V2 and V3 distribution is the norm (occurring in approximately 80% of patients) but is typically mild and often improves with time to the point that it is not a major problem. Most patients have some degree of jaw or pterygoid weakness, which is usually mild and often resolves over weeks to months. In rare cases, the unilateral symptomatic jaw weakness is permanent. Because of the possibility of permanent jaw weakness, this procedure is contraindicated for patients with preexisting contralateral jaw weakness because "drop jaw" can result. Theoretically, this complication can also be a problem when this procedure is performed bilaterally, such as for some patients with multiple sclerosis. Other, rarer complications include diplopia from compression of the fourth or sixth cranial nerve.

Pain relief is immediate in 92% to 100% of patients, and recurrence rates are reported as 19% to 32% over 5 to 20 years.[71,72] Severe sensory loss or dysesthesia occurs in 3% to 20% of patients.[71,72] Three to 16% of patients develop masseter or jaw weakness, although most improve or resolve after 1 year.[71,72] Transient diplopia has been reported to occur in 1.6% of patients.[72] Corneal anesthesia and anesthesia dolorosa have not been reported.

RF trigeminal (retrogasserian) rhizotomy is the third percutaneous procedure used to treat trigeminal neuralgia. The theory behind the use of RF to lesion the trigeminal nerve is that it may selectively injure or destroy the unmyelinated or poorly myelinated nociceptive nerve fibers and spare the (heavily) myelinated fibers that serve touch, proprioception, and motor function. The procedure consists of low-current stimulation to determine the proper position of the electrode in the offending trigeminal nerve fibers, followed by the creation of a permanent lesion using higher current to generate enough temperature to destroy the selected nerve fibers.

Mild paresthesia in the distribution of the facial pain is the goal of RF treatment of trigeminal neuralgia. Significant dysesthesia or sensory loss is reported in approximately 6% to 28% of patients, and loss of the corneal reflex may occur in 3% to 8% of patients, depending on the technique employed.[73–75] Certainly, when treating ophthalmic distribution trigeminal neuralgia, the risk of corneal anesthesia and keratitis is greater. Trigeminal nerve motor weakness has been reported following RF treatment in up to 14% of patients; however, this weakness is most often mild and transient.[73–75] Anesthesia dolorosa has been reported in 0.5% to 1.6% of patients.[73–75] Rare complications of carotid artery injury, stroke, diplopia, meningitis, seizures, and death have been reported.

Investigators have reported that 88% to 99% of patients obtain immediate pain relief following RF, with 20% to 27% recurrence rates over a 9- to 14-year follow-up.[73,74] Patients with a more dense sensory loss from the RF lesion tend to have a lower rate of recurrence, but they are subject to greater complications from dysesthesias and analgesia. One investigators reported that, following recurrence of pain, 81% of patients obtained "good or excellent" pain relief with a second RF treatment.[73]

Gamma Knife Radiosurgery

GKRS is the only noninvasive "surgical" treatment for trigeminal neuralgia. This same-day procedure is performed in the outpatient radiosurgery center. Treatment delivery can take 45 to 90 minutes, depending on the age of the cobalt sources in the Gamma Knife system used. After treatment is completed, the head frame is removed, and bandages are placed over the pin sites. The patient is observed in the radiosurgery center to allow complete recovery from any residual intravenous sedation and is discharged the same day.

Although GKRS can be performed using general anesthesia, a particular advantage of this technique is that it can be done with minimal intravenous sedation. The drawbacks are the cost of purchasing and maintaining the radiosurgery device and the latency period between treatment and facial pain improvement. Pain relief typically occurs after a latency period of 4 to 12 weeks following treatment, with a reported range of 1 day to 13 months following treatment. The rates of pain control and recurrence of trigeminal neuralgia have been somewhat variable between reports. The variability likely reflects different pain scales used to report outcome, follow-up duration, number of patients lost to follow-up, prior surgical treatment, the size and placement of the radiation dosage, and the maximal radiation dose. Investigators have reported that an excellent (complete pain relief without medication) or good (50% to 90% improved pain with or without medication) response is achieved in 57% to 86% of patients at 1 year following radiosurgery treatment.[76,77]

As with most surgical treatments for trigeminal neuralgia, recurrence of facial pain following GKRS increases with time after treatment. Pain recurrence rates of 23%, 33%, 39%, and 44% have been reported 1, 2, 3, and 5 years following radiosurgery treatment, respectively.[78,79] Mild or tolerable facial numbness occurs in up to 25% to 29% of patients and significant numbness or dysesthesia is reported in 12% to 18% of patients.[76,80] Complications of facial weakness, trigeminal motor weakness, and anesthesia dolorosa have not been reported. Greater doses of radiation correlate with both higher rates of pain control and higher rates of complications, which mostly consist of facial numbness and bothersome facial dysesthesias. Patients who experience more facial numbness seem to have a better chance of pain control.[76] Repeat radiosurgery for patients with recurrent pain has also been reported; approximately 50% reported excellent or good pain relief and an increased rate of facial sensory loss within a limited follow-up period.[81] Long-term follow-up studies of more than 10 to 20 years are needed. The ideal Gamma Knife dose and treatment strategy, as well as the role of other radiosurgery modalities, such as linear accelerator, remain to be determined.

Microvascular Decompression

MVD is the only medical or surgical intervention that directly addresses the presumed underlying pathologic features of classic trigeminal neuralgia: focal vascular compression of the trigeminal nerve near the brainstem root entry zone. The procedure requires a general anesthetic. Under intraoperative microscopic guidance, the arachnoid membrane surrounding the trigeminal nerve is opened, and the nerve is explored from the brainstem to the entrance of the nerve to Meckel's cave, where the trigeminal nerve ganglion (gasserian ganglion) is located. Under microscopic and endoscopic visualization, microdissection is performed to mobilize any arteries or veins compressing the trigeminal nerve. One or more Teflon sponges are then placed between the dissected blood vessels and the trigeminal nerve to prevent continued vascular compression of the trigeminal nerve. Veins compressing the trigeminal nerve can frequently be cauterized and divided. The compression is usually arterial, most commonly a branch of the superior cerebellar artery.[82] However, venous compression alone or a combination of arterial and venous compression may also occur.[83,84]

When offending vessels are identified and decompressed, most patients obtain immediate relief from their facial pain. Rates of immediate pain relief as high as 90% to 98% have been reported following MVD. Barker et al[85] reported on Dr. Jannetta's large series of MVD procedures with up to 10-year follow-up and defined the outcome as "excellent" if at least 98% pain relief was achieved without the need for medications and "good" if at least 75% pain relief was achieved with only intermittent need for pain medication. In that series, excellent or good early postoperative outcome was achieved in 98% of patients. This number decreased to approximately 84% and 67% after 1- and 10-year follow-up, respectively. Tronnier et al[86] reported that 64% of their patients were pain free 20 years following MVD. Whether continued recurrence of facial pain will occur in time is debated. Some investigators reported the majority of recurrences early, within 2 years of MVD, whereas others reported a more constant rate of recurrence, 3.5% annually in one series.[87,88]

Surgical complications associated with MVD have diminished since the regular use of brainstem and cranial nerve intraoperative neurophysiologic monitoring. Complications of MVD have included cerebellar injury (0.45%), transient facial numbness (15%), mild persistent facial numbness (12%), significant facial numbness (1.6%), facial dysesthesia (0% to 3.5%), hearing loss (<1%), transient or permanent facial weakness (<1%), cerebrospinal fluid leakage (1.5% to 2.5%), hematoma (0.5%), and mortality (0.3%).[82,89,90] In addition, lower morbidity rates have been reported from high-volume centers and from high-volume surgeons.[90]

When no arterial or venous compression is identified, the trigeminal nerve may be "traumatized" by stroking or squeezing the nerve with microinstruments, yet the resulting pain relief is only temporary. Such manipulation can be associated with trigeminal dysesthesias. Some surgeons have advocated partial sectioning of the sensory portion of the trigeminal nerve for negative explorations or during repeat surgical exploration of the nerve for recurrent pain following MVD.[87,91,92]

For several decades, MVD has been the standard to which each of the other surgical treatments for classic trigeminal neuralgia has been compared. In an experienced surgeon's hands, however, any of the techniques outlined in this chapter may be used to manage trigeminal neuralgia successfully. Each procedure has its own attributes and limitations, and the procedure selected must be based on the patient's individual situation. Therefore, from a surgical perspective, patients with trigeminal neuralgia are probably best managed at centers that are able to offer various interventions, including one or more percutaneous techniques (i.e., GKRS, and MVD).

Complications and Pitfalls

Diagnosis is extremely important in the treatment of trigeminal neuralgia. A thorough history, clinical examination, and diagnostic imaging are the mainstays of diagnosing facial pain. When all information has been collected, a treatment plan can be formulated. Pharmacotherapy must be engaged in a systematic manner, by testing each medication to its fullest potential. All cases should be evaluated from both a medical and surgical standpoint soon after the diagnosis is made, to ensure that the patient fully understands all available options before he or she makes an ultimate choice. Problems arise with one-sided approaches that may delay the ultimate goal of relieving the patient's pain. Multiple therapies are discussed here, and navigating these options must be done on a case-by-case basis with the patient, the physician, and the surgeon all working together.

Conclusion

Although arriving at a clinical diagnosis is often flawed and results in multiple consultations, misguided treatments, and in some cases unnecessary procedures, once a diagnosis of trigeminal neuralgia is made, many therapeutic options become available. The initial treatment is medical management, and with newer agents becoming available, many possibilities exist for monotherapy or even polypharmacy to reduce the patient's pain greatly. Surgical interventions are available for patients who are intolerant of medication therapy or whose pain is extreme and unremitting. Secondary causes must be explored in all patients because, if such causes are discovered, surgical interventions may supersede medical options.

Each of the medications and each of the surgical procedures is associated with side effects and potential risks. These pitfalls must be weighed based on each individual's medical conditions, lifestyle, age, personal preference, and past therapies. Further reviews of the literature are helping guide the clinical treatment with evidence-based recommendations.[93] The patient must be well-informed about both medical and surgical options as soon as the diagnosis is made. This allows time for the patient and the physicians to tailor the treatment plan to each individual. Withholding surgical or medical options until one modality has failed is inappropriate. As part of the initial evaluation, the patient should be required to consult with both surgical and medical practitioners. This approach allows for a planned therapeutic attack, with all parties seeking timely and effective pain relief for the patient.

References

Full references for this chapter can be found on www.expertconsult.com.

Glossopharyngeal Neuralgia

Steven D. Waldman

Glossopharyngeal neuralgia is a rare condition characterized by paroxysms of pain in the sensory division of the ninth cranial nerve. Clinically, the pain of glossopharyngeal neuralgia resembles that of trigeminal neuralgia, but the incidence rate of this painful condition is significantly less. The pain of glossopharyngeal neuralgia is rarely complicated by associated cardiac dysrhythmias and asystole. This chapter reviews the clinical features of glossopharyngeal neuralgia and discusses the current recommended treatment options for this uncommon pain syndrome.

Historical Considerations

Weisenburg[1] first described pain in the distribution of the glossopharyngeal nerve in a patient with a cerebellopontine angle tumor in 1910. In 1921, Harris[2] reported the first idiopathic case and coined the term glossopharyngeal neuralgia. Early attempts at treatment of glossopharyngeal neuralgia were primarily aimed at the extracranial surgical section of the glossopharyngeal nerve.[3] This approach met with limited success. Intracranial section of the glossopharyngeal nerve was first performed by Adson in 1925 and was refined by Dandy. The intracranial approach appeared to yield better results but was a riskier procedure.[4]

Clinical Syndrome

Demographic Considerations

The demographics of glossopharyngeal neuralgia are summarized in **Table 51.1**. Glossopharyngeal neuralgia is a rare disease with an incidence rate of 0.7 cases per 100,000 population.[5] Although the pain of glossopharyngeal neuralgia resembles that of trigeminal neuralgia, it occurs 100 times less frequently than trigeminal neuralgia.[6] Glossopharyngeal neuralgia occurs more commonly in patients older than 50 years but can occur at any age. The quality of pain associated with glossopharyngeal neuralgia is often described as shooting, stabbing, or needle-like, occurring in paroxysms that last from a few seconds to a minute. These paroxysms of pain are triggered by swallowing, chewing, coughing, or talking.

Location of the Pain

The localization of pain in the 217 patients with glossopharyngeal neuralgia reviewed by the Mayo Clinic is summarized in **Fig. 51.1**.[5] Otalgia was present in 155 patients, tonsillar pain in 147, laryngeal pain in 69, and tongue pain in 43. Sixty-eight patients had both ear and tonsillar pain, bilateral in approximately 2% of patients with glossopharyngeal neuralgia. Investigators at the Mayo Clinic also noted the spread of pain beyond the usual sensory distribution of the glossopharyngeal nerve to areas innervated by the vagus and trigeminal nerves and upper cervical segments. This phenomenon is termed overflow pain. Overflow pain occurs in approximately 20% of patients with glossopharyngeal neuralgia and was first noted by Keith[7] in 1932. The overflow pain associated with glossopharyngeal neuralgia has been postulated to be related to the spillover of intense impulses from the glossopharyngeal nerve through the tractus solitarius of the medulla to the vagus.[8] Fibers of the glossopharyngeal nerve may also join the descending portion of the trigeminal nerve, thereby contributing to this phenomenon.

An alternative hypothesis to account for overflow pain holds that an artificial synapse exists between the glossopharyngeal and vagus nerves at the level of the proximal glossopharyngeal and vagus nerves.[9] The overflow of neural impulses to the vagus nerve is most likely responsible for the bradycardia and cardiac arrest observed in patients with glossopharyngeal neuralgia associated with syncopal episodes. The coexistence of glossopharyngeal pain and cardiovascular abnormalities is extremely rare; only 35 patients have been reported to have this potentially lethal combination of symptoms.

Table 51.1 Demographics of Glossopharyngeal Neuralgia

1. Incidence rate is 0.7 cases per 100,000 population.
2. Occurs 100 times less frequently than trigeminal neuralgia.
3. Occurs more commonly in patients older than 50 years but can occur at any age.
4. Quality of pain described as shooting, stabbing, or needle-like.
5. Episodes of pain occur in paroxysms that last from a few seconds to a minute.
6. Paroxysms of pain are often triggered by swallowing, chewing, coughing, or talking.

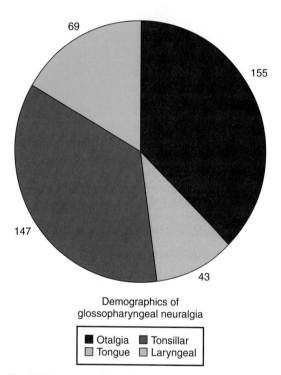

Demographics of glossopharyngeal neuralgia

- ■ Otalgia ■ Tonsillar
- ▨ Tongue ▨ Laryngeal

Fig. 51.1 **Demographics of glossopharyngeal neuralgia.**

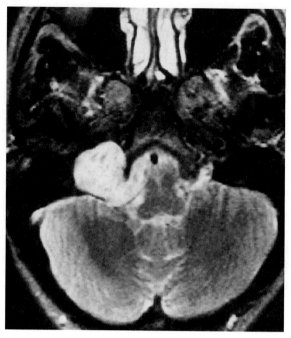

Fig. 51.2 **Jugular fossa schwannoma in a 32-year-old woman.** Axial T2-weighted magnetic resonance scan. The sharply defined tumor centered in the right jugular foramen is well seen. The tumor represents a benign schwannoma with smooth expansion of the skull base but no involvement of the right internal auditory canal. *(From Stark DD, Bradley WG: Magnetic resonance imaging, ed 3, St Louis, 1999, Mosby, p 1217.)*

Evaluation

As with most other head and facial pain syndromes, the diagnosis of glossopharyngeal neuralgia is made by performing a targeted history and physical examination.[10,11] Most cases of glossopharyngeal neuralgia are idiopathic; however, care must be taken to exclude tumors of the head and neck, especially those that occur at the cerebellopontine angle that may be the cause of the patient's symptoms (**Fig. 51.2**). Although the condition is exceedingly rare, a careful cardiac examination is indicated to rule out glossopharyngeal neuralgia with associated syncope.

Idiopathic glossopharyngeal neuralgia has four major characteristics that include: (1) a history of shooting, stabbing, shock-like pain in the neck, throat, or ear that occurs in paroxysms and is triggered by talking, chewing, drinking or coughing; (2) the neurologic examination results are normal, and the ear, pharynx, hypopharynx, piriform sinuses, and larynx are free from objective disease; (3) the patient is relatively pain free between attacks and can carry out normal activities; and (4) the pain is markedly improved or relieved by blockade of the glossopharyngeal nerve with local anesthetic.[12] Dull, aching, poorly localized pain that persists between paroxysms of tic-like pain is strongly suggestive of a space-occupying lesion and requires a thorough evaluation.[13]

Testing

Clinical laboratory tests that consist of a complete blood count, erythrocyte sedimentation rate, antinuclear antibody, and automated serum chemistry are indicated to rule out occult systemic diseases, including temporal arteritis, inflammatory conditions, infection, and malignant disease that may mimic glossopharyngeal neuralgia.[13]

Magnetic resonance imaging of the head helps rule out intracranial tumor and demyelinating disease that may be responsible for the patient's symptomatology.[14] Imaging of the neck is also indicated, if tumor of the hypopharynx, larynx, or piriform sinus is considered. Differential neural blockade with local anesthetic aids in establishing the diagnosis of glossopharyngeal neuralgia.

Treatment

In most patients, the pain of glossopharyngeal neuralgia can be controlled. In the acute, uncontrolled attack of glossopharyngeal neuralgia, hospitalization is indicated to facilitate the relief of pain and to monitor for side effects from the treatments chosen.

Table 51-2 Guidelines for Use of Carbamazepine in Treatment of Glossopharyngeal Neuralgia

1. Order baseline complete blood count, blood chemistry, and urinalysis before initiation of therapy.

2. Start therapy slowly if the pain is not out of control.

3. Begin with a 200-mg bedtime dose for 2 nights.

4. Drug is increased in 200-mg increments in equally divided doses every 2 days, as side effects allow, until pain relief is obtained or a total dose of 1200 mg daily is reached.

5. Patient is cautioned regarding side effects, including dizziness, sedation, confusion, and rash.

6. Carefully monitor laboratory data to avoid life-threatening blood dyscrasias.

7. Discontinue drug at the first sign of blood count abnormality or rash.

8. After pain relief is obtained, the patient should be left at this dose of carbamazepine for at least 6 months before tapering.

9. Patient should be informed that under no circumstances should the dose of drug be changed or the prescription refilled or discontinued without consultation with the pain management specialist.

10. Patient should be aware that premature tapering or discontinuation may lead to recurrence of pain with subsequent pain control being more difficult.

11. Hospitalize patients for pain emergencies.

Pharmacologic Treatment

Carbamazepine

Carbamazepine (Tegretol) represents the first line of treatment for glossopharyngeal neuralgia.[15] A rapid response to this drug helps confirm the clinical diagnosis of glossopharyngeal neuralgia. In spite of the efficacy and safety of this drug relative to other treatments for glossopharyngeal neuralgia, much confusion and unfounded anxiety surround the use of carbamazepine. Practical guidelines for the use of carbamazepine are summarized in **Table 51.2**.[16] Baseline clinical laboratory tests that consist of a complete blood count, blood chemistry, and urinalysis are obtained before initiation of carbamazepine. This pretreatment testing avoids the need to discontinue carbamazepine because of an unsuspected laboratory abnormality that is erroneously attributed to the carbamazepine.

If the pain is not out of control, carbamazepine should be initiated slowly. Therapy begins with a 200-mg bedtime dose for 2 nights. The patient is cautioned regarding side effects, including dizziness, sedation, confusion, and rash. The drug is increased in 200-mg increments (in equally divided doses) every 2 days, as side effects allow, until pain relief is obtained or a total dose of 1200 mg daily is reached. Careful monitoring of laboratory parameters is mandatory to avoid the (rare) possibility of life-threatening blood dyscrasias. At the first sign of blood count abnormality or rash, this drug should be discontinued. Failure to monitor patients started on carbamazepine can lead to disaster. When pain relief is obtained, the patient should be maintained on this dose of carbamazepine for at least 6 months before tapering is considered. The patient should be informed that under no circumstances should the dosage of drug be changed or the drug refilled or discontinued without consultation with the pain management specialist. The patient should be aware that premature tapering or discontinuation of carbamazepine may lead to recurrence of pain with subsequent pain control being more difficult.

With treatment of a patient in whom the pain of glossopharyngeal neuralgia is unbearable, carbamazepine may be initiated in the inpatient setting at a dose of 200 mg three to four times a day with careful observation for central nervous system side effects.

Table 51.3 Guidelines for Use of Gabapentin in Treatment of Glossopharyngeal Neuralgia

1. Order baseline complete blood count, blood chemistry, and urinalysis.

2. Begin treatment with 300-mg bedtime dose for 2 nights.

3. Increase drug in 300-mg increments in equally divided doses every 2 days, as side effects allow, until pain relief is obtained or a total dose of 300 mg daily is reached.

4. If patient has experienced partial pain relief, blood level is drawn and the drug is carefully titrated upward with 100-mg tablets.

5. Rarely is more than 2400 mg needed to control pain.

6. Patient is cautioned regarding side effects, including dizziness, sedation, confusion, and rash.

Gabapentin

In the patient in whom carbamazepine does not adequately control the pain of glossopharyngeal neuralgia, gabapentin (Neurontin) is a reasonable next step.[13] Practical guidelines for the use of gabapentin are summarized in **Table 51.3**.[16] Baseline clinical laboratory tests that consist of a complete blood count, blood chemistry, and urinalysis are obtained before beginning treatment with gabapentin. Treatment is initiated with a 300 mg bedtime dose for 2 nights and is increased in 300-mg increments (in equally divided doses) every 2 days, as side effects allow, until pain relief is obtained or a total dose of 1800 mg daily is reached. At this point, if the patient has experienced partial relief of pain, the drug is carefully titrated upward in 100-mg doses. Rarely is more than 2400 mg necessary. The patient is cautioned regarding side effects including dizziness, sedation, confusion, and rash. Pregabalin may also be a reasonable alternative to gabapentin.

Baclofen

Baclofen (Lioresal) has been reported to be of value in some patients with glossopharyngeal neuralgia who do not obtain relief from carbamazepine and gabapentin.[17] Practical guidelines for the use of baclofen are summarized in **Table 51.4**.[16] Baseline clinical laboratory tests that consist of a complete blood count, blood chemistry, and urinalysis are obtained before beginning treatment with baclofen. Treatment is initiated with a 10-mg bedtime dose for 2 nights. The drug is increased in 10-mg increments (in equally divided doses) every 5 days, as side effects allow, until pain relief is obtained or a total dose of 80 mg daily is reached. The patient is cautioned regarding side effects including dizziness, sedation, confusion, and rash. Baclofen has significant central nervous system and hepatic side effects and is poorly tolerated by most patients. As with carbamazepine, careful monitoring of laboratory data is indicated during the initial use of this drug.

Neural Blockade

Glossopharyngeal Nerve Block

The use of glossopharyngeal nerve block with a local anesthetic and a steroid serves as an excellent adjunct to the pharmacologic treatment of glossopharyngeal neuralgia.[11,12] The use of this technique allows rapid palliation of pain while oral medications are titrated to effective levels.

CLINICALLY RELEVANT ANATOMY

The glossopharyngeal nerve exits from the jugular foramen in proximity to the vagus and accessory nerve and the internal jugular vein.[18] All three nerves lie in the groove between the internal jugular vein and internal carotid artery (**Fig. 51.3**). Inadvertent puncture of either vessel during glossopharyngeal nerve block can result in intravascular injection or hematoma formation. Even small amounts of local anesthetic injected into the carotid artery at this location can produce profound local anesthetic toxicity. The landmarks for glossopharyngeal nerve block involve location of the styloid process of the temporal bone. This osseous process represents the calcification of the cephalad end of the stylohyoid ligament. Although the process is usually easy to identify, if ossification is limited, location with the exploring needle may be difficult.

TECHNIQUE

The patient is placed in the supine position. An imaginary line is visualized running from the mastoid process to the angle of the mandible (**Fig. 51.4**). The styloid process

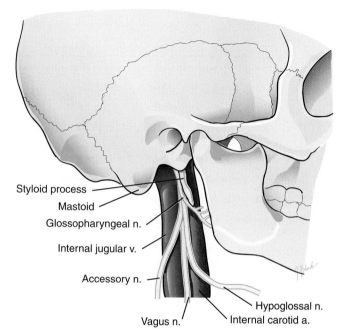

Fig. 51.3 **Clinically relevant anatomy for glossopharyngeal nerve block.** *(From Waldman SD:* Atlas of interventional pain management, *ed 2, Philadelphia, 2003, Saunders, p 69.)*

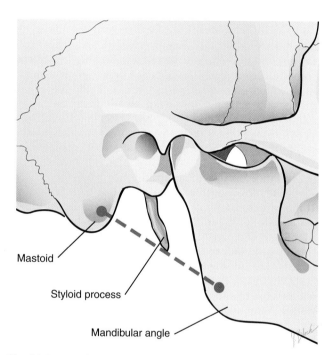

Fig. 51.4 For a glossopharyngeal nerve block, the patient is placed in the supine position and an imaginary line is visualized running from the mastoid process to the angle of the mandible. *(From Waldman SD:* Atlas of interventional pain management, *ed 2, Philadelphia, 2003, Saunders, p 71.)*

should lie just below the midpoint of this line. The skin is prepped with antiseptic solution. A 22-gauge 1½-inch needle attached to a 10-mL syringe is advanced at this midpoint location in a plane perpendicular to the skin. The styloid process should be encountered within 3 cm (**Fig. 51.5**). After contact is made, the needle is withdrawn and walked off the styloid process posteriorly. As soon as bony contact is lost and

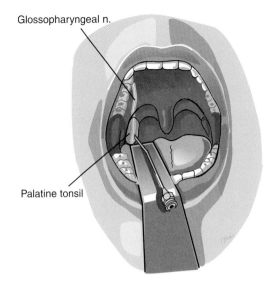

Fig. 51.6 **Intraoral technique for glossopharyngeal nerve block.** *(From Waldman SD: Atlas of interventional pain management, ed 3, Philadelphia, 2009, Saunders, p 98.)*

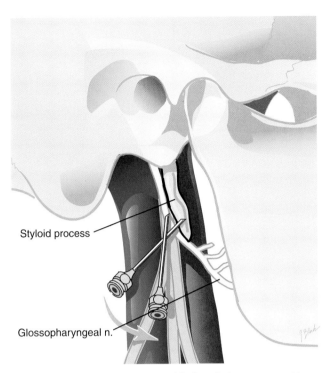

Fig. 51.5 **Glossopharyngeal nerve block technique.** *(From Waldman SD: Atlas of interventional pain management, ed 3, Philadelphia, 2009, Saunders, p 94.)*

careful aspiration reveals no blood or cerebrospinal fluid, 7 mL of 0.5% preservative-free lidocaine combined with 80 mg of methylprednisolone is injected in incremental doses. Subsequent daily nerve blocks are carried out in a similar manner, substituting 40 mg of methylprednisolone for the initial 80-mg dose.[19] The nerve may also be blocked via an intraoral approach (**Fig. 51.6**). Either approach may be used for breakthrough pain in patients who previously experienced adequate pain control with oral medications.

Potential complications of glossopharyngeal nerve block are related to trauma of the internal jugular and carotid arteries.[19] Hematoma formation and intravascular injection of local anesthetic with subsequent toxicity can represent significant problems for the patient.

Neurodestructive Procedures

The injection of small quantities of alcohol, phenol, and glycerol into the area of the glossopharyngeal nerve has been shown to provide long-term relief for patients with glossopharyngeal neuralgia that has not responded to optimal trials of the previously mentioned therapies.[18] Destruction of the glossopharyngeal nerve can also be carried out with creation of a radiofrequency lesion, with biplanar fluoroscopic guidance.[20] This procedure is reserved for patients in whom all the treatments described for intractable

glossopharyngeal neuralgia have failed and whose physical status otherwise precludes more invasive neurosurgical treatments.

Microvascular Decompression of the Glossopharyngeal Root

Microvascular decompression of the glossopharyngeal root (Jannetta technique) is the neurosurgical procedure of choice for intractable glossopharyngeal neuralgia.[21] The theoretical basis of the operation is that glossopharyngeal neuralgia is, in fact, a compressive mononeuropathy. The operation consists of identification of the glossopharyngeal root close to the brainstem and isolation of the offending compressing blood vessel.[22] A sponge is interposed between the vessel and nerve, thereby effecting a cure.

Conclusion

The pain specialist should be aware of the severity of pain associated with glossopharyngeal neuralgia and the psychologic effects of persistent, uncontrolled, severe pain. Correctly used, pharmacologic therapy combined with neural blockade should control the pain of glossopharyngeal neuralgia in most cases. Surgical therapy should be considered if conservative therapy fails to provide long-lasting relief for patients with glossopharyngeal neuralgia.

References

Full references for this chapter can be found on www.expertconsult.com.

Chapter **52**

Giant Cell Arteritis

Brian L. Hazleman

Historical Considerations

The earliest description of giant cell arteritis (GCA) may have been in the tenth century in the Tadkwat of Ali Iba Isu, where removal of the temporal artery was recommended as treatment. Jan Van Eyck's work depicting the Holy Virgin with Canon Van der Paele (1436) and Pieri di Cosimo's portrait of Fracesco Gamberti (1505) both show signs of prominent temporal arteries. Contemporary accounts document rheumatic pains and difficulty attending morning service with possible stiffness and general ill health. No further evidence for the existence of GCA exists until the late nineteenth century, when recognizable descriptions were documented in the British Isles. Jonathan Hutchinson in 1890 described "a peculiar form of thrombotic arteritis of the aged, which is sometimes productive of gangrene." For 40 years, no published reports are found until Horton et al[1] (1932) described the typical histologic evidence of temporal artery biopsy. In 1960, a report of 67 patients emphasized the occurrence of anarthritic rheumatism (an earlier title for polymyalgia rheumatica [PMR]) in GCA, providing clinical evidence for the relationship between PMR and GCA.[2]

The Clinical Syndrome

Key clinical features of GCA are the following:

1. A wide range of symptoms is seen, but most patients have clinical findings related to involved arteries.
2. Frequent features include fatigue, headaches, jaw claudication, loss of vision, scalp tenderness, PMR, and aortic arch syndrome (decreased or absent peripheral pulses, discrepancies of blood pressure, arterial bruits).
3. Unlike other forms of vasculitis, GCA rarely involves the skin, kidneys, and lungs.

4. The erythrocyte sedimentation rate (ESR) is usually highly elevated but may infrequently be normal.

The mean age of onset is approximately 70 years; the condition is rare in those younger than 50 years. Women are affected about three times as often as men. The onset can be dramatic but is usually insidious. The constitutional symptoms, including fever, anorexia, weight loss, and depression, are present in most patients, may be an early or even an initial finding, and can lead to a delay in diagnosis. Patients may present with a pyrexia of unknown origin and be subjected to many investigations. The condition causes a wide range of symptoms, but most patients have clinical features related to affected arteries. Common features include headache and tenderness of the scalp, particularly around the temporal and occipital arteries (**Fig. 52.1**).

The most common symptom of GCA is headache, which is present in more than two thirds of patients. It usually begins early in the course of the disease and may be the presenting symptom. The pain is severe and localized to the temple. However, it may be occipital or be less defined and precipitated by brushing the hair. Headache can be severe even when the arteries are clinically normal and, conversely, may subside even when the disease remains active. The nature of the pain varies; some patients describe it as shooting, and others as a more steady ache. Scalp tenderness is common, particularly around the temporal and occipital arteries, and may disturb sleep. Tender spots, or nodules, or even small skin infarcts may be present for several days. The vessels are thickened, tender, and nodular with absent or reduced pulsation. Occasionally they are red and clearly visible (**Fig. 52.2**).

Visual disturbances have been described in 25% to 50% of cases, although the incidence rate of visual loss is now regarded as much lower, about 6% to 10% in most series, which is probably the result of earlier recognition and treatment.[3] Visual symptoms are an ophthalmic emergency; if they are identified and treated urgently, blindness is almost entirely preventable. The variety of ocular lesions essentially results from occlusion of the various orbital or ocular arteries. Blindness is the most serious and irreversible feature. The visual loss is usually sudden, painless, and permanent; it may vary from mistiness of vision, or involvement of a part of the visual field, to complete blindness. The second eye is at risk of involvement if the patient is not treated aggressively. Involvement of the second eye can occur within 24 hours. Blindness may be the initial presentation in cases of GCA, but it tends to follow other symptoms by several weeks or months.

The incidence of various ocular manifestations given in the literature varies widely because the incidence depends on a number of factors—the most important of which is how early the diagnosis of GCA is established and the treatment started. It also depends on the rigor with which cases are diagnosed. The most common cases are optic nerve ischemic lesions. These are usually anterior and are associated with partial or more frequently complete visual loss. They can occasionally be posterior, which can lead to partial or complete loss. Extraocular mobility disorders are usually transient and not associated with visual loss. Pupillary abnormalities can be seen as a result of visual loss. Cerebral ischemic lesions producing visual loss are rare, as are anterior segment ischemic lesions and choroidal infarcts. Retinal ischemic lesions can affect the central retinal artery, which is associated with severe visual loss. The cilioretinal artery can be occluded but is invariably associated with anterior ischemic optic neuropathy (AION).

Pain on chewing, from claudication of the jaw muscles, occurs in up to two thirds of patients. Tingling in the tongue, loss of taste, and pain in the mouth and throat can also occur, presumably as a result of vascular insufficiency. The widespread nature of the vasculitis has been previously mentioned. Clinical evidence of large artery involvement is present in 10% to 15% of cases, and in some instances, aortic dissection and rupture occur.

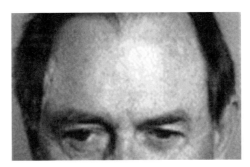

Fig. 52.2 **Patient with untreated giant cell arteritis.** The temporal artery is visibly swollen. It was tender to palpation and somewhat nodular on physical examination. Any visibly or palpably abnormal area of artery should be included in the biopsy specimen when temporal artery biopsy is performed to increase diagnostic yield. *(From Evans JM, GG Hunder: Polymyalgia rheumatica and giant cell arteritis, Rheumatic Dis Clin North Am 26:493, 2000.)*

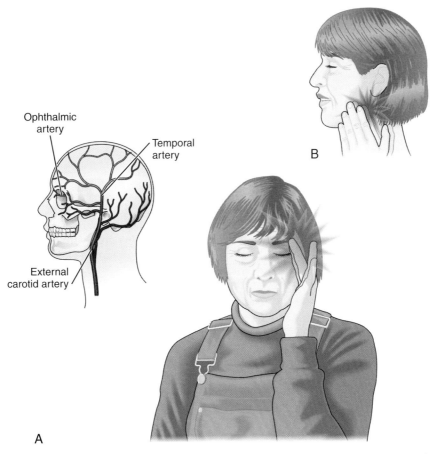

Fig. 52.1 **A,** Temporal arteritis is a disease of the sixth decade that occurs almost exclusively in whites, with a predilection of 3:1 for women. **B,** The *sine qua non* of temporal arteritis is jaw claudication.

Less common features of GCA include hemiparesis, peripheral neuropathy, deafness, depression, and confusion. Involvement of the coronary arteries may lead to myocardial infarction. Aortic regurgitation and congestive cardiac failure may also occur. Abnormalities of thyroid and liver function are well described. An association between carpal tunnel syndrome and PMR has been noted by several authors. Local corticosteroid injection or surgical decompression is sometimes necessary.

Epidemiology

GCA almost exclusively affects the white population. Most reports originate from northern Europe and parts of the northern United States; however, the diseases are recognizable worldwide. Both PMR and GCA affect elderly people and are seldom diagnosed before the age of 50 years (**Table 52.1**). A study of biopsy-proven GCA diagnosed from 1950 to 1985 in Olmsted County, Minn, showed average annual incidence and prevalence rates of 17 and 223, respectively, per 100,000 inhabitants aged 50 years or more.[4] The age-adjusted incidence rates were approximately three times higher in women than in men.[4] In addition, the incidence rate increased with age in both genders.[4] The incidence rate also increased significantly during the period 1950 to 1985 for females but decreased for males over the same period.[4] The incidence rates reported from Olmsted County are similar to those in Göteborg, Sweden.[5] Between 1970 and 1975, the incidence rate was 16.8 per 100,000 inhabitants in Sweden versus 18.3 per 100,000 in Minnesota.[4,5]

The temporal arteries and aortas of all adults who died in Malmö throughout 1 year were examined, and although active GCA was not found, evidence of previous arteritis was found in 1.7% of the 889 cases.[6] Either biopsy evidence or a clinical history suggestive of GCA was found in 75% of these subjects.[6] This study certainly suggests that GCA may be underdiagnosed, but further studies are needed.

Cyclic patterns and seasonal variations have been reported and suggest that infective agents may trigger the disease, although none have been isolated.

Relationship Between Polymyalgia Rheumatica and Giant Cell Arteritis

In recent years, GCA and PMR have increasingly been considered as closely related conditions.[7,8] The two syndromes form a spectrum of diseases and affect the same types of patients. The conditions may occur independently or may occur in the same patient, either together or separately.

In patients with PMR who have no symptoms or signs of GCA, positive temporal biopsy results are found in 10% to 15%. Those investigators who wish to preserve the identity of the two diseases base their argument on the latter figure and on the failure to find evidence of arteritis in many patients followed for many years with polymyalgia. Conversely, many similarities are seen between the two conditions. The age and gender distributions are similar, the biopsy findings show an identical pattern, and the laboratory features are similar, although many are nonspecific inflammatory changes. In addition, similarity is found in the myalgia, in the associated systemic features, and in the response to corticosteroid therapy.

The onset of myalgic symptoms may precede, coincide with, or follow that of the arteritic symptoms. No difference has been found between the characteristics for those patients with myalgia with positive biopsy results and those with no histologic evidence of arteritis. Mild aching and stiffness may persist for months after other features of GCA have remitted. Little evidence is found to suggest that the musculoskeletal symptoms are related to vasculitis. Many patients with GCA do not have PMR, even when large vessels are involved. In addition, the finding of joint swelling in some patients and the production of pain with the injection of 5% saline solution into the acromioclavicular, sternoclavicular, and manubriosternal joints suggests that PMR in some patients may be a particular form of proximal synovitis.

Clinical Testing

One of the most frequently performed diagnostic tests in suspected cases of GCA is temporal artery biopsy (**Table 52.2**). The choice of patients for biopsy depends on local circumstances, but a pragmatic policy is selection of only patients with suspected GCA (not those with obvious clinical features). Patients with PMR alone need to be monitored carefully for development of clinical GCA and do not need a biopsy.

One third of patients with signs and symptoms of cranial arteritis may have negative temporal artery biopsy results, which may be the result of the localized involvement of arteries in the head and neck. Temporal artery biopsy may show arteritis even after 14 days of corticosteroid treatment, so biopsy may be worthwhile for up to 2 weeks of treatment. However, the biopsy should be obtained as soon as possible, and treatment for suspected GCA should not be delayed simply to allow a biopsy to be carried out.

Clinicians vary greatly in their approach to temporal artery biopsy. Some believe it emphasizes the value of a positive

---

Table 52.1 Epidemiologic Features of Giant Cell Arteritis

Peak incidence rate at ages 60 to 75 years.

Gender distribution of three women to one man.

Annual incidence and prevalence rates of biopsy-proven GCA are 17 and 223 of 100,000, respectively.

Mainly affects white people but can occur worldwide.

Familial aggregation has been reported, which suggests a genetic association.

GCA, giant cell arteritis.

Table 52.2 Diagnostic Value of Temporal Artery Biopsy for Giant Cell Arteritis

Perform biopsy if diagnosis is in doubt, particularly if systemic symptoms predominate.

Biopsy is most useful within 24 hours of starting treatment, but do not delay treatment for sake of biopsy.

A negative biopsy result does not exclude GCA.

A positive result helps to prevent later doubts about diagnosis, particularly if treatment causes complications.

GCA, giant cell arteritis.

histologic diagnosis, especially months or years later when side effects of the steroid treatment have developed. Others believe that a high false-negative rate diminishes the value of the procedure. In most instances, the high false-negative rate can be attributed to the focal nature of involvement of the superficial temporal artery by the inflammatory process.

The histologic appearance of GCA is one of the most distinctive of vascular disorders (**Table 52.3**). The dense granulomatous inflammatory infiltrates that characterize the acute stages of the disease resemble those of Takayasu's arteritis, but the clinicopathologic features in patients with positive temporal artery biopsy results are diagnostic. The arteritis is histologically a panarteritis with giant cell granuloma formation, often in close proximity to a disrupted internal elastic lamina. Large and medium-sized arteries are affected; the involvement is patchy, and skip lesions are often found. More patients with skip lesions have normal arteries to palpation but do not have a more benign disease.

The gross features are not characteristic. The vessels are enlarged and nodular and have little or no lumen. Thrombosis often develops at sites of active inflammation. Later, these areas may recanalize. The lumen is narrowed by intimal proliferation, which is a common finding in arteries and may result from advancing age, nearby chronic inflammation, or low blood flow. The adventitia is usually invaded by mononuclear and occasionally polymorphonuclear inflammatory cells, often cuffing the vasa vasorum; here, fibrous proliferation is frequent. The changes in the media are dominated by the giant cells, which vary from small cells with two to three nuclei up to masses of 100 nm containing many nuclei. Invasion by mononuclear cells that resemble histiocytes is found here. Fibrinoid necrosis is infrequent. Giant cells are not seen in all sections and, therefore, are not required for the diagnosis if other features are compatible. The more sections that are examined in the area of arteritis, the more likely it is that giant cells will be found. Fragments of elastic tissue can be seen within giant cells, which are surrounded with plasma cell and lymphocytic infiltration (**Fig. 52.3**).

Corticosteroids reduce the inflammatory cell infiltrate so temporal artery biopsy should, if possible, be carried out before treatment is started. Therapy should not be delayed until a biopsy has been performed. Involvement of the aorta and its branches, the abdominal vessels, and the coronary arteries has been described. GCA as a cause of aortic dissection has been recorded rarely at autopsy, and most exceptionally during life, which probably reflects the relatively low incidence of aortic involvement in GCA. Of note is that most patients have a history of hypertension in life or features of hypertensive disease at autopsy.

The ESR is usually greatly elevated and provides a useful means of monitoring treatment, although it must be appreciated that some elevation of the ESR may occur in otherwise healthy elderly people. A normal ESR is occasionally found in patients with active biopsy-proven disease. Repeated measurements may show raised ESRs after an initial normal value.

Anemia, usually of a mild hypochromic type, is common and resolves without specific treatment, but more marked normochromic anemia occasionally occurs and may be a presenting symptom. Leukocyte and differential counts are generally normal; platelet counts are also usually normal but may be increased. Protein electrophoresis may show a nonspecific rise in alpha$_2$ globulin, with less frequent elevation of alpha$_1$ globulin and gamma globulin. Quantification of acute-phase proteins and alpha$_1$-antitrypsin, orosomucoid, haptoglobin, and C-reactive protein (CRP) are no more helpful than the ESR in the assessment of disease activity.

Abnormalities of thyroid and liver function have also been well described. In a retrospective survey of 59 cases of GCA, five patients with hyperthyroidism were identified.[9] The arteritis followed the thyrotoxicosis by intervals of 4 to 15 years in three cases, and in two, it occurred simultaneously. In 250 patients with autoimmune thyroid disease, seven cases of PMR or GCA were identified. All cases occurred in women older than age 60 years, for a prevalence rate of 9.3% in this age group.[10]

Raised serum values for alkaline phosphatase were found in up to 70% of patients with PMR, and transaminases in some cases were mildly elevated. Liver biopsies have shown portal and intralobular inflammation with focal liver cell necrosis and small epithelioid cell granuloma. The pathologic significance of these abnormalities is unclear.

Etiology and Pathogenesis

Cell-mediated immune responses are key mechanisms in the pathogenesis of GCA. Dendritic cells with an activated phenotype have been identified in the wall of the temporal arteries from patients with GCA engrafted into immunodeficient mice. Once activated, dendritic cells acquire the capacity to release chemokines, which recruit CD4T cells and macrophages through the vasa vasorum into the vessel wall (**Fig. 52.4**).

Table 52.3 **Histologic Features of Giant Cell Arteritis**
Histologically, a panarteritis is found with giant cell granuloma.
The involvement is patchy, and skip lesions are often found.
Clinically, the artery is enlarged and nodular with a reduced or absent lumen.
The aorta and other arteries are involved.

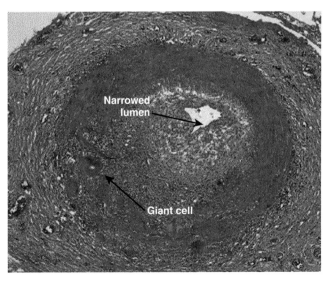

Fig. 52.3 **Arterial biopsy shows giant cells.**

PATHOGENESIS OF GIANT CELL ARTERITIS

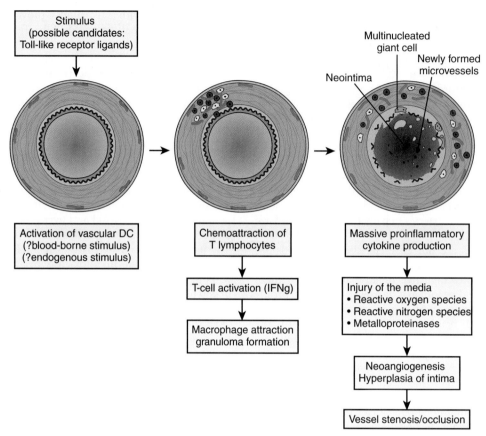

Fig. 52.4 **Pathogenesis of giant cell arteritis.** *DC,* dendritic cells; *IFNg,* interferon gamma.

Activated dendritic cells are also able to provide costimulatory signals needed to trigger T-cell activation. In turn, activated CD4T cells and macrophages start secreting proinflammatory cytokines. In particular, in the media, they release metalloproteinases that lead to fragmentation of the internal elastic lamma. In the adventitia, macrophages release interleukin-1 (IL-1) and IL-6.

Inflammatory cytokines synthesized by macrophages are thought to cause systemic manifestations in both PMR and GCA.[11]

Imaging in Giant Cell Arteritis

High-resolution color duplex ultrasound scan has gained widespread acceptance in diagnosis. Inflamed temporal arteries show a concentric hypoechogenic mural thickening "halo" that is thought to represent inflammatory wall edema. A positive halo sign is considered to rule in the diagnosis of GCA in the presence of clinical features, but a negative halo sign does not rule it out.

Typical changes in GCA on magnetic resonance imaging (MRI) include thickening and edema of the vessel wall. It can be used to diagnose early large-vessel vasculitis while angiography is still negative. MRI and computed tomographic (CT) scan are useful in evaluation of deep large vessels, such as thoracic and abdominal aorta.

Positron emission tomography (PET) with fluorodeoxyglucose (FDG) is being increasingly used because of its capacity to reveal inflammatory cell infiltration of the vessel wall. However, PET does not give information about wall structure or luminal flow.[12]

Treatment

Corticosteroids are mandatory in the treatment of GCA; they reduce the incidence of complications, such as blindness, and rapidly relieve symptoms (**Table 52.4**). Nonsteroidal anti-inflammatory drugs (NSAIDs) lessen the painful symptoms, but they do not prevent arteritic complications. The response to corticosteroids is usually dramatic and occurs within days. Corticosteroid treatment has improved the quality of life for patients, although no evidence shows that therapy reduces the duration of the disease. A fear of vascular complications in those patients with positive biopsy results often leads to the use of high doses of corticosteroids. Recent studies have emphasized the importance of adopting a cautious and individual treatment schedule and have highlighted the efficacy of lower doses of prednisolone.

Initially, the corticosteroids should be given in a sufficient dosage to control the disease and then maintained at the lowest dose that controls the symptoms and lowers the ESR. In patients with GCA, corticosteroids should preferably be given

Table 52.4 Treatment of Giant Cell Arteritis

Initial dose: Prednisolone 20 to 40 mg daily for 8 weeks. Patients with ocular symptoms may need up to 80 mg daily.

Reduce dose by 5 mg every 3 to 4 weeks until dose is 10 mg daily; then as for PMR (see Table 45.4).

Maintenance dose: About 3 mg daily may be needed.

Comment: Recurrence of symptoms necessitates an increase in the prescribed dose.

after the diagnosis has been confirmed histologically. However, when GCA is strongly suspected, there should be no delay in starting therapy because the artery biopsy will still show inflammatory changes for several days after corticosteroids have been started and the result is unlikely to alter therapeutic decisions. If the temporal artery (or other artery) biopsy shows no arteritis but the suspicion of disease is strong, corticosteroid treatment should be started. The great danger is delay in therapy because blindness may occur at any time.

Few clinical trials exist to help decide the correct initial dose. Most clinicians have strong views on the dose needed, but some views are based on tradition and anecdote. The recommended initial dose for PMR/GCA varies from 10 mg to 100 mg prednisolone daily. Intravenous corticosteroids are occasionally used if there are visual complications. In practice, most clinicians use 10 to 20 mg prednisolone daily to treat PMR and 40 to 60 mg for GCA because of the higher risk of arteritic complications in cases of GCA. Some ophthalmologists suggest an initial dose of at least 60 mg because they have seen blindness occur at a lower dose. However, this has to be balanced against the potential complication of high dosage in this older age group. Patients should be advised that although they are taking a maintenance dose of steroids, any sudden exacerbation of symptoms, particularly sudden visual deterioration, necessitates an immediate increase in dose.

Glucocorticoid therapy is adequate for most patients with GCA, but in those with long-standing glucocorticoid-resistant disease and those at risk of glucocorticoid-related adverse events, glucocorticoid-sparing agents should be considered (these include methotrexate and tumor necrosis factor α [TNFα] blockers).

Methotrexate appears to be effective in GCA but does not have a rapid onset of action and cannot be recommended as a replacement for glucocorticoids at disease onset. TNFα inhibition is to some extent effective in long-standing, refractory GCA but is not effective in new-onset GCA.[13]

Prognosis

Rapid reduction or withdrawal of corticosteroids has been reported to contribute to deaths in patients with GCA. Fortunately, complications are rare, and the activity of the disease seems to decline steadily. Relapses are more likely during the initial 18 months of treatment and within 1 year of withdrawal of corticosteroids. No reliable method of predicting those most at risk exists, but arteritic relapses in patients who presented with pure PMR are unusual. Temporal artery biopsy does not seem helpful in predicting outcome.

Controversy exists over the expected duration of the disease. Most European studies within the last 20 years report that between one third and one half of the patients are able to discontinue corticosteroids after 2 years of treatment. Studies from the Mayo Clinic in the United States have reported a shorter duration of disease for both PMR (11 months was the median duration of treatment, and three quarters of patients had stopped taking corticosteroids by 2 years) and GCA (most patients had stopped taking corticosteroids within 2 years).[14] The consensus seems to be that stopping treatment is feasible from 2 years onward.

Patients who are unable to reduce the dosage of prednisolone because of recurring symptoms or who have serious corticosteroid-related side effects develop pose particular problems. Drugs such as azathioprine and methotrexate have not been shown to exert a corticosteroid-sparing effect in corticosteroid-resistant cases of PMR/GCA.

Between one fifth and one half of patients may experience serious treatment-related side effects. Serious side effects are significantly related to high initial doses, maintenance doses, cumulative doses, and increased duration of treatment. Side effects can be minimized with use of low doses of prednisolone whenever possible.

In elderly people, corticosteroid treatment carries the risk of increasing osteoporosis. Glucocorticoids have more effect on the spine than on the femur. Bisphosphonates, such as etidronate and alendronate, have been shown to be useful in retarding bone loss in the setting of prolonged corticosteroid use.

Conclusion

GCA is the prime medical emergency in ophthalmology because it may result in loss of vision in one or both eyes. This vision loss is preventable if patients are diagnosed early and treated immediately with high doses of corticosteroids.

References

Full references for this chapter can be found on www.expertconsult.com.

Chapter **53**

Pain of Ocular and Periocular Origin

Steven D. Waldman and Corey W. Waldman

Pain of ocular and periocular origin represents a special challenge to the pain management physician. Pain in this anatomic region is unique because: (1) most diseases of the eye and periocular regions that cause blindness are relatively painless, yet the fear of blindness is ever present in any patient with eye pain; (2) most painful conditions of the eye and periocular region do not cause blindness in spite of the aforementioned fear to the contrary; (3) both lay persons and most health care professionals approach any problem involving the eye with great fear and trepidation because of the potential for disastrous consequences if a mistake in diagnosis or treatment is made; (4) the rich innervation of the cornea, conjunctiva, and periocular region means that even minor problems such as a superficial corneal abrasion can result in severe pain that is completely out of proportion to the scope and risk of the injury; and (5) if the pathologic process responsible for the patient's pain resides in the eye, an ophthalmologist is needed, and if it does not involve the eye, the ophthalmologist has little to offer, thus leaving the pain management physician to sort out the cause and provide the treatment for the patient's pain. In the author's experience, an element of each of these factors is present in almost every patient presenting with the symptoms of ocular and periocular pain. Thus, the care of such patients is more challenging in comparison with patients with less-threatening painful conditions such as low back pain. That said, as a practical matter, the management of most patients with ocular and periocular pain is relatively straightforward. For the purposes of this chapter, we must accept the simple fact that primary diseases of the eye are best treated by an ophthalmologist and the pain

management specialist's role in this setting is to attempt to identify those patients with primary eye disease and timely refer them to the ophthalmologist for definitive treatment of the ocular pathologic process responsible for the pain. For those patients with ocular and periocular pain that is unrelated to primary eye disease, identification and treatment of the painful condition usually becomes the responsibility of the pain management specialist. The following chapter provides an overview of primary eye diseases that require the treatment by an ophthalmologist and a discussion of those diseases that may cause ocular and periocular pain that do not find the nidus of their symptomatology in the eye and are best treated by the pain management specialist.

The Sensory Innervation of the Eye

The primary sensory innervation of the eye is mediated via the trigeminal ganglion.[1] The first division of the trigeminal nerve (V_1 ophthalmic division) carries the bulk of the pain impulses from the eye itself via the long ciliary branches of the nasociliary nerve (**Fig. 53.1**). The infratrochlear branch of the nasociliary nerve also provides sensory innervation to the medial portion of the eyelids, the adjacent nose, and the lacrimal sac. Trigeminal fibers intimately associated with the intraorbital parasympathetic ganglion and its parasympathetic fibers and the second cervical ganglion and its postganglionic sympathetic fibers may also subserve ocular and periocular pain. Other branches of the first division of the trigeminal nerve, the frontal and lacrimal nerves, provide sensory innervation to the upper eyelid, forehead, and the frontal sinus and the lacrimal gland and portions of the conjunctiva, respectively. Numerous fibers from the sphenopalatine ganglion also interact with trigeminal somatic fibers and the sympathetic and parasympathetic ganglia and fibers just mentioned and may serve an important role in some painful conditions that involve the eye, such as Sluder's neuralgia and cluster headache. The second division of the trigeminal nerve (V₂ maxillary) provides sensory innervation to the lower eyelid and conjunctiva via the infraorbital nerve.

Interestingly, the cornea receives most of the sensory innervation of the eye, with the density of sensory innervation of the cornea rivaled only by that of the anal mucosa.[2] Teleologically, this density of sensory innervation presumably serves to enhance the mechanisms to protect our most important sense organ by allowing the blink response and the convergence avoidance reflex to protect the eye.

In addition to the dense concentration of pain receptors to transmit the afferent sensation of pain via the trigeminal ganglion to higher centers, thermal receptors for cold and heat are also found throughout the eye. These mechanoreceptors are found in both the cornea and iris and may be responsible for afferent traffic carried via the trigeminal system that may be perceived by the patient as ocular pain even when no actual ocular tissue damage has occurred. Stretching of the extraocular muscles and the dural covering of the optic nerve by mass or tumor may also result in a sensation of ocular pain, even in the absence of actual nerve damage.

Common Causes of Ocular Pain

The following section presents a brief description of the most common causes of eye pain encountered in clinical practice. The patient with eye pain often presents in an anxious state armed with a detailed history of symptoms. The pain management specialist should begin the evaluation of such patients first by offering reassurance and a calm demeanor and second by rapidly assessing whether the clinical condition presents immediate risk to the patient's vision so that immediate ophthalmologic referral can be undertaken.

Styes (Hordeolums)

Styes, or hordeolums, are probably the most common cause of eye pain encountered in clinical practice. Styes are the result of bacterial infection of the small oil-producing meibomian glands or the eyelash follicles at the margin of the eyelid (**Fig. 53.2**).[3] More than 98% of styes are caused by *Staphylococcus aureus*.[4] These pus-filled abscesses can appear quite suddenly and can run the gamut from small self-limited infections that produce little pain and resolve on their own to rapidly growing, extremely painful abscesses that require immediate surgical incision and drainage and systemic antibiotics for resolution. If the condition is identified early, the use of non–neomycin-containing antibiotic ointment such as gentamicin or polymyxin-B and bacitracin ophthalmic ointment combined with frequent applications of warm moist packs usually resolves the problem.[4] If fever is present or the stye does not drain with conservative therapy, systemic antibiotics and immediate ophthalmologic referral for surgical incision and drainage is indicated.[5] If untreated, what begins as a simple localized folliculitis or meibomianitis can evolve into a vision-threatening and life-threatening periorbital cellulitis that has the potential to spread to the adjacent central nervous system.

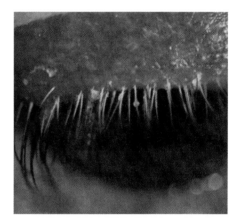

Fig. 53.2 **Blepharitis.** *(From Swartz MH: Textbook of physical diagnosis, ed 4, Philadelphia, 2002, Saunders, p 215.)*

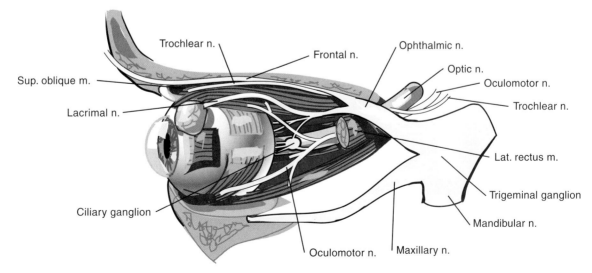

Fig. 53.1 **The sensory innervation of the eye.**

Corneal Abrasions

Corneal abrasions are another frequent cause of eye pain that prompts patients to seek urgent medical attention. The unique nature of the sensory innervation of the cornea results in the patient's perception of a foreign body in the eye any time the superficial corneal stroma is injured, and the C-type polymodal nociceptors that richly innervate the cornea are stimulated. A foreign body sensation is usually felt by the patient as being located under the upper eyelid even when no foreign body is present, and damage is limited to the corneal stroma. The continued firing of the polymodal receptors and recruitment of the corneal mechanoreceptors are probably responsible for this foreign body sensation, which occurs in almost all patients with corneal abrasion, even in the absence of a foreign body.

Patients with corneal abrasion usually relate a history of grit or a foreign body being blown into the eye or of minor mechanical trauma to the cornea during the insertion of contact lens or while playing sports.[6,7] Fluorescein staining usually reveals the damage to the corneal stroma; rarely is a foreign body seen.[8] The patient reports severe pain that is out of proportion to the apparent injury and insists that something is trapped under the upper eyelid, even after repeated attempts to convince the patient to the contrary. Photophobia and excessive lacrimation and scleral and conjunctival injection are often present, as is a significant substrate of anxiety.

In the presence of corneal abrasion, the clinician should evert the upper eyelid and rinse the eye with copious amounts of sterile saline solution to remove any residual foreign body that may not be readily apparent on initial investigation. If the corneal abrasion is the result of an accident that occurred during hammering or the use of power tools, a careful search for a metallic foreign body should be undertaken and a plain radiograph or computed tomographic (CT) scan of the orbit and orbital contents should be obtained to rule out occult intraocular metallic foreign body, which can present a significant risk to vision if undetected (**Figs. 53.3** and **53.4**). Treatment with non–neomycin-containing antibiotic ointment such as gentamicin or polymyxin-B and bacitracin ophthalmic ointment combined with patching of the eye and a large dose of reassurance usually resolves the problem.[9]

Conjunctivitis

Infection of the conjunctiva is a common cause of eye pain. Caused by bacteria, fungus, or virus, conjunctivitis can range from a mild self-limited disease that requires no treatment to a purulent eye infection that can be quite painful and upsetting to the patient.[10] Bacterial and viral conjunctivitis, which is also known as pink eye, can be contagious, and all patients with conjunctivitis should be instructed in good hand-washing techniques and informed of the need to sterilize fomites that they have in common with the family and coworkers (e.g., copy machines, faucets, telephones, computer keyboards). In addition to infectious causes, conjunctivitis can also be caused by environmental irritants, including pollen, dust, smog, and fumes.[11]

The patient with conjunctivitis presents with a red, irritated, and painful eye that is often associated with excessive lacrimation and some degree of photophobia (**Fig. 53.5**). A purulent

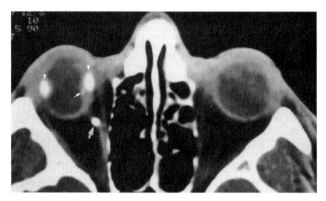

Fig. 53.4 CT scan shows intraconal, metallic foreign bodies just medial to the medial rectus *(large arrow)* and intraocular *(small arrow)*. Scleral band is in place at the right *(arrowheads)*. *(From Haaga JR, Lanzieri C: CT and MR imaging of the whole body, ed 4, vol 1, St Louis, 2003, Mosby, p 479.)*

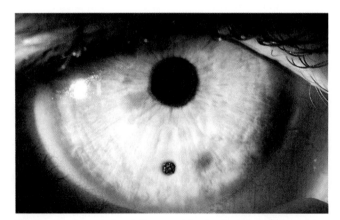

Fig. 53.3 An impacted metallic corneal foreign body is a common injury associated with drilling or grinding steel without protective goggles. These particles normally have insufficient energy to pass through the cornea and so lodge superficially. They become surrounded by a ring of rust within a few days, which should be lifted off with a sharp needle or dental burr with use of topical anesthesia, to prevent delayed healing. *(From Spalton DJ: Atlas of clinical ophthalmology, ed 3, Philadelphia, 2005, Mosby, p 170.)*

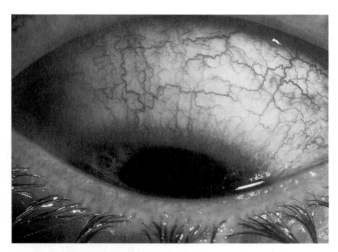

Fig. 53.5 Hyperemia of the conjunctiva may occur as part of any acute inflammatory process or in response to chronic irritative factors. An increase is seen in the number, caliber, and tortuosity of the vessels, producing a characteristic bright red appearance. Hyperemia is often associated with increased vascular permeability and edema or cellular infiltration. *(From Spalton DJ: Atlas of clinical ophthalmology, ed 3, Philadelphia, 2005, Mosby, p 65.)*

discharge is also often present. If the discharge is severe, the patient may awaken with the eyelids stuck together, resulting in extreme anxiety for the patient and often resulting in a trip to the nearest emergency department for treatment. Treatment of acute conjunctivitis begins with reassurance and the use of a warm moist pack to the affected eye to afford symptomatic relief. Non–neomycin-containing antibiotic eye drops or ointment such as gentamicin or polymyxin-B and bacitracin should be used, with care being taken to avoid touching the affected eye with the dropper or the tip of the tube of antibiotic ointment to avoid reinfection.[12] If the possibility of sexually transmitted conjunctivitis is present, a culture should be taken, and systemic antibiotics and ophthalmologic consultation on an urgent basis are indicated.[13]

Glaucoma

Glaucoma is the most common eye disease that results in blindness in the United States. It is not a single disease but a group of diseases that have in common dysfunction of the circulation and drainage of the aqueous humor inside the eyeball.[14] Glaucoma is rarely seen in the absence of trauma or a congenital abnormality of the globe before the age of 40 years. It occurs more commonly in blacks and those with a family history of glaucoma. Any severe trauma to the globe increases the risk of glaucoma.

For purposes of this discussion, the pain management specialist must be aware of the two types of glaucoma: (1) open-angle glaucoma; and (2) angle-closure glaucoma.[15] A comparison of both types of this vision-threatening disease is provided in **Table 53.1**. Open-angle glaucoma has been called the "silent thief" in that the disease presents with little or no symptoms and gradually causes permanent eye damage from increased intraocular pressure, which causes ischemic damage to the optic nerve. Open-angle glaucoma is caused by an inability of aqueous humor to drain from the anterior chamber of the eye even though the angle between the iris and cornea is opened (**Fig. 53.6**). Initially, only the peripheral vision is affected, but as the disease progresses, the patient may present with painless

vision loss and tunnel vision. Fundoscopic examination reveals disc cupping (**Fig. 53.7**). Because of the lack of pain associated with open-angle glaucoma, patients with this disease rarely present to the pain management physician, although one should remember that all patients older than age 60 years are at risk for glaucoma and thus an inquiry regarding visual loss should be part of every pain management assessment in this age group.

In contradistinction to open-angle glaucoma, the pain management physician will in all likelihood encounter patients with eye pain and visual loss that may be the result of angle-closure glaucoma. Angle-closure glaucoma occurs when the angle between the iris and the cornea becomes blocked, impeding the drainage of aqueous humor (**Fig. 53.8**). Angle-closure glaucoma represents a true ophthalmologic emergency, and failure to rapidly identify the disease and help the patient receive immediate ophthalmologic care invariably results in permanent visual loss.[16] The patient with acute angle-closure glaucoma presents with the acute onset of severe eye pain, blurred vision,

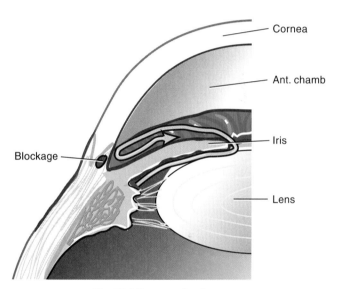

Fig. 53.6 **Open-angle glaucoma.**

Table 53.1 Comparison of Open-Angle and Angle-Closure Glaucoma

	Open-Angle Glaucoma	Angle-Closure Glaucoma
Occurrence	85% of all glaucoma	15% of all glaucoma
Cause	Unknown	Closed angle prevents aqueous drainage
Age at onset	Variable	Age 50 years or older
Anterior chamber	Usually normal	Shallow
Chamber angle	Normal	Narrow
Symptoms	Insidious loss of vision, no pain early in disease	Acute pain, halos around lights, vomiting, headache
Cupping of disc	Progressive if untreated	After untreated attacks
Visual fields	Peripheral visual fields affected early, central vision affected later	Loss occurs as disease progresses
Ocular pressure	Progressively higher as disease progresses	High as disease progresses
Other signs	None	Fixed, partially dilated pupil, red eye, steamy cornea
Treatment	Medical, laser surgery	Surgical
Prognosis	Good if diagnosed early, poor if treatment delayed	Good if treated early, poor if treatment delayed

(Modified from Swartz MH: *Textbook of physical diagnosis*, ed 4, Philadelphia, 2002, Saunders, p 235.)

a halo effect around lights, nausea and vomiting, and a red eye. The cornea may appear steamy, like looking though a steamy window. The pupil may be poorly reactive or fixed in mid position, and the iris may have a whorled appearance (**Fig. 53.9**). The patient appears acutely ill in contradistinction to the chronically ill-appearing patient with temporal arteritis, which

can also present in this age group. The onset of angle-closure glaucoma frequently occurs at night when the pupil dilates, further impeding the flow of aqueous humor by further narrowing or closing the angle between the iris and the cornea.

The first step in the diagnosis of glaucoma is for the clinician to think of it. The diagnosis of both types of glaucoma can be made with simple measurements of intraocular pressure.[17] Although a rare low-pressure glaucoma exists, most patients with glaucoma can be identified with simple ocular applanation or air-puff tonometry.

Uveitis

Uveitis is a term used to describe inflammation of the uvea that is not the result of infection.[18] The uvea is divided into anterior and posterior parts. The anterior uvea consists of the ciliary body and iris, and the posterior uvea consists of the choroidal layer. Uveitis is a common cause of eye pain, and the pain is frequently associated with a red eye. Uveitis is frequently associated with the autoimmune diseases (e.g., rheumatoid arthritis, Behçet's disease), although the causes of uveitis may defy specific diagnosis.[19] Patients with uveitis present with eye pain, red eye, photophobia, blurred vision, and "floaters" (**Figs. 53.10** and **53.11**).[20] The pain of uveitis can be exacerbated by shining a bright light into the eye, causing the inflamed iris to constrict. Uveitis is an ophthalmologic emergency, and immediate ophthalmologic evaluation and treatment with corticosteroids is mandatory if permanent visual loss is to be avoided.[21]

Optic Neuritis

Optic neuritis is another common cause of eye pain. Although pain is invariably present, it is the acute visual loss associated with the disease that usually prompts the patient to seek medical attention. The most common cause of optic neuritis is multiple sclerosis, with approximately 20% of patients with multiple sclerosis having optic neuritis as the initial symptom.[22] Approximately 70% of patients with multiple sclerosis have optic neuritis at some point in the disease.[23]

Other causes of optic neuritis include temporal arteritis, tuberculosis, HIV, hepatitis B, Lyme disease, and cytomegalovirus (**Fig. 53.12**).[24] Whether the optic neuritis is from actual infection

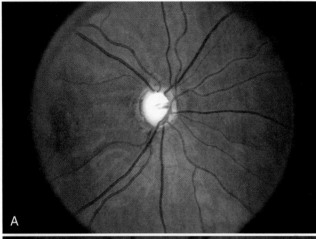
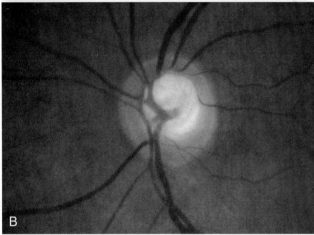

Fig. 53.7 **A** and **B,** Glaucomatous cupping of the optic nerve head. The cup-to-disc ratio is 50% to 60%. *(From Swartz MH: Textbook of physical diagnosis, ed 4, Philadelphia, 2002, Saunders, p 234.)*

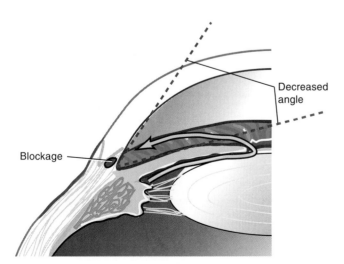

Fig. 53.8 **Angle-closure glaucoma.**

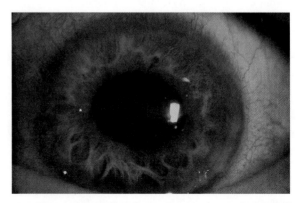

Fig. 53.9 After an episode of symptomatic angle closure, the iris may have suffered a sectorial infarction of the sphincter muscle, causing distortion and recognized clinically by its whorled appearance. If this condition is severe, the eye is left with a poorly reactive ovoid pupil. *(From Spalton DJ: Atlas of clinical ophthalmology, ed 3, Philadelphia, 2005, Mosby, p 210.)*

of the optic nerve or from part of a complex inflammatory response is the subject of debate. Optic neuritis is also seen as a sequela to sinus infection and occurs after radiation therapy.

The incidence rate of optic neuritis is approximately 7 cases per 100,000 patients. It occurs most commonly in whites of northern European ancestry. Blacks and Asians are rarely affected in the absence of an infectious cause. Optic neuritis occurs more often in females and usually presents between the ages of 20 and 50 years. In patients older than 50 years with

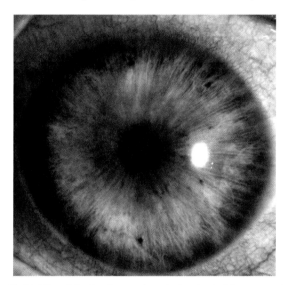

Fig. 53.10 Ciliary injection is seen here in its classical form as a dusky red circumlimbal vasodilation in the area around the cornea where the ciliary and scleroconjunctival circulations anastomose. Its degree reflects the acuteness and severity of inflammation in the anterior uveal tract. With very severe inflammation, the whole of the bulbar conjunctiva can be involved and the appearance may be difficult to distinguish from the diffuse appearance of conjunctival inflammation. *(From Spalton DJ: Atlas of clinical ophthalmology, ed 3, Philadelphia, 2005, Mosby, p 290.)*

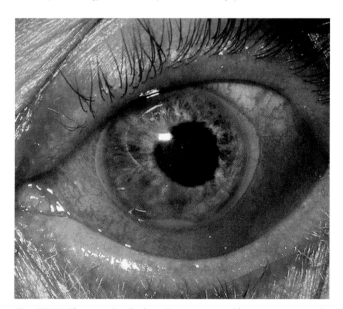

Fig. 53.11 The massive leukocytic response with an acute anterior uveitis can lead to cells precipitating as a hypopyon. This is typical of HLA-B27–positive anterior uveitis but is also seen with other causes of severe anterior uveitis such as Behçet's disease. Hypopyon may also be the presenting sign of retinoblastoma in children, ocular lymphoma, and bacterial or fungal endophthalmitis. *(From Spalton DJ: Atlas of clinical ophthalmology, ed 3, Philadelphia, 2005, Mosby, p 292.)*

acute vision loss in one eye, ischemic optic neuritis is a more likely diagnosis.

Patients with optic neuritis present with a triad of symptoms, including: (1) acute vision loss; (2) eye pain; and (3) dyschromatopsia, which is impairment of accurate color vision. Some patients with optic neuritis also report sound-induced or sudden movement–induced flashing lights, which are known as phosgenes, and heat-induced visual loss. Approximately 70% of patients with optic neuritis have unilateral symptoms. On physical examination, the patient with optic neuritis exhibits a pale, swollen, optic disc (**Fig. 53.13**). Magnetic resonance imaging (MRI) and visual evoked responses confirm the clinical diagnosis (**Fig. 53.14**).[25]

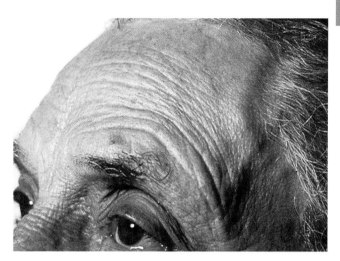

Fig. 53.12 The temporal arteries of this woman were tender, inflamed, thickened, and nonpulsatile, although frequently the signs are more subtle. The diagnosis is suggested with finding a high erythrocyte sedimentation rate and C-reactive protein level and confirmed with temporal artery biopsy. Prompt treatment with corticosteroids is necessary because of a grave risk of fellow eye involvement or stroke. *(From Spalton DJ: Atlas of clinical ophthalmology, ed 3, Philadelphia, 2005, Mosby, p 591.)*

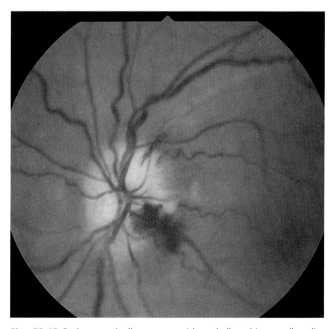

Fig. 53.13 Patients typically present with a chalky white, swollen disc with few hemorrhages. *(From Spalton DJ: Atlas of clinical ophthalmology, ed 3, Philadelphia, 2005, Mosby, p 592.)*

Urgent ophthalmologic referral for treatment with intravenous corticosteroids or alpha-interferon therapy is indicated in all patients suspected of having optic neuritis.[26,27]

Referred Eye Pain

What all of the following disease entities have in common is their ability to cause eye pain. Given the broad range of anatomic structures that are either directly innervated by the first division of the

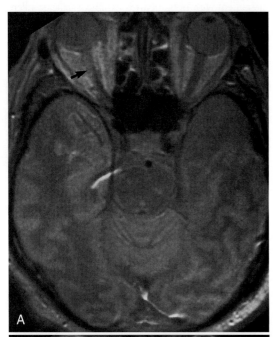

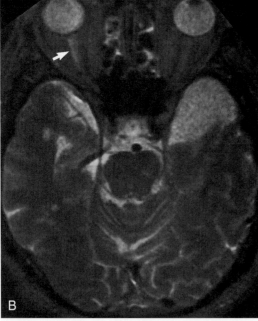

Fig. 53.14 High signal intensity is shown in the right optic nerve in a patient with multiple sclerosis and optic neuritis *(arrow)*. When the classic spin-echo technique is used, the lesion is seen on the spin-echo density-weighted image **(A)** but more clearly on the T2-weighted image **(B)** because of decreased signal from adjacent intraorbital fat. With modern fast imaging techniques, these lesions are better seen with T2-weighted fast spin-echo imaging with fat suppression or fast STIR imaging. *(From Stark DD, Bradley WG Jr: Magnetic resonance imaging, ed 3, St Louis, 1999, Mosby, p 393.)*

trigeminal nerve (e.g., the orbit, the cavernous sinus) or that interact with the trigeminal ganglion via sympathetic or parasympathetic fibers (e.g., carotid artery, sphenopalatine ganglion), that many pathologic processes are perceived by the patient as ocular or periocular pain is not surprising. As mentioned previously, the patient's firm belief that the pathologic process resides within the eye makes the evaluation and treatment of ocular and periocular pain challenging. A discussion of diseases that can have eye pain as a prominent presenting feature follows.

Cluster Headache

Cluster headache is a common cause of referred ocular and periocular pain. The presumption is that interplay between the sphenopalatine ganglion and the trigeminal ganglion is responsible for the patient's perception of eye pain with cluster headache. Cluster headache derives its name from the pattern of its occurrence: namely, the headaches occur in clusters followed by headache-free remission periods.[28] Unlike other common headache disorders that affect primarily females, cluster headache occurs much more often in males by a ratio of 5:1. Much less common than tension-type headache or migraine headache, cluster headache is thought to affect approximately 0.5% of the male population.

The onset of cluster headache occurs in the late third or early fourth decade, in contradistinction to migraine, which almost always manifests itself by the early second decade. Unlike migraine, cluster headache does not appear to run in families, and cluster headache sufferers do not experience aura. Attacks of cluster headache generally occur approximately 90 minutes after the patient falls asleep. This association with sleep is reportedly maintained when a shift worker changes to and from nighttime to daytime hours of sleep. Cluster headache also appears to follow a distinct chronobiologic pattern that coincides with the seasonal change in the length of daylight. This results in an increased frequency of cluster headaches in the spring and fall.

During a cluster headache period, attacks occur two to three times a day and last for 45 minutes to an hour. Cluster headache periods usually last for 8 to 12 weeks, interrupted by remission periods of less than 2 years. In rare cases, the remission periods become shorter and shorter and the frequency may increase up to tenfold. This situation is termed chronic cluster headache and differs from the more common episodic cluster headache described previously.

Cluster headache is characterized as a unilateral headache that is ocular, retroorbital, and temporal. The pain has a deep burning or boring quality. Physical findings during an attack of cluster headache may include Horner's syndrome, consisting of ptosis, abnormal pupil constriction, facial flushing, and conjunctival injection (**Fig. 53.15**). In addition, profuse lacrimation and rhinorrhea is often present. The ocular changes may become permanent with repeated attacks. Peau d'orange skin over the malar region, deeply furrowed and glabellar folds, and telangiectasia may be observed.

Attacks of cluster headache may be provoked by small amounts of alcohol, nitrates, histamines, and other vasoactive substances and occasionally by high altitude. When the attack is in progress, the patient may not be able to lie still and may pace or rock back and forth in a chair. This behavior contrasts to that in other headache syndromes, during which patients seeking relief lie down in a dark quiet room.

The pain of cluster headache is said to be among the worst pain that mankind suffers. Because of the severity of pain associated with cluster headaches, the clinician must watch closely for medication overuse or misuse. Suicides have been associated with prolonged, unrelieved attacks of cluster headaches.

No specific test for cluster headache exists. Testing is aimed primarily at identifying occult pathology or other diseases that may mimic cluster headache. All patients with a recent onset of headache thought to be cluster headache should undergo MRI testing of the brain. If neurologic dysfunction accompanies the patient's headache symptomatology, the MRI should be performed with and without gadolinium contrast medium, and magnetic resonance (MR) angiography should also be considered. MRI testing should also be performed in those patients with previously stable cluster headache who are experiencing an inexplicable change in headache symptoms. Screening laboratory testing including erythrocyte sedimentation rate, complete blood cell count, and automated blood chemistry should be performed if the diagnosis of cluster headache is in question. Ophthalmologic evaluation including measurement of intraocular pressures is indicated in those patients with headache who experience significant ocular symptom.

In contradistinction to migraine headache, where most patients experience improvement with the implementation of therapy with beta-adrenergic blockers, patients with cluster headache usually need more individualized therapy. A reasonable starting place in the treatment of cluster headache is to begin treatment with prednisone combined with daily sphenopalatine ganglion blocks with local anesthetic.[29] A reasonable starting dose of prednisone is 80 mg given in divided doses tapered by 10 mg per dose per day. If headaches are not rapidly brought under control, the inhalation of 100% oxygen is added via a close-fitting mask.

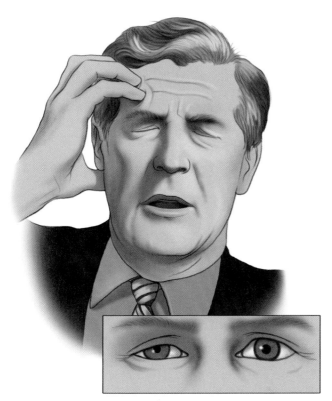

Fig. 53.15 Horner's syndrome may be present during acute attacks of cluster headache. (From Waldman S: Atlas of common pain syndromes, Philadelphia, 2002, Saunders, p 17.)

If headaches persist and the diagnosis of cluster headache is not in question, a trial of lithium carbonate may be considered. Note that the therapeutic window of lithium carbonate is small and thus this drug should be used with caution. A starting dose of 300 mg at bedtime may be increased after 48 hours to 300 mg twice a day. If no side effects are noted, after 48 hours, the dose may again be increased to 300 mg three times a day. The patient should be continued at this dosage level for a total of 10 days, and the drug should then be tapered downward over a 1-week period. Other medications that can be considered if the aforementioned treatments are ineffective include methysergide, sumatriptan, and sumatriptan-like drugs.

Tolosa-Hunt Syndrome

Tolosa-Hunt syndrome is another disease with a primary presenting symptom of unilateral eye pain. The exact cause of Tolosa-Hunt syndrome is unknown, but the ocular and periocular symptoms are the result of nonspecific inflammation of the cavernous sinus or superior orbital fissure.[30] In addition to severe eye pain, which often heralds the onset of this disease, dysfunction of cranial nerves III, IV, and VI occurs as a result of granulomatous inflammatory damage to the nerves.[31] This results in ophthalmoparesis, which can be quite distressing to the patient. In some patients, the ophthalmoparesis may precede the pain, further confusing the diagnosis. Pupillary dysfunction from inflammation of the sympathetic fibers and third cranial nerve may also be seen in patients with Tolosa-Hunt syndrome. If the inflammation extends beyond the cavernous sinus and affects the optic nerve, blindness may result. Paresthesias into the forehead presumably via the supraorbital branch of the trigeminal nerve may also be present as part of the inflammatory response. Tolosa-Hunt syndrome rarely occurs before the second decade and affects males and females equally. The extent of physical findings is a direct function of which cranial nerves are affected by the inflammatory process. Although ophthalmopareses is a hallmark of Tolosa-Hunt syndrome, papillary abnormalities and ptosis may also be present. Fundoscopic examination may reveal edema of the optic disc.[32] The corneal reflex may be diminished or lost if significant trigeminal nerve involvement occurs.

Because Tolosa-Hunt syndrome mimics many other diseases, laboratory testing, including a complete blood cell count and determination of erythrocyte sedimentation rate, glucose level, Lyme disease titer, rapid plasma reagin, antinuclear antibody, HIV titer, and thyroid function, is indicated.[33] MRI of the brain and orbit may reveal findings suggestive of a local inflammatory response but may be normal even in the presence of significant disease.[34] Biopsy of the region of inflammation may ultimately be necessary to confirm the diagnosis of Tolosa-Hunt syndrome. Tolosa-Hunt syndrome represents an ophthalmologic emergency and should be treated as such. Rapid treatment with high doses of intravenous corticosteroids may prevent loss of vision and cranial nerve function. Although spontaneous remissions have been reported, early treatment is key to avoiding disastrous results. Thirty percent to 40% of patients with Tolosa-Hunt syndrome experience a relapse of symptoms after successful treatment with corticosteroids.

The Cavernous Sinus Syndromes

The cavernous sinus syndromes are a heterogeneous groups of diseases that have in common their ability to produce ocular and periocular pain and a variety of neurologic symptoms, including ophthalmoplegia, pupillary abnormalities, orbital and conjunctival congestion, proptosis, and, if severe, visual loss.[35] Also known as the parasellar syndromes, the evaluation of all patients with cavernous sinus syndrome should include a complete blood cell count and determination of erythrocyte sedimentation rate, glucose level, Lyme disease titer, rapid plasma reagin, antinuclear antibody, HIV titer, and thyroid function. MRI of the brain, sinuses, cavernous sinus, and orbit is also indicated as is MR angiography of the carotid artery. Diseases that comprise the cavernous sinus syndrome include cavernous sinus aneurysms, carotid-cavernous sinus fistulas, tumors, and cavernous sinus thrombosis, and the idiopathic inflammatory syndromes that involve the cavernous sinus (e.g., Tolosa-Hunt syndrome).[36,37] Each is briefly discussed individually.

Cavernous Sinus Aneurysms

Aneurysms of the carotid artery as it passes through the cavernous sinus can cause all of the symptoms associated with cavernous sinus syndrome. Unlike intracranial aneurysms, which carry the risk of intracranial hemorrhage, unruptured carotid artery aneurysms in this region create symptoms with pressure on the various neural structures in proximity to the aneurysm. When the aneurysm ruptures, a direct carotid artery–cavernous sinus fistula results (**Fig. 53.16**). Such fistulas can cause only limited symptoms or can result

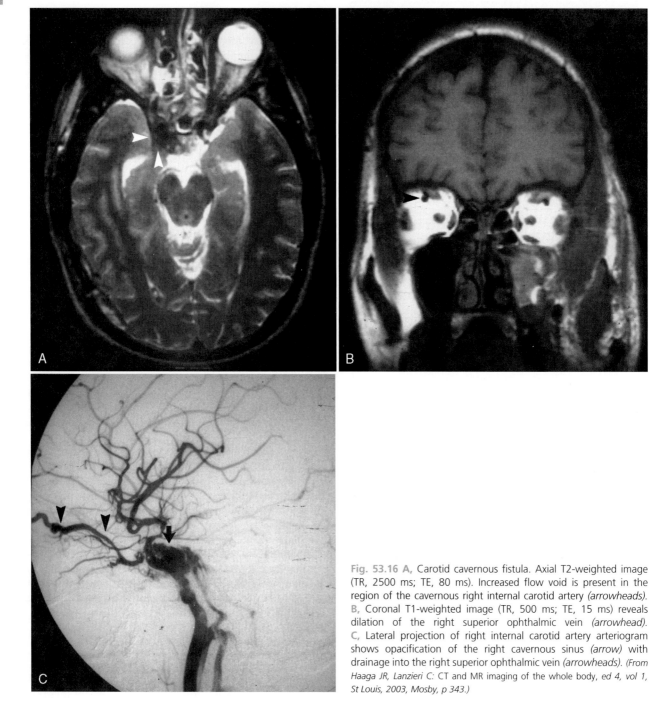

Fig. 53.16 A, Carotid cavernous fistula. Axial T2-weighted image (TR, 2500 ms; TE, 80 ms). Increased flow void is present in the region of the cavernous right internal carotid artery *(arrowheads)*. **B,** Coronal T1-weighted image (TR, 500 ms; TE, 15 ms) reveals dilation of the right superior ophthalmic vein *(arrowhead)*. **C,** Lateral projection of right internal carotid artery arteriogram shows opacification of the right cavernous sinus *(arrow)* with drainage into the right superior ophthalmic vein *(arrowheads)*. *(From Haaga JR, Lanzieri C: CT and MR imaging of the whole body, ed 4, vol 1, St Louis, 2003, Mosby, p 343.)*

in massive neurologic dysfunction. A loud carotid and ocular bruit is often present. Treatment with endovascular occlusion has been attempted with some success.[38]

Cavernous Sinus Tumors

Tumors that involve the cavernous sinus can be either primary or metastatic in origin. Primary tumors including meningiomas and neurofibromas are the most common primary tumors seen that involve the cavernous sinus.[39] Metastatic breast, prostate, lung, and craniopharyngeal tumors can also involve the cavernous sinus, often with disastrous results (**Fig. 53.17**).[40] Occasionally, large pituitary tumors may extend into the cavernous sinus (**Fig. 53.18**). Symptoms associated with tumors of this region vary with the neurologic structures affected as the tumor grows, and the onset of symptoms can be either acute or insidious. Treatment is primarily limited to palliative radiotherapy, and the results in most cases are poor at best, with the type of tumor the major determinant of outcome. The exception to this rule is endocrine-responsive pituitary tumors, which often respond to antiendocrine drug therapy.

Carotid-Cavernous Fistulas

Fistulas between the carotid artery and the cavernous sinus can be the result of either a rupture of a preexisting carotid artery aneurysm or direct trauma to the carotid artery and cavernous sinus (**Fig. 53.19**).[41] Direct fistulas between the carotid artery and the cavernous sinus occur when a carotid artery aneurysm ruptures directly into the cavernous sinus or trauma to the region damages the artery. The onset of symptoms is immediate and often quite severe. Misdiagnosis is common, and prognosis if untreated is poor. A loud carotid and ocular bruit is often present. The patient may report hearing "water running" in the head. Indirect aneurysms between branches of the internal or external carotid arteries tend to be less symptomatic. Both types of fistulas can be treated with endovascular occlusion techniques and carotid artery ligation.

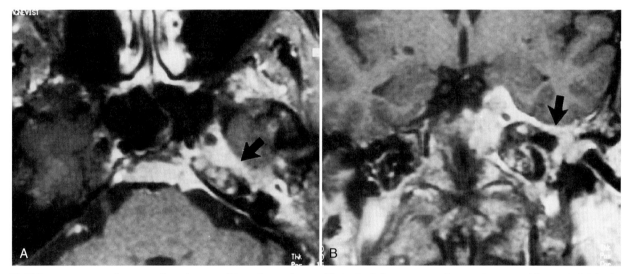

Fig. 53.17 **Recurrent nasopharyngeal carcinoma with perineural spread into the left cavernous sinus and temporal bone.** A, Axial enhanced image with fat saturation. Tumor surrounds the left trigeminal ganglion and extends from Meckel's cave into the left petrous apex *(arrow)*. B, Coronal enhanced image with fat saturation. The tumor extends laterally along the left greater superficial petrosal nerve and enters the temporal bone through the geniculate ganglion *(arrow)*. *(From Stark DD, Bradley WG Jr: Magnetic resonance imaging, ed 3, St Louis, 1999, Mosby, p 1223.)*

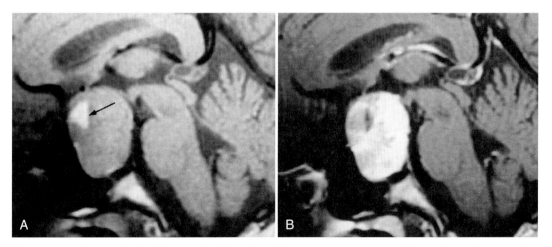

Fig. 53.18 **Pituitary macroadenoma.** A, Sagittal precontrast T1-weighted image shows oval mass with smooth border and sellar enlargement—typical MR features of macroadenoma. Hemorrhage-fluid level *(arrow)* is visible. B, Postcontrast T1-weighted image shows intense but heterogeneous enhancement of tumor. *(From Stark DD, Bradley WG Jr: Magnetic resonance imaging, ed 3, St Louis, 1999, Mosby, p 1226.)*

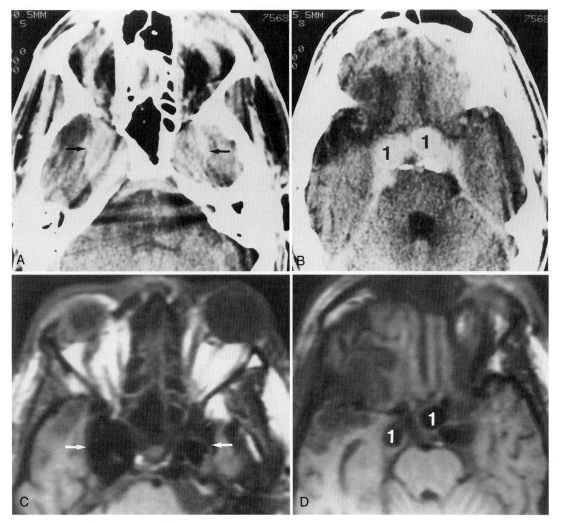

Fig. 53.19 Traumatic carotid cavernous fistula. A, Axial contrast medium–enhanced CT scan. **B,** Axial contrast medium–enhanced CT scan. **C,** Axial head surface-coil, short-TR, short-TE MR image. **D,** Axial head surface-coil, short-TR, short-TE MR image. Greatly distended superior ophthalmic veins and cavernous sinuses *(arrows)* are seen as enhancement in **A** and as signal void in **C.** Note that the enhancing suprasellar "masses" (1) in **B** are definitively diagnosed as massively dilated venous channels by MRI **(D),** obviating the need for intravenous contrast. *(From Stark DD, Bradley WG Jr:* Magnetic resonance imaging, *ed 3, St Louis, 1999, Mosby, p 1660.)*

Cavernous Sinus Thrombosis

A common sequela to periorbital or frontal or maxillary sinusitis in the preantibiotic era, cavernous sinus thrombosis is now primarily seen in patients with immunocompromise (e.g., patients with HIV).[42] The patient with an infectious etiology to cavernous sinus thrombosis appears septic, and the nidus of the infection may be clinically evident. Severe ocular and retroocular pain is often the first symptom, followed by diplopia and ptosis. Ophthalmoplegia and signs of meningeal irritation may also be present. Immediate treatment with antibiotics and corticosteroids combined with surgical drainage of any abscess formation is crucial to avoid blindness or, in some cases, death.

Other Inflammatory Conditions Associated with Cavernous Sinus Syndrome

Acute herpes zoster and sarcoidosis have both been implicated in the development of cavernous sinus syndrome (**Fig. 53.20**).

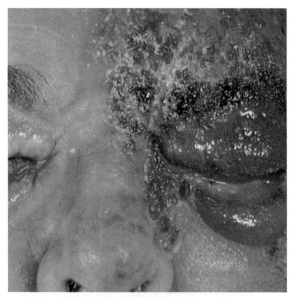

Fig. 53.20 Herpes zoster ophthalmicus. *(From Swartz MH:* Textbook of physical diagnosis, *ed 4, Philadelphia, 2002, Saunders, p 214.)*

The lesions of acute herpes zoster usually make the diagnosis a relatively straightforward endeavor, but the diagnosis of sarcoidosis can be much more subtle.[43] If uveitis is present as a component of ocular pain, sarcoidosis should always be included in the differential diagnosis.

Conclusion

Ocular and periocular pain represent a challenge for the pain management physician in both diagnosis and treatment. Familiarity with the more common pathologic processes that cause ocular and periocular pain allows the pain management physician to more readily identify those diseases that present a risk to vision and allows more immediate ophthalmologic referral. More self-limited causes of ocular and periocular pain can often be managed with simple treatment and reassurance.

References

Full references for this chapter can be found on www.expertconsult.com.

Chapter 54

Pain of the Ear, Nose, Sinuses, and Throat

Steven D. Waldman

Pain that originates from the ear, nose, sinuses, and throat accounts for a significant number of visits to primary care physicians and specialists each year. Although most of the painful conditions responsible for these visits are easy to diagnose and treat and, in general, will not harm the patient with proper treatment, a significant number of painful conditions of the ear, nose, and throat have the potential to cause considerable morbidity and mortality (**Table 54.1**). The clinician should also remain vigilant for diseases of this anatomic region that do not cause pain but have the potential, if undiagnosed, to create significant problems for the patient, such as acoustic neuroma, thyroid carcinoma, and malignant melanoma. This chapter provides the clinician with a concise road map for the evaluation of painful conditions of the ear, nose, sinuses, and throat.

Otalgia

Ear pain can result from local pathology, such as cellulitis or tumor, or can be referred from distant sites, most commonly the nasopharynx.[1,2] Because of the complex functions of the ear, local disease may cause disturbances in hearing and balance that can be quite distressing for the patient and may serve as a harbinger of serious diseases, such as acoustic neuroma. As mentioned, many of these conditions do not have pain as a predominant symptom.

Functional Anatomy of the Ear As It Relates to Pain

The ear and surrounding tissues are innervated by both cranial nerves and branches of nerves that have as their origin the spinal nerves (**Fig. 54.1**). The auricle is innervated by the greater auricular nerve, and the lesser occipital nerve, the auricular branch of the vagus nerve, and the auriculotemporal branch of the mandibular nerve. The external auditory canal receives innervation from branches of the glossopharyngeal and facial nerves. The inferoposterior portion of the tympanic membrane receives its innervation from the auriculotemporal branch of the mandibular nerve, the auricular branch of the vagus nerve, and the tympanic branch of the glossopharyngeal nerve. The structures of the middle ear receive innervation from the tympanic branch of the glossopharyngeal nerve along with the caroticotympanic nerve and the superficial petrosal nerve. It is the overlap of these nerves, and their diverse origin, that can make localization of the pathology responsible for the patient's pain quite challenging.

Painful Diseases of the Ear
Auricular Pain

The skin of the auricle is richly innervated and is frequently the source of local ear pain. Auricular cartilage is poorly innervated, and diseases that are limited to cartilage may produce little or no pain until distention or inflammation of the overlying skin develops. Most painful conditions involving the auricle are the result of infection, trauma, connective tissue disease, or tumor.

Superficial infections of the auricle include folliculitis, abscess, cellulitis, and infection by herpes simplex and zoster, including Ramsay Hunt syndrome[3] (**Fig. 54.2**). Deep infections that involve the cartilage, once uncommon, now occur with much greater frequency because of the current increase in body piercing involving auricular cartilage.

Both superficial and deep infections of the auricle are quite painful. Early incision and drainage, débridement of nonviable cartilage, and aggressive use of antibiotics are necessary to avoid spread of infection to the middle ear, bone, and intracranial structures, including the central nervous system.

Trauma to the auricle can be quite painful and, if not appropriately treated, can result in loss of cartilage and disfigurement. Blunt trauma to the auricle can cause superficial ecchymosis

Table 54.1 Painful Conditions of the Ear, Nose, Sinuses, and Throat

EAR PAIN

The Auricle

Superficial infections

Folliculitis

Cellulitis

Herpes simplex

Ramsay Hunt syndrome

Deep infections involving cartilage

Trauma

Ecchymosis of the auricle

Perichondral hematoma

Lacerations

Thermal injuries

Heating pad burns

Ice pack burns

Frostbite

Chondritis-associated and perichondritis-associated connective tissue diseases

Primary tumors

Metastatic tumors

The External Auditory Canal

Otitis media

Cholesteatoma

The Tympanic Membrane and Middle Ear

Myringitis

Otitis media

Mastoiditis

PAIN OF THE NOSE AND SINUSES

Superficial infection

Folliculitis

Vestibulitis

Intranasal foreign body

Acute sinusitis

Osteomyelitis

Primary tumors of the nose and sinuses

Metastatic tumors involving the nose and sinuses

THROAT PAIN

Superficial infection

Acute pharyngitis

Tonsillitis

Dental pain

Deep infection

Parapharyngeal abscess

Retropharyngeal abscess

Primary tumors of the throat and aerodigestive tract

Metastatic tumors involving the throat and aerodigestive tract

Carotidynia

Eagle syndrome

Hyoid syndrome

or, if severe enough, perichondral hematoma or cauliflower ear (**Fig. 54.3**).[4] Lacerations of the lobule, tragus, and cartilage from body piercings that have been torn from the ear are increasingly common occurrences at local emergency rooms and urgent care centers. Prompt débridement and repair with careful observation for infection are crucial if disfiguring sequelae are to be avoided.

Thermal injuries from heat or cold are also common painful traumatic injuries to the ear that usually follow the use of heating pads or cold packs in patients who are also taking pain medications or self medicating with alcohol, or both. Frostbite injuries that affect the auricle are likewise common and are frequently related to alcohol or drug use (or both). Thermal injuries can initially appear less severe than they really are. Initial treatment with topical antibiotics such as silver sulfadiazine and sterile dressings should be followed with reevaluation and redressing of the affected area on a daily basis until the thermal injury is well on the way to healing.

Connective tissue diseases can cause inflammation of the auricular cartilage. Usually manifested as bilateral, acutely inflamed, and painful swelling of the auricle, chondritis, and perichondritis may initially be misdiagnosed as cellulitis (**Fig. 54.4**). The bilateral nature of the disease, and involvement of other cartilage, should alert the clinician to the possibility of a noninfectious cause of the pain, rubor, and swelling.[5] Because many of the connective tissue diseases affect other organ systems, prompt diagnosis and treatment are essential.

Primary tumors of the auricle are generally basal cell or squamous cell carcinoma caused by actinic damage of the skin (**Fig. 54.5**). Rarely, primary tumors of the cartilage can occur. Metastatic lesions to the auricle are uncommon, but not unheard of.

The External Auditory Canal

Far and away the most common painful condition of the external auditory meatus is otitis externa. Usually the result of swimming or digging in the ear with a fingernail, cotton swab, or hairpin, the initial symptom of otitis media is generally pruritus, followed by pain that is made worse by yawning or chewing. On physical examination, a reddened, wet-appearing, edematous canal may reveal abraded areas from previous digging or itching as a result of the patient's attempt to relieve the symptoms (**Fig. 54.6**).[6] Pulling on the auricle posteriorly usually exacerbates the pain of otitis media. The pain of this disease is often out of proportion to the findings on physical examination. Treatment of otitis media consists of cleaning any debris from the acoustic auditory canal and instilling topical antibiotic drops or solution. If significant edema is present, the use of topical antibiotic drops or solution containing corticosteroid speeds recovery.

Another cause of external auditory canal pain is cholesteatoma, which most often occurs after trauma to the bone of the external auditory canal. Caused by invasion of the external auditory canal wall by exuberant tissue growth, cholesteatoma can become quite invasive if left untreated, despite its benign tissue elements.[7] A patient with cholesteatoma has a ball-like growth in the external auditory canal that has an onion skin–like appearance (**Fig. 54.7**). Unless infected, the pain most often is dull and aching. Secondary infection may cause a foul-smelling purulent exudate to drain from the affected ear. Computed tomographic (CT) scanning helps the clinician determine the

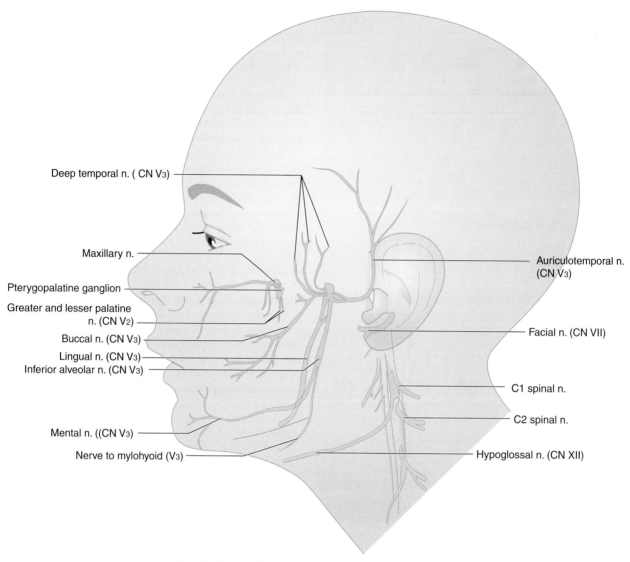

Deep temporal n. (CN V₃)

Maxillary n.

Pterygopalatine ganglion

Greater and lesser palatine n. (CN V₂)

Buccal n. (CN V₃)

Lingual n. (CN V₃)

Inferior alveolar n. (CN V₃)

Mental n. ((CN V₃)

Nerve to mylohyoid (V₃)

Auriculotemporal n. (CN V₃)

Facial n. (CN VII)

C1 spinal n.

C2 spinal n.

Hypoglossal n. (CN XII)

Fig. 54.1 **Innervation of the ear and surrounding tissues.**

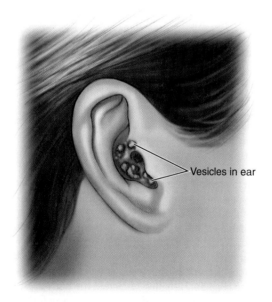

Vesicles in ear

Fig. 54.2 Ramsay Hunt syndrome is the result of infection of the geniculate ganglion by varicella-zoster virus. *(From Waldman SD:* Atlas of uncommon pain syndromes, *ed 2, Philadelphia, 2008, Saunders.)*

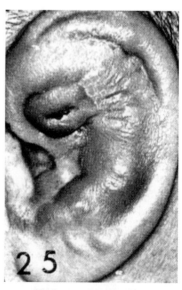

Fig. 54.3 **Cauliflower ear.** *(Courtesy of Roy Sullivan, PhD.)*

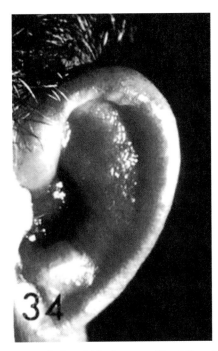

Fig. 54.4 **Polychondritis.** *(Courtesy of Roy Sullivan, PhD.)*

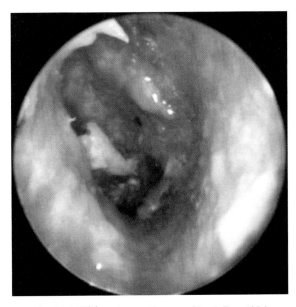

Fig. 54.6 **Otitis externa.** *(Courtesy of Roy Sullivan, PhD.)*

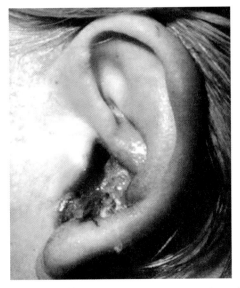

Fig. 54.5 **Basal cell carcinoma.** *(Courtesy of Roy Sullivan, PhD.)*

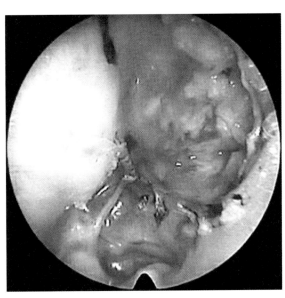

Fig. 54.7 **Cholesteatoma.** *(Courtesy of Roy Sullivan, PhD.)*

amount of bone destruction and helps guide microsurgical resection of this not uncommon cause of ear pain.

In younger patients and those with impaired mentation, foreign bodies are a frequently overlooked cause of ear pain originating from the external auditory meatus. Most problematic is vegetable matter, such as dried peas and beans, which swells once inside the acoustic auditory canal and makes removal quite difficult. If the foreign body remains in the external auditory canal for any period, secondary infection invariably occurs. Insects may also fly or crawl into the external auditory meatus and cause the patient much distress (**Fig. 54.8**). If the insect remains alive, instillation of lidocaine or mineral oil stops the insect from moving around and makes removal easier.[8]

The Tympanic Membrane and Middle Ear

Myringitis is a painful condition that may be caused by viral infection of the tympanic membrane. Vesicles or blebs of the tympanic membrane may be present on physical examination, or the tympanic membrane may appear normal. Antibiotic drops containing local anesthetic usually provide symptomatic relief, although in the absence of physical findings, the diagnosis of idiopathic myringitis is one of exclusion and other diseases of the middle ear or referred pain remain an ever-present possibility.

Acute otitis media is perhaps the second most common cause of otalgia after otitis externa. Although more common in children, otitis media can occur at any age. The pain of otitis media

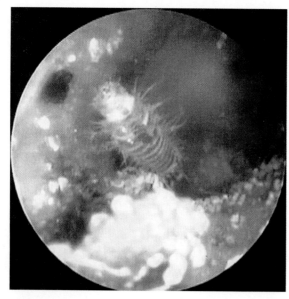

Fig. 54.8 **Insect in the external auditory canal.** *(Courtesy of Roy Sullivan, PhD.)*

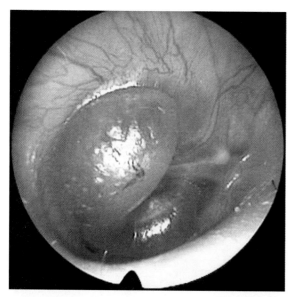

Fig. 54.9 **Otitis media.** *(Courtesy of Roy Sullivan, PhD.)*

is caused primarily by distention and inflammation of the tympanic membrane (**Fig. 54.9**).[9] Young children with otitis media may pull on the ear, whereas older patients report a deep, severe, unremitting pain. Fever is also usually present. Untreated, the pain becomes increasingly severe as the tympanic membrane becomes more distended until the tympanic membrane ruptures. Although the pain may dramatically improve after spontaneous rupture, infection of the mastoid air cells can occur. Treatment of acute otitis media is based on the administration of oral antibiotics and decongestants. Topical local anesthetic drops administered via the external auditory canal may provide symptomatic relief while waiting for the antibiotics and decongestants to work. For otitis media that does not promptly resolve, therapeutic tympanocentesis with the placement of myringotomy tubes should be considered.

As mentioned previously, acute mastoiditis is often the result of untreated or undertreated otitis media. Mastoiditis is characterized by pain, tenderness, and rubor in the posterior auricular region.[10] The condition is often misdiagnosed initially as recurrent otitis media because examination of the tympanic membrane often reveals findings of the unresolved otitis media. Fever is invariably present, and the patient generally appears more ill than with otitis media alone. Radiographic examination of the mastoid air cells reveals opacification of the normally aerated structure and, as the disease progresses, bony destruction. Untreated, mastoiditis can become life threatening as the infection spreads to the central nervous system (**Fig. 54.10**). The findings of headache, stiff neck, and visual disturbance are warning signs of central nervous system involvement and constitute a medical emergency. Surgical treatment combined with aggressive antibiotic therapy is necessary on an emergency basis for patients with signs of central nervous system infection.

A word of caution is in order whenever the clinician is unable to identify the cause of a patient's ear pain. Idiopathic otalgia, especially if unilateral, is a diagnosis of exclusion that should generally be resisted because it is invariably wrong.[11] Repeat physical examination and careful retaking of the history, with special attention directed to areas where occult tumor might cause pain that is referred to the ear, are essential if disaster is to be avoided. This clinical situation is one in which serial magnetic resonance imaging (MRI) of the brain and soft tissues of the neck, and CT scan of these areas, often yields results. All patients with unexplained ear pain should undergo careful endoscopic examination of the aerodigestive tract, with special attention paid to the region of the piriform sinuses to identify any occult pathology responsible for the pain (see subsequent discussion).

Pain of the Nose and Sinuses

Infection of the nose is the most common cause of nasal pain absent trauma. Superficial soft tissue infections can be quite painful and have the potential to spread to deep structures if left untreated. Folliculitis of the vestibule of the nose can also be very painful and, when caused by *Staphylococcus*, can be quite difficult to treat.[12] This condition has been occurring more commonly as the use of intranasal steroid sprays to treat atrophic rhinitis increases, and the early use of topical intranasal antibiotics, such as mupirocin, at the first sign of intranasal tenderness can help prevent more severe disease. Persistent foul-smelling discharge from the nose should alert the physician to the possibility of an intranasal foreign body, especially in children or mentally impaired individuals.

Acute sinusitis is another painful condition of the mid face that can be caused by all infectious agents. Blockage of the ostia of the sinus is usually the cause of acute sinusitis, with the pressure within the sinuses increasing because mucus from the affected sinuses cannot flow into the nose. The maxillary sinuses are most commonly affected, and the pain associated with this disease can be quite severe. The pain is usually localized to the area over the sinus and may be worse with recumbency.

The diagnosis of acute sinusitis is usually made on clinical grounds and then confirmed with plain radiographs or CT scan (**Fig. 54.11**).[13,14] Treatment with decongestant nasal sprays and antibiotics resolves most cases of acute sinusitis.

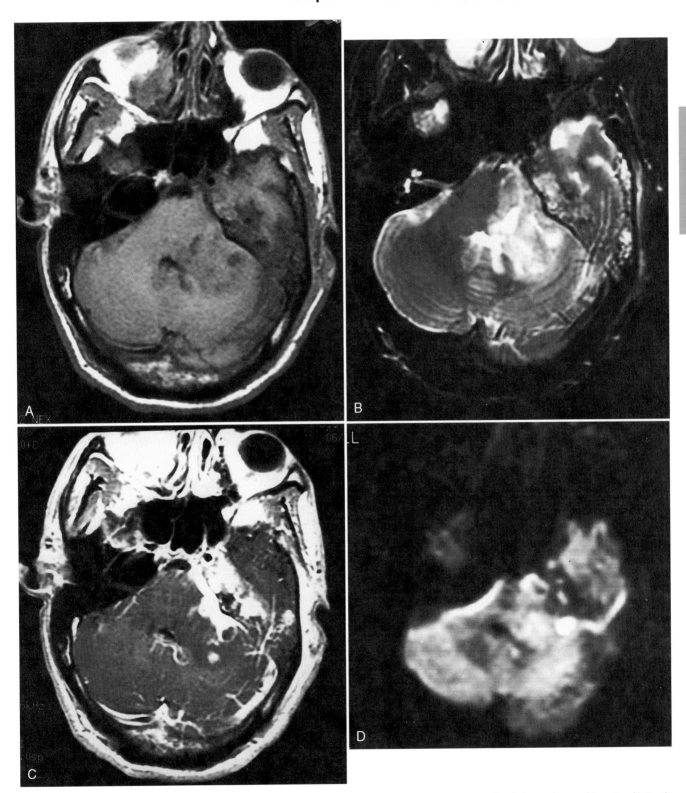

Fig. 54.10 Mastoiditis, cerebritis, and abscess formation. A, A T1-weighted magentic resonance image (MRI) shows abnormal low signal intensity in the left temporal lobe, left brachium pontis, and left mastoid. B, A T2-weighted MRI shows heterogeneous high signal intensity involving the left temporal lobe, left brachium pontis, and left mastoid. C, A gadolinium-enhanced image shows abnormal enhancement involving the left temporal lobe, left brachium pontis, and left mastoid. Note the presence of a small ring-like enhancement in the posterior aspect of the brachium pontis. D, A diffusion-weighted image reveals a focal area of increased signal intensity corresponding to the ring-like enhancement, consistent with restricted diffusion in an abscess. *(From Haaga JR, Lanzieri CF, Gilkeson RC, editors: CT & MR imaging of the whole body, ed 4, Philadelphia, 2002, Mosby.)*

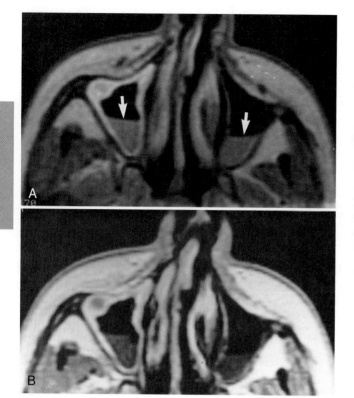

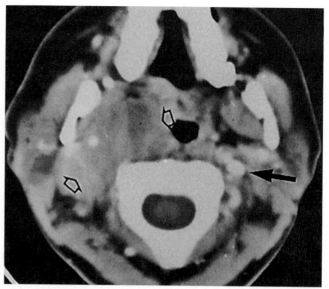

Fig. 54.12 **Coronal computed tomography scan showing a maxillary antral cholesterol granuloma (black arrow).** The antrum is expanded and occupied by material of soft tissue density *(open arrows). (From Grainger RG, Allison DJ:* Grainger and Allison's diagnostic radiology: a textbook of medical imaging, *ed 3, New York, 1996, Churchill Livingstone.)*

Fig. 54.11 Acute maxillary sinusitis on (A) T2-weighted (SE 2000/80) and (B) T1-weighted (SE 400/20) post–Gd-diethylenetriaminepentaacetic acid scans. Note the bilateral air-fluid levels *(arrows)* and mucosal thickening on the right. *(From Grainger RG, Allison DJ:* Grainger and Allison's diagnostic radiology: a textbook of medical imaging, *ed 3, New York, 1996, Churchill Livingstone.)*

Untreated, osteomyelitis may occur. Surgery may ultimately be necessary for recurrent disease, for disease that remains unresponsive to conservative therapy, or when radiographs reveal obstructive polyps or tumors.

Malignant diseases of the nose and sinuses can be notoriously difficult to diagnose. The most common tumors of the nose are basal cell and squamous cell carcinoma.[15] Usually not painful unless infection intervenes or a painful structure is invaded, these tumors can become quite large before detection (**Fig. 54.12**). Squamous cell carcinoma of the sinuses is manifested in a manner identical to sinusitis, so the diagnosis is often delayed. Nasopharyngoma occurs most commonly in patients of Asian descent. Thought to be caused by Epstein-Barr virus, these tumors frequently cause referred pain to the face, neck, and retroauricular area. Other lesions known for their ability to cause referred nose and facial pain are tumors that involve the parapharyngeal space.[16] Almost always causing unilateral symptoms such as facial paralysis and pain, parapharyngeal tumors are frequently of neural origin (**Fig. 54.13**). As previously mentioned, delay in diagnosis of these tumors can complicate treatment and worsen the prognosis.

Throat Pain

Pain that emanates from this region is poorly localized because of mixed innervation of the anatomic structures by the trigeminal, glossopharyngeal, and vagus nerves, and rich innervation by the sympathetic nervous system. For this reason, referred pain from this region is not the exception, but the rule. Because of the patient's difficulty in accurately localizing the source of the pain when pathology affects this anatomic region, extra vigilance on the part of the clinician is needed.

Both superficial and deep infections are a common source of throat pain. Acute pharyngitis and laryngotracheobronchitis are among the most common reasons that patients seek medical attention.[17] Dental infections are also common causes of pain in this anatomic region and often cause pain referred to the ear.[18] Generally self-limited, these infections can become problematic if they spread to the deep structures of the neck and aerodigestive tract or if they occur in patients with immunocompromise. In particular, parapharyngeal and retropharyngeal space abscesses after acute pharyngitis and tonsillitis can become life threatening if not promptly diagnosed and treated.[19] Patients with these disorders appear acutely ill and talk with a characteristic muffled "hot potato voice." With the increased availability of MRI and CT scan, early diagnosis of parapharyngeal and retropharyngeal abscesses is much easier (**Fig. 54.14**).

In addition to infections, tumors of this region can produce both local and referred pain.[20] These tumors are often hard to diagnose, and by the time that the pain is so severe that it causes the patient to seek medical attention, the tumors are already extremely problematic and in many cases have already metastasized. Most primary tumors in this region are squamous cell tumors, although primary tumors of the neural structures and craniopharyngiomas occur with sufficient frequency to be part of the differential diagnosis. Metastatic lesions can also cause local and referred pain in this anatomic area. Given the silent nature of this area insofar as symptoms are concerned, the clinician should make early and frequent use of MRI and CT scan to identify occult tumors and other pathology (see Fig. 54.13).[21] In particular, the clinician should never attribute pain in this region to an idiopathic or psychogenic etiology

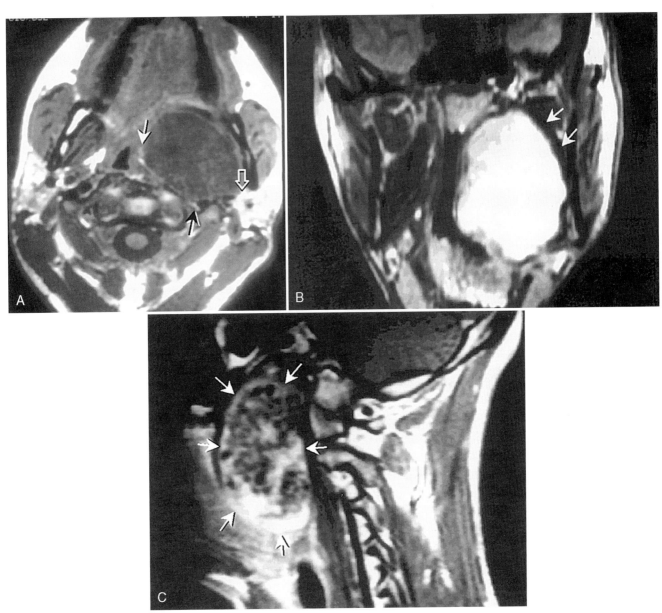

Fig. 54.13 Pleomorphic adenoma. A, A nonenhanced, T1-weighted axial MRI (TR = 540 msec; TE = 12 msec) shows a well-defined mass of lower signal intensity than adjacent muscle that is replacing the prestyloid parapharyngeal fat; in addition, the minimal residual fat is displaced medially *(white arrow)* and the internal carotid artery is displaced posteriorly *(black arrow)*. No intact fat plane can be seen between the lesion and the deep lobe of the parotid gland *(open arrow)*. **B,** An intermediate-weighted (TR = 2540 msec; TE = 30 msec) coronal magnetic resonance image (MRI) shows the mass as relatively homogeneous, of increased signal intensity relative to adjacent muscles and lymphoid tissue, and well defined. The oropharyngeal mucosa is displaced medially. The left medial pterygoid muscle is compressed and displaced superolaterally *(arrows)*. **C,** A contrast-enhanced, T1-weighted (TR = 540 msec; TE = 15 msec) sagittal MRI shows marked heterogeneity of the mass, with multiple low–signal intensity regions that may represent areas of calcification or fibrosis. Both sagittal and coronal images are useful in revealing the craniocaudal extent of the lesion, which fills most of the prestyloid parapharyngeal space *(arrows)*. The mass is inseparable from the deep lobe of the parotid gland and must be considered as arising from the deep lobe for surgical planning. However, the deep lobe of the parotid gland has been compressed and displaced laterally, with no visible connection to the mass at surgery. *(From Haaga JR, Lanzieri CF, Gilkeson RC, editors:* CT & MR imaging of the whole body, *ed 4, Philadelphia, 2002, Mosby.)*

without serial physical examinations, laboratory evaluations, and imaging. In particular, unilateral otalgia in the absence of demonstrable ear pathology should be taken seriously and considered to be referred pain from occult tumor until proved otherwise.

Other painful conditions unrelated to infection and tumor can also occur in this anatomic region, including Eagle syndrome, carotidynia, and hyoid syndrome.

Eagle syndrome is caused by calcification of the stylohyoid ligament and is characterized by paroxysms of pain with movement of the mandible during chewing, yawning, and talking (**Fig. 54.15**).[22] Carotidynia consists of deep neck pain in the region of the carotid that radiates to the ear and jaw. It is made worse with palpation of the area overlying the carotid artery. Hyoid syndrome is characterized by sharp paroxysms of pain with swallowing or head turning.

The pain radiates to the ear and the angle of the jaw and can be reproduced with movement of the hyoid bone. In most cases, these unusual causes of ear, throat, and anterior neck pain are self limited and produce no long-lasting harm to the patient. However, before they are diagnosed, the clinician must rule out other pathologic processes that may harm the patient because on a statistical basis they are much more common.

Conclusion

Pain of the ear, nose, sinuses, and throat is commonly encountered in clinical practice. For the most part, the pathologic process responsible for the patient's pain symptomatology is easily identifiable after the physician performs a targeted history and physical examination. Unfortunately, the nature of this anatomic region makes it possible for the most thorough physician to miss pathology that may ultimately harm the patient. For this reason, the following rules for the treatment of ear, nose, sinus, and throat pain serve both the patient and the clinician well: (1) take a targeted history; (2) perform a careful, targeted physical examination; (3) heed the warning signs of serious disease, such as fever, constitutional symptoms, or weight loss; (4) image early and frequently if the diagnosis remains elusive; (5) perform laboratory tests that help identify "sick from well," such as erythrocyte sedimentation rate, hematology, and blood tests; (6) avoid attributing the patient's pain to idiopathic or psychogenic causes; and (7) always assume that you have missed the diagnosis.

References

Full references for this chapter can be found on www.expertconsult.com.

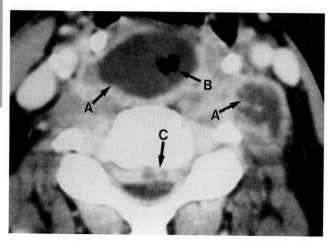

Fig. 54.14 Contrast-enhanced computed tomography scan of a retropharyngeal abscess. Two locules (A and A) are shown in this section, along with a gas bubble (B). An anterior epidural abscess (C) is also seen. *(From Grainger RG, Allison DJ:* Grainger and Allison's diagnostic radiology: a textbook of medical imaging, *ed 3, New York, 1996, Churchill Livingstone.)*

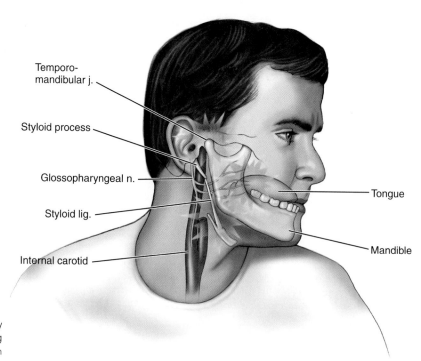

Fig. 54.15 The pain of Eagle syndrome is triggered by swallowing, movement of the mandible, or turning of the neck. *(From Waldman SD:* Atlas of uncommon pain syndromes, *ed 2, Philadelphia, 2008, Saunders.)*

Occipital Neuralgia

Steven D. Waldman

Perhaps one of the most overdiagnosed headache syndromes, occipital neuralgia represents a diagnostic and therapeutic challenge to the clinician. Further complicating any discussion of this painful condition is the contention by some headache specialists that the syndrome does not exist and represents a variant of cervicogenic headache emanating from the C1-C4 nerve roots.[1] Assuming that occipital neuralgia is a clinical entity distinct from cervicogenic headache, it is usually the result of blunt trauma to the greater and lesser occipital nerves.[2] Repetitive microtrauma from working with the neck hyperextended (e.g., painting ceilings, or working for prolonged periods with computer monitors whose focal point is too high, causing extension of the cervical spine) may also cause occipital neuralgia. The pain of occipital neuralgia is characterized as persistent pain at the base of the skull with occasional sudden shock-like paresthesias in the distribution of the greater and lesser occipital nerves (**Fig. 55.1**). Tension-type headache, which is much more common than occipital neuralgia, occasionally mimics the pain of occipital neuralgia.[3] Less commonly, primary or metastatic tumors involving this anatomic region may cause pain that may be misdiagnosed as occipital neuralgia.

Signs and Symptoms

The greater occipital nerve arises from fibers of the dorsal primary ramus of the second cervical nerve and to a lesser extent fibers from the third cervical nerve. The greater occipital nerve pierces the fascia just below the superior nuchal ridge along with the occipital artery. It supplies the medial portion of the posterior scalp as far anterior as the vertex.

The lesser occipital nerve arises from the ventral primary rami of the second and third cervical nerves. The lesser occipital nerve passes superiorly along the posterior border of the sternocleidomastoid muscle, dividing into cutaneous branches that innervate the lateral portion of the posterior scalp and the cranial surface of the pinna of the ear (see Fig. 55.1).

The patient with occipital neuralgia experiences neuritic pain in the distribution of the greater and lesser occipital nerve when the nerves are palpated at the level of the nuchal ridge.[2] Some patients can elicit pain with rotation or lateral bending of the cervical spine.

Testing

No specific test for occipital neuralgia exists. Testing is aimed primarily at identification of occult pathology or other diseases that may mimic occipital neuralgia (see subsequent section Differential Diagnosis). All patients with the recent onset of headache thought to be occipital neuralgia should undergo magnetic resonance imaging (MRI) testing of the brain and of the cervical spine (**Fig. 55.2**). MRI testing should also be performed in those patients with previously stable occipital neuralgia who have experienced a recent change in headache symptomatology or in whom traditional therapeutic interventions fail to provide long-lasting pain relief. Screening laboratory testing consisting of complete blood count, erythrocyte sedimentation rate, and automated blood chemistry testing should be performed if the diagnosis of occipital neuralgia is in question.

Neural blockade of the greater and lesser occipital nerves can serve as a diagnostic maneuver to help confirm the diagnosis and separate it from tension-type headache (see subsequent discussion). The greater and lesser occipital nerves can easily be blocked at the nuchal ridge.

Differential Diagnosis

Occipital neuralgia is an infrequent cause of headaches and rarely occurs in the absence of blunt trauma to the greater and lesser occipital nerves. More often, the patient with headaches that involve the occipital region does in fact have tension-type or cervicogenic headaches. Tension-type headaches do not respond to occipital nerve blocks but are amenable to treatment with antidepressant compounds such as amitriptyline in conjunction with cervical steroid epidural nerve blocks.[4] Therefore, the clinician should reconsider the diagnosis of occipital neuralgia in those patients whose symptoms are consistent with occipital neuralgia but do not respond to greater and lesser occipital nerve blocks. As mentioned previously, occult tumor may rarely mimic the pain of occipital neuralgia (see Fig. 55.2).

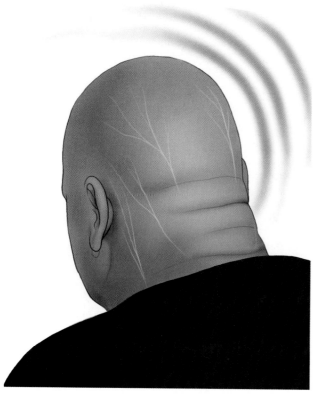

Fig. 55.1 Occipital neuralgia is caused by trauma to the greater and lesser occipital nerves. *(From Waldman SD: Atlas of common pain syndromes, Philadelphia, 2002, Saunders, p 23.)*

Treatment

The treatment of occipital neuralgia consists primarily of neural blockade with local anesthetic and steroid combined with the judicious use of nonsteroidal anti-inflammatory drugs, muscle relaxants, tricyclic antidepressants, and physical therapy. Neural blockade of the greater and lesser occipital nerve is carried out with the following technique: The patient is placed in a sitting position with the cervical spine flexed and the forehead on a padded bedside table. A total of 8 mL of local anesthetic is drawn up in a 12-mL sterile syringe. With treatment of occipital neuralgia or other painful conditions that involve the greater and lesser occipital nerve, a total of 80 mg of depot steroid is added to the local anesthetic with the first block and 40 mg of depot steroid is added with subsequent blocks.[5]

The occipital artery is then palpated at the level of the superior nuchal ridge. After preparation of the skin with antiseptic solution, a 22-gauge 1½-inch needle is inserted just medial to the artery and is advanced perpendicularly until the needle approaches the periosteum of the underlying occipital bone. A paresthesia may be elicited, and the patient should be warned of such. The needle is then redirected superiorly, and after gentle aspiration, 5 mL of solution is injected in a fan-like distribution, with care taken to avoid the foramen magnum, which is located medially (**Fig. 55.3**).

The lesser occipital nerve and a number of superficial branches of the greater occipital nerve are then blocked by directing the needle laterally and slightly inferiorly. After gentle aspiration, an additional 3 to 4 mL of solution is injected

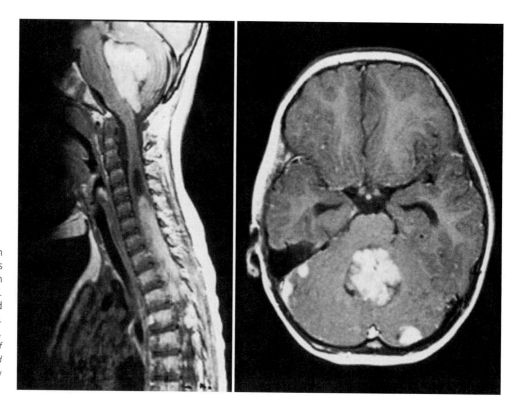

Fig. 55.2 Medulloblastoma with metastatic spread to the meninges within the posterior fossa and with a large intramedullary deposit. Sagittal and axial MRI, T1-weighted gadolinium contrast enhancement. *(From Alba A, Brandes EF, Tosoni A, et al: Adult neuroectodermal tumors of posterior fossa (medulloblastoma) and of supratentorial sites (stPNET), Crit Rev Oncol Hematol 71:167, 2009, p 167.)*

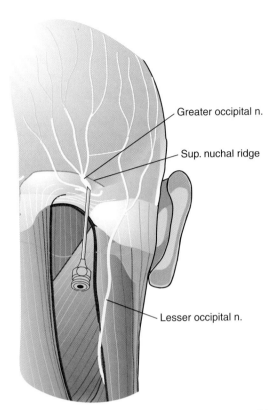

Fig. 55.3 **Technique for greater and lesser occipital nerve block.**

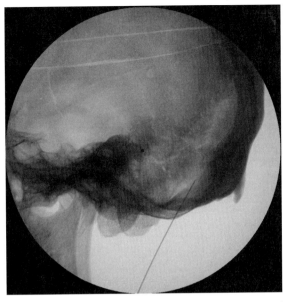

Fig. 55.4 Proper needle position for radiofrequency lesioning of the greater occipital nerve. *(From Waldman SD: Atlas of interventional pain management, ed 3, Philadelphia, 2009, Saunders, p 30.)*

(see Fig. 55.3). In rare cases, radiofrequency lesioning of the occipital nerves may be necessary to provide long-lasting pain relief (**Fig. 55.4**).[6]

Complications and Pitfalls

The scalp is highly vascular, and this—coupled with the fact that both the greater and the lesser occipital nerves are in close proximity to arteries—means that the clinician should carefully calculate the total milligram dosage of local anesthetic that may be safely given, especially if bilateral nerve blocks are being performed. This vascularity and proximity to the arterial supply gives rise to an increased incidence of postblock ecchymosis and hematoma formation. These complications can be decreased if manual pressure is applied to the area of the block immediately after injection. Application of cold packs for 20-minute periods after the block also decrease the amount of postprocedure pain and bleeding the patient may experience. Care must be taken to avoid inadvertent needle placement into the foramen magnum because the subarachnoid administration of local anesthetic in this region results in an immediate total spinal anesthetic.

Conclusion

As with other headache syndromes, the clinician must be sure that the diagnosis is correct and that no coexisting intracranial pathology or diseases of the cervical spine may be erroneously attributed to occipital neuralgia.

The most common reason that greater and lesser occipital nerve block fails to relieve headache pain is that the headache syndrome being treated has been misdiagnosed as occipital neuralgia. Any patient with headaches bad enough to need neural blockade as part of the treatment plan should undergo an MRI scan of the head to rule out unsuspected intracranial pathology. Furthermore, cervical spine radiographs should be considered to rule out congenital abnormalities, such as Arnold-Chiari malformations, which may be the hidden cause of the patient's occipital headaches.

References

Full references for this chapter can be found on www.expertconsult.com.

Chapter 56

Reflex Sympathetic Dystrophy of the Face

Kenneth D. Candido and Alon P. Winnie

Reflex sympathetic dystrophy (RSD) of the face is an unusual and rarely reported disease entity. Although the syndrome of RSD typically affects the distal upper or lower extremities, some patients present with facial pain of a nature reminiscent of that of extremity RSD: that is, pain not limited to the territory of a single peripheral nerve and pain that is spontaneous and associated with allodynia and hyperalgesia, edema, and abnormal skin blood flow. A recent review of the literature revealed that 14 cases had been described that loosely meet the International Association for the Study of Pain (IASP) criteria for complex regional pain syndrome type I (CRPS [RSD]; **Table 56.1**),[1] even though eight of those case reports predate the 1994 IASP publication and the earliest is from 1947.[2] However, Behrman,[3] in the commentary section of his single 1949 case report, stated that he had "encountered about ten cases" (of facial RSD), usually always after a difficult dental extraction. If his description is even partially accurate, it may perhaps indicate that many cases of unusual or atypical facial pain have simply gone unrecognized as representing RSD or that they may have gone unreported.

Clinical Presentation

The main features of RSD of the face are burning pain with allodynia, hyperalgesia, dysesthesias, hyperesthesia, and hyperpathia typically starting after some type of trauma to the craniofacial region, including dental extractions, vascular reconstructive surgery, gunshot wounds, and other insults. Physical signs are reported less often than the aforementioned symptoms (**Table 56.2**).[2] The pain of facial RSD appears to follow the topography of the sympathetically innervated vascular system rather than a radicular or dermatomal pattern. However, according to the actual case reports in the literature, facial RSD is infrequently associated with vasomotor and sudomotor changes and rarely progresses to a dystrophic or atrophic stage. The influence of the autonomic nervous system is considered separately from the type of CRPS (CRPS I [RSD] or CRPS II [causalgia]). Response to a sympatholytic procedure, such as a stellate ganglion block (**Figs. 56.1** and **56.2**), is used to differentiate between sympathetically mediated pain and sympathetically independent pain; this is in addition to and independent of the diagnosis of CRPS types I or II.

The literature describes 14 cases of RSD of the face and neck from 1947 to 2010 (**Table 56.3**).[2–13] The male:female ratio of these cases was 9:5, and the mean age of patients at the time of presentation was 45.5 years.

Trauma was the inciting factor in five of the cases (35.7%), whereas surgery (including neurolytic trigeminal nerve block) was the cause in five cases (35.7%) and dental extraction in three cases (21.4%).

Traumatic injury or surgery of the face and neck may damage postganglionic sympathetic fibers distributed along the external carotid artery plexus. Sympathetic innervation to the facial skin, and the submandibular ganglion, is derived from the external carotid artery plexus (**Figs. 56.3 [online only]** and **56.4**). Adventitial trauma or irritation at this location is consistent with the clinical signs noted. Facial pain was consistently present, unlike the clinical reports of somatic RSD in which pain is described about 75% of the time (see Table 56.2).[2] Pain was usually of a burning quality and was associated with hyperalgesia or hyperesthesia. Skin color changes, temperature changes, numbness, and hypoesthesia were reported less frequently. In rare cases, edema and trophic changes involving the skin of the face have been noted.[2] The profound bony, vascular, and trophic changes associated with advanced RSD of the extremities are not typical of facial RSD.[4] This lack of physical signs severely inhibits the assignation of the IASP criteria to confirm the diagnosis in all cases. However, this is typical of articles purporting to describe CRPS in general. Indeed,

Table 56.1 IASP Classification of Complex Regional Pain Syndrome Type 1 (RSD)

DIAGNOSTIC CRITERIA FOR CRPS I (RSD)

1. The presence of an inciting noxious event or a cause of immobilization.

2. Continuing pain, allodynia, or hyperalgesia with which the pain is disproportionate to any inciting event.

3. Evidence at some time of edema, changes in skin blood flow, or abnormal sudomotor activity in the region of the pain.

4. This diagnosis is excluded by the existence of conditions that would otherwise account for the degree of pain and dysfunction.

Note: Criteria 2 to 4 must be satisfied.
From Merskey H, Bogduk N, editors: *Classification of chronic pain: descriptions of chronic pain syndromes and definitions of pain terms,* ed 2, Seattle, 1994, IASP Press.

Table 56.2 Comparison of the Signs and Symptoms of Facial RSD versus Those of Somatic Reflex Sympathetic Distrophy (CRPS Type I)

Signs/Symptoms	Facial RSD (%)	Somatic RSD (%)
Pain	100	75
Hyperalgesia/ hyperesthesia	54	70 to 80
Allodynia	38	70 to 80
Dysesthesia	8	70
Edema	23	50
Sweating abnormalities	15	50
Skin color changes	46	75 to 98
Skin temperature changes	46	75 to 98

(From Melis M, Zawawi K, Al-Badawi E, et al: Complex regional pain syndrome in the head and neck: a review of the literature, *J Orofac Pain* 16:93, 2002.)

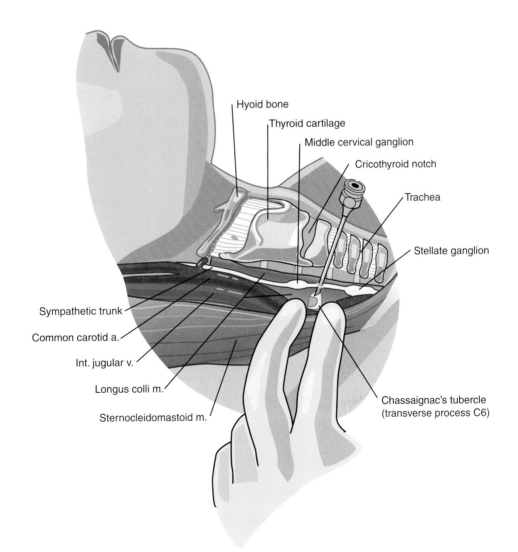

Fig. 56.1 **Stellate ganglion block—anterior approach.** *(From Waldman SD, editor:* Atlas of interventional pain management, *Philadelphia, 1998, Saunders, p 103.)*

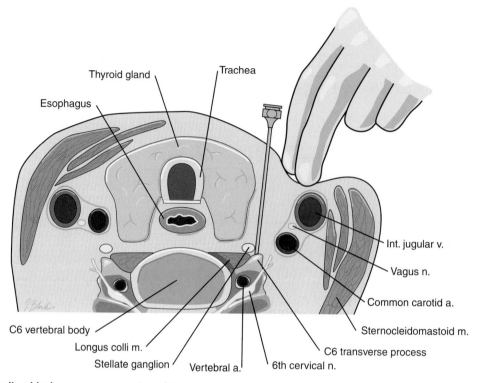

Fig. 56.2 Stellate ganglion block—transverse section of the anterior approach. *(From Waldman SD, editor:* Atlas of interventional pain management, *Philadelphia, 1998, Saunders, p 103.)*

Reinders, et al[1] after performing a MEDLINE search, found 66 publications between January 1996 and January 2010 incorporating "complex regional pain syndrome," or "reflex sympathetic dystrophy" in their descriptions. IASP criteria were used scarcely in describing the syndrome in those 66 articles.[1] None of the articles reviewed fulfilled the strict IASP criteria for CRPS type I. The conclusion was that the validity of the consensus diagnostic criteria is debatable.[1]

Although diagnostic tests may assist in confirmation of the diagnosis, the ultimate determination of whether CRPS is present lies with the clinical evaluation and with a high index of suspicion after elimination of other factors comprising the differential diagnosis. In the 14 cases reported, a successful analgesic response to sympathetic stellate ganglion block (SGB) with local anesthetic was noted in 79% (11 of 14 cases); and in one case each, morphine SGB and phenol SGB were successfully used for treatment. One patient each was successfully treated with amitriptyline, oral clonidine, oral methylprednisolone, oral *N*-acetylcysteine, and intravenous guanethidine plus physical therapy, and intravenous ketamine/midazolam. Two patients in the earliest report were successfully treated with cervical sympathectomies after analgesic SBGs were performed.[5] Ultimate pain relief after treatment ranged from 50% to 100% in all cases noted.[2]

Pain is the cardinal symptom of RSD, whether of the face or of the periphery (see Table 56.2). Pain is typically spontaneous, but it may be evoked by stimuli and may be episodic, paroxysmal, or continuous. The quality of pain may be burning, shooting, throbbing, pressing, or aching or some combination of these qualities. The intensity of the pain is typically out of proportion to the inciting event. Also noted are mechanical and thermal hyperalgesia, dysesthesias, hyperesthesias, allodynia, and hyperpathia. Signs of inflammation may or may not be present. Edema and abnormalities in sudomotor and vasomotor function experienced as increased (hyperhidrosis: warm, moist skin) or decreased (hypohidrosis: cool, dry skin) sweating from autonomic dysfunction may be present. The skin may appear mottled and discolored (reddish, bluish, or purplish), or it may be pale. In the case report by Saxen and Campbell,[6] the patient presented with noninflammatory atypical telangiectasia in the left infraorbital area and cheek. The size and color of the skin lesion varied throughout the treatment period, although the burning pain in that area remained unchanged for much of that time. The skin on the affected side may be warmer or colder than that of the nonaffected side. Facial hair may become coarser and thick or thin and sparse. Combing the hair on the scalp may be extremely painful.[4] Stiffness and ankylosing of the facet joints of the cervical spine or of the temporomandibular joint may be reported. Facial muscles may droop or become notably weaker on the affected side. In the case report of Veldman and Dunkl Jacobs,[7] the patient noted that the right side of her mouth and the right upper eyelid drooped, in a distribution that was unrelated to the anatomic innervation area of a peripheral nerve. Hypersalivation may be present, as noted by Arden and associates.[8] Postganglionic fibers are distributed to approximately the same cutaneous areas as those supplied with sensory fibers by the corresponding radicular nerve (i.e., oral tongue–jaw–V$_3$ dermatome). Considering that 71% of resting salivation is provided by the submandibular glands, with the observation that copious secretions from this gland can be elicited in response to sympathetically stimulated alterations in vasomotor tone, it is plausible to presume a causal relationship between symptoms of hypersalivation and heightened sympathetic activity in the submandibular ganglion.[8]

Table 56.3 Summary of Reflex Sympathetic Dystrophy Cases of the Face and Neck: 1947 to 2010

Author	Year	Age/Gender	Etiology	Symptoms	Signs	Treatment	Outcomes
Bingham[5]	1947	28/M	Shell fragment in (R) cheek	Burning pain V1-V3 distribution	Hyperalgesia V1-V3	SGB, then cervical sympathectomy	Pain free at 3-mo follow-up
Bingham[5]	1947	23/M	Mortar wounds (L) cheek	Burning pain V2	Hyperesthesia in cheek	SGB, then cervical sympathectomy	Symptoms resolved
Behrman[3]	1949	?/F	Tooth extraction	Mandibular pain	Not reported	SGB	Not reported
Hanowell/Kennedy[10]	1979	59/M	Cancer of tongue; radical neck dissection	Phantom tongue pain; burning in cheeks and temples	Hyperemia on side of face; hyperesthesia; stabbing pain	SGB; aimtriptyline (Elavil)	Complete pain relief after 3 blocks
Khoury et al[11]	1980	60/M	Cancer: maxillectomy	Burning pain; eyelid, nose, face, lip	Skin edema, erythema; coolness, side of face	SGB	75% to 85% improved; still some lip sensitivity
Teeple et al[9]	1981	38/F	Trauma, side of face (sail boom)	Pain; left shoulder, arm	Papillary dilatation; face coolness	SGB; aspirin	Pain free at 6-mo; pupils equal
Jaeger et al[4]	1986	33/F	Tooth extraction	Facial pain; preauricular area to orbit, zygoma, mandible; photophobia	Facial swelling; trismus, temperature change	SGB	Pain free at 15-mo follow-up
Jaeger et al[4]	1986	31/M	Subtotal resection frontal sinus; reoperation	Burning in forehead radiating to orbits and maxilla	Tender scar; suprabrow; hyperesthesia	SGB with morphine	66% improved facial pain; scar pain persists
Veldman/Jacobs[7]	1994	47/F	Motor vehicle accident; zygomatic arch impaction; orbital floor fracture	Dull pain side of face and head	Hyperesthesia; facial paresis; swelling; erythema; warmth; hyperhidrosis	N-acetylcysteine, 600 mg tid	Partial decrease in face pain; decreased warmth, redness
Saxen/Campbell[6]	1995	32/F	Tooth extraction	Constant burning pain infraorbital area	Hyperesthesia on cheek; erythema	SGB; clonidine, 0.1 mg bid	Pain relief for 24hr; long-term follow-up not specified
Arden et al[8]	1998	69/M	External carotid to distal vertebral artery transposition	Sharp cheek pain; excess salivation	Hyperesthesia lower part of face	SGB with LA and phenol	80% to 85% relief at 3-yr follow-up
Arden et al[8]	1998	69/M	External carotid to distal vertebral artery transposition	Burning cheek pain; excess salivation; tongue claudication	Hyperesthesia lower part of face	SGB with LA	50% to 70% relief at 2.5-yr follow-up
Figueroa et al[12]	2000	37/M	Motor vehicle accident; head and neck injury	Burning pain; hyperpathia; side of face	Increased skin temperature, pallor, side of face; allodynia	Steroids (methyl-prednisolone, 60 mg/kg/day)	100% pain relief at 6 days
Sakamoto et al[13]	2010	68/M	Trigeminal nerve gangliolysis side of face; right mandibular hypesthesias; nerve injury hyperalgesia tongue atrophy	Burning pain	Allodynia	Ketamine bolus (10 mg) followed by midazolam (2 mg) LA, local anesthetics.	Slow, gradual improvement

bid, twice daily; F, female; L, left; LA, local anesthetics; M, Male; R, right; SGB, stellate ganglion blocks; tid, three times daily.

Summary

Total cases: 14
Male/female: 9:5
Mean age: 45.5 years (13 cases)
Trauma: 5/14 (35.7%)
Surgery: 5/14 (35.7%)
Tooth extraction: 3/14 (21.4%)
Stellate ganglion blocks: 12/14 (85%)

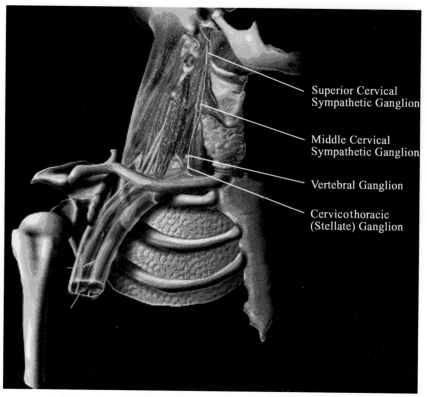

Superior Cervical
Sympathetic Ganglion

Middle Cervical
Sympathetic Ganglion

Vertebral Ganglion

Cervicothoracic
(Stellate) Ganglion

Fig. 56.4 Pharmacologic and physiologic pathways at the site of nerve injury. *(From Khoury R, Kennedy SF, MacNamara TE: Facial causalgia: report of a case, J Oral Surg 38:782, 1980.)*

Pathophysiology

The mechanism by which pain and other physical abnormalities develop in CRPS has not been clearly elucidated. Several theories have been devised to attempt to correlate the physical and biochemical findings with accepted mechanisms of peripheral and central nervous system functioning. Trauma usually precedes the syndrome, resulting in derangements in peripheral nerve functioning and inducing neurobiologic changes in both the peripheral and central nervous systems.[14] Simply stated, a deafferentation mechanism ensues that becomes self perpetuating via the central sensitization syndrome involving activation of wide-dynamic range (WDR) or multireceptive neurons.[15] The initiation of this central sensitization is peripheral tissue injury that activates lightly myelinated A-delta or unmyelinated C-nociceptors, which in turn activate and sensitize WDR neurons in the dorsal horn whose axons ascend to higher centers. This sensitization persists, so that the WDR neurons now respond to mechanical activity in large-diameter, low-threshold A-mechanoreceptor afferents, which are activated by brushing or light touch. A painful sensation results (allodynia), independent of and not proportional to any actual noxious stimulus applied to the nociceptors. Moreover, these sensitized WDR neurons respond to mechanoreceptive activity initiated by sympathetic efferent action on sensory receptors in the absence of cutaneous stimulation, thus producing spontaneous "sympathetically mediated pain." In this hypothetical model, the only abnormal neuronal state required is a persistent sensitization or increase gain of WDR neurons.

Although this hypothesis only focuses on central changes in sensitivity to afferent impulses, accumulating experimental evidence shows that the following changes take place. After peripheral nerve injury occurs, large-diameter myelinated axons sprout from their site of termination in lamina III or deeper into the upper laminae, a region normally only innervated by small-diameter, high-threshold afferents. Indeed, Woolf, et al[16] described sprouting of A-fibers into lamina II of the dorsal horn of the spinal cord. Thus, low-threshold afferents gain access to a pool of dorsal horn neurons involved in nociceptive processing that were originally accessed only by high-threshold afferent input. Some WDR neurons send their axons to the thalamus or to the reticular formation through the ventrolateral fasciculus in the company of axons from nociceptor-specific neurons.[15] This accounts, at least in part, for the development of allodynia after peripheral nerve injury.[14] One scenario postulated is that this neural rewiring alters lamina II recognition, so that this zone, which normally recognizes only nociceptive inputs, now receives non-nociceptive inputs that may be misinterpreted as noxious. Allodynia results when light touch or pressure is applied to the skin. Activation of second-order neurons in the dorsal horn might result from release of substance P and calcitonin gene–related peptide (CGRP) from normally non-nociceptive A-fibers after a phenotypic change occurs in those fibers after nerve injury.[2]

In addition, after some types of nerve injury, primary afferent neurons undergo biologic changes that lead to abnormal sensitization and spontaneous ectopic discharge. This phenomenon resembles attempts of nerves to sprout after nerve injury and also resembles the formation of a neuroma on the cut end of a nerve.[14] Ephaptic (nonsynaptic) transmission, nerve collaterals, or nerve sprouting after injury has been suggested to perhaps account for abnormal nerve functioning.[14] Total axonal disruption is not a prerequisite for a sprout to develop, but the nerve injury does result in a breakdown of the blood-nerve barrier (vaso-nervorum) and facilitates the entry of chemical mediators or blockers. These sprouts or "growth cones" seek to track down the original neural channels; however, such regrowth is often thwarted, leading to local collections of sprouts with chaotic organization, or neuromas. A neuroma is not a true neoplasm but is a disorganized structure that includes axoplasmic elements, myelin, Schwann cells, and connective tissue elements.[2] Neuromas can produce spontaneous continuous pain or episodic pain triggered by external pressure or tension.[2] Many myelinated and unmyelinated afferents that innervate these neuromas can be excited by epinephrine and norepinephrine, thus raising the question of whether damaged sensory fibers may express adrenergic receptors. Devor and Jänig[17] demonstrated that afferent fibers from a neuroma are activated by sympathetic stimulation or by intravenous norepinephrine and that this activation can be blocked by the alpha-adrenergic antagonist phentolamine but not by the beta-antagonist propranolol. These findings have led to the hypothesis that nociceptors (A-delta and C fibers) develop sensitivity to norepinephrine through expression of $alpha_1$-adrenergic receptors on their terminals. Indirect mechanisms supporting this hypothesis include activation of alpha-adrenergic receptors on mast cells, leukocytes, and platelets by norepinephrine, which then release chemical mediators (histamine, bradykinin, prostaglandins), which in turn activate nociceptive afferents. Norepinephrine released by activity of sympathetic postganglionic axons excites primary afferent neurons by activating alpha-adrenergic receptors. According to the theory of Roberts,[15] a vicious cycle develops when nociceptive input to the trigeminal ganglion stimulates sympathetic efferent responses as a result of tonic release of norepinephrine. The combination of tonic norepinephrine release and sympathetic efferent responses results in further norepinephrine release, which perpetuates the pain.[6] Although compelling and theoretically plausible, the neuroma model is not relevant to those cases of sympathetically mediated pain in which the nerve is not injured. Furthermore, it cannot explain the efficacy of nerve blocks distal to the site of nerve injury or the immediate onset of RSD pain after nerve injury in some individuals.[17]

Another theory suggests that in sympathetically mediated pain, a short-circuiting phenomenon may develop in which collateral sympathetic efferents synapse with afferent sensory fibers at the site of peripheral injury. After peripheral nerve injury, sensory axons may express alpha-adrenergic or beta-adrenergic receptors on their membranes. These axons might subsequently become sensitized to circulating catecholamines. The same modification may be occurring at the dorsal root ganglion neurons.[14] The influence of the heightened sympathetic activity on peripheral afferent fibers may also occur from norepinephrine-induced stimulation of prostaglandin synthesis, an effect reversible with the administration of anti-inflammatory medications. Prostaglandins are known to sensitize sensory afferents, and this information led investigators to experiment with the use of intravenous regional blocks with use of ketorolac (a cyclooxygenase-1 [COX-1] and COX-2 nonselective, nonsteroidal anti-inflammatory drugs [NSAIDs]) for treatment of RSD of the extremity.[14] Ketorolac inhibits the enzyme cyclooxygenase and subsequently reduces prostaglandin synthesis, suggesting that because prostaglandins sensitize pain receptors to both chemical and mechanical stimuli, reduction of prostaglandin levels should reduce this sensitivity.[14] NSAIDs may also interfere with the vasoconstriction produced by thromboxanes. Reduction in prostaglandin levels may lead to the inhibition of norepinephrine release and, in addition, may result in direct vasodilation. At a cellular level, RSD is characterized, then, by cellular hypoxia, decreased oxygen extraction at the tissue level, and increased permeability for macromolecules, supporting a role for toxic oxygen radicals as a cause for the syndrome.[7] Sudek's[18] theory of more than 60 years ago may indeed be true, that RSD is a pathologic course of a physiologic inflammatory response to an injury.[7,18]

In addition to pain, other abnormalities are seen in CRPS, some of which may be related to altered function of the sympathetic nervous system. Edema, abnormalities in skin blood flow, and abnormal sudomotor activity may all be blocked by sympathetic nervous system blockade. Vasculature in the vicinity of the insult may develop an increased sensitivity to local cold-temperature stimuli and catecholamines, demonstrated experimentally by testing the thermoregulatory response to skin cooling and warming, suggesting that both an inhibition and activation of sympathetic reflexes may be evident.[19] Trophic changes (not typically seen in facial RSD or CRPS) such as abnormal nail growth, increased hair growth, palmar and plantar fibrosis, thin glossy skin, and hyperkeratosis, have been hypothesized to have an inflammatory pathogenesis. Scintigraphic investigations strongly support an inflammatory component in CRPS, hence the rationale for anti-inflammatory medication use in treatment as described previously.[2,14]

Diagnostic Tests

The diagnosis of CRPS is a clinical one, based on careful analysis of signs, symptoms, and exclusion of other factors in the differential diagnosis. Objective tests, however, are described in the literature that, although not specific, tend to confirm the diagnostic impression of autonomic, sensory, and motor dysfunction, as follows:

- Quantitative sensory tests (QST): These tests measure subjective responses to superficial stimulation and provide information regarding peripheral nerve function of afferent fibers in response to tactile, pressure, thermal, and noxious stimuli.[19] QST can also test the functional status of large myelinated fibers with the dorsal columns by testing vibratory threshold activity.[20]
- Laser Doppler flowmetry: This test measures skin blood flow in the area tested; results may be compared with those from the contralateral side.[6,19]
- Infrared thermography: This modality records the distribution of skin temperature. Each area is subsequently compared with the contralateral side's equivalent area.[19]
- Quantitative sudomotor axon reflex test (QSART): This is a measure of evoked sweat response. QSART provides information on the function of the sudomotor reflex loops. Although it examines axon reflex response, it cannot be used to measure the effect of sympatholysis.[19]
- Bone scintigraphy: Changes in bone vascularity are noted with this test. Only an indication of changes that occur in the subacute period may be determined. A three-phase bone scan provides more discriminative scintigraphic description of the disease.[21]

- Plain radiographs: These may show the status of bone demineralization of the bones of the face, in contradistinction to those of the nonaffected side.[22]
- Sympathetic nerve blocks: A sympathetic nerve block (SGB) may be used for diagnostic and therapeutic purposes for individuals with CRPS of the face and neck (see Figs. 56.1 and 56.2). A reduction of pain concomitant with signs of sympathetic block of the face (ipsilateral ptosis, miosis, anhidrosis, apparent enophthalmos—Horner's syndrome) and an elevation of the temperature of the ipsilateral hand are sought. Care must be taken to interpret results of the block in light of underlying pathology because Horner's syndrome may be caused by interruption of the preganglionic fibers at any point between their origin in the intermediolateral cell column of C8-T1 spinal segments and the superior cervical ganglion or by interruption of the descending, uncrossed hypothalamospinal pathway in the tegmentum of the brain stem or cervical cord. Causes of Horner's syndrome are tumorous or inflammatory involvement of cervical lymph nodes, surgical and other types of trauma to cervical structures, neoplastic invasion of the proximal part of the brachial plexus, basilar skull fractures, tumor, syringomyelia or traumatic lesions of the first and second thoracic spinal segments, and infarcts or other lesions of the lateral part of the medulla (Wallenberg's syndrome). There is also an idiopathic variety that may be hereditary. A superior sulcus tumor of the lung may produce a chronic Horner's syndrome as well. With preganglionic lesions, flushing may develop on the side of the sympathetic disorder; this effect may be brought on in some instances by exercise (harlequin effect).[23]

Treatment

The purpose of therapy is to relieve pain and improve function. Along with interventions, physical therapy is essential to help restore function and improve muscle strength. In the early stages of RSD, gentle controlled stimulation with use of heat, massage, pressure, cold, vibration, and movement may all help restore normal sensory processing. Appropriate counseling is essential to help deal with issues of depression, denial, anxiety, anger, and fear. A cognitive-behavioral approach is often helpful to overcome pain avoidance, overprotection, movement phobia, and bracing.[2]

Nonpharmacologic modalities attempted for pain relief have included the use of transcutaneous electrical nerve stimulation (TENS), peripheral nerve stimulation, or biofeedback. Biofeedback has been touted as a means of enabling the patient to alter sympathetic activity and increase blood flow to the affected area.

Medication management has included NSAIDs, corticosteroids, opioids, and membrane stabilizers acting on sodium channels, such as phenytoin, carbamazepine, mexiletine, and local anesthetics, with the purpose of reducing the normal and ectopic firing of neurons. Some success has been shown with phenytoin and carbamazepine in the treatment of painful diabetic polyneuropathy syndromes, and these agents have been tried in RSD cases as well.[20] Mexiletine, the oral congener of lidocaine hydrochloride, may have beneficial effects in chronic persistent neuropathic pain states and may be attempted in

facial RSD if patients have a positive response to an intravenous lidocaine test. Tricyclic antidepressants, particularly amitriptyline, have been used with some success in neuropathic pain.[20] The drugs of this class work at the central nervous system (CNS) brainstem/dorsal horn nociceptive-modulating system, where they alter 5-hydroxytryptamine and norepinephrine activity.[20] They also bind to other receptor sites, including histaminergic, cholinergic, and adrenergic. Other types of antidepressants have not shown the kind of success seen with amitriptyline for neuropathic pain states, but venlafaxine, a serotonin and norepinephrine reuptake inhibitor, has been suggested in the treatment paradigm.[20,24] Venlafaxine is a strong uptake inhibitor of both serotonin and norepinephrine with minimal muscarinic, histaminergic, and adrenergic activity.[20] Venlafaxine may produce analgesia similar to that of the tricyclic antidepressants without their frequent anticholinergic and histaminergic side effects. Gabapentin has been successfully used in the treatment of neuropathic pain states and has also been used in CRPS.[9,20] A major benefit of gabapentin use is its excellent safety profile, permitting repetitive escalating dose use without fear of catastrophic consequences. Clonidine, a peripheral alpha$_2$-receptor agonist with CNS activity, is available in an oral form, as a transdermal preparation, and for intrathecal use. Transdermal clonidine has been used successfully in the treatment of painful diabetic neuropathy and was successfully used in the facial RSD case report of Saxen and Campbell.[6] Capsaicin has been used topically in an effort to reduce peripheral inputs. The advantages of topical application of medications over oral administration include a directed activity at a mechanistic site of pain generation in the periphery with minimal risk of significant systemic side effects, no drug-drug interactions, and no need for dose titration.[20] In one case of facial RSD, N-acetylcysteine was used with significant reduction in allodynia.[7] Other modalities used have included scavengers of oxygen free radicals, deep brain stimulation in the sensory thalamus and medial lemniscus, and spinal cord stimulators. Pregabalin, duloxetine, milnacipran and other newer agents used for treating chronic neuropathic pain conditions have not been assessed in terms of efficacy for use in facial RSD, largely because of the obvious difficulties of encountering appropriate populations of patients for study.

Repeated SGBs have been used most frequently when a sympathetic component is present for RSD of the face and neck. SGB may be efficacious by removing sympathetic excitation of A-fiber mechanoreceptors. A reduction in tonic mechanoreceptor activity after sympathetic block should result in a disfacilitation of WDR neurons, and therefore a reduction in the allodynia and hyperpathia that accompanies sympathetically mediated pain if those symptoms are mediated by mechanoreceptors.[15] The sympathetic fibers that serve the orofacial structures arise from the upper thoracic (primarily the first and second) spinal segments (see Figs. 56.3 [online only] and 56.4). These fibers course upward through the stellate (fused inferior cervical and upper thoracic) and middle cervical ganglia to synapse in the superior cervical ganglion before leaving the chain to supply the face (see Figs. 56.3 [online only] and 56.4).[4] The cervicothoracic chain can be injected via anterior, posterior, or paravertebral approaches with local anesthetics or adjuvant medications (see Figs. 56.1 and 56.2). These medications tend to spread along the ganglia. Interruption of any of these levels can cause Horner's syndrome. In the 13 case studies, SGB was used in 11 (85%). In one study, cervical plexus block was added to SGB to relieve muscle spasms in the neck.[9] Based on an atypical response to treatment, Arden and colleagues[8] suggest implementing contralateral SGB when symptomatic improvement with ipsilateral blocks plateaus. Although the mechanism for this idiosyncratic response is unclear, observations of crossed lateral radiation responses (particularly of the hand) favorably influenced by ipsilateral injections have been documented.[1] Typically, local anesthetics such as bupivacaine or mepivacaine have been used. Mepivacaine, an amino-amide local anesthetic, may be the safest amide in terms of systemic toxicity and has a shorter duration of action at sodium channels than does bupivacaine. Because the actual duration of sympathetic block resulting from local anesthetic stellate ganglion block does not correlate with overall outcome,[14] it makes little sense to use long-acting agents. If a complication results from the misplacement of such agents in a blood vessel or in the central neuraxis during performance of the block, significantly greater morbidity may result from the longer acting, highly protein bound, highly lipophilic action of such drugs.

Other agents used for stellate ganglion block have included neurolytics, such as phenol or alcohol, and opioids, such as morphine and fentanyl. Other sympatholytics that act on the norepinephrine receptor may be used, including drugs such as guanethidine and reserpine. Guanethidine decreases the presynaptic release of norepinephrine at neuronal sites. Phentolamine reduces the action of norepinephrine on receptors by blocking both $beta_1$ and $beta_2$ receptors peripherally. The $alpha_2$-agonist clonidine, a centrally acting agent, decreases the release of norepinephrine from presynaptic neurons.

A somewhat more aggressive intervention, surgical cervical sympathectomy, may be reserved for refractory cases.[5]

Conclusion

RSD of the face is an uncommon and rarely reported clinical entity. Comparison between this syndrome and RSD (CRPS type I) in other parts of the body may not be valid because of the small number of reported cases of CRPS in the head and neck. Many of the older case summaries are notably brief, and the authors have probably not included the entire constellation of symptoms and signs. Indeed, in the report of Behrman[3] from 1949, even the patient's age was not included. In any event, only 14 cases were reported between 1947 and 2010. It is entirely possible that facial RSD may be a variant or atypical presentation of a more common disorder such as myofascial pain with concomitant involvement of the autonomic nervous system.[2] An additional hypothesis is that the orofacial region, being overrepresented in a neurologic homunculus, may respond differently to trauma than other somatic areas. The rich collateral and anastomotic vascular supply of the face may minimize the development of the signs seen with extremity RSD.[4] This phenomenon of differential response to trauma between the head and other body areas has some support in nonhuman models.[25,26] In a rat model, peripheral nerve injury–induced sprouting of sympathetic nerve fibers occurred less frequently in the trigeminal ganglion than it did in spinal nerve regions, perhaps suggesting that the face is somewhat more resistant to development of RSD-related physiologic derangements than are the distal extremities.[25,26] A recently reported case of suspected RSD of the face in the orofacial region (CRPS type II) demonstrated the potential utility of using N-methyl-D-aspartate (NMDA)-receptor antagonists (ketamine) in cases refractory to the effects of sympathetic blocks.[26] A high index of suspicion, combined with a broad-based differential diagnosis, is essential to identifying and treating this group of patients. Ignoring or misdiagnosing these cases may ultimately result in overmedication with opioids with the attendant addiction issues, potential for severe psychologic disturbances, and possibly suicidal ideation. In that regard, it remains essential, when treating these patients, to not dismiss the important role that depression or anxiety plays in perpetuating the illness. Maladaptive coping skills need to be addressed as well. Prompt initiation of physical therapy, once the acute stage has resolved, remains a logical and intuitive mainstay of treatment.

References

Full references for this chapter can be found on www.expertconsult.com.

Part B

Pain Emanating From the Neck and Brachial Plexus

Chapter 57

Cervical Facet Syndrome

Khuram A. Sial, Thomas T. Simopoulos, Zahid H. Bajwa, and Carol A. Warfield

Historical Considerations

Cervical facet joints have gained considerable attention as a potential origin for head and neck pain. In 1911, lumbar facet joints were first identified as a source of back pain.[1] In 1977, Pawl[2] reported the reproduction of pain in patients with headache and neck pain after injections of hypertonic saline solution into the cervical facet joints. Similar findings were published by Hadden[3] in 1940, Raney and Raney[4] in 1948, Taren and Kahn[5] in 1962, Brain and Wilkinson[6] in 1967, and McNab[7] and Mehta[8] in 1973. Bogduk and Marsland[9] were pioneers in the use of diagnostic cervical medial branch blocks and facet joint injections to study the role of cervical facet joints in causation of idiopathic neck pain. Specific referral patterns of neck pain were mapped out by Dwyer et al[10] with facet joint injections performed in healthy volunteers. The accuracy of this pain chart by Dwyer et al[10] was confirmed with anesthetization of the medial branches of the dorsal rami above and below the symptomatic joint. Similar results were obtained by Fukui and associates[11] when they studied the referred pain distribution of cervical facet joints and cervical dorsal rami. Windsor and coworkers[12] also studied cervical medial branch referral patterns with use of electrical stimulation.

Clinical Syndrome

Few reliable epidemiologic studies report the prevalence of neck pain; a study in Finland and a Norwegian study estimated the prevalence rate of neck pain in the general population to be approximately 14%. Ghormley[13] coined the term facet syndrome in 1933 to describe a constellation of symptoms associated with degenerative changes of the lumbar spine. Facet joint morphology varies with regions of the cervical spine, gender, and location. Because of the lack of intervertebral disks in this region, variations in these geometric characteristics affect the biomechanical behaviors of the human spine secondary to external loads.[14] The term cervical facet syndrome

(CFS) implies axial pain from involvement of posterior spinal column elements. Degenerative changes in the cervical facet joints have been well documented in the literature with skeletal spinal column remains, with the C2-C3 facet joints showing the highest rate of changes.[15,16]

The classic clinical presentation of CFS includes neck pain from the cervical facet joints with referred pain in the head and upper extremities. The facet joint is an important structure in resisting compression at higher loads, anterior shear, extension, lateral bending, and torsion.[17] Usually, no other cause is evident. The numerous other pain generators in the neck include the intervertebral discs, ligaments, muscles, nerve roots, and bony tissue, which includes the facet joints. The diagnosis of CFS is often one of exclusion. Facet joints are extensively innervated, and the presence of neuropeptides, such as substance P and calcitonin gene–related peptide, lends credence to the cervical facet joint capsules as a key source of neck pain.[18] Patients may present with headaches and limited range of motion associated with classic neck pain. The quality of the pain is described as a dull ache in the posterior neck region, which sometimes radiates to the shoulder or the midback region or both areas. A history of whiplash injury always should be suspected and noted during history taking. Clinical features that may be present include tenderness to palpation over the facet joints or paraspinal muscles, accentuation of pain with cervical extension or rotation, and the absence of any neurologic deficits.[16] CFS should be strongly considered in the differential diagnosis if these symptoms are present.

Patients with CFS may not respond to conservative management, including physical therapy, heat, cryotherapy, ultrasound scan, transcutaneous electrical nerve stimulation, stretching and range-of-motion exercises, cervical traction, manual manipulation, chiropractic treatment, massage, phonophoresis, iontophoresis, acupuncture, muscle relaxants, nonsteroidal anti-inflammatory drugs (NSAIDs), and other analgesics. The average pain level with use of the visual analog scale is usually greater than 5 on a scale of 0 to 10. The pain commonly may be severe enough to cause functional impairments as well. Referral pain patterns may resemble the patterns described in healthy volunteers via provocation or stimulation of facet joints. Radicular symptoms are not associated with CFS, although patients may have coexisting upper extremity pain.

Imaging usually is not helpful and is devoid of evidence of disk herniation or radiculitis, although it can help to rule out a fracture or tumors. One may visualize cervical facet hypertrophic changes on cervical spine magnetic resonance imaging (MRI) films. Friedenberg and Miller[19] published an article in 1963 that stated that signs of cervical spondylosis, narrowing of the intervertebral foramina, osteophytes, and other degenerative changes are equally prevalent in individuals with and without neck pain. Neurophysiologic abnormalities are absent as well. Patients also may present with cervicogenic headache and upper back pain. The duration of pain is at least 3 months.

In compliance with the criteria established by the International Association for the Study of Pain,[20] the prevalence rate of CFS was determined with controlled diagnostic blocks of cervical facet joints and found to be 54% to 67% of patients with chronic neck pain.[21-24] Aprill and Bogduk[25] reviewed the records of 318 patients who had neck pain for at least 6 months to estimate the prevalence rate of cervical facet joint pain. These studies indicate that the prevalence rate of cervical facet joint pain ranges from 26% to 65%. Of those who underwent both discography and facet joint medial branch nerve blocks, 62% had painful facet joints. Manchikanti and associates[23] completed a large study with 500 patients with chronic, nonspecific spine pain to obtain an epidemiologic prevalence rate. They used controlled comparative local anesthetic blocks with 1% lidocaine and repeat confirmatory blocks with 0.25% bupivicaine, with the latter yielding longer lasting relief for a positive diagnosis. This study indicated the prevalence rate of cervical facet joint pain was 55%. Because of the subjective nature of diagnostic blocks and the lack of specificity, a wide range in found in studies that attempt to estimate the prevalence rate of CFS.

Cervical facet joint pain is a common sequela of whiplash injury. Numerous studies have been performed to estimate the prevalence rate of CFS as the cause of post-traumatic neck pain, which ranges from 63% to 100%, with a mean of approximately 70%.[26-32] With use of double-blind, controlled, diagnostic blocks of the facet joints of 38 patients with whiplash injury, Barnsley and colleagues[26] used a double-blind controlled study to perform diagnostic blocks with short-acting or long-acting anesthetics; if complete relief was obtained, the joint was blocked with the other agent 2 weeks later. They found that cervical facet joint pain had a prevalence rate of 54%, making cervical facet joint pain the most common cause of chronic neck pain after whiplash injury in this population. Lord and colleagues[27] studied a sample of 41 patients with neck pain of 3 months duration after a motor vehicle accident. These investigators used another double-blind, placebo-controlled protocol and found the prevalence rate of cervical facet joint pain after whiplash injury to be 60%; the most common levels were C2-C3 and C5-C6.

The referral patterns for cervical facet joint pain vary; however, particular radiation patterns have been identified for each facet joint level on painful stimulation. Even in asymptomatic subjects, provocation by capsular distention of the facet joints

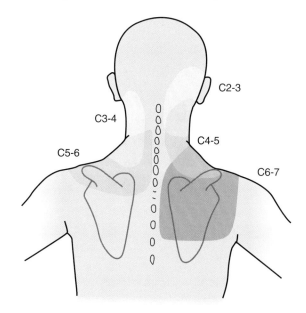

Fig. 57.1 **Diagram of cervical zygapophyseal joint pain distribution in volunteers.**

with contrast material produces neck pain in a specific pattern corresponding to a particular facet joint. Dwyer et al[10] mapped out the referral patterns in five subjects (**Fig. 57.1**). The C2-C3 facet joint refers pain to the posterior upper cervical region and head, whereas the C3-C4 facet joint refers pain to the posterolateral cervical region but does not radiate to the head or shoulder. The C5-C6 joint refers pain to the posterolateral middle and primarily lower cervical spine and the top and lateral parts of the shoulder and caudally to the spine of the scapula. The C6-C7 facet joint refers pain to the top and lateral parts of the shoulder and radiates caudally to the inferior border of the scapula. In patients with cervical pain, these pain referral maps may be powerful diagnostic tools. Fukui and associates[11] studied 61 patients with neck pain and used two methods to stimulate their facet joints (**Fig. 57.2**). They compared pain referral maps constructed from injection of contrast medium into the joints with electrical stimulation of the medial branches and found that they correlated relatively well.

Testing

The optimal method for diagnosis of CFS includes putting everything together, including a thorough history and physical examination, imaging techniques, and use of diagnostic blocks. Numerous attempts by investigators to correlate neurophysiologic findings, physical findings, radiologic findings, and other signs and symptoms with the diagnosis of facet joint syndrome have been unsuccessful.[28-30] Because no formal effective diagnostic study exists, the frequency of pain from CFS has been estimated by subjective relief in response to local anesthetic injections. Radiographs should be obtained in the neutral, flexed, and extended positions, and the range of motion should be documented. The angular displacement of one body on the next should be less than 11 degrees, and the horizontal movement of one vertebral body on the next

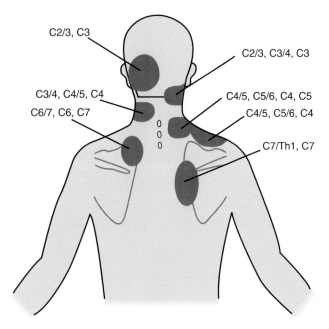

Fig. 57.2 Referred pain distributions for the zygapophyseal joints from C1 to T7-Th1 and the dorsal rami C3 to C7.

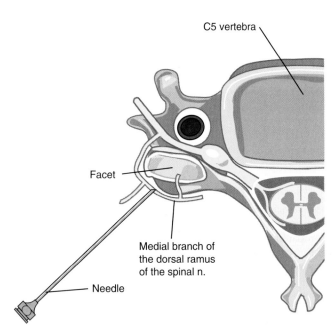

Fig. 57.3 Medial branch block technique used for the diagnosis and treatment of cervical facet syndrome.

should not exceed 3.5 mm. Cervical spine MRI may reveal degenerative changes consistent with cervical facet arthropathy. Imaging alone does not reveal that the facet joints are the true source of pain.

Cervical facet joint blocks can be performed to test the hypothesis that the target joint is the source of the patient's pain.[28,29,31] The cervical facet joints can be anesthetized with local anesthetic injected directly into the intra-articular joint space or with anesthetizing the medial branches of the dorsal rami that innervate the corresponding joint (**Fig. 57.3**).[28,29] Below C2-C3, each cervical facet joint is supplied by the medial branches above and below the joint; the C2-C3 joint is

innervated primarily by the third occipital nerve (a small and variable contribution may derive from the greater occipital nerve). The joint may be considered the source of the pain if the pain is relieved.[28,29] The range of motion often improves, specifically rotation and extension. Controlled blocks are confirmed as true-positive responses in the form of placebo injections with normal saline solution or comparative local anesthetic blocks, in which the same joint is anesthetized with local anesthetics with differing durations of action on two separate occasions.[28,29] In practice, placebo injections are replaced by a series of local anesthetic blocks to confirm the pain generator and dissipate the placebo response.

Differential Diagnosis

The cervical spine includes many pain generators, including intervertebral disks, facet joints, ligaments, muscles, and nerve roots. Regarding cervical spine motion, an intimate relationship exists between the cervical intervertebral discs and the facet joints above and below them. Many patients with cervical facet joint pain also have painful cervical intervertebral discs. For evaluation of the contribution of cervical pain from degenerative discs, Manchikanti et al evaluated a sample of 56 patients from the previous study population with neck pain who had undergone a cervical discography and facet joint nerve blocks at the same level as part of the diagnostic process.[32] Disk disease identified with diskography was present in 64% of patients with a positive cervical medial branch test for facet joint pain. Results revealed that 41% of the patients had a symptomatic disk and a symptomatic facet joint at the same segment, and an additional 23% had a painful facet joint, but not a painful disk at the same segment. Degenerative changes to the facet joint include hypertrophic arthropathy, which may impinge on nerve roots and may irritate afferents on the posterolateral aspect of the disk. In patients with incidental abnormalities of the facet joints, multiple other structures and pain generators could be the cause of pain, or at least may contribute to a condition more complex than a facet origin of pain. Blockade of medial branches denervates not only the joints they supply but also the muscles, ligaments, and periosteum. Sources of pain in these alternative sites are relieved with medial branch block. Other painful conditions can overlap with signs and symptoms of CFS, including cervicodynia, cervical myofascial pain syndrome, cervical degenerative disk disease, ligamentous laxity, neck strain, compression fracture, cervical radiculopathy, and cervical stenosis.

Treatment

A comprehensive rehabilitation program is pertinent to a thorough and complete treatment program for patients with CFS. Three phases of rehabilitation are illustrated as defined by Cole et al.[33] Reducing pain and inflammation and increasing the pain-free range of motion are the primary goals of the first phase. Application of ice during the acute phase decreases blood flow and subsequent hemorrhage into injured tissues, which ultimately reduces local edema. It also can relieve painful muscle spasms. Therapeutic modalities, such as ultrasound scan and electrical stimulation, also may be beneficial in terms of pain and muscle spasm. Manual therapy, joint mobilization, soft tissue massage, and muscle

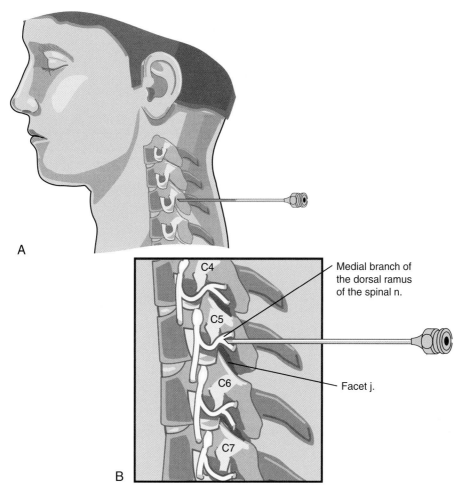

Fig. 57.4 A and B, Radiofrequency ablation of the medial branch of the dorsal ramus of the spinal nerve. Radiofrequency energy is applied to the tip of the ablative probe to denature the medial branch nerve, preventing signals from entering the brain.

stretching often are helpful. Passive range of motion followed by active range of motion exercises in a pain-free range should be initiated in this phase. Finally, strengthening should begin with isometric exercises, progressing to isotonic exercises as tolerated. The recovery phase is entered as the patient is approaching pain relief. The goals of this second phase are improved range of motion, complete pain relief, and improved strength and neuromuscular control. The maintenance phase is the third and final phase, which entails balancing strength and flexibility while increasing endurance.

If a conservative approach does not suffice, more invasive procedures should be considered and used. A significant role has been described for therapeutic facet joint injections, with intra-articular facet joint injections, medial branch blocks, or medial branch neurotomy (**Fig. 57.4 A** and **B**).[34] According to one randomized controlled trial, however, the evidence is poor for short-term and long-term relief of intra-articular injections of the cervical spine.[34] Manchikanti and associates[34] reviewed the literature extensively and concluded that except for one negative randomized control trial[35] for intra-articular injections, no other nonobservational trials qualified to be included for evidence-based practice.

Barnsley and colleagues[35] studied the efficacy of intra-articular facet joint injections for the treatment of chronic cervical facet pain after whiplash injury and found a 50% reduction in pain compared with the preinjection level. The duration of pain relief from intra-articular facet joint injections varies among different investigators. Some studies of intra-articular joint injections report only minor pain relief lasting days to weeks,[35,36] whereas others report substantial relief for weeks to months.[37–39]

Medial branch blocks also have been used for therapeutic purposes in the cervical spine (see Fig. 57.3). In one prospective, nonrandomized, and observational study,[40] significant effectiveness of medial branch blocks was shown in management of chronic neck pain. Barnsley and Bogduk[41] studied 16 patients with chronic neck pain who underwent repeated cervical medial branch blocks with 0.5 mL of local anesthetic in a double-blind, controlled protocol to obtain an estimated sensitivity and specificity of medial branch block in the diagnosis of CFS. The sensitivity of a single uncontrolled block was estimated to be 95%, and the specificity was 73%.[41] A high false-positive rate (27%), however, is found for single, uncontrolled blocks.[42] Medial branch blocks also have been performed with comparative local anesthetics. In one study, 34 patients (77%) correctly identified the longer acting agent when they received a series of injections with bupivacaine or lidocaine.[30]

In a related study, the sensitivity and specificity of comparative local blocks were evaluated.[43] These blocks were compared with placebo-controlled blocks in a randomized, double-blind trial. A low sensitivity of 54% indicated many false-negative results (46%). The specificity was 88%, indicating few false-positive results (12%). When surgical decisions are based on the results of the medial branch blocks, placebo-controlled triple blocks may be prudent.

Barnsley and Bogduk[41] used contrast material in another study to show that 0.5 mL of local anesthetic followed by 0.5 mL of contrast medium was an appropriate volume that does not spread far enough to affect structures other than the intended nerve. No spread of contrast material occurred above or below the intended level, no spread occurred anterior to the ventral ramus, and no spread occurred laterally beyond the semispinalis muscle. The anesthetic blocked only the facet joint and did not anesthetize any other structures that might be a source of chronic neck pain. Traditionally, therapeutic facet joint injections are performed only in patients in whom controlled diagnostic blocks establish a diagnosis of facet joint pain.

In suspected cases of CFS in our clinic, a diagnostic medial branch block technique is first used. If a positive response is seen, a series of three medial branch blocks is performed over 12 to 18 weeks to dissipate the placebo response and document length of time with good response. Patients with significant relief lasting 2 to 3 months may need a maintenance program of cervical medial branch blocks thereafter with a maximum of four to six repeat procedures per year. An evanescent response to diagnostic medial branch blocks may be an indication for radiofrequency ablation in hopes for longer term relief with a maximum of four treatments per year.

Medial branch neurotomy also has been described with well-controlled trials (see Fig. 57.4). The effectiveness has been described in systematic reviews, observational studies, randomized trials, and case reports, although inconclusive results were reported.[44–51] Most investigators have found that radiofrequency thermocoagulation of medial branches for facet arthropathy is a safe and efficacious modality with the potential for long-term benefit. Radiofrequency lesioning is performed with continuous or pulsed mode radiofrequency. Radiofrequency neurotomy denervates the facet joint by coagulating the medial branch of the dorsal ramus, which denatures the proteins in the nerve.[52] In doing so, nerve impulses sending electrical messages of pain to the dorsal root ganglion are inhibited. Because the dorsal root ganglion is preserved, however, the nerve is not destroyed, and the medial branch cell bodies are intact. Also, depending on the radiofrequency lesion site, the nerve may grow back to its target joint in 6 to 9 months, which could reproduce the facet joint pain. In this case, repeating the neurotomy is a viable option. One should use caution in denervating multiple segments bilaterally because this can lead to an increased risk of cervical muscular fatigue with activities of daily living.[46]

A randomized double-blind trial with 24 patients was used by Lord and colleagues[53] to evaluate the efficacy of radiofrequency neurotomy. After confirmation of painful facet joints with placebo-controlled, diagnostic blocks, the patients were randomized to treatment and control groups. The treatment group was subjected to heating of the medial branch to 80°C (176°F) for 90 seconds; in the control group, the temperature probe was maintained at 37°C (99°F). The 12 patients in the treatment group reported an average of 263 days before the pain level returned to 50% of the preoperative level. The 12 patients in the control group perceived this in just 8 days. At 27 weeks, one patient in the control group and seven in the treatment group remained pain free.[53]

Long-term efficacy of radiofrequency neurotomy was evaluated in 28 patients with neck pain from motor vehicle accidents.[46] After the initial procedure, 71% of the patients reported complete relief of pain; the mean duration was 422 days. The patients benefited from 219 days of relief when the procedure was repeated, and some patients maintained pain relief for years after multiple repeat procedures.

Cervical fusion should be considered only after aggressive nonsurgical care has failed. In patients with CFS, the outcome for surgical fusion is significantly less propitious than for radicular pain.[54,55] In a few medical centers, cervical pain without neurologic deficit with degenerative changes of the facet joints may represent a delicate indication for cervical fusion.[56] Spondylotic changes on plain films are not an indication for surgical fusion because these changes are evident in patients with and without symptoms and do not correspond to neck pain.[19] In some cases, cervical facet joint pain can occur even after anterior cervical fusion or may become increasingly more painful after surgery. This may be related to small movement in the joints or intrinsic mechanisms that are not motion dependent.[9] Immobilization of specific levels renders the remaining joints responsible to take on the burden of the mechanical stresses. Cervicodynia also may be the result of intrinsic mechanisms that are not motion dependent or may be related to small movements in the joints.[9] NSAIDs also can help to reduce pain and inflammation, although long-term use can lead to gastric irritation or ulceration in many individuals.

Complications and Pitfalls

As with all invasive medical procedures, potential risks and complications are associated with facet joint injections. In general, the risk is low, and complications are rare. Disastrous complications with cervical facet joint injections may occur, however, including complications related to technique with needle placement and those related to the administration of various drugs (**Table 57.1**). Patients who are undergoing anticoagulant therapy (e.g., warfarin [Coumadin]) or have an active infection may not be able to have this procedure. These situations should be discussed with the treating physician.

Okada,[57] in a series of facet joint injections, showed a communicating pathway was found in 80% of subjects from the facet joint to the interlaminar portion, interspinous portion, contralateral facet joint, paraextradural space, and cervical extradural space. Dreyfuss et al[58] showed that 7% of cases were found to have extra-articular leaks even with low volumes. Rare but potential complications include vertebral artery and ventral ramus damage and a risk of embolus resulting in serious neurologic sequelae with spinal cord damage and cerebral infarction. Other minor complications include headaches, pain at the injection site, syncope, hypotension, nausea, sweating, flushing, and lightheadedness.

Complications of radiofrequency thermoneurolysis are rare and include worsening of the usual pain and possible deafferentation pain, local pain (including myofascial, symptomatic hematoma, non-neuritic), neuritic pain, sensory or motor deficits, burning pain or dysesthesias, decreased sensation and allodynia in the paravertebral skin or the denervated facets, transient leg pain, and persistent leg weakness.[33,59,60] Spinal cord injury can lead to infarction, bowel and bladder dysfunction, proprioception and sensory loss, loss of motor function, Brown-Séquard syndrome, and paraplegia.

Table 57.1 Risks Related to Cervical Facet Joint Injections

Potential Complications from Facet Joint Injection	Potential Side Effects of Steroid Medications
Allergic reaction: Usually to x-ray contrast or steroid; rarely to local anesthetic. A history of allergies should be elicited before any procedure	Transient flushing with a feeling of warmth ("hot flashes")
Bleeding: A rare complication; typically occurs in patients with underlying bleeding disorders. Proximity to the vertebral artery makes the injection highly vulnerable. Intravascular injection into the veins also can occur	Fluid retention, weight gain, or increased appetite
Infection: Minor infections occur in <1% to 2% of all injections; severe infections are rare and occur in 0.1% to 0.01% of injections. Infectious complications include epidural abscess and bacterial meningitis	Elevated blood pressure
Worsening of pain symptoms	Mood swings, irritability, anxiety, insomnia
Discomfort at the point of injection	High blood glucose: Patients with diabetes should inform their primary care physician about the injection before their appointment
Nerve or spinal cord damage or paralysis: Although rare, damage can occur from direct trauma from the needle or from infection, bleeding resulting in compression, or injection into an artery causing blockage	Transient decrease in immunity
Dural puncture, subdural injection, injection into the intervertebral foramen, and intervertebral formation	Cataracts: A rare result of excessive or prolonged steroid usage Severe arthritis of the hips or shoulders (avascular necrosis): A rare result of excessive or prolonged steroid usage Separation of pituitary-adrenal access Hypocorticism Cushing's syndrome Osteoporosis Avascular necrosis of the bone Steroid myopathy Epidural lipomatosis

Conclusion

CFS occurs as a result of facet joint pain that manifests with neck pain and referral patterns in the head, shoulders, and upper extremities. The medial branches innervate these facet joints, transmitting pain signals via the spinal cord to higher central regions. Numerous studies have shown that blocks of cervical facet joints or medial branches with local anesthetics, steroids, or a combination of both can significantly relieve the pain of CFS. Although limited evidence exists for cervical intra-articular facet joint injections, a moderate amount of evidence is found for cervical medial branch blocks and even more evidence is found for radiofrequency thermoneurolysis. Multiple effective and therapeutic modalities are available for management of cervical facet joint pain. Although complications are rare, serious disastrous events are possible. Proper technique, adequate training and experience, meticulous observance of safety guidelines, and use of proper fluoroscopic imaging equipment are indispensable for safe and effective injection of cervical anatomy.

References

Full references for this chapter can be found on www.expertconsult.com.

Chapter 58

Cervical Radiculopathy

Laxmaiah Manchikanti, Vijay Singh, and Mark V. Boswell

Historical Considerations

Cervical radiculopathy is a term applied when a nerve root is irritated and inflamed, but it also implies that damage to the root has produced a clinically appreciable motor or sensory neurologic deficit in the nerve root's distribution. In contrast, cervical radiculitis implies irritation and inflammation of a nerve root. Cervical radicular pain is a condition that poses several problems in clinical practice. Problems arise in recognizing the condition, how it should be investigated, and how best it should be treated. Failure to recognize the condition accurately can result not only in misdiagnosis but also in overdiagnosis, leading to unnecessary and ineffective treatment.

When the early clinicians wrote about the cervical spine, they were almost totally concerned with injuries rather than acquired nontraumatic disk disease.[1] Hippocrates[2,3] described cervical injuries in his book, *On the Articulations*. In general, he was pessimistic about the value of treatment. Hippocrates emphasized the cervical spine's importance of involvement in head injuries. Early clinicians also appreciated the principle of traction to the cervical spine. The use of traction for neck injuries was reported as early as 1887 by Bontecou.[4] The Egyptians performed cervical laminectomies as part of the mummification process.[1] Paulus of Aegina[5] performed laminectomies for spinal cord compression. Around 1646, Fabricus Hildanus[6] of Padua described his attempt to replace a fractured disk by clamping the spinous processes and manipulating the cervical spine. The first successful laminectomy in modern times was performed by Alban Smith of Danville, Ky (**Fig. 58.1**). By the 1930s, otolaryngologists were approaching the front of the cervical vertebra to remove osteophytes at about the C5 level, which made swallowing difficult. However, little interest was evidenced by neurosurgeons or orthopedic surgeons until 1955, when Robinson and Smith[7] reported anterior disk

removal and fusion. The official description of cervical disk herniation with radiculopathy was by Semmes (**Fig. 58.2**) and Murphey[8] (**Fig. 58.3**) in 1943—9 years after Mixter and Barr[9] (**Fig. 58.4**) described lumbar disk herniation with radiculopathy. Subsequently, Spurling and Scoville,[10] Michelsen and Mixter[11], and Stookey[12] published additional reports of cervical disk herniation in 1928 and in 1944. In 1953, Mair and Druckman[13] provided a classic description of cervical spinal cord compression from protruded disks in the neck, which they said caused clinical symptoms by compression of the anterior spinal artery.

Cervical spinal stenosis also has been recognized for about as long as lumbar spinal stenosis. The earliest mention of what was certainly cervical spinal stenosis was by Stookey[12] in 1928. The first attempts at cervical spinal stenosis treatment in humans was with massive bony posterior decompression, opening of the dura, and often cutting of the dentate ligaments.[1] However, later treatments included anterior interbody fusion popularized by Robinson and Smith.[7] Whiplash injury was first described by Harold Crowe[14] of Los Angeles in 1928.

The Clinical Syndrome

Definition

Cervical radicular pain is a term applied to describe pain that results from the stimulation of, or a disorder of, a cervical nerve root.[15] Thus, cervical radicular pain and cervical radiculitis appear to be synonymous because cervical radiculitis is a term applied when a nerve root is irritated and inflamed. In contrast, the extension of both terms is cervical radiculopathy, which implies that damage to the root has produced a clinically appreciable motor or sensory neurologic deficit in

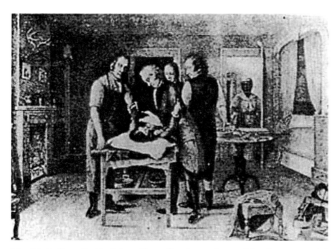

Fig. 58.1 Alban Smith, MD, of Danville, Ky, performed the first successful laminectomy after those of Paulus of Aegina in 1829. *(©2004 American Association of Neurological Surgeons.)*

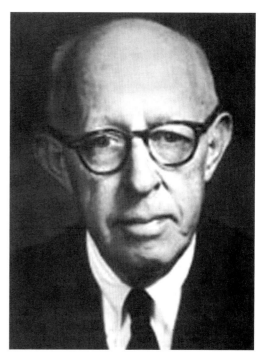

Fig. 58.3 **Francis Murphey, MD, originating Member of the American Academy of Neurological Surgery.**

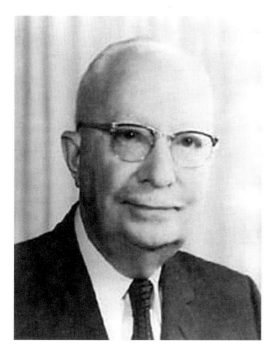

Fig. 58.2 **R. Eustace Semmes, MD, Professor of Neurosurgery in 1932 at the University of Tennessee.**

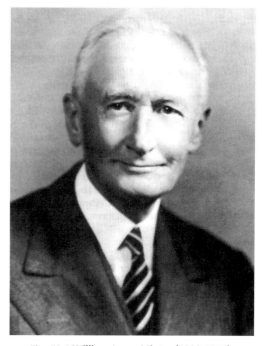

Fig. 58.4 **William Jason Mixter (1880-1958).**

the distribution of the nerve root. Thus, radiculopathy is a disorder in which conduction along a nerve root is blocked, resulting in objective neurologic signs such as numbness or weakness; or in which the blood supply to a nerve root is compromised, resulting in paresthesia.[16] The general belief is that cervical radicular pain is perceived along the distribution of the affected nerve root in a dermatomal distribution.[17] However, cervical spinal nerves are distributed to deep structures, such as muscles, joints, ligaments, and skin. Thus, radicular pain is felt in deep structures in areas remote from the expected dermatome. Combining all the experimental data, Bogduk[15] arrived at a workable definition of cervical radicular pain, which is consonant with the definition offered by the International Association for the Study of Pain (IASP).[16] Bogduk's definition incorporates these many various aspects

as follows: "Cervical radicular pain is produced by the stimulation of cervical nerve roots; it may be perceived in some or all of the tissues supplied by the affected nerve, both deep and cutaneous; radicular pain cannot be distinguished from somatic referred pain in either quality or distribution in the proximal upper limb; but pain in the forearm and/or hand is far more likely to be of radicular origin; and pain that radiates into the upper limb, and is shooting or electric in quality, is bound to be radicular in origin."

Prevalence

The annual incidence rate has been described as approximately 64 to 107 per 100,000 population; the most common causes are disk prolapse or spondylitic spurs at the corresponding level.[18–20] In a Swedish study, neck pain with transient radicular abnormalities was reported in almost 40% of the population at some time during their lives.[21] In a neuroepidemiologic study in 1997, pain in the neck and cervical radiculopathy were the most frequently occurring neurologic disorders in an indigenous tribe.[22] Although degeneration of the cervical disk structures is a normal consequence of the aging process, it undoubtedly plays a significant role in the production of neck pain, nerve root pathology, and spinal cord compression.[23–43] However, herniated nucleus pulposus in the cervical region is much less common than in the lumbar region.[44–46] The most common areas of disk herniation are C5-C6 and C6-C7, with involvement of the 6th and 7th cervical nerve roots.[17,23,47–51]

Recurrence, defined as the reappearance of symptoms of radiculopathy after a symptom-free interval of at least 6 months, was seen in 32% of patients during a median follow-up period of 4.9 years.[20]

Etiology

The most common causes of cervical radicular pain and cervical radiculopathy are disk protrusion and cervical spondylosis. Other rare causes include facet joint pathology; vertebral body pathology; meningeal pathology; and pathology from the involvement of blood vessels, nerve sheath, and nerve.[52] Disk protrusions are described as soft and hard, with soft protrusions extruding into the vertebral canal.[53] Disk protrusions are also described as medial and lateral, with medial protrusions affecting primarily the spinal cord and typically producing myelopathy, whereas lateral lesions protrude toward the intervertebral foramina and impinge on the spinal nerves and nerve roots causing radicular pain.[17,53] However, pain is an uncommon or inconspicuous feature of medial protrusions. In contrast to soft protrusions, hard protrusions are typically features of cervical spondylosis, accompanied by osteophytes from the facet joints, causing central or foraminal stenosis.

The present view is that radiculopathy's clinical features are produced by compression of the affected nerve. Compression accounts for numbness, paresthesia, weakness, and hyporeflexia by blocking conduction in nerves and causing ischemia. However, radicular pain may have explanations in addition to compression. Lumbar disks and nerve roots have been studied extensively to explain lumbar radicular pain. Extensive studies have shown unique properties of spinal nerves and inflammatory mechanisms in the lumbar spine, explaining various mechanisms other than mechanical compression and compression affecting dorsal root ganglion.[54] However, these mechanisms have not been confirmed in cervical radicular pain. Only one study[55] has shown that herniated cervical intervertebral disks also produce metalloproteinases, nitric oxide, interleukin-6, and prostaglandin E_2. All these substances are considered as potential irritants of spinal nerves or marks of inflammation.

Signs and Symptoms

Symptoms and signs of cervical radiculopathy are related to pain and neurologic features. The typical patient has a history of intermittent neck pain with the sudden onset of radicular pain, which might follow a traumatic incident. Radicular pain is aggravated by coughing, sneezing, neck movement (especially extension), and the Spurling test. However, patients with radiculopathy may have pain in the neck, in the shoulder girdle, in the anterior chest wall, and in the arm, forearm, or hand.[56] The reported prevalence of various types of neck and upper limb pain differs in different studies.[23,48,57–60]

Neurologic Features

The neurologic features of radiculopathy are numbness, weakness, paresthesia, and hyporeflexia.[23,48,57–60] Pain in the forearm associated with paresthesia has been inferred to be the cardinal feature of cervical radicular pain.[56,58] **Table 58.1** summarizes various signs and symptoms of nerve root compression in the cervical region and describes location of the lesion, referred pain, motor dysfunction, sensory dysfunction, and reflex changes. Cervical radiculopathy is suggested clinically by the presence of numbness or paresthesia in a dermatomal distribution, or weakness in a myotomal distribution. However, hyporeflexia alone is a not a diagnostic sign. Hyporeflexia is a feature that arises as a result of sensory block or motor block and is, therefore, not independent of numbness or weakness as primary signs.[56] Finally, cervical radicular pain is most strongly suggested by pain in the forearm and hand, particularly if associated with paresthesia.[56] Although this distribution of pain is consistent with the classic notion of pain in a dermatomal distribution, pain radiating from the neck, through the shoulder region, and into the upper limb is also consistent with the experimental evidence on radicular pain.[56] Neck pain alone, or pain in the shoulder girdle or proximal regions of the upper limb, is *not* diagnostic of radicular pain and suggests somatic referred pain.

Primary tumors of spinal nerves may present with radicular pain. However, this type of pain typically is characterized by profound sensory loss.[61] Thus, presentation dominated by neurologic signs warrants consideration of a primary neurologic disorder. Neurofibroma is usually associated with cutaneous phakomata.[61] Involvement of C8 or T1 spinal nerves may indicate apical lung tumors because these levels are involved very rarely by disk protrusion. The pulmonary masses are also associated with Horner's syndrome.[56]

Cervical radiculopathy as a result of intracranial tumor progresses rapidly.[62] For inflammatory disorders, systemic signs with fever and malaise are the hallmarks, with elevated blood count and erythrocyte sedimentation rate.[63] Sarcoidosis also has been described, with profound sensory and motor loss dominating the clinical presentation.[64]

Physical Examination

For a patient with symptoms of neck pain with or without upper extremity pain, suspected disk herniation, or radicular pain or radiculopathy, the neurologic examination should address the neck, trunk, upper extremities, and lower

Table 58-1 Signs and Symptoms of Nerve Root Compression of the Cervical Region

Root Involvement	Location of Lesion	Referred Pain	Motor Dysfunction	Sensory Dysfunction	Reflex Changes
C5	C4/5	Shoulder and upper arm	Shoulder muscles (deltoid-supraspinatus-infraspinatus ↓ abduction and external rotation	↓ Upper and lateral aspect of the shoulder	↓ Biceps reflex
C6	C5/6	Radial aspect of forearm	Biceps and brachialis muscles ↓ flexion of the elbow and supination ↓ wrist extensors	Radial aspect of forearm	↓ Thumb reflex and brachioradialis reflex
C7	C6/7	Dorsal aspect of forearm	Triceps muscle ↓ extension of the elbow	↓ Index and middle digits	↓ Triceps reflex
C8	C7/T1	Ulnar aspect of forearm	Intrinsics of the hand ↓ adduction and abduction	↓ Ring and little digits	No change

extremities. Lower extremity examination is necessary to determine the presence or absence of long-tract signs evident with myelopathy. Further, in myelopathy, tests of proprioception, vibration, and two-point discrimination are also important. Additional appropriate tests include compression test, manual traction, abduction test, or a combination thereof.

Local neck pain has been described with an extremely high prevalence rate of more than 90%. Numbness in the upper limbs is a reasonably reliable sign.[65,66] However, it is not a universal feature in patients with radiculopathy. The prevalence rate has varied significantly from 24%,[58] to 48%,[60] to as high as 86%.[23] Numbness is most often seen in the C6 and C7 dermatomes, indicating the most frequent involvement of these nerve roots. The predictive validity of numbness was calculated to be 0.7 for the C6 dermatome, whereas it was 4.4 for the C7 dermatome.[65] Bogduk[65] described the likelihood of numbness in the C7 dermatome as diagnostic of 87% of the involvement of the C7 nerve root, whereas it was 73% for C6 dermatomal involvement.

Weakness has been considered as a better and more reliable sign than numbness. Weakness has been reported in about 70% of patients in older studies.[58,60] However, more recent studies have reported it in only one third of patients.[23] Biceps weakness has been reported as very specific for C6 radiculopathy; however, its sensitivity was low.[65] In contrast, triceps weakness is very sensitive for C7 radiculopathy, although it is not very specific. Bogduk[65] described that objective motor weakness provides a diagnostic confidence interval of 77% for C6 radiculopathy, whereas diagnostic confidence was 67% for C7 radiculopathy. However, the weakness of wrist extensor and wrist flexors is not a discriminating sign[58] because it is seen with radiculopathy of C6, C7, or C8. Weakness of the hand muscles is seen only with C8 radiculopathy.[58]

Reflex abnormalities are seen in 70% of patients.[23,58,60] However, these data are limited to biceps or triceps, whereas the data with brachioradialis are unconvincing. A strong correlation has been established between reflex inhibition of the biceps with C6 and the triceps with C7.[58,60,65]

Provocative Tests

Many specialized provocative tests have been described for neck and cervical spine physical examination. Most relate to identification of radiculopathy, spinal cord pathology, or brachial plexus pathology. These include Spurling neck compression test, shoulder abduction test, neck distraction test, Lhermitte's sign, Hoffmann's sign, and Adson's test.[67] However, these tests are often performed routinely by many providers with variable methods and interpretations. The existing literature appears to indicate high specificity, low sensitivity, and good-to-fair interexaminer reliability for Spurling neck compression test, the neck distraction test, and shoulder abduction (relief) test when performed as described. For Hoffmann's sign, the existing literature does not address interexaminer reliability but appears to indicate fair sensitivity and fair-to-good specificity. For Lhermitte's sign and Adson's test, not even tentative statements can be made with regard to interexaminer reliability, sensitivity, and specificity, based on the existing literature.[67] In fact, Wainner and Gill[68] stated that with regard to cervical radiculopathy, many investigators believe that, "Given the paucity of evidence, the true value of the clinical examination… is unknown at this time." Malanga, Landes, and Nadler[67] examined the historical basis and scientific analysis of multiple provocative tests in cervical spine examination. Their summary, as shown in **Table 58.2**, includes multiple examination maneuvers, original descriptions, reliability analyses, and validity studies of each test.[69–72]

Diagnostic Testing

Diagnostic tests may be helpful in differentiating neck and arm pain causes, along with localizing the level of the lesion. Among the multiple tests available, including imaging, electrodiagnostics and diskography, imaging is the most useful.

Imaging

Plain radiography is not of any significant use in radiculopathy. Myelography is an invasive and stressful investigation. However, this can show the deformations produced by intradural, dural,

Table 58-2 Examination Maneuvers for Cervical Radiculopathy

Text	Original Description	Reliability Studies	Validity Studies
Spurling/neck compression test	Passive lateral flexion and compression of head. Postive test is reproduction of radicular symptoms distant from neck.	Viikari-Juntura[66] 1987 Seated position. Kappa = 0.40-0.77 Proportion specific agreement = 0.47-0.80	Viikari-Juntura et al, 1989[69] Seated position Sensitivity: 40-60% Specificity: 92-100%
Shoulder abduction (relief) sign	Active abduction of symtomatic arm, placing patient's hand on head. Postive test is relief or reduction of ipsilateral cervical radicular symptoms	Viikari-Juntura[66] 1987 Seated position. Kappa = 0.21-0.40 Proportion specific agreement = 0.57-0.67	Viikari-Juntura et al, 1989[69] Seated position Sensitivity: 43%-50% Specificity: 80%-100%
Neck distraction test	Examiner grasps patient's head under occiput and chin and applies axial traction force. Postive test is relief or reduction of cervical radicular symptoms	Supine postion. 10-15kg traction force applied. Kappa = 0.50 Proportion specific agreement = 0.71	Viikari-Juntura et al, 1989[69] Supine position 10-15kg traction force applied Sensitivity: 40%-43% Specificity: 100%
Lhermitte sign	Passive anterior cervical flexion. Postive test is presence of "electric-like sensations" down spine or extremities	Not reported	Uchihara et al, 1994[77] Sensitivity: <28% Specificity: high
Hoffman sign	Passive snapping flexion of middle finger distal phalanx. Positive test is flexion-adduction of ipsilateral thumb and index finger	Not reported	Glaser et al, 2000[71] Sensitivity: 58% Specificity: 75% Positive predictive value: 62% Negative predictive value 75%
Adson test	Inspiration, chin elevation, and head rotation to affected side. Positive test is alteration or obliteration of radial pulse.	Not reported	Not reported

From Walnner RS, Gill H: Diagnosis and nonoperative management of cervical radiculopathy. *J Orthoped Sports Phys Ther* 30: 728, 2000, reproduced with permission from authors and pubilsher.

and some extradural lesions of the cervical vertebral canal. It does not demonstrate a lesion directly, and it demonstrates those affecting the lateral reaches of the cervical spine nerves poorly, if at all.[72] Conventional computed tomographic (CT) scan provides axial images, in which the lateral reaches of the intervertebral foramina can be seen. CT myelography is considered as an accurate and reliable test and has proven to be superior to myelography in the diagnosis of cervical disk protrusions; however, it is an expensive and invasive test.

Magnetic Resonance Imaging

Magnetic resonance imaging (MRI) is the choice of imaging in the modern era—replacing myelography, CT scan, and CT myelography.[73–75] MRI is considered to be as accurate as CT myelography for detection of cervical nerve root compression,[75,76] even though it may be slightly inferior for detection of bony impingements of nerve roots.[75–77] The prevalence of numerous abnormalities on MRI of the cervical spine in asymptomatic individuals is a concern.[77–80]

Neurophysiologic Testing

Electromyography and nerve conduction studies offer no advantage in radiculopathy. However, they are of significant value in identification and differentiation of cervical radiculopathy with a peripheral lesion.

Diskography

Diskography is a diagnostic procedure designed to determine whether a disk is intrinsically painful. Although originally introduced as a technique for the study of disk herniation, diskography is no longer used in this way. Thus, cervical diskography has no role in cervical radiculopathy; its usefulness is limited to diskogenic pain.

Differential Diagnosis

The most common causes of cervical nerve root compression are cervical spondylosis, disk degeneration, and disk herniation. However, numerous other causes exist. Radiculopathy is a shooting, radiating pain that extends into the hand, accompanied by objective neurologic signs with sensory loss, objective motor weakness, or hyporeflexia.

Spinal cord compression in the neck may result in cervical myelopathy, which produces radicular symptoms in the upper extremities and long-tract signs in the lower extremities. Sensory impairment, muscle weakness, and loss of tendon reflexes may be found in the upper extremities. In the lower extremities, spastic weakness, hyporeflexia, clonus, extensor plantar reflexes, and impaired vibratory and position sense may be observed. Bowel and bladder function are usually intact. Pain associated with degenerative disk disease, facet joint arthropathy, or myofascial syndrome is somatic in nature with referred characteristics. Pain referred to the upper back, shoulders, and upper extremities with somatic characteristics without reflex changes and without radiation into distal upper extremities indicates causes other than radiculopathy. Myelopathy is characterized by symptoms and signs of long-tract impairment affecting the lower limbs and trunk. However, such features may be absent in the lower limbs and manifest only in the upper limbs. In that event, the distinction from radiculopathy is made by the nonradicular distribution of features, the absence of lower motor neuron signs, and the presence of upper motor neuron features.[80] Bilateral neurologic features that are present with myelopathy are most likely absent with radiculopathy.

Spinal cord lesions typically affect the lower extremities and trunk in a similar manner to cervical myelopathy. However, if the manifesting features are limited to the upper extremities, they are differentiated by their diffuse nature and bilateral presence for cord lesions.

Pancoast syndrome and thoracic outlet syndrome manifest with involvement of C8 or T1 radiculopathy that is rarely caused by disk herniation. Characteristic features of thoracic outlet syndrome and Pancoast syndrome are not diagnostic of cervical radiculopathy.

Peripheral neuropathies of the upper extremity are present with shooting pain, paresthesia, and numbness. However, the distribution of this symptomatology is different from cervical radiculopathy without a dermatomal pattern. Nerve conduction studies, rather than imaging studies, are discriminating with peripheral neuropathies or a combination of cervical radiculopathy and peripheral neuropathy. Other conditions include brachial neuritis, multiple sclerosis, and postherpetic neuralgia.

Differential Diagnosis of a Symptomatic Level

For the purposes of differential diagnosis, indication of symptomatic level is also crucial. A symptomatic level may be identified by pain distribution, sensory loss, motor weakness, and reflex inhibition.

Radicular pain alone has been shown to be poorly predictive of the involved level. Nevertheless, pain in the lateral arm or the posterior arm is most likely to be encountered in patients with C7 radiculopathy, whereas pain or paresthesia in the medial or posterior forearm distinguishes C6 radiculopathy from C7. However, the pain in the medial or posterior forearm does not distinguish between C7 and C8. Pain or paresthesia in the lateral forearm distinguishes C6 and C7 radiculopathy from C5 and C8, but does not discriminate between C6 and C7.

Paresthesias are considered as more valid contributions in identifying the level of the lesion than dermatomal distribution. Bogduk[80] reported that involvement of the C6 nerve root affects the thumb or index finger; the C7 nerve root affects the middle finger; and the C8 nerve root affects the little finger. Other fingers may also be involved. However, the cardinal features for the C8 dermatome are the little fingers, with or without involvement of the ring fingers, whereas the features for the C7 dermatome are the middle fingers, with or without involvement of the index

fingers. Motor dysfunction, sensory dysfunction, and reflex changes are shown in **Table 58.1**.

Treatment

Various treatment methods include conservative management with drug therapy or noninterventional modalities, interventional pain management, and surgical management.

Conservative Therapy

Conservative therapy includes drug therapy, physical therapy, traction, collar, bed rest, exercise, and TENS.[81,82] Saal, Saal, and Yurth[81] extensively described conservative management in cervical disk herniation. Although numerous reports are found of treatments in managing chronic neck pain, very few have studied cervical radiculopathy. During the past decades, an increasing interest has been seen in summarizing and analyzing the available evidence on the conservative management of neck pain. Hoving and coworkers[83] critically appraised review articles on the effectiveness of conservative treatment for neck pain. They evaluated 25 review articles; 12 were systematic reviews from more than 100 articles identified. They recommended that review articles should avoid bias in the selection of articles, explicitly describe the population and symptoms reviewed, detail the number of treatments and their specific characteristics, use accepted classifications if possible, and use systematic techniques in conducting the review. They also concluded that consumers should consider reports of reviews both carefully and critically, given the wide variety of review methodology, descriptive information, and conclusions. They considered the majority of the reviews to be of low quality.

van Tulder, Goossens, and Hoving[82] concluded that, because of methodologic problems, they believed it was not opportune to make any recommendations in favor of any chronic neck pain treatment. The conservative treatment methods they included were drug therapy with muscle relaxants, manual therapy, physical therapy, behavioral therapy, acupuncture, traction, pillows, laser therapy, electromagnetic therapy, and proprioceptive exercises.

Interventional Pain Management

Epidural injections for management of chronic neck pain are one of the most commonly performed interventions in the United States.[4,48–54,84]

Access to the epidural space is available via caudal, interlaminar, and transforaminal approaches.[54,84–102] Substantial differences with the technique and outcomes have been described among the three approaches. Thus, because of the inherent variations, differences, advantages, and disadvantages applicable to each technique (including the effectiveness and outcomes), caudal epidural injections, interlaminar epidural injections (cervical, thoracic, and lumbar epidural injections), and transforaminal epidural injections (lumbosacral) are considered as separate entities.

In addition, the response to epidural injections for various pathologic conditions (disk herniation or radiculitis, diskogenic pain without disk herniation, spinal stenosis, and postsurgery syndrome) is variable.

Benyamin and colleagues,[84] in a systematic review, assessed multiple randomized and observational studies and showed moderate evidence.[103–110] Transforaminal epidural injections also have been recommended to manage neck pain for diagnosis and treatment; however, these have been associated with significant complications.[111–131]

Surgery

Surgery is considered for patients with intractable symptoms and signs of cervical radiculopathy. However, no current data exist regarding the proper timing for surgery.[23,132,133] Surgery indications differ, based on whether a patient exhibits only radiculopathy or whether spinal cord impairment is also present.

Surgery is typically indicated for cervical radiculopathy absent of myelopathy when every one of the following are present: MRI or CT myelography visualization of definite cervical root compression; coinciding cervical root-related dysfunction, pain, or both; pain persistence after 6 to 12 weeks of nonsurgical treatment; and a progressive, functionally important motor deficit.[134] No randomized trials are found to compare these approaches. Surgery is also indicated when imaging shows cervical spinal cord compression and when clinical evidence of moderate-to-severe myelopathy is present.

Research shows that 2 years after surgery for cervical radiculopathy without myelopathy, 75% of patients have substantial relief from radicular symptoms such as pain, numbness, and weakness.[135,136] In patients treated for cervical myelopathy, relief of radicular arm pain after surgery appears to be comparable.[137]

Surgery complications are uncommon for cervical radiculopathy with or without myelopathy, including spinal cord injury (<1%), nerve root injury (2% to 3%), recurrent nerve palsy (hoarseness, 2% after anterior cervical surgery), esophageal perforation (<1%), and instrumentation failure (e.g., breakage, screw loosening, plate loosening, or nonunion, <5% for single-level surgery).[134–136]

Surgical Versus Nonsurgical Management

A Cochrane review summary[138] showed few good-quality studies comparing surgical and nonsurgical cervical radiculopathy treatments.[139,140] Consequently, nonsurgical treatment is reasonable for patients with mild cervical myelopathy signs who do not meet the surgery criteria.

Complications

Disk herniation complications include nerve damage and spinal cord compression, apart from long-lasting disability. Cervical disk herniation may produce Brown-Séquard syndrome.[141] Conservative management, and surgical management, is associated with side effects. All types of analgesics, both narcotic and nonnarcotic, have a multitude of side effects. Acetaminophen is associated with hepatic toxicity. NSAIDs can have serious side effects, particularly at high doses and in elderly patients. Opioids cause dizziness, respiratory depression, CNS dysfunction, and dependency and addiction. Muscle relaxants have significant adverse effects, including drowsiness, and carry a significant risk of habituation and dependency. Bed rest is associated with deconditioning, whereas traction also adds to other complications of immobilization, including muscle wasting, loss of bone density, pressure sores, and thromboembolism. Although risks of manipulation are low, serious complications could occur, resulting in severe or progressive neurologic deficit. Manipulation with use of anesthesia is also associated with an increased risk of serious neurologic damage.

Interventional techniques are also associated with multiple complications.[83,142–154] The most common and worrisome complications of interlaminar and transforaminal epidural injections are related to needle placement and drug administration. Complications include dural puncture, spinal cord trauma, infection, hematoma formation, abscess formation, subdural injection, intracranial air injection, epidural lipomatosis, pneumothorax, nerve damage, headache, death, brain damage, increased intracranial pressure, intravascular injection, vascular injury, cerebrovascular pulmonary embolus, and effects from steroids.

Surgical technique complications include infection, nerve damage, spinal cord trauma, death, epidural fibrosis, and postlumbar laminectomy syndrome.

References

Full references for this chapter can be found on www.expertconsult.com.

Brachial Plexopathy

Divya Patel and C.R. Sridhara

History

Obstetric brachial plexopathy was first described in 1779 by Smellie (**Fig. 59.1**). In the 1870s, Duchenne reported a series of infants with upper brachial plexus injury resulting in primary involvement of the proximal upper limb and leading to a characteristic upper limb posture. Around the same time, Erb also reported on upper brachial plexopathy. Since then, neonatal upper brachial plexopathy has been commonly known as *Erb-Duchenne palsy*. In the 1880s, Klumpke described lower brachial plexopathy affecting mainly the distal limb and pupil (Horner's syndrome).

Anatomy

The word *brachial* means "arm," and *plexus* means "network of nerves." The brachial plexus is one of the most complex structures in the peripheral nervous system. It is a triangular structure that extends anteriorly and inferiorly from the neck to the axilla. The brachial plexus is usually 15 to 18 cm long in adults. It travels posterior to the anterior scalene muscle and anterior to the middle scalene muscle in the proximal portion. In the distal part, it travels posterior to the clavicle and pectoralis minor muscle and anterior to the first rib (**Fig. 59.2**). The brachial plexus is subdivided into five components for better description and understanding: (1) anterior primary rami of C5-T1 spinal roots; (2) trunks: superior, middle, and inferior; (3) anterior and posterior divisions of each trunk; (4) cords: medial, lateral, and posterior; and (5) multiple peripheral nerves from rami, trunks, and cords (**Fig. 59.3**).

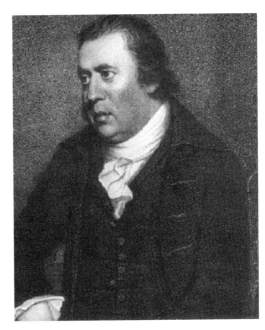

Fig. 59.1 **Mr. William Smellie.**

Multiple dorsal and ventral rootlets arise from each spinal cord segment. Rootlets join to form dorsal and ventral roots, respectively, which unite to become a spinal nerve. Each spinal nerve gives rise to anterior and posterior primary rami. Posterior rami innervate the paraspinal muscles.

Axilla (Dissection): Anterior View

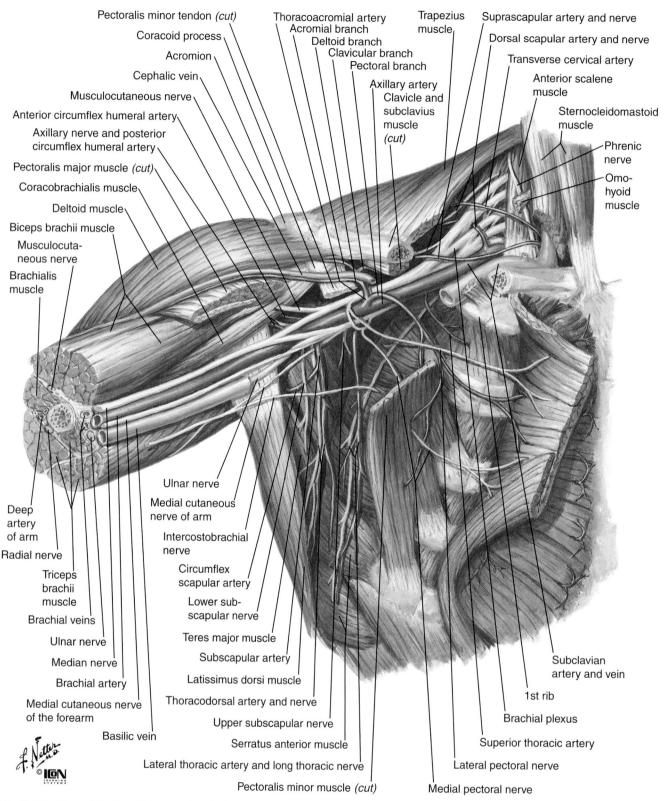

Pectoralis minor tendon *(cut)*
Coracoid process
Acromion
Cephalic vein
Musculocutaneous nerve
Anterior circumflex humeral artery
Axillary nerve and posterior circumflex humeral artery
Pectoralis major muscle *(cut)*
Coracobrachialis muscle
Deltoid muscle
Biceps brachii muscle
Musculocutaneous nerve
Brachialis muscle

Thoracoacromial artery
Acromial branch
Deltoid branch
Clavicular branch
Pectoral branch
Axillary artery
Clavicle and subclavius muscle *(cut)*

Trapezius muscle
Suprascapular artery and nerve
Dorsal scapular artery and nerve
Transverse cervical artery
Anterior scalene muscle
Sternocleidomastoid muscle
Phrenic nerve
Omo-hyoid muscle

Deep artery of arm
Radial nerve
Triceps brachii muscle
Brachial veins
Ulnar nerve
Median nerve
Brachial artery
Medial cutaneous nerve of the forearm
Basilic vein

Ulnar nerve
Medial cutaneous nerve of arm
Intercostobrachial nerve
Circumflex scapular artery
Lower sub-scapular nerve
Teres major muscle
Subscapular artery
Latissimus dorsi muscle
Thoracodorsal artery and nerve
Upper subscapular nerve
Serratus anterior muscle
Lateral thoracic artery and long thoracic nerve
Pectoralis minor muscle *(cut)*

Subclavian artery and vein
1st rib
Brachial plexus
Superior thoracic artery
Lateral pectoral nerve
Medial pectoral nerve

Fig. 59.2 Position of the brachial plexus in relation to other structures in the neck and upper chest. *(From Netter F: Atlas of human anatomy, ed 2, Philadelphia, 1997, Saunders, plate 400.)*

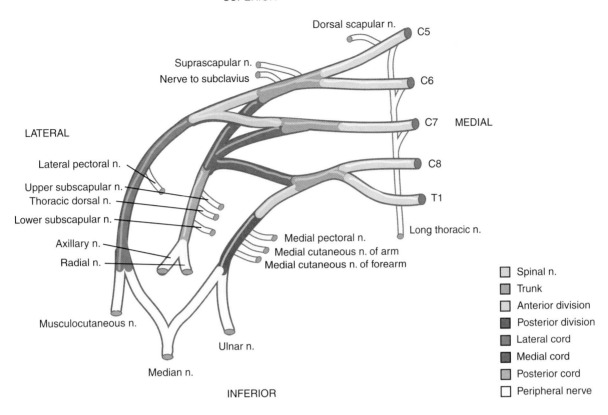

Fig. 59.3 **Brachial plexus.**

Each spinal nerve from T1 to L2 gives rise to the white ramus communicans, which carries preganglionic sympathetic fibers that, in turn, end in sympathetic ganglia. Postganglionic fibers from ganglia enter the spinal nerve through the gray ramus communicans or travel along the blood vessels to reach the target organs (**Fig. 59.4**). Head and neck sympathetic supply emerges from the T1 spinal nerve to reach cervical sympathetic ganglia. Thus, lesions of the lower brachial plexus may result in Horner's syndrome.

Usually, C5-6 anterior rami join to form the upper trunk, the C7 anterior ramus forms the middle trunk, and the C8-T1 anterior rami unite to form the lower trunk. When the brachial plexus has more contribution from the C4 anterior ramus and very little from the T1 level, it is called a *prefixed plexus*. In contrast, when the T2 rami contribute more with little or no contribution from the C5 level, it is known as a *postfixed brachial plexus*. The trunks are named for their relationship with each other. The lower trunk is adjacent to the subclavian artery and the apex of the lung.

Each trunk divides into anterior and posterior divisions. Anterior divisions of the upper and middle trunk unite to form the lateral cord. The anterior division of lower trunk continues as the medial cord, while the posterior divisions of all three cords join to form the posterior cord. The cords are named according to their relationship with the second segment of the axillary artery. The cords end by dividing into terminal branches. The medial and lateral cords innervate the pectoral region and flexors or anterior upper limb muscles; the posterior cord innervates the shoulder, posterior arm, and forearm muscles.

Branches are given at each subcomponent of the brachial plexus, except at the level of divisions, as follows:

At the primary ramus level: The dorsal scapular nerve arises from the C5 anterior ramus to supply the levator scapulae and the major and minor rhomboid muscles. The C5 spinal segment also has some contribution to the phrenic nerve to supply the ipsilateral dome of the diaphragm. The long thoracic nerve is formed by union of branches from C5, C6, and C7 anterior rami and supplies the serratus anterior (see Fig. 59.3).

At the trunk level: The upper trunk gives rise to two branches. The suprascapular nerve innervates the supraspinatus and infraspinatus muscles. The nerve to the subclavius supplies the subclavius muscle (see Fig. 59.3).

At the cord level: Many preterminal nerves exit from all three cords. The medial cord gives rise to the medial pectoral nerve, which innervates the sternal part of the pectoralis major and minor muscles. The medial brachial cutaneous nerve and medial antebrachial cutaneous nerve innervate the skin of the medial arm and forearm, respectively. Then the medial cord ends by dividing into two main branches: the ulnar nerve and the medial division of the median nerve. The ulnar nerve, along with the median nerve, supplies the anterior forearm and hand muscles, as well as the cutaneous innervation to palm, digits, and medial half of the dorsal hand and one and a half digits. The lateral cord gives rise to the lateral pectoral nerve, which supplies the clavicular head of the pectoralis major muscle. Then the lateral cord ends by dividing into the musculocutaneous nerve and the lateral division of the median nerve, which joins the medial division to form the median nerve. The musculocutaneous nerve supplies the anterior arm muscles and lateral forearm

skin. The posterior cord gives the upper and lower sub-scapular nerves that supply the subscapularis and teres major muscles. The thoracodorsal nerve innervates the latissimus dorsi muscle. Finally, the posterior cord divides into axillary and radial nerves. The axillary nerve inner-vates the deltoid and teres minor muscles, as well as the skin over the upper lateral arm. The radial nerve supplies the posterior muscles of arm and forearm, as well as the skin over the posterior arm, forearm, lateral half of the dorsal hand, and three and a half digits.

The upper trunk has the most cutaneous sensory repre-sentation, followed by the lower trunk and then the middle trunk. The posterior cord has the most cutaneous sensory representation, followed by the lateral cord and the medial cord. The radial nerve has the most cutaneous sensory repre-sentation, and the least is in the ulnar nerve. The upper trunk and posterior cord have the most motor representation, and the least motor representation is in the middle trunk.

Pathophysiology

Nerve injury varies from mild to severe. Mild injury results in physiologic conduction block and is known as *neurapraxia,* in which only the myelin is damaged with no axon injury (**Fig. 59.5**). In such an injury, symptoms are only of short

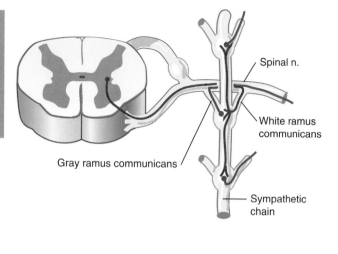

Fig. 59.4 **Cervical sympathetic chain.**

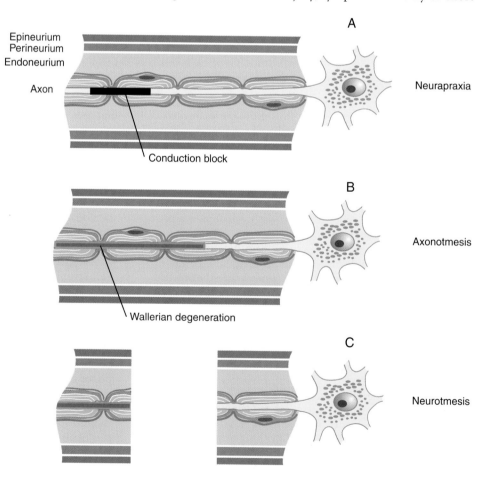

Fig. 59.5 **Seddon's classification of nerve injury.** A, Neurapraxia: physiologic conduction block. B, Axonotmesis leading to wallerian degeneration of axon distal to the site of injury. Note, all three neural supporting structures are intact. C, Neurotmesis: axonotmesis with injury to one or more neural supporting structures.

duration, and the prognosis for recovery of function is best. Examples of this type of an injury include burner or stinger and Saturday night palsy of the radial nerve. Moderate nerve injury at one or multiple places in the brachial plexus, in which individual axons are damaged with intact surrounding tissue, is called *axonotmesis*. This injury leads to degeneration (wallerian) of the axon distal to the site of insult. The axon regrows from the injury site in the endoneurium at a rate of 1 mm per day, thus, on average, 1 inch per month, to reach the end organ again. Examples of this type of injury include Erb-Duchenne palsy and Klumpke's palsy resulting from fast progression of birth. The most severe type of neural injury results in damage to the nerve axon, as well as the surrounding connective tissue, and is known as neurotmesis Endoneurium may be blocked by scar tissue to cause neuroma formation, or it may grow in multiple directions leading to aberrant pathways. Therefore, this injury has the worst prognosis. Examples of this type of injury include a gunshot wound or knife injuries to the area of the brachial plexus.

Classification

Brachial plexopathy can be classified according to cause or site of lesion (**Table 59.1**).

Clinical Presentation
Upper Brachial Plexopathy

In upper brachial plexopathy, weakness is noted in the shoulder abductors, external rotators, elbow flexors, forearm supinators, and wrist extensor muscles. This pattern of weakness causes the upper limb to stay on the side of the body with the shoulder in adduction and internal rotation with the elbow hyperextended, forearm pronated, and wrist hyperflexed. This posture is well known as porter's tip or waiter's tip hand. Loss of muscle stretch reflexes is noted in the biceps, brachioradialis, triceps, and pronators. Sensation is lost in the involved dermatomes and in the peripheral nerve distribution.

Lower Brachial Plexopathy

In lower brachial plexopathy, weakness is noted in the distal limb, involves hand muscles, and may mimic one or more of the distal nerve lesions. The hand position typically includes hyperextension of the metacarpophalangeal joints, flexion of the proximal and distal interphalangeal joints, and derotation of the thumb and is known as a *simian hand* or *monkey hand*. It may be accompanied by a stellate ganglion injury leading to Horner's syndrome. The findings in Horner's syndrome include ptosis (drooping of eyelid), miosis (pupil constriction), anhidrosis (loss of perspiration on ipsilateral face),

Table 59.1 Classification of Brachial Plexopathy

Etiology	Site of Lesion

A. Traumatic
  1. Traction or stretch injury: fast progression: birth injury, motor vehicle accident, sports related (burner/stinger), fall, hanging from a height to prevent fall
  2. Penetrating injury: gunshot wound, knife cut, chainsaw injury, animal bites
  3. Slow progression: compression from muscle, fibrous band, cervical rib (thoracic outlet syndrome), enlarging aneurysm or hematoma, arteriovenous malformation, postfracture callus of clavicle, rucksack paralysis
B. Infectious: herpes zoster
C. Neoplastic
  1. Primary
    a. Benign: schwannoma, neurofibroma, dermoids
    b. Malignant: neurofibrosarcoma, malignant schwannoma
  2. Secondary: metastasis from breast cancer, lung cancer, and lymphoma
D. Iatrogenic
  1. Radiation
  2. Surgical: shoulder area surgery, medial sternotomy
  3. Anesthesia: postnarcosis paralysis or anesthesia paralysis
  4. Chiropractic manipulation
  5. Neuralgic amyotrophy, also known as Parsonage-Turner syndrome, brachial plexitis, idiopathic brachial plexopathy, and brachial amyotrophy
	A. Supraclavicular (usually involves anterior rami and trunks)
	  1. Upper plexus
	    a. Erb-Duchenne palsy
	    b. Burner (stinger)
	    c. Rucksack (backpack) paralysis
	    d. Radiation plexopathy
	  2. Lower plexus
	    a. Klumpke's palsy
	    b. Thoracic outlet syndrome
	    c. Neoplastic
	    d. Hanging from height to prevent fall
	B. Infraclavicular (usually involves cords and terminal branches)
	  1. Needle-induced plexopathy
	    a. Axillary angiography: medial branchial fascial compartment syndrome
	    b. Venous cannulation
	    c. Regional anesthesia
	C. Panplexopathy: trauma and neuralgic amyotrophy can involve any part of the plexus

Modified from Dumitru D: *Common brachial plexopathies: findings and prognosis*, course C,1994 Amercian Academy of Emergency Medicine.

and enophthalmos (retracted eyeball). Loss of muscle strength reflexes is noted mainly in the finger flexors. Sensation is lost in the corresponding dermatomes and in the peripheral nerve distribution.

Traumatic Brachial Plexopathy

The basic mechanism of injury in traumatic brachial plexopathy varies from stretching to avulsion and from focal injury to panplexus involvement, depending on the amount of force applied and the anatomy of the individual. Commonly, when the shoulder is adducted, contralateral cervical lateral hyperflexion leads to upper plexus injury (**Fig. 59.6**). An example of this injury is in a motorcycle accident when the rider falls and separates the head and the shoulder. A fall on an abducted shoulder with the upper limb over the head, thus separating the body and the upper limb, predominantly causes lower plexus injury. In patients with bilateral upper limb weakness involving the distal limb muscles, the clinician must rule out cervical spinal cord injury. Clinical features that strongly correlate with root avulsion include severe pain in an anesthetic limb and Horner's syndrome.

The incidence of Erb-Duchenne palsy and Klumpke's palsy is 4 per 1000 full-term deliveries. Many infants improve rapidly unless they have root avulsion. Permanent morbidity varies from 3% to 25%. Male and female infants are affected equally. Risk factors for these injuries include shoulder dystocia, weight more than 4 kg, breech presentation, prolonged second stage of delivery for more than 60 minutes, a previous child with obstetric brachial plexopathy, and multiparity (**Fig. 59.7**).[1] The right side is more frequently involved, and 4% of infants have bilateral symptoms. Infants with brachial plexopathy must be evaluated for associated injuries and pathologic processes such as clavicle or humerus fractures, facial nerve or phrenic nerve palsy, cephalhematoma, and shoulder dystocia. The differential diagnosis includes hemiparesis and central hypotonia. An infant with hemiparesis has exaggerated muscle strength reflexes with the Moro reflex, and results of electromyography (EMG) are normal. In central hypotonia, muscle strength reflexes may not be present, and the results of EMG are normal.

Stingers or burners are common in athletes, especially football players. These injuries represent traction, compression, or a direct blow to the upper roots of the brachial plexus that causes abrupt intense burning dysesthesia, sometimes with weakness involving the entire limb. Stingers or burners are usually transient and resolve within minutes (**Fig. 59.8**). Cervical spinal canal stenosis with concurrent degenerative disk disease may predispose an athlete to persistent weakness and sensory changes. Return-to-play criteria are largely based on the number of previous episodes and the duration of symptoms. Appropriate counseling, including modification of tackling for a football player and the addition of protective gear, in conjunction with complete rehabilitation, may be effective in preventing this condition or in decreasing the rate of recurrence. The athlete, family, and coaches need to understand that the risk of recurrence remains unpredictable.[2]

Thoracic outlet syndrome (TOS) is an all-encompassing title for multiple entities including neurologic, vascular, and neurovascular conditions, with true neurologic TOS, disputed neurologic TOS, and traumatic TOS as subcomponents. The neurovascular bundle can become entrapped at different levels when it enters the upper limb. The subclavian artery and trunks of the brachial plexus pass through a triangle called the *scalene interval,* which is bounded by the anterior and middle scalene muscles and the first rib. This interval can be narrowed by the cervical rib, anterior scalene spasm, or injury, which encroaches on an artery or plexus. TOS is also

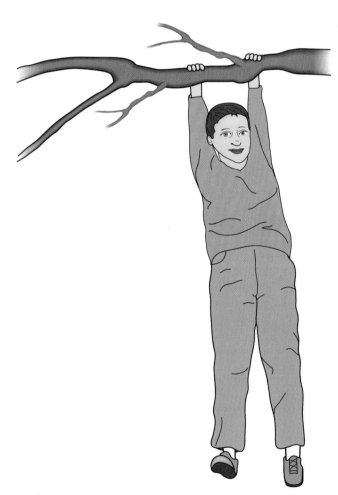

Fig. 59.6 Overstretching of the upper limb can lead to lower brachial plexus injury.

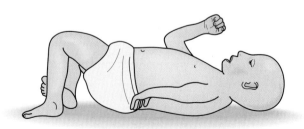

Fig. 59.7 **Classic porter's tip hand in Erb's palsy.**

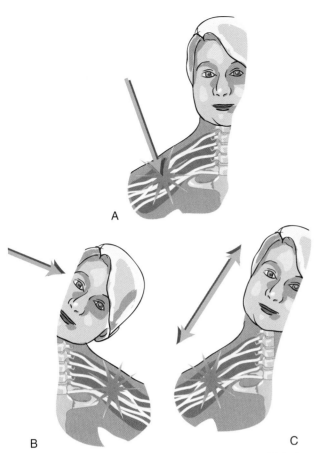

A

B   C

Fig. 59.8 A to C, Mechanisms of injury for upper brachial plexus stingers.

known as *thoracic inlet syndrome, scalene interval syndrome,* and *anterior scalene syndrome* (**Fig. 59.9**). Further down, the subclavian vessels and plexus can be compressed between the clavicle and first rib, and this is called the *costoclavicular syndrome*. Once the vessels and cords of the plexus cross the first rib, they pass under the pectoralis minor and coracoid process. When the shoulder is fully abducted or flexed, this neurovascular bundle is tethered under these structures and produces paresthesias and other neurovascular symptoms. This is called *pectoralis minor syndrome* or the *coracopectoral syndrome*.

Another entity that may occur is *rucksack (backpack) paralysis*. A rucksack is a cloth sack designed to carry 20 lb on the shoulder. A backpack is bigger than a rucksack and has a metal frame supported by a waist belt. Waist belts prevent pack palsies because the weight is shifted to the hips, and the shoulder straps are used only to keep the pack in position. Soldiers, hikers, campers, and children who carry books use these articles. Symptoms are gradual in onset and include weakness and numbness. Pain is usually rare.[3] The upper plexus is commonly involved. To prevent this condition, one should use wider and well-padded shoulder straps and secure the waist belt appropriately. Even then, frequent stops while hiking should be made to rest the shoulders and recover from any transient physiologic block.

Iatrogenic Brachial Plexopathy

Patients lose muscle tone during anesthesia, and they also lose the sensibility of stretch and any pain related to it. Patients who are positioned with their shoulders abducted 90 degrees or more and externally rotated in this setup stretch

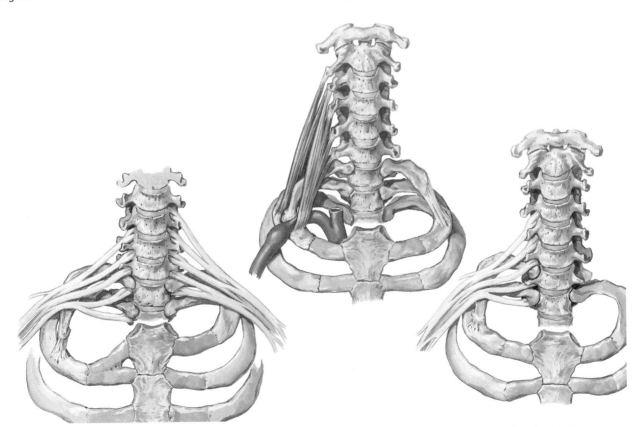

Fig. 59.9 **Thoracic outlet syndrome.** *(From Netter F:* Atlas of human anatomy, *ed 2, Philadelphia, 1997, Saunders, plate 173.)*

the brachial plexus.[4] If the upper limb is extended at the same time (hanging from the table) or if the patient is put in the Trendelenburg position, the trauma is compounded. Adding rotation and lateral flexion of the head to the opposite side of the arm being abducted may cause added trauma to the brachial plexus. Another positions that puts the brachial plexus at risk is prone positioning with the shoulder in 90 degrees of abduction and external rotation.[5] When the patient is placed in the side-lying position with the upper limb in shoulder abduction and elbow extension, with the arm suspended from a pole or overhead frame in the operating room for axillary or lateral chest wall skin grafting or in bed to decrease limb edema or to prevent axillary contracture, traction injury to the brachial plexus can result. To prevent such an injury, with the patient supine, adduction of the shoulder to 15 degrees can avoid traction. In a prone patient, placement of two pillows under the chest avoids traction. In cardiothoracic surgery (median sternotomy), prolonged or substantial retraction of the sternum or hematomas from the internal jugular catheter may put stress on the lower trunk or medial cord of the brachial plexus and cause a neurapraxic-type injury.[6]

Radiation Plexopathy

Three types of syndromes are recognized after radiation treatment:

1. Transient plexus injury occurs in 1% of patients treated with 5000 cGy to the area. Symptoms usually start after 4 months.
2. Acute ischemic brachial neuropathy follows subclavian artery occlusion resulting from prior radiation. This acute, nonprogressive disorder causes painless weakness with sensory loss.
3. Symptoms of radiation fibrosis appear months to years later. Risk factors include previous radiation, concomitant chemotherapy, and radiation doses higher than 5700 rad.

Symptoms of radiation plexopathy are chronic before the condition is diagnosed.[7] Radiation fibrosis is by far the most common type of radiation-induced brachial plexopathy. Magnetic resonance imaging (MRI) shows postradiation changes in the soft tissue or bone. MRI with gadolinium contrast enhances the recurrent tumor. Patients who have undergone radiation may have chronic enhancement of the area on MRI (**Table 59.2**).[8]

Neoplastic Brachial Plexopathy

Primary tumors of the brachial plexus are less common than are secondary neoplasms. Most primary tumors are benign. The most common primary tumor is neurofibroma, which is solitary, fusiform, and supraclavicular. Female patients are more often affected than male patients. The second most common primary tumor is benign schwannoma. Less common are primary malignant tumors of the neural sheath, such as neurogenic sarcomas and fibrosarcomas. Secondary tumors include Pancoast's tumor, lymphoma, small cell lung cancer, and breast cancer. MRI is the modality of choice for diagnosis (**Fig. 59.10**; see Table 59.1).[9]

Table 59.2 Neoplastic versus Radiation Plexopathy

Recurrent Neoplasm	Sequela of Radiation
Severe pain predominant; Horner's syndrome present	Painless paresthesias; lymphedema present
Lower plexus commonly involved	Upper plexus commonly involved
Myokymia usually absent	Myokymia and fasciculation; motor conduction block on Erb's point stimulation
Rapid onset of symptoms; <6 months after radiation	Insidious onset of symptoms; symptom duration >4 years
MRI with gadolinium enhances the recurrent tumor	May have chronic enhancement of the area on MRI

MRI, magnetic resonance imaging.

Parsonage-Turner Syndrome (Neuralgic Amyotrophy)

Viral illness, immunization, or surgical intervention commonly precedes this Parsonage-Turner syndrome. The patient usually has a history of waking up at night from severe shoulder pain, which improves in 1 to 2 weeks. Once the pain is better, atrophy with weakness of the shoulder or upper limb becomes obvious. This disorder can involve any nerve in the brachial plexus, but long thoracic, axillary, anterior interosseous, and suprascapular nerves are most commonly affected (**Figs. 59.11** and **59.12**). Sometimes, nerve branches to the individual muscles may be affected (e.g., infraspinatus, pronator teres).[10] Parsonage-Turner syndrome can be properly described as mononeuritis multiplex. It mostly occurs unilaterally, but needle EMG may detect involvement of the asymptomatic, contralateral side. The clinician should rule out a rare, dominantly inherited disorder known as *hereditary neuralgic amyotrophy* in patients with multiple episodes of painful brachial plexitis.

Diagnosis

Electrodiagnosis

Electromyography and Nerve Conduction Studies

Diagnosis of the exact site of the lesion in brachial plexopathy is a challenge even for an experienced physician (**Table 59.3**). Most of the changes noted on EMG and nerve conduction studies (NCSs) are more pronounced 2 to 4 weeks after injury. The differential diagnosis of involvement of muscles versus nerves is shown in **Table 59.4**.

C5-6 root avulsion differs from upper trunk injury as follows: In root avulsion, on sensory NCS, the sensory nerve action potential (SNAP) from the median first or second digit, radial SNAP from the first digit, and lateral antebrachial cutaneous nerve SNAP are normal (in a preganglionic lesion, one sees continuation of the cell body that is in the dorsal root ganglion to the peripheral axon). On needle EMG, involvement of the serratus anterior rhomboids and cervical paraspinals at the C5-6 area is evident. Clinically, involvement of these

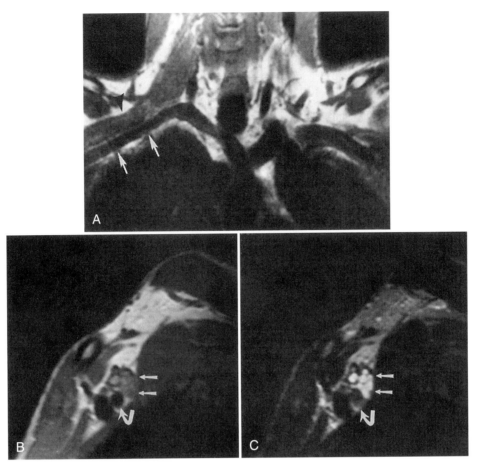

Fig. 59.10 **MRI appearance of brachial plexus neurofibroma.** A, Coronal T1-weighted image including the right brachial plexus demonstrates diffuse thickening and enlargement of the brachial plexus components *(arrowheads)* coursing just above the right subclavian artery *(arrows)*. Sagittal proton-density (B) and sagittal T2-weighted (C) images demonstrate the enlarged brachial plexus in cross section *(arrows)* located just above the subclavian artery *(curved arrow)*. *(From Braddom R, Buschbacher D, Dumitru D, et al, editors:* Textbook of physical medicine and rehabilitation, *ed 2, Philadelphia, 2000, Saunders.)*

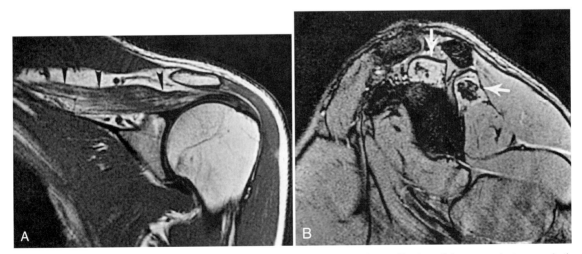

Fig. 59.11 **Inflammatory neuritis.** A, T1-weighted coronal image of shoulder. There is fatty infiltration of the supraspinatus muscle *(arrowheads)* without a tear of the rotator cuff, indicating a nerve abnormality. This patient had profound weakness and pain that was believed to be from a viral neuritis (Parsonage-Turner syndrome). B, T2-weighted sagittal image of shoulder. Higher signal intensity is present in both the supraspinatus and infraspinatus muscles *(white arrows)*, rather than in the other musculature of the shoulder girdle, from muscle atrophy secondary to the brachial neuritis. *(From Kaplan PA, Helms CA, Dussault R, et al, editors:* Musculoskeletal MRI, *Philadelphia, 2001, Saunders, p 99.)*

muscles is noted, in addition to those muscles involved in the upper trunk lesion.

C7 root avulsion differs from middle trunk injury as follows: In root avulsion, on sensory NCS, SNAP from the median third digit and radial SNAP from the posterior antebrachial cutaneous nerve are normal. On needle EMG, involvement of the C7 area paraspinal muscles is evident. Clinically, C7 root avulsion and middle trunk injury are identical.

C8-T1 root avulsion differs from lower trunk injury as follows: In root avulsion, on sensory NCS, SNAP from the ulnar fifth digit, the ulnar dorsal cutaneous nerve, and the medial antebrachial cutaneous nerve is normal. Involvement of the C8-T1 paraspinal level is observed in needle EMG. Clinically, C8-T1 root avulsion and lower trunk injury are identical.

The presence of myokymia on EMG favors the diagnosis of radiation plexopathy, rather than recurrent neoplastic plexopathy. Fibrillations and positive sharp waves suggest a diagnosis of neoplastic plexopathy.

When brachial plexopathy is mild, motor and sensory conduction study may not reveal obvious abnormalities at the same time, and needle EMG may require a complete and detailed examination to record subtle abnormalities. Low limb temperature increases SNAP amplitude, thus masking reduced amplitude from a postganglionic injury. Concomitant lesions such as carpal tunnel syndrome may make the sensory responses small and may thereby complicate the diagnosis of root avulsion.

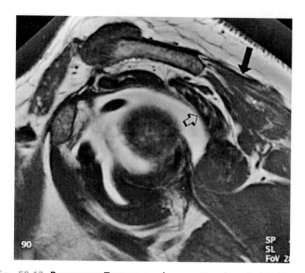

Fig. 59.12 Parsonage-Turner syndrome. Atrophy of deltoid and infraspinatus muscles. T1-weighted sagittal oblique MR arthrogram of shoulder. There is fat streaking in the deltoid (*solid arrow*), and the infraspinatus (*open arrow*) muscles. The patient had pain and weakness. The tendons were not torn. This was presumably from a viral brachial neuritis. (*From Kaplan PA, Helms CA, Dussault R, et al, editors: Musculoskeletal MRI, Philadelphia, 2001, Saunders, p 217.*)

Somatosensory Evoked Potentials

As the name *somatosensory evoked potentials* (SSEPs) suggests, this test evaluates somatic sensory fibers only. When terminal branches (median, ulnar, or radial nerves) of the brachial plexus are stimulated in the distal limb, a response is recorded from the supraclavicular fossa at Erb's point (the negative wave obtained is called *N9*), at the C2 cervical spinous process over the posterior column (N13), and at the contralateral scalp over the parietal cortex (N19). When the N9 amplitude is reduced more than 30% as compared with a contralateral N9 with a normal amplitude of N13, this finding is interpreted as a postganglionic lesion of the respective spinal nerve. In other words, when the ulnar nerve is stimulated, the loss of N9 amplitude indicates a postganglionic lesion of C8-T1; for the median nerve, it represents a lesion at C5-6 (**Table 59.5**).

In one study, lesion localization with SSEPs correlated with surgical localization in only 50% of cases.[11] Because SSEPs are more complex than are sensory NCSs and provide far less information about the status of the brachial plexus than a thorough electrodiagnostic examination, SSEPs are of limited usefulness.[3]

Table 59.3 Diagnosis of Brachial Plexopathy

	Preganglionic Lesion as Seen in Root Avulsion or Radiculopathy	Postganglionic Lesion	Preganglionic and Postganglionic Lesion
CLINICAL EXAMINATION			
Sensation	Decreased or absent	Decreased or absent	Decreased or absent
Motor	Weakness	Weakness	Weakness
NERVE CONDUCTION STUDIES			
SNAP amplitude	Normal	Decreased or absent	Decreased or absent
CMAP amplitude	Decreased or absent	Decreased or absent	Decreased or absent
ELECTROMYOGRAPHY			
At rest: increased insertional activity, PSW, fibrillation potentials	Present	Present	Present
Recruitment of motor unit potentials	Decreased or absent	Decreased or absent	Decreased or absent

CMAP, compound motor nerve action potential; PSW, positive sharp waves; SNAP, sensory nerve action potential.

Plain Radiography

Severe trauma that results in brachial plexopathy can also involve the cervicobrachial bones, with dislocation or fracture of the cervical vertebrae, clavicle, or upper humerus. The C5-7 anterior rami are closely related to the transverse processes; therefore, a displaced fracture of the cervical transverse process usually causes severe brachial plexus injury.[12]

Myelography

With root avulsion, the dural covering of the root is also pulled through the intervertebral foramen. After a few weeks, this dural cover forms a diverticulum, which is easily seen on a cervical myelogram. This test is no longer used for this purpose, however, because of the availability of MRI.

Computed Tomography

Computed tomography (CT) can be used to see a fracture that is not visible on plain radiography. CT myelography is better than conventional myelography, but MRI provides even clearer anatomic detail of the brachial plexus and its branches. CT myelography is useful in detecting fracture of the first rib, as may happen with medial sternotomy that predominantly causes brachial plexopathy involving the C8 root or lower trunk.

Magnetic Resonance Imaging

MRI is noninvasive, and its soft tissue resolution is much better than that of other diagnostic studies. Therefore, MRI is the study of choice for the evaluation of neural tissue. MRI can show signal intensity changes in denervated muscles a few days after injury. The findings are those of muscle edema with high signal intensity on T2-weighted images (see Figs. 59.10 and 59.11).[13] Three-dimensional MR myelography has a 92% diagnostic accuracy, 89% sensitivity, and 95% specificity.[14,15] MR neurography has been developed to evaluate peripheral nerves, but its accuracy has yet to be established.

Treatment

Rehabilitation

A comprehensive rehabilitation program includes the following: joint range of motion (varying among passive, assisted, and active); strengthening exercises; exposure to various sensory modalities; proper positioning of the affected limb; a home exercise program; and the use of various modalities, such as transcutaneous electric nerve stimulation (TENS) to help in pain management and ultrasound for stretching contracted

Table 59.5 Somatosensory Evoked Potentials in Brachial Plexopathy

	Amplitude of N9	Amplitude of N13
Preganglionic lesion	Normal or reduced <30%	Reduced >30% or absent
Postganglionic lesion	Reduced >30%	Normal
Preganglionic and postganglionic lesion	Reduced >30%	Absent or reduced >N9 amplitude reduction

Table 59.4 Differential Diagnosis of Nerve versus Muscle Involvement in Brachial Plexopathy

Abnormal Electrodiagnostic Study	Motor Nerve	Sensory Nerve	Involved Muscles on Electromyography
Upper trunk	Axillary Musculocutaneous Suprascapular	Lateral antebrachial cutaneous (terminal branch of musculocutaneous) Radial: thumb Median: first or second digit	Deltoid Biceps Brachioradialis Supraspinatus Infraspinatus Teres minor
Middle trunk	Radial	Radial: posterior antebrachial cutaneous Median: third digit	Triceps Pronator teres Flexor carpi radialis Extensor carpi radialis
Lower trunk	Median Ulnar Radial	Ulnar: fifth digit Ulnar: dorsal cutaneous nerve Medial antebrachial cutaneous	All muscles supplied by ulnar nerve; hand muscles supplied by median nerves Distal muscles supplied by radial nerve: extensor indicis, carpi ulnaris, and pollicis brevis
Lateral cord	Musculocutaneous	Lateral antebrachial cutaneous (terminal branch of musculocutaneous) Median: first, second, or third digit	Biceps Pronator teres Flexor carpi radialis
Posterior cord	Radial Axillary	Radial: posterior antebrachial cutaneous Radial: thumb	All muscles supplied by radial nerve in arm and forearm Latissimus dorsi Deltoid Teres major
Medial cord	Median Ulnar	Ulnar: fifth digit Ulnar: dorsal cutaneous nerve Medial antebrachial cutaneous	All hand muscles supplied by ulnar and median nerves All ulnar forearm muscles

tendon. The use of appropriate orthoses to prevent contracture, maintain proper position, or improve functional gain is usually tailored to the patient's need. Rehabilitation therapy also addresses various activities of daily living with the use of adaptive equipment and functional orthoses. Recreational therapy provides compensatory techniques for arm use in various leisure activities.

Rehabilitation therapy for the child with neonatal brachial plexopathy begins in infancy. Gentle range-of-motion exercises are started in the first month. Parents are taught different exercises, as well as how to give care without worsening the injury. A wrist extension splint is necessary to prevent contracture.

Edema control, with retrograde massage, compressive garments, and elevation, is important in postradiation plexopathy and in some cases of recurrent neoplastic plexopathy.

Surgery

Surgical exploration and repair of brachial plexus lesions are technically feasible, and favorable outcomes can be achieved if patients are thoroughly evaluated and appropriately selected.[16] Surgery is indicated when the deficit does not improve with conservative treatment, except in clean, lacerating wounds with neural symptoms, for which immediate surgical exploration and repair may be indicated. For traumatic plexopathy, surgery gives better results when performed by 3 months after the injury. If this approach fails, tendon transfer or osteotomy can improve function.[17] Common tendon transfers include triceps or pectoralis major or latissimus dorsi to biceps procedures and may be good options for patients with an encapsulated primary neoplasm.

Surgical procedures varying from placement of spinal cord stimulators, morphine pump implantation, or creation of a dorsal root entry zone (DREZ) lesion may be used for pain control in brachial plexopathy.[18]

Pharmacologic Treatment

Nonsteroidal anti-inflammatory agents, antiepileptic agents, tricyclic antidepressants, opiates, muscle relaxants, and antispasticity medications including botulinum A or B are used in various combinations to help reduce pain, paresthesias, muscle spasms, and spasticity.

Complications

Like any other peripheral nerve injury, brachial plexopathy of any origin can lead to complex regional pain syndrome type II (reflex sympathetic dystrophy). Myofascial pain syndromes, joint and muscle contracture, subluxation, and heterotopic ossification may complicate the recovery. Scoliosis from muscle imbalance is a possible complication in children. The sequelae commonly seen in children are the results of muscle imbalance or contractures and may include osseous deformities of the shoulder and elbow, dislocation of both shoulder and elbow, and dislocation of both the humeral and radial heads. Patients with postradiation brachial plexopathy are at risk for lymphangiitis and cellulitis.

In general, the prognosis of lower trunk lesions is poor, for two reasons: (1) because C8-T1 roots have weak connective tissue support, these structures are more vulnerable to avulsion (preganglionic) injury compared with other roots; and (2) even in a postganglionic lesion, the target organs for motor and sensory nerves are farthest to reach. Muscle contracture, joint

capsulitis, and fibrosis of the endoneural tube work against the functional recovery. The prognosis of complete lesions is poor because the unaffected neural fibers are not available for collateral sprouting. Connective tissue disruption in the lesion site causes fibrosis and impedes advancement of the axon that leads to a poor prognosis for recovery of function. The prognosis is best in patients with upper trunk lesions.

Conclusion

Brachial plexus injury represents a complex clinical challenge from both diagnostic and treatment standpoints. Nerve grows 1 mm per day, hence an average of 1 inch per month. Most postanesthetic or surgical brachial plexopathy improves rapidly. Supraclavicular brachial plexopathy is more common than infraclavicular plexopathy. Upper plexus lesions have a better prognosis than lower plexus lesions. Practitioners from multiple specialties, including physical medicine and rehabilitation, pain medicine, neurosurgery, orthopedics, plastic surgery, pediatrics, oncology, and radiation oncology, should be consulted as appropriate. A list of organizations to consult for additional information is provided in **Box 59.1**.

References

Full references for this chapter can be found on www.expertconsult.com.

Box 59.1 Organizations

Brachial Plexus Palsy Foundation
c/o 210 Springhaven Circle
Royersford, PA 19468
email: Brachial@aol.com; website: http://membrane.com/bpp
telephone: 610-792-4234

National Institute on Disability and Rehabilitation Research (NIDRR)
600 Independence Avenue, SW
Washington, DC 20013-1492
website: http://www.ed.gov/offices/OSERS/NIDRR
telephone: 202-205-8134

National Organization for Rare Disorders (NORD)
P.O. Box 1968 (55 Kenosia Avenue)
Danbury, CT 06813-1968
email: orphan@rarediseases.org; website: http://www.rarediseases.org
telephone: 203-744-0100; voice mail: 800-999-NORD (6673); fax: 203-798-2291

National Rehabilitation Information Center (NARIC)
4200 Forbes Boulevard, Suite 202
Lanham, MD 20706-4829
email: naricinfo@heitechservices.com; website: http://www.naric.com
telephone: 301-562-2400 or 800-346-2742; fax: 301-562-2401

United Brachial Plexus Network
1610 Kent Street
Kent, OH 44240
email: info@ubpn.org; website: http://www.ubpn.org
telephone: 866-877-7004

Cervical Myelopathy

Yoshiharu Kawaguchi

Based on neurologic findings in cervical spine disease, the pathologic entity is divided into two categories, cervical myelopathy and cervical radiculopathy. As for cervical disk herniation (**Fig. 60.1**), when disk prolapse occurs in the central part of the spinal canal and the cervical spinal cord is involved, the patient usually has cervical myelopathy. Conversely, when disk prolapse develops in the lateral part of the spinal canal and the herniated disk compresses the spinal nerve, cervical radiculopathy may occur. Patients with cervical radiculopathy often complain of unilateral radicular pain in an upper extremity. In contrast, patients with cervical myelopathy rarely have pain. They have clumsiness or loss of fine motor skills in the hand, gait disturbance, and vesicoureteral disturbance. Thus, pain is treatable in patients with cervical radiculopathy. However, one fourth of the patients with cervical degeneration have both myelopathy and radiculopathy.[1,2] Further, neck pain from degenerative change in the cervical spine may be associated with cervical myelopathy and radiculopathy. Neck pain is regarded as a nonspecific complaint in these patients.

Cervical myelopathy implies spinal cord dysfunction in the cervical spine. The causes are numerous and are divided into extrinsic and intrinsic neurogenic conditions (**Table 60.1**). Extrinsic neurogenic conditions are caused by spinal cord compression. Structural abnormalities surrounding the spinal cord contribute to encroachment on the available space in the spinal canal and result in spinal cord compression. Investigators have reported that spinal cord compression entities are some of the most common conditions in myelopathic patients who are more than 55 years of age, because these abnormalities generally result from degeneration of the cervical spine.[3] Intrinsic neurogenic conditions are caused by the primary spinal cord disorder. These intrinsic disorders are important in the differential diagnosis of compressive myelopathy.[4] Patients with cervical myelopathy do not always complain of pain. However, they may feel a type of pain resembling electric shock when the neck is in extension or flexion. This symptom is known as Lhermitte's sign.[5] This chapter reviews the pathology, diagnosis, and therapeutic strategy of compressive myelopathy in the cervical spine.

Pathology of Compressive Cervical Myelopathy

Pathologic Change in the Spinal Cord

In the degenerative stage of the cervical spine, spinal canal narrowing is caused by intervertebral disk bulging, deformity of the uncovertebral joint, hypertrophy of the facet joints, and hypertrophy of the ligamentum flavum (**Fig. 60.2**). In the presence of these degenerative changes, spinal cord compression may occur. Macroscopically, the spinal cord with myelopathy shows anteroposterior flatness and becomes atrophic as a result of compression. According to morphologic studies using computed tomography myelography (CTM), the spinal cord sometimes has either a boomerang shape or is triangular. Histopathologic studies have shown that damage to neuronal components is mild in the spinal cord with a boomerang shape, whereas such damage is marked in patients with a triangular spinal cord.[6] Ono et al[7] reported the

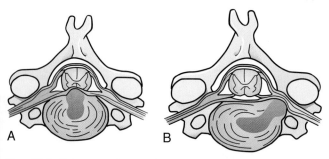

Fig. 60.1 Patterns of neurologic impairment resulting from cervical disk herniation. A, The cause of cervical myelopathy. B, The cause of cervical radiculopathy.

Table 60.1 Causes of Cervical Myelopathy

EXTRINSIC NEUROLOGIC CONDITIONS

Cervical spondylotic myelopathy

Ossification of the posterior longitudinal ligament (OPLL)

Cervical disc herniation

Rheumatoid arthritis (RA)

Spinal tumors

Epidural abscess

Anomaly in the cervical spine

Destructive spondyloarthropathy (DSA)

INTRINSIC NEUROLOGIC CONDITIONS

Viral infections

Neoplasms

Vascular diseases

Motor neuron diseases

Radiation myelopathy

Nutritional myelopathy

Syringomyelia

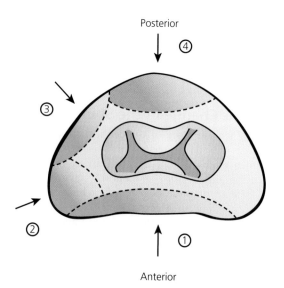

Fig. 60.2 Causes of spinal canal narrowing resulting from degeneration of the cervical spine: ① intervertebral disk, ② uncovertebral joint, ③ facet joint, and ④ ligamentum flavum.

clinicopathologic findings in five necropsy cases with cervical spondylotic myelopathy. These investigators found extensive destruction in both the gray matter and the white matter at the most damaged segment. Ogino et al[8] revealed that in mild compression, limited demyelination and spongy degeneration are seen in the posterolateral white column, whereas in severe compression, extensive degeneration and infarction of the gray matter with diffuse degeneration of the lateral white columns are observed. Ito et al[9] also noted marked atrophy and neuronal loss in the gray matter in severely degenerated white matter columns.

Patients with severe cases usually have accompanying developmental spinal stenosis. These pathologic changes are localized not only at the most markedly compressed site, but also at the craniocaudal regions in addition to the compression. Ascending degenerative demyelination is consistently seen in the cuneate and gracilis fasciculi of the posterior white columns in the spinal cord cranial to the compression site. Distinct descending demyelination of the lateral corticospinal tract is generally observed in the caudal site of the spinal cord. The pathologic changes in the spinal cord vary depending on age and extent and duration of compression.

Causes of Spinal Cord Compression

Various disorders have the potential for encroachment in the spinal canal.[3,10–13] The conditions discussed in the following subsections increase the risk of spinal cord involvement.

Cervical Spondylosis

Cervical spondylotic myelopathy is the most common cause of spinal cord dysfunction in patients with compressive myelopathy (**Fig. 60.3**). Cervical spondylosis initially results from degeneration of the intervertebral disk. Disk

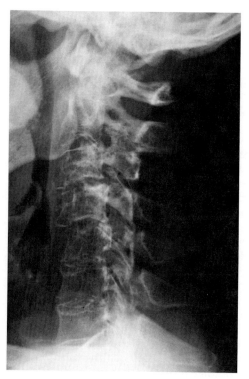

Fig. 60.3 **Radiologic features of cervical spondylotic myelopathy.**

degeneration increases mechanical stress at the end plate, and this condition causes subperiosteal bone formation. By such a mechanism, osteophytes develop at the upper or lower edge of the vertebral body. Osteophytes at the posterior margin of the vertebral body, which is called *posterior bony spur,* have the potential risk of encroaching on the spinal cord, followed by deformity of the uncovertebral joint, hypertrophy of facet joints, and hypertrophy of the ligamentum flavum. These findings are termed *spondylotic changes in the cervical spine.* These spondylotic changes are often observed at multiple levels in the cervical spine. However, the presence of cervical spondylosis alone does not generally lead to myelopathy. The pathology of cervical myelopathy is multifactorial. The clinician should consider the context of static and dynamic mechanical factors as well as ischemic factors.[14,15]

STATIC MECHANICAL FACTORS

The size of the spinal canal plays an important role in the development of cervical myelopathy.[16,17] Spinal canal size is the distance between the posterior margin of the vertebral body and the anterior edge of the spinous process (**Fig. 60.4**). The normal spinal canal diameter from C3 to C7 is 17 to 18 mm in white persons and 15 to 17 mm in Japanese persons.[6,18] The spinal canal size in patients with cervical myelopathy is smaller than in those without the disorder.[18] A sagittal diameter of 12 mm[14,15,19] (or 13 mm in some reports)[13,20,21] or less is believed to be a critical factor in the development of cervical spondylotic myelopathy. Younger patients, less than 50 years of age, with cervical myelopathy usually have a developmentally narrow cervical spinal canal.

The Pavlov ratio is also used to identify cervical spinal stenosis.[22] This is the ratio of the anteroposterior diameter of the spinal canal to the anteroposterior diameter of the vertebral body at the same level as measured on a lateral radiograph (**Fig. 60.5**). The merit of this measurement is that the ratio is not affected by variations in radiologic magnification. A normal ratio is 1.0, and a ratio of less than 0.82 indicates cervical spinal stenosis. The Torg ratio is the same as the Pavlov ratio. Torg described that a ratio of less than 0.8 indicates cervical stenosis.[23]

DYNAMIC MECHANICAL FACTORS

In cervical spondylosis, movement of the cervical spine may have an impact on spinal cord compression. During extension of the cervical spine, the ligamentum flavum buckles and thus narrows the spinal canal. The spinal cord is compressed between the posterior margin of one vertebral body and the lamina or ligamentum flavum of the next caudal level. During flexion, spinal cord compression occurs by the posterior margin of caudal vertebral body and the lamina or ligamentum flavum of the cranial level. This mechanism has been called the "pincer effect" of spinal cord compression (**Fig. 60.6**).[24] Dynamic magnetic resonance imaging (MRI) clearly shows the pathologic features of cervical cord compression in flexion and extension (**Fig. 60.7**). As for the pathomechanism of cervical myelopathy in older patients, retrolisthesis of C4 results from intervertebral disk degeneration, which is the likely cause the spinal cord compression.[25,26] During flexion of the cervical spine, the spinal cord must lengthen or move anteriorly within the spinal canal, and the result is axial tension. Bulged disk or anterior osteophytes can stretch the spinal cord in flexion. Anterolisthesis of the vertebral body can cause spinal cord compression. These local conditions lead to the onset of myelopathy.

Investigators have reported that some patients with athetoid cerebral palsy show evidence of cervical myelopathy at an early age (30 to 40 years old).[27] This condition results

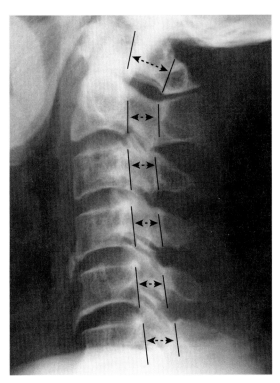

Fig. 60.4 Measurement of the spinal canal. The *dotted lines* and *arrows* show the width of the spinal canal.

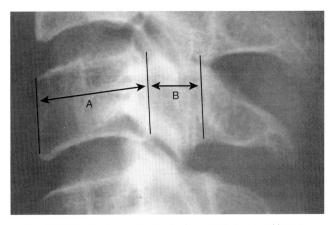

Fig. 60.5 **The Pavlov ratio.** The Pavlov ratio is measured by A/B.

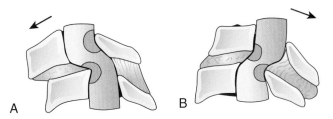

Fig. 60.6 The pincer effect of the spinal cord in flexion (A) and extension (B).

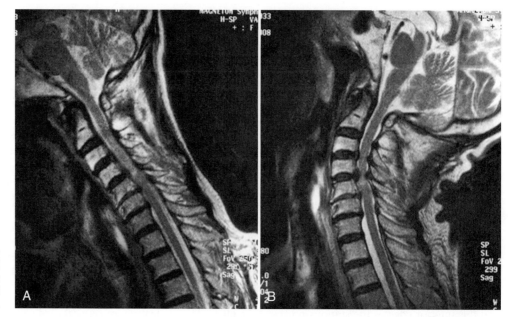

Fig. 60.7 Dynamic magnetic resonance imaging (MRI) showing sagittal views of T2-weighted MRI in flexion (**A**) and extension (**B**). Spinal cord compression is marked in extension.

from excessive movement of the cervical spine. These typical cases show the importance of dynamic factors in cervical cord dysfunction.

ISCHEMIC FACTORS

Spinal cord compression leads to ischemia of the spinal cord.[28] Histopathologic examination reveals the occurrence of ischemic injury in the gray matter and the white matter in patients with myelopathy.[14] In addition, several animal models showed that disturbance in the vascular supply to the spinal cord plays an important role in the pathophysiology of spinal cord dysfunction.[6]

Ossification of the Posterior Longitudinal Ligament

Ossification of the posterior longitudinal ligament (OPLL) often causes narrowing of the spinal canal as a result of the replacement of spinal ligamentous tissue by ectopic new bone formation (**Fig. 60.8**).[29,30] This disease is more common among Japanese persons and other nonwhite ethnic groups than among white persons. The incidence of OPLL among Japanese people is reported to be 3%, whereas it is 0.2% to 1.8% in Chinese persons, 0.95% in Koreans, 0.12% in residents of the United States, and 0.1% in Germans.[31]

Although the origin of OPLL remains obscure, investigators have reported that genetic background is a contributory factor. Studies using molecular biology have revealed that the collagen 11 α 2 gene *(COL11A2)*,[32,33] the retinoic X receptorβgene *(RXRβ)*,[34] the nucleotide pyrophosphatase gene *(NPPS)*,[35] and transforming growth factor-β3 (TGFβ3)[36] may be responsible for OPLL. It is widely recognized that severe myelopathy and radiculopathy may be caused by OPLL. Matsunaga and Sakou[37] reported that cervical myelopathy was seen in all patients with more than 60% of the spinal canal compromised by OPLL. These investigators also found that dynamic factors were important in patients with less than 60% of OPLL-related spinal canal compromise.[37]

Ossification in OPLL is classified as continuous type, segmental type, mixed type, and other type, according to the

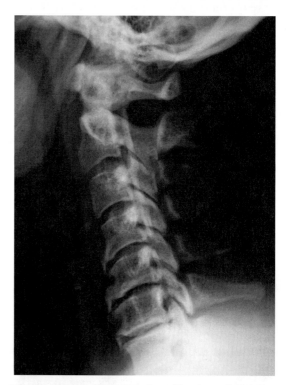

Fig. 60.8 Radiologic features of ossification of the posterior longitudinal ligament (OPLL). This 46-year-old woman has mixed-type OPLL.

criteria proposed by the Investigation Committee on the Ossification of the Spinal Ligaments of the Japanese Ministry of Public Health and Welfare (**Fig. 60.9**).[38] Among these types, cervical myelopathy frequently develops in patients with the continuous or mixed type of OPLL. The progression of OPLL is often observed in long-term follow-up after cervical laminoplasty, and OPLL can cause recurrent cervical myelopathy.[39] The risk of OPLL progression after posterior surgery is highest in patients in their 40s who have continuous and mixed types of ossification.[40,41]

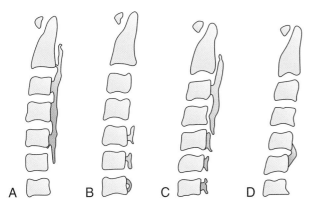

Fig. 60.9 **Classification of ossification of the posterior longitudinal ligament by the Investigation Committee on the Ossification of the Spinal Ligaments, Japanese Ministry of Public Health and Welfare.** **A,** Continuous type. **B,** Segmental type. **C,** Mixed type. **D,** Other type. *Adapted from Tsuyama N, Terayama K, Ohtani K, et al: The ossification of the posterior longitudinal ligament (OPLL): the investigation committee on OPLL of the Japanese Ministry of Public Health and Welfare,* J Jpn Orthop Assoc 55:425, 1981.

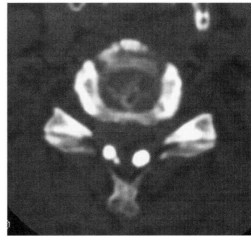

Fig. 60.11 **Radiologic features of calcification of the ligamentum flavum.** Computed tomography image obtained at the C5-6 level.

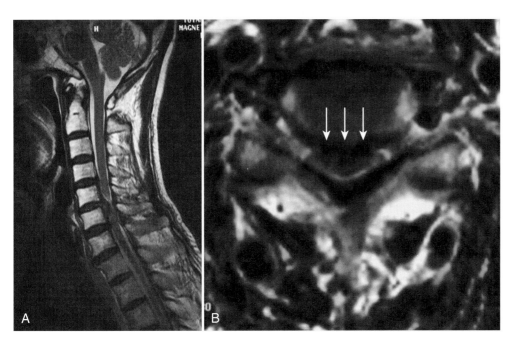

Fig. 60.10 **Radiologic features of cervical disk herniation.** Centrally located disk herniation *(arrows)* compresses the spinal cord at the C5-6 level. Sagittal (A) axial (B) images.

Cervical Disk Herniation

Cervical disk herniation is one of the compressive lesions that may cause cervical myelopathy (**Fig. 60.10**). Investigators proposed that nuclear herniation or anulus protrusion compresses the spinal cord, but precise histopathologic examination revealed that disk herniation associated with the cartilaginous end plate is the predominant type of herniation in the cervical spine.[42] Patients with myelopathy resulting from disk herniation are relatively young, compared with patients who have cervical spondylotic myelopathy. The spinal canal is narrower in patients with herniation, and this configuration leads to myelopathy. A history of cervical spinal trauma appears to be a predisposing factor for disk herniation.[43] In some patients with the median or diffuse type of disk herniation, spontaneous regression of the herniated mass is observed on MRI.[44] The symptoms often resolve during such regression, and,

therefore, conservative treatment can be an option for mild myelopathy caused by cervical disk herniation.[45]

Calcification of the Ligamentum Flavum

A few cases have been reported in which calcification of the ligamentum flavum narrowed the cervical spinal canal and resulted in myelopathy (**Fig. 60.11**). In the literature, most cases are Japanese. Kokubun et al[46] reported that 4% (11 patients) of 306 patients with cervical myelopathy in northern Japan had calcification of the ligamentum flavum. CT is the most useful diagnostic tool for detecting this disease. Although the cause of calcification of the ligamentum flavum is unknown, calcium phosphate deposition in the ligamentum flavum is observed. The calcification can be absorbed after administration of cimetidine or etidronate. Experience indicates that the calcification disappears after cervical laminoplasty.

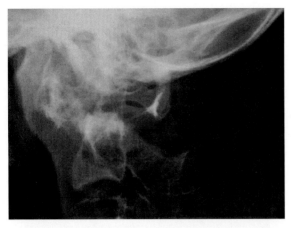

Fig. 60.12 **Atlantoaxial su bluxation in rheumatoid arthritis.**

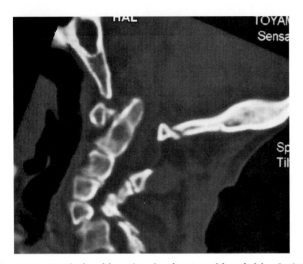

Fig. 60.13 **Vertical subluxation in rheumatoid arthritis.** Sagittal computed tomography image.

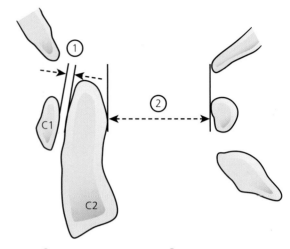

Fig. 60.14 ① Atlas dental interval and ② space available for the spinal cord.

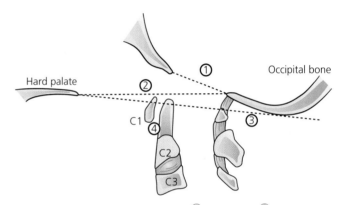

Fig. 60.15 Analysis of vertical subluxation: ① McRae's line, ② Chamberlain's line, ③ McGregor's line, and ④ Ranawat's line.

Rheumatoid Arthritis

Involvement of the cervical spine in rheumatoid arthritis (RA) has been well studied.[47–52] Compression of the spinal cord may result from direct compression by synovial pannus or from indirect compression caused by cervical subluxation. Upper cervical lesions, identified as atlantoaxial subluxation (**Fig. 60.12**) and vertical subluxation (**Fig. 60.13**), can cause cervical myelopathy.[47,48] The atlas dental interval (ADI) is a useful marker for the analysis of atlantoaxial subluxation. In patients with an ADI exceeding 5 mm, the space available for the spinal cord (SAC) becomes narrow, and these patients are at risk of developing cervical myelopathy (**Fig. 60.14**).

Several methods for analysis of vertical subluxation have been reported (**Fig. 60.15**). McGregor's line connects the posterior margin of the hard palate to the most caudal point of the occiput. The tip of the odontoid should not project more than 4.5 mm above this line. Ranawat's baseline measurement is another method. Ranawat's line is from the center of the sclerotic ring of C2 to the line between the center of the anterior and posterior arches of C1. A distance of less than 13 mm

is abnormal. Lower cervical lesions, such as subaxial subluxation (**Fig. 60.16**) and swan-neck or goose-neck deformity, also cause myelopathy.[53]

Although the cervical spine is affected in 36% to 86% of patients with RA, the incidence of myelopathy is reported to be 4.9% to 32%.[47] Neck pain is the most common symptom in patients with RA and cervical spine involvement. Erosive changes along the apophyseal joints and surrounding soft tissues may be a source of pain. Cervical instability at C1-2 may cause secondary impingement of the posterior rami of the occipital nerve and may lead to occipitalgia.[48] The Ranawat grading system provides useful information on the clinical status of patients with RA (**Table 60.2**).[54] In patients with severe neck pain resulting from cervical instability or subluxation, fusion surgery is usually necessary.

Spinal Tumors

Spinal tumors are classified as intramedullary, intradural extramedullary, and extradural. Meningioma, neurofibroma,

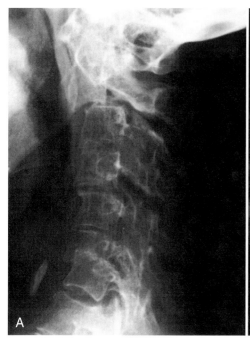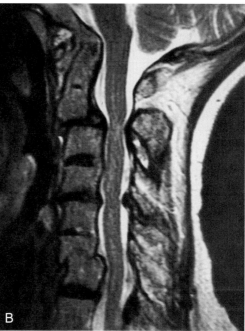

Fig. 60.16 **Subaxial subluxation in rheumatoid arthritis.** This 54-year-old woman had anterior subluxation of C2, C4, and C6. **A,** Plain radiograph. **B,** T2-weighted sagittal magnetic resonance image.

Table 60.2 The Ranawat Criteria for Pain and Neural Assessment

PAIN ASSESSMENT

Grade 0: None

Grade 1: Mild; intermittent, requiring only aspirin analgesia

Grade 2: Moderate; a cervical collar was needed

Grade 3: Severe; pain could not be relieved by either aspirin or collar

NEURAL ASSESSMENT

Class I: No neurologic deficit

Class II: Subjective weakness, hyperreflexia, dysesthesias

Class III: Objective weakness, long tract signs

Class IIIa: Ambulatory (walking possible)

Class IIIb: Nonambulatory (quadriparesis with resultant inability to walk or feed oneself)

Adapted from Ranawat CS, O'Leary P, Pellici P, et al: Cervical spine fusion in rheumatoid arthritis, *J Bone Joint Surg Am* 61:1003, 1979.

neurilemoma, and schwannoma are common examples of intradural extramedullary tumors.[55-57] Intradural extramedullary tumors may cause cervical myelopathy. Meningioma grows from the cells in the arachnoid. Neurofibroma, neurilemoma, and schwannoma usually arise from the dorsal sensory roots. Neurofibroma occurs in von Recklinghausen's disease and sometimes follows the nerve root out of the spinal canal, with a resulting dumbbell tumor. Intradural extramedullary tumors are typically eccentric and lead to Brown-Séquard–type myelopathy. Gadolinium-enhanced MRI is very useful for detecting intradural extramedullary tumors.

Metastasis to the cervical spine is another entity that may cause compression myelopathy, although such lesions are rare in the cervical spine.[58,59] The most likely primary tumors to metastasize to the cervical spine are breast, prostate, and lung cancers. Because these metastases frequently occur in the vertebral bone, most cases of spinal metastasis are classified as extradural tumors. The symptoms of myelopathy are sometimes acute and gradually progressive. Neck pain is frequently observed in patients who have destructive changes in the cervical spine caused by the tumors. Kyphotic deformity resulting from vertebral collapse, direct tumor invasion in the epidural space, and insufficiency of the anterior spinal artery system may produce cervical myelopathy.

Epidural Abscess

Spinal epidural abscess can cause a mass to develop in the spinal canal (**Fig. 60.17**) that can lead to acute myelopathy and quadriplegia.[60-62] In patients with epidural abscess, fever and severe neck pain are usually observed. *Staphylococcus aureus* is the etiologic agent in more than 50% of cases of acute epidural abscess. Spondylodiskitis may be accompanied by epidural abscess as a local pathology, whereas epidural infection may occur hematogenously from a distant site.

Anomaly in the Cervical Spine

Anomalies in the cervical spine are frequently seen at the craniovertebral junction or at the upper cervical spine. In most patients, the anomalies are usually found in childhood congenital malformations. However, abnormal structures in the cervical spine are sometimes found in adulthood. Cervical myelopathy can develop in patients with basilar impression, Arnold-Chiari malformation, and atlantoaxial instability, which is associated with Down's syndrome.[63,64] Klippel-Feil syndrome and os odontoideum (**Fig. 60.18**) with instability also may cause myelopathy. Severe neck pain is less common in these conditions.

Destructive Spondyloarthropathy

Destructive change in the cervical spine is often seen in patients undergoing long-term hemodialysis. The disease entity destructive spondyloarthropathy (DSA) was first reported by Kuntz et al in 1984.[65] Radiologic features of this disease are disk space narrowing and irregularity of the cartilaginous end plate without osteophyte formation. The C5-6 level is involved in more than half these patients, but involvement of multiple levels is common. The prevalence

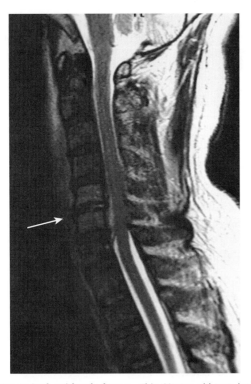

Fig. 60.17 **Spinal epidural abscess.** This 69-year-old-man had acute onset of cervical myelopathy. The T2-weighted sagittal magnetic resonance image shows an epidural abscess *(arrow)* from C5-6 diskitis.

of DSA is 4% to 20% in patients undergoing hemodialysis and is higher in patients who undergo hemodialysis for more than 10 years.[66] Causes of myelopathy are spinal cord compression resulting from spinal instability, intervertebral subluxation, intracanal amyloid deposition, and hypertrophy of the ligamentum flavum.[67,68] In patients with marked destructive change and instability in the cervical spine, neck pain is frequently a symptom. Although the pathology of DSA has not been clearly elucidated, investigators have reported that hyperparathyroidism and amyloidosis play important roles in the progression of DSA.[67]

Diagnosis of Cervical Myelopathy

Clinical Symptoms

Clinical symptoms of cervical myelopathy vary from patient to patient. Thus, history taking is very important for the diagnosis. Symptoms depend on the stage of myelopathy and the impaired pattern of the spinal cord. In the upper extremities, numbness, paresthesia, and clumsiness are often observed. The typical manifestations of numbness and paresthesia represent a global and nondermatomal pattern in the upper extremities. Patients often complain of clumsiness. Their symptoms include difficulties with handwriting, manipulating buttons or zippers, and using a knife and fork or chopsticks. The "myelopathy hand,"[69,70] which is defined as "loss of power of adduction and extension of the ulnar two or three fingers and an inability to grip and release rapidly with these fingers," is one of the characteristic findings in patients with cervical myelopathy.

In the lower extremities, subtle changes in gait and balance occasionally progress to spastic gait. Patients with cervical myelopathy have difficulties walking down stairs smoothly. These patients are often frightened to use steps without a handrail. Singh and Crockard[71] reported that a simple walking test is useful to detect cervical myelopathy. These investigators found that both the time taken and the number of steps in a 30-m walk test in patients with cervical spondylotic myelopathy were significantly greater than in controls. Significant recovery in these parameters was reported after decompressive surgery. Patients occasionally complain of urinary urgency, hesitation, or frequency. In the advanced stage, they may have incontinence or retention of urine, although the incidence is very rare.

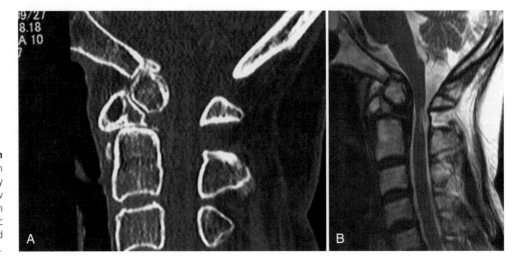

Fig. 60.18 **Os odontoideum with instability.** This 67year-old woman had moderate cervical myelopathy at the C1 level. **A,** Sagittal view on computed tomography. **B,** With T2-weighted sagittal magnetic resonance imaging, spinal cord atrophy is marked at the C1-2 level.

Neck pain is noted as a nonspecific symptom in patients with cervical myelopathy. Neck pain may be caused by degeneration of the intervertebral disk and facet joint in the cervical spine.[15,72] Pain in the upper or lower extremities is also rarely found in patients with pure cervical myelopathy. Patients with both myelopathy and radiculopathy may have radiating pain in upper extremities. In contrast, Lhermitte's sign may be characteristic in patients with cervical myelopathy. Lhermitte's sign consists of a sensation resembling electricity that radiates from the head to the upper or lower extremities and is induced by forward flexion of the neck. The sign was first described by Babinski and Dubois and was emphasized by Lhermitte as a symptom of multiple sclerosis.[5] The phenomenon is believed to be caused by the lesion in the posterior and lateral columns of the spinal cord. Investigators have reported that this sign is present in patients with cervical spondylosis, neoplasms, radiation myelopathy, and subacute combined degeneration,[73,74] although the incidence of the sign is unclear in these disorders.

Opinions diverge on the presenting symptoms of cervical myelopathy. Gorter[75] reported that cervical myelopathy usually first manifests as a subtle gait disturbance. In contrast, Kokubun et al[47] stated that the most common initial symptom is numbness or tingling in the upper extremities, especially in the hand. Although investigators have believed that these symptoms gradually worsen, one study suggested that most patients with mild myelopathy have a stable condition for a long time.[45]

Guidelines for the surgical management of cervical degenerative disease, published in the *Journal of Neurosurgery Spine* in 2009,[76] state that the natural history of cervical spondylotic myelopathy is mixed. The disorder may manifest as a slow, stepwise decline, or the patient may note a long period of quiescence (class III). The classification of evidence is as follows: class I, evidence derived from well-designed, randomized controlled trials (RCTs); class II, evidence derived from RCTs with design problems or from well-designed cohort studies; and class III, evidence derived from case series or poorly designed cohort studies. In patients with severe or long-lasting symptoms of cervical spondylotic myelopathy, the likelihood of improvement with nonoperative treatment is low. Objectively measurable deterioration is rarely seen in patients less than 75 years of age with mild cervical spondylotic myelopathy.[76] Patients with severe, progressive cervical myelopathy cannot walk without a cane, even on a flat road, at the late stage of the disorder. Bowel or bladder dysfunction accompanies extremely severe myelopathy.

Several attempts have been made to classify the symptoms of spinal cord dysfunction in patients with cervical myelopathy. In 1966, Crandall and Batzdorf [77] devised a classification system based on the differential susceptibility of various spinal cord tracts (**Table 60.3**). In 1975, Hattori and Kawai[78] categorized spinal cord symptoms into three types based on clinical experience (**Fig. 60.19**). Ferguson and Caplan[79] categorized spondylosis with nerve involvement into four distinct but overlapping syndromes (lateral or radicular syndrome, medial or spinal syndrome, combined medial and lateral syndrome, and vascular syndrome) in 1985.

Physical Examination

The most characteristic findings in cervical myelopathy are segmental signs and long tract signs. Segmental signs indicate lower motor findings at the level of the compressive lesion. Long tract signs signify upper motor findings observed below the lesion. Neurologic findings vary, depending on the level and nature of compression. Further, cervical spondylotic myelopathy is frequently combined with lumbar spinal stenosis. This combination of disorders renders the neurologic findings more complex.

Careful physical examination should be carried out to ascertain the presence or absence of cervical myelopathy.[80,81] If myelopathy is present, the clinician will need to detect the precise lesion.[82] The finding of myelopathy hand[70,71] strongly

Table 60.3 Crandall and Batzdorf Classification of Cervical Myelopathy

1. Transverse Lesion Syndrome
Patients with a transverse lesion, with involvement of the appropriate neurologic tracts (corticospinal, spinothalamic, posterior columns), have severe spasticity and frequent sphincter involvement, and one third exhibit Lhermitte's sign.

2. Motor System Syndrome
Patients with motor system lesions (anterior horn cells, corticospinal tract) show spasticity but relatively innocuous or absent sensory disturbance.

3. Central Cord Syndrome
Patients with central cord syndrome have severe motor and sensory disturbances, with greater expression in the upper extremities (Lhermitte's sign characterizes this group).

4. Brown-Séquard Syndrome
Patients with Brown-Séquard syndrome have typical contralateral sensory deficits and ipsilateral motor deficits.

5. Brachialgia Cord Syndrome
Patients with brachialgia cord syndrome demonstrate lower motoneuron and upper extremity involvement and upper motoneuron and lower extremity involvement.

Adapted from Crandall PH, Batzdorf U: Cervical spondylotic myelopathy, *J Neurosurg* 25:57, 1966.

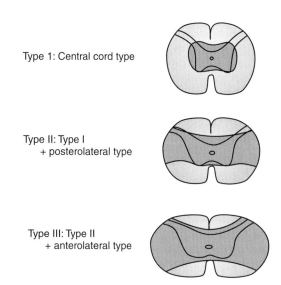

Type 1: Central cord type

Type II: Type I + posterolateral type

Type III: Type II + anterolateral type

Fig. 60.19 Classification of cervical myelopathy by Hattori and Kawai. (*Adapted from Hattori S, Kawai S: Diagnosis of cervical spondylosis [in Japanese], Orthop Mook 6:13, 1979.*)

suggests the presence of cervical myelopathy. The diagnosis of myelopathy hand is made by two simple tests, the finger escape sign and the rapid grip and release test. The finger escape sign is positive when the patient is asked to hold all digits of the hand in an adducted and extended position and the two ulnar digits fall into flexion and abduction within 30 seconds. In the rapid grip and release test, a neurologically normal person can make a fist and rapidly release it 20 times in 10 seconds, but patients with cervical myelopathy are unable to do this with rapid motion. Hosono et al[83] developed quantitative methods to evaluate the severity of myelopathy hand by the video-recorded 15-second test of rapid grip and release of fingers.

The gait becomes wide-based and jerky. Patients have difficulty in toe walking and heel walking. These provocative tests are useful to detect subtle gait disturbance resulting from cervical myelopathy. Patients with cervical myelopathy have impaired proprioception below the lesion.[84] Impairment in the lower extremities may lead to gait disturbance. A full neurologic examination is performed, with careful evaluation of reflex change, motor weakness, and sensory disturbance.

Reflex Change

Reflex changes are extremely important in making a diagnosis of cervical myelopathy. Hyperreflexia is found as a long tract sign in the upper and lower extremities below the lesion. However, hyporeflexia in the upper extremity may result from a segmental sign of spinal cord compression. Further, hyporeflexia in the lower extremity may be accompanied by lumbar spinal stenosis. As for provocative tests, not many patients have clonus in their lower extremity, and this finding indicates the typical condition of hyperreflexia.

Pathologic reflexes, such as Hoffman's reflex, Trömner's reflex, Wartenberg's reflex, and inverted radial reflex in the upper extremity and Babinski's reflex, Chaddock's reflex, and Oppenheimer's reflex in the lower extremity also indicate abnormal long tract signs consistent with spinal cord compression. One report noted a low incidence of hyperreflexia and provocative signs; thus, the absence of these signs does not preclude the diagnosis of cervical myelopathy.[85] The scapulohumeral reflex[86] is useful for detecting lesions cranial to the C3 vertebral body level. The reflex is hyperactive when elevation of the scapula or abduction of the humerus is found during tapping of the spine of the scapula or tapping of the acromion in a caudal direction. More than 95% of patients with high cervical spinal cord compression have a hyperactive scapulohumeral reflex.

Motor Weakness

Generalized weakness and extremity weakness are found in some patients with cervical myelopathy. Muscle atrophy, muscle wasting, and fasciculation can be observed in the upper extremity of patients with cervical myelopathy. These findings are caused by lower motoneuron dysfunction and are regarded as segmental signs of a compressive lesion. Conversely the weakness in the lower extremity has been speculated to be caused by dysfunction of the corticospinal tract.

Sensory Disturbance

The changes in senses of pain, touch and vibration, and proprioception are important to differentiate because the tracts of each sensation vary. In cervical myelopathy, sensory change is global and ill-defined, compared with radiculopathy. A *cervical line* is typical for cervical myelopathy. This is the sensory change around the clavicle. Patients have sensory disturbance below the level of the clavicle and normal sensation above it. Investigators have speculated that the phenomenon of cervical line results from the distinct change of sensory lamination shown by Keegan's dermatome. Loss of vibration and proprioception signifies involvement of the posterior columns and is an indicator of poor prognosis of cervical myelopathy.[84] Disturbance of proprioception is found in both upper and lower extremities.[87,88]

Evaluation System

Various systems, including Odom's criteria[89] and Nurick's score,[90] have been suggested for evaluating the severity of cervical myelopathy. In 1975, the Japanese Orthopaedic Association (JOA)[91] proposed a scoring system for cervical myelopathy as a basis for treatment of this disorder. In 1990, the JOA proposed a modified, 17-point scoring system (**Table 60.4**).[92] This JOA system is reliable because of its high interobserver and intraobserver reliabilities,[92] and it is used not only in Japan, but also in other countries. A patient-based scoring system for cervical spine disease was established in 2006 by the JOA (**Table 60.5**).[93]

Radiologic Evaluation

X-ray studies, CT, three-dimensional CT, myelography, CTM, scintigraphy, MRI, and positron emission tomography (PET) are radiologic tools used in the evaluation of cervical myelopathy. Each imaging type has its own features and specificities. Thus, it is important to understand the purpose of the study before choosing an imaging modality.

When patients are suspected of having cervical lesions, plain x-ray films should be taken at first. Plain x-ray films of the cervical spine in these patients include the following: the anteroposterior view; lateral views in neutral position, flexion, and extension; and oblique views.[94] On the anteroposterior view, findings such as scoliotic deformity, tilting of cervical vertebrae, spondylotic change of uncovertebral joints (Luschka's joints), cervical ribs, and destructive changes are examined. Lateral views usually give the most useful information in patients with cervical myelopathy. Sagittal alignment, whether straight, lordotic, or kyphotic, is checked. Swan-neck deformity or goose-neck deformity can be observed in patients with RA. Destruction of the vertebral body may be caused by DSA or by metastasis from a malignant tumor.

In the analysis of degenerative findings in the cervical spine, it is reasonable to categorize spinal canal findings as static factors or dynamic factors (previously described in this chapter). Static factors include the degree of disk space narrowing, the size of end-plate osteophyte, sagittal alignment, the size of the spinal canal, and ossified lesions such as OPLL and calcification of the ligamentum flavum. Dynamic factors can be determined by lateral views taken in flexion and extension. Instability and retrolisthesis or anterolisthesis of cervical vertebrae are checked on flexion and extension views. Foraminal stenosis is shown on oblique views. In contrast, the finding of a wide foramen may indicate the existence of a dumbbell

Table 60.4 Modified Japanese Orthopaedic Association Scoring System for Cervical Myelopathy*

MOTOR FUNCTION

Fingers

0	Unable to feed oneself with any tableware including chopsticks, spoon, or fork, and/or unable to fasten buttons of any size
1	Can manage to feed oneself with a spoon and/or fork but not with chopsticks
2	Either chopstick feeding or writing is possible but not practical, and/or large buttons can be fastened
3	Either chopstick feeding or writing is clumsy but practical, and/or cuff buttons can be fastened
4	Normal

Shoulder and Elbow (Evaluated by MMT Score of the Deltoid or Biceps Muscles, Whichever Is Weaker)

−2	MMT2 or below
−1	MMT3
−0.5	MMT4
0	MMT5

Lower Extremity

0	Unable to stand and walk by any means
0.5	Able to stand but unable to walk
1	Unable to walk without a cane or other support on a level
1.5	Able to walk without support but with a clumsy gait
2	Walks independently on a level but needs support on stairs
2.5	Walks independently when going upstairs, but needs support when going downstairs
3	Capable of fast but clumsy walking
4	Normal

SENSORY FUNCTION

Upper Extremity

0	Complete loss of touch and pain sensation
0.5	≤50% normal sensation and/or severe pain or numbness
1	>60% normal sensation and/or moderate pain or numbness
1.5	Subjective numbness of slight degree without any objective sensory deficit
2	Normal

Trunk

0	Complete loss of touch and pain sensation
0.5	≤50% normal sensation and/or severe pain or numbness
1	>60% normal sensation and/or moderate pain or numbness
1.5	Subjective numbness of slight degree without any objective sensory deficit
2	Normal

Lower Extremity

0	Complete loss of touch and pain sensation
0.5	≤50% normal sensation and/or severe pain or numbness
1	>60% normal sensation and/or moderate pain or numbness
1.5	Subjective numbness of slight degree without any objective sensory deficit
2	Normal

BLADDER FUNCTION

0	Urinary retention and/or incontinence
1	Sense of retention and/or dribbling and/or thin stream and/or incomplete continence
2	Urinary retardation and/or pollakiuria
3	Normal

*Total score for a healthy patient = 17.
MMT, manual muscle test.

Table 60.5 Japanese Orthopaedic Association Cervical Myelopathy Evaluation Questionnaire

With regard to your health condition during the last week, please circle the number of *one* answer that best applies for each of the following questions. If your condition varies depending on the day or time, circle the number of the answer that applies when your condition was its *worst*.

Q1-1. While in the sitting position, can you look up at the ceiling by tilting your head upward?
1. Impossible
2. Possible to some degree (with some effort)
3. Possible without difficulty

Q1-2. Can you drink a glass of water without stopping despite the neck symptoms?
1. Impossible
2. Possible to some degree
3. Possible without difficulty

Q1-3. While in the sitting position, can you turn your head toward the person who is seated to the side but behind you and speak to that person while looking at his or her face?
1. Impossible
2. Possible to some degree
3. Possible without difficulty

Q1-4. Can you look at your feet when you go down the stairs?
1. Impossible
2. Possible to some degree
3. Possible without difficulty

Q2-1. Can you fasten the front buttons of your blouse or shirt with both hands?
1. Impossible
2. Possible if I spend time
3. Possible without difficulty

Q2-2. Can you eat a meal with your dominant hand using a spoon or fork?
1. Impossible
2. Possible if I spend time
3. Possible without difficulty

Q2-3. Can you raise your arm? (Answer for the weaker side.)
1. Impossible
2. Possible up to shoulder level
3. Possible although the elbow and/or wrist is a little flexed
4. I can raise it straight upward

Q3-1. Can you walk on a flat surface?
1. Impossible
2. Possible but slowly even with support
3. Possible only with the support of a handrail, a cane, or a walker
4. Possible but slowly without any support
5. Possible without difficulty

Q3-2. Can you stand on either leg without the support hand? (Do you need to support yourself?)
1. Impossible with either leg
2. Possible on either leg for more than 10 seconds
3. Possible on both legs individually for more than 10 seconds

Q3-3. Do you have difficulty going up stairs?
1. I have great difficulty
2. I have some difficulty
3. I have no difficulty

Q3-4. Do you have difficulty with one of the following motions: bending forward, kneeling, or stooping?
1. I have great difficulty
2. I have some difficulty
3. I have no difficulty

Q3-5. Do you have difficulty walking more than 15 minutes?
1. I have great difficulty
2. I have some difficulty
3. I have no difficulty

Q4-1. Do you have urinary incontinence?
1. Always
2. Frequently
3. When retaining urine over a period of more than 2 hours
4. When sneezing or straining
5. No

Q4-2. How often do you go to the bathroom at night?
1. Three times or more
2. Once or twice
3. Rarely

Table 60.5 Japanese Orthopaedic Association Cervical Myelopathy Evaluation Questionnaire—cont'd

Q4-3. Do you have a feeling of residual urine in your bladder after voiding?
1. Most of the time
2. Sometimes
3. Rarely

Q4-4. Can you initiate (start) your urine stream immediately when you want to void?
1. Usually not
2. Sometimes
3. Most of the time

Q5-1. How is your present health condition?
1. Poor
2. Fair
3. Good
4. Very good
5. Excellent

Q5-2. Have you been unable to do your work or ordinary activities as well as you would like?
1. I have not been able to do them at all.
2. I have been unable to do them most of the time.
3. I have sometimes been unable to do them.
4. I have been able to do them most of the time.
5. I have always been able to do them.

Q5-3. Has your work routine been hindered because of the pain?
1. Greatly
2. Moderately
3. Slightly (somewhat)
4. Little (minimally)
5. Not at all

Q5-4. Have you been discouraged and depressed?
1. Always
2. Frequently
3. Sometimes
4. Rarely
5. Never

Q5-5. Do you feel exhausted?
1. Always
2. Frequently
3. Sometimes
4. Rarely
5. Never

Q5-6. Have you felt happy?
1. Never
2. Rarely
3. Sometimes
4. Almost always
5. Always

Q5-7. Do you think you are in decent health?
1. Not at all (my health is very poor)
2. Barely (my health is poor)
3. Not very much (my health is average)
4. Fairly (my health us better than average)
5. Yes (I am healthy)

Q5-8. Do you feel your health will get worse?
1. Very much so
2. A little bit at a time
3. Sometimes yes and sometimes no
4. Not very much
5. Not at all

On a scale of 0 to 10, with 0 meaning "no pain (numbness) at all" and 10 meaning "the most intense pain (numbness) imaginable," mark a point between 0 and 10 on the lines below to show the degree of your pain or numbness when your symptom was at its worst during the week.

If you feel pain or stiffness in your neck or shoulders, mark the degree.

0 ———————————————————————— 10

If you feel tightness in your chest, mark the degree.

0 ———————————————————————— 10

If you feel pain or numbness in your arms or hands, mark the degree. (If there is pain in both limbs, judge the worse of the two.)

0 ———————————————————————— 10

If you feel pain or numbness from chest to toe, mark the degree.

0 ———————————————————————— 10

Adapted from Fukui M, Chiba K, Kawakami M, et al: JOA back pain evaluation questionnaire (JOABPEQ)/JOA cervical myelopathy evaluation questionnaire (JOACMEQ): the report on the development of revised version April 16, 2007, *J Orthop Sci* 14:348, 2009.

tumor. Further, the open-mouth anteroposterior view is used to detect lesions of the upper cervical spine.

In 1970s and 1980s, myelography was the most useful and reliable tool for detecting lesions of the spinal canal. However, myelography was supplanted by the widespread use of MRI. CTM is clearly beneficial in its ability to detect atrophy of the spinal cord (**Fig. 60.20**). CT provides better information on bony lesions, such as bony spur and ossified ligament. Three-dimensional CT is clinically useful not only in the diagnosis of myelopathy, but also in the decision process and safety promotion for surgical procedures in patients with cervical myelopathy.

MRI has become the most important tool for detecting characteristic lesions in patients with cervical myelopathy.[95] However, MRI is not indicated for everyone who is suspected to have cervical lesions. This imaging technique is recommended for patients who have obvious neurologic findings and persistent or worsening symptoms. The standard screening

cervical spine MRI includes sagittal and axial sequences with T1- and T2-weighted images. The T1-weighted image provides superior spatial resolution and a survey of bone marrow signal intensity, whereas the T2-weighted study has the advantage of imaging the central canal and thecal sac. Because the cerebrospinal fluid and spinal cord are shown to be white and black, respectively, on the T2-weighted image, spinal cord compression is easily identified by the disappearance of cerebrospinal fluid. MRI can detect the extent of pathologic changes of the soft tissues, such as disk herniation and hypertrophy of the ligamentum flavum and posterior longitudinal ligament. Further, MRI is useful for visualizing various aspects of the spinal cord. The size and shape of the spinal cord are evident on both sagittal and transverse images. Long-lasting severe compression leads to spinal cord atrophy. Investigators have speculated that the size of the spinal cord is related to postoperative prognosis. In addition, MRI can show the intramedullary pathologic features of the spinal cord.

The presence of high signal intensity on the T2-weighted image is considered to reflect a wide spectrum of pathologic changes of the spinal cord including reversible changes, such as edema, and irreversible changes, such as gliosis, myelomalacia, cystic necrosis, and syrinx formation (**Fig. 60.21**). Matsumoto et al[96] reported that increased signal intensity is not related to a poor prognosis or the severity of myelopathy. In contrast, Mizuno et al[97] examined the pathologic features of snake-eye appearance (a unique finding characterized as nearly symmetrical, round high signal intensity of the spinal parenchyma resembling the face of a snake; see Fig. 60.21) and noted that this finding revealed cystic necrosis of the spinal cord that led to poor recovery of upper extremity motor strength. Yukawa et al[98] prospectively analyzed high signal intensity in the spinal cord on T2-weighted images. These investigators classified signal changes in the spinal cord into three grades: grade 0, none; grade 1, light (obscure); and grade 2, intense (bright). The result was that patients with greatest increased signal intensity in the spinal cord had the worst postoperative recovery.[98] Therefore, the precise pathology of high signal intensity on T2-weighted images should be carefully analyzed.

An attempt has been made to assess the utility of [18]fluorodeoxyglucose ([18]FDG) PET in the evaluation of patients with

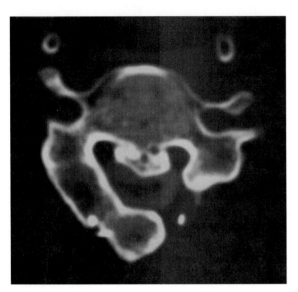

Fig. 60.20 Spinal cord atrophy shown by computed tomography myelography. This 60-year-old man had ossification of the longitudinal ligament after cervical laminoplasty.

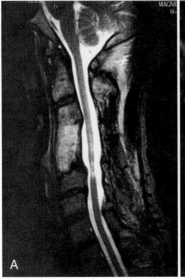
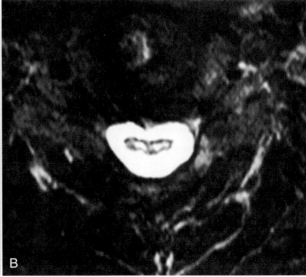

Fig. 60.21 High intensity in the spinal cord at the C5-6 level on T2-weighted sagittal (A) and axial (B) magnetic resonance images. The snake-eye appearance in the spinal cord is obvious on the axial image.

cervical myelopathy. Uchida et al[99] analyzed the glucose metabolic rate (standardized uptake value) in the spinal cord and found that postoperative neurologic improvement is correlated with the mean standardized uptake value.

Therapeutic Strategies for Cervical Compressive Myelopathy

The therapeutic strategy for cervical myelopathy should be based on the patient's symptoms, the severity of the disorder, and the patient's general condition. Given that 5% of patients have a rapid onset of symptoms followed by a long period of quiescence, 20% show gradual but steady progression of signs and symptoms, and 75% show stepwise deterioration of clinical function with intervening variable periods of quiescent disease,[2] careful observation is essential in the treatment of cervical compressive myelopathy. Emery[15] noted that reevaluation every 6 to 12 months to assess deterioration of neurologic function or a change in symptoms may be appropriate during follow-up for patients with cervical compressive myelopathy.

When the patient has a slight complaint, such as neck pain and mild myelopathy, conservative treatment should be considered. Conservative treatment consists of medication, cervical immobilization in a soft collar, active discouragement of high-risk activity, and avoidance of overloading, manipulation therapies, and vigorous or prolonged flexion and extension of the neck. When the patient complains of neck pain or radiculopathy mainly, narcotic analgesics, nonsteroidal anti-inflammatory agents, corticosteroids, muscle relaxants, and antidepressants are commonly recommended. A prospective randomized study by Kadanka and Bednarik et al[100,101] revealed that surgery is not superior to conservative treatment for patients with mild or moderate forms of spondylotic cervical myelopathy, whereas surgery is more suitable for patients with a clinically worse status.

Indications for Surgery

Patients with severe or progressive cervical myelopathy associated with concordant radiologic findings, such as spinal cord compression, are candidates for operative treatment. However, the clinician must consider the definition of severe myelopathy. A patient with spastic gait and myelopathy hand may be considered to have severe myelopathy, although no clear definition exists for the severity of this disease. Guidelines for the surgical management of cervical degenerative disease in the *Journal of Neurosurgery Spine* in 2009 stated that patients with more severe cervical spondylotic myelopathy (modified JOA score $\leq$ 12) should be considered for surgery, on a case-by-case basis.[76] One study reported that 12 patients with severe disability showed significant improvement after surgical intervention; however, in patients with mild or moderate myelopathy, no difference between the operative group and the nonoperative group was evident at 12 and 24 months after treatment.[102,103]

Surgical intervention is not generally recommended when the sole symptom is neck pain, because surgical treatment is not always effective in patients whose predominant complaint is pain.[2,72] However, in patients with severely limiting pain caused by cervical degenerative disease, surgical intervention may be considered.[104] Provocative diskography may

be recommended to improve the clinical success rate in such cases. When the results of provocative diskography are positive, anterior diskectomy and fusion surgery are usually performed at the affected segment.[2]

Surgical Approaches

With regard to the surgical management of cervical spondylotic myelopathy, controversy remains about whether the anterior or posterior technique is preferable because both techniques have been used successfully. The anterior option includes diskectomy with fusion and corpectomy with strut graft fusion techniques, which are performed with or without anterior instrumentation (plate or intervertebral cage) and cervical arthroplasty with artificial disk placement. The posterior option includes laminectomy, as well as laminoplasty with or without instrumentation (miniplate and ceramic spacer for opening the lamina or facet screw and screw and rod system for posterior fusion). Posterior foraminotomy can be added.

The choice of approach is based on the local pathologic features, the patient's general condition, and the surgeon's skill. As for the local pathologic features of cervical myelopathy, the factors important in decision making are as follows: (1) the sagittal cervical alignment, (2) the width of the spinal canal, (3) the number of affected segments, (4) the location of the compressive abnormality, and (5) the presence of instability.[2] The various surgical approaches, anterior cervical diskectomy, with fusion, anterior cervical corpectomy with fusion, laminectomy, laminoplasty, and laminectomy with arthrodesis, all provide near-term functional improvement in patients with cervical spondylotic myelopathy. The advantages, disadvantages, and possible early and late complications are described in **Table 60.6**.

Anterior Approach

Anterior decompression and arthrodesis are performed through the anterior approach. This approach is advantageous for patients who have anterior compressive factors, such as bony spur behind the vertebral bodies, intervertebral disk herniation, and OPLL, because this approach allows direct decompression of the spinal cord. Further, in patients with cervical segmental instability, defined as excessive segmental motion according to the criteria proposed by White et al[105] or anterolisthesis or retrolisthesis exceeding 3.5 mm,[106] arthrodesis should be considered. Arthrodesis may also be effective for the management of axial pain. Studies have indicated that anterior fusion procedures provide good axial pain relief.[2,19,72] However, the anterior approach is technically demanding, especially in patients with multilevel stenosis. Yonenobu et al[107] reported that patients with one- or two-level involvement were managed with anterior cervical diskectomy or corpectomy and fusion, patients with involvement of four levels or more were managed with the posterior approach, and patients with involvement of three levels were managed with either the anterior or the posterior approach. When patients have a developmentally narrow spinal canal, posterior decompression is recommended because these patients generally have multilevel spinal stenosis.

Autograft, allograft, titanium cage, polymethylmethacrylate (PMMA), hydroxyapatite, polyetheretherketone (PEEK), and recombinant human bone morphogenic protein-2 (rhBMP-2)

Table 60.6 Advantages, Disadvantages, and Possible Early and Late Complications of Anterior and Posterior Surgical Approaches in Cervical Myelopathy

Approach	Advantages	Disadvantages	Early Complications	Late Complications
Anterior approach	Direct decompression of the spinal cord Stabilization with fusion Correction of deformity Axial pain relief	Technically demanding Graft complication Need for a rigid brace after surgery	Dysphagia Recurrent laryngeal nerve palsy Bone graft dislodgment C5 palsy Horner's syndrome	Adjacent segment disease Loss of motion
Posterior approach	Not technically demanding Less need for a brace Avoidance of graft complications Applicable for multiple segments Applicable for developmental stenosis	Indirect decompression Not applicable for preoperative kyphosis	C5 palsy Postoperative axial pain Limited range of motion Shoulder stiffness	Late instability OPLL progression Postoperative kyphosis

OPLL, ossification of the posterior longitudinal ligament.

have been used for interbody grafting. These multiple strategies have been successful, and class II evidence supports the use of autograft, allograft, and titanium cage.[108] Cervical spondylotic myelopathy has also been managed with cervical arthroplasty and the use of an artificial disk. Several types of artificial disks have been developed,[109] and on the basis of biomechanical and clinical studies,[110,111] favorable results have been reported.[112] Cervical disk replacement seems to be successful in the management of single-level cervical spinal radiculopathy, but not myelopathy. Effectiveness during long-term follow-up is still uncertain. Strict selection criteria and adherence to scientific evidence are necessary.[113]

One of the disadvantages of the anterior approach is the long-term application of a rigid orthosis. Patients must wear a rigid brace until fusion is complete. Further, postoperative complications such as recurrent laryngeal nerve palsy, sympathetic nerve injury resulting in Horner's syndrome, dysphagia, and vertebral artery injury are associated with the anterior surgical approach. Dislodgment of grafted bone may occur in the postoperative period. During long-term follow-up, it is important to be aware of possible adjacent segment disease above or below the fusion levels.[114]

Posterior Approach

Posterior surgery is divided into laminoplasty and laminectomy with posterior fusion. Laminectomy alone has become uncommon because many surgeons believe that postlaminectomy kyphosis is a possible complication. Because the spinal cord shifts dorsally after posterior decompressive surgery, posterior surgery causes indirect decompression of the spinal cord.[115] Based on this background, posterior decompression is generally contraindicated for patients who have neutral or kyphotic cervical alignment. In fact, patients with lordotic alignment have better clinical results after cervical laminoplasty compared with patients with neutral or kyphotic alignment.[116]

Although the procedure has many modifications, cervical laminoplasty consists of two types, the French door type and the unilateral hinge type.[117,118] No difference is reported in the postoperative results of these two types of laminoplasty. Because both of the posterior approaches are technically less demanding than the anterior approach, posterior surgery is indicated in patients with multilevel cervical stenosis.

Further, when patients have a developmentally narrow spinal canal, posterior decompression is recommended. In patients with cervical radiculopathy, posterior foraminotomy can be added at the affected level. When patients have cervical instability, segmental fusion with instrumentation can be considered. In particular, posterior fusion surgery is very effective in patients with RA and severe neck pain resulting from cervical instability.[48,49] Procedures include occipitocervical fusion, occipitothoracic fusion, C1-2 fusion, cervical fusion, and cervical laminoplasty with posterior fusion.

Fixation techniques using facet screws and pedicle screws or lateral mass screws with rod system fixation have been developed. Halo vest or rigid orthoses are required for posterior cervical fusion. In contrast, braces are less necessary after cervical laminoplasty. A soft collar is generally used for comfort after laminoplasty. A soft collar should be used for less than 1 month postoperatively. Based on data and experience,[119] early muscle exercise with a short period (1 month) of soft collar use is beneficial postoperatively for patients who undergo cervical laminoplasty.

Few complications are associated with the posterior surgical approach. However, when posterior instrumentation is used, especially fixation using pedicle screws, care must be taken not to penetrate the vertebral artery. Postoperative radiculopathy, motor palsy of the C5 nerve root, is a well-known occasional complication of posterior decompression of the spinal cord. This complication can occur after anterior surgery. Postoperative C5 palsy is reported to occur in 5% to 8% of patients after surgery for cervical compressive myelopathy.[120] No significant differences were noted between patients undergoing anterior decompression and fusion and laminoplasty, nor were distinctions apparent between the French door type and unilateral hinge type. Several causes, including a tethering effect of the nerve root and thermal or mechanical damage, have been suggested.[121,122] However, the cause of this complication has not been clarified. The two mechanisms that may account for postoperative segmental motor paralysis are nerve root impairment and segmental spinal cord disorder.

In a prospective study using MRI, Sakaura et al[122] found that linear T2-weighted high-intensity areas in the spinal cord were significantly more likely to appear in the paralyzed segments after laminoplasty. Based on the findings, these investigators proposed that some of the motor paralysis seen in these patients may be caused by spinal cord disease. Although definite preventive measures have not been developed, a previous report stated that foraminotomy and durotomy may be effective for releasing the tethering effect of the nerve root after laminoplasty.[121] The prognosis is usually favorable, and investigators have reported that postoperative motor palsy spontaneously resolves within 12 months.[121–123]

Another common postoperative problem associated with the posterior approach is the presence of axial symptoms, such as axial pain and limited range of motion of the cervical spine. Regarding postoperative axial pain, the incidence was reported to be as high as 60% to 80% in early studies.[124,125] However, the cause of this pain remains largely uncertain. Hosono et al[126] reported that axial pain was prevented by avoiding inclusion of C7 in laminoplasty. This finding suggests that the pain originates from the neck muscle, because the C7 spinous process is connected to the scapula by the trapezius and rhomboideus minor muscles and has critically important biomechanical functions. Patients also complain of limited ROM of the neck after posterior surgery. The reduction in ROM is reported to range from 30% to 70% of preoperative ROM after cervical laminoplasty.[127] Avoidance of postoperative laminar fusion and early mobilization after surgery are recommended.[119]

Conclusion

1. Patients with cervical myelopathy rarely have pain. However, neck pain from degenerative change in the cervical spine may be associated with cervical myelopathy.

2. Cervical myelopathy is caused by various pathologic conditions, such as cervical spondylosis, OPLL, cervical disk herniation, calcification of the ligamentum flavum, RA, spinal tumors, epidural abscess, anomaly of the cervical spine, and DSA.

3. The diagnosis of cervical myelopathy is based on history taking, physical examination, and radiologic evaluation.

4. The therapeutic strategy should be based on the patient's symptoms, severity of myelopathy, and general condition.

5. When patients complain of mild myelopathy and neck pain, conservative treatment, including medications (e.g., nonsteroidal anti-inflammatory drugs) and cervical immobilization should be provided, and therapeutic advice should be given.

6. Patients with severe or progressive cervical myelopathy associated with concordant radiologic findings are candidates for operative treatment.

7. Either an anterior or a posterior decompressive surgical procedure effectively improves symptoms of cervical myelopathy.

8. Both anterior and posterior approaches have specific advantages and disadvantages.

9. Anterior decompression and fusion may be effective for the management of axial pain when the patient has lesions at one or two intervertebral levels.

References

Full references for this chapter can be found on www.expertconsult.com.

Chapter **61**

Cervical Dystonia

H. Michael Guo, James A. MacDonald, and Martin K. Childers

Cervical dystonia (CD), one of the most common forms of focal dystonia, is characterized by simultaneous and sustained involuntary contraction of the cervical muscles that leads to twisting and repetitive head movements and abnormal postures.[1,2] CD is also known as spasmodic torticollis and torsion dystonia. The prevalence of CD was reported to be 8.9 per million population in 1988.[3] One study in Europe reported an annual prevalence for CD of 57 per million,[4] and the Dystonia Medical Research Foundation estimated that no less than 300,000 people suffer from CD in North America. Patients with CD tend to be women in their fourth or fifth decades of life.[5] In a study involving 266 patients, Chan et al[6] found that the median age of onset was 41 years and the male-to-female ratio was 1:1.9. Sixty-six percent to 75% of the patients with CD are believed to be disabled from the pain associated with this disorder.[3,6–8] Dauer et al[9] reported that CD is most often idiopathic, and it slowly develops over several years in patients 30 to 50 years old. Jankovic et al[10] noted that approximately 12% of the patients with CD have a family history of the condition.

Historical Considerations

As early as in the sixteenth century, the term *torty colly* was used by Rabelaris to elucidate wry neck.[11] The term *dystonia* is attributed to the German neurologist Hermann Oppenheim who, in 1911, shortened the term *dystonia musculorum deformans* (reflecting the deforming nature of the syndrome). In his original article, Oppenheim (**Fig. 61.1**) described a childhood syndrome characterized by twisting of the torso, muscle spasms, jerky movements, and eventually progression of symptoms leading to fixed, contracted postures.[12] Today, *dystonia* is defined as a clinical syndrome characterized by sustained, involuntary muscular contractions that frequently lead to twisting and repetitive movements or abnormal postures.[2,13] Therefore, the term *cervical dystonia* refers to focal dystonia of the neck muscles that often leads to twisting or turning of the head and is more commonly known by the name *torticollis* or *spasmodic torticollis*.

Pathogenesis

CD was described by Meige as a disorder originating in "the mind itself." In the 1960s, psychiatrists postulated that the disorder resulted from castration anxiety or a symbolic "turning away from the world." Thanks to modern imaging technology, electrophysiologic methods, and genetic analysis, the putative cause of CD has evolved from being a purely psychiatric disorder to a syndrome with links to a genetic origin and objective features. The pathogenesis of CD is still unknown, although evidence suggests a role for genetic factors. In 2001, a polymorphism in the dopamine D5 receptor *(DRD5)* gene was associated with CD in a British population, a finding suggesting that *DRD5* is a susceptibility gene for CD.[14] These findings were independently replicated by an Italian group of investigators who performed a large case-control study of the microsatellite deoxyribonucleic acid (DNA) region containing a polymorphism (CT/GT/GA)(n) at the *DRD5* locus.[15] The frequency of allele 4 was higher in the CD patients compared with controls, and this finding provided further evidence of an association between *DRD5* and CD and supported the involvement of the dopamine pathway in the pathogenesis of CD.

Several other lines of evidence point to a relationship between dopamine and CD. For example, primary torsion dystonia, a genetically heterogeneous group of movement disorders that includes CD, is inherited in an autosomal dominant fashion and is reported to be caused by a protein encoded by the *DYT1* gene, torsion A, mutated in some forms of primary torsion dystonia. At least two other primary torsion dystonia gene loci have been mapped. The *DYT6* locus on chromosome 8 is associated with a mixed phenotype, whereas the *DYT7* locus on chromosome 18p is associated with adult-onset focal CD. A novel primary torsion dystonia locus *(DYT13)* was identified on chromosome 1 in a large Italian family with 11 affected members who displayed cervical, cranial, and upper limb dystonic symptoms.[16] At present, 13 genes have been identified as causes for various forms of dystonia.[17]

In another line of research, electrophysiologic tests were used to evaluate three patients with hereditary dopa-responsive

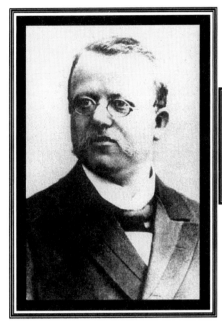

I. Originalmitteilungen.

1. Über eine eigenartige Krampfkrankheit des kindlichen und jugendlichen Alters (Dysbasia lordotica progressiva, Dystonia musculorum deformans).

Von H. Oppenheim.

Im Laufe der letzten 5 Jahre ist mir wiederholentlich ein Leiden entgegengetreten, dessen Deutung und Klassifizierung große Schwierigkeit bereitete. In

Fig. 61.1 German neurologist Hermann Oppenheim and the title page of his original article describing cervical dystonia. *(From Goetz CG, Chmura TA, Lanska DJ: History of dystonia: part 4 of the MDS-sponsored history of movement disorders exhibit, Barcelona, June, 2000,* Mov Disord 16:339, 2001.)

dystonia, before and during treatment with levodopa.[18,19] Results were compared with those in a group of 48 healthy subjects. In the patients before levodopa treatment, the soleus H-reflex recovery curve showed increased late facilitation and depressed late inhibition, a finding reflecting alterations in postsynaptic interneuronal activity. The inhibition of the H-reflex caused by vibration (presumably reflecting presynaptic inhibition) was depressed. Normalization of these test results occurred during levodopa treatment, concurrent with a clear clinical response. Because the H-reflex tests are thought to reflect mechanisms operating at the spinal level, the investigators concluded that spinal aminergic or dopaminergic systems are probably involved in dopa-responsive dystonia. Alternatively, patients with Parkinson's disease, when treated with levodopa, can develop dystonic symptoms (dyskinesias), and antipsychotic drugs that inhibit dopamine receptors are well known for their dystonic side effects.

Hypothesized causes of CD include basal ganglia dysfunction, loss of motor cortex inhibition, and sensorimotor mismatch.[20] Zhuang et al[21] demonstrated abnormal firing rates within the basal ganglia in patients with dystonia. Those patients with focal dystonia had abnormal discharge rates in segmental distributions, whereas patients with generalized dystonia had involvement of the entire basal ganglia. The basal ganglia and its connections with the motor cortices are important in motor planning and movement. Disruption anywhere along the pathway from the basal ganglia to the motor cortex may lead to dystonia.[22] Sensorimotor mismatch may also lead to the agonist and antagonist muscle contractions that occur in CD.[23]

Clinical Presentation

Most patients with CD present with a combination of neck rotation (torticollis, the most common form), flexion (anterocollis), extension (retrocollis), side tilt (laterocollis), or lateral shift.[24-26] These distinctive observable features of CD make the diagnosis fairly easy for the experienced clinician.[27] Neck posturing may be static, but more commonly the head moves in a rhythmic or continuous pattern. Over time, sustained

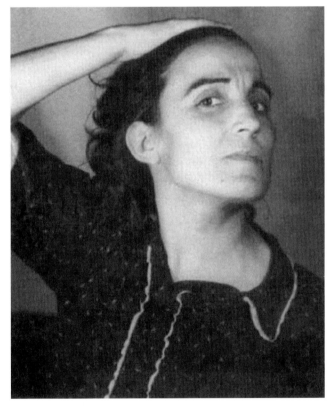

Fig. 61.2 Touching the top or back of the head is one of the common sensory tricks in patients with cervical dystonia. *(From Goetz CG, Chmura TA, Lanska DJ: History of dystonia: part 4 of the MDS-sponsored history of movement disorders exhibit, Barcelona, June, 2000,* Mov Disord 16:339, 2001.)

abnormal postures can result in permanent and fixed contractures. The duration of the disease is variable, ranging from months to decades. Sensory tricks (geste antagonistique) may temporarily improve symptoms. Sensory tricks commonly used by patients with CD include touching the chin, the back of the head, or the top of the head (**Fig. 61.2**).[24] Symptoms of

Table 61.1 Clues Suggesting Psychogenic Origin of Cervical Dystonia

MOVEMENTS

Abrupt onset

Inconsistent movements (changing characteristics over time)

Incongruous movements and postures (movements do not fit with recognized patterns or with normal physiologic patterns)

Presence of additional types of abnormal movements that are not consistent with the basic abnormal movement pattern or are not congruous with a known movement disorder, particularly rhythmical shaking, bizarre gait, deliberate slowness carrying out requested voluntary movement, bursts of verbal gibberish, and excessive startle (bizarre movements in response to sudden, unexpected noise or threatening movement)

Spontaneous remissions

Movements that disappear with distraction

Response to placebo, suggestion, or psychotherapy

Presence as a paroxysmal disorder

Dystonia beginning as a fixed posture

OTHER OBSERVATIONS

False weakness

False sensory complaints

Multiple somatizations or undiagnosed conditions

Self-inflicted injuries

Obvious psychiatric disturbances

Employment in the health profession or in insurance claims

Presence of secondary gain, including continuing care by a "devoted" spouse

Litigation or compensation pending

Adapted from Fahn S: The varied clinical expressions of dystonia, *Neurol Clin* 2:541, 1984.

CD stabilize over time, and remission rates of 10% to 20% are reported, usually within the first few years. Symptoms of dystonia can spread to other parts of the body, most typically to the face, jaw, arms, or trunk.[9] For example, in a study of 72 British patients who were followed up for 7 years, dystonia progressed to areas other than the neck (mainly the face and upper limbs in approximately one third of patients). Only 20% of patients experienced remission of symptoms.[28]

Patients with CD generally report insidious onset of symptoms that gradually worsen with time. Sleep helps relieve symptoms, whereas tasks such as driving, reading, or working at the computer exacerbate the unwanted movements. Stressful situations such as meeting others in social gatherings, giving a presentation, or concentrating on a difficult task also tend to make the symptoms worse. Because the diagnosis of CD depends on clinical examination without confirmatory laboratory tests, one of the most difficult tasks for the clinician treating these patients is to distinguish psychogenic CD from idiopathic CD. Sudden onset of symptoms or relentless progression of movements without abatement or change suggests a psychogenic disorder. Fahn listed "situations" (**Table 61.1**) that may provide clues to identifying a patient with psychogenic CD.[13]

Patients with CD do not attribute any particular head position to discomfort.[27] Myofascial trigger points are not present. Patients with CD describe unpleasant sensations accompanied by "pulling" or "tugging." Headaches are common[25] and may respond to local injections with botulinum toxin (BoNT). Pain attributed to CD differs from pain described by patients with diskogenic pain or fibromyalgia. The severity of the pain is usually related to the intensity of the dystonia and muscle spasms.[6] Jahanshahi et al[28] reported progression of dystonic symptoms to extranuchal but still cervical innervated sites such as the hand, arm, oromandibular region in one third of 72 patients with adult-onset CD. Patients with CD may develop neck pain from the muscle contraction and muscle strain resulting from correcting the abnormal posture. The chronic abnormal posture may also lead to degenerative changes in the cervical spine, with consequent facet pain, radiculopathy, or spinal stenosis.

Acute post-traumatic CD is different, and symptoms include immediate local pain followed by significant cervical range of motion, abnormal head and shoulder posture, and possible trapezius hypertrophy. Those changes often result in abnormal muscle contraction and pain,[6,10] which contribute to functional limitations in these patients and interfere with activities of daily living.[10] Rondot et al[29] revealed that 99% of the 220 patients they studied had various functional difficulties. Dysphasia and subclinical swallowing motility disturbances were also reported in patients with CD.[30] Permanent disability from the decreased cervical range of motion, involuntary movements, and intractable pain may occur in these patients.[31] Although the diagnosis of CD is clinical, and inspection is usually enough, a thorough physical examination should be conducted to rule out "pseudodystonia," caused by structural abnormalities,[32] and secondary dystonia.

Adolescents or children, particularly those patients with a sudden onset of symptoms, should be evaluated for other disorders. These disorders are discussed in the next paragraph.

Differential Diagnosis

Torticollis is the observable feature of a twisted neck, and it may result from underlying causes other than CD.[9] Therefore, the differential diagnosis (**Table 61.2**) includes other disease states associated with abnormal postures, movement disorders, alterations in the dopaminergic system, and neurodegenerative processes. Rarely, CD with dystonic components occurs in the context of Parkinson's disease. Head tremors may suggest an underlying cause of essential tremor but should not occur with the fixed abnormal postures seen in CD. Patients with acquired (congenital) CD of childhood should not display alternating hypertonia and hypotonia, and no palpable muscle hypertrophy or geste antagonistique should be present.

Testing

A family history of movement disorders may suggest familial dystonia rather than idiopathic CD. Therefore, genetic tests based on DNA analysis for specific hereditary dystonias are available that use polymerase chain reaction to detect and amplify DNA in blood samples. However, no simple

Table 61.2 Differential Diagnosis of Cervical Dystonia

Idiopathic torsion dystonia

Corticobasal ganglionic degeneration
  Cerebral palsy
  Huntington's disease
  Stroke
  Spinal cord ependymoma

Wilson's disease

Essential tremor

Multiple sclerosis

Myasthenia gravis

Tardive dyskinesia

Psychogenic torticollis

Posterior fossa tumor

Parkinson disease

Multiple sclerosis

Syrinx

Congenital dystonia

Side effects of psychogenic drugs

Electrical injury

test confirms the diagnosis of CD or excludes a psychogenic component. Further research is needed before genetic testing becomes widely available in the clinic to identify patients at risk or to confirm a clinical diagnosis of idiopathic CD.

Cervical radiographs may identify structural changes of the spine caused by scoliosis or spondylosis secondary to long-standing CD. Similarly, magnetic resonance imaging (MRI) of the cervical spinal cord is useful for determining the presence of spinal cord impingement secondary to bony changes from chronic CD. Contrast medium–enhanced swallowing studies can be performed in consultation with a speech pathologist to evaluate and treat patients for swallowing disorders that accompany CD. One treatment for CD, BoNT injection, may weaken the muscles surrounding the larynx. Thus, patients at risk for aspiration should be evaluated by a speech pathologist or a swallowing study before they are treated with BoNT. Brain imaging (by computed tomography or MRI) is indicated when the physical examination demonstrates findings consistent with an upper motoneuron syndrome, dementia, or pigmented corneal rings (e.g., Kayser-Fleischer rings seen in Wilson's disease).

Electromyography (EMG) can help exclude the diagnosis in patients in whom the diagnosis is in question. For example, an EMG study of the sternocleidomastoid and splenius capitis muscles of eight patients with CD and of eight age-matched controls demonstrated that all control subjects but one showed a peak in splenius capitis EMG at 1 to 12 Hz, a finding that was absent in all subjects with CD.[33] Frequency analysis between patients with CD and controls demonstrated differences suggesting that EMG may provide data to help distinguish CD from psychogenic torticollis. More commonly, EMG is used as a tool for mapping injection patterns for patients treated with BoNT. Identifying muscles by EMG, particularly those muscles deep to the surface that are contracting involuntarily, is useful before injection. The use of palpation alone to identify

tight or contracting muscles may bias the examiner to identify only the most superficial muscles, whereas the use of EMG can assist the clinician in identifying deeper muscles that can contribute to dystonic postures.[27]

Treatment

In general, oral medications are not very effective for CD, and only a few have been systematically evaluated in clinical trials.[34–36] Anticholinergic medications such as trihexyphenidyl or benztropine are worth a trial for patients with CD, but these medications are more useful in patients with generalized dystonias. Mexiletine was reported as helpful in the treatment of both CD and generalized dystonia.[37,38] Glutamate receptor blockers such as amantadine, riluzole, and lamotrigine and spasmolytic agents such as clonazepam and baclofen have all been reported to be useful in some patients with CD.[39,40]

A subset of patients may respond to biofeedback training[41] or muscle relaxation training. A soft cervical collar can reproduce the sensory tricks that reduce head turning, but effects usually wane after a few hours of wear. In patients who are refractory to all other conservative treatments, including BoNT injections, surgical resection of cervical muscles, peripheral selective denervation, or deep brain stimulation is a treatment option, and positive results are reported.[42–55] Because many patients with CD find that specific postures, positions, or physical activities exacerbate symptoms, evaluation of workplace or household ergonomics can be helpful. Occupational or physical therapists can assist in the evaluation and make strategic recommendations for ergonomic aids. Patients often discover their own coping strategies to diminish physical stress, such as reducing the number of hours spent in front of a computer, working at a standing desk instead of a conventional desk, standing to the left or right of a person while carrying on a conversation, or making automobile seat adjustments.

Patients with CD often seek treatment for pain other than for motor symptoms, and headache and neck pain are the main complaints. Therefore, it is advisable to examine new patients with neck pain or headache for physical findings consistent with CD. One theory[27] attributed CD pain to the "relentless contraction of neck muscles" and theorized that one of the beneficial effects of BoNT is that it causes local muscle relaxation and thereby relieving pain. The most effective therapy for patients with CD is local injections of BoNT, the treatment supported by evidence-based reviews and meta-analysis.[35,56–59] The United States Food and Drug Administration approved the indication for CD treatment in 2000.

Three membrane proteins (collectively known as SNAREs)—synaptobrevin (Sbr), synaptosome-associated protein of molecular weight 25,000 (SNAP-25), and syntaxin—mediate the process of exocytosis of synaptic vesicles containing the neurotransmitter acetylcholine. Vesicle membrane fusion at the neuromuscular junction transfers the contents of secretory proteins and transmitters. SNARE proteins provide the substrate for at least one of the seven serotypes (A to G) of BoNT or tetanus toxin (TeTx), which are bacterial proteases that act to block neurotransmitter release.[60] The family of BoNTs is also responsible for illness resulting from food contamination or wound infection. Botulinum neurotoxin type A (BoNT-A, Botox, Allergan, Inc., Irvine, CA; Dysport, Ipsen Pharmaceuticals, Boulogne-Billancourt, France) and type B (Myobloc, Solstice Neurosciences, San Francisco, CA) are produced by the anaerobic bacteria *Clostridium botulinum*, an organism found in soil and water. Only BoNT-A and BoNT-B are clinically available for therapeutic use in the United States. BoNT-A and BoNT-E cleave the carboxyl terminus of SNAP-25,[61] whereas BoNT-B cleaves Sbr. The time course of functional motor recovery after synaptic BoNT intoxication differs among serotypes.[61] Thus, the major assumption regarding the mechanism by which BoNTs decrease muscular contraction involves blocking acetylcholine release from presynaptic motor nerve terminal synapses. It is generally assumed that conditions such as dystonia and spasticity may be relieved subsequent to decreased muscular force in the areas injected, but this hypothesis has not been directly tested. Moreover, preclinical data may not necessarily apply to humans, because physiologic differences exist in the density, distribution, and morphology of the neuromuscular junction between species, age,[62] and disease states.[63,64]

Indeed, chemodenervation by BoNT is generally considered the treatment of choice for patients with CD,[65–67] and 63% of patients report benefit at 5 years.[68] Jankovic and Schwartz[69] followed up 202 of 232 patients who received BoNT injection for CD that was resistant to medical treatments. Seventy-one percent of those patients had improved symptoms, and 76% had almost complete relief of pain. Success is determined by the following clinical outcome measures: prevalence of complications (e.g., dysphagia),[70] score on the Tsui scale,[71–73] pain scores,[72,74] the Toronto Western Spasmodic Torticollis Rating Scale (TWSTRS),[57,75,76] and the relative cost of treatment.[77] However, because neurologic impairments may have only a small impact on the functional health of patients with CD, other outcome measures that include disability, handicap, and global disease scales may increase the relative response rate of patients with CD who are treated with BoNT.[73] The American Academy of Neurology[78] performed an extensive evidence-based review in 2008 on the use of BoNT for the treatment of movement disorders. Academy investigators stated that level A evidence confirmed that BoNT should be offered for the treatment of CD by the Therapeutics and Technology Assessment Subcommittee of the American Academy of Neurology.[78]

No clear guidelines are available for the appropriate dose of BoNT for the treatment of CD. The reason is that the most appropriate dose depends on several clinical and logistical considerations. First, the dose of BoNT should be individualized. Koller et al[79] noted that fixed-dose fixed-muscle controlled studies of BoNT for the clinical management of CD did not produce the same effects as studies (or case reports) in which the dosages and muscles were individualized according to the patient. Second, clinicians should strive to administer the lowest effective dosage of BoNT for treatment of CD, to protect the patient from becoming immune to the agent's therapeutic effect.[24,80] In general, patients should receive as few doses of toxin over the life span as possible, so long as their symptoms are manageable and until further studies of long-term effects of toxin therapy are completed.

Because of the complexity of the neck, it is critical for the clinician to be familiar with anatomic landmarks, vital structures, and muscles for successful treatment of CD with BoNT injection. Attention should be paid to the following structures and organs when injecting BoNT: brachial plexus, carotid sheath, pharynx, esophagus, and apex of the lung. The muscles involved in various forms of CD are listed in **Table 61.3**. EMG guidance may play a role in determining dosage, in that

Table 61.3 Typical Muscle Involvement in Cervical Dystonia

Type of Cervical Dystonia	Muscles Involved
Torticollis	Ipsilateral splenius/semispinalis capitis Contralateral sternocleidomastoid
Laterocollis	Ipsilateral sternocleidomastoid Ipsilateral splenius/semispinalis capitis Ipsilateral scalene complex Ipsilateral levator scapulae Ipsilateral posterior paravertebrals
Retrocollis	Bilateral splenius/semispinalis capitis Bilateral upper trapezius Bilateral deeper paravertebrals
Anterocollis	Bilateral sternocleidomastoid Bilateral scalene complex Bilateral submental complex
Shoulder elevation	Ipsilateral levator scapulae Ipsilateral trapezius

Adapted from Brashear A: Botulinum toxin type A in the treatment of patients with cervical dystonia, *Biologics* 3:1, 2009.

it may help with both effectively targeting affected muscles[81] and also with targeting motor end plates within those muscles,[82–84] thereby potentiating neurotoxin effects. However, when palpation alone is used to identify affected muscles, injection into either the midbelly or several sites of the muscle is generally recommended.

Finally, conversion of equivalent units among BoNT serotypes (or even different formulations of the same serotype) may not be a simple matter of mathematical calculation.[85] Two formulations of BoNT-A, marketed as Botox (Allergan, Inc.) and Dysport (Ipsen, Inc.), are available for clinical use. Although they are the same serotype, controversy exists regarding the conversion of units between available commercial formulations. Reviews[65–67] suggested that 200 U Botox are roughly equivalent to 500 U Dysport (i.e., a 2:5 ratio or a conversion factor of 2.5), as indicated by results of a comparison trial.[86] Only one formulation of BoNT-B, marketed as Myobloc, is commercially available for the treatment of patients with CD.[57] Although it was not possible to make a definitive comparison between BoNT type A and type B for treatment of CD,[87] Costa et al[57,88] concluded in the *Cochrane Review* that single injections of BoNT type A and type B are effective and safe for treating CD and that further injection cycles continue to work for most patients, based on long-term uncontrolled studies. **Table 61.4** lists published doses of BoNT-B for CD that range from 2500 to10,000 U. Fewer data are available on efficacy, safety, and dosing for BoNT-B. The *Cochrane Review* suggested that uncontrolled comparisons of BoNT-A and BoNT-B should be regarded "with suspicion."[57] Therefore, dosing conversions between A and B serotypes may be speculative. Another serotype, BoNT-F, may be a future option for patients who are immunoresistant to serotypes A and B, although less literature exists for BoNT-F.[89,90]

The effects of long-term treatment of CD with BoNT are not well studied. Three studies of long-term effects of BoNT-A in CD suggested that safety and efficacy persist over time. Brans et al[91] reported improvements in disability, handicap, and perceived general health after 12 months of treatment.

Table 61.4 Prospective Trials of Botulinum Neurotoxin in Cervical Dystonia

Serotype	Product	No. of Patients	Dose	Injection Site	Reference
A	Botox	55	30–250 U	SCM, trapezius, splenius capitis	Greene et al, 1990[94]
A	Oculinum	7	50–100 U	SCM, trapezius	Jankovic and Orman, 1987[95]
A	Botox	242	~222 U	Splenius capitis, SCM, trapezius, scalenus	Jankovic and Schwartz, 1991[70]
A	Botox	23	150 U	SCM, splenius capitis, trapezius	Lorentz et al, 1991[96]
A	Botox	20	500 U	Active muscles	Moore and Blumhardt, 1991[97]
A	Botox	35	152 U (SD ± 45)	One or more clinically indicated muscles	Odergren et al, 1998[98]
A	Botox	54	NS	Individualized	Ranoux et al, 2002[82]
A	Dysport	32	262–292 U	Individualized	Brans et al, 1996[71]
A	Dysport	303	778 (SD ± 253)	SCM, trapezius, splenius capitis, levator scapulae	Kessler et al, 1999[92]
A	Dysport	38	477 U (SD ± 131)	One or more clinically indicated muscles	Odergren et al, 1998[98]
A	Dysport	75	500–1000 U	Splenius capitis and SCM	Poewe et al, 1998[72]
A	Dysport	54	NS	Individualized	Ranoux et al, 2002[82]
A	N/A	19	480 U	SCM, splenius capitis, trapezius	Blackie and Lees, 1990[99]
A	N/A	20	100–140 U	SCM, splenius capitis, trapezius	Gelb et al, 1998[100]
B	Myobloc	109	5,000–10,000 U	2–4 cervical muscles	Brashear et al, 1999[101]
B	Myobloc	76	10,000 U	2–4 cervical muscles	Brin et al, 1999[102]
B	Myobloc	122	2,500–10,000 U	2–4 cervical muscles	Lew et al, 1997[103]
F	BoNT-F*	5	520–780 MU	Affected neck muscles	Houser et al, 1998[90]

*BoNT-F is not commercially available in the United States.
SCM, sternocleidomastoid muscle; NS, not specified; SD, standard deviation.

Kessler et al[92] reported disease severity improvement over 5 years, and Haussermann et al[93] reported safety and efficacy data on BoNT treatment of 100 consecutive CD patients over 10 years. This line of evidence suggests that long-term treatment of CD with BoNT is both safe and effective, but further longitudinal studies will be required.

Complications and Pitfalls

Children or adults with fixed contractures of the neck caused by other problems (e.g., congenital torticollis) may be misdiagnosed with CD. Because a distinctive feature of CD is that the neck moves almost continually,[27] patients with no active neck movement may not have true CD but rather a fixed contracture and will not respond to BoNT injections. Rarely, torticollis or torsion dystonia accompanies an upper motoneuron syndrome. In these cases when the neurologic examination reveals abnormalities, the patient should be referred to a neurologist or neurosurgeon for appropriate workup to determine the underlying cause. Finally, for patients with CD who are treated with BoNT injections, dysphagia can result from BoNT-induced weakening of the laryngeal muscles and may place the patient at risk for aspiration. Any patient with an underlying swallowing disorder should be approached with caution when BoNT treatment is contemplated. Swallowing studies are helpful in determining proper nutritional strategies for patients at risk or for those patients who develop dysphagia after injections.

Conclusion

CD causes involuntary head turning or tilting, it may be painful, and it most often affects women in the third or fourth decade of life. The diagnosis is based on clinical examination and the finding of abnormal head and neck position. A diagnosis of idiopathic CD is made in the presence of an otherwise normal physical examination, normal family history, and normal results of laboratory and imaging studies. Local injection of BoNT is the treatment of choice for CD. Dysphagia is a potential complication of the injections.

References

Full references for this chapter can be found on www.expertconsult.com.

Part C

Shoulder Pain Syndromes

Degenerative Arthritis of the Shoulder

Steven D. Waldman

The shoulder joint is susceptible to the development of arthritis from a variety of conditions that have in common the ability to damage the joint cartilage.[1] Osteoarthritis is the most common cause of shoulder pain and functional disability.[2] It may occur following seemingly minor trauma or may be the result of repeated microtrauma. Pain around the shoulder and upper arm that is worse with activity is present in most patients suffering from osteoarthritis of the shoulder. Difficulty in sleeping is also common, as is progressive loss of motion (**Fig. 62.1**).

Most patients presenting with shoulder pain secondary to osteoarthritis, rotator cuff arthropathy, and post-traumatic arthritis pain complain of pain that is localized around the shoulder and upper arm.[3] Activity makes the pain worse, whereas rest and heat provide some relief. The pain is constant and characterized as aching. The pain may interfere with sleep. Some patients complain of a grating or popping sensation with use of the joint, and crepitus may be present on physical examination.

In addition to the aforementioned pain, patients suffering from arthritis of the shoulder joint often experience a gradual decrease in functional ability with decreasing shoulder range of motion that render simple, everyday tasks such as combing hair, fastening a brassiere, or reaching overhead quite difficult.[4] With continued disuse, muscle wasting may occur, and a frozen shoulder may develop (**Fig. 62.2**).

Testing

Plain radiographs are indicated in all patients who present with shoulder pain (**Fig. 62.3**).[5] Based on the patient's clinical presentation, additional testing, including complete blood count, erythrocyte sedimentation rate, and antinuclear antibody testing, may be indicated. Magnetic resonance imaging scan of the shoulder is indicated if rotator cuff tear is suspected (**Fig. 62.4**). Radionuclide bone scan is indicated if metastatic disease or primary tumor involving the shoulder is being considered.

Differential Diagnosis

Osteoarthritis of the joint is the most common form of arthritis that results in shoulder joint pain (**Table 62.1**).[6] However, rheumatoid arthritis, post-traumatic arthritis, and rotator cuff tear arthropathy are also common causes of shoulder pain secondary to arthritis. Less common causes of arthritis-induced shoulder pain include the collagen vascular diseases, infection,

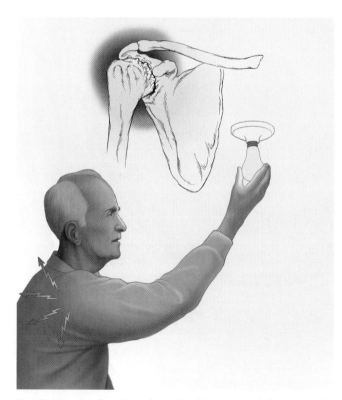

Fig. 62.1 **Range of motion of the shoulder can precipitate the pain of osteoarthritis of the shoulder.** *(From Waldman SD: Atlas of common pain syndromes, ed 2, Philadelphia, 2008, Saunders, p 75.)*

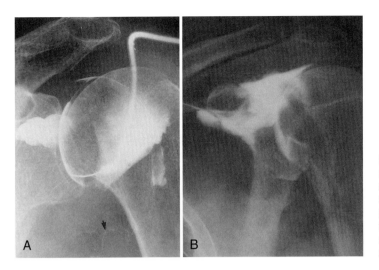

Fig. 62.2 **Adhesive capsulitis: Arthrography.** **A,** Frontal radiograph obtained after the injection of 5 mL of radiopaque contrast material into the glenohumeral joint reveals a tight-appearing articulation with lymphatic filling *(arrow)*. No axillary pouch is seen. **B,** In a second patient, incomplete opacification of the glenohumeral joint is indicative of adhesive capsulitis. *(From Resnick D:* Diagnosis of bone and joint disorders, *ed 4, Philadelphia, 2002, Saunders, p 3108.)*

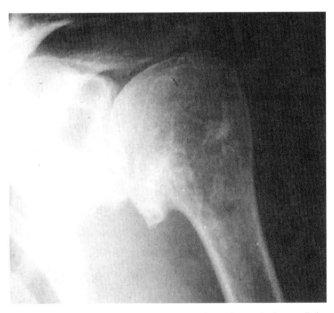

Fig. 62.3 **Osteoarthritis of the shoulder.** The radiograph shows all the features of a "hypertrophic" form of osteoarthritis of the glenohumeral joint, with joint space narrowing, subchondral sclerosis, large cysts in the glenoid, and the massive inferior osteophytosis that is characteristic of this condition. *(From Klippel JH, Dieppe PA:* Rheumatology, *ed 2, London, 1998, Mosby.)*

villonodular synovitis, and Lyme disease. Acute infectious arthritis is usually accompanied by significant systemic symptoms including fever and malaise. This form of arthritis should be easily recognized by the astute clinician and treated appropriately with culture and antibiotics, rather than injection therapy. The collagen vascular diseases generally manifest with polyarthropathy rather than monoarthropathy limited to the shoulder joint, although shoulder pain secondary to collagen vascular disease responds exceedingly well to the intra-articular injection technique described in the next section.

Treatment

Initial treatment of the pain and functional disability associated with osteoarthritis of the shoulder should include a combination of the nonsteroidal anti-inflammatory drugs

(NSAIDs) or cyclooxygenase-2 (COX-2) inhibitors and physical therapy. The local application of heat and cold may also be beneficial. For patients who do not respond to these treatment modalities, an intra-articular injection of local anesthetic and steroid may be a reasonable next step.[7]

Intra-articular injection of the shoulder is performed by placing the patient in the supine position and preparing with antiseptic solution the skin overlying the shoulder, subacromial region, and joint space. A sterile syringe containing 2.0 mL of 0.25% preservative-free bupivacaine and 40 mg of methylprednisolone is attached to a 1½ inch 25-gauge needle, and strict aseptic technique is used. With strict aseptic technique, the midpoint of the acromion is identified, and at a point approximately 1 inch below the midpoint, the shoulder joint space is identified. The needle is then carefully advanced through the skin and subcutaneous tissues, through the joint capsule, and into the joint (**Fig. 62.5**). If bone is encountered, the needle is withdrawn into the subcutaneous tissues and is redirected superiorly and slightly more medially. Once the joint space is entered, the contents of the syringe are gently injected. The clinician should feel little resistance to the injection. If resistance is encountered, the needle is probably located in a ligament or tendon and should be advanced slightly into the joint space until the injection proceeds without significant resistance. The needle is then removed, and a sterile pressure dressing and ice pack are placed at the injection site.

The major complication of intra-articular injection of the shoulder is infection. This complication should be exceedingly rare if strict aseptic technique is followed. Approximately 25% of patients will complain of a transient increase in pain following intra-articular injection of the shoulder joint, and patients should be warned of this possibility.

Conclusion

Osteoarthritis of the shoulder is a common condition encountered in clinical practice. It must be separated from other causes of shoulder pain including rotator cuff tears. Intra-articular injection of the shoulder is extremely effective in the treatment of pain secondary to the aforementioned causes of arthritis of the shoulder joint. Coexisting bursitis

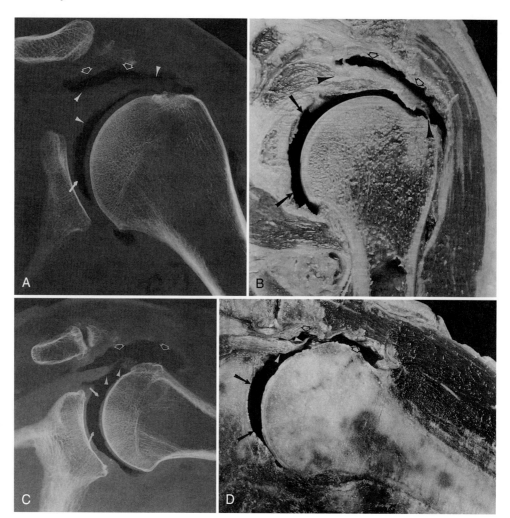

Fig. 62.4 **Full thickness rotator cuff tears: Glenohumeral joint arthography.** These coronal sections were prepared after air arthography of the glenohumeral joint in cadavers of older persons. A and B, On a corresponding radiograph and photograph, note the irregular and torn rotator cuff *(arrowheads)*, allowing communication of the glenohumeral joint *(solid arrows)* and the subacromial (subdeltoid) bursa *(open arrows)*. C and D, In a different cadaver, note the irregular rotator cuff *(arrowheads)* with communication of the glumohumeral joint *(solid arrows)* and the subacromial (subdeltoid) bursa *(open arrows)*. The articular cartilage is eroded. *(From Resnick D: Diagnosis of bone and joint disorders, ed 4, Philadelphia, 2002, Saunders, p 3090.)*

Table 62.1 Causes of Shoulder Pain

Localized Bony or Joint Space Disorders	Periarticular Disorders	Systemic Disease	Sympathetically Mediated Pain	Pain Referred from Other Body Areas
Fracture	Bursitis	Rheumatoid arthritis	Causalgia	Brachial plexopathy
Primary bone tumor	Tendinitis	Collagen vascular	Reflex sympathetic	Cervical radiculopathy
Primary synovial tissue	Rotator cuff tear	disease	dystrophy	Cervical spondylosis
tumor	Impingement	Reiter's syndrome	Shoulder-hand	Fibromyalgia
Joint instability	syndromes	Gout	syndrome	Myofascial pain syndromes such
Localized arthritis	Adhesive capsulitis	Other crystal	Dressler's syndrome	as scapulocostal syndrome
Osteophyte formation	Joint instability	arthropathies	Postmyocardial	Parsonage-Turner syndrome
Joint space infection	Muscle strain	Charcot's	infarction adhesive	(idiopathic brachial neuritis)
Hemarthrosis	Periarticular	neuropathic	capsulitis of the	Thoracic outlet syndrome
Villonodular synovitis	infection not	arthritis	shoulder	Entrapment neuropathies
intra-articular foreign	involving joint			Intrathoracic tumors
body	space			Pneumothorax
				Subdiaphragmatic disorders such
				as subscapular hematoma of the
				spleen with positive Kerr's sign

Adapted from Waldman SD: *Physical diagnosis of pain,* ed 2, Philadelphia, 2010, Saunders, p 42.

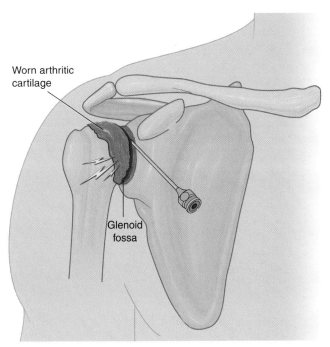

Worn arthritic cartilage

Glenoid fossa

Fig. 62.5 Injection technique for intra-articular injection of the shoulder. *(From Waldman SD: Atlas of pain management injection techniques, ed 2, Philadelphia, 2007, Saunders, p 58.)*

and tendinitis may also contribute to shoulder pain and may require additional treatment with more localized injection of local anesthetic and depot steroid. The foregoing technique is a safe procedure if careful attention is paid to the clinically relevant anatomy of the areas to be injected. Care must be taken to use sterile technique to avoid infection and universal precautions to avoid risk to the operator. The incidence of ecchymosis and hematoma formation can be decreased if pressure is placed on the injection site immediately following injection. The use of physical modalities, including local heat and gentle range-of-motion exercises, should be introduced several days after the patient undergoes the injection for shoulder pain. Vigorous exercises should be avoided because they will exacerbate the patient's symptoms. Simple analgesics and nonsteroidal anti-inflammatory agents or a COX-2 inhibitor may be used concurrently with this injection technique.

References

Full references for this chapter can be found on www.expertconsult.com.

Chapter **63**

Disorders of the Rotator Cuff

D. Ross Henshaw and Edward V. Craig

Disorders of the rotator cuff, ranging from tendon inflammation to rupture, are a common source of anterior shoulder pain. The etiology of rotator cuff disease is a subject of debate between those who believe in extrinsic causes of cuff injury and those who favor intrinsic causes. Although many extrinsic and intrinsic mechanisms have been described, the actual cause in each patient is likely multifactorial. Whatever the origin, cuff disorders from tendinosis to tearing have certain characteristic clinical and radiographic features that aid in diagnosis. Both operative and nonoperative treatments have their place in the definitive treatment of cuff disorders.

Historical Considerations

The rotator cuff is a composite of four tendons that insert circumferentially on the proximal humerus and is one of the largest tendinous structures in the body (**Fig. 63.1**). The unconstrained bony architecture of the glenohumeral joint allows for the highest range of motion of any joint, and it sacrifices stability to do so. Along with labroligamentous restraints, the rotator cuff contributes to maintaining a delicate balance between mobility and stability by providing crucial dynamic stability throughout the arch of motion. These demands make the rotator cuff susceptible to overload and failure.

The diagnosis and treatment of shoulder disorders were first described by Codman in his text *The Shoulder*, which represented 25 years of dedication to understanding and treating painful and stiff shoulders.[1] In 1941, Bosworth[2] described the supraspinatus syndrome, and our understanding of this was amplified by McLaughlin in 1944.[3] Other investigators focused on the biceps tendon as a source of shoulder pain.[4,5] However, until Neer[6] introduced his concept of "impingement syndrome" in 1972, the etiology and treatment of shoulder pain were poorly understood, and the condition was often unsuccessfully treated. Neer's landmark articles clarified the source of rotator cuff injuries and how to treat them. He described the concept of primary impingement as an external source of mechanical injury to the rotator cuff, its pathologic

stages, clinical diagnosis, and surgical treatment. Narrowing of the supraspinatus outlet is most frequently the result of anterolateral subacromial spurring; however, hypertrophy of the coracoacromial ligament, acromioclavicular joint spurring, or greater tuberosity malunion can also lead to impingement with mechanical cuff abrasion.[7–9] Neer's concept of the acromion as a primary cause of cuff injury unified much of the thinking on rotator cuff surgery and led to anterior acromioplasty as the definitive surgical treatment. This operation has reported success rates ranging from 80% to 90%. However, disappointing results obtained with young athletes who throw overhand after acromioplasty and improved understanding of shoulder biomechanics led several investigators to offer alternative explanations to primary impingement as the cause of shoulder pain in athletes.

Overuse syndromes are common in unconditioned athletes and occur when repetitive eccentric contractions lead to microtrauma within the tendon and inflammation.[10,11] Secondary impingement occurs in athletes who use their shoulders repetitively at the extremes of motion, a situation that leads to gradual attenuation of static stabilizers and may result in instability. This microinstability causes the humeral head to sublux anteriorly and superiorly, thus creating secondary impingement as the cuff is compressed on the undersurface of the coracoacromial arch.[12,13] Internal impingement is another source of rotator cuff injury. This entity, as described by Jobe et al,[14] occurs when anterior subluxation leads to contact and abrasion of the undersurface of the supraspinatus tendon against the posterosuperior glenoid labrum. Impingement occurs within the joint rather than in the subacromial space.[14] Treatment of these injuries in throwers thus focuses on reducing inflammation and, if necessary, on correcting the instability through either strengthening of scapular stabilizers and rotator cuff or retensioning of the capsuloligamentous complex.

In contrast to the theory of an extrinsic, mechanical cause of rotator cuff disease, Codman[1] was the first to introduce the concept of an intrinsic tendon degeneration as a source of

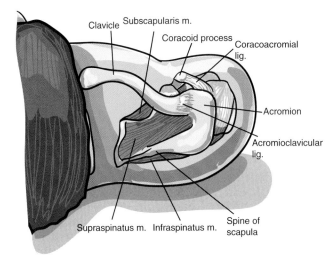

Fig. 63.1 A superior view of the rotator cuff shows the four cuff tendons inserting circumferentially around the proximal humerus: subscapularis, supraspinatus, infraspinatus, and teres minor. The coracoclavicular ligament and the acromion are also labeled.

rotator cuff disorders. From his anatomic dissections, Codman observed a "critical" zone near the insertion of the rotator cuff on the greater tuberosity of the proximal humerus that was both hypovascular and the common location of tears. Further work by Rathbun and Macnab[15] on the vascularity of the rotator cuff supported this observation and led some investigators to emphasize primary anatomic pathologic features of the tendon itself that make the tendon prone to degeneration and tears. This finding contrasted with the concept by Neer of mechanical impingement as the primary cause of rotator cuff injuries. However, changes within the cuff can occur without accompanying stenosis of the subacromial space. Uhtoff et al[16] showed that most tears begin inside the joint on the articular surface, rather than externally in the subacromial space. Ozaki et al[17] looked at 200 anatomic shoulder specimens and correlated pathologic changes on the undersurface of the acromion with cuff tears. Subacromial spurring was present only with cuff tears, and, with partial tears, the acromion was almost always nonpathologic. These investigators concluded that primary cuff degeneration leads to tendon rupture. Nirschl and Pettrone[18] called this degeneration *angiofibroblastic hyperplasia* and theorized that it led to diminished tissue perfusion. More recently, Yuan et al[19] showed apoptotic cells in areas of tendon degeneration, a finding implicating uncontrolled apoptosis in the pathogenesis of intrinsic rotator cuff degeneration.

Although the primary etiology of rotator cuff disease may still be debated, it is likely that for each individual patient the cause is multifactorial and probably includes some component of extrinsic and intrinsic injury. If the origin is multifactorial, then treatments should be tailored toward whichever cause is thought to dominate the clinical picture.

Clinical Presentation

Rotator cuff disease usually manifests as anterior shoulder pain. The signs and symptoms, however, can often be vague and difficult to interpret. The diagnosis of rotator cuff injury therefore requires a systematic approach, including history of presentation, physical examination, and diagnostic testing.

History

Patients with rotator cuff disorders most often present complaining of pain with an insidious onset and progressive course. These patients often have no history of trauma and frequently cannot clearly define when the pain started. Night pain, when present, is frequently associated with tendon tearing. Other symptoms include crepitus, catching, clunking, weakness, and loss of motion. Although weakness with loss of motion is characteristic of rotator cuff tears, this condition needs to be differentiated from strength deficiencies resulting from pain inhibition. The pain most commonly radiates to the anterolateral aspect of the shoulder to the deltoid insertion. However, significant overlap with other shoulder conditions occurs in this region. Labral injury, biceps inflammation, glenohumeral arthritis, joint stiffness, and acromioclavicular arthropathy can also cause shoulder pain. Radicular pain with motion crossing the elbow to the hand and wrist may indicate lower cervical involvement. However, C5 root involvement may manifest as isolated shoulder pain. It is essential to have a high index of suspicion for cervical spine disease as a cause of the painful shoulder.

The age, occupation, and handedness of the patient and the onset, duration, timing, severity, quality, exacerbation, and relief of symptoms are important differentiating factors. Younger patients should be asked about their sports and activities and the relation of their symptoms to specific activities. A younger patient is more likely to have an underlying instability, whereas an older patient is more likely to have a mechanical or degenerative source of pain. Therapeutic history, whether with pain medication, physical therapy, or corticosteroid injections, should also be elicited to determine whether conservative therapy has been exhausted. Previous surgical treatment can also have an important impact on diagnosis and future management.

Physical Examination

The physical examination includes inspection, palpation, range of motion, and special provocative testing. The cervical spine, elbow, wrist, hand, and neurovascular status should also be thoroughly assessed as potential pathologic sources.

Cervical spine disease, particularly when it involves the C5 root, may manifest as shoulder pain. This is particularly true if neck pain with palpation, range of motion, and provocative maneuvers such as a Spurling test duplicates and reproduces the patient's presenting symptoms. Unlike in a patient who has a cuff tear, C5 root involvement may produce biceps weakness, and this may be a distinguishing feature.

Visual inspection of both shoulders should be performed on every patient. The shoulders are examined from the front and back in a search for previous scars, discoloration, swelling, deformity, asymmetry, muscle atrophy, acromioclavicular prominence, and biceps rupture (**Fig. 63.2**). Scapular winging may accompany underlying scapulothoracic dysfunction and can be related to shoulder instability, muscle fatigue, muscle imbalance, scoliosis, kyphosis, and neurologic injury. The bony prominences of the neck, scapula, acromion, acromioclavicular joint, clavicle, and sternoclavicular joints are palpated. Acromioclavicular joint pain is an often overlooked but common source of anterior shoulder pain. Tenderness over the greater tuberosity and in the bicipital groove can be helpful to differentiate between bicipital and cuff inflammation. Pain in the suprascapular notch or the quadrilateral space may be associated with suprascapular and axillary nerve entrapment, respectively.

Range of motion should be performed with the patient in the standing and supine positions in all planes, and the painful and nonpainful extremities should be compared. In the supine position, compensatory movements of the scapula and torso are removed and give a more precise measurement of range of motion. Discrepancies between active and passive range of motion may be secondary to pain inhibition, cuff tears, glenohumeral arthritis, volitional factors, muscle disease, and neurogenic factors. Patients with rotator cuff tears frequently have less range of motion actively than passively because of weakness. This situation differs from the loss of motion in arthritis and stiffness resulting from capsular contraction or inflammation, in which patients frequently have both active and passive reduced mobility. Excessive passive external rotation may indicate subscapularis rupture. However, in throwing athletes, excessive external rotation and decreased internal rotation are common and are secondary to stretched anterior structures and a contracted posterior capsule.

Muscle strength testing of the deltoid, teres minor, infraspinatus, supraspinatus, subscapularis, and biceps should be conducted. However, these tests may be unreliable in the presence of pain. Several tests enable the examiner to isolate the individual muscles of the rotator cuff and to record results separately.[20]

Because the subscapularis is less frequently torn than the supraspinatus tendon, the diagnosis is often overlooked and may be delayed. Two reliable clinical tests for subscapularis function are available. For the *liftoff test* described by Gerber and Krushell,[21] the arm is internally rotated, and the hand rests on the lower back or buttock. The patient then pushes his or her hand away in the horizontal plane, a maneuver that isolates the subscapularis.[21] This test can be inaccurate when the patient recruits the triceps to move the hand away. To avoid

this situation, a modification of the test can be done in which the examiner holds the patient's hand away from the small of the back and asks the patient to maintain the position. If the patient cannot do this, weakness or a tear of the subscapularis is suspected. Because the liftoff test is painful for many patients, the *belly-press test* may be used, as described by Tokish et al.[22] With this test, the patient places his or her hands on the abdomen and rotates the elbows forward with and without resistance. The subscapularis is responsible for the ability to press against the abdomen and push the elbows away from the body. An inability to do this suggests tendon discontinuity.

Jobe and Bradley[23] described a useful test to isolate supraspinatus strength. Both arms are abducted to 90 degrees in the scapular plane and then are fully pronated to point the thumbs toward the ground. Side-to-side comparison to resisted downward force gives an accurate indication of function. Pain and weakness are indicators of partial- or full-thickness tears. The infraspinatus and teres minor are external rotators contributing approximately 90% and 10% rotational force, respectively. Their strength is best measured with the arm at the side in 0 degrees of abduction and the elbow flexed to 90 degrees. In this position, the patient externally rotates his or her hand and forearm against resistance. Weakness suggests a tear. This maneuver is perhaps the best clinical test for cuff discontinuity. This test is particularly useful because both arms may be simultaneously tested and compared. The *hornblower's sign* or *drop sign* is an attempt to isolate the teres minor (**Fig. 63.3**). The patient's arm is placed in 90 degrees of abduction and 90 degrees of forward elevation in maximal external rotation, and the patient is asked to maintain the position of the arm.[24] Insufficient strength of the muscle or tendon is suggested if the patient cannot maintain this position.

Assessing each muscle individually enables the examiner to determine the size and location of a tear. Complete ruptures of four tendons are rare. Most commonly, tears originate in the supraspinatus and enlarge to involve the tendons of the infraspinatus and teres minor. Small tears of the supraspinatus cause pain and weakness with the Jobe test, but external rotation usually remains strong. Patients with large tears involving

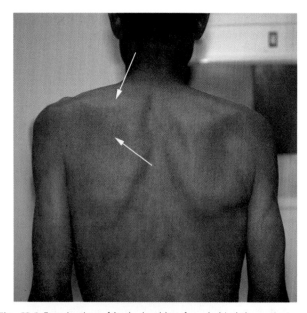

Fig. 63.2 Examination of both shoulders from behind the patient may reveal muscle asymmetry. In this patient, atrophy of the supraspinatus and infraspinatus muscles is present, as evidenced by wasting in the infraspinatus and supraspinatus fossae *(arrows)* on the right as compared with the left side.

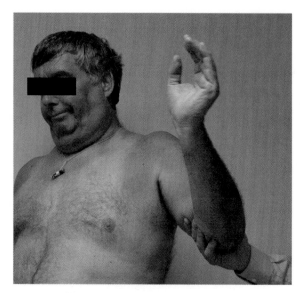

Fig. 63.3 **Hornblower's sign.** The inability to hold the forearm in 90 degrees of abduction indicates injury of the teres minor tendon.

the supraspinatus and infraspinatus have positive Jobe signs and weak external rotation, but an intact hornblower's sign. Patients with massive tears have weakness in the supraspinatus and infraspinatus, and because the teres is involved, they will not be able to hold the arm in the 90/90-degree position in maximal external rotation. Patients with massive cuff tears often use accessory muscles to elevate their arms. A common physical finding is the *shrug sign,* in which the patient activates the trapezius and deltoid when attempting forward elevation (**Fig. 63.4**). Less common are isolated subscapularis

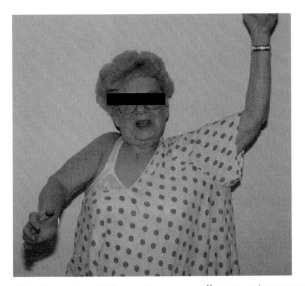

Fig. 63.4 Shrug sign. With massive rotator cuff tears, patients recruit accessory muscles when attempting forward elevation. When this patient tries to elevate her arm, her shoulder shrugs as her trapezium and deltoid fire to compensate for a massive cuff tear.

tears, and patients often report a history of prior surgery or trauma. These patients have intact supraspinatus, infraspinatus, and teres minor strength with isolated subscapularis weakness and excessive external rotation.

After the shoulder musculature has been assessed, provocative tests can be used to identify specific disorders.[20] These tests include maneuvers that reproduce pain associated with impingement, instability, labral disease, and bicipital involvement. Not all of these tests are applicable for each patient, and the history and physical findings guide the examiner's choice of tests.

Impingement signs are not specific and point only to the cause of pain within the subacromial space (subacromial spurs, bursitis, or cuff tear). In his description of impingement lesions, Neer described his classic impingement maneuver. While the scapula is stabilized, the arm is elevated in the plane of the scapula. As the arm reaches the limit of forward elevation, the greater tuberosity is jammed underneath the acromion and thus produces pain. Hawkins and Hobeika[25] described another test for subacromial inflammation. With the arm at 90 degrees of forward elevation and slight adduction, and with the elbow flexed at 90 degrees, the shoulder is internally rotated, a maneuver that impales the greater tuberosity under the acromion.[25] In the presence of cuff disease, this maneuver may elicit pain (**Fig. 63.5**).

A simple adjunct used to confirm the location is the *injection test.* Local anesthetic is injected into the subacromial space, and the Neer and Hawkins tests are repeated. Significant reduction or elimination of pain within the subacromial space confirms that the pain originates in the subacromial space. If the patient reports pain relief, range of motion and muscle testing should be repeated. Weakness resulting from pain inhibition is minimized, and range of motion is improved. In this way, this test is highly effective at both localizing the source of pain and differentiating between weakness resulting from

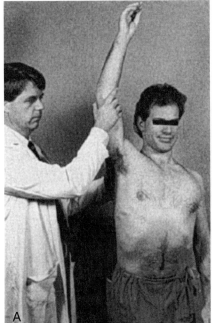
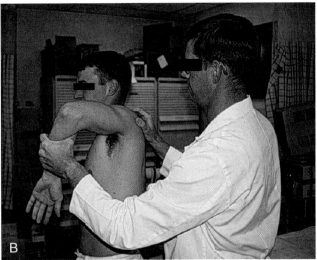

Fig. 63.5 Neer and Hawkins tests. For the Neer test (A), the scapula is stabilized and the arm is elevated in the plane of the scapula. As the arm reaches the limit of forward elevation, the greater tuberosity is jammed underneath the acromion and thus produces pain. The Hawkins test (B) is performed with the arm at 90 degrees of forward elevation, in slight adduction; with the elbow flexed at 90 degrees, the shoulder is internally rotated, a maneuver than impales the greater tuberosity under the acromion.

pain and weakness secondary to rotator cuff tear. Internal impingement can be assessed with Jobe's *relocation test*.[14] With the patient supine, the arm is placed in the abducted externally rotated position (the same as for testing anterior apprehension when instability is suspected). The result of the test is positive if the patient experiences pain or discomfort. This position puts the undersurface of the supraspinatus in contact with the posterosuperior labrum, the site of internal impingement. This pain can be relieved with gentle posterior pressure placed on the anterior aspect of the arm to minimize

contact. When the examiner's hand is withdrawn, the contact and pain return.

The most common direction of clinical instability is anterior. The *anterior apprehension sign* is performed by placing the patient's arm at 90 degrees of abduction and 90 degrees of external rotation. In this position, the patient may feel the sensation of shoulder subluxation anteriorly. The examiner should beware that patients often refuse to let the arm be put in this compromising position and are thus "apprehensive" about this arm position (**Fig. 63.6**).

Other assessments of instability are the load and shift sign and the sulcus sign (**Fig. 63.7**). For the *load and shift sign*, the examiner places axial pressure along the humerus with one hand to center the humeral head and with the other hand translates the humerus anteriorly and posteriorly. Laxity is graded from 1 to 3. Grade 1 laxity is translation of the humeral head to the rim. For grade 2 laxity, the humeral head translates over the rim but is reducible. Grade 3 laxity manifests as translation over the rim and a humeral head that remains dislocated after pressure is removed. Inferior traction on the arm tests inferior translation and is noted by the presence of a sulcus under the lateral acromion: the *sulcus sign*. Anterior instability is called unidirectional if the instability is in one plane, and multidirectional laxity is increased translation in two or more directions when compared with the normal side. Generalized ligamentous laxity is not uncommon and should be assessed in every patient with multidirectional instability. Laxity should also be distinguished from instability. Many asymptomatic patients have loose or lax shoulders, but unless laxity causes pain or discomfort, it is not considered to reflect clinical instability. Instability therefore is symptomatic laxity.

Involvement of the superior labrum and biceps anchor is best evaluated with the O'Brien *active compression test*.[26]

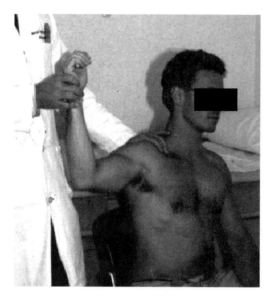

Fig. 63.6 Patients with anterior instability often feel a sense of instability and apprehension when the arm is placed in 90 degrees of abduction and 90 degrees of external rotation.

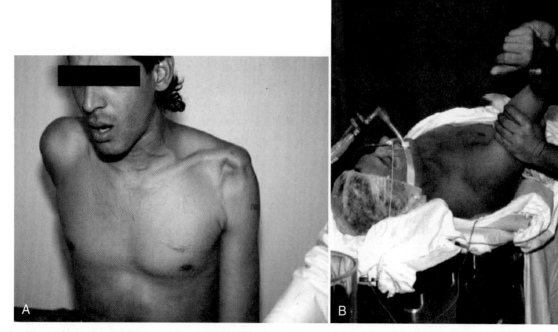

Fig. 63.7 In the load and shift maneuver, an axial load is placed along the humerus, and the humeral head is then shifted anteriorly and posteriorly (**A**). Inferior traction of the arm causing inferior subluxation produces a sulcus under the acromion (**B**).

The patient's arm is flexed, with the elbow kept straight and adducted to 15 degrees. In full pronation with the patient's palm facing down, an inferior force is applied to the arm. In the presence of superior labral disease, this position will elicit pain; and when the arm is fully supinated with the palm upward, the pain with downward pressure is relieved. In internal rotation with arm adduction, the biceps anchor is impinged by the humeral head; and with supination, which externally rotates the humeral head, the biceps pressure is relieved.

Acromioclavicular disease is often overlooked as a common cause of failed rotator cuff treatment. The clinical diagnosis is usually not difficult because most patients are "point tender" over the joint. To test this source of pain, the examiner palpates the joint with one finger and with the other hand adducts the shoulder. It is also useful to palpate both the involved and uninvolved acromioclavicular joints simultaneously to compare the degree of tenderness. This maneuver often reproduces acromioclavicular symptoms.

Diagnosis

Studies such as plain radiography, ultrasound, and magnetic resonance imaging (MRI) can be extremely helpful to confirm the clinical diagnosis of rotator cuff disease and in some cases to rule out other pathologic conditions. In some cases, these diagnostic studies can also help to determine the severity of the disease, the size of tears, and prognosis.

Plain Radiology

Five standard radiographs are recommended for every patient with shoulder pain. These include a "true" anteroposterior view to evaluate the integrity of the glenohumeral joint articulation and anteroposterior views with the arm in internal and external rotation to show Hill-Sachs lesions and greater tuberosity sclerosis, respectively. Hill-Sachs and reverse Hill-Sachs lesions are indicative of anterior and posterior instability, respectively. With the patient's arm in external rotation, the greater tuberosity is rotated orthogonal to the x-ray, to allow better evaluation of its bony contour and to assess for the presence of sclerosis indicative of chronic injury from tendinosis or tear. The anteroposterior views also show resting state glenohumeral articulation. In patients with chronic large cuff tears, the centering effect of the cuff is lost, and the humeral head may migrate superiorly, thus decreasing the acromial humeral interval, which is normally 7 to 10 mm.[27] An "outlet" view, which is a lateral view taken with 10 degrees of caudal tilt, allows evaluation of acromial morphology (**Fig. 63.8**) [**online only**]. In 1986, Bigliani and April[7] described three types of acromial morphology: type 1 is smooth, type 2 is curved, and type 3 is hooked. Impingement and tears are more likely with curved and hooked acromions. Moreover, the presence of acromial spurring and calcification of the coracoacromial ligament can also be seen and indicate impingement. Finally, axillary radiographs show articular congruity and integrity of the glenoid bony architecture.

Ultrasound

The potential use of ultrasound to evaluate rotator cuff disease has been recognized since the early 1980s.[28,29] Even though sonography of the rotator cuff is more difficult than ultrasound imaging of other large tendons, a concerted effort has been made to develop and refine shoulder sonography, primarily because the shoulder is a common site of symptoms and clinical evaluation is challenging. Ultrasound is rapid, inexpensive, and comprehensive, and comparison with the asymptomatic shoulder is possible. Dramatic improvements since 2000 include newer high-resolution transducers, advances in the understanding of the technique of shoulder sonography, and more widespread agreement of the findings seen in patients with rotator cuff tears. All these factors have contributed to making the examination easier to perform and to interpret (**Fig. 63.9**).

Ultrasound has evolved into a mature modality for evaluating rotator cuff tears and bicipital inflammation.[30,31] Yamaguchi et al[30] and Middleton et al[31] reported their results of 100 shoulders evaluated preoperatively with ultrasound as compared with their arthroscopic findings. These investigators reported 100% sensitivity and 85% specificity, with an overall accuracy of 96% for full-thickness rotator cuff tears. Ultrasound, however, was less sensitive in detecting partial-thickness tears and biceps tendon ruptures. Although ultrasound has become a more sensitive and accurate diagnostic tool, its use is still not widespread, and results depend on the operator's experience.

Magnetic Resonance Imaging

MRI is the modality of choice for assessing rotator cuff integrity. MRI is a noninvasive tool offering multiplanar analysis of not only the rotator cuff muscles and tendons but also the cartilage, cortical and medullary bone, and labral and acromioclavicular disease. Although sensitivities approach 100% and specificity is 95% for detecting full-thickness tears, MRI is less reliable for diagnosing partial-thickness tears. The size, shape, and amount of retraction and muscle atrophy are characterized by MRI and determine the repair potential (**Fig. 63.10**). The use of higher-resolution magnetic fields and improved pulse sequencing has made MRI arthrography with gadolinium contrast less routine.[32] However, MRI arthrography may be useful in some instances for the identification of labral tears.

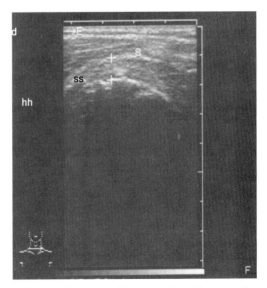

Fig. 63.9 Ultrasound has evolved into a useful tool for evaluating rotator cuff disorders. This image depicts a normal rotator cuff. Note the deltoid (d), supraspinatus (ss), and humeral head (hh).

Treatment

The cause of rotator cuff disease is multifactorial, and the disorder affects patients of different ages and activity levels. Therefore, treatment should be individualized and tailored to meet the demands of each individual patient. Specifically, the physician should consider the patient's age, disability, and expectations and should carefully review the risks and benefits of both nonsurgical and surgical treatment. For instance, the incidence of cuff tears in patients who are more than 60 years old has been reported as high as 40%, and not all these patients are symptomatic.[30] An active, healthy patient with acute rotator cuff tear should have acute surgical repair to restore function and to prevent retraction and secondary muscle atrophy, which can make repair more difficult and can adversely affect prognosis. Patients with chronic (≥3 months) symptomatic cuff tears who do not have precluding medical conditions should also have their tears repaired.

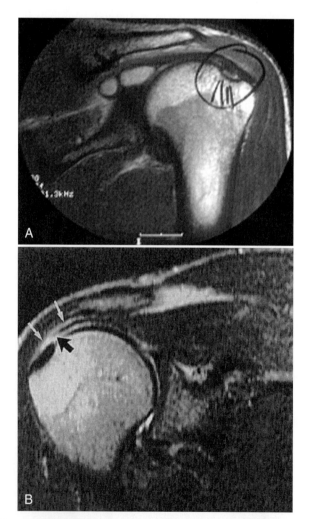

Fig. 63.10 **Magnetic resonance imaging evaluation of rotator cuff tears.** **A,** Partial-thickness tear is demonstrated by high signal intensity through the articular half of the supraspinatus tendon *(lines)*. The intact tendon has characteristic low signal intensity and is shown inserting onto the greater tuberosity. **B,** Full-thickness tear is demonstrated by the low-signal tendon that is detached from its insertion and is retracted medially *(arrows)*.

Nonoperative Management

The effectiveness of nonoperative management was recognized by Neer, who found that many patients with impingement responded to nonoperative management. Nonoperative management may also improve symptoms in patients with cuff tears; however, complete pain relief is uncommon without surgical intervention.[33] The principles of rehabilitation are to allow healing of inflamed tissue, to maintain motion, and to restore function. Generally, the earlier a rehabilitation program is begun, the more successful it is likely to be. Various nonoperative rotator cuff programs have been described, and all emphasize phases of therapy and recovery. Wirth et al[33] described three phases of rotator cuff therapy: pain control, range of motion, and muscle strengthening. A fourth phase should also include modification of work or sport to avoid reinjury.[33]

Pain control and reduction of inflammation are the primary goals of the first phase. They are accomplished by rest and working with the therapist to avoid aggravating activities. This may involve avoiding overhead activities, and for athletes it may involve changing throwing mechanics or technique. For the worker who must work over his or her head, it may involve changing the work environment or, if that is not possible, job retraining or vocational change. Pain modification techniques such as cryotherapy, infrared therapy, ultrasound, transcutaneous electric nerve stimulation, and acupuncture can provide symptomatic relief. A course of nonsteroidal anti-inflammatory medication can be helpful, but these drugs should be used with caution in older patients and in those with peptic ulcer disease or hypertension. Subacromial corticosteroid injections can also be useful in patients with refractory cases, but this treatment should be limited to two to three injections spaced 2 to 3 months apart because of the possible adverse effects of catabolic steroids on tendons.

After the patient's pain has been adequately controlled, the second phase begins with gentle stretching programs and restoration of range of motion to match that of the unaffected shoulder. The goal is to stretch out all area of tightness, with particular emphasis on the posterior capsule. Exercises progress variably from pendulum and wall walking to pulleys and often achieve capsular stretching.

When near-normal passive flexibility of the shoulder is restored, the third phase, focusing on muscle strengthening, is initiated. Scapular strengthening is an essential and often overlooked component of shoulder therapy and should be initiated early. Internal and external rotator strengthening exercises are carried out with the arm at the side to strengthen the anterior and posterior cuff muscles while avoiding the position of impingement, as can occur with flexion and abduction exercises. These strengthening exercises are most conveniently performed using rubber tubing anchored to a door knob. The resistance is increased as the patient's muscle strength improves. Deltoid and supraspinatus strengthening exercises are added when they can be performed comfortably. The role of strength is in part to augment the resting tension of the humeral head "depressors" and, in effect, dynamically open the subacromial space.

Finally, to return the patient to the comfortable pursuit of normal activities, analysis and modification of working environment or recreational techniques should be made, when necessary. Modifications include simple aids such as the use of a stepstool for patients needing to reach for high items. For throwing athletes, modification of body mechanics may prevent relapse and may return the athlete to the previous level of competition. When a patient's occupation requires vigorous or repeated use of the shoulder in provocative positions, job retraining may be required.

Operative Management

Surgical intervention is generally reserved for rotator cuff disease refractory to a 3- to 6-month period of conservative therapy. The precise surgical technique depends on the cause of rotator cuff injury and disease. Impingement and cuff tears caused by a narrowed subacromial space benefit from decompression or widening of the subacromial space through anterior acromial resection, whereas restoration of capsuloligamentous restraint is required for disorders secondary to instability.

Arthroscopic surgery has permitted more accurate diagnosis and treatment of shoulder injuries. Because techniques and instrumentation have improved, most rotator cuff tears can be successfully treated arthroscopically. Traditional open procedures are gradually being replaced by arthroscopic techniques, but the type of procedure chosen depends both on the nature and severity of the disorder and, to some extent, the surgeon's experience and preference. The initial aims of surgical treatment are to relieve pain and to restore functional deficits. With arthroscopic techniques, less tissue injury occurs, with resulting improvements in postoperative pain and therapy.

Classic impingement syndrome caused by a subacromial spur, thickened coracoacromial ligament, or other lesion is best treated with arthroscopic subacromial decompression. Decompression as described by Neer involved an open procedure with removal of up to 1 cm of anterolateral acromion.[6] Modern arthroscopic techniques allow for accurate diagnosis of the source, location, and removal of the offending lesion (**Fig. 63.11**). Arthroscopic subacromial decompression has been shown to have success rates equal to those of open procedures, with faster recovery time.[34] Another advantage of arthroscopic surgery is the ability to view both sides of the rotator cuff. In cases of impingement caused by subtle instability, capsular laxity or labral injury may be identified and treated.

For partial- and full-thickness rotator cuff tears, surgical intervention is also based on treating both the cause of the injury and the tear itself. Decompression should be performed for impingement-associated tears, whereas a stabilization

procedure may be necessary to treat tears associated with microinstability. The treatment of partial-thickness tears is controversial, and no clear guidelines exist. In general, tears involving than 50% of the thickness are treated with decompression and débridement, and those involving more than 50% are treated by resecting the damaged tendon and repairing the defect as though the tear were full thickness (**Fig. 63.12**) [**online only**].[35–38] Treatment of full-thickness tears is moving progressively more toward entirely arthroscopic techniques (**Fig. 63.13**). Arthroscopically assisted, mini-open procedures are also widely used as surgeons transition toward less invasive surgery (**Fig. 63.14**). As always, the choice of treatment is multifactorial, depending on the size, location, chronicity, and quality of the muscle and tendon. Many surgeons have reported success with mini-open and arthroscopic repairs that are equal or superior to open repair.[39,40] The goal of surgery is to relieve pain. This can usually be achieved even in patients with large tears. However, improved strength and function, although desirable and often achievable, are less predictable than pain relief because tear size, quality of tissue, biologic healing potential, and irreversible muscle atrophy are not controllable.[41]

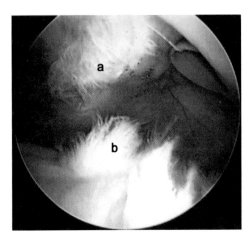

Fig. 63.11 **Subacromial impingement.** Arthroscopic evaluation of the subacromial space shows a subacromial spur (a) and fraying of the rotator cuff underneath (b).

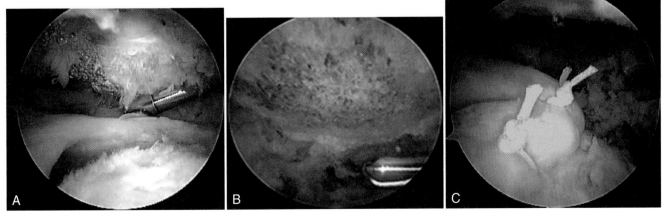

Fig. 63.13 Example of a full-thickness tear and a subacromial spur (A) treated with arthroscopic acromioplasty (B) and rotator cuff repair (C).

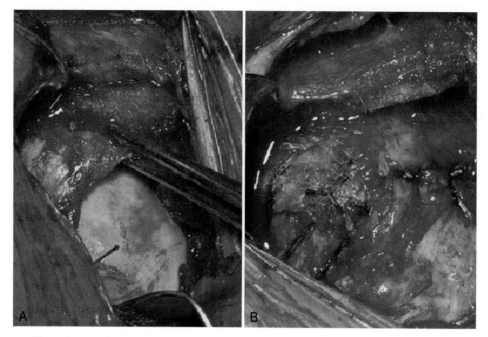

Fig. 63.14 Mini-open cuff repair. A and B, In arthroscopy-assisted rotator cuff repair, bursectomy, acromioplasty, and cuff mobilization can be achieved with arthroscopic techniques. Through a mini-open incision, the cuff is repaired to the greater tuberosity.

Conclusion

Disorders of the rotator cuff are a common cause of anterior shoulder pain. Although the primary etiology of rotator cuff disease may still be debated, it is likely that for each individual patient the cause is multifactorial and probably includes some components of extrinsic and intrinsic injury. If the origin is multifactorial, then treatments should be tailored toward whichever cause is thought to dominate the clinical picture.

A careful history and physical examination are crucial for diagnosing the source of injury. The age, occupation, and handedness of the patient and the onset, duration, timing, severity, quality, exacerbation, and relief of symptoms are important differentiating factors. Night pain and weakness are associated with tendon tears. Younger patients should be asked about their sports and activities and the relation of their symptoms to specific activities. A younger patient is more likely to have an underlying instability, whereas an older patient is more likely to have a mechanical or degenerative source of pain. Physical examination can test for specific cuff muscle weakness and intra-articular disease, as opposed to extra-articular sources of pain. Radicular pain from the cervical spine should always be considered as a source of shoulder symptoms. Adjunctive studies including plain radiographs and MRI are an integral part of the evaluation and help determine the source and extent of injury. Ultrasound is also a useful, noninvasive method for diagnosing rotator cuff disease.

Treatment is tailored to each individual patient's pathologic process. Although nonoperative modalities such as physical therapy, anti-inflammatory agents, and corticosteroid injections are successful, some patients require operative intervention. Both open and arthroscopic surgical procedures are highly successful for treating rotator cuff disease. Arthroscopy has improved clinicians' ability to define the pathologic features and treat many lesions more precisely, and it has become the technique of choice for most shoulder specialists.

References

Full references for this chapter can be found on www.expertconsult.com.

Acromioclavicular Joint Pain

Steven D. Waldman

The acromioclavicular joint is a common source of shoulder pain (**Fig. 64.1**).[1] This joint is vulnerable to injury from acute trauma and repeated microtrauma. Acute injuries frequently take the form of falls directly onto the shoulder when playing sports or falling from bicycles. Repeated strain from throwing injuries or working with the arm raised across the body also may result in trauma to the joint. After trauma, the joint may become acutely inflamed; if the condition becomes chronic, arthritis and osteolysis of the acromioclavicular joint may develop.[2]

Signs and Symptoms

A patient with acromioclavicular joint dysfunction frequently complains of pain when reaching across the chest (**Fig. 64.2**). Often the patient is unable to sleep on the affected shoulder and may complain of a grinding sensation in the joint, especially on first awakening. Physical examination may reveal enlargement or swelling of the joint with tenderness to palpation. Downward traction or passive adduction of the affected shoulder may cause increased pain (**Fig. 64.3**). If the ligaments of the acromioclavicular joint are disrupted, these maneuvers may reveal joint instability.

Testing

Plain radiographs of the joint may reveal narrowing or sclerosis of the joint consistent with osteoarthritis. Magnetic resonance imaging is indicated if disruption of the ligaments is suspected. The injection technique described subsequently is both a diagnostic and a therapeutic maneuver. If polyarthritis is present, screening laboratory testing, including complete blood count, erythrocyte sedimentation rate, and antinuclear antibody testing, should be performed.

Differential Diagnosis

Osteoarthritis of the acromioclavicular joint is a frequent cause of shoulder pain. This condition is usually the result of trauma. Rheumatoid arthritis and rotator cuff tear arthropathy also are common causes of shoulder pain that may mimic the pain of acromioclavicular joint pain and may confuse the diagnosis.[3] Less common causes of arthritis-induced shoulder pain include collagen vascular diseases, infection, and Lyme disease. Acute infectious arthritis usually is accompanied by significant systemic symptoms, including fever and malaise, and should be recognized easily by the astute clinician and treated appropriately with culture and antibiotics, rather than by injection therapy. The collagen vascular diseases generally manifest with polyarthropathy, rather than with monoarthropathy limited to the shoulder joint, although shoulder pain secondary to collagen vascular disease responds well to the intra-articular injection technique described subsequently.

Treatment

Initial treatment of pain and functional disability associated with the acromioclavicular joint should include a combination of the nonsteroidal anti-inflammatory drugs (NSAIDs) or cyclooxygenase-2 (COX-2) inhibitors and physical therapy. The local application of heat and cold also may be beneficial. For patients who do not respond to these treatment modalities, an intra-articular injection of local anesthetic and steroid may be a reasonable next step.[4]

Intra-articular injection of the acromioclavicular joint is performed by placing the patient in the supine position and preparing with antiseptic solution of the skin overlying the superior shoulder and distal clavicle. A sterile syringe containing 1 mL of 0.25% preservative-free bupivacaine and 40 mg of methylprednisolone is attached to a 1½-inch 25-gauge needle, and strict aseptic technique is used. With strict aseptic technique, the top of the acromion is identified, and at a point approximately 1 inch medially, the acromioclavicular joint space is identified. The needle is carefully advanced through the skin and subcutaneous tissues, through the joint capsule, and into the joint (**Fig. 64.4**). If bone is encountered, the needle is withdrawn into the subcutaneous tissues and is redirected slightly more medially. After the joint space is entered, the contents of the syringe are gently injected. Some resistance to injection should be felt because the joint space

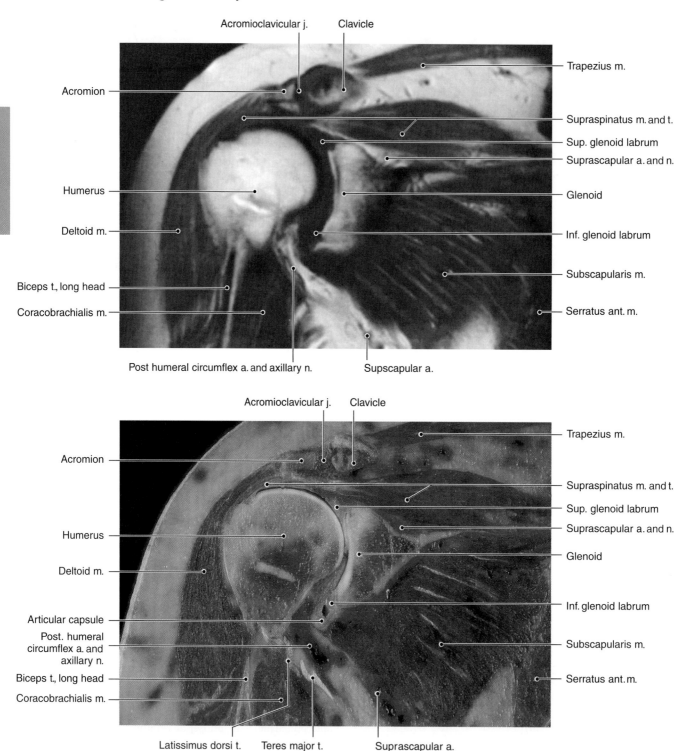

Acromioclavicular j.   Clavicle

Acromion

Humerus

Deltoid m.

Biceps t., long head

Coracobrachialis m.

Post humeral circumflex a. and axillary n.   Supscapular a.

Trapezius m.

Supraspinatus m. and t.

Sup. glenoid labrum

Suprascapular a. and n.

Glenoid

Inf. glenoid labrum

Subscapularis m.

Serratus ant. m.

Acromioclavicular j.   Clavicle

Acromion

Humerus

Deltoid m.

Articular capsule

Post. humeral circumflex a. and axillary n.

Biceps t., long head

Coracobrachialis m.

Latissimus dorsi t.   Teres major t.   Suprascapular a.

Trapezius m.

Supraspinatus m. and t.

Sup. glenoid labrum

Suprascapular a. and n.

Glenoid

Inf. glenoid labrum

Subscapularis m.

Serratus ant. m.

Fig. 64.1 **Acromioclavicular joint.** *(From Kang HS, Ahn JM, Resnick D: Shoulder. In MRI of the extremities, ed 2, Philadelphia, 2002, Saunders, p 8.)*

is small, and the joint capsule is dense. If significant resistance is encountered, the needle is probably in a ligament and should be advanced slightly into the joint space until the injection proceeds with only limited resistance. If no resistance is encountered on injection, the joint space is probably not intact, and magnetic resonance imaging is recommended. The needle is removed, and a sterile pressure dressing and ice pack are placed at the injection site.

The major complication of intra-articular injection of the acromioclavicular joint is infection. This complication should be exceedingly rare if strict aseptic technique is followed. Approximately 25% of patients complain of a transient increase in pain after intra-articular injection of the shoulder joint, and patients should be warned of this possibility.

This injection technique is extremely effective in the treatment of pain secondary to the foregoing causes of arthritis of

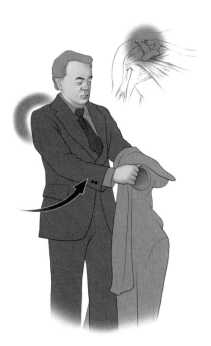

Fig. 64.2 A patient with acromioclavicular joint dysfunction frequently complains of pain when reaching across the chest. *(From Waldman SD: Acromioclavicular joint pain.* In Atlas of common pain syndromes, *ed 2, Philadelphia, 2008, Saunders, p 78.)*

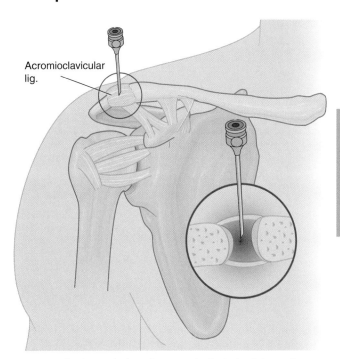

Acromioclavicular lig.

Fig. 64.4 **Injection technique for acromioclavicular joint pain.** *(From Waldman SD: Acromioclavicular joint pain.* In Atlas of pain management injection techniques, *ed 2, Philadelphia, 2007, Saunders, p 63.)*

the acromioclavicular joint. Coexistent bursitis and tendinitis also may contribute to shoulder pain and may require additional treatment with more localized injection of local anesthetic and depot steroid.[2] This technique is a safe procedure if careful attention is paid to the clinically relevant anatomy in the areas to be injected. Care must be taken to use sterile technique to avoid infection and universal precautions to avoid risk to the operator. The incidence of ecchymosis and hematoma formation can be decreased if pressure is placed on the injection site immediately after injection. The use of physical modalities, including local heat and gentle range-of-motion exercises, should be introduced several days after the patient undergoes this injection technique for shoulder pain. Vigorous exercises should be avoided because they exacerbate the patient's symptoms. Simple analgesics and NSAIDs or COX-2 inhibitors may be used concurrently with this injection technique.

Conclusion

Acromioclavicular joint pain is commonly encountered in clinical practice. It may manifest as an independent diagnosis after trauma to the shoulder, but more frequently it is a component of more complex shoulder dysfunction, including impingement syndromes and rotator cuff disease. Careful physical examination and confirmatory radiographic imaging usually confirm the diagnosis. If conservative treatment fails, injection of the acromioclavicular joint with local anesthetic and steroid is a reasonable next step.

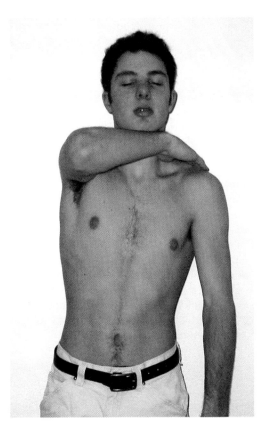

Fig. 64.3 **The chin adduction test for acromioclavicular joint dysfunction.** *(From Waldman SD:* Physical diagnosis of pain: an atlas of signs and symptoms, *Philadelphia, 2006, Saunders, p 105.)*

References

Full references for this chapter can be found on www.expertconsult.com.

Chapter 65

Subdeltoid Bursitis

Steven D. Waldman

Inflammation of the subdeltoid bursa is a common cause of shoulder pain and functional disability.[1] The subdeltoid bursa is vulnerable to injury from both acute trauma and repeated microtrauma. Acute injuries frequently take the form of direct trauma to the shoulder when playing sports or falling from bicycles. Repeated strain from throwing injuries, bowling, carrying a heavy briefcase, working with the arm raised across the body, rotator cuff injuries, or repetitive motion associated with assembly line work may result in inflammation of the subdeltoid bursa. The subdeltoid bursa lies primarily under the acromion and extends laterally between the deltoid muscle and the joint capsule under the deltoid muscle. It may exist as a single bursal sac or in some patients may exist as a multisegmented series of sacs that may be loculated (**Fig. 65.1**). If the inflammation of the subdeltoid bursa becomes chronic, calcification of the bursa may occur.

The patient suffering from subdeltoid bursitis frequently complains of pain with any movement of the shoulder, but especially with abduction.[2] The pain is localized to the subdeltoid area, with referred pain often noted at the insertion of the deltoid at the deltoid tuberosity on the upper third of the humerus (**Fig. 65.2**). Often, the patient is unable to sleep on the affected shoulder and may complain of a sharp, catching sensation when abducting the shoulder, especially on first awakening.

Signs and Symptoms

Physical examination may reveal point tenderness over the acromion, and occasionally swelling of the bursa gives the affected deltoid muscle an edematous feel.[1] Passive elevation and medial rotation of the affected shoulder reproduce the pain, as do resisted abduction and lateral rotation. Sudden release of resistance during this maneuver markedly increases the pain. Rotator cuff tear may mimic or coexist with subdeltoid bursitis and may confuse the diagnosis (see the later section on differential diagnosis).

Testing

Plain radiographs of the shoulder may reveal calcification of the bursa and associated structures consistent with chronic inflammation (see Fig. 65.1). Magnetic resonance imaging scan is indicated if tendinitis, partial disruption of the ligaments, or rotator cuff tear is suspected. Based on the patient's clinical presentation, additional testing including complete blood count, erythrocyte sedimentation rate, and antinuclear antibody testing may be indicated. Radionucleotide bone scan is indicated if metastatic disease or primary tumor involving the shoulder is being considered. The injection technique described later serves as both a diagnostic and a therapeutic maneuver.

Differential Diagnosis

Subdeltoid bursitis is one of the most common forms of arthritis that results in shoulder joint pain. However, osteoarthritis, rheumatoid arthritis, post-traumatic arthritis, and rotator cuff tear arthropathy are also common causes of shoulder pain secondary to arthritis. Less common causes of arthritis-induced shoulder pain include the connective tissue diseases, infection, villonodular synovitis, and Lyme disease.[3,4] Acute infectious arthritis is usually accompanied by significant systemic symptoms including fever and malaise and should be easily recognized by the astute clinician and treated appropriately with culture and antibiotics, rather than by injection therapy. The connective tissue diseases generally manifest with polyarthropathy rather than monoarthropathy limited to the shoulder joint, although shoulder pain secondary to connective tissue disease responds exceedingly well to the injection technique described subsequently.

Treatment

Initial treatment of the pain and functional disability associated with osteoarthritis of the shoulder should include a combination of the nonsteroidal anti-inflammatory drugs

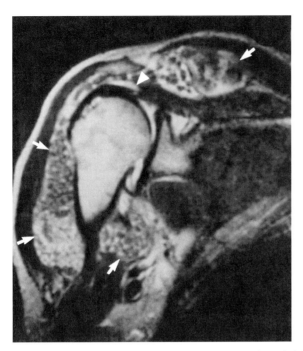

Fig. 65.1 **Abnormalities of bursae in rheumatoid arthritis.** Subdeltoid-subacromial bursitis. T2-weighted (TR/TE, 2000/80) coronal oblique spin-echo magnetic resonance image reveals a markedly distended bursa (*arrows*). Note the increase in signal intensity of fluid in the joint and in the bursa; however, regions of low signal density remain in the bursa. At surgery, these areas were found to be small fibrous nodules, or rice bodies. Also note the tear of the supraspinatus tendon (*arrowhead*), which may represent a complication of rheumatoid arthritis. *(Courtesy of J Hodler, MD, Zurich, Switzerland. From Resnick D, Kransdorf MJ, editors: Bone and joint imaging, ed 3, Philadelphia, 2004, Saunders, p 214.)*

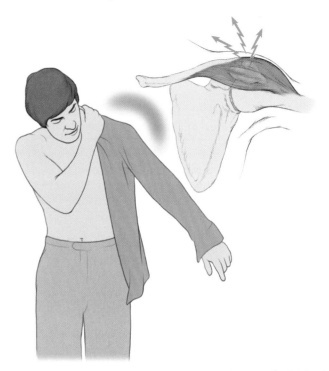

Fig. 65.2 Abduction of the shoulder exacerbates the pain of subdeltoid bursitis. *(From Waldman SD: Atlas of common pain syndromes, ed 2, Philadelphia, 2008, Saunders, p 82.)*

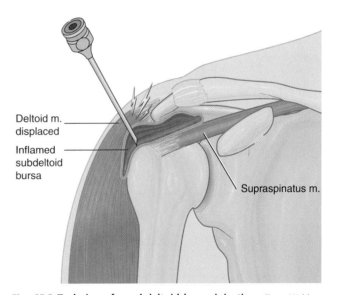

Deltoid m. displaced

Inflamed subdeltoid bursa

Supraspinatus m.

Fig. 65.3 **Technique for subdeltoid bursa injection.** *(From Waldman SD: Atlas of pain management injection techniques, ed 2, Philadelphia, 2007, Saunders, p 110.)*

(NSAIDs) or cyclooxygenase-2 (COX-2) inhibitors and physical therapy. The local application of heat and cold may also be beneficial. For patients who do not respond to these treatment modalities, an intra-articular injection of local anesthetic and steroid may be a reasonable next step.[5]

Injection of the subdeltoid bursa is performed by placing the patient in the supine position; proper preparation with antiseptic solution of the skin overlying the superior shoulder, acromion, and distal clavicle is performed. A sterile syringe containing 4.0 mL of 0.25% preservative-free bupivacaine and 40 mg of methylprednisolone is attached to a 1½-inch 25-gauge needle, and strict aseptic technique is used. With strict aseptic technique, the lateral edge of the acromion is identified, and at the midpoint of the lateral edge, the injection site is identified. At this point, the needle is carefully advanced in a slightly cephalad trajectory through the skin and subcutaneous tissues beneath the acromion capsule into the bursa (**Fig. 65.3**). If bone is encountered, the needle is withdrawn into the subcutaneous tissues and is redirected slightly more inferiorly. After the bursa has been entered, the contents of the syringe are gently injected while the operator slowly withdraws the needle. Resistance to injection should be minimal unless calcification of the bursal sac is present. Calcification of the bursal sac is identified as resistance to needle advancement with an associated gritty feel. Significant calcific bursitis may ultimately require surgical excision to effect complete relief of symptoms.

The needle is then removed, and a sterile pressure dressing and ice pack are placed at the injection site.

The major complication of injection of the subdeltoid bursa is infection. This complication should be exceedingly rare if strict aseptic technique is followed. Approximately 25% of patients complain of a transient increase in pain following injection of the subdeltoid bursa, and patients should be warned of this possibility.

This injection technique is extremely effective in the treatment of pain secondary to subdeltoid bursitis. Coexistent arthritis and tendinitis may also contribute to shoulder pain and may require additional treatment with more localized injection of local anesthetic and depot steroid. This technique is a safe procedure if careful attention is paid to the clinically relevant anatomy in the areas to be injected. Care must be taken to use sterile technique to avoid infection and to use universal precautions to avoid risk to the operator. The incidence of ecchymosis and hematoma formation can be decreased if pressure is placed on the injection site immediately following injection. The use of physical modalities including local heat and gentle range-of-motion exercises should be introduced several days after the patient undergoes this injection technique for shoulder pain. Vigorous exercises should be avoided because they exacerbate the patients' symptoms. Simple analgesics and NSAIDs may be used concurrently with this injection technique.

Conclusion

The pain of subdeltoid bursitis is commonly encountered in clinical practice. It may manifest as an independent diagnosis following trauma to the shoulder, but more frequently it occurs as a component of more complex shoulder dysfunction including arthritis, impingement syndromes, and rotator cuff disease. Careful physical examination combined with confirmatory radiographic imaging usually confirms the diagnosis. If conservative treatment fails, injection of the subdeltoid bursa with local anesthetic and steroid is a reasonable next step.

References

Full references for this chapter can be found on www.expertconsult.com.

Biceps Tendinitis

Robert Trout

Historical Considerations

The role of the biceps tendon in shoulder pain was controversial in the literature for most of the twentieth century. The earliest descriptions of bicipital tendinitis as a clinical entity were a series of articles by Meyer in the 1920s,[1,2] in which he reported spontaneous subluxations and degeneration of the tendon. Many investigators remained skeptical regarding the concept of the biceps tendon as a primary source of pain in the shoulder, and numerous articles were published that either supported or refuted the idea.[3,4] In hindsight, both groups may have been partly correct. In the 1970s, Neer[5] was the first to describe biceps tendinitis as a secondary manifestation of impingement syndrome. Thus, the biceps tendon does not usually act as a primary pain generator in the shoulder, but rather acts in association with other shoulder diseases, most notably rotator cuff disorders. Numerous later studies supported this finding and eventually led to the classification of primary and secondary bicipital tendinitis.[6,7] Secondary tendinitis, occurring in association with other underlying shoulder problems, is the most common type and may account for approximately 95% of cases.[8] Primary tendinitis, in which the patient has an isolated problem of the biceps tendon, is often seen in younger patients and may be related to abnormality of the bicipital groove, possibly from previous trauma. These patients are at high risk for eventual rupture of the tendon.

Initially, articles focused on tenodesis of the tendon as the definitive treatment of the problem.[9] However, this approach eventually fell out of favor because of the high failure rate.[10] More recently, arthroscopy was combined with tenodesis and acromioplasty, with better results. However, the main focus has been on early conservative treatment, with surgery considered in selected cases only.

Signs and Symptoms

Although tendinitis implies an inflammatory condition, biceps tendinitis is usually a primarily degenerative problem because the tendon is subject to wear and tear under the coracoacromial arch, similar to the process observed in the rotator cuff (**Fig. 66.1**).[5] The most common symptom is pain in the anterior shoulder that may radiate to the biceps muscle and worsen with overhead activities. Patients often report significant nighttime pain. Usually, they have no history of a specific traumatic event. Throwing athletes, in particular, also develop instability of the biceps tendon. They experience an audible pop or snap while moving through their throwing motion.

On physical examination, the most common finding is point tenderness in the bicipital groove. The point of tenderness should move as the shoulder is passively internally and externally rotated. Other provocative tests that are specific for bicipital tendinitis include the Speed test and the Yergason test. In the Speed test, the patient holds the elbow in extension with the forearm supinated and then flexes the shoulder against resistance, thus reproducing the patient's pain (**Fig. 66.2**).[8] When performing the Yergason test, the patient supinates the forearm against resistance with the forearm flexed (**Fig. 66.3**). A positive test result occurs when pain refers to the bicipital groove.[8] Instability should be evaluated by placing the arm in abduction and external rotation and then slowly bringing it down to the patient's side. A palpable snap signifies a positive test result as the tendon subluxes.

Because of the high percentage of other common shoulder disorders that occur in association with bicipital tendinitis, a full shoulder examination should always be performed. This examination should include passive and active range of motion, subdeltoid bursal and acromioclavicular joint tenderness, and other provocative testing for impingement syndrome and rotator cuff tears.

Testing

Initial testing consists of plain films of the shoulder. These radiographs are usually unremarkable, but they can detect glenohumeral arthritis, fracture, or articular abnormalities from previous trauma. In addition, calcific tendinitis of the biceps tendon has been reported rarely and may be visible on plain films. If this finding is present, arthroscopic débridement of the tendon may be required.[11] A biceps groove view can also be performed to evaluate for spurring of the groove, which many predispose a patient to primary tendinitis.

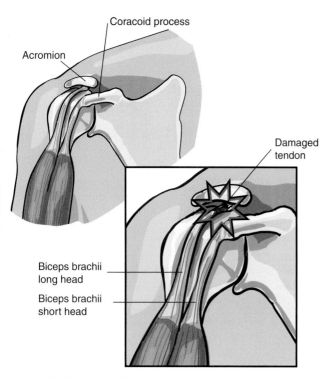

Fig. 66.1 The long head of the biceps may be subjected to wear and tear under the acromion arch.

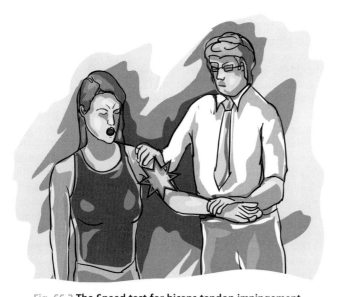

Fig. 66.2 **The Speed test for biceps tendon impingement.**

For patients with persistent symptoms or when tendon rupture is suspected, magnetic resonance imaging (MRI) is the most sensitive and specific test. Although MRI is expensive, it is the standard for imaging of the joint and surrounding tendons. It can elucidate both edema and full and partial tears of the biceps tendon while also identifying rotator cuff and labral disorders.

For patients unable to undergo an MRI scan, other possible alternatives include computed tomography (CT) scan, ultrasound, and arthrography. CT is useful to evaluate for bony lesions when ruling out other possible causes of pain, such as humeral fractures or acromioclavicular joint disease, but this imaging technique cannot adequately detect soft tissue damage. As a result, it has only limited use during attempts to make a definitive diagnosis. Arthrography and CT arthrography

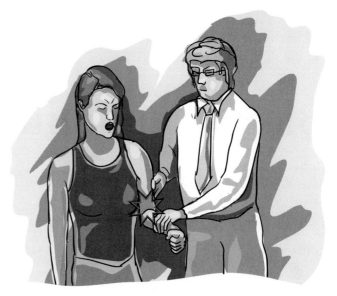

Fig. 66.3 **The Yergason test for biceps tendon impingement.**

may detect full-thickness tendon tears, but they lack sensitivity for partial-thickness tears, particularly if the joint does not adequately fill with contrast material. These methods are also invasive. Ultrasound is noninvasive and inexpensive and may have a role in initial testing. Ultrasound is able to reveal both rotator cuff and bicipital tendon tears. However, its sensitivity varies widely among institutions because the technique is highly operator dependent. Ultrasound is also unable to reveal labral disease.

Rarely, primary tendinitis may occur secondary to a generalized inflammatory or autoimmune condition. If the patient's shoulder symptoms are accompanied by signs of synovitis or arthritis in other joints, routine laboratory tests should also be considered including erythrocyte sedimentation rate, antinuclear antibody, and rheumatoid factor.

Differential Diagnosis

The temptation to diagnose a case of anterior shoulder pain rapidly as tendinitis should be resisted because biceps tendinitis is often secondary to other types of shoulder disorders such as impingement syndrome and rotator cuff disorders. **Table 66.1** lists the differential diagnosis of bicipital tendinitis. Patients with other neuropathic and neoplastic conditions may also exhibit radiating or referred pain to the anterior shoulder that may mimic a simple case of tendinitis. Fortunately, these problems can usually be identified with an adequate history and physical examination.

Impingement syndrome is typified by the "painful arc" of 60 to 120 degrees of active abduction. A helpful test is the *Neer sign,* in which the patient's pronated arm is brought into full flexion, thus causing impingement under the acromion and reproducing the painful symptoms. Patients with adhesive capsulitis and glenohumeral osteoarthritis exhibit decreased passive and active range of motion in all planes. Some patients with long-standing bicipital tendinitis may eventually develop adhesive capsulitis.

Clicking of the shoulder with overhead movements or a positive *clunk sign* may indicate labral disease. Provocative tests, such as the *Hawkins test,* may identify a rotator cuff

Table 66.1 **Differential Diagnosis of Bicipital Tendinitis**
Bicipital rupture
Impingement syndrome/rotator cuff tear
Glenohumeral arthritis
Adhesive capsulitis
Acromioclavicular joint arthritis
Cervical radiculopathy
Brachial plexitis
Autoimmune/systemic inflammatory disorders
Pancoast's tumor/metastatic disease

disorder by eliciting pain when the patient's arm is raised to 90 degrees and the shoulder is then internally rotated.

Pain that localizes more to the top of the shoulder may be an indication of acromioclavicular joint arthritis and often worsens with abduction of greater than 120 degrees. This pain can be reproduced with the *cross-arm test,* in which the patient raises the arm to 90 degrees and then actively adducts it.

Pain radiating distal to the elbow or other associated symptoms of numbness and paresthesias are typical of a radicular origin or brachial plexitis. Radicular pain is often exacerbated by coughing or sneezing, whereas a common presentation of brachial plexitis is acute pain followed within 2 weeks by weakness in the upper extremity. If these diagnoses are suspected, electrodiagnostic studies or cervical imaging may be considered.

Treatment

Initial treatment for both primary and secondary bicipital tendinitis is conservative, with rest, icing, and anti-inflammatory medications. Several studies advocated the use of subacromial and glenohumeral steroid injections. This approach is logical given the high incidence of associated impingement syndrome and that the tendon of the long head is intra-articular.

For patients with primary tendinitis, injection into the biceps tendon sheath can be beneficial (**Fig. 66.4**). The technique for this injection is not difficult, but the procedure should be performed carefully to avoid direct injection into the tendon, which can increase the potential for tendon rupture. The patient is placed in the supine position with the shoulder externally rotated 45 degrees. Doses for the injection can vary among specialties, particularly between surgeons and nonsurgeons.[12] However, in a typical injection, a small volume of fluid is used, with 1.0 mL of 0.25% bupivacaine and 40 mg methylprednisolone in a sterile syringe attached to a 1½-inch 25-gauge needle. The insertion of the bicipital tendon is found by first identifying the coracoid process and then palpating the lesser tuberosity slightly lateral to it. The needle is slowly advanced until it hits bone, and then it is withdrawn 1 to 2 mm. The medication is injected, and the operator should feel a small amount of resistance. If no resistance is felt, the needle is probably in the joint space. If resistance is significant, the needle may be within the tendon itself and should be withdrawn slightly.[13]

Once symptoms improve, physical therapy is initiated with range-of-motion exercises progressing to rotator cuff

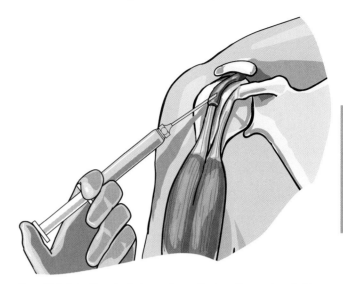

Fig. 66.4 **Injection technique for relieving the pain of biceps tendinitis.**

strengthening for patients with impingement syndrome. For patients with significant instability or with recalcitrant symptoms despite appropriate treatment, referral to an orthopedist may be needed for possible arthroscopy of the shoulder with or without tenodesis of the tendon.

Complications and Pitfalls

The most likely pitfall that should be avoided is bicipital tendon rupture. Most tendon ruptures occur in tendons previously degenerated and frayed from prolonged wear and tear under the acromial arch. These patients are most often older and will give a history of chronic shoulder pain that improved after a sudden and brief episode of severe pain in the anterior shoulder. A large amount of bruising may be present, as well as a palpable lump in the biceps region. Tendon rupture purely secondary to acute trauma is rare.

Complications after injection, such as infection and hematoma, are rare if proper aseptic technique is used. The incidence of hematoma can be reduced by applying direct pressure immediately after the injection and by taking extra precautions with patients who take anticoagulants or have clotting disorders.

Conclusion

Bicipital tendinitis is a common cause of anterior shoulder pain that is seen mostly in individuals who have some other type of intra-articular disorder or abnormality. Patients exhibit tenderness at the insertion of the tendon, and they report increased pain with active shoulder movements, most significantly flexion. Radiographs are most often unremarkable, although an MRI scan may demonstrate an inflamed or degenerated tendon and rule out other problems such as labral disease or rotator cuff tear. Response to conservative treatment is generally excellent with anti-inflammatory medication, relative rest, injections, and gradual return to activity with physical therapy.

References

Full references for this chapter can be found on www.expertconsult.com.

Chapter 67

Scapulocostal Syndrome

Bernard M. Abrams

The scapulocostal syndrome, also known as the levator scapulae syndrome, is a common painful musculoskeletal syndrome that mainly affects the posterior shoulder area; however, because of the pattern of pain radiation, it can mimic numerous other conditions including cervical radicular pain, intrinsic shoulder joint disease, and even visceral pain. This syndrome can be diagnosed clinically with a careful history and physical examination. No blood test abnormalities or neurophysiologic or imaging abnormalities are associated with the syndrome, but these tests may be useful in eliminating other entities from diagnostic consideration.

Historical Considerations

The scapulocostal syndrome was first described by Michele et al in 1950.[1] These investigators pointed out that, during the preceding 3 years, 30% of all middle-aged individuals presenting with shoulder complaints had this syndrome. Michele et al also described the syndrome's protean manifestations and pain radiation patterns. They noted that pain could radiate to the occiput or spinous processes of C3 and C4, it could appear to originate at the root of the neck and radiate into the shoulder joint, or it could radiate down the arm into the hand, usually along the posteromedial aspect of the upper arm and along the ulnar distribution in the forearm and hand. These investigators pointed out that the pain alternatively could radiate along the course of the fourth and fifth intercostal nerves and could mimic angina pectoris on the left and cholecystitis on the right. Finally, the patient could present with any combination of the foregoing symptoms and signs (**Fig. 67.1**). After some initial interest in this syndrome between 1956 and 1968,[2–5] interest languished until the 1980s and early 1990s, when attention turned to the anatomy of this region.

The Clinical Syndrome: Signs, Symptoms, and Physical Findings

The hallmark of the scapulocostal syndrome is pain. The pain may be localized to the medial superior border of the scapula, or it may radiate up into the neck and cause headache. It can

also cause pain into the root of the shoulder that simulates rotator cuff syndrome or other shoulder disorders. It can radiate around the chest wall or down the arm, usually in an ulnar nerve distribution. The characteristic pattern is that of acute pain localized in the upper trunk. The patient may complain of radicular-type pain, with or without sensory features.[4,6] Although weakness of the arm and shoulder may be offered as complaints, this weakness is usually a result of guarding, without atrophy or neurophysiologic evidence of denervation on electromyography. The pain has been described variously as aching, burning, or gnawing, and rarely as sharp or radicular. The symptoms may be intermittent, but a nagging, constant quality is not uncommon. Insomnia is a frequent complaint because patients cannot find a comfortable sleeping position.

The original article by Michele et al[1] cited an equal distribution between the sexes. Since that time, most observers have noted a female predominance, as well as a predominance in the dominant shoulder. Clerical occupation, rounded shoulders, large and pendulous breasts, and the carrying of personal items including handbags are often implicated.

Russek[7] classified the syndrome into three types: (1) primary, probably postural in origin; (2) secondary, a complication of preexisting neck or shoulder lesions; and (3) static, occurring in severely disabled patients who are unable to control the scapulothoracic relationship.

Muscular, reflex, or sympathetic, or sensory findings are usually absent in the examination. The classic finding is a trigger point elicited by digital pressure at the medial scapular border in a line extending from the scapular spine. This trigger point (**Fig. 67.2**) may be missed (both diagnostically and therapeutically), unless the arm is adducted, with the palm of the affected hand flat on the opposite shoulder and crossing in front of the chest (**Fig. 67.3**). Alternatively, extension and internal rotation of the arm also elicit the pain (**Fig. 67.4**) Secondary trigger points may be found in the trapezius and rhomboid muscles (**Fig. 67.5**).[1] Diffuse tenderness over the chest wall is usually mild.

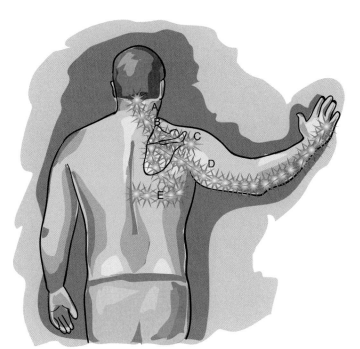

Fig. 67.1 **Patterns of pain radiation.** A, The pain radiates into the occiput. B, The pain is originating at the root of the neck and radiates into the shoulder joint. C and D, The pain radiates along the posteromedial aspect of the upper arm and the ulnar distribution of the forearm. Traction on the lower trunk of the brachial plexus as it passes over the first rib produces pain and numbness in the ulnar distribution of the hand and fingers. E, The pain may radiate into the fourth and fifth thoracic nerves because of the exaggerated lumbar lordosis. *(Adapted from Michele AA, Davies JJ, Krueger FJ, et al: Scapulocostal syndrome [fatigue-postural paradox], N Y J Med 50:1353, 1950.)*

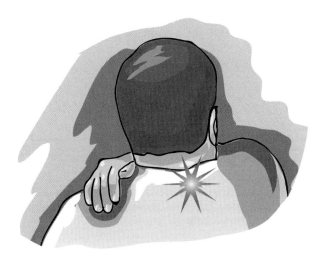

Fig. 67.2 **The trigger point.** *(Adapted from Ormandy L: Scapulocostal syndrome, Va Med Q 121:105, 1994.)*

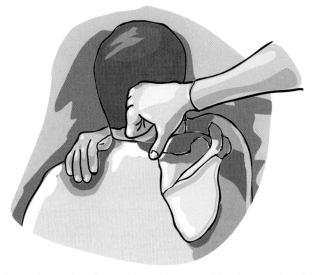

Fig. 67.3 Location of the trigger point area of tenderness when the scapula has been retracted from the posterior chest wall. *(Adapted from Michele AA, Davies JJ, Krueger FJ, et al: Scapulocostal syndrome [fatigue-postural paradox], N Y J Med 50:1353, 1950.)*

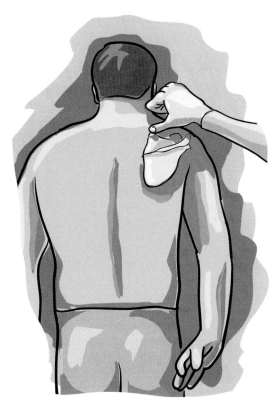

Fig. 67.4 Deep pressure over the superior medial angle of the scapula with compression of the posterior chest wall in conjunction with backward extension of the internally rotated arm. *(Adapted from Michele AA, Davies JJ, Krueger FJ, et al: Scapulocostal syndrome [fatigue-postural paradox], N Y J Med 50:1353, 1950.)*

Consistent biochemical, rheumatologic, radiologic, or neurophysiologic (electromyographic) findings have not been reported. One study reported increased heat emission from the upper medial angle of the affected shoulder on thermography in more than 60% of patients.[8] Reproduction of the pain by palpation and relief by local anesthetic infiltration are the essential elements of this syndrome.

Clinically Relevant Anatomy

The constant location of the pain in the deep trigger point seems to indicate that the levator scapulae muscle is involved in this syndrome (**Fig. 67.6**). Considerable controversy exists about the constancy of a bursa in connection with the levator scapulae,

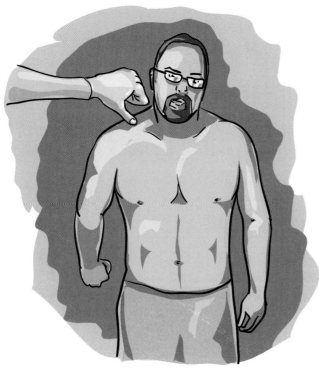

Fig. 67.5 Digital pressure underneath midbelly of the descending fibers of the trapezius toward the anterior surface of the superior medial angle of the scapula. Reinforcement by internal rotation and backward flexion of the arm. (*Adapted from Michele AA, Davies JJ, Krueger FJ, et al: Scapulocostal syndrome [fatigue-postural paradox], N Y J Med 50:1353, 1950.*)

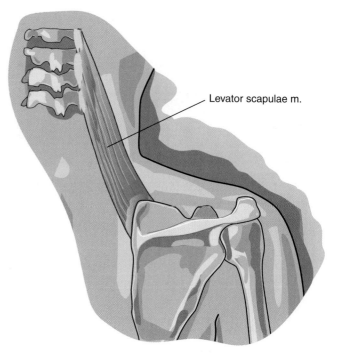

Fig. 67.6 **Levator scapulae.** Origin: transverse process of C1-C4 vertebrae; insertion: vertebral border of scapula between the medial angle and root of the spine. (*Adapted from Quiring DP, Boyle BA, Boroush EL, et al: The extremities, with 106 engravings, Philadelphia, 1945, Lea & Febiger.*)

Table 67.1 Three Layers of the Scapulothoracic Articulation

Structure	Superficial	Intermediate	Deep
Muscles	Latissimus dorsi Trapezius	Levator scapulae Rhomboid minor Rhomboid major	Subscapularis Serratus anterior
Bursae	Inferior angle (number 1) 4 of 8 specimens	Superomedial angle (number 2) 8 of 8 specimens	Serratus space (number 3) 8 of 8 specimens Subscapularis space (number 4) 5 of 8 specimens
Nerves		Spinal accessory	

From Williams GR, Shakil M, Klimkiewicz J, et al: Anatomy of the scapulothoracic articulation, *Clin Orthop Relat Res* 359:237, 1999.

which may be inserted in two layers enfolding the medial border of the scapula, with a second bursa found in the areolar tissue between the two layers.[8] Williams et al[9] undertook a dissection of four frozen human cadavers and also noted that the surgical anatomy of the scapulothoracic region was described infrequently. These investigators pointed out that the scapulothoracic articulation had three layers (**Table 67.1**).[9] They described a superficial layer composed of the trapezius and latissimus dorsi muscles and an inconsistent bursa, which they found in four of eight specimens, between the inferior angle of the scapula and the superior fibers of the latissimus dorsi. These investigators then observed that the intermediate layer contained the rhomboid minor, rhomboid major, and levator scapulae muscles, along with the spinal accessory nerve, and a consistent bursa found in eight of eight specimens, between the superior medial scapula and the overlying trapezius. The deep layer consisted of the serratus anterior and subscapularis muscles in addition to two bursae. One of the two bursae was consistently located between the serratus anterior muscle and the thoracic cage, whereas the other was inconsistently located between the serratus anterior and subscapularis muscles. These relationships probably account for the clinical finding that turning the head opposite the affected limb reproduces the pain.

Differential Diagnosis

The differential diagnosis of pain in and about the scapula is extensive. Shoulder problems including rotator cuff disease, adhesive capsulitis, instability or arthritis of the glenohumeral joint, and vascular or neurogenic thoracic outlet syndrome may be at play.[10] The pain in these individuals is generally exacerbated by scapulothoracic movement, as well as by movements at the glenohumeral joint. Restriction of range of motion is frequent. Imaging of the shoulder with plain radiographs generally shows degenerative changes. Findings on magnetic resonance imaging or computed tomography arthrography may be definitive.

An entity known as the "snapping scapula" has been used to describe the clinical situation of tenderness at the superomedial angle of the scapula, painful scapulothoracic motion, and scapulothoracic crepitus.[10] Causes of snapping scapula include scapular exostosis, malunion of scapula or rib fracture, and Sprengel's deformity.[11,12]

Cervical radiculopathy can produce an aching pain into the scapula (protopathic pain), especially with C7 radiculopathy, which is associated with sharp (epicritic) pain down into the appropriate segment of the upper limb. In the case of C7 radiculopathy, pain usually descends the posterior aspect of the upper arm (triceps muscle) into the middle finger and is associated with weakness of the triceps and wrist extensors, diminution of the triceps reflex, and hypesthesia in the C7 dermatome.

Suprascapular nerve entrapment may produce deep, poorly circumscribed pain.[13] Because the suprascapular nerve is a motor nerve, the pain resulting from its irritation is deep and poorly circumscribed. This pain is roughly localized to the posterior and lateral aspects of the shoulder. When patients have an appreciable traction stress element on the upper trunk, they also have pain down the radial nerve axis. If the neuropathy has been present for a sufficient time, atrophy of the supraspinatus and infraspinatus muscles will be visible and palpable. This weakness is confirmed when patients have difficulty in initiating abduction and rotation at the glenohumeral joint. Most cases of suprascapular neuropathy are associated with an earlier motion impediment at this joint. Deep pressure toward the region of the suprascapular notch is painful. Motion of the scapula causes pain. The *cross-body adduction test,* performed by adducting the extended arm passively across the midline, is extremely painful because it lifts the scapular nerve away from the thoracic nerve and thereby tenses the suprascapular nerve. A suprascapular nerve block may be necessary for diagnosis. The region involved is somewhat lateral to the medial superior scapular border (at least three to four finger breadths in an average-sized person), so the tender area is clearly differentiated from the medial angle of the scapula where the levator scapulae muscle inserts in the scapulocostal syndrome (**Fig. 67.7**).

Treatment

Nonoperative treatment is sometimes successful in these patients. This treatment consists of activity modification, physical therapy, use of systemic anti-inflammatory medications, and injection into the region of the medial superior scapular border. Mixtures of 2 to 8 mL of plain 1% lidocaine HCl, in addition to 1 mL of betamethasone, followed by physical therapy exercises, have been advocated (**Fig. 67.8**).[14] Ormandy[14] treated 190 patients, 43% with one block, 40% with two blocks, and 17% with three blocks. On completion of treatment, approximately 98% of patients were relieved of pain and returned to their original occupations. Fourie[15] invoked the serratus posterior superior muscle, a member of the third muscle layer of the back. He used 1 mL of steroid and 1.8 mL of local anesthetic. In his report of 201 cases, conservative treatment was successful in

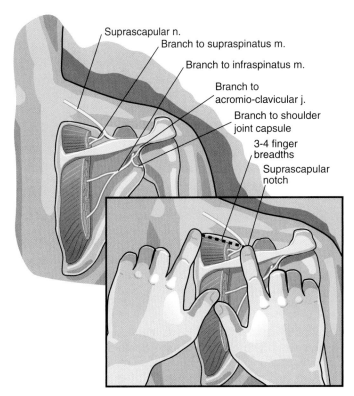

Fig. 67.7 Suprascapular nerve: motor and joint distribution. *(Adapted from Kopell HP, Thomspon WAL: Suprascapular entrapment neuropathy, Surg Gynecol Obstet 109:92, 1959.)*

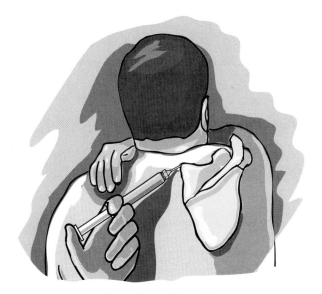

Fig. 67.8 Infiltration of the subscapular region. *(Adapted from Ormandy L: Scapulocostal syndrome, Va Med Q 121:105, 1994.)*

95.9% of patients. Very few writers on this subject mention that the arm needs to be cross-adducted or internally rotated and extended to move the scapula out of the way and expose the levator scapulae muscle at its insertion into the medial border of the scapula. If this maneuver is done, success is much more likely. The recommended approach is to use a 25-gauge needle at a 90-degree angle to reach underneath the scapula, to place the needle in the most lateral excursion of the scapula, and then to infiltrate while withdrawing the needle toward the medial superior scapula border.

Surgical options for patients who do not respond to nonoperative management include scapulothoracic bursectomy, excision of the superomedial angle of the scapula, and combined bursectomy and superior angle resection.[9,16,17] One report described the operative treatment of scapulothoracic bursitis in professional baseball pitchers, four of whom were operated on and returned to their pitching careers.[18] Endoscopic surgery has also been performed in the scapulothoracic region.[19,20] Results of surgery have been reported infrequently and inconsistently.[9]

Complications and Pitfalls

The major pitfall is a failure to diagnose this common and easily overlooked syndrome. A thorough history and a few simple physical diagnostic maneuvers involving the crossed adduction of the affected arm with palpation should be sufficient to make the diagnosis. Treatment can be unsuccessful if a similar posture for injection is not maintained, because one would be attempting to inject through the scapula itself, to reach the levator scapulae insertion or the putative bursa in this area. Once the clinician attempts to inject in this area, the possibility of pneumothorax should be kept in mind at all times, and the patient should be warned of this possibility and its potential consequences, including traction pneumothorax. Patients should be instructed to go the emergency room with any chest pain on inspiration. Operative techniques have their own associated risks and morbidity. However, inconclusive results up to this point have clouded the issue.

Conclusion

Scapulocostal syndrome is a common occurrence, especially in posturally compromised, middle-aged individuals, usually women, in particular persons with desk jobs or those whose vocations force them to extend their arms in front of them for prolonged periods. This syndrome has no definitive biologic markers. The differential diagnosis rests largely on ruling out cervical radiculopathy, intrinsic shoulder disease, osseous disease of the bony skeleton, and other afflictions of the scapula, including the snapping scapula syndrome and Sprengel's deformity. Scapulocostal syndrome is easily diagnosed and may be treated with a relative degree of success by injection therapy, which should be combined with physical therapy and alteration of lifestyle. Surgical treatment may be considered in refractory cases, but whether it is successful remains largely controversial.

References

Full references for this chapter can be found on www.expertconsult.com.

Part D

Elbow Pain Syndromes

Chapter 68

Tennis Elbow

Steven D. Waldman

Tennis elbow, also known as lateral epicondylitis, is caused by repetitive microtrauma to the extensor tendons of the forearm.[1] The pathophysiology of tennis elbow is initiated by micro-tearing at the origin of extensor carpi radialis and extensor carpi ulnaris (**Fig. 68.1**).[2] Secondary inflammation may occur and can become chronic as the result of continued overuse or misuse of the extensors of the forearm. Coexisting bursitis, arthritis, and gout may also perpetuate the pain and disability of tennis elbow.

Tennis elbow occurs in patients engaged in repetitive activities that include hand grasping (e.g., politicians shaking hands) or high-torque wrist turning (e.g., scooping ice cream at an ice cream parlor) (**Fig. 68.2**). Tennis players develop tennis elbow by two separate mechanisms: (1) increased pressure grip strain as a result of playing with too heavy a racquet and (2) making backhand shots with a leading shoulder and elbow rather than keeping the shoulder and elbow parallel to the net (**Fig. 68.3**). Other racquet sport players are also susceptible to the development of tennis elbow.

Signs and Symptoms

The pain of tennis elbow is localized to the region of the lateral epicondyle. It is constant and is made worse by active contraction of the wrist. Patients note the inability to hold a coffee cup or a hammer. Sleep disturbance is common. On physical examination, patients report tenderness along the extensor tendons at, or just below, the lateral epicondyle.[1] Many patients with tennis elbow have a bandlike thickening within the affected extensor tendons. Elbow range of motion is normal. Grip strength on the affected side is diminished. Patients with tennis elbow demonstrate a positive response to the *tennis elbow test*. The test is performed by stabilizing the patient's forearm and then having the patient clench his or her fist and actively extend the wrist. The examiner then attempts to force the wrist into flexion (**Fig. 68.4**). Sudden, severe pain is highly suggestive of tennis elbow.

Testing

Electromyography helps to distinguish cervical radiculopathy and radial tunnel syndrome from tennis elbow. Plain radiographs are indicated in all patients who present with tennis elbow, to rule out joint mice and other occult bony disorders. Based on the patient's clinical presentation, additional testing including complete blood count, uric acid, sedimentation rate, and antinuclear antibody testing may be indicated. Magnetic resonance imaging scan of the elbow is indicated if joint instability is suspected or if the patient's pain fails to respond to traditional treatment modalities (**Fig. 68.5**). The injection technique described subsequently serves as both a diagnostic and a therapeutic maneuver.

Differential Diagnosis

Radial tunnel syndrome and occasionally C6-7 radiculopathy can mimic tennis elbow. Radial tunnel syndrome is an entrapment neuropathy that results from entrapment of the radial nerve below the elbow. Radial tunnel syndrome can be distinguished from tennis elbow in that, in radial tunnel syndrome, the maximal tenderness to palpation is distal to the lateral epicondyle over the radial nerve, whereas in tennis elbow, the maximal tenderness to palpation is over the lateral epicondyle.[3]

The most common nidus of pain from tennis elbow is the bony origin of the extensor tendon of extensor carpi radialis brevis at the anterior facet of the lateral epicondyle. Less commonly, tennis elbow pain can originate from the extensor carpi radialis longus at the supracondylar crest or, rarely, more distally at the point where the extensor carpi radialis brevis overlies the radial head. As mentioned earlier, bursitis may accompany tennis elbow. The olecranon bursa lies in the posterior aspect of the elbow joint and may also become inflamed as a result of direct trauma or overuse of the joint. Other bursae susceptible to the development of bursitis exist between the insertion of the biceps and the head of the radius, as well as in the antecubital and cubital area.[4]

Treatment

Initial treatment of the pain and functional disability associated with tennis elbow should include a combination of the nonsteroidal anti-inflammatory agents or cyclooxygenase-2

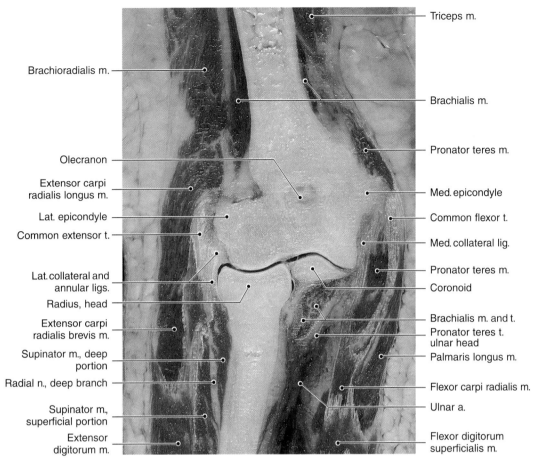

Brachioradialis m.

Olecranon

Extensor carpi
radialis longus m.

Lat. epicondyle

Common extensor t.

Lat. collateral and
annular ligs.

Radius, head

Extensor carpi
radialis brevis m.

Supinator m., deep
portion

Radial n., deep branch

Supinator m.,
superficial portion

Extensor
digitorum m.

Triceps m.

Brachialis m.

Pronator teres m.

Med. epicondyle

Common flexor t.

Med. collateral lig.

Pronator teres m.

Coronoid

Brachialis m. and t.

Pronator teres t.
ulnar head

Palmaris longus m.

Flexor carpi radialis m.

Ulnar a.

Flexor digitorum
superficialis m.

Fig. 68.1 **Anatomy of the lateral epicondyle.** *(From Kang SH, Ahn JM, Resnick D: MRI of the extremities, ed 2, Philadelphia, 2002, Saunders, 2002, p 87.)*

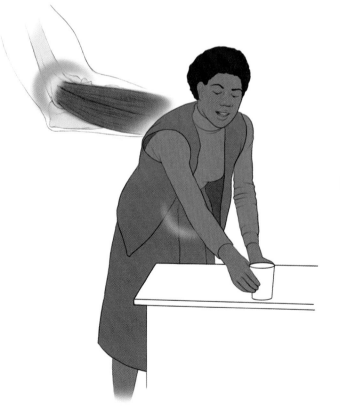

Fig. 68.2 **The pain of tennis elbow is localized to the lateral epicondyle.** *(From Waldman SD: Atlas of common pain syndromes, ed 2, Philadelphia, 2008, Saunders, p 110.)*

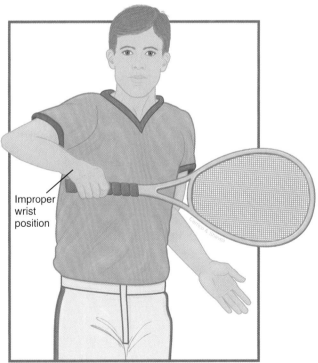

Improper
wrist
position

Fig. 68.3 **Improper wrist position causes tennis elbow syndrome.** *(From Waldman SD: Atlas of pain management injection techniques, ed 2, Philadelphia, 2007, Saunders, p 138.)*

inhibitors and physical therapy. The local application of heat and cold may also be beneficial. Any repetitive activity that may exacerbate the patient's symptoms should be avoided.[5] For patients who do not respond to these treatment modalities, the following injection technique may be a reasonable next step.[6]

Injection technique for tennis elbow is performed by placing the patient in a supine position with the arm fully adducted at the patient's side and the elbow flexed with the dorsum of the hand resting on a folded towel to relax the affected tendons. A total of 1 mL of local anesthetic and 40 mg of methylprednisolone is drawn up in a 5-mL sterile syringe.

After sterile preparation of skin overlying the posterolateral aspect of the joint, the lateral epicondyle is identified. Using strict aseptic technique, the operator inserts a 1-inch 25-gauge

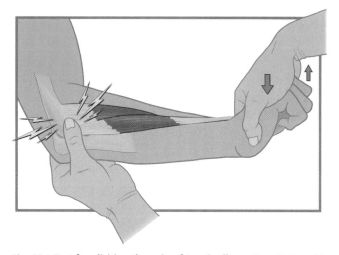

Fig. 68.4 **Test for eliciting the pain of tennis elbow.** (From Waldman SD: Atlas of pain management injection techniques, ed 2, Philadelphia, 2007, Saunders, p 239.)

needle perpendicular to the lateral epicondyle through the skin and into the subcutaneous tissue overlying the affected tendon (**Fig. 68.6**). If bone is encountered, the needle is withdrawn into the subcutaneous tissue. The contents of the syringe are then gently injected. Little resistance to injection should be felt. If resistance is encountered, the needle is probably in the tendon and should be withdrawn until the injection proceeds without significant resistance. The needle is then removed, and a sterile pressure dressing and ice pack are placed at the injection site.

Side Effects and Complications

The major complication associated with tennis elbow is rupture of the affected inflamed tendons, either from repetitive trauma or from injection directly into the tendon. Inflamed and previously damaged tendons may rupture if they are directly injected, and the needle position should be confirmed outside the tendon before injection, to avoid this complication. Another complication of this injection technique is infection. This complication should be exceedingly rare if strict aseptic technique is followed. The ulnar nerve is especially susceptible to damage at the elbow, and care must be taken to avoid this nerve when injecting the elbow. Approximately 25% of patients will complain of a transient increase in pain following this injection technique, and patients should be warned of this possibility.

Conclusion

This injection technique is extremely effective in the treatment of pain secondary to tennis elbow. Coexistent bursitis and tendinitis may also contribute to elbow pain and may require additional treatment with more localized injection of local anesthetic and depot steroid. This technique is a safe procedure if careful attention is paid to the clinically relevant

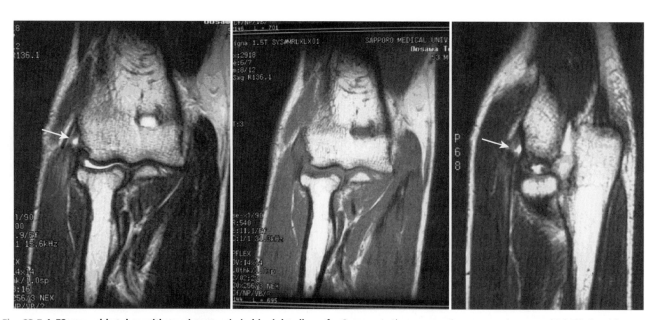

Fig. 68.5 **A 53-year-old stoker with persistent pain in his right elbow for 2 years.** In these magnetic resonance images, a high T2 signal focus was found in the origin of the extensor carpi radialis brevis in the coronal and oblique planes (arrows). Intra-articular effusion was observed. Left image, T2; center image, T1; right image, T2 oblique.

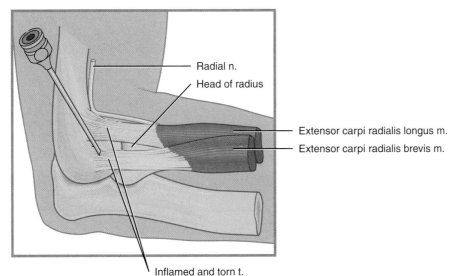

Radial n.

Head of radius

Extensor carpi radialis longus m.

Extensor carpi radialis brevis m.

Inflamed and torn t.

Fig. 68.6 **Injection technique for relieving the pain of tennis elbow.** *(From Waldman SD:* Atlas of pain management injection techniques, *Philadelphia, 2000, Saunders, p 83.)*

anatomy of the areas to be injected. The use of physical modalities including local heat, as well as gentle range-of-motion exercises, should be introduced several days after the patient undergoes this injection technique for tennis elbow pain. A Velcro band placed around the extensor tendons may also help relieve the symptoms of tennis elbow. Vigorous exercises should be avoided because they will exacerbate the patient's symptoms. Simple analgesics and nonsteroidal anti-inflammatory agents may be used concurrently with this injection technique. As mentioned earlier, cervical radiculopathy and radial tunnel syndrome may mimic tennis elbow and must be ruled out to treat the underlying disorder effectively.

References

Full references for this chapter can be found on www.expertconsult.com.

Chapter **69**

Golfer's Elbow

Steven D. Waldman

Although 15 times less common than tennis elbow, golfer's elbow remains one of the most common causes of elbow and forearm pain.[1] Golfer's elbow, also known as medial epicondylitis, is caused by repetitive microtrauma to the flexor tendons of the forearm in a manner analogous to tennis elbow.[2] The pathophysiology of golfer's elbow is initiated by micro-tearing at the origin of the pronator teres, flexor carpi radialis, flexor carpi ulnaris, and the palmaris longus. Secondary inflammation may occur and can become chronic as the result of continued overuse or misuse of the flexors of the forearm. The most common nidi of pain from golfer's elbow are the bony origin of the flexor tendon of flexor carpi radialis and the humeral heads of the flexor carpi ulnaris and pronator teres at the medial epicondyle of the humerus (**Fig. 69.1**). Less commonly, golfer's elbow pain can originate from the ulnar head of the flexor carpi ulnaris at the medial aspect of the olecranon process. Coexisting bursitis, arthritis, and gout may also perpetuate the pain and disability of golfer's elbow.[3]

Golfer's elbow occurs in patients engaged in repetitive flexion activities that include throwing baseballs or footballs, carrying heavy suitcases, and driving golf balls (**Fig. 69.2**). These activities have in common repetitive flexion of the wrist and strain on the flexor tendons resulting from excessive weight or sudden arrested motion. Many of the activities that can cause tennis elbow can also cause golfer's elbow.[1]

Signs and Symptoms

The pain of golfer's elbow is localized to the region of the medial epicondyle (see Fig. 69.1). It is constant and is made worse with active contraction of the wrist. Patients note the inability to hold a coffee cup or a hammer. Sleep disturbance is common. On physical examination, the patient reports tenderness along the flexor tendons at or just below the medial epicondyle. Many patients with golfer's elbow have a bandlike thickening within the affected flexor tendons. Elbow range of motion is normal. Grip strength on the affected side is diminished. Patients with golfer's elbow demonstrate a positive response to the *golfer's elbow test*.[2] The test is performed by stabilizing the patients forearm and then having the patient actively flex the wrist (**Fig. 69.3**). The examiner then attempts to force the wrist into extension. Sudden, severe pain is highly suggestive of golfer's elbow.

Testing

Plain radiographs are indicated in all patients who present with golfer's elbow to rule out joint mice and other occult bony disorders. Based on the patient's clinical presentation, additional testing including complete blood count, uric acid, sedimentation rate, and antinuclear antibody testing may be indicated. Magnetic resonance imaging scan of the elbow is indicated if joint instability is suspected. Electromyography is indicated to diagnose entrapment neuropathy at the elbow and to help distinguish golfer's elbow from cervical radiculopathy. The injection technique described subsequently serves as a diagnostic and a therapeutic maneuver.

Differential Diagnosis

Occasionally, C6-7 radiculopathy can mimic golfer's elbow. The patient suffering from cervical radiculopathy usually has neck pain and proximal upper extremity pain in addition to symptoms below the elbow. Electromyography helps to distinguish radiculopathy from golfer's elbow. Bursitis, arthritis, and gout may also mimic golfer's elbow and may confuse the diagnosis. The olecranon bursa lies in the posterior aspect of the elbow joint and may also become inflamed as a result of direct trauma or overuse of the joint. Other bursae susceptible to the development of bursitis exist between the insertion of the biceps and the head of the radius, as well as in the antecubital and cubital area (**Fig. 69.4**).

Treatment

Initial treatment of the pain and functional disability associated with golfer's elbow should include a combination of the nonsteroidal anti-inflammatory drugs (NSAIDs) or cyclooxygenase-2 inhibitors and physical therapy.[4] The local application of heat and cold may also be beneficial. Any repetitive

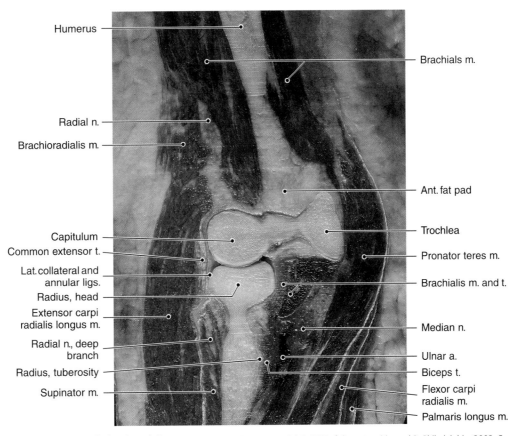

Fig. 69.1 **Anatomy of the medial epicondyle.** *(From Kang SH, Ahn JM, Resnick D:* MRI of the extremities, *ed 2, Philadelphia, 2002, Saunders, p 91.)*

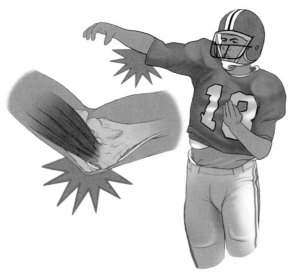

Fig. 69.2 **The pain of golfer's elbow occurs at the medial epicondyle.** *(From Waldman SD:* Atlas of common pain syndromes, *ed 2, Philadelphia, 2008, Saunders, p 114.)*

activity that may exacerbate the patient's symptoms should be avoided. For patients who do not respond to these treatment modalities, the following injection technique may be a reasonable next step.[5]

Injection for golfer's elbow is carried out by placing the patient in a supine position with the arm fully adducted at the patient's side and the elbow fully extended with the dorsum of the hand resting on a folded towel to relax the affected tendons.

A total of 1 mL of local anesthetic and 40 mg of methylprednisolone is drawn up in a 5-mL sterile syringe.

After sterile preparation of skin overlying the medial aspect of the joint, the medial epicondyle is identified. Using strict aseptic technique, the operator inserts a 1-inch, 25-gauge needle perpendicular to the medial epicondyle through the skin and into the subcutaneous tissue overlying the affected tendon (**Fig. 69.5**). If bone is encountered, the needle is withdrawn into the subcutaneous tissue. The contents of the syringe are then gently injected. Little resistance to injection should be felt. If resistance is encountered, the needle is probably in the tendon and should be withdrawn until the injection proceeds without significant resistance. The needle is then removed, and a sterile pressure dressing and ice pack are placed at the injection site.

Side Effects and Complications

The major complications associated with this injection technique are related to trauma to the inflamed and previously damaged tendons. Such tendons may rupture if they are directly injected, and the needle position should be confirmed outside the tendon before injection, to avoid this complication. Another complication of this injection technique is infection. This complication should be exceedingly rare if strict aseptic technique is followed. The ulnar nerve is especially susceptible to damage at the elbow, and care must be taken to avoid this nerve when injecting the elbow. Approximately 25% of patients will complain of a transient increase in pain following intra-articular injection of the elbow joint, and patients should be warned of this possibility.

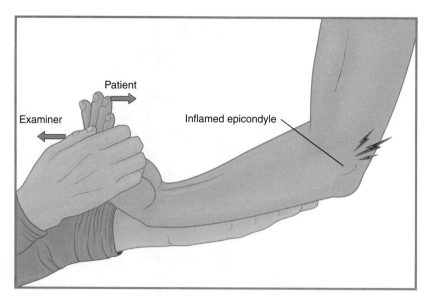

Fig. 69.3 **Test for eliciting the pain of golfer's elbow.** *(From Waldman SD: Atlas of pain management injection techniques, ed 2, Philadelphia, 2007, Saunders, p 149.)*

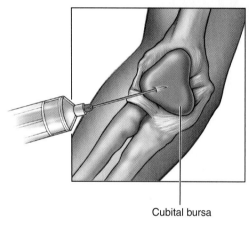

Fig. 69.4 **Proper needle placement for injection for cubital bursitis.** *(From Waldman SD: Atlas of common pain syndromes, ed 2, Philadelphia, 2008, Saunders, p 92.)*

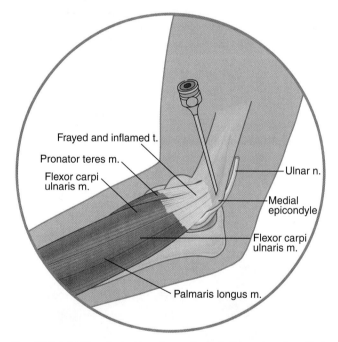

Fig. 69.5 **Injection technique for relieving the pain of golfer's elbow syndrome.** *(From Waldman SD: Atlas of pain management injection techniques, ed 2, Philadelphia, 2007, Saunders, p 150.)*

This injection technique is extremely effective in the treatment of pain secondary to golfer's elbow. Coexisting bursitis and tendinitis may also contribute to elbow pain and may require additional treatment with more localized injection of local anesthetic and depot steroid. This technique is a safe procedure if careful attention is paid to the clinically relevant anatomy of the areas to be injected. The use of physical modalities including local heat, as well as gentle range-of-motion exercises, should be introduced several days after the patient undergoes this injection technique for elbow pain. A Velcro band placed around the flexor tendons may also help relieve the symptoms of golfer's elbow. Vigorous exercises should be avoided because they will exacerbate the patient's symptoms. Simple analgesics and NSAIDs may be used concurrently with this injection technique. As mentioned earlier, cervical radiculopathy may mimic golfer's elbow and must be ruled out to treat the underlying disorder effectively.

Conclusion

Golfer's elbow is a common cause of elbow and forearm pain encountered in clinical practice. This painful condition frequently coexists with other elbow disorders including tendinitis, lateral epicondylitis, and bursitis. Entrapment neuropathy may also complicate the clinical picture. Identification of the activities responsible for the pathophysiology of golfer's elbow is paramount if rapid relief of pain and functional disability are to be achieved.

References

Full references for this chapter can be found on www.expertconsult.com.

Olecranon and Cubital Bursitis

Steven D. Waldman

Olecranon bursitis and cubital bursitis are common causes of elbow pain encountered in clinical practice. Bursae are formed from synovial sacs that exist to allow easy sliding of muscles and tendons across one another at areas of repeated movement. These synovial sacs are lined with a synovial membrane invested with a network of blood vessels that secrete synovial fluid. Inflammation of the bursa results in an increase in the production of synovial fluid, with swelling of the bursal sac. With overuse or misuse, these bursae may become inflamed, enlarged, and, on rare occasions, infected. Although intrapatient variability is significant with regard to the number, size, and location of bursae, anatomists have been able to identify some clinically relevant bursae, including the olecranon and cubital bursae. The olecranon bursa lies in the posterior aspect of the elbow, whereas the cubital bursa lies in the anterior aspect. Both may exist as a single bursal sac or, in some patients, as a multisegmented series of sacs that may be loculated.

Olecranon Bursitis

Olecranon bursitis may develop gradually as a result of repetitive irritation of the olecranon bursa or acutely in response to trauma or infection.[1] The swelling associated with olecranon bursitis may, at times, be quite impressive, and the patient may complain about difficulty in wearing a long-sleeved shirt (**Fig. 70.1**).

The olecranon bursa is vulnerable to injury from both acute trauma and repeated microtrauma. Acute injuries frequently take the form of direct trauma to the elbow when playing sports such as hockey or falling directly onto the olecranon process. Repeated pressure from leaning on the elbow to arise from bed or from working long hours at a drafting table may result in inflammation and swelling of the olecranon bursa (**Fig. 70.2**). Gout or bacterial infection may rarely precipitate acute olecranon bursitis.[2] If the inflammation of the olecranon bursa becomes chronic, calcification of the bursa with residual nodules called *gravel* may occur.

Clinically Relevant Anatomy

The elbow joint is a synovial hinge-type joint that serves as the articulation of the humerus, radius, and ulna (**Fig. 70.3**). The joint's primary function is to position the wrist to optimize hand function. The joint allows flexion and extension at the elbow as well as pronation and supination of the forearm. The joint is lined with synovium. The entire joint is covered by a dense capsule that thickens medially to form the ulnar collateral ligament and medially to form the radial collateral ligament (**Fig. 70.4**). These dense ligaments, coupled with the elbow joint's deep bony socket, makes this joint extremely stable and relatively resistant to subluxation and dislocation. The anterior and posterior joint capsule is less dense and may become distended in the presence of joint effusion.

The elbow joint is innervated primarily by the musculocutaneous and radial nerves. The ulnar and median nerves provide varying degrees of innervation. At the middle of the upper arm, the ulnar nerve courses medially to pass between the olecranon process and the medial epicondyle of the humerus. The nerve is susceptible to entrapment and trauma at this point. At the elbow, the median nerve lies just medial to the brachial artery and is occasionally damaged during brachial artery cannulation for blood gas determination.

Signs and Symptoms

The patient suffering from olecranon bursitis frequently complains of pain and swelling during any movement of the elbow, but especially extension. The pain is localized to the olecranon area, and referred pain is often noted above the elbow joint.[3] The patient is frequently more concerned about the swelling around the bursa than about the pain. Physical examination reveals point tenderness over the olecranon and swelling of the bursa that can be quite extensive (see Figs. 70.1 and 70.2).[4] Passive flexion and resisted extension of the elbow reproduce the pain, as does any pressure over the bursa. Fever and chills usually accompany infection of the bursa. If infection is suspected, aspiration, Gram stain, and culture of the bursa followed by treatment with appropriate antibiotics are indicated on an emergency basis.

Testing

The diagnosis of olecranon bursitis is usually made on clinical grounds alone. Plain radiographs of the posterior elbow are indicated if the patient has a history of elbow trauma or if arthritis of the elbow is suspected. Plain radiographs may also reveal calcification of the bursa and associated structures consistent with chronic inflammation (**Fig. 70.5**). Magnetic resonance imaging (MRI) scan is indicated if infection or joint instability is suspected (**Fig. 70.6**). Complete blood count and an automated chemistry profile including uric acid, sedimentation rate, and antinuclear antibody are indicated if collagen vascular disease is suspected. When infection is considered, aspiration, Gram stain, and culture of bursal fluid are indicated on an emergency basis.

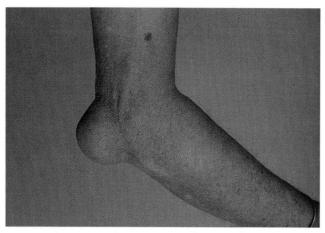

Fig. 70.1 **Olecranon bursitis in early rheumatoid arthritis.** *(From Groff GD: Olecranon bursitis. In Klippel JH, Dieppe PA, editors:* Rheumatology, *ed 2, London, 1998, Mosby, p 4.14.3.)*

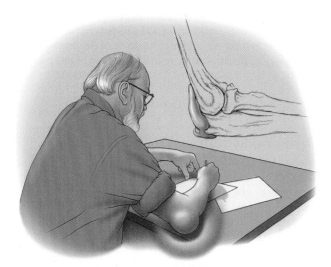

Fig. 70.2 Olecranon bursitis is often caused by repeated pressure on the elbow. *(From Waldman SD: Olecranon bursitis. In* Atlas of common pain syndromes, *ed 2, Philadelphia, 2007, Saunders, p 131.)*

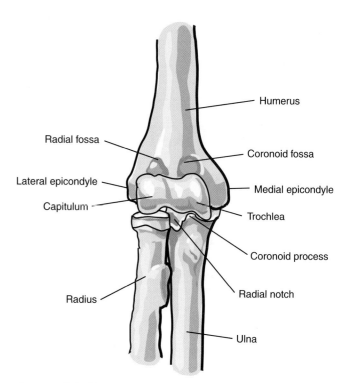

Fig. 70.3 **Clinically relevant anatomy of the elbow.** The elbow joint is a synovial hinge-type joint that serves as the articulation of the humerus, radius, and ulna.

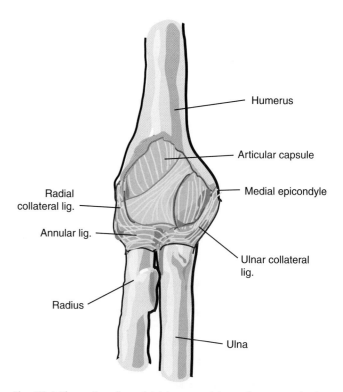

Fig. 70.4 The entire elbow joint is covered by a dense capsule that thickens medially to form the ulnar collateral ligament and medially to form the radial collateral ligament.

Differential Diagnosis

Olecranon bursitis is usually a straightforward clinical diagnosis. Occasionally, rheumatoid nodules or gouty arthritis of the elbow may confuse the clinician. Synovial cysts of the elbow may also mimic olecranon bursitis. Coexisting tendinitis, (e.g., tennis elbow and golfer's elbow) may require additional treatment.

Treatment

A short course of conservative therapy consisting of simple analgesics, nonsteroidal anti-inflammatory drugs (NSAIDs)

or cyclooxygenase-2 (COX-2) inhibitors, and an elbow protector to prevent further trauma is a reasonable first step in the treatment of patients suffering from olecranon bursitis. If the patient does not experience rapid improvement, the following injection technique is a logical next step.[5]

The patient is placed in a supine position with the arm fully adducted at the patient's side and the elbow flexed with the palm of the hand resting on the patient's abdomen. A total of 2 mL of local anesthetic and 40 mg of methylprednisolone is drawn up in a 5-mL sterile syringe. After sterile preparation of skin overlying the posterior aspect of the joint, the olecranon process and overlying bursa are identified. Using strict aseptic technique, the operator inserts a 1-inch, 25-gauge needle through the skin and subcutaneous tissues directly into the bursa in the midline (**Fig. 70.7**). If bone is encountered, the needle is withdrawn into the bursa. After entering the bursa, the operator gently injects the contents of the syringe. Resistance to injection should be minimal. The needle is then removed, and a sterile pressure dressing and ice pack are placed at the injection site.

Cubital Bursitis

The cubital bursa is vulnerable to injury from both acute trauma and repeated microtrauma. Acute injuries frequently take the form of direct trauma to the anterior aspect of the elbow. Repetitive movements of the elbow, including throwing javelins and baseballs, may result in inflammation and swelling of the cubital bursa. Gout or rheumatoid arthritis may rarely precipitate acute cubital bursitis. If the inflammation of the cubital bursa becomes chronic, calcification of the bursa may occur.

The patient suffering from cubital bursitis frequently complains of pain and swelling with any movement of the elbow (**Fig. 70.8**). The pain is localized to the cubital area, and referred pain is often noted in the forearm and hand. Physical examination reveals point tenderness in the anterior aspect of the elbow over the cubital bursa and swelling of the bursa. Passive extension and resisted flexion of the shoulder reproduce the pain, as does any pressure over the bursa. Plain radiographs of

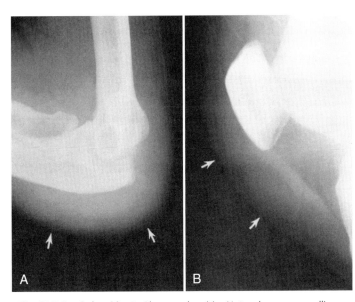

Fig. 70.5 **Septic bursitis.** A, Olecranon bursitis. Note olecranon swelling (*arrows*) and soft tissue edema resulting from *Staphylococcus aureus* infection. Previous surgery and trauma are the causes of the adjacent bony abnormalities. B, Prepatellar bursitis. This 28-year-old carpenter who had worked on his knees for prolonged periods developed tender swelling in front of the knee (*arrows*). Inflammatory fluid that was culture positive for *S. aures* was recovered from the bursa. *(From Resnick D, editor: Diagnosis of bone and joint disorders, ed 4, Philadelphia, 2002, Saunders, p 2438.)*

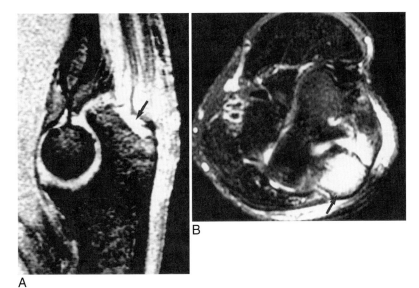

Fig. 70.6 **Septic olecranon bursitis.** A sagittal multiplanar gradient (MPGR; TR/TE, 500/11; flip angle, 15 degrees) magnetic resonance imaging (MRI) scan (A) reveals abnormal high signal intensity in the region of the olecranon bursa with bone involvement (*arrow*), also of high signal intensity. A transaxial fat-suppressed fast spin echo (TR/TE, 5000/108) MRI scan (B) confirms bone involvement (*arrow*). *(From Resnick D, editor: Diagnosis of bone and joint disorders, ed 4, Philadelphia, 2002, Saunders, p 2439.)*

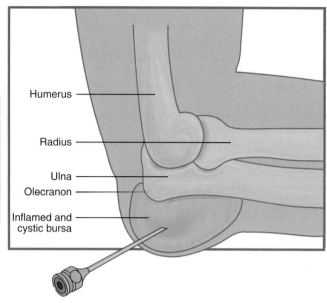

Fig. 70.7 **Injection technique for olecranon bursitis pain.** *(From Waldman SD: Olecranon bursitis pain. In* Atlas of pain management injection techniques, *ed 2, Philadelphia, 2007, Saunders, p 181.)*

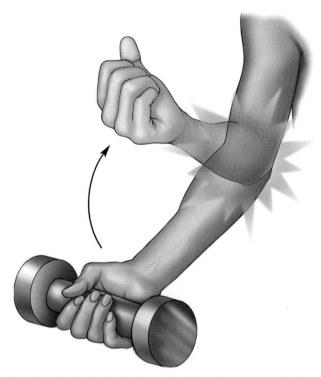

Fig. 70.8 A patient suffering from cubital bursitis complains of pain and swelling on movement of the elbow. *(From Waldman SD: Cubital bursitis. In Atlas of uncommon pain syndromes, ed 2, Philadelphia, 2008, Saunders, p 92.)*

the posterior elbow may reveal calcification of the bursa and associated structures consistent with chronic inflammation.

Clinically Relevant Anatomy

The elbow joint is a synovial hinge-type joint that serves as the articulation of the humerus, radius, and ulna (see Fig. 70.3). The joint's primary function is to position the wrist to optimize

hand function. The joint allows flexion and extension at the elbow, as well as pronation and supination of the forearm. The joint is lined with synovium. The entire joint is covered by a dense capsule that thickens medially to form the ulnar collateral ligament and medially to form the radial collateral ligaments (see Fig. 70.4). These dense ligaments coupled with the elbow joint's deep bony socket make this joint extremely stable and relatively resistant to subluxation and dislocation. The anterior and posterior joint capsule is less dense and may become distended if joint effusion is present.

The cubital fossa lies in the anterior aspect of the elbow joint and is bounded laterally by the brachioradialis muscle and medially by the pronator teres. The cubital fossa contains the median nerve, which is susceptible to irritation and compression from a swollen, inflamed cubital bursa. The elbow joint is innervated primarily by the musculocutaneous and radial nerves. The ulnar and median nerves provide varying degrees of innervation. At the middle of the upper arm, the ulnar nerve courses medially to pass between the olecranon process and the medial epicondyle of the humerus. The nerve is susceptible to entrapment and trauma at this point. At the elbow, the median nerve lies just medial to the brachial artery and is occasionally damaged during brachial artery cannulation for blood gas measurement. The median nerve may also be injured during injection of the cubital bursa.

Signs and Symptoms

The patient suffering from cubital bursitis frequently complains of pain and swelling with any movement of the elbow, but especially flexion. The pain is localized to the cubital fossa, and referred pain is often noted above the elbow joint.[6] The patient is frequently more concerned about the swelling around the bursa than about the pain. Physical examination reveals point tenderness over the cubital bursa and swelling of the bursa that, at times, can be quite extensive.[6] Passive extension and resisted flexion of the elbow reproduce the pain, as does any pressure over the bursa. Fever and chills usually accompany infection of the bursa. When infection is suspected, aspiration, Gram stain, and culture of the bursa followed by treatment with appropriate antibiotics are indicated on an emergency basis.

Testing

The diagnosis of cubital bursitis is usually made on clinical grounds alone. Plain radiographs of the posterior elbow are indicated if the patient has a history of elbow trauma or if arthritis of the elbow is suspected. Plain radiographs may also reveal calcification of the bursa and associated structures consistent with chronic inflammation. MRI scan is indicated if infection or joint instability is suspected. Complete blood count and an automated chemistry profile including uric acid, sedimentation rate, and antinuclear antibody testing are indicated if collagen vascular disease is suspected. When infection is considered, aspiration, Gram stain, and culture of bursal fluid are indicated on an emergency basis.

Differential Diagnosis

Cubital bursitis is usually a straightforward clinical diagnosis. Occasionally, rheumatoid nodules or gouty arthritis of the elbow may confuse the clinician. Synovial cysts of the

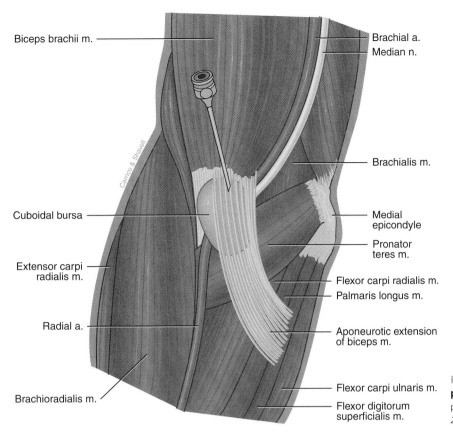

Biceps brachii m.

Brachial a.
Median n.

Brachialis m.

Cuboidal bursa

Medial epicondyle

Pronator teres m.

Extensor carpi radialis m.

Flexor carpi radialis m.
Palmaris longus m.

Radial a.

Aponeurotic extension of biceps m.

Brachioradialis m.

Flexor carpi ulnaris m.

Flexor digitorum superficialis m.

Fig. 70.9 **Injection technique for cubital bursitis pain.** *(From Waldman SD: Cubital bursitis pain. In Atlas of pain management injection techniques, ed 2, Philadelphia, 2007, Saunders, p 189.)*

elbow may also mimic cubital bursitis. Coexistent tendinitis (e.g., tennis elbow and golfer's elbow) may require additional treatment.

Treatment

A short course of conservative therapy consisting of simple analgesics, NSAIDs or COX-2 inhibitors, and an elbow protector to prevent further trauma is a reasonable first step in the treatment of patients suffering from cubital bursitis. If the patient does not experience rapid improvement, the following injection technique is a logical next step.[7,8]

The patient is placed in a supine position with the arm fully adducted at the patient's side and the elbow extended with the dorsum of the hand resting on a folded towel. A total of 2 mL of local anesthetic and 40 mg of methylprednisolone is drawn up in a 5-mL sterile syringe. The clinician identifies the pulsations of the brachial artery at the crease of the elbow. After preparation of the skin with antiseptic solution, a 1-inch, 25-gauge needle is inserted just lateral to the brachial artery at the crease and is slowly advanced in a slightly medial and cephalad trajectory through the skin and subcutaneous tissues (**Fig. 70.9**). If bone is encountered, the needle is withdrawn into the subcutaneous tissue. The contents of the syringe are then gently injected. Resistance to injection should be minimal. If resistance is encountered, the needle is probably in the tendon and should be withdrawn until the injection proceeds without significant resistance. The needle is then removed, and a sterile pressure dressing and ice pack are placed at the injection site.

Injection of the cubital bursa at the elbow is a relatively safe block. The major complications are inadvertent intravascular injection and persistent paresthesia secondary to needle trauma to the median nerve. This technique can safely be performed in patients receiving anticoagulants with the use of a 25- or 27-gauge needle, albeit at an increased risk of hematoma, if the clinical situation dictates a favorable risk-to-benefit ratio. These complications can be decreased if manual pressure is applied to the area of the block immediately following injection. The application of cold packs for 20-minute periods following the block also decreases the amount of postprocedure pain and bleeding.

Conclusion

Olecranon bursitis and cubital bursitis are common causes of elbow pain encountered in clinical practice. Coexistent tendinitis and epicondylitis often contribute to elbow pain and may require additional treatment with more localized injection of local anesthetic and depot steroid. Failure to treat olecranon and cubital bursitis adequately may result in the development of chronic pain and loss of range of motion of the affected elbow.

References

Full references for this chapter can be found on www.expertconsult.com.

Entrapment Neuropathies of the Elbow and Forearm

Steven D. Waldman

Entrapment neuropathies of the elbow and forearm provide significant diagnostic and therapeutic challenges to the clinician. Although reasonably common in clinical practice, these disorders are frequently misdiagnosed and mistreated. This chapter provides the clinician with a concise review of these clinical syndromes and presents a step-by-step guide to treatment.

Tardy Ulnar Palsy

Ulnar nerve entrapment at the elbow is one of the most common entrapment neuropathies encountered in clinical practice.[1] Causes include compression of the ulnar nerve by an aponeurotic band that runs from the medial epicondyle of the humerus to the medial border of the olecranon, direct trauma to the ulnar nerve at the elbow, and repetitive elbow motion (**Fig. 71.1**). Ulnar nerve entrapment at the elbow is also called *tardy ulnar palsy, cubital tunnel syndrome,* and *ulnar nerve neuritis.* This entrapment neuropathy manifests as pain and associated paresthesias in the lateral forearm that radiate to the wrist and to the ring and little fingers (**Fig. 71.2**). Some patients suffering from ulnar nerve entrapment at the elbow may also notice pain referred to the medial aspect of the scapula on the affected side. Untreated, ulnar nerve entrapment at the elbow can result in a progressive motor deficit and, ultimately, flexion contracture of the affected fingers. The onset of symptoms usually occurs after repetitive elbow motion or results from repeated pressure on the elbow, such as using the elbows to arise from bed. Direct trauma to the ulnar nerve as it enters the cubital tunnel may also cause a similar clinical presentation. Patients with vulnerable nerve syndrome (e.g., patients with diabetes or alcoholism) are at greater risk for the development of ulnar nerve entrapment at the elbow (**Fig. 71.3**).

Signs and Symptoms

Physical findings include tenderness over the ulnar nerve at the elbow. A positive Tinel sign over the ulnar nerve as it passes beneath the aponeuroses is usually present. Weakness of the intrinsic muscles of the forearm and hand that are innervated by the ulnar nerve may be identified by careful manual muscle testing, although early in the evolution of cubital tunnel syndrome, the only physical finding other than tenderness over the nerve may be the loss of sensation on the ulnar side of the little finger. Muscle wasting of the intrinsic muscles of the hand can best be identified by viewing the hand with the palm down. The Tinel sign at the elbow is often present when the ulnar nerve is stimulated.

Testing

Electromyography with nerve conduction velocity testing is an extremely sensitive test. The skilled electromyographer can diagnose ulnar nerve entrapment at the elbow with a high degree of accuracy, as well as help sort out other neuropathic causes of pain that may mimic ulnar nerve entrapment at the elbow including radiculopathy and plexopathy. Plain radiographs are indicated in all patients who present with ulnar nerve entrapment at the elbow to rule out occult bony disease. If surgery is contemplated, a magnetic resonance imaging (MRI) scan of the affected elbow may help further delineate that pathologic process responsible for the nerve entrapment

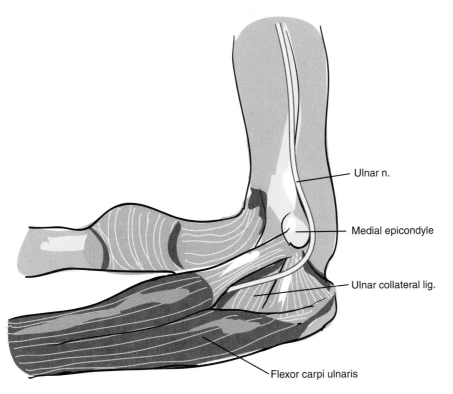

Fig. 71.1 The causes of ulnar nerve entrapment at the elbow include compression of the ulnar nerve by an aponeurotic band that runs from the medial epicondyle of the humerus to the medial border of the olecranon, direct trauma to the ulnar nerve at the elbow, and repetitive elbow motion.

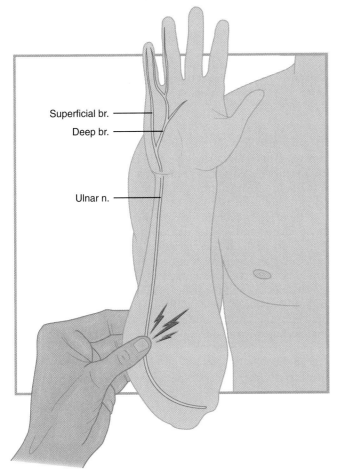

Fig. 71.2 Ulnar nerve entrapment at the elbow manifests as pain and associated paresthesias in the lateral forearm that radiate to the wrist and to the ring and little fingers. *(From Waldman SD: Cubital tunnel syndrome. In Atlas of pain management injection techniques, ed 2, Philadelphia, 2007, Saunders, p 196.)*

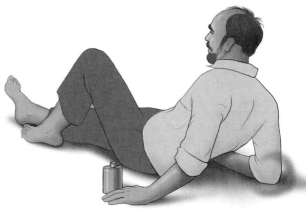

Fig. 71.3 The ulnar nerve is susceptible to compression at the elbow. *(From Waldman SD: Ulnar nerve entrapment at the elbow. In Atlas of common pain syndromes, ed 2, Philadelphia, 2007, Saunders, p 125.)*

(e.g., bone spur, tumor, or aponeurotic band thickening) (**Fig. 71.4**). If Pancoast's tumor or other tumors of the brachial plexus are suspected, chest radiographs with apical lordotic views may be helpful. Screening laboratory testing consisting of complete blood count, erythrocyte sedimentation rate, antinuclear antibody testing, and automated blood chemistry testing should be performed if the diagnosis of ulnar nerve entrapment at the elbow is in question, to help rule out other causes of the patient's pain. The injection technique described subsequently serves as both a diagnostic test and a therapeutic maneuver.[2]

Differential Diagnosis

Ulnar nerve entrapment at the elbow is often misdiagnosed as golfer's elbow, and this error accounts for the many patients whose "golfer's elbow" fails to respond to conservative measures.[3]

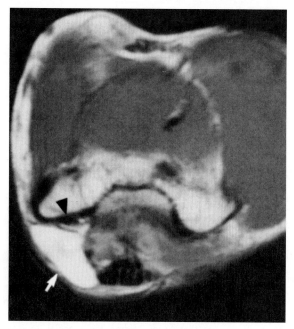

Fig. 71.4 Entrapment of the ulnar nerve: cubital tunnel syndrome. A lipoma (*arrow*) adjacent to the ulnar nerve (*arrowhead*) is well shown in these transverse intermediate-weighted (TR/TE 2000/20) spin-echo magnetic resonance images. The lipoma led to clinical findings of ulnar nerve entrapment in this 36-year-old man. (*Courtesy of Z. Rosenberg, MD, New York.*)

Ulnar nerve entrapment at the elbow can be distinguished from golfer's elbow in that in cubital tunnel syndrome, the maximal tenderness to palpation is over the ulnar nerve 1 inch below the medial epicondyle, whereas in golfer's elbow, the maximal tenderness to palpation is directly over the medial epicondyle. Ulnar nerve entrapment at the elbow should also be differentiated from cervical radiculopathy involving the C7 or C8 roots. Cervical radiculopathy and ulnar nerve entrapment may coexist as the *double-crush syndrome*. The double-crush syndrome is seen most commonly with median nerve entrapment at the wrist or carpal tunnel syndrome.[4]

Treatment

A short course of conservative therapy consisting of simple analgesics, nonsteroidal anti-inflammatory drugs (NSAIDs) or cyclooxygenase-2 (COX-2) inhibitors, and splinting to avoid elbow flexion is indicated in patients who present with ulnar nerve entrapment at the elbow. If the patient does not experience marked improvement in symptoms within 1 week, careful injection of the ulnar nerve at the elbow with the following technique is a reasonable next step.[2]

Ulnar nerve injection at the elbow is carried out by placing the patient in the supine position with the arm fully adducted at the patient's side and the elbow slightly flexed with the dorsum of the hand resting on a folded towel. A total of 5 to 7 mL of local anesthetic is drawn up in a 12-mL sterile syringe. A total of 80 mg of depot steroid is added to the local anesthetic with the first block, and a 40-mg dose of depot steroid is added with subsequent blocks.

The clinician then identifies the olecranon process and the medial epicondyle of the humerus. The ulnar nerve sulcus between these two bony landmarks is then identified. After preparation of the skin with antiseptic solution, a ⅝-inch,

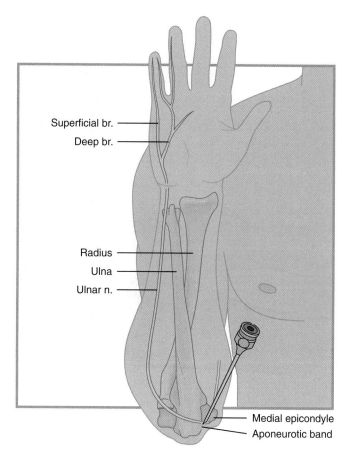

Fig. 71.5 Injection technique for relieving pain resulting from ulnar nerve entrapment at the elbow. (*From Waldman SD: Cubital tunnel syndrome. In Atlas of pain management injection techniques, ed 2, Philadelphia, 2007, Saunders, p 199.*)

25-gauge needle is inserted just proximal to the sulcus and is slowly advanced in a slightly cephalad trajectory (**Fig. 71.5**). As the needle advances approximately ½ inch, strong paresthesia in the distribution of the ulnar nerve is elicited. The patient should be warned that paresthesia will occur and to say "there!!!!" as soon as the paresthesia is felt. After paresthesia is elicited and its distribution is identified, gentle aspiration is carried out to identify blood. If the aspiration test result is negative and no persistent paresthesia into the distribution of the ulnar nerve remains, a total of 5 to 7 mL of solution is slowly injected, and the patient is monitored closely for signs of local anesthetic toxicity. If no paresthesia can be elicited, a similar amount of solution is slowly injected in a fanlike manner just proximal to the notch, with care taken to avoid intravascular injection.

If the patient does not respond to the aforementioned treatments or if the patient is experiencing progressive neurologic deficit, strong consideration to surgical decompression of the ulnar nerve is indicated. As mentioned earlier, MRI scanning of the affected elbow should help to clarify the disorder responsible for compression of the ulnar nerve.

Complications and Pitfalls

Failure to identify and treat ulnar nerve entrapment at the elbow promptly can result in permanent neurologic deficit. It is also important to rule out other causes of pain and

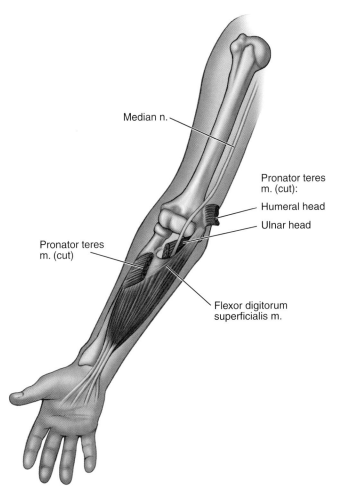

Fig. 71.6 The symptoms of pronator syndrome result from compression of the median nerve by the pronator teres muscle. *(From Waldman SD: Pronator syndrome. In Atlas of uncommon pain syndromes, ed 2, Philadelphia, 2008, Saunders, p 87.)*

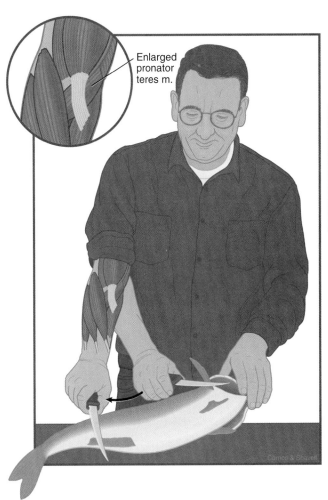

Fig. 71.7 The onset of pronator syndrome usually occurs after repetitive elbow motions such as chopping wood, sculling, or cleaning fish, although occasionally the onset is more insidious, without apparent antecedent trauma. *(From Waldman SD: Pronator syndrome. In Atlas of pain management injection techniques, ed 2, Philadelphia, 2007, Saunders, p 187.)*

numbness that may mimic the symptoms of ulnar nerve entrapment at the elbow, such as Pancoast's tumor, to avoid harm to the patient.

Ulnar nerve block at the elbow is a relatively safe block. The major complications are inadvertent intravascular injection into the ulnar artery and persistent paresthesia secondary to needle trauma to the nerve. Care should be taken to inject just proximal to the sulcus slowly, to avoid additional compromise of the nerve because, as the nerve passes through the ulnar nerve sulcus, it is enclosed by a dense fibrous band.

Pronator Syndrome

Entrapment of the median nerve in the forearm occurs at several sites. The median nerve may be entrapped at the lacertus fibrosus, at the lateral edge of the flexor digitorum superficialis, by fibrous bands of the superficial head of the pronator teres muscle, or, most commonly, by the pronator teres muscle itself (**Fig. 71.6**). Compression of the median nerve by the pronator teres muscle is called *pronator syndrome.*[5] The onset of symptoms usually occurs after repetitive elbow

motions such as chopping wood, sculling, or cleaning fish, although occasionally the onset is more insidious, without apparent antecedent trauma (**Fig. 71.7**). Clinically, pronator syndrome manifests as a chronic aching sensation localized to the forearm with pain occasionally radiating into the elbow. Patients with pronator syndrome may complain about a tired or heavy sensation in the forearm during minimal activity, as well as clumsiness of the affected extremity. The sensory symptoms of pronator syndrome are identical to those of carpal tunnel syndrome. However, in contradistinction to carpal tunnel syndrome, nighttime symptoms are unusual in pronator syndrome.[5]

Signs and Symptoms

The physical findings of pronator syndrome include tenderness over the forearm in the region of the pronator teres muscle. Unilateral hypertrophy of the pronator teres muscle may be identified. A positive Tinel sign over the median nerve as it passes beneath the pronator teres muscle may also be present. Weakness of the intrinsic muscles of the forearm and hand that are innervated by the median nerve may be identified

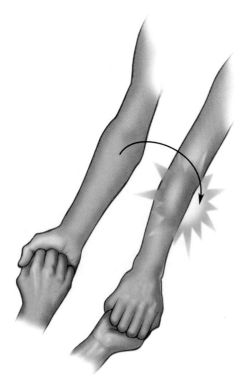

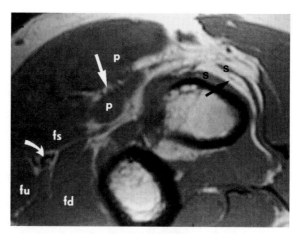

Fig. 71.9 **Median nerve anatomy.** Transverse T1-weighted (TR/TE 500/20) spin-echo magnetic resonance image at the level of the proximal portion of the forearm of an extended elbow shows the following: the median nerve (*straight white arrow*) located between the two heads of the pronator teres (p) muscles; the ulnar nerve (*curved white arrow*) between the flexor digitorum profundus (fd), flexor digitorum superficialis (fs), and flexor carpi ulnaris (fu) muscles; and the radial nerve (*black arrow*) between the two heads of the supinator (s) muscle. (*From Kim YS, Yeh LR, Trudell D, et al: MR imaging of the major nerves about the elbow: cadaveric study examining the effect of flexion and extension of the elbow and pronation and supination of the forearm,* Skeletal Radiol *27:419, 1998.*)

with careful manual muscle testing. A positive pronator syndrome test result, characterized by pain on forced pronation of the patient's fully supinated arm, is highly suggestive of compression of the median nerve by the pronator teres muscle (**Fig. 71.8**).

Testing

Electromyography helps to distinguish cervical radiculopathy, thoracic outlet syndrome, and carpal tunnel syndrome from pronator syndrome. Plain radiographs are indicated in all patients who present with pronator syndrome, to rule out occult bony disease. Based on the patient's clinical presentation, additional testing including complete blood count, uric acid, sedimentation rate, and antinuclear antibody testing may be indicated. MRI scan of the forearm is indicated if a primary elbow disorder or a space-occupying lesion is suspected (**Fig. 71.9**). The injection of the median nerve at the elbow serves as both a diagnostic test and a therapeutic maneuver.

Differential Diagnosis

Median nerve entrapment by the ligament of Struthers manifests clinically as unexplained persistent forearm pain caused by compression of the median nerve by an aberrant ligament that runs from a supracondylar process to the medial epicondyle. Clinically, this disorder is difficult to distinguish from pronator syndrome. The diagnosis is made by electromyography and nerve conduction velocity testing, which demonstrate compression of the median nerve at the elbow, combined with the radiographic finding of a supracondylar process.

Both of these entrapment neuropathies can be differentiated from isolated compression of the anterior interosseous nerve that occurs some 6 to 8 cm below the elbow. These syndromes should also be differentiated from cervical radiculopathy involving the C6 or C7 roots that may, at times, mimic median nerve compression. Cervical radiculopathy and median nerve entrapment may coexist as the double-crush syndrome. The double-crush syndrome is seen most commonly with median nerve entrapment at the wrist or carpal tunnel syndrome. Thoracic outlet syndrome may also cause forearm pain and be confused with pronator syndrome. However, the pain of thoracic outlet syndrome radiates into the ulnar rather than the median portion of the hand.

Treatment

Use of NSAIDs or COX-2 inhibitors represents a reasonable first step in the treatment of pronator syndrome. The administration of tricyclic antidepressants (e.g., nortriptyline, at a single bedtime dose of 25 mg, with upward titration as side effects allow) is useful, especially if sleep disturbance is also present. Avoidance of repetitive trauma thought to contribute to this entrapment neuropathy is also important. If these maneuvers fail to produce rapid symptomatic relief, injection of the median nerve at the elbow with local anesthetic and steroid is a reasonable next step (**Fig. 71.10**).[6] If symptoms continue to persist, surgical exploration and release of the median nerve will be indicated.

Complications and Pitfalls

Median nerve block at the elbow is a relatively safe block. The major complications are inadvertent intravascular injection and persistent paresthesia secondary to needle trauma to the nerve. This technique can safely be performed in patients

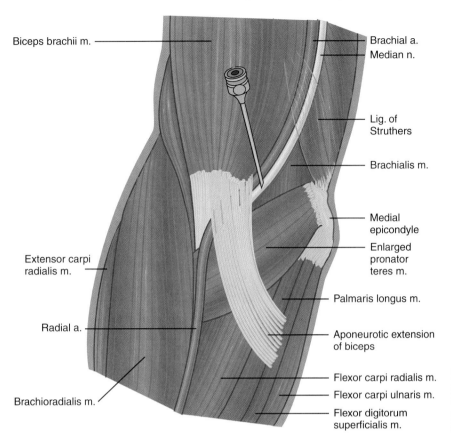

Biceps brachii m.

Brachial a.

Median n.

Lig. of Struthers

Brachialis m.

Medial epicondyle

Enlarged pronator teres m.

Extensor carpi radialis m.

Palmaris longus m.

Radial a.

Aponeurotic extension of biceps

Flexor carpi radialis m.

Brachioradialis m.

Flexor carpi ulnaris m.

Flexor digitorum superficialis m.

Fig. 71.10 **Injection technique for relieving pain resulting from pronator syndrome.** *(From Waldman SD: Pronator syndrome. In* Atlas of pain management injection techniques, *ed 2, Philadelphia, 2007, Saunders, p 189.)*

receiving anticoagulants by using a 25- or 27-gauge needle, albeit at increased risk of hematoma, if the clinical situation dictates a favorable risk-to-benefit ratio. These complications can be decreased if manual pressure is applied to the area of the block immediately following injection. The application of cold packs for 20-minute periods following the block also decreases the amount of postprocedure pain and bleeding.

Anterior Interosseous Syndrome

Anterior interosseous syndrome is characterized by pain and muscle weakness secondary to median nerve compression syndrome below the elbow by the tendinous origins of the pronator teres muscle and flexor digitorum superficialis muscle of the long finger or by aberrant blood vessels (**Fig. 71.11**). The onset of symptoms is usually after acute trauma to the forearm or following repetitive forearm and elbow motions such as using an ice pick. An inflammatory origin analogous to that of Parsonage-Turner syndrome has also been suggested as a cause of anterior interosseous syndrome.

Clinically, anterior interosseous syndrome manifests as an acute pain in the proximal forearm.[7] As the syndrome progresses, patients with anterior interosseous syndrome may complain about a tired or heavy sensation in the forearm during minimal activity, as well as the inability to pinch items between the thumb and index fingers because of paralysis of the flexor pollicis longus and flexor digitorum profundus muscles (see Fig. 71.11).

Physical findings include the inability to flex the interphalangeal joint of the thumb and the distal interphalangeal joint

of the index finger because of paralysis of the flexor pollicis longus and flexor digitorum profundus muscles.[8] Tenderness over the forearm in the region of the pronator teres muscle is seen in some patients suffering from anterior interosseous syndrome. A positive Tinel sign over the anterior interosseous branch of the median nerve approximately 6 to 8 cm below the elbow may also be present.

The anterior interosseous syndrome should also be differentiated from cervical radiculopathy involving the C6 or C7 roots that may mimic median nerve compression. Furthermore, cervical radiculopathy and median nerve entrapment may coexist as the double-crush syndrome. The double crush syndrome is seen most commonly with median nerve entrapment at the wrist or carpal tunnel syndrome.

Clinically Relevant Anatomy

The median nerve is composed of fibers from C5-T1 spinal roots. The nerve lies anterior and superior to the axillary artery. Exiting the axilla, the median nerve descends into the upper arm along with the brachial artery. At the level of the elbow, the brachial artery is just medial to the biceps muscle. At this level, the median nerve lies just medial to the brachial artery. As the median nerve proceeds downward into the forearm, it gives off numerous branches that provide motor innervation to the flexor muscles of the forearm, including the anterior interosseous nerve. These branches are susceptible to nerve entrapment by aberrant ligaments, muscle hypertrophy, and direct trauma. The nerve approaches the wrist overlying the radius. It lies deep to and between the tendons of the palmaris longus muscle and the flexor carpi radialis muscle at the wrist. The terminal branches of the median nerve provide

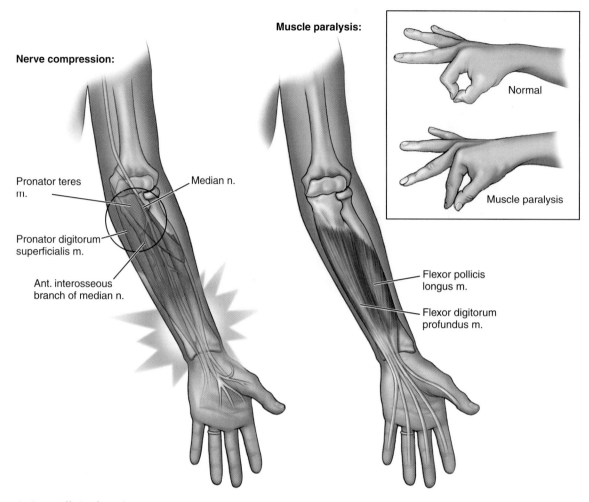

Nerve compression:

Pronator teres
m.

Median n.

Pronator digitorum
superficialis m.

Ant. interosseous
branch of median n.

Muscle paralysis:

Normal

Muscle paralysis

Flexor pollicis
longus m.

Flexor digitorum
profundus m.

Fig. 71.11 Patients suffering from the anterior interosseous syndrome exhibit acute forearm pain and progressive weakness of pinch. *(From Waldman SD: Anterior interosseous syndrome. In* Atlas of uncommon pain syndromes, *ed 2, Philadelphia, 2008, Saunders, p 107.)*

sensory innervation to a portion of the palmar surface of the hand, as well as to the palmar surface of the thumb and the index, and middle fingers and the radial portion of the ring finger. The median nerve also provides sensory innervation to the distal dorsal surface of the index and middle fingers and the radial portion of the ring finger.

Treatment

Use of the NSAIDs or COX-2 inhibitors represents a reasonable first step in the treatment of pronator syndrome. The administration of a tricyclic antidepressant (e.g., nortriptyline, at a single bedtime dose of 25 mg, with upward titration as side effects allow) is useful, especially if sleep disturbance is also present. Avoidance of repetitive trauma thought to contribute to this entrapment neuropathy is also important. If these maneuvers fail to produce rapid symptomatic relief, injection of the median nerve at the forearm with local anesthetic and steroid is a reasonable next step.[7] If symptoms continue to persist, surgical exploration and release of the median nerve will be indicated.

The patient is placed in a supine position with the arm fully adducted at the patient's side and the elbow slightly flexed with the dorsum of the hand resting on a folded towel. A total

of 5 to 7 mL of local anesthetic and 40 mg of methylprednisolone is drawn up in a 12-mL sterile syringe. The patient is then asked to flex his or her forearm against resistance to identify the biceps tendon at the crease of the elbow. A point 6 to 8 cm below the biceps tendon is then identified and marked with a sterile skin marker.

After preparation of the skin with antiseptic solution, a 1½-inch, 25-gauge needle is inserted at the previously marked point and is slowly advanced in a slightly cephalad trajectory (**Fig. 71.12**). As the needle advances approximately ½ to ¾ inch, strong paresthesia in the distribution of the median nerve is elicited. If no paresthesia is elicited and the needle contacts bone, the needle is withdrawn and is redirected slightly more medially until paresthesia is elicited. The patient should be warned that paresthesia will occur and to say "there!!!!" as soon as the paresthesia is felt. After paresthesia is elicited and its distribution is identified, gentle aspiration is carried out to identify blood. If the aspiration test result is negative and no persistent paresthesia into the distribution of the median nerve remains, a total of 5 to 7 mL of solution is slowly injected, and the patient is monitored closely for signs of local anesthetic toxicity. If no paresthesia can be elicited, a similar amount of solution is injected in a fanlike manner, with care taken not to inadvertently inject into the anterior interosseous artery.

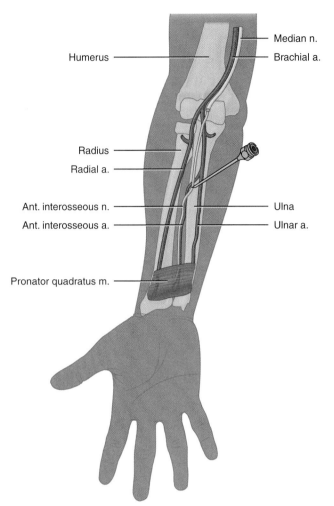

Fig. 71.12 Injection technique for relieving pain resulting from anterior interosseous syndrome. *(From Waldman SD: Anterior interosseous syndrome.* In *Atlas of pain management injection techniques, ed 2, Philadelphia, 2007, Saunders, p 193.)*

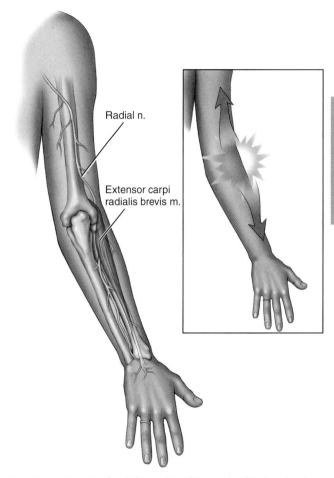

Fig. 71.13 The pain of radial tunnel syndrome is localized to the deep exterior muscle mass and may radiate proximally and distally into the upper arm and forearm. *(From Waldman SD: Radial tunnel syndrome.* In *Atlas of uncommon pain syndromes, ed 2, Philadelphia, 2008, Saunders, p 102.)*

Complications and Pitfalls

Median nerve block below the elbow is a relatively safe block. The major complications are inadvertent intravascular injection and persistent paresthesia secondary to needle trauma to the nerve. This technique can safely be performed in patients receiving anticoagulants by using a 25- or 27-gauge needle, albeit at increased risk of hematoma, if the clinical situation dictates a favorable risk-to-benefit ratio. These complications can be decreased if manual pressure is applied to the area of the block immediately following injection. The application of cold packs for 20-minute periods following the block also decreases the amount of postprocedure pain and bleeding.

Radial Tunnel Syndrome

Radial tunnel syndrome is an entrapment neuropathy of the radial nerve that is often clinically misdiagnosed as resistant tennis elbow.[9,10] In radial tunnel syndrome, the posterior interosseous branch of the radial nerve is entrapped by various mechanisms that share a similar clinical presentation.

These mechanisms include aberrant fibrous bands in front of the radial head, anomalous blood vessels that compress the nerve, and a sharp tendinous margin of the extensor carpi radialis brevis (see Fig. 71.11). These entrapments may exist alone or in combination.

Regardless of the mechanism of entrapment of the radial nerve, the common clinical feature of radial tunnel syndrome is pain just below the lateral epicondyle of the humerus.[9] The pain of radial tunnel syndrome may develop after an acute twisting injury or direct trauma to the soft tissues overlying the posterior interosseous branch of the radial nerve, or the onset may be more insidious, without an obvious inciting factor (**Fig. 71.13**). The pain is constant and is made worse by active supination of the wrist. Patients often note the inability to hold a coffee cup or hammer. Sleep disturbance is common. On physical examination, the patient will report tenderness to palpation of the posterior interosseous branch of the radial nerve just below the lateral epicondyle[11] (**Fig. 71.14**). Elbow range of motion is normal. Grip strength on the affected side may be diminished. Patients with radial tunnel syndrome exhibit pain on active resisted supination of the forearm.

Cervical radiculopathy and tennis elbow can mimic radial tunnel syndrome.[10] Radial tunnel syndrome can

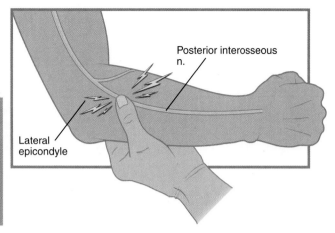

Fig. 71.14 Radial tunnel syndrome can be distinguished from tennis elbow by careful identification of the point of maximal tenderness. *(From Waldman SD: Radial tunnel syndrome. In Atlas of uncommon pain syndromes, ed 2, Philadelphia, 2008, Saunders, p 103.)*

be distinguished from tennis elbow in that in radial tunnel syndrome, the maximal tenderness to palpation is distal to the lateral epicondyle over the posterior interosseous branch of the radial nerve, whereas in tennis elbow, the maximal tenderness to palpation is over the lateral epicondyle (see Fig. 71.12). Electromyography helps to distinguish cervical radiculopathy and radial tunnel syndrome from tennis elbow. Plain radiographs are indicated to rule out occult bony disease in all patients who present with radial tunnel syndrome. Based on the patient's clinical presentation, additional testing including complete blood count, uric acid, sedimentation rate, and antinuclear antibody testing may be indicated. MRI scan of the elbow is indicated if joint instability is suspected. The injection technique described here serves as both a diagnostic test and a therapeutic maneuver.[12]

Clinically Relevant Anatomy

The radial nerve is made up of fibers from C5-T1 spinal roots. The nerve lies posterior and inferior to the axillary artery. Exiting the axilla, the radial nerve passes between the medial and long heads of the triceps muscle. As the nerve curves across the posterior aspect of the humerus, it supplies a motor branch to the triceps. Continuing its downward path, it gives off numerous sensory branches to the upper arm. At a point between the lateral epicondyle of the humerus and the musculospiral groove, the radial nerve divides into its two terminal branches. The superficial branch continues down the arm along with the radial artery and provides sensory innervation to the dorsum of the wrist and the dorsal aspects of a portion of the thumb, index, and middle finger. The deep posterior interosseous branch provides most of the motor innervation to the extensors of the forearm.

Treatment

Use of the NSAIDs or COX-2 inhibitors represents a reasonable first step in the treatment of pronator syndrome. The administration of the tricyclic antidepressants (e.g., nortriptyline, at a single bedtime dose of 25 mg, with upward titration as side effects allow) is also useful, especially if sleep disturbance is also present. Avoidance of repetitive trauma thought to contribute to this entrapment neuropathy is also important. If these maneuvers fail to produce rapid symptomatic relief, injection of the median nerve at the forearm with local anesthetic and steroid is a reasonable next step.[7] If symptoms continue to persist, surgical exploration and release of the radial nerve will be indicated.

Conclusion

The myriad and overlapping clinical presentations of the entrapment neuropathies at the elbow and forearm present a diagnostic challenge to the clinician. To make the correct diagnosis, a targeted history and physical examination are mandatory. Electromyography and nerve conduction studies combined with judicious use of diagnostic imaging techniques will help to confirm the diagnosis. Failure to diagnose and treat in a timely manner the entrapment neuropathies discussed here can lead to significant suffering and disability for the patient.

References

Full references for this chapter can be found on www.expertconsult.com.

Part E

Wrist and Hand Pain Syndromes

Chapter **72**

Arthritis of the Wrist and Hand

Richard M. Keating

General Considerations

Pain in the wrist and hand is a relatively common symptom that patients bring to a clinician. The pain may emanate from any of the numerous bones or joints in the hand, from periarticular soft tissue sites (subcutaneous tissues, palmar fascia, tendon sheaths), from vascular structures, or from peripheral nerves. The pain may even be referred pain from anomalies in the cervical spine, thoracic outlet, shoulder, or elbow. **Table 72.1** provides a list of the differential diagnoses of painful disorders of the wrist and hand, based on location. Many of these entities are discussed more fully in other chapters. As always, an accurate diagnosis depends on a detailed history and on a careful physical examination of the joints, the tenosynovial sheaths and periarticular structures, the cervical spine, and the nerve and blood supplies to the hand. Laboratory testing and imaging studies supplement the history and physical examination, to arrive at a correct diagnosis.[1]

The onset of many painful, nontraumatic hand disorders is often insidious, with the exception of crystalline disease, which usually has an abrupt onset. A history of unaccustomed, repetitive, or excessive hand activity is particularly important in the diagnosis of wrist, thumb, or finger arthritis or tenosynovitis when the cause is an overuse syndrome. A detailed occupational history is important for determining whether the hand tenosynovitis is work related, either as a cumulative trauma disorder or as an acute injury.

A working knowledge of the anatomy of the wrist joint, the metacarpophalangeal (MCP) joints, the proximal interphalangeal (PIP) and distal interphalangeal (DIP) joints of the fingers, and the tendon sheaths (**Figs. 72.1** and **72.2**) is important for precise diagnosis. The back of the hand is called the *dorsum*, the palmar aspect is called the *volar side*, and each finger has three joints: the MCP, PIP, and DIP. The thumb has an MCP and an interphalangeal joint (IP) but no DIP joint. The base of the thumb, where the metacarpal bone meets the carpal row, is the carpometacarpal (CMC) joint.

The ability to localize the area of pain accurately in the hand quickly narrows the differential diagnosis. For example,

most pain in the CMC joint results from osteoarthritis (OA), whereas pain with swelling in the MCP joints is often a sign of rheumatoid arthritis (RA) or another inflammatory arthritis.

Correct localization of the pain allows the clinician to make the correct diagnosis. Most disorders of the hand and wrist can be diagnosed without the need for laboratory analysis. Diagnostic studies may include a complete blood count, erythrocyte sedimentation rate, chemistry studies, and rheumatoid factor and antinuclear antibody determinations (if the overall history and physical examination suggest a diffuse connective tissue disease). Hand radiographs are useful for diagnosing certain forms of arthritis, if the arthritis has been present for long enough to result in bony changes. Synovial fluid analysis (if joint effusion is present) may be diagnostic of crystalline disease, and this analysis is also necessary to differentiate inflammatory from noninflammatory arthritis. Additional studies are sometimes required and may include skeletal scintigraphy, ultrasonography, nerve conduction studies, noninvasive vascular (Doppler) studies, arteriography, computed tomography, magnetic resonance imaging, arthrography, and even synovial biopsy.

Arthritis of the Wrist

Etiology

The radiocarpal (wrist) joint is a common site for inflammatory arthritides, such as RA, systemic lupus erythematosus (SLE), crystalline arthritis (gout and pseudogout), psoriatic arthritis (PsA), ankylosing spondylitis, reactive arthritis, and enteropathic arthritis.[1] Primary OA of the wrist is rare, but the joint can be affected by secondary OA brought on by trauma, hemochromatosis, ochronosis, osteonecrosis, or past infection.

Clinical Features and Differential Diagnosis

Arthritis of the wrist is associated with pain and stiffness just distal to the radius and ulna. Movements are often restricted, and crepitus may be appreciated with both active and passive range of motion. Inflammatory arthritis is usually accompanied by joint capsule–based swelling (synovitis), along with reduced function and even deformity. Inflammatory arthritis effusions may be appreciated when pressure with one hand on one side of the joints produces a fluid wave transmitted to the second hand placed on the opposite side of the joint. Wrist deformities are common in RA and other chronic inflammatory arthritides. Findings may include volar subluxation of the carpus with a visible step opposite the radiocarpal joint, carpal collapse (loss of carpal height to less than half the length

Table 72.1 Differential Diagnoses of Wrist and Hand Pain

Articular	
Wrist	RA, SLE, crystalline disease
MCP	RA, SLE, crystalline disease
PIP	Nodal OA, RA, SLE, psoriatic arthritis
DIP	Nodal OA, SLE, psoriatic arthritis
Periarticular	
Subcutaneous	RA nodule, gouty tophus, glomus tumor
Palmar fascia	Dupuytren's contracture
Tendon sheath	de Quervain's tenosynovitis Wrist volar flexor tenosynovitis Thumb or finger flexor tenosynovitis (trigger or snapping thumb or finger) Pigmented villonodular tenosynovitis (giant cell tumor of the tendon sheath)
Acute calcific periarthritis	Wrist, MCP, and rarely PIP and DIP
Ganglion	Attached to joint capsule, tendon sheath, or tendon
Osseous	Fractures, neoplasms, infection (osteomyelitis) Osteonecrosis including Kienböck's disease (lunate bone) and Preiser's disease (scaphoid bone)
Nerve Entrapment Syndromes	
Median nerve	Carpal tunnel syndrome (at wrist) Pronator teres syndrome (at pronator teres) Anterior interosseous nerve syndrome
Ulnar nerve	Cubital tunnel syndrome (at elbow) Guyon canal (at wrist)
Posterior interosseous	Radial nerve palsy (spiral groove syndrome)
Lower brachial plexus	Thoracic outlet syndrome, Pancoast's tumor
Cervical nerve roots	Herniated cervical disk, tumors
Spinal cord lesion	Spinal tumors, syringomyelia
Vascular	
Vasospastic disorders (Raynaud's)	Scleroderma, occupational vibration syndrome
Vasculitis	Digital ischemia and ischemic ulcers, SLE, RA
Referred Pain	
Cervical spine disorders	Referred radicular pain syndromes
Complex regional pain syndrome*	Shoulder-hand syndrome and causalgia
Cardiac	Angina pectoris

*Formerly called reflex sympathic dystrophy.

DIP, distal interphalangeal; MCP, metacarpophalangeal; OA, osteoarthritis; PIP, proximal interphalangeal; RA, rheumatoid arthritis; SLE, systemic lupus erythematosus.

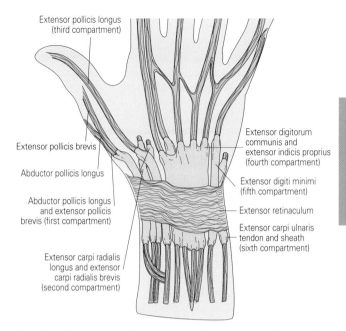

Fig. 72.1 **Extensor tendons and tendon sheaths of the wrist, fingers, and thumb.** *(From Hochberg M, Silman A, editors: Rheumatology, ed 3, Philadelphia, 2003, Mosby, p 642.)*

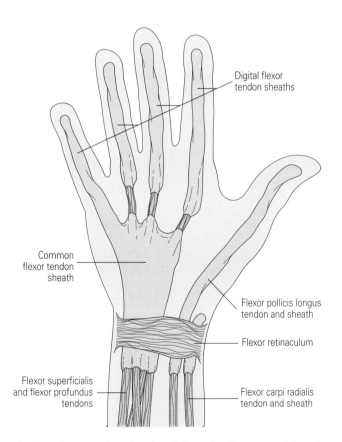

Fig. 72.2 **Flexor tendon sheaths of the wrist, fingers, and thumb.** *(From Hochberg M, Silman A, editors: Rheumatology, ed 3, Philadelphia, 2003, Mosby, p 642.)*

of the third metacarpal), and radial deviation of the carpus from the axis of the wrist and hand. Chronic inflammatory arthritis of the distal radioulnar joint is associated with local swelling, painful restriction of pronation and supination, and often instability with dorsal subluxation of the ulnar head and a "piano key sign" on the distal ulna (it sits higher than the distal radius and can be easily moved up and down because of ligamentous laxity).

Extensor wrist tenosynovitis, by contrast, manifests as a superficial, linear or oval, dorsal swelling localized to the distribution of the affected tendon sheath and extending well beyond the joint margins, seemingly to involve the entire dorsum of the hand. When the fingers are actively extended, the distal margin of the swelling moves proximally and folds inward, like a sheet being tucked under a mattress (the "tuck sign"). Tenosynovitis of the common flexor tendon sheath manifests as a swelling over the volar aspect of the wrist just proximal to the carpal tunnel (volar "hot dog sign").[1] Ganglia are mucinous structures with a jelly-like consistency on palpation that arise in the hand. They may be attached to various structures including the joint capsule, tendon sheath, or tendons themselves. The cause of ganglia is not known. Most ganglia are found on the dorsal aspect of the wrist. Often painless, they can sometimes interfere with smooth mechanical function. Although aspiration diminishes their size, they often recur following the procedure, and surgical excision is required.[2]

Arthritis of the Metacarpophalangeal Proximal Interphalangeal, and Distal Interphalangeal Joints

Inflammatory arthritis of the MCP and PIP joints is most often associated with RA and SLE. These same joints can be affected by PsA, but PsA may also affect the DIP joints, especially when the nails are affected by psoriasis. MCP synovitis produces diffuse, tender swelling of the joint that may obscure the valleys between the knuckles and that is sometimes referred to as "the mogul sign."[1] Swelling of the PIP joint produces a fusiform or spindle-shaped finger. To detect PIP or DIP joint effusion, compression of the joint by one hand produces ballooning or a hydraulic lift sensed by the other hand ("balloon sign"). Unlike PIP synovitis, dorsal knuckle pads are a subcutaneous tissue thickening that produces nontender thickening of the skin localized to the dorsal surface overlying the PIP joints. Both the PIP and DIP joints are commonly affected in primary "nodal" OA, which manifests as Bouchard's nodes and Heberden's nodes, respectively. Digital flexor tenosynovitis, by contrast, produces a linear tender swelling over the volar aspect of the finger ("sausage finger"), often associated with thickening, nodules, and fine crepitus of the flexor tendon sheath.

Deformities of the MCP, PIP, and DIP joints are relatively common in inflammatory arthritis.[1] MCP joint deformities include ulnar drift, volar subluxation (often visible as a step), and fixed flexion deformity. The term *boutonnière deformity* describes a finger with flexion of the PIP joint and hyperextension of the DIP joint (**Fig. 72.3**). The term *swan-neck deformity* describes the appearance of a finger with hyperextension of the PIP joint and flexion of the DIP joint (**Fig. 72.4**). A Z-shaped deformity of the thumb consists of flexion of the MCP joint and hyperextension of the IP joint (see Fig. 72.4). Telescoped

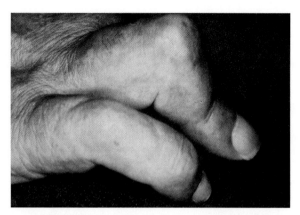

Fig. 72.3 Boutonnière deformity of the right ring finger. *(From Hochberg M, Silman A, editors:* Rheumatology, *ed 3, Philadelphia, 2003, Mosby, p 644.)*

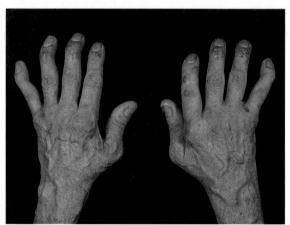

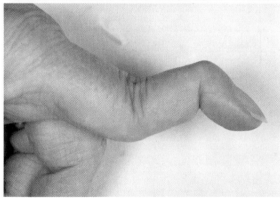

Fig. 72.4 Swan-neck deformities of the fingers and Z-shaped deformities of the thumbs. *(From Hochberg M, Silman A, editors:* Rheumatology, *ed 3, Philadelphia, 2003, Mosby, p 644.)*

shortening of the digits, produced by partial resorption of the phalanges secondary to PsA, RA, or other destructive arthritis, is often associated with concentric wrinkling of the skin ("opera-glass hand").

Treatment

Treatment of arthritis of the wrist, MCP, PIP, or DIP joints depends on identifying the underlying cause and addressing treatment to that disorder. For example, RA should be treated with methotrexate, other disease-modifying agents, or a biologic agent. OA should be treated with pain control, physical therapy, and possibly the use of assistive devices when the hand is affected. General measures include resting of the affected joint by splinting and physical and occupational therapies. Soft tissue causes of hand and wrist pain are treated in a specific fashion, depending on type. Specific disorders are described in separate chapters.

For persistent inflammatory synovitis, intra-articular corticosteroids are often helpful. The radiocarpal (wrist) joint can be injected through a dorsoradial approach.[3] With the wrist slightly palmar flexed, the needle is inserted perpendicularly to a depth of 1 to 2 cm at a point distal to Lister's tubercle of the distal radius (a bony prominence palpated along the distal radius) and just ulnar to the extensor pollicis longus tendon. The MCP, PIP, and DIP joints can be readily entered through a dorsoradial or a dorsoulnar approach using a 28-gauge needle.[3] It is sometimes necessary to tease the needle tip into the joint space while the operator applies slight traction to the finger, to pull the articulating surfaces apart. A correctly placed intra-articular injection produces fluid distention of the joint on all sides.

References

Full references for this chapter can be found on www.expertconsult.com.

Chapter 73

Carpal Tunnel Syndrome

Richard M. Keating

The carpal tunnel is an anatomic region in the wrist and the site of the body's most common entrapment neuropathy. The true carpal tunnel is bounded on its dorsal and lateral aspects by the carpal bones and the intercarpal joints and on its volar aspect by the transverse carpal ligament (flexor retinaculum).[1] Passing through this canal are nine flexor tendons that include the flexor digitorum profundus, flexor digitorum sublimis, and flexor pollicis longus, along with the median nerve. In 1854, James Paget first reported what is now considered carpal tunnel syndrome (CTS).[2]

Etiology

Any process that can result in swelling of the flexor tendons or in infiltration of the carpal tunnel space can cause the symptoms of CTS by pressure on the median nerve. Most often, nonspecific tenosynovitis in an otherwise healthy person is thought to be the cause of CTS.[3] Synovitis from rheumatoid arthritis, inflammation from a gout attack or tophi deposition, inflammation from systemic lupus erythematosus, a pseudogout attack, or any other inflammatory process can also result in CTS. In addition, infiltrative diseases such as amyloid can cause CTS. Obesity, hypothyroidism, acromegaly, diabetes, and pregnancy are all recognized risk factors for CTS.

More commonly, however, CTS is idiopathic and is believed to be caused by repetitive motion, whether occupational or recreational. On rare occasion, CTS may be attributable to a space-occupying lesion in the carpal tunnel such as a ganglion, lipoma, or even a fracture callus.

Clinical Features and Physical Examination

The typical CTS sufferer is a woman between 40 and 60 years old.[4] The usual symptoms include burning pain, paresthesias, numbness, or even sensory loss along the median nerve distribution: fingers 1, 2, 3, and the radial aspect of finger 4 (the thumb, first two fingers, and the radial half of the ring finger). Nocturnal awakening with symptom exacerbation is a characteristic and frequent complaint, and the presence of symptoms on first awakening is also common. Many patients awaken to find themselves shaking their hand or forearm to alleviate the symptoms. Some patients experience pain or paresthesia radiation more proximally up the forearm, to the elbow region or even toward the shoulder. Repetitive flexion and extension at the wrist worsen the symptom complex.

Physical examination findings, especially early in the course of CTS, are entirely normal. With a longer duration of symptoms, one can see flattening of the thenar eminence from muscle loss.[5] Provocative maneuvers employed by the clinician to reproduce symptoms and to help make the diagnosis of CTS include *Tinel's sign.* The volar aspect of the wrist, at the level of the carpal tunnel, is percussed in a tapping manner. The proper site for percussion is at the flexor retinaculum, just radial to the palmaris longus tendon at the distal wrist crease. This maneuver is performed with the patient's wrist in slight extension. A positive test result is characterized by reproduction of paresthesia in the median nerve distribution (along fingers 1, 2, 3, and the radial aspect of finger 4)[4] (**Fig. 73.1**). Another provocative test is the *Phalen maneuver.* The wrist is flexed for 30 to 60 seconds; this maneuver may well reproduce finger paresthesias (**Fig. 73.2**). Wrist extension narrows the carpal tunnel, increases pressure within the canal, and thereby reproduces the symptoms. This test is termed the *reverse Phalen maneuver.* Simply elevating the affected hand for 1 or 2 minutes may also reproduce the patient's symptoms. A good sensory examination may demonstrate diminished touch, two-point discrimination, or vibratory sense in the median nerve distribution. Chronic symptoms may result in loss of thenar muscle bulk, with resultant weakness in the abductor pollicis brevis (weakness of resisted palmar abduction of the thumb) and opponens pollicis muscles (inability to maintain a pinch between tip of thumb and tip of little finger against resistance).[4] The reported sensitivity and specificity of these maneuvers varies widely, and the diagnosis should always still be considered if the history is consistent with CTS but no particular maneuver reproduces the pain or paresthesias.

Median nerve entrapment at the elbow, known as *pronator teres syndrome,* can cause weakness of the intrinsic muscles in the second and third fingers with hyperextension at the MCP joints and can sometimes be confused with CTS. Pronator teres syndrome can be distinguished from CTS by a positive

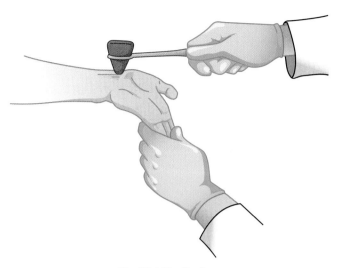

Fig. 73.1 **Tinel's sign.**

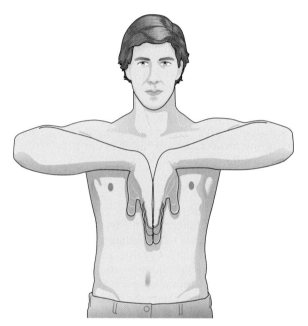

Fig. 73.2 **Phalen's test.**

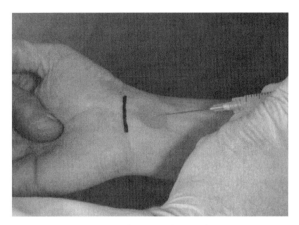

Fig. 73.3 **Injection for carpal tunnel syndrome.**

Tinel sign at the elbow instead of at the wrist. Other conditions that can be confused with CTS include diabetic neuropathy and cervical radiculopathy.

Diagnostic Studies

CTS is a *clinical* diagnosis. The clinician usually makes the diagnosis based on history, with possibly some support from physical examination maneuvers. The diagnosis can be confirmed by an electrodiagnostic study that demonstrates slowing of sensory conduction through the median nerve as it traverses the carpal tunnel, but this test is not absolutely required to make the diagnosis. CTS may also be associated with prolonged distal motor latency, although sensory conduction is far more often affected than is motor conduction.[3] Electrodiagnostic studies may also be useful in localizing the entrapment site. However, false-negative results can occur in up to 10% of patients.[6] Occasionally, magnetic resonance imaging or ultrasonography demonstrates swelling within the flexor tendons from tenosynovitis.

Treatment

Treatment of CTS can start conservatively, with avoidance of repetitive action, volar splinting (especially at night) of the wrist in a slightly extended position, and judicious use of nonsteroidal anti-inflammatory drugs (NSAIDs) for pain and inflammation.[7] However, a 2003 systematic review found no significant benefit from using NSAIDs as compared with placebo.[8] In the setting of CTS and concomitant first carpometacarpal joint osteoarthritis, splinting of both the wrist and the first carpometacarpal may be preferred. The purpose of referral to a hand occupational therapist is to instruct the patient on stretching exercises for the volar carpal ligaments may be helpful.

A local corticosteroid injection of the carpal tunnel may be useful if the condition is of shorter duration (<1 year) and the patient has no evidence of thenar atrophy or obvious muscle weakness. The median nerve, lying radial to and below the palmaris longus tendon, must be avoided during injection. Therefore, a 28-guage needle should be inserted tangentially, directed toward the palm, and placed ulnar to the palmaris longus tendon and just proximal to the distal wrist crease. The needle is advanced through the transverse carpal ligament to a depth of 2 to 4 mm until the sheath is entered, followed by injection of 20 to 40 mg methylprednisolone acetate (**Fig. 73.3**). Although this procedure may give some temporary relief, its long-term effect on CTS is unclear. A 2007 meta-analysis of glucocorticoid injection treatment for CTS concluded that these injections did improve symptoms at 1 month, but no evidence had established the benefit of this treatment beyond 1 month.[9] A 2-week course of oral prednisone, at 20 mg daily for 10 to 14 days, may be considered as an alternative to corticosteroid injection.

Surgical treatment consists of releasing the carpal tunnel by sectioning the transverse carpal ligament through a volar incision.[10] Closed (endoscopic) CTS release may also be employed.[11] A more limited incision release has been introduced with comparable efficacy to endoscopic or standard open procedures.[12] The timing of any of these procedures is critical. Once muscle atrophy or weakness or neurologic deficit is established, surgical care cannot guarantee a return of function. Early referral to a hand surgeon is encouraged.

References

Full references for this chapter can be found on www.expertconsult.com.

de Quervain's Tenosynovitis

Richard M. Keating

An excessive load or repetitive movement of a tendon within its tendon sheath can result in tenosynovitis with subsequent fibrosis, stenosis, sheath thickening, and edema or swelling of the tendinous structures.[1] This tenosynovitis is an impediment to the smooth motion of the tendon within its tendon sheath and eventually manifests as pain during motion, in addition to localized swelling and stiffness. One particular form of tenosynovitis is de Quervain's tenosynovitis. *de Quervain's tenosynovitis* was first described in 1895 as fibrosing tenosynovitis at the first extensor compartment with involvement of the sheath that envelops both the abductor pollicis longus and extensor pollicis brevis tendons of the thumb.

Clinical Features

de Quervain's tenosynovitis is most common in women 30 to 50 years of age. Patients typically report several weeks of pain, often severe, on the radial aspect of the wrist at about the level of the radial styloid. Wrist pain and grip weakness are the hallmarks of de Quervain's tenosynovitis. Pinch grip, thumb extension or abduction, and wrist motion exacerbate and reproduce the pain. The pain of de Quervain's tenosynovitis can extend proximally up the forearm from the region of the anatomic "snuff box." Repetitive activities, especially activities that involve pinching with the thumb while moving the wrist in either the radial or ulnar direction, result in inflammation and pain within the shared tendon sheath of the abductor pollicis longus and extensor pollicis brevis.

de Quervain's tenosynovitis can occur in isolation. It can also occur in conjunction with rheumatoid arthritis or psoriatic arthritis, after traumatic injury, secondary to calcium apatite deposition, during pregnancy, and in the postpartum period.[2]

The differential diagnosis of de Quervain's tenosynovitis includes osteoarthritis of the first carpometacarpal joint and the intersection syndrome. It is not unusual to see de Quervain's tenosynovitis and carpometacarpal osteoarthritis at the same time. The *intersection syndrome* is caused by tenosynovitis of the second extensor compartment (extensor carpi radialis longus and brevis) at its intersection with the tendons of the first extensor compartment (abductor pollicis longus and extensor pollicis brevis). The intersection syndrome usually results from repetitive motion of the wrist (flexion and extension) and is associated with pain and swelling over the dorsoradial aspect of the forearm, approximately 4 cm proximal to the wrist joint itself.[3]

Diagnosis

The affected tendon sheath is tender and swollen maximally 1 to 2 cm proximal to the radial styloid in the vicinity of the anatomic snuff box. Crepitus can often be appreciated. The definitive physical examination maneuver for the diagnosis of de Quervain's tenosynovitis is *Finkelstein's test*[4] (**Fig. 74.1**). The examiner puts the patient's wrist into passive ulnar deviation while the patient flexes the fingers over the thumb and encircles the thumb (the patient is asked to grab his or her thumb with fingers 2 to 5 and to squeeze the thumb into the palm of the hand). This maneuver stretches the affected tendons and reproduces the characteristic pain.

Treatment

Initial treatment for de Quervain's tenosynovitis should consist of local heat, a nonsteroidal anti-inflammatory agent if no contraindications exist, and a splint to immobilize both the wrist and the thumb.[5] An ideal splint is the radial gutter splint because it immobilizes the wrist in slight extension and radial deviation, the first carpometacarpal joint in slight abduction, and the first metacarpophalangeal joint in slight extension. Even if the patient is not wearing a splint, he or she should avoid tasks that require repetitive thumb movement or pinch grasping. Patients with more severe or persistent symptoms

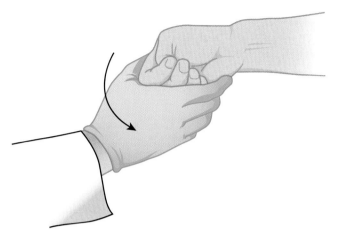

Fig. 74.1 **Finkelstein's test.**

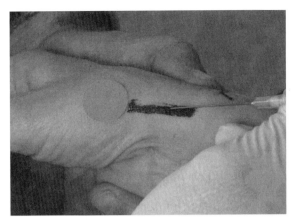

Fig. 74.2 **Injection for de Quervain's tenosynovitis.**

may require local corticosteroid injection into the affected tendon sheath. This maneuver is often quite dramatic in the relief it can provide. A 28-gauge needle is inserted tangentially into the distal end of the abductor pollicis longus and extensor pollicis brevis tendon sheath approximately 1 cm proximal to the radial styloid and aimed distally. The operator then instills 7.5 to 10 mg of methylprednisolone into the tendon sheath (**Fig. 74.2**). Surgical decompression is indicated for those patients with continued symptoms despite a trial of conservative and corticosteroid injection treatments. Decompression of the first extensor compartment, possibly with tenosynovectomy and compartment reconstruction, should be considered if symptoms persist for more than 6 months.[1]

References

Full references for this chapter can be found on www.expertconsult.com.

Chapter **75**

Dupuytren's Contracture

Richard M. Keating

Clinical Features

Dupuytren's contracture is a relatively common, painless palmar disorder characterized by painless nodular thickening, fibrosis, and contraction of the palmar fascia, with a resultant drawing up of one or more fingers with flexion at the metacarpophalangeal (MCP) joint (see **Fig. 75.1**).[1] Nodules and cords develop along the course of the flexor tendons, although the tendons themselves are not intrinsically involved. The fourth finger is usually affected first, followed in descending order by the fifth finger, third finger, and second finger.[2] The thumb is usually not affected. The condition is seen more frequently in those of Celtic or Scandinavian background and in association with diabetes, smoking, alcohol abuse, aging, complex regional pain syndrome, malignant disease, and male gender. Often, the process proceeds to a certain point and then stops, leaving the patient with essentially preserved hand function. Other patients experience a rapid and progressive course with an inability to place the palm flat on a tabletop (a positive "tabletop" test result). Thickened knuckle pads over the proximal interphalangeal joints are more common in Dupuytren's contracture but are also a normal variant. Prediction of progression with such a variable course is not possible.

Diagnosis

The diagnosis of Dupuytren's contracture depends on recognition of the typical physical examination findings. Dermal puckering overlying the flexor tendons proximal to the MCP joints is an early finding and is followed by passive flexion of the fingers at the MCP joints, nodule formation along the track of the flexor tendons in the palm, and an absence of any features of a systemic, inflammatory disease. The differential diagnosis includes diabetic cheiroarthropathy (this condition does not usually give any nodularity, only limited finger mobility that involves all fingers) and scleroderma (this condition causes tightening of the extensor skin surface and often distal digital ulcerations). Palmar fibromatosis or palmar fasciitis may be seen as a paraneoplastic process and can cause flexion contractures in all fingers of both hands simultaneously. It is brought about by tethering of the palmar fascia and skin to the flexor tendons, without any nodularity.

Etiology

The inciting event that sets the development of Dupuytren's contracture in motion has not been identified. A link between repetitive injury and occupational trauma is still unfounded, although considered a strong possibility. Lesions are characterized by fibroblastic proliferation, and dense, disordered collage deposition results in thickening of the palmar fascia with nodularity. The flexor tendons themselves are not involved. The involved fascia shows an increase in the total collagen with increased content of reducible cross links and hydroxylysine. Nodules form as a result of contraction of fibroblasts in the superficial palmar fascia with fibroblasts, and myofibroblasts are also present in the nodules.[3]

Treatment

Management needs to be individualized, with integration of the tempo of disease progression and the functional limitations imposed on the patient. Some patients, with minimally progressive disease, adapt quite well to the change in anatomy and need no specific intervention.[4] Referral to hand occupational therapist for local modality therapy, such as heat, stretching exercises, or issuance of protective gloves, may be beneficial. Adaptive devices can help the patient avoid a tightened grip with use of common tools or objects.

An intralesional corticosteroid injection may be useful if the previously mentioned efforts prove to be of no benefit. Local corticosteroid injection may reduce the rate of fibroblastic and myofibroblastic proliferation, increase apoptosis among inflammatory cells, and decrease the expression within Dupuytren's tissue of transforming growth factor-β1 and fibronectin.[5]

Another nonsurgical option is injection of clostridial collagenase into Dupuytren's lesions monthly for 3 months, with each injection followed by closed manipulation the next day.[6] This newer approach to treatment has shown encouraging early results and may spare the patient an open surgical procedure.

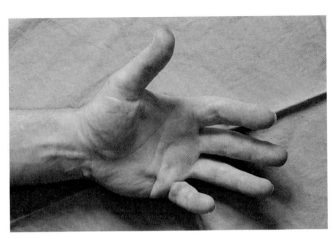

Fig. 75.1 **Dupuytren's contracture of the palmar fascia.**

In patients with significant functional decline in hand use, surgery may be considered. Some hand surgeons recommend a percutaneous needle fasciotomy. This procedure does give prompt relief, but recurrence is common.[7] A limited or complete palmar fasciectomy can be performed, although recurrence rates are high.[8]

References

Full references for this chapter can be found on www.expertconsult.com.

Trigger Finger and Trigger Thumb

Richard M. Keating

Trigger finger or trigger thumb (when the condition affects the first digit) has been variously called stenosing digital tenosynovitis, stenosing tenosynovitis, snapping finger, or snapping thumb (when the condition affects the first digit).

Usually brought on by overuse, the anatomic lesion is a tenosynovitis within the flexor tendons of the finger or thumb, with eventual fibrosis, thickening, and constriction. On occasion, one can see fibrocartilaginous metaplasia localized to the first (A1) annular pulley that overlies the metacarpophalangeal joint. A nodular consistency to the tendon often develops at the site of the stenosis.[1,2]

The condition is more frequent in middle-aged women than in men and is often a sequela of overuse. The condition affects the digits in the following rank order: thumb (first digit), ring (fourth digit), middle (third digit), little (fifth digit), and index (second digit; **Fig. 76.1**).

Etiologies of trigger finger and trigger thumb, other than simple overuse, include rheumatoid arthritis (RA), psoriatic arthritis, diabetes mellitus, Dupuytren's contracture, amyloidosis, hypothyroidism, sarcoidosis, pigmented villonodular tenosynovitis, and even infections, such as mycobacterium tuberculosis and spirotrichosis.[2]

The differential diagnosis includes slipping of an extensor tendon, as in RA, a collateral ligament catching on a bony prominence, or even a benign tendon tumor.

Clinical Features

A patient has symptoms of painful locking, snapping, clicking, catching, or, less often described, triggering with movement of the thumb or finger, frequently noticed when the bent proximal interphalangeal (PIP) joint is passively returned to full extension with an accompanying snapping sensation. The symptom is most noticeable on first awakening but may come on unpredictably with normal use.[2] Pain is maximal over the A1 pulley site, at about the level of the metacarpophalangeal (MCP) joint on the flexor surface, but pain may course along the entire tendon sheath length. Extension of the digit brings on the pain and, in extreme cases, a catching, but with force, the nodule is pulled free and the finger clicks and then extends. This is known as the catching tendon sign (**Fig. 76.2**). More subtle cases may be associated with a slight sensation of the finger "giving way" with extension. Some nodularity may be appreciated in the palm proximal to the MCP joint with finger motion.

Treatment

The nonoperative approach to the trigger finger includes splinting, nonsteroidal anti-inflammatory drugs, heat, and physical therapy. Splinting of the affected digit is often helpful, with the MCP joint at 10 to 15 degrees of palmar flexion and free motion at the PIP and distal interphalangeal joints allowed.[2] A corticosteroid injection via 28-gauge needle into the affected flexor tendon sheath, just proximal to the A1 pulley and opposite the volar aspect of the metacarpal head, is often effective and even curative.[3] The needle is advanced until gentle passive movements of the affected digit produce a crepitant sensation, indicating that the needle tip is rubbing against the surface of the tendon. The needle is then withdrawn 0.5 to 1 mm to a level above the tendon but within the synovial space. This is followed by injection of 10 to 20 mg of methylprednisolone acetate into the sheath. One should not inject against pressure. The syringe contents should flow smoothly. Intratendon sheath corticosteroid injections for trigger finger are superior to the injection of lidocaine alone for symptom relief of up to 4 months.[4] Splinting should definitely be continued after the injection itself. A corticosteroid injection is indicated if splinting has not improved the symptoms after 4 to 6 weeks.

Surgical therapy involves a "release" with transaction of the A1 pulley. Surgical treatment should be considered if two corticosteroid injections have been attempted without benefit.

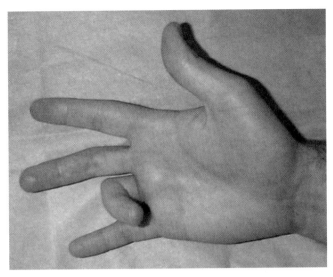

Fig. 76.1 **Trigger finger involving the forth digit.**

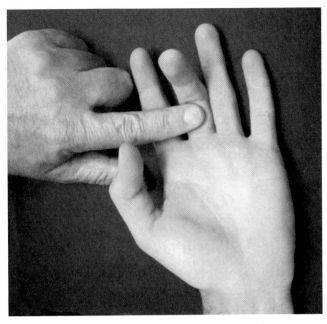

Fig. 76.2 **The catching tendon sign for trigger finger.** *(From Waldman SD: Physical diagnosis of pain: an atlas of signs and symptoms, Philadelphia, 2006, Saunders, p 195.)*

References

Full references for this chapter can be found on www.expertconsult.com.

Glomus Tumor of the Hand

Richard M. Keating

Presentation

A patient, usually a middle-aged woman, has a painful "burning" sensation, often under the fingernail. The pain may be paroxysmal in nature and insidious in onset. Temperature sensitivity is often a predominant feature, typically aggravated by cold and relieved by warming. A small, subcutaneous nodule may be palpated beneath the nail or in the finger pulp. The area around the nodule is often quite tender.[1,2]

Pathology

Glomus tumor (paraganglioma or glomangioma) is a rare, benign hamartoma that represents 1% to 5% of soft neoplasms of the hand.[1] These tumors are derived from the neuromyoarterial glomus body, a smooth muscle neuromyoarterial receptor that is sensitive to temperature changes and so governs microvascular blood flow. The tumor itself consists of an arteriole, a venule, and an anastomotic vessel (Sucquet-Hoyer canal) surrounded by smooth muscle fibers, without an intervening capillary bed. These lesions are usually solitary and found under the nail or in the pulp space of the fingers, more so than in the toes. They are far more common in the digit tips than elsewhere in the body but have been found in widespread body areas.

Clinical Features

A glomus tumor often presents insidiously with the noted episodic pain exacerbations and temperature sensitivity. The pain may migrate along the affected digit proximally and distally but more frequently is focal. Handling of a cold object or a cooler ambient temperature may worsen the pain, and warming often gives some relief. Sometimes, a reddish purple mass can be visualized or palpated, but this finding is not consistent. The overlying nail may be discolored and distorted if the lesion is subungual. Hildreth's test is performed by applying a tourniquet to the base of the digit and then applying pressure to the nail plate overlying the suspected lesion. When there is blood flow to the lesion, pressure on the lesion is quite painful. In Hildreth's test, when there is no flow to the lesion, pressure on the lesion is painless. Positive test results are indicated by a reduction in pain and tenderness at the site of the lesion with return of symptoms with deflation of the cuff.[2,3] Cold immersion of the affected finger or limb often accentuates the symptoms (**Fig. 77.1**).

The differential diagnosis for a glomus tumor might include a melanoma, neuroma, angioma, arteriovenous malformation (AVM), mucoid cyst, or pigmented nevus. The exact incidence rate of glomus tumors is unknown. The multiple variant is rare, accounting for less than 10% of all cases. The probable misdiagnosis of many of these lesions as hemangiomas or venous malformations also makes an accurate assessment of incidence rate difficult. Malignant glomus tumors, or glomangiosarcomas, are extremely rare and usually represent a locally infiltrative malignant disease. Solitary glomus tumors, particularly subungual lesions, are more common in females than in males. Multiple lesions are slightly more common in males.

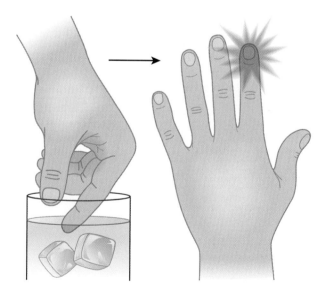

Fig. 77.1 Glomus tumor is characterized by (1) excruciating distal digit pain, (2) ability to trigger the pain with palpation, and (3) marked intolerance to cold.

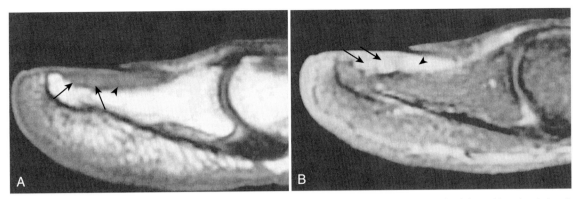

Fig. 77.2 **Glomus tumor: Magnetic resonance imaging (MRI) abnormalities.** A, On a sagittal T1-weighted (repetition time/echo time [TR/TE], 350/25), spin-echo MRI, a glomus tumor *(arrows)* has led to subtle erosion of the dorsal surface of the distal phalanx. Its signal intensity is identical to that of the nail bed *(arrowhead)*. B, After intravenous gadolinium administration, a sagittal fat-suppressed T1-weighted (TR/TE, 500/25) spin-echo MRI shows the glomus tumor *(arrows)* and nail bed *(arrowhead)* as regions of high signal intensity. *(From Resnick D, editor: Diagnosis of bone and joint disorders, ed 4, Philadelphia, 2002, Saunders, p 3999.)*

Diagnostic Studies

Transillumination may help identification of a glomus tumor if light through the lesion is diminished. Plain film x-ray results may be normal or may show some cortical erosion of the distal phalanx. Ultrasound scan may reveal a well-demarcated, hypoechoic oval or round mass in the finger.[4] Magnetic resonance imaging (MRI) is a more sensitive modality for identification of glomus tumors. Most glomus tumors show high signal intensity on T2-weighted spin-echo MRIs and strong enhancement after gadolinium injection (**Fig. 77.2**).[5–7]

Treatment

Treatment of glomus tumors is invariably surgical.[1,2]

References

Full references for this chapter can be found on www.expertconsult.com.

Part F

Pain Syndromes of the Chest Wall, Thoracic Spine, and Respiratory System

Chapter **78**

Chest Wall Pain Syndromes

Steven D. Waldman

Patients commonly seek medical attention for noncardiogenic chest pain syndromes. Often, these calls for help are as middle-of-the-night visits to the emergency department because patients fear they are having a heart attack. Such emergency visits are increasing as a result of the increased marketing efforts by hospitals regarding chest pain centers and cardiology services. Although these painful conditions are common, they are frequently misdiagnosed as cardiogenic pain, which leads to unnecessary invasive cardiac catheterizations, expensive nuclear medicine studies, and much needless anxiety for patient and their families. This chapter provides the clinician with a clear roadmap for identification and treatment of most common musculoskeletal causes of noncardiac chest pain (**Table 78.1**). The ability to diagnose and treat these problems rapidly represents a cost-effective endeavor and helps alleviate much anxiety and suffering.

Costosternal Syndrome

The costosternal joints can serve as a source of pain that often may mimic pain of cardiac origin. These joints are susceptible to the development of arthritis, including osteoarthritis, rheumatoid arthritis, ankylosing spondylitis, Reiter's syndrome, and psoriatic arthritis. The joints often are traumatized during acceleration and deceleration injuries and blunt trauma to the chest. With severe trauma, the joints

may subluxate or dislocate. Overuse or misuse also can result in acute inflammation of the costosternal joint, which can be debilitating for the patient. The joints also are subject to invasion by tumor from primary malignant diseases, including thymoma, and metastatic disease.

Functional Anatomy

The cartilage of the true ribs articulates with the sternum via the costosternal joints (**Fig. 78.1**). The cartilage of the first rib articulates directly with the manubrium of the sternum and is a synarthrodial joint, which allows a limited gliding movement. The cartilage of the second through sixth ribs articulates with the body of the sternum via true arthrodial joints. These joints are surrounded by a thin articular capsule. The costosternal joints are strengthened by ligaments but can be subluxated or dislocated by blunt trauma to the anterior chest. Posterior to the costosternal joint are the structures of the mediastinum.

Signs and Symptoms

On physical examination, the patient with costosternal syndrome vigorously attempts to splint the joints by keeping the shoulders stiffly in neutral position (**Fig. 78.2**). Pain is reproduced with active protraction or retraction of the shoulder, deep inspiration, and full elevation of the arm. Shrugging of the shoulder also may reproduce the pain.[1] Coughing may be difficult, which can lead

Table 78.1 Common Chest Wall Pain Syndromes

Costosternal syndrome
Tietze's syndrome
Sternalis syndrome
Fractured ribs
Post-thoracotomy pain syndrome
Intercostal neuralgia
Xiphisternal syndrome
Sternoclavicular syndrome

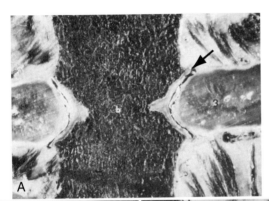

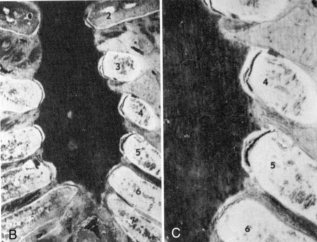

Fig. 78.1 **Sternal, sternocostal, and intercostal joints: normal anatomy.** A, Third sternocostal articulation (coronal section). Observe sternal body *(b)*, third costal cartilage *(3)*, and intervening synovial articulation *(arrow)*. B and C, Sternocostal articulations. Coronal section of a cadaveric sternum, showing second through seventh *(2-7)* sternocostal joints. *(From Resnick D, editor:* Diagnosis of bone and joint disorders, *ed 4, Philadelphia, 2002, Saunders, p 785.)*

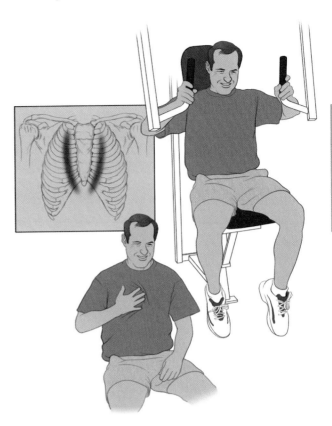

Fig. 78.2 Irritation of the costosternal joints from overuse of exercise equipment can cause costosternal syndrome. *(From Waldman SD: Costosternal syndrome. In* Atlas of common pain syndromes, *ed 2, Philadelphia, 2008, Saunders, p 175.)*

Testing

Plain radiographs are indicated in all patients with pain thought to emanate from the costosternal joints to rule out occult bony pathology, including tumor. If trauma is present, radionucleotide bone scanning may be useful to rule out occult fractures of the ribs or sternum or both. On the basis of the patient's clinical presentation, additional testing, including complete blood count, prostate-specific antigen, sedimentation rate, and antinuclear antibody, may be indicated. Magnetic resonance imaging (MRI) of the joints is indicated if joint instability or occult mass is suspected. The following injection technique serves as a diagnostic and a therapeutic maneuver.

Treatment

Initial treatment of the pain and functional disability associated with costosternal syndrome should include a combination of simple analgesics and nonsteroidal anti-inflammatory drugs (NSAIDs) or cyclooxygenase-2 (COX-2) inhibitors. Local application of heat and cold also may be beneficial. The use of an elastic rib belt may help provide symptomatic relief and protect the costosternal joints from additional trauma. For conditions that do not respond to these treatment modalities, the following injection technique with local anesthetic and steroid may be a reasonable next step.[2]

For intra-articular injection of the costosternal joint, the patient is placed in the supine position. Proper preparation with antiseptic solution of the skin overlying the affected costosternal joints is carried out. A sterile syringe containing 1 mL

to inadequate pulmonary toilet in patients who have sustained trauma to the anterior chest wall. The costosternal joints and adjacent intercostal muscles also may be tender to palpation. The patient may have a clicking sensation with movement of the joint.

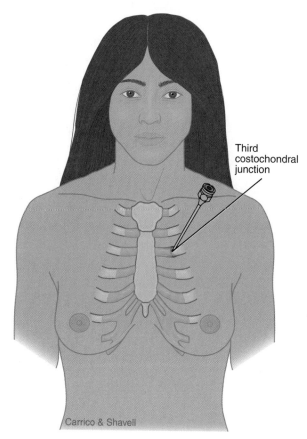

Third costochondral junction

Carrico & Shavell

Fig. 78.3 **Injection technique for relief of pain from costosternal syndrome.** *(From Waldman SD: Costosternal syndrome. In* Atlas of pain management injection techniques, *ed 2, Philadelphia, 2007, Saunders, p 302.)*

of 0.25% preservative-free bupivacaine for each joint to be injected and 40 mg of methylprednisolone is attached to a 1.5-inch 25-gauge needle with strict aseptic technique.

With use of strict aseptic technique, the costosternal joints are identified. The costosternal joints should be easily palpable as a slight bulging at the point where the rib attaches to the sternum. The needle is advanced carefully through the skin and subcutaneous tissues medially with a slight cephalad trajectory into proximity with the joint (**Fig. 78.3**). If bone is encountered, the needle is withdrawn out of the periosteum. After the needle is in proximity to the joint, 1 mL of solution is gently injected. Limited resistance to injection should be found. If significant resistance is encountered, the needle should be withdrawn slightly until the injection proceeds with only limited resistance. This procedure is repeated for each affected joint. The needle is removed, and a sterile pressure dressing and ice pack are placed at the injection site.

Tietze's Syndrome

Tietze's syndrome is a common cause of chest wall pain encountered in clinical practice. Distinct from costosternal syndrome, Tietze's syndrome was first described in 1921 and is characterized by acute painful swelling of the costal cartilages.[3] The second and third costal cartilages are most commonly involved. In contrast to costosternal syndrome, which usually occurs no earlier than 40 years of age, Tietze's syndrome is a disease of 20-year-olds to 30-year-olds.[4] The onset is acute and

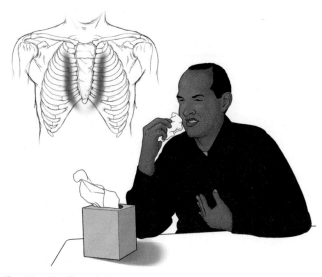

Fig. 78.4 Swelling of the second and third costochondral joints is the hallmark sign of Tietze's syndrome. *(From Waldman SD: Tietze's syndrome. In* Atlas of common pain syndromes, *ed 2, Philadelphia, 2008, Saunders, p 188.)*

is often associated with a concurrent viral respiratory tract infection (**Fig. 78.4**). Microtrauma to the costosternal joints from severe coughing or heavy labor has been postulated as the cause of Tietze's syndrome. Painful swelling of the second and third costochondral joints is the sine qua non of Tietze's syndrome. Such swelling is absent in costosternal syndrome, which occurs much more frequently than Tietze's syndrome.

Functional Anatomy

The cartilage of the true ribs articulates with the sternum via the costosternal joints. The cartilage of the first rib articulates directly with the manubrium of the sternum and is a synarthrodial joint, which allows a limited gliding movement. The cartilage of the second through sixth ribs articulates with the body of the sternum via true arthrodial joints. These joints are surrounded by a thin articular capsule. The costosternal joints are strengthened by ligaments but can be subluxated or dislocated by blunt trauma to the anterior chest. Posterior to the costosternal joint are the structures of the mediastinum.

Signs and Symptoms

On physical examination, a patient with Tietze's syndrome vigorously attempts to splint the joints by keeping the shoulders stiffly in neutral position. Pain is reproduced with active protraction or retraction of the shoulder, deep inspiration, and full elevation of the arm. Shrugging of the shoulder also may reproduce the pain. Coughing may be difficult, which can lead to inadequate pulmonary toilet in patients with Tietze's syndrome. The costosternal joints, especially the second and third joints, are swollen and exquisitely tender to palpation. The adjacent intercostal muscles also may be tender to palpation. The patient may have a clicking sensation with movement of the joint.

Testing

Plain radiographs are indicated in all patients with pain thought to emanate from the costosternal joints to rule out occult bony pathology, including tumor. If trauma is present, radionucleotide bone scanning should be considered to rule out occult fractures of the ribs or sternum or both. On the

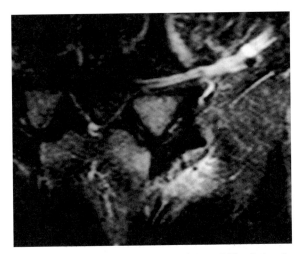

Fig. 78.5 **Tietze's syndrome.** A coronal STIR MRI of the thorax, showing high-intensity signal at the costosternal joint. *(From Resnick D, editor:* Diagnosis of bone and joint disorders, *ed 4, Philadelphia, 2002, Saunders, p 2605.)*

basis of the patient's clinical presentation, additional testing, including complete blood count, prostate-specific antigen, sedimentation rate, and antinuclear antibody, may be indicated. MRI of the joints shows costosternal joint inflammation on short tau inversion recovery sequences and is indicated if joint instability or an occult mass is suspected (**Fig. 78.5**). The following injection technique serves as a diagnostic and a therapeutic maneuver.[5]

Treatment

Initial treatment of the pain and functional disability associated with Tietze's syndrome should include a combination of simple analgesics and NSAIDs or COX-2 inhibitors. Local application of heat and cold also may be beneficial. The use of an elastic rib belt may help provide symptomatic relief and protect the costovertebral joints from additional trauma. For conditions that do not respond to these treatment modalities, the following injection technique with local anesthetic and steroid may be a reasonable next step.

For injection for Tietze's syndrome, the patient is placed in the supine position. Proper preparation with antiseptic solution of the skin overlying the affected costosternal joints is carried out. A sterile syringe containing 1 mL of 0.25% preservative-free bupivacaine for each joint to be injected and 40 mg of methylprednisolone is attached to a 1.5-inch 25-gauge needle with strict aseptic technique.

With use of strict aseptic technique, the costosternal joints are identified. The costosternal joints should be easily palpable as a slight bulging at the point where the rib attaches to the sternum. The needle is advanced carefully through the skin and subcutaneous tissues medially with a slight cephalad trajectory into proximity with the joint (**Fig. 78.6**). If bone is encountered, the needle is withdrawn out of the periosteum. After the needle is in proximity to the joint, 1 mL of solution is gently injected. Limited resistance to injection should be found. If significant resistance is encountered, the needle should be withdrawn slightly until the injection proceeds with only limited resistance. This procedure is repeated for each affected joint. The needle is removed, and a sterile pressure dressing and ice pack are placed at the injection site.

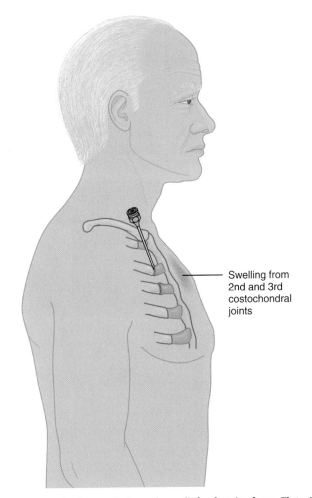

Swelling from 2nd and 3rd costochondral joints

Fig. 78.6 **Injection technique for relief of pain from Tietze's syndrome.** *(From Waldman SD: Tietze syndrome. In* Atlas of pain management injection techniques, *ed 2, Philadelphia, 2007, Saunders, p 311.)*

Sternalis Syndrome

Chest wall pain syndromes are commonly encountered in clinical practice. Some syndromes occur with relatively greater frequency and are more readily identified by the clinician (e.g., costochondritis, Tietze's syndrome). Others occur so infrequently that they are often misdiagnosed, resulting in less than optimal outcome. Sternalis syndrome is an infrequent cause of anterior chest wall pain. Sternalis is a constellation of symptoms that consist of midline anterior chest wall pain that can radiate to the retrosternal area and the medial aspect of the arm.[5]

Sternalis syndrome can mimic the pain of myocardial infarction and frequently is misdiagnosed as such. Sternalis syndrome is a myofascial pain syndrome and is characterized by trigger points in the midsternal area (**Fig. 78.7**). In contradistinction to costosternal syndrome, which also presents as midsternal pain, the pain of sternalis syndrome is not exacerbated by movement of the chest wall and shoulder. The intensity of the pain associated with sternalis syndrome is mild to moderate and described as having a deep, aching character. The pain of sternalis syndrome is intermittent.

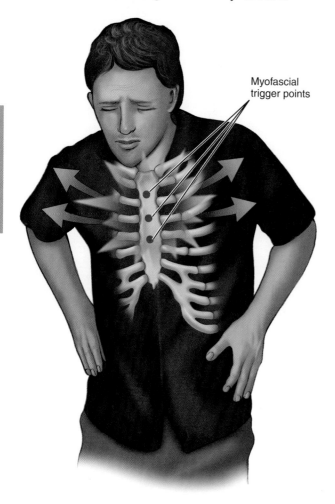

Myofascial
trigger points

Fig. 78.7 Patients with sternalis syndrome exhibit myofascial trigger points at the midline over the sternum. *(From Waldman SD: Sternalis syndrome. In Atlas of uncommon pain syndromes, ed 2, Philadelphia, 2008, Saunders, p 157.)*

Functional Anatomy

The sternalis muscle lies anterior to the sternal end of the pectoralis major muscle. The sternalis muscle runs parallel to the sternum and is not present in all individuals. Some anatomists believe that the sternalis muscle is a developmental abnormality and represents an aberrant portion of the pectoralis muscle. The sternalis muscle is innervated by the anterior thoracic nerves.

Signs and Symptoms

On physical examination, a patient with sternalis syndrome exhibits myofascial trigger points at the midline over the sternum. Occasionally, a coexistent trigger point in the pectoralis muscle or sternal head of the sternocleidomastoid muscle is seen. Pain is reproduced with palpation of these trigger points, rather than movement of the chest wall and shoulders. A positive jump sign is present when these trigger points are stimulated. Trigger points at the lateral border of the scapula also may be present and amenable to injection therapy. As mentioned previously, movement of the shoulders and chest wall does not exacerbate the pain.

Testing

Plain radiographs are indicated in all patients with suspected sternalis syndrome to rule out occult bony pathology, including metastatic lesions. On the basis of the patient's clinical presentation, additional testing, including complete blood count, prostate-specific antigen, sedimentation rate, and antinuclear antibody, may be indicated. MRI of the chest is indicated if a retrosternal mass, such as thymoma, is suspected. Electromyography is indicated in patients with sternalis syndrome to help rule out cervical radiculopathy or plexopathy, which may be considered because of the referred arm pain. Injection of the sternalis muscle with local anesthetic and steroid serves as a diagnostic and therapeutic maneuver.

Treatment

Initial treatment of sternalis syndrome should include a combination of simple analgesics and NSAIDs or COX-2 inhibitors. Local application of heat and cold also may be beneficial to provide symptomatic relief of the pain of sternalis syndrome. The use of an elastic rib belt may help provide symptomatic relief in some patients. For conditions that do not respond to these treatment modalities, injection of the trigger areas located in the sternalis muscle with local anesthetic and steroid may be a reasonable next step.[6]

The goals of the injection technique are explained to the patient. The patient is placed in the supine position with the arms resting comfortably at the patient's side. The midline of the sternum is identified and is palpated for identification of myofascial trigger points in the sternalis muscle. A positive jump sign should be noted when a trigger point is identified. Each trigger point is marked with a sterile marker.

Proper preparation with antiseptic solution of the skin overlying the trigger points is carried out. A sterile syringe containing 1 mL of 0.25% preservative-free bupivacaine for each trigger point and 40 mg of methylprednisolone is attached to a 1.5-inch 25-gauge needle with strict aseptic technique. With use of strict aseptic technique, each previously marked point is palpated, and the trigger point is identified again with the gloved finger. The needle is carefully advanced at this point through the skin and subcutaneous tissues into the trigger point in the underlying sternalis muscle (**Fig. 78.8**). The needle is fixed in place, and the contents of the syringe are gently injected. Minimal resistance to injection should be found. The needle is removed, and a sterile pressure dressing and ice pack are placed at the injection site. Other trigger points at the lateral border of the sternum and pectoralis major are identified and injected in an analogous manner.

Rib Fractures

Rib fractures are a common cause of chest wall pain. Fractures are associated most commonly with trauma to the chest wall. In osteoporotic cases or in patients with primary tumors or metastatic disease involving the ribs, fractures may occur with coughing (tussive fractures) or spontaneously.

The pain and functional disability associated with fractured ribs are determined in large part by the severity of injury (e.g., the number of ribs involved), the nature of the injury (e.g., partial or complete fractures), the presence of free-floating fragments, and the amount of damage to surrounding structures

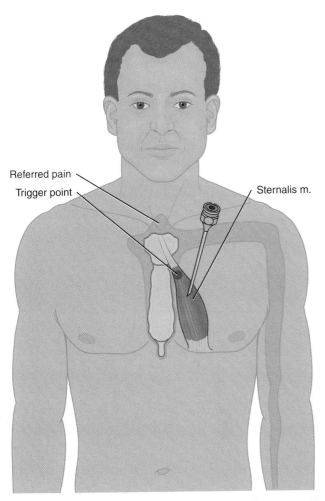

Fig. 78.8 **Injection technique for relief of pain from sternalis syndrome.** *(From Waldman SD: Sternalis syndrome. In Atlas of pain management injection techniques, ed 2, Philadelphia, 2007, Saunders, p 317.)*

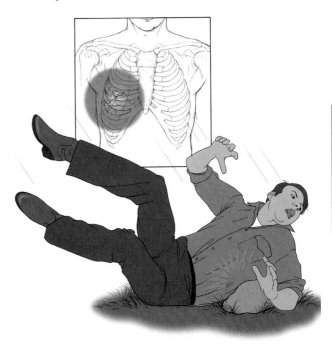

Fig. 78.9 The pain of fractured ribs is amenable to intercostal nerve block with local anesthetic and steroid. *(From Waldman SD: Fractured ribs. In Atlas of common pain syndromes, ed 2, Philadelphia, 2008, Saunders, p 193.)*

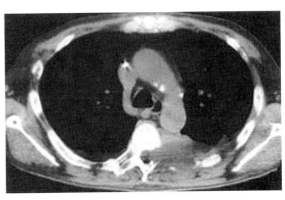

Fig. 78.10 **Adenocarcinoma metastatic to rib and chest wall.** CT scan shows the bone destruction and the soft tissue component inside and outside the rib and the invasion of the vertebra where tumor tissue reaches the spinal canal. *(From Grainger R, Allison DJ, editors: Grainger and Allison's diagnostic radiology, ed 4, Philadelphia, 2002, Churchill Livingstone, p 322.)*

(e.g., the intercostal nerves and pleura).[7] The severity of pain associated with fractured ribs may range from a dull, deep ache with partial osteoporotic fractures to severe sharp, stabbing pain that limits the patient's ability to maintain adequate pulmonary toilet.

Signs and Symptoms

Rib fractures are aggravated by deep inspiration, coughing, and any movement of the chest wall. Palpation of the affected ribs may elicit pain and reflex spasm of the musculature of the chest wall. Ecchymosis overlying the fractures may be present (**Fig. 78.9**). The clinician should be aware of the possibility of pneumothorax or hemopneumothorax. Damage to the intercostal nerves may produce severe pain and result in reflex splinting of the chest wall, further compromising the patient's pulmonary status. Failure to treat this pain and aggressive splinting may result in a negative cycle of hypoventilation, atelectasis, and ultimately, pneumonia.

Testing

Plain radiographs of the ribs and chest are indicated in all patients with pain from fractured ribs to rule out occult fractures and other bony pathology, including tumor, and pneumothorax and hemopneumothorax (**Fig. 78.10**). If trauma is present, radionucleotide bone scanning may be useful to rule out occult fractures of the ribs or sternum or both. If no trauma is present, bone density testing to rule out osteoporosis is appropriate, as is serum protein electrophoresis and testing for hyperparathyroidism. On the basis of the patient's clinical presentation, additional testing, including complete blood count, prostate-specific antigen, sedimentation rate, and antinuclear antibody, may be indicated. Computed tomographic (CT) scan of the thoracic contents is indicated if an occult mass or significant trauma to the thoracic contents is suspected. Electrocardiogram to rule out cardiac contusion is indicated in all patients with traumatic sternal fractures or significant anterior chest wall trauma. The following injection technique should be used early on to avoid the previously mentioned pulmonary complications.

Treatment

Initial treatment of rib fracture pain should include a combination of simple analgesics and NSAIDs or COX-2 inhibitors. If these medications do not adequately control the patient's symptoms, short-acting potent opioid analgesics, such as hydrocodone, represent a reasonable next step. Because opioid analgesics have the potential to suppress the cough reflex and respiration, the clinician must be careful to monitor the patient closely and to instruct the patient in adequate pulmonary toilet techniques. Local application of heat and cold also may be beneficial to provide symptomatic relief of the pain of rib fracture. The use of an elastic rib belt may help provide symptomatic relief. For conditions that do not respond to these treatment modalities, the following injection technique with local anesthetic and steroid should be implemented to avoid pulmonary complications.[8]

The patient is placed in the prone position with the patient's arms hanging loosely off the side of the cart. Alternatively, this block can be done with the patient in the sitting or lateral position. The rib to be blocked is identified with palpation of its path at the posterior axillary line. The index and middle fingers are placed on the rib bracketing the site of needle insertion. The skin is prepared with antiseptic solution. A 1.5-inch 22-gauge needle is attached to a 12-mL syringe and is advanced perpendicular to the skin, aiming for the middle of the rib between the index and middle fingers (**Fig. 78.11**). The needle should impinge on bone after being advanced approximately 3/4 inch. After bony contact is made, the needle is withdrawn into the subcutaneous tissues, and the skin and subcutaneous tissues are retracted with the palpating fingers inferiorly, which allows the needle to be walked off the inferior margin of the rib. As soon as bony contact is lost, the needle is slowly advanced approximately 2 mm deeper; this advancement places the needle in proximity to the costal groove, which contains the intercostal nerve and the intercostal artery and vein. After careful aspiration reveals no blood or air, 3 to 5 mL of 1% preservative-free lidocaine is injected. If an inflammatory component to the pain is present, the local anesthetic is combined with 80 mg of methylprednisolone and injected in incremental doses. Subsequent daily nerve blocks are carried out in a similar manner substituting 40 mg of methylprednisolone for the initial 80-mg dose. Because of the overlapping innervation of the chest and upper abdominal wall, the intercostal nerves above and below the nerve suspected of subserving the painful condition have to be blocked.

Post-Thoracotomy Pain

Essentially all patients who undergo thoracotomy have acute postoperative pain. This acute pain syndrome invariably responds to the rational use of systemic and spinal opioids and intercostal nerve block. A small percentage of patients who undergo thoracotomy have persistent pain beyond the usual course of postoperative pain. This post-thoracotomy pain syndrome can be difficult to treat. The causes of post-thoracotomy pain (**Table 78.2**) include direct surgical trauma to the intercostal nerves, fractured ribs from the rib spreader, compressive neuropathy of the intercostal nerves from direct compression to the intercostal nerves, cutaneous neuroma formation, and stretch injuries to the intercostal nerves at the costovertebral junction.[9] With the exception of fractured ribs, which produce

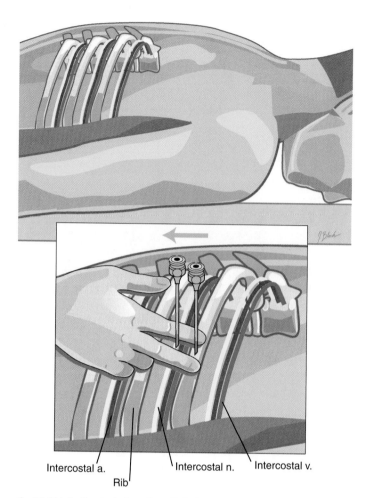

Fig. 78.11 Injection technique for relief of pain from fractured ribs. *(From Waldman SD: Intercostal nerve block. In Atlas of interventional pain management, ed 2, Philadelphia, 2004, Saunders, p 296.)*

Intercostal a.   Intercostal n.   Intercostal v.   Rib

Table 78.2 Causes of Post-Thoracotomy Pain Syndrome

Direct surgical trauma to the intercostal nerves

Fractured ribs from the rib spreader

Compressive neuropathy of the intercostal nerves from direct compression to the intercostal nerves by retractors

Cutaneous neuroma formation

Stretch injuries to the intercostal nerves at the costovertebral junction

characteristic local pain that is worse with deep inspiration, coughing, or movement of the affected ribs, the other causes of post-thoracotomy pain result in moderate to severe pain that is constant in nature and follows the distribution of the affected intercostal nerves. The pain may be characterized as neuritic and occasionally may have a dysesthetic quality.

Signs and Symptoms

Physical examination of a patient with post-thoracotomy syndrome generally reveals tenderness along the healed thoracotomy incision. Occasionally, palpation of the scar elicits

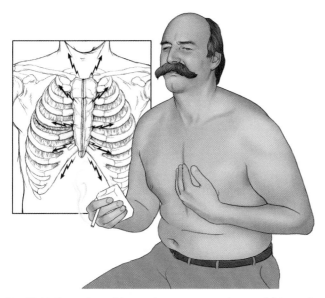

Fig. 78.12 The patient with post-thoracotomy syndrome exhibits tenderness to palpation of the scar. *(From Waldman SD: Post-thoracotomy pain. In* Atlas of common pain syndromes, *ed 2, Philadelphia, 2008, Saunders, p 196.)*

paresthesias suggestive of neuroma formation (**Fig. 78.12**). A patient with post-thoracotomy syndrome may attempt to splint or protect the affected area. Careful sensory examination of the affected dermatomes may reveal decreased sensation or allodynia. With significant motor involvement of the subcostal nerve, the patient may report that the abdomen bulges out. Occasionally, patients with post-thoracotomy syndrome have development of a reflex sympathetic dystrophy of the ipsilateral upper extremity. If the reflex sympathetic dystrophy is left untreated, frozen shoulder may develop.

Testing

Plain radiographs are indicated in all patients with pain thought to emanate from the intercostal nerve to rule out occult bony pathology, including tumor. Radionucleotide bone scanning may be useful to rule out occult fractures of the ribs or sternum or both. On the basis of the patient's clinical presentation, additional testing, including complete blood count, prostate-specific antigen, sedimentation rate, and antinuclear antibody, may be indicated. CT scan of the thoracic contents is indicated if occult mass or pleural disease is suspected. The following injection technique serves as a diagnostic and therapeutic maneuver. Electromyography is useful in distinguishing injury of the distal intercostal nerve from stretch injuries of the intercostal nerve at the costovertebral junction.

Treatment

Initial treatment of post-thoracotomy syndrome should include a combination of simple analgesics and NSAIDs or COX-2 inhibitors. If these medications do not control the patient's symptoms adequately, a tricyclic antidepressant or gabapentin should be added.

Traditionally, tricyclic antidepressants have been a mainstay in the palliation of pain from post-thoracotomy syndrome. Controlled studies have shown the efficacy of amitriptyline for this indication. Other tricyclic antidepressants, including nortriptyline and desipramine, also have been shown to be

clinically useful. This class of drugs is associated with significant anticholinergic side effects, including dry mouth, constipation, sedation, and urinary retention. These drugs should be used with caution in patients with glaucoma, cardiac arrhythmia, and prostatism. To minimize side effects and encourage compliance, the primary care physician should start amitriptyline or nortriptyline at a 10-mg dose at bedtime. The dose can be titrated upward to 25 mg at bedtime as side effects allow. Upward titration of dosage in 25-mg increments can be carried out each week as side effects allow. Even at lower doses, patients generally report a rapid reduction in sleep disturbance and begin to experience some pain relief in 10 to 14 days. If the patient does not experience any improvement in pain as the dose is titrated upward, the addition of gabapentin alone or in combination with nerve blocks with local anesthetics or steroid or both is recommended (see subsequent discussion). The selective serotonin reuptake inhibitors, such as fluoxetine, also have been used to treat the pain of diabetic neuropathy. Although better tolerated than the tricyclic antidepressants, selective serotonin reuptake inhibitors seem to be less efficacious.

If the antidepressant compounds are ineffective or contraindicated, gabapentin is a reasonable alternative. Gabapentin should be started with a 300-mg dose at bedtime for 2 nights. The patient should be cautioned about potential side effects, including dizziness, sedation, confusion, and rash. The drug is increased in 300-mg increments, given in equally divided doses over 2 days, as side effects allow, until pain relief is obtained or a total dose of 2400 mg daily is reached. At this point, if the patient has experienced partial relief of pain, blood values are measured, and the drug is carefully titrated upward with 100-mg tablets. More than 3600 mg daily rarely is needed.

Local application of heat and cold may be beneficial to provide symptomatic relief of the pain of post-thoracotomy syndrome. The use of an elastic rib belt may help provide symptomatic relief. For conditions that do not respond to these treatment modalities, the following injection technique with local anesthetic and steroid may be a reasonable next step.

The patient is placed in the prone position with the patient's arms hanging loosely off the side of the cart. Alternatively, this block can be done with the patient in the sitting or lateral position. The rib to be blocked is identified with palpation of its path at the posterior axillary line. The index and middle fingers are placed on the rib bracketing the site of needle insertion. The skin is prepared with antiseptic solution. A 1.5-inch 22-gauge needle is attached to a 12-mL syringe and is advanced perpendicular to the skin, aiming for the middle of the rib between the index and middle fingers. The needle should impinge on bone after being advanced approximately 3/4 inch. After bony contact is made, the needle is withdrawn into the subcutaneous tissues, and the skin and subcutaneous tissues are retracted with the palpating fingers inferiorly, which allows the needle to be walked off the inferior margin of the rib. As soon as bony contact is lost, the needle is slowly advanced approximately 2 mm deeper; this advancement places the needle in proximity to the costal groove, which contains the intercostal nerve and the intercostal artery and vein. After careful aspiration reveals no blood or air, 3 to 5 mL of 1% preservative-free lidocaine is injected. If an inflammatory component to the pain is present, the local anesthetic is combined with 80 mg of methylprednisolone and is injected in incremental doses. Subsequent daily nerve blocks are carried out in a similar manner substituting 40 mg of methylprednisolone for the initial 80-mg dose. Because of the overlapping innervation of the chest and upper abdominal wall, the intercostal nerves above and below the nerve suspected of subserving the painful condition have to be blocked.

Intercostal Neuralgia

In contradistinction to most other causes of pain involving the chest wall that are musculoskeletal in nature, the pain of intercostal neuralgia is neuropathic.[10] Similar to costosternal joint pain, Tzietze's syndrome, and rib fractures, many patients who have intercostal neuralgia first seek medical attention because they believe they are having a heart attack. If the subcostal nerve is involved, patients may believe they have gallbladder disease. The pain of intercostal neuralgia is the result of damage or inflammation of the intercostal nerves. The pain is constant and burning in nature and may involve any of the intercostal nerves and the subcostal nerve of the 12th rib. The pain usually begins at the posterior axillary line and radiates anteriorly into the distribution of the affected intercostal and subcostal nerves (**Fig. 78.13**). Deep inspiration or movement of the chest wall may increase the pain of intercostal neuralgia slightly but much less compared with the pain associated with the musculoskeletal causes of chest wall pain (e.g., costosternal joint pain, Tietze's syndrome, or broken ribs).

Signs and Symptoms

Physical examination of a patient with intercostal neuralgia generally reveals minimal physical findings, unless there is a history of thoracic or subcostal surgery or cutaneous findings

of herpes zoster involving the thoracic dermatomes. In contrast to the previously mentioned musculoskeletal causes of chest wall and subcostal pain, a patient with intercostal neuralgia does not attempt to splint or protect the affected area. Careful sensory examination of the affected dermatomes may reveal decreased sensation or allodynia. With significant motor involvement of the subcostal nerve, the patient report that the abdomen bulges out.

Testing

Plain radiographs are indicated in all patients with pain thought to emanate from the intercostal nerve to rule out occult bony pathology, including tumor (**Fig. 78.14**). If trauma is present, radionucleotide bone scanning may be useful to rule out occult fractures of the ribs or sternum or both. On the basis of the patient's clinical presentation, additional testing, including complete blood count, prostate-specific antigen, sedimentation rate, and antinuclear antibody, may be indicated. CT scan of the thoracic contents is indicated if occult mass is suspected. The following injection technique serves as a diagnostic and therapeutic maneuver.

Initial treatment of intercostal neuralgia should include a combination of simple analgesics and NSAIDs or COX-2 inhibitors. If these medications do not control the patient's symptoms adequately, a tricyclic antidepressant or gabapentin should be added.

Traditionally, tricyclic antidepressants have been a mainstay in the palliation of pain from intercostal neuralgia. Controlled studies have shown the efficacy of amitriptyline for this indication. Other tricyclic antidepressants, including

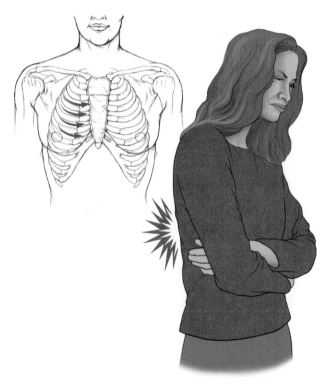

Fig. 78.13 The pain of intercostal neuralgia is neuropathic rather than musculoskeletal in origin. *(From Waldman SD: Intercostal neuralgia. In Atlas of common pain syndromes, ed 2, Philadelphia, 2008, Saunders, p 181)*

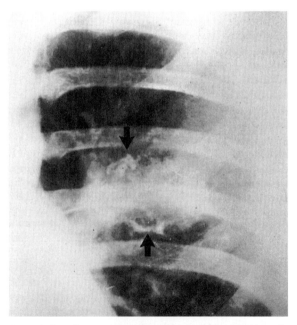

Fig. 78.14 **A chondroma arising from the costochondral junction of the left third rib.** This tumor commonly arises from the costochondral junction. It contains typical cartilaginous calcification *(arrows). (From Grainger R, et al, editors: Grainger and Allison's diagnostic radiology, ed 4, Philadelphia, 2002, Churchill Livingstone, p 322.)*

nortriptyline and desipramine, also have been shown to be clinically useful. This class of drugs is associated with significant anticholinergic side effects, including dry mouth, constipation, sedation, and urinary retention. These drugs should be used with caution in patients with glaucoma, cardiac arrhythmia, and prostatism. To minimize side effects and encourage compliance, the primary care physician should start amitriptyline or nortriptyline as a 10-mg dose at bedtime. The dose can be titrated upward to 25 mg at bedtime as side effects allow. Upward titration of dosage in 25-mg increments can be carried out each week as side effects allow. Even at lower doses, patients generally report a rapid reduction in sleep disturbance and begin to experience some pain relief in 10 to 14 days. If the patient does not experience any improvement in pain as the dose is titrated upward, the addition of gabapentin alone or in combination with nerve blocks with local anesthetics or steroid or both is recommended (see subsequent discussion). The selective serotonin reuptake inhibitors, such as fluoxetine, also have been used to treat the pain of diabetic neuropathy. Although better tolerated than tricyclic antidepressants, selective serotonin reuptake inhibitors seem to be less efficacious.

If the antidepressant compounds are ineffective or contraindicated, gabapentin is a reasonable alternative. Gabapentin should be started with a 300-mg dose at bedtime for 2 nights. The patient should be cautioned about potential side effects, including dizziness, sedation, confusion, and rash. The drug is increased in 300-mg increments, given in equally divided doses over 2 days, as side effects allow, until pain relief is obtained or a total dose of 2400 mg daily is reached. At this point, if the patient has experienced partial pain relief, blood values are measured, and the drug is carefully titrated upward with 100-mg tablets. More than 3600 mg daily is rarely needed.

The local application of heat and cold also may be beneficial to provide symptomatic relief of the pain of intercostal neuralgia. The use of an elastic rib belt may help provide symptomatic relief. For conditions that do not respond to these treatment modalities, the following injection technique with local anesthetic and steroid may be a reasonable next step.[9]

The patient is placed in the prone position with the patient's arms hanging loosely off the side of the cart. Alternatively, this block can be done in the sitting or lateral position. The rib to be blocked is identified with palpation of its path at the posterior axillary line. The index and middle fingers are placed on the rib bracketing the site of needle insertion. The skin is prepared with antiseptic solution. A 1.5-inch 22-gauge needle is attached to a 12-mL syringe and is advanced perpendicular to the skin, aiming for the middle of the rib between the index and middle finger. The needle should impinge on bone after being advanced approximately 3/4 inch. After bony contact is made, the needle is withdrawn into the subcutaneous tissues, and the skin and subcutaneous tissues are retracted with the palpating fingers inferiorly, which allows the needle to be walked off the inferior margin of the rib. As soon as bony contact is lost, the needle is slowly advanced approximately 2 mm deeper; this advancement places the needle in proximity to the costal groove, which contains the intercostal nerve and the intercostal artery and vein. After careful aspiration reveals no blood or air, 3 to 5 mL of 1% preservative-free lidocaine is injected. If an inflammatory component to the pain is present,

the local anesthetic is combined with 80 mg of methylprednisolone and injected in incremental doses. Subsequent daily nerve blocks are carried out in a similar manner substituting 40 mg of methylprednisolone for the initial 80-mg dose. Because of the overlapping innervation of the chest and upper abdominal wall, the intercostal nerves above and below the nerve suspected of subserving the painful condition have to be blocked.

Xiphisternal Syndrome

The xiphisternal joint can serve as a source of pain that often may mimic the pain of cardiac and upper abdominal origin. The xiphisternal joint is susceptible to the development of arthritis, including osteoarthritis, rheumatoid arthritis, ankylosing spondylitis, Reiter's syndrome, and psoriatic arthritis. The joint is often traumatized during acceleration and deceleration injuries and blunt trauma to the chest. With severe trauma, the joint may subluxate or dislocate. The joint also is subject to invasion by tumor from primary malignant diseases, including thymoma, and metastatic disease (**Fig. 78.15**). This joint seems to serve as the nidus of pain for xiphodynia syndrome. Xiphodynia syndrome, also known as xiphodynia, is a constellation of symptoms that consists of severe intermittent anterior chest wall pain in the region of the xiphoid process that is made worse with overeating, stooping, and bending.[11] The patient report a nauseated feeling associated with the pain of xiphodynia syndrome.

On physical examination, the pain of xiphodynia syndrome is reproduced with palpation or traction on the xiphoid.[12] The xiphisternal joint may feel swollen. Stooping or bending may reproduce the pain (**Fig. 78.16**). Coughing may be difficult, which may lead to inadequate pulmonary toilet in patients who have sustained trauma to the anterior chest wall. The xiphisternal joint and adjacent intercostal muscles also may be tender to palpation. The patient report a clicking sensation with movement of the joint.

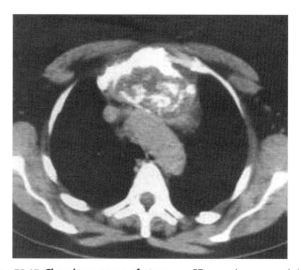

Fig. 78.15 **Chondrosarcoma of sternum.** CT scan shows manubrial irregularity and the preaortic soft tissue mass with its chondral calcification. Nearly all sternal tumors are malignant. (*From Grainger R, et al, editors:* Grainger and Allison's diagnostic radiology, *ed 4, Philadelphia, 2002, Churchill Livingstone, p 323.*)

Plain radiographs are indicated in all patients with pain thought to emanate from the xiphisternal joint to rule out occult bony pathology, including tumor. On the basis of the patient's clinical presentation, additional testing, including complete blood count, prostate-specific antigen, sedimentation rate, and antinuclear antibody, may be indicated. MRI of the joint is indicated if joint instability or occult mass is suspected. The following injection technique serves as a diagnostic and therapeutic maneuver.

Functional Anatomy

The xiphoid process articulates with the sternum via the xiphisternal joint (**Fig. 78.17**). The xiphoid process is a plate of cartilaginous bone that becomes calcified in early adulthood. The xiphisternal joint is strengthened by ligaments but can be subluxated or dislocated with blunt trauma to the anterior chest. The xiphisternal joint is innervated by the T4-T7 intercostal nerves and the phrenic nerve. This innervation by the phrenic nerve is thought to be responsible for the referred pain associated with xiphodynia syndrome. Posterior to the xiphisternal joint are the structures of the mediastinum. These structures are susceptible to needle-induced trauma during injections for xiphisternal syndrome if the needle is placed too deep. The pleural space may be entered if the needle is placed too deep and laterally, and pneumothorax may result.

Treatment

Initial treatment of the pain and functional disability associated with xiphisternal syndrome should include a combination of simple analgesics and NSAIDs or COX-2 inhibitors. The local application of heat and cold also may be beneficial. The use of an elastic rib belt may help provide symptomatic relief and protect the xiphisternal joint from additional trauma. For conditions that do not respond to these treatment modalities, the following injection technique with local anesthetic and steroid may be a reasonable next step.[12]

The goals of this injection technique are explained to the patient. The patient is placed in the supine position, and proper preparation with antiseptic solution of the skin overlying the affected xiphisternal joint is carried out. A sterile syringe containing 1 mL of 0.25% preservative-free bupivacaine and 40 mg of methylprednisolone is attached to a 1.5-inch 25-gauge needle with strict aseptic technique.

The xiphisternal joint is identified with strict aseptic technique. It should be easily palpable as a slight indentation at the point where the xiphoid process attaches to the body of the sternum. The needle is carefully advanced at the center of the xiphisternal joint through the skin and subcutaneous tissues with a slight cephalad trajectory into proximity with the joint (**Fig. 78.18**). If bone is encountered, the needle is withdrawn out of the periosteum. After the needle is in proximity to the joint,

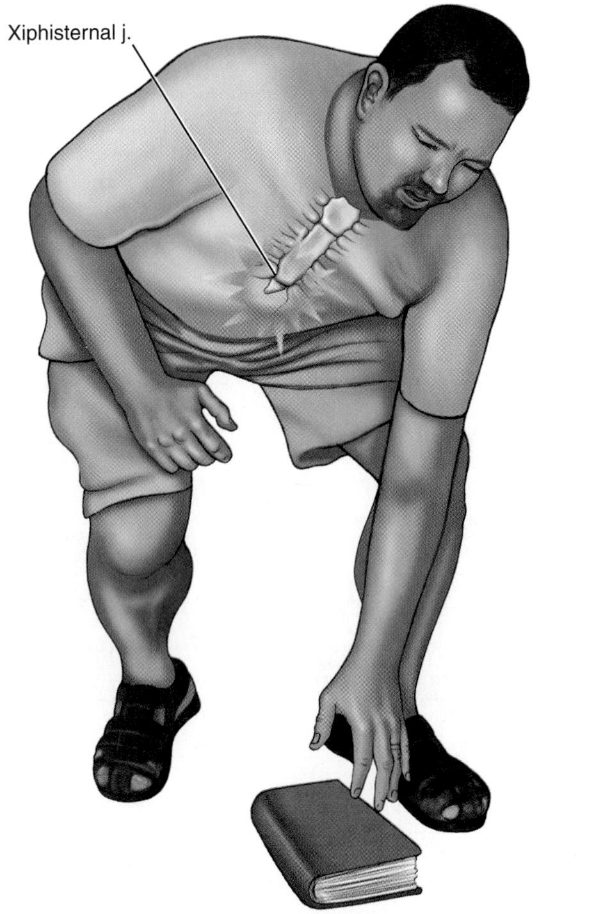

Xiphisternal j.

Fig. 78.16 The xiphisternal joint is swollen in patients with xiphodynia. *(From Waldman SD: Xiphodynia. In Atlas of uncommon pain syndromes, ed 2, Philadelphia, 2008, Saunders, p 159.)*

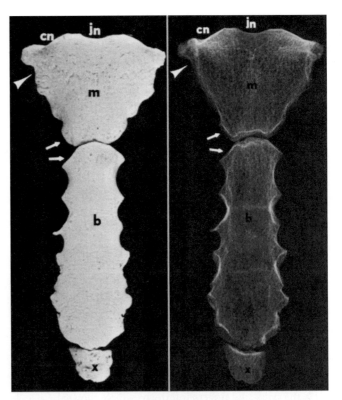

Fig. 78.17 **Sternum: osseous anatomy.** Anterior aspect. The three segments of the sternum are the manubrium *(m)*, body *(b)*, and xiphoid process *(x)*. Additional landmarks are the clavicular notch *(cn)* and jugular notch *(jn)*. A sternal facet for articulation with the first costal cartilage *(arrowheads)* and hemifacets for articulation with the second costal cartilage *(arrows)* are indicated. Other articular facets also are apparent on the body of the sternum. *(From Resnick D, editor: Diagnosis of bone and joint disorders, ed 4, Philadelphia, 2002, Saunders, p 731.)*

1 mL of solution is gently injected. Limited resistance to injection should be found. If significant resistance is encountered, the needle should be withdrawn slightly until the injection proceeds with only limited resistance. This procedure is repeated for each affected joint. The needle is removed, and a sterile pressure dressing and ice pack are placed at the injection site.

The major complication of this injection technique is pneumothorax if the needle is placed too laterally or too deep and invades the pleural space. Infection, although rare, can occur if strict aseptic technique is not followed. Trauma to the contents of the mediastinum remains an ever-present possibility. This complication can be greatly decreased if the clinician pays close attention to accurate needle placement.

Sternoclavicular Joint Syndrome

The sternoclavicular joint can serve as a source of pain that often may mimic the pain of cardiac origin. The sternoclavicular joint is a true joint and is susceptible to the

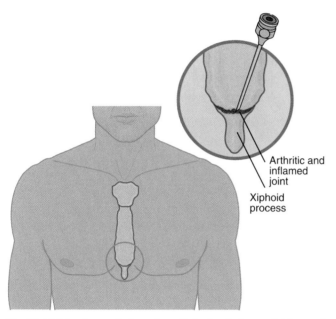

Fig. 78.18 Injection technique for relief of pain from xiphisternal syndrome. *(From Waldman SD: Xiphodynia syndrome. In Atlas of pain management injection techniques, ed 2, Philadelphia, 2007, Saunders, p 320.)*

development of arthritis, including osteoarthritis, rheumatoid arthritis, ankylosing spondylitis, Reiter's syndrome, and psoriatic arthritis. The joint is often traumatized during acceleration and deceleration injuries and blunt trauma to the chest. With severe trauma, the joint may subluxate or dislocate. Overuse or misuse also can result in acute inflammation of the sternoclavicular joint, which can be debilitating for the patient. The joint also is subject to invasion by tumor from primary malignant diseases, including thymoma, and metastatic disease (**Fig. 78.19**).

On physical examination, the patient vigorously attempts to splint the joint by keeping the shoulders stiffly in neutral position. Pain is reproduced with active protraction or retraction of the shoulder and full elevation of the arm. Shrugging of the shoulder also may reproduce the pain. The sternoclavicular joint may be tender to palpation and feel hot and swollen if acutely inflamed.[13] The patient also may report a clicking sensation with movement of the joint.

Plain radiographs are indicated in all patients with pain thought to emanate from the sternoclavicular joint to rule out occult bony pathology, including tumor. On the basis of the patient's clinical presentation, additional testing, including complete blood count, prostate-specific antigen, sedimentation rate, and antinuclear antibody, may be indicated. MRI of the joint is indicated if joint instability is suspected. The following injection technique serves as a diagnostic and therapeutic maneuver.

Functional Anatomy

The sternoclavicular joint is a double gliding joint with an actual synovial cavity (**Fig. 78.20**). Articulation occurs between the sternal end of the clavicle, the sternal manubrium, and the cartilage of the first rib. The clavicle and sternal manubrium are separated by an articular disk. The joint is reinforced in front and back by the sternoclavicular ligaments. Additional support is provided by the costoclavicular ligament, which runs from the junction of the first rib and its costal cartilage to the inferior surface of the clavicle. The joint is dually innervated by the supraclavicular nerve and the nerve supplying the subclavius muscle. Posterior to the joint are numerous large arteries and veins, including the left common carotid and brachiocephalic vein and on the right, the brachiocephalic artery. These vessels are susceptible to needle-induced trauma if the needle is placed too deep.

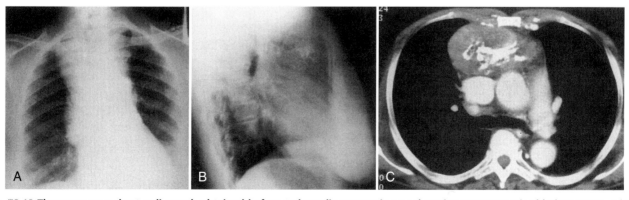

Fig. 78.19 Thymoma on a chest radiograph obtained before orthopedic surgery in an otherwise asymptomatic elderly woman. A large anterior mediastinal mass (A) with coarse calcification visible on the lateral view (B) and the contrast-enhanced CT scan (C). *(From Grainger R, et al, editors: Grainger and Allison's diagnostic radiology, ed 4, Philadelphia, 2002, Churchill Livingstone, p 357.)*

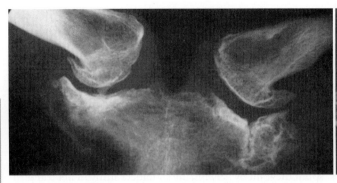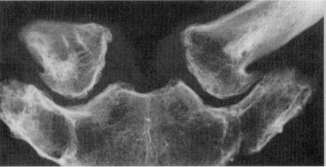

Fig. 78.20 Osteoarthritis of the sternoclavicular joint. Radiographs of coronal sections through the sternoclavicular joints in two different cadavers show the spectrum of osteoarthritis. Changes include subchondral osseous irregularity and osteophytosis of the medial ends of the clavicle and sternum. Note the large excrescences that extend laterally from the inferior aspect of the clavicular heads. *(From Resnick D, editor: Diagnosis of bone and joint disorders, ed 4, Philadelphia, 2002, Saunders, p 1324.)*

The serratus anterior muscle produces forward movement of the clavicle at the sternoclavicular joint, with backward movement at the joint produced by the rhomboid and trapezius muscles. Elevation of the clavicle at the sternoclavicular joint is produced by the sternocleidomastoid, rhomboid, and levator scapulae. Depression of the clavicle at the joint is produced by the pectoralis minor and subclavius muscles.

Treatment

Initial treatment of sternoclavicular syndrome pain should include a combination of simple analgesics and NSAIDs or COX-2 inhibitors. If these medications do not control the patient's symptoms adequately, short-acting potent opioid analgesics, such as hydrocodone, represent a reasonable next step. Because opioid analgesics have the potential to suppress the cough reflex and respiration, the clinician must be careful to monitor the patient closely and to instruct the patient in adequate pulmonary toilet techniques. The local application of heat and cold also may be beneficial to provide symptomatic relief of the pain of sternoclavicular syndrome. For conditions that do not respond to these treatment modalities, the following injection technique with local anesthetic and steroid should be implemented to avoid pulmonary complications.[14]

The goals of the injection technique are explained to the patient. The patient is placed in the supine position, and the skin overlying the root of the neck anteriorly and the skin overlying the proximal clavicle are prepared with antiseptic solution. A sterile syringe containing 1 mL of 0.25% preservative-free bupivacaine and 40 mg of methylprednisolone is attached to a 1.5-inch 25-gauge needle with strict aseptic technique.

With use of strict aseptic technique, the sternal end of the clavicle is identified. The sternoclavicular joint should be easily palpable as a slight indentation at the point where the clavicle meets the sternal manubrium. The needle is advanced carefully through the skin and subcutaneous tissues medially at a 45-degree angle from the skin through the joint capsule into the joint (**Fig. 78.21**). If bone is encountered, the needle is withdrawn into the subcutaneous tissues and redirected slightly more medially. After the joint space is entered, the contents of the syringe are gently injected. Some resistance to injection should be encountered because the joint space is small and the joint capsule is dense. If significant resistance is encountered, the needle is probably in a ligament and should

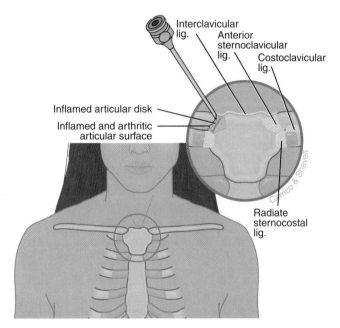

Fig. 78.21 Injection technique for relief of pain from sternoclavicular joint syndrome. *(From Waldman SD: Sternoclavicular syndrome. In Atlas of pain management injection techniques, ed 2, Philadelphia, 2007, Saunders, p 285.)*

be advanced or withdrawn slightly into the joint space until the injection proceeds with only limited resistance. The needle is removed, and a sterile pressure dressing and ice pack are placed at the injection site.

Differential Diagnosis of Chest Wall Pain Syndromes

The pain associated with the previously mentioned chest wall pain syndromes is often mistaken for pain of cardiac origin and can lead to visits to the emergency department and unnecessary cardiac workups. If trauma has occurred, these chest wall pain syndromes may coexist with fractured ribs or fractures of the sternum itself, which can be missed on plain radiographs and may necessitate radionucleotide bone scanning for proper identification. Because a patient with one of these chest wall pain syndromes may be in acute pain and may be experiencing anxiety, careful physical examination is

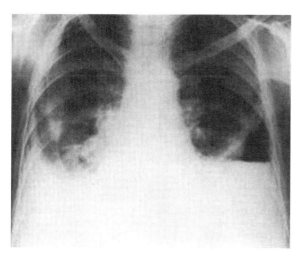

Fig. 78.22 **Right pleural effusion and left hydropneumothorax.** The pleural effusion obscures the hemidiaphragm and the right costophrenic angle. It has a curvilinear upper margin concave to lung and is higher laterally than medially. This contrasts with the straight horizontal upper border of the fluid in the left hydropneumothorax. The meniscus on the right has a second, faint medial component caused by intrusion of fluid into the oblique fissure. *(From Grainger R, Allison DJ, editors: Grainger and Allison's diagnostic radiology, ed 4, Philadelphia, 2002, Churchill Livingstone, p 325.)*

mandatory to help identify the exact chest wall pain syndrome and to allow reassurance that the pain is noncardiac in nature.

Neuropathic pain involving the chest wall also may be confused or coexist with the aforementioned musculoskeletal causes of chest wall pain. Examples of such neuropathic pain include diabetic polyneuropathies and acute herpes zoster involving the thoracic nerves. The possibility of diseases of the structures of the mediastinum is ever present, and at times, diagnosis can be difficult. Pathologic processes that inflame the pleura (e.g., pulmonary embolus, infection, Bornholm disease) also can confuse the clinical picture and make diagnosis more difficult (**Fig. 78.22**). In addition, most of the joints of the chest wall are subject to the development of osteoarthritis and inflammation and destruction by the collagen-vascular diseases, including rheumatoid arthritis, ankylosing spondylitis, Reiter's syndrome, and psoriatic arthritis (**Fig. 78.23**). The joints also are subject to invasion by tumor from primary malignant diseases, including thymoma, and metastatic disease.

Complications and Pitfalls in the Care of Patients with Chest Wall Pain Syndromes

The major problem in the care of patients thought to have chest wall pain syndromes is the failure to identify potentially serious pathology of the thorax or upper abdomen or occult

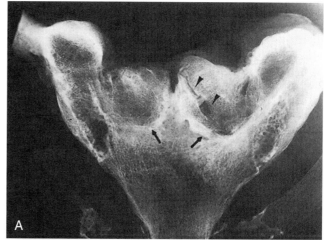

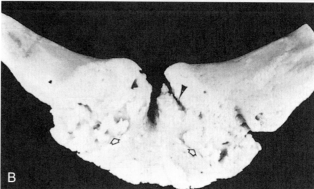

Fig. 78.23 **Abnormalities of the sternoclavicular joint. A,** Radiograph of a coronal section of the sternoclavicular joints indicates intra-articular osseous fusion *(arrows)* between the medial aspect of each clavicle and the sternum. A remnant of the articular space on one side can be identified *(arrowheads).* **B,** Photograph of the anterior aspect of the coronal section in A shows the extent of intra-articular ankylosis. Note an identifiable segment of the articular space *(arrowhead)* and the irregular anterior bony excrescences *(open arrows). (From Resnick D, editor: Diagnosis of bone and joint disorders, ed 4, Philadelphia, 2002, Saunders, p 1056.)*

cardiac conditions. Because of the proximity to the pleural space and mediastinum intercostal nerve and artery, the potential for iatrogenic complications from the previously mentioned nerve block techniques remains ever present. Although uncommon, infection after trauma or nerve block remains an ever-present possibility, especially in an immunocompromised cancer patient. Early detection of infection is crucial to avoid potentially life-threatening sequelae.

References

Full references for this chapter can be found on www.expertconsult.com.

Chapter **79**

Thoracic Radiculopathy

Steven D. Waldman

Thoracic radiculopathy is a common source of chest wall and upper abdominal pain that emanates from the thoracic nerve roots. In addition to the dorsal spine pain, which radiates in a thoracic dermatomal distribution, a patient with thoracic radiculopathy may have associated paresthesias, numbness, weakness, and rarely, loss of superficial abdominal reflexes. The causes of thoracic radiculopathy include herniated disk, foraminal stenosis, tumor, osteophyte formation, vertebral compression fractures, and rarely, infection.[1]

Signs and Symptoms

A patient with thoracic radiculopathy has pain, numbness, tingling, and paresthesias in the distribution of the affected nerve root or roots.[2] Muscle spasms of the paraspinous musculature also are common. Decreased sensation, weakness, and rarely, superficial abdominal reflex changes are shown on physical examination.[3] Patients with thoracic radiculopathy commonly have a reflex shifting of the trunk to one side, which is called *list*. Occasionally, a patient with thoracic radiculopathy also has compression of the thoracic spinal cord that results in myelopathy. Thoracic myelopathy is most commonly the result of midline herniated thoracic disk, spinal stenosis, demyelinating disease, tumor, or rarely, infection.[4] Patients with thoracic myelopathy have varying degrees of neurologic disturbance based on the level and extent of cord compression. Significant compression of the thoracic spinal cord results in Brown-Séquard syndrome, with spastic paralysis of the ipsilateral muscles below the lesion and loss of sensation on the contralateral side (**Fig. 79.1**). Thoracic myelopathy represents a neurosurgical emergency and should be treated as such.

Testing

Magnetic resonance imaging (MRI) of the thoracic spine provides the clinician with the best information regarding the thoracic spine and its contents. MRI is highly accurate and helps with identification of abnormalities that may put the patient at risk for the development of thoracic myelopathy

(**Figs. 79.2 and 79.3**). In patients who cannot undergo MRI (e.g., patients with pacemakers), computed tomographic (CT) scan or myelography followed by CT scan of the affected area is acceptable. Radionucleotide bone scanning and plain radiographs are indicated if fractures or bony abnormalities, such as metastatic disease, are being considered.

Although the aforementioned testing provides the clinician with useful neuroanatomic information, electromyography and nerve conduction velocity testing provide the clinician with neurophysiologic information that can delineate the actual status of each individual nerve root and the thoracic plexus. Screening laboratory testing, consisting of complete blood count, erythrocyte sedimentation rate, and automated blood chemistry, should be performed if the diagnosis of thoracic radiculopathy is in question.

Differential Diagnosis

Thoracic radiculopathy is a clinical diagnosis that is supported by a combination of clinical history, physical examination, radiographs, and MRI. Pain syndromes that may mimic thoracic radiculopathy include dorsal spine strain; thoracic bursitis; thoracic fibromyositis; inflammatory arthritis; mononeuritis multiplex; infectious lesions, such as epidural abscess; and disorders of the thoracic spinal cord, roots, plexus, and nerves (see Fig. 79.3).[5] MRI of the thoracic spine should be done on all patients with suspected thoracic radiculopathy. Screening laboratory testing, consisting of complete blood count, erythrocyte sedimentation rate, antinuclear antibody testing, human leukocyte antigen (HLA)–B27 antigen screening, and automated blood chemistry, should be performed if the diagnosis of thoracic radiculopathy is in question to help rule out other causes of the patient's pain.

Treatment

Thoracic radiculopathy is best treated with a multimodality approach. Physical therapy, including heat modalities and deep sedative massage, combined with nonsteroidal

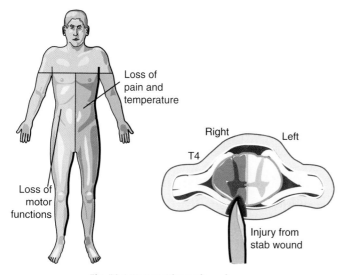

Fig. 79.1 **Brown-Séquard syndrome.**

anti-inflammatory drugs and skeletal muscle relaxants represents a reasonable starting point. The addition of thoracic steroid epidural nerve blocks is a reasonable next step. Thoracic epidural blocks with local anesthetic and steroid have been shown to be extremely effective in the treatment of thoracic radiculopathy. Underlying sleep disturbance and depression are best treated with a tricyclic antidepressant, such as nortriptyline, which can be started at a single bedtime dose of 25 mg.

Complications and Pitfalls

A failure to diagnose thoracic radiculopathy accurately may put the patient at risk for the development of thoracic myelopathy, which, if untreated, may progress to paraparesis or paraplegia. Electromyography helps in differentiation of mononeuritis multiplex from radiculopathy, which can confuse the diagnosis because the conditions may coexist in patients with diabetes.

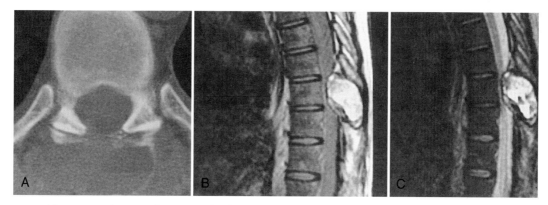

Fig. 79.2 **Aneurysmal bone cyst. Computed tomography (CT) scan and magnetic resonance image (MRI) showing abnormalities in the spine. A,** In a 52-year-old man, transaxial CT scan shows an expansile lesion of the spinous process of the ninth thoracic vertebra. A calcified or ossified shell is evident about a portion of this lesion. **B,** Sagittal intermediate-weighted (TR/TE, 2000/30) and, **C,** T2-weighted (TR/TE, 2000/90) spin-echo MRIs show the lesion, which is inhomogeneous, but mainly of high signal intensity. Fluid levels are present in **A** and **C.** *(From Resnick D, editor:* Diagnosis of bone and joint disorders, *ed 4, Philadelphia, 2002, Saunders, p 4046.)*

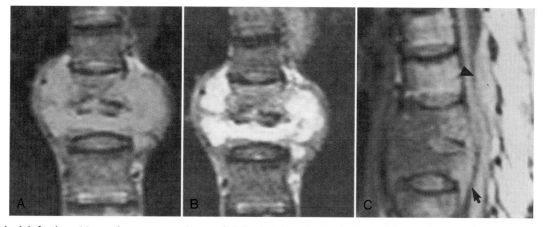

Fig. 79.3 **Spinal infection. Magnetic resonance image (MRI) of tuberculosis. A,** Coronal intermediate-weighted (TR/TE, 1800/50) and, **B,** T2-weighted (TR/TE, 1800/100) spin-echo MRIs reveal spinal and paraspinal involvement in the midthoracic region. The infectious process is of higher signal intensity in **B. C,** Sagittal T1-weighted (TR/TE, 450/30) spin-echo MRI in the same patient reveals tuberculosis involvement of contiguous vertebral bodies with extension anteriorly. Also, note the anterior *(arrow)* and posterior *(arrowhead)* extradural disease. *(Courtesy of T. Mattsson, MD, Riyadh, Saudi Arabia. From Resnick D, editor:* Diagnosis of bone and joint disorders, *ed 4, Philadelphia, 2002, Saunders, p 2497.)*

Conclusion

Thoracic radiculopathy is a common cause of chest and upper abdominal pain. It is often overlooked in the attempt to attribute the patient's pain symptoms to intrathoracic or intra-abdominal pathology. Mononeuritis multiplex can mimic the signs and symptoms of thoracic radiculopathy, but both clinical syndromes may coexist, especially in patients with diabetes. The clinician always must rule out causes of thoracic radiculopathy that if undiagnosed may result in neurologic disaster, including primary tumors, metastatic disease, infection, syringomyelia, multiple sclerosis, and spinal cord disease.

References

Full references for this chapter can be found on www.expertconsult.com.

Painful Disorders of the Respiratory System

Paul T. King

This chapter reviews the causes of chest pain that occur with lung (and pleural) disease. Respiratory chest pain, with the exception of pleuritic pain (in association with pulmonary embolism or pneumonia), is generally not considered to be an important clinical feature. When faced with a patient with chest pain, a clinician often first excludes cardiac causation and then gastrointestinal disease before considering a respiratory cause. However, the lungs have a complex network of sensory fibers, and chest pain is a prominent symptom of most forms of respiratory disease. An accurate history and examination is usually used to determine the underlying etiology of respiratory system pain.

A description of the sensory innervation of the respiratory system is followed by a classification of different types of chest pain and a suggested clinical approach. Individual causes are then described in detail. A section on cough, which is a closely related symptom, is also included.

Sensory Innervation of the Respiratory System

The sensations that originate from the respiratory system include those of pain and related sensations, such as cough, dyspnea, and chest tightness.[1,2] The complex and dense sensory innervation of the lungs is often not appreciated. Respiratory chest pain may arise from: (1) involvement of the parietal pleura/adjacent chest wall; or (2) the airways and the lung viscera. Pulmonary malignant disease may have features of both pleural and visceral pain.

Pleuritic/Chest Wall Chest Pain

The chest wall and parietal pleura have a rich innervation, supplied by the costal nerves. The stimulation of these areas causes pain referred to the adjacent chest wall. The central portion of the diaphragmatic pleura is innervated by the phrenic nerve, and the pain is referred to the ipsilateral shoulder.[3] This form of pain is generally sharp and well localized.

Visceral Chest Pain

The visceral pleura and the lung parenchyma are generally considered to be pain insensitive.[4] The passage of a needle into the lung for biopsy does not cause any sensation, and significant traumatic lung injury is painless.[5,6] Lung cancer is not thought to cause pain unless it involves the parietal pleura or bronchi. However, the lung airways have a dense sensory network. Irritation of the larynx, upper airway, and tracheobronchial tree (e.g., by inhaled irritants or mucosal inflammation) induces a sensation of burning, rawness, and chest discomfort most often described by patients to involve the retrosternal and midthoracic areas.[1,7,8]

The visceral sensations from the respiratory system go through afferent fibers that travel within the vagus nerve to its nuclei located in the medulla oblongata. The fibers reach the lung via the thoracic branches of the vagus and the trachea in its upper portion via the recurrent laryngeal nerve.[4] The sensory pathway originates in close contact with the epithelium, submucosa, interstitium, smooth muscles, and pulmonary vessels, in three main groups of sensory receptors.[4,9]

The slowly adapting stretch receptors (SARs), mechanoreceptors connected to small myelinated afferent fibers, are thought to be located in the smooth muscle of the extrapulmonary and large intrapulmonary airways, respond to moderate lung inflation, and are responsible for the inflation and expiration Hering-Breuer reflexes. The inflation reflex consists of a reduction in the inspiratory time and prolongation of expiration with increased inflation; the expiration reflex is an increase in the respiratory rate associated with lung deflation.[1,7,8,10,11]

The rapidly adapting stretch receptors (RARs), also known as irritant receptors, are located in the lung parenchyma, bronchioles, and distal bronchi and are connected to small myelinated fibers.[8] The main stimuli for these receptors are rapidly adapting lung deflation, bronchial deformation, and mucosal irritation. They are involved in the cough reflex, bronchoconstriction, and mucus production.[1,9,10,12] The general agreement is that pain from irritation of the airways is the result of the activation of the rapidly adapting stretch receptors.[4]

The C-fiber endings associated with the type J receptor, a term coined by Paintal,[13] referring to the juxtapulmonary capillary location, reside close to the pulmonary capillaries and within the bronchi. They are chemosensitive[14] but also are activated by mechanical stimuli and are connected to unmyelinated afferent fibers. As described by Coleridge and Coleridge,[15] these receptors are involved in responses, such as bronchoconstriction, secretion of mucus, bradycardia, and hypotension, and can influence breathing rate. The organization of the nerves for visceral chest pain is shown in **Fig. 80.1**.

In contrast to pleuritic chest pain, stimulation of the visceral pathway generally produces deep-seated, diffuse, and poorly localized pain. This particularly applies when the C fibers are stimulated.

Clinical Features of Chest Pain

The clinical features of pleuritic/chest wall pain and visceral pain differ, and other specific features are characteristic of different causes of chest pain.

Pleuritic/Chest Wall Pain

The pain associated with pleuropulmonary disorders is usually described as "pleuritic" in nature and usually increases with forced maneuvers, respiratory movements, coughing, or sneezing; however, it must be separated from respirophasic chest pain of musculoskeletal origin.[14,16,17] Pleuritic chest pain may be acute in onset, sharp, often severe, and unilateral. It usually is made worse by deep breathing and coughing and is ameliorated by splinting of the affected side.[16] Musculoskeletal pain also may vary with respiration but is not as intense; is

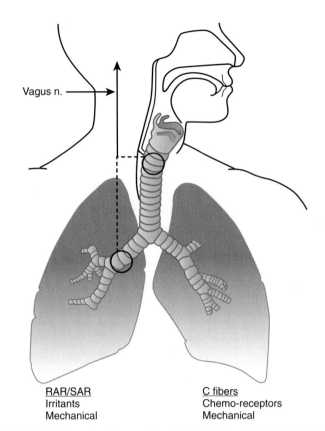

Fig. 80.1 Visceral pain sensation in the lung. Pain receptors are diffusely present in the lung but are most concentrated in the upper airways and bifurcations of the bronchi. The three main sensory receptors are: (1) rapidly adapting receptors (RARs); (2) slowly adapting receptors (SARs); and (3) C fibers. These receptors respond to mechanical, irritant, and chemical stimuli. Impulses are then conducted via the vagus nerve to the brainstem.

made worse by extension, abduction, or adduction of the arms and shoulders; and usually is accompanied by tenderness of the muscle group involved.[16] Most reviews state that potential musculoskeletal causes of chest pain represent 10% to 20% of the patients with chest pain of noncardiac origin.[18] The sternum and its articulation with the ribs and clavicle are recognized as sites of involvement in some seronegative arthropathies, in particular those associated with pustular skin disease.[18] In addition, rheumatoid arthritis (RA) has been reported to affect the chest wall and cause chest pain, and pleuritic chest pain is the most common symptom in lupus pleuritis and occurs in 86% to 100% of cases of lupus pleurisy.[16,19] Tzietze syndrome is an uncommon but well-described chest wall syndrome.[19] Initially reported in 1921, Tzietze syndrome is defined as a benign, painful, nonsuppurative localized swelling of the costocondral, sternoclavicular, or costosternal joints in the area of the second and third ribs (see chapter 78).[19]

Visceral Pain

In contrast to the well-defined and localized pain that occurs with involvement of the parietal pleura and chest wall pain, visceral pain is less defined. Generally, this pain arises from stimulation of the bronchi and most commonly is associated with a burning discomfort that is localized to the retrosternal area. Pain localized to areas with atelectasis or collapse may also occur.[20,21]

Clinical Features of Specific Conditions

A large number of causes of respiratory chest pain need to be considered. Some clinical features may suggest specific etiologies.

Pain that has a very acute onset is most commonly the result of pulmonary embolism. Another important cause is pneumothorax.

Severe and unrelenting pain that is present for a prolonged period (i.e., at least a month) is consistent with malignant disease. This is particularly the case with pain that prevents sleep.[22] Progressive weight loss is also suggestive of cancer.

Fever, productive cough, and localized crackles suggest lower respiratory tract infection.

Patients who have pain on touching of the chest or who have focal tenderness on examination are likely to have chest wall involvement as the cause.

Specific Causes of Chest Pain

No generally accepted classification exists for causes of respiratory chest pain. Pain can be considered to be arising from involvement of the parietal pleura/chest wall, from the lung viscera, or in the context of cancer (which often has visceral and parietal/chest wall components). Specific causes are listed in **Table 80.1**. Some conditions (e.g., cancer and pneumonia) are associated with both visceral and pleural pain.

Visceral Causes of Chest Pain

A large number of lung conditions have pain that is predominantly sensed through the vagal nerve afferents. Some of these conditions, such as asthma and infective bronchitis, are extremely common, and pain is generated through inflammation of the bronchi. Rarer systemic diseases that cause pain, including sickle cell anemia, lymphangioleiomyomatosis (LAM), and sarcoidosis, have less well-defined mechanisms. Many of these conditions are inflammatory and associated with the production of mediators, which stimulate the pain receptors.

Most commonly, the pain is not severe, and therapy is primarily directed at treatment of the underlying condition (e.g., with corticosteroids or with antibiotics).

Bronchial Inflammation: Bronchitis and Asthma

Asthma and chronic bronchitis are extremely common and cause bronchial inflammation. Asthma is an inflammatory disease of the airways that is characterized by increased responsiveness of the tracheobronchial tree to a variety of stimuli. Chronic bronchitis is defined by chronic cough and sputum production (for at least 6 months) and occurs particularly in smokers and those with chronic obstructive pulmonary disease (COPD). Asthma and chronic bronchitis produce bronchial inflammation, which causes the release of mediators (e.g., bradykinin, which stimulate the pain pathway).

An important feature is the occurrence of exacerbations in which increased airway inflammation (e.g., after exposure to an allergen or establishment of bacterial infection) leads to increased symptoms. Patients typically have a burning retrosternal chest pain that is of mild severity. Exacerbations are treated with standard medications that

Table 80.1 **Causes of Respiratory Chest Pain**
VISCERAL
Asthma/bronchitis
Pneumonia/lung abscess
Atelectasis/lobar collapse
Lymphangioleiomyomatosis
Pulmonary Langerhans cell histiocytosis
Sarcoidosis
Pulmonary hypertension
PARIETAL PLEURA/CHEST WALL
Pulmonary embolism
Pleurisy in association with local infection
Pleurisy in association with systemic inflammatory conditions
Trauma to chest wall from coughing
Operative chest pain (e.g., thoracotomy)
Traumatic injury to chest wall
Pneumothorax
Sickle cell disease
CANCER
Primary bronchogenic lung tumor
Mesothelioma
Metastatic tumor

include corticosteroids, bronchodilators, and antibiotics. **Fig. 80.2** shows an inflamed airway in a subject with bronchitis.

Subjects with inflamed airways produce secretions or mucous, which may cause partial (atelectasis) or complete collapse of a lobe.[20,21] This is not a well-recognized entity but, in the author's experience, is associated with distinctive chest pain. Subjects have a deep-seated continuous pain of acute onset and moderate severity of the area of the collapsed lung that resolves when the lung reinflates. The mechanism of pain involved is not clear but may involve the stretch and mechanoreceptors of the SAR and RAR nerve sensors. **Fig. 80.3** shows an x-ray of a subject with lung collapse and localized chest pain.

Lymphangioleiomyomatosis

Lymphangioleiomyomatosis (LAM) is a rare disease that affects mainly premenopausal women and results from the proliferation of an atypical smooth muscle–like cell involving the small airway, pulmonary microvasculature, and intrathoracic and extrathoracic lymphatic systems.[23] The proliferation of these LAM cells produces airway obstruction, cystic changes, and pulmonary hemorrhage.[23] LAM is associated with the development of pneumothorax and chylothorax, both pleural complications that usually present as chest pain and breathlessness.

Patients with LAM most commonly present with dyspnea on exertion and nonproductive cough, but chest pain can be the initial symptom in 12% to 14% of the cases, according to different series.[24,25] In patients with LAM, the frequency of spontaneous pneumothorax ranges from 60% to 81%, with a recurrence rate of 64% without pleurodesis or surgery.[25–27]

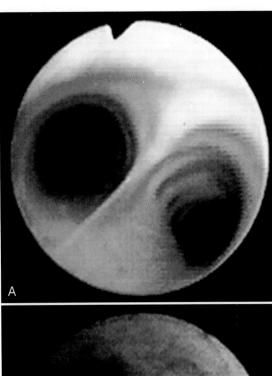

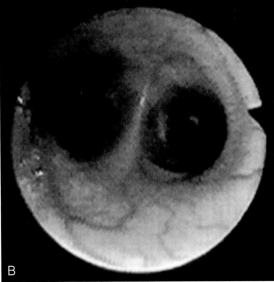

Fig. 80.2 Picture of inflamed airway as visualized with bronchoscopy. **A,** Shows a normal airway in contrast to **B,** an inflamed airway (as may occur with bronchitis). The inflammation causes the release of mediators, which cause pain. Typically a patient has poorly localized retrosternal pain of moderate severity.

A chylous pleural effusion or chylothorax is the accumulation of chyle within the pleural space usually caused by a disruption in the thoracic duct or in the lymphatic flow within the chest.[28] Treatment is primarily supportive.

Pulmonary Langerhans Cell Histiocytosis

Pulmonary Langerhans cell histiocytosis (PLCH) is a rare interstitial lung disease that forms part of a spectrum of diseases characterized by the proliferation and infiltration of different organs by cells known as Langerhans cells.[29] Strongly associated with cigarette smoking, this disorder also has been previously referred to as primary pulmonary histiocytosis X, pulmonary eosinophilic granuloma, and pulmonary Langerhans cell granulomatosis. It usually affects young adults and has a variable and unpredictable course, ranging

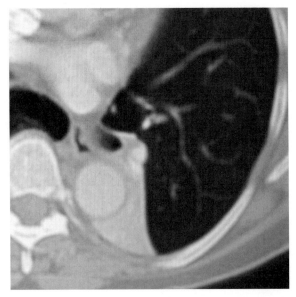

Fig. 80.3 Computed tomography scan of left lower lobe collapse. This subject presented with recurrent left lower lobe collapse, which produced moderately severe continuous chest pain localized over this part of the lung.

from asymptomatic to progressive disease with respiratory failure and death over months.[29–34] Secondary spontaneous pneumothorax, a complication with a reported mortality rate in the literature of 16%, occurs in 4% to 17% of patients with PLCH during the course of the disease.[32–34] Patients with PLCH are predisposed to the development of pneumothorax based on destructive changes in the lung parenchyma resulting from the disease. Thin-walled cysts, nodules (with or without cavitation), or a combination of these are present in the lungs of patients with PLCH.[29] Although dyspnea and cough are common presenting features, spontaneous pneumothorax and chest pain can be the initial manifestation of PLCH, as occurred in 11% of a cohort of 102 patients with PLCH examined over a 23-year period at the Mayo Clinic.[29,31,35]

Sarcoidosis

Sarcoidosis is a multisystem disorder of unknown etiology characterized by noncaseating, epithelioid granulomas in affected organs.[36] It most commonly affects the lungs and associated lymph nodes, although any organ may be involved. Important extrapulmonary manifestations include skin, cardiac, eye, and neurologic involvement. The pathogenesis involves cytokine production by type 1 T-helper lymphocytes and macrophages, which form noncaseating granulomas.[37] A diagnosis is established by a compatible clinical picture with the presence of granulomas on biopsy (and the exclusion of other causes). The clinical course of sarcoid is highly variable, ranging from asymptomatic disease to progressive respiratory failure. Most subjects have a good outcome but have acute flares of disease periodically.

The range of pulmonary manifestations includes pulmonary lymphadenopathy, bronchial sarcoidosis, and pulmonary fibrosis.[37] **Fig. 80.4** shows pulmonary changes of sarcoidosis. Chest pain is a frequent manifestation of sarcoidosis. This chest pain is not well described in the literature, but there seem to be several different forms. It may manifest as retrosternal chest pain

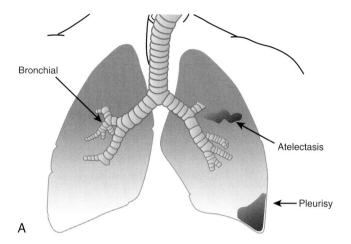

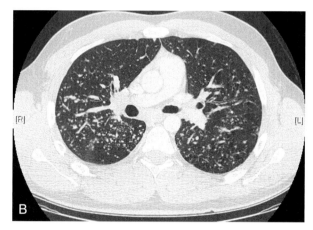

Fig. 80.4 **Sarcoidosis. A,** Shows different mechanisms of lung pathology. **B,** Computed tomography scan of patient with sarcoid and changes of nodular infiltrate and mediastinal lymphadenopathy. This subject had both bronchial irritation and atypical fleeting sharp chest pain.

that occurs with bronchial sarcoidosis[38] with a mechanism that may be similar to that described in asthma or bronchitis. This form may occur with chest tightness and wheezing. Fleeting episodes of deep-seated pain may also occur, sometimes associated with general exacerbations. Pleuritic and chest wall pain may also occur in sarcoidosis.

Acute manifestations of sarcoidosis generally respond well to treatment with corticosteroids. Whether treatment with immunosuppressive medications like cortisol changes long-term outcome (e.g., in pulmonary fibrosis) is not clear.

Pulmonary Hypertension

Patients with pulmonary hypertension may present with significant chest pain that radiates to the neck and arms.[39] This pain has been described in patients with acute and chronic conditions associated with pulmonary hypertension.[14] About half of patients who have primary pulmonary hypertension have chest pain.[40] The mechanism involved in this pain is unclear, but acute dilation of the pulmonary artery and mechanoreceptors has been postulated to be involved in acute pulmonary hypertension resulting from a massive pulmonary embolism.[14] Likewise for chronic primary pulmonary hypertension, the pain has been hypothesized to be induced over the right ventricle by the pressure overload,

relative ischemia, or supply-demand imbalance and by compression of the coronary arteries by the dilated pulmonary artery.[14,41] Pulmonary artery aneurysms are dilations of more than 4 to 5 cm that can be congenital or acquired and present with or without pulmonary hypertension and chest pain.[42,43]

Pleuritic and Chest Wall Pain

As with visceral pain, a number of respiratory conditions may cause pleuritic or chest wall pain. This form of pain is often severe and nearly always well localized. Inflammation, trauma, and malignant invasion of tissue are the main mechanisms involved.

Chest Wall Trauma Caused by Coughing

Chest wall trauma caused by coughing is common but (similar to asthma and chronic bronchitis) is often not considered by clinicians. Severe, persistent, or paroxysmal coughing may cause damage to intercostal muscles and connecting ligaments and occasionally fractures.[44,45] The pain may be quite severe and also prolonged, particularly if the patient is still coughing.

Treatment is aimed at the underlying cause (usually of cough) and simple analgesics. Unfortunately, cough suppressants are rarely better than placebo.

Pulmonary Embolism

Pulmonary embolism (PE) is a respiratory condition that is commonly considered to be associated with pleuritic chest pain. Approximately 250,000 patients are hospitalized annually in the United States because of venous thromboembolism.[46]

Pleuritic chest pain with or without hemoptysis, dyspnea, and circulatory collapse has been classically associated with pulmonary thromboembolic disease.[47] In the Prospective Investigation of Pulmonary Embolism Diagnosis study, more than half of the patients with chest pain or hemoptysis (56%) had pleural effusions.[47–49] Reports are that 75% of patients with pleural effusion associated with pulmonary emboli have pleuritic chest pain.[49] Dyspnea, when present, is usually out of proportion with the size of the pleural effusion.[42,47] Patients with pulmonary emboli and associated pleural effusions may or may not have an associated parenchymal infiltrate; when present, these are more common in the lower lobes and are pleural based and convex toward the hilum (Hampton's hump).[50] Pleural fluid analysis is nonspecific but can help rule out other causes, such as malignant disease, tuberculosis, or pneumonia with a parapneumonic effusion.[50,51] The fluid may be transudative or exudative, sometimes bloody, and the white blood cell count usually ranges from 100 to more than 50,000 cells/mm^3 and may reveal large numbers of eosinophils and mesothelial cells.

The clinical diagnosis of pulmonary embolism is inaccurate, and some controversy exists in the literature over the diagnostic value and sensitivity of certain signs and symptoms, such as dyspnea and pleuritic chest pain.[52–54] The diagnosis usually is based on the history and clinical suspicion plus finding of an unmatched ventilation-perfusion defect in a lung scan or with computed tomographic (CT) angiography (increasingly the test of choice).[55] **Fig. 80.5** shows a CT pulmonary angiogram of a saddle embolus.

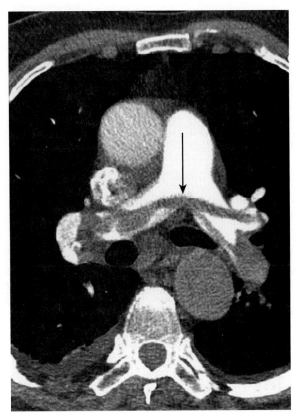

Fig. 80.5 **Computed tomography angiogram showing pulmonary saddle embolus.**

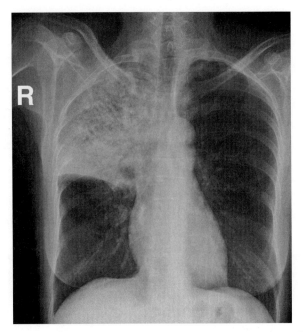

Fig. 80.6 **Chest x-ray showing right upper lobe pneumonia.** This condition was associated with local pleuritic pain.

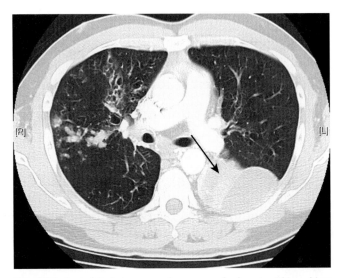

Fig. 80.7 **Computed tomography scan of abscess.** This subject presented with malaise and left-sided pleuritic chest pain that necessitated operative drainage.

Anticoagulation therapy to prevent recurrent embolism is the cornerstone of treatment for pulmonary emboli. Therapy initially with heparin (standard or low–molecular weight) is instituted before the patient's condition is stabilized with oral anticoagulation. In life-threatening circumstances, the clot may be removed with fibrinolytic therapy or embolectomy.[55]

Pleurisy from Adjacent Pulmonary Infection

The most common cause of pleurisy is pulmonary infection, particularly from bacterial pneumonia. The main common organisms that cause pneumonia in adults are *Streptococcus pneumoniae, Moxarella catarrahalis,* and *Haemophilus influenzae.*[56] *Staphylococcus aureus* and *Pseudomonas aeruginosa* are important causes of nosocomial pneumonia.[56]

Pneumonia may produce pleurisy with localized chest pain (**Fig. 80.6**). A parapneumonic effusion occurred in 90 of 203 patients (44%) with pneumonia studied prospectively by Light and coworkers[57]; the investigators reported 10 patients who had a complicated pleural effusion based on positive cultures, a pleural fluid pH of less than 7.00, or glucose lower than 40 mg/100 mL.

Some less common infections have a relatively high incidence of pleuritic chest pain. The fungus *Histoplasma capsulatum,* endemic in Ohio and the Mississippi River Valleys,[58] may cause symptomatic disease in 5%, with most subjects having pleuritic chest pain.[58,59] Other fungal conditions associated with pleurisy include histoplasmosis,[60] blastomycosis,[60] and coccidioidomycosis.[60]

Lung abscess is a pus-containing necrotic lesion of the lung, often with an air-fluid level.[61] A long list of pulmonary pathology, mainly infectious, but also noninfectious, may lead to the formation of an abscess. Bacterial pneumonia and mycobacterial, fungal, and parasitic infections have been reported as causes of lung abscesses. Pulmonary infarction after emboli, lung tumor, and necrotic lesions of silicosis may appear as a lung abscess. **Fig. 80.7** shows a CT scan of a lung abscess. The treatment of pleurisy in this context is primarily directed at the underlying infection. Appropriate antibiotics to cover relevant organisms are necessary, usually given parenterally. Subjects with an infected effusion, empyema (pus on pleural tap), or abscess generally need drainage with a chest tube and may need thoracotomy and decortications.[56] Simple analgesics are generally the only specific medication necessary.

Table 80.2 **Causes of Pneumothorax**
SPONTANEOUS
Primary (usually in thin young males)

Secondary—many potential causes, including:
    Chronic obstructive pulmonary disease
    Asthma
    Pulmonary fibrosis
    Pulmonary Langerhans cell histiocytosis
    Sarcoidosis
    Congenital cyst

IATROGENIC
Penetrating chest wound
Chest compression injury

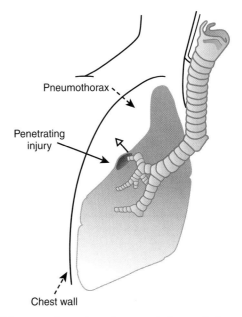

Fig. 80.8 A pneumothorax is most commonly the result of spontaneous rupture of a pleural bleb (or pleural abnormality) that connects with a bronchus. Less commonly, pneumothorax may occur as a complication of an external penetrating injury. *Open arrow*, air from a bronchus.

Pleurisy in Association with Systemic Inflammatory Conditions

Systemic inflammatory conditions may cause pleurisy with associated pain. This is most common in autoimmune diseases, such as RA, systemic lupus erythematosus (SLE), Sjögren's syndrome, scleroderma, polyarteritis nodosa, and Wegener's granulomatosis. The general mechanism appears to be deposition of autoantibodies, which cause a local inflammatory response and pleurisy.

Pleural involvement is the most common lung manifestation in RA (most commonly asymptomatic), and symptomatic pleurisy is a relatively common manifestation of RA that occurs in 3% to 5%.[62] The effusion is characterized by very low glucose level and elevated rheumatoid factor. Pleurisy is an important finding in SLE.[63]

Treatment primarily involves immunosuppression, particularly with high-dose corticosteroids. The pain with these conditions may be quite severe, and strong pain relief may be needed.

Pneumothorax

Pneumothorax refers to the presence of free air between the visceral and parietal pleura. Pneumothoraces are classified as spontaneous or iatrogenic. The vast majority are spontaneous.[64]

Primary spontaneous pneumothorax most commonly occurs in young adults (especially male smokers) and appears to commonly arise from rupture of a pleural bleb on the surface of the lung, which causes an air leak. Secondary spontaneous pneumothorax occurs in subjects with an underlying lung disease, most commonly COPD. Iatrogenic pneumothorax occurs in the context of a penetrating chest wound that allows air to access the pleural space through the rib cage. Important causes of pneumothorax are listed in **Table 80.2**. Pneumothorax is also shown in **Fig. 80.8**.

The clinical manifestations are determined by the size of the pneumothorax.[64] Complete lung collapse and mediastinal shift may occur in severe cases. Most commonly, subjects describe the very acute onset of chest pain and dyspnea. The chest pain may be pleuritic or continuous in nature and can be severe. The mechanism of the pain is not well understood but may relate to pressure on the parietal pleura. The acute lung collapse could itself contribute to pain (as suggested previously).

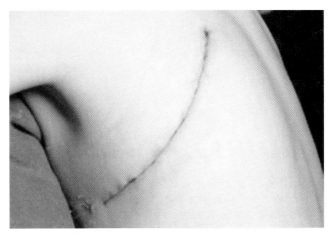

Fig. 80.9 **Thoracotomy scar.** Incision of the chest wall is associated with a high incidence of chronic chest wall pain.

A pneumothorax of moderate size or causing significant clinical problems necessitates drainage by a variety of techniques, ranging from needle aspiration to thoracotomy.

Chest Pain After Thoracotomy

Thoracic surgery in which there is division of the intercostal muscles (e.g., thoracotomy) generally is associated with significant postoperative pain; inadequate treatment may result in complications that include atelectasis, pneumonia, and respiratory failure.

In addition, such subjects often have pain for prolonged periods (commonly for year) after such procedures. Chronic pain after thoracic surgery occurs in 25% to 60% of patients.[65,66] Typically, this pain is moderately severe, continuous in nature, and localized. The pain may be the result of intercostal nerve damage or local muscle damage and may be resistant to treatment. **Fig. 80.9** shows a thoracotomy scar.

Sickle Cell Disease

Sickle cell disease is one of the most prevalent genetic disorders. This hemoglobinopathy derives from a substitution of glutamic acid by valine in the beta subunit of the hemoglobin molecule.[67] The deoxygenated hemoglobin S forms large polymers that aggregate, leading to a change in the red blood cell shape, affecting its deformability and inducing vascular occlusion and hemolysis.

The pulmonary manifestations of this disorder include acute chest syndrome and chronic restrictive pulmonary disease characterized mainly by pulmonary hypertension.[67] The Cooperative Study of Sickle Cell Disease followed the clinical course of sickle cell disease in 3751 patients at 23 centers from 1979 through 1988.[68] The incidence rate of acute chest syndrome in the Cooperative Study of Sickle Cell Disease population was reported to be higher for patients with homozygous sickle cell disease (SS; 12.8/100 patient-years) and in patients with sickle cell β-thalassemia (9.4/100 patient-years).[68,69] The incidence of acute chest syndrome was inversely related to age and was higher in children and lower in adults.[69]

Lung Cancer

A number of different forms of lung cancer all may cause pain. Primary bronchogenic lung cancer is the leading cause of cancer death. Primary tumors from other organs frequently metastasize to the lung. Mesothelioma characteristically involves the lung pleura. Other less common thoracic tumors are sarcomas and thymomas. Lung cancer may cause pain by invasion of the bronchi, parietal pleura, chest wall, or adjacent structures, such as nerves.

Most patients with primary lung cancer (86%)[70] and virtually all patients with mesothelioma die of the disease, so appropriate pain management is important.[71] There is a lack of randomized trials that assess the use of pain relief in lung cancer. Approximately 75% of patients with advanced lung cancer have pain; however, effective management can be achieved in about 80% to 90% of subjects.[72]

The World Health Organization (WHO) has developed a three-stage analgesic ladder for the management of cancer pain (**Fig. 80.10**).[72] If pain occurs, prompt oral administration of drugs should occur in the following order: nonopioids (aspirin and paracetamol); then, as necessary, mild opioids (codeine); and then, strong opioids, such as morphine, until the patient is free of pain. For calming of fears and anxiety, additional drugs, adjuvants, should be used. Adjuvant drugs include corticosteroids (to reduce edema and inflammation) and anticonvulsants and tricyclic antidepressants for neuropathic pain. For maintenance of freedom from pain, drugs should be given "by the clock," that is, every 3 to 6 hours, rather than "on demand." This three-step approach of administration of the right drug in the right dose at the right time is inexpensive and 80% to 90% effective. Surgical intervention on appropriate nerves may provide further pain relief if drugs are not wholly effective. Also, a number of other nonpharmacologic approaches may be useful. Reassurance to patient and family is important. Metastatic disease is usually treated with palliative radiotherapy.

Primary Lung Cancer

Primary lung cancer arises from the airways or pulmonary parenchyma. It is classified into two types: (1) small cell lung cancer (SCLC); and (2) non–small cell lung cancer (NSCLC). Approximately 75% of cancers are the NSCLC type; 20% are SCLC, and 5% are other types, including carcinoids, lymphoma, and sarcoma. The dominant risk factor is smoking; other factors include asbestos exposure and air pollution.[70]

Most patients with lung cancer present with advanced disease. Chest pain is seen is 35% of patients at presentation.[22,72] Persistent, deep-seated pain may arise from mediastinal, bronchial, pleural, or chest wall extension. Pleuritic pain may occur with pleural extension, obstructive pneumonitis, or pulmonary embolism.

Limited-stage small cell cancer is curable with chemotherapy, and limited-stage NSCLC is curable with resection. For most patients who do not have curable disease, a combination of chemotherapy and radiotherapy may be offered.

Superior Sulcus Tumors and Pancoast-Tobias Syndrome

Superior sulcus tumors represent a variety of benign and malignant tumors with apical extension into the superior thoracic inlet.[73] The involvement of the first and second ribs and lower brachial plexus nerve roots T1, T2, and C8 and cervical stellate ganglion is associated with the Pancoast-Tobias syndrome, characterized by shoulder and arm pain radiating down to the inner aspect of the arm and forearm, weakness and atrophy of the hand muscles, and Horner's syndrome. Superior sulcus tumors include adenocarcinoma, large cell carcinoma, and squamous cell carcinoma of the lung.[73] Sarcomas, metastatic disease, bacterial and fungal pneumonia, parasitic infections, tuberculosis, hematologic malignant diseases, and amyloidosis also can be associated with this syndrome.[73,74]

The usual initial symptom is shoulder pain that radiates to the arm and neck. This pain is usually from the involvement of the brachial plexus, endothoracic fascia, ribs, and parietal pleura. The confusion of this syndrome with arthrosis or bursitis of the shoulder leads to common

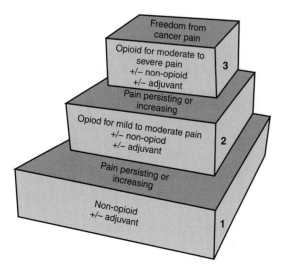

Fig. 80.10 **Pain relief ladder for lung cancer as described by the World Health Organization.**

delays in diagnosis of 10 months, as reported in the literature.[75] X-rays of a subject with Pancoast-Tobias syndrome are shown in **Fig. 80.11**.

Mesothelioma

Mesothelioma is a malignant tumor that arises from serosal surfaces, such as the pleura and peritoneum. The primary risk factor is exposure to asbestos. Often, a very long delay (>40 years) is seen between exposure and the development of cancer. It most commonly arises in the lung, although it may occur in the peritoneal cavity.

Patients with mesothelioma have a mean age of 60 years (range, 40 to 70 years) and a history of exposure to asbestos 20 or more years in the past.[76] The most common presentation is a pleural effusion with dyspnea and in 60% chest pain.[71,77] The chest pain tends to be severe and continuous and is not classically pleuritic. The pain may be referred to the shoulder or upper abdomen because of diaphragmatic involvement. Cough and weight loss are late manifestations. The chest radiograph shows a large pleural effusion in 75% to 90% of the cases.[78,79] Pleural plaques are seen in the opposite hemithorax in about one third of patients. CT scan may show pleural involvement that is not visible in the plain radiograph because of effusion. The pleura is thickened with an irregular, nodular internal margin that is characteristic of this tumor.[80] A CT scan of mesothelioma is shown in **Fig. 80.12**.

At presentation, 40% of patients have dyspnea, and more than 50% have a large pleural effusion.[80] Patients without large effusions are more likely to have chest pain as the predominant symptom. Pleural fluid analysis reveals an exudate, serosanguineous in half of the patients; glucose and pH may be reduced, particularly in patients with large tumors.[81] Cytologic examination of the pleural fluid is diagnostic in approximately 25% of cases. The diagnosis of malignant mesothelioma usually is made with thoracoscopy.[82] Therapy for mesothelioma is rarely curative and is mainly palliative.[71]

Tumors of the Mediastinum

Mediastinal tumors are symptomatic in 50% to 65% of the cases, according to different series.[83–85] The most frequent symptoms are chest pain, cough, dyspnea, dysphagia, and recurrent respiratory infections. Additional conditions are syndromes from the compression of the specific structures, such as Horner's syndrome, superior vena cava syndrome, and spinal cord compression or bone erosion. Between them, the neurogenic tumors, arising from the sympathetic ganglia, intercostal nerves, and chemoreceptor cells, are common and can be benign or malignant. They usually appear on the chest radiograph as unilateral paravertebral masses.[86] Benign tumors should be surgically resected; neuroblastomas are

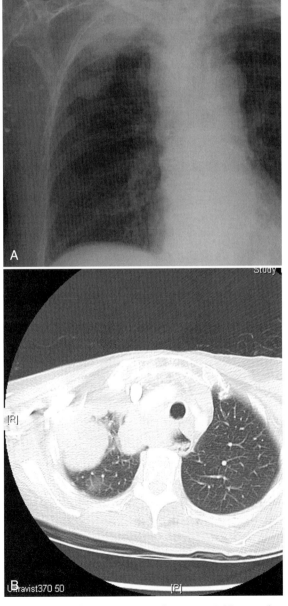

Fig. 80.11 Tumor of the lung apex (Pancoast-Tobias syndrome). A, Chest x-ray shows tumor in right lung apex. B, Computed tomography scan of same patient. This lesion may produce severe neuropathic pain from invasion of the brachial plexus.

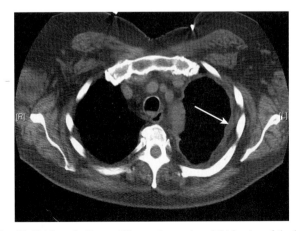

Fig. 80.12 Mesothelioma. CT scan shows pleural thickening of the left pleura. The subject presented with the rapid onset of weight loss and intractable chest pain. Biopsy confirmed mesothelioma.

usually unresectable. A combined coordinated surgical effort including neurosurgeons, orthopedic surgeons, and thoracic surgeons is often necessary to approach some of these tumors, particularly when the spinal cord is involved.

Traumatic Chest Pain

Chest trauma is present in 60% of patients with multisystem injuries.[87] A major clinical feature is the presence of pain usually severe in association with injury.

On arrival in the emergency department, and after a brief history and vital signs evaluation, a physical examination should be done to look for additional posterior wounds and injuries. If no breath sounds are heard on one side of the chest, and the patient's condition is hemodynamically unstable, a chest x-ray should be ordered and a thoracostomy tube should be considered.[88] The output from the chest tube is noted, and the subsequent hours dictate whether or not a thoracotomy is needed. More than 100 mL of blood per hour of output usually indicates a lesion of a major pulmonary vessel or bronchial artery. Interventional radiology procedures are now available for embolization of arteries and vessels in the pulmonary circulation in cases of significant posttraumatic pulmonary hemorrhage. The most serious injuries that need immediate attention are airway obstruction, tension pneumothorax, open pneumothorax, massive hemothorax, flail chest, and cardiac tamponade, as detailed by Owens et al.[87] When these have been ruled out, a second survey should consider the possibilities of simple pneumothorax, hemothorax, pulmonary contusion, traumatic aortic rupture, tracheobronchial disruption, esophageal disruption, traumatic diaphragmatic injury, and wounds penetrating to the mediastinum.

The treatment of rib fractures is directed toward pain control, effective clearance of secretions, and preservation of lung function to avoid complications.[87] Complications and greater severity of injury are seen when more than three ribs are involved. Clearance of secretions and pain control are crucial. Although oral or intravenous narcotics, patient-controlled analgesia, and intrapleural catheters are common methods for pain management in these cases, epidural catheters have been suggested to be superior in controlling the pain and maintaining lung function.[89,90] Special consideration should be given to fractures of the first and second ribs because of the common association with lesions of the great vessels seen with these fractures. Flail chest is the result of multiple rib fractures with chest wall instability that leads to abnormal or paradoxic movements with respiration (inward during inspiration and outward in expiration).

Patients with traumatic flail chest are usually in severe respiratory distress.[91] For more than four decades, internal stabilization of flail chest has been advocated with mechanical ventilation, pain control, and muscle relaxants to prevent paradoxic motion of the chest wall.[91] Positive end-expiratory pressure is used to treat the underlying contusion. Controversy has existed over whether improvement with use of positive-pressure ventilation, and expanding the lung, is the result of the pneumatic fixation of the chest wall or improved gas exchange and protective effect of positive end-expiratory pressure over the lung parenchyma.[91] More recently, pain control and secretion management has been shown to decrease complications and

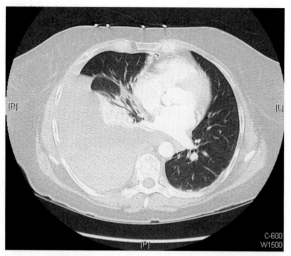

Fig. 80.13 **Computed tomography scan shows large right hemothorax.** This subject fell and fractured multiple ribs posteriorally and transverse sinus processes (of the vertebra). The subject had moderately severe pain and respiratory distress. Operative drainage was necessary.

need for mechanical ventilatory support in flail chest cases.[92,93] Internal fixation is of value in patients with severe chest wall instability. **Fig. 80.13** shows a CT scan of a traumatic hemothorax.

Cough

Cough is a major clinical problem; postviral cough and chronic cough (lasting more than 8 weeks) may be the most common reasons to seek medical attention.[94,95]

The cough reflex has three components: (1) an inspiratory phase; (2) a forced expiratory phase against a closed glottis; and (3) opening of the glottis with subsequent rapid expiration that clears the larynx, trachea, and large bronchi.[95,96] This reflex is modified by input from the cerebral cortex.[97,98] The afferent pathway is activated through receptors concentrated in the bronchial bifurcations, larynx, and esophagus, and impulses are conveyed through the vagus nerve (and also superior laryngeal nerve) to the brainstem. Relay neurons in the nucleus tractus solitaries transmit to the central cough generator.

A cough can be triggered by inflammatory/mechanical changes in the airways and by inhalation of chemical and mechanical irritants. The upper airways are particularly sensitive to stimuli. As in the pain pathway, there are three main types of sensory nerve receptors for cough: (1) RARs; (2) SARs; and (3) C fibers. These sensory nerve receptors receive input from ion channels and metaboreceptors for mechanical, irritant, and chemical stimuli. The afferent pathways of cough and pain overlap to a large degree, with the same receptors and nerves involved. In addition, mediation of pain and cough in the cerebral cortex also overlaps.[99,100] Like pain, the cough reflex can be sensitized by chronic stimulation.[101,102] The sensory pathways of cough are shown in **Fig. 80.14**.

Thus, cough and visceral respiratory pain can be considered to be closely related entities. Therapy for cough has recently emphasized the role of treatment of pain.[103–105]

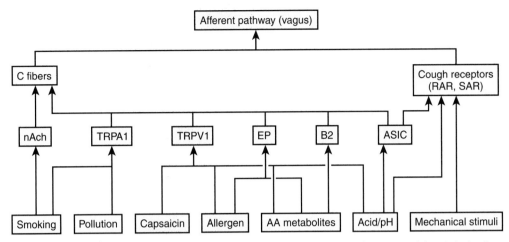

Fig. 80.14 **Cough sensory pathway.** The cough pathway is similar to the pain pathway. Mechanical, irritant, and chemical stimuli act on a variety of ion channels and metaboreceptors. The three main sensory receptors are: (1) RARs; (2) SARs; and (3) C fibers, which conduct impulses via the vagus nerve to the brainstem. AA, arachidonic acid; ASIC, acid sensing ion channel; B2, bradykinin2 receptor; EP, E prostanoid receptor; nAch, nicotine acetylcholine; RAR, rapidly adapting stretch receptors; SAR, slowly adapting stretch receptors; TRPA1, transient receptor potential channel A1.

Conclusion

Chest pain is a major feature of respiratory disorders but has a relatively low profile for most practicing clinicians when compared with other causes, such as cardiac or gastrointestinal disease. Significant spectrum is found in the respiratory chest pain, but it can be considered to arise either from visceral pathways or involvement of the parietal pleura/chest wall. Visceral pain is generally less well defined. Successful management of this form of chest pain is dependent on an accurate diagnosis of the underlying cause.

References

Full references for this chapter can be found on www.expertconsult.com.

Chapter 81

Postmastectomy Pain

Mirjana Lovrincevic, Mark J. Lema, and Bernard H. Hsu

Historical Considerations

Postmastectomy pain syndrome reportedly affects up to 47% of patients who undergo breast surgery.[1] Lumpectomy, mastectomy, and sentinel or complete lymph node dissection can all produce this chronic pain condition. The underlying pathophysiologic mechanism seems to be damage to the intercostobrachial nerve,[2,3] a cutaneous sensory branch of T1, T2, and T3, although the nerve damage may be difficult or impossible to document with conventional neurophysiologic methods (**Fig. 81.1**). The pain is usually felt in the region innervated by the damaged nerves, in the axilla, arm, or shoulder of the affected side, and is described as burning, stabbing, tingling, or electric shock-like. In addition, patients may have neuroma pain,[4] which is described as pain in the region of the scar that is exacerbated with percussion. Phantom breast pain can also occur and is described as the painful sensation of the removed breast as if it were still there. All these symptoms are distressing and may be difficult to treat.

The mechanisms of chronic pain after surgery are complex. Oftentimes, the patient blames the surgeon for doing something wrong, which is usually not the case. Patients who attribute blame for chronic pain after surgery report increased behavioral disturbance and distress and a poor response to pain treatments and have lower expectations of the success of future treatments.[5] Preoperative depression and anxiety were found to place a patient at risk for postmastectomy pain, although statistical significance was not achieved.[6,7] The increased frequency of postmastectomy pain seems to be influenced by marital status, employment status, housing conditions, and educational status of patients who report typical symptoms. Younger patients, increased body weight, and increased height are all associated with an increased frequency of postmastectomy pain syndrome.[8] The greater frequency with younger patients may be associated with their larger tumors.

Intraoperative factors, such as the type of surgery, are probably the most important predictive factors. The large retrospective study by Tasmuth and colleagues[7] showed that postmastectomy pain syndrome was more common in patients who had mastectomy combined with implantation of breast prosthesis (53%) than in patients who had mastectomy alone (31%). Three months after axillary lymph node dissection, 61% of patients with preservation of the intercostobrachial nerve reported sensory deficits compared with 80% of patients in whom the nerve was divided.[9] Postoperative factors thought to be the best predictors for the development of postmastectomy pain syndrome include the extent of immediate postoperative pain, the number of doses of postoperative analgesics received, and immediate adjuvant postoperative radiation therapy.[10]

Clinical Syndrome: Signs, Symptoms, and Physical Findings

Neuropathic pain refers to a chronic disorder of the central or peripheral nervous system (or both) that is poorly responsive to standard therapeutic approaches and standard doses of analgesics. In essence, the loss of normal somatosensory input and the increased input from sensitized peripheral nerve endings induce a central sensitization in the dorsal horn of the spinal cord. Ectopic impulses may be generated at sites other than the damaged nerve endings. When a peripheral nerve is damaged, a region near the dorsal root ganglion, which is distant from the site of injury, becomes capable of generating spontaneous impulses.[11]

The definition of postmastectomy pain syndrome is based on three criteria: (1) character of the pain; (2) location of the pain; and (3) timing of the pain. This definition was developed on the basis of numerous studies.[8,12,13] The pain usually is described as shooting, sharp, stabbing, pulling, tight,

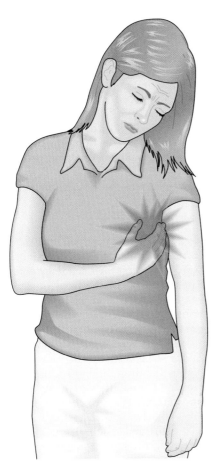

Fig. 81.1 The pain of postmastectomy syndrome is from damage of the intercostobrachial nerve.

or burning, and it significantly interferes with daily activities. It is located in the axilla, arm, shoulder, or chest wall ipsilateral to the side of the surgery. The pain persists beyond the usual healing time of 3 months. Most studies have shown that straining, sudden movements, tiredness, rubbing of clothes, cold weather, and coughing aggravate the pain, whereas resting and lying down relieve the pain. The most important risk factor according to the studies is younger age. Taller and heavier patients and patients with increased body mass index also showed increased frequency of postmastectomy pain syndrome. Complete lymph node dissection was noted to increase the incidence of postmastectomy pain syndrome, as opposed to sentinel lymph node dissection, probably because of a smaller incidence of nerve injury associated with the surgical procedure.[14] Numerous studies examined pain and sensory abnormalities in women after breast surgery. These studies showed an increased evoked pain intensity after repetitive pinprick and thermal stimulation and lower pressure pain threshold in patients in whom chronic neuropathic pain developed after breast surgery compared with patients in whom it did not.[15,16] One large study also found that 58% of women experience sensory disturbances in the surgical region 1 to 3 years after surgery.[1]

A striking similarity is found between the pathophysiologic and biochemical mechanisms that are observed in neuropathic pain and in epilepsy: increased expression of sodium channels in the neural membrane and activation of N-methyl-D-aspartate (NMDA) receptors (wind-up phenomenon) in chronic pain, and hippocampal neurons kindling in epilepsy.[17] Antiepileptic medications are widely used to treat neuropathic pain. Increased monoamine activity (dopamine, norepinephrine, and serotonin) may inhibit nociception at the thalamic, brainstem, and spinal cord levels, which supports the use of tricyclic antidepressants and serotonin reuptake inhibitors in the treatment of neuropathic pain.

Testing

The selection of an objective pain assessment tool should be based on the care setting, patient characteristics (e.g., age, cognitive ability, functional status), and other relevant considerations. Unidimensional pain scales (verbal descriptor scale, numeric rating scale, and visual analog scale) are useful in assessment of pain intensity, whereas multidimensional pain scales (e.g., Brief Pain Inventory, Pain Disability Index) provide information on pain history, intensity, location, quality, and functional status.

Diagnostic studies and tests are often used to determine an etiology and to confirm a diagnosis suggested by the history and physical examination.[18] Patients with chronic pain typically undergo many tests to determine a diagnosis. Very few patients have an alteration in treatment, however. Pain is a subjective experience, but the final diagnosis of the etiology and the decision to pursue specific treatment are clinical ones and can be supported only by relevant data, including electromyographic findings.[19] In the case of postmastectomy pain syndrome, there is an obvious clue to a causative relationship between surgery and onset of pain. Determination of the relevance of an established peripheral neuropathic lesion to the subjective symptom, however, might be important in selected cases. These studies are best for separating neuropathy from myopathy and determining whether a neuropathy is generalized axonal, demyelinating, mixed, or focal.

Psychologic evaluation is often an important assessment strategy. When pain persists, psychosocial and behavioral factors affect the individual's personal and social relationships. The assessment determines the factors that contribute to pain, suffering, and disability and helps to formulate treatment plans. The patient's social support, caregivers, family relationships, work history, cultural considerations, spirituality, and access to health care also are important contributors to the psychologic response to persistent pain. The West Haven–Yale Multidimensional Pain Inventory, the Survey of Pain Attitudes, and the Barriers Questionnaire assess several dimensions related to patient beliefs about pain and pain treatment.

Differential Diagnosis

At the conclusion of the patient's assessment, the clinician should be able to make a diagnosis of a pain syndrome on which to base treatments. Cancer patients often experience mixed pain syndromes. In addition to what seems like a pure neuropathic postmastectomy pain syndrome, they may experience myofascial pain with distinctive trigger points, transient somatic pain at the site of the skin incision, or pain resulting from neuroma formation near the incision site. Because these other conditions all necessitate different therapeutic modalities for successful treatment, one must take into consideration the typical "neuropathic" symptoms of the patient, such as

Table 81.1 Sensory Abnormalities Seen in Postmastectomy Pain Syndrome

Allodynia	Pain from a touch or temperature stimulus that normally does not provoke pain
Dysesthesia	Unpleasant sensation that is spontaneous or evoked
Hyperalgesia	Excessive response to a painful stimulus
Hyperpathia	Increased reaction to a stimulus, especially a painful stimulus
Paresthesia	Abnormal sensation in the distribution of a nerve that is spontaneous or evoked

allodynia (pain from non-noxious stimuli applied to the symptomatic cutaneous area), dysesthesia (spontaneous or evoked unpleasant sensation), hyperalgesia (an exaggerated pain response to a mildly noxious stimulus applied to the symptomatic area), hyperpathia (a delayed and explosive pain response to a noxious stimulus applied to the symptomatic area), and paresthesias (spontaneous intermittent painless abnormal sensations; **Table 81.1**).

Treatment

Based on a comprehensive assessment, a multimodality approach can be devised for the treatment of postmastectomy pain syndrome. The most important treatments in most cases are pharmacologic. Some patients benefit from interventional strategies, however, which may involve neural blockade or sophisticated neuraxial stimulation or infusion.

Pharmacologic therapies for neuropathic pain include antiepileptics, antidepressants, local anesthetics, and other adjuvant analgesics. Opioid analgesics also have shown efficacy against neuropathic pain, although in higher doses than those usually necessary for treatment of nociceptive pain.

Antiepileptics

Antiepileptics have been used for many years to treat neuropathic pain, especially when it is lancinating, episodic, or burning. The exact mechanism by which these drugs prevent spread of abnormal activity is unknown but may involve post-tetanic potentiation, reductions in movement of sodium or calcium ions, potentiation of presynaptic or postsynaptic inhibition, or reduction of responsiveness of various monosynaptic or polysynaptic pathways. Inhibition of postsynaptic neurons by some drugs may reflect binding to γ-aminobutyric acid (GABA) receptors and may lead to greater chloride ion influx through chloride channels.

Neuropathic pain, whether of peripheral or central origin, is characterized by a neuronal hyperexcitability in damaged areas of the nervous system. In peripheral neuropathic pain, damaged nerve endings exhibit abnormal spontaneous and increased evoked activity, mainly as a result of an increased and novel expression of sodium channels.[20] The fact that the neuronal hyperexcitability and corresponding molecular changes are underlying mechanisms in certain forms of epilepsy has led to the use of anticonvulsant drugs for the treatment of neuropathic pain, including postmastectomy pain syndrome.

First-line agents in this class for neuropathic pain typically include gabapentin and pregabalin.[21] Carbamazepine and phenytoin were the first anticonvulsants to be used for this purpose, although today, oxcarbazepine, lamotrigine, and zonisamide are used more often. Antiepileptics can produce adverse effects that range from mild to serious. The most common side effects are drowsiness, dizziness, and gait disturbance. The side effects are usually dose dependent and can be minimized with a careful dose reduction. The most troublesome effects are hepatic toxicity and dermatologic effects that range from rashes to life-threatening erythema, desquamation, and mucositis similar to Stevens-Johnson syndrome.

Tricyclic Antidepressants

Tricyclic antidepressants have been found to be useful in the treatment of a variety of painful syndromes, including postmastectomy pain. They exert their action by potentiation and prolongation of the effects of the biogenic amines, norepinephrine or serotonin or both, in the central nervous system and by interfering with the reuptake of these amines into postganglionic sympathetic nerve endings.

Appropriate use of tricyclic antidepressants requires a good understanding of their pharmacologic features and actions,[22] careful selection of the drug to be used, slow adjustment of the dosage given, and close attention to the time of the day the medication is taken. Failure to consider these factors can make the difference between a successful response and failure. The evidence for analgesic efficacy is greatest for the tertiary amine tricyclic drugs, such as amitriptyline, doxepine, and imipramine. The secondary amine tricyclic antidepressants, such as desipramine and nortriptyline,[23] have fewer side effects and are preferred when concern about sedation, anticholinergic effects, or cardiovascular toxicity is high. The starting dose of a tricyclic antidepressant should be low, and doses can be increased every few days. Analgesia usually occurs within 1 week after an effective dosing level is achieved (**Table 81.2**).

Opioids

The use of opioids to treat chronic neuropathic pain is controversial. Although opioids traditionally have been avoided in treatment of neuropathic pain, more recent trials and reports have led practitioners to reconsider this position.[24] For the most part, opioids are considered second-line medications in the treatment of neuropathic pain because of concerns with long-term safety, especially compared with first-line agents like antidepressants and antiepileptics.[21] The current theories postulate that not all persistent pain syndromes respond to opioid therapy and that opioid response needs to be assessed in a therapeutic titration trial. The titration is necessary because the initial prescribed dose may be too low or too high to achieve the optimal balance of analgesia and acceptable side effects.

Local Anesthetics

Topical lidocaine patches have proven efficacy and safety in the treatment of refractory neuropathic pain.[25] They are considered a first-line treatment of neuropathic pain syndromes.[21] EMLA cream (eutectic mixture of local anesthetics) has also been shown to provide some efficacy for postmastectomy pain.[26,27]

Table 81.2 Commonly Used Tricyclic Antidepressants and Their Side Effects

Drug	Sedation	Anticholinergic Effects	Orthostatic Hypotension	Dysrhythmia Potential
Doxepin	+++	++	++	++
Amitriptyline	+++	++++	+++	++
Imipramine	++	++	+++	++
Protriptyline	+	+++	+	++
Nortriptyline	+	+	+	++
Desipramine	+	+	+++	++

+, Low; ++, moderate; +++, high; ++++, marked.

Several studies were performed on mexiletine, a class Ib antiarrhythmic agent that blocks sodium channels,[28] and showed that it was effective in treatment of neuropathic pain mostly characterized by lancinating dysesthesias.[29] Because mexiletine is prone to many drug interactions, especially interactions from the cytochrome P-450 2D6 system, it should be used with caution in patients already receiving tricyclic antidepressants and serotonin reuptake inhibitors. The most commonly encountered side effects are nausea, heartburn, dizziness, tremor, nervousness, and headache, although they tend to disappear with long-term use. The biggest concern is, however, propensity toward arrhythmias, and it should not be used in patients with second-degree or third-degree heart block.

Capsaicin

Many painful neuropathies that involve small afferent fibers are resistant to the analgesic agents already mentioned. Capsaicin, the vanilloid compound derived from hot peppers, acutely and chronically depletes the neurotransmitter substance P from sensory nerves.[28] This effect suggests that long-term use of the drug could reduce central transmission of information about noxious stimuli. The choice to use a therapy must take into account the adverse event profile versus potential benefit: degranulation of primary afferent fibers can cause a burning sensation that can worsen the existing cutaneous hyperalgesia.[30]

Clonidine

Clonidine, an alpha-adrenergic agonist, exhibits analgesic efficacy when administered intrathecally or epidurally, probably by several different mechanisms, including reduction in peripheral norepinephrine release with stimulation of prejunctional inhibitory alpha$_2$-adrenoreceptors, inhibition of noxious neural transmission in the dorsal horn by presynaptic and postsynaptic mechanisms, and direct inhibition of spinal preganglionic sympathetic neurons.[31] Adverse reactions include hypotension, bradycardia, sedation, and dry mouth.

Neurostimulation

Transcutaneous electrical nerve stimulation (TENS) has been shown to give the best results for deafferentation pain, for precisely localized pain, and for treatment that may be applied closely to the nervous structure supplying the painful area.[32] Nevertheless, a TENS trial needs to be conducted in patients to ensure that the pain is not aggravated by TENS, to ensure that

the patient is responding to the treatment, and to determine the amount of stimulation time needed to achieve pain relief. The few contraindications to TENS are pregnancy, presence of a pacemaker, and patient noncompliance. Interestingly, one study showed that TENS can decrease the amount of skin flap necrosis after mastectomy in patients with breast cancer.[33] This finding may have implications in regards to long-term pain development.

Spinal cord stimulation generally is considered to be a treatment of last resort. It is usually reserved for cases when conservative measures have failed to control the patient's pain. It also is a method of diminishing returns because the probability of reduced effectiveness increases with time; this can be attributed to several causes, including fibrosis around the stimulation arrays, disease progression in some cases, and lead migration, particularly in the cervical area. The mechanism of action is based on partial painful stimuli blockage and its ability to control the neuropathic component of a pain syndrome and is relatively ineffective against the nociceptive component.[34] To improve success, several requirements need to be met, including localized pain, overlapping stimulation paresthesiae with painful area, positioning of electrodes above pain segments, and absence of psychologic disease in a patient.

Intraspinal Therapies

When pain control cannot be achieved with oral medications, the intraspinal route is considered.[35] With opioids alone, profound analgesia can be achieved at a much lower dose, without the motor, sensory, or sympathetic block associated with intraspinal local anesthetic administration. In patients with postmastectomy pain, addition of a local anesthetic, clonidine, or both may be necessary to achieve more complete pain relief. In the future, the use of adenosine, ziconotide, neostigmine, ketorolac, or midazolam may become viable alternatives for patients with intractable pain.[36-38]

Surgically implanted catheters with implanted infusion pumps at a fixed rate or constant flow pumps are made of titanium and silicone rubber and are available in different reservoir sizes. Changes in dosing are accomplished by modifying the concentration of the drugs placed in the pump.

Regional Anesthesia

Various studies have shown the benefits of regional anesthesia in regards to acute postoperative pain from surgical procedures, including breast surgery.[39,40] The effects of regional anesthesia, more specifically a thoracic paravertebral nerve block, have also been shown to produce a reduction in the development of chronic pain after breast surgery. Kairaluoma et al[41] studied 60 patients and concluded that preoperative paravertebral nerve block performed before incision reduced the prevalence and severity of chronic pain 1 year after breast cancer surgery. Although paravertebral nerve block can be used solely as an anesthetic for breast surgery, it is usually performed before general anesthesia induction as an adjunct for intraoperative and acute postoperative pain control. Adequate and effective acute pain relief has a positive association with the prevention of chronic pain development.[10] In addition to nerve blocks, some role may exist for radiofrequency treatment of the thoracic paravertebral nerve for relief of chronic postmastectomy pain.[42] However, the use of radiofrequency for pain management, in general, is still being investigated.

Interestingly, an association can be found with regional anesthesia in patients undergoing breast surgery and decreased progression, spread, and recurrence of tumors.[43] Regional anesthesia seems to decrease the stress response to surgery, thereby affecting the release of certain tumor-promoting cells. Other mechanisms also suggest that anesthetic technique affects the concentration of immune molecules which can promote or suppress the growth of tumor cells.

Conclusion

Although any surgical incision may result in chronic pain, only a few syndromes have been clearly recognized as sequelae of specific surgical procedures. Postmastectomy pain syndrome is one. Considering that one in eight women has development of breast cancer, of which roughly 60% are treated with mastectomy, and that the incidence rate of chronic pain after this procedure is 47%, this problem clearly warrants prompt attention and aggressive treatment. The underlying mechanism is believed to be neuropathic, related to damage to the intercostobrachial nerve.

Treatment of postmastectomy pain syndrome requires a multidisciplinary approach in which each member of the team addresses a specific problem the patient faces. The team usually includes a pain physician, psychologist or psychiatrist, and physical therapist with the objectives to rationalize medications, teach coping skills, and help return to previous level of physical functioning. Strong consideration should be given to invasive approaches when conservative pharmacologic measures fail to provide pain control.

References

Full references for this chapter can be found on www.expertconsult.com.

Postthoracotomy Pain

Bassem Asaad and Vitaly Gordin

Introduction

Postthoracotomy pain is one of the most severe forms of postoperative pain. Pain management after thoracotomy is vital not only for patient comfort but also for minimized postoperative pulmonary complications, improved ventilation-perfusion ratio, and overall surgical outcome. Adequate deep breathing, coughing with minimal splinting, and postoperative ambulation are hard to achieve when pain is poorly controlled. The postoperative pain may not be limited to the acute interval but may evolve, in up to 52% of patients, into chronic pain syndrome known as postthoracotomy pain syndrome (PTPS)[1] that invariably affects quality of life. The International Association of the Study of Pain defines chronic pain after thoracotomy as "pain that recurs, or persists along a thoracotomy scar at least 2 months after a surgical procedure."[2]

Pathogenesis

The exact causality of PTPS is still unclear. With the different surgical approaches, consideration of the likely implications of positioning and surgical trauma is always important. Many surgical and nonsurgical factors may predispose and influence the occurrence of PTPS. Injury of intercostal nerves by retractors, suturing, and the possibility of development of an intercostal neuroma are likely causes.[3] Injury of intercostal muscles, the serratus anterior, the latissimus dorsi, and the shoulder girdle muscles may cause significant myofascial pain that may even results in frozen shoulder.[3] Costochondral or costovertebral junction disarticulations from extensive retraction are possible causes.[4] Pleurectomy is a strong risk factor for chronic pain development.[5] Sternal osteomyelitis, sternal fracture, incomplete healing, sternocostal chondritis, brachial plexus injury, entrapment of nerves from sternal wires, and

even hypersensitivity reaction against the metal wires were found to be other possible factors for development of PTPS after thymectomy and coronary artery bypass surgery.[6] Bachiocco et al found that personality traits play a strong modulatory role.[7]

Relevant Clinical Anatomy and Surgical Approaches

The pain impulses from the skin, ribs, and parietal pleura are transmitted through the intercostal nerves, from the visceral pleura through autonomic nerves, from the lung through the vagus nerve, and from the mediastinum, pericardial pleura, and diaphragm through the phrenic nerves.[8] Several surgical approaches to the content of the thoracic cage have been described. The type and degree of damage to the regional tissues depend on the chosen surgical approach. Lateral thoracotomy provides good exposure of the pleural cavity and the hilar structures. Other approaches to the thoracic cavity include a supine thoracotomy, video-assisted thoracoscopic surgery (VATS), and muscle-sparing thoracotomy. These approaches have different impacts on the incidence, prevalence, and severity of PTPS. Extensive surgery and pleurectomy were found to be predictive factors for development of postthoracotomy chronic pain, suggesting also a visceral component.[9]

Epidemiology

The overall incidence rate of chronic PTPS is about 52%; of those patients, 3% to 16% have moderate to severe pain develop.[1] Orcroch et al[10] found certain differences in the analgesic requirement in men and women. They reported that women had more pain after major thoracotomy, with a higher rate of nonsteroidal anti-inflammatory drug

(NSAID) consumption, but not opioid consumption, in comparison with men; the same study showed that older patients reported less pain after discharge than did younger patients.[10]

Predictive and Preventive Factors

The impact of the acute pain phase and its management on the development of chronic PTPS is still controversial. Preemptive thoracic epidural analgesia appears to reduce the severity of acute pain but has no effect on the incidence of chronic pain.[11] A multimodal pain management approach is advocated. When cryoanalgesia was used in conjugation with thoracic epidural analgesia, a decrease was found in pain associated with movement during the acute stage with earlier recovery of pulmonary function. However, this combined technique failed to decrease the incidence of chronic pain.[12] In another randomized controlled study, Ju et al[13] found that cryoanalgesia increases the incidence of postthoracotomy neuropathic chronic pain.

Clinical Presentation

During the acute postoperative phase, patients experience sharp pain that increases with breathing and coughing. The pain is also associated with numbness, especially along the scar site. If the pain persists, or recurs at least 2 months after the surgical procedure, it is considered a chronic pain.[1] Chronic pain after thoracotomy is typically a combination of neuropathic and nociceptive pain. In a retrospective study with a Pain DETECT Questionnaire developed and validated by the German Research Network on Neuropathic pain, neuropathic pain was found to be absent in 47% of patients who underwent either open thoracotomy or VATS.[9] Patients present with different types of pain symptoms. They may have burning pain and allodynia along the thoracotomy scar but may also have aching chest or back pain. Significant myofascial pain may be present, and referred shoulder pain may occur, especially after procedures that cause injury to the diaphragm or the phrenic nerve.

Differential Diagnosis

A key to the differential diagnosis of PTPS is identification of the nature of pain, whether nociceptive or neuropathic. Primary or recurrent malignant diseases to any of the structures in the rib cage or the thoracic cavity must be ruled out. The differential diagnosis of PTPS is broad. Any etiology of nociceptive or neuropathic pain should be considered. Causes of radicular pain in the thoracic area, such as pain from a herniated disc, neuroforaminal stenosis, or rib pathology, should be excluded. Neuropathic pain may also result from postherpetic neuralgia that may give rise to a similar clinical picture of severe pain in a thoracic dermatome with a history of rash in the dermatomal distribution. Nociceptive chronic chest pain may be related to such conditions as slipping rib syndrome; costochondritis; Tietze's syndrome, which is a form of costochondritis accompanied by swelling of the costal cartilages; and myofascial pain syndrome.

Management

Acute Phase

A full understanding is needed between the patient, anesthesiologist, and surgeon regarding the desired level of pain control, with the risk-benefit ratio of any chosen pain management technique taken into consideration. Individual physician's experience and the availability of the appropriate facility equipped to accommodate any potential complication are critical factors in any pain management plan.

Thoracic epidural anesthesia (TEA) is the gold standard modality for pain control, not only in reduction of postoperative pain but also in improvement of respiratory function and outcome after thoracotomy. When prospectively compared with patient-controlled opioid analgesia (PCA), epidural analgesia was found to be a superior modality in improved quality of life (QOL) as reflected by Short Form- (SF-)8 and SF-36 QOL health surveys for up to 1 week after surgery.[14] Epidural fentanyl 5 µg/mL combined with bupivacaine 0.1% provided an optimal balance between pain relief and side effects.[15] TEA was effective in control of the incision pain but not effective in alleviation of postthoracotomy shoulder pain, which is most likely related to irritation of the pericardium or the pleura.[16] In a prospective randomized double-blind placebo controlled study performed on 50 patients receiving thoracic epidural analgesia for postthoracotomy pain, phrenic nerve infiltration with 10 mL of ropivacaine just before lung expansion and chest closure reduced the incidence and delayed the onset of ipsilateral shoulder pain by about 50% during the first 24 hours after open lung resection, with no clinically relevant adverse effects on respiratory function.[17] Thoracic epidural analgesia has its potential complications that may result from insertion or removal of the catheter, or from the medications administered in the epidural space. Hypotension and urinary retention are common side effects related to TEA. An important factor is also the timing of insertion and removal in patients with anticoagulated or coagulopathic conditions and its possible interference with the surgical management plan.

Another modality for management of acute postthoracotomy pain is paravertebral block. In a review article of randomized trials that evaluated regional techniques for management of postthoracotomy pain, paravertebral block was found to be as effective as epidural block with local anesthetic.[18] Davies, Myles, and Graham[19] reported that paravertebral block and epidural analgesia provided comparable pain relief after thoracic surgery; however, paravertebral block had a better side effect profile. In a review article, Conlon, Shaw, and Grichnik[20] found no difference in analgesic efficacy between paravertebral and epidural techniques, but paravertebral block was associated with a better postoperative function and a significant reduction in side effect profile. Unlike epidural catheterization, paravertebral blockade is not associated with serious neurologic complications and is specifically useful when epidural catheter insertion is contraindicated.[20] Both bupivacaine 0.25% and ropivacaine 0.3% with fentanyl 3 µg/mL were found to be equally effective for postthoracotomy pain control when used via continuous paravertebral blockade.[21] One limitation to this technique is that not all anesthesiologists are as experienced in performing paravertebral blocks as they are with epidural blocks.

Interpleural block is another modality for control of pain after thoracotomy. The end result is significantly affected by the amount of medication that remains in the interpleural space. Not only does the local anesthetic get lost through unclamped chest drain, but it can be also diluted in pleural effusions. In addition, it binds to blood proteins in bloody effusion. An uneven distribution of the local anesthetic in the pleural cavity may also be seen, especially in pnemonectomy cases.[22] Yildirim et al[23] conducted a prospective randomized study on 60 young patients scheduled for elective correction of aortic coarctation and patent ductus arteriosis. One group of 30 patients received TEA, and the other group received interpleural (IP) catheter. In both groups, ropivacaine 0.2% was administered through the corresponding catheter. TEA was found to have a more beneficial effect on respiratory function and postoperative pain control after thoracotomy than IP catheters.[23] One limitation to this study is that the TEA group received the local anesthetic before the incision whereas the other group received it after the incision.

Although PCA with an opioid analgesic is among the most frequently used pain management modalities, its benefits could be offset by the potential for the opioid-induced respiratory depression. Adjuvant analgesics can play an important role when combined with opioid PCA. A prospective randomized controlled study was done on 24 patients to investigate the effect of intravenous magnesium on the management of postthoracotomy pain. In that study, 1 hour after the procedure, the magnesium group received 30 mg/kg bolus of magnesium sulfate followed by 10 mg/kg/hr infusion for 48 hours combined with intravenous morphine PCA (0.5 mg/h, 0.3-mg patient-controlled anesthesia dose, 15-min lockout time). The control group received the same PCA protocol. The conclusion was that the addition of magnesium was associated with decreased morphine requirements during the first 48 hours after thoracotomy without adverse effects.[24]

Kobas and Yedicocuklu[25] reported in a prospective controlled study done on 50 patients that infiltration of the sternotomy incision and the medaistianal tube sites with 0.25% levobupivacaine in addition to administration of PCA with morphine resulted in decreased morphine consumption during the first 24 hours after cardiac surgery when compared with the control group that did not receive the infiltration with bupivacaine.

Transcutaneous electrical nerve stimulation (TENS) was shown to be a safe and effective modality in alleviation of postoperative pain and improvement in patient recovery.[26]

Osteopathic manipulations can be helpful in the subset of patients with a strong musculoskeletal component by increasing joint mobility and normalizing autonomic output.[27]

Chronic Phase

As in any chronic pain condition, pain management should include a multimodal approach consisting of medications, possible interventions, cognitive behavioral therapy, and physical therapy.

Medical Management

The choice of medications should be tailored to the type of pain and the patient's medical history. More than 45% of patients do not have neuropathic symptoms, and reliance mainly on medications that target neuropathic pain may

not result in a satisfactory result. In those cases of chronic postthoracotomy pain in which neuropathic pain plays a significant role, gabapentin appears to be both safe and effective with minimal side effects and high patient compliance.[28] Patients whose conditions fail to respond to NSAIDs or acetaminophen might benefit from tramadol for moderate pain or opioid analgesics for severe pain. As in any chronic pain condition, normalization of sleep and mood disturbance plays an important role and can be achieved with addition of an antidepressant. Antidepressants that inhibit norepinephrine reuptake, such as tricyclic ones and selective serotonin norepinephrine reuptake inhibitors, might offer additional benefits because of their analgesic properties, especially in the presence of neuropathic pain.[29,30]

Glantz et al[31] conducted an open-label prospective clinical trial to study the effect of combining transdermal nitroglycerin (NTG) with etodolac for chronic postthoracotomy pain. In 30 of 129 patients with chronic postthoracotomy pain who did not respond to etodolac, NTG 5 mg/day was added. A significant reduction in visual analogue scale was observed on the 14th day of treatment. Similar changes were noted in breakthrough pain intensity and sleep efficiency. The only side effect reported was self-limited headache that occurred during the first few days of the study. A known limitation to this study is the lack of a placebo group, but the delayed response to NTG makes the placebo effect unlikely.[31] The mechanism of action of NTG is still not well understood. NTG is metabolized to nitric oxide, which may result in increasing the intracellular concentration of cyclic guanosine monophostate that is thought to have a modulatory effect on pain neurotransmission.

Interventional Procedures

Trigger point injections can be helpful in patients with myofascial pain. Also, scar neuroma injection may be attempted, especially in patients with pain over the scar site.

Moore et al[32] conducted a retrospective study on 18 patients to determine whether computed tomographic (CT) scan intercostal cryoneurolysis is an effective method of reducing pain in patients with PTPS. The patients were followed for an average of 51 days. With acknowledgement of the limitation of their small sample size, they concluded that CT scan–guided cryoneurolysis of intercostal nerves is a safe and effective pain management modality. They reported a statistically significant difference in numeric pain score 7.5 ± 2 before procedure that decreased to 1.2 ± 1.9 immediately after the procedure and 4.1 ± 1.7 51 days after the procedure.[32]

Cohen et al[33] conducted a retrospective data analysis that involved 49 patients with postthoracotomy pain to study the difference in outcome between radiofrequency of the dorsal root ganglia, pulsed radiofrequency ablation of intercostals nerves, and pharmacotherapy. They concluded that radiofrequency ablation (RFA) of the dorsal root ganglia is superior to pulsed radiofrequency ablation of intercostal nerves and to pharmacotherapy. Because of the risk of RFA on the dorsal root ganglia, they recommended that such procedure be reserved for patients with intractable pain with failure of other conservative pain management approaches.[33]

The authors of this chapter performed peripheral nerve stimulation along the thoracotomy scar in two patients, which resulted in more than 60% reduction in the pain score in each patient. Both patients have been followed for more than 12 months after

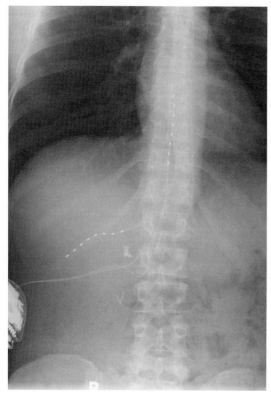

Fig. 82.1 Epidural and peripheral stimulator lead 1.

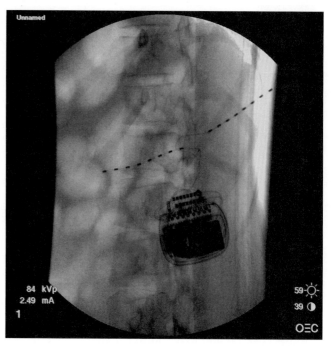

Fig. 82.2 Peripheral nerve stimulator.

the placement of the peripheral nerve stimulator, and the benefits of the procedure have not diminished (**Figs. 82.1** and **82.2**).

Physical Therapy

Physical therapy, including such modalities as ultrasound scan, TENS, and moist heat, can be helpful in patients with significant myofascial pain component. It should be considered when a comprehensive treatment plan is being formulated for any patient with PTPS. Early introduction of physical therapy may decrease the incidence of certain complications, such as frozen shoulder syndrome.

Conclusion

The management of postthoracotomy pain in the acute stage is essential to decrease the incidence of atelectasis and pneumonia. The pain commonly evolves into a chronic phase. Patients usually present with more than one type of pain.

The differential diagnosis of that pain is broad and might originate from any anatomic structure in the area affected by thoracotomy. Preemptive analgesia might be helpful in decreasing the pain in the acute stage but has not shown to be helpful in decreasing the incidence or the severity of pain in the chronic stage. Thoracic epidural analgesia and paravertebral blockade are the two most effective pain management modalities in the acute stage. In the chronic stage, as in any chronic pain condition, management includes medical management, interventional procedures, cognitive behavior modification, and physical therapy. PTPS pain was earlier thought to be mainly neuropathic, and most of the management approaches were targeted towards that. In fact, a significant number of patients experience mainly nociceptive pain, which warrants a different management approach. PTPS is difficult to manage, and a multimodal approach tailored to the individual patient is the key to a better outcome.

References

Full references for this chapter can be found on www.expertconsult.com.

Mononeuritis Multiplex

Steven D. Waldman

Although the term *mononeuritis multiplex* is often incorrectly used in clinical medicine as a term of art to describe what is more correctly called diabetic truncal neuropathy, it is in fact the name that is used to describe a myriad group of disorders that share a common clinical presentation. This clinical presentation is characterized by a painful, multifocal, asymmetrical peripheral neuropathy that affects both the sensory and the motor nerves.[1] Mononeuritis multiplex is associated with a heterogeneous group of diseases that each shares the ability to damage nerves. These diseases include diabetes mellitus, Hansen's disease, the connective tissue diseases, amyloidosis, acquired immunodeficiency syndrome (AIDS), Lyme disease, sarcoidosis, paraneoplastic syndromes, cryoglobulinemias, acute viral hepatitis, and the macroglobulinemias (**Table 83.1**).[2-5]

The pathophysiology responsible for the pain and motor dysfunction associated with mononeuritis multiplex is damage to the neuronal axon must commonly from vasculitis-induced ischemia (**Fig. 83.1**).[6,7] However, the exact etiology responsible for the nerve destruction may remain elusive in approximately 20% to 25% of those patients with mononeuritis multiplex.

The most common neurologic presentation of diabetic neuropathy is mononeuritis multiplex. Diabetic neuropathy is now thought to be the most common form of peripheral neuropathy in the world, affecting an estimated 220 million people worldwide. Diabetic neuropathy has for the first time outstripped leprosy as the leading cause of peripheral neuropathy.[2] The onset of symptoms of mononeuritis multiplex in diabetics frequently coincides with periods of extreme hypoglycemia or hyperglycemia or with weight loss or weight gain.[8] With other diseases associated with mononeuritis multiplex, no clear association is found with the severity of the underlying disease state and the onset of neurologic symptoms.

Signs and Symptoms

The patient with mononeuritis multiplex often presents with severe dysesthetic pain with patchy sensory deficits and associated motor dysfunction. A deep, aching component to the pain may be seen, with the onset of this aching pain often preceding clinically apparent motor and sensory deficits. The pain of mononeuritis multiplex is often worse at night, and significant sleep disturbance may result, further worsening the patient's pain symptoms. Although by definition mononeuritis multiplex must affect at least two isolated nerve segments, the initial clinical presentation of the pain symptoms and neurologic findings may appear to be a localized condition only to rapidly progress to a constellation of multifocal neurological symptoms that can initially confuse the unsuspecting clinician. As the disorder progresses, the pain and neurologic dysfunction often become more symmetrical, which makes diagnosis more straightforward. The severity of the functional disability of mononeuritis multiplex varies from mild motor dysfunction to complete motor deficits.

The pain of mononeuritis multiplex can be quite severe and debilitating, and early intervention is universally recommended. In some patients, the pain of mononeuritis multiplex tends to "burn itself out" as the damage to the sensory axons becomes more extensive; in other patients, the resulting deafferentation pain remains a devastating problem. In general, the symptoms of mononeuritis multiplex often spontaneously resolve in 6 to 12 months. Because of the severity of symptoms associated with this condition, however, aggressive symptomatic relief with pharmacotherapy and neural blockade with local anesthetics and steroids is indicated.

Physical examination of a patient with mononeuritis multiplex generally reveals minimal physical findings early in the course of the disorder, with sensory and motor findings developing as the axonal damage progresses. Deep tendon reflexes tend to be preserved, except in those patients with severe neurologic

Table 83.1 Causes of Mononeuritis Multiplex

VASCULAR INSUFFICIENCY

Vasculitic neuropathy

Diabetic proximal neuropathy (amyotrophy)

IMMUNE-MEDIATED

Multifocal motor neuropathy*

Lewis-Sumner syndrome*

Chronic inflammatory demyelinating polyneuropathy (CIDP)*

Neuralgic amyotrophy (idiopathic brachial plexitis)

Idiopathic lumbosacral plexitis

NEOPLASTIC

Leukemia/lymphoma

Neurolymphomatosis

INFECTIOUS/INFLAMMATORY

Leprosy

Lyme disease

Herpes zoster

Sarcoidosis

INHERITED

Hereditary neuropathy with liability to pressure palsy (HNPP)*

Hereditary neuralgic amyotrophy

Hereditary high-density lipoprotein deficiency (Tangier disease)

Neurofibromatosus

COMPRESSIVE/TRAUMATIC

Multiple nerve entrapments

Multiple peripheral nerve injury

From Katirji B: *Electromyography in clinical practice*, ed 2, Philadelphia, 2002, Mosby, pp 397.
* Demyelinating neuropathies.

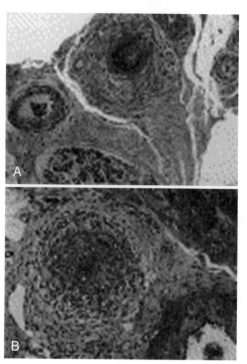

Fig. 83.1 A, Superficial peroneal nerve biopsy specimen showing classic necrotizing vasculitis of epineurial artery, characterized by transmural mononuclear inflammatory cell infiltration and circumferential fibrinoid necrosis (epoxy resin embedded). B, Peroneus brevis muscle biopsy revealing more chronic vasculitic lesion of perimysial vessel, with intimal and adventitial thickening, disorganization of vessel wall, obliteration of lumen, vascular inflammation, and focal fibrinoid necrosis (hematoxylin and eosin). *(From Collins MP, Kissel JT: Neuropathies with systemic vasculitis. In Dyck PJ II and Thoman PK, editors: Peripheral neuropathy, ed 4, Philadelphia, 1994, Saunders, pp 2335–2404.)*

dysfunction. Although mononeuritis multiplex often initially manifests as deep muscle aching that may be erroneously attributed to musculoskeletal etiologies, unlike the pain of musculoskeletal etiologies in which the patient may attempt to splint or protect the painful area, the patient with pain from mononeuritis multiplex does not attempt to splint or protect the affected area. Careful sensory examination of the affected dermatomes or peripheral nerves should reveal decreased sensation or allodynia. Careful motor examination of the affected area may reveal subtle weakness early in the course of the disorder.

Testing

If a diagnosis of mononeuritis multiplex is entertained on the basis of the targeted history and physical examination, screening laboratory testing, including a complete blood count, chemistry profile, sedimentation rate, thyroid function, hepatitis screen, human immunodeficiency virus (HIV), antinuclear antibody, and urinalysis, should help rule out the most common causes of mononeuritis multiplex and those that are more easily treatable. Electromyography and nerve conduction velocity testing are indicated in all patients with neurologic dysfunction to help identify treatable causes of nerve damage and the surgically treatable entrapment neuropathies.[9] Electromyography and nerve conduction velocity testing also helps further delineate the type of peripheral neuropathy that is present.[10] Electromyography and

nerve conduction velocity testing may help quantify the severity of peripheral nerve damage or entrapment neuropathy. Additional laboratory testing is indicated as the clinical situation dictates (e.g., Lyme disease titers, heavy metal screens, biopsies for amyloidosis, etc). Magnetic resonance imaging (MRI) of the spinal canal and cord should be performed if myelopathy is suspected. Nerve or skin biopsy (or both) occasionally is indicated if no etiology for the patient's neurologic dysfunction can be ascertained. Lack of response to the therapies discussed subsequently should cause the clinician to reconsider the working diagnosis and repeat testing as clinically indicated (see Fig. 83.1).

Differential Diagnosis

As mentioned previously, mononeuritis multiplex is not a specific disease but the name given to a specific constellation of symptoms caused by a diverse group of diseases. These causative diseases may exist alone or in combination, making identification and subsequent treatment more difficult. Because some of the more common diseases that cause mononeuritis multiplex are easily treatable, early correct diagnosis is important to avoid sequella.[11]

Although uncommon in the United States, globally, Hansen's disease is a common cause of mononeuritis multiplex and should be considered in patients who have lived or traveled in areas where this disease is endemic. Other infectious etiologies of peripheral neuropathies include Lyme disease and HIV. Substances that are toxic to nerves also may cause peripheral neuropathies that are indistinguishable from mononeuritis multiplex on clinical grounds. Such substances include alcohol, heavy metals, chemotherapeutic agents, and hydrocarbons. Heritable disorders, such as Charcot-Marie-Tooth disease and other familial diseases of the peripheral nervous system, also must be considered, although treatment options are limited. Metabolic and endocrine causes of peripheral neuropathy that must be ruled out include vitamin deficiencies, pernicious anemia, hypothyroidism, uremia, and acute intermittent porphyria. Other causes of peripheral neuropathy that may confuse the clinical picture include Guillain-Barré syndrome, amyloidosis, entrapment neuropathies, carcinoid, paraneoplasitc syndromes, and sarcoidosis. Because many of these causes of peripheral neuropathy are treatable (e.g., pernicious anemia), the clinician must rule out these treatable diagnoses before attributing a patient's symptoms to an occult cause.

Treatment

Pharmacologic Treatment

Analgesics

In general, neuropathic pain such as mononeuritis multiplex responds poorly to analgesic compounds. The simple analgesics, including acetaminophen and aspirin, can be used in combination with antidepressant and anticonvulsant compounds, but care must be taken not to exceed the recommended daily dose, or renal or hepatic side effects may occur. Nonsteroidal anti-inflammatory drugs also may provide pain relief when used with antidepressants and anticonvulsant compounds, but given the nephrotoxicity of this class of drugs, they should be used with extreme caution in patients with diabetes because of the high incidence of diabetic nephropathy, even early in the course of the disease. The role of cyclooxygenase-2 inhibitors in the palliation of the pain has not been adequately studied, and given the incidence of undiagnosed cardiac disease in patients with diabetes, this class of drugs should be used with caution if at all.

Opioid analgesics treat neuropathic pain such as mononeuritis multiplex poorly. Given the significant central nervous system and gastrointestinal side effects coupled with the problems of tolerance, dependence, and addiction, opioid analgesics rarely, if ever, should be used as a primary treatment for the pain of mononeuritis multiplex. If an opioid analgesic is considered in this setting, consideration should be given to the analgesic tramadol, which binds weakly to the opioid receptors and may provide some symptomatic relief. Tramadol should be used with care in combination with antidepressant compounds to avoid the increased risk of seizures.

Antidepressant Compounds

Traditionally, tricyclic antidepressants have been a mainstay in the palliation of pain from mononeuritis multiplex. Controlled studies have shown the efficacy of amitriptyline for this indication. Other tricyclic antidepressants, including nortriptyline and desipramine, also have shown to be clinically useful. This class of drugs is associated with significant anticholinergic side effects, including dry mouth, constipation, sedation, and urinary retention. These drugs should be used with caution in patients with glaucoma, cardiac arrhythmia, and prostatism. To minimize side effects and encourage compliance, the primary care physician should start amitriptyline or nortriptyline at a 10-mg dose at bedtime. The dose can be titrated up

to 25 mg at bedtime as side effects allow. Upward titration of dosage in 25-mg increments can be done each week as side effects allow. Even at lower doses, patients generally report a rapid improvement in sleep disturbance and begin to experience some pain relief in 10 to 14 days. If the patient does not experience any improvement in pain as the dose is titrated upward, the addition of gabapentin or pregabalin alone or in combination with nerve blocks with local anesthetics or steroid or both is recommended (see subsequent discussion). The selective serotonin reuptake inhibitors, such as fluoxetine, also have been used to treat the pain of mononeuritis multiplex, and although better tolerated than the tricyclic antidepressants, they seem to be less efficacious.

Anticonvulsants

Anticonvulsants have long been used to treat neuropathic pain, including mononeuritis multiplex. Phenytoin and carbamazepine have been used with varying degrees of success alone or in combination with the antidepressant compounds. The side-effect profiles of these drugs have limited their clinical utility. More recently, the anticonvulsant gabapentin has been shown to be highly efficacious in the treatment of a variety of neuropathic painful conditions, including postherpetic neuralgia and mononeuritis multiplex. Used properly, gabapentin is extremely well tolerated compared with other drugs, including the aforementioned antidepressant compounds and anticonvulsants, which previously had been used routinely to treat mononeuritis multiplex. In most pain centers, gabapentin has become the adjuvant analgesic of choice in treatment of mononeuritis multiplex.

Gabapentin has a large therapeutic window, but the primary care physician is cautioned to start this medication at the lower end of the dosage spectrum and titrate upward slowly to avoid central nervous system side effects, including sedation and fatigue. The following recommended dosage schedule minimizes side effects and encourages compliance. A single bedtime dose of 300 mg for two nights can be followed with a 300-mg dose twice daily for an additional 2 days. If the patient tolerates this twice-daily dosage, the dosage may be increased to 300 mg three times a day. Most patients begin to experience pain relief at this dosage range. Additional titration upward can be done in 300-mg increments as side effects allow. Daily doses greater than 3600 mg in divided doses are not currently recommended. For simplification of maintenance dosing after titration has been completed, 600-mg and 800-mg tablets have been made available.

Pregabalin at an initial dose of 50 mg three times daily (tid) increasing to 100 mg tid as side effects dictate may be another reasonable choice in the management of the pain associated with mononeuritis multiplex. Topiramate at a daily initial dose of 50 mg titrated slowly upward to a target dose of 200 mg twice daily (bid) may also worth a try. Topiramate has a large therapeutic window, and a maximum dose of 1600 mg/day has been shown to be useful in some patients with refractory pain from mononeuritis multiplex.

Antiarrhythmics

Mexiletine is an antiarrhythmic compound that has been shown to be possibly effective in the management of mononeuritis multiplex. Some pain specialists believe that mexiletine is especially useful in patients with mononeuritis multiplex with pain that manifests primarily as sharp lancinating or burning pain. This drug is poorly tolerated by most patients, however, and should be reserved for patients who have not had a response to first-line pharmacologic treatments, such as gabapentin or nortriptyline alone or in combination with neural blockade.

Topical Agents

Some clinicians have reported success in the treatment of mononeuritis multiplex with topical application of capsaicin. An extract of chili peppers, capsaicin is thought to relieve neuropathic pain by depleting substance P. The side effects of capsaicin include significant burning and erythema and limit the use of this substance by many patients.

Topical lidocaine administered via transdermal patch or in a gel also has been shown to provide short-term relief of the pain of mononeuritis multiplex. This drug should be used with caution in patients who are taking mexiletine because of the potential for cumulative local anesthetic toxicity. Whether topical lidocaine has a role in the long-term treatment of mononeuritis multiplex remains to be seen.

Prednisone and Immunosuppressives

The use of prednisone and immunosuppressives to treat the vasculitis frequently responsible for the nerve damage associated with mononeuritis multiplex should be considered sooner rather than later if an inflammatory etiology is suspected. Prednisone 60 mg given in daily divided doses in a tapering dose over 2 weeks is a reasonable starting place in this clinical situation. For patients that do not have a response to or cannot tolerate prednisone, intravenous immune globulin may be considered.

Neural Blockade

Neural blockade with local anesthetics alone or in combination with steroids has been shown to be useful in the management of acute and chronic pain associated with mononeuritis multiplex. For truncal neuropathic pain, thoracic epidural or intercostal nerve block with local anesthetic or steroid or both may be beneficial.[2] Occasionally, neuroaugmentation via spinal cord stimulation may provide significant relief of the pain of mononeuritis multiplex in patients who have not had a response to more conservative measures. Neurodestructive procedures rarely, if ever, are indicated to treat the pain of mononeuritis multiplex because they often worsen the patient's pain and cause functional disability.

Physical and Occupational Therapy

Early treatment of the motor and sensory deficits associated with mononeuritis multiplex is crucial to avoid prolonging the patient's functional disability. Initial treatment should be aimed at preserving range of motion and residual function and at the same time protecting insensate areas. Therapeutic heat and cold to provide symptomatic relief should be used with extreme caution because of sensory deficits.

Control of Blood Glucose

Current thinking suggests that the better the glycemic control, the less severe the symptoms of mononeuritis multiplex associated with diabetes mellitus.[7] Significant swings in blood glucose values seem to predispose patients with diabetes to the development of clinically significant mononeuritis multiplex. Some investigators believe that oral hypoglycemic agents, while controlling blood glucose, do not protect the patient from the development of mononeuritis multiplex as well as insulin. Some patients with mononeuritis multiplex who are on hypoglycemic agents experience improvement in symptoms when switched to insulin.

Conclusion

The major problem in the care of patients thought to have mononeuritis multiplex is the failure to identify potentially treatable diseases responsible for this constellation of signs and symptoms. Early correct diagnosis is necessary to treat this painful condition properly and to avoid overlooking serious underlying pathology. The use of pharmacologic agents discussed in this chapter, including gabapentin, allows the clinician to control the pain of mononeuritis multiplex adequately. Intercostal or epidural nerve blocks are simple techniques that can produce dramatic relief for patients with mononeuritis multiplex.

References

Full references for this chapter can be found on www.expertconsult.com.

Part G

Syndromes of the Abdomen, Retroperitoneum, and Groin

Chapter 84

Abdominal Wall Pain Syndromes

Steven D. Waldman

Abdominal wall pain syndromes are a common reason that patients seek medical attention. Often these calls for help take the form of middle-of-the-night visits to the emergency room and the like because patients fear that they have appendicitis, a heart attack, an ulcer, or acute gallbladder disease. Unfortunately, although these painful conditions are common, they are frequently misdiagnosed, which can lead to unnecessary invasive cardiac and gastrointestinal studies and result in much needless anxiety for the patient and family. This chapter provides the clinician with a clear roadmap of how to identify and treat the more common musculoskeletal causes of abdominal wall pain. The ability to rapidly diagnose and treat these problems is a cost-effective endeavor and helps alleviate much of the patient's anxiety and suffering.

Anterior Cutaneous Nerve Entrapment Syndrome

Anterior cutaneous nerve entrapment syndrome is a constellation of symptoms consisting of severe knife-like pain that emanates from the anterior abdominal wall and associated point tenderness over the affected anterior cutaneous nerve.[1] The pain radiates medially to the linea alba but in almost all cases does not cross the midline. Anterior cutaneous nerve entrapment syndrome occurs most commonly in young females. The patient can often localize the source of pain quite accurately by pointing to the spot at which the anterior cutaneous branch of the affected intercostal nerve pierces the fascia of the abdominal wall at the lateral border of the rectus abdominis muscle. At this point, the anterior cutaneous branch of the intercostal nerve turns sharply in an anterior direction to provide innervation to the anterior wall (**Fig. 84.1**).

The nerve passes through a firm fibrous ring as it pierces the fascia, which is where the nerve is subject to entrapment. The nerve is accompanied through the fascia by an epigastric artery and vein. The potential exists for small amounts of abdominal fat to herniate through this fascial ring and become incarcerated, which results in further entrapment of the nerve (**Fig. 84.2**). Contraction of the abdominal muscles or an increase in intra-abdominal pressure places additional traction on the nerve and may elicit sudden, sharp, lancinating pain in the distribution of the affected anterior cutaneous nerve (**Fig. 84.3**).

Physical examination reveals that the patient attempts to splint the affected nerve by keeping the thoracolumbar spine slightly flexed to avoid increasing tension on the abdominal musculature (**Fig. 84.4**). Pain is reproduced with pressure on the anterior cutaneous branch of the affected intercostal nerve at the point at which the nerve pierces the fascia of the abdominal wall at the lateral border of the abdominis rectus muscle. Having the patient do a sit-up often reproduces the pain, as does the Valsalva's maneuver.

Plain radiographs are indicated in all patients with pain thought to emanate from the lower costal cartilage and ribs to rule out occult bony pathology, including rib fracture and tumor. Radiographic evaluation of the gallbladder is indicated if cholelithiasis is suspected. On the basis of the patient's clinical findings, additional testing may be indicated, including a complete blood count, rectal examination with testing for the presence of occult blood, sedimentation rate, and antinuclear antibody testing. Computed tomographic (CT) scan of the abdomen is indicated if intra-abdominal pathology or an occult mass is suspected (**Fig. 84.5**). The injection technique discussed in the section on treatment serves as both a diagnostic and a therapeutic maneuver.

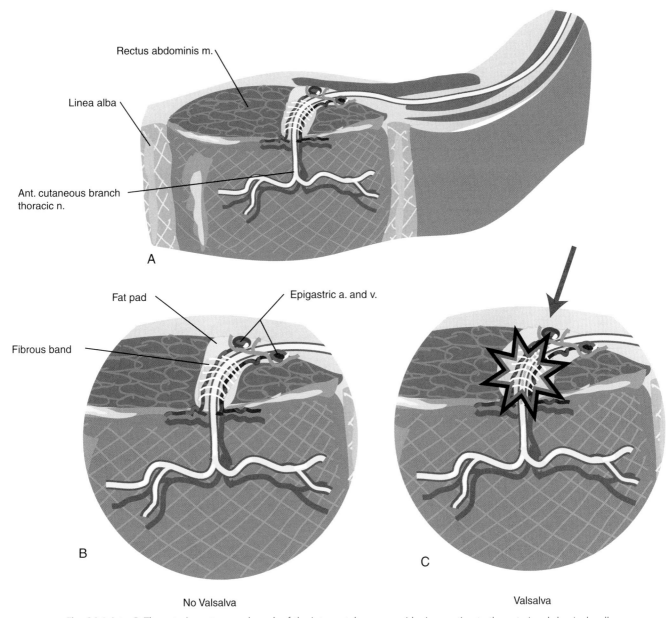

Fig. 84.1 A to C, The anterior cutaneous branch of the intercostal nerve provides innervation to the anterior abdominal wall.

Clinically Relevant Anatomy

The intercostal nerves arise from the anterior division of the thoracic paravertebral nerve. A typical intercostal nerve has four major branches. The first branch is the unmyelinated postganglionic fibers of the gray rami communicantes, which interface with the sympathetic chain. The second branch is the posterior cutaneous branch, which innervates the muscles and skin of the paraspinal area. The third branch is the lateral cutaneous division, which arises in the anterior axillary line. The lateral cutaneous division provides the majority of the cutaneous innervation of the chest and abdominal wall. The fourth branch is the anterior cutaneous branch that supplies innervation to the midline of the chest and abdominal wall (see Figs. 84.1 and 84.2). The anterior cutaneous branch pierces the fascia of the abdominal wall at the lateral border of the rectus abdominis muscle. The nerve turns sharply in an anterior direction to provide innervation to the anterior wall.

The nerve passes through a firm fibrous ring as it pierces the fascia, which is where the nerve is subject to entrapment. The nerve is accompanied through the fascia by an epigastric artery and vein. Occasionally, the terminal branches of a given intercostal nerve may actually cross the midline to provide sensory innervation to the contralateral chest and abdominal wall. The 12th nerve is called the subcostal nerve and is unique in that it gives off a branch to the first lumbar nerve, thus contributing to the lumbar plexus.

Treatment

Initial treatment of the pain and functional disability associated with anterior cutaneous nerve entrapment syndrome should include a combination of nonsteroidal anti-inflammatory drugs (NSAIDs) or cyclooxygenase-2 (COX-2) inhibitors. Local application of heat and cold may likewise be beneficial.

The use of an elastic rib belt may also help provide symptomatic relief and protect the affected nerves from additional irritation. For patients who do not respond to these treatment modalities, the following injection technique with local anesthetic and steroid may be a reasonable next step.[2]

Injection of the anterior cutaneous nerve is performed by placing the patient in the supine position; proper preparation with the application of antiseptic solution to the skin overlying the affected nerves as they pierce the abdominal wall is carried out. A sterile syringe containing 1.0 mL of 0.25% preservative-free bupivacaine for each nerve to be injected and 40 mg of methylprednisolone is aseptically attached to a 1½–inch, 25-gauge needle.

The affected nerves are identified with strict aseptic technique and should be easily palpable; pressure on them should elicit a positive jump sign in most patients. The needle is then carefully advanced through the skin and into subcutaneous tissue through the anterior fascia of the rectus abdominis muscle (**Fig. 84.6**). The needle should be advanced just beyond the fascia but no further, or damage to the abdominal viscera could result. After careful aspiration to ensure that the needle tip is not in a vein or artery, 1 mL of solution is gently injected. Limited resistance to injection should be seen, but the patient may experience paresthesia as the solution is injected. If significant resistance is encountered, the needle should be advanced slightly until the injection proceeds

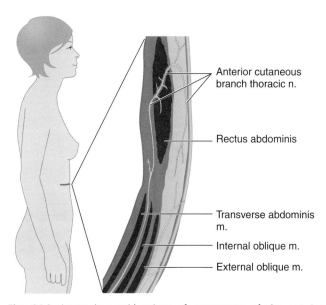

Fig. 84.2 Anatomic considerations of entrapment of the anterior cutaneous branch of the intercostal nerve.

Anterior cutaneous branch thoracic n.

Rectus abdominis

Transverse abdominis m.

Internal oblique m.

External oblique m.

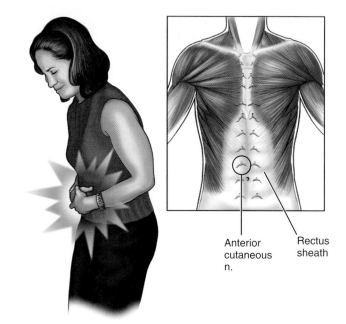

Fig. 84.4 Patients often attempt to splint the affected nerve by keeping the thoracolumbar spine slightly flexed to avoid increasing tension on the abdominal musculature. (*From Waldman SD, editor:* Atlas of uncommon pain syndromes, *ed 2, Philadelphia, 2008, Saunders, p 174.*)

Anterior cutaneous n.

Rectus sheath

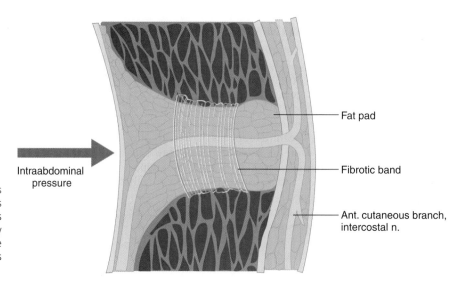

Fig. 84.3 Contraction of the abdominal muscles or an increase in intra-abdominal pressure puts additional traction on the anterior cutaneous branch of the intercostal nerve and may elicit sudden, sharp, lancinating pain in the distribution of the affected anterior cutaneous nerve.

Intraabdominal pressure

Fat pad

Fibrotic band

Ant. cutaneous branch, intercostal n.

with only limited resistance. This procedure is repeated for each affected nerve. The needle is then removed, and a sterile pressure dressing and ice pack are placed at the injection site.

The major complication of this injection technique is damage to the abdominal viscera and, rarely, pneumotho-rax if the needle is placed too deeply and invades the peritoneal cavity or pleural space. Infection, although rare, can occur if strict aseptic technique is not adhered to. These complications can be greatly decreased if the clinician pays close attention to accurate needle placement. Because this technique blocks the anterior cutaneous nerve, the patient should be warned to expect some transient numbness of the abdominal wall and bulging of the abdomen in the region injected as a result of blockade of the motor innervation to these muscles.

Slipping Rib Syndrome

Slipping rib syndrome is a constellation of symptoms consisting of severe knife-like pain that emanates from the lower costal cartilages associated with hypermobility of the anterior end of the lower costal cartilages.[3] The 10th rib is most commonly involved, but the eighth and ninth ribs can also be affected.[4] This syndrome is also known as rib-tip syndrome. Slipping rib syndrome is almost always associated with trauma to the costal cartilage of the lower ribs. This cartilage is often traumatized during acceleration or deceleration injuries and blunt trauma to the chest. With severe trauma, the cartilage may subluxate or dislocate from the ribs. Patients with slipping rib syndrome may also have a clicking sensation with movement of the affected ribs and associated cartilage.

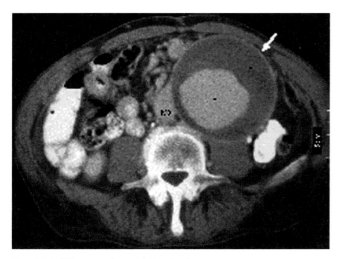

Fig. 84.5 CT scan of an abdominal aneurysm. *(From Grainger RG, Allison DJ, editors: Grainger and Allison's diagnostic radiology, ed 3, Philadelphia, 1999, Churchill Livingstone, p 2378.)*

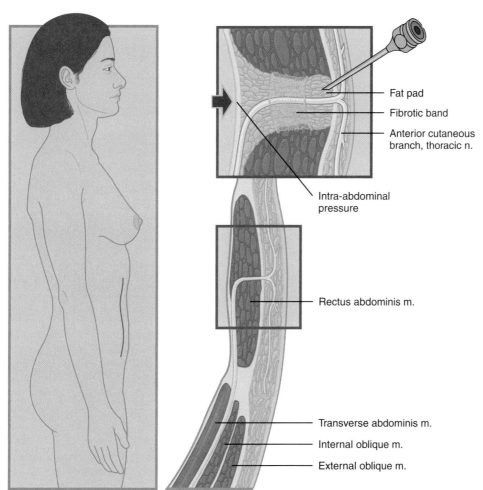

Carrico & Shavell

Fat pad
Fibrotic band
Anterior cutaneous branch, thoracic n.
Intra-abdominal pressure
Rectus abdominis m.
Transverse abdominis m.
Internal oblique m.
External oblique m.

Fig. 84.6 Injection technique for anterior cutaneous nerve entrapment syndrome. *(From Waldman SD, editor: Atlas of pain management injection techniques, ed 2, Philadelphia, 2007, Saunders, p 327.)*

Physical examination reveals that the patient vigorously attempts to splint the affected costal cartilage joints by keeping the thoracolumbar spine slightly flexed. Pain is reproduced with pressure on the affected costal cartilage. Patients with slipping rib syndrome exhibit positive hooking maneuver test results. The hooking maneuver test is performed by having the patient lie in the supine position with the abdominal muscles relaxed while the clinician hooks his or her fingers under the lower part of the rib cage and pulls gently outward (**Fig. 84.7**). Pain and a clicking or snapping sensation of the affected ribs and cartilage indicate positive test results.

Plain radiographs are indicated in all patients with pain thought to emanate from the lower costal cartilage and ribs to rule out occult bony pathology, including rib fracture and tumor. On the basis of the patient's clinical findings, additional testing may be indicated, including a complete blood count, prostate-specific antigen, sedimentation rate, and antinuclear antibody testing. Magnetic resonance imaging (MRI) of the affected ribs and cartilage is indicated if joint instability or an occult mass is suspected.

Clinically Relevant Anatomy

The cartilage of the true ribs articulates with the sternum via the costosternal joints. The cartilage of the first rib articulates directly with the manubrium of the sternum and is a synarthrodial joint that allows a limited gliding movement. The cartilage of the second through sixth ribs articulates with the body of the sternum via true arthrodial joints. These joints are surrounded by a thin articular capsule. The costosternal joints are strengthened by ligaments.

The 8th, 9th, and 10th ribs attach to the costal cartilage of the rib directly above. The cartilages of the 11th and 12th ribs are called floating ribs because they end in the abdominal musculature. The pleural space and peritoneal cavity may be entered when performing the following injection technique if the needle is placed too deeply and laterally, and pneumothorax or damage to abdominal viscera may result.

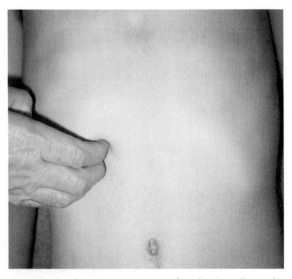

Fig. 84.7 **The hooking maneuver test for slipping rib syndrome.** *(From Waldman SD, editor:* Physical diagnosis in pain: an atlas of signs and symptoms, *Philadelphia, 2005, Saunders, p 197.)*

Treatment

Initial treatment of the pain and functional disability associated with sleeping rib syndrome should include a combination of NSAIDs or COX-2 inhibitors. Local application of heat and cold may likewise be beneficial. The use of an elastic rib belt may also help provide symptomatic relief and protect the affected nerves from additional irritation. For patients who do not respond to these treatment modalities, the following injection technique with local anesthetic and steroid may be a reasonable next step.[5]

The goals of this injection technique are explained to the patient. The patient is placed in the supine position, and proper preparation with the application of antiseptic solution to the skin overlying the affected costal cartilage and rib is carried out. A sterile syringe containing 1.0 mL of 0.25% preservative-free bupivacaine for each joint to be injected and 40 mg of methylprednisolone is aseptically attached to a 1 ½-inch, 25-gauge needle.

The distal rib and costal cartilage are identified with strict aseptic technique. The lower margin of each affected distal rib is identified and marked with a sterile marker. The needle is then carefully advanced at the point marked through the skin and subcutaneous tissue until the needle tip impinges on the periosteum of the underlying rib (**Fig. 84.8**). The needle

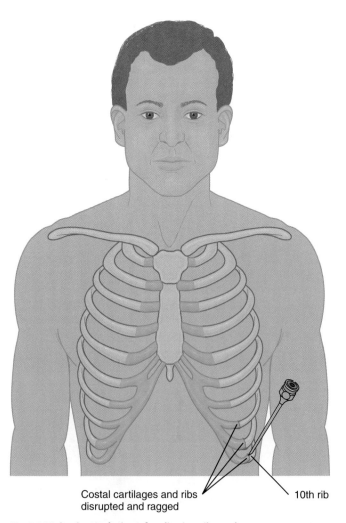

Costal cartilages and ribs disrupted and ragged

10th rib

Fig. 84.8 **Injection technique for slipping rib syndrome.** *(From Waldman SD, editor:* Atlas of pain management injection techniques, *ed 2, Philadelphia, 2007, Saunders, p 325.)*

is then withdrawn back into subcutaneous tissue and walked inferiorly off the inferior rib margin. The needle should be advanced just beyond the inferior rib margin but no further, or pneumothorax or damage to the abdominal viscera could result. After careful aspiration to ensure that the needle tip is not in an intercostal vein or artery, 1 mL of solution is gently injected. Limited resistance to injection should be seen. If significant resistance is encountered, the needle should be withdrawn slightly until the injection proceeds with only limited resistance. This procedure is repeated for each affected rib and associated cartilage. The needle is then removed, and a sterile pressure dressing and ice pack are placed at the injection site.

The major complication of this injection technique is pneumothorax or damage to the abdominal viscera if the needle is placed too medially or deeply and invades the pleural space or peritoneal cavity. Infection, although rare, can occur if strict aseptic technique is not adhered to. These complications can be greatly decreased if the clinician pays close attention to accurate needle placement. Because this technique blocks the intercostal nerve corresponding to the rib injected, the patient should be warned to expect some transient numbness of the chest and abdominal wall and bulging of the abdomen in the subcostal region as a result of blockade of the motor innervation to these muscles.

Liver Pain

Liver pain is a common clinical occurrence, but it is often poorly diagnosed and treated. The liver can serve as a source of pain in and of itself via the sympathetic nervous system and be a source of referred pain from peritoneal irritation via the intercostal and subcostal nerves.[6] Pain that emanates from the liver itself tends to be ill defined and may be referred primarily to the epigastrium. It is dull and aching in character and mild to moderate in severity. It can be related to swelling of the liver and concomitant stretching of the liver capsule or result from distention of the veins, as seen with portal obstruction. This pain is carried via sympathetic fibers from the celiac ganglion, which enter the liver along with the hepatic artery and vein. This type of liver pain responds poorly to adjuvant analgesics. Occasionally, hepatic enlargement causes diaphragmatic pain that is referred to the supraclavicular region (**Fig. 84.9**). This referred pain is transmitted via the phrenic nerve and is often misdiagnosed.

Referred liver pain is caused by mechanical irritation and inflammation of the inferior pleura and peritoneum. This pain is somatic in nature and is carried primarily via the lower intercostal and subcostal nerve. This somatic pain is sharp and pleuritic in nature and moderate to severe in intensity. This pain responds more favorably to NSAIDs and opioid analgesics than sympathetically mediated liver pain does.

Signs and Symptoms

The clinical manifestations of liver pain are directly related to whether the pain is mediated via the sympathetic or somatic nervous system, or both. In patients with sympathetically mediated pain, the abdominal examination may reveal hepatomegaly with tenderness to palpation of the

liver. Primary tumor or metastatic disease may also be identified. The remainder of the abdominal examination is bland. Auscultation over the liver fails to reveal a friction rub in most cases. As mentioned previously, the patient may have ill-defined pain in the supraclavicular region.

Patients with somatically mediated liver pain respond in an entirely different manner. The patient often splints the right lower portion of the chest wall and abdomen and takes small short breaths to avoid exacerbating the pain. The patient may avoid coughing because the pain and accumulated upper airway secretions and atelectasis may be a problem. The abdominal examination may reveal signs of peritoneal irritation over the right upper quadrant. A friction rub is often present with auscultation over the liver. The liver may be extremely tender to palpation. Primary tumor or metastatic disease (or both) may be present.

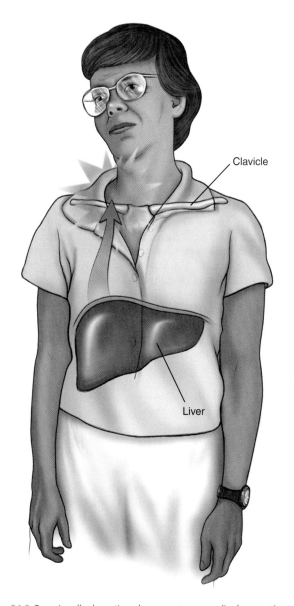

Fig. 84.9 Occasionally, hepatic enlargement causes diaphragmatic pain that is referred to the supraclavicular region. (*From Waldman SD, editor: Atlas of uncommon pain syndromes, ed 2, Philadelphia, 2008, Saunders, p 179.*)

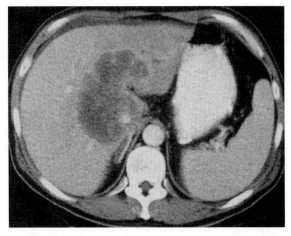

Fig. 84.10 Intrahepatic cholangiocarcinoma in a 45-year-old man. A contrast-enhanced CT scan shows a large central, predominantly hypointense mass with peripheral enhancement. The lobulated mass encases the inferior vena cava, which remains patent. *(From Haaga JR, Lanzieri CF, Gilkeson RC, editors: CT & MR imaging of the whole body, ed 4, Philadelphia, 2002, Mosby, p 1290.)*

Testing

Testing of patients with liver pain should be aimed at identification of the primary source of liver disease responsible for the pain and at ruling out of other pathologic processes that may be responsible for the pain (**Fig. 84.10**). Plain radiographs of the chest and abdomen, including an upright abdominal film, are indicated in all patients with pain thought to emanate from the liver. Radiographs of the ribs are indicated to rule out occult bony pathology, including tumor. On the basis of the patient's clinical findings, additional testing may be indicated, including a complete blood count, automated chemistry panels, liver function test, sedimentation rate, and antinuclear antibody testing. CT scan of the lower thoracic contents and abdomen is indicated in most patients with liver pain to rule out occult pulmonary and intra-abdominal pathology, including cancer of the gallbladder and pancreas. Differential neural blockade on an anatomic basis can serve as both a diagnostic and therapeutic maneuver (see the Treatment section).

Differential Diagnosis

Pain of hepatic origin must be taken seriously. It is often the result of an underlying serious disease, such as biliary malignancy disease, portal hypertension, or hepatic metastatic disease. Pain that emanates from the liver is often mistaken for pain of cardiac or gallbladder origin and can lead to visits to the emergency department and unnecessary cardiac and gastrointestinal workups. If trauma has occurred, liver pain may coexist with fractured ribs or fractures of the sternum itself, which can be missed on plain radiographs and may necessitate radionuclide bone scanning for proper identification.

Neuropathic pain that involves the chest wall may also be confused or coexist with liver pain. Examples of such neuropathic pain include diabetic polyneuropathies and acute herpes zoster involving the lower thoracic and upper

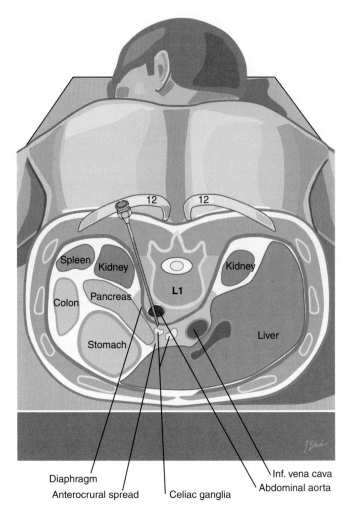

Fig. 84.11 Technique for transaortic celiac plexus block. *(From Waldman SD, editor: Atlas of interventional pain management, ed 3, Philadelphia, 2009, Saunders, p 343.)*

lumbar nerves. The possibility of diseases of the structures of the inferior mediastinum and retroperitoneum remain ever present, and at times, these conditions can be difficult to diagnose. Pathologic processes that inflame the pleura, such as pulmonary embolism, infection, and Bornholm disease, may also mimic or coexist with pain of hepatic origin.

Treatment

Initial treatment of liver pain should include a combination of simple analgesics and NSAIDs or COX-2 inhibitors. If these medications do not adequately control the patient's symptomatology, an opioid analgesic may be added.

Local application of heat and cold may also be beneficial and provide symptomatic relief of liver pain. The use of an elastic rib belt over the liver may likewise help provide symptomatic relief. For patients who do not respond to these treatment modalities, an injection of local anesthetic and steroid may be a reasonable next step. If the pain is thought to be sympathetically mediated, a celiac plexus block is a reasonable next step (**Fig. 84.11**). This technique provides both diagnostic and therapeutic benefit. If the pain is thought to be somatic in nature, intercostal nerve blocks should be the next step (**Fig. 84.12**). Remember that pain of hepatic origin may be both somatic and sympathetic in nature and may necessitate both celiac plexus and intercostal nerve blocks for complete control.

The major problem in the care of patients thought to have liver pain is failure to identify potentially serious pathology of the thorax or upper part of the abdomen. Given the proximity of the pleural space, pneumothorax is a distinct possibility after an intercostal nerve block. The incidence rate of the complication is less than 1%, but it occurs with greater frequency in patients with chronic obstructive pulmonary disease. Although uncommon, infection, including liver abscess, remains an ever-present possibility, especially in a cancer patient with immunocompromise. Early detection of infection is crucial to avoid potentially life-threatening sequelae.

Conclusion

Patients with the pain syndromes discussed in this chapter often attribute their pain symptomatology to appendicitis, a gallbladder attack, ulcer disease, or on occasion, a heart attack. Reassurance is needed if the source of the pain is from the abdominal wall, although one should remember that musculoskeletal pain syndromes and intra-abdominal pathology can coexist. Failure to diagnose occult pathology can lead to disastrous outcomes.

References

Full references for this chapter can be found on www.expertconsult.com.

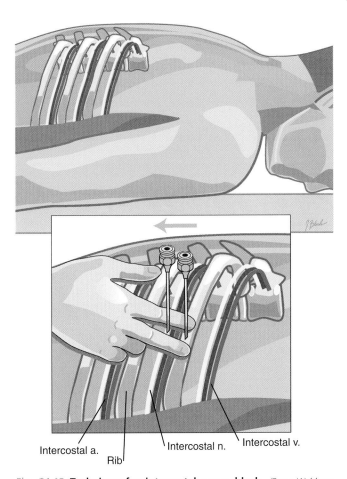

Intercostal a.
Rib
Intercostal n.
Intercostal v.

Fig. 84.12 **Technique for intercostal nerve block.** *(From Waldman SD, editor:* Atlas of interventional pain management, *ed 2, Philadelphia, 2003, Saunders, p 286.)*

Evaluation and Treatment of Acute and Chronic Pancreatitis

Steven D. Waldman

It has been said that if one knows pancreatitis, one knows medicine. Anyone who has had experience in the care of a patient with acute or chronic pancreatitis is likely to agree. This chapter familiarizes the clinician with the broad scope of problems associated with pancreatitis and provides a concise roadmap for the management of associated pain.

Acute Pancreatitis

Acute pancreatitis is one of the most common causes of abdominal pain. The incidence rate of acute pancreatitis is approximately 0.5% of the general population, with a mortality rate of 1% to 1.5%.[1] In the United States, acute pancreatitis is most commonly caused by alcohol; gallstones are the most common cause in most European countries.[2,3] Acute pancreatitis has many causes (**Table 85.1**). In addition to alcohol and gallstones, other common causes of acute pancreatitis include viral infections, tumor, and medications.

Abdominal pain is a common feature in acute pancreatitis.[4] Pain may range from mild to severe and is characterized by steady, boring epigastric pain that radiates to the flanks and chest. The pain is worse with the supine position, and a patient with acute pancreatitis often prefers sitting with the dorsal spine flexed and the knees drawn up to the abdomen (**Fig. 85.1**). Nausea, vomiting, and anorexia also are common features of acute pancreatitis.

Signs and Symptoms

A patient with acute pancreatitis appears ill and anxious. Tachycardia and hypotension resulting from hypovolemia are common, as is low-grade fever.[5] Saponification of subcutaneous fat is seen in approximately 15% of patients with acute pancreatitis, as are pulmonary complications, including pleural effusions and pleuritic pain that may compromise respiration.

Diffuse abdominal tenderness with peritoneal signs is invariably present.[6] A pancreatic mass or pseudocyst from pancreatic edema may be palpable (**Fig. 85.2**). If hemorrhage occurs, periumbilical ecchymosis (Cullen's sign) and flank ecchymosis (Turner's sign) may be present (**Figs. 85.3** and **85.4**). Both of these findings suggest severe necrotizing pancreatitis and indicate a poor prognosis. If hypocalcemia is present, Chvostek's or Trousseau's signs may be present.

Testing

Elevation of the serum amylase level is the sine qua non of acute pancreatitis.[7] Levels tend to peak at 48 to 72 hours and then begin to drift toward normal. Serum lipase level remains elevated and may correlate better with the actual severity of the disease. Because elevated serum amylase levels may be caused by other diseases (e.g., parotitis), amylase isoenzmes may be necessary to confirm a pancreatic basis for this laboratory finding. Plain radiographs of the chest are indicated in all patients who present with pain from acute pancreatitis to identify pulmonary complications, including pleural effusion, which result from the acute pancreatitis. Given the extrapancreatic manifestations of acute pancreatitis (e.g., acute renal or hepatic failure), serial complete blood count, serum calcium, serum glucose, liver function tests, and electrolytes are indicated in all patients with acute pancreatitis. Computed tomographic (CT) scan of the abdomen helps in identification of pancreatic pseudocyst and may help the clinician gauge the severity and progress of the disease. Gallbladder evaluation with radionucleotides is indicated if gallstones are being considered as a cause of acute pancreatitis. Arterial blood gases help in identification of respiratory failure and metabolic acidosis.

The differential diagnosis should consider perforated peptic ulcer, acute cholecystitis, bowel obstruction, renal calculi, myocardial infarction, mesenteric infarction, diabetic ketoacidosis, and pneumonia. Rarely, connective tissue diseases, including systemic lupus erythematosus and polyarteritis nodosa, may mimic pancreatitis. Because the pain of acute herpes zoster may precede the rash by 24 to 72 hours, the pain may be attributed erroneously to acute pancreatitis.

Treatment

Most cases of acute pancreatitis are self limited and resolve within 5 to 7 days. Initial treatment of acute pancreatitis is aimed primarily at putting the pancreas at rest. This is accomplished by keeping the patient at NPO ("nothing per mouth") status to decrease serum gastrin secretion and, if ileus is present, by instituting nasogastric suction. Short-acting potent opioid analgesics, such as hydrocodone, represent a reasonable next step if conservative measures do not control the patient's pain. If ileus is present, parenteral narcotics, such as meperidine, are a good alternative. Because the opioid analgesics have the potential to suppress the cough reflex and respiration, the clinician must be careful to monitor the patient closely and to instruct the patient in adequate pulmonary toilet techniques. If symptoms persist, CT scan–guided

celiac plexus block with local anesthetic and steroid is indicated and may help decrease the mortality and morbidity associated with the disease (**Fig. 85.5**). As an alternative, continuous thoracic epidural block with local anesthetic or opioid or both may provide adequate pain control and allow

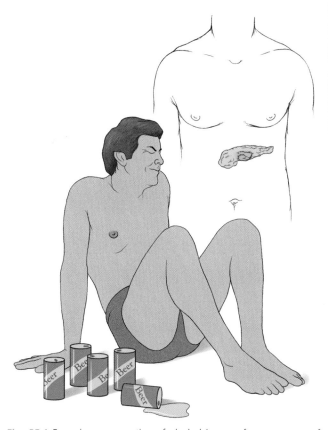

Fig. 85.1 Excessive consumption of alcohol is one of many causes of acute pancreatitis. *(From Waldman SD: Acute pancreatitis. In* Atlas of common pain syndromes, *ed 2, Philadelphia, 2008, Saunders, p 215.)*

Table 85.1 Common Causes of Acute Pancreatitis

Alcohol abuse
Gallstones
Viral infections
Medications
Metabolic causes
Connective tissue diseases
Tumor obstruction of ampulla of Vater
Hereditary disease

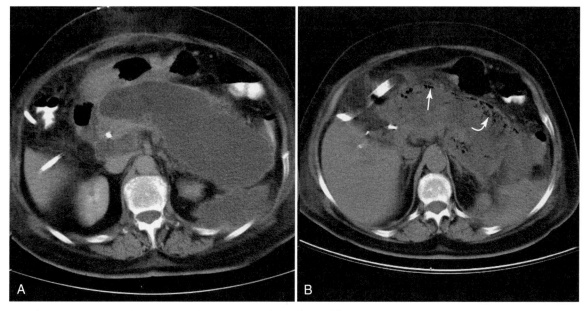

Fig. 85.2 A and **B,** In acute pancreatitis, a pancreatic mass or pseudocyst *(arrows)* from pancreatic edema may be present. *(From Haaga JR, Lanzieri CF, Gilkeson RC:* CT and MR imaging of the whole body, *ed 4, Philadelphia, 2003, Mosby, p 1443.)*

the patient to avoid the respiratory depression associated with systemic opioid analgesics.

Hypovolemia should be treated aggressively with crystalloid and colloid infusions. For prolonged cases of acute pancreatitis, parenteral nutrition is indicated to avoid malnutrition. Surgical drainage and removal of necrotic tissue may be necessary in severe necrotizing pancreatitis that fails to respond to the previously mentioned treatment modalities.

Complications and Pitfalls

The major problem in the care of patients with acute pancreatitis is a failure of the clinician to recognize the severity of the patient's condition and to identify and treat aggressively the extrapancreatic manifestations of acute pancreatitis.

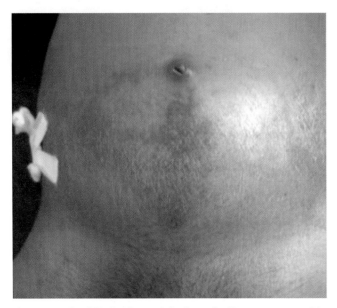

Fig. 85.3 Periumbilical ecchymosis (Cullen's sign) in acute pancreatitis. *(Courtesy of Vikram Kate, Jawaharlal Institute of Postgraduate Medical Education and Research, Pondicherry, India.)*

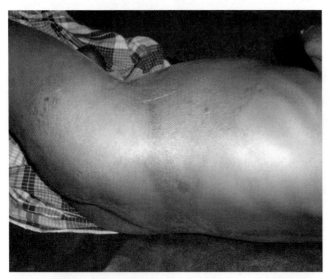

Fig. 85.4 Flank ecchymosis (Turner's sign) in acute pancreatitis. *(Courtesy of Vikram Kate, Jawaharlal Institute of Postgraduate Medical Education and Research, Pondicherry, India.)*

Hypovolemia, hypocalcemia, renal failure, and respiratory failure occur with enough frequency that the clinician must look actively for these potentially fatal complications and manage them aggressively.[8]

Chronic Pancreatitis

Chronic pancreatitis has numerous causes; alcohol abuse and gallstones account for approximately 85% of all cases (**Table 85.2**). Chronic pancreatitis may manifest as recurrent episodes of acute inflammation of the pancreas superimposed on chronic pancreatic dysfunction or as a more constant problem.[9] As the exocrine function of the pancreas deteriorates, malabsorption with steatorrhea develops. Abdominal pain is usually present, but it may be characterized by exacerbations and remissions. In the United States, chronic pancreatitis is caused most commonly by alcohol, followed by cystic fibrosis and pancreatic malignant diseases.[10] Hereditary causes, such as alpha$_1$-antitrypsin deficiency, also are common causes of chronic pancreatitis.[11] In the developing countries, the most common cause of chronic pancreatitis is severe protein calorie malnutrition.

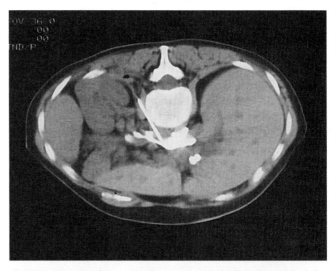

Fig. 85.5 Computed tomography scan–guided celiac plexus block for acute pancreatitis. *(From Waldman SD: Neural blockade and neurolytic blocks. In Interventional pain management, ed 2, Philadelphia, 2001, Saunders, p 500.)*

Table 85.2 **Common Causes of Chronic Pancreatitis**
Alcohol abuse
Gallstones
Medications
Abdominal trauma
Hereditary diseases (e.g., cystic fibrosis and alpha$_1$-antitrypsin deficiency)
Post–endoscopic retrograde cholangiopancreatography
Viral infections (e.g., mumps)
Abnormalities of the pancreas or intestine (e.g., pancreatic divisum)
Hyperlipidemia

Abdominal pain is a common feature in chronic pancreatitis.[12] It mimics the pain of acute pancreatitis and may range from mild to severe. It is characterized by steady, boring epigastric pain that radiates to the flanks and chest (**Fig. 85.6**). The pain is worse with alcohol and fatty meals. Nausea, vomiting, and anorexia also are common features of chronic pancreatitis, but as mentioned, the clinical symptoms frequently encountered in chronic pancreatitis are characterized by exacerbations and remissions.

Signs and Symptoms

A patient with chronic pancreatitis presents similar to a patient with acute pancreatitis but may appear more chronically ill than acutely ill. Tachycardia and hypotension resulting from hypovolemia are much less common in chronic pancreatitis and if present represent an extremely ominous prognostic indicator or suggest that another pathologic process, such as perforated peptic ulcer, is present.[13] Diffuse abdominal tenderness with peritoneal signs may be present if acute inflammation occurs. A pancreatic mass or pseudocyst from pancreatic edema may be palpable.

Testing

Although elevation of serum amylase levels is the sine qua non of acute pancreatitis, amylase levels in chronic pancreatitis may be only mildly elevated or normal. Amylase levels tend to peak at 48 to 72 hours and then begin to drift toward normal.[12] Serum lipase levels also are attenuated in chronic pancreatitis compared with the findings seen in acute pancreatitis. Serum lipase levels may remain elevated longer than serum amylase levels in this setting and may correlate better with the actual severity of the disease. Because elevated serum amylase levels may be caused by other diseases, such as parotitis, amylase isozymes may be necessary to confirm a pancreatic basis for this laboratory finding. Plain radiographs of the chest are indicated for all patients who present with pain from chronic pancreatitis to identify pulmonary complications, including pleural effusion, that result from the chronic pancreatitis.

Given the extrapancreatic manifestations of chronic pancreatitis (e.g., acute renal or hepatic failure), serial complete blood count, serum calcium, serum glucose, liver function tests, and electrolytes are indicated in all patients with chronic pancreatitis. CT scan of the abdomen helps in identification of pancreatic pseudocysts, calcifications, or pancreatic tumor that may have been previously overlooked and may help the clinician gauge the severity and progression of the disease (**Fig. 85.7**). Gallbladder evaluation with radionucleotides

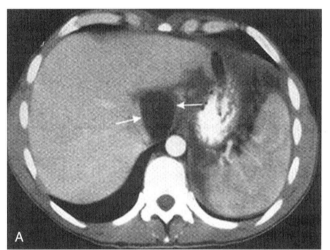
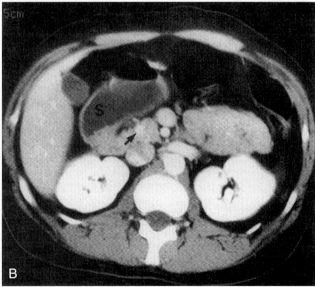

Fig. 85.7 **A,** Pancreatic pseudocyst. A well-defined fluid collection with a thin wall *(arrows)* lies superior to the pancreas. **B,** Pancreatic calcification. Computed tomography scan at the level of the head of the pancreas shows a dominant calcification site in the main pancreatic duct *(arrow). (From Feeny PC: The pancreas. In Grainger RG, Allison DJ, Adam A, et al, editors: Grainger and Allison's diagnostic radiology, ed 4, Philadelphia, 2002, Churchill Livingstone.)*

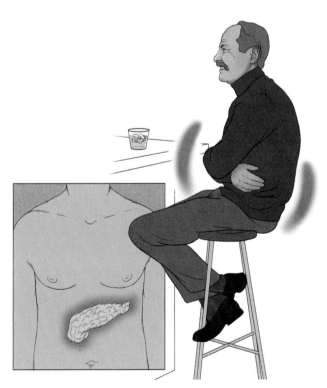

Fig. 85.6 Chronic pancreatitis may manifest in a manner analogous to the presentation of acute pancreatitis but can be more challenging to treat. *(From Waldman SD: Chronic pancreatitis. In Atlas of common pain syndromes, ed 2, Philadelphia, 2008, Saunders, p 189.)*

is indicated if gallstones are being considered as a cause of chronic pancreatitis.[14] Arterial blood gases help in identification of respiratory failure and metabolic acidosis.

Differential Diagnosis

The differential diagnosis should include perforated peptic ulcer, acute cholecystitis, bowel obstruction, renal calculi, myocardial infarction, mesenteric infarction, diabetic ketoacidosis, and pneumonia. Rarely, collagen-vascular diseases, including systemic lupus erythematosus and polyarteritis nodosa, may mimic chronic pancreatitis. Because the pain of acute herpes zoster may precede the rash by 24 to 72 hours, the pain may be erroneously attributed to chronic pancreatitis in patients who have had previous bouts of the disease. The clinician always should consider the possibility of pancreatic malignancy disease in patients who are thought to have chronic pancreatitis (**Fig. 85.8**).

Treatment

Initial management of chronic pancreatitis should be focused on the treatment of the pain and malabsorption. Similar to acute pancreatitis, the treatment of chronic pancreatitis is aimed primarily at putting the pancreas at rest. This is accomplished by keeping the patient on NPO status to decrease serum gastrin secretion and, if ileus is present, by instituting nasogastric suction. Short-acting potent opioid analgesics, such as hydrocodone, represent a reasonable next step if conservative measures do not control the patient's

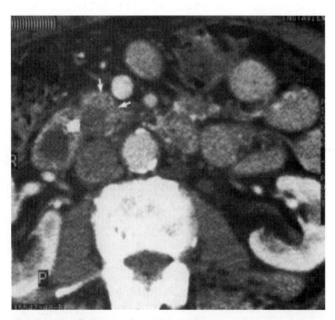

Fig. 85.8 **Small pancreatic carcinoma.** Computed tomography scan shows a relatively poorly enhancing mass within normally enhancing pancreatic parenchyma *(arrows)*. *(From Grainger RG, Allison DJ, Adam A, et al, editors: Grainger and Allison's diagnostic radiology, ed 4, Philadelphia, 2002, Churchill Livingstone, p 1357.)*

pain. If ileus is present, parenteral opioids, such as meperidine, are a good alternative. Because opioid analgesics have the potential to suppress the cough reflex and respiration, the clinician must be careful to monitor the patient closely and to instruct the patient in adequate pulmonary toilet techniques. As with all chronic diseases, the use of opioid analgesics must be monitored carefully because the potential for misuse and dependence is high. If the symptoms persist, CT scan–guided celiac plexus block with local anesthetic and steroid is indicated and may help decrease the mortality and morbidity rates associated with the disease (see Fig. 85.5). If the relief from this technique is short lived, neurolytic CT scan–guided celiac plexus block with alcohol or phenol is a reasonable next step. As an alternative, continuous thoracic epidural block with local anesthetic, opioid, or both may provide adequate pain control and allow the patient to avoid the respiratory depression associated with systemic opioid analgesics.

Hypovolemia should be treated aggressively with crystalloid and colloid infusions. For prolonged cases of chronic pancreatitis, parenteral nutrition is indicated to avoid malnutrition. Surgical drainage and removal of necrotic tissue may be necessary in patients with severe necrotizing pancreatitis that fails to respond to the previously mentioned treatment modalities.[15]

Complications and Pitfalls

Similar to patients with acute pancreatitis, the major problem in the care of patients with chronic pancreatitis is a failure of the clinician to recognize the severity of the patient's condition and to identify and treat aggressively the extrapancreatic manifestations of chronic pancreatitis. Hypovolemia, hypocalcemia, and renal and respiratory failure occur with sufficient frequency that the clinician must actively seek these potentially fatal complications and treat them aggressively. If opioids are used, the clinician must watch constantly for overuse and dependence, especially if the underlying cause of the chronic pancreatitis is alcohol abuse.

Conclusion

Pancreatitis is a commonly encountered cause of abdominal pain. Correct diagnosis is necessary to treat this painful condition properly and to avoid overlooking serious extrapancreatic complications associated with this disease. The use of the previously mentioned treatment modalities, including the judicious use of opioid analgesics to treat the pain of acute exacerbations, allows the clinician to control the pain of chronic pancreatitis adequately. Celiac plexus block and thoracic epidural block are straightforward techniques that can produce dramatic relief for patients with chronic pancreatitis.

References

Full references for this chapter can be found on www.expertconsult.com.

Ilioinguinal, Iliohypogastric, and Genitofemoral Neuralgia

Steven D. Waldman

Ilioinguinal, iliohypogastric, and genitofemoral neuralgias are among the most common causes of lower abdominal and pelvic pain encountered in clinical practice. The anatomic variability of these nerves often leads to overlapping patterns of innervation, which can confuse the unsuspecting clinician. This chapter reviews the clinical presentation of ilioinguinal and genitofemoral neuralgia and provides the reader with a concise approach to the evaluation and treatment of these painful conditions.

Ilioinguinal Neuralgia

Ilioinguinal neuralgia is caused by compression of the ilioinguinal nerve as it passes through the transverse abdominis muscle at the level of the anterior superior iliac spine.[1] The most common causes of compression of the ilioinguinal nerve at this anatomic location involve injury to the nerve induced by trauma, including direct blunt trauma to the nerve and damage during inguinal herniorrhaphy or pelvic surgery.[2,3] Rarely, ilioinguinal neuralgia occurs spontaneously.

Signs and Symptoms

Ilioinguinal neuralgia presents as paresthesias and burning pain, and occasionally as numbness over the lower abdomen that radiates into the scrotum or labia and sometimes into the inner upper thigh.[2] The pain does not radiate below the knee. The pain of ilioinguinal neuralgia is worsened by extension of the lumbar spine, which puts traction on the nerve. Patients with ilioinguinal neuralgia often assume a bent-forward novice skier's position (**Fig. 86.1**). If the condition is left untreated, progressive motor deficit consisting of bulging of the anterior abdominal wall muscles may occur. This bulging may be confused with inguinal hernia.

Physical findings include sensory deficit in the inner thigh, scrotum, or labia in the distribution of the ilioinguinal nerve (**Fig. 86.2**). Weakness of the anterior abdominal wall musculature may be present. A Tinel's sign may be elicited with tapping over the ilioinguinal nerve at the point it pierces the transverse abdominis muscle.

Testing

Electromyography helps in distinguishing ilioinguinal nerve entrapment from lumbar plexopathy, lumbar radiculopathy, and diabetic polyneuropathy. Plain radiographs of the hip and pelvis are indicated in all patients who present with ilioinguinal neuralgia to rule out occult bony pathology. On the basis of the patient's clinical presentation, additional testing may be indicated, including complete blood count, uric acid, sedimentation rate, and antinuclear antibody testing. Magnetic resonance imaging (MRI) of the lumbar plexus is indicated if tumor or hematoma is suspected. The injection technique described subsequently serves as a diagnostic and therapeutic maneuver.

Differential Diagnosis

Lesions of the lumbar plexus resulting from trauma, hematoma, tumor, diabetic neuropathy, or inflammation can mimic the pain, numbness, and weakness of ilioinguinal neuralgia and must be included in the differential diagnosis. Significant intrapatient variability is found in the anatomy of the ilioinguinal nerve, which can result in significant variation in patients' clinical presentation. The ilioinguinal nerve is a branch of the L1 nerve root with contribution from T12 in some patients. The nerve follows a curvilinear course, which takes it from its origin of the L1 and occasionally T12 somatic nerves to inside

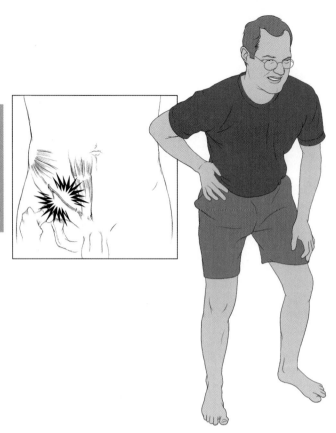

Fig. 86.1 A patient with ilioinguinal neuralgia often bends forward in the novice skier's position to relieve the pain. *(From Waldman SD: Ilioinquinal neuralgia. In* Atlas of common pain syndromes, *ed 2, Philadelphia, 2008, Saunders, p 193.)*

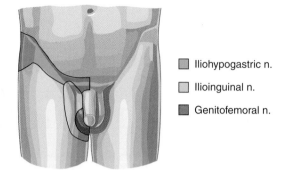

Iliohypogastric n.
Ilioinguinal n.
Genitofemoral n.

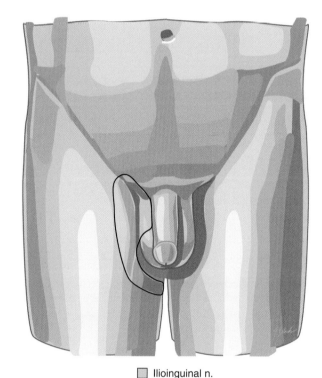

Ilioinguinal n.

Fig. 86.2 **Sensory distribution of the ilioinguinal nerve.** *(From Waldman SD: Ilioinquinal nerve block. In* Atlas of interventional pain management, *ed 3, Philadelphia, 2009, Saunders, p 360.)*

the concavity of the ilium. The ilioinguinal nerve continues anteriorly to perforate the transverse abdominis muscle at the level of the anterior superior iliac spine. The nerve may interconnect with the iliohypogastric nerve as it continues to pass along its course medially and inferiorly, where it accompanies the spermatic cord through the inguinal ring and into the inguinal canal. The distribution of the sensory innervation of the ilioinguinal nerves varies among patients because considerable overlap with the iliohypogastric nerve may occur. In general, the ilioinguinal nerve provides sensory innervation to the upper portion of the skin of the inner thigh and the root of the penis and upper scrotum in men or the mons pubis and lateral labia in women.

Treatment

Pharmacologic management of ilioinguinal neuralgia is generally disappointing, and a general nerve block is necessary to provide pain relief. Initial management of ilioinguinal neuralgia should consist of treatment with simple analgesics, nonsteroidal anti-inflammatory drugs (NSAIDs), or cyclooxygenase-2 (COX-2) inhibitors. Avoidance of repetitive activities thought to exacerbate the symptoms of ilioinguinal neuralgia (e.g., squatting or sitting for prolonged periods) also helps ameliorate the patient's symptoms. If the patient's condition fails to respond to these conservative measures, a next reasonable step is ilioinguinal nerve block with local anesthetic and steroid.[4]

Ilioinguinal nerve block is performed with placement of the patient in the supine position, with a pillow under the knees if lying with the legs extended increases the patient's pain because

of traction on the nerve. The anterior superior iliac spine is identified with palpation. A point 2 inches medial and 2 inches inferior to the anterior superior iliac spine is identified and prepared with antiseptic solution. A 1½–inch 25-gauge needle is advanced at an oblique angle toward the pubic symphysis (**Fig. 86.3**), and 5 to 7 mL of 1% preservative-free lidocaine in solution with 40 mg of methylprednisolone is injected in a fanlike manner as the needle pierces the fascia of the external oblique muscle. Care must be taken not to place the needle too deep so as to enter the peritoneal cavity and perforate the abdominal viscera. This technique can also be performed with ultrasound scan guidance (**Fig. 86.4**).

Because of overlapping innervation of the ilioinguinal and iliohypogastric nerves, it is not unusual to block branches of each nerve when performing ilioinguinal nerve block. After injection of the solution, pressure is applied to the injection site to decrease the incidence of postblock ecchymosis and hematoma formation, which can be quite dramatic, especially in a patient undergoing anticoagulation therapy.

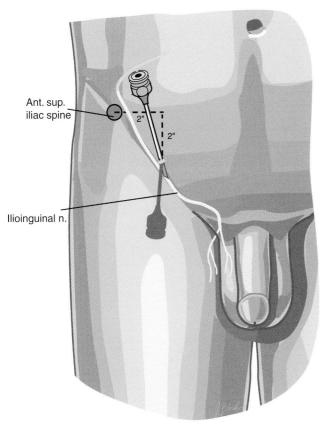

Fig. 86.3 **Ilioinguinal nerve block technique.** *(From Waldman SD: Ilioinquinal nerve block. In* Atlas of interventional pain management, *ed 3, Philadelphia, 2009, Saunders, p 360.)*

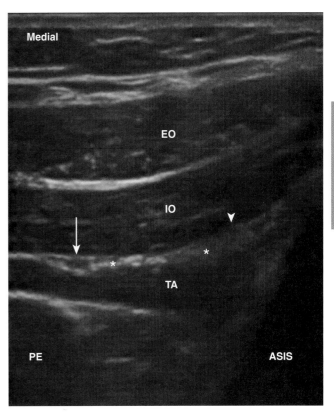

Fig. 86.4 Ultrasound scan image of the muscular layers of the abdomen and the ilioinguinal *(arrowhead)* and iliohypogastric *(arrow)* nerves. *The ideal sites of injection between the muscular layers, adjacent to the nerves. *EO,* External oblique muscle; *IO,* internal oblique muscle; *TA,* transversus abdominus muscle; *PE,* peritoneum; *ASIS,* anterior superior iliac spine. *(From Bellingham GA, Peng PWH: Ultrasound-guided interventional procedures for chronic pelvic pain,* Tech Regional Anesth Pain Manage *13:171, 2009.)*

The clinician should be aware that because of the anatomy of the ilioinguinal nerve, damage or entrapment of the nerve anywhere along its course can produce a similar clinical syndrome. A careful search for pathology at the T12-L1 spinal segments and along the path of the nerve in the pelvis is mandatory in all patients who present with ilioinguinal neuralgia without a history of inguinal surgery or trauma to the region.

The major side effect of ilioinguinal nerve block is postblock ecchymosis and hematoma formation. If needle placement is too deep and enters the peritoneal cavity, perforation of the colon may result in the formation of intra-abdominal abscess and fistula. Early detection of infection is crucial to avoid potentially life-threatening sequelae.

Iliohypogastric Neuralgia

Iliohypogastric neuralgia is caused by compression of the iliohypogastric nerve as it passes through the transverse abdominis muscle.[5] The iliohypogastric nerve is a branch of the L1 nerve root with a contribution from T12 in some patients. The nerve follows a curvilinear course that takes it from its origin of the L1 and occasionally T12 somatic nerves to inside the concavity of the ilium (**Fig. 86.5**). The iliohypogastric nerve continues anteriorly to perforate the transverse abdominis muscle to lie between it and the external oblique muscle. At this point, the iliohypogastric nerve divides into an anterior and a lateral branch. The lateral branch provides cutaneous sensory innervation to the pos-

terolateral gluteal region. The anterior branch pierces the external oblique muscle just beyond the anterior superior iliac spine to provide cutaneous sensory innervation to the abdominal skin above the pubis (see Fig. 86.2). The most common causes of compression of the iliohypogastric nerve at this anatomic location involve injury to the nerve induced by trauma, including direct blunt trauma to the nerve and damage during inguinal herniorrhaphy and pelvic surgery.[2,3] Rarely, iliohypogastric neuralgia occurs spontaneously. The nerve may interconnect with the ilioinguinal nerve along its course, resulting in variation of the distribution of the sensory innervation of the iliohypogastric and ilioinguinal nerves.

Signs and Symptoms

Ilioinguinal neuralgia presents as paresthesias, burning pain, and occasionally numbness of the abdominal skin above the pubis. The pain and paresthesia sometimes radiate into the posterior gluteal region.[5] The pain does not radiate below the knee. The pain of iliohypogastric neuralgia is worsened by extension of the lumbar spine, which puts traction on the nerve. Patients with iliohypogastric neuralgia often assume a bent-forward novice skier's position. If the condition is left untreated, progressive motor deficit in the distribution of the nerve may occur.

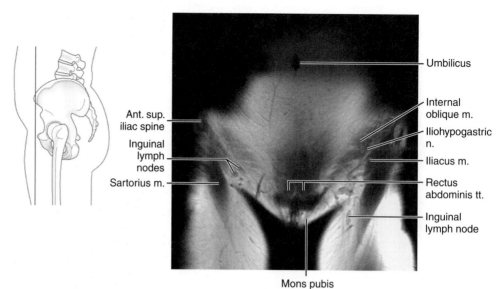

Umbilicus

Internal
oblique m.

Iliohypogastric
n.

Iliacus m.

Rectus
abdominis tt.

Inguinal
lymph node

Ant. sup.
iliac spine

Inguinal
lymph
nodes

Sartorius m.

Mons pubis

Fig. 86.5 MRI of the female pelvis: coronal.

Physical findings include sensory deficit of the abdominal skin above the pubis in the distribution of the iliohypogastric nerve (see Fig. 86.2). Weakness of the anterior abdominal wall musculature may be present. A Tinel's sign may be elicited with tapping over the iliohypogastric nerve at the point where it pierces the transverse abdominis muscle.

Treatment

Pharmacologic management of iliohypogastric neuralgia is generally disappointing, and a general nerve block is necessary to provide pain relief. Initial treatment of iliohypogastric neuralgia should consist of treatment with simple analgesics, NSAIDs, or COX-2 inhibitors. Avoidance of repetitive activities thought to exacerbate the symptoms of iliohypogastric neuralgia (e.g., squatting or sitting for prolonged periods) also helps ameliorate the patient's symptoms. If the patient's condition fails to respond to these conservative measures, a next reasonable step is iliohypogastric nerve block with local anesthetic and steroid.[6]

The patient is placed in the supine position, with a pillow under the knees if extending the legs increases the patient's pain because of traction on the nerve. The anterior superior iliac spine is identified with palpation. A point 1 inch medial and 1 inch inferior to the anterior superior iliac spine is identified and prepared with antiseptic solution. A 1½-inch 25-gauge needle is advanced at an oblique angle toward the pubic symphysis (**Fig. 86.6**), and 5 to 7 mL of 1% preservative-free lidocaine is injected in a fanlike manner as the needle pierces the fascia of the external oblique muscle. Care must be taken not to place the needle too deep to avoid entering the peritoneal cavity and perforating the abdominal viscera. This technique can also be performed with ultrasound scan guidance (see Fig. 86.4).

If the pain has an inflammatory component, the local anesthetic is combined with 80 mg of methylprednisolone and is injected in incremental doses. Subsequent daily nerve blocks are performed similarly, substituting 40 mg of methylprednisolone for the initial 80-mg dose. Because of overlapping innervation of the ilioinguinal and iliohypogastric nerves, it is not unusual to block branches of each nerve when performing iliohypogastric nerve block. After injection of the solution, pressure is

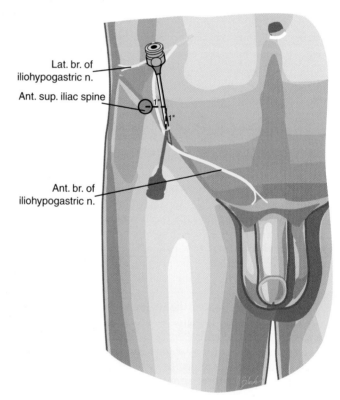

Lat. br. of
iliohypogastric n.

Ant. sup. iliac spine

Ant. br. of
iliohypogastric n.

Fig. 86.6 Iliohypogastric nerve block technique. *(From Waldman SD: Iliohypogastric nerve block. In Atlas of interventional pain management, ed 2, Philadelphia, 2004, Saunders, p 364.)*

applied to the injection site to decrease the incidence of post-block ecchymosis and hematoma formation, which can be dramatic, especially in a patient undergoing anticoagulation therapy.

The main side effect of iliohypogastric nerve block is post-block ecchymosis and hematoma formation. If needle placement is too deep and enters the peritoneal cavity, perforation of the colon may result in intraabdominal abscess and fistula formation. Early detection of infection is crucial to avoid potentially life-threatening sequelae.

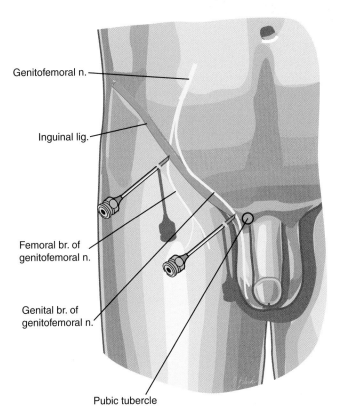

Genitofemoral n.

Inguinal lig.

Femoral br. of
genitofemoral n.

Genital br. of
genitofemoral n.

Pubic tubercle

Fig. 86.7 Genitofemoral nerve block technique. *(From Waldman SD: Genitofemoral nerve block. In* Atlas of interventional pain management, *ed 3, Philadelphia, 2009, Saunders, p 367.)*

Genitofemoral Neuralgia

Genitofemoral neuralgia is a common cause of lower abdominal and pelvic pain encountered in clinical practice.[7] Genitofemoral neuralgia may be caused by compression or damage to the genitofemoral nerve anywhere along its path. The genitofemoral nerve arises from fibers of the L1 and L2 nerve roots. The genitofemoral nerve passes through the substance of the psoas muscle, where it divides into a genital and a femoral branch. The femoral branch passes beneath the inguinal ligament along with the femoral artery and provides sensory innervation to a small area of skin on the inside of the thigh.[8] The genital branch passes through the inguinal canal to provide innervation to the round ligament of the uterus and labia majora in women. In men, the genital branch of the genitofemoral nerve passes with the spermatic cord to innervate the cremasteric muscles and provide sensory innervation to the bottom of the scrotum.

The most common causes of genitofemoral neuralgia involve injury to the nerve induced by trauma, including direct blunt trauma to the nerve and damage during inguinal herniorrhaphy and pelvic surgery. Rarely, genitofemoral neuralgia occurs spontaneously.

Signs and Symptoms

Genitofemoral neuralgia presents as paresthesias, burning pain, and occasionally numbness over the lower abdomen, which radiate into the inner thigh in men and women, into the labia majora in women, and into the bottom of the scrotum and cremasteric muscles in men. The pain does not radiate below the knee. The pain of genitofemoral neuralgia is worsened by extension of the lumbar spine, which puts traction on the nerve. Patients with genitofemoral neuralgia often assume a bent-forward novice skier's position.

Physical findings include sensory deficit in the inner thigh and base of the scrotum or labia majora in the distribution of the genitofemoral nerve. Weakness of the anterior abdominal wall musculature occasionally may be present. A Tinel's sign may be elicited with tapping over the genitofemoral nerve at the point it passes beneath the inguinal ligament.

Testing

Electromyography helps in distinguishing genitofemoral nerve entrapment from lumbar plexopathy, lumbar radiculopathy, and diabetic polyneuropathy. Plain radiographs of the hip and pelvis are indicated in all patients who present with genitofemoral neuralgia to rule out occult bony pathology. On the basis of the patient's clinical presentation, additional testing may be indicated, including complete blood count, uric acid, sedimentation rate, and antinuclear antibody. MRI of the lumbar plexus is indicated if tumor or hematoma is suspected. The injection technique described subsequently serves as a diagnostic and a therapeutic maneuver.

Differential Diagnosis

Lesions of the lumbar plexus resulting from trauma, hematoma, tumor, diabetic neuropathy, or inflammation can mimic the pain, numbness, and weakness of genitofemoral neuralgia and must be included in the differential diagnosis. Significant interpatient variability is found in the anatomy of the genitofemoral nerve, which can result in significant variation in patients' clinical presentation.

Treatment

Pharmacologic management of genitofemoral neuralgia is generally disappointing, and a general nerve block is necessary to provide pain relief. Initial management of genitofemoral neuralgia should consist of treatment with simple analgesics, NSAIDs, or COX-2 inhibitors. Avoidance of repetitive activities thought to exacerbate the symptoms of genitofemoral neuralgia (e.g., squatting or sitting for prolonged periods) also helps ameliorate the patient's symptoms. If the patient's condition fails to respond to these conservative measures, a next reasonable step is genitofemoral nerve block with local anesthetic and steroid.[9]

Genitofemoral nerve block is performed with placement of the patient in supine position, with a pillow under the knees if lying with the legs extended increases the patient's pain because of traction on the nerve. The genital branch of the genitofemoral nerve is blocked as follows. The pubic tubercle is identified with palpation. A point just lateral to the pubic tubercle is identified and prepared with antiseptic solution. A 1½–inch 25-gauge needle is advanced at an oblique angle toward the pubic symphysis (**Fig. 86.7**), and 3 to 5 mL of 1% preservative-free lidocaine and 80 mg of methylprednisolone is injected in a fanlike manner as the needle pierces the inguinal ligament. Care must be taken not to place the needle too deep to avoid entering the peritoneal cavity and perforating the abdominal viscera.

The femoral branch of the genitofemoral nerve is blocked with identification of the middle third of the inguinal ligament. After preparation of the skin with antiseptic solution, 3 to 5 mL of 1% lidocaine is infiltrated subcutaneously just below the ligament (see Fig. 86.7). Care must be taken not to enter the femoral artery of vein or inadvertently block the femoral nerve. The needle must be kept subcutaneous because too deep of placement may allow the needle to enter the peritoneal cavity and perforate the abdominal viscera. If the pain has an inflammatory component, the local anesthetic is combined with 80 mg of methylprednisolone and is injected in incremental doses. Subsequent daily nerve blocks are carried out in a similar manner, substituting 40 mg of methylprednisolone for the initial 80-mg dose.

Because of overlapping innervation of the ilioinguinal and iliohypogastric nerves, it is not unusual to block branches of each nerve when performing a genitofemoral nerve block. After injection of the solution, pressure is applied to the injection site to decrease the incidence of postblock ecchymosis and hematoma formation, which can be quite dramatic, especially in an patient undergoing anticoagulation therapy.

Conclusion

Ilioinguinal, iliohypogastric, and genitofemoral neuralgia are common causes of lower abdominal and pelvic pain encountered in clinical practice. The anatomic variability of these nerves often leads to overlapping patterns of innervation, which can confuse an unsuspecting clinician. The clinician should be aware that because of the anatomy of the ilioinguinal, iliohypogastric, and genitofemoral nerves, damage or entrapment of the nerves anywhere along their course can produce a similar clinical syndrome. A careful search for pathology at the T12-L2 spinal segments and along the path of the nerve in the pelvis is mandatory in all patients who present with neuralgia of the groin without a history of inguinal surgery or trauma to the region.

References

Full references for this chapter can be found on www.expertconsult.com.

Part H

Pain Syndromes of the Lumbar Spine and Sacroiliac Joint

Chapter 87

Low Back Pain

David Borenstein

Low back pain is defined as an acute, subacute, or chronic discomfort localized to the anatomic area below the 12th rib posteriorly and above the lower margins of the buttock. Low back pain is second only to the common cold as the most common affliction of humans. The lifetime prevalence rate of back pain is greater than 70% in most industrialized countries.[1] National statistics from the United States indicate a 1-year prevalence rate of 15% to 20%.[2] In the last 3 months, 59 million Americans have had an episode of low back pain.[3] Low back pain is the fifth most common reason for visiting a physician, according to a US National Ambulatory Care survey.[4]

Low back pain is a symptom that is associated with a wide range of clinical disorders.[5] Most patients with back pain have the symptom on a mechanical basis. Nachemson[6] suggested that 90% of individuals have a mechanical reason for back pain. Mechanical low back pain may be defined as pain that results from overuse of a normal anatomic structure (e.g., muscle strain) or pain that results from trauma or deformity of an anatomic structure (e.g., herniated nucleus pulposus). Characteristically, mechanical disorders are exacerbated by physical activities, such as lifting, and are relieved by other activities, such as assuming a supine position. The remaining 10% of adults with back pain have the symptom as a manifestation of a systemic illness. In some systemic illnesses (i.e., nonmechanical), back pain is noted in almost every individual who has the disorder (e.g., ankylosing spondylitis). In other illnesses, back pain is a rare symptom (e.g., infective endocarditis). Mechanical and systemic disorders associated with low back pain are listed in **Table 87.1**.

The natural history of low back pain is one of improvement. More than 50% of all conditions improve after 1 week, and 90% are better at 8 weeks. Recurrence of spinal pain occurs in 75% of individuals, however, over the next year. Back pain persists for 1 year or longer in 10% of patients with spinal pain.[7]

The challenge for the practicing physician is to separate individuals with mechanical disorders from patients with systemic illnesses. The patient's symptoms and signs help differentiate

mechanical from systemic causes of localized axial pain. In addition, these clinical findings, along with radiographic and laboratory data, designate specific disorders in these two major groups. This chapter focuses on the process of identifying the factors that define the most likely cause of the symptom of low back pain.

Another symptom frequently associated with low back pain is sciatica or radicular pain. Individuals who have radicular pain to the lower extremity have disorders associated with neural impingement (e.g., herniated intervertebral disk, spinal stenosis) or referred pain (e.g., facet syndrome). These illnesses with pain that affects structures beyond the lumbosacral spine are subjects of other chapters in this book.

Initial Evaluation

Guidelines have been proposed for the evaluation and treatment of low back pain.[8] The recommendations agree with a focused history and physical examination to differentiate patients with localized, nonspecific mechanical low back pain, from those with radicular symptoms and those with systemic diseases. Recent reports have suggested that systemic illnesses are so rare as not to be considered in the initial evaluation of patients with back pain.[9] The most common systemic illness is vertebral fracture associated with osteoporosis. Physicians should consider mechanical problems first in the differential diagnosis but should remain aware of nonmechanical possibilities for those conditions that do not improve in the expected timeframe.

The initial diagnostic evaluation for low back pain includes a focused history and physical examination. The history concentrates on the onset of pain. Was the onset associated with a specific trauma or an unusual period of strenuous physical activity? What are the duration and frequency of the pain? Systemic disorders cause chronic pain that is more persistent than episodic. Location and radiation help in identification of the structures that are possible pain generators. Aggravating

Table 87.1 Disorders Associated with Low Back Pain

MECHANICAL
Muscle strain
Herniated disk
Osteoarthritis
Spinal stenosis
Spondylolysis
Adult scoliosis

RHEUMATOLOGIC
Ankylosing spondylitis
Reactive arthritis
Psoriatic arthritis
Enteropathic arthritis
DISH syndrome
Vertebral osteochondritis
Polymyalgia rheumatica
Fibromyalgia
Behçet's syndrome
Whipple's disease
Hidradenitis suppurativa

HEMATOLOGIC
Hemoglobinopathies
Myelofibrosis
Mastocytosis

ENDOCRINOLOGIC
Osteoporosis
Osteomalacia
Parathyroid disease
Microcrystalline disease
Ochronosis
Fluorosis
Heritable genetic disorders

MISCELLANEOUS
Paget's disease
Vertebral sarcoidosis
Infective endocarditis
Retroperitoneal fibrosis

NEOPLASTIC/INFILTRATIVE
Benign Tumors
Osteoid osteoma
Osteoblastoma
Osteochondroma
Giant cell tumor
Hemangioma
Eosinophilic granuloma
Aneurysmal bone cyst
Gaucher's disease
Sacroiliac lipoma
Malignant Tumors
Skeletal metastases
Multiple myeloma
Chondrosarcoma
Chordoma
Lymphoma
Intraspinal Lesions
Metastases
Meningioma
Gliomas
Vascular malformations
Syringomyelia

INFECTIOUS
Vertebral osteomyelitis
Diskitis
Pyogenic sacroiliitis
Herpes zoster
Lyme disease

REFERRED PAIN
Vascular
Abdominal aorta
Gastrointestinal
Pancreas
Gallbladder
Intestine
Genitourinary
Kidney
Ureter
Bladder
Uterus
Ovary
Prostate

NEUROLOGIC/PSYCHIATRIC
Neuropathic arthropathy
Neuropathies
Tumors
Vasculitis
Compression
Psychogenic rheumatism
Malingering

DISH, diffuse idiopathic skeletal hyperostosis.

and alleviating factors characterize the mechanical quality of the disorder. Mechanical and systemic disorders may be worsened or improved with a change of activity. Pain improvement with immobility helps define specific disorders (e.g., muscle injury, vertebral compression fracture) in either group. The time of day associated with the maximum degree of pain also is characteristic of certain disorders. Inflammatory arthritis of the lumbar spine causes most symptoms in the morning, whereas mechanical disorders are most problematic at the end of the day. The quality of the pain helps separate musculoskeletal pain (aching) sources from sources associated with neural injuries (burning). Documentation of the intensity of pain is important in determination of patient improvement but does not discriminate between mechanical and systemic disorders.

Physical examination includes a complete evaluation of the musculoskeletal system, including palpation of the axial skeleton and assessment of range of motion and alignment of the spine. Neurologic examination to detect evidence of spinal cord, spinal root, or peripheral nerve dysfunction is essential. In most patients, radiographic and laboratory tests are not indicated. Erythrocyte sedimentation rate and plain radiographs are most informative in patients who are 50 years old or older, who have a history of cancer, or who have constitutional symptoms. Most guidelines advise against the use of radiographs or laboratory tests for the initial evaluation of patients with low back pain exclusively.

The initial evaluation should eliminate the presence of cauda equina syndrome, a rare condition that necessitates emergency intervention. Cauda equina compression is characterized by low back pain, bilateral motor weakness of the lower extremities, bilateral sciatica, saddle anesthesia, and bladder or bowel incontinence. Common causes of cauda equina compression include central herniation of an intervertebral disk, epidural abscess or hematoma, and tumor masses. If cauda equina syndrome is suspected, immediate radiographic evaluation is necessary. Magnetic resonance imaging (MRI) is the most sensitive radiographic technique for visualization of the spine. Surgical decompression must be completed within 48 hours for the best opportunity for recovery of neurologic function.[10]

Nonmechanical Disorders

Most individuals with spinal pain and nonmechanical illnesses can be identified with the presence of one or more of the following: fever or weight loss, pain with recumbency, prolonged morning stiffness, localized bone pain, or visceral pain.

Fever or Weight Loss

Patients with a history of fever or weight loss are likely to have an infection as the cause of low back pain. Patients with vertebral osteomyelitis may have pain that develops gradually over time. In a review of 142 patients with vertebral osteomyelitis, 66% had symptoms for 3 months or longer before diagnosis.[11] The pain becomes constant, is present at rest, and is exacerbated by motion. Physical findings include a decreased range of spinal motion, muscle spasm, and percussion tenderness over the vertebral column. Fever is present in 58% of patients. Approximately 40% of patients with vertebral osteomyelitis have an unequivocal extraspinal primary source of infection, including the skin, lungs, or urinary tract.[12]

Plain radiographs should be reviewed for localized areas of osteopenia. Early abnormalities that appear after 1 to 2 months of infection in pyogenic vertebral osteomyelitis include subchondral bone loss, narrowing of disk space, and loss of definition of the vertebral body (**Fig. 87.1**). If radiograph results are normal, a bone scintiscan is indicated because abnormalities appear at an earlier stage of disease.[13] Bone scintiscan is a sensitive but not specific test for bone lesions. Computed tomographic (CT) scan may show bone changes before their appearance on routine radiographs; however, alterations of bony architecture are not specific for osteomyelitis and may be confused with severe degenerative disk disease or vertebral malignancy disease. MRI is the most useful radiographic technique for identification of osteomyelitis.[14] The involvement of the vertebral bodies, the intervening disk, and the extent of the extraosseous infection into the surrounding soft tissues can be determined.

The definitive diagnosis of osteomyelitis is based on the recovery and identification of the causative organism from aspirated material, biopsy of the bony lesion, or blood cultures. Blood culture results may be positive in 50% of patients with osteomyelitis and obviate the need for bone biopsy. *Staphylococcus aureus* is the bacterium associated with vertebral osteomyelitis in 60% of patients.[15] Gram-negative organisms (*Escherichia coli, Proteus, Pseudomonas*) are often grown from parenteral drug abusers

and elderly patients with urinary tract infections. Cultures from peripheral sources of infection should be obtained from patients suspected to have vertebral infection.

Therapy of vertebral osteomyelitis includes antibiotics, bed rest, and immobilization. The choice of antibiotic therapy is based on the organism that causes the infection and its sensitivity to specific agents. Patients are treated with 4 to 6 weeks of parenteral antibiotics followed by a course of oral antibiotics that may have a duration of 6 months. Bed rest is useful in decreasing pain by limiting motion. Some patients need braces when spinal instability is present.

Pain with Recumbency

Tumors of the spinal column are the prime concern in patients with nocturnal pain or pain with recumbency. The mechanism of increased nocturnal pain with benign or malignant tumors is unknown. Increased pressure associated with increased blood flow at night has been suggested as one possible mechanism of nocturnal pain.[16] An example of a benign bone tumor associated with nocturnal pain is an osteoid osteoma. The nocturnal pain with an osteoid osteoma is slowly progressive over months. The pain may be responsive to nonsteroidal anti-inflammatory drugs (NSAIDs) but recurs with discontinuance of the medication. Stretching of spinal nerves over an expanding mass is a potential mechanism that mediates increased pain with recumbency.

Metastatic lesions in the skeleton are the most common neoplastic lesion of bone, with a 25:1 ratio of metastatic to primary tumor.[17] Metastases occur more commonly in the axial skeleton

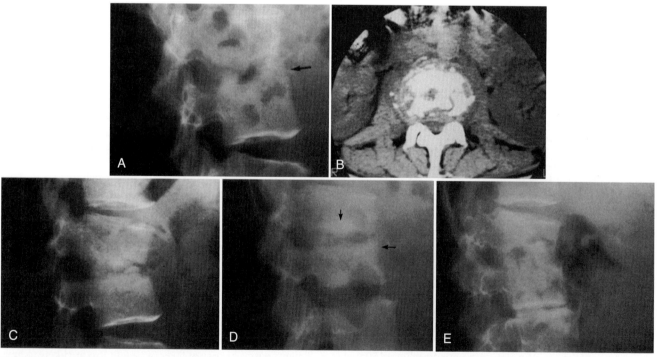

Fig. 87.1 **Serial radiographs of a 41-year-old man with staphylococcal osteomyelitis of the lumbar spine.** A, Radiograph obtained November 8, 1985. Erosion of the L2 and L3 end plates is associated with destruction of the intervertebral disk *(arrow)*. B, Computed tomography (CT) scan obtained November 20, 1985. CT scan reveals marked bony destruction associated with soft tissue extension of the infection. C, Radiograph obtained November 27, 1985. Further collapse of the L2 vertebral body is seen with reactive sclerosis. D, Radiograph obtained November 4, 1986. Reactive sclerosis is noted in the vertebral body *(arrow)*, and osteophytes are forming *(arrowhead)* at the body margin. E, Radiograph obtained January 13, 1987. Total fusion of the L2 and L3 vertebral bodies has occurred. The duration of infection from onset to total fusion was 12 to 14 months. *(From Borenstein D, Wiesel S, Boden S: Low back and neck pain: comprehensive diagnosis and management, ed 3, Philadelphia, 2004, Saunders, p 416.)*

than in the appendicular skeleton. The lumbar and thoracic spines are affected in approximately 46% and 49% of cases, with the remainder affecting the cervical spine. Suspicion for the presence of metastasis is increased in individuals older than age 50 years with back pain unassociated with a trauma. These patients have progressive back pain that increases in intensity over time. Radicular pain may increase at night as the spine lengthens with recumbency. Pain with recumbency is a symptom associated with spinal tumors. Examples of benign and malignant vertebral column tumors are listed in Table 87.1.

Physical examination shows localized tenderness over the vertebral column and neurologic dysfunction if the spinal cord is compressed by benign or malignant lesions. Radiographic evaluation of the lumbosacral spine is useful in identification of characteristic changes in the bony and soft tissue areas of the spine associated with neoplastic lesions. The finding of a lucent nidus, a lesion about 1.5 cm in diameter with a surrounding well-defined area of dense sclerotic bone, is virtually pathognomonic of osteoid osteoma. Osteomas arise in the posterior elements of a vertebra. The size and location of these lesions make detection with plain radiographs difficult. Bone scintiscans are useful in localization of the lesion if plain radiograph results are negative. CT scan is the most useful test for precise localization of the lesion and differentiation from other bone lesions. MRI adds little in regard to clarification of bone architecture and is not used routinely in the evaluation of this primary bone tumor.

Radiographic abnormalities of metastatic lesions include osteolytic, osteoblastic, and mixed lytic and blastic lesions. Osteolytic lesions are associated with carcinomas of the lung, kidney, breast, and thyroid. Multiple osteoblastic lesions are associated with prostate, breast, and colon carcinomas and bronchial carcinoid (**Fig. 87.2**). Vertebral lesions that contain lytic and blastic metastases are associated with carcinoma of the

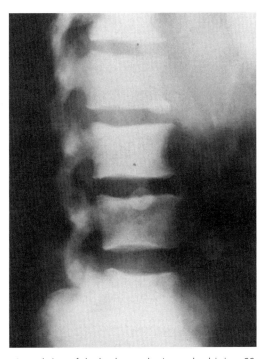

Fig. 87.2 Lateral view of the lumbosacral spine and pelvis in a 66-year-old man with a 3-month history of back pain reveals multiple, discrete osteoblastic lesions that proved to be metastatic prostatic carcinoma on biopsy. *(From Borenstein D, Wiesel S, Boden S: Low back and neck pain: comprehensive diagnosis and management, ed 3, Philadelphia, 2004, Saunders, p 534.)*

breast, lung, prostate, or bladder. Vertebral body destruction is not associated with alterations in the intervertebral disk. The presence of vertebral body and intervertebral disk destruction is more closely associated with infection. Early in the course of a metastatic lesion, plain radiograph results are unremarkable because 30% to 50% of bone must be destroyed before a lesion is evident on plain radiographs.[18] Bone scintiscan is more sensitive than plain radiographs and can detect areas of bone involvement in 85% of patients with metastases. Bone scintiscan may be the more useful diagnostic test in differentiation of pain caused by metastatic disease from pain caused by a benign lesion. CT scan normally is reserved for assessment of patients with positive scan results but negative radiograph results. CT scan differentiates among bony metastases, benign lesions, and no abnormality.[19] CT scan is particularly useful in showing small areas of bone destruction and of bone and tumor impingement on the spinal canal. CT scan should not be used as a screening procedure because of the exposure to high levels of radiation. MRI is better at showing the extent of tumor inside the spinal canal, the size of extraosseous extension, and bone marrow invasion, whereas CT scan is better at showing the degree of cortical bone loss.[20] A study of 40 patients with metastatic disease revealed that patients with breast, kidney, or prostatic cancer or multiple myeloma had abnormal MRI results but normal CT scan and bone scintiscan results.[21] Gadolinium diethylenetriaminepentaacetic acid, an MRI contrast agent, enhances the capability of MRI to differentiate the size, location, configuration, and characteristics of spinal tumors from normal tissues.[22]

The diagnosis of a primary tumor of the lumbosacral spine necessitates biopsy of the lesion. The diagnosis is confirmed with histologic examination of biopsy material. For patients with metastatic disease with no known primary neoplasm, biopsy of the lesion for tissue diagnosis is necessary. Closed needle biopsy of the lesions in the lumbar spine can yield definitive information safely. The therapy for benign lesions is excisional biopsy completed for histologic examination of the lesion. Benign lesions that are not entirely removed may grow and cause recurrent pain. Treatment of metastatic disease of the spine is directed toward palliation of pain. Cure is not possible because most solitary metastatic lesions are accompanied by asymptomatic deposits that become evident over time. Surgical intervention to prevent progression of structural instability can result in a mean survival time of 26 months after operation.[23]

Local Vertebral Column Pain

Patients with pain over the vertebral column have fractures of the vertebral body or expansion of the bone marrow space. Any systemic process that increases mineral loss from bone (e.g., osteoporosis, hyperparathyroidism, Paget's disease) or hypertrophy or replacement of bone marrow cells with inflammatory or neoplastic cells (multiple myeloma, hemoglobinopathy) weakens vertebral bone to the degree that fracture may occur spontaneously or with minimal impact. Although many patients with these disorders have acute bone pain develop, patients with osteoporosis may experience microfractures that cause chronic pain. Severe pain usually lasts 3 to 4 months and then resolves; however, some patients are left with persistent, dull spinal pain without any evidence of vertebral fracture. The source of pain may be microfractures too small to be detected with radiographs or biomechanical effects of the deformity on the lumbar spine below. Recurrent pain, increased deformity,

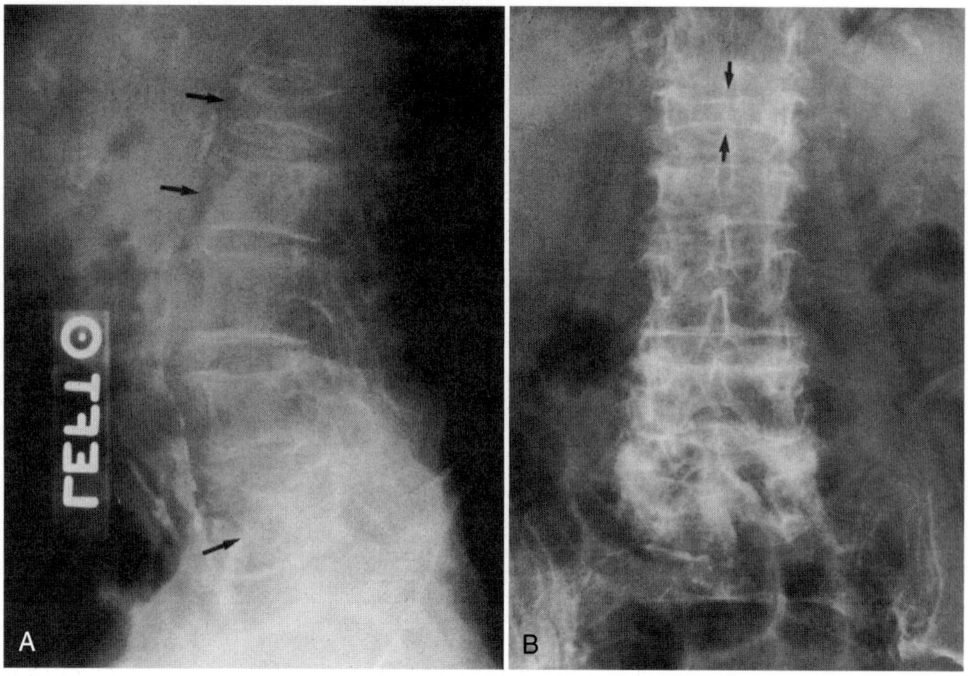

Fig. 87.3 An 83-year-old woman presented with a history of acute low back pain localized to the thoracolumbar junction. **A,** Lateral view reveals generalized osteoporosis with diminished height of L1, L2, and L5 *(arrows).* **B,** Anteroposterior view reveals marked loss of height of the L1 vertebral body *(arrows). (From Borenstein D, Wiesel S, Boden S:* Low back and neck pain: comprehensive diagnosis and management, *ed 3, Philadelphia, 2004, Saunders, p 575.)*

and loss of height suggest new fractures. With hemoglobinopathies, marrow hyperplasia causes loss of bone trabeculae in the axial skeleton. Acute crises associated with bone infarctions cause acute pain. Between crises, back pain may persist from alterations of bony architecture.

Physical examination is remarkable for pain with palpation localized to the affected area of the lumbar spine. If present, muscle spasm tends to surround the area of bony tenderness. This phenomenon is particularly noticeable in the setting of sacral fractures.

Radiographic evaluation concentrates on the area of the spine that is tender with palpation. Plain radiographs may pinpoint skeletal abnormalities but may have normal results because greater than 30% of the bone calcium must be lost before decreased bone content is recognized (**Fig. 87.3**).[24] Microfractures may not be detected with plain radiographs. Bone scintiscans are useful to detect increased bone activity soon after a fracture occurs. CT scans also may identify the location of a fracture or area of bone that has been replaced with hypertrophied or inflammatory tissue. MRI is helpful in identification of the disease processes that complicate the course of patients with hemoglobinopathies, such as infections.[25]

Laboratory evaluation is helpful for differentiation of the myriad of systemic illnesses that cause localized vertebral bone pain. Screening tests that heighten the physician's suspicion of a systemic illness include an elevated erythrocyte sedimentation rate or decreased hematocrit value. Abnormalities of complete blood count may indicate a primary hemoglobinopathy or replacement of bone marrow elements with neoplastic cells. Serum chemistries may detect abnormalities of calcium metabolism associated with elevated parathyroid hormone levels (hyperparathyroidism). The diagnosis of osteoporosis should be considered in an individual with normal laboratory values and decreased bone mineral content. A variety of radiographic techniques are available to quantify vertebral bone mineral.[26]

The treatment for patients with local vertebral column pain is specific for the underlying disorder causing alterations in bone calcium or vertebral bone marrow. Most of these patients need analgesic therapy for extended periods to diminish the degree of spinal pain.

Prolonged Morning Stiffness

Morning stiffness of the lumbosacral spine is a frequent symptom of patients with mechanical and nonmechanical low back pain. Mechanical back pain is associated with morning stiffness of short duration (≤1 hour). Morning stiffness lasting more than 1 hour is a common symptom of spondyloarthropathy. The spondyloarthropathies include ankylosing spondylitis, reactive arthritis, psoriatic arthritis, and enteropathic arthritis. Patients with a spondyloarthropathy may have a history of bilateral sacroiliac joint pain associated with morning stiffness that may be present for years without a specific diagnosis.[27] Patients with reactive arthritis and psoriatic spondylitis may have development of unilateral sacroiliac disease associated with low back pain that is lateralized to the affected side. Patients with reactive arthritis and psoriatic spondylitis also may have development of spondylitis (lumbar spine inflammation) without sacroiliitis.

Physical examination of patients with spondyloarthropathy shows various degrees of decreased motion in the lumbosacral spine corresponding to the extent and severity of disease. Plain radiographs of the lumbosacral spine are helpful for identification of early changes of spondyloarthropathy. Radiographic abnormalities include loss of lumbar lordosis, joint erosions in the lower one third of the sacroiliac joints, and squaring of the vertebral bodies (**Fig. 87.4**). CT scan of the sacroiliac joints is more sensitive for recognition of sacroiliitis than conventional radiographs. The test should be reserved for patients with normal or equivocal radiograph results in whom a diagnosis of spondyloarthropathy is suspected. MRI also may be able to detect alterations of sacroiliac joints that are not shown with conventional radiographs but incurs a greater expense.

Treatment of spondyloarthropathy includes a combination of NSAIDs with physical therapy to maximize the motion of the spine. Tumor necrosis factor (TNF) inhibitors are indicated for patients with severe disease associated with serum

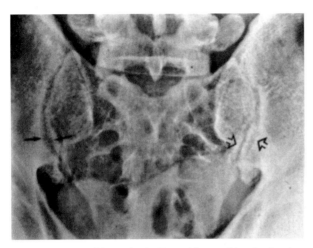

Fig. 87.4 A 35-year-old man had a 5-year history of low back pain and morning stiffness. He previously had not sought medical care for back pain. Posteroanterior view of the sacroiliac joints reveals early joint margin erosions on both sides of the joints *(black arrows)* and sclerosis *(open arrows)*. Bilateral sacroiliac joint disease was compatible with a diagnosis of ankylosing spondylitis. *(From Borenstein D, Wiesel S, Boden S: Low back and neck pain: comprehensive diagnosis and management, ed 3, Philadelphia, 2004, Saunders, p 200.)*

inflammatory markers. These drugs represent a major advance for the treatment of ankylosing spondylitis (AS).[28] Of interest, NSAIDs, not TNFs, are the pharmacologic agents that prevent the development of syndesmophytes over time in AS.[29]

Visceral Pain

Disorders of the vascular, genitourinary, and gastrointestinal systems can cause stimulation of sensory nerves that results in the perception of pain in the damaged area and in superficial tissues supplied by the same segments of the spinal cord. The duration and sequence of visceral pain follows the periodicity of the involved organ. Colicky pain occurs in peristaltic waves and is associated with a hollow viscus, such as the colon, gallbladder, uterus, or ureter. Throbbing pain is associated with vascular structures. Somatic pain frequently is exacerbated by activity and improved by rest. Patients with viscerogenic pain get little relief from bed rest. Many patients prefer to be moving in an attempt to achieve a comfortable position.

Back pain is rarely the only symptom of visceral disease. Kidney pain is felt in the costovertebral angle. Ureteral pain from nephrolithiasis may cause dull flank pain with chronic distention or colic if obstruction occurs at the ureteropelvic junction. Patients with bladder infections may have development of diffuse low back pain centered over the sacrum. Pain from genital organs may occur locally or in a referred pattern. Endometriosis causes recurrent low back pain on a monthly basis corresponding to menstrual periods. The severity of endometrial pain is not particularly modified by changes in position. Pain may be related to pancreatitis, peptic ulcer disease, or colon or rectal disorders. The diagnosis of an aortic aneurysm should be suspected in an elderly individual with chronic nondescript back pain that does not improve with rest or is not exacerbated with activity. Vascular lesions cause dull, steady abdominal pain that is unrelated to activity. Throbbing or tearing back pain also may be associated with vascular abnormalities, including an expanding abdominal aneurysm. Any change in the frequency, intensity, or location of the pain suggests expansion in the size of the aneurysm. Patients with an abdominal aneurysm are usually older individuals with a history of lower extremity claudication. Irritation of retroperitoneal structures causes back pain associated with epigastric discomfort that may radiate to the hips or thighs. Rupture or acute expansion of the aneurysm is associated with tearing pain and circulatory collapse.

Physical examination of the abdomen may help in identification of the source of maximal pain. Tenderness with palpation of the abdomen may localize over the epigastrium (aorta) or lower quadrant (uterus). Physical examination has adequate sensitivity to identify individuals with a large enough aneurysm to warrant elective intervention.[30] Ovarian tenderness and enlargement also may be palpated. Range of motion of the lumbar spine is unaffected. Palpation of the lumbar spine is painless.

Ultrasound scan and CT scan of the abdomen readily identify aortic aneurysms. Abdominal ultrasound scan detects aneurysms with sensitivity that approaches 100%.[31] The longitudinal and transverse diameters can be determined without radiation or contrast medium. The effectiveness of ultrasound scan is diminished by excessive bowel gas that obscures the infrarenal abdominal aorta and by the pancreas, which hides the suprarenal aorta. Ultrasound scan is inadequate for a plan of vascular surgery. CT scan is highly sensitive and specific for identification of aneurysms. In contrast to ultrasound scan, CT scan visualizes aortic anomalies, horseshoe kidney, and involvement of the iliac and hypogastric arteries. CT scan is a most effective test for planning of surgery.

MRI is the radiographic technique best used in identification of endometriosis. MRI is 98% sensitive for the identification of endometriosis. MRI may find deposits in the pouch of Douglas, ureterosacral ligaments, ovaries, uterine surface, retrovaginal septum, fallopian tubes, bowel, or appendix.

Therapy for visceral disorders that cause back pain is directed toward the organ system associated with the disorder. The therapy of abdominal aneurysm is surgical. Improved survival is documented for individuals with elective surgery for intact aneurysms. If an aneurysm is smaller than 5.5 cm in diameter, elective repair has a 30-day operative mortality rate of 5.4%. At 3 years, surgery has no better advantage than surveillance does with regard to survival.[32] At 8 years, patients who undergo surgery have a lower mortality rate than patients monitored with ultrasound scan every 6 months.[33]

Mechanical Low Back Pain

Most individuals with mechanical low back pain have symptoms localized to the lumbar region demarcated from the 12th rib to the crease of the buttock. In general, mechanical pain is relieved by certain motions and exacerbated by opposite actions.

Lumbosacral Strain

Many individuals with pain in the lumbar spine have back strain. The cause of back strain is unclear. Possible causes of pain associated with back strain include muscular or ligamentous injuries, continuous mechanical stress from poor posture, or a small tear in an annulus fibrosus.

Damage may occur in lumbar spine structures if the force generated in a task does not match the stress placed on the spine.[34] If the force is too great or too little, paraspinous muscles are at risk of being damaged, resulting in muscle contraction and pain. Excess fatigability and paraspinal weakness occur in patients with low back pain. Muscle wasting and weakness arises rapidly as a result of reduced motor unit recruitment because of fear of pain or reflex inhibition of motion.[35]

Patients with muscle strain have pain limited to a local area. In others, the distribution of pain may follow the referred pattern of muscles of the same mesenchymal origin. These individuals have myofascial pain. Most individuals experience pain simultaneously with an injury. Subsequently, increased pain occurs with tissue edema and associated reflex contraction of the surrounding muscles and limitation of motion. Exacerbation of pain occurs with motion that contracts the injured muscle. Certain motions may be painless, whereas others cause incapacitating pain.

On physical examination, any active motion of the involved muscle against resistance causes pain. The damaged muscle may be tender on palpation. The muscle may have increased contraction and firmness compared with the surrounding muscles under normal tension. Neurologic examination results are normal.

Therapy for back strain includes controlled physical activity, NSAIDs, and muscle relaxants. The recommendation to maintain activity as tolerated is an important component of muscle strain therapy.[36] A short period of 2 days has been shown to be effective in relief of back pain. Cherkin and colleagues[37] conducted a longitudinal observational study of the efficacy of medications at 7 days for the treatment of acute low back pain in 219 patients. Patients who received a muscle relaxant and NSAIDs had the best self-reported outcomes. Muscle relaxants have a beneficial role in relief of pain associated with muscle spasm in the absence of sedation.[38]

Lumbar Spondylosis (Osteoarthritis)

Osteoarthritis affects the apophyseal joints of the lumbar spine. The same pathology that affects the appendicular joints, such as the knees, also can damage the axial joints. Major changes occur in the lumbar spine between the third and fifth decades of life. The first manifestations of aging develop in the intervertebral disks. The nucleus loses its turgor, and the annulus fissures and degenerates. Disk degeneration itself may not be a painful process. Patients with disk degeneration may be asymptomatic until alterations in facet joint alignment result in the onset of articular pain. In response to disk degeneration, the apophyseal joints narrow, resulting in osteoarthritis.[39] The resulting biomechanical insufficiency results in transfer of stresses posteriorly to the facet joints.[40] Capsular strains, hypermobility, and degenerative changes develop. Traction spur, and redundancy of the ligamentum flavum manifest these changes radiographically. Progression of this process results in spinal stenosis.

Patients with osteoarthritis of the facet joints have pain over the lower lumbar spine. Any body movements that compress the joints (extension) exacerbate symptoms of dull, aching pain. Stiffness of the lumbar spine is another common symptom.

Radiographs of the lumbar spine reveal loss of disk height, traction osteophytes, decreased interpedicular distance, and facet degeneration (**Fig. 87.5**). CT scan can be used to identify the irregularity of articular surfaces and alterations in positional orientation of the facet joints but are necessary for diagnosis in a minority of patients.

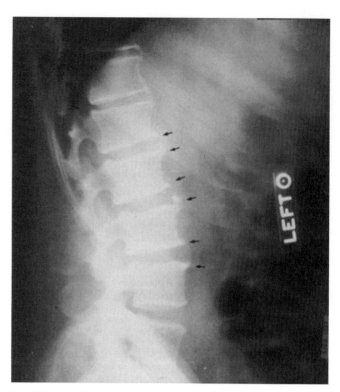

Fig. 87.5 Lateral view shows traction osteophytes (arrows) at multiple levels associated with disk degeneration. The osteophytes are horizontally oriented and emerge slightly above or below the disk space. A claw osteophyte is noted at the fourth arrow from the top; a traction osteophyte is located at the fifth arrow from the top. (From Borenstein D, Wiesel S, Boden S: Low back and neck pain: comprehensive diagnosis and management, ed 3, Philadelphia, 2004, Saunders, p 262.)

The therapy of osteoarthritis, whether in the knee or lumbar spine, consists of analgesics, NSAIDs, and exercises. The choice of these therapies is a trial-and-error process. Ideal therapies may not be tolerated by patients. Maximum doses of medications may be ineffective. An ongoing dialogue between the patient and physician is the best method to identify the ideal regimen for an individual patient.

Conclusion

The evaluation of a patient with pain localized to the lumbar spine is a daunting task. The disease possibilities are numerous. The diagnostic options are complicated and expensive. Most patients have mechanical disorders. Therapies have the potential to relieve significant amounts of suffering when chosen appropriately. Inappropriate therapies may be ineffective at best and harmful at worst. The prognosis ranges from total recovery to life-threatening illness. This chapter clarifies the evaluation and treatment of the patient with low back pain. Disorders of the lumbar spine have characteristic symptoms and signs that help organize the illnesses into specific categories. Appropriate therapies can be selected when these specific categories are identified. A successful outcome is most likely when these basic rules are followed.

References

Full references for this chapter can be found on www.expertconsult.com.

Osteoporosis

F. Michael Gloth III

Osteoporosis generally is not classified as a painful diagnosis. The sequelae, however, can be very painful and can lead to significant functional disability, morbidity, and even mortality.[1] In addition, other causes of secondary osteoporosis are also associated with pain. Vitamin D deficiency is probably most noteworthy, and this chapter deals with this in some detail. Also, some treatments of osteoporosis may cause pain; this is discussed as well.

The annual rate of hip fractures from osteoporosis is expected to reach 2.3 million worldwide by 2020.[1] In the long-term care setting, osteoporosis prevalence rate hovers around 85%.[2] Any fracture is painful, and aggressive intervention that involves open or closed repair necessitates sufficient analgesics. This almost always includes opioids, especially in older adults in whom adequate pain control is needed to optimize participation in therapy. Quick participation in rehabilitation is of vital concern because, even when healthy, bed rest for an 85-year-old patient for a few days may require weeks to recover the associated loss in strength and function. With treatment with opioids, older adults also need attention to the development of adverse effects. Any chronic opioid use is likely to be complicated by constipation. This can be handled with chronic laxative use, although the peripheral opioid antagonist, methylnaltrexone, at the time of this writing, is the only drug with an indication for this problem. Because of its relatively predictable response time, this can be helpful in maintenance of dignity during amelioration of constipation, if prescribed appropriately (ideally when staffing is optimal and most likely to be available to assist).[3] Because of the complications related to nonsteroidal anti-inflammatory drugs (NSAIDs), these agents should not be used beyond a few days in older adults.[4]

One half or more of the world's population is estimated to have a vitamin D deficiency. In the United States, more than a third of women have low blood levels of vitamin D. Overall, women are more than twice as likely as men to have low levels of this important vitamin.[5] Older adults are particularly susceptible if exposure to sunlight is impaired.[6,7] A vitamin D deficiency syndrome appears to be associated with intense pain with even light pressure over large muscle groups and greater tenderness of pressure sores than normally seen. This pain resolves within 5 to 7 days of 100,000 IU of oral vitamin D.[8] The most recent guidelines advise that every adult receive, on average, at least 4000 IU of vitamin D input daily. This includes contributions from sunlight and diet. If monthly supplementation is used, 100,000 IU of vitamin D_3 (cholecalciferol) is recommended.

Vitamin D supplementation has also been associated with reduction of fracture risk. Prevention of fracture is, of course, the best way to prevent pain associated with a fracture!

Addressing the underlying etiologies of bone pain often requires management of disorders associated with calcium and bone metabolism in addition to the practice of good pain principles. Although similar principles of pain management apply, in general, optimal control of bone pain requires expertise both in bone conditions and in pain relief. A vertebral compression fracture for example may also be accompanied by nerve root impingement, producing pain from the bone destruction and inflammation locally and that of a neuropathic origin from nerve injury. In such a circumstance, the treatment regimen may involve multiple modalities. In addition to treatment of the pain itself, the cause of bone loss needs to be addressed, with recognition of the higher risk for additional skeletal events.

Prevalence

A recent review of data from the United States Centers for Medicare and Medicaid Services (CMS) revealed that 29% of nursing home residents who had experienced a fracture in the prior 6 months continued to have daily pain.[9] It is, of course, not only nursing home residents who suffer in pain. Every patient with osteoporosis-related fracture in any setting can be expected to experience pain for weeks unless adequate analgesia is provided. Other bone-related diseases can also produce suffering even in the absence of fracture. Paget's disease, hypoparathyroidism, vitamin D deficiency, and malignant diseases involving bone are but a few such examples. See **Table 88.1**.

Table 88.1 Nonmacro Fracture Examples of Bone Disease Associated with Pain

Vitamin D deficiency (osteomalacia, vitamin D deficiency pain syndrome)

Skeletal metastasis

Primary bone malignant diseases

Paget's disease

Hypoparathyroidism

Tuberculosis (and other infections)

Medications (including bisphosphonates and granulocyte-colony stimulating factor)

Rheumatoid arthritis and other connective tissue disorders (e.g., ankylosing spondylitis)

Leukemia

Acute cholinergic dysautonomia

Albers-Schönberg disease

Amyloidosis

Aseptic osteitis

Celiac disease

Aseptic necrosis

Erdheim-Chester disease

Gaucher's disease

Hypercalcemia

Hyperphosphatemia

Myelofibrosis

Osteitis condensans

Multiple myeloma

Nasu-Hakola disease

Mastocytosis

Schnitzler's syndrome

Sickle cell disease

Histiocytosis

Sclerosis

Osteoradionecrosis

Kissing rib syndrome

Blast crisis

Aneurysmal bone cysts

Cholestasis

Fibrous dysplasia

Vitamin A toxicity

Chemical poisoning (e.g., hydrogen fluoride)

Cytomegalic inclusion body disease

Di Guglielmo's I syndrome

Ehlers-Danlos syndrome

Haferkamp's syndrome

Hand-Schüller-Christian syndrome

Weber-Christian disease

Sarcoidosis

WT limb blood syndrome

Insufficient assessment, fear of use of certain medications appropriate for pain control (e.g., opioids), and inadequate knowledge have been identified as reasons for poor pain management.[10]

Issues with Assessment

One reason that assessment is such an issue in pain management is that few people use standardized instruments of assessment. Even when standardization has been performed, such tests often were not conducted in a population similar to those most likely to have bone pain, in particular, the older adults with such pain. A young cognitively intact patient after fracture is likely to be very different than the 85-year-old patient, who has a minimal trauma fracture after a fall.

Assessment, of course, involves much more than abbreviated pain instruments. The initial evaluation of pain should include a good history and physical examination. Documentation should reflect a methodical history. The manifestation of the pain should be described, including onset, duration, location, description, relieving and exacerbating factors, ineffective prior interventions, and psychologic components (e.g., secondary gain, depression, mental focus, prior experience, and anxiety). Any physical findings should also be recorded. Bone pain in particular, necessitates sensitivity to direct pathology to bone and remote origins of pain, which ultimately take up residence in bone (i.e., nonskeletal primary malignant diseases, thyroid disease, parathyroid disease, vitamin D deficiency, etc.)

Assessment also should include appropriate laboratory testing and imaging as dictated by the history and physical findings (**Table 88.2**). For bone pain, the clinician must be especially astute in conceiving of remote etiologies behind bone or joint discomfort.

The final point to be made about assessment is that once is never enough. Reassessment is absolutely necessary in achieving and maintaining adequate pain relief. Preferably, an appropriately standardized instrument with good reliability, validity, *and* responsiveness testing in population similar to the patient is available. One scale that is particularly useful in an older population is the Functional Pain Scale (FPS: **Fig. 88.1**).[11] This scale has been tested with a subject population that includes individuals with Mini-Mental State Examination scores as

Table 88.2 Suggested Baseline Blood Testing for Evaluation of Bone Pain

Comprehensive metabolic profile

Liver function tests (with alkaline phosphatase, albumin, and gamma glutamyl transferase)

Albumin

Calcium

Phosphorous

Complete blood count

Thyroid function studies

Serum protein electrophoresis

Erythrocyte sedimentation rate

Fasting 25-hydroxyvitamin D and 1,25-dihydroxyvitamin D serum levels

Intact PTH serum level

low as 17 and, with a more objective functional component to the assessment, is more responsive that other instruments that have not been designed specifically for frail older adults so commonly encountered when dealing with bone pain.

Treatment

The key to unlocking appropriate treatment for bone pain is found in the identification of the etiology of the pain. Once a plan of treatment is identified, compliance and success are more likely if patient education rests in the center of the treatment strategy. A patient should be informed about how much time can be anticipated before some degree of pain relief. Any adverse symptoms that are likely to be associated with the treatment should be discussed as well.

Nonpharmacologic Interventions

Bone pain is transmitted along two types of fibers: A-delta and C fibers. The larger and faster A-delta fibers are associated with acute-onset, localized, sudden noxious perturbations (e.g., the pain associated with an acute fracture). In treatment of most bone-related pain, the strategy confronts transmission of noxious stimulation along slower, amyelenic, nociceptive C fibers. By modulating the signal to and along these afferent receptors, we can reduce the sensation of pain. Although medications can be used to achieve some degree of relief, simple nonpharmacologic interventions can be useful as well. Also, some strategies rely on a feedback loop with a descending neuralgic pathway that stimulates release of endogenous opioids capable of providing pain relief as well (**Fig. 88.2**).

The simplest of nonpharmacologic interventions is the application of cold or warmth to the local area of injury or discomfort. Although evidence is scant, cold seems to decrease the release of tissue damage products (e.g., histamines, prostaglandins, substance P, bradykinins, and potassium) that stimulate neurotransmission of C fibers.

Heat and cold may stimulate descending pathways associated with endogenous opioid production as appears to be likely with vibration, transcutaneous electrical nerve stimulation (TENS), massage, and acupuncture.[12,13] Space precludes more than a mention of other modalities, such as radiation, either by external beam or through oral radionuclide treatment, which are often reserved for refractory cases of pain

---

Functional Pain Scale

ID#: _____   Date: _____

Name: _____   Unit: _____

RA: _____   Score: _____

1. Are you in pain?
   No pain = 0   If yes, continue.

2. Is pain tolerable?
   Yes = continue to question 3.
   No = continue to question 4.

3. Does it prevent you from doing activities?
   No = 1   (pain tolerable)
   Yes = 2   (pain tolerable)

4. Can you use the telephone, watch television, or read?
   Yes = 3   (pain tolerable)
   No = 4

5. Pain is intolerable and you can't use telephone, watch television, or read?
   Yes = 4
   Unable to verbally communicate because of pain = 5

Ideally, all patients should reach a 0 to 2 level, preferably 0 to 1. It should be made clear to the respondent that limitations in function only apply if limitations are due to the pain being evaluated.

First determine whether or not pain is present. If subject replies that pain exists, the other two categories in the assessment are evaluated–subjective and functional.
Second is to have the patient rate the pain subjectively as tolerable or intolerable.
Third, if pain is tolerable, the next step is to determine whether pain interferes with any activity.
If pain is intolerable, the next step is to ascertain whether pain is so intense as to prevent passive activities (e.g. using telephone, watching television, or reading).

Fig. 88.1 **Functional Pain Scale.** *(Copyright © F. Michael Gloth, III. Used with permission.)*

THE PAIN PATHWAY

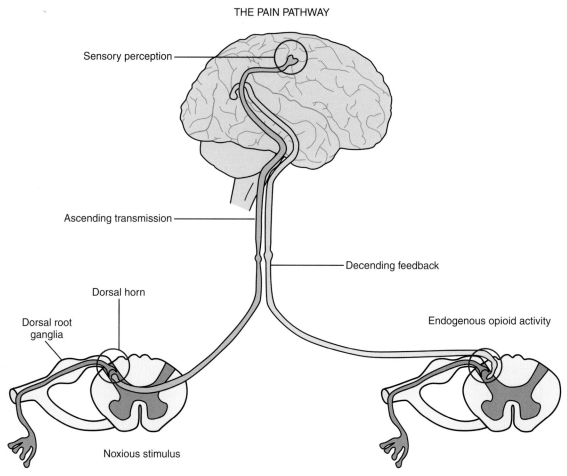

Fig. 88.2 **Pain pathway.**

because of their high costs and usual requirement of multiple repeat dosing along with the use of adjuvants. Nerve blocks and other neurochemical interventions may be used in refractory cases of pain, as well, but usually require specialty consultation and are beyond the scope and space of this chapter.

During conceptualization of nonpharmacologic interventions for bone pain, physical and occupational therapy must be recognized and incorporated into the treatment plan as an integral part of the pain management plan. In addition to splinting and local modalities, rehabilitative therapies can help to optimize exercise, something consistently shown to help reduce pain.[14,15] In addition, therapists play an important role in helping to restrengthen deconditioned muscles that have atrophied from disuse in association with pain. Thus, a sudden increase in activity may make one susceptible to local irritation or even reinjury. This concept is illustrated in **Fig. 88.3** as part of the Pain Pentagon.[16]

Pharmacologic Intervention
Nonopioids

Initial pharmacologic options should focus on nonopioid drugs. Acetaminophen is often cited as an initial agent to consider because it is perceived as well tolerated. However, acetaminophen is recognized for adverse events as well, particularly as it relates to liver toxicity. Although daily dosing beyond 4 g/day, particularly in older patients, has long been recognized

Pain-Treatment-Pain Pentagon

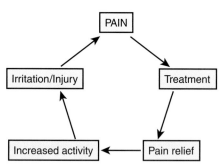

Fig. 88.3 The Pain Pentagon represents a cycle of pain, treatment, improved function, and activity that produces further local irritation or remote injury that results in new or recurrent pain. This illustrates the risk of reinjury and the potential impact of increased activity accompanying successful pain intervention, which paradoxically may strain deconditioned areas of the body after long periods of rest because of prior underlying discomfort. *(Copyright © 2003 F. Michael Gloth, III, MD. Used with permission.)*

as markedly increasing the risk for toxicity, more recent data indicate that lower doses used chronically also are linked to abnormalities in liver function testing.[17] Nonetheless, acetaminophen remains one of the preferred agents in initial pain management, even that which is related to bone pathology.[18,19]

Another agent to consider is tramadol, which is likely to be even more effective at lower doses when combined with another agent, such as acetaminophen.[20] Regardless, the lowest dose of this agent should be used and gradually increased over time to avoid more common manifestation of adverse events.[21]

For bone pain and inflammation, the NSAID class has been preferred by some. For all of these agents, data warrant caution over renal and cardiovascular effects, particularly with older patients.

Calcitonin, known to most people who see patients in the bone arena, also has analgesic properties. Although the mechanism of action is debatable, both a central and a peripheral role for the analgesia have been shown in controlled settings.[22–25] Regardless, unless another reason is seen to prescribe calcitonin, there are generally less expensive and better studied options available for control of pain.

Although not specifically classified as an analgesic, bisphosphonate also should be a recognized medication option for bone pain. Currently, the US Food and Drug Administration (FDA) has approved only intravenous (IV) forms of bisphosphonates for skeletal events, but little reason is found to believe that oral agents are not also effective.[26] Usually, better results occur when doses more comparable with recommendations for Paget's disease treatment are used rather than doses used commonly in osteoporosis therapy.

Vitamin D also must be mentioned here. Besides an association with musculoskeletal pain in rickets, a vitamin D deficiency pain syndrome has been described that produces intense localized tenderness with light pressure, especially over large muscle groups.[27,28] This condition does not respond well to opioids or tricyclic antidepressants but resolves within 5 to 7 days of vitamin D replacement of 100,000 IU orally. Vitamin D and calcium have also been shown to decrease fracture rates, and of course, fractures are a source of pain as well.[29]

In addition to oral and inhaled agents is an ever-growing list of topical and injectable agents. Capsaicin, derived from the pepper plant family, has received accolades for its analgesic effect. It should be initiated in the lowest, 0.025%, dose because of its tendency to be accompanied by a local burning sensation (which warrants caution during administration to others as well). This medication inhibits the uptake of substance P and must be applied every 6 hours to prevent substance P from reaccumulating with a reappearance of pain. Beyond the over-the-counter capsaicin, a variety of local anesthetics, usually containing lidocaine, are also available topically.

The management of joint discomfort related to connective tissue diseases, especially rheumatoid arthritis, has seen an influx of products recently. Some are disease-modifying agents like leflunamide, which inhibits the formation of pyrimidines by inhibiting the formation of orotate from dihydroorotate. Others include hyaluronanate injections that are designed to stimulate endogenous hyaluronanate synthesis. Although the improvement in pain is better than with placebo, the medications are expensive and may themselves cause an inflammatory response.[30] Etanercept is another of many agents now approved for rheumatoid arthritis.[31] Usually, this is administered as a 25-mg subcutaneous injection twice weekly. A local reaction may occur but usually dissipates over time.

Other agents such as tricyclic antidepressants, some antiepileptics (e.g., clonazepam, carbamazepine, gabapentin, phenytoin, and pregabalin), and mexilitine have also been recommended for neuropathic pain.[32–36] Selective serotonin reuptake inhibitors with norepinephrine activity have also been recognized as having efficacy in neuropathic pain, and duloxetine has recently been approved by the FDA for such an indication. Although duloxetine for neuropathy is usually titrated to doses higher than commonly used for depression, initial doses of antidepressants and antiepileptics in pain therapy are usually below those needed for the treatment of depression or seizures. Depression is very common in patients with chronic pain and necessitates treatment independently from the pain intervention.

Opioids

Very severe pain (e.g., level 4 or 5 on the FPS) may warrant opioid intervention as an initial intervention, with attempts to reduce or remove the opioids once pain is under control. Usually, however, opioids are initiated for chronic pain after nonopioids have proved to be inadequate for pain management.

For chronic skeletal pain, a controlled release opioid is preferred to more frequent dosing with immediate release formulations. In addition to promoting uninterrupted opportunities for sleep, the reduced fluctuations in therapeutic levels reduce chances of development of tolerance.[37,38]

The use of opioids has long been an area of interest and confusion due, in part, to regulatory oversight and misconceptions about addiction. At the outset, it is important to explain that even chronic use of morphine rarely leads to addiction when used to control pain.[39,40] An individual who has nausea and vomiting on morphine is likely to have those symptoms resolve as tolerance develops over the course of a few days to weeks. For this reason, it is important to work on palliating the nausea and vomiting through antiemetic medications (and possibly opioid dose reduction), rather than trying to switch to different opioids.[41]

Tolerance does not develop to opioid-induced constipation; the condition may be exacerbated for patients at risk for osteoporosis, who are often taking calcium carbonate. In such circumstances, an alternate form of calcium is recommended, and an emphasis on adequate hydration, activity, and the use of agents to facilitate bowel mobility (e.g., senna or sorbitol) is warranted.

A general rule is to avoid only "as needed" (prn) dosing to control pain and to increase regular dosages if prn medication is used three times over a 24-hour period.[42] Concomitantly, patients should be told that they may refuse a regularly scheduled medication if they do not need it or if they are having undesired side effects.

Greater amounts of analgesic may be necessary to initially bring pain under control than to maintain control of pain. The anxiety that is associated with inadequate pain control may be a factor that makes pain management more difficult as noted previously. Once the anxiety is eliminated, less opioid is likely necessary to maintain pain control than was necessary to initially resolve the patient's pain.

Additional Points for Better Pain Relief

As noted previously, vigilance for adverse events is important in dealing with pain medications. However, some observations may be misinterpreted as side effects from medication when such is not the case at all. For example, a patient who has been in pain for a long period of time may fall asleep from exhaustion once pain is finally relieved. All too often, this is mistaken as a side effect from morphine. Normally, if respirations are found to be 12 breaths per minute or greater, the prescriber can rest more comfortably as well.

In pain relief, where greater effect may be obtained with synergy among medications, use of multiple drugs at lower dosing ranges actually may be preferable to pushing the dose on each individual analgesic before adding an adjuvant.[43] Adjuvant use is particularly important with use of opioids to control pain from bone compressing a nerve because such neuropathic pain rarely responds adequately to opioids alone.

Preemptive analgesia is a concept of providing a medication before a procedure or episode likely to induce pain. With analgesia before surgery for spinal fusion, for example, a patient uses less opioid after surgery and have better pain control.[44,45]

Conclusion

Osteoporosis with minimal trauma and other metabolic bone diseases can produce bone pain. Attention to astute clinical review and targeting of the underlying etiology, in conjunction with a focus on the symptom of pain, pay great rewards in pain relief. Nonopioids and opioids should be part of the armamentarium used to fight pain. Frequent assessment with appropriately standardized instruments and a thoughtful strategy of preventive measures should allow for continued relief in an otherwise challenging clinical arena.

References

Full references for this chapter can be found on www.expertconsult.com.

Lumbar Radiculopathy

Laxmaiah Manchikanti, Vijay Singh, and Mark V. Boswell

Historical Considerations

Solid lumbar radiculopathy descriptions date back to the Hippocratic collection, where the condition was described as sciatica (**Fig. 89.1**).[1] Sciatica was described as, "hipache at the end of the sacrum and the buttocks with radiation into the thigh." In 1543, Andreas Vesalius[2,3] provided a detailed account of the anatomy of the disk. In 1764, Cortugno,[4] an Italian physician, implicated the sciatic nerve as the cause and described sciatica as follows: "for it seems to be an acrid and irritating matter, which lying on the nerve, preys on the stamina, and gives rise to pain."[4] Cortugno's description distinguished sciatica from generalized low back pain. In 1824, Bell[5] provided a model description of posttraumatic disk herniation. In 1841, Valleix[3,6] described the gross and microscopic details of the intervertebral disk in autopsy findings of a patient who died after a severe injury with a fractured disk. In 1858, Von Luschka[7] provided the first descriptions of a posterior protrusion of a disk, although he attached no clinical significance to this finding and made no correlation to sciatica. Brissaud[3,8] coined the term *sciatic scoliosis*.

The first diskectomy dates back to 1908 by Krause.[9] In 1911, Middleton and Teacher,[10,11] a practicing physician and a pathologist at Glasgow University, described classic disk extrusion in a man after a lifting incident with the "feeling of a crack" in the small of his back. Goldthwait,[12] commonly known for his description of facet joint arthropathy, in 1911 showed that the anulus fibrosus with pulpi nucleus may produce paralysis by loosening and backward projection. Since then, multiple physicians from all over the world have described their experiences with various types of disk surgery.[3,13–18] As a result of mistakes in semantics and descriptions, the final credit for disk herniation went to Mixter and Barr[19] in 1934 (**Figs. 89.2 and 89.3**). In their classic publication, they described a herniated lumbar disk as the cause of radiculopathy. In 1948, Hirsch[20] confirmed the disk as the cause of sciatica by injecting procaine into a patient's disk, which resulted in sciatica. Spinal fusion for disk disease was first attempted in 1891 by Hadra.[21]

In 1880, Forst[22] described the Lasègue test (**Fig. 89.4**).[23] In 1885, Roentgen,[24] a Holland-born physicist of German ancestry, received a Nobel prize for discovering the x-ray (**Fig. 89.5**). Dandy[25] introduced the myelogram in 1918. Sicard discovered the importance of spinal myelography.[26] Lindblom[27] first reported diskography in 1948. In 1961, Oldendorf,[28] a neurologist at the University of California, Los Angeles, envisioned computed tomography (CT; **Fig. 89.6**), with rapid developments by others.[29,30] CT scan was followed by the development of magnetic resonance imaging (MRI).[3]

After the descriptions of Mixter and Barr,[19] it was assumed that the mechanical deformation of the nerve root induced by displaced disk material was the primary cause of the symptoms, and the surgical removal of the herniated mass was the preferred treatment. Since then, however, numerous experimental studies have indicated the complex mechanism of pathogenesis of sciatica or lumbar radiculopathy.[31–34] Now, radicular pain is recognized to be evoked by stimulation of the sensory (dorsal) root of a spinal nerve, or its dorsal root ganglion.[31–41] Radicular pain is not synonymous with radiculopathy, however.[42] In contrast to radicular pain, radiculopathy pertains to a pathologic state in which a disorder affects the function of nerve roots.[33,42]

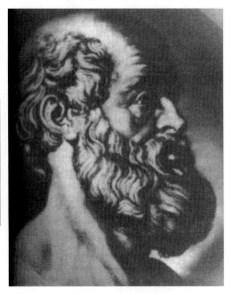

Fig. 89.1 **Hippocrates (1460-1375 BC).**

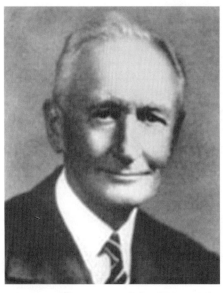

Fig. 89.2 **William Jason Mixter (1880-1958), Boston.**

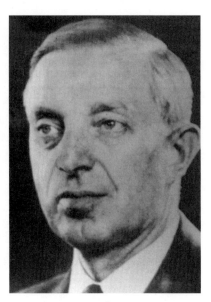

Fig. 89.3 **Joseph Seaton Barr (1901-1964), Boston.**

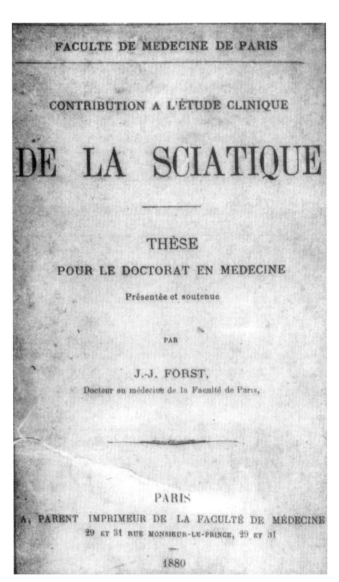

Fig. 89.4 **Title page of Forst's thesis on the "Lasègue" test.**

Clinical Syndrome

Etiology

Radicular pain is a single and subjective clinical feature.[42] It can be a feature of radiculopathy, along with numbness or weakness or both, but it can occur alone. Radiculopathy is separate from radicular pain, with a combination of numbness, motor loss, and pain, depending on which fibers in the nerve roots are affected and how they are affected.[33,42] Any lesion that affects the lumbosacral nerve roots may cause radiculopathy, radicular pain, or both.[42] The most common lesion that causes radiculopathy or radicular pain is lumbar disk herniation; it accounts for 98% of radicular pain or radiculopathy. Multiple other causes account for approximately 2% of cases of radiculopathy or radicular pain. They include vertebral causes (e.g., spinal stenosis, spondylolisthesis, osteophytosis, vertebral subluxation); neuromeningeal causes (e.g., meningeal cysts, ossification of dura, nerve root anomalies); neoplastic causes of radicular pain (e.g., benign and malignant tumors); and infectious, vascular, cystic, and miscellaneous causes.

Experimental studies have indicated that the epidural presence of the herniated part of the disk, the nucleus pulposus, may induce structural and functional changes in the adjacent nerve roots and sensitize the nerve root to produce pain when deformed mechanically.[35–40] The intervertebral disk and posterior longitudinal ligament have been shown to contain free nerve endings.[42–47] The outer third of the anulus is richly innervated,[44–46] and nerve fibers may extend as deeply as the middle third of the anulus. In patients with chronic low back pain and abnormal disks, however, the nerve supply may extend even more deeply into the anulus and nucleus.[47–50]

Pain from disk herniation can arise from nerve root compression and stimulation of nociceptors in the anulus or posterior longitudinal ligament. A simple compression or mass effect cannot be the mechanism of pain from disk disease. Several studies that evaluated progressive disk herniation showed that even though the resolution of symptoms tends to be associated with diminution of a disk herniation's size, it is not always the case because compression may continue

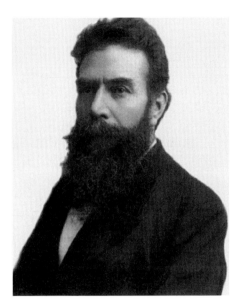

Fig. 89.5 **William Conrad Roentgen (1845-1923).**

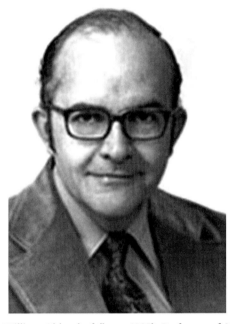

Fig. 89.6 **William Oldendorf (born 1925), Professor of Neurology and Psychiatry, University of California at Los Angeles.**

despite the resolution of symptoms.[51–55] In 1935, Mixter and Ayers,[56] only a year after the landmark description of Mixter and Barr,[19] showed that radicular pain can occur without disk herniation. The pathophysiology of lumbar radicular pain is a subject of not only ongoing research, but also controversy.

Proposed etiologies include neural compression with dysfunction, vascular compromise, inflammation, and biochemical influences.[31] Spinal nerve roots have unique properties that might explain their proclivity to produce symptoms.[57] Spinal nerve roots, in contrast to peripheral nerves, lack a well-developed intraneural blood-nerve barrier, which probably makes them more susceptible to symptomatic compression injury than peripheral nerves and makes them more vulnerable to endoneural edema formation.[58–60] Endoneural edema can be induced by increased vascular permeability, which is caused by mechanical nerve root compression.[58,59] Elevated

endoneural fluid pressure, caused by intraneural edema, also can impede capillary blood flow and might cause intraneural fibrosis,[58] which may play a crucial role in lumbar radiculopathy because spinal nerve roots receive approximately 58% of their nutrition from the surrounding cerebrospinal fluid (CSF).[57–60] Perineural fibrosis, by interfering with CSF-mediated nutrition, might render nerve roots hyperesthetic and hypersensitive to compressive forces.[57–59] In addition, reports have shown that venous and capillary stasis with congestion also might contribute to symptomatic nerve root syndromes.[58,59] Consequently, nerve root ischemia or venous stasis, or both, might generate pathologic biochemical changes, which cause radicular pain.[58]

Another complicating factor has been that the occlusion pressure for radicular arterioles is significantly higher in experimentally induced ischemia through nerve root compression, whereas compensatory nutrition from CSF diffusion during low-pressure radicular compression is probably inadequate in the presence of either epidural inflammation or fibrosis.[57,59] Rapid onset of neural and vascular compromise also was shown to be more likely to produce symptomatic radiculopathy than gradual mechanical deformity.[59–63] Inflammation has taken a central role in recent years since the description by McCarron and colleagues[64] of nucleus pulposus producing a marked epidural inflammatory reaction in dogs. Since then, many investigators have shown the inflammatogenic properties of the nucleus pulposus and its role in producing spinal pain.[36–38,40,41,65–74] Studies after exposure to autologous nucleus pulposus have shown myelin and axonal injury to the nerve roots and reduced nerve conduction velocities.[38,59] Some of these descriptions are contradicted, however, with more recent studies that suggest that normal frozen and hyaluronidase-digested nucleus pulposus in experimentally degenerated nucleus pulposus failed to produce similar changes in nerve root function.[75,76] An autoimmune or chemical basis for lumbar radicular pain was postulated in 1977.[77,78] Extensive literature has been published focusing attention on multiple agents, such as phospholipase A_2, metalloproteinase, interleukin-6, prostaglandin E_2, and tumor necrosis factor.[79]

Signs and Symptoms

Bogduk and Govind[80] stated that finding a comprehensive definition of radicular pain's clinical features in the literature is difficult. Classically, radicular pain has been described as following a dermatomal distribution. Research has shown, however, that radicular pain, whether caused by disk herniation or spinal stenosis, may not follow a dermatomal distribution.[80–82] Typical radicular pain is described with a distribution pattern of the entire length of the lower extremity, specifically below the knee; with a pattern describing a narrow band, traveling quasisegmentally but not dermatomally, and not distinguishable by segment; with a shooting, lancinating quality, perhaps like an electric shock; and with a depth described as both deep and superficial.[80] The distinguishing features of lumbar radicular pain and somatic referred pain are shown in **Table 89.1**. Haldeman, Shouka, and Robboy[83] showed that pain below the knee is neither a valid indicator of radiculopathy nor of abnormalities on electrodiagnostic studies and findings of nerve root compression on CT scan.

Table 89.1 Features of Somatic and Radicular Pain

	Somatic or Referred Pain	Radicular Pain
SEGMENT CAUSES	Posterior segment or element Facet joint pain Sacroiliac joint pain Myofascial syndrome Internal disk disruption	Anterior segment Disk herniation Annular tear Spinal stenosis
SYMPTOMS QUALITY	Dull, aching, deep Like an expanding pressure Poorly localized Back worse than leg No paresthesia Covers a wide area No radicular or shooting pain	Sharp, shooting, superficial, lancinating Like an electrical shock Leg worse than back Paresthesia present Well-defined and localized Radicular distribution
MODIFICATION	Worse with extension Better with flexion No radicular pattern	Worse with flexion Better with extension Radicular pattern
RADIATION	Low back to hip, thigh, groin Radiation below knee unusual Quasisegmental	Follows nerve root distribution Radiation below knee common Radicular pattern
SIGNS		
Sensory Alteration	Uncommon	Probable
Motor Changes	Only subjective weakness Atrophy rare	Objective weakness Atrophy possibly present
REFLEX CHANGES	None	Commonly described, but seen only occasionally
STRAIGHT LEG RAISES	Only low back pain No root tension signs	Reproduction of leg pain Positive root tension signs

Lumbosacral radicular pain is felt in the lower extremity when L4, L5, S1, or S2 nerve roots are involved. The pain typically radiates along the back of the thigh, into the leg, and into the foot. In contrast, radicular pain from L1, L2, and L3, is felt in the lower abdominal wall, groin, and anterior thigh. The pain might not follow the corresponding dermatomes, however, and it might not be distinguishable on the basis of the distribution.[81] Lumbar radicular pain has been described as radiating into the lower extremity along a narrow band not more than 5 to 8 cm wide.[84] This narrow band is one of the more distinguishing characteristics separating it from somatic referred pain. In contrast to radicular pain, somatic pain is felt in a wide region described in the patterns of a patch or a region rather than a band.[85] Experimental studies have shown that radicular pain is shooting or lancinating in character,[84-86] rather than dull or aching.[80] Although somatic pain may be felt deeply, radicular pain is the only pain felt superficially in the skin (see Table 89.1).[85,87] Radicular pain is most likely to travel below the knee, and somatic referred pain is most often limited to above the knee, but radicular pain may be restricted to the thigh or posterior hip, and somatic pain may radiate below the knee.[88,89] Symptoms may be confusing because radicular and somatic pain may coexist.

Deyo, Rainville, and Kent[90] analyzed the sensitivity and specificity of a patient's history for the diagnosis of tumors, spinal stenosis, spinal osteomyelitis, herniated disks, and compression fractures. They showed that a history of malignancy disease was the most specific information for tumor (0.98) but had comparatively low sensitivity, whereas pain when resting in bed had high sensitivity (0.90) and low specificity. Sciatica was highly sensitive for a clinically important herniated disk, as was old age for spinal stenosis and compression fractures.

Subjective symptom of numbness is considered reasonably sensitive (0.76), but not specific (0.33), as a sign of radiculopathy.[83] The objective sensory loss may indicate the segment involved more appropriately if the radicular pain is accompanied by sensory loss. Objective signs of numbness are reasonably sensitive, although numbness is not specific as a sign of radiculopathy.

Physical findings involving straight leg raising are reasonably specific for radicular pain from disk herniation.[90] Cross-leg straight leg raising is superior to ipsilateral straight leg raising. Straight leg raising and objective sensory loss correlate well with positive findings on electrodiagnostic tests and compressive features on CT scan.[83] Deyo, Rainville, and Kent[90] showed that in older age groups, spinal stenosis becomes a more significant problem. Neurologic impairment identification is important to diagnosis and treatment. Ipsilateral imitation of straight leg raising is common, but nonspecific. In contrast, cross-leg straight leg raising is less sensitive, but more specific. Other neurologic signs include impairment of ankle dorsiflexor weakness, with a sensitivity of 0.9 and specificity of 0.54; great toe extensor weakness, with a sensitivity of 0.2 to 0.57 and specificity of 0.71 to 0.82; ankle reflex, with a sensitivity of 0.52 and specificity of 0.62; patellar reflex, with a sensitivity of 0.04 and specificity of 0.93 to 0.97; quadriceps weakness, with a sensitivity of approximately 0.5 and specificity of 0.99; and ankle plantar flexor weakness with a sensitivity of 0.06 and specificity of 0.95.

Physical Examination

A neurologic and musculoskeletal examination is carried out in evaluation of a patient with symptoms of radiculopathy or radicular pain. **Fig. 89.7** illustrates the clinical features of disk herniation at various levels.[91] Objective neurologic signs of radiculopathy, with dermatomal abnormalities, myotomal weakness, reflex inhibition, and positive straight leg raising, indicate radiculopathy. The clinical examination does not differentiate, however, among a multitude of causes in disk herniation even though a few of the causes were described previously from all the tests; straight leg raising has the best sensitivity, but low specificity.[92] The other clinical tests have modest to poor sensitivities and specificities. Combinations of multiple tests considered together also have not been shown to improve likelihood ratios.[92] During the history and physical examination, the following three elements are important in the diagnosis of lumbar disk herniation:

1. Predominant leg or radicular pain below the knee in a dermatomal distribution
2. Nerve root tension signs with straight leg raising between 30 and 70 degrees or a positive cross-leg straight leg raising
3. Corroboration of neurologic signs with muscle weakness and wasting, sensory impairment, and reflex suppression

The physical findings may be corroborated with imaging or electrophysiologic studies.

Diagnostic Tests

Imaging

Imaging's objective is to show pain's cause and location.[93] Although plain radiography is the most common imaging technique, it does not satisfy the objective of identification of the cause of the pain. The major utility of plain films is exclusion of systemic pathology. Plain radiography's value, if any, is limited to the demonstration of foraminal stenosis, tumors, and infections.

In contrast to plain radiography, CT scan and MRI are powerful and reliable tools for the investigation of lumbar radicular pain. Both tests are reasonably reliable and valid. Because of its greater resolution of soft tissues and intraosseous tissues, MRI is considered superior to CT scan for the demonstration of conditions such as nerve tumors, cysts, infection, and other disorders. In contrast, CT scan is superior to MRI in the demonstration of bone and is the preferred modality for diagnosing of complex fractures or deformities. Studies show, however, that sensitivity and specificity for plain CT, CT myelography, and MRI are the same, with an approximate sensitivity of 0.90 and specificity of 0.70. A positive and negative predictive value of 0.82 is also the same for all three modalities.[94,95] Compared with surgical findings, CT has an accuracy of 77% to 92%, and MRI has an accuracy of 76% to 90%.[96–99] Studies in asymptomatic volunteers also have shown a high prevalence of disk abnormalities.

On CT scan, a herniated nucleus pulposus was evident in 20% of individuals younger than 40 years and in 27% of individuals older than 40 years.[95] On MRI, disk bulges and disk herniations occurred with increasing frequency with age, with a high prevalence of asymptomatic disk herniations.[100,101] A positive relationship with symptoms and disk herniation has been

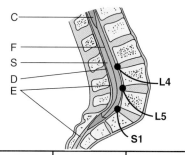

Herniation	L3–4	L4–5	L5–S1
Nerve root	**L4**	**L5**	**S1**
Pain	Low back ► hip ► antero-lateral thigh ► medial leg	Above S-1 joint ► hip ► lateral thigh and leg ► dorsum of foot	Above S-1 joint ► hip ► posterolateral thigh and leg ► heel
Numbness	Anteromedial thigh and knee	Lateral leg and first 3 toes	Back of calf ► lateral heel and foot ► toe
Atrophy	Quadriceps	Minor or non-specific	Gastrocnemius and soleus
Motor weakness	Extension of quadriceps	Dorsiflexion of great toe and foot	Plantar flexion of great toe and foot
Screening exam	Squat and rise	Heel walking	Walking on toes
Reflexes	Knee jerk diminished	None reliable	Ankle jerk diminished

Fig. 89.7 **Clinical features of a posterolateral lumbar intervertebral disk herniation.** *C,* Conus medullaris; *D,* dural tube; *E,* epidural space; *F,* filum terminale; *S,* subarachnoid space. *(Modified from Wilkinson JL: Neuroanatomy for medical students, Bristol, 1986, John Wright & Sons, p. 46; Keim HA, Kirkaldy-Willis WH: Low back pain, Clin Symp 39:18, 1987; and Bigos S, Bowyer O, Braen G, et al: Acute low back problems in adults: practice guideline, quick reference guide number 14: AHCPR Pub. No. 95-0643, Rockville, MD, 1994, US Department of Health and Human Services, Public Health Service, Agency for Health Care Policy and Research, 1994. Adapted from Giles LG: Diagnosis of mechanical low back pain with or without referred leg pain. In Giles LG and Singer KP, editors: Clinical anatomy and management of low back pain, vol 1, Oxford, 1997, Butterworth-Heinemann, p 322.)*

shown in some cases, but not all.[52,54,96,102–104] Symptoms from large disk herniations tend to improve better than symptoms from small herniations, and resolution of symptoms correlates with reduction in size of the large herniations. Large herniations are reduced in size to a greater extent than smaller herniations.

Contrast-enhanced MRI shows inflammatory changes surrounding affected nerve roots. No consistent relationship, however, is found between enhancement and the presence or severity of clinical symptoms or signs.[93,96] Although no major differences are seen between CT and MRI, the use of CT myelography has been attractive for spinal stenosis even though it has not been presented in sufficient detail in the literature to allow calculation of sensitivity and specificity.

Neurophysiologic Studies

Electromyography identifies signs of denervation and muscles innervated by the affected nerve root. The utility of electrophysiologic studies has been based on the ability to objectify abnormalities of nerve conduction resulting from radiculopathy and to identify the particular segment. Andersson and colleagues,[105] in a consensus summary on the diagnosis and treatment of lumbar disk herniation, concluded that "although neurophysiological testing is frequently used to diagnose patients with radiculopathy associated with disk herniation, these tests are not clinically necessary to confirm the presence of radiculopathy." These investigators added that neurophysiologic testing can determine the chronicity and severity of spinal nerve root lesions and differentiate the nervous system level of involvement (i.e., cord, peripheral nerve, and muscle). Neurophysiologic testing might be appropriate when the clinical situation is less clearly delineated and for differentiation of a disk herniation from other neurologic disorders, such as neuropathy or peripheral nerve entrapment.

Differential Diagnosis

An important differential diagnosis to consider in radiculopathy is compression or irritation of the nerve root by sources other than disk herniation, spinal stenosis, or diskogenic pain with disk herniation. Although prevalence of all these conditions is extremely low, the list is long, and the exercise is tedious. The list is detailed in a monograph by Bogduk and Govind.[32]

Kirkaldy-Willis and Hill[106] described five nerve entrapment sites as follows:

1. Anterior to the dura and nerve sleeves: the sinuvertebral and spinal nerves from the disk
2. In the medial part of the nerve canal: the spinal nerves
3. In the posterolateral part of the main spinal canal: the cauda equina from enlarged posterior joints
4. In the lateral part of the nerve canal: spinal and sinuvertebral nerves from subluxed and enlarged superior articular processes
5. At the posterior joints: the medial branches of the posterior primary rami

The five frequently seen syndromes are:

1. Herniation of the nucleus pulposus
2. Central spinal stenosis
3. Nerve entrapment in the lateral recess
4. Sacroiliac and piriformis syndromes
5. Facet joint pain

Facet joint pain is the easiest to identify based on somatic and radicular pain and diagnostic blocks; however, sacroiliac and piriformis syndromes, herniated disk, spinal stenosis, and lateral recess entrapment have similar features and warrant differential diagnosis.

Sacroiliac and piriformis syndromes might manifest with lower extremity pain but without low back pain. The usual presentation is buttock, trochanteric, and posterior thigh pain, which rarely radiates as far as the ankle.[106] Sensory changes are rarely described.

Central spinal stenosis resulting in lumbar radiculopathy is differentiated by pain on walking that is relieved by rest, the feeling that the legs are going to give way, a feeling of cold or numbness in the legs, a feeling that the legs are made of rubber and do not belong to the patient, and night pain that is relieved by walking. Radiologic evaluation often differentiates this from disk herniation.[106]

Lateral recess stenosis with nerve entrapment mostly resembles facet joint pain or sacroiliac syndrome. Low back pain is often absent, and muscle weakness is rare. The pain may radiate all the way into the ankle and occasionally into toes. Radiologic examination often differentiates it from lumbar radiculopathy from disk herniation.

Disk herniation has a typical presentation as described previously. Atypical presentations have been described in which the herniation is central and does not entrap the L5 or S1 nerves; L3-L4 herniation produces anterior thigh pain, quadriceps weakness, and the sensation that the legs are missing. A higher lesion with lateral herniation produces lower abdominal and scrotal pain, occasionally confused with renal or ureteric disorders. **Table 89.2** illustrates the diagnostic features for various levels of nerve root involvement.

Treatment

Lumbar radicular pain or radiculopathy may be treated with conservative management, interventional techniques, or surgical treatment.

Conservative Management

Conservative treatments include back school, exercises to teach spinal stabilization, strengthening exercises, flexibility exercises, and drug therapy. In management of acute and subacute radicular pain, limited evidence shows that nonsteroidal anti-inflammatory drugs (NSAIDs) do not provide effective pain relief for nerve root pain.[107] Strong evidence also shows that different types of NSAIDs are equally effective. NSAIDs can have serious adverse effects, particularly at high doses and in elderly patients.

Muscle relaxants have not been studied in radicular pain. Strong evidence, however, shows that muscle relaxants effectively reduce acute low back pain; the different types of muscle relaxants are equally effective. Muscle relaxants also have significant adverse effects, including drowsiness, and carry a significant risk of habituation and dependency, even after relatively short courses. Systemic steroids have been shown to have the same effectiveness as a placebo in management of radicular pain.[108]

Only limited evidence indicates that bed rest is effective in management of acute disk prolapse or nerve root pain.[109] Limited evidence shows that bed rest with traction is not effective. Traction essentially may add complications to immobilization

Table 89-2 Diagnostic Features for Various Levels of Nerve Root Involvement

Herniation	Nerve Root	Pain	Numbness	Atrophy	Motor Weakness	Screening Examination	Relexes
L3-4	L4	Low back; hip anterolateral thigh; medial leg	Anteromedial thigh and knee	Quadriceps	Extension of quadriceps	Squat and rise	Knee jerk diminished
L4-5	L5	Above S1 joint; hip; lateral thigh and leg; dorsum of foot	Lateral leg and first 3 toes	Minor or nonspecific	Dorsiflexion of great toe and foot	Heel walking	None reliable
L5-S1	S1	Above S1 joint; hip; posterolateral and thigh leg; heel	Back of calf; lateral heel and foot; toe	Gastrocnemius and soleus	Plantar flexion of great toe and foot	Walking on toes	Ankle jerk diminished

with deleterious effects, in particular, joint stiffness, muscle wasting, loss of bone mass, pressure sores, and thromboembolism.[110]

Strong evidence is found that most types of specific back exercises (e.g., flexion, extension, aerobics, or strengthening exercises) are not more effective than alternative treatments for acute low back pain, with which they have been compared, including no intervention.[107] Conflicting evidence, however, is seen that McKenzie's exercises might produce some short-term symptomatic improvement in acute low back pain.[107] Back schools have been shown to have conflicting evidence on their effectiveness in management of low back pain.

Manipulation has been shown to have moderate evidence that it is more effective than a placebo treatment for short-term pain relief of acute low back pain.[107] Transcutaneous electrical nerve stimulation (TENS) was shown to have conflicting evidence regarding its effectiveness in the treatment of acute low back pain.[107] Other modalities, including ice, heat, short-wave diathermy, massage, and ultrasound scan, for the treatment of acute low back pain have been shown to be ineffective.[107]

For chronic low back pain, the following modalities have been studied:

1. Exercise therapy: Strong evidence shows that exercise therapy is effective, and moderate evidence shows that various exercises are equally effective.[111]
2. Back schools: Limited evidence showed that an intensive back school program in an occupational setting in Scandinavia was more effective than no actual treatment. Conflicting evidence is found on the effectiveness of back schools in nonoccupational settings and outside Scandinavia.
3. Behavioral therapy: Multidimensional programs that include cognitive behavioral therapy programs are statistically and clinically superior to control groups on key outcome variables. Compared with active treatment, however, cognitive behavioral treatment has a small to moderate effect on outcome variables. Cognitive behavioral treatment programs seem to have their largest effects on psychologic function, pain, physical function, and medication intake.[112]
4. Multidisciplinary pain treatment programs: Strong evidence is seen that a multidisciplinary treatment program aimed at functional restoration is useful for patients with long-lasting, severe, chronic low back pain.[111]
5. Manual therapy: Moderate evidence shows that manual therapy is more effective than usual care by the general practitioner, bed rest, analgesics, and massage for short-term pain relief. Limited and conflicting evidence is found of any long-term effect.[111]
6. Traction: Strong evidence is seen that traction has no effect in treatment of chronic low back pain.[111]
7. Arthrosis: Limited evidence shows that a lumbar corset with support may produce some subjective improvement.[111]
8. TENS: Inconsistent evidence is found regarding whether TENS is effective.[111]
9. *Acupuncture:* Inconsistent evidence is found regarding whether acupuncture is effective.

Interventional Techniques

Epidural steroids in the lumbar spine are administered transforaminally, caudally, or via interlaminar route.[113–115] Synthesis of evidence on epidural steroid injections by Manchikanti and colleagues[79] was comprehensive. Evidence from other reviews was conflicting, however.[116–120] Manchikanti and colleagues[79] evaluated the evidence based on short-term relief (≤6 months) or long-term relief (>6 months). The results were as follows:

The indicated evidence was Level I for caudal epidural injections in management of disk herniation or radiculitis and diskogenic pain without disk herniation or radiculitis.[113] The evidence was Level II-1 or II-2 for caudal epidural injections in management of pain of post–lumbar surgery syndrome and lumbar spinal stenosis and for lumbar transforaminal epidural injections.[113]

Surgical Treatment
Percutaneous Disk Decompression

The primary goal of surgical treatment of a disk prolapse, protrusion, or extrusion is the relief of nerve root compression with removal of the herniated nuclear material.[121–123] Surgical interventions include surgical diskectomy, chemonucleolysis (not available in the United States), and microdiskectomy. Several alternative techniques to open diskectomy and microdiskectomy include automated percutaneous laser diskectomy (APLD), percutaneous lumbar laser diskectomy (PLLD), mechanical disk decompression with a high rotation-per-minute (RPM) device or DeKompressor (Stryker, Kalamazoo, MI), and nucleoplasty. All the techniques were assessed systematically.[124–127]

Automated Percutaneous Lumbar Diskectomy

According to Hirsch et al,[124] the indicated level of evidence is Level II-2 for short-term and long-term relief for APLD.

Percutaneous Lumbar Laser Diskectomy

Singh et al[125] showed the indicated level of evidence as Level II-2 for short-term and long-term relief.

Nucleoplasty

Manchikanti et al[127] showed the indicated evidence for nucleoplasty as Level II-3 in management of predominantly lower extremity pain from contained disk herniation. No evidence was available for axial low back pain. Gerges et al[128] also found similar results.

Mechanical High Rotation-per-Minute Device

Singh et al[126] showed the indicated evidence for Dekompressor as Level III for short-term and long-term relief.

Surgical Diskectomy

Limited direct evidence was found on the efficacy of surgical diskectomy for lumbar disk prolapse.[121,122,129]

Chemonucleolysis

Strong indirect evidence from randomized controlled trials of chemonucleolysis showed that diskectomy is more effective than chemonucleolysis, which in turn is more effective than placebo.[122] Diskectomy provided faster relief from an acute attack, although any positive or negative effects on the lifetime natural history of disk problems are unclear.[122]

Strong evidence was found that chemonucleolysis with chymopapain produced better clinical outcomes than placebo.[122]

Microdiskectomy

Strong evidence showed that microdiskectomy and standard diskectomy give broadly comparable clinical outcomes.[122]

Side Effects and Complications

Apart from long-lasting disability, disk herniation complications include nerve damage and cauda equina syndrome. Other complications are related to treatment; conservative management and surgical management alike have multiple side effects. All types of narcotic and non-narcotic analgesics have a multitude of side effects. Acetaminophen is associated with hepatic toxicity. NSAIDs can have serious side effects, particularly at high doses and in elderly patients. Opioids cause dizziness, respiratory depression, central nervous system dysfunction, and dependency and addiction. Significant adverse effects of muscle relaxants include drowsiness and a significant risk of habituation and dependency. Bed rest is associated with deconditioning; traction adds to other complications of immobilization, including muscle wasting, loss of bone density, pressure sores, and thromboembolism. Although manipulation risks are low, serious complications could occur and result in severe or progressive neurologic deficit. Manipulation with anesthesia also is associated with an increased risk of serious neurologic damage.[111]

Interventional techniques also have multiple complications.[79] Needle placement and drug administration are the most common and worrisome complications of caudal, interlaminar, and transforaminal epidural injections. Complications include dural puncture, spinal cord trauma, infection, hematoma formation, abscess formation, subdural injection, intracranial air injection, epidural lipomatosis, pneumothorax, nerve damage, headache, death, brain damage, increased intracranial pressure, intravascular injection, vascular injury, cerebrovascular pulmonary embolus, and effects from steroids. Surgical technique complications include infection, nerve damage, spinal cord trauma, death, epidural fibrosis, and post–lumbar laminectomy syndrome.

Conclusion

Lumbar radiculopathy descriptions date back to the Hippocratic collection describing sciatica. Since the early descriptions of sciatica, numerous experimental studies have indicated the complex mechanism of sciatic pathogenesis or lumbar radiculopathy. Radicular pain is a subjective clinical feature; however, it can be a feature of radiculopathy, along with neurologic symptoms and signs.

Lumbar disk herniation is reliably diagnosed with three history examination elements, including predominant leg or radicular pain below the knee in a dermatomal distribution, nerve root tension signs, and corroborating neurologic signs. Imaging with CT scan and MRI seems to be equally beneficial. Neurophysiologic studies are indicated to differentiate a disk herniation from other neurologic disorders, such as neuropathy or peripheral nerve entrapment.

Among the numerous modalities of treatments available in management of lumbar radiculopathy, the effectiveness of physical modalities, manipulation, and traction in patients with lumbar disk herniation is inadequately studied and controversial. Similarly, the effectiveness of different types of exercise programs for the treatment of patients with lumbar disk herniation has not been determined. Moderate evidence is found that caudal epidural steroids are effective in disk herniation and radiculopathy, whereas strong evidence shows that transforaminal epidural steroids are effective. Microdiskectomy and open diskectomy are effective modalities in management of radiculopathy from disk herniation.

Key Points

- Radicular pain is evoked by the stimulation of the sensory (dorsal) root of the spinal nerve, or its dorsal root ganglion. It is not synonymous with radiculopathy.
- Radiculopathy is associated with radicular pain and any combination of numbness or motor loss.
- Radicular and somatic referred pain may differ in distribution, pattern, quality, and depth, along with causation.
- Nerve root or radicular pain, root irritation signs, and root compression signs are important in the diagnosis of radiculopathy.
- Imaging should be undertaken only if warranted by the patient's clinical condition. In the absence of clinical indicators of a "red flag" condition, medical imaging is neither indicated nor warranted.

- Neurophysiologic testing is used to differentiate a disk herniation from other neurologic disorders, such as neuropathy or peripheral nerve entrapment.
- The efficacy of physical modalities, manipulation, and traction in patients with lumbar disk herniation is inadequately studied and controversial.
- The efficacy of different types of exercise programs for the treatment of patients with lumbar disk herniation has not been determined.
- Moderate evidence shows that caudal epidural steroids are effective in disk herniation and radiculopathy; strong evidence shows that transforaminal epidural steroids are effective.
- Microdiskectomy and open diskectomy are effective modalities of treatment in managing radiculopathy from disk herniation.

References

Full references for this chapter can be found on www.expertconsult.com.

Chapter 90

Lumbar Facet Syndrome

Nikolai Bogduk

Lumbar facet syndrome does not exist. A syndrome is a clinical entity defined, and recognized, by a specific constellation of clinical features. Reiter's syndrome is defined by the combination of urethritis, uveitis, and spondyloarthropathy. Tolosa-Hunt syndrome is headache combined with palsy of one or more of the third, fourth, or sixth cranial nerves.

No combination of clinical features defines lumbar facet syndrome. Although some proponents contended that aggravation of pain by certain movements of the back is indicative of facet syndrome,[1,2] this has been refuted by studies using controlled diagnostic blocks.[3–6] Even the features proposed by Revel et al[7] do not define a facet syndrome; they may serve to identify patients who do not have facet pain,[8] but they fail to identify those who do.[9,10]

No syndrome exists. Instead, what patients have is lumbar zygapophysial joint pain. This is an entity defined not by clinical features, but by a specific source of pain. In many circles, it is a diagnosis that is rejected or disdained, but ironically it is one of the best studied, and most strongly validated, entities in pain medicine. Those who deny this condition either simply do not want to know or are unaware of the literature and its strength.

Few, if any, other conditions in pain medicine satisfy the following theoretical and practical criteria.

- The pain has an anatomic basis.
- The pain has been produced experimentally in normal volunteers.
- The pain can be diagnosed by a test that has been validated.
- The test used to diagnose the condition protects normal volunteers from experimentally induced versions of the condition.
- When tested, patients with the condition obtain complete relief of their pain.
- When diagnosed with the condition, patients can be treated.
- When treated, patients obtain complete relief of pain.
- When pain recurs, it can again be completely relieved.

Anatomy

The lumbar zygapophysial joints are formed by the superior and inferior articular processes of consecutive lumbar vertebrae (**Fig. 90.1**). Each joint is named according the segmental numbers of the vertebrae that form it. The joint between L5 and the sacrum is known as the lumbosacral, or L5-S1 zygapophysial, joint. Each has the typical structure of a synovial joint.

The joints are innervated by the medial branches of the lumbar dorsal rami. Each joint receives articular branches from the ipsisegmental medial branch, as well as from the medial branch above[11,12] (see Fig. 90.1). The joints are therefore endowed with the necessary neurologic apparatus to be a potential source of pain.

Confusion arises around the names of the nerves that innervate each joint. The segmental numbers of the nerves are one segment less than the name of the joint. Thus, the L4-5 joint is innervated by the L3,4 medial branches, and the L5-S1 joint is innervated by the L4,5 nerves. As a matter of discipline, for clarity in communication, practitioners should take care when referring to a segment, whether they are referring to the joint or to the nerves that innervate the joint. One device is to use a hyphen (L4-5) when naming a joint but a comma (L4,5) when naming its nerves. A hyphen indicates conjunction and therefore a joint; a comma indicates a sequence and therefore a pair of nerves.

Normal Volunteers

When lumbar zygapophysial joints are stimulated experimentally with a noxious stimulus, normal volunteers suffer and describe pain that resembles that reported in patients with low back pain. The experimental stimuli that have been used include injections of hypertonic saline into the joints,[13,14] injections of contrast medium to distend the capsules of the joints,[15] and electrical stimulation of the nerves that innervate the joints.[15,16]

In all studies that have been conducted, noxious stimulation of the zygapophysial joints has produced low back pain and some degree of referred pain. Studies have differed with respect to the distribution of referred pain (**Fig. 90.2**). As a rule, the referred pain tends to radiate inferolaterally from the site of stimulation. Pain from upper lumbar zygapophysial joints extends into the loin or toward the posterior iliac crest from above. Pain from lower lumbar joints extends across the iliac crest into the buttock.

The pattern of referred pain is segmental insofar as pain from higher levels tends to be perceived in more cephalad regions than is pain from lower levels, but the pattern is not distinctive. Within and between studies, the distribution of pain from particular segments overlaps with the distribution of pain from adjacent and lower segments. Consequently, the location of referred pain cannot be used reliably to infer the exact location of its source. Although not quantified, investigators have noted qualitatively that the distance of referral appears to be proportional to the intensity of stimulation. When stronger noxious stimuli are applied, the referred pain spreads further.[13]

Also not rigorously studied, but noted in one study, experimentally induced referred pain from the lumbar zygapophysial joints can be associated with increased electromyographic activity in the hamstring muscles.[13] This finding is in accord with the more general observation that pain from structures innervated by the lumbar dorsal rami can be accompanied by involuntary activity in muscles of the lower limb.[17]

Diagnostic Blocks

Pain from a lumbar zygapophysial joint can be relieved temporarily by anesthetizing the joint. This procedure can be done by injecting local anesthetic into the cavity of the joint or by anesthetizing the medial branches that innervate the joint.

Intra-articular blocks constitute a direct test of zygapophysial joint pain and were originally promoted in orthopedic and radiologic circles.[18–34] Intra-articular blocks have face validity, in that it can be shown, by injecting contrast medium into the joint, that the local anesthetic accurately and exclusively targets the joint. However, although still used by some operators, intra-articular blocks have not been validated further. In particular, these blocks have not been subjected to controls and have not been shown to have predictive validity or therapeutic utility. Provocation of pain during injection of a joint is not diagnostic of joint pain. Provocation is not associated with subsequent relief when the joint is anesthetized.[35]

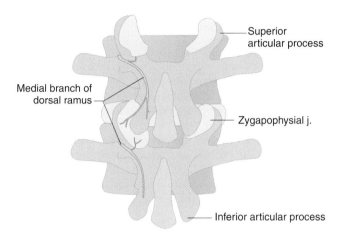

Fig. 90.1 Sketch of a posterior view of a lumbar segment that illustrates the structure and innervation of the zygapophysial joints. The zygapophysial joint is formed by the adjacent superior articular process and inferior articular process. Each is innervated by articular branches from the medial branch of the same segment and the one above.

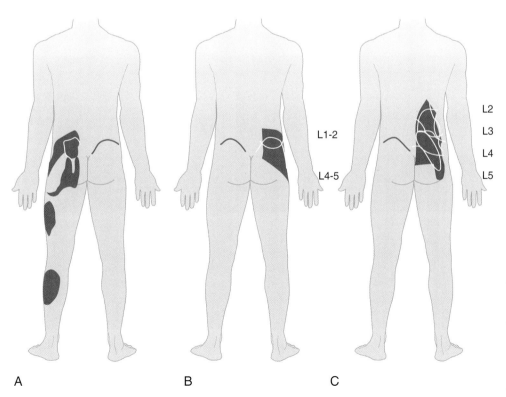

Fig. 90.2 Maps of referred pain patterns elicited from the lumbar zygapophysial joints in normal volunteers. A, Following injection of hypertonic saline into the lower lumbar joints, with segments not specified. **B,** Following injection of hypertonic saline into the L1-2 and L4-5 joints. **C,** Following electrical stimulation of the medial branches at the segments indicated. (*A, Adapted from Mooney V, Robertson J: The facet syndrome,* Clin Orthop Relat Res *115:149–156, 1976; B, adapted from McCall IW, Park WM, O'Brien JP: Induced pain referral from posterior elements in normal subjects,* Spine *4:441, 1979; and C, adapted from Windsor RE, King FJ, Roman SJ, et al: Electrical stimulation induced lumbar medial branch referral patterns,* Pain Physician *5:347, 2002.)*

In contrast, medial branch blocks have been extensively tested. They involve injecting a tiny amount of local anesthetic (0.3 mL), under fluoroscopic control, onto each of the medial branches that innervate the target joint. The blocks require a preliminary test dose of contrast medium, because in approximately 8% of cases the injection can be into the vena comitans of the medial branch.[36] Venous uptake is not a complication, given the small volume of local anesthetic injected, but it risks producing a false-negative response.

The face validity of lumbar medial branch blocks has been established. Provided that correct target points are used, the local anesthetic covers the target nerve and does not spread to affect other structures that may be alternative sources of pain. The correct target point lies midway between two points[36]: the notch between the superior articular process and the transverse process, where the medial branch enters the posterior compartment of the spine, and the mammilloaccessory notch, where it hooks medially beneath the mammilloaccessory ligament[37] (**Fig. 90.3**). When deposited in the correct location, local anesthetic surrounds the nerve reliably. It may spread dorsally into the cleavage plane between the multifidus and longissimus lumborum, or between fascicles of the multifidus at lower lumbar levels, but it does not indiscriminately anesthetize the back muscles. Target points more rostral on the transverse process risk spread of some of the local anesthetic to the intervertebral foramen, where, theoretically, the drug may affect the spinal nerve and compromise the specificity of the block. Pointing the bevel of the needle caudally guards against this direction of spread.

The L5 medial branch cannot be selectively anesthetized. At this segmental level, the target nerve is the L5 dorsal ramus itself, which runs over the ala of the sacrum. The target point is nevertheless analogous to that at typical lumbar levels. It lies opposite the middle of the base of the superior articular process of S1. Placement of the needle further rostrally risks flow of injectate to the L5-S1 intervertebral foramen. More caudal placement risks flow to the S1 posterior foramen.

The face validity of medial branch blocks was established by stimulating the lumbar zygapophysial joints, in normal volunteers, with injections of hypertonic saline, before and after medial branch blocks of the target joint. Medial branch blocks protect volunteers from experimentally induced zygapophysial joint pain.[38]

Single, uncontrolled blocks of lumbar medial branches are not valid. They have a false-positive rate of between 25% and 41%.[39-41] This means that investigators who encounter a positive response to a block cannot be certain whether the response is truly positive or falsely positive. The diagnostic confidence depends both on the false-positive rate and on the prevalence of zygapophysial joint pain. For most prevalence estimates, the diagnostic confidence is low, and the positive response is more likely to be false than true (**Table 90.1**). To achieve clinically useful diagnostic confidence, some form of control needs to be applied in all cases. Unless this is done, the diagnosis will be wrong more often than correct.

In the past, comparative local anesthetic blocks were used. These procedures involved the same block on each of two, separate occasions, with a different local anesthetic agent used on each occasion. The agents typically used were lignocaine and bupivacaine. Under these conditions, a true-positive response was defined as one in which the patient reported longer-lasting relief when the longer-acting agent was used and shorter-lasting relief when the shorter acting agent was used.

The validity of comparative blocks was established for cervical medial branch blocks.[42,43] That validity was subsequently extrapolated and applied to lumbar medial branch blocks. However, investigators have since shown that this extrapolation creates an illusion of diagnostic confidence.[44] Comparative blocks remain valid for cervical medial branch blocks because the prevalence of cervical zygapophysial joint pain is high. Comparative blocks are not valid for lumbar medial branches because the prevalence of lumbar zygapophysial joint pain is low.

Comparative blocks are not perfect. They have a sensitivity of 100% but a specificity of only 65%.[44] When applied to

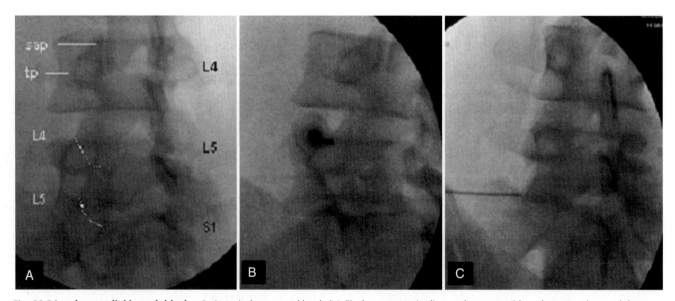

Fig. 90.3 Lumbar medial branch blocks. A, At typical segmental levels (L1-5), the target point lies on the nerve midway between the notch between the superior articular process (sap) and the transverse process (tp) and where the nerve hooks medially under the mammilloaccessory ligament. At L5, a homologous point applies lateral to the superior articular process. The numbering of the nerves *(white)* is one less than their respective vertebrae *(black)*. **B,** Oblique view of a needle in position for an L4 medial branch block. **C,** Anteroposterior view of a needle in position for an L5 dorsal ramus block.

low prevalence rates, these values yield low diagnostic confidence (**Table 90.2**). For typical prevalence rates of 15% or 5%, the diagnostic confidence is so low that the diagnosis will be wrong twice or seven times as often as correct.

The only means by which to be confident of a correct diagnosis of lumbar zygapophysial joint pain is to perform placebo controls. This procedure requires three blocks. The first block is with a local anesthetic agent, to establish prima facie that the joint is putatively symptomatic. The second block uses either an inactive agent or another local anesthetic. The third block uses the agent not used for the second block. Under these conditions, the response is considered positive when the patient obtains complete relief of pain whenever a local anesthetic is used but no relief when the placebo is used.

Some practitioners, and some insurers, object to controlled blocks. Mistaken, or misguided, they believe that they can diagnose zygapophysial joint pain with a single block, and that controlled blocks simply increase costs. This attitude overlooks the cost of false-positive responses. If only single blocks are used, diagnosis will be false in more than 60% of cases, and all subsequent decisions about these patients will be founded on a false premise. Cost saving pays for diagnostic noise and therapeutic failure. Meanwhile an economic study showed that, even at modest rates of reimbursement, controlled blocks are cost effective.[45]

Clinical Features

Lumbar zygapophysial joint pain has no clinical diagnostic features. The patient has lumbar spinal pain and may have somatic referred pain into the lower limb. Most often, the pain is referred only to the region of the buttock or proximal thigh, but it can extend beyond the knee and even into the foot. It is not true that pain below the knee always represents sciatica. Pain distal to the knee has successfully been relieved, in some patients, by anesthetizing lower lumbar zygapophysial joints.[13,25]

No associated features, however, are unique to lumbar zygapophysial joint pain. Aggravation of pain by any movements or by any applied, clinical maneuver does not distinguish lumbar zygapophysial joint pain from pain stemming from other sources.[3–6] This finding should not be surprising. All the elements of the lumbar spine share a similar segmental innervation. Therefore, the symptoms that they produce should be similar. No movement selectively stresses just the zygapophysial joints. The disk is also stressed by movement, along with ligaments and muscles. Therefore, all sources of pain should be aggravated in a similar manner by movement.

Nevertheless, this lack of distinctive clinical features is not an indictment of the condition. Demands for a distinctive, clinical syndrome are based on the cynical and artificial expectation that all disorders in medicine must have distinctive features, and that if they do not, they cannot exist. Elsewhere in medicine, conditions abound that do not constitute distinctive clinical syndromes. Most causes of chest pain cannot be determined unless and until investigations such as radiography are performed. Most causes of abdominal pain are not distinctive until imaging, laboratory tests, ultrasound scans, or endoscopic examinations are performed. For lumbar zygapophysial joint pain, the definitive test consists of placebo-controlled, diagnostic blocks.

Prevalence

Multiple studies have provided estimates of the prevalence of lumbar zygapophysial joint pain. The prevalence estimates differ according to the population studied and the criteria used to define a positive response.

Table 90.1 Selected Examples of How Different Prevalence Rates and Different False-Positive Rates Affect the Diagnostic Confidence that a Positive Response to a Single Diagnostic Block Is Truly Positive

Prevalence (%)	False-Positive Rate (%)	Single Block	Joint Pain* Yes	Joint Pain* No	Diagnostic Confidence (%)
30	25	Positive	30	18	63
		Negative	0	52	
	41	Positive	30	29	51
		Negative	0	41	
15	25	Positive	15	21	42
		Negative	0	64	
	41	Positive	15	35	30
		Negative	0	50	
5	25	Positive	5	24	17
		Negative	0	71	
	41	Positive	5	39	9
		Negative	0	56	

*Percent of patients who experience joint pain.

Table 90.2 Selected Examples of How Different Prevalence Rates Affect the Diagnostic Confidence that a Positive Response to a Comparative Diagnostic Block Is Truly Positive

Prevalence (%)	Comparative Block	Joint Pain* Yes	Joint Pain* No	Diagnostic Confidence (%)
30	Positive	30	24	55
	Negative	0	46	
15	Positive	15	30	33
	Negative	0	55	
5	Positive	5	33	13
	Negative	0	62	

*Percent of patients who experience joint pain.

Among injured workers, with a median age of 38 years, the prevalence was found to be 15% (95% confidence interval, 10% to 20%).[4] In an older population, without a history of trauma, it was found to be 40% (27% to 53%).[5] A similar prevalence (45%; 39% to 54%) was found in a heterogeneous population attending a pain clinic.[40]

These figures, however, may constitute an overestimate, because the studies often used a generous criterion for a positive response to blocks. These studies considered that results were positive for anyone who had greater than 50% relief of pain. This response falls short of 100% relief, which would be more compelling evidence that the zygapophysial joint tested was the sole source of pain.

When complete relief of pain has been the required criterion for a positive response to blocks, the prevalence in general populations has been 7% or 5%.[9,10,46,47] This finding suggests that the prevalence of lumbar zygapophysial joint pain is substantially lower than commonly believed.

A modifying factor is the nature of the population tested. Whereas lumbar zygapophysial joint pain seems uncommon in younger, injured workers, it may be more common in older persons. Using placebo controls and a criterion of 90% relief, a study of older patients reported a prevalence of 32%.[5]

Pathology

The pathologic basis of lumbar zygapophysial joint pain is not known. Lumbar zygapophysial joint pain is an entity with an established source but elusive pathogenesis.

Although evident as a disease of the lumbar zygapophysial joints,[48,49] osteoarthrosis cannot be blamed. The radiologic features of osteoarthrosis, as seen radiographically,[50,51] or on computed tomography (CT),[52] do not correlate with the presence or absence of pain in the affected joint. Osteoarthrosis is a normal age change and does not constitute a basis for zygapophysial joint pain.

At postmortem examination, investigators showed that the lumbar zygapophysial joints can sustain small fractures, which are not evident in radiographs.[53,54] In principle, such lesions could be construed as likely causes of pain. Such lesions have been detected stereoradiographically in living patients.[55] However, these lesions have not been investigated with CT, or other imaging tests, and have not been correlated with zygapophysial joint pain.

Disorders that can rarely affect the lumbar zygapophysial joints are rheumatoid arthritis,[56] infection,[57-60] and pigmented villonodular synovitis.[61,62] These conditions, however, do not explain the large numbers of patients whose pain is relieved when their zygapophysial joints are anesthetized.

Treatment

Although readily diagnosed, lumbar zygapophysial joint pain is not easily treated. Few treatments, explicitly for diagnosed lumbar zygapophysial joint pain, have been tested, let alone validated. No evidence indicates that conservative therapy of any kind relieves zygapophysial joint pain, nor does evidence suggest that fusing a segment relieves zygapophysial joint pain. The tested treatments are limited to minimally invasive procedures.

Intra-articular Steroids

Perhaps the most prolific treatment for lumbar zygapophysial joint has been intra-articular injection of corticosteroids.[18-22,27-34] This treatment has a checkered past and a vexatious future.

A review of the literature showed an abundance of descriptive and observational studies on the use of intra-articular steroids for lumbar zygapophysial joint pain.[63] In none of these studies, however, was injection of steroids tested in patients with proven zygapophysial joint pain. Steroids were injected presumptively, and without controls. The reported success rates are therefore meaningless.

No rationale exists for the use of intra-articular steroids. No evidence indicates that lumbar zygapophysial joint pain is caused by inflammation. Steroids were adopted for zygapophysial joint pain simply on the strength that they appeared to be effective for osteoarthritis in joints of the limbs.

Two controlled studies denied any efficacy of intra-articular steroids. One studied patients with a presumed diagnosis of zygapophysial joint pain and found no differences in outcome among patients treated with intra-articular steroids, extra-articular steroids, or intra-articular saline solution.[64-66] The other study attempted a diagnosis and recruited patients who responded to a single diagnostic block.[47] The outcomes after intra-articular injection of steroids were no different from those after injection of normal saline solution.[47,63]

Despite the objections that have been raised about these studies, no other study has produced data that refute these negative results. Intra-articular steroids are no more effective than sham treatment.

Radiofrequency Neurotomy

Radiofrequency neurotomy is a procedure in which pain from a zygapophysial joint can be relieved by percutaneous coagulation of the nerves that innervate the joint. It, too, is a treatment with a checkered past.

This treatment was originally described as facet denervation,[67-71] and astounding results were claimed for it.[67-87] Anatomic studies showed, however, that no nerves were located where the electrode was placed.[88,89] Nonetheless, this finding did not dissuade some operators, who continued to use the discredited technique,[90,91] even in controlled trials.[92]

Anatomic studies showed that the articular branches to the zygapophysial joints could not be selectively coagulated, but their parent nerves—the medial branches of the dorsal rami—could be.[88,89] Because these nerves ran a constant course across the root of the transverse process at each segmental level, electrodes placed on that bony landmark could be relied on to incur the target nerve. These realizations converted the procedure from facet denervation to lumbar medial branch neurotomy.[88,89]

Using the modified surgical anatomy, some studies claimed successful results,[93,94] but even that technique was flawed. A laboratory study showed that electrodes do no coagulate distally from their tip.[95] Therefore, an electrode placed perpendicular to the course of the nerve would not reliably coagulate it. Because electrodes coagulate circumferentially (i.e., sideways), to coagulate the nerve, the electrode must be placed parallel to it.

This explanation has not been heeded. Operators still insist on placing electrodes perpendicular or semiperpendicular to

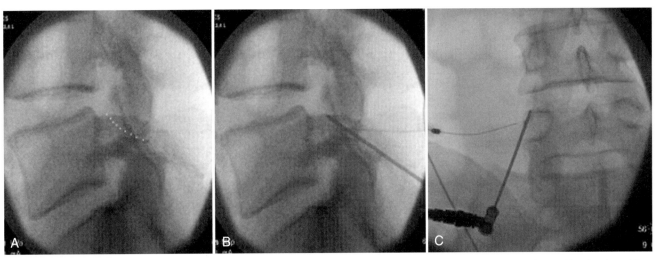

Fig. 90.4 **Lumbar radiofrequency neurotomy.** A, Lateral view of the target zone. The course of the medial branch is depicted by the *dotted lines*. B, Lateral view of the electrode in place, parallel to and on the nerve. C, Anteroposterior view of the electrode, inserted obliquely from below to lie parallel to the nerve.

the target nerve, in the manner in which block needles are introduced onto the nerve.[96–101] Doing so limits the chances of coagulating the nerve thoroughly. If the nerve is incompletely coagulated, pain may not be relieved. If only a short length of nerve is coagulated, pain relief may be only brief. Accurate technique is paramount. An anatomically accurate technique requires placing the electrode parallel to the target nerve and creating either a lesion of sufficient magnitude or a sufficient number of lesions to encompass all possible locations of the nerve[102,103] (**Fig. 90.4**).

Medial branch neurotomy is not a permanent cure. The coagulated nerve will regenerate. Pain will recur. In that event, however, the procedure can be repeated, and relief can be reinstated. One study[104] showed that, in patients whose pain recurred after an initially successful neurotomy, repeating the treatment reinstated relief. Two, three, and even four repetitions continued to provide relief. The median duration of relief following each repetition was just short of a calendar year.

Multiple systematic reviews cast doubts on the efficacy of lumbar medial branch neurotomy,[105–108] as did several practice guidelines.[109–112] In all instances, however, the procedure was misrepresented. The reviews did not recognize the importance of technical accuracy. As a result, they included studies that used refuted or flawed techniques. Not surprisingly, these studies yielded negative results. This amounts to selection bias: choosing studies for their negative results rather than studies that used correct technique. When only studies that used correct or reasonable techniques were reviewed, the evidence supported lumbar medial branch neurotomy.[113] The results of controlled trials did not refute the results of observational studies.

Three observational studies reported success rates of 80%,[114] 56%,[115] and 43%,[116] for relief of pain at up to 1 year. All three studies showed that relief of pain was associated with improvement of disability, and two studies showed reduced requirements for analgesia.[115,116]

Similar success rates were encountered in three controlled trials, two using sham treatment as the control[100, 117] and one using pulsed radiofrequency as the control.[118] All three studies showed that relief of pain was associated with reduced need for analgesics, and two studies showed improvements in disability.[100,118]

Conclusion

An irony applies. Lumbar zygapophysial joint pain is one of the best-studied and best-validated entities in pain medicine. At the same time, it is one of the most abused. Few other conditions have an established anatomic basis, have a validated diagnostic test, and have a treatment that can abolish the pain. Nonetheless, few practitioners practice according to the evidence. They do not use diagnostic blocks. They do not use placebo-controlled blocks so that their diagnosis is valid. They use treatments that do not work, yet ignore treatments that do. They claim to use a procedure that has been proven to work, but use the wrong technique. It is difficult to find another realm of medicine with so much dissonance between science and practice.

It is no wonder therefore that insurers and others are so opposed to lumbar facet syndrome and its management. They are justified in being opposed to what is practiced, but they are not justified in opposing the science. Unfortunately, those who follow the science responsibly are compromised by those who abuse it. Lack of recognition of lumbar facet syndrome is not a scientific issue; it is a social one, in which the lack of responsibility and discipline by medical practitioners is to blame.

References

Full references for this chapter can be found on www.expertconsult.com.

Chapter **91**

Occupational Back Pain

Brian McGuirk and Nikolai Bogduk

The literature on back pain is abundant. Most of it, however, is descriptive or anecdotal. Only a small proportion of it constitutes evidence. Occupational back pain may be considered a particular subset of back pain, defined by its context. It is back pain sustained at work or attributed to injury at work. It is perhaps the largest subset of back pain. This subset is also served by an extensive literature, but ironically an even smaller proportion of that literature constitutes evidence than for back pain in general.

It is not possible to compose a chapter on occupational back pain that is based exclusively on evidence. Too many issues that apply to occupational back pain have simply not been studied scientifically. Therefore, to address this problem, this chapter combines the resources of an occupational physician of some 30 years' standing with those of an academic. The chapter is based on the formula (EBM)², which stands for (Experienced-Based Medicine) × (Evidence-Based Medicine).

Overview

Occupational back pain differs from back pain in the general community because it is confounded by extraneous influences (**Fig. 91.1**). In the occupational setting, the progression from acute back pain to chronic back pain (and the prevention of progression) is governed by how the condition is managed medically, but this process is also affected by issues of certification, attribution, and compensation. Indeed, it is a common prejudice that pursuit of financial compensation is the critical driving factor that causes acute back pain to persist and become chronic. An analysis of the literature shows that this not typically the case.[1-3]

The factors that most profoundly affect the outcome of acute occupational back pain are the way in which it is managed medically and the way in which it is certified. When the pain becomes chronic, medical management remains a factor, but attribution and compensation arise as confounding issues.

Another perception is that occupational back pain is a growing problem (**Fig. 91.2**). The number of patients with chronic pain continues to increase. This increase can be attributed to inadequate or incorrect management of acute back pain. Patients present with fears and misunderstandings that are not properly addressed. Once it becomes chronic, back pain persists because no treatment is effective or because available treatments that can work are not applied. Meanwhile, authorities battle to suppress the growth of chronic back pain, not by medical means, but by legislating against it or by bringing false witness to bear when disputes reach legal circles.

Medical Management

The medical management of occupational back pain should be no different from that of back pain in general. From a biologic perspective, back pain occurring at work is usually the same as back pain sustained in the general community. Therefore, in the first instance, the literature on back pain in general can be applied to the management of occupational back pain specifically. Care needs to be taken, however, to distinguish acute from chronic back pain. The two differ in their biologic features; the evidence concerning each is distinctly different, as is the treatment of each.

OCCUPATIONAL BACK PAIN

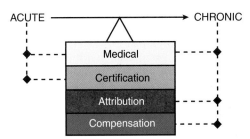

Fig. 91.1 **Extraneous factors that confound occupational back pain.** The links show where particular factors are most influential.

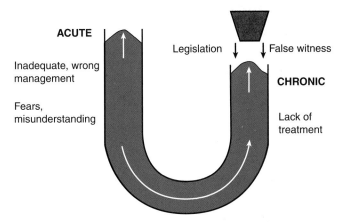

Fig. 91.2 **The U-tube of occupational back pain.** Patients with acute back pain present with fears and misunderstandings but are subjected to inadequate or wrong management. Like an increased pressure, increased numbers of poorly managed patients with acute pain drives an increase in the number with chronic pain. Treatment for those patients is lacking. Meanwhile, authorities try to plug the rise in chronic pain by legislative measures and by false witness.

Acute Low Back Pain

For the management of acute low back pain, multiple evidence-based guidelines are available.[4,5] Some have been formulated specifically in the context of occupational back pain.[6–8] These guidelines are uniform in their recommendations.

The guidelines emphasize that patients should be assessed foremost for possible but rare serious causes of back pain, the so-called red flag conditions. To this end, a compact checklist has been devised to address all the possible indicators for red flag conditions (**Fig. 91.3**).[9] If the patient answers "no" to all the questions, the practitioner can be more than reasonably assured that the patient does not have a serious cause of back pain, and no further investigations are required. Answering "yes" does not necessarily incriminate a serious cause, but rather it invites the practitioner to explore what is suggested by the positive response. The checklist has been tested and found to be effective and efficient in clinical practice.[10]

In particular, routine medical imaging, especially plain radiography, is not indicated. The indications for medical imaging are specific and explicit. Plain radiographs are indicated only in patients at risk of having had a fracture. These risks are severe trauma and the possibility of pathologic fracture secondary either to metastases or osteoporosis, in older persons, or in patients taking corticosteroids.[11] In the absence of these indications, plain radiography is not indicated, and its use amounts to irresponsible professional practice and poses a biologic hazard to the patient.

As a screening test for tumors or infections, the investigation of choice is magnetic resonance imaging (MRI) because of its high sensitivity and specificity for these conditions.[11] MRI is indicated only if the red flag assessment reveals clinical indicators of a possible serious disorder, however. For patients with acute low back pain, MRI is not indicated "just in case."

Once red flags have been excluded, the guidelines emphasize that medical assessment should be thorough. This requires exploration of the patient's beliefs and fears about the pain. Those fears and beliefs need to be addressed as much as, if not

Name:					Low Back Pain		
D.O.B					M.R.N.		
Presence of			**Cardiovascular**			**Endocrine**		
Trauma	Y	N	Risk factors?	Y	N	Corticosteroids?	Y	N
Night sweats	Y	N	**Respiratory**			**Musculoskeletal**		
Recent surgery	Y	N	Cough?	Y	N	Pain elsewhere?	Y	N
Catheterization	Y	N	**Urinary**			**Neurological**		
Venipuncture	Y	N	UTI?	Y	N	Symptoms/signs	Y	N
Occupational	Y	N	Hematuria?	Y	N	**Skin**		
Hobby exposure	Y	N	Retention?	Y	N	Infections?	Y	N
Sporting exposure	Y	N	Stream problems?	Y	N	Rashes?	Y	N
(Overseas) travel	Y	N	**Reproductive**			**G.I.T.**		
Illicit drug use	Y	N	Menstrual	Y	N	Diarrhea?	Y	N
Weight loss	Y	N	**Hematopoietic**			**Signature:**		
History of cancer	Y	N	Problems?	Y	N			
Comments							
					Date:		

Fig. 91.3 **A checklist for red flag clinical indicators suitable for inclusion in medical records used in general practice.** D.O.B., date of birth; G.I.T., gastrointestinal tract; M.R.N., medical record number. *(From Bogduk N, McGuirk B, editors: Medical management of acute and chronic low back pain: an evidence-based approach, Amsterdam, 2002, Elsevier.)*

more than, the more conventional medical aspects of their problem. Unfortunately, this domain of the patient's problem is commonly neglected. In one audit of workers' compensation patients, only 28% of reports made any mention of psychosocial factors; the assessment was poor, and in less than half of the cases was any action taken.[12]

In the context of occupational back pain, those fears and beliefs may pertain to work. Patients who have been injured at work may blame work at large, rather than the specific accident, for their problem. They may fear a recurrence of the accident. They may fear that continuing to work will make their condition worse. Because of their propensity to impede full rehabilitation, these fears and beliefs need to be addressed.

The guidelines recommend explanation, assurance, and activation as the key components of management. Passive interventions are discouraged. Bed rest is to be avoided, and it can be explained to patients that it has been shown that bed rest is less effective than remaining active. Patients who retire to bed have pain for longer, and are less likely to recover, than those who remain active.[13,14] Providing such explanations constitutes evidence-based practice and is a critical component of management.

Simple analgesics may be used for pain relief. Nonsteroidal anti-inflammatory drugs are not indicated. For the relief of pain, these drugs are no more effective than placebo.[15] Simple exercises may be used to encourage and maintain movement, but formal or named exercises are not required.[16]

Several studies have shown that such measures are effective. Indahl et al[17,18] showed that a single, prolonged consultation that focused on fears and activation was enough to double the return-to-work rate. Other investigators[19] confirmed this finding. A study by McGuirk et al[10] showed that complete recovery could be achieved in more than 70% of patients simply by providing explanation, assurance, and support.

A comprehensive plan of management, and instructions on how to pursue one, cannot be explained in a single textbook chapter. Readers interested in descriptions, explanations, and justifications of an evidence-based algorithm or readers interested in instructions on how to implement a management plan should consult sources where this is described.[20]

Prompt return to work is an imperative. Investigators have shown that patients who return to work, or who remain at work, recover sooner and have fewer recurrences.[7,8] The longer patients spend away from work, the less chance they have of recovering.[7] This can, and should, be explained to patients as part of their management. Most patients are able to return to work.[7,8] Most will comply with advice to return to work and will remain at work.[7,21] Return to work is not simply a matter of ordering the patient to do so, however. Return to work is achieved by identifying barriers and assisting the patient to overcome them.

Pertinent in this regard is workplace intervention. Investigators have shown that adding a work site visit to the management regimen improves outcomes.[22] It results in reduced absence from work, faster return to work, less disability, less sickness impact, and reduced pain. The effects are greater, and statistically significant, when clinical intervention is combined with occupational intervention than when occupational intervention or clinical intervention is used in isolation.

Significantly, workplace intervention is not tantamount to ergonomic intervention. By and large, formal ergonomic intervention has not been vindicated by research studies. Rather, work site intervention is a psychosocial intervention.

Not all patients who present with acute low back pain have a problem with work. Once they have been properly assessed, have had their condition explained, and have been empowered with a plan of management, some patients can resume their normal work. Others may do so tentatively and be surprised, yet relieved, that they can successfully resume work.

For other patients, matters pertaining to work may be important factors in delaying or preventing rehabilitation. The possible problems can range from inappropriate beliefs and fears on the part of the patient to clearly unsafe and even outrageous work practices that oppressively are imposed on the patient. Whether or not serious workplace issues exist in a particular case is a matter of judgment on the part of the practitioner and the patient, but it can be determined only if work is examined in a concerted manner during consultations with the patient.

In assessing work matters, a practitioner may be at a significant disadvantage if he or she does not really understand what is involved in a particular job. Without a knowledge of the workplace, practitioners may appear foolish or elitist to the patient and therefore unconvincing when giving advice (e.g., "What would you know?"). Uninformed advice just to be careful tends to promote fear avoidance and invalidism. Specific ergonomic instruction is probably neither required nor valid. Instead, the practitioner can ask what the job involves and learn from the patient. With the patient, the practitioner can reconstruct the workstation and mimic the worker's activities. It is better still when the practitioner is actually familiar with the work practices, by having visited the workplace, if not by having experienced the work practices. With some insight into what the worker does, the practitioner can assist by explaining how the worker can reasonably execute the required tasks.

Rural practitioners may well be better able to engage in workplace intervention. If they are faced with large or regular numbers of patients with back pain, it would be profitable for them to become familiar with the various work sites of their patients. This familiarity with the sites and their practices provides rural practitioners with valuable knowledge, and it also establishes social contact during management that can be beneficial should the need arise, in the future, for the practitioner to intervene on behalf of a patient. When advocacy is required, it is potentially impressive and reassuring to the patient when it emerges, in the course of a consultation, that the practitioner knows not only what the job entails but also the key personnel.

For urban practitioners, this approach may not be practicable. Their patients may work far afield, and practitioners may not be able to visit and experience all the possible work sites of their patients. Beyond learning what they can about the job from the patient, the urban practitioner may need to collaborate with a colleague or specialist practitioner trained in occupational medicine, if concerted workplace intervention is required.

The workplace intervention should not be misrepresented or misconstrued as an adversarial occupational health and safety visit. Rather, it involves several dimensions, both overt and subtle.

Foremost, the patient's practitioner, or a surrogate representative (e.g., rehabilitation provider, occupational therapist, or occupational medicine physician) should become familiar with the patient's work and work environment, so that he or she can help the patient return to work in an informed and insightful manner.

Second, on behalf of the worker, the practitioner can negotiate the following with the employer:

- Any amendments to the workplace specifically to prevent recurrences of accidents of the type in which the worker may have been injured
- Modifications to the workplace to prevent or avoid recurrences of back pain problems
- Mutually acceptable modified duties that allow the worker to return to work and therein feel welcome

Guidelines for the management of occupational back pain emphasize that communication and cooperation among workers, supervisors, managers, and the primary care provider are fundamental to successful outcome.[7]

Third, the practitioner can be seen to have been the patient's advocate. In this regard, it is not so much what the practitioner does in terms of actual ergonomic changes but that he or she is seen to have done something. Although the full implications of this dimension have never been evaluated, its power should not be underestimated, given the extent to which fear of work and dissatisfaction with the workplace are prognostic of poor outcome.

A pragmatic review[23] emphasized the virtue and importance of modified duties (as opposed to so-called light duties). Such duties consist of appropriately modified work according to the injured worker's physical capacity, developed in the context of sympathetic communication with the worker, and nonadversarial handling of the worker's compensation claim. A critical issue in this regard is to return the worker to his or her preinjury job, as far as possible, with restrictions if required, rather than allotting the worker to different and usually more menial duties. Moreover, it is recommended that a supportive workplace response to injury needs to start when the pain is first reported, and that an individualized and accommodative approach to return to work should follow promptly.[23] Such measures can reduce both the incidence and the duration of disability resulting in time lost from work by up to 50%.[23]

Understated in the literature is the significance of return to work to the dignity of these patients. By not returning to work, not only do patients risk becoming chronic invalids, but also they lose their personal dignity and the social recognition of their peers. While away from work, they are alone and isolated. They risk becoming victims of an impersonal and impassionate system that engulfs their lives. As objects, they are directed from assessment to assessment, from treatment to treatment, and no longer have control of their destiny. Some patients come to feel that they are treated like criminals who are required to prove their innocence. All these factors sow the seeds of depression and resentment.

Equally important, in this respect, is the type of work that is provided. When patients are physically unable to return to their preinjury duties, it is nevertheless important that they feel that they are contributing. Being given what is obvious to these patient and others, especially work colleagues, as being nothing more than "made-up" jobs (e.g., counting paper clips) is demeaning, particularly when the reason for such an approach is purely to minimize workers' compensation costs or to keep some specious safety record intact. Doing so

is almost certainly guaranteed to cause these patients to take time off from work.

Guidelines and reviews recommend that if acute pain persists and becomes subacute (i.e., lasting longer that 7 weeks), the patient should be referred to a multidisciplinary rehabilitation program that can provide workplace intervention.[7,8] Indeed, the evidence shows that such programs are not indicated and are not effective for patients with acute back pain,[24] but they are demonstrably effective for patients with subacute pain.[25,26] This line of action is not the only one, however, because investigators have shown that the same outcomes can be achieved by a single practitioner, provided the treatment is appropriate.[17-19] The key factor is that the intervention must be closely related to the workplace or tied explicitly to the specific goal of return to work.[23]

Euphemistic Back Pain

Patients with occupational back pain are often misrepresented and are accused or suspected of being malingerers. Malingering is rare, with a probable incidence of less than 5%.[27] However, some patients present ostensibly with back pain but for other reasons. They are not actually malingering; they are not being fraudulent. Euphemistic back pain is a considerate neologism without prejudice that can be applied to such patients.

These patients do indeed have back pain, but their back pain is not the true reason that they present for treatment. Under other circumstances, their pain would not be of sufficient gravity to seek medical care. Rather, these patients have another agenda, and they use their back pain euphemistically to seek attention. They may be dissatisfied with their employer or supervisor; they may be dissatisfied with their job. They may have a social problem at work that they feel unable to solve. They use a complaint of back pain as a potential means of escaping their dissatisfaction. Viewed another way, these patients are calling for intervention on matters that they are not directly espousing.

Rather than simply asking a series of questions purporting to address these issues, the "secret" is to *listen* to these patients. Why did they present? What are their expectations? For their back pain, most are looking for reassurance that nothing is seriously wrong, and having received that advice, they seek a "quick fix." They usually have their own perceptions about what constitutes appropriate management, often obtained, in this day and age, from information available on the Internet. Their interpretation of this information varies widely and often necessitates further appropriate explanation and advice.

Unfortunately, but in reality, this takes *time*. It is most unlikely that patients will volunteer any of the so-called psychosocial issues at the first consultation unless they are relaxed and comfortable and are presenting to their own general practitioner, usually of long standing. These patients perceive these issues as personal and usually do not realize their implications. When the general practitioner is overscheduled and is therefore unable or unwilling to spend time with patients, these issues are rarely discussed, and thus the seeds of chronicity are sown at an early stage.

All is not lost, however. Often certain key words or points are volunteered that can be acted on by an alert physician. In this regard, these clues may be considered the equivalent, at the history stage of the consultation, to Waddell's signs.

They all invite consideration and management of what amounts to a parallel or hidden agenda.

Examples of these key points include the following:

- An unsupportive work environment: "I came to see you because my supervisor didn't believe me when I told him [or her] that I had developed back pain and wouldn't consider giving me some less strenuous activities."
- A perception or belief that work is harmful or that all pain must be abolished before attempting to return to work: "I need time off work because until my pain has settled if I try to continue working I can only make things worse."
- Catastrophizing usually associated fear avoidance and other behaviors: "I told them at work that the job was too heavy, but they wouldn't listen. Now my back is so bad I won't be able to work again. I can't do anything because the pain is so bad, and when I try it only makes the pain worse. I've been to the pharmacy, and the painkillers don't help. All I do is lie around, but this doesn't help, either. I can't sleep unless I have several beers."
- Personal issues: "Doctor, is it serious? My mother developed back pain and eventually they diagnosed cancer, and she only lasted 3 months."
- Overprotective spouse or avoidance of normal activity: "I brought my partner along so he [or she] could help me. I don't know what I would do without him [or her]. He [or she] does everything for me so I can rest."

By no means is this list intended to be complete, but it represents some of the issues that can become evident in the course of a consultation in which the patient has the opportunity to voice these concerns.

Very significant can be the patient who says very little, responds to direct questions in monosyllables, and often is disheveled, with lack of personal grooming. Almost invariably, these patients are severely depressed. These signs may indicate an unrelated (and often undiagnosed) psychiatric disorder that has been heightened by the back injury.

If these patients are recognized, medical management can be channeled toward dealing with the psychosocial problems that the patients harbor and, one hopes, reveal on inquiry. Doing so addresses the real problem instead of mistakenly trusting that treating the back pain will solve the problem. Whether or not the psychosocial problem is soluble depends on the individual circumstances. However, failing to recognize these problems, or ignoring them, eliminates any chance of resolving the problem when it is solvable. Furthermore, not recognizing these patients and channeling them into conventional management will simply add to the population of medicalized patients who will not, and do not, recover.

Certification

Certification is the earliest of several processes that distinguish occupational back pain from back pain in the general community. Although specific requirements differ in different countries, states, and provinces, some form of certification is usually required for a patient who presents with occupational back pain.

The most innocuous form of paperwork is certification required simply to record the case, essentially for archival or administrative purposes. Recording an event should not interfere with medical management or with prognosis. The practitioner remains free to implement a plan of management as he or she would for a patient for whom no paperwork is required.

Yet even this seemingly innocuous exercise can be hazardous. Practitioners need to take care how they label the patient. Certain diagnostic labels are not only incorrect, but they also can be disturbing to patients.[28,29] "Disk degeneration" may seem an accepted rubric to fellow practitioners, but to some patients it evokes images of inexorable deterioration. This label is not compatible with assurances of prompt recovery. "Instability" conveys connotations of fragility and possible catastrophe. It is not compatible with encouragement to resume normal activities. "Arthritis" implies an incurable chronic condition. It is not compatible with rapid recovery. Although used with impunity within the medical profession, these terms are potentially alarming to patients and may compromise a rehabilitation plan. Moreover, they should not be used because none is a legitimate diagnosis. The use of false terms whose only effect is the potential to engender or reinforce fears has no merit.

No universally accepted, alternative labels have been developed for a diagnosis of nonspecific back pain. Even that term potentially conveys an impression that the physician does not know the cause and therefore may not be competent or sufficiently interested. As an offer in this regard, Bogduk and McGuirk proposed a unique and challenging set of terms. "Red back pain" is used for conditions associated with red flag indicators. "Yellow back pain" denotes pain associated with evident psychosocial features. "Green back pain" is used for back pain about which the patient should have no concerns and through which they can proceed with confidence. Bogduk and McGuirk[29] defined and justified these terms and demonstrated how they can be explained to patients.

In many areas, certification can mean providing a management plan. Completing the paperwork may be tedious, but that should not interfere with good medical management. The report should simply state the proposed plan of management. Efficient practitioners may prepare a generic plan on the computer, to save time in preparing plans or reports individually for each new patient (Appendix 91.1). Due consideration, however, must be given to any relevant restrictions required by privacy legislation.

The most vexatious forms of certification, however, are certification for time off from work and certification for light duties. If these are used injudiciously, they can corrupt the patient's prognosis and outcome.

Simply giving patients time off from work, reflexly, routinely, or because the patient expects it, can be deleterious to prognosis. Practitioners cannot expect, and cannot rely on the presumption, that the passage of time, while the patient is idle, alone, and unsupervised, will cure the patient's back pain or solve his or her problems. Indeed, such a passive intervention is contrary to established evidence concerning the management of back pain and can be deleterious. Certificates should therefore be viewed as potentially toxic to the patient.

All patients should be encouraged and helped to return to work. In most instances, patients do not require time off from work. If time away from work is required, it should be for explicit and specifiable purposes. Giving patients time off from work should be treated in the same manner as admitting a patient to the hospital. It is done for a therapeutic purpose.

Something the practitioner prescribes must be done during the time off from work, and the patient should be constantly monitored for progress. It becomes an irresponsible, and dangerous, practice when practitioners give patients a certificate for time off from work just to get them out of their office; and if this is rationalized on the basis of a perceived need of the patient to rest, it reflects an ignorance of the evidence base.

Related to the writing of certificates is the absurdity of so-called light duties. This concept is absurd on three counts. First, no medical formula is available to calculate what a patient can and cannot do. It is not a professional concept. Anyone who prescribes light duties is inventing them as a layperson. Second, it is a dismissive, not a therapeutic, intervention. Instead of assisting patients to return to work, patients are relegated to menial tasks that offend their dignity. In some jurisdictions, workers are returned to the workplace simply to enhance workers' compensation performance data. Yet at the workplace, the worker does nothing and is treated with resentment. The third absurdity is perhaps the most crucial. Most employers simply cannot accommodate employees on light duties. No light duties are available. Compelling employers to take on such workers breeds resentment and, in practice, often means that the employer sends the patient home.

Not to be confused with light duties is modification of work practices. By negotiation with the employer, injured workers can be returned to useful employment if practices can be modified. This may entail retaining the worker in his or her accustomed role, but having the worker perform his or her duties in another way. It may involve reassigning the worker temporarily to other duties while he or she recovers from the episode of back pain. An important and often underestimated facet of this is that by keeping an employee in the preinjury work environment, he or she continues to have access to colleagues at work. If reassignment is used, however, it should prospectively be temporary. Progress and recovery should be monitored assiduously, and the worker should return to his or her former role as soon as able to do so. Not monitoring patients is tantamount to neglect, and the abandoned patient is unlikely to return to the former role. Prescribing and monitoring modified activities should be part of the concerted medical intervention. This intervention cannot be left to its own devices. When it appears to fail, it is not because the intervention does not intrinsically work. It fails when the patient is not assiduously monitored. It fails when practitioners forget that they put the patient on modified duties and neglect to bring them up to conventional duties. It fails when practitioners neglect to titrate and monitor their intervention.

Certification is susceptible to confounding, competing, and interfering influences. A proper and concerted medical plan can be confounded when other physicians, who are less responsible, disagree and provide the patient with certificates for time off from work. Medical treatment plans can be confounded when friends of the patient provide incorrect and deleterious lay advice. They can also be confounded when management or insurance physicians fail to understand the merits of a proper rehabilitation plan and demand instant fixes. Under those circumstances, it is important that a single physician be responsible for, and in charge of, the patient's management and certification. Some jurisdictions,

recognizing the importance of this view, have legislated to include this requirement.[30]

Even so, this approach may not always be practical. Management by the individual practitioner can be unduly complicated by legislation whereby others (e.g., rehabilitation providers) are given a legal responsibility to be involved in the development of plans to return the patient to work. The singular recourse in this regard is for the practitioner to lead by example. By persevering, the prospects arise that successes will be noticed and that others will support the practitioner's efforts. The practitioner can enlist the cooperation of employers by explaining the merits of the plan of management. Unfortunately, until that occurs, the practitioner and the patient risk being continually frustrated by interference from other physicians, allied health professionals, insurers, and managers who do not understand the evidence concerning the management of back pain and who prefer to impose their own often misguided notions on the process.

Evidence

All the precepts outlined previously for the management of acute low back pain have been tested in a workers' compensation situation.[31] The study was conducted in an area health service in Australia, which encompassed three hospitals and their ancillary services such as laundry, kitchen, cleaning, and engineering. All workers who believed that they had injured their back and had thereby incurred back pain were eligible for compensation if they registered their precipitating event. On registering their event, all patients were invited to see either their own general practitioner, who provided usual care, or a staff specialist in staff health. This staff specialist was a musculoskeletal occupational physician who provided evidence-based care, as described earlier, including the guidelines for certification and light duties. During the period of study, a total of 253 patients presented with a complaint of back pain, ostensibly incurred at work. Of these patients, 62 elected to pursue usual care immediately. Initially, 191 patients saw the staff specialist, but only 164 elected to remain under the specialist's care; 27 elected to pursue usual care after their first consultation.

The outcomes in the three groups of the foregoing study varied (**Table 91.1**).[31] The outcomes of those patients who transferred to usual care did not differ from the outcomes of those who pursued usual care from the start. However, the outcomes of those patients who remained under evidence-based care were significantly better. A greater proportion retained their normal duties (i.e., agreed that they did not require time off from work). A smaller proportion required modified duties, and virtually none lost time from work. Far fewer patients suffered recurrence or developed chronic pain. With close monitoring of their progress, most patients receiving evidence-based care required only 2 weeks or less on modified duties.

Among the patients who remained under evidence-based care, three types were identified in the course of the study.[31] Patients classified as "uncomplicated" were those who promptly understood the plan of management and complied with it. Patients classified as "informed" were those who brought to the initial consultation their own ideas or expectations about how they should be managed. Typically, these patients were nurses or other health care professionals who

Table 91.1 Outcomes of Patients with Back Pain Treated by Evidence-Based Care, and by Usual Care, and Those Who Transferred from Evidence-Based Care to Usual Care*

	Evidence-Based Care	Transferred to Usual Care	Usual Care
Number	164	27	62
Normal duties			
Proportion	0.63	0.00	0.00
95% CI	0.56–0.70	0.00–0.12	0.00–0.06
Modified duties			
Proportion	0.37	0.67	0.92
95% CI	0.30–0.44	0.59–0.85	0.86–0.92
Lost time			
Proportion	0.01	0.33	0.35
95% CI	0.00–0.02	0.15–0.51	0.23–0.46
Recovered			
Proportion	0.98	0.81	0.84
95% CI	0.96–1.00	0.66–0.96	0.75–0.93
Recurrence			
Proportion	0.06	0.52	0.27
95% CI	0.02–0.10	0.33–0.71	0.12–0.42
Chronic pain			
Proportion	0.02	0.15	0.10
95% CI	0.00–0.04	0.02–0.28	0.03–0.17

*Outcomes achieved by patients under evidence-based care that are significantly different from those achieved by patients under usual care are highlighted in bold.
95% CI, 95% confidence interval of the proportion.
From McGuirk B, Bogduk N: Evidence-based care for low back pain in workers eligible for compensation, *Occup Med* 57:36, 2007.

Table 91.2 Outcomes under Evidence-Based Care of Uncomplicated and Informed Patients and Those with Psychosocial Issues*

	Uncomplicated	Informed	Psychosocial
Number	61	32	71
Normal duties			
Proportion	0.87	0.72	0.38
95% CI	0.79–0.95	0.56–0.98	0.27–0.49
Modified duties			
Proportion	0.11	0.28	0.62
95% CI	0.03–0.19	0.02–0.54	0.51–0.63
Lost time			
Proportion	0.02	0.00	0.00
95% CI	0.00–0.05	0.00–0.11	0.00–0.05
Recovered			
Proportion	0.98	1.00	0.96
95% CI	0.95–1.00	0.89–1.00	0.91–1.00
Recurrence			
Proportion	0.02	0.00	0.13
95% CI	0.00–0.06	0.00–0.11	0.05–0.21
Chronic pain			
Proportion	0.02	0.00	0.04
95% CI	0.00–0.05	0.00–0.11	0.00–0.09

*Although a greater proportion required a period on modified duties, patients with psychosocial issues had subsequent outcomes that were as good as those of other patients under evidence-based care.
95% CI, 95% confidence interval of the proportion.

suggested the possible need for physical therapy or acupuncture or who had read Internet sites about how to manage back pain. Pivotal in the management of these patients were acute awareness of the literature and the ability to explain to the patient the difference between actual evidence and unsubstantiated claims or common, but discredited, beliefs. Once this was done, these patients understood evidence-based care and complied.

The largest subgroup consisted of patients classified as "psychosocial." These were patients with euphemistic back pain who typically had problems with workplace relations. They required longer or repeated consultations to elicit their psychosocial complaints and more concerted care to address these complaints. Nevertheless, the basic plan for evidence-based care was followed.

A greater proportion of patients with psychosocial issues required modified duties for a limited period, and, therefore, fewer returned immediately to normal duties (**Table 91.2**). However, in other outcome measures, they did not differ from the other patients. In all subgroups, lost time was next to zero, recovery rates were high, and recurrence rates were low. Thus, although patients with psychosocial issues required more concerted care, they eventually responded to evidence-based care as well as did patients who were easier to manage.

It is not evident from this study whether evidence-based care produced better outcomes or whether usual care was simply responsible for poorer outcomes. Nevertheless, the study provided evidence that stark differences in outcome occur. Among the observations pertinent to this chapter are ones that emerged in usual care. Apparently, it is easier to provide a patient with a certificate for time off from work than to explain to a patient why he or she does not need one.[31] Furthermore, once certified, patients languished without being monitored. However, these patients could be returned to work when the primary care physician was contacted and urged to review their cases with the objective of returning them to work. Conspicuous was the greater proportion of patients under usual care who suffered recurrences and developed chronic back pain.

Chronic Back Pain

When a patient's pain persists despite good medical management, there is no point in persevering with the same interventions. Continuing to ply analgesics and exercises will not suddenly abolish the pain when these measures have not done so to date. Continuing to explore and modify the patient's fears and beliefs will not suddenly change the patient's attitudes.

In contrast, if the patient has not been managed well during the acute phase of the condition, the prospect exists that implementing good management, albeit late, may still help the patient. It is unfortunate that most patients do not undergo good management from the start. Much of medical practice in patients with chronic back pain therefore amounts to salvaging the patient from the efforts of others.

Nevertheless, even with good management, not all patients recover. Some 10% to 30% can be expected to have persistent pain.[10] Some of these patients may have only minor pain and no disabilities (e.g., a pain score of only 15 out of 100). These patients may not require further intervention. Some, however, remain in pain and become disabled by it.

The foremost question is whether the persistence is caused by an unrecognized lesion or whether it stems from psychosocial factors. The tendency, to date, has been to attribute all chronic back pain to psychosocial factors, to the neglect of medical factors.

The belief in psychosocial factors is founded on epidemiologic data showing that these factors are poor prognostic indicators. The fashion has therefore been to commit patients with chronic back pain to behavioral therapy. However, the epidemiologic data themselves account for no more than 30% of the variance between patients whose back pain remains chronic and those who recover. Some 70% of the variance remains unexplained.[6,7] Psychosocial factors are not the cardinal determinant of chronicity. They are simply the most publicized.

Psychosocial Treatment

Despite, or contrary to, the predictions of psychosocial theories of back pain, psychological treatment has not proved to be the answer. As a sole intervention, behavioral therapy has not proved effective.[32] It may have a place as a component in multidisciplinary pain therapy, but even multidisciplinary pain therapy, which focuses on education, cognitive therapy, and exercise, is not the solution for chronic back pain. It may be what is currently promoted as the preferred intervention, but it does not produce results.

A systematic review[33] found the following:

- Strong evidence indicates that intensive multidisciplinary biopsychosocial rehabilitation with functional restoration improves function when compared with inpatient or outpatient non-multidisciplinary rehabilitation.[34-36]
- Moderate evidence indicates that intensive multidisciplinary biopsychosocial rehabilitation with functional restoration reduces pain when compared with outpatient non-multidisciplinary rehabilitation or usual care.[34-36]
- The evidence regarding vocational outcomes of intensive multidisciplinary biopsychosocial rehabilitation is contradictory. Whereas Bendix et al[34] reported improvements in "work-readiness," Alaranta et al[36] and Mitchell and Carmen[37] showed no benefit on sick leave.
- Regarding less intensive multidisciplinary biopsychosocial rehabilitation, five trials could not show improvements in pain, function, or vocational outcomes when compared with non-multidisciplinary outpatient rehabilitation or usual care.[34,38-41]

With respect to the two major of these conclusions, an inspection of the published data provides an insight into the effect size. In the first study of Bendix et al,[34] the intensive functional restoration program reduced disability from 15.5, on a 30-point scale, to 8.5 at 4 months; this program reduced back pain from 5.3, on a scale of 0 to 10, to 2.7. These results would seem to represent reasonable improvements, although few patients were rendered pain free or fully rehabilitated.

The second study of Bendix et al[35] reported more modest gains. Function improved from 16.9 to only 12.1, and pain improved from 6.1 to 5.7. Alaranta et al[36] achieved an average reduction in pain of only 17 points on a 100-point scale. With respect to functional capacity, the significant gain reported by Alaranta et al[36] was that a smaller proportion of their index patients suffered back problems during light activities or at rest; however, no differences from control patients were noted with respect to the proportion of patients who were pain free or who had problems only during moderate activities. Bendix et al[34,35] achieved significantly greater reductions in sick leave and contacts with the health care system. However, this was not the experience of Alaranta et al[36] or of Mitchell and Carmen.[37]

Of the studies not covered by systematic reviews, one study[42] showed that a group of patients receiving multidisciplinary management achieved no greater reduction in pain than did an untreated control group; the major gains were reduction in use of medication and a 48% return to work rate. Another study[43] found no consistent advantages of multidisciplinary treatment over usual care with respect to pain, but the index patients were slightly more satisfied with their jobs and were slightly less distressed psychologically. However, return-to-work rates were not better.

Practitioners, insurers, and employers should understand what these data show:

- Multidisciplinary, behavioral therapy does not eliminate back pain and does not achieve a greater rate of return to work than usual care.
- Psychologically based programs are not effective. Psychologically based programs have palliative effects in that they may reduce distress and prevent deterioration, but no evidence indicates that they restore patients to normal activities, including work. In this regard, these programs may be appropriate when complete restoration and return to work are not the intended goals or when those goals are considered unachievable.
- Intensive programs focused on exercises are more effective than less intensive programs or programs that focus on behavior. Even so, the improvements achieved are limited. Patients can expect to have less pain and be able to function somewhat better, but their problems are not eliminated. In essence, multidisciplinary treatment is tantamount to palliative care.

Medical Treatment

Medical treatments in the form of drug therapies and physical treatments in the form of physical therapy, exercises, or manual therapy are abjectly unsuccessful in the resolution of chronic low back pain.[44,45] Persisting with such interventions when they fail to resolve the patient's problems is intellectually and professionally irresponsible. The only justification for continuing with these interventions is that these interventions constitute some form of palliative care, but that is not the same as representing them as desirable treatments.

Investigations

Conventional investigations, such as radiography and computed tomography, are inappropriate for chronic low back pain. Such investigations can reveal nothing that is known to cause back pain. The one useful test is MRI.[46]

The foremost role of MRI is as a screening test to clear patients of serious disorders. Of all investigations, MRI is best able to detect or exclude conditions such as occult tumors or indolent infections that have not produced any clinical features by which they may be suspected.

To some extent, MRI also has a positive role. It is able to reveal high-intensity zones in the posterior anulus fibrosus of the lumbar disks. This uncommon sign occurs in only approximately 30% of patients with chronic low back pain, but it is highly specific.[46] This sign indicates that the affected disk is internally disrupted and painful. Its likelihood ratio in this regard is 6. On average, this likelihood ratio allows practitioners to be 80% certain that the affected disk is the source of the patient's pain.

Invasive Investigations

Although conventional medical imaging cannot reveal the source or cause of pain in most patients with chronic low back pain, other tests can. They are all tests performed with an injection of some form.

Zygapophysial joint pain can be pursued using controlled diagnostic blocks[47] (see Chapter 90). Diskogenic pain can be pursued using disk stimulation and diskography[47] (see Chapter 14). Sacroiliac joint pain can be pursued using intra-articular blocks[47] (see Chapter 95).

Given the availability of these tests, patients can be investigated to establish the source of their chronic back pain. Pinpointing a diagnosis, at the very least, serves to establish that these patients do, indeed, have a genuine source of pain and refutes the accusation that they are malingering or suffering from psychogenic pain. Pinpointing the source of pain can also serve to direct treatment to that source.

Contrary to the prevailing, but unsubstantiated, notion that 80% of chronic back pain cannot be diagnosed, the opposite holds true. Among patients with chronic low back pain, zygapophysial joint pain accounts for 10% or 40% (depending on the population); sacroiliac joint pain accounts for some 20%; and internal disk disruption accounts for at least 39%.[47] These sources of pain, however, cannot be determined other than by invasive investigations. Failure to investigate patients by these means leaves them with an undetermined diagnosis and at the mercy of a system that does not want them to exist.

Precision Treatment

Lumbar zygapophysial joint pain can be treated with percutaneous lumbar medial branch neurotomy[48] (see Chapter 90). Diskogenic pain can be treated with disk excision and arthrodesis or perhaps by a variety of percutaneous procedures, such as intradiskal electrothermal therapy[47] (see Chapter 181). Of the known sources of chronic low back pain, the sacroiliac joint is the most difficult to treat. No means of relieving sacroiliac joint pain have been validated. Emerging, however, are various ways of denervating this joint.[48]

Attribution

In some jurisdictions, a patient who cannot return to work because of back pain may be entitled to compensation in the form of income replacement or some other financial benefit. In other jurisdictions, such provisions do not apply, and patients continue to suffer their pain and are unable to work.

Pivotal to any claim for compensation is attribution. It must be shown that work was responsible for the patient's problem. In different countries, states, and provinces, the laws differ. In some, all that is required is for the patient to have developed the problem at work. In others, work has to be shown to have been a substantial contributory factor. Much of the process in establishing attribution is legal and is determined by the laws and practices where the case occurred. From a medical perspective, however, two issues arise: medical opinion that work was the cause and medical opinion that it was not.

In a given case, no absolute way exists to prove that work was the cause of injury and subsequent back pain. At the time of the alleged injury, medical witnesses were not present to perform real-time fluoroscopy, which could demonstrate the biomechanics of injury. Patients are not monitored with regular MRI, which could have demonstrated that a lesion was not present before injury but developed soon after injury.

From a positivist perspective, all that an expert witness can testify is that the patient's clinical features are consistent with the occurrence of an injury. If the source of pain has been pinpointed by MRI, or by invasive investigations, an expert witness can testify that the source of pain, or lesion found, is consistent with an injury at work.

Epidemiologic data can support, but not confirm, such testimony. Epidemiologic studies can demonstrate, in populations, whether certain activities or work practices are significantly associated with an increased risk of injury or an increased incidence of back pain. In this regard, the literature is extensive and is beyond the scope of this chapter. That literature was reviewed by the Occupational Safety and Health Administration of the US Department of Labor,[49] which found that, overall, many occupations and several occupational activities are significantly associated with a genuine, increased risk of back pain.

A problem with epidemiologic data, however, is that they cannot be directly applied to individual cases. The finding of an average increased risk does not in itself prove that work was responsible for an individual patient's back pain. At best, when the epidemiologic data are positive, they provide only a background of likelihood that work was responsible. Conversely, if correlations are absent in the epidemiologic data, it becomes more difficult to sustain the argument that work was responsible. A more direct line of evidence, or argument, is required.

Thus, if heavy lifting, or twisting, has been established as a risk factor for back pain, and if the patient's work has involved sustained heavy lifting or twisting, it can be argued that those activities are likely to have been responsible for the patient's complaint. In this regard, the cardinal occupational risk factors for back pain are as follows[49]: heavy physical work (notably in health care, manufacturing, and construction); prolonged exposure to heavy work; and forward bending, lifting and forceful movements, bending and twisting, and working in a bent position.

Conversely, epidemiologic evidence can be used to refute assertions made pejoratively to discredit patients. In this regard, the legal system has been slow to catch up with scientific evidence. Sometimes, it even prefers to shun scientific evidence because it disturbs the way in which lawyers and the courts have been accustomed to dealing with claims. Two examples arise.

By word of mouth, spondylolysis and spondylolisthesis are regarded, in some circles, as causes of back pain. Indeed, the American Medical Association guides to evaluation of impairment reward patients with an automatic increase in total person impairment if their radiographs demonstrate spondylolysis or spondylolisthesis.[50] However, this practice flies in the face of the available evidence. A systematic review of the literature established that, in adults, these conditions are not associated with back pain.[51]

Similar arguments apply to spondylosis. A common retort from witnesses for insurers is that work was not responsible for the patient's pain; rather, the patient's pain results from preexisting degenerative joint disease. Such a statement is false and is contrived simply to deny claims.

Multiple studies demonstrated minimal to no association between back pain and spondylosis (**Table 91.3**).[52-63] The data from individual studies, and the pooled data, yield likelihood ratios barely greater than 1.0 and odds ratios less than 2.0, both of which are neither statistically nor clinically significant. In colloquial terms, one could say that a patient with back pain is only 5% more likely to have degenerative changes than by chance alone. Degenerative changes are normal features of aging and do not constitute a diagnosis of the cause of back pain.

Under those conditions, the argument cannot be sustained that a worker's back pain was simply the result of preexisting degenerative changes. This argument is contrary to the available scientific data, yet it is still often used to deny claims.

Compensation

In different jurisdictions, different entitlements are available to injured workers. Those entitlements may be adjudicated by tribunals, by judges, or by juries. It is therefore neither possible nor appropriate to provide an internationally relevant synopsis of these administrative and legal provisions. Nevertheless, certain principles and phenomena are common to all systems.

Compensation was originally devised to support genuinely injured workers who were no longer able to work. The compensation served to replace the income that these workers had lost, in order that they could maintain a livelihood. In a sense, it was a charitable and compassionate benefaction, but not a reward for having been injured.

For genuinely injured workers who are permanently disabled, compensation is a reasonable recourse. If society cannot solve their medical problems, it may at least ensure that these workers are not left destitute because they cannot work. However, compensation can be abused. Individuals may pursue compensation for reasons other than the intended purpose.

Claimants may be under the misapprehension that compensation is an easy means of securing a cash sum, like winning the lottery, that otherwise in their life they could never expect. Such a sum amounts to a means of escape from the working class. (This situation can be magnified in rural areas, which often have limited options for employment and high

Table 91.3 Validity of Degenerative Changes on Plain Radiographs as a Diagnosis of Low Back Pain

Reference	Degenerative Changes	Back Pain Present	Back Pain Absent	SENS	SPEC	LR	OR
Symmons et al[52,53]	Present	130	92	0.55	0.61	1.4	1.9
	Absent	106	142				
Symmons et al[52,53]	Present	170	135	0.72	0.44	1.3	2.0
	Absent	66	106				
Horal[54]	Present	90	61	0.46	0.68	1.4	1.8
	Absent	105	127				
Frymoyer et al[55]	Present	45	19	0.23	0.80	1.2	1.2
	Absent	151	77				
Biering-Sorensen et al[56]	Present	115	71	0.32	0.77	1.4	1.6
	Absent	243	237				
Wiikeri et al[57]	Present	39	42	0.58	0.70	1.9	3.3
	Absent	28	100				
Lawrence[58]	Present	462	360	0.59	0.52	1.1	1.6
	Absent	320	390				
Kellgren and Lawrence[59]	Present	55	77	0.75	0.37	1.2	1.8
	Absent	18	45				
Sairanen et al[60]	Present	139	51	0.80	0.45	1.5	3.2
	Absent	35	41				
Hult[61]	Present	177	35	0.81	0.36	1.3	2.5
	Absent	41	20				
Magora and Schwartz[62]	Present	217	164	0.58	0.24	0.8	0.5
	Absent	155	53				
Torgerson and Dotter[63]	Present	208	102	0.54	0.53	1.2	1.3
	Absent	179	115				
Pooled	Present	1847	1209	0.56	0.55	1.2	1.5
	Absent	1447	1453				

LR, positive likelihood ratio; OR, odds ratio; SENS, sensitivity; SPEC: specificity.

unemployment rates.) This misapprehension may be reinforced by peers who share that perception.

Claimants may feel aggrieved because they believe that they were innocently injured, and the pursuit of compensation is tantamount to the pursuit of justice. They may feel wronged because the system has not fixed their problem. Under those conditions, compensation amounts to a penalty against the system for having failed the worker.

Lawyers may be responsible. Perhaps with the best of intentions, lawyers advise clients of what they are entitled to and encourage them to pursue their maximum entitlements. (Particularly relevant in this respect is when employees in the older age groups, usually those with more menial jobs, perceive such an approach as a means of supplementing their superannuation entitlements, as well as an early retirement.) When lawyers work on commission, questions can be raised about the motivation of lawyers who influence clients to maximize claims.

Each of these factors may be counterproductive to recovery. The worker seeking a windfall will not be motivated to recover; without the pain, the worker cannot lay claim to compensation. The aggrieved worker will not recover, or will deny recovery, until he or she feels that justice has been served. Overtly or indirectly, lawyers may direct their clients to retain their complaint to maximize the entitlement.

Unfortunately, no one has determined the extent to which any or all of these factors operate either to prolong the compensation process or to discourage recovery. Also unfortunately, each of the cynical reasons for pursuing compensation disenfranchises honest injured workers who have a genuine disability. These workers find themselves caught in a cynical system that deals with every claim as potentially fraudulent. The genuinely injured worker is then treated as a criminal, with the burden of proof placed on him or her.

It is almost pointless to appeal that more research needs to be conducted in this arena to determine how often patients are honest or misguided and to ascertain the extent to which their recovery is impeded by confounding influences. The problem is obvious, but means for its solution are not readily available. We have no test for honesty. The courts are not a substitute, because the outcome of a court case may depend as much on successful rhetoric as on objective evidence.

However, one avenue is immediately available. If legal matters, or personal issues such as vengeance, are counterproductive to recovery, they become part of the patient's medical problems. It is possible and therefore appropriate for the treating physician to explore these issues with the patient. Just as patients can have mistaken and inappropriate beliefs about the biology of their pain, they may have inappropriate beliefs about compensation. These beliefs can be addressed. That is not to say that patients should be dissuaded from seeking compensation. Rather, patients need to understand what is involved and to what they will be subjected as they pursue their claim. They need to reconcile the extent to which recovery is compromised by the pursuit of a claim. The treating physician can assist with these issues. No guarantee exists that addressing these issues will improve the patient's condition, but unless they are explored there is no hope that it will improve.

Unfortunately, many physicians do not appear to be any more aware of these issues and potential implications than are their patients, and this situation reflects a need for further training. Alternatively, some practitioners choose, based on their own political and social biases, to act as surrogate lawyers.

These practitioners not only advocate such approaches, but also go so far as to provide obviously biased reports to the legal fraternity in support of their perception of their patient's entitlement. What these practitioners fail to recognize, or refuse to acknowledge, are the full ramifications of their actions. In most jurisdictions, the acceptance of a compensation claim by the courts is no longer the "pot of gold" it may once have been. Once the claim has been settled and all outstanding accounts (including the lawyer's fees) have been paid, the patient may end up in a parlous state in the long term, with little money, no job, and no prospects.

Innuendos

Certain myths pervade the medicolegal system. They are the notions of secondary gain and malingering and the belief that Waddell's tests can detect patients with so-called nonorganic back pain.

Purportedly, patients eligible for compensation fabricate or maintain their back pain to obtain financial gain. Variably, this behavior has been described as secondary gain or malingering. Technically, secondary gain is a reward that the patient obtains as a result of being ill, but nevertheless the illness is basically genuine. What cynics argue is that patients would not be as ill as they claim if secondary gain were not available. Malingering differs in that the patient is not genuinely ill, but rather invents a false complaint of illness to obtain financial reward. As applied in clinical practice at large (i.e., not by experts), both concepts are essentially colloquial and abused. Secondary gain and malingering are terms used to describe patients in a pejorative manner, usually to deny their compensation claims. The scientific literature about them is extremely sobering.

A systematic review showed that evidence is lacking on secondary gain as a determinant of behavior by injured workers with back pain.[64] Indeed, when looked for, secondary gain has proved difficult to detect. Lawyers, insurers, and employers should therefore be advised that this phenomenon lacks scientific evidence and, when used pejoratively, is essentially only a lay point of view.

As for malingering, a systematic review of the literature was particularly damning.[27] Although commonly referred to, malingering has proved to be rare when sought. Moreover, it is not a medical diagnosis and has no valid diagnostic criteria. A medical practitioner may believe that a patient is malingering, but no medical test can prove that he or she is. Malingering is a social or legal diagnosis and requires lay techniques, such a video surveillance, to support it.

When Waddell developed his nonorganic signs, they were designed to alert physicians to patients who were communicating something more than the simple signs of back injury.[65] The objective was to cue physicians into pursuing something more than conventional medical management. Positive Waddell's signs constituted an invitation to the physician to explore the patient's fears, beliefs, and attitudes about the pain and about the circumstances. The tests were introduced to enrich medical practice. They did not.

Many practitioners abused the tests. They interpreted, portrayed, and applied them as tests of malingering or of psychogenic pain. For having positive Waddell's signs, patients were abused in medicolegal reports and had legitimate claims denied. Discourteously and conveniently, those practitioners who abused the tests did not commit themselves to print.

Therefore, no conveniently citable evidence of their behavior exists. However, the improper practice became sufficiently commonplace, widespread, and evident that Waddell was prompted to publish again, to deprecate the practice and to restate the legitimate purpose of the tests.[66]

Waddell's tests are not for detecting malingerers; they do not detect nonorganic pain. If used in this way, the tests should not be accepted by fellow practitioners or by courts. The tests echo the pivotal principles concerning the management of back pain. Patients are often distressed by their pain. They harbor fears and may behave in strange ways when in strange circumstances, such as being interrogated by an independent medical examiner. Positive responses to Waddell's tests do not invalidate the patient. They are only signs that something more than simply back pain is occurring with the patient, and that those other factors should be addressed.

A structured review of all the literature on Waddell's signs provided illuminating conclusions.[67] Consistent evidence indicated that Waddell's signs were associated with decreased functional performance, poor nonsurgical treatment outcome, and greater levels of pain. Generally consistent evidence indicated that Waddell's signs were not associated with psychological distress, abnormal illness behavior, or secondary gain. Moreover, generally consistent evidence showed that Waddell's signs are an organic phenomenon and that they cannot be used to discriminate organic from nonorganic problems.

Prevention

A final distinguishing feature of occupational back pain is the notion of primary prevention. In the past, experts or consultants optimistically believed that the incidence of occupational back pain could be reduced if ergonomic, and related, measures were taken to prevent it. As a result, campaigns were initiated to teach workers safe lifting techniques and otherwise to educate them about back pain.

Reviews of the literature showed that classical measures have not succeeded in preventing occupational back pain.[7,68–70] Safe handling does not prevent it. Education does not prevent it. Exercises have a positive but modest effect. Back pain occurs nonetheless.

Intriguingly to some, but obvious to those intimately involved with industry, studies showed gains in another domain. If management (i.e., the employer) is made responsible for the welfare of patients, and if management expresses compassion and encouragement to the worker, the incidence of back pain diminishes, and the duration of sick leave decreases.[71] There seems to be more power in an employer's checking a patient and inviting him or her back to work than in a physician's telling the patient that he or she should go back to work.

The same can be achieved if management is engaged from day 1 and cooperates with a sensible rehabilitation plan. In a mining company in Australia, dramatic decreases in compensation claims were achieved by two measures, each reflecting an important sociologic dimension.[72] First, a physical therapist cooperated with the work site nurse to develop an efficient system of triage and first aid. At the coalface (literally and figuratively), the nurse and the physical therapists treated injured workers on site but encouraged and supported them not to stop work. Only patients with ostensibly serious injuries were referred to an orthopedic surgeon, who saw them promptly.

Meanwhile, at another social level, it was the orthopedic surgeon who met prospectively with management, peer to peer as it were, to engage the employer's cooperation and support. With that secured, the nurse and physical therapist continued their medical treatment unhindered.

McGuirk applied a somewhat similar approach as occupational physician to a large health service in Australia. What became evident from his discussions with management was the lack of training (and perhaps empathy) of many immediate supervisors in managing such patients at a work site level. Often their personal attitudes to the patient, which could have reflected interpersonal prejudices, delayed recovery.

Ten Confounders

Occupational back pain does not deserve to be any more difficult than back pain in the general community. The prognosis should be good. Yet it continues to be a problem, and the reasons are multiple.

1. Back pain cannot be assessed and treated in 5 or even 25 minutes. Good initial assessment may take 50 minutes. General practitioners, however, are typically not geared for such consultations or are unaccustomed to providing them. Inadequate consultation becomes the *first* confounder.
2. Early assessment and early management require focus on psychosocial factors. General practitioners are not accustomed, or are not prepared, to pursue this area. It appears too time consuming to talk to patients, to discover what they do and do not understand and what they fear. It is too time consuming to explain to them what is wrong with their back and why they need not be afraid. It is too time consuming to explore vocational issues. It is not conventional to visit the workplace and to be the patient's trusted advocate. It seems that medical practitioners believe, or expect, that back pain should be something that has a simple "quick fix." The irony is that it does not. The management of acute back pain is time consuming. If that time is provided, management of the condition is eminently successful.[10,17,18,19,31] If the time is denied, management becomes suboptimal. That becomes the *second* confounder.
3. Occupational back pain requires certification. That can be tedious if it is seen as an imposition, but it can become expeditious if it is based on a regular, sensible plan of management that is evidence based. Certification can be abused, however. "Time off from work" and "light duties" can be expedient entries by which to complete certificates rapidly, but neither recommendation is justified by the evidence. On the contrary, certificates should be used as an integral part of the management plan. What they describe should be treated as a prescription, with all the responsibilities that follow. Misuse of certificates becomes the *third* confounder.
4. Return to work and workplace intervention are paramount components of the management of occupational back pain. Both provide for better outcomes. However, both are demanding of aptitude, inclination, and time. Failure to become engaged with the workplace becomes the *fourth* confounder.

5. Whereas most patients with back pain should recover, provided they are managed well, some will have suffered a genuine and substantial injury from which they do not recover. These patients will not recover if treatments are prescribed that are known not to work. Practitioners should be aware of what works and what does not work. Continuing to prescribe treatments destined to fail and blaming the patient when they do become the *fifth* confounder.

6. Conventional investigations do not provide for a diagnosis of chronic back pain. If a diagnosis is required, invasive tests need to be undertaken. Denying patients these tests and leaving them without a diagnosis become the *sixth* confounder.

7. Even if a diagnosis can be made, proven treatments are the exception rather than the rule. Entrenched and socially accepted interventions do not cure these patients. Innovative treatments have unknown efficacy. Lack of proven treatments for chronic back pain becomes the *seventh* confounder.

8. Left with no treatment for persisting pain, the patient with occupational back pain will, in all probability, lodge a claim for (financial) compensation in those countries where legislation allows for such entitlements. This claim will be resisted, if not denied, by employers and their insurers on the basis of concerns they have about the impact of such claims on the employer's premiums. Statements, although not evidence, will often be brought to bear that the complaint and claim are not genuine. Lack of integrity and dishonesty on the part of expert witnesses who compile reports become the *eighth* confounder.

9. Pursuit of a claim may dominate over pursuit of recovery. Tension may develop between doctors and lawyers, with each claiming to act in the interests of the worker. The lawyer's imperative is to maximize the entitlement. This requires maximizing disability. The doctor's imperative is to eliminate or reduce disability. This conflict becomes the *ninth* confounder.

10. When claims are resisted, the matter may come to trial. Statements, although not evidence, will be brought to bear that the complaint and claim are not genuine. False witness becomes the *tenth* confounder.

The system does not want these patients to exist. It blames the patient for presenting for treatment in the first instance and for persisting if the pain persists. Against the background of 10 confounders, the blame lies not with the patient but with the system.

References

Full references for this chapter can be found on www.expertconsult.com.

Appendix 91.1
A Matrix for Preparing a Succinct Medical Report from a General Practitioner

Principles

For administrative purposes, a medical report from the treating physician does not need to be lengthy. It is not a report from an expert witness to defend or contest the cause of pain, its prognosis, or its attribution. It needs only to communicate succinctly the facts as the treating physician found them and what is happening to the patient. Those who use the report, in the first instance, want to know only what to expect:

- A short or protracted course
- Requiring few or multiple services
- Return to work or not

All this information can be compiled into a short report (1 to 2 pages) that outlines the typical algorithm for management of acute low back pain.[1]

Components

[Enter your letterhead]
[Enter address of insurer]
[Enter date of report]
Dear [Insurer]
[Title and name of patient] presented to me on [date of consultation] with a complaint of low back pain that [he or she] attributed to [circumstances of onset] on [date of incident].

Assessment

I obtained a history and performed a physical examination.
EITHER
The history, supplemented by a red flag checklist, revealed no evidence of a serious cause for the pain.
OR
The history revealed that [patient's name] … [stipulate any red flags]. Accordingly, I have arranged for [patient's name] to undergo [state investigations ordered], and I am awaiting the results of these investigations before adjusting my plan of management. In the meantime I [proceed to plan of management, as outlined here].
Physical examination revealed tenderness in/at [briefly state the location of any tenderness]. [List movements] were restricted by pain to approximately [75%, 50%, 25%] of expected normal range for age.
EITHER
In taking the history, I found no suggestion of any psychosocial problems.
OR

In taking the history, I found the [patient's name] expressed certain psychosocial, yellow flag, risk factors for chronicity, which I will address in my management plan.
OPTION
For the purposes of completing the certificate I recognize the problems associated with how to label low back pain.[2,3] Accordingly I have not entered on the certificate any specious or counterproductive labels. Instead, in accordance with expert suggestions,[1] I have provided a diagnosis of
EITHER
Red Back Pain
to indicate that [patient's name] exhibits certain features that need to be taken seriously.
OR
Yellow Back Pain
to indicate that I have found no evidence of any serious physical cause for the pain but that [patient's name] exhibits certain fears, beliefs, and behaviors that would constitute poor prognostic factors if left unattended and which I propose to address.
OR
Green Back Pain
to indicate that I have found no evidence of any serious physical cause for the pain and no psychosocial impediments to recovery. Wherefore, there is no reason why [patient's name] should not proceed promptly and confidently to resume normal activities while the back pain recovers naturally.

Management

For pain management, I have explained to [patient's name] what the likely causes are of [his or her] pain, and have reassured [him or her] that this is nothing to worry about. I have explained the natural history of this condition and how we can expect a good outcome. I have prescribed [name drug] on a time-contingent basis, to provide analgesia while natural recovery takes its course.

To restore movement, I have mobilized [his or her] back muscles with some soft tissue techniques [if done], and have instructed [patient's name] in some simple exercises. I have explained how resuming normal activities and remaining active provide for a good prognosis. I will continue to assist [patient's name] to regain normal daily activities. [if relevant] I have set modest goals in the first instance that I expect [patient's name] can achieve over [insert time: day or so, few days].

I plan to review [patient's name] in [2 days/1 week] to assess [his or her] progress, at which time I shall check [his or her] compliance with my suggested interventions. I will then have the opportunity to correct any misunderstandings and reinforce what I have done already. If required, I can implement other interventions that are not immediately indicated at this stage. Should a change in the management plan occur at that time, I will inform you of those changes if they significantly alter the prognosis and anticipated return to work.

EITHER

[patient's name] has no inappropriate beliefs or fears about [his or her] pain and requires no intervention in this regard.

OR

Because [patient's name] has certain fears and inappropriate beliefs about [his or her] pain, I will seek to engage [him or her] about these, with every prospect of allaying these fears and promoting an appropriate optimistic outlook.

With respect to work,

EITHER

[patient's name] feels able and encouraged to return to work. Accordingly, I have completed the certificate for administrative purposes but have not provided any time off.

OR

[patient's name] should be able to return to work promptly, and I have encouraged [him or her] to do so. Therefore, I have completed the certificate to allow time off from work only to obtain this medical consultation.

OR

I have explained to [patient's name] the benefits of returning to work promptly, and I will assist [him or her] to do so.

This will not require restricted duties but should entail modified duties. These I have explained to [patient's name]. I [have negotiated/will negotiate] these modifications on [his or her] behalf with [patient's name]'s employer. I expect that [patient's name] should be able to embark on this return to work plan within [stipulate time]. I have provided [him or her] with a certificate for the intervening period, during which time I expect [patient's name]'s pain to settle, and [he or she] will improve movements and activities with a brief course of home rehabilitation.

OR

We may have some problems returning to work, because [list reasons]. Accordingly I propose to

EITHER

[outline personal plan of intervention, e.g.; discussion, explanation]

OR

engage the assistance of [stipulate assistance, e.g., occupational medicine consultant or occupational therapist]. However, I will remain pivotal to the management of [patient's name] and will keep you informed of any plan that we devise and how it progresses.

I have issued a certificate for a period of [insert duration], which should allow for the additional assessment and consultations required.

My account for this report is enclosed.

Yours truly,

[signature]

Infections of the Spine

Steven D. Waldman

Infections of the spine are the result of spread of infection from a distant source most commonly through the bloodstream or by extension into the spinal elements of an adjacent infection. Spinal infections can be divided into two main categories: (1) infective spondylitis and epidural abscess; and (2) infections of the subdural space, meninges, and spinal cord. Occasional elements of both types of spinal infection are present in the same patient making diagnosis and treatment more challenging. Many infectious agents can cause infections of the spine further complicating diagnosis and treatment. This chapter will focus on the first category of spinal infections as these infections are more commonly encountered by the pain management specialist.

Infective Spondylitis and Epidural Abscess

Infective spondylitis is defined as an infection involving the boney vertebra, intervertebral disk, or the spinal extradural ligaments (**Fig. 92.1**).[1] *Epidural abscess* is defined as a localized collection of purulent material made up of destroyed tissue and leukocytes surrounded by an inflammatory reaction in the epidural space (**Fig. 92.2**).[2] Infective spondylitis and epidural abscess, although relatively uncommon, are extremely important clinically because of the significant associated morbidity and mortality. Death rates in older persons with epidural abscess approach 20%. Infective spondylitis most commonly affects the thoroacolumbar spine, whereas isolated epidural abscess is slightly more common in the cervical epidural space (**Figs. 92.3** and **92.4**).[3,4] Patients who have a compromised immune system (e.g., individuals infected with human immunodeficiency virus) as well as intravenous drug abusers and patients who have undergone spinal interventions (e.g., surgery and epidural blocks) are at greatest risk for developing spinal infections (**Table 92.1**).[5-7]

For purposes of diagnosis and treatment, infective spondylitis and epidural abscess are best divided into two distinct groups: (1) pyogenic infections and (2) nonpyogenic infections.[8]

More than 60% of pyogenic infections of the spine are caused by *Staphylococcus aureus*. An additional 30% of pyogenic infections are caused by *Enterococcus* species, and *Enterococcus faecalis* and *Enterococcus faecium* are the most common isolates.[9-11] In patients suffering from sickle cell disease, *Salmonella* is the most common cause of pyogenic spine. Immunocompromised patients are susceptible to infection from almost any pathogen, with *Serratia, Pseudomonas,* and occasionally *Candida* the most common (**Fig. 92.5**).[12,13]

Because children have a much more robust blood supply to the intervertebral disk and surrounding structures through the paravertebral and interosseous arteries as compared with adults, hematogenous spread of infectious agents to the spine is thought to be the most common source of infective spondylitis and epidural abscess in the pediatric age group and to

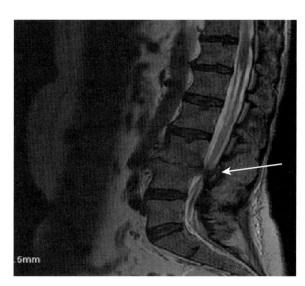

Fig. 92.1 Magnetic resonance imaging T2-weighted sagittal section showing narrowing of the L3-4 disk space with end-plate destruction *(black arrow). (From Purushothaman B, Lakshmanan P, Gatehouse S, et al: Spondylodiscitis due to Prevotella associated with ovarian mass: a rare case report and review of literature,* World Neurosurg *73:119, 2010.*

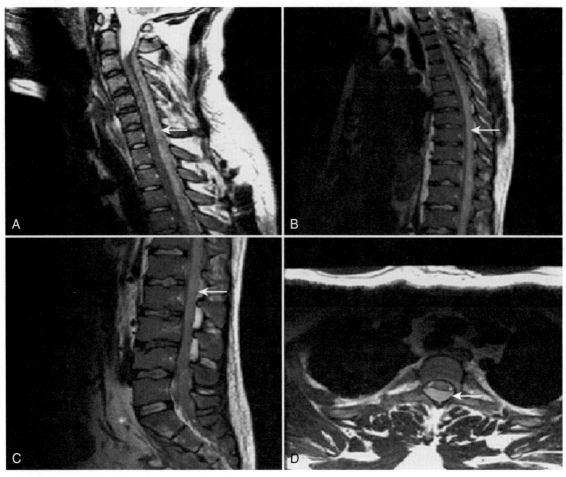

Fig. 92.2 Sagittal T2-weighted magnetic resonance imaging (MRI) scan of the spine showing an extensive spinal epidural abscess *(arrows)* involving cervical **(A)**, thoracic **(B)**, and lumbar **(C)** regions. A presacral collection is also visible **(C,** *asterisk).* **D,** An axial MRI scan defines the extent of spinal canal involvement *(arrow). (From Smith C, Kavar B: Extensive spinal epidural abscess as a complication of Crohn's disease,* J Clin Neurosci *17:144, 2010.)*

a lesser extent in adults[14,15] (see **Fig. 92.4** for an example of hematogenous seeding of a cervical epidural abscess from a distant site). In children, such infections tend to be more localized to the intervertebral disk, and adult infections tend to be initially more localized to the vertebral end plates, with the less vascular intervertebral disks affected later in the course of the disease. Infected urinary, spinal, or intravenous catheters, as well as infected heart valves, have also been implicated as common nidi of pyogenic spinal infections (see **Table 92.1**).[16] Urinary tract and intra-abdominal infections are also frequently associated with hematogenously spread pyogenic spinal infections.[10, 11,13] In addition, epidural steroid injections have been associated with an increased incidence of spinal infections, in particular epidural abscess.[6] Whereas infections involving the vertebral body and intervertebral disk are generally more localized, because of the nature of the epidural space, epidural abscess may spread over several spinal segments, especially in the posterior epidural space. As a result of the more tightly confined anterior epidural space, epidural abscess formation in this area tends to be more localized and is often seen in conjunction with infection of the anterior vertebral end plates and intervertebral disk.

Nonpyogenic infections are most commonly caused by *Mycobacterium tuberculosis,* although infections with fungi such as *Candida, Nocardia, Aspergillus, Cryptococcus,* and *Coccidioides* species are also seen, especially in immunocompromised patients.[17–19] Unlike the pathogens commonly implicated in pyogenic spinal infections that produce proteolytic enzymes that facilitate the spread of infection, nonpyogenic *Mycobacterium tuberculosis* and fungal infections tend to spread much more slowly and remain more localized. This slower spread contributes to the delay in diagnosis of many nonpyogenic spinal infections and is responsible for the formation of the characteristic large paravertebral abscesses.

Nonpyogenic tuberculous spondylitic infection occurs most commonly in the thoracic spine and is known as Pott's disease (**Fig. 92.6**).[17,18] Initially, the infection involves the anterior subchondral portion of the vertebral bodies and produces a characteristic abnormality known as a *corner lesion,* which is highly suggestive of tuberculous spondylitis (**Fig. 92.7**). As the disease slowly and often silently progresses, the neural arch and cortical portion of the vertebral body are affected, and vertebral compression fractures and resultant kyphosis are common sequelae. As mentioned earlier, large paravertebral abscess formation is quite characteristic of tuberculous spondylitic infection, as is adjacent soft tissue calcification. Spread of the infection under the anterior longitudinal ligament with

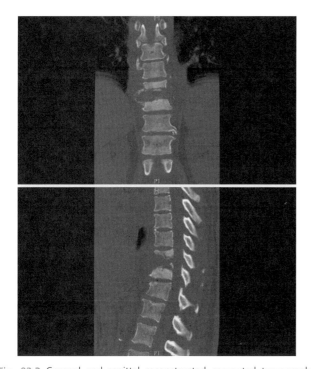

Fig. 92.3 Coronal and sagittal reconstructed computed tomography images of the thoracic spine revealing bone destruction involving the inferior surface of the T9 vertebral body and superior surface of the T10 vertebral body with paraspinal mass consistent with diskitis and osteomyelitis. *(From Lee SW, Manahan M, Fast A: Thoracic osteomyelitis: an easily missed diagnosis, PM R 1:889, 2009.)*

sparing of the intervertebral disk is also a common radiographic finding (**Fig. 92.8**).

Many nonpyogenic fungal infections may mimic the clinical and radiographic findings of nonpyogenic tuberculous spondylitic infection, and biopsy and culture may be required for specific diagnosis. Spinal infection with *Brucella* species is seen in regions where brucellosis is endemic (e.g., the Mediterranean and Saudi Arabia).[20] The source of the infection is most commonly unpasteurized dairy products or undercooked meat that have been infected with *Brucella*. *Brucella* spine infections have a predilection for the L5-S1 interspace (**Fig. 92.9**). Although rare, echinococcal infections of the spine do occur and are associated with more extensive destruction of the bony spinal elements[21] (**Fig. 92.10**).

Signs and Symptoms

The clinical presentations of infective spondylitis and epidural abscess are based on a variety of factors including the pathogen responsible for the infection and the immune status of the patient.[22] In general, pyogenic epidural abscess manifests and progresses more quickly than infective spondylitis.[23] Immunocompetent patients with pyogenic epidural abscess appear acutely ill, are almost always febrile, and develop neurologic findings early in the course of the illness. Ill-defined back pain quickly progresses to radicular symptoms and then to myelopathy. If the condition remains untreated, progressive and often permanent paraplegia or quadriplegia may result. Delays in treatment of pyogenic epidural abscess are associated with a 20% to 25% mortality rate. For this reason, the clinician should

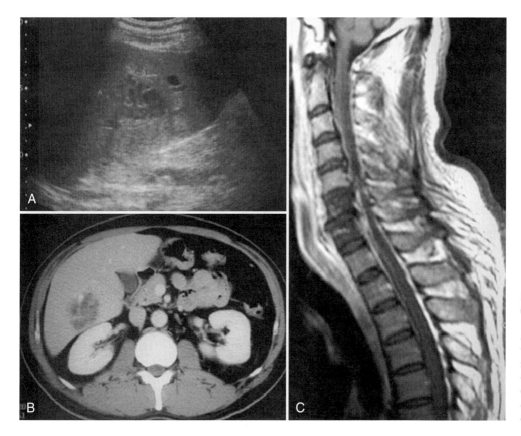

Fig. 92.4 Abdominal sonography (A) and computed tomography scanning (B) showing a 4.7 × 2.8-cm liver abscess with multiple septations at the right hepatic lobe. C, T2-weighted sagittal magnetic resonance imaging of the spine showing abnormal signal enhancement over C5, C6, and C7 and a peridural and prevertebral abscess.

Table 92.1 Predisposing Factors and Their Associations with Patients with Spinal Sepsis Compared with Control Patients, Reported as Odds Ratios

Variable	Percentage of Patients (No. of Patients; n = 72)	Percentage of Controls (No. of Controls; n = 80)	Odds Ratio (95% CI)	P Value
PREDISPOSING FACTORS				
Diabetes mellitus	21 (15)	8 (6)	3.2 (1.2–8.9)	.022
Immunodeficiency*	38 (27)	14 (11)	3.8 (1.7–8.3)	.001
Intravenous drug use	15 (11)	6 (5)	2.7 (0.9–8.2)	.079
Cancer or therapy	17 (12)	6 (5)	3.0 (1.0–9.0)	.050
Splenomegaly	4 (3)	0 (0)	NE	.104[†]
Other immunodeficiency	3 (2)	0 (0)	NE	.223[†]
PRIOR NONVIRAL INFECTION				
Related[‡§]	8 (6)	1 (1)	7.2 (0.8–61.2)	.071
Unrelated[‡]	21 (15)	8 (6)	3.2 (1.2–8.9)	.022
Spinal trauma[‡]	10 (7)	23 (18)	0.4 (0.1–0.9)	.039
Spinal procedure[‡{ParaMarks}]	15 (11)	13 (10)	1.3 (0.5–3.2)	.621
Spinal nerve block[‡]	3 (2)	1 (1)	2.3 (0.2–25.4)	.510
Degenerative spinal disease	25 (18)	19 (15)	1.4 (0.7–3.1)	.352
Alcoholism	15 (11)	4 (3)	4.6 (1.2–17.3)	.023
Obesity	11 (8)	1 (1)	9.9 (1.2–81.0)	.033
Any predisposing factor[¶]	93 (67)	56 (45)	10.4 (3.8–28.6)	<.001
PRESENTING SYMPTOMS				
Classic triad**	15 (11)	0 (0)	NE	<.001[†]
Fever	51 (37)	0 (0)	NE	<.001[†]
Neurologic deficit	54 (39)	28 (22)	3.1 (1.6–6.1)	.001
Muscle weakness	36 (26)	6 (5)	8.5 (3.0–23.6)	<.001
Radiating pain	42 (30)	48 (38)	0.8 (0.4–1.5)	.470
Vertebral tenderness	19 (14)	11 (9)	1.9 (0.8–4.7)	.164

*Includes below listed factors and human immunodeficiency virus infection/acquired immunodeficiency syndrome and long-term steroid use.
[†]Calculated using Fisher's exact χ2 test.
[‡]Within the past year.
[§]Includes vertebral osteomyelitis, diskitis, and paravertebral infections.
{ParaMarks}Not including spinal nerve block.
[¶]Includes all of the above listed factors and other nonspinal surgery, end-stage renal disease, congenital spinal anomaly, and recent pregnancy.
**Comprises fever, spine pain, and neurologic deficit.
CI, confidence interval; NE, not estimable.
From Angsuwat M, Kavar B, Lowe AJ: Early detection of spinal sepsis, *J Clin Neurosci* 17:59, 2010.

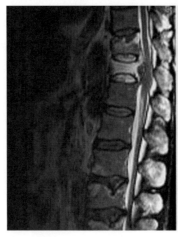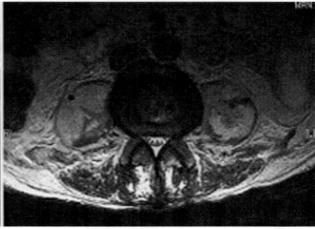

Fig. 92.5 Magnetic resonance imaging of the thoracolumbar spine showing destruction and compression of T12 with large bilateral psoas muscle abscesses; the signals of the disk above and below T12 were high in T2-weighted and short T1-weighted inversion recovery (STIR) images. *Left*, T2-weighted fast spin-echo sagittal image. *Right*, T2-weighted fast spin-echo axial image. Cultures of the abscess grew *Salmonella*. (From Zheng X, Wang J, Wu C, et al: Salmonella osteomyelitis of multiple ribs and thoracic vertebra with large psoas muscle abscesses, *Spine J* 9:e1, 2009.)

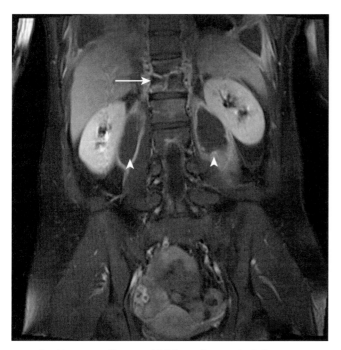

Fig. 92.6 **Pott's disease with bilateral paraspinal abscesses.**

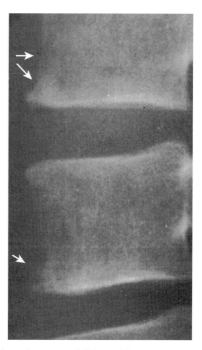

Fig. 92.8 **Tuberculous spondylitis: subligamentous extension.** The findings, although subtle, include erosion of the anterior surface of the vertebral bodies (arrows). (Courtesy of C. Resnik, MD, Baltimore, Maryland.)

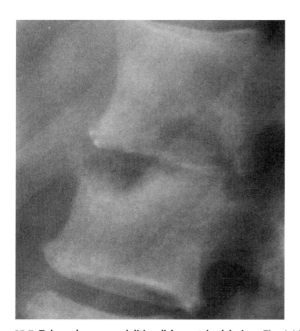

Fig. 92.7 **Tuberculous spondylitis: diskovertebral lesion.** The initial radiograph reveals subchondral destruction of two vertebral bodies with mild surrounding eburnation and loss of intervertebral disk height. The appearance is identical to that of pyogenic spondylitis.

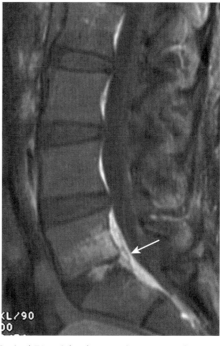

Fig. 92.9 Sagittal T1-weighted magnetic resonance image of a patient with brucellosis shows posterior longitudinal ligament elevation (arrow) and marked enhancement of the disk and vertebral end plate after gadolinium administration. (From Bozgeyik Z, Ozdemir H, Demirdag K, et al: Clinical and MRI findings of brucellar spondylodiscitis, Eur J Radiol 67:153, 2008.)

have a high index of suspicion for this diagnosis in any patient with back pain and fever, especially if the patient falls into a high-risk category. Careful neurologic examination should be carried out, with special attention paid to physical findings suggestive of myelopathy, such as Babinski's sign, clonus, and Chaddock's sign (**Figs. 92.11** and **92.12** [**online only**]) Nonpyogenic epidural abscess tends to manifest more slowly in immunocompetent patients, and the onset of neurologic symptoms may not be appreciated by either the patient or the clinician until significant neurologic damage has occurred. Immunocompromised patients may have a more fulminate course.

In the immunocompetent patient, infective spondylitis generally follows a clinical course more similar to that of nonpyogenic epidural abscess. Back pain is invariably present, and a low-grade fever accompanied by a flulike illness is often seen.[24] Neurologic findings early in the course of the disease may be

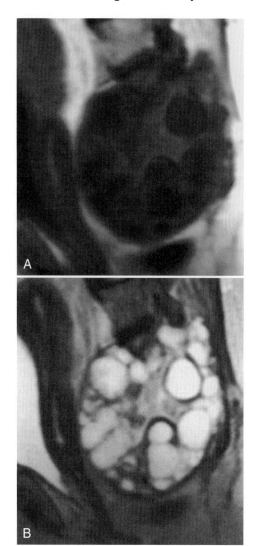

Fig. 92.10 Echinococcosis. A, Sagittal T1-weighted (TR/TE, 650/20) spin-echo magnetic resonance imaging (MRI) scan reveals a large mass predominantly involving the sacrum with anterior extension leading to displacement of pelvic viscera. Note the circular regions of low signal intensity within the mass, consistent with fluid-filled cysts. **B,** Sagittal T2-weighted (TR/TE, 4348/150) spin-echo MRI scan reveals the cysts as regions of high signal intensity. *(Courtesy of J. Kramer, MD, Vienna, Austria.)*

absent or very subtle, and as in patients suffering from non-pyogenic epidural abscess, these findings may not be appreciated by either the patient or the clinician.

Testing

Some clinicians believe that myelography is still the best test to ascertain compromise of the spinal cord and exiting nerve roots by an extrinsic mass such as an epidural abscess. However, in this era of readily available magnetic resonance imaging (MRI) and high-speed computed tomography (CT) scanning, it may be more prudent to obtain this noninvasive testing first rather than wait for a radiologist or spine surgeon to perform a myelogram.[25, 26] Both MRI with gadolinium enhancement and, to a lesser extent, CT with contrast are highly accurate in the diagnosis of epidural abscess and infective spondylitis and are probably more accurate than myelography in the diagnosis of intrinsic disease of the spinal cord or spinal tumor.[27] All patients suspected

of having an epidural abscess or infective spondylitis should undergo laboratory testing consisting of complete blood cell count, sedimentation rate, and automated blood chemistry studies. Blood and urine cultures should be immediately obtained in all patients thought to be suffering from epidural abscess, to allow immediate implementation of antibiotic therapy while the diagnostic workup is in progress.[28] Gram stain and cultures of the abscess material should also be obtained, but antibiotic treatment should not be delayed while awaiting this information.

Treatment

The rapid initiation of treatment of epidural abscess or infective spondylitis is mandatory if the patient is to avoid the sequelae of permanent neurologic deficit or death. Treatment of epidural abscess or infective spondylitis has two goals: (1) treatment of the infection with antibiotics and (2) drainage of the abscess to relieve compression on neural structures. Because most pyogenic epidural abscesses are caused by *Staphylococcus aureus* or *Enterococcus* species, antibiotics such as vancomycin that will treat staphylococcal infection and a third- or fourth-generation cephalosporin to treat gram-negative infections should be started immediately after blood and urine culture samples are taken.[29,30] Daptomycin has been reported to be useful in patients with methicillin-resistant staphylococcal infection of the spine.[31] Antibiotic therapy can be tailored to the culture and sensitivity reports as they become available. As mentioned, antibiotic therapy should not be delayed while waiting for definitive diagnosis if epidural abscess or infective spondylitis is considered in the differential diagnosis.

Antibiotics alone rarely successfully treat an epidural abscess unless the diagnosis is made very early in the course of the disease; thus, drainage of the abscess is required to affect full recovery.[31] Drainage of the epidural abscess is usually accomplished by decompression laminectomy and evacuation of the abscess.[32,33] More recently, interventional radiologists have been successful in draining epidural abscesses percutaneously using drainage catheters placed with the use of CT or MRI guidance.[34] Serial CT or MRI scans are useful in following the resolution of epidural abscess and should be repeated immediately at the first sign of negative change in the patient's neurologic status.

Conclusion

Infections of the spine continue to present a diagnostic challenge for the clinician. Delays in diagnosis often result in permanent neurologic sequelae and, in 25% of cases, death. A high index of suspicion of spinal infection is indicated in any patient presenting with low back pain and fever, especially in those patients who have identifiable risk factors. Unusual spinal infections can occur in immunocompromised patients, and the usual sign of fever may be minimal or absent. Immediate imaging of the spine in any patient suspected of having a spinal infection is imperative to avoid disaster. Antibiotic treatment appropriate to cover staphylococcal and enterococcal infection should be initiated and then adjusted as Gram stain and culture results become available.

References

Full references for this chapter can be found on www.expertconsult.com.

Arachnoiditis and Related Conditions

J. Antonio Aldrete

Arachnoiditis is usually identified as a spinal illness characterized by motor and sensory symptoms in the lower extremities. These symptoms generally appear after invasive interventions in the vertebral canal such as spinal tap, intradural and extradural anesthesia, laminectomy, and fusion. However, arachnoiditis may also affect the normal dynamics of the cerebrospinal fluid (CSF) and thus alter proprioceptive, hearing, and visual functions. These effects confirm that arachnoiditis is an entity far more complex than its name implies. Although arachnoiditis appears more often in the lumbosacral region, it may appear in the thoracic and cervical spine and intracranially.

Currently, the most common causes of arachnoiditis include the following:

- Surgical interventions, chiefly laminectomies and spinal fusions, with or without hardware, can cause arachnoiditis.[1] The pathogenic mechanism is related to the entry of blood into the subarachnoid space, because patients are usually in the prone position and the dural sac is at the bottom of the wound. Incidental durotomies, especially when they are not recognized and not repaired, are ominous events,[2] leading to significant CSF leaks and pseudomeningoceles,[3] as well as to the possible initiation of a severe inflammatory reaction of the arachnoid.[4] A second alternative occurs in cases in which large hematomas accumulate extradurally. The degradation of old blood may liberate cytokines and leukotrienes that cross the dural barrier, thus resulting in the same end product. Unsatisfactory results have ensued in a progressively increased population of patients with the dreadful diagnosis of "failed back surgery syndrome."[5]

- Similar pathophysiologic processes can be considered as the cause of arachnoiditis when blood enters the subarachnoid or the epidural space, such as when neuraxial anesthesia is performed in anticoagulated patients or in patients who receive antithrombin preparations. In addition, large volumes of blood injected to seal dural tears may, by a pressure gradient, permit the entry of blood into the CSF compartment. Furthermore, extradural hematomas and granulomas may compress the spinal cord and nerve roots to the point of leaving permanent neurologic deficits (cauda equina) coexisting with arachnoiditis only when blood gains access to the CSF.

- During neuraxial anesthesia, injuries may occur from direct needle or catheter trauma and from chemical substances that may irritate the spinal cord or the nerve roots, such as local anesthetics (5% lidocaine, 3% chloroprocaine), additives such as sodium bicarbonate and preservatives (sodium bisulfate), and blood (traumatic taps or epidural blood patches whenever the intradural compartment is breached). Paresthesia from needle trauma is an ominous sign because it may allow the passage of otherwise innocuous concentrations of local anesthetics (2% lidocaine, 0.5% bupivacaine, or 1% tetracaine) to come into contact with the endoneurium, with resulting axon demyelination.[6] Similarly, certain neurolytic substances such as injected phenol and alcohol, injected extradurally, may cross the dural barrier and enter the subarachnoid space.

- Interventional procedures for pain relief such as incidental intradural injection of corticosteroids, all of which contain preservatives (polyethylene glycol, benzilic alcohol, or benzalkonium),[7] misguided radiofrequency electrode application,[8] diskography,[9] intradiskal electrotherapy probes,[10] failed attempts to inject neurolytic substances near sympathetic chains, methylmethacrylate injected intrathecally[11] while attempting vertebroplasty, and epidural neurolysis[12] with 10% saline solution may have serious consequences if the substances end up intradurally.

■ Infections of the spine can be caused by common bacteria such as *Neisseria meningitides, Haemophilus influenzae,* viridans streptococci, *Enterococcus faecalis,* and *Klebsiella.* However, investigators have expressed concern regarding infections following regional anesthesia or interventional procedures, caused by organisms such as *Staphylococcus aureus, Pseudomonas aeruginosa,* and methicillin-resistant *S. aureus* (MRSA)[13] and in ambulatory patients by *Staphylococcus epidermidis.*[14] In certain regions, arachnoiditis may be caused in the spine by tuberculosis, human immunodeficiency virus infection, and West Nile virus infection; parasitosis such as cysticercosis, trichinosis, and malaria may occur in the brain.[15] Severe chronic sinus infections may penetrate the floor of the skull and appear in dependent areas of the cranium, around the optic chiasma or the mastoid region. Unexpectedly, infections occurring in parturients undergoing neuraxial anesthesia were noted to be on the rise.[16] Some of these infections were traced to bacteria and fungi grown from oronasal cultures out of anesthesia personnel, and investigators concluded that a casual approach surrounding the birthing experience may have allowed personnel to relax the expected sterile environment. Recommendations are to wear caps, masks, and shoe covers properly.[17] The need to wear sterile gowns during the insertion of extradural and intradural catheters used for infusions and reinjections is under study.[18]

■ Repeated intrathecal injections with antibiotics or chemotherapeutic agents (e.g., amphotericin, methotrexate) or antimetabolites (cytarabine), depending on the dose, concentration, and state of hydration of the patient, may cause arachnoiditis.[19]

Pain Mechanisms

Most patients with arachnoiditis usually experience severe, constant pain with typical neuropathic features that may be exacerbated by motion of the lower spine and extremities. The actual anatomic and pathologic mechanisms responsible for the pain and related symptoms are initiated by peripheral nociceptive afferent fibers that terminate in the dorsal horn of the spinal cord.[20] Because the thinly laminated A-delta fibers end in lamina I and lamina V, the unmyelinated C fibers enter the outer lamina I and II and activate large numbers of second-order interneurons within the dorsal horn,[21] including two main groups of dorsal horn cells: (1) the nociceptive-specific cells that respond mostly to noxious stimuli and to innocuous stimuli[22] and (2) the multireceptive convergent cells that are usually activated by innocuous stimuli.

Some networks communicating with various types of spinal cord neurons modulate nociceptive information and transmit it to neurons that project to the brain. Certain stimuli sensitize these projecting neurons and increase nociceptive transmission, whereas others produce inhibition. This relationship between the excitatory and the inhibitory processes has confirmed the "gate theory" of pain transmission.[23] When temporal summation of postsynaptic, excitatory potentials exceeds the action potential threshold, it may produce another phenomenon observed in neuropathic pain called "central sensitization." After an injurious event, the arachnoid usually responds with an acute inflammatory reaction in which repetitive C-fiber input evokes a state of spinal facilitation similar to what has been labeled "wind-up," characterized by repeated stimuli evoking progressively greater responses in dorsal horn neurons, as well as a gradual increase in extension of the size of their respective fields.[24]

In addition, other receptors and transmitters intervene in this phenomenon, including the following:

■ Calcitonin gene–related peptide
■ *N*-methyl-d-aspartate (NMDA) (participates in the wind-up phenomenon and in central sensitization)
■ Nerve growth factor
■ Substance P of the neurokinin type
■ Neurokinin A
■ Nitric oxide (especially contributing to hyperalgesia and allodynia)
■ Eicosanoids including prostaglandins, thromboxanes, and leukotrienes[25]

In neuropathic pain, C fibers and large A-beta fibers mediate the information from low-threshold mechanoreceptors interacting with dynamic range neurons. It appears that histologic changes that occur in post-traumatic total or partial section of peripheral nerves differ from injuries on nerve roots caused by irritant chemical agents, as shown by Romero-Figueroa et al.[26] These investigators injected 22% phenol intrathecally in rats, and the result was almost complete demyelination of some nerve roots; intravascular thrombosis was a consistent feature, whereas nonaffected nerve roots had their vessels patent (**Fig. 93.1**). Sprouting was noted within 2 weeks after phenol administration, and by 2 months, recovery was nearly complete, although the pattern of myelin distribution in the axons was obviously abnormal.

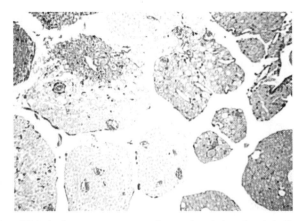

Fig. 93.1 Lesions on nerve roots produced by the intrathecal injection of 22% phenol in rats. Two days after injection, marked demyelinization of axons in nerve roots with thrombosed vessels is noted. Normal myelination of the axons is evident in nerve roots with patent vessels (hematoxylin-eosin stain ×30). *(From Romero-Figueroa S, Aldrete JA, Martinez-Cruz A, et al: Ischemic axon degeneration in nerve roots after intrathecal phenol with evidence of atypical regeneration,* J Peripher Nerv Syst *11:1, 2006.)*

Diagnosis

Laboratory Diagnosis

Efforts to identify a laboratory test that would indicate the presence or the progress of arachnoiditis have been unsuccessful. Exceptions may be certain infections in which immune reactivity to certain microorganisms has been determined within the meningeal layers by using specific antibody synthesis.[27]

Although CSF leukocytosis and hyperproteinemia have been noted in the early stage, pleocytosis, high levels of proteins, and a reduced amount of β-endorphin (in monkeys) have been found in the late stages of arachnoiditis.[28] Other observations suggest that plasma and CSF C-reactive protein values are elevated in the inflammatory phase of this disease with peaks during flare-ups.

Electrodiagnostic Studies

Nerve conduction, electromyographic, and somatosensory evoked potential studies have been considered helpful in the diagnosis of radiculitis and in cases of radiculopathy and peripheral neuropathy. However, in neither the early nor the late stage of arachnoiditis has a specific pattern been identified.

Epiduroscopy and Myeloscopy

The information obtained from epidural endoscopy is limited in terms of the extent of the disease (several levels) and the ability to diagnose intrathecal disease with an extradurally placed scope. However, experience with a thecaloscope has shown diffuse arachnoiditis, although attempts to separate clumped nerve roots by high-pressure irrigation[29] have not provided evidence that this traumatic method is innocuous. Thus far, the use of thecaloscopy may confirm the diagnosis of arachnoiditis, but the assertion that it is a more effective diagnostic tool than magnetic resonance imaging (MRI) remains unsubstantiated.[30]

Radiologic Diagnosis

MRI has been accepted as the gold standard.[31] However, it requires the administration of the intravenous enhancing agent gadolinium to identify most clearly the presence of edema or clumping of nerve roots in all its varieties (**Fig. 93.2**) and intradural fibrosis. MRI also has the advantage of enabling the examiner to differentiate between scar tissue and nerve roots.[32]

Contrast-enhanced nerve roots are usually found in the inflammatory stage of arachnoiditis and are noted as swollen and thicker; in the axial views, they sometimes have a stellar appearance (**Fig. 93.3**). This feature may be visible in patients with the transient nerve root irritation syndrome, which in fact represents an inflammatory response[33] manifested as radicular edema (**Fig. 93.4**). In cases of myelopathic syringomyelia from a needle puncture (**Fig. 93.5**), the extent (several intervertebral levels) and communication with the subarachnoid compartment may be identified.[34]

In some instances, when patients have implanted metal objects (e.g., surgical staples, screws, plates), MRI is contraindicated (unless these objects are made of titanium). An alternative approach is to obtain a myelogram using a water-soluble dye, followed by a computed tomography (CT) scan that allows the visualization of intrathecal disease. Plain radiographic films are helpful to identify intrathecal calcifications or other disease (spondylolisthesis). Although water-soluble dyes are currently used, excessive volumes, paresthesias, or bloody taps may exacerbate arachnoiditis by igniting another inflammatory reaction.[35]

Epidurography may reveal dural sac deformities and peridural scarring, but intrathecal lesions cannot be visualized. Pantopaque droplets (**Fig. 93.6**) may be trapped in the distal portion of the dural sac and in Tarlov's cysts. Considered by some investigators to be a pathognomonic lesion, intrathecal calcification can be seen by CT or on plain radiographs (**Fig. 93.7**).

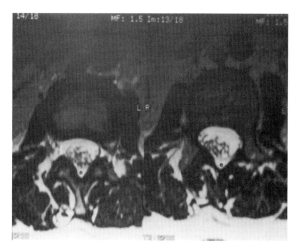

Fig. 93.2 Two axial magnetic resonance imaging views of the lumbar spine with clumped nerve roots mostly on the right side of the dural sac at the L3-4 level. Epidural spaces are patent (e).

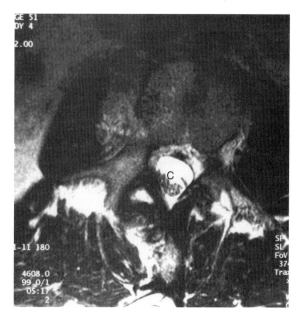

Fig. 93.3 Axial view at the L4 level, showing clumped nerve roots (C) mostly on the right side of the dural sac, 2 years after a laminectomy. The paravertebral muscles have been separated from their bone insertions and are being substituted by adipose tissue.

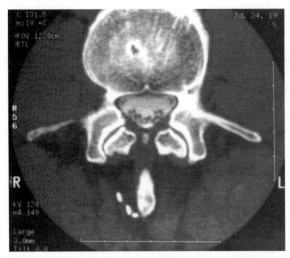

Fig. 93.4 Computed tomography scan after myelogram at the L3-4 level demonstrating "enhanced" nerve roots mostly on the posterior half of the dural sac. They are edematous and stellar in aspect.

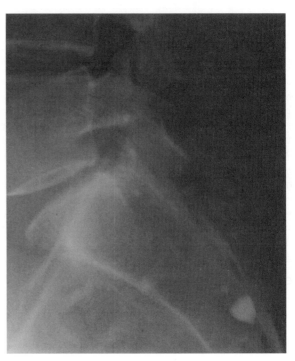

Fig. 93.6 Lateral radiograph of lumbosacral spine showing Pantopaque present in a Tarlov cyst at the S2 level, 9 years after a myelogram.

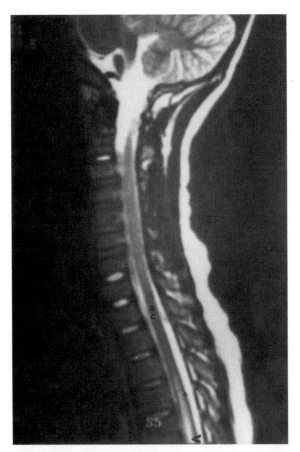

Fig. 93.5 Sagittal magnetic resonance image of the cervical spine and thoracic spine showing syringomyelia (arrows) in the spinal cord (sc) from T6 down.

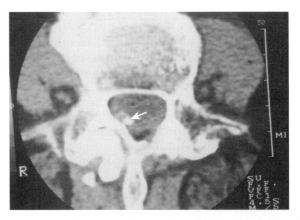

Fig. 93.7 Computed tomography scan of L4 with an osteophyte on the right side of the vertebral body and an intrathecal calcification shown by the arrow. Evidence of an attempted fusion is shown against the right lamina.

A scale has been introduced for the quantitative evaluation of (1) changes in the distribution of the nerve roots, (2) the number of interspaces involved, and (3) the aggregated lesions (pseudomeningocele, intrathecal cysts, syringomyelia, obliterative arachnoiditis, and cervical or thoracic location).[36] By grading each of these lesions into five parameters, the scale allows a numeric quantification of the disease and permits the examiner to determine the progression of the disease after a diagnostic or therapeutic procedure or its improvement in response to a certain therapeutic modality (**Fig. 93.8**).[36]

Clinical Diagnosis

No one single symptom identifies arachnoiditis clinically. Nevertheless, from the examination of patients with radiologically diagnosed arachnoiditis, it is apparent that the predominant symptoms are related to neuropathic pain, although the distribution is not classically "in dermatome," as may be expected in sciatica.[37]

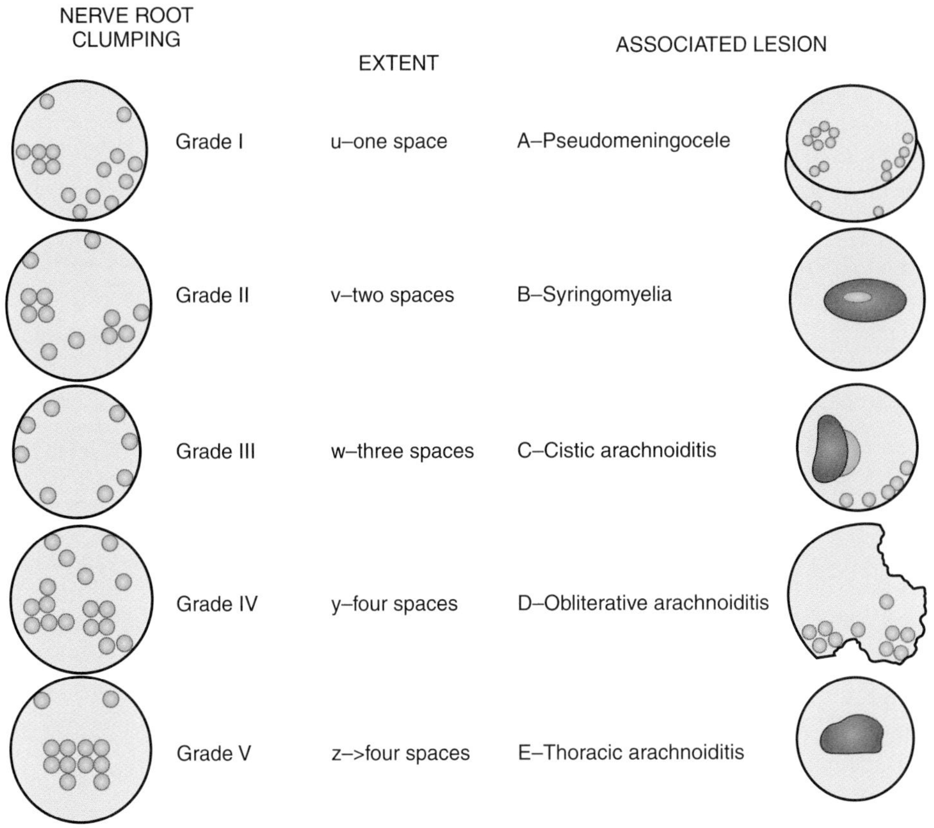

NERVE ROOT
CLUMPING

EXTENT

ASSOCIATED LESION

Grade I   u–one space   A–Pseudomeningocele

Grade II   v–two spaces   B–Syringomyelia

Grade III   w–three spaces   C–Cistic arachnoiditis

Grade IV   y–four spaces   D–Obliterative arachnoiditis

Grade V   z–>four spaces   E–Thoracic arachnoiditis

Fig. 93.8 Quantitative scale to estimate and compare the degree of extent and severity brought by the pattern of distribution and clumping of the nerve roots. The scale lists the number of interspaces involved and includes other associated lesions.

Burning pain is indeed the characteristic manifestation on one or both lower extremities, with or without hyperalgesia and allodynia and usually accompanied by sensory disturbances including hypoesthesia, dysesthesia, and a tingling sensation. Hyperreflexia may be noted, although it depends on the presence of other lesions. Muscle spasms are common. Peculiarly enough, most patients also have autonomic nervous system manifestations, such as low-grade fever, frequent diaphoresis and nocturnal sweating, and chronic fatigue. Most patients with cauda equina nerve root involvement have considerable bladder dysfunction; incontinence and incomplete emptying are more common in women, whereas dysuria, frequency, and residual urine after micturition occur more often in men. Rectal dysfunction is more commonly manifested as constipation, with or without rectal incontinence, and it is present in both genders in approximately 40% of patients.

In most clinical settings, seldom are patients asked about changes in sexual function after the onset of arachnoiditis. In this same group of patients, investigators found that loss of libido and difficulty in arousing were the most frequent dysfunctions in both men and women. Men reported impotence, penel pain at erection, and low back pain during sexual intercourse, and women reported pain during and after intercourse.[38]

Needless to say, considerable depression is present in most patients with arachnoiditis. Some patients also have anxiety and feelings of loss, guilt, and despair because no cure is available. These symptoms contribute to intramarital and interfamily conflicts, as well as social dysfunction, ending in separation or divorce in more than one third of the patients. Cigarette smoking is prevalent, as are isolation and disability. This perspective implies a population group with several disabling clinical manifestations that impair the ability to remain in a functional family, preclude participation in social interactions, and make it impossible to support themselves and their families. These patients become dependent on the health care system or on their close relatives, and the result is a sense of permanent loss.[39]

Correlative Diagnosis

In a group of patients seen from 1989 to 2008, Aldrete attempted to identify suggestive features that would indicate the apparent injurious event that produced arachnoiditis (confirmed by radiologic diagnosis). Patients who had undergone surgical procedures by far exceeded those whose arachnoiditis was caused by neuraxial anesthesia, epidural steroid injections, and other irritant substances (e.g., neurolytics, dyes, local anesthetics containing preservatives or enzymes). The numbers of cases attributed to the intrathecal injection of Pantopaque for myelograms declined. Usually, the localization of symptoms to one or both sides corresponded to the intervertebral level affected and the findings of the neurologic examination. Numerous patterns of nerve root clumping exist, and no single pattern signifies the typical representation of arachnoiditis. Nevertheless, it is important to determine the location of the clumping as well as the intervertebral levels affected.[31–34,36] In cases of arachnoiditis caused by surgical interventions, in addition to finding some of the nerve roots clumped and the dural sac retracted or dilated at the level of the operated intervertebral space, these patients also had peridural scarring and fibrosis (see Fig. 93.8). Not uncommonly, distal ectasia or pseudomeningocele may be present (see Chapters 96 and 98). A scale to grade the extent of clumping, the levels included, and other related lesions has been proposed. However, because the same patient may have undergone myelographies, laminectomies, and various invasive procedures, in some cases it is not clearly evident which intervention caused the lesions unless a sudden appearance of clumped nerve roots (see Figs. 93.2 and 93.3) at MRI corresponds to the relevant clinical neurologic findings and the level at which the intervention was done.

Prevention

In this disease, prevention is a primordial concern that would reduce the number of cases of arachnoiditis. Although the recommendations for prevention appear to be simple, they are crucial.

In the case of suspected infections, associated symptoms or findings may be helpful to define the cause. An MRI scan confirms the diagnosis of peridural or intrathecal location. Although the use of spinal taps to sample CSF appears reasonable, a postdural puncture headache in a patient with increased CSF pressure would increase the persistence of postural cephalalgia. It is suggested that an MRI scan be obtained first, especially with the present availability of MRI. Thereafter, dural puncture may be necessary only to obtain a specimen for culture and sensitivity.

The occurrence of paresthesias during an interventional procedure of the spine may be a reason for stopping the procedure and choosing a different technique, because perforation of the dura and arachnoid is implied, as well as penetration of the perineural layer of a nerve root. Furthermore, the injection of local anesthetics, even at their usual concentrations, may, under these circumstances, irritate the endoneurial structures and initiate an inflammatory response.[6,22,23] Because the posterior epidural space has no nerve trunks, eliciting paresthesias implies that the tip of the needle was in the subarachnoid space. Strict aseptic technique is essential when the vertebral canal is to be invaded; currently, the injection of neuroirritant or neurolytic substances into the canal is best avoided.

Treatment

Because different disease mechanisms are involved in the two phases of arachnoiditis, the therapeutic approach needs to be tailored to each of these stages. The presence of blood or serosanguineous CSF usually implies the puncture of a vessel within the intrathecal compartment. The injection of any chemical substances, including local anesthetics or dyes,[1,2,28] may, under these circumstances, appear to increase the likelihood of arachnoidal inflammation. Similarly, the concomitant peridural administration of certain additives such as sodium bicarbonate, vasoconstrictors (epinephrine or phenylephrine), or therapeutic agents such as corticosteroids or blood in the presence of an incidental penetration of the dura may initiate intrathecal inflammation, even when small volumes of these substances have been administered.

The decision to postpone these procedures is not easy, and it needs to be practical. If feasible, however, a delay may be considered before proceeding, in view of the added risk weighed against rescheduling the procedure for another day. As alternatives, one may consider proceeding but using an extraspinal (paravertebral) or caudal technique or a peripheral nerve block, if indicated.

Treatment of the Acute Phase of Arachnoiditis

Because of the critical interval when proper diagnosis and treatment may reduce or stop the inflammatory process, treatment is urgent. If a neurologic deficit, uncontrollable severe burning pain, or loss of bladder or bowel control occurs after an invasive or surgical procedure, the following steps are recommended[34,40,41]:

- Perform a complete neurologic examination.
- Obtain a neurology consultation.
- Perform an MRI scan to search for specific lesions that may need to be treated promptly (e.g., intrathecal or extradural hematoma, dural leaks).

Once the clinical diagnosis of arachnoiditis, cauda equina syndrome, pseudomeningocele, or any other neurologic deficit is made and is confirmed by the typical appearance of enhanced nerve roots, and if the patient is considered to be in the inflammatory stage of the disease (estimated to last 8 to 10 weeks after the injurious event; see Fig. 93.4), treatment is indicated to prevent the condition from evolving into the permanent proliferative phase. The following protocol is recommended:

- Limit physical activities.
- Administer steroids intravenously.
- Administer magnesium oxide.
- Use anti-inflammatory agents such as indomethacin.
- Use an anticonvulsant.
- Administer an antidepressant.
- Monitor improvement by repeating the neurologic examination every 3 days and the MRI scan every 3 to 4 weeks.
- In the event that radiologic confirmation is inconclusive but the clinical manifestations are evident, treating physicians may consider proceeding with this protocol.
- For information, consult www.arachnoiditis.com.

Preliminary observations have indicated that the sooner this protocol is initiated, the better the chances will be for having the symptoms subside completely or partially. This study, still in progress, appears to suggest that procrastination is not helpful, whereas prompt treatment may offer the possibility of reversing the neurologic deficits and burning pain. Once the third month passes, usually the symptoms are permanent. Interventional procedures during this phase of arachnoiditis are best avoided.

Treatment of Chronic Arachnoiditis

Most patients with the diagnosis of arachnoiditis have features of neurogenic pain; therefore, the concepts already described in Chapters 2 to 6, 32 to 38, and 98 apply to its mechanisms, pathophysiology, and proposed treatment. However, some special characteristics in this disease merit mention.[32,40] Considering that the intensity of burning pain, hyperalgesia, and allodynia is severe and continuous, the initiation of opioid medications is not one to be undertaken lightly. Because tolerance to this group of medications and the dependency syndrome most likely will develop, it is preferable to initiate treatment with schedule III opiates.[40,42] Apparent increases in pain intensity, usually accompanied by requests to increase the dosage, usually imply a reduction of the drug's efficacy, owing to tachyphylaxis rather than to progression of the disease, given that arachnoiditis tends to evolve very slowly.[43] Moreover, the development of hyperalgesia with progressive doses of opioids[44] has been recognized as a detractor to the indiscriminate use of these medications. Naturally, other associated conditions such as spondylolisthesis, spondylosis, recurrent herniated nucleus pulposus, and so on, must be ruled out because their symptoms may be superimposed on those of arachnoiditis. These other disorders manifest with similar symptoms but require a different type of treatment.

Whenever possible and as early as feasible, an anticonvulsant medication is indicated. Gabapentin has been the most effective in taming the pain. Pregabalin, topiramate, and phenytoin are possible alternatives if side effects to gabapentin develop.

Psychological counseling is usually required in most patients to help them to cope with the sense of loss and specifically the depression,[39] which can become severe. Psychiatric consultation is required in patients with severe cases and to define selectively the type of antidepressant best for each of these patients, as well as to determine the need for anxiolytic medications, hypnotics, and so on.

Muscle relaxants are indicated if severe muscle spasms appear. The usual physical therapy modalities may actually increase the pain; however, because it is crucial to maintain some type of fitness, it is preferred to institute a program of isometric exercises, together with hydrotherapy and a stationary bike program for cardiovascular fitness. Selectively, other treatments are designed for each patient. In cases of neurogenic bladder, patients are taught to reduce fluids at certain times (evening) to prevent sleep disturbances. If necessary, women with marked sphincter dysfunction may be taught self-catheterization, as well as how to prevent urinary tract infections. Medications indicated for erectile dysfunction may be tried, although their effectiveness is usually meager.

Other measures have been proposed to help with some of the autonomic nervous system symptoms, such as anticholinergic medications to reduce the profuse diaphoresis experienced by these patients. Because of its effective relaxing action on striated muscle, magnesium oxide assists with the treatment of muscle spasms and also appears to be effective in the treatment of constipation occurring from the ingestion of opiates or rectal neurogenic malfunction. In cases of impairment of CSF ascending return from either surgical interventions resulting in dural sac ectasia or massive clumping of nerve roots, propranolol, 40 to 80 mg/day, has been shown to reduce the pressure sensation experienced by some patients in the most dependent region of the spine when the cephalic return of the CSF is impeded by the clumped nerve roots, scar tissue, or intrathecal cysts. That is why most patients with arachnoiditis have been found to have elevated CSF pressure. Therefore, the concurrent administration of acetazolamide, 250 to 500 mg/day, appears to tame the pain, presumably by changing the CSF pH. In both instances, the effects on the heart rate from the former agent and on plasma potassium concentration from the latter agent must be monitored.

Acupuncture, in its various modalities, has had limited use and ambiguous results. Nevertheless, it is worth trying, although its efficacy appears to depend greatly on the experience and expertise of the practitioner.

Interventionism

Most invasive procedures have no application in cases of arachnoiditis because most of these procedures are aimed at extradural structures. Even so, most of them have been tried. Undoubtedly, these procedures may provide partial and short-lasting pain relief because in many cases procedures such as epidural corticosteroid, facet, or sacroiliac joint injections may address concomitant disease but have little significant and longer-lasting effect on arachnoiditis. The same commentary applies to diagnostic procedures such as differential spinal procedures and diskograms, for example.

Spinal Cord Stimulation

Two other modalities appear to have a more realistic indication, one of which is spinal cord stimulation, which supposedly acts by one or more of the following mechanisms:

- Interruption of stimuli traveling through spinothalamic fibers
- Expand descending dorsolateral funiculus pathways
- Supraspinal gating mechanisms
- Alteration of spinal neurotransmitter pools by disinhibition at supraspinal sites

Undoubtedly, technologic advances have improved since this modality was first proposed. Although assessments of this modality reported that the efficacy was similar to that of placebo, most other publications included patients with various diagnoses, some of them subgroups of patients with arachnoiditis. Results varied, but one concept seems to have been constant: after 6 months from implantation, only 50% of the patients had 50% of pain relief; the rest had either unsatisfactory results or had left the study. Problems with infection, fibrosis around the tip of the electrode, and lead migration still plague this technique. Two different studies showed that improvement after use of this modality differs little from the effect produced by placebo.[45,46] Although these latter studies included patients with chronic pain, these commentaries apply solely to the indications for arachnoiditis. Moreover, Carter[45] assessed the evidence from the published articles on spinal cord stimulation by meta-analysis and found significant problems with the methodology of most studies, including patient selection, lack of comparative methods of treatment, lack of randomization, and blinding. Carter[45] concluded that the absence of quality evidence in the literature prevents recommendation of this modality at present.

Nonimplantable and Implantable Pumps

Although implantable and nonimplantable pumps were initially proposed for patients with terminal cancer, the application of these devices to patients with chronic nononcologic pain has become customary. Specially designed catheters that are surgically implanted are used for this pain management approach. Although these infusions temporarily reduce the pain in most patients, their effect is palliative because the drugs do nothing to improve the arachnoiditis. Patients are provided a vacation from pain, and many patients feel that it is worth it. The concern about infection and the frequent occurrence of epidural fibrosis make this location and the limited period of implantation an alternative only for short-lasting therapy.[48,49]

Implantable infusion pumps that deliver smaller doses of opiates into the subarachnoid space appear to provide more effective pain relief. This therapeutic approach seems to be especially indicated in patients with chronic arachnoiditis. These pumps require refills every 6 to 8 weeks. Undoubtedly, they produce analgesia and allow for physical activities that otherwise would be impossible. Infusates combining morphine with baclofen, bupivacaine, clonidine, or ketamine allow for reduction in the dose of the opiate or another opioid such as hydromorphone.[50] Infections are rare after the initial implantation; however, dependency develops gradually. Patients believe that their disease is advancing, whereas they are developing a tolerance that necessitates increases in the dosage.[51] Larger doses of morphine produce significant sexual dysfunction in both men[52] and women,[53] with hyperalgesia, allodynia, and hyperreactivity that is not reversible with naloxone, possibly related to the formation of morphine-3-glucuronide.[34,51] Lower extremity edema has been reported in approximately 20% of the patients receiving intrathecal infusions of opiates, purportedly because of sympathetic blockade from these medications.[54,55] Most patients with this problem have had varicose veins or pedal edema before implantation, and such a condition becomes a relative contraindication to this therapeutic modality.

However, the main concern has been the reports of granulomas forming at the tip of the catheter. These granulomas seem to occur mostly with opiate infusions,[51,56] starting within 6 months and from doses higher than 10 mg/day. As the catheter tip becomes gradually obstructed, the tendency has been to increase the dosage or the concentration, an approach that in fact accelerates granuloma formation. Multifocal accumulation of neutrophils, monocytes, macrophages, and plasma cells is characterized by high protein and normal glucose levels in the CSF.[57,58] Opiates have been shown to initiate release of nitric oxide in human endothelial cells; the continued exposure of immunocytes to morphine may lead to an exaggerated response of monocytes to other proinflammatory stimuli that activate nitric oxide synthase in the arachnoid vasculature and increase local capillary permeability.[59] The absence of positive stains for bacteria, the failure to obtain CSF or infusate cultures, and the finding of normal CSF glucose levels imply the presence of granuloma, which is confirmed by the finding of a soft mass with a necrotic center at surgery.[59,60] Currently, the N-type blocker ziconotide, which interrupts the transmission of pain by closing the calcium channels, is being infused for this purpose, although its elevated cost and side effects have limited its application. Because of possible liability,[61] these complications have reduced the previously wide use of these devices. In an attempt to avoid granulomas, ziconotide has been used more; however, its toxic effects in some patients[61] and its high cost have discouraged some practitioners.

Nonconventional Treatment of Chronic Arachnoiditis

In addition to the use of propranolol, indomethacin, and acetazolamide, it appears prudent to continue a sensible strategy that, although not specific, is tangibly applicable to this disease. Medications that have been approved by the US Food and Drug Administration have been reevaluated for different indications. When drug studies have suggested an apparent beneficial effect on one of the pathologic processes in patients with arachnoiditis, it seems logical and justified to assess the value of these drugs, as long as they are demonstrated to have minimal risk. Some of the medications include the following: probenecid,[62] a drug used to treat gout that has been shown to facilitate the transfer of certain medications across the dural barrier; the cholesterol-lowering simvastatin, which has revealed itself as a notable anti-inflammatory drug; and the antioxidant lipoidic acid, already known and available in alternative medicine.

This sensible approach of giving a second look to medications that may be considered "off label" has been legitimized by the use of the erythropoietin as a protector of neural tissue in stroke,[63,64] diabetic neuropathy,[65] and other neurologic conditions.[64] Similarly, antioxidants such as *N*-acetylcysteine, neurotrophic peptides such as nerve growth factor, and prosaposin have been tried, without consistent effect. The tumor necrosis factor-α inhibitor etarnecept,[66] injected paraspinally, has been claimed to reduce cervical disk pain and arachnoiditis.[65] The neurotransmitter memantine[47] is being tried in multiple sclerosis, amyotrophic lateral sclerosis, and diabetic neuropathy and is showing only some light benefit to patients with diseases that have, in the past, been considered incurable.

References

Full references for this chapter can be found on www.expertconsult.com.

Spondylolysis and Spondylolisthesis

Nikolai Bogduk

Fundamental to the stability of the lumbar spine is the architecture of the posterior elements of the lumbar vertebrae. The inferior articular processes project downward and act like hooks to engage the superior articular processes of the vertebra below (**Fig. 94.1A**). This arrangement provides for stability against anterior translation. If the upper vertebra in a segment attempts to translate forward (**Fig. 94.1B**), its inferior articular processes impact the superior articular processes of the lower vertebra and thus prevent translation.

The inferior articular processes are suspended from the lamina on each side (**Fig. 94.2A**). The superolateral portion of the lamina can be perceived as lying between the superior articular process and the inferior articular process of the parent vertebra. Accordingly, this portion is known as the pars interarticularis: the part between the joints (see Fig. 94.2A). Defects can occur in the pars interarticularis in which the inferior articular process becomes disconnected from the rest of its parent vertebra (see **Fig. 94.2B**). Traditionally, this condition is known as *spondylolysis* because it was originally attributed to dissolution of the pars interarticularis.

The perceived threat to the stability of the lumbar spine is that when a pars defect develops, the vertebra is denied the restraining function of the inferior articular processes, and it can dislocate into forward translation (**Fig. 94.3**). The resultant dislocation is known as *spondylolisthesis*: slipping of the vertebra.

These abnormalities may have some relevance in the assessment of instability and deformity in children, but they have little relevance in adult pain medicine. Arcane is the belief that radiographic abnormalities of the lumbar spine constitute or provide a diagnosis of low back pain. Nonetheless, spondylolysis and spondylolisthesis are still promoted as causes of low back pain in some medical circles. They are still promoted as causes of pain in medicolegal circles. Indeed, according to the *American Medical Association Guides to the Evaluation of Permanent Impairment,*[1] patients are rewarded with higher total person impairment scores if they exhibit spondylolysis. Nothing could be so undeserving. Nothing could be so dissonant with the scientific evidence.

Spondylolysis

An early belief concerning spondylolysis was that it constituted a congenital defect, produced by failure of ossification centers in the lamina to fuse with those of the pedicle and vertebral body. This belief is incompatible with the embryology of the lumbar spine. No separate ossification center arises in the lamina.[2] Consequently, the lamina has no ossification center that can fail to fuse with that of the pedicle body and produce a defect. The pars interarticularis develops from a single ossification center that produces the lamina, pedicle, and articular

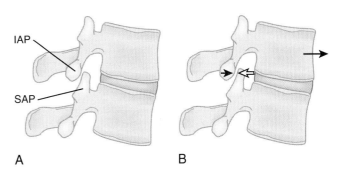

A   B

Fig. 94.1 **Structure and function of the inferior articular processes of lumbar vertebrae.** A, In a lateral view, the inferior articular processes (IAP) hang down like hooks to engage the superior articular processes (SAP) of the vertebra below. B, If the upper vertebra attempts to translate forward, its inferior articular processes impact the superior articular processes of the vertebra below, whereby translation is prevented.

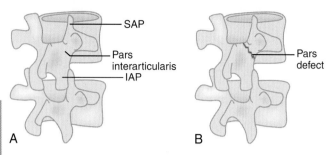

Fig. 94.2 Defect in the pars interarticularis. **A,** An oblique view showing the superior articular process (SAP), the inferior articular process (IAP) of a lumbar vertebra, and the pars interarticularis. **B,** The same view showing a pars defect.

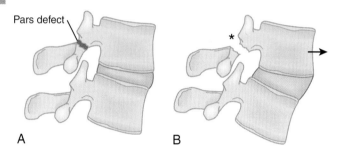

Fig. 94.3 Spondylolisthesis. **A,** A defect in the pars interarticularis prevents the inferior articular process from protecting the vertebra from forward translation. **B,** Disconnected from its posterior elements by the defect (*), the vertebral body is able to translate forward, thus leaving its inferior articular processes, laminae, and spinous processes behind.

Table 94.1 Prevalence of Spondylolysis in Athletes		
Category	**Prevalence (%)**	**Reference**
Contact sports	>20	Ichikawa et al[11]
Gymnasts	11	Jackson et al[12]
Various sports	>20	Hoshina[13]
Football	13	McCarroll et al[14]
Fast bowlers in cricket	50	Foster et al[15]

hatchback, and this bending stresses the pars. Under repeated loading, the pars will fracture.

These biomechanical data correlate with the available epidemiologic data. Pars fractures are more common in athletes, particularly, although not exclusively, in those whose sports involve twisting of the lumbar spine or forced extension (**Table 94.1**).[11–15] Among Native Alaskans, these fractures are more common in individuals who live on ice and who use kayaks.[4] However, pars fractures are not restricted to such individuals. Some 7% of the asymptomatic adult population has spondylolysis.[16] The prevalence is higher (7.7%) in men than in women (4.6%), but it varies by geographic region and by the nature of work and the number of pregnancies.[17]

Pathology

Overwhelmingly, the epidemiologic and biomechanical evidence indicates that pars defects are stress fractures. This view is consonant with pars morphology.

If studied early, spondylolysis has all the features of an acute fracture: hyperemia and a jagged fracture line. When the fracture does not heal, the appearance of the defect is that of a pseudarthrosis. The bony margins are eburnated and smooth. The defect is filled with fibrous tissue, thus forming a syndesmosis.[18] The fibrous tissue may contain fragments of bone,[19] a finding that underscores the traumatic origin of the defect. The defect may undercut the capsules of one or both of the adjacent zygapophysial joints.[18] Under those conditions, it can communicate with the cavities of those joints, as may become evident on arthrography of the joints.[20]

When pars fractures are bilateral, the entire lamina and its inferior articular processes are effectively disconnected from the pedicles and vertebral body. The lamina becomes flail, for which reason it has been described as the "rattler." The multifidus muscle still acts on the spinous process of the lamina and draws it into extension. However, only the fibrous tissue of the defect resists this motion. Consequently, the flail lamina can exhibit excessive motion during normal movements of the lumbar spine.

Diagnosis

The traditional means of diagnosing a pars fracture has been plain radiography. The fractures can be difficult to see on anteroposterior or lateral films, and for that reason the oblique view of the lumbar spine was introduced. In an oblique view, the posterior elements of a lumbar vertebra assume the appearance of a Scottie dog (**Fig. 94.4**). The pars interarticularis corresponds to the neck of the dog. In a patient with a

processes on each side. The possibility of failure to fuse applies only to the midline posteriorly, where the ossification centers of each side can fail to meet (spina bifida), or to the neurocentral junction, between the pedicles and the vertebral centrum. Furthermore, investigators have shown that pars defects do not occur in infants,[2] and they do not occur in individuals paralyzed from birth, who have never used their lumbar spine in weight bearing.[3]

Spondylolysis has also been viewed as a genetic problem, largely because it was found to have an inordinately high prevalence among Native Alaskans.[4] Later studies, however, showed that this prevalence was not the result of race. Not all Native Alaskans exhibit the high prevalence. Rather, the prevalence of this condition is related to differences in lifestyle; the defect is therefore an acquired abnormality.[4] In all races, the prevalence increases with age,[5] and it is related to repeated activities that involve hyperextension, rotation, or flexion of the lumbar spine.[5]

Anatomic studies have shown that the pars interarticularis is the weakest region of bone in a lumbar vertebra.[6] Ironically, however, it is subject to enormous stresses during activities of daily living. Whereas most individuals are endowed with a pars interarticularis that is thick enough to withstand the stress put on it, others have a less than adequate pars and are susceptible to acquired injuries.

Biomechanical studies have shown that the pars interarticularis is susceptible to stress failure. This can occur if the vertebra is loaded in repeated torsion or repeated extension.[7–10] In all these movements, impaction of the inferior articular process, as it resists movement, causes it to bend backward, like a

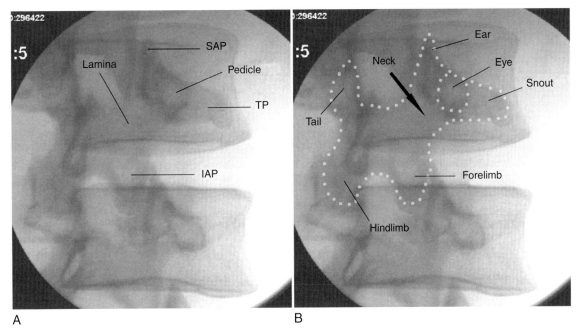

Fig. 94.4 **Radiographic appearance of the pars interarticularis. A,** An oblique view with the posterior elements labeled. iap, inferior articular process; SAP, superior articular process; TP, transverse process. **B,** How the posterior elements can be likened to the appearance of a Scottie dog.

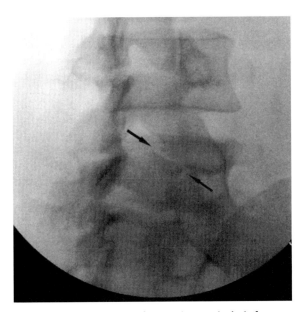

Fig. 94.5 **Oblique radiograph of a pars interarticularis fracture.** The fracture appears as a *white line,* across the neck of the "Scottie dog," between the *arrows.*

Table 94.2 Relationship between History and Bone Scan in Patients with a Radiographically Evident Pars Defect

History	Bone Scan	
	Positive*	Negative*
Trauma within 1 year	9	4
Repeated minor trauma	9	20
Chronic back pain	5	35
No pain	0	14

*Number of patients.
Data from Lowe J, Schachner E, Hirschberg E, et al: Significance of bone scintigraphy in symptomatic spondylolysis, *Spine* 9:654–655, 1984.

pars fracture, the fracture appears as a necklace around the neck (**Fig. 94.5**).

Radiography, however, can detect only an established fracture. A greater imperative is to detect abnormalities that precede actual fracture, so that fracture can be averted. This is possible with bone scanning.

Bone scans show hyperemia, and therefore scan results are positive for stress reactions, recent fracture, or a healing fracture.[3,21] Typically, scan results are not positive in chronic pars fractures, because the hyperemia has settled.

Once a pars fracture has occurred, however, the role and utility of bone scan are questionable, given that the relationship between clinical features and bone scans is imperfect (**Table 94.2**). Pars defects do not produce positive results on bone scan in asymptomatic individuals. Scan results may be positive in patients with chronic back pain or in patients with a history of repeated minor trauma and are more likely to be positive in patients with a history of a traumatic incident, but not reliably so.[22]

In athletes with back pain who are suspected of having a pars fracture, the correlations between bone scan and radiography are varied and differ from study to study (**Table 94.3**).[23-26] Most of these patients have negative results of both investigations. Only a few have positive results of both. Some have a positive bone scan but a negative radiograph, a finding consistent with a stress reaction without actual fracture. Some have a positive radiograph but a negative bone scan, a finding consistent with an old fracture.

The virtue of bone scan lies in being able to detect stress reactions before fracture occurs. Investigators have been found that athletes with positive bone scan results but negative radiographic results were able to return to their sports, and follow-up radiographs revealed no detects.[25] In athletes with positive results of both tests, bone scans resolved, but radiographs revealed persisting defects.

Magnetic resonance imaging (MRI) is a suitable, and perhaps preferable, alternative to bone scan. On MRI, five grades of abnormality can be detected, ranging from completely normal, through stress reactions without fracture, incipient or partial fracture, overt fracture, and fracture without reactive edema.[27] In this regard, MRI has the advantage over bone scan in that it can simultaneously show bone marrow reaction and fracture. Its cost effectiveness has not been calculated, but the cost of a single MRI scan would seem competitive with that of a bone scan in addition to plain radiography.

The data suggest that in individuals at risk of a stress fracture, bone scan or MRI is the investigation of choice to screen for stress reactions before fracture. However, only a few patients suspected of fracture actually have a fracture. Plain radiography has no role as the initial test. If bone scan is used, it is the critical test. Radiography is indicated only if the bone scan result is positive. If MRI is used, plain radiography becomes superfluous.

These guidelines, however, apply to individuals at risk of a pars fracture. They do not apply to patients in general with back pain. In those patients, pars fractures are an uncommon and unlikely source of pain.

Relationship with Pain

Most vexatious is the relationship of spondylolysis with pain. Whereas detecting stress reactions to avert fracture and to preserve the integrity of the lumbar spine has merit, this does not amount to establishing a diagnosis for the cause of pain.

Detecting a pars fracture does not constitute making a diagnosis. The confounding factor is that pars fractures are very common in individuals with no pain. Moreton[16] reviewed the radiographs of 32,600 asymptomatic individuals and found pars fractures in 7.2%. Consequently, pars fractures can be expected to occur as an incidental finding in 7% of patients presenting with back pain. Their pain arises from sources other than the pars defect. Other studies directly compared symptomatic and asymptomatic individuals and found no difference in the prevalence of spondylolysis (**Table 94.4**).[28,29]

Finding a pars fracture in a patient has no diagnostic validity. The positive likelihood ratio is essentially 1.0, which means the test contributes nothing to diagnosis. The data of Magora and Schwartz[29] actually indicate that pars fractures are more common in asymptomatic individuals. The likelihood ratio of 0.14, less than 1.0, means that finding a pars fracture actually detracts from making a diagnosis.

These conclusions have been reinforced by a systematic review.[30] Multiple studies have confirmed an equivalent prevalence of spondylolysis in symptomatic and asymptomatic individuals. The odds ratios for spondylolysis as a risk factor for pain are nonsignificant.

Nevertheless, it is possible for a pars fracture to become symptomatic. The fibrous tissue of the defect contains nerve endings,[31] ostensibly derived from the dorsal rami that innervate the affected segment, and so has the necessary apparatus to be a source of pain. What is required is the application of a means, other than radiography, by which to incriminate the fracture as a source of pain.

The definitive test is to anesthetize the defect.[32] Pars blocks are the only means available by which to determine whether a radiographically evident defect is symptomatic or asymptomatic. Such a test is imperative in view of the high prevalence of defects in asymptomatic individuals. Relief of

Table 94.3 Correlation Between Bone Scan and Radiography in the Detection of Pars Fractures

Bone Scan	Radiography Positive*	Radiography Negative*	Reference
Positive	9	4	Elliott et al[23]
Negative	9	16	
Positive	18	5	Jackson et al[24,25]
Negative	7	7	
Positive	5	1	Van den Oever et al[26]
Negative	22	38	

*Number of patients.

Table 94.4 Validity of Radiography in the Diagnosis of Painful Spondylolysis

Pars Fracture	Pain*	No Pain*	Sensitivity	Specificity	+Likelihood Ratio	Reference
Unilateral	2	26	0.03	0.97	1.08	Lisbon et al[28]
None	660	910				
Bilateral	62	65	0.09	0.93	1.3	
None	600	871				
Any	64	91	0.10	0.90	1.0	
None	598	845				
Any	44	64	0.07	0.83	0.14	Magora and Schwartz[29]
None	604	312				

*Number of patients.

pain implies that the defect is actually the source pain and predicts surgical success.[32] Patients who do not respond to blocks preoperatively are less likely to respond to fusion of the defect, even if the fusion is technically satisfactory.[32]

Unfortunately, no systematic population studies have been conducted to establish just how often pars fractures are responsible for back pain, either in general patients or in athletes. Too many practitioners are satisfied, despite the scientific evidence, that finding a fracture radiographically is sufficient to establish a diagnosis.

Also untested is the contention that the pain could arise not from the fracture, but from the zygapophysial joints of the flail lamina. Medial branch blocks of the suspected joint would be a valid test for this contention, but no study has reported the prevalence of pain from the zygapophysial joints in patients with pars fractures.

Treatment

The ideal opportunity for treatment is before fracture occurs. Finding a stress reaction allows the affected part to be rested. Athletes can modify their training regimens. If that is done, the prospect obtains that fracture can be avoided. Bone scan is the only means by which an early diagnosis can be established.

In principle, if and once a fracture has occurred, healing and complete resolution are possible. Radiographic union can be expected in some 37% of patients, especially if the fracture is unilateral.[33]

In practice, most pars fractures pass unnoticed and are undetected at inception. They do not need to be detected because most remain asymptomatic and become incidental radiographic findings. If and when pars fractures become symptomatic, however, their optimal management has not been established. Bracing is recommended, supplemented by hamstring stretching, pelvic tilts, and abdominal strengthening, as the patient becomes pain free during activities of daily living,[33] but this regimen has not been controlled for natural history.

Local anesthetic blocks of the pars fracture may be diagnostic, but they have not been established as therapeutic. In principle, radiofrequency neurotomy of the medial branches of the lumbar dorsal rami of the affected segment should relieve the pain of a pars fracture, but this treatment has not been formally tested for this condition.

For persistent pain, the mainstay of treatment has been arthrodesis of the pars fracture, by various means.[34-36] For some procedures, success rates of 80% have been reported. However, the efficacy of surgery, at large, is elusive because the treatment of pars fractures has often been confounded by, or confused with, the treatment of spondylolisthesis.

Spondylolisthesis

Spondylolisthesis is an obvious structural abnormality of the lumbar spine that typically affects the fifth or fourth lumbar vertebra. It is characterized by anterior displacement of the affected vertebra in relation to the one below (**Fig. 94.6**). The displacement implies that the vertebra has slipped forward. Formally, spondylolisthesis is classified according to etiology (**Table 94.5**).[37] Of the various forms, isthmic, lytic spondylolisthesis is the most common and constitutes the archetypical form.

Although other methods have been used to quantify the magnitude of vertebral slippage,[38] the most commonly used are variants of the method of Taillard.[39] Spondylolisthesis is graded according to the extent to which the affected vertebra has moved across the superior surface of the vertebra below (**Fig. 94.7**). Four grades are recognized (I to IV) according to whether the posterior corner of the affected vertebra lies opposite one, two, three, or four quarters of the way across the supporting vertebra.

A perception is that segments affected by spondylolisthesis are unstable and that the slippage will progress. Longitudinal studies deny this as a rule. In a study of 27 children followed into adulthood, no female patient exhibited an increase in slip of greater than 10%, and only 4 male patients exhibited progression, which ranged in magnitude from 10% to 28%.[5] That study concluded that slippage occurs largely at the time

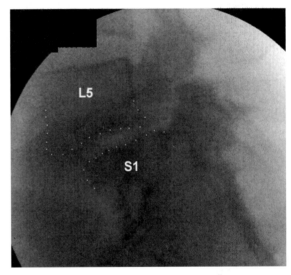

Fig. 94.6 **Lateral radiograph of an L5 vertebra that exhibits spondylolisthesis.** For clarity, the inferior margin of L5 and the superior margin of S1 have been traced with *dots*.

Table 94.5 **Classification of Spondylolisthesis by Etiology**

Type	Etiology
Dysplastic	Congenital abnormality of upper sacrum
Isthmic	
Lytic	Fatigue fracture of pars interarticularis
Elongated pars	Congenital
Acute fracture	Acute trauma
Degenerative	Loss of cartilage and/or progressive deformation of zygapophyseal joints
Traumatic	Fracture in posterior elements other than pars
Pathologic	Intrinsic bone disease

Data from Wiltse LL, Newman PH, Macnab I: Classification of spondylolysis and spondylolisthesis, *Clin Orthop Relat Res* 117:23–29, 1976.

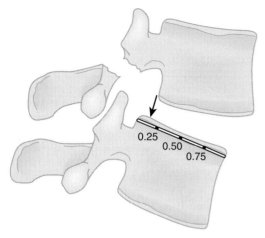

Fig. 94.7 Grading of spondylolisthesis. The grade is expressed in terms of whether the posterior corner of the affected vertebra lies opposite the first, second, third, or fourth quarter of the anteroposterior width of the supporting vertebra.

of acquisition of bilateral pars fractures. No patient exhibited disease progression after the age of 18 years. These conclusions were echoed by another study of 311 adolescents.[40] Only 3% exhibited progression greater than 20%.

Another study[41] confirmed some but disputed others of these findings. During follow-up of 272 adolescent patients, the mean progression of slip was only 3.5%, a finding indicating that, as a rule, spondylolisthesis does not progress appreciably. However, 23% of patients exhibited progression of 10% or more. (The proportion who exhibited progression of more than 20% was not reported.) Greater amounts of disease progression occurred in patients who had larger slips at presentation. However, in all cases, the greatest amount of slipping (90%) had already occurred at the time of presentation. Subsequent progression accounted for only 10% of the final slip, on average. This calculation reinforces the rule that most of the slip occurs when the pars fracture is acquired.

Relationship with Pain

Spondylolisthesis is not related to back pain. This was resoundingly established in a systematic review.[30] For an association with back pain, the odds ratios range between 1 and 2 for half the studies conducted and are less than 1 for the remainder. These values preclude any diagnostic significance of finding spondylolisthesis. One study[42] found that women with spondylolisthesis were more likely to report pain during the previous day, but no association was reported with pain during the previous year, previous month, or previous week. No association at all was found for men. Pain intensity was not related to the magnitude of slip.

Treatment

It is somewhat ironic that a condition known not to be associated with back pain has such an abundance of literature on its treatment. Proponents of conservative therapy advocate flexion exercises, other exercises,[43-45] traction,[43] braces,[43,46] casts,[43] corsets,[43] and manipulation.[47,48] However, arthrodesis is the longest-established treatment, with claimed success rates of 70% to 80%.[49-60] The one randomized study established that operative treatment was more effective than exercises.[61]

Although the literature celebrates the success of treatment, it is not consistently clear from that literature what was being treated. Investigators treated patients for low back pain only,[47] low back pain or back pain with radiculopathy,[55] low back pain with or without radiculopathy,[56] low back pain and sciatica,[53,58] low back pain or leg pain,[59] low back pain and leg pain,[52] low back pain with or without nerve root irritation,[53] or radicular pain only.[49] Some investigators did not specify the clinical features of their patients and so ostensibly treated patients for the lesion.[43,46,48]

Mechanisms of Pain

The literature on treatment fails to provide evidence on the mechanism by which spondylolisthesis may cause pain. Indeed, it seems to have paid no attention to this issue, and patients have been treated without regard to differing symptoms or their cause. The lesion, rather than the symptoms, has attracted treatment.

It is credible that spondylolisthesis could cause radicular pain, by stretching nerve roots, by narrowing the intervertebral foramen, or by the flail lamina's impinging on the nerve roots. The one study that explicitly addressed the last phenomenon showed that radicular pain could be relieved simply by removing the loose lamina.[49] Conversely, the mechanisms by which spondylolisthesis may cause back pain are no more than speculative. It is conceivable that the patient may have back pain stemming from the disk of the affected segment, or that the patients may have pain from the pars fracture or from the zygapophyseal joints of the flail lamina. None of these contentions, however, has been formally tested, let alone proven.

The one piece of circumstantial evidence was reported in a small retrospective study. The investigators claimed that progression of spondylolisthesis was associated with the onset of marked degeneration of the disk.[62] The study implied that the pain the patients suffered arose in the affected disk, but this concept was not explicitly tested and proved.

An alternative interpretation, consistent with the epidemiologic evidence, is that spondylolisthesis is irrelevant to the patient's symptoms. Affected patients have back pain regardless of their spondylolisthesis. Circumstantial evidence to this effect comes from one study that showed that the clinical pattern and functional disability were similar in patients with spondylolisthesis and in patients with nonspecific low back pain.[63] Furthermore, when treated in the same way, patients with spondylolisthesis and patients with nonspecific back pain responded in the same way.[47]

If this is the case, spondylolisthesis is immaterial to the diagnosis and immaterial to outcome. Even surgery may have a nonspecific, serendipitous effect. Surgery does not only fuse the affected segment. It involves extensive débridement of the lumbar spine, with denervation of the zygapophyseal joints, the pars fracture, or disk, depending on the technique used. These procedures may be the active components of surgical treatment, rather than the arthrodesis.

References

Full references for this chapter can be found on www.expertconsult.com.

Sacroiliac Joint Pain and Related Disorders

Steven Simon

The sacroiliac joint (SIJ) has been a source of pain to both sufferers of low back pain (LBP) and those who refuse to recognize its contribution to this common problem.[1] Many of the frustrations experienced by patients who hurt but continually have "negative" examinations and studies can be traced to this overlooked synovial joint and its maladies. In this chapter, the anatomy, motion, pain generators, evaluation, and treatment of the SIJ and its relation to LBP are explored. Historically, Meckel described motion within the SIJ in 1816, and before Mixter and Barr recognized the contribution of herniated lumbar disks to LBP in 1934, SIJ motion was believed to be a main generator of LBP.

Anatomy

The axial spine rests on the sacrum, a triangular fusion of vertebrae arranged in a kyphotic curve and ending with the attached coccyx in the upper buttock. Iliac wings (innominate bones [IBs]) attach on either side, to form a bowl with a high back and a shallow front. Three joints result from this union: the pubic symphysis in the anterior midline and the left and right SIJs on the posterior (**Fig. 95.1**). Multiple ligaments and fascia attach across these joint spaces, thus limiting motion and providing stability (**Figs. 95.2** and **95.3**).[2] The hip joints are formed by the femoral heads and the acetabular sockets deep within the IBs. The hips create a direct link between the lower extremities and the spine to relay ground reaction forces from weight bearing and motion. A physiologic balance between lumbar lordosis and sacral curvature exists both at rest and in motion. Changes of pelvic tilt and lumbar lordosis occur in the anteroposterior (AP) plane and rely on attached muscles and fascia, but they do not have significant effects on the SIJs, owing to a self-bracing mechanism

created by friction from the ligaments. The sacrum, positioned between the IBs, functions as the keystone of an arch assembly and allows cephalocaudad (CC) and AP motion.[3] Innervation is varied and quite extensive because of the overall size of the joint, which includes outflow from anterior to posterior rami of L3-S1.[4]

The SIJ is a synovial (diarthrodial) joint that is more mobile in youth than later in life, when the upper two thirds of the joint will become fibrotic. As the capsule thickens, sacral ossification occurs, and the distinct propeller shape of the joint becomes more pronounced (**Fig. 95.4**). The adult female pelvis is five times more mobile than the male pelvis, and to accommodate pregnancy and parturition, it will increase another 2.5 times because of the effects of relaxin on fascia and ligaments. Ligament and muscle attachments help to maintain stability of the pelvic ring and allow movement within limits. Further motion is also limited by the irregular shape of the joint articulation, in which ridges and grooves increase resistance friction and add to the keystone arch structure. Prolonged loading, such as standing or sitting for long periods, and alterations of the sacral base (leg asymmetry or ligamentous injury) are associated the joint hypermobility and resultant LBP.[3,8,9]

Multiple muscle attachments cross the SIJs and contribute to pelvic stability and force transfer.[3] These include the lower trapezius, latissimus dorsi, and extensor abdomen obliques, which attach cephalad to the SIJ, thoracolumbar fascial attachments to the twelfth rib, lumbar spinous and lateral processes, and pelvic brim. Fascial and muscle attachments expand to include the erector spinae, internal obliques, serratus posterior inferior, sacrotuberous ligament, dorsal SI ligament, and iliolumbar ligaments, which attach to the posterior iliac spine, pelvic brim, and sacral crest. Major movement and stabilizing muscles also attach to the SIJ, including the gluteus maximus,

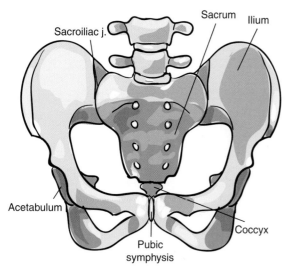

Fig. 95.1 **Bony pelvis.**

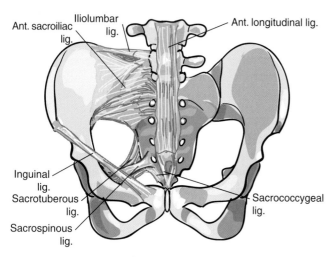

Fig. 95.2 **Anterior ligaments of the pelvis.**

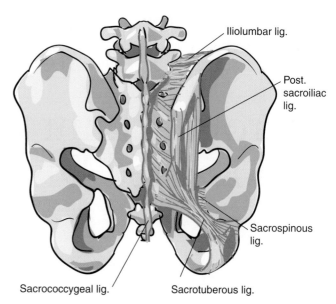

Fig. 95.3 **Posterior ligaments of the pelvis.**

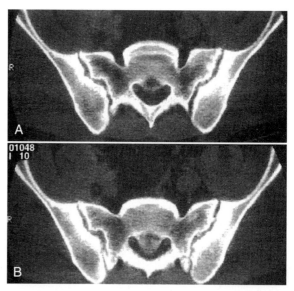

Fig. 95.4 **Computed tomography scans of the traverse section of the sacroiliac joint.** A, Male. B, Female. Note the thicker sacral cartilage, typical of female patients. *(From Paradise LE: Sacroiliac joint blocks. In Raj PP, Lou L, Erdine S, et al, editors:* Interventional pain management: image-guided procedures, *ed 2, Philadelphia, 2008, Saunders.)*

gluteus medius, latissimus dorsi, multifidus, biceps femoris, psoas, piriformis, obliquus, and transversus abdominis. Vleeming et al[10] concluded that the purpose of these muscles is not for motion, but for stability, to balance the forces of walking and running, and the friction of joint surfaces allows both shock absorption and transfer of bending forces.[5,11]

Motion

Movement of the SIJ is performed in a stable environment, governed by muscle ligaments and the joint shape and cartilage, which increase friction and limit mobility by creating a self-locking mechanism.[10,12,13] Motion is allowed in three dimensions: AP, CC, and left-right (LR). The major ligaments and their actions are listed here (see Figs. 95.2 and 95.3). These ligaments can be divided into four distinct layers from superficial to deep, but they are discussed relative to their function.

1. The interosseous ligament resists joint separation and motion in the cephalad and AP direction.
2. The dorsal sacral ligament covers and assists the interosseous ligament.
3. The anterior SI ligament is a thickening of the anterior inferior joint capsule and resists CC and LR motion.
4. The sacrospinous ligament resists rotational motion of the pelvis around the axial spine.
5. The iliolumbar ligaments resist motion between the distal lumbar segments and the sacrum and help to stabilize the sacral position between the IBs.
6. The sacrotuberous ligament resists flexion of the iliacs on the axial spine.
7. The pubic symphysis resists AP motion of the IBs, shear, and LR forces.

Next, actual movement of the pelvis and SIJs and their integrated functions are reviewed. That ground reaction forces from weight bearing pass through the legs and pelvis to the spine has already been established. The point in the body where these forces are in balance is termed the *center of gravity* and has been determined to be 2 cm below the navel. Gravity can also be considered a force line that produces different effects on the pelvic girdle as it shifts from anterior to posterior relative to the center of the acetabular fossae.[14] Body posture and positioning, muscle strength, and weight distribution determine alterations in the force lines. An anterior force line (e.g., a protuberant abdomen) produces anterior (downward) rotation of the pelvis over the femoral heads and decreases tension in the sacrotuberous ligament while maintaining pressure on posterior ligaments. This situation creates an overuse strain on the spinal support muscles and a resultant painful condition. As the line of gravity moves posterior to the acetabula, the pelvis rotates posteriorly (i.e., the anterior rib tilts upward), and the sacrotuberous and posterior interosseous ligaments tighten. This is easier to visualize if one imagines a line between the femoral heads on which the pelvis rotates. The vertical distance of motion is approximately 2.5 cm in each direction at L3.[15] The pelvis also rotates in relation to the spine during gait. As the legs alternately move forward, the pelvic IBs rotate forward and toward the midline, but the spine and sacrum counter-rotate, although to a lesser degree.[16] The SIJ lies between these moving planes and forces, central to vertical, horizontal, and rotational activity. Hula and belly dancers have perfected rhythmic pelvic motion, much to the delight of their audiences.

Dysfunction of the joint without direct trauma commonly arises from an imbalance in the anterior pelvis without adequate stabilization of posterior (sacrotuberous and interosseous) ligaments. Lifting or bending while leaning forward produces an anterior pelvic tilt that slightly separates the IBs from the sacrum and makes unilateral AP shift more likely, especially if proper ergonomic technique is not used.[17,18] The net effect of such a unilateral anterior rotation on the ipsilateral side would be to raise the pelvic brim and posterior superior iliac spine (PSIS) and cause apparent leg lengthening in supine positions and shortening in long sitting. (*"Apparent"* means that the affected leg is not necessarily longer, but appears to be so, owing to its attachment to the hip socket, which is rotated forward, or caudad in a supine position. Long sitting in this situation positions the acetabulum posterior to the SIJ and results in apparent shortening). This provides a simple test during the physical examination to determine stability of ligament structures within the SIJ. Bilateral anterior SI rotation would not produce leg length asymmetry but would stretch the iliopsoas muscles, thus simulating tight and tender hip flexors. Posterior unilateral rotation would produce ipsilateral PSIS and brim drop, as well as a shortening of the supine leg and lengthening with long sitting.

Pain Generators

The net effect of this type of sustained unilateral force is to create an imbalance of attached myofascial insertions. Pain may result from periosteal irritation or circulatory congestion on the shortened side and loss of strength and tenderness on the elongated side. The joint line becomes stressed by the combined muscle and ligament pull that resists resolution and physiologic positioning and creates a painful strain. The patient should be examined to determine the possible presence of physiologic, restricted, or excessive joint motion.

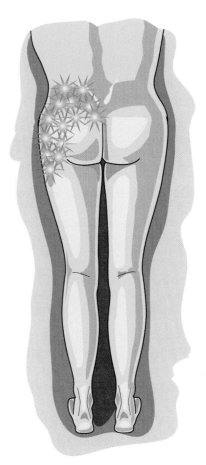

Fig. 95.5 **Distribution of pain emanating from the sacroiliac joint.**

Surgical fusions of the lumbosacral spine may present special problems in this regard, and radiographic examination must be included to determine fully whether malpositioning is a contributing factor. Other conditions that produce acute or chronic discomfort must be considered and include *trauma* (seat belt injury, falls with pelvic ring fractures), *inflammatory conditions* (ankylosing spondylitis, rheumatoid arthritis, Reiter's syndrome, psoriatic arthritis, inflammatory bowel disease), *infections* (bacterial or mycobacterial [tuberculosis]), *metabolic imbalance* (gout), *neoplastic disease* (prostate, bowel, pulmonary), or *degenerative changes* within the joint.[19–21]

The SIJ line is densely innervated by several levels of spinal nerves (L3-S1) that, when stimulated, may produce symptoms resembling those caused by lumbar disks.[4] Muscle insertions near the area, such as gluteus maximus and hamstrings, refer pain to the hip and ischial areas, respectively, when stressed. Fortin et al[1,22] examined asymptomatic and symptomatic patients to generate a pain map of SI symptoms. The most common discomfort was described as aching or hypersensitivity along the joint line to the ipsilateral hip and trochanter (**Fig. 95.5**).[1,22]

Other pains, reported less frequently, occur approximately 5 cm lateral to the umbilicus on a line between the navel and the anterior superior iliac spine or referred into the groin or testicles. Sitting may become painful when anterior rotation of the pelvis changes the relationship of the acetabulum with the femoral head. Because the ischial tuberosity cannot move while a person is seated, balanced support for the pelvic "bowl" is lost, and the effect is aggravated by the tendency to sit in a lopsided way or on the sacrum, instead of on the ischial tuberosities. The resultant forces produce AP or LR torque on the SIJ. Standing decreases this pain because the femoral heads and are repositioned and thus buttress the pelvis. Sciatic nerve stretch may also be relieved by allowing the pelvis to rotate, a maneuver that shifts weight to the opposite leg.

Evaluation

A thorough history must be taken to seek preexisting disease or injury or new trauma and to evaluate the patient's general health status. Bladder, bowel, or sexual dysfunction or numbness often suggests an emergency that requires immediate care. The pain history should also include the duration of the problem and previous treatments, including medications, injections, thermal or electrical modalities, bracing, or manipulations and their outcomes. Provocative and palliative positions or activity can be guides to aid in treatment planning. Functional loss is significant because it can be an indication of suffering and a measure of treatment success as the patient begins to resume normal activities.

Radiographic testing is indicated to investigate fractures, osteophytes, fusion of the SIJ, or lumbosacral lesions. Inflammatory changes in the SIJ are characteristic of rheumatoid spondylitis (Marie-Strumpell spondylitis) and can be verified with blood tests for human leukocyte antigen (HLA)-B27 or rheumatoid markers. Male patients in their 20s to 30s generally present with atraumatic LBP and marked stiffness. Although x-ray films may show negative results on initial reading, and although fuzziness over the SIJ region and stiffness in the lumbar spine may be the only early signs of this progressive disease, many of the tests listed later yield positive results. Quantitative radionuclide bone scanning has also been helpful in early diagnosis.[23]

Because many pain physicians now have access to fluoroscopy, a comparison series of traditional tests (Patrick's maneuver, Gaenslen's test, midline sacral thrust) with diagnostic SIJ infiltration suggested that infiltration may be a more reliable indicator of pain generator and should be incorporated into the testing if possible.[24]

How the patient walks reveals important information on antalgic gait, weight shifting, and asymmetry of the pelvic brim or of shoulder height. Spinal examination for range of motion, scoliosis, myospasm, and ligamentous irritation will localize pain generators. Familiarity with the anatomy of this region (i.e., muscles and their insertions and actions) is essential to understanding mechanical relationships with pelvic girdle positioning and the necessity of balancing forces to cure, rather than just to palliate, an SIJ syndrome. Various tests have been developed to detect SI dysfunction, and most can be performed quickly and simply during the regular examination and then verified by provocation.

1. *Fortin's finger test:* The patient points to the area of pain with one finger. The result is positive if the site is within 1 cm of the PSIS; generally it is inferomedial to the PSIS.
2. *Fabere maneuver* (*f*lexion, *ab*duction, *e*xternal *ro*tation, and *e*xtension of the hip, also known as Patrick's test): The patient lies supine. One heel is placed on the opposite knee, and the elevated leg is guided toward the examining table. The result is positive if pain is elicited along the SIJ. (This maneuver also stresses the

hip joint and may result in trochanteric or groin pain from the hip.)
3. *Gaenslen's test:* The patient is supine. The hip and knee are maximally flexed toward the trunk, and the opposite leg is extended. Some examiners perform this test with the patient's extended leg off the examination table, to force the SIJ through maximal range of motion. The result is positive if pain is felt across the SIJ. (This maneuver also stresses the hip and can produce trochanteric or groin pain.)
4. *Compression test:* The patient lies on one side. The examiner applies pressure on one pelvic brim in the direction of the other. The results are positive if pain is felt across the SIJ.
5. *Compression test at SIJ:* The patient is prone. The examiner places a palm along the SIJ or on the sacrum and makes a vertical downward thrust. The results are positive if pain is felt at the SIJ.
6. *Pubic symphysis test:* The patient is supine. Pressure is applied with the examining finger at the left or right pubic bone adjacent to the symphysis pubis. The results are positive if pain is felt at the site. (Most patients are not aware of this tenderness before it is elicited. The examiner should ask permission before applying pressure and should have other staff in the room to witness the examination, to avoid the misconception of inappropriate sexual contact.)
7. *Distraction test:* The patient is supine. The examiner alternately presses each anterior superior iliac spine in a posterolateral direction. The results are positive if pain is felt at the SIJ or if movement is asymmetrical.
8. *Fade test:* The patient is supine. The hip is flexed and adducted to midline. The examiner applies pressure to the long axis of the femur to push the ilium in a posterior direction. The results are positive if pain is felt at the SIJ.
9. *Passive straight leg raising test:* The patient is supine. The examiner grasps the patient's heel and lifts the leg vertically from the examining table with the knee extended. The patient is asked to hold the leg elevated and then slowly lower it. The result is positive if ipsilateral pain is elicited at the SIJ, a finding that suggests anterior rotation.
10. *One-legged stork test:* The patient is standing. The examiner is positioned behind the patient with thumbs placed on the PSIS and the sacrum at S2. The patient then flexes the palpated hip to 90 degrees. The results are positive if the examining thumb is moved upward instead of inferomedially.
11. *Van Dursen's standing flexion test:* The patient is standing. The examiner is positioned behind the patient with thumbs on the PSIS. The patient flexes the trunk forward without bending the knees. The results are positive with upward motion at the involved side.
12. *Piedallu's or seated flexion test:* The patient is seated. The examiner is positioned behind with thumbs placed just inferior to the PSIS. The patient flexes the trunk in a forward position. The results are positive with asymmetrical motion, elevated on the involved side.
13. *Rectal examination:* Although not specific for SIJ, a thorough rectal examination is recommended to search for referred pain from the prostate or uterus

or from spasm of the rectal or pelvic floors. Piriformis muscle spasm can be identified at the 2- or 10-o'clock positions. The results are positive if pain is felt at the SIJ, and this must be differentiated from anal discomfort, associated with the examination itself.

Treatment

Correct diagnosis is the first part of successful treatment because it focuses therapy toward the pain generator. Control of pain early in the treatment course encourages better patient cooperation. Structural attempts to correct for mechanical malpositioning can start and then move to education, modalities, exercises, and interventions.

Education

Descriptions of pelvic anatomy and rotational motion at the pelvic brim help the patient to understand what forces are continuing to stress the SIJ and cause pain. Proper ergonomic training for gait, bending, lifting, and stretching prevents repeated injury from undermining the overall treatment program and increases the patient's interest and participation.

Modalities

Deep heat is tolerated better than ice and is more likely to reach affected areas. Hot packs feel good and may relax or "soften" muscles before stretching or massage. Ultrasound along the SIJ is palliative. The addition of 10% steroid gel, which can replace electrode gel required for ultrasonography, can also be used to reduce inflammation by phonophoresis.

Electricity can be curative by relaxing muscle spasm electrogalvanic stimulation, functional electrical stimulation, or electrical acupuncture, or it can be palliative by blocking the pain signal (transcutaneous electrical nerve stimulation). The pain practitioner can choose from larger office-based units that follow preset cycles of stimulation or portable units that the patient can either operate at home or wear for convenient use.

Traction has not been helpful for SIJ dysfunction, but it has benefited patients with LBP from spinal causes. Braces provide a form of traction that applies direct pressure and stabilization over a movable area, which can be palliative in SIJ dysfunction. The SI belt has a pad that fits over the upper sacrum, to cover both SIJs and provide support. The belt should cross the pelvic brims, fasten in the abdominal area, and fit tightly enough to resist AP motion. Ground reaction forces, however, are very strong and eventually overcome most bracing attempts. Some investigators argue that the real purpose of bracing is to remind the patient to use proper body mechanics and limit rotational forces, but pelvic support in pregnant patients has been especially helpful when pain is present and options are limited. Whatever the source of its benefit, bracing is a patient-friendly means to provide stability and some relief when the SIJs are hypermobile.

Mobilization

Mobilization is helpful for restoring anatomic SIJ alignment and sacral or coccyx position. Many osteopathic, chiropractic, and physical therapy resistance techniques are used to perform these maneuvers. The reader is directed to other texts for full mechanical descriptions. Simple office manipulations are safe, effective, and immediately palliative for SI dysfunction, but efforts may be frustrated by muscle spasm along the pelvic floor or spinal attachments. One simple technique that can be performed in the office, or with a helper at home, is "leg lengthening" to correct anterior rotation shortening. To perform this maneuver in the office, the patient should lie supine on an examination table with the examiner standing at the foot of the table with thumbs on the medial malleoli to evaluate for leg length discrepancy. The patient is asked to sit up (long sitting), and leg length is observed. If one leg appears to shorten, it can grasped at the ankle by the examiner and gently pulled toward the foot of the table. Leg length is tested following this manipulation, and the procedure can be repeated until the legs are of equal length.

Self-manipulation is key in allowing the patient an opportunity to correct recurrent malpositioning secondary to ligament laxity. Even proper seating can help to maintain a self-bracing system for the SIJ. A small cushion beneath the proximal thighs distributes weight directly to the ischium, and a second cushion in the lumbar lordotic curve supports the spine and allows even distribution of reaction forces.

Injections

Injections may be the best option for providing quick assessment and relief of inflammation and painful SIJs.[25] Typical injections contain both analgesic and corticosteroid and are placed in the lower third of the joint (the true synovial portion).

Although these injections have been performed "blind" for many years, the new standard has become the use of guidance by fluoroscopy, ultrasound, or computed tomography scan. Other injections to the upper two thirds of the joint can also be very effective in relieving pain by reducing ligament irritation. Ketorolac has been substituted for steroids on repeated injections with beneficial results. Contraindications to injection are local infection, sepsis, possible fracture, coagulopathy, and allergy to medications used for procedure.

PROCEDURE FOR SACROILIAC JOINT INJECTION

1. Explain the goals and general procedure to the patient.
2. The patient is place supine, preferably over a pelvic pillow, which helps to open the SIJ.
3. Sterile technique is employed over the SIJ.
4. A wheal of analgesic is placed first at the PSIS, and then a sterile syringe containing 4 mL of 0.25% preservative-free bupivacaine and 40 mg of methylprednisolone is attached to a 3-inch 25-gauge needle under strict aseptic technique.
5. The PSIS is identified, and the needle is advanced through the wheal at a 45-degree angle toward the affected SIJ (**Fig. 95.6**). If bone is encountered, the needle tip is withdrawn into subcutaneous tissue and is redirected superiorly and slightly more laterally. When the needle is correctly positioned in the joint space, the contents of the syringe are gently injected. If resistance is encountered, the needle is probably in a ligament and may be advanced or withdrawn a bit to achieve better position.
6. The needle is withdrawn, and a sterile pressure dressing and ice pack are placed on the site.[26]

PROLIFERANT INJECTIONS

Proliferant injections attempt to create inflammation in an area to allow the body's natural healing mechanisms to repair the initial mobility dysfunction. An irritant such as dextrose

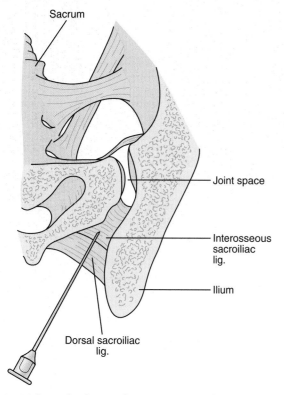

Fig. 95.6 Schematic picture of a cross section of a sacroiliac joint injection. Note that the needle enters at the dorsal inferior aspect of the joint. *(From Paradise LE: Sacroiliac joint blocks. In Raj PP, Lou L, Erdine S, et al, editors:* Interventional pain management: image-guided procedures, *ed 2, Philadelphia, 2008, Saunders.)*

is often injected along the entire joint line. The desired results are thickening of muscle attachments or ligaments, and the goal is to stabilize a hypermobile joint. Physicians should be familiar with the technique and complications before they attempt this procedure.[27]

Radiofrequency Ablation

Radiofrequency ablation is a technique for creating lesions (deafferentation) along sensory afferent nerves in the L4-S2 distribution. When successful, this procedure can create a longer-lasting block to painful nerve transmissions, but occasional complications have developed including gluteal, hip, or posterior thigh pain. As a result, specialized training is recommended before this procedure is attempted by the physician.[21]

Surgery

Surgery should be considered only when pain is intractable and disabling and all other conservative treatments have failed. Screw fixation of the ilium to the sacrum has been described to benefit some patients.[28]

Exercises

The goals of exercise programs are to provide stretch and strength to connecting muscles, to enhance posture, and to introduce means of self-manipulation for the patient. These exercises can be done alone or with a helper.

Strengthening Exercises

A "six pack" of repetitions of these isometric strengthening maneuvers are recommended: six sets of six, 6 seconds on and 6 seconds off, six times daily.

ABDOMINAL CRUNCHES

The patient lies supine with hip and knee flexed and feet flat on the floor. A partial sit-up is performed and held according the six-pack regimen.

HIP ABDUCTION, ADDUCTION, AND EXTENSION

The patient may be standing, sitting, or lying. Isometric exercises are performed by resisting the direction of motion, using furniture or hands to push against, according to the six-pack regimen.

PELVIC TILT, ANTERIOR AND POSTERIOR

The patient stands with hands on hips. The pelvis is tilted anteriorly (upward) then posteriorly (downward) according to the six-pack regimen.

ISOMETRIC HIP EXTENSION

The patient may be sitting, standing or lying. One foot is elevated and braced on a pedestal in a vertical position. The hip and knee are flexed maximally against the trunk, held in the flexed position with both hands. Isometric extension is then resisted by the arms according to the six-pack regimen. Men seem to prefer a variation of this maneuver that involves standing against the inside of a door frame with one foot against the opposite side. Resisted extension of the hip and knee from pressure against the sole of the foot produces a similar effect.

Posture Enhancement

Correct trunk posture enhances force distribution by maintaining correct spinal alignment. Holding the abdomen "in" (contracting the abdominal and rectus muscles) creates an internal brace against the lower back and helps to maintain adequate pelvic tilt and lumbar lordosis. Holding shoulders and head in proper alignment also enhances spinal positioning and distribution of forces.

References

Full references for this chapter can be found on www.expertconsult.com.

Failed Back Surgery Syndrome

J. Antonio Aldrete

In the 1980s, the complex diagnosis of "failed back surgery syndrome (FBSS)" entered the medical literature. This unusual nomenclature refers to an unfortunate group of patients who, having undergone surgical treatment for a back problem, usually end up in worse condition than when they first sought medical care for the disorder.[1] This chapter deals with a paradoxical deviation from the expected benefit obtained from surgical care because in most cases, in spite of considerable expense and substantial attention given by competent physicians, many of these care seekers achieve not only little improvement, but also, in some instances, a hopelessly worse progression of their spinal condition. The process is disappointing. Once in pain management, after many visits to physicians' offices, undergoing various procedures at pain clinics, spending days or weeks as hospital inpatients, receiving hundreds of hours of care, and incurring great expenses, these patients end up with greater disability, with several more scars, still in considerable pain and discomfort, unable to support their families or even to sit still for half an hour, and with little chance of ever riding a bicycle, returning to their jobs, having sexual intercourse when they wish, or even playing with their children. Most of these patients have no chance of ever finding a cure for their back problem.

The rationale for this nomenclature is not clear, but it seems to be related to patients who, after by virtue of having some type of (low) back pain, sought to achieve full health by consulting their physicians and then their respective specialists. For whatever reason, these patients may have been subjected to one or multiple operations in the spine, but their initial complaints appear to have been made worse. At that point, the possibility of continuing employment becomes an illusion. In hope, these patients apply for disability in the belief that they will be taken care of completely. After going through a humiliating process, however, these patients find out that disability is not what they thought it would be. It usually consists of a minimal income with limited follow-up care. For some patients, being disabled is like being less than a second-class citizen because they have limited rights and are considered by some to be a burden to society.

Literally, this vague diagnosis implies that the patient's back failed to get better. However, it is the treatment chosen by the patient's care providers that failed to restore anatomic perfection and optimal function. The appearance of this syndrome and the progressive increase in the numbers of patients receiving this denomination defy all the predictions that technology, if properly applied, may achieve a cure for most pathologic entities. A specific diagnosis for the patient with FBSS is not listed, and a precise evaluation of the effectiveness of each procedure is not performed. Moreover, this approach does not allow a determination of the optimal operation for certain conditions, nor does it ascertain which operations should be contraindicated for any one specific spinal condition. It is not clear whether the term FBSS is included in the Medicare rule or whether it is an exemption to the Medicare rule necessary to list all the diagnoses present in the admission and discharge notes. Such omission would essentially fail to mention in the postoperative notes such incriminating diagnoses as the following:

- Recurrent disk herniation
- Dural tear
- Incomplete removal of disk
- Loose disk fragment in vertebral canal
- Wrong interspace
- Failure to explore the foramen
- Intradural pseudocyst
- Entrapped nerve root
- Cerebrospinal fluid (CSF) fistula

The presence of one or more of these diagnoses may reveal a failure of treatment (including spinal surgery). It seems that for lack of a better global term that would encompass every one of these diagnoses, or "by default," FBSS has been incorporated into the medical jargon.[1,2] In a way, this attribution is not fair to patients because they do not understand this negative term. Moreover, the designation casts a stigma that assumes that nothing else favorable or positive can be done to help these patients. What is worse, in the current era of paying for results, someone must decide which among the treatments given was the one that failed to provide the proper outcome. When these patients are referred to pain management, the illusion that they are going to be free of pain eventually turns into a cruel reality because this treatment "manages the pain," but rarely eliminates it.

In their search for the dream of "no pain," these patients accept procedures that are painful, while being only sedated. Soon these patients seek refuge in drugs, prescribed but dangerous drugs that are allowed in certain amounts and in certain doses, which are sometimes not enough for pain relief lasting more than a few hours and at the cost of dependency. These drugs produce hyperalgesia, allodynia, hyperpathia,[3] and the very grave conclusion, opioid dependence.[4]

These diagnoses were not present initially, but in the postoperative period these conditions are difficult to treat successfully. Governmental agencies have gone from developing piety to advocating the relief of pain as the fifth vital sign.[5,6] They suggest that opioid-tolerant patients require at least 60 mg of morphine daily, 8 mg of hydromorphone, 30 mg of oxycodone, and so on,[5,7] only to have inspectors persecute and apprehend doctors because some patients overdosed.[6] What does one expect when doctors are directed by the US Food and Drug Administration not to undertreat patients[6,7] in pain, are professionally obligated by the Hypocratic oath to relieve pain, and provide their patients with prescriptions for large numbers of lethal pills. Pharmacists gladly oblige and fill the prescriptions, only to denounce doctors for overprescribing, although it is the pharmacists who sell and hand the drugs to the patients.

Each case varies, but they all have some common denominators. After one or more laminectomies, spinal fusion, artificial disk implantation, bone growth electrical stimulation, and other operative procedures,[8] these factors may include one or more of the following diagnoses:

- Recurrent disk herniation
- Peridural scarring
- Nerve root compressed by scarring
- Deformity of the dural sac
- Herniation of adjacent disk

- Spinal instability
- Facetectomy
- Pseudomeningocele
- Arachnoid cysts
- Arachnoiditis
- Foraminal restenosis

Not uncommonly after one or two laminectomies, the spine becomes "destabilized" as portions of disks are removed and laminectomies are extended laterally, thus rendering the facet joints dysfunctional and painful.[8] The sequence follows with a spinal fusion to stabilize that portion of the spine. Although spinal fusions are supposed to convert two or more vertebrae into one bony (with or without hardware) union, they may result in one or more of the following:

- Pseudarthrosis
- Malposition of screws
- Protrusion of screws through the vertebral body
- Protrusion of screws into the vertebral canal
- Fracture of screws
- Displacement of hardware (cages)
- Intrathecal scarring
- Intrathecal calcification
- Impingement of nerve roots
- Pedicular pain
- Paravertebral muscle dysfunction and atrophy

Historical Perspective

The historical events that brought the visualization of the spinal canal are mentioned in Chapter 161. The operative resection of extruded lumbar disks was popularized in 1934 by Mixter and Barr,[9] who identified herniated disks as the main cause of sciatica, demonstrated that diskectomy could be performed through a laminectomy incision, and initiated the trend for elective surgical operations of the spine. The precise diagnosis of radiculopathy was facilitated by the introduction of Pantopaque (ethyl iodophenyl undecylate), which was first administered to patients in 1944[10] and provided good definition and contrast of images. The use of this contrast medium established myelography as the standard test for identifying spinal disease. An oil-soluble dye, Pantopaque was used extensively in spite of evidence that it caused arachnoiditis.[11,12] When disk disease reappeared at the same level or on another interspace, laminectomies were repeated. However, when surgeons found evidence of instability, spinal fusions were indicated. Initially, bone grafts were used, but after 1993, pedicular screws, bars, and rods[13] were preferred, followed later by intervertebral cages. More recently, various artificial disks[14] have been tried, with limited success.[15] The use of water-soluble dyes made myelography safer, and both computed tomography (CT) and magnetic resonance imaging (MRI) have allowed more precise visualization of extradural and intradural disease, respectively. Minimally invasive approaches to laminectomy have become popular; these operations are attempted through a small incision, but results remain inconclusive.[16] The other, less common but still frequent lesion corrected surgically is malalignment of the vertebrae or spondylolisthesis.[17] These procedures may have given the impression that extensive interventions in the spine are feasible and uneventful. However, reports of these procedures indicate that these procedures are currently overused in the United States.[18] Criteria for indications are lacking, and overuse is especially common in certain age groups.[19]

Rationalization for Laminectomy and Fusions

The removal of a compressive lesion from a tubular osseous structure containing delicate neural elements such as the spinal cord, nerve roots, dural sac, and CSF more often than not eliminates the pain and dramatically improves the affected function. However, surgical access into the spine does not occur without risks and consequences.

Zeidman and Long[20] defined FBSS as "the condition resulting from one or more surgical interventions, with disastrous results with persistence of back pain and exacerbation of the preexisting complaints, characterized by a constellation of symptoms, including referred pain to the lower extremities, sphincter dysfunction and psychological alterations associated to the disease of the spine." Even though the syndrome has been clearly defined, not all surgeons accept the criterion for failure. Patients seek medical attention and request help for lower back pain. If the procedure performed for this purpose does not relieve the back pain, then the operation should be considered a failure. This fact is pertinent to laminectomies and especially to spinal fusions, even when solid arthrodesis is achieved. If the patient's pain continues, the operation has not succeeded in its primary objective of relieving that pain. According to Cherkin et al,[21] based on this premise, the objectives of spinal operations need to be redefined to include only those therapeutic modalities that have proven effective in relieving the specific cause of the pain experienced by that specific patient. This lack of selectivity was evident in the early stages of some clinical trials that are reported as ongoing studies, but the final conclusions have not yet appeared in the literature.[13–15]

Epidemiology

Considering that low back pain is one of the most prevalent diseases of middle and older age, the iatrogenic component of this entity adds a threatening dimension. If more than 300,000 spinal fusions are performed annually in the United States,[18] and if 20% to 40% of these patients end up with FBSS,[1,2,19,21] the outcomes of these interventions need to be reviewed and the indications revised. This is especially important given that the lifetime incidence of back pain includes approximately 80% of the general population. These numbers are also substantial in terms of cost, because by the time the diagnosis of FBSS is reached, it is estimated that more than $300,000 has already been spent on the care of each patient. By that time, these patients face the prospect of persistent pain and suffering for the remainder of their life.

The frequency of surgical operations of the spine for comparative populations in industrialized countries has been estimated to be 8 to 10 times more in the United States than in the Scandinavian countries, 8 times more than in the United Kingdom, and 7 times more than in Germany.[16] The reasons for these disparities are numerous, but the most relevant are as follows:

- Labor protection is given to workers in other countries, where lifting, pulling, and carrying are done mechanically rather than by humans. Lifting in industry, offices, hospitals, and so on is done by pulleys that have been placed strategically to avoid back injuries.[22] Back-saving education is a subject taught in middle schools and is taken seriously by students, supervisors, and workers.
- The financial incentive is undoubtedly an uncontrollable factor that influences excessive surgical intervention in the private practice of medicine, in contrast to conservative therapy in institutional medicine.
- Specific clinical guidelines are lacking on when and what operations are indicated for each specific condition that produces low back pain.[23]
- Inadequate control is exercised by governmental agencies over new surgical procedures and the implantation of medical devices.
- Implementation of evidence-based medicine as necessary proof that new treatments truly benefit patients is lacking.

Most cases start with low back pain. After a variable degree of conservative therapy, patients are offered laminectomy to remove the herniated portion of a disk, supposedly because the corresponding nerve root is compressed by such herniation.[24] For insurance approval of these procedures, symptoms and signs of radiculopathy must be evident, and conservative therapies must be proved to have failed. The most common access into the spinal canal is through the posterior approach, and it usually requires laminectomy or laminotomy. Even then, access to the degenerated disk is narrow and is frequently complicated by swelling of the affected nerve root that has been compressed for some time.[20] This swelling may improve soon thereafter, but in some cases the distal end of the root can actually become more swollen,[25] depending on the radicular vascular response to the surgical manipulation.

The consequences of spinal surgery must be taken seriously. The outcomes in patients younger than 30 years old who have a single degenerated intervertebral disk are more favorable than the outcomes in middle-aged patients with two or three affected disks; outcomes are worse when patients have some degree of spondylosis or when they are smokers.[26,27] The outcomes are less hopeful in older patients who have multiple levels and degrees of disk disease, facet joint arthritis, osteoporosis, and spinal stenosis. Because of work-related injuries, motor vehicle accidents, and possibly other factors such as insurance coverage, however, a greater proportion of the middle-aged group undergoes spinal surgery more often.[2,18,21]

In his follow-up treatise, Wilkinson[28] admitted that "the conclusion that in America many failed back syndromes result from excessive surgical intervention seems difficult to avoid." He went on to list several culprits:

- *Incorrect diagnosis,* which may include misdiagnosed neoplasms, the so-called flabby back syndrome common in affluent societies where obesity is prevalent, rheumatoid arthritis, osteoarthritis, ankylosing spondylitis, and so on.
- *Unnecessary surgery,* such as operations on a bulging disk without radiculopathy symptoms; slight sensory loss does not necessarily mandate operation. To perform fusions in grade I spondylolisthesis is still under debate.[13]
- *Improper or inadequate surgery,* such as disk excision performed at the wrong level or the wrong side, leaving of a loose fragment of disk, or selection of the wrong hardware to execute a fusion.[13,14,20]

To these items, at least three more predisposing factors may be added:

- Short pedicles, lumbarization of S1, sacralization of L5, and arachnoid cysts may be present.
- Inadequate imaging or inconclusive interpretation may offer a misleading diagnosis or may fail to recognize associated diseases, such as vertebral hemangiomas and scoliosis. The value of diagnostic invasive tests such as differential spinal blocks, epidurography, diskography, and others is still in doubt because most disease can be identified by MRI. For example, in diskography, 1.0 mL of dye produces little pain in normal and ruptured disks alike, but 2 mL of dye will produce pain in every disk injected, a finding that casts doubt on this procedure.[29]
- Cigarette smoking has been found to decrease the threshold of pain,[26] increase perioperative opioid requirements,[30] affect wound healing,[31] increase postoperative pulmonary morbidity,[32] and add to a patient's stress response.[33] Furthermore, it increases dural sac pressure during bouts of coughing and thus facilitates CSF leaks.[29–34] Nevertheless, this factor is rarely considered a contraindication to surgery in patients who refuse to stop smoking.

What Has Failed in the "Failed Back" Syndrome?

The reasons are multiple, and at any given time, one or more may cause the reappearance of pain and neurologic symptoms after these operations. The following causes are not listed in order of frequency or seriousness of their occurrence.

Incidental Durotomy

Perhaps one of the most underrated complications, incidental durotomy may occur in 6% to 8% of first-time laminectomies, in 12% to 20% of repeat laminectomies, and in 14% to 30% of spinal fusions.[35] Recognition of these tears allows them to be repaired on site. Unrecognized tears not only result in CSF leak but also allow for blood accumulated at the bottom of the wound (in patients in the prone position) to enter the subarachnoid space.[36,37] This usually unexpected development may have serious consequences because blood is an active irritant of nerve tissue and may initiate an arachnoiditic inflammatory response. Depending on the amount of CSF lost, postural headache and even meningismus may occur, with a bulging mass under the incision. Occasionally, serosanguineous fluid, which can be tested for glucose content with a glucose strip, may leak through the incision. Ultimate confirmation can be obtained by MRI of the lumbar spine. If CSF is contained in the retrospinal tissues, eventually a soft, thin pseudomembrane will form around it. If not initially repaired, it may give rise to a pseudomeningocele.[37,38] Puncture is not recommended because CSF may leak persistently.[39]

Further discussion on durotomies is included in Chapter 98.

Loose Disk Fragments

With an incidence of 2% to 7%, loose disk fragments of nucleus pulposus may be "dragged out" of the anulus fibrosus cavity by the rongeurs employed to remove the loose portions of the nucleus.[40] Less commonly, loose fragments can also

be dislodged from the disk cavity later on, when the patient is mobilized. Pain is sharp, severe, and localized to the dermatome corresponding to the compressed nerve root that is being pressured by the 0.5- to 1.4-cm fibrocartilaginous mass.[40] Confirmation is again done with MRI. This condition requires immediate surgical reintervention because patients are in severe, constant pain and may also have bladder dysfunction.[41] Initially, interventions were performed with bone graft and later with hardware.

Intrathecal or Peridural Hematoma

Both intrathecal hematoma and peridural hematoma are serious events. A substantial amount of blood in the subarachnoid space is manifested by severe, burning low back pain, with or without radicular symptoms, immediately on the patient's awakening from the anesthetic.[42] This pain usually requires high doses of opiates to control it. More common are extradural hematomas (**Fig. 96.1**), which initially manifest as mild to moderate back pain but with moderate to severe paravertebral muscle spasm. Depending on the size of the hematoma and its proximity to the dural sac, back pain and neurologic symptoms may appear 2 or 3 weeks postoperatively. This delay may result from the degradation of blood elements and products and the subsequent liberation of leukotrienes and cytokines that are able to cross the dural barrier.[43] After 10 days, intrathecal hemosiderin may be recognized on MRI.

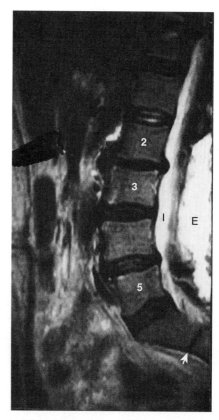

Fig. 96.1 Sagittal view of a magnetic resonance imaging scan of the lumbar spine 2 weeks after multiple laminectomies, with blood intrathecally (I) and extradurally (E) and a posterior and anteriorly herniated L2-3 disk. A vestigial S1-2 disk is noted *(arrow)*.

Nerve Root Cysts

Leg pain with minimal back pain may be caused by postoperative cystic outpouchings when dural tears occur in the dural cuff that accompanies the emerging nerve roots (**Fig. 96-2**) during their intraspinal canal passage. These cysts should be differentiated from the congenital Tarlov or arachnoid cysts that occur at the same location, but these are located along the nerve root dural cuffs. At myelography, these cysts fill immediately. Postoperative arachnoidal cysts are formed at the time of surgery when a small dural tear occurs in this same sheath location. If the tear is not repaired, the arachnoid may herniate through this dural tear to form a primary cyst, which is usually reinforced by an outer wall of fibrous tissue.[44] These cysts may be identified by fluid pulsations. In any case, at surgery the ostium or opening communicating with the subarachnoid space is very small and difficult to find.

Epidural Fibrosis

Epidural fibrosis is perhaps the most dreaded complication of spinal surgery and the most frequent cause of FBSS.[45] Most laminectomies are usually followed by a short period (3 to 6 months) of improvement because excision of the herniated portion of the disk and removal of a portion of the lamina and the ligamentum flavum provide relief from the stenotic compression, with a satisfactory result as the patient's symptoms subside or are markedly improved.[46] All along, as the wound heals, an inflammatory response is occurring around the dural sac and the paravertebral muscles (**Fig. 96.3**). Eventually, the cellular infiltrate gives way to collagen deposition that proliferates for months, and the incision heals, as all tissues in every organ do, with scar tissue. The operated intervertebral space heals with collagen and fibrous tissue that lead to scarring in the peridural space and fibrous adhesions to dura, nerve roots, bone, muscles, and fascia where the operation took place.[47] Guizar-Sahagun et al[48] demonstrated that the administration of steroids before spinal cord injury not only did not help to prevent the inflammatory changes but also actually exacerbated them. In some cases, this proliferation of fibrotic tissue and adhesions is exaggerated, and eventually it may indent or compress the dural sac and even encircle a nerve root. If foreign bodies (e.g., Surgicel, Gelfoam,[49] cotton pads),[50] glues, sealants[51] (e.g., ADPL), or natural materials[51] are left in the wound or if access was difficult or traumatic or a large extradural hematoma was present, this reaction may be accelerated. Fatal anaphylaxis has occurred after fibrin glue application.[44] Symptoms of radiculopathy may appear and depend on the nerve root affected. However, not uncommonly, all these materials may provoke more inflammation, with resulting greater fibrosis and scarring. In this regard, meticulous surgical technique makes a difference.

The gradual surrounding of a nerve root by scar tissue produces radicular pain and sensory disturbances as it elicits traction and a compressive effect on the root.[52] At that point, it becomes difficult to determine whether the radiculopathy is caused by a recurrent herniated disk or by peridural fibrosis. In this case, the nerve root is displaced. Nerve root involvement may be defined by electrodiagnostic studies and by MRI with gadolinium that enhances the scar tissue by transfer of the dye from the intravascular to the interstitial compartment, as would occur from inflammation or scarring.[53] Conversely, disks usually do not enhance.[54] Caution in the interpretation is advised because high doses of contrast agent (0.3 mmol/kg) have been demonstrated to increase the conspicuity of the disk.[54] Repeated attempts to prevent peridural scarring have not been successful.[55–57]

Insufficient Decompression

Insufficient decompression may be lateral when it occurs after a decompressive attempt within the lateral foramina that may have compressed the nerve root by an osteophyte within the

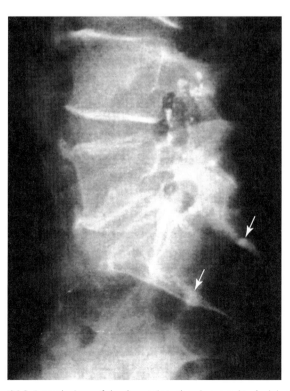

Fig. 96.2 Lateral view of lumbar spine showing previously injected residual pantopaque lodged in nerve root cuffs *(arrows)*.

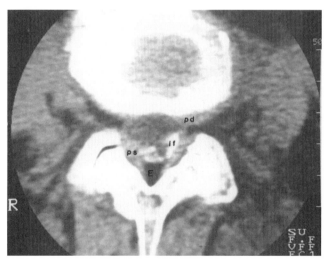

Fig. 96.3 Computed tomography scan of the lumbar spine depicting intrathecal fibrosis (if) on the left inside of the dural sac wall. Peridural scarring and fibrosis (ps) adhering to the right lamina are abundant. The epidural space (E) is preserved. A broad protruding disk (pd) mostly to the left, narrows the lateral foramen, and bilateral facet joint hypertrophy is present.

lumen, soft tissue, or even bone residues from bony spurs. Within the spinal canal, central stenosis may result from a hypertrophic ligamentum flavum, short pedicles, a loose disk fragment, or a herniated disk, in which case wider decompression, such as obtained from bilateral laminotomy or lateral foraminectomy, may be necessary to gain ample access to the lesion that is generating the pain.[46,48,51]

Minimally Invasive Access

In more recent and popular access, procedures are performed through a 3-cm skin incision with the use of a tubular amplifier that provides limited exposure. Guided by fluoroscopy, procedures such as limited minimal laminectomy, diskectomy, removal of osteophytes, and other operations are performed.[58] Although these procedures are feasible to perform, the success of these operations is difficult to confirm in subsequent MRI studies. A definite objection to this approach is the practice of these procedures by nonsurgeons and in outpatient facilities. Moreover, the recurrence of disk herniation usually occurs 2 years later, as opposed to 12 years later when ample and multiple laminectomies are performed (**Fig. 96.4**).

Residual, Recurrent, or Adjacent Herniated Nucleus Pulposus

An incompletely removed herniation may be extruded again because the anulus fibrosus is usually left open, thus liberating a free fragment in the vertebral canal.[44] A single herniated nucleus pulposus is more frequent in young patients (see **Fig. 96.4**), whereas in middle-aged and older patients, several lumbar disks may have various degrees of degeneration. Thus, when a herniated portion of the most severely degenerated disk is removed, the protruding[31,33,38,52] or slightly herniated disks may not be able to tolerate the new undue pressures applied while in the erect position or during flexion.

Therefore, adjacent disks continue to degenerate in an accelerated process, and soon another disk is fully ruptured, thereby producing radiculopathy.[54] Depending on its extent (>4 mm) or whether its location is lateral (**Fig. 96.5**) or broad based, the nerve root is more likely to be compressed against a hypertrophic facet joint; this finding suggests an apparent need for another laminectomy, in sort of a domino effect.[56]

Mechanical Instability

Certain preexisting abnormalities predispose patients to lumbosacral spine instability. Among them are sacralization of L5 or lumbarization of S1 and scoliosis from 5 to 15 degrees, which, if present, may render that portion of the spine unstable. Usually, these congenital variances can be recognized in sagittal MRI views.[57] Prior facetectomies, extensive bilateral laminotomies, and severe unilateral spondylosis destabilize the adjacent segments of the spine. Malalignment of adjacent vertebrae may occur after extensive diskectomy, thus leading to spondylolisthesis. Alteration of the usually even axial surface of each vertebra, whether by scoliosis, a degenerated disk, an osteophyte, or one-sided spondylosis, may change the individual support given by each segment. In addition, an unstable spinal segment prevents the normal dissipation of the load sharing and thus changes the distribution of stress forces throughout the axial topography of each vertebra.[51,53]

Depending on which lesion predominates, spinal stenosis, spondylolisthesis, or ligament stretching may result, reducing and morphologically changing the transverse diameter of the vertebral canal or the neural foramen. During the aging process, these changes occur gradually. In severe trauma, some of these changes may appear suddenly. Diskectomies, as helpful as they may be in reducing the compression of neural elements under certain circumstances, may affect the stability of the spine sufficiently to precipitate the need for a stabilizing fusion.[57]

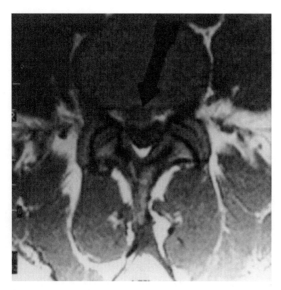

Fig. 96.4 Axial magnetic resonance image of the lumbar spine (L3-4 level) demonstrating a centrally located herniated nucleus pulposus *(arrow)* compressing the dural sac (darker semilunar structure). The posterior epidural space is shown to be accessible.

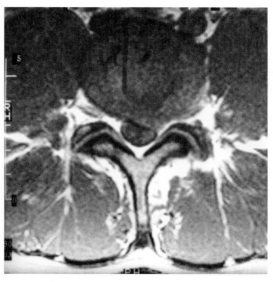

Fig. 96.5 Axial magnetic resonance image of the lumbar spine showing a paracentral L4-5 herniated disk, toward the left, narrowing the lateral foramen. Impingement of the dural sac is present, with reduction in size of the posterior epidural space.

Pseudarthrosis

After spinal fusions, it is essential to monitor the stability of the fused unit; however, the usual plain films on flexion and extension show only extreme causes of instability.[58] To determine whether bone growth is taking place between vertebrae, either CT or MRI[59] is required to detect the presence of any vacuum phenomena or spaces (**Fig. 96.6**) in between where new bone growth should be.[60] In all fairness, a maximum of 2 years is suggested as a waiting period for fusion to be successful. If no bone pockets persist, most likely the pseudarthrosis is permanent. If hardware was applied, then as long as the screws and plates are in place and are not causing side effects, they can be left in place. However, if pain persists and the screw head sites are tender, or if the screws are bending or fractured, the screws may have to be removed. This may leave an unstable spine that is sometimes worse than it was before because the disks usually have been removed.[53] Occasionally, when bone fragments are placed in between the vertebral bodies, close to the posterior edge, growing graft bone eventually may protrude into the vertebral canal and acting as an osteophyte and impinge on the dural sac. Repeat fusion procedures are usually less likely to succeed than is the first attempt.[61–63]

Spondylolisthesis

The overriding of a vertebra over the posterior plate of the one below results in undue compression of the posterior end of the intervertebral disk, narrowing of the lateral foramen, and possible impingement of the corresponding nerve root. This condition produces moderate constant pain that is exacerbated by standing and walking.[53,59] According to the degree of disparity of the alignment of the two vertebrae involved, spondylolisthesis is given one of four grades (I to IV) (**Fig. 96.7**).[55] Grade I may be treated with conservative measures; a higher level of deviation usually requires surgical stability (**Fig. 96.8**). It is desirable not only to stabilize the two adjacent vertebrae but also to attempt to correct the misalignment and relieve the pain.[56,61] However, patients may need to be informed that with the fusion, the "slip vertebra" will be prevented from mobilizing any further, but usually it is not possible to return it to its previous aligned position.

Infections

Infections can occur in the soft tissue as cellulitis, fasciitis, epidural abscess (**Fig. 96.9**), or meningitis, with delayed clinical manifestations for up to 1 month.[64] Diskitis may also be present and produce localized pain, low-grade fever, and malaise for months.[63] Ultrasound or radiologic imaging[64] usually identifies the location of the infections.[65] Most of these infections can be treated conservatively,[66] but if a neurologic deficit persists, surgical drainage and evacuation may be necessary.[62]

Infections with methicillin-resistant *Staphylococcus aureus* (MRSA) have become more common after laminectomy. These infections are characterized by a prolonged period of purulent discharge through the surgical incision, and they require an infectious disease consultation and intravenous antibiotic therapy for months. Needless to say, if this complication occurs in a patient with spinal fusion with metal hardware, the hardware may need to be removed prematurely, and this situation presents a disastrous dilemma.

Spinal Stenosis

Repeated operations may produce both axial and radicular pain that may be caused by a herniated disk, hypertrophy of the facet joints (**Fig. 96.10**), progression or overgrowth of a previous spinal fusion, or hypertropic osteophyte, which may coexist with peridural scarring that significantly compressed the dural elements.[67] Although bony and ligamentum compression may be mechanically reduced, pain relief may be minimal.

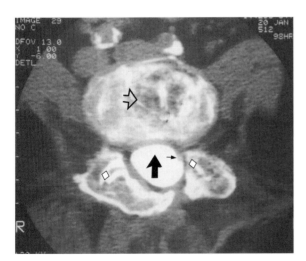

Fig. 96.6 Lumbar spine computed tomography scan at the L4-5 level showing areas of nonsolidification implying pseudarthrosis *(open arrow)*. In addition, a dilated dural sac with a cluster of nerve roots adhering to the left wall of the dural sac *(black arrow)* is present, indicative of arachnoiditis. Bilateral spondylosis *(open diamonds)* and evidence of a left laminectomy are visible.

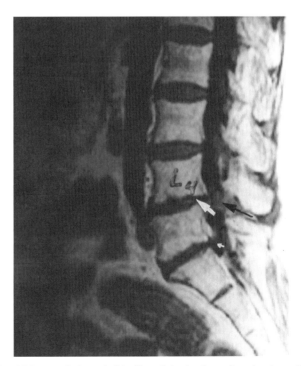

Fig. 96.7 Lateral view of plain film of the lumbar spine showing mild spondylolisthesis of L5 on S1 with reduction of the lateral foramen (x). Residual Pantopaque is shown at the end of the dural sac *(white arrow)* and at the L4 and L5 levels.

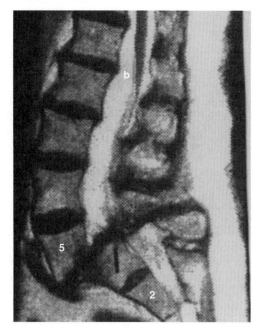

Fig. 96.8 Sagittal magnetic resonance image of the lumbar spine showing a IV grade spondylolisthesis of L5 on S1 with expansion of the dural sac cephalad. From L2 down, the lumbar nerve roots appear to be tethered posteriorly. The S1-2 vestigial disk is well developed, allowing for considerable instability of the L4-5-S1-2 segment of the spine.

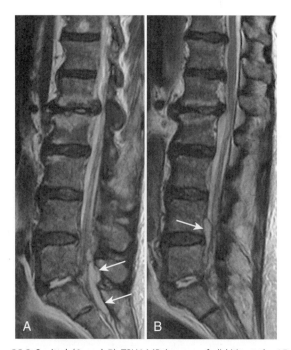

Fig. 96.9 Sagittal (A and B) T2W MR images of diskitis at the L5-S1 disk level showing high-S1 fluid within the disk. There are high-S1 fluid collections (*white arrows*) in the epidural space consistent with abscesses.

Pseudomeningocele

Pseudomeningoceles and other postoperative dilatations of the dural sac are discussed in detail in Chapter 98. One early typical CSF leak after minimally invasive surgery is shown in **Figure 96.11**.

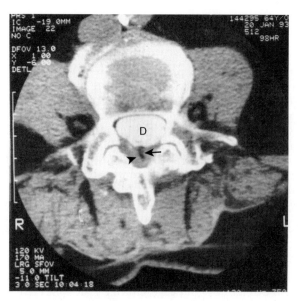

Fig. 96.10 Computed tomography scan of the lumbar spine depicting spinal canal stenosis as result of hypertrophy of the ligamentum flavum (*black arrowhead*); also, the epidural space (*black arrow*) has become rather narrowed by it. D, Dural sac.

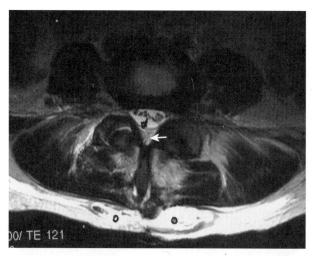

Fig. 96.11 Six days after laminectomy, an axial magnetic resonance image of the lumbosacral spine depicts an infiltration of the paravertebral muscles probably with cerebrospinal fluid, also present in the subcutaneous tissue (O). Within the dural sac (d), the nerve roots are enhanced and located in the anterior half of the sac with an asymmetrical distribution. The posterior epidural space (*white arrow*) also contains fluid.

Surgery at the Wrong Level

Indeed, the surgeon's nightmare can occur because sometimes the S1-2 space is mobile or the L5-S1 space is immobile, thus misleading the surgical team.[35] The only way to avoid operating in the wrong space is to follow the routine that the whole operating team must "wait 1 minute" before starting the operation. In addition, once the lumbar fascia is reached, the level at which the operation is to be conducted must be verified by placing a metal object (hemostat) in the intended space and then taking a lateral radiograph or, best

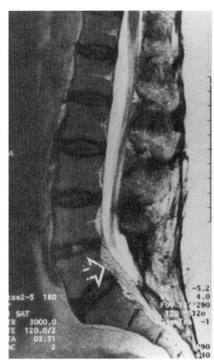
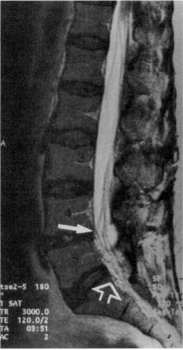

Fig. 96.12 Sagittal magnetic resonance image of the lumbosacral spine with extensive scarring on the anterior epidural space from the L4-5 disk caudad, 7 months after laminectomies, at L4-5 and L5-S1 *(open arrow)*. Thickened nerve roots are noted displaced anteriorly in the dural sac *(white arrow)*, a finding suggestive of arachnoiditis.

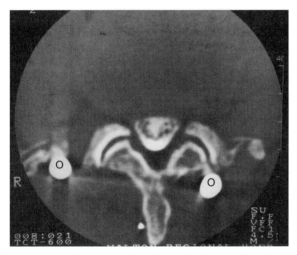

Fig. 96.13 Postmyelogram computed tomography scan of L3 illustrating clumped nerve roots, suggestive of arachnoiditis in the chronic phase. Evidence of asymmetrically placed vertical bars *(O)* is present.

practice, two fluoroscopic views (anteroposterior and lateral).[67] This error may be more likely to occur when microdiskectomies are performed when exposure is marginal and when fluoroscopy guidance depends on the interpretation of the operator.

Arachnoiditis

Arachnoiditis is recognized as one of the most common and serious complications of spinal operations. Only the postoperative aspects of this disease are discussed here. A complete description of arachnoiditis from other causes is contained in Chapter 93. A definite incidence has not been determined, but isolated series have indicated that arachnoiditis occurs in 5% to 22% of patients who undergo lumbar laminectomies and in 8% to 24% of patients who undergo spinal fusions.[19,28,62] One of the most revealing studies was conducted by Matsui et al,[68] who performed lumbar spine MRI on the third, seventh, twenty-first, and forty-second days in 10 patients (7 with herniated nucleus pulposus and 3 with spinal stenosis) who underwent spinal surgery by a posterior approach. In axial views, intrathecal adhesions to the cauda equina were prevalent at the "laminectomized" levels in all patients. Partial adhesions were found at 9 levels 6 weeks after the surgical procedures. Most of these adhesions had resolved by the forty-second day, but in 5 of 14 spaces exposed, partial nerve root adhesions were still present. An initial shrinking or indentation of the dural sac returned to nearly normal levels at the end of the observation period. This study showed that although some of these changes are transitory, intradural lesions (enhanced or clumped nerve roots) may occur, even when only extradural surgery is performed (**Figs. 96.12** and **96.13**). The possible mechanisms for these events are described in the section on intrathecal hematoma and extradural hematoma (see Fig. 96.1).[43]

Nakano et al[69] reported that laminectomy in rats consistently induced an increase in vascular permeability in the cauda equina, as well as an increase in the vesicular transport of the endothelial cells with opening of the "tight junction." This finding suggests a breakdown of the blood-nerve barrier that facilitates the formation of adhesions. Furthermore, the same group[70] was able to show that the administration of the anti-inflammatory agents indomethacin and methylprednisolone, 24 hours after laminectomy, suppressed the formation of such adhesions and the leakage from the nutrient vessels. Moreover, as shown by Guizar et al,[48] the same steroid medication, when given to rats preoperatively, exerted no protective effect, but the formation of adhesions was considerably reduced when these drugs were given 3 or 6 weeks after laminectomy.

Conducting serial neurologic examinations and obtaining imaging studies (preferably an MRI with contrast) of the operated region are crucial in patients who develop severe pain and neurologic deficits after laminectomy. This premise also applies to cases of arachnoiditis in patients who had a fusion with bone or titanium hardware. When the devices are made of other metals, a myelogram, followed by CT, is necessary to visualize the intrathecal structures. Early manifestations are swollen, enhanced nerve roots that may be located in their normal position or in the anterior half of the sac (**Fig. 96.14**).[72] Depending on the extent and intensity of the inflammatory reaction, clumping of nerve roots is not seen clearly until 2 or 3 months after the adverse event (**Fig. 96.15**; see also Fig. 96.13). Thereafter, the swelling gradually subsides, and the nerve roots remain adhered to each other in clumps or to the interior wall of the dural sac.[73,74] This condition is permanent. Although arachnoiditis is not present in every case of FBSS, it nevertheless complicates the clinical features of FBSS and makes the differential diagnosis difficult, especially if metal hardware has been implanted,[75] as shown in **Figure 96.16**.

Distal Dural Sac Ectasia

This complication is discussed in Chapter 98.

Diagnosis

Practitioners need to have a precise understanding of FBSS because it usually includes numerous diagnoses that have been globalized in the definition. Because adequate noninvasive procedures are available, to subject these patients to invasive tests such as differential spinal or epidural blocks, diskograms, and neuroplasty is not only futile and wasteful but also hazardous.[76–79]

A complete, detailed history, including diagnostic tests, adverse events, and attempted therapeutic modalities, described chronologically, is desirable. Minor injuries and work accidents, as trivial as they may appear, may give clues to the patient's actual complaints. Monitoring spinal evoked potentials in the perioperative period may prevent permanent injury.[80] Specific tracking[81] of the time of appearance of symptoms in relation to one of the operations performed not only may help to determine the cause of the FBSS but also may assist in considering certain therapeutic modalities that have not been of benefit in the past (**Fig. 96.17**). Repeated operations may produce both axial and radicular pain that may be caused by progression or overgrowth of a previous spinal fusion or hypertrophic osteophyte that may coexist with peridural scarring, thus significantly compressing the dural contents.[60,61] Although bony and ligamentum compression may be mechanically reduced, pain relief would likely be minimal.

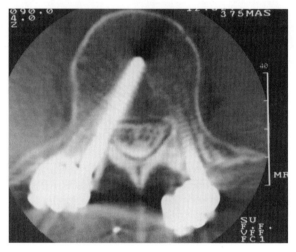

Fig. 96.15 Postmyelogram computed tomography scan at the L4 vertebra with pedicular screws, bilaterally. The right screw is misplaced, invading the vertebral canal and impinging on the dural sac. The nerve roots are mostly clustered in two clumps, indicative of arachnoiditis in the chronic proliferative phase.

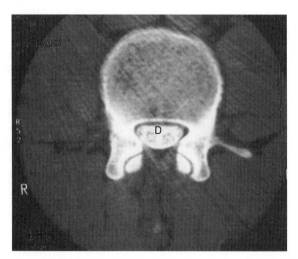

Fig. 96.14 Postmyelogram computed tomography scan of the lumbar spine showing enhanced (edematous) nerve roots located in the dural sac (D), at the level of the L3 vertebra, a finding suggesting arachnoiditis in the early inflammatory phase.

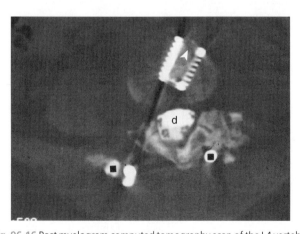

Fig. 96.16 Post myelogram computed tomography scan of the L4 vertebra showing a right laminectomy and evidence of an attempted fusion by replacing the intervertebral disk with one cage (white arrowhead) and vertical bars (black squares) asymmetrically placed. The dural sac (d) is deformed and contains enhanced nerve roots. The posterior epidural space has been replaced by fibrosis.

Symptoms may be classified as follows:

- *Mechanical,* noted as increased back pain when standing, walking, or sitting
- *Related,* including referred pain, muscle spasms, pain in the hips or sacroiliac joints, and bone friction, as in pseudarthrosis
- *Neurologic,* including headaches, electrical shock–like pain, burning, lacerating pain from stretching of the dural sac or the nerve roots, numbness, and weakness not following a dermatome path; symptoms indicate alterations of proprioception such as dizziness, tinnitus, a positive Romberg sign, and loss of balance
- *Functional,* implying dysfunction of bladder, bowel, sexual activities, and autonomic dysfunction (e.g., excessive sweating, heat intolerance, hypertension)

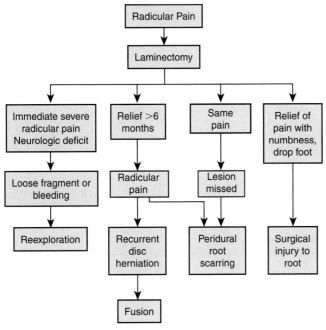

Fig. 96.17 Algorithm for the diagnosis of postlaminectomy complications.

- *Aggregated,* caused by other related illnesses such as diabetic neuropathy, rheumatoid arthritis, and lupus erythematosus
- *Psychogenic,* such as fears, depression, anxiety, hopelessness, insomnia, and suicidal ideation
- *Radicular,* including pain and sensory alteration (e.g., numbness, tingling, formication) and weakness along a specific dermatome, usually resulting from extradural compression of a nerve root

Patients usually have several of these clinical manifestations requiring early consultation, understanding, and guidance. A detrimental trend has been the globalization of the radiologic findings referred to by radiologists as "surgical changes" or "peridural enhancement." These statements are difficult to understand and to interpret by nonradiologists. It is imperative to have a detailed and precise description of all the abnormal findings, even if they have been described before, level by level, in the narrative and a complete listing of the various diagnoses with opinions regarding their possible occurrence, at the end of the report. A retrospective review was conducted of the medical records of 684 patients diagnosed with FBSS.[76] After a history was obtained and a physical examination was performed, followed by a review of imaging studies, specific possible pain generators were identified. By correlating these possible pain generators with the location, extent, and side of the clinical symptoms, their frequency in these patients was noted (**Table 96.1**).

Because some of these pain generators are not surgically correctable, patients with FBSS need to be informed that the presenting symptom, *pain,* will likely continue after any subsequent operation. A list of specific diagnoses is preferable, to avoid the generalized and imprecise diagnosis of FBSS.

Because of the current availability of objective radiologic findings as evidence, the "Waddell signs evaluation" may be discarded, given that it was based on nonorganic, attitudinal, and preconceived notions.[82] Earlier, Waddell and Richardson[83] had already cast certain doubts regarding the reliability of this evaluation. These doubts were reinforced by the report of Polatin et al,[84] who conducted a prospective study in patients with low back pain and noted inconsistencies in the evaluation processes performed by the participating physicians.

Table 96.1 Guide to Diagnosis and Therapy for Failed Back Surgery Syndrome

Presumptive Diagnosis	Diagnostic Tests	Initial Therapy	Extended Therapy
Retained disk fragment	H&P, MRI	Reexploration	Analgesics, protocol
Foreign body fragment	CT, MRI	Removal	Repeat CT or MRI
Periradicular fibrosis	H&P, electrodiagnostics, MRI	IV protocol	Protocol, muscle relaxants
Pseudomeningocele	H&P, MRI	Bed rest, binder	Propranolol, acetazolamide
Nerve root cyst	H&P, MRI, myelogram	Analgesics, binder	Surgical resection, disk plication
Spinal stenosis	H&P, radiographs, MRI, or CT	Analgesics, MgO_2, muscle relaxants	Peridural steroid, bilateral laminotomy
Arachnoiditis	H&P, MRI	IV protocol	Analgesics, oral steroids for flare-ups, protocol

CT, computed tomography; ESI, epidural steroid injection; H&P, history and physical examination; IV, intravenous; MgO_2, magnesium peroxide; MRI, magnetic resonance imaging

Prognosis

This prediction relates only to patients who have already been assigned the diagnosis of FBSS. Unfortunately, the prognosis is not hopeful because, by definition, the label implies a hopeless condition, essentially condemning these patients to severe chronic pain, dysfunction, and disability.

Attempts to identify the factors with a greater effect on the eventual symptoms noted after herniated nucleus pulposus resection showed that men usually had more spinal canal compromise than women,[22,84] as well as more positive sciatic nerve tension,[85–87] both of which correlated with larger disk herniations. In nonoperated groups, a shorter duration of sciatica symptoms predicted good outcomes.[88] Moreover, younger patients with symptoms that lasted less than 6 months and had no litigation also had better outcomes. In contrast, larger disks in relation to the vertebral canal diameter, cigarette smoking, involvement in litigation, and age were predictors of a poor outcome. In the operated groups, larger anteroposterior diameter and smaller central and paracentral herniations indicated better outcomes, whereas concurrent and preexistent diseases, cigarette smoking, spondylosis, worker's compensation claims, middle age, and female gender led to the worst outcomes.[18,89] These findings confirm that morphometric features of disk herniation as they relate to the dimensions of the spinal canal, examined by MRI, appear to be the most reliable predictors of prognosis.[13,84,90]

The volume of complex operations performed by one specific surgeon in one specific hospital has been shown to affect the outcomes of most operations.[13–15] In addition, patients with obesity, patients who smoke tobacco products, patients with osteoporosis, or patients with certain congenital anatomic variances (e.g., short vertebral pedicles, spondylosis, the presence of a rudimentary disk at S1-2, lateral recess stenosis, or mild scoliosis of the lumbar region) have a greater predisposition to postlaminectomy complications ending in FBSS.[19,63,91]

Treatment

Prevention is the best treatment, although a constellation of therapeutic modalities has been used in efforts to relieve pain, which is the most significant manifestation of this disease. Most of these techniques, however, have proven not only to be merely palliative but also to have been inadequately evaluated according to determinations of evidence-based effectiveness.[13] In most cases, therapeutic approaches have been less than satisfactory, including intrathecal[92] or epidural infusions of opiates,[93] spinal cord stimulation,[94,95] sympathetic blocks,[96] epidural injections of corticosteroids,[97] and anti-inflammatory drugs.[98] Other forms of therapy using neurolytic substances[78,99] are associated with a high risk of injury and have a low benefit ratio.[79,100–102] Further surgical interventions are indicated only when precisely necessary, such as in the case of a loose disk fragment compressing a nerve root, a sudden sensory or motor deficit, or a severe infection. A guideline for treatment based on clinical diagnosis is depicted in Table 96.1.

When fusions include implanted hardware, a screw may be pressing on a nerve root. Moreover, if a screw is malpositioned or if a screw is fractured, screw removal may be indicated. If screws protruding through the S1 vertebral body produce pelvic pain, they may have to be removed or replaced. Because fusions have not been proven to be cost effective and given their high incidence of complications and failure to relieve the patient's chief complaint of pain, Deyo et al[13,94] emphasized that research should address who should undergo fusion rather than how to perform another fusion.[103] Destructive or neuroablative procedures are not recommended because they may result in added morbidity and neural deficit.[95] The treating physician must determine whether the pain originates in the fusion elements (e.g., protruding or loose screws, compressed nerve root) or intrathecally (e.g., arachnoiditis, pseudocyst, syringomyelia). Then specific treatment may be directed to the source of the pain. For further information, readers are directed to Chapters 93 and 98 for in-depth details on these therapeutic modalities.

The selection of patient candidates for spinal surgery is crucial, to avoid further increasing the population of patients with FBSS. The aims of the operation should be reevaluated, and the surgeon should focus on the elimination of pain, rather than on the technical success of the operation.[103] Implantation of hardware and spinal interventions must be proven beneficial for at least 2 years in 400 patients before the application of these techniques can be generalized to a larger population.

References

Full references for this chapter can be found on www.expertconsult.com.

Pelvic Girdle and Low Back Pain in Pregnancy

Colleen M. Fitzgerald and Cynthia A. Wong

Epidemiology and Definitions

Low back pain is a common complaint in pregnancy. Up to 76% of women experience low back pain during pregnancy,[1] and as many as 50% of these women take time off from work or have reduced social interactions as a result of their pain. In one cohort study, 37% of women with back pain in pregnancy continued to report back pain at 18 months post partum.[2] A population survey study found that 68% of women with moderate to severe pain continued to have pain after pregnancy.[3] In a follow-up study of women prospectively identified with severe low back pain during pregnancy, 19% stated that they had refrained from another pregnancy because of fear of recurrent low back pain.[4] Variations in reported prevalence and incidence rates of low back pain during pregnancy likely reflect variable definitions of low back pain.

Pelvic girdle pain is a specific form of low back pain. It may occur separately or in conjunction with low back pain.[5] Some studies include lumbar and pelvic pain in the same group. Other studies suggest that pelvic girdle pain in pregnancy is a distinct diagnosis. *Pelvic girdle pain* is defined as pain experienced between the posterior iliac crest and the gluteal fold, particularly in the region of the sacroiliac (SI) joint. The pain may radiate to the posterior thigh and may also occur in conjunction with or separately in the symphysis. Endurance capacity for standing, walking, and sitting is diminished. Most commonly, the pain arises in relation to pregnancy, trauma, or reactive arthritis. Pelvic girdle pain is a diagnosis of exclusion after ruling out lumbar causes of pain.

The pain or functional disturbances should be reproducible by specific clinical tests.[5]

The single greatest risk factor for developing pelvic girdle pain during pregnancy is a history of low back pain.[5] Pelvic trauma may predispose a patient to pelvic girdle pain in pregnancy. A history of oral contraceptive use, time interval since last pregnancy, height, weight, smoking, and age are not risk factors.[5] Elite athletes were not protected against low back and pelvic girdle pain compared with controls.[6]

In a Danish cohort study of 1789 consecutive women whose pregnancies were at 33 weeks' gestational age, 24% of these women had daily pelvic girdle pain diagnosed by history and an objective clinical examination.[7] The investigators classified pelvic girdle pain into four distinct groups—double-sided SI syndrome (6.3%), pelvic girdle syndrome defined as daily pain in both SI joints and the pubic symphysis (6%), one-sided SI syndrome (5.5%), symphysiolysis (2.3%)—and a fifth miscellaneous group characterized by a daily report of pelvic joint pain with inconsistent objective findings (1.6%). The investigators also found that women with pelvic girdle syndrome during pregnancy had a markedly worse postpartum prognosis for long-term pain than did women with single joint pain.[7]

Musculoskeletal Changes During Pregnancy

A woman's body goes through tremendous changes that affect all organ systems during pregnancy, and the musculoskeletal system is no exception. Overall weight gain averages 9 to 18 kg.

A 20% weight gain may double the force on joints.[8–11] The center of gravity shifts to a more upward and forward position.[12,13] Hyperlordosis, rotation of the pelvis on the femur, an increase in the anterior flexion of the cervical spine, and adduction of the shoulders also occur.[14] The abdominal muscles stretch as the gravid uterus grows while the muscles of the low back work harder to maintain upright posture. The muscles of the pelvic floor bear the weight of the growing uterus and eventually allow passage of the fetus. This process creates a natural disruption of the "core" musculature. Inherent pelvic asymmetry associated with pregnancy may have effects on muscle length that lead to suboptimal biomechanical alterations. These changes may cause the pelvic floor muscles to have a less protective effect on the pelvic joints they surround.

The hormone relaxin has been identified as the major contributor to joint laxity during pregnancy.[15] Evidence showing that elevated serum relaxin levels correlate with pain is inconsistent.[16–21] Relaxin levels increase during the first trimester, decline early in the second trimester to a level that remains stable throughout the pregnancy, and then decline sharply after delivery. Widening of the symphysis pubis and increased mobility of the SI synchondroses begin as early as the 10th through the 12th week of pregnancy as a result of relaxin.[8] The strong SI ligament, which normally resists forward flexion of the sacral ala, becomes lax in response to the effects of relaxin.[8] Studies using an animal model showed that relaxin has a potent effect on the amount of collagen in the nonpregnant rat pubic symphysis.[22] A clear relationship exists between asymmetric laxity of the SI joints and pregnancy-related pelvic pain.[23] Asymmetric laxity of the SI joints in pregnancy is believed to increase the presence of postpartum pelvic pain by as much as threefold.[24]

Differential Diagnosis of Low Back and Pelvic Pain

Many potential pathoanatomic pain generators may lead to low back pain or pelvic girdle pain in pregnant women. The cause may be musculoskeletal (joint, ligament, muscle, bone), hormonal (ligamentous laxity), inflammatory, neural (peripheral or central), or related to changes in tissue composition (collagen).[25] Any cause of musculoskeletal pain in the nonpregnant state may also occur in pregnancy. The SI joint is thought to be the most common source of pelvic girdle pain in pregnancy because most patients present with posterior pain.[26] Myofascial pain of the low back, pelvis, hip, or lower extremities may be seen in conjunction with other musculoskeletal diagnoses. Weakness and deconditioning of one muscle group may lead to pain and dysfunction in another. Up to 52% of pregnant women with low back and pelvic pain have been found to have pelvic floor dysfunction.[27]

SI joint pain is often mistaken for sciatica. Lumbar disk herniation, an unusual cause of low back pain in pregnancy, occurs in only 1 of 10,000 pregnant women.[28] True sciatica in pregnancy is rare.[13] The differential diagnosis of musculoskeletal causes of low back and pelvic girdle pain is listed in **Table 97.1**.

Clinical History

The onset of low back pain or pelvic girdle pain in pregnancy typically occurs between 18 and 36 weeks' gestation. Patients may complain of low back pain or buttock, tailbone, hip, or groin pain of varying characteristics and intensity. Many women say the pain began in pregnancy and that they never experienced anything like this in the past. The pain often radiates from the low back into the buttock and posterior thigh past the knee and occasionally into the calf. It is typically better at rest or in sitting and worse with changing positions such us moving from a sit to a stand or turning in bed. It may also worsen with increasing the speed of walking or with stair climbing. Patients may complain of pain at night or difficulty lying on their side. Some patients describe numbness or tingling or giveaway weakness of the lower extremities.

Pain may vary from mild to disabling. Disabling pain not only limits mobility but also may interfere with job performance, child care, and attempts at exercise. Pregnant women may also complain of urinary urgency and frequency, as well as constipation. Some women experience urinary incontinence particularly with coughing, laughing, or sneezing. The patient's signs and symptoms are often nonspecific, and it may be difficult to differentiate between SI joint pain and true radiculopathy related to lumbar disease. The onset of sudden urinary retention, fecal incontinence, or numbness in the perineal area should prompt the physician to consider cauda equina syndrome. Physical examination can help differentiate these potential diagnoses.

Table 97.1 Differential Diagnosis of Low Back Pain and Pelvic Girdle Pain in Pregnancy

Category	Diagnoses
Pelvic (skeletal/joint)	Sacroiliac joint dysfunction, sacroiliitis Pelvic obliquity or derangement, pelvic asymmetry Pubic symphysitis, osteitis pubis, pubic symphysis separation Coccydynia Pelvic insufficiency, stress fracture Bony metastasis
Lumbar	Lumbar degenerative disk disease, spondylosis, or spondylolisthesis (with referral to posterior pelvis: L4/L5/S1)
Hip	Hip osteoarthritis Hip fracture Acetabular labral tears Chondrosis Developmental hip dysplasia Femoral acetabular impingement Avascular necrosis of the femoral head
Muscular/fascial	Pelvic floor myofascial pain Levator ani syndrome Tension myalgia Myofascial pain syndromes of associated extrinsic muscles (iliopsoas, adductor, piriformis) Dyssynergia of the pelvic floor muscles Vaginismus, dyspareunia
Neurologic	Radiculopathy Plexopathy Peripheral neuropathy (pudendal neuropathy)

Physical Examination

A directed examination of the pregnant patient is an important part of the workup of low back and pelvic pain in pregnancy, especially because diagnostic tests are limited. A detailed neurologic examination, a lumbar examination including range of motion, and hip range of motion testing are the initial steps. Abdominal examination, particularly of the rectus abdominis musculature to assess for diastasis, and an internal pelvic floor muscle examination to assess for pelvic floor myofascial pain or dysfunction may also be appropriate. Certain provocation tests for pelvic instability have been investigated; in general, the tests have high specificity (80% to 100%) and variable sensitivity (40% to 90%).[5] These tests are designed to provoke a painful response in an affected pelvic joint region (SI joint or pubic symphysis), although they do not definitively identify the anatomic pain generator (bone, joint, ligament, tendon, muscle).

Patrick's Fabere Test

The patient is placed supine, with one leg flexed, abducted and externally rotated so that the heel rests on the opposite kneecap. This test result is positive with production of pain anywhere in the pelvic girdle (**Fig. 97.1**).

Posterior Pelvic Pain Provocation Test (or Thigh Thrust)

The patient is placed supine, the femur is flexed so that it is perpendicular to the table and the knee is flexed at 90 degrees. A gentle force is applied to the femur in the direction of the examination table. The test result is positive when the patient experiences pain in the gluteal region or ipsilateral leg (**Fig. 97.2**).

Long Dorsal Sacroiliac Ligament Palpation

The patient lies on her side with slight flexion in both hip and knee joints. The areas above both SI joints are palpated. Specifically, the long dorsal SI ligament is palpated directly caudomedially from the posterior iliac spine to the lateral dorsal border of the sacrum. If palpation causes pain that persists 5 seconds after removal of the examiner's hand, it is recorded as pain. If the pain disappears within 5 seconds, it is recorded as tenderness. When the identical pain is felt directly in the vicinity, but outside the borders of the ligament, the test result is not deemed positive.

Pubic Symphysis Palpation

The examiner palpates the subject's pubic symphysis joint and checks for tenderness while the patient is lying supine. If palpation causes pain that persists 5 seconds after removal of the examiner's hand, it is recorded as pain. If the pain disappears within 5 seconds, it is recorded as tenderness.

Modified Trendelenburg's Test

The standing woman turns her back to the examiner and, standing on one leg, flexes the other leg at 90 degrees (hip and knee). The test result is considered positive if pain is experienced in the symphysis (**Fig. 97.3**).

Gaenslen's Test

The patient lies on her side with the upper leg (test leg) hyperextended at the hip. The patient holds the lower leg flexed against the chest, and the examiner stabilizes the patient's pelvis while extending the hip of the test leg. A positive test result is pain provoked in the ipsilateral (upper) pelvic girdle.

Active Straight Leg Raise Test (for Assessing Lumbopelvic Stability)

The test is performed with the patient supine with straight legs extended on the table, feet 20 cm apart. The patient raises the each leg one at a time 30 degrees above the table without bending the knee. The test result is positive when the patient describes a heaviness or difficulty in performing the task. In the second part of the maneuver, posterior compression is applied at the iliac crests in a lateral to medial direction, and the patient is then asked to perform a straight leg raise actively. The test result is considered positive if ease of motion is greater (**Fig. 97.4**).

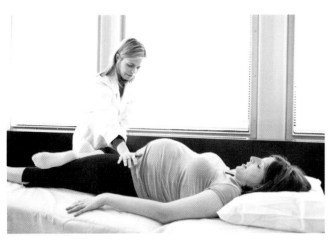

Fig. 97.1 **Patrick's Fabere test.** The patient is supine, with one leg flexed, abducted and externally rotated so that the heel rests on the opposite kneecap. The test result is positive with production of pain anywhere in the pelvic girdle.

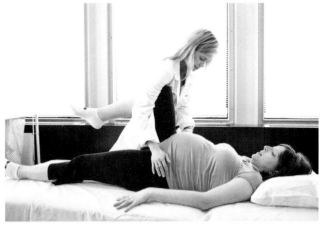

Fig. 97.2 **Posterior pelvic pain provocation test.** The patient is supine, the femur is flexed so that it is perpendicular to the table, and the knee is flexed at 90 degrees. Gentle force is applied to the femur in the direction of the examination table. The test result is positive when the patient experiences pain in the gluteal region of the ipsilateral leg.

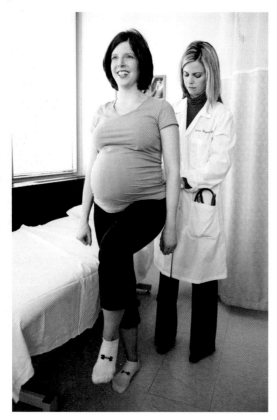

Fig. 97.3 **Modified Trendelenburg's test.** The standing woman turns her back to the examiner and, standing on one leg, flexes the other leg at 90 degrees (hip and knee). The test result is considered positive if pain is experienced in the symphysis.

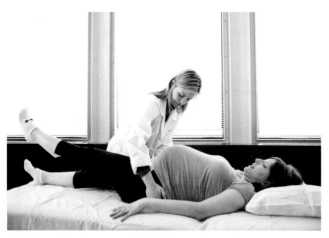

Fig. 97.4 **Active straight leg raise test.** The patient is supine with straight legs extended on the table, feet 20 cm apart. The patient raises the each leg one at a time 30 degrees above the table without bending the knee. The test result is positive when the patient describes a heaviness or difficulty in performing the task. In the second part of the test, posterior compression is applied at the iliac crests in a lateral to medial direction, and the patient is then asked to perform a straight leg raise actively. The test result is positive if the ease of motion is greater.

Imaging

Imaging in pregnancy may be limited because of the potential for radiation exposure of the fetus. However, most single diagnostic radiologic procedures are associated with little, if any,

known fetal risk.[29] In deciding whether to perform an imaging procedure on a pregnant woman, the risk to the fetus must be weighed against the risk to the mother of making the wrong or delayed diagnosis by avoiding imaging. Ultrasonography and magnetic resonance imaging (MRI), which do not use ionizing radiation, are the imaging modalities of choice during pregnancy.[29] No adverse effects of diagnostic ultrasound on the fetus, including duplex Doppler imaging, have been documented, although concern exists that tissue temperature elevation (a function of the intensity, frequency, beam width, exposure time, and tissue composition) could have adverse effects.[29-31] The United States Food and Drug Administration (FDA) has set an upper limit of 94 mW/cm^2 for the spatial-peak temporal average intensity of the ultrasound beam used for obstetric imaging.[31]

No evidence indicates harmful effects to the fetus from MRI, although current data are derived from studies using 1.5 T or lower magnetic field strength.[30] Some investigators have raised concern about potential fetal harm resulting from the heating effects of radiofrequency pulses and the acoustic effects of noise.[32] The American College of Radiologists stated that MRI may be used in pregnant women at any gestational age if the test is considered necessary by referring physicians.[33] Written informed consent is recommended. Animal studies of gadolinium showed potential fetal toxic effects, although demonstration of fetal harm in humans is lacking (FDA category C drug).[30] After maternal administration, gadolinium rapidly crosses the placenta, appears in the fetal bladder, and then moves into the amniotic fluid, from which it is potentially swallowed by the fetus and absorbed through the gastrointestinal tract.[34] The fetal half-life of gadolinium is not known, but it is potentially prolonged. The American College of Radiologists recommended a "well documented and thoughtful risk-benefit analysis" before using gadolinium in pregnancy.[33] Fortunately, gadolinium is not necessary for most pelvic imaging.[34]

Fetal exposure to ionizing radiation may result in (1) cell death and teratogenic effects, (2) carcinogenesis, and (3) mutations in germ cells. High-dose radiation exposure (much greater than that of a normal diagnostic procedure) before embryo implantation will likely result in embryo death. Strong evidence indicates that in utero radiation exposure increases the risk of childhood cancers, particularly leukemia, although the extent of the risk of controversial.[30] The most common human teratogenic effects of ionizing radiation are growth restriction, mental retardation, and microcephaly.[30] The risk appears greatest for exposures between 8 and 15 weeks' gestation. Data based on animal studies and epidemiologic studies of atomic bomb victims suggested that the risk to intelligence is linear based on dose, although the threshold for risk of severe mental retardation has been estimated at 60 to 310 mGy.[30] Natural background radiation dose to the fetus during pregnancy is approximately 1 mGy. Computed tomography (CT) outside the pelvis or abdomen is associated with minimal fetal exposure, and CT scans may be safely performed at any gestational age, provided the pelvis is shielded. The estimated mean fetal absorbed dose of an abdominal or pelvic CT scan is 30 mGy, although this dose can be reduced by altering parameters such as the slice thickness and pitch.

In the 2008 European guidelines for diagnosis and treatment of pelvic girdle pain, MRI was recommended for use in discriminating changes in and around the SI joint and for excluding ankylosing spondylitis and traumatic injuries (post partum) or tumor.[5] The guidelines stated that conventional radiography, CT, or scintigraphy (bone scan) had no role in the diagnosis of pelvic girdle pain.

Treatment

Physical Therapy

Treatment options for low back pain and pelvic girdle pain during pregnancy include physical therapy, bracing, other treatment modalities (e.g., cold, transcutaneous electrical nerve stimulation), oral medications, and injection therapy. Surgery is reserved for patients with progressive neurologic disease such as cauda equine syndrome related to acute disk herniation and is rarely necessary.

After activity modification, physical therapy may offer significant relief to patients with low back pain. A 2007 systematic review of treatment options for back and pelvic pain in pregnancy suggested that pregnancy-specific exercises, physical therapy programs, acupuncture, and the use of special pillows resulted in better outcomes than did usual care.[35] Adverse effects appeared minor or transient. However, the investigators emphasized that most studies had moderate to high potential for bias and that further study was required. No studies have addressed the *prevention* of back and pelvic pain.

In general, studies show that women with low back pain who receive education and physical therapy report lower pain intensities and disability, better quality of life, and improved results of physical tests. Physical therapy focuses on postural modifications, stretching, manual therapy, self-mobilization techniques, awareness of symmetrical body mechanics, functional rehabilitation, and core strengthening. Core strengthening involves strengthening of the muscles around the lumbar spine to maintain functional stability.[36] These core muscles include the diaphragm and the transversus abdominis, multifidus, and gluteal and pelvic floor muscles. Transversus abdominis contraction decreases SI joint laxity to a greater degree than does general abdominal exercise,[37] and strengthening the pelvic floor musculature increases the stiffness and stability of the pelvic ring.[38] Pelvic floor muscle training in pregnancy not only encompasses Kegel exercises but also includes endurance muscle training, relaxation and biofeedback, and functional retraining. In the postpartum period, pelvic floor muscle training may broaden to include electrical stimulation, weighted cones, and pressure biofeedback.

A multicenter Swedish study of 386 pregnant women with pelvic girdle pain compared standard therapy (education and home exercise) with stabilizing exercises, with and without acupuncture.[39] Women who received stabilizing exercises in addition to standard therapy had less pain, and the addition of acupuncture to standard therapy and stabilizing exercises resulted in even further reduction in pain.[39] Acupuncture is generally considered safe during pregnancy, although certain acupuncture points that stimulate the cervix and uterus should be avoided.

Other modalities to treat back and pelvic pain have not been well studied in the setting of pregnancy. Deep heat is contraindicated in pregnancy (hyperthermia is teratogenic); therefore, cold modalities are preferred. Transcutaneous electrical nerve stimulation has not been studied in pregnancy. Bracing in the form of a SI joint belt may be used for SI joint

or pubic symphysis pain during pregnancy and post partum. The belt facilitates motor control of core stabilizing muscles and provides a sense of stability through joint approximation. Placement of the belt just caudal to the anterior superior iliac spines decreases SI joint laxity to a greater degree than when the belt is placed lower at the level of the pubic symphysis.[40] Studies showed that the combination of a pelvic belt with muscle training improved pelvic stability; the belt decreased sagittal rotation in the SI joints by 19%.[41]

Physical therapy may also be of benefit post partum. In a randomized controlled trial in postpartum women with pelvic girdle pain, women randomized to receive pelvic stabilizing exercises in additional to routine physical therapy had less disability 2 years after delivery than did women who received physical therapy alone.[42]

Medical Therapy

Almost all drugs cross the placenta from the maternal to the fetal circulation. The medical management of pain during pregnancy is complicated by the need to limit the transfer of drugs across the placenta, particularly during the first trimester. Unfortunately, placental transfer of drugs and drug effects on the fetus are difficult to measure.

Drug teratogenicity is species specific and depends on timing of exposure, dose and duration of exposure, maternal physiology, embryology, and genetics. The classic period of structural teratogenicity coincides with the period of organogenesis, between 31 and 71 days' gestation (starting the first day of the last menstrual period), although the central nervous system continues to develop throughout gestation and indeed during the first several years of life. Therefore, behavioral teratogenicity is a possible consequence of drug exposure at any gestational age.

The FDA uses a five-category pregnancy drug classification system (categories A, B, C, D, X); however, this classification has some major limitations. There are very few controlled studies in humans in which lack of fetal harm has been demonstrated. All new drugs are classified as category C (either animal studies have revealed adverse effects, but no controlled studies in women have been reported, or studies in women and animals are not available). Unfortunately, this situation does not help the practitioner or patient assess the drug's safety during pregnancy. Several Internet databases offer information on drug use during pregnancy and lactation, as does a well-known reference book.[43] Some drug companies maintain pregnancy registries for specific drugs.

No studies of drug use for the treatment of back and pelvic girdle pain during pregnancy have been reported. Acetaminophen is the first-line analgesic drug of choice for the treatment of mild pain during pregnancy, although it has no anti-inflammatory effect and therefore is unlikely to be effective for low back and pelvic girdle pain. Low-dose aspirin is considered safe; however, higher doses should be avoided because they may be associated with an increased risk for placental abruption and other bleeding problems, as well as fetal gastroschisis.[43,44] Nonsteroidal anti-inflammatory drugs (NSAIDs) may cause constriction of the ductus arteriosus and may have adverse effects on fetal renal function, leading to oligohydramnios. These drugs are not recommended for use for more than 2 days beyond the first trimester.[44] Opioids are considered safe during pregnancy, although the potential exists for neonatal abstinence syndrome after delivery.

Cyclobenzaprine, a muscle relaxant, is a class B drug. Data are inconsistent on whether benzodiazepines are associated with increased risk of cleft lip and palate and other congenital defects, and most practitioners try to avoid long-term benzodiazepine use during pregnancy. Diazepam is a class D drug. Lidocaine patches (class B) are presumably safe. Prednisone and prednisolone are inactivated by the placenta, and only a small amount crosses the placenta. Use in early pregnancy may be associated with an increased risk of orofacial clefts, and treatment of asthmatic patients with oral steroids during pregnancy is associated with an increased risk of preeclampsia and prematurity.[45] The safety of a low dose of tapering steroids is uncertain.

Interventional Injections

Interventional injections have gained popularity in the treatment of low back and pelvic girdle pain. No studies have addressed their efficacy in pregnancy. Fluoroscopy-guided injections require exposure to ionizing radiation. Alternatives include blind injections, MRI-guided injections, and ultrasound-guided injections. Clinically guided blind SI joint injections are usually not successful; in one study, only 22% of blind injections were placed intra-articularly.[46] MRI-guided SI joint injection is safe and effective.[47] Ultrasound-guided caudal epidural injections had 100% accuracy in one study.[48] Ultrasound-guided SI joint injection may require more technical skill, however. In a study in nonpregnant patients, the percentage of successful injections increased with greater experience.[49] Local anesthetics appear to be safe for joint injection; the safety of glucocorticoid injection during pregnancy has not been established. For radicular pain, ultrasound-guided selective nerve root block is preferable to a caudal approach, and if ultrasound is not available, a blind interlaminar or caudal approach may be used. For axial back pain, an ultrasound-guided caudal or interlaminar approach is recommended.

Labor and Delivery

No data suggest that a history of low back pain or pelvic girdle pain will have a positive or negative effect on labor or delivery. Patients are advised to assume positions during childbirth that are most comfortable for them. Patients with a history of herniated disk are advised not to assume a flexed position while pushing because this position contributes to further disk herniation.

Neuraxial analgesia may effectively block low back and pelvic pain, and women with effective analgesia should not assume positions that cause pain in the absence of neural blockade.

Postpartum Pelvic Girdle Pain and Low Back Pain and Prognosis

Pelvic girdle pain is usually self-limiting and resolves within several weeks to months after delivery; however, 8% to 10% of women may continue to have pain for 1 or more years.[7,50,51] The process of childbirth adds to disruption of core musculature; abdominal muscles are disrupted by cesarean delivery, and pelvic floor muscles are disrupted by vaginal delivery. In an MRI study of 80 nulliparous and 160 primiparous women, none of the nulliparous and 20% of the primiparous women exhibited damage to the levator ani muscles.[52] Although not well studied, trauma to the pelvic floor during childbirth likely has an impact on the persistence of postpartum pelvic girdle pain or the new onset of pelvic girdle pain, particularly in the setting of an instrumental delivery. Clearly, musculoskeletal changes persist post partum, including pelvic floor muscle defects, rectus abdominis diastasis, pelvic asymmetry or obliquity, and impaired load transfer with overall decreased core strength. Additionally, scar tissue (perineal or abdominal) may interfere with fascial support. Breast-feeding causes notable thoracic kyphosis and poor posture. Risk factors for persistent pelvic girdle pain include prepregnancy back pain, prolonged duration of labor,[51] a high number of positive pain provocation test results, a low mobility index,[7] the onset of pain in early gestation, and the inability to lose weight after delivery.[50] Emotional well-being may also play a role in recovery from pelvic girdle pain.[53,54]

Low back pain may also persist after delivery. In several studies, the incidence of persistent back pain ranged from 21% to almost 50%.[54-56] Risk factors for postpartum back pain included prepregnancy back pain and an inability to lose weight after delivery.[54]

Treatment options for postpartum low back and pelvic pain do not differ from the options available to pregnant patients but now include oral NSAIDs and fluoroscopically guided injections.

References

Full references for this chapter can be found on www.expertconsult.com.

Postoperative Deformities of the Dural Sac

J. Antonio Aldrete

The dural sac has an important role in the protection of the central nervous system. This delicate wrap not only involves and surrounds these vital organs, but also contains the cerebrospinal fluid (CSF). The CSF lubricates these organs and their constituents and also acts as a transporter. Circulation of the CSF starts from the brain; the CSF then descends behind the spinal cord toward the distal end of the dural sac and finally ascends anterior to the dural sac. In essence, the CSF communicates with all organs as it lubricates their surface and transports enzymes, drugs, neurotransmitters, proteins, glucose, and other ingredients.[1] The CSF also reaches adjacent structures such as the eyes, through the canaliculus present within the optic nerve, and the inner ear, by way of the labyrinth. While being eliminated, the CSF passes not only through the arachnoid villi into the venous system but also through the lymphatic system of the neck and even into the retroperitoneal space (**Fig. 98.1**).

Not uncommonly, after undergoing spinal surgery, patients continue to experience symptoms, either similar to or different from those present preoperatively. Commonly, these patients are referred to pain management specialists for evaluation and treatment. However, not infrequently, the cause of the postoperative symptoms has not been precisely determined. In this chapter, some of the possible postoperative complications affecting the dural sac, its surroundings, and its contents are discussed. This discussion is a warning to pain practitioners not to assume the diagnosis, but rather to attempt to define the cause of the new clinical manifestations. This issue may also have considerable medicolegal importance.

Pseudomeningoceles

The dural sac deformity known as pseudomeningocele usually originates as an intraoperative complication following an incidental dural tear that may or may not have been recognized intraoperatively.[2] When the tear is observed intraoperatively,

an attempt to repair it is usually conducted while the surgeon has complete exposure of the surgical field. Such repair is usually difficult because the delicate dura may be torn, even by the passage of a fine needle; thus, the dural repair may need to be reinforced with tissue (muscle or fascia) or by a patch of synthetic material.[3-5] If the tear is not repaired or if the repair ruptures in the first postoperative days, leakage of CSF may be abundant, and CSF may permeate the soft tissues posterior to the spine (**Fig. 98.2**). Patients who have a continuous CSF leak tend to remain recumbent because the postural headache can be severe.[2,3]

Such leakage may exit through a wound that has not yet healed. If the skin incision has healed, then the fluid will accumulate posteriorly in a single pseudosac (**Fig. 98.3**). Occasionally, however, patients may have two or more communicating sacs that are evident only on magnetic resonance imaging (MRI) or computed tomography (CT) postmyelographic studies (**Fig. 98.4**). Wound healing is usually delayed, but in most instances, it eventually takes place, although the sac remains as a pseudomeningocele. If the communicating ostium is large, occasionally a nerve root of the cauda equina may be trapped.[6]

In addition to conducting the usual history, a comparison of the patient's current complaints with those present preoperatively is helpful. The appearance of clear or serosanguineous fluid in the wound dressing may suggest possible leakage of CSF, which, in turn, implies a dural rent that has continued to leak after the wound was apparently closed. This complication may be confirmed by the presence of a posture-dependent headache occurring in the first postoperative days. Once the wound has closed, a moderately tender and fluctuating "bulge" may be evident. This bulge may increase in size when the patient remains standing for a while.

Removal of the posterior bone support of the vertebral canal (laminae and spinous processes) may allow the dural sac to bulge through the canal, as seen after extensive laminectomies, bilateral laminotomies, and facetectomies

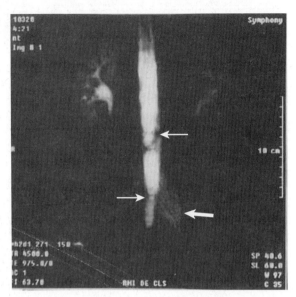

Fig. 98.1 Scintillogram of the lumbosacral dural sac depicting two partial obstructions *(thin white arrows)*. Dye is seen leaving through the retroperitoneal lymphatic system *(thick white arrow)*.

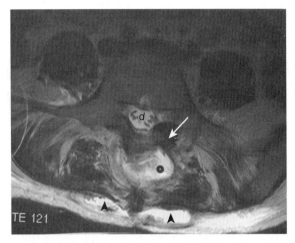

Fig. 98.2 Axial magnetic resonance view of the L5 vertebra showing a left laminectomy *(white arrow)*, the dural sac (d) containing clumped nerve roots, and free cerebrospinal fluid in the paravertebral muscles (O) and in the subcutaneous tissue *(black arrowheads)*.

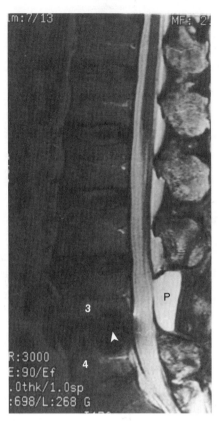

Fig. 98.3 Sagittal magnetic resonance view showing a single pseudomeningocele (P) posterior and communicating with the dural sac. Evidence of diskitis is noted at the L3-4 intervertebral disk *(white arrowhead)*.

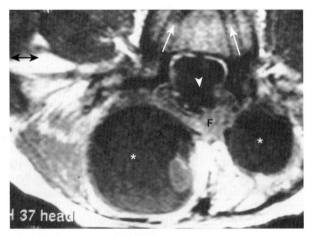

Fig. 98.4 Axial magnetic resonance view of the lumbar spine showing tracts of pedicular screws in the body of the vertebra with a deformed and dilated dural sac *(white arrowhead)* containing enhanced nerve roots *(white dots)*, some of them clumped and adherent to the dural sac wall; inflammation and fibrosis are noted (F) posterior to it. A bilateral laminotomy has been performed. Two pseudomeningoceles *(white asterisks)* are visible.

(Fig. 98.5). Pseudomeningoceles are thought to be related to dural injuries, but they have also been attributed to a spontaneous burst of the dural wall during early postoperative ambulation, strenuous physical therapy, or vigorous and repeated coughing, chiefly in smokers.[7] Moreover, glues, hemostatic powders, or synthetic materials containing chemical solvents have also been suspected.[8] However, this assumption remains to be proven.

Dural Sac Ectasia

Dural sac ectasia is an isolated dilatation of the dural sac that may occur several months after single disk excision through a laminectomy. This procedure tends to elicit considerable fibrosis at the most cephalad and the most caudad points of the operative procedure and creates an isolated, but well-circumscribed widening of the dural sac with fibrotic rings just above and below the site of the operation **(Fig. 98.6)**. Usually, the rest of the dural sac appears to be normal, but the CSF dynamics may be mildly affected.[9] Attempts to liberate

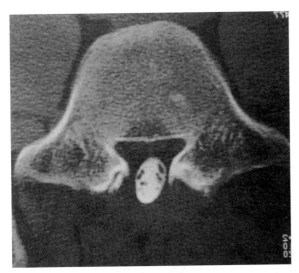

Fig. 98.5 Postmyelogram computed tomography scan at the L5 vertebra level showing a bilateral laminotomy and facetectomy, with posterior extrusion of the dural sac that contains enhanced and clumped nerve roots.

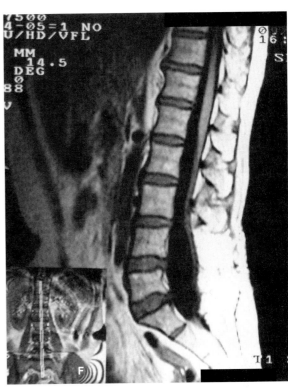

Fig. 98.7 Sagittal magnetic resonance view of the lumbar spine depicting distal dural sac dilatation following L3-4, L4-5, and L5-S1 bilateral laminectomies. The nerve roots appear adherent to the posterior wall of the dural sac.

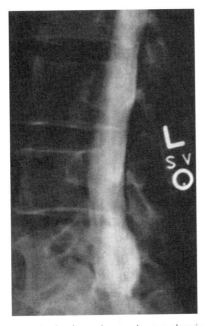

Fig. 98.6 Postoperative lumbar spine myelogram showing a dural sac ectasia at the L5 level, after diskectomies at L4-5 and L5-S1.

the sac from the surrounding fibrotic rings may be hazardous because the wall of the sac, at these points, is usually hardened, but friable, and easy to damage by traction or pressure. These lesions are best left alone, unless the fibrosis surrounding the sac produces enough constriction to produce a serious impediment to the normal circulation of the CSF.

Distal Dural Sac Dilatation

Distal dural sac dilatation usually appears after operations (laminectomies, laminotomies, or fusions) performed at the L4-5 or the L5-S1 levels that leave a substantial constricting ring above the upper point where the surgical procedure was performed. Symptoms, which begin to appear 5 or 6 months

postoperatively, are weakness, alterations of sensibility in the lower extremities but not necessarily with a radicular distribution, and the sensation of pressure in the lower back, usually including the sacral region. Radiologic imagines delineate the extent of the dilatation, as well as nerve roots within the cavity that may be subjected to undue pressure (**Fig. 98.7**).

Arachnoid Webs

Also labeled "focal arachnoiditis," arachnoid webs are membranous extensions of the subdural arachnoid. These webs extend toward the pia and may resemble intradural arachnoid cysts with an inward retracting point at the internal wall of the dural sac and a protrusion of the external dural wall just above it (**Fig. 98.8**). This specific point of localized inflammation is usually caused by traumatic needle puncture or suture or by the application of chemical glues, sealants,[10,11] or hemostatic pads[12] placed at the site of a repaired dural tear. Intrathecally, these webs may form a septum-like partial barrier to the normal flow of CSF that may give the radiographic impression of a pseudocyst.[13,14] These apparent barriers are truly well-defined septa, as described in the sagittal plane by Roche and Vignanendra,[15] who believed that these webs split the subarachnoid space without being in continuity with the peridural fibrosis and without involving the spinal cord.

Dural Cuff Diverticula

Dural cuff diverticula are usually expansions of one or more localized dural cuffs of the nerve roots as they pass through the lateral foramen. Generally, these diverticula are caused by

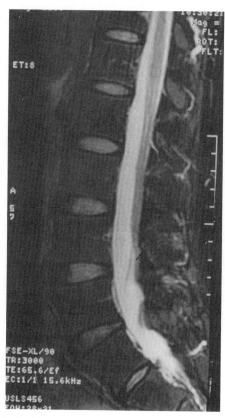

Fig. 98.8 Sagittal magnetic resonance view of the lumbar spine with arachnoid webs and buckling the posterior wall of the dural sac, typical of "focal" arachnoiditis.

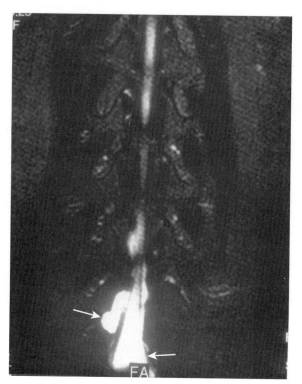

Fig. 98.9 Coronal magnetic resonance view of the lumbar spine depicting a dilated, right dural cuff and a distal dural sac diverticula (white arrows) after an L5-S1 laminectomy and diskectomy.

postoperative fibrosis around the dural cuff within the lateral foramen and often are present during surgical exploration, after the removal of an osteophyte in the foramen, or during facetectomies (**Fig. 98.9**). Occasionally, dilatation of multiple dural cuffs may be noted, distal to the application of Harrington rods or other similar devices that tend to partial compression of the dural sac with the hooklike attachments usually placed under the transverse processes or the ribs (**Fig. 98.10**). In both cases, symptoms may resemble those of radiculopathy and localized tenderness. Removal of the osteophyte or fibrosis inside the foramen is usually difficult; besides, these diverticula are prone to recur, and traction placed on adjacent tissues may further damage the dura. The transforaminal approach[16] for the injection of steroid and other medications may lead to puncture of the nerve root, the radicular artery, and even the intraforaminal dural cuff.

Diagnosis

Pain on and around the healed incision is common. Patients occasionally note a bulge that fluctuates on palpation that is slightly tender but shows no signs of an abscess. In any of these postoperative complications, spasms of the lower extremity muscles, paresthesias, photophobia, phonophobia, headache, loss of balance, altered gait, tinnitus, and muscle weakness may also be present. These findings suggest alteration of proprioception.

These lesions may be easily identified (see Figs. 98.2 to 98.4) by MRI. However, if hardware has been used, unless it is made of titanium, the only approach possible is myelography

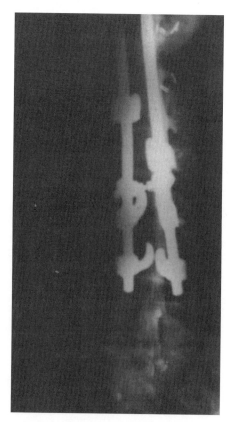

Fig. 98.10 Myelogram of the thoracolumbar spine showing dilatation of distal dural cuffs after bilateral Harrington rod implantation.

followed by CT, which may not be desirable in the early postoperative period. As an alternative, ultrasound may be used to identify the presence of any of these lesions.[3] For complicated cases and when several lesions are suspected, a scintillogram (see Fig. 98.1) can define the precise morphology of the dural sac, the presence of CSF leaks, stenosis, and morphologic deviations.

Treatment

Unless a major defect is present and even though dural leaks secondary to surgical interventions may initially diffuse into the posterior soft tissues (see Fig. 98.2), approximately 50% of these dural leaks gradually coalesce into a cystlike, rounded structure (see Fig. 98.3) adherent to and in communication with the dural sac at the level where the intervention took place. An elastic low thoracoabdominal corset may be helpful in reducing the size of the extra sac.[15] In persistent cases, decompression may be achieved by continuous drainage of CSF through a catheter inserted above the pseudomeningocele for 8 to 10 days. This temporary catheter implantation requires that the patient remain in bed for this period because it is essential to reduce the internal pressure within the sac, to allow its closure.[16] Reoperation to close the pseudomeningocele is not easy because the ostium that connects the pseudomeningocele to the main dural sac is difficult to locate. Attempts to find the ostium by injection of colorant dyes (methylene blue or indigo red) may result in severe inflammatory reaction with intradural cyst and pseudocyst formation and arachnoiditis. Pseudomeningocele after spinal surgery at any level remains a serious and common liability from these interventions.[5,8,9,17]

Small pseudomeningoceles, dural sac ectasias, and distal dilatations may be treated conservatively with an elastic low back support,[18] in addition to acetazolamide, 500 mg twice daily, and propranolol, 1 mg once daily.[17] These drugs are reported to reduce the volume of CSF,[18,19] and they can be used if no medical contraindications to these medications are present.

Insertion of a spinal or epidural needle near or into the scar of a previous spinal operation should be done only after a clinical examination has been conducted and imaging studies have been carefully examined.[20] These scars usually have considerable fibrosis, and the posterior epidural space is absent. Moreover, the posterior surgical entry into the spine usually abolishes the posterior epidural space (see Figs. 98.1 to 98.8), and the dural sac may be closer to the skin than under normal circumstances (see Figs. 98.3 and 98.8). Further, the nerve roots and the spinal cord may be tethered to the posterior wall of the sac (see Fig. 98.9) and may thus be at risk of direct injury.[20] Excessive intradural pressure for a prolonged period may exacerbate the existing neural injury.[21,22] As an alternative, a one-way valve may be implanted to prevent the buildup of intradural pressure; however, these devices need frequent revisions and replacement.

Attempting any interventional procedures that may incidentally puncture any of the dural sac defects mentioned in this discussion is ill advised, not only because CSF leakage may be reinitiated, but also because gravity promotes the persistence of this leakage, given that these defects are usually at the distal end of the spinal canal.[13,14]

References

Full references for this chapter can be found on www.expertconsult.com.

Part I

Pain Syndromes of the Pelvis and Genitalia

Chapter 99

Osteitis Pubis

Steven D. Waldman

A common cause of anterior pelvic pain, osteitis pubis is relatively straightforward to diagnose if the clinician thinks of it. This disease of the second through fourth decades affects female patients more frequently than male patients.[1] Osteitis pubis is a constellation of symptoms consisting of localized tenderness over the symphysis pubis, pain radiating into the inner thigh, and a waddling gait.[2,3] The characteristic radiographic changes of erosion, sclerosis, and widening of the symphysis pubis are pathognomonic for osteitis pubis[4] (**Figs. 99.1** and **99.2**). Osteitis pubis occurs most commonly following bladder, inguinal, or prostate surgery and pregnancy and is thought to result from hematogenous spread of infection to the relatively avascular symphysis pubis.[5–7] This condition is often seen in athletes involved in kicking sports because of the stresses placed on the pubic symphysis[8–10] (**Fig. 99.3**). Osteitis pubis can appear without an obvious inciting factor or infection.[1,8]

Signs and Symptoms

On physical examination, the patient exhibits point tenderness over the symphysis pubis. The patient may be tender over the anterior pelvis and may note that the pain radiates into the inner thigh with palpation of the symphysis pubis.[1,2] Patients may adopt a waddling gait to avoid movement of the symphysis pubis.[3] This dysfunctional gait may result in lower extremity bursitis and tendinitis, which may confuse the clinical picture and further increase the patient's pain and disability.

Testing

Plain radiographs are indicated in all patients who present with pain thought to be emanating from the symphysis pubis, to rule out occult bony disease and tumor. Based on the patient's clinical presentation, additional testing including complete blood count, prostate specific antigen, sedimentation rate, serum protein electrophoresis, and antinuclear antibody testing may be indicated.[1,2] Magnetic resonance imaging

of the pelvis is indicated if an occult mass or tumor is suspected. Radionuclide bone scanning may be useful to rule out stress fractures not seen on plain radiographs[4] (**Fig. 99.4**). The injection technique described subsequently serves as both a diagnostic and a therapeutic maneuver.

Differential Diagnosis

A pain syndrome clinically similar to osteitis pubis can be seen in patients suffering from rheumatoid arthritis and ankylosing spondylitis. However, these patients lack the characteristic radiographic changes of osteitis pubis. Multiple myeloma and metastatic tumors may also mimic the pain and radiographic changes of osteitis pubis. Insufficiency fractures of the pubic rami should also be considered if generalized osteoporosis is present.

Treatment

Initial treatment of the pain and functional disability associated with osteitis pubis should include a combination of nonsteroidal anti-inflammatory drugs (NSAIDs) or cyclooxygenase-2 inhibitors and physical therapy. The local application of heat and cold may also be beneficial. For patients who do not respond to these treatment modalities, the following injection technique with local anesthetic and steroid may be a reasonable next step.[11]

Injection for osteitis pubis is carried out by placing the patient in the supine position. The midpoint of the pubic bones and the symphysis pubis is identified by palpation. Proper preparation with antiseptic solution of the skin overlying this point is then performed. A syringe containing 2.0 mL of 0.25% preservative-free bupivacaine and 40 mg of methylprednisolone is attached to a 3½-inch, 25-gauge needle.

The needle is then carefully advanced through the previously identified point at a right angle to the skin directly toward the center of the pubic symphysis. The needle is advanced very slowly until it impinges on the fibroelastic cartilage of the joint

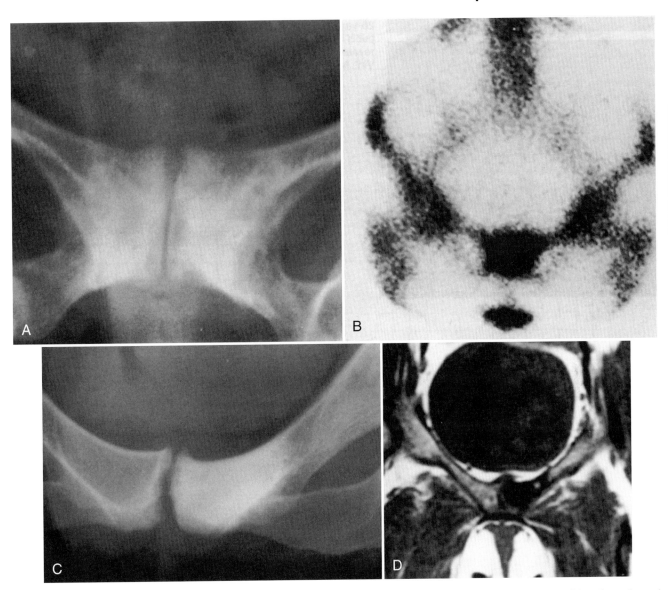

Fig. 99.1 In this 61-year-old woman, local pain and tenderness about the symphysis pubis were the major clinical abnormalities. The radiograph (A) reveals considerable bone sclerosis on both sides of the symphysis with narrowing of the joint space. Marked increased accumulation of the bone-seeking radiopharmaceutical agent (B) is observed. In this 34-year-old woman, a routine radiograph (C) shows unilateral osteitis pubis. A coronal T1-weighted (TR/TE, 633/17) spin-echo magnetic resonance image (D) shows low signal intensity in the involved bone. *(A and B, Courtesy of M. Austin, MD, Newport Beach, Calif. C and D, Courtesy of S. Eilenberg, MD, San Diego, Calif. From Resnick D, editor: Diagnosis of bone and joint disorders, ed 4, Philadelphia, 2002, Saunders, p 2132.)*

(Fig. 99.5). The needle is then withdrawn slightly back out of the joint, and, after careful aspiration for blood and if no paresthesia is present, the contents of the syringe are then gently injected. Resistance to injection should be minimal.

The proximity to the pelvic contents makes it imperative that this procedure be carried out only by clinicians well versed in the regional anatomy and experienced in performing injection techniques. Many patients also complain of a transient increase in pain following the aforementioned injection technique. Reactivation of latent infection, although rare, can occur, and careful attention to sterile technique is mandatory. In rare patients, surgical wedge resection of the demineralized portion of the pubic symphysis with internal fixation is required for relief of symptoms.[12]

Conclusion

Osteitis pubis should be suspected in patients presenting with pain over the pubic symphysis in the absence of trauma. The foregoing injection technique is extremely effective in the treatment of osteitis pubis. This technique is a safe procedure if careful attention is paid to the clinically relevant anatomy in the areas to be injected. Care must be taken to use sterile technique to avoid infection and universal precautions to avoid risk to the operator. Most side effects of this injection technique are related to needle-induced trauma to the injection site and underlying tissues. The incidence of ecchymosis and hematoma formation can be decreased if pressure is placed on the injection site immediately following injection.

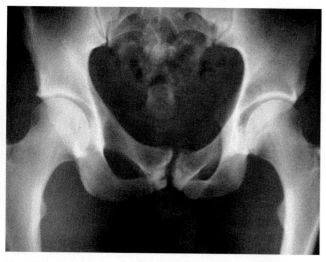

Fig. 99.2 Anteroposterior pelvis radiograph showing classic findings of osteitis pubis. *(From Mandelbaum B, Mora S: Osteitis pubis, Oper Tech Sports Med 13:62, 2005.)*

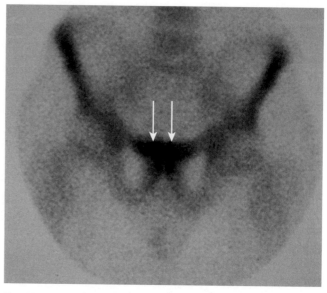

Fig. 99.4 Isotope bone scan shows concentration of radiotracer activity at the symphysis pubis in a patient with increased marginal osteoblastic activity in a 27-year-old soccer player with osteitis pubis *(arrows)*. *(MacMahon PJ, Hogan BA, Shelly MJ, et al: Imaging of groin pain, Magn Reson Imaging Clin N Am 17:655, 2009.)*

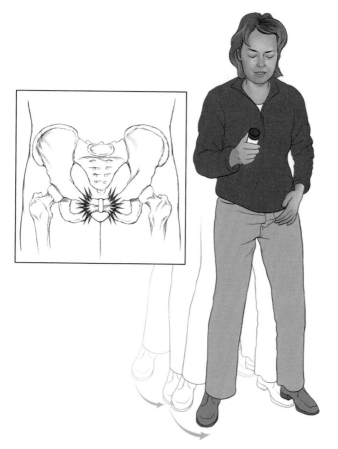

Fig. 99.3 Patients with osteitis pubis often develop a waddling gait. *(From Waldman SD: Osteitis pubis. In Waldman SD, editor: Atlas of common pain syndromes, Philadelphia, 2002, Saunders.)*

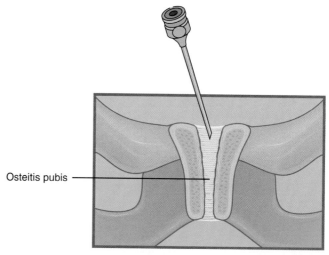

Osteitis pubis

Fig. 99.5 Injection technique for osteitis pubis. *(Waldman SD: Osteitis pubis. In Waldman SD, editor: Atlas of pain management injection techniques, ed 2, Philadelphia, 2007, Saunders, p 401.)*

The use of physical modalities including local heat and gentle stretching exercises should be introduced several days after the patient undergoes this injection technique. Vigorous exercises should be avoided because they will exacerbate the patient's symptoms. Simple analgesics, NSAIDs, and antimyotonic agents such as tizanidine may be used concurrently with this injection technique.

References

Full references for this chapter can be found on www.expertconsult.com.

Piriformis Syndrome

Lowell W. Reynolds and Thomas F. Schrattenholzer

Historical Considerations

Initially described in 1928, piriformis syndrome is thought to be responsible for as much as 6% of sciatica.[1,2] Piriformis syndrome may be even more common, because it is often underdiagnosed and undertreated.[3–5] Misdiagnosis frequently occurs because piriformis syndrome can resemble more common pain syndromes such as lumbar radiculopathy, sacroiliac joint dysfunction, and greater trochanteric bursitis.[4,5] It is usually caused by compression or irritation of the proximal sciatic nerve by the piriformis muscle.[6]

Clinically Relevant Anatomy

The piriformis is a flat, pyramid-shaped muscle. It originates anterior to the S2-4 vertebrae, near the sacroiliac capsule and the upper margin of the greater sciatic foramen. This muscle passes through the greater sciatic notch and inserts on the superior surface of the greater trochanter of the femur. As the piriformis courses through the sciatic notch, it comes in close proximity to the sciatic nerve (**Fig. 100.1**). With the hip extended, the piriformis muscle is primarily an external rotator. When the hip is flexed, however, this muscle helps to abduct the hip. The muscle is innervated by branches of the L5, S1, and S2 nerve roots. Lower lumbar radiculopathy can also cause secondary irritation of the piriformis muscle.[7,8]

Many developmental variations exist between the sciatic nerve and the piriformis muscle. In approximately 20% of the population, the muscle belly is split by the sciatic nerve. In 10% of the population, the tibial and peroneal divisions are not enclosed in a common sheath. The peroneal portion splits the piriformis muscle belly, whereas the tibial division rarely splits the muscle belly.[9–11]

Etiology

Approximately 50% of patients with piriformis syndrome have a history of direct trauma to the buttock, hip, or lower back.[2] Blunt injury causes hematoma formation and subsequent scarring between the sciatic nerve and the piriformis muscle. Sciatic nerve injury can also occur with prolonged pressure on the nerve. Other causes of spontaneous piriformis syndrome are the following[12,13]

- Pseudoaneurysms of the inferior gluteal artery adjacent to the piriformis muscle
- Bilateral piriformis syndrome resulting from prolonged sitting during an extended neurosurgical procedure
- Cerebral palsy
- Total hip arthroplasty
- Myositis ossificans
- Vigorous physical activity

Differential Diagnosis

The differential diagnosis includes the following:

- Lumbosacral radiculopathy
- Lumbar degenerative disk disease
- Lumbar facet arthropathy
- Lumbar spondylolysis and spondylolisthesis
- Myofascial pain
- Trochanteric bursitis
- Ischial tuberosity bursitis

Clinical Presentation

When the piriformis muscle spasms or becomes inflamed, the condition may mimic sacroiliac joint dysfunction, greater trochanteric bursitis, or lumbar radiculopathy. Generally, the patient complains of low back, buttock, and hip pain that radiates down the ipsilateral leg.[4] Physical examination shows tenderness over the sacroiliac joint region and the superior aspect of the greater trochanter of the femur.[6] Palpation of the muscle belly is difficult because of the overlying gluteal muscles. A more reliable way of palpating the piriformis muscle is during a rectal examination. A sausage-shaped mass may be felt laterally that can reproduce the patient's pain.[14]

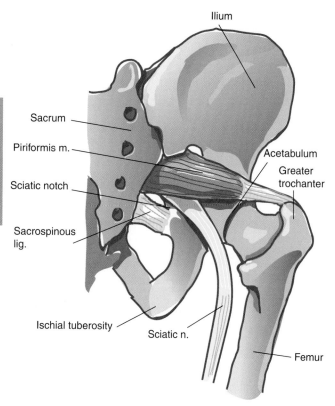

Fig. 100.1 **Clinically relevant anatomy for piriformis syndrome.**

Other findings on examination may include the following:

- The Pace test reproduces pain with weakness to resisted abduction and external rotation.[2]
- The Freiberg test elicits pain on forced internal rotation of the extended thigh.[15]
- Shortening of the involved lower extremity may be observed.[16]

Treatment

A trial of nonsteroidal anti-inflammatory and muscle relaxant medications should be given to reduce inflammation and spasm of the piriformis muscle. Patients should be educated about the possible causes of piriformis syndrome and ways in which to prevent further injury. Measures may include avoiding or reducing aggravating physical activity until the current flare-up has subsided. Applying heat, massage, and stretching to the muscle in spasm may also significantly reduce the patient's discomfort.

Physical Therapy

Patients with piriformis syndrome often respond to a trial of physical therapy. Stretching exercises are intended to lengthen the contracted piriformis muscle. The most common stretching exercise is to have the patient lie supine with the affected knee bent and pulled into the chest and toward the midline. This position should be held for 30 seconds and should be repeated several times a day. A similar stretch can be performed in the standing position.[5] Care should be taken not to pull the affected knee toward the contralateral chest, because this maneuver may cause stretching at the sacroiliac joint. Ultrasound, electric stimulation, and the use of vapor-coolant spray over the area in combination with stretching have produced good results.

Acupuncture

Acupuncture has been used for centuries to reduce muscle spasm and to promote healing. Several techniques can be used such as needling, cupping, and electrical stimulation of inserted needles. Improving blood flow to the affected region seems to be an important component.[17]

Injections

Various injection techniques and injectates may be used for treating piriformis syndrome. Traditionally, injection procedures have been done using a blind technique. With the patient in a lateral decubitus position with the affected side upward, the patient's ipsilateral leg is flexed until the knee rests on the treatment table. A line is then drawn from the greater trochanter to the posterior superior iliac crest. The injection site is then located approximately 5 cm below the midpoint of this line. A 22-gauge spinal needle is then inserted slowly until paresthesias are identified. After negative aspiration, 40 mg methylprednisolone and 10 mL 0.25% bupivacaine may be injected. Care must be taken not to inject into the sciatic nerve.[18]

Alternative techniques such those using fluoroscopy,[19] electromyographically assisted fluoroscopy,[20] ultrasound guidance,[21] computed tomography guidance,[22] or magnetic resonance imaging guidance may be used.[23] These techniques may improve the reliability of proper needle placement and may allow definitive diagnosis and treatment. Botulinum toxin (Botox) is an alternative to the local anesthetic and corticosteroid injectate therapy just described. Botulinum toxin can prolong the relaxation of the piriformis muscle and reduce the associated radicular symptoms.[24,25]

Dry needling, synonymous with acupuncture, may also have a role in the treatment of piriformis syndrome. Unlike with trigger points, however, the efficacy of this technique has not been adequately studied.

Surgery

If more conservative treatments prove ineffective, persistent piriformis syndrome may be treated by surgical intervention. Patients who have objective pathologic changes or dysfunction tend to be more responsive to surgical intervention. The procedure involves dissecting the piriformis muscle and the sciatic nerve. The section of the piriformis muscle overlying the sciatic nerve is often removed. Most patients ambulate 1 day after surgery and progress to weight bearing within a week. Although patients often have persistent paresthesias in the distribution of the sciatic nerve for several weeks postoperatively, many patients report immediate relief of their sciatic pain.[26,27]

Conclusion

Piriformis syndrome often masquerades as lumbar radiculopathy, sacroiliac joint dysfunction, or greater trochanteric bursitis. Performing a careful history and physical examination is imperative for differentiating this disorder from other common ailments. Correct diagnosis significantly improves the patient's chances of responding to appropriate therapies.

References

Full references for this chapter can be found on www.expertconsult.com.

Orchialgia

Lowell W. Reynolds and Shawn M. Sills

Historical Considerations

One of the most frustrating clinical situations for the physician and for the patient is the management of *orchialgia,* or testicular pain. Also known as orchiodynia or orchidalgia, this syndrome frequently has no obvious identifiable, causative factors.[1] In addition, the male psyche, strongly influenced by the genitalia, brings a strong psychological dimension to the management of this problem.[2]

Orchialgia can be classified in various ways. These include time course (acute or chronic), age at onset (pediatric or adult), anatomic site (referred or nonreferred), pathology (mechanical or infectious), severity (severe or mild), treatment (surgical or supportive), mechanism (traumatic or nontraumatic), whether it is medication induced, whether it is physical versus psychiatric (pain disorder resulting from a general medical condition or pain disorder associated with psychological factors), or whether it is reality based (malingering or real).[3]

Chronic orchialgia is defined as intermittent or constant, unilateral or bilateral testicular pain lasting 3 months or longer that interferes with the daily activities of a patient sufficiently to prompt him to seek medical intervention.[4] This chapter provides an explanation of the nerve supply and innervation of the testis, develops a differential diagnosis for orchialgia, highlights the key components of the history and physical examination, and discusses the common therapeutic approaches.

Pathophysiology

The innervation of the testis is poorly understood (**Fig. 101.1**).[5] However, the autonomic supply to the testes and epididymis is mostly sympathetic and originates from the T10-L1 segments.[6] Approximately 10% of the autonomic supply is parasympathetic and originates from the S24 segments.[7] The term *spermatic plexus* describes the group of autonomic fibers that accompany the internal spermatic vessels (the testicular artery and vein) and vas deferens to the epididymis and the testis.[6]

Three nerve groups contribute to this plexus: (1) the superior spermatic nerves, (2) the middle spermatic nerves, and (3) the inferior spermatic nerves.[8,9] The superior spermatic nerves, composed of fibers from the intermesenteric and renal plexuses, run toward the testicular artery and follow its course to the testis. This association between the intestinal and testicular nerves may account for the visceral symptoms of a "sick stomach" associated with testicular trauma. The middle spermatic nerves arise from fibers of the *superior hypogastric plexus.* The middle spermatic nerves pass to the midureter and then travel inferiorly and laterally along the vas deferens to the internal abdominal ring, where they join the spermatic cord and plexus.[10] The inferior spermatic nerves originate from the *pelvic plexus,* or *inferior hypogastric plexus,* and may provide the predominant sympathetic input to the testis.[7] Hypogastric nerves entering the plexus from the superior hypogastric plexus are joined by pelvic and sacral splanchnic nerves at the prostatovesical junction anterior to the rectum. The inferior spermatic nerves then join the vas deferens to exit the internal abdominal ring. Some afferent and efferent fibers cross over to the contralateral pelvic plexus.[11] This neural crosscommunication may explain how pathologic processes in one testis affect the function of the contralateral testis.

The somatic supply to the testes and scrotum originates from the L1 and L2 nerve roots through the iliohypogastric, ilioinguinal, and genitofemoral nerves.[12] The iliohypogastric nerve is a branch of the L1 nerve root, with a contribution from T12 in some patients.[13] It follows a curvilinear course along the ilium until it perforates the transversus abdominis muscle to lie between it and the external oblique muscle. The anterior branch goes on to provide cutaneous sensory innervation to the abdominal skin above the pubis. The nerve may interconnect with the ilioinguinal nerve along its course, and this feature results in the variable sensory distribution of these nerves. The ilioinguinal nerve is a branch of the L1 nerve root, with a contribution from T12 in some patients.[14] It follows a curvilinear course along the ilium, until it perforates the transversus abdominis muscle at the level of the anterior

SOMATIC

AUTONOMIC

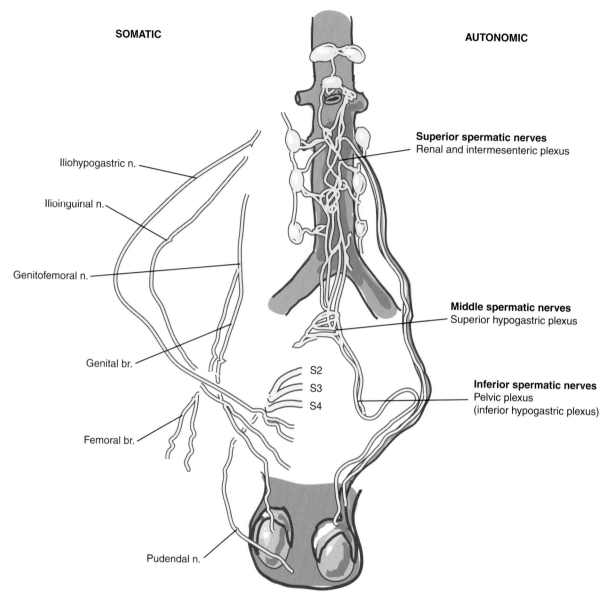

Iliohypogastric n.

Ilioinguinal n.

Genitofemoral n.

Genital br.

S2
S3
S4

Femoral br.

Pudendal n.

Superior spermatic nerves
Renal and intermesenteric plexus

Middle spermatic nerves
Superior hypogastric plexus

Inferior spermatic nerves
Pelvic plexus
(inferior hypogastric plexus)

Fig. 101.1 **Innervation of the testis.**

superior iliac spine. In general, this nerve supplies sensory innervation to the upper portion of the skin of the inner thigh, the root of the penis, and the upper scrotum. The genitofemoral nerve arises from fibers of the L1 and L2 nerve roots.[15] This nerve passes through the psoas muscle, where it divides into a genital and a femoral branch. The femoral branch passes beneath the inguinal ligament along with the femoral artery and provides sensory innervation to a small area of skin on the inside of the thigh. The genital branch passes through the inguinal canal and travels with the spermatic cord to provide innervation to the cremaster muscle, as well as the parietal and visceral tunica vaginalis. The S2-4 nerve roots provide innervation to the posterior and inferior scrotum through the pudendal nerve.[16]

Damage to the testes or epididymis or to the nerve supply of these structures results in orchialgia. In addition, lesions affecting somatic structures in the same segmental nerve supply as the testes, namely, L1 and L2, may refer pain to this area. As in other neuropathic pain syndromes, sympathetically

maintained and mediated pain may occur after injury to these structures. Thus, patients who do not respond to inguinal denervation or subcutaneous blockade may respond to application of local anesthetics to the pelvic plexus.[17]

Differential Diagnosis

Orchialgia may result from a host of processes that have nothing to do with intrascrotal disease (**Table 101.1**).[3] Somatic structures in the same segmental nerve supply as the testis (L1, L2) may refer pain to this area. Radiculitis is the most likely cause of referred orchialgia.[18] Degenerative lesions of the lower thoracic and upper lumbar spine refer an "aching" pain to the groin and testis.[19] Nephrolithiasis masquerades as orchialgia when a midureteric stone is present. This occurs by two mechanisms. First, the ureteric autonomic afferents arising from the same somatic segment at L1 and L2 cross over to the testis afferents in the autonomic ganglia. Second, the

Table 101.1 Differential Diagnosis of Orchialgia

REFERRED PAIN

Radiculitis

Nephrolithiasis

Ilioinguinal, genitofemoral neuralgia

Inguinal hernia

Tendinitis of the inguinal ligament

Abdominal aortic aneurysm

Appendicitis

Epilepsy

CAUSATIVE FACTORS

Testicular torsion

Torsion of the testicular appendage

Infection: scrotitis, epididymitis

Trauma

Surgery (herniorrhaphy, vasectomy)

Inguinal hernia

Tumor

Vasculitis, Henoch-Schönlein purpura

Idiopathic scrotal edema

"Blue balls" (sexual frustration)

Self-palpation orchitis

Hydrocele

Varicocele

Spermatocele

Table 101.2 Diagnostic Workup for Orchialgia

HISTORY AND PHYSICAL EXAMINATION

Past medical history: nephrolithiasis, low back pain, hernia

Past surgical history: herniorrhaphy, scrotal surgery

LABORATORY TESTS

Complete blood cell count with differential

Urinalysis with culture and sensitivity

OTHER TESTS

Testicular ultrasonography

Color flow Doppler imaging

Radionuclide scans

Magnetic resonance imaging of testes or low back

Electromyography

genitofemoral nerve lying in contact with the ureter at the L4 vertebral level can become irritated and refer pain along its distribution.[20] Ilioinguinal neuralgia and genitofemoral neuralgia not uncommonly follow inguinal herniorrhaphy.[21] These complications are usually caused by the entrapment of neural tissue by suture placement, surgical clips, fibrous adhesions, or a cicatricial neuroma.[18] A small indirect inguinal hernia may irritate the genital branch of the genitofemoral nerve.[19] Tendinitis at the insertion of the inguinal ligament into the pubic tubercle may cause testicular pain,[4] as can pelvic floor dysfunction.[22] Even acute abdominal aortic aneurysm rupture or leakage may produce testicular pain,[23] as may aneurysm of the common iliac artery.[24]

Causative factors for orchialgia include torsion, ischemia, infection, trauma, tumor, inguinal hernia, hydrocele, spermatocele, varicocele, vasculitis, polyarteritis nodosa,[25] edema, and previous surgery (e.g., herniorrhaphy, vasectomy, or other scrotal procedures).[26,27]

In the acute setting, and especially in the pediatric population, acute testicular pain should be considered testicular torsion until proven otherwise.[28] The prognosis of testicular torsion is poor; up to 55% of affected boys will lose a testis, even with immediate surgical exploration.[29] Typically, this poor outcome is the result of the slow response of the patient or the patient's parents to present to a physician. Torsion of the testicular appendage may also occur and is sometimes associated with the "blue dot" sign, which is a blue discoloration beneath the skin of the scrotum.[30] Intermittent torsion may manifest with recurrent severe pain. These patients usually have a "bell-clapper" deformity that puts them at risk for torsion.[31] Any man with a history of recurrent pain and a horizontal testicular lie, even in the absence of pain at the time of physical examination, should have exploration and bilateral testicular fixation.[32] Autoimmune testicular vasculitis, with involvement of medium-sized arteries, may manifest in the absence of any systemic symptoms.[33]

Acute scrotitis, which is usually bacterial, may also cause acute orchialgia and should especially be considered in the diabetic patient or otherwise immunocompromised patient. When bacterial infection becomes fulminant, gangrene can set in (Fournier's gangrene).[27] Epididymitis or orchitis often occurs secondary to chlamydial or *Ureaplasma* infection.[26]

Trauma is a leading cause of acute testicular pain and may lead to hematocele, ruptured testes, or sperm granuloma.[34,35] Self-palpation orchitis, caused by frequent squeezing of the testis by a neurotic man overly concerned about developing testis cancer, may manifest as orchialgia.[36] Malignant disease may manifest as persistent scrotal pain. If malignant disease is suspected, this possibility should be investigated with magnetic resonance imaging (MRI) or scrotal ultrasonography.[37]

Hydrocele, spermatocele, and varicocele are amenable to surgical management, which may be highly effective.[38] However, these lesions may be incidental findings, and surgical intervention may exacerbate the pain.[39] Indeed, surgery is often the cause of orchialgia.[4] During herniorrhaphy, if the vascular supply is compromised, acute ischemic orchitis and testicular atrophy may follow.[40] Vasectomy with distention of the epididymis is commonly associated with orchialgia.[41,42] However, the cause of orchialgia may never be identified. Up to 25% of patients with chronic orchialgia have no obvious cause of the pain.[4] A strong clinical depressive abnormality is often evident on psychological tests.[43]

Diagnosis

A complete history and physical examination performed with careful attention to the scrotal region comprise the cornerstone of proper evaluation (**Table 101.2**).[44] The history should include the typical questions regarding onset, duration, exacerbating and alleviating factors, associated symptoms, and so on, but it should also include a sexual history with questions about sexual dysfunction, sexually transmitted disease risk factors, and history of sexual abuse.[3] The past medical history is vital and often suggests a potential cause, such as a history of nephrolithiasis, lumbar disk disease, or hernia. The past surgical history may reveal prior inguinal surgery, such as herniorrhaphy, or other urologic procedures. The patient's complaint is usually of a squeezing, deep ache in the testis, often bilateral or alternating from one side to the other, that is intermittent and commonly associated with low back pain.[43] Sometimes the patient reports that it feels as though the testis is pinched in the underwear but that trouser readjustment does not help. The onset of pain is commonly related to particular activities (e.g., long automobile journeys or unsupported seating posture).[43]

Occasionally, a physical examination may reveal an obvious source of pain, but usually the patient has no abnormality on physical examination. A thorough physical examination should be done to help rule out causes of radicular pain. Palpation of the testes while the patient is standing should be performed as part of the routine examination. Palpation may reveal a varicocele that classically resembles a "bag of worms." These patients may benefit from semen analysis, because as many as 40% of patients seen in infertility clinics have an associated varicocele.[3] A hydrocele may be diagnosed by transillumination of the testes.

Simple laboratory tests include a complete blood cell count with differential, urinalysis, and cultures. If pyuria or hematuria is detected, these conditions are investigated in the same way as they would be in the absence of pain. If results of these laboratory studies are normal, a good next step would be scrotal ultrasound. An obvious abnormality would prompt surgical consultation and intervention. If a tumor is suspected, tumor markers, such fetoprotein, human chorionic gonadotropin, and lactate dehydrogenase, should be obtained. Other potentially useful tests are color flow Doppler imaging, radionuclide (technetium-99m pertechnetate) scans, MRI, and needle aspiration.[45–49] Electromyography may be useful to distinguish ilioinguinal nerve entrapment from lumbar plexopathy, lumbar radiculopathy, and diabetic polyneuropathy.[50] MRI of the thoracic and lumbar spines should be considered if radiculitis is suspected.

Conservative Management

Initial relief may be obtained by implementation of modified exertional and postural habits, use of a scrotal suspension sling or jock strap, heat and cold therapy, and a trial of anti-inflammatory agents and oral antibiotics (**Fig. 101.2**). A minimum 1-month trial of at least two nonsteroidal anti-inflammatory agents is recommended.[4] Even in the presence of normal laboratory findings, a course of oral antibiotics (either from the tetracycline or the quinolone group) is indicated to treat possible chlamydial or *Ureaplasma* infection.[26]

If this management regimen fails, a multidisciplinary approach, as used in other chronic pain syndromes, is best.[39] This may include the addition of a low-dose antidepressant, such as doxepin or amitriptyline of the tricyclic antidepressant class. It is important to start with a low dose at bedtime and to titrate the dose to the patient's response. This approach helps to decrease the side effects of sedation and disorientation,

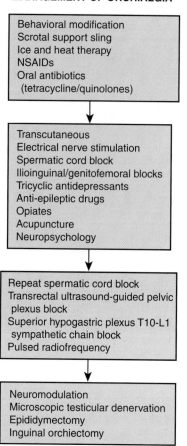

MANAGEMENT OF ORCHIALGIA

Behavioral modification
Scrotal support sling
Ice and heat therapy
NSAIDs
Oral antibiotics
(tetracycline/quinolones)

↓

Transcutaneous
Electrical nerve stimulation
Spermatic cord block
Ilioinguinal/genitofemoral blocks
Tricyclic antidepressants
Anti-epileptic drugs
Opiates
Acupuncture
Neuropsychology

↓

Repeat spermatic cord block
Transrectal ultrasound-guided pelvic
plexus block
Superior hypogastric plexus T10-L1
sympathetic chain block
Pulsed radiofrequency

↓

Neuromodulation
Microscopic testicular denervation
Epididymectomy
Inguinal orchiectomy

Fig. 101.2 **Algorithm for the management of orchialgia.** NSAIDs, nonsteroidal anti-inflammatory drugs.

factors that cause many patients to stop taking the medication before any therapeutic effect is achieved. Long-term opiate therapy may also be indicated. Antiepileptic drugs, such as gabapentin, may be beneficial.[51,52] Transcutaneous electrical nerve stimulation (TENS) has been useful in many patients with chronic scrotal pain. A trial of TENS for 1 to 3 months is safe and may be beneficial.[39] Biofeedback, acupuncture, and psychotherapy are other adjunctive therapies.

Should pain continue, consultation should be sought with an interventional pain specialist for a selective nerve block. Access to a pain management clinic is a strong asset. A spermatic cord block can be tried by using a mixture of epinephrine-free local anesthetic and corticosteroid. Patients who obtain temporary pain relief may be considered for repeated spermatic cord blocks.[4] Patients with ilioinguinal or genitofemoral neuralgia may be treated with similar blocks to these nerves. Pulsed radiofrequency has been used successfully for chronic groin pain or orchialgia originating from these nerves.[53]

For patients unresponsive to spermatic cord blockade, local anesthetic and corticosteroid applied to the pelvic plexus may be beneficial.[17,54] The pelvic plexus lies anterior to the rectum at the prostatovesical junction. These periprostatic nerves are localized under transrectal ultrasound guidance. The location of these nerves may explain the association of testicular pain with prostatic inflammation or postsurgical status. As shown by the success of this block, the pelvic plexus may provide the predominant sympathetic and parasympathetic efferent input to the testis. Alternatively, the superior hypogastric plexus may be blocked. In the case of testicular cancer, neurolysis of this plexus using 8 to 10 mL of 10% aqueous phenol or 50% alcohol may produce long-lasting pain relief.[55] A lumbar sympathetic chain block at the T10-L1 level is a third approach.

Occasionally, tendinitis caused by insertion of the inguinal ligament into the pubic tubercle may masquerade as testicular pain. This condition usually responds well to injection of the tubercle and ligament with a mixture of local anesthetics and corticosteroid.[1]

Surgical Treatment

Surgical treatment may ultimately be necessary if medical management proves unsuccessful. Orchidectomy, with the inguinal approach favored over the scrotal approach, is usually a last resort. The response to this procedure is unpredictable, and the impact on the male psyche may be profound. Consequently, other testis-sparing procedures have been advocated. Neuromodulation, such as spinal cord stimulation, has proven effective in treating groin and testicular pain. This approach may be indicated in select patients. Many urologists prefer epididymectomy as the initial surgical treatment, especially when the pain seems to be localized to the epididymis.[4] Alternatively, microscopic testicular denervation or laparoscopic testicular denervation may offer patients a significant reduction in pain with a technique that is minimally invasive and causes minimal morbidity.[56–60] In these procedures, the spermatic plexus and adventitia are stripped away from the vas deferens and vessels and are divided, or the vessels with nerves themselves are simply divided. Spermatic cord block should be performed before these procedures and is a prognostic indicator of surgical success.

Conclusion

Chronic orchialgia is a difficult problem to manage. The clinician should be aware of the unique relationship of the genitalia and the male psyche. Behavioral and psychological issues should be addressed concurrently with medical therapy. Despite the often unclear cause of orchialgia, the possibility of testicular cancer remains ever present and should be carefully sought in all patients suffering from orchialgia. The ultimate goal of therapy is the patient's return to gainful activity, with minimal loss of function and sparing of the testes. Improved interventional techniques, such as transrectal ultrasound–guided pelvic plexus blockade and microsurgical denervation of the spermatic cord, are helping in achieving this goal.

References

Full references for this chapter can be found on www.expertconsult.com.

Chapter 102

Vulvodynia

Lowell W. Reynolds and Brett T. Quave

Historical Considerations

Vulvodynia is a complex syndrome of vulvar pain, sexual dysfunction, and psychological distress. Multiple attempts have been made to categorize varying types of vulvodynia. Some of these classifications include primary vulvodynia, secondary vulvodynia, vulvar pain syndrome, essential vulvodynia, vulval vestibulitis, dysesthetic vulvodynia, and cyclic vulvitis.

Clinically Relevant Anatomy

When addressing a patient with vulvodynia, the clinician must remember to educate the patient. This includes using the appropriate anatomic vocabulary with the patient and even giving her an illustration of relevant anatomy to take home and study (**Fig. 102.1**). Not only does this approach improve the physician's ability to outline a treatment plan with the patient, but it also allows the patient to communicate more comfortably with the physician. Having said this, the vulva consists of the mons pubis, the labia majora, the labia minora, the vestibule of the vagina, the clitoris, the bulb of the vestibule, and the greater vestibular glands.[1] The ilioinguinal and genitofemoral nerves supply the mons pubis, labia majora, and labia minora.[1,2] Any of these structures may be involved in a chronic pain condition. However, the vestibule, vestibular glands, and labia are frequently involved in vulvodynia.

Clinical Presentation

As noted earlier, this painful condition has many differing terms. *Vulvodynia* is either primary (or essential) or secondary. *Primary* or *essential vulvodynia* is idiopathic. *Secondary vulvodynia* results from an infection or other known cause. Regardless of the primary or secondary classification, vulvodynia typically is described as a burning or aching sensation that is painful to the touch.[3] Patients frequently scratch and wash the affected area, thus leading to excoriations and extensive drying.

Vulvar vestibulitis is a painful condition that occurs when something is inserted into the opening of the vagina. This may occur with insertion of a tampon or during sexual activity. *Dysesthetic vulvodynia* is a painful condition that persists even in the absence of touch or pressure. These burning and aching sensations can be constant, or they can be caused by light, normally nonpainful touch. These findings are similar to complex regional pain syndrome, which is known for such conditions as allodynia and hyperalgesia.[4] Pain that occurs with contact seems to lessen with age, but the overall prevalence of vulvodynia remains fairly consistent at approximately 16% of the female population regardless of age. Hispanic women tend to have an 80% higher likelihood of having chronic vulvar pain than do African American or white women.[5]

Some women experience worsening symptoms before menses or after sexual intercourse, a disorder referred to as *cyclic vulvitis*. This condition may have an infectious origin, or it may simply reflect an increased sensitivity to hormone replacement therapy. These patients may be completely pain free at other times of the month.

Depression frequently is found in conjunction with vulvodynia but is rarely the cause. The opposite, in fact, is true. Usually, the chronic pain of vulvodynia leads to depression. This depression may manifest as depressed mood and loss of interest in work, recreation, and sexual activity. Sleep disturbances are also common with depression and lead to further reduced function and worsening pain.[6]

Diagnosis

A thorough history and physical examination are essential in making a diagnosis of vulvodynia (**Table 102.1**). Various sensory and pain testing modalities can be used to make the diagnosis and to assess for severity.[7,8] Biopsy results consistently reveal a low-grade chronic inflammatory process that is not pathognomonic. Histologic studies may illustrate neural hyperplasia. Infection should be excluded as the cause of vulvodynia. This is frequently difficult, especially if a fungus is the

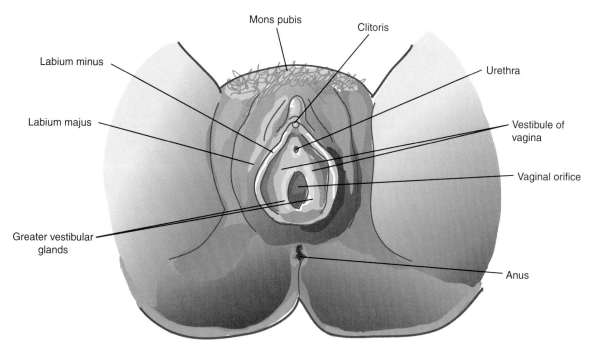

Fig. 102.1 **Female external genitalia.**

Mons pubis

Clitoris

Urethra

Labium minus

Labium majus

Vestibule of vagina

Vaginal orifice

Greater vestibular glands

Anus

Table 102.1 **Diagnosis of Vulvodynia**

History: illnesses, hygiene, pain, depression

Physical examination: vulva, vagina, pelvis

Biopsy lesions

Microscopic examination

Culture

infective agent. Two of the more common causes of secondary vulvodynia are *Candida albicans* and group B *Streptococcus*. Cultures can be performed to help make this diagnosis. Once infections have been ruled out or treated, neuropathic vulvodynia can be addressed.[4,9]

Treatment

Education

Educating the patient about her condition is imperative. This education may involve discussing the condition with the patient, giving her handouts, and referring her to support groups. Avoiding harmful habits, such as scratching and overcleansing the vulva, should be stressed. Most importantly, ways to maintain a normal sex life, exercise regimen, and work routine should also be discussed.[10,11]

Pharmacology

Agents to fight *C. albicans* or other types of infections should be administered if vulvodynia secondary to infection is suspected. The avoidance of estrogen and progesterone used in hormone replacement therapies should be considered because these agents have been implicated in vulvodynia. Other irritants should also be avoided, such as abrasive wash cloths and irritating cleansers. If these agents are thought to be the cause, they should be removed from the patient's daily regimen. Topical lidocaine,

benzocaine, doxepin, amitriptyline, baclofen, capsaicin, atropine, or nitroglycerin cream may be applied at bedtime.[12]

Amitriptyline and other antidepressants should be used as first-line therapy for primary vulvodynia. Typically, this approach involves slowly escalating the dose until the patient achieves pain relief or must stop because of side effects of the medication. The dose of amitriptyline may be as high as 300 mg at bedtime. Night-time dosing is preferred because amitriptyline can be very sedating. Thus, this drug not only serves as a simple analgesic but also may improve the sleep pattern of the patient. This improvement in the sleep-wake cycle may be one reason that vulvodynia sufferers, like other patients with chronic pain, respond well to tricyclic antidepressants. Other tricyclic antidepressants have also been used successfully to treat vulvodynia, but selective serotonin reuptake inhibitors generally do not seem to offer the same analgesic qualities. However, all antidepressants may reduce the depressive component of the patient's suffering.[12,13]

Antiepileptic medications have been used for years to treat various neuropathic pain syndromes. For instance, medications such as phenytoin, carbamazepine, and valproic acid have all been used with varying success and side effects. Some newer medications arguably work equally well and have fewer side effects. Gabapentin has been used successfully in treating postherpetic neuralgia, complex regional pain syndrome, and vulvodynia. Like most antiseizure medications, gabapentin is slowly titrated upward to find a balance of the lowest effective dose for the patient and the fewest side effects. Frequently, the dose of gabapentin may be as high as 1200 mg three times a day. Common side effects include dizziness, nausea, and sedation.[14] Other antiepileptic medications such as topiramate, oxcarbazepine, lamotrigine, and pregabalin may also be effective in cases of vulvodynia caused by a neuropathic process.[12,15,16]

Injections

The ilioinguinal and genitofemoral nerves supply the external genitalia. In the setting of vulvodynia, blocking these nerves may prove diagnostic or even therapeutic. For pain of the mons pubis

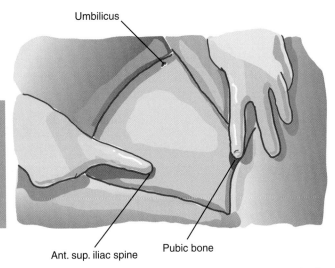

Fig. 102.2 Anterior view shows important anatomic landmarks for ilioinguinal iliohypogastric-genitofemoral nerve blocks. ASIS, anterior superior iliac spine.

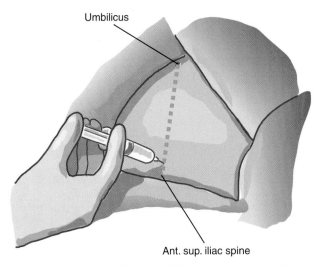

Fig. 102.3 **Technique of ilioinguinal-iliohypogastric nerve block.**

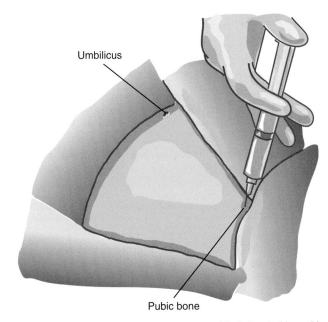

Fig. 102.4 **Technique of genitofemoral nerve block (genital branch).**

or labium majora, the ilioinguinal nerve can be blocked with the patient lying supine. A mark is made on the skin 2 cm medial and 2 cm cephalad to the anterior superior iliac spine. After the skin is sterilely prepared, a 1.5-inch 25-gauge needle connected to a syringe is advanced perpendicular to the skin. When the tip of the needle reaches the fascia of the external oblique muscle, 2.5 mL of 0.25% bupivacaine and 20 to 40 mg of methylprednisolone are injected. An equal amount of solution is then injected in a fanlike manner in the surrounding area[2] (**Figs. 102.2 and 102.3**).

Blocking the genital branch of the genitofemoral nerve may reduce pain of the labia majora and labia minora. This procedure is done by placing the patient in a supine position. The pubic tubercle is then palpated. After sterile preparation, a 1.5-inch, 25-gauge needle is advanced perpendicular to the skin, just lateral to the pubic tubercle below the inguinal ligament. Infiltration of 5 mL of 0.25% bupivacaine and 20 to 40 mg of methylprednisolone is used for the nerve block[2] (**Fig. 102.4**).

Other procedures may prove effective and should be considered in treating vulvodynia. Two of these include hypogastric plexus blockade and spinal cord stimulation.[17,18] A discussion of these procedures is beyond the scope of this chapter.

Psychology

Depression and anxiety are very common in patients suffering from vulvodynia. These patients should have their psychological issues addressed while they are receiving ongoing treatment for the primary physiologic disease.[19] A referral to a psychologist or psychiatrist should be made early in the diagnosis and treatment phase. These referrals should not be made only when an organic cause for a patient's illness is excluded. This either-or mentality should be avoided, so as not to give the patient the impression that she is being written off as a "mental case." Patients should be informed about the power of a cognitive-behavioral approach to chronic pain. Through biofeedback, visual imagery, and other powerful psychological tools, the patient can be expected to improve her pain management and coping skills.[12,20] Medications prescribed by the psychiatrist not only may lessen depression and anxiety, but also, as mentioned earlier, may directly reduce pain as adjuvant analgesics.

Surgery

Various surgical approaches have been employed after nonoperative treatments have failed. Pudendal nerve decompression has been shown to be very effective for suspected pudendal canal syndrome, as supported by temporary pain relief after pudendal nerve block.[21] Procedures involving resection of the hymen and vestibule with mobilization of the lower vagina to cover the resulting defect have been helpful in cases of intractable vulvar vestibulitis.[22]

Conclusion

Understanding and treating vulvodynia are only the first steps in reducing the patient's pain. A return to a normal, active lifestyle and a reduction in depression and anxiety should also be treatment goals. These objectives can be met most easily by using a stepwise approach to diagnosis, treatment, and adjunctive psychological therapy.

References

Full references for this chapter can be found on www.expertconsult.com.

Coccydynia

Steven D. Waldman

Coccydynia is a common pain syndrome characterized by pain localized to the tailbone that radiates into the lower sacrum and perineum.[1,2] It affects female patients more frequently than male patients. Coccydynia occurs most commonly after direct trauma to the coccyx from a kick or a fall directly onto the coccyx (**Fig. 103.1**). It can also occur after difficult vaginal delivery.[2,3] The pain of coccydynia is thought to result from strain of the sacrococcygeal ligament or occasionally from fracture of the coccyx.[2,3,4] Less commonly, arthritis of the sacrococcygeal joint can result in coccydynia, as can tumors affecting the coccyx and adjacent soft tissue.[3,5]

Clinical Presentation

On physical examination, the patient exhibits point tenderness over the coccyx; the pain increases during movement of the coccyx.[1,2,3] Movement of the coccyx may also cause sharp paresthesias into the rectum, which can be quite distressing to the patient. On rectal examination, the levator ani, piriformis, and coccygeus muscles may feel indurated, and palpation of these muscles may induce severe spasm.[2] Sitting may exacerbate the pain of coccydynia, and the patient may attempt to sit on one buttock to avoid pressure on the coccyx (**Fig. 103.2**).

Diagnosis

Plain radiographs are indicated in all patients who present with pain thought to be emanating from the coccyx, to rule out occult bony disease and tumor.[5] Based on the patient's clinical presentation, additional testing including complete blood cell count, prostate-specific antigen, sedimentation rate, and antinuclear antibody testing may be indicated. Magnetic resonance imaging of the pelvis is indicated if an occult mass or tumor is suggested (**Fig. 103.3**). Radionuclide bone scanning may be useful to rule out stress fractures not seen on plain radiographs. The injection technique presented later serves as both a diagnostic test and a therapeutic maneuver.

Differential Diagnosis

Primary disease of the rectum and anus may occasionally be confused with the pain of coccydynia. Primary tumors or metastatic lesions of the sacrum or coccyx may also manifest as coccydynia.[3,5] Proctalgia fugax may mimic the pain of coccydynia, but in proctalgia fugax, movement of the coccyx does not reproduce the pain.[6] Insufficiency fractures of the pelvis and sacrum may, on occasion, also mimic coccydynia, as can disorders of the sacroiliac joints.

Treatment

A short course of conservative therapy consisting of simple analgesics, nonsteroidal anti-inflammatory agents or cyclooxygenase-2 inhibitors, and use of a foam donut to prevent further irritation to the sacrococcygeal ligament is a reasonable first step in the treatment of patients suffering from coccydynia. If the patient does not experience rapid improvement, the following injection technique is a reasonable next step.[7]

To treat the pain of coccydynia, the patient is placed in the prone position. The legs and heels are abducted to prevent tightening of the gluteal muscles, which can make identification of the sacrococcygeal joint more difficult. Preparation of a wide area of skin with antiseptic solution is then carried out so that all the landmarks can be palpated aseptically. A fenestrated sterile drape is placed to avoid contamination of the palpating finger. The middle finger of the operator's nondominant hand is placed over the sterile drape into the natal cleft with the fingertip palpating the sacrococcygeal joint at the base of the sacrum. After the sacrococcygeal joint is located, a 1.5-inch, 25-gauge needle is inserted through the skin at a 45-degree angle into the region of the sacrococcygeal joint and ligament (**Fig. 103.4**).

If the sacrococcygeal ligament is penetrated, a "pop" will be felt, and the needle should be withdrawn back through the ligament. If contact with the bony wall of the sacrum occurs, the needle should be withdrawn slightly. This maneuver

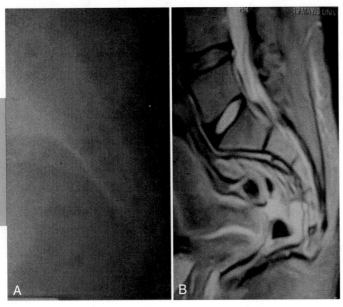

Fig. 103.1 Radiographic (A) and magnetic resonance imaging (MRI) (B) views of anterior luxation of the coccyx with accompanying L4-5 disk bulging (bulging is seen in the sagittal plane on MRI). *(From Cebesoy O, Guclu B, Kose KC, et al: Coccygectomy for coccygodynia: do we really have to wait? Injury 38:1183, 2007.)*

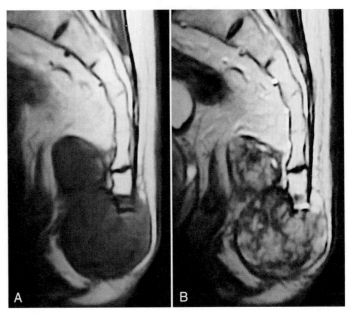

Fig. 103.3 **Chordoma: magnetic resonance imaging (MRI) abnormalities.** Sagittal T1-weighted (TR/TE, 470/10) spin-echo (A) and T2-weighted (TR/TE, 5000/136) fast spin-echo (B) MRI scans document a sacrococcygeal tumor with a large soft tissue mass. *(Courtesy of Y. Kakitsubata, MD, Miyazaki, Japan; in Resnick D: Tumors and tumor like lesions of bone: imaging and pathology of specific lesions. In Diagnosis of bone and joint disorders, ed 4, Philadelphia, 2002, Saunders, p 4017.)*

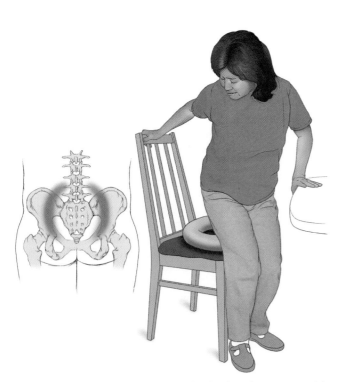

Fig. 103.2 The pain of coccydynia is localized to the coccyx and is made worse by sitting. *(From Waldman SD: Atlas of common pain syndromes, Philadelphia, 2002, Saunders, p 227.)*

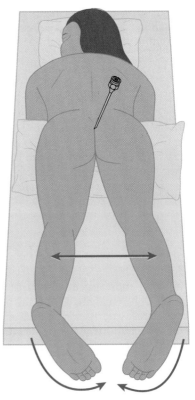

Fig. 103.4 **Injection technique for relieving pain in coccydynia.** *(From Waldman SD: Coccydynia syndrome. In Atlas of pain management injection techniques, Philadelphia, 2000, Saunders, p 244.)*

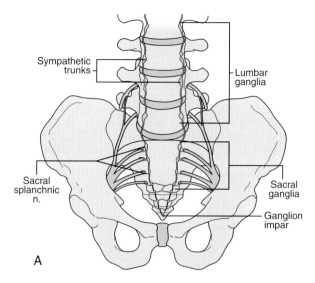

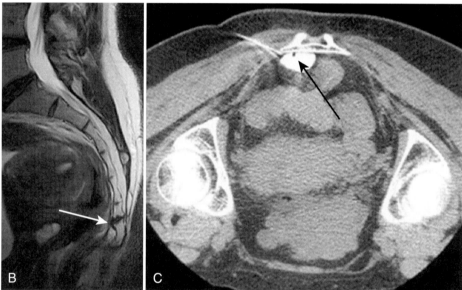

Fig. 103.5 **Anatomic location of the ganglion impar.** A, Ganglion impar represents the termination of the paravertebral sympathetic chains, converging at the sacrococcygeal level. B, Sagittal, T2-weighted magnetic resonance imaging shows the ganglion impar as a small, isointense signal structure anterior to the sacrococcygeal level *(white arrow)*. C, Contrast medium outlines the ganglion impar, seen as a filling defect *(black arrow)* in the pool of contrast. *(From Datir DC: CT-guided injection for ganglion impar blockade: a radiological approach to the management of coccydynia, Clin Radiol 65: 21A, 2010.)*

disengages the needle tip from the periosteum. When the needle is satisfactorily positioned, a syringe containing 5 mL of 1.0% preservative-free lidocaine and 40 mg of methylprednisolone is attached to the needle.

Gentle aspiration is carried out to identify cerebrospinal fluid or blood. If the aspiration test result is negative, the contents of the syringe are slowly injected. Resistance to injection should be minimal. Any significant pain or sudden increase in resistance during injection suggests incorrect needle placement, and the clinician should stop injecting immediately and reassess the position of the needle. The needle is then removed, and a sterile pressure dressing and ice pack are placed at the injection site. Occasionally, a ganglion impar block **(Fig.103.5)** may be used in patients who fail to respond to the foregoing injection technique.[8] In rare patients, surgical coccygectomy may be required to provide long-lasting pain relief.[9]

Conclusion

Coccydynia should be considered a diagnosis of exclusion in the absence of trauma to the coccyx and its ligaments. Failure to diagnose an underlying tumor can have disastrous consequences. As with all pelvic pain syndromes, careful evaluation of behavioral abnormalities that may be contributing to the patient's pain and functional disability should be considered.

References

Full references for this chapter can be found on www.expertconsult.com.

Chapter **104**

Proctalgia Fugax

Steven D. Waldman and Jennifer E. Waldman

Proctalgia fugax is a nonmalignant pain syndrome of unknown origin that is characterized by paroxysms of rectal pain with pain-free periods between attacks.[1] The pain-free periods between attacks can last seconds to minutes.[2] As in cluster headache, spontaneous remissions of the disease occur and may last from weeks to years. The pain of proctalgia fugax is localized to the anus and lower rectum.[3] Studies attempting to elucidate the pathologic mechanism responsible for the pain of proctalgia fugax implicated spasm of the levator ani muscles, anal sphincter, and sigmoid colon. Proctalgia fugax is more common in female patients, as well as in patients suffering from irritable bowel syndrome. The symptoms of proctalgia fugax are not typically present before puberty.

The pain of proctalgia fugax is sharp or gripping and is severe. As in other urogenital focal pain syndromes such as vulvodynia and prostadynia, the causes remain obscure.[1-3] Stressful life events often increase the frequency and intensity of attacks of proctalgia fugax, as does sitting for prolonged periods. However, a specific factor or activity does not typically trigger the exact onset of pain. Patients often feel an urge to defecate with the onset of the paroxysms of pain (**Fig. 104.1**). Depression frequently accompanies the pain of proctalgia fugax but is not thought to be the primary cause. The symptoms of proctalgia fugax can be severe enough to limit the patient's ability to carry out activities of daily living.

Clinical Presentation

Results of the physical examination of the patient suffering from proctalgia fugax are usually normal. The patient may be depressed or may appear anxious. Patients suffering from proctalgia fugax often exhibit perfectionistic, neurotic, and hypochondrial personality traits. Results of rectal examination are normal, although deep palpation of the surrounding musculature may trigger paroxysms of pain. Patients suffering from proctalgia fugax often report that they can abort the attack of pain by placing a finger in the rectum. Rectal suppositories may also interrupt the attacks.

Diagnosis

As with the physical examination, results of diagnostic tests in patients suffering from proctalgia fugax are usually within normal limits. Because of the risk of overlooking rectal malignant disease that may be responsible for pain that could be attributed to a benign cause, by necessity proctalgia fugax must be a diagnosis of exclusion[4,5] (**Fig. 104.2**). Rectal examination is mandatory in all patients thought to be suffering from proctalgia fugax. Sigmoidoscopy or colonoscopy is also strongly recommended in such patients. Hereditary forms of proctalgia fugax have been described and are associated with hypertrophy and hypertonia of the internal anal sphincter.[6]

Testing of the stool for occult blood is also indicated. Screening laboratory tests consisting of a complete blood cell count, automated blood chemistry studies, and erythrocyte sedimentation rate should also be performed. Magnetic resonance imaging or computed tomography of the pelvis should also be considered if the diagnosis is in doubt. If psychological problems are suspected, or if the patient has a history of sexual abuse, psychiatric evaluation should be included with laboratory and radiographic testing.[3]

Differential Diagnosis

As mentioned earlier, because of the risk of overlooking serious disease of the anus and rectum, proctalgia fugax must be a diagnosis of exclusion. First and foremost, the clinician must rule out rectal cancer, to avoid disaster. Proctitis can mimic the pain of proctalgia fugax and can be diagnosed on sigmoidoscopy or colonoscopy. Hemorrhoids usually manifest with bleeding associated with pain and can be distinguished from proctalgia fugax on physical examination. Prostadynia may sometimes be confused with proctalgia fugax, but the pain is more constant and is duller and aching.

Treatment

Several simple methods have proven effective for aborting the pain after the onset of a proctalgia fugax attack. For many patients, ingesting food or drink at the immediate onset of the

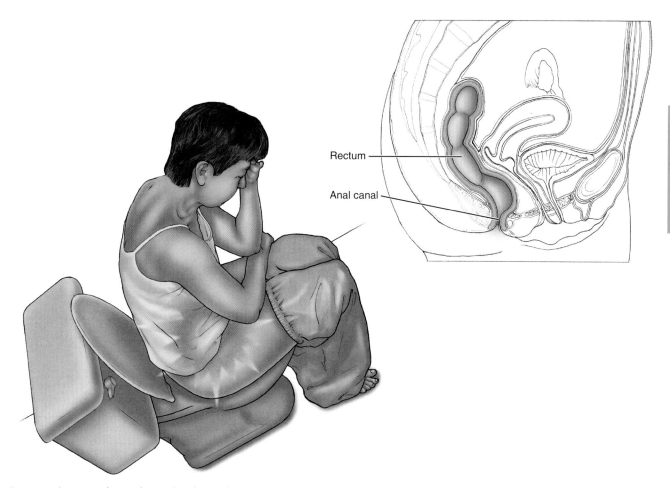

Rectum

Anal canal

Fig. 104.1 The onset of pain of proctalgia fugax often causes the patient to feel an urge to defecate. *(From Waldman SD:* Atlas of common pain syndromes, *Philadelphia, 2002, Saunders, p 177.)*

attack helps to stop the pain.[7] In addition, dilatation of the rectum either digitally or by inserting an enema or rectal suppository also aborts the pain. Patients may also find relief by attempting a bowel movement or by applying direct pressure to the perineum.

Initial treatment of proctalgia fugax should include a combination of simple analgesics and nonsteroidal anti-inflammatory agents or cyclooxygenase-2 inhibitors. If these medications do not adequately control the patient's symptoms, a tricyclic antidepressant or gabapentin should be added.

Traditionally, the tricyclic antidepressants have been a mainstay in the palliation of pain secondary to proctalgia fugax. Controlled studies have demonstrated the efficacy of amitriptyline for this indication. Other tricyclic antidepressants including nortriptyline and desipramine have also shown to be clinically useful. Unfortunately, this class of drugs is associated with significant anticholinergic side effects, including dry mouth, constipation, sedation, and urinary retention. These drugs should be used with caution in patients suffering from glaucoma, cardiac arrhythmia, and prostatism. To minimize side effects and to encourage compliance, the primary care physician should start amitriptyline or nortriptyline at a 10-mg dose at bedtime. The dose can be then titrated upward to 25 mg at bedtime as side effects allow. Upward titration of dosage in 25-mg increments can be carried out each week as side effects allow. Even at lower doses, patients generally report

rapid improvement in sleep disturbance and begin to experience some pain relief in 10 to 14 days.

The selective serotonin reuptake inhibitors such as fluoxetine have also been used to treat the pain of diabetic neuropathy. Although the selective serotonin reuptake inhibitors are better tolerated than the tricyclic antidepressants, they appear to be less efficacious for treatment of proctalgia fugax.

If the patient does not experience any improvement in pain as the dose is increased, the addition of gabapentin alone or in combination with pudendal nerve blocks using local anesthetics or corticosteroid is recommended. If the antidepressant compounds are ineffective or are contraindicated, gabapentin represents a reasonable alternative. Gabapentin should be started with a 300-mg dose at bedtime for 2 nights. The patient should be cautioned about potential side effects, including dizziness, sedation, confusion, and rash. The drug is then increased in 300-mg increments, given in equally divided doses over 2 days, as side effects allow, until pain relief is obtained or a total dose of 2400 mg daily is reached. At this point, if the patient has experienced partial relief of pain, blood values are measured, and the drug dose is carefully titrated upward using 100-mg tablets. Rarely is a dose larger than 3600 mg daily required.

The local application of heat and cold may be beneficial to provide symptomatic relief of the pain of proctalgia fugax. The use of bland rectal suppositories may also help to relieve symptoms. For patients who do not respond to these treatment

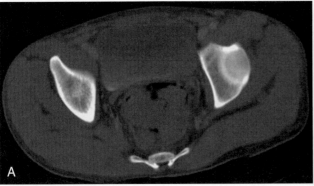

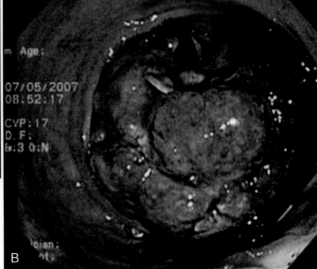

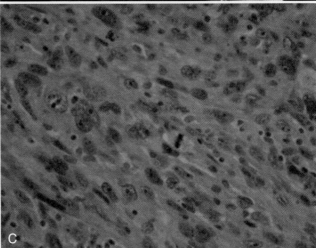

Fig. 104.2 **A,** This 19-year-old man with a 2-month history of lower abdominal pain and a 10-kg weight loss during the past year presented with difficulty in passing stool and blood in his stool for 2 days. Computed tomography of abdomen and pelvis, with and without contrast medium, showed a nonenhancing mass in the rectum, compatible with fecal impaction. **B,** A colonoscopy revealed a large, intraluminal, polypoid hard mass starting about 5 cm above the anal verge and extending upward about 12 cm. **C,** A biopsy taken of the mass showed a neoplastic rectal tumor. Histopathologic examination revealed infiltrative sheets of bizarre cells ulcerating the rectal mucosa. The tumor cells had epithelioid, oval, and spindled shapes, with pleomorphic nuclei, clumped chromatin, prominent nucleoli, and abnormal mitotic figures, admixed with a moderate inflammatory component (hematoxylin-eosin stain, original magnification ×400).

modalities, injection of the peroneal nerves or caudal epidural nerve block using local anesthetic and corticosteroid may be a reasonable next step.[7] The clinician should be aware that anecdotal reports have noted that the calcium channel blockers, topical nitroglycerin, and inhalation of albuterol will provide symptomatic relief of the pain of proctalgia fugax.

The major problem in the care of patients thought to suffer from proctalgia fugax is the failure to identify potentially serious disease of the anus or rectum related to primary tumor or invasion of these structures by pelvic tumor.[3,7] Although uncommon, occult rectal infection remains a possibility, especially in the immunocompromised patient with cancer (see Fig. 104.2). Early detection of infection is crucial to avoid potentially life-threatening sequelae. Given the psychological implications of pain involving the genitalia and rectum, the clinician should not overlook the possibility of psychological abnormality in patients with pain in the rectum. Both behavior modification and biofeedback can be used to treat proctalgia fugax related to a psychological abnormality. In patients whose symptoms occur infrequently, prevention of the attacks is difficult, if not impossible. For such patients, an understanding of the condition and reassurance by the physician can be very important.

References

Full references for this chapter can be found on www.expertconsult.com.

Part J

Pain Syndromes of the Hip and Proximal Lower Extremity

Chapter 105

Gluteal and Ischiogluteal Bursitis

Steven D. Waldman

Gluteal bursitis and ischiogluteal bursitis are among the myriad causes of buttock pain that are frequently misdiagnosed as primary hip disease. Frequently coexisting with tendinitis and sacroiliac joint pain, these painful types of bursitis require not only treatment of the acute symptom of pain and the decreased range of motion but also correction of the functional abnormalities that perpetuate the patient's symptoms.

Gluteal Bursitis

A patient suffering from gluteal bursitis frequently complains of pain at the upper outer quadrant of the buttock and with resisted abduction and extension of the lower extremity. The pain of gluteal bursitis, also known as *weaver's bottom,* is localized to the area over the upper outer quadrant of the buttock, with referred pain noted into the sciatic notch.[1] Often, the patient is unable to sleep on the affected hip and may complain of a sharp, catching sensation when extending and abducting the hip, especially on first awakening.

The gluteal bursae lie between the gluteus maximus and medius and minimus muscles as well as between these muscles and the underlying bone (**Fig. 105.1**). These bursae may exist as a single bursal sac or in some patients as a multisegmented series of sacs that may be loculated. The gluteal bursae are vulnerable to injury from both acute trauma and repeated microtrauma. The action of the gluteus maximus muscle includes the flexion of trunk on thigh when maintaining a sitting position, such as when riding a horse (**Fig. 105.2**). This action can irritate the gluteal bursae and can result in pain and inflammation. Acute injuries frequently take the form of direct trauma to the bursa from falls directly onto the buttocks or from repeated intramuscular injections, as well as from overuse such as running for long distances, especially on soft or uneven surfaces. If inflammation of the gluteal bursae becomes chronic, calcification of the bursae may occur.

Clinical Presentation

Physical examination of patients suffering from gluteal bursitis may reveal point tenderness in the upper outer quadrant of the buttocks. Passive flexion and adduction, as well as active resisted extension and abduction of the affected lower extremity, reproduce the pain. Sudden release of resistance during this maneuver markedly increases the pain.

Results of examination of the hip and the sacroiliac joint are within normal limits. Careful neurologic examination of the affected lower extremity should reveal no neurologic deficits. If neurologic deficits are present, evaluation for plexopathy, radiculopathy, or entrapment neuropathy should be undertaken.[2] These neurologic symptoms can coexist with gluteal bursitis and can thus confuse the clinical diagnosis.

Differential Diagnosis

Gluteal bursitis is often misdiagnosed as sciatica or is attributed to primary hip disease. Radiography of the hip and electromyography help to distinguish gluteal bursitis from radiculopathy emanating from the hip. Most patients suffering from lumbar radiculopathy have back pain associated with reflex, motor, and sensory changes associated with back pain, whereas patients with gluteal bursitis have only secondary back pain and no neurologic changes. Piriformis syndrome may sometimes be confused with gluteal bursitis but can be distinguished by the presence of motor and sensory changes involving the sciatic nerve.[3] These motor and sensory changes are limited to the distribution of the sciatic nerve below the sciatic notch. Lumbar radiculopathy and sciatic nerve entrapment may coexist as the *double-crush syndrome.* The pain of gluteal bursitis may cause alteration of gait that may result in secondary back and radicular symptoms and may coexist with this entrapment neuropathy.

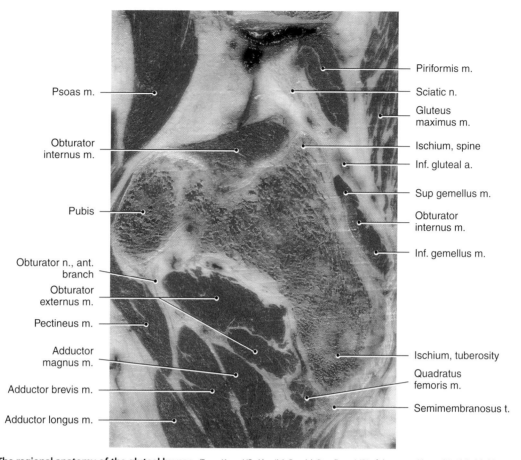

Psoas m.

Obturator
internus m.

Pubis

Obturator n., ant.
branch

Obturator
externus m.

Pectineus m.

Adductor
magnus m.

Adductor brevis m.

Adductor longus m.

Piriformis m.

Sciatic n.

Gluteus
maximus m.

Ischium, spine

Inf. gluteal a.

Sup gemellus m.

Obturator
internus m.

Inf. gemellus m.

Ischium, tuberosity

Quadratus
femoris m.

Semimembranosus t.

Fig. 105.1 **The regional anatomy of the gluteal bursae.** *(From Kang HS, Ahn JM, Resnick D, editors: MRI of the extremities, ed 2, Philadelphia, 2002, Saunders.)*

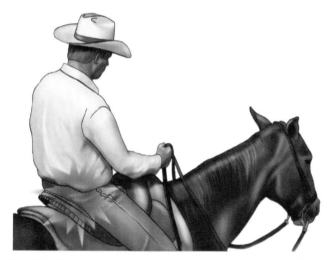

Fig. 105.2 The action of the gluteus maximus muscle includes the flexion of trunk on thigh when maintaining a sitting position, such as while riding a horse. This action can irritate the gluteal bursae and result in pain and inflammation. *(From Waldman SD: Gluteal bursitis. In Atlas of uncommon pain syndromes, ed 2, Philadelphia, 2008, Saunders, p 231.)*

Diagnosis

Plain radiographs of the hip may reveal calcification of the bursa and associated structures consistent with chronic inflammation. Magnetic resonance imaging (MRI) is indicated if occult

mass or tumor of the hip is suspected. Electromyography should be performed in patients with neurologic findings, to rule out plexopathy, radiculopathy, or nerve entrapment syndromes of the gluteal nerve or of the lower extremity nerves **(Fig. 105.3)**. Based on the patient's clinical presentation, additional testing including complete blood cell count, human leukocyte antigen-B27 (HLA-B27) testing, automated serum chemistry studies including uric acid, sedimentation rate, and antinuclear antibody testing may be indicated. The injection technique described later serves as both a diagnostic test and a therapeutic maneuver for patients suffering from gluteal bursitis.[4]

Treatment

Initial treatment of the pain and functional disability associated with gluteal bursitis should include a combination of nonsteroidal anti-inflammatory drugs (NSAIDs) or cyclooxygenase-2 (COX-2) inhibitors and physical therapy. The local application of heat and cold may also be beneficial. Repetitive movements that incite the syndrome should be avoided. For patients who do not respond to these treatment modalities, injection of the gluteal bursa with local anesthetic and corticosteroid may be a reasonable next step.

To inject the gluteal bursae, the patient is placed in the lateral position with the affected side upward and the affected leg flexed at the knee. Proper preparation with antiseptic solution of the skin overlying the upper outer quadrant of the buttocks is then performed. A syringe containing 4.0 mL of 0.25% preservative-free bupivacaine and 40 mg of methylprednisolone is attached to a 1.5-inch, 25-gauge needle. The point of maximal tenderness within the upper outer quadrant of the buttocks is then identified with a sterile-gloved finger. Before needle placement, the patient should be advised to say "there" immediately if he or she feels paresthesia into the lower extremity; this symptom indicates that the needle has impinged on the sciatic nerve. Should paresthesia occur, the needle should be immediately withdrawn and repositioned more medially. The needle is then carefully advanced perpendicular to the skin at the previously identified point until it impinges on the wing of the ilium (**Fig. 105.4**). Care must be taken to keep the needle in a medial position and not to advance it laterally, to avoid impinging on the sciatic nerve. After careful aspiration and if no paresthesia is present, the contents of the syringe are then gently injected into the bursa. Resistance to injection should be minimal.

Ischiogluteal Bursitis

The ischial bursa lies between the gluteus maximus muscle and the bone of the ischial tuberosity. This bursa may exist as a single bursal sac or in some patients may be a multisegmented series of sacs that may be loculated. The ischial bursa is vulnerable to injury from both acute trauma and repeated microtrauma. Acute injuries frequently take the form of direct trauma to the bursa from direct falls onto the buttocks and from overuse such as prolonged riding of horses or bicycles. Running on uneven or soft surfaces such as sand may also cause ischial bursitis (**Fig. 105.5**). If inflammation of the ischial bursa becomes chronic, bursal calcification may occur.

Clinical Presentation

A patient suffering from ischial bursitis frequently complains of pain at the base of the buttock during resisted extension of the lower extremity. The pain is localized to the area over the ischial tuberosity, with referred pain noted into the hamstring

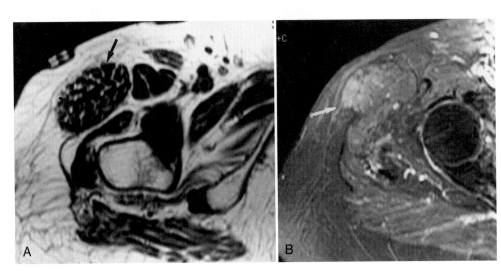

Fig. 105.3 Possible entrapment of the superior gluteal nerve. Note the denervation hypertrophy of the tensor fasciae latae muscle (*arrow*), as shown on a transverse T1-weighted (TR/TE, 416/14) spin-echo magnetic resonance imaging (MRI) scan (**A.**), and similar hypertrophy of and high signal intensity in this muscle (*arrow*) on a transverse fat-suppressed T1-weighted (TR/TE 500/14) spin-echo MRI scan obtained after intravenous administration of gadolinium (**B**). *(From Resnick D: Neuromuscular disorders. In Diagnosis of bone and joint disorders, ed 4, Philadelphia, 2002, Saunders, p 3351.)*

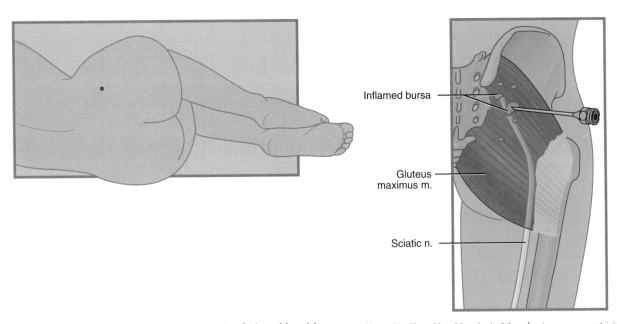

Fig. 105.4 **Injection technique for relieving the pain of gluteal bursitis.** *(From Waldman SD: Gluteal bursitis pain. In Atlas of pain management injection techniques, ed 2, Philadelphia, 2007, Saunders, p 351.)*

muscle, which may also develop coexistent tendinitis.[5] Often, the patient is unable to sleep on the affected hip and may complain of a sharp, catching sensation when extending and flexing the hip, especially on first awakening. Physical examination may reveal point tenderness over the ischial tuberosity. Passive straight-leg raising and active resisted extension of the affected lower extremity reproduce the pain. Sudden release of resistance during this maneuver markedly increases the pain.

Diagnosis

Plain radiographs of the hip may reveal calcification of the bursa and associated structures consistent with chronic inflammation. MRI is indicated if disruption of the hamstring musculotendinous unit is suspected. The injection technique described later serves as both a diagnostic test and a therapeutic maneuver and also treats hamstring tendinitis. Screening laboratory tests consisting of a complete blood cell count, erythrocyte sedimentation rate, and antinuclear antibody level are indicated if collagen vascular disease is suspected. Plain radiographs and radionuclide bone scanning are indicated in the presence of trauma or if tumor is a possibility.

Differential Diagnosis

Although the diagnosis of ischiogluteal bursitis is usually straightforward, this painful condition can occasionally be confused with sciatica, primary hip disease, insufficiency fractures of the pelvis, and tendinitis of the hamstrings. Tumors of the hip and pelvis may be overlooked and should be considered in the differential diagnosis of ischiogluteal bursitis.

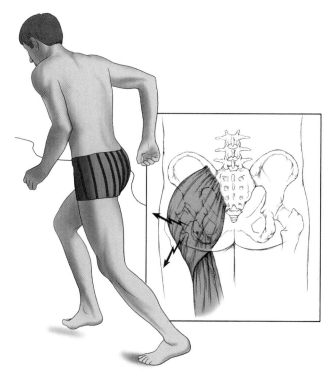

Fig. 105.5 Ischiogluteal bursitis is often perpetuated by running on soft, uneven surfaces, such as sand. *(From Waldman SD: Ischiogluteal bursitis. In* Atlas of common pain syndromes, *ed 2, Philadelphia, 2007, Saunders, p 258.)*

Treatment

Initial treatment of the pain and functional disability associated with ischiogluteal bursitis should include a combination of NSAIDs or COX-2 inhibitors and physical therapy. The local application of heat and cold may also be beneficial. Any repetitive activity that may exacerbate the patient's symptoms should be avoided. For patients who do not respond to these treatment modalities, the following injection technique may be a reasonable next step.[6]

To inject the ischiogluteal bursa, the patient is placed in the lateral position with the affected side upward and the affected leg flexed at the knee. Proper preparation with antiseptic solution of the skin overlying the ischial tuberosity is then performed. A syringe containing 4.0 mL of 0.25% preservative-free bupivacaine and 40 mg of methylprednisolone is attached to a 1.5-inch 25-gauge needle. The ischial tuberosity is then identified with a sterile-gloved finger. Before needle placement, the patient should be advised to say "there" immediately if he or she feels paresthesia into the lower extremity; this symptom indicates that the needle has impinged on the sciatic nerve. Should paresthesia occur, the needle should be immediately withdrawn and repositioned more medially. The needle is then carefully advanced at that point through the skin, subcutaneous tissues, muscle, and tendon until it impinges on the bone of the ischial tuberosity (**Fig. 105.6**). Care must be taken to keep the needle in the midline and not to advance it laterally, to avoid impinging on the sciatic nerve. After careful aspiration and if no paresthesia is present, the contents of the syringe are then gently injected into the bursa.

The proximity to the sciatic nerve makes it imperative that the injection procedure be carried out only by clinicians well versed in the regional anatomy and experienced in performing injection techniques. Many patients complain of a transient increase in pain after injection of the bursa and tendons. Patients should be warned that improvement will be limited if they continue the repetitive activities responsible for the evolution of the ischiogluteal bursitis.

Conclusion

Gluteal bursitis and ischiogluteal bursitis are among the myriad causes of buttock pain that are encountered in clinical practice. Frequently coexisting with tendinitis and sacroiliac joint pain, these painful types of bursitis require not only treatment of the acute symptoms of pain and the decreased range of motion but also correction of the functional abnormalities that perpetuate the patient's symptoms. The clinician should be sure to consider occult tumors of the hip joint, pelvis, and surrounding soft tissues when evaluating the patient with pain thought to have gluteal or ischiogluteal bursitis.

Although the treatment is the same, ischial bursitis can be distinguished from hamstring tendinitis by the following: ischial bursitis manifests with point tenderness over the ischial bursa, whereas the tenderness of hamstring bursitis is more diffuse over the upper muscle and tendons of the hamstring. The foregoing injection technique is extremely effective in the treatment of ischial bursitis

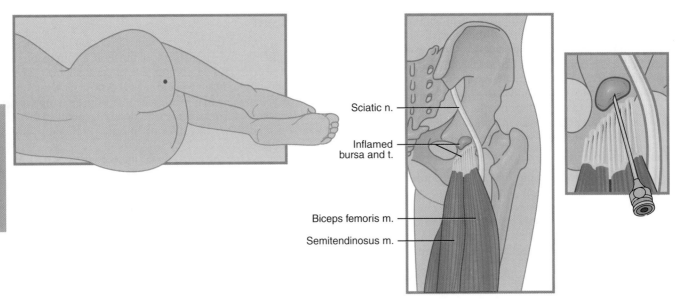

Fig. 105.6 **Injection technique for relieving the pain of ischial bursitis.** *(From Waldman SD: Ischial bursitis pain. In* Atlas of pain management injection techniques, *ed 2, Philadelphia, 2007, Saunders, p 247.)*

and hamstring tendinitis. This procedure is safe if careful attention is paid to the clinically relevant anatomy of the areas to be injected.

The use of physical modalities including local heat and gentle stretching exercises should be introduced several days after the patient undergoes this injection technique. Vigorous exercises should be avoided because they will exacerbate the patient's symptoms. Simple analgesics, NSAIDs, and antimyotonic agents such as tizanidine may be used concurrently with this injection technique.

References

Full references for this chapter can be found on www.expertconsult.com.

Trochanteric Bursitis

H. Michael Guo and Martin K. Childers

Trochanteric bursitis is a common painful condition caused by the irritation or inflammation of the trochanteric bursa. It is also known as the *greater trochanteric pain syndrome* (GTPS). This type of bursitis is mostly associated with repetitive microinjuries in the soft tissue and bursae around the greater trochanter (e.g., iliotibial band friction), but trauma (e.g., fall to the lateral hip) has also been implicated.[1] The incidence of trochanteric bursitis peaks between the fourth and sixth decades of life and has a female-to-male ratio of 4:1.[2,3] The difference is thought to result from female and male biomechanics.[4] The prevalence of patients with trochanteric bursitis referred to an orthopedic spine clinic was reported to be 20.2%, and the mean age was 54 years.[5] In the same study, 20% of patients referred for low back pain were found to have trochanteric bursitis, with higher incidences reported elsewhere.[2,6] Thus, trochanteric bursitis appears to be a relatively common condition among middle-aged or older women who are evaluated by specialists for the treatment of hip or low back pain.

Historical Considerations

Calcifications of the gluteal tendons associated with the trochanteric bursae were reported as early as 1930 by Nilsonne[7] and were generally considered to be caused by tuberculosis.[8] The condition was also thought to be acute rather than chronic until 1952, when Spear and Lipscomb[9] published a case series of 64 patients. In the late 1950s and early 1960s, several journal articles[8,10–13] challenged the traditional notion that trochanteric bursitis was an acute, rare condition[14] and instead indicated that the condition was a discrete, and often chronic, clinical entity. However, as Anderson pointed out in 1957,[8] trochanteric bursitis is a complex diagnosis usually associated with other disorders.

Etiology

Historically, the general assumption regarding the origin of trochanteric bursitis involves one or more of three relatively constant bursae associated with the greater trochanter: two major bursae (subgluteus maximus and subgluteus medius) and one minor bursa (gluteus minimus) (**Fig. 106.1**).[2,15] Whether disease of one or more trochanteric bursae directly results in trochanteric bursitis is not entirely clear. During hip replacement surgery in a patient with hip pain and osteoarthritis, the trochanteric bursa was reported to be enlarged and contained calcium pyrophosphate dihydrate (CPPD) crystals.[16] However, prospective data from magnetic resonance imaging (MRI) and physical findings in patients with chronic lateral hip pain indicate that fluid distention of the trochanteric bursae is uncommon,[17] whereas gluteus medius tendon disease appears to be much more common. Nevertheless, tendon disease and bursae distention are not mutually exclusive because one report[18] noted that both tendinopathy and partial tears of the gluteus medius occurred in the presence of bursae fluid distention. In a series of 250 MRI studies of the hip, Kingzett-Taylor et al[19] reported that 14 of 35 patients with gluteal tendon disease also had discrete fluid collections within the trochanteric bursae. Indeed, in 1961, Gordon[11] proposed that the primary lesion in trochanteric bursitis was injury to the gluteal tendons at their insertion onto the greater trochanter and that the adjacent bursae were damaged as a consequence. Thus, trochanteric bursitis is probably caused by gluteal tendinitis in a manner analogous to that of shoulder joint bursitis and rotator cuff tendinitis. Accordingly, Walsh and Archibald[18] have urged prompt review of the tendon insertions for signs of tendinopathy and tears when MRI findings demonstrate gluteus medius and minimus atrophy and fatty replacement in patients with chronic lateral hip pain.

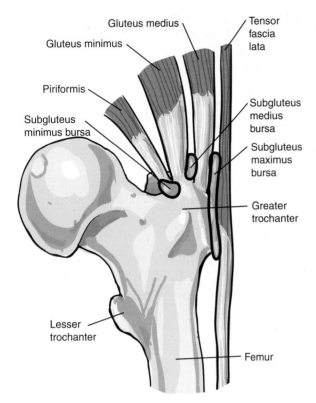

Fig. 106.1 **The bursae associated with the greater trochanter.**

Clinical Presentation

Patients with trochanteric bursitis generally present with chronic intermittent aching pain over the lateral aspect of the affected hip.[5,8,10] Pain is worsened by hip abduction or external rotation, prolonged lower extremity weight bearing, sitting in a deep chair or car seat,[20] bicycling, golfing, climbing stairs,[17] or lying on the affected side.[21] The condition also occurs as a result of a running injury, most commonly in female athletes with a wide pelvis[22] or a cavus foot.[23] In contrast, in patients with hip osteoarthritis, pain is usually relieved by sitting.[24] Clinical criteria for trochanteric bursitis have been proposed,[8,25,26] and they include the first and second and at least one of the remaining findings: (1) history of lateral aching hip pain; (2) localized tenderness over the greater trochanter; (3) radiation of pain over the lateral thigh; (4) pain of resisted hip abduction; and (5) pain at extreme ends of rotation, particularly a positive Patrick (FABER) test result.

Occasionally, pain may extend from the hip to include the lateral thigh[11] and may radiate down the leg to the level of the insertion of the iliotibial tract on the proximal tibia,[18] with associated paresthesia[6] that does not follow a dermatomal pattern. In fact, Ege and Fano[25] included "pseudoradiculopathy" as an inclusion criterion for trochanteric bursitis. Groin pain was reported in 10% of patients with trochanteric bursitis who presented to a Dutch rheumatology clinic.[27] Indeed, the finding that patients complain of pain in areas of the body at sites far removed from the hip is one of the more fascinating aspects of trochanteric bursitis.

Diagnosis

Physical Examination

The examiner should try to localize the patient's usual hip pain by performing careful palpation of the hip area followed by active and passive range-of-motion testing. Trochanteric

bursitis is one cause of hip pain that Roberts and Williams[28] categorized into one of three areas: (1) anterior groin pain, (2) posterior buttock pain, or (3) lateral trochanteric pain. Anterior groin pain should alert the clinician of the likelihood of an intra-articular cause, such as a septic joint or fracture. The most consistent physical finding in patients with trochanteric bursitis is localized tenderness over the greater trochanter, usually on the posterosuperior aspect over the tendinous insertion of the gluteus medius.[8,10] With the patient in the lateral decubitus position with the painful hip facing the examiner, the clinician should palpate the hip with one fingertip in a caudal to cephalad direction, from below the greater trochanteric eminence to the area of maximal tenderness.[2] While the patient is still in the lateral decubitus position, the examiner can typically reproduce the patient's usual lateral hip pain by resistive active hip abduction and external rotation. The examiner should also check for hip pain on active resisted hip extension and flexion, because this maneuver should not elicit pain in patients with trochanteric bursitis but rather indicates intra-articular hip disease.[2,26]

On observation of gait, a "gluteal limp" is frequently present.[13] Disease (tears or inflammation) of the gluteus medius tendon results in a positive Trendelenburg sign (upward movement of the pelvis on the weight-bearing side while the pelvis moves downward on the non–weight-bearing side during gait) and is a more accurate predictor of tendon disease (assessed with MRI) as compared with two other physical signs (pain elicited by resisted hip abduction or pain in response to internal rotation).[17] Leg-length discrepancy may be assessed by visual inspection of the height of the iliac crests or by comparing the side-to-side difference between the distance from the anterior superior iliac spine to the medial malleolus. However, standing plain radiographs of the pelvis to determine differences in leg length are considered more accurate than clinical measurements.[28]

Testing

The diagnosis of trochanteric bursitis is based on clinical evidence. No radiographic findings are necessarily diagnostic, although imaging studies may help to distinguish trochanteric bursitis from an intra-articular cause of hip pain. Gordon[11] reported calcifications of the tendons associated with the greater trochanter in 40% of patients with trochanteric bursitis, but these data may have reflected tuberculous involvement of the bursa, a diagnosis rarely seen today.[29] Such calcifications may be identified in radiographic images of the hip as linear or small, rounded masses of varying size.[2] After hip arthroplasty, some patients may develop bursitis within communicating cavities or "psuedobursae."[30] For these patients, arthrography may be useful to distinguish pain from causes other than loosening and infection.

Plain radiographs may help to distinguish rare causes of trochanteric bursitis. For example, few (1% to 3%) of patients with tuberculosis have skeletal involvement.[31] Moreover, patients with tuberculosis rarely present with trochanteric bursitis. Nonetheless, tuberculous involvement of the greater trochanter bursa or its associated tendons may be identified based on imaging features, with a pattern of tendon tethering suggestive of tuberculosis. For instance, in a case series of patients with tuberculous tenosynovitis and bursitis, Jaovisidha et al[31] found soft tissue swelling on plain radiographs with calcification in 3 of 9 cases. When the tendon sheath was replaced by vascular tuberculous granulation tissue, high signal intensity was observed in T2-weighted MRI scans. In 6 of 12 cases of tuberculous tenosynovitis, pulmonary tuberculosis was evident on plain chest radiographs.

More advanced imaging methods, such as MRI, computed tomography, or bone scans, have characteristic features of trochanteric bursitis and have also been used to rule out other causes of lateral hip pain. MRI may demonstrate fluid distention of the trochanteric bursae and associated gluteus medius tendon disease[18] represented by high signal intensity on short-echo time-inversion recovery sequences in the greater trochanteric region.[2] Ultrasound also detects this type of bursa fluid distention and enlargement.[32] MRI may demonstrate gluteus medius and minimus atrophy with fatty replacement. Radioisotope bone scanning may demonstrate a characteristic linear uptake[29] in the lateral aspect of the greater trochanter generally seen in the early blood-pooling phase and on delayed images.[2]

Differential Diagnosis

Tendinopathy of the gluteal tendons is thought to be responsible for trochanteric bursitis, but the pathogenesis of trochanteric bursitis is unclear and is probably multifactorial. Numerous common musculoskeletal conditions have been reported in association with trochanteric bursitis, including leg-length discrepancy, cavus foot,[23] mechanical low back pain, hip osteoarthritis,[33] gluteal tendinitis, and lumbar radiculopathy,[34] but a cause-and-effect relationship between any of these conditions and trochanteric bursitis has not been definitively established. Infection of the bursae can occur,[35] although reports in the literature are infrequent. In a series of 100 patients with rheumatoid arthritis, 15 patients were found to have trochanteric bursitis, a finding suggesting a casual association.[34] Biomechanical alteration in gait and associated forces may predispose some patients to trochanteric bursitis.[19] Gordon[11] postulated that a strain of the hip results in a slight tear in the relatively avascular tendon of the gluteus medius or minimus muscle with subsequent hemorrhage, local necrosis, and organization of scar tissue and tendon calcification. The cause of injury to the gluteal tendons may originate from iliotibial band friction on the tendons and their respective bursae.[19]

The differential diagnosis of trochanteric bursitis is listed in **Table 106.1**. Common conditions associated with trochanteric bursitis include degenerative processes of the hip and spine. For this reason, patients may initially present with low back pain. Symptoms of trochanteric bursitis may be confused with those of lumbosacral strain, osteoarthritis of the hip, or herniated lumbar disk.[11] Because of the overlap of the iliotibial tract and the lumbar dermatomes, back and associated lower limb pain can mimic lumbar radiculopathy.[5,36] Collee et al[6,27] diagnosed trochanteric bursitis in 35 of 100 consecutive patients who presented to a rheumatology clinic with a primary complaint of low back pain. Distinguishing trochanteric bursitis from lumbar radiculopathy requires a careful history and physical examination, in which pain and tenderness are most often elicited in the hip rather than in the back.

Treatment

Reported benefits of treatment for trochanteric bursitis are myriad, but few treatment protocols have been rigorously tested using scientific methods. A series of "deep x-ray therapy" was recommended in the 1950s,[37] but it is no longer

Table 106.1 Differential Diagnosis of Trochanteric Bursitis

Iliotibial band syndrome
Lumbosacral strain
Osteoarthritis of the hip
Lumbar radiculopathy
Septic joint
Hip fracture
Avascular necrosis of the femur head
Synovitis
Lumbar facet syndrome
Iliohypogastric nerve entrapment
Tuberculosis with skeletal involvement
Neoplasms

Table 106.2 Treatment of Trochanteric Bursitis

CONSERVATIVE TREATMENT

Rest
Ice or heat
Nonsteroidal anti-inflammatory drugs
Bisphosphonates
Local corticosteroid injection
Miscellaneous modalities (e.g., ultrasound, shock wave, iontophoresis)

SURGERY

Release of iliotibial band
Removal of trochanteric osteophytes
Débridement of gluteus maximus bursae

suggested. In 1959, Krout and Anderson[12] reported that short-wave diathermy applied to the trochanteric and low back region was effective in 41 of 50 cases. Furia et al[38] reported that shock wave therapy was an effective treatment for GTPS, and the treatment group had significant visual analog score reductions.

Table 106.2 lists the routine treatment regimen consisting of rest, ice or heat, nonsteroidal anti-inflammatory drugs (NSAIDs), and local injection of a corticosteroid[20] such as methylprednisolone (40 to 80 mg) or triamcinolone hexacetonide (20 to 40 mg) or mixtures of betamethasone sodium phosphate and betamethasone acetate suspension with 1% lidocaine.[25,26] Ultrasound or fluoroscopic guidance may increase the precision of needle placement.[14,39,40] Clinical evidence supports the use of corticosteroids in trochanteric bursitis. A favorable dose-response relationship with betamethasone was reported in a series of 75 patients with trochanteric bursitis.[26] As early as 1958, Leonard[13] reported that local injection of hydrocortisone acetate resulted in "complete relief of symptoms in all instances." Gordon's 1961 description[11] outlined the process of local injection for trochanteric bursitis: "The most successful method of treatment was local infiltration and needling of the bursa, selecting the point of maximum tenderness behind or above the greater trochanter as the point of entry.... The tip of the needle was directed against the posterosuperior point of the greater trochanter, and then the solution infiltrated in fan-like fashion adjacent to and above the trochanter."

Conservative treatment that decreases forces placed on the painful hip is generally thought to be helpful in trochanteric bursitis. Use of a cane that is held in the hand on the side opposite the painful hip reduces forces placed on the affected side equivalent to one half of the body weight.[41] Correction of leg-length discrepancy with a shoe lift may similarly work to relieve pain.[20] In support of this idea, Swezey[36] noted an association between hip disease and leg-length discrepancies in a group of older patients with trochanteric bursitis. Swezey speculated that gait alterations resulting from back pain or prolonged bed rest could predispose patients to trochanteric bursitis. Alternatively, active exercise is considered to be the cornerstone of treatment for friction-induced bursitis in athletes. Increased flexibility and symmetrical strengthening of the muscle involved in adjacent joint motion are thought to improve faulty joint mechanics that may induce excessive tension over the greater trochanter.[42] Exercises that stretch the external rotators of the hip and the iliotibial band were suggested to prevent recurrences of trochanteric bursitis in young adults.[36] Alternative therapies proposed for trochanteric bursitis include identification and injections of fibrofatty nodules with corticosteroid and lidocaine.[43]

NSAIDs and acetaminophen have also been reported to be effective for trochanteric bursitis. Monteforte et al[44] compared pain relief obtained with the use of paracetamol (known as acetaminophen in the United States) (a 500-mg oral dose twice daily for 15 days, followed by 500 mg daily for 15 days) with pain relief obtained with the bisphosphonate disodium clodronate (100-mg daily intramuscular injection for 30 days) in an open-label comparison trial of 10 patients with trochanteric bursitis who were previously unresponsive to conservative treatment. Patients treated with the bisphosphonate demonstrated better pain relief compared with those in the paracetamol-treated group, a finding suggesting that an increase in bone turnover may be implicated in the pathogenesis of trochanteric bursitis.

In refractory cases, surgical release of tight fascia has been reported.[11,20,45,46] In seven athletes with chronic disabling hip pain caused by a snapping iliotibial band and secondary trochanteric bursitis, partial excision of the iliotibial band with excision of the trochanteric bursa resulted in long-term pain relief and a return to athletic acitivity.[44] Arthroscopy has been used for treating refractory trochanteric bursitis, and arthroscopic procedures have included bursectomy and iliotibial band release.[47,48]

Complications and Pitfalls

Fatal necrotizing fasciitis in a non–insulin-dependent diabetic man was reported as a complication of a single corticosteroid injection of the greater trochanteric bursa.[49] Accordingly, the clinician should be wary of performing similar procedures in patients with diabetes or any other condition that could predispose them to infection from a corticosteroid injection. Because other syndromes including entrapment neuropathies, radiculopathies, and lumbar facet syndromes can mimic trochanteric bursitis, the astute clinician should carefully consider the differential diagnoses. Entrapment neuropathy of the iliohypogastric nerve can mimic the lateral thigh pain that is commonly observed in trochanteric bursitis. Perineural injection with local anesthetic over the superior margin of the ilium where the terminal branches of the iliohypogastric nerve cross the iliac crest should confirm the diagnosis.[50] For patients with a presumptive diagnosis of trochanteric bursitis but who do not respond to local peritrochanteric injection of corticosteroid and local anesthetic, selective neural blockade may help to determine the underlying cause. Electromyography or transforaminal nerve root blocks may identify lumbar radiculopathy. Lumbar facet blockade may elucidate lumbar facet syndrome as the cause of lateral hip pain.

Conclusion

Trochanteric bursitis, also known as GTPS, is a common cause of lateral hip pain in middle-aged or older women. This condition is readily diagnosed by finding localized tenderness over the greater trochanter, with radiation of pain over the lateral thigh and increased pain with resistive hip abduction and external rotation. The differential diagnosis includes tendinopathy of the gluteal muscles, degenerative processes of the hip and spine, lumbosacral strain, herniated lumbar disk, and, rarely, tuberculosis or infection. Treatment of this condition usually consists of rest, ice, heat, and local corticosteroid injection into the most tender area around the greater trochanter, although double-blind placebo-controlled trials have yet to demonstrate the efficacy of a particular treatment paradigm.

References

Full references for this chapter can be found on www.expertconsult.com.

Iliopsoas Bursitis

Robert Trout

Historical Considerations

Although it is often overlooked in the standard evaluation of hip pain, the iliopsoas bursa is the largest in the body and measures up to 7 cm in length (**Fig. 107.1**).[1] Also known as the iliopectineal or iliofemoral bursa, this bursa has been studied as a source of hip pain since 1834, when Fricke[2] described painful bursitis in a case report. In 1917, a distended bursa was identified with arthrography by Kummer and De Senarclens,[3] and for many years arthrography remained the only helpful imaging study for diagnosis until the advent of computed tomography (CT) and magnetic resonance imaging (MRI) scanning.

In 1967, Melamad et al[4] described the following clinical triad for iliopsoas bursitis: a mass in the inguinal region, the effects of pressure on other structures nearby, and osteoarthritis of the hip as visualized on radiographs. This triad has become less relevant because patients with only the most significant symptoms present with such findings. Along with better imaging techniques, greater emphasis has been placed on earlier conservative treatment that can help to prevent these symptoms from occurring.

Signs and Symptoms

Two types of patients present with iliopsoas bursitis. First, this disorder most commonly occurs in older individuals who have some type of underlying hip disease, such as degenerative or rheumatoid arthritis. Investigators have theorized that increased intra-articular pressure causes the bursa to act as a reservoir for fluid that leaks through the anterior joint capsule, similar to the formation of Baker's cyst in the knee.[5,6] Eventually, the bursa becomes distended and inflamed. Because these patients are likely to exhibit physical signs and radiographic findings of other types of articular problems, a thorough hip examination is essential to differentiate between pain from bursitis and pain related to arthritis or other bony disease.

The second category of patient is younger and has completely normal radiographs. These patients are often athletes who perform repetitive or forceful flexion and extension of the hip. They are at risk for developing bursitis as a result of the friction of the iliopsoas tendon that overlies it because the purpose of this bursa is to reduce the friction between the tendon and the hip capsule. Thus, for a patient who presents with persistent hip pain and normal hip films, iliopsoas bursitis should remain near the top of a differential diagnosis list.

Patients present with pain in the inguinal or hip regions, and this the pain often radiates to the anterior thigh. Aggravating activities include walking up stairs, putting on shoes and socks, and moving from a sitting to a standing position. Some patients may also describe abdominal pain. Although not as common, edema in the lower extremity or numbness may occur if the bursa is large enough to compress the femoral vein or nerve.

Gait should be observed because a common initial finding is a shortened stride length when the patient attempts to minimize flexion and extension of the hip. A mass in the area of the inguinal ligament may be palpable and is sometimes mistaken for a hernia, a lymph node, or even an aneurysm. The mass may be pulsatile because of its proximity to the femoral artery.[7] Pain can be reproduced by placing the hip in flexion, abduction, and external rotation and then moving it into extension (**Fig. 107.2**).[8] A palpable or audible snap may occur as the bursa passes underneath the tendon; thus, this disorder is sometimes called *snapping hip syndrome* or *iliotibial band syndrome.*

The Thomas test is helpful to evaluate for tight hip flexors. The patient lies supine and fully flexes one knee and hip. If the contralateral hip rises off the examination table, then a contracture is present.

Testing

Initial testing with plain radiographs of the hip often demonstrates intra-articular disease such as degenerative change, effusion, or calcification. The diagnostic yield for this specific disorder is limited, however, because plain radiographs do not show an inflamed bursa unless calcification of the bursa occurs.

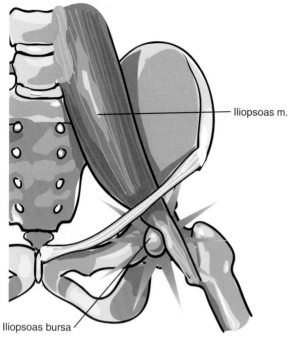

Fig. 107.1 **Iliopsoas bursa, also known as the iliopectineal or iliofemoral bursa.**

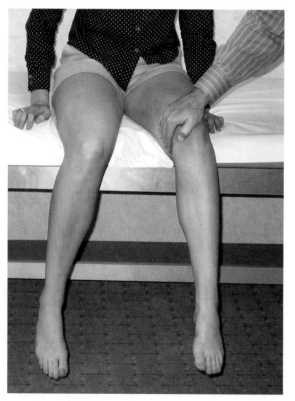

Fig. 107.2 **Resisted hip adduction test for iliopsoas bursitis.**
(From Waldman SD: Physical diagnosis in pain: an atlas of signs and symptoms, *Philadelphia, 2005, Saunders, p 313.)*

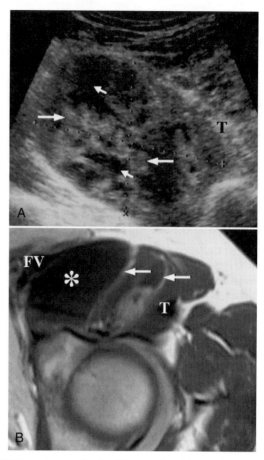

Fig. 107.3 **Imaging studies for iliopsoas bursitis. A,** Ultrasound. *Small arrows,* fluid-filled bursa; *large arrows,* loculations; T, inguinal ligament. **B,** Magnetic resonance imaging. *Asterisk,* fluid-filled bursa; *arrows,* loculations; FV, femoral vessel; T, inguinal ligament.

vessels), arthrography has become essentially obsolete for this purpose.

Ultrasound is fast and noninvasive, and it has the advantage of ruling out other possible causes of a palpable inguinal mass, including hernia and aneurysm. In patients with bursitis, ultrasound studies show a well-defined mass between the anterior hip capsule and the iliopsoas muscle (**Fig. 107.3A**), although ultrasound has often been found to underestimate the size of the mass. CT scan also demonstrates an encapsulated mass that has a water density and, if present, a communication with the hip joint. Surrounding structures are well visualized, and displacement of the femoral vessels may be observed. MRI is the most sensitive and accurate test in evaluating the characteristics of the bursa such as its size and shape and its relation to the adjacent soft tissues and structures (see **Fig. 107.3B**).[8] MRI is also valuable in ruling out other potential causes of hip pain such as avascular necrosis or stress fracture.

Differential Diagnosis

The differential diagnosis includes both intra-articular and extra-articular causes of pain around the hip joint (**Table 107.1**). Differentiating bursitis from osteoarthritis of the hip may be difficult because many patients have arthritic hip changes visible on plain films. The pain of osteoarthritis

For many years, arthrography was the only available means to diagnose a distended iliopsoas bursa, which would fill with contrast material if the bursa communicated with the hip joint. However, because of its invasiveness and its inability to visualize other nearby structures (e.g., the femoral

Table 107.1 Differential Diagnosis of Iliopsoas Bursitis

Osteoarthritis

Rheumatoid arthritis

Avascular necrosis

Femoral stress fracture

Osteitis pubis

Pelvic abscess or hematoma

Lymphadenopathy or aneurysm

Metastatic disease

Radiculopathy

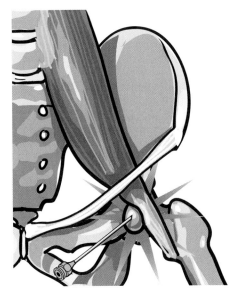

Fig. 107.4 **Injection technique for iliopsoas bursitis.**

typically occurs during standing and weight bearing, and these patients more often demonstrate a Trendelenburg gait in which they lean toward the affected side during the stance phase. On examination, range of motion (ROM) is reduced by pain when these patients internally or externally rotate the hip.

Avascular necrosis should also remain in the differential diagnosis for patients with significant hip or groin pain, particularly if they have a history of steroid use. These patients also report worsened pain with weight bearing and have a significantly antalgic gait, to avoid placing any weight on the hip joint. Avascular necrosis can be excluded by a bone scan or MRI.

For athletes, primarily long-distance runners, femoral neck stress fracture causes an aching pain in the groin or thigh that is exacerbated by activity and improved with rest. ROM is reduced and painful. Radiographs may show callus formation or an actual fracture line, but early results may be negative. If such a fracture is suspected clinically, a bone scan should be performed because it is sensitive within 2 to 8 days of the injury.

Osteitis pubis, or inflammation of the pubic bone, is another condition seen in athletes who perform repetitive side-to-side motions, such as in hockey or soccer. This disorder is also common in pregnant women because of the instability of the pubic symphysis. These patients report pain in the groin or thigh areas, but the pain is most tender at the pubic symphysis. Radiographs show resorption or sclerosis of the pubic bones, but results may be negative initially. A bone scan may also be needed for an early diagnosis.

Radicular pain may manifest with symptoms similar to those of bursitis, with pain extending into the anterior thigh. The mass effect of an enlarged bursa on the femoral nerve may cause numbness or paresthesias. Usually, the clinician can distinguish between the two conditions by means of adequate hip and lumbar physical examinations; however, electrodiagnostic studies may be helpful if the diagnosis is unclear.

For the patient who presents with a palpable inguinal mass, the other possibilities include hernia, aneurysm, and lymphadenopathy. Although these other diagnoses may also produce pain, the pain is usually not clearly related specifically to hip flexion and extension, and the patient should otherwise have a normal hip examination. Ultrasound is a good first-line test in this situation when one of these other causes is suspected.

Treatment

Initial treatment for most cases of iliopsoas bursitis is conservative and includes relative rest and avoidance of aggravating activities, anti-inflammatory medications, and physical therapy for localized hip flexor stretching. Johnston and Wiley[9] also advocated a hip rotation strengthening program, with good results, to correct subtle muscle imbalances that may lead to the problem over time.

Corticosteroid injection to the bursa is often quite helpful for rapid relief of pain symptoms. A solution of 40 mg methylprednisolone is diluted in 0.25% bupivacaine or similar equivalent in a syringe attached to a 3.5-inch, 25-gauge needle. The patient is placed in the supine position, and the femoral artery pulse is palpated. The needle is placed at a point 2.5 inches below and 3.5 inches lateral to the femoral pulse. It is then advanced superiorly at a 45-degree angle (**Fig. 107.4**). The patient should be advised to tell the clinician if he or she feels paresthesia into the thigh on advancement of the needle; this is a sign that the needle has impinged on the femoral nerve. If no paresthesia occurs, the needle is advanced slowly until it hits bone and then is withdrawn slightly. After initial aspiration, the medication is injected into the bursa with very little resistance.[10] For patients with a significantly distended bursa or if infection is suspected, an empty syringe may be used first to aspirate the excess synovial fluid from the sac. Obviously, if the fluid appears cloudy or infected, the corticosteroid is not injected. If the clinician has difficulty in aspirating a palpable bursa, a CT scan or ultrasound-guided procedure may be performed.

Although most patients respond very well to a regimen of medications, injections, and therapy, those with recalcitrant cases may still require surgical treatment. This treatment usually consists of bursectomy with possible release of the iliopsoas tendon, and it has a good outcome rate.

Complications and Pitfalls

The most common pitfall of this process is a delay in making the proper diagnosis. Often, the condition is mistaken for osteoarthritis or radicular pain. Iliopsoas bursitis should always be considered in patients with persistent hip pain who have negative radiographic results and an unremarkable lumbar examination.

Patients commonly experience soreness or increased pain for 1 to 2 days after an injection to the bursa, but major complications are rare with proper technique. The most serious complication is abscess or hematoma formation, and it manifests with progressively worsening hip or flank pain, guarding of hip movements, and possibly fever. Weakness occurs when the lumbosacral plexus is compressed. If these symptoms occur after injection, a pelvic CT scan should be obtained immediately. To reduce this risk, patients should be asked about clotting disorders, immune dysfunction, or use of anticoagulants before any injection.

Conclusion

Iliopsoas bursitis is an often overlooked cause of hip pain that occurs in older patients with other underlying hip disease and in young athletes. The diagnosis is usually made clinically, with point tenderness in the iliopsoas tendon and reproduction of pain during flexion and extension of the hip. When further information is needed, a CT scan, ultrasound scan, or MRI scan may demonstrate the presence of a distended bursa and rule out other potential causes of hip pain. Patients typically respond well to conservative treatment and a well-placed injection, although surgery is a possible option for patients with severe or persistent cases.

References

Full references for this chapter can be found on www.expertconsult.com.

Meralgia Paresthetica

Steven D. Waldman

Meralgia paresthetica is caused by compression of the lateral femoral cutaneous nerve by the inguinal ligament as it passes through or under the inguinal ligament.[1,2] This entrapment neuropathy manifests as pain, numbness, and dysesthesias in the distribution of the lateral femoral cutaneous nerve.[3] These symptoms often begin as a burning pain in the lateral thigh with associated cutaneous sensitivity. Patients suffering from meralgia paresthetica note that sitting, squatting, and wearing wide belts or low-rider trousers that compress the lateral femoral cutaneous nerve cause their symptoms to worsen (**Figs. 108.1 to 108.3**).[1,4,5] Weight gain and weight loss, as well as pregnancy, have also been implicated as inciting events for meralgia paresthetica.[6,7] Although traumatic lesions to the lateral femoral cutaneous nerve have been implicated in the onset of meralgia paresthetica, no obvious antecedent trauma can be identified in most patients.[8–10]

Clinical Presentation

Physical findings include tenderness over the lateral femoral cutaneous nerve at the origin of the inguinal ligament at the anterior superior iliac spine.[2] A positive Tinel sign over the lateral femoral cutaneous nerve as it passes beneath the inguinal ligament may be present[11] (**Fig. 108.4**). Careful sensory examination of the lateral thigh reveals a sensory deficit in the distribution of the lateral femoral cutaneous nerve. A burning thigh sign may be present[12] (**Fig. 108.5**). No motor deficit should be evident. Sitting or the wearing of tight waistbands or wide belts or low-rider trousers that compress the lateral femoral cutaneous nerve may exacerbate the symptoms of meralgia paresthetica.

Diagnosis

Electromyography helps to distinguish lumbar radiculopathy and diabetic femoral neuropathy from meralgia paresthetica. Plain radiographs of the back, hip, and pelvis are indicated in all patients who present with meralgia paresthetica, to rule out occult bony disease. Based on the patient's clinical presentation, additional testing including complete blood cell count, uric acid, sedimentation rate, and antinuclear antibody

testing may be indicated. Magnetic resonance imaging (MRI) of the back is indicated if herniated disk, spinal stenosis, or a space-occupying lesion is suspected. The injection technique described later serves as both a diagnostic test and a therapeutic maneuver.

Differential Diagnosis

Meralgia paresthetica is often misdiagnosed as lumbar radiculopathy or trochanteric bursitis or is attributed to primary hip disease.[13,14] Radiography of the hip and electromyography help to distinguish meralgia paresthetica from radiculopathy or pain emanating from the hip. Most patients suffering from lumbar radiculopathy have back pain associated with reflex, motor, and sensory changes accompanied by neck pain, whereas patients with meralgia paresthetica have no back pain and no motor or reflex changes. The sensory changes of meralgia paresthetica are limited to the distribution of the lateral femoral cutaneous nerve and should not extend below the knee (see Fig. 108.4). Lumbar radiculopathy and lateral femoral cutaneous nerve entrapment may coexist as the *double-crush syndrome*. Occasionally, diabetic femoral neuropathy may produce anterior thigh pain that may confuse the diagnosis.

Treatment

The patient suffering from meralgia paresthetica should be instructed in avoidance techniques to help reduce the unpleasant symptoms and pain associated with this entrapment neuropathy. A short course of conservative therapy consisting of simple analgesics, nonsteroidal anti-inflammatory agents, or cyclooxygenase-2 inhibitors is a reasonable first step in the treatment of patients suffering from meralgia paresthetica.[1,2] If the patient does not experience rapid improvement, the following injection technique is a reasonable next step.[15,16]

To treat the pain of meralgia paresthetica, the patient is placed in the supine position with a pillow under the knees. Lying with the legs extended increases the patient's pain because of traction on the nerve. The anterior superior iliac spine is identified by palpation. A point 1 inch medial to the

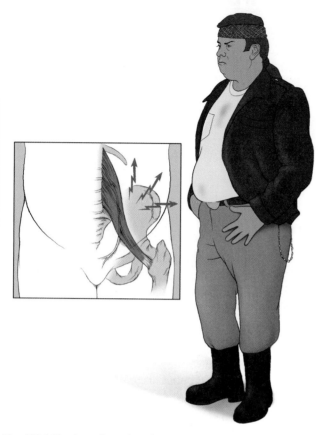

Fig. 108.1 Obesity and wearing of wide belts may cause compression of the lateral femoral cutaneous nerve and result in meralgia paresthetica. *(From Waldman SD: Atlas of common pain syndromes, Philadelphia, 2002, Saunders, p 235.)*

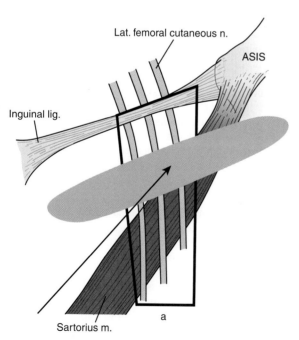

Fig. 108.2 Area of compression of the lateral femoral cutaneous nerve by low-cut "taille basse" trousers (danger zone) *(a)*, site of compression within the muscle; ASIS, anterior superior iliac spine. *(From Moucharafieh R, Wehbe J, Maalouf G: Meralgia paresthetica: a result of tight new trendy low cut trousers ["taille basse"], Int J Surg 6:164, 2008.)*

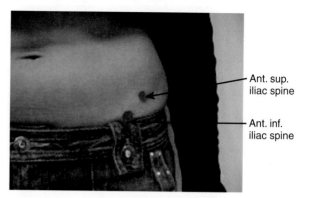

Fig. 108.3 Direct compression of the lateral femoral cutaneous nerve is caused by the waistband of low-cut "taille basse" trousers. *(From Moucharafieh R, Wehbe J, Maalouf G: Meralgia paresthetica: a result of tight new trendy low cut trousers ["taille basse"], Int J Surg 6:164, 2008.)*

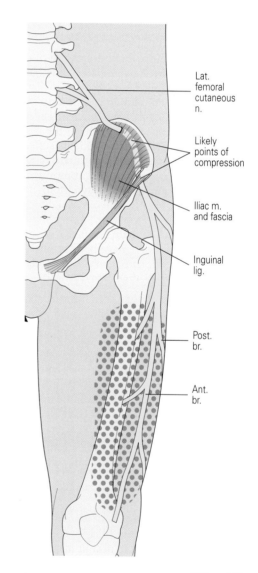

20 Rheum 5.13

Fig. 108.4 **Course of the lateral femoral cutaneous nerve.** The potential for entrapment of the lateral femoral cutaneous nerve can be seen by its course just under the inguinal ligament and medial to the anterior superior iliac spine. *(From Klippel JH, Dieppe PA, editors: Rheumatology, ed 2, London, 1998, Mosby.)*

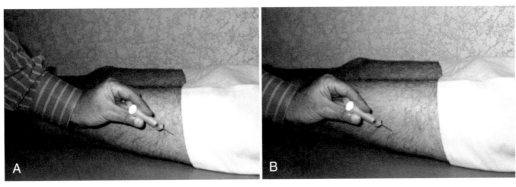

Fig. 108.5 A and B, Eliciting the burning lateral thigh sign for meralgia paresthetica.

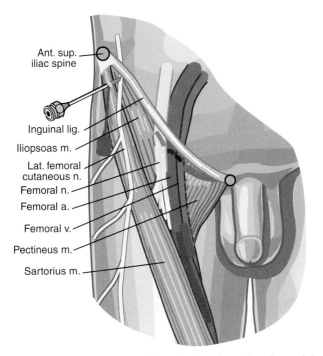

Fig. 108.6 **Injection technique for relieving the pain of meralgia paresthetica.** *(From Waldman SD: Atlas of interventional pain management,* ed 3, *Philadelphia, 2009, Saunders, p 522.)*

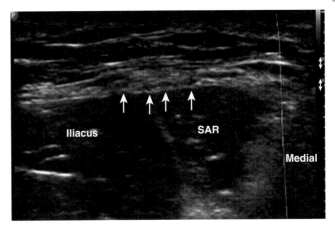

Fig. 108.7 Ultrasonographic image of the lateral femoral cutaneous nerve *(solid arrows),* which has already branched into smaller nerves and appears as hypoechoic structures. SAR, sartorius muscle. *(From Seib RK, Peng PWH: Ultrasound-guided peripheral nerve block in chronic pain management,* Tech Reg Anesth Pain Manag *13:110, 2009.)*

anterior superior iliac spine and just inferior to the inguinal ligament is then identified and is prepared with antiseptic solution (**Fig. 108.6**). A 1.5-inch 25-gauge needle is then advanced perpendicular to the skin slowly until the needle is felt to pop through the fascia. Paresthesia is often elicited. After careful aspiration, a total of 5 to 7 mL of 1.0% preservative-free lidocaine and 40 mg of methylprednisolone is injected in a fanlike manner as the needle pierces the fascia of the external oblique muscle. Care must be taken not to place the needle too deeply, to avoid entering the peritoneal cavity and perforating the abdominal viscera. After injection of the solution, pressure is applied to the injection site to decrease the incidence of postblock ecchymosis and hematoma formation, which can be quite dramatic, especially in the anticoagulated patient. Ultrasound guidance (**Fig. 108.7**) may be beneficial in patients whose anatomic landmarks are difficult to identify.[17]

Care must be taken to rule out other conditions that may mimic the pain of meralgia paresthetica. The main side effects of the just-described nerve block are postblock ecchymosis and

hematoma formation. If needle placement is too deep and enters the peritoneal cavity, perforation of the colon may result in the formation of intra-abdominal abscess and fistula. Early detection of infection is crucial to avoid potentially life-threatening sequelae. If the needle is placed too medially, blockade of the femoral nerve may occur and may make ambulation difficult.

Conclusion

Meralgia paresthetica is a common pain complaint encountered in clinical practice. It is often misdiagnosed as lumbar radiculopathy. If a patient presents with pain suggestive of lateral femoral cutaneous neuralgia and does not respond to lateral femoral cutaneous nerve blocks, a diagnosis of lesions more proximal in the lumbar plexus or L2-3 radiculopathy should be considered. Such patients often respond to epidural steroid blocks. Electromyography and MRI of the lumbar plexus are indicated in this patient population to help rule out other causes of lateral femoral cutaneous pain, including malignant disease invading the lumbar plexus or epidural or vertebral metastatic disease at L2-3.

References

Full references for this chapter can be found on www.expertconsult.com.

Femoral and Saphenous Neuropathies

Bernard M. Abrams

Femoral and saphenous neuropathies are uncommon pain-producing conditions. Femoral neuropathy can produce pain of the anterior thigh and midcalf and is associated with weakness of the quadriceps muscle. This disorder can be caused by myriad factors.[1] The saphenous nerve, a pure sensory nerve and anatomic extension of the femoral nerve, can produce medial calf pain that may be confused with medial calf claudication.[2]

Historical Considerations

In 1960, Kopell and Thompson[3] described entrapment of the saphenous nerve, but undoubtedly saphenous nerve dysfunction and injury have been known for many years as a result of experience with trauma and surgery in the region of the medial thigh. Descriptions of diabetic neuropathy as early as 1890 recognized cases characterized by asymmetrical lower extremity pain and weakness.[4] This concept dates back to 1798, when John Rollo mentioned neurologic disorders in his book *Cases of Diabetes Mellitus,* and it persisted through the eighteenth, nineteenth, and twentieth centuries until, at least, 1976.[5] Then it became recognized that what had previously been termed *femoral neuropathy* was much more frequently lumbar plexopathy. Asbury[6] clarified the issue advocating the term *proximal diabetic neuropathy* in view of the ambiguities associated with the earlier term *diabetic amyotrophy.* Unfortunately, the

association of the relatively uncommon femoral neuropathy with diabetes mellitus persisted when, in fact, diabetes is much more commonly associated with lumbar plexopathy. The long history of this erroneous association terminated only with the advent of modern meticulous electrodiagnostic methods and should serve as a cautionary note not to neglect the multiple possible causes of true femoral neuropathy.[7]

Femoral Neuropathy

Anatomy

The femoral nerve arises from the lumbar plexus within the psoas major muscle. It is formed from the posterior divisions of the ventral rami of the L2-4 spinal nerve roots (**Fig. 109.1**). After emerging from the lateral border of the psoas muscle, the femoral nerve lies in a groove between the psoas and iliacus muscles. As it approaches the external iliac artery (which is anteromedial to it), the nerve and artery descend toward the pelvis. In its descent, the nerve gives off some branches to innervate the iliacus and psoas muscles.[7] The psoas is also innervated by branches of the L2 and L3 spinal nerve roots. Authorities differ on whether clinically significant innervation of the iliacus and psoas muscles arises from the beginning of the femoral nerve or from fibers of the lumbar plexus proximal to the origin of the femoral nerve. Therefore, weakness of hip

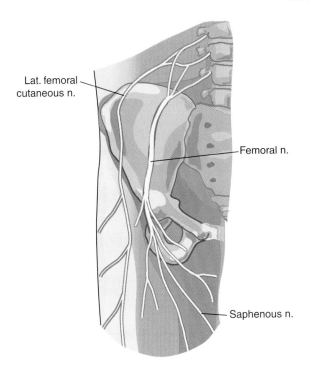

Lat. femoral cutaneous n.

Femoral n.

Saphenous n.

Fig. 109.1 **Anatomy of the femoral nerve.**

Table 109.1 **Causes of Femoral Neuropathy**

Retroperitoneal and Iliacus Compartment Hemorrhage
    Spontaneous
    Associated with anticoagulants (e.g., heparin, warfarin [Coumadin])
    Traumatic iliacus muscle avulsion
    Hemophilia and other coagulopathies
    Traumatic pseudoaneurysm and iliacus hematoma

Iliacus abscess
Abdominal aortic aneurysm and pseudoaneurysm
Trauma, stretch, or compression
Idiopathic
Tumors, enlarged lymph nodes, complications of radiation, and chemotherapeutic injection
Diabetes mellitus (usually as part of lumbar plexopathy)
Pregnancy and labor

Iatrogenic
    Hip arthroplasty
    Neural blockade and tourniquet use
    Abdominal hysterectomy including retractor injury
    Renal transplants and other urologic and pelvic surgery
    Lithotomy position for delivery and surgery, including vaginal hysterectomy
    Inguinal and femoral herniorrhaphies

flexion resulting from involvement of the psoas and iliacus may or may not be included in the definition of the femoral nerve syndrome, depending on which viewpoint is espoused.

The femoral nerve, the psoas muscle, the iliacus muscle, and the iliolumbar vessels, roofed over by the iliacus fascia, form a tight *iliacus compartment*. This compartment accounts for femoral nerve lesions resulting from space-occupying processes in this area.

The femoral nerve then passes beneath the inguinal ligament, gives off a branch to the pectineus muscle, and then enters the femoral triangle lateral to the femoral artery and separated from the artery by some psoas fibers. Approximately 4 cm distal to the inguinal ligament, the artery bifurcates into an anterior division and a posterior division. The anterior division innervates the sartorius muscle and forms the medial and intermediate femoral cutaneous nerves that give sensory innervation to the skin of the medial and anterior surfaces of the knee, the medial surface of the lower leg, medial malleolus, and part of the arch of the foot and great toe. The anterior division also gives motor branches to the quadriceps muscles composed of the rectus femoris, vastus lateralis, vastus intermedius, and vastus medialis muscles. It continues as the saphenous nerve (see later).

Clinical Presentation

Patients with femoral neuropathies usually complain that their lower extremity buckles at the knee and they cannot maintain their stance, especially when trying to descend stairs.[8] These patients may have pain, numbness, and paresthesias in the entire femoral nerve and saphenous nerve distribution, or sensory abnormalities may be mild or even absent entirely. When pain is felt, it may be in the inguinal region or in the iliac fossa. When flank pain is severe in patients with other symptoms and signs of femoral neuropathy, hemorrhage in the iliacus compartment should be strongly suspected, especially in circumstances conducive to hemorrhage, such

as anticoagulation. Severe femoral nerve lesions produce weakness and eventually wasting of the quadriceps group of muscles, loss of the knee reflex (although this may also be seen in high lumbar radiculopathies [L3-4]), and sensory abnormalities over the anterior aspect of the thigh and the medial part of the lower leg. In proximal diabetic neuropathy[8,9] (actually lumbar plexopathy in most cases), patients characteristically have severe pain radiating from the groin into the anterior thigh. This pain is usually worse at night and at rest (in contrast to a lumbar radiculopathy), and it subsides over several days to weeks, followed by severe painless weakness of the quadriceps group of muscles. This pain may be severe enough to require opioids for relief.

During examination of a patient with suspected femoral neuropathy, the iliopsoas muscle and hip adductor strength must be evaluated to differentiate among femoral neuropathy, combined obturator and femoral neuropathy, and upper lumbar plexopathy or L2, L3 radiculopathy.[10]

Etiology

Numerous conditions, many of them iatrogenic, can produce femoral neuropathies. The most common causes are listed in **Table 109.1.**

Iliac Hemorrhage

A hemorrhage in the tight iliacus compartment can compress the femoral nerve. Causes range from the common hemorrhage resulting from anticoagulation to hemophilia and other coagulopathies. The characteristic clinical picture consists of femoral nerve dysfunction and severe pain and swelling. The pain is generally located in the iliac fossa and groin and is associated with a flexed posture of the leg at the hip. Ecchymoses may be present in the upper thigh.[9] Hematomas within the psoas muscle characteristically cause widespread lumbar plexopathy, but occasionally patients have only femoral dysfunction. False aneurysms may form within the psoas muscle.[10-30] Traumatic avulsion of the iliacus muscle may occur in otherwise healthy people, occasionally after only minor trauma.[31,32,34]

Iliac Abscess

Iliac abscess may develop independently or may result from infection of a hematoma. With the addition of the signs of infection, the signs are the same as in hemorrhage.[33]

Abdominal Aortic Aneurysms

Sometimes, abdominal aortic aneurysms rupture into the psoas muscle and produce false aneurysms that compress the femoral nerve. Other arteries, including the profunda femoral artery and the iliac artery, may have aneurysms or false aneurysms that compress the femoral nerve.[35-42]

Trauma, Stretch, or Compression

Direct injury by bullet wounds, stab wounds, blunt injuries, and hip and pelvic fractures can compromise the femoral nerve. Gymnasts and dancers have been reported to incur femoral nerve injuries during hyperextension of the hip. Damage during coma and drunken stupors has also been reported, and alcoholism itself has been reported as a cause.[43-49]

Idiopathic Etiology

One report in 1970[49] found that 18 of 50 patients had no demonstrable cause of their neuropathy. Given that most of these patients were men who were more than 50 years old and who had eventual resolution of the neuropathy over months, some may of these patients have had occult diabetic plexopathy.

Tumors, Complications of Cancer Therapy, and Other Space-Occupying Lesions

Tumors may arise primarily from the nerve sheath, they may arise from the iliopsoas muscle or the ilium itself, or rarely they may be primary malignant neoplasms or metastases and cause femoral neuropathy.[50-60] Infusions of chemotherapeutic agents into the femoral artery may also cause femoral neuropathy.[5]

Diabetes Mellitus

Although the older literature described diabetes as the most common cause of femoral neuropathy, current electrodiagnosis has clearly identified the lumbosacral plexus as the primary pathologic site of the lesion. The femoral nerve is often the most severely affected structure involved, although other portions of the lumbosacral plexus can clearly be shown to be affected.[7] An association with renal failure has been noted.[61]

Pregnancy and Delivery

Femoral neuropathy has been reported as a result of pregnancy and delivery, even in patients with uncomplicated situations.[62-68] During pregnancy and before delivery, pressure on the femoral nerve in the pelvis is presumably implicated.[64]

Iatrogenic Causes

Unfortunately, iatrogenic femoral neuropathy is all too frequent. It has been associated with many different surgical procedures in the abdomen, pelvic inguinal, and hip areas.[69] This complication has most frequently been associated with abdominal hysterectomy and the use of self-retaining retractors that compress the femoral nerve directly or within the iliopsoas muscle and the lateral wall of the pelvis. The incidence of iatrogenic femoral neuropathy is significantly lower when these retractors are not used. Hip replacement and repair have also been reported as common causes of femoral neuropathy, although sciatic neuropathy occurs more frequently in these situations.

Other circumstances in which femoral neuropathy may occur are renal transplantation, inguinal or femoral herniorrhaphy, lymph node resection in the groin, femoral artery surgery, cardiac catheterization, and angioplasty. Suturing of the femoral nerve may occur during surgery, as may extrusion of cement, adverse effects of tourniquet use, and untoward effects of neural anesthetic blockage.

Hip Arthroplasty

Following hip arthroplasty, femoral neuropathy occurs much less frequently than does sciatic neuropathy (0.1% to 2.3%). When femoral neuropathy occurs, it is usually the result of retractor compression, heat from bone cement or nerve encasement in cement, laceration, and complicating iliac hematoma. The onset of the disorder may be delayed by scar formation. Iliacus hemorrhage following prophylactic anticoagulation postoperatively has also been reported.[70-80]

Neural Blockade and Tourniquet Use

Both neural blockade in the psoas compartment and ilioinguinal block for hernia repair have been associated with transient or permanent femoral nerve damage. Use of a tourniquet has damaged both the femoral and saphenous nerves.[81-83]

Abdominal Hysterectomy and Tuboplasty

Abdominal hysterectomy has been the operation most strongly associated with intraoperative femoral nerve palsies. Two studies in the 1980s gave statistical incidences of 11.6% and 7.5%, respectively.[84,85]

Based on cadaver anatomic studies and clinical experience, the lateral blade of self-retaining retractors was ascribed to be the likely cause of femoral neuropathy. The abandonment of this instrument led to a reduction in femoral neuropathies from 7.5% to 0.7%.[86] Other possible situations conducive to femoral neuropathy include suturing of the nerve and attempts at tubal ligation and reanastomosis.[87-100]

Laparoscopy

Laparoscopy and suprapubic interventions have been implicated in the development of femoral neuropathy.

Renal Transplantation

Femoral neuropathy has been reported with some frequency in renal transplants that involve retroperitoneal placement of the donated kidney. Again, self-retaining retractors have been implicated, but even without the use of these instruments, delayed femoral neuropathy resulting from compression of the nerve by hematoma has been seen and confirmed at autopsy. In addition, surgical procedures for genitourinary malignant diseases and other pelvic urologic operations have been complicated by femoral neuropathies.[101–116]

Lithotomy Positions

Prolonged and, rarely, even brief intervals in the lithotomy position have produced femoral neuropathies, possibly because of kinking and compression of the nerve below the inguinal ligament. Prolonged lithotomy position for obstetric delivery and for surgical procedures such as laparoscopy may produce femoral neuropathy.[117–119]

Inguinal and Femoral Herniorrhaphies

Femoral neuropathy may complicate inguinal or femoral herniorrhaphies when suture material is cut or placed around the nerve. Delayed onset of the neuropathy may result from later development of scar tissue.[120–122]

Diagnosis and Testing

The cause of femoral neuropathy may be obvious because of the setting in which it arose, such as immediately postoperatively following a surgical procedure well known to be associated with this complication. Renal transplants, abdominal hysterectomy, and prolonged lithotomy positions head this category. Injections, catheterizations, and hernia surgery in the groin provide clear causality on many occasions. Confusion may arise in cases of delayed onset resulting from scarring or hemorrhage, although hemorrhage is generally associated with severe pain in the iliacus fossa. Again, circumstances may clearly show the cause in patients with hemorrhagic lesions, such as patients who undergo anticoagulation or those who have hemophilia or another coagulopathy.

One of the maneuvers necessary when evaluating more occult causes is strict delineation of the anatomic boundaries of the patient's deficits. Often, what appears to be pure femoral neuropathy clinically may actually be part of a radiculoplexopathy. In patients with radiculoplexopathy, the anatomic site of the lesion is more proximal, and the diagnostic possibilities of diabetes mellitus and other processes such as malignant disease in the pelvis must be considered. Electromyography is well suited for this task, and testing should include sufficient interrogation of the quadriceps muscle group and the paraspinal, iliopsoas, and hip adductor muscles, to differentiate femoral neuropathy from more extensive lesions. Motor nerve conduction tests of the femoral nerve (stimulation point above the inguinal ligament and recording from the quadriceps muscle) may be performed, but these tests are generally less informative than needle electromyography[123] and may need to be followed up with laboratory tests for diabetes mellitus and imaging of the pelvis by computed tomography (CT) or magnetic resonance imaging (MRI) scans.[124–128]

CT scan has long been shown to image the femoral nerve clearly, as have MRI and ultrasound. CT scan is indicated for suspected iliacus hemorrhages and other masses affecting the femoral nerve. Ultrasound and MRI are also effective in diagnosing iliacus hemorrhage and other masses.[129–137]

Treatment

Obvious inciting lesions should be treated with such curative measures as are available. Exploration of the femoral nerve should be undertaken if complete disruption of the nerve, unintentional suturing, or stapling of the nerve is suspected. Management of retroperitoneal or iliopsoas hemorrhage may constitute a surgical emergency.[138–140] Percutaneous relief of hemorrhage has been reported.[140] In acute hemorrhage, anticoagulation, when present, must be reversed. Fluid and blood replacement may be necessary. Persistent pain requires pharmacologic treatment such as with gabapentin, pregabalin, other membrane stabilizers (newer anticonvulsants), tricyclic antidepressants, or other medications useful in neuropathic pain. Nerve blocks of the femoral nerve may be helpful to relieve pain. Physical therapy, bracing, and assistive devices may be necessary. Mobility and range of motion should be maintained.

Prognosis

In iatrogenic femoral neuropathy, recovery is the usual outcome. The prognosis is better in incidents induced by the lithotomy position than it is in hip or inguinal surgical untoward events. The only significant prognostic factor is the percentage of axon loss in the vastus lateralis; this value is derived by a comparison of the vastus lateralis compound muscle action potential on the affected and unaffected sides.[10]

Saphenous Neuropathy

Saphenous neuropathies can occur in the thigh as a result of lacerations, arterial surgery, compression by fibrous bands, and entrapment at the subsartorial canal exit.[3] At the knee, saphenous neuropathies result from surgery, including arthroscopy or external compression. In the lower leg, this disorder is a complication of surgery. The infrapatellar branch can be injured by direct compression or by knee surgery, including arthroscopy and possibly entrapment in the sartorius muscle tendon.

Anatomy

The saphenous nerve is the distal sensory continuation of the femoral nerve. It descends in the thigh through the quadriceps muscle in the subsartorial canal of Hunter lateral to the femoral artery. The saphenous nerve gives off an infrapatellar branch that supplies sensation to the anterior skin of the patella before it enters a fascial layer between the sartorius and gracilis muscles (**Fig. 109.2**). It emerges from the canal and becomes subcutaneous approximately 10 cm proximal to the knee.[10]

The nerve crosses the pes anserine bursa at the upper medial portion of the tibia and then runs distally along the medial aspect of the tibia. The saphenous vein is closely apposed to the nerve along most of its descent in the calf, especially in the distal third of the leg. At the lower third of the leg, the saphenous nerve divides into two main branches. One branch continues along the medial border of the tibia and terminates at the ankle. The other branch passes anteriorly with the vein to cross the medial surface of the tibia and in front of the medial malleolus to reach the foot; it then continues along the medial surface to the ball of the great toe. The saphenous nerve innervates the medial and anterior sensory portions of the knee and the medial surface of the lower leg, the medial malleolus, and a minor part of the medial arch of the foot and great toe.[10]

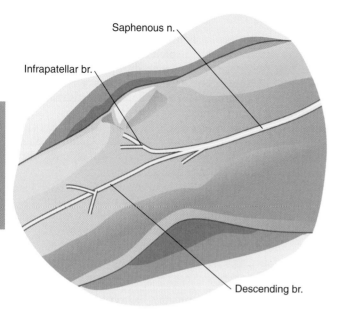

Fig. 109.2 **Anatomy of the saphenous nerve.**

Table 109.2 **Causes of Saphenous Neuropathy**
THIGH
Lacerations
Arterial surgery (femoral artery)
Compression
Schwannoma
Subsartorial canal entrapment
KNEE
Surgery: arthroscopy; medial meniscectomy
External compression (stirrups)
LOWER LEG
Surgical injury (varicose vein operations, vein harvest for arterial surgery)
Cannulation of saphenous vein
INFRAPATELLAR BRANCH
Compression and other direct injuries
Arthroscopy
POSSIBLE ENTRAPMENT IN THE SARTORIUS TENDON

Etiology

Causes of saphenous neuropathy are outlined in **Table 109.2**. The differential diagnosis of saphenous neuropathy depends on the anatomic location. In the thigh, because of its proximity to the femoral artery in the subsartorial canal, the saphenous nerve can be damaged by arterial surgery, lacerations, compression by fibrous bands, schwannoma, or nerve entrapment in which the nerve pierces a fascial layer to leave the subsartorial canal.[3] At the knee, saphenous nerve injury results from arthroscopic surgery, medial meniscectomy, and external compression from knee-supporting stirrups. It also occurs in surfers, who habitually grasp the board between their knees. In the lower leg, surgical damage or saphenous nerve cannulation can produce neuropathy. Spontaneous paresthesia of the infrapatellar branch has been termed *gonyalgia paresthetica*.[141,142] The infrapatellar branch can be injured by direct compression, by knee surgery (arthroscopy), and questionably by entrapment in the sartorius tendon.

Clinical Presentation

In saphenous neuropathy, patients may report trivial numbness, but severe neuropathic pain may also occur. The course of the nerve should be palpated for tenderness, a neuroma, or Tinel's sign. The pain may be present at the medial aspect of the knee and may radiate downward to the medial side of the foot. Patients often state that negotiating stairs causes significant aggravation of the pain.[3] The sensory abnormality in the medial calf that may extend to the medial foot and the great toe may take the form of numbness or paresthesia.

Diagnosis and Testing

Electromyography provides an anatomic method of differentiating plexopathy from radiculopathy or combined lesions. Saphenous nerve conduction studies are technically challenging but may be useful for confirming damage to the sensory fibers of the saphenous nerve.[143–145]

Somatosensory evoked potentials may document dysfunction of the saphenous nerve but may not localize the lesion.[141,146,147] CT scan of the abdomen is mandatory in patients with suspected lesions of the psoas muscle or retroperitoneal space. MRI has supplemented CT because of superior tissue resolution. Focal lesions of the saphenous nerve can be confirmed by nerve conduction studies, which may be technically difficult. Somatosensory evoked potentials have been used for saphenous nerve studies. If a differential diagnosis between L4 radiculopathy and a saphenous nerve lesion is under consideration, electromyography of the L4-innervated muscles should be performed. Suspicion of a schwannoma should lead to an MRI scan of the thigh, with and without gadolinium enhancement.[7]

Treatment

Treatment depends on accurate diagnosis that, in turn, depends on setting up and resolving the diagnostic dilemma. Surgical correction of any lesion, when possible, is ideal. When residual pain and disability persist, rehabilitative efforts must be made. Although medical knowledge is constantly changing, neuropathic pain at this juncture is best dealt with by pharmacologic treatment such as with nonsteroidal anti-inflammatory drugs, mild analgesics, gabapentin, pregabalin, other membrane stabilizers (newer anticonvulsants), and tricyclic antidepressants, as well as by avoidance of precipitating factors for pain.

References

Full references for this chapter can be found on www.expertconsult.com.

Obturator Neuropathy

Bernard M. Abrams

Obturator neuropathy is an uncommon affliction that can cause medial thigh pain.[1] Although its description as an entrapment neuropathy is historically interesting,[2] the most frequent etiologic agent by far is trauma; and, unfortunately, iatrogenic trauma is the most common cause.

Anatomy

Anatomically, the obturator nerve is formed within the psoas muscle by the ventral divisions of the ventral primary rami of the L2, L3, and L4 nerve roots (**Fig. 110.1**). It shares fibers from the same nerve roots as the femoral nerve. After descending through the psoas muscle, it emerges from the medial border of the psoas at the pelvic brim immediately anterior to the sacroiliac joint. In the female, it is separated from the ovary by a thin layer of peritoneum. The nerve then curves downward and forward around the pelvic cavity wall to emerge through the obturator foramen, where it is in company with the obturator vessels. The obturator canal is an osseofibrous canal formed by a hiatus in the obturator membrane up against the pubic bone. Of the anatomic structures in the canal, the nerve is the closest to the bone, which leads to its purported involvement in osteitis pubis (**Fig. 110.2**).[3] In the canal, it divides into anterior and posterior branches.[4] The anterior branch innervates the adductor longus, adductor brevis, and gracilis muscles. The supply to the pectineus muscles is variable. The posterior branch supplies the obturator externus and adductor magnus muscles. The adductor brevis muscle may be supplied by either branch. Articular branches are given off to the hip joint.[4] Sensory innervation of a limited area of the upper medial thigh is found. Because of its position, the nerve is seldom directly traumatized.

Clinical Presentation

Although seldom damaged alone in extensive trauma, the hallmarks of obturator neuropathy are pain and weakness of the adductor musculature. The patient cannot stabilize the hip joint, and leg weakness is usually the predominant symptom, but paresthesias, often painful, may be the main symptom.

Maneuvers that stretch the nerve such as extension or lateral leg movement may increase the pain. In an obturator hernia, if still mobile, an increase in abdominal pressure, as in coughing, sneezing, or straining, increases the pain.[5]

Careful examination of the strength of the hip adductors and quadriceps muscle, the patella reflexes, and the sensory deficit (**Fig. 110.3**) may serve to differentiate obturator neuropathy from femoral neuropathy, but the two nerves are often damaged together because of their shared nerve root and lumbar plexus origin and course in pelvic trauma or hip surgery. Lumbar radiculopathy of L3 or L4 may also account for the weakness and shifts the focus to the lumbar spine for pathology.

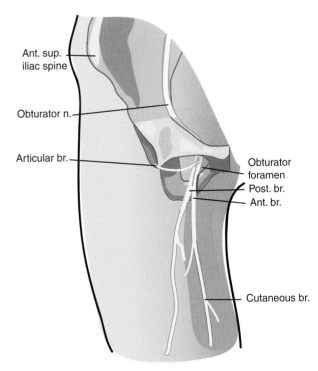

Fig. 110.1 **Anatomy of the obturator nerve.**

Ant. sup. iliac spine
Obturator n.
Articular br.
Obturator foramen
Post. br.
Ant. br.
Cutaneous br.

Etiology

Broad categories of etiology are pelvic fractures, complications of hip replacements, malignant pelvic mass or endometriosis (note its proximity to the ovary in the female), obturator hernia, complications of labor, lithotomy position, entrapment, and as a complication in the newborn (**Table 110.1**).

As stated previously, isolated obturator nerve injuries are relatively rare, and pelvic fractures and penetrating injuries such as gunshot wounds much more frequently injure multiple nerves or other neural structures, such as nerve roots or the lumbar plexus.[6–9] The obturator nerve can be injured during hip or pelvic surgery as a result of stretch, retractor compression, injury from cement (encasement or thermal injury), or electrocautery.[10–14] Massive pelvic hemorrhage, either spontaneous or during gynecologic surgery, can cause obturator neuropathy.[15,16] Obturator hernias can cause pain down the medial thigh, especially with Valsalva's maneuvers.[17,18] The lithotomy position has been implicated in obturator neuropathies, both in urologic

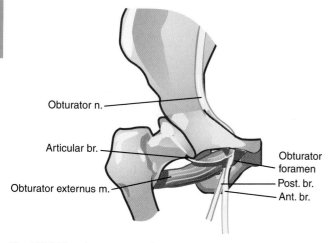

Fig. 110.2 **The obturator canal.** *(Redrawn from Kopell HP, Thompson WAL: Obturator nerve entrapment, N Engl J Med 262:56, 1960.)*

Table 110.1 Causes of Obturator Neuropathy
Pelvic fractures
Direct penetrating injuries
Pelvis malignant diseases
Endometriosis
Complications of hip arthroplasty, including encasement by cement
Obturator hernia
Obturator nerve entrapment
Lithotomy position
Pregnancy and labor (multiple mechanisms)
Pelvic hemorrhage (including as a complication of procedures such as cardiac catheterization)
Obturator palsy of the newborn

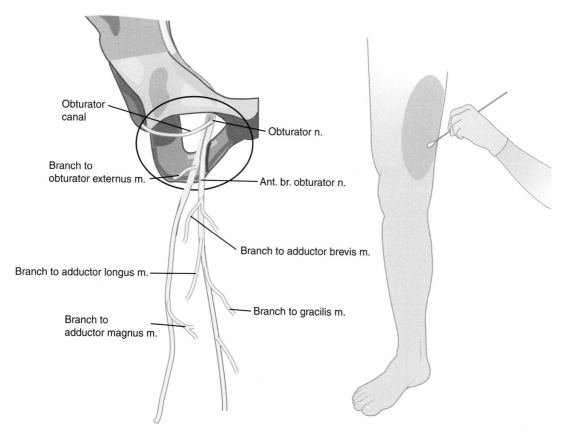

Fig. 110.3 **Sensory testing of the obturator nerve.**

and in gynecologic surgeries.[19–23] It also has been reported during pregnancy and delivery, but here, multiple factors are at play, including the fetal head, forceps application, hematoma, or other trauma occasioned by cesarean section or improper lithotomy position.[24,25] Malignant tumors can compress or invade the obturator nerve, as can endometriosis and laparoscopic pelvic lymphadenectomy, making visualization of the nerve mandatory during electrocautery.[26,27] Aneurysm of the hypogastric artery can also produce compression of the obturator nerve.[6,28,29]

Obturator neuropathy caused by cardiac catheterization is a special case of retroperitoneal hematoma formation compressing the nerve.[30,31] Bradshaw and associates[32] reported on 32 athletes who had entrapment of the obturator nerve by fascial entrapment of the nerve entering the thigh with distal pain radiating along the medial thigh induced by exercise with surgical relief from excision of the thickened fascia over the short adductor muscle. All of the afflicted athletes participated in sports with a "leg predominance," such as soccer and rugby. Idiopathic obturator neuropathy has also been described.[33] Finally, infants are not immune to obturator neuropathy, and one case possibly related to prolonged abnormal intrauterine leg position has been reported.[34]

Diagnosis

The clinical examination and the setting in which the neuropathy arose generally suggest its cause. Electromyography is essential for confirmation of anatomic location, and the differential diagnosis includes much more common multiple neuropathies, lumbar plexopathies, and L3-L4 nerve root lesions. For possible retroperitoneal hemorrhage or tumor, computed tomographic scan, magnetic resonance imaging, and ultrasound scan are helpful.[35,36] Angiography may be necessary in the patient suspected of having a hypogastric artery aneurysm.

The question of the possible relationship to diabetes mellitus arises in the same context as that for femoral neuropathy. Muscles innervated by the obturator nerve are almost invariably affected by so-called diabetic amyotrophy. Two reports in the literature[37,38] invoke diabetes as a cause of obturator neuropathy, but this, as in the case of femoral neuropathy, remains problematic. The reader is referred to a recent retrospective study that analyzed causes and outcomes.[39]

Treatment

Obvious inciting lesions should be treated with such curative measures as are available, that is, surgery for management of tumors, hemorrhage, or entrapment as indicated. In particular, when hip arthroplasty has been carried out, after a period of observation, reexploration may be indicated because of the possibility of the nerve being encased in cement. Persistent pain necessitates pharmacologic treatment, such as with gabapentin, pregabalin, other membrane stabilizers (newer anticonvulsants), tricyclic antidepressants, or other medications useful in neuropathic pain. One report in the literature seems to indicate some promise in the treatment of intractable pain, but further evaluation is warranted.[40]

References

Full references for this chapter can be found on www.expertconsult.com.

Part K

Pain Syndromes of the Knee and Distal Lower Extremity

Chapter 111

Painful Conditions of the Knee

Steven D. Waldman

Knee pain is one of the most common reasons that patients seek medical attention from their primary care physicians, orthopedists, rheumatologists, and pain management specialists. Knee pain can arise from the joint or the periarticular tissues (e.g., the bursae and tendons) or may be referred from the hip joint, femur, or proximal tibia and fibula. The largest joint in the body, the knee is subject to an amazing array of forces and injuries.[1] In this chapter, an overview is presented of some of the more common knee pain syndromes encountered in clinical practice.

Functional Anatomy of the Knee

For accurate diagnosis and treatment of knee pain, the clinician must have a clear understanding of the functional anatomy of the knee. The knee is not just a simple hinge joint that flexes and extends. The largest joint in the body in terms of articular surface and joint volume, the knee is capable of amazingly complex movements that encompass highly coordinated flexion and extension.[2] The knee joint is best thought of as a cam capable of locking in a stable position. Even the simplest movements of the knee involve an elegantly coordinated rolling and gliding movement of the femur on the tibia. Because of the complex nature of these movements, the knee is extremely susceptible to functional abnormalities with relatively minor alterations in the anatomy from arthritis or damage to the cartilage or ligaments.

Although both clinicians and laypersons think of the knee joint as a single joint, from the viewpoint of understanding its functional anatomy, it is more helpful to think of the knee

as two separate but interrelated joints: the femoral-tibial and the femoral-patellar joints (**Fig. 111.1**). Both joints share a common synovial cavity, and dysfunction of one joint can easily affect the function of the other.

The femoral-tibial joint is made up of the articulation of the femur and the tibia. Interposed between the two bones are two fibrocartilaginous structures known as the medial and lateral menisci (**Fig. 111.2**). The menisci serve to help transmit the forces placed on the femur across the joint onto the tibia. They possess the property of plasticity in that they are able to change their shape in response to the variable forces placed on the joint through its complex range of motion. The medial and lateral menisci are relatively avascular and receive the bulk of their nourishment from the synovial fluid, which means that little potential for healing exists when these important structures are traumatized.

The femoral-patellar joint's primary function is to use the patella, which is a large sesamoid bone embedded in the quadriceps tendon, to improve the mechanical advantage of the quadriceps muscle. The medial and lateral articular surfaces of the sesamoid interface with the articular groove of the femur (**Fig. 111.3**). In extension, only the superior pole of the patella is in contact with the articular surface of the femur. As the knee flexes, the patella is drawn superiorly into the trochlear groove of the femur.

Most of the knee joint's stability comes from the ligaments and muscles surrounding it, with little contribution from the bony elements. The main ligaments of the knee are the anterior and posterior cruciate ligaments, which provide much of the

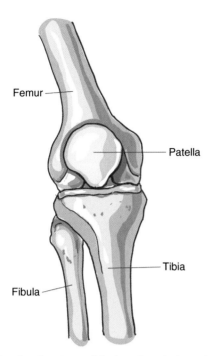

Fig. 111.1 Functional anatomy of the knee is easier to understand if it is viewed as two separate but interrelated joints: the femoral-tibial and the femoral-patellar joints. *(From Waldman SD:* Physical diagnosis of pain: an atlas of signs and symptoms, *ed 2, Philadelphia, 2010, Saunders, p 322.)*

anteroposterior stability of the knee, and the medial and lateral collateral ligaments, which provide much of the valgus and varus stability (**Fig. 111.4**). All of these ligaments also help prevent excessive rotation of the tibia in either direction. A number of secondary ligaments also add further stability to this inherently unstable joint.

The main extensor of the knee is the quadriceps muscle, which attaches to the patella via the quadriceps tendon. Fibrotendinous expansions of the vastus medialis and vastus lateralis insert into the sides of the patella and are subject to strain and sprain. The hamstrings are the main flexors of the hip, along with help from the gastrocnemius, sartorius, and gracilis muscles. Medial rotation of the flexed knee is via the medial hamstring muscle, and lateral rotation of the knee is controlled by the biceps femoris muscle.

The knee is well endowed with a variety of bursa to facilitate movement. Bursae are formed from synovial sacs whose purpose it is to allow easy sliding of muscles and tendons across one another at areas of repeated movement. These synovial sacs are lined with a synovial membrane that is invested with a network of blood vessels that secrete synovial fluid. Inflammation of the bursa results in an increase in the production of synovial fluid with swelling of the bursal sac. With overuse or misuse, these bursae may become inflamed, enlarged, and, on rare occasions, infected (**Fig. 111.5**). Given that the knee shares a common synovial cavity, inflammation of one bursa can cause significant dysfunction and pain of the entire knee.

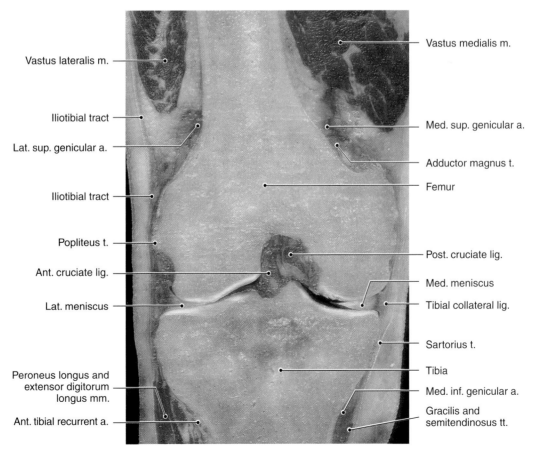

Fig. 111.2 **Coronal view of the knee.** *(From Kang HS, Joong AM, Resnick D:* MRI of the extremities, *Philadelphia, 2002, Saunders, p 301.)*

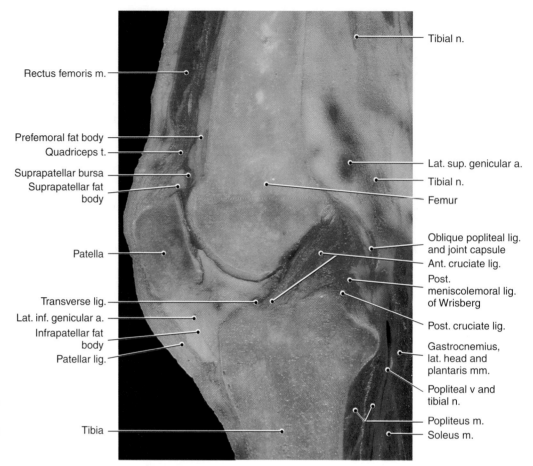

Rectus femoris m.

Tibial n.

Prefemoral fat body
Quadriceps t.
Suprapatellar bursa
Suprapatellar fat body

Lat. sup. genicular a.
Tibial n.
Femur

Patella

Oblique popliteal lig. and joint capsule
Ant. cruciate lig.
Post. meniscolemoral lig. of Wrisberg

Transverse lig.
Lat. inf. genicular a.
Infrapatellar fat body
Patellar lig.

Post. cruciate lig.

Gastrocnemius, lat. head and plantaris mm.

Popliteal v and tibial n.

Tibia

Popliteus m.
Soleus m.

Fig. 111.3 **Sagittal view of the knee.** *(From Kang HS, Joong AM, Resnick D: MRI of the extremities, Philadelphia, 2002, Saunders, p 341.)*

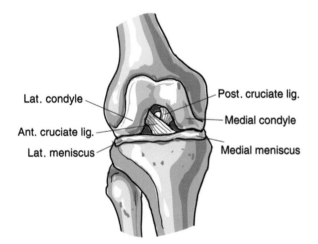

Lat. condyle
Ant. cruciate lig.
Lat. meniscus

Post. cruciate lig.
Medial condyle
Medial meniscus

Fig. 111.4 **The main ligaments of the knee.** *(From Waldman SD: Physical diagnosis of pain: an atlas of signs and symptoms, ed 2, Philadelphia, 2010, Saunders, p 325.)*

Common Painful Conditions of the Knee

The initial general physical examination of the knee guides the clinician in narrowing his or her differential diagnosis and helps suggest which specialized physical examination maneuvers and laboratory and radiographic testing will aid

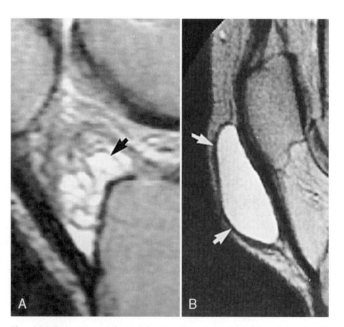

Fig. 111.5 **A,** Deep infrapatellar bursitis. A sagittal T2-weighted (TR/TE, 2300/70) spin-echo MRI shows fluid of high signal intensity *(arrow)* in the deep infrapatellar bursa. **B,** Prepatellar bursitis. A sagittal T2-weighted (TR/TE, 2000/80) spin-echo MRI shows fluid of high signal intensity *(arrows)* in the prepatellar bursa. *(A, Courtesy of M Zlatkin, MD, Hollywood, FL. B, Courtesy of EM Bellon, MD, Cleveland, OH. From Resnick D, editor: Diagnosis of bone and joint disorders, ed 4, Philadelphia, 2002, Saunders, p 3285.)*

in confirming the cause of the patient's knee pain and dysfunction.[3] For the clinician to make best use of the initial information gleaned from the general physical examination of the knee, a grouping of the common causes of knee pain and dysfunction is exceedingly helpful. Although no classification of knee pain and dysfunction can be all inclusive or all exclusive because of the frequently overlapping and multifactoral nature of knee pathology, **Table 111.1** should help improve the diagnostic accuracy of the clinician confronted with the patient with knee pain and dysfunction and help the clinician avoid overlooking less common diagnoses.

The list of disease processes in Table 111.1 is by no means comprehensive, but it does aid the clinician in organizing the potential sources of pathology that manifest as knee pain and dysfunction. The most commonly missed categories of knee pain and the categories that most often result in misadventures in diagnosis and treatment are the last three categories. The knowledge of this potential pitfall should help the clinician keep these sometimes overlooked causes of knee pain and dysfunction in the differential diagnosis.

A Rational Approach to Knee Pain

The Targeted History

The starting point for the clinician faced with the patient with knee pain is to obtain a targeted history and perform a targeted physical examination of the affected knee or knees based on that history. Salient features of the targeted history are summarized in **Table 111.2**. The relevance of each is discussed briefly.

Acute or Chronic?

The onset of acute knee pain in the absence of trauma is a cause for concern in that many of the diseases associated with acute knee pain can cause significant damage to the joint if not promptly diagnosed and treated.[4] The connective tissue diseases, septic arthritis, the crystal arthropathies, and hemarthrosis in the patient undergoing anticoagulation therapy are just a few of the diseases that can permanently damage a knee. Any acute knee pain associated with fever or constitutional symptoms or occurring in a patient on anticoagulation therapy should be taken seriously and not automatically attributed to "arthritis."

Age of the Patient

The age of the patient can provide significant direction to the clinician's search for a diagnosis. **Table 111.3** provides a grouping of the most common causes of knee pain in different age groups. The presence of knee pain in childhood and early adolescence in the absence of trauma is a cause for concern and should not be attributed to "growing pains."

Presence of Trauma

Traumatic knee pain is common. Many knee pain syndromes after trauma can be managed conservatively. However, the clinician should remember that many cannot. Early use of magnetic resonance imaging (MRI) of the traumatic knee serves two purposes: (1) it allows the clinician to aggressively rehabilitate those knees in which no internal derangement has be identified; and (2) it allows rapid surgical treatment of those patients with significant ligamentous and cartilaginous injuries before they do more damage to an already compromised joint.[4–6]

Table 111.1 Classification of Painful Conditions That Affect the Knee

KNEE PAIN FROM LOCALIZED BONY OR JOINT SPACE PATHOLOGY

Fracture

Primary bone tumor

Primary synovial tissue tumor

Joint instability

Localized arthritis

Osteophyte formation

Joint space infection

Hemarthrosis

Villonodular synovitis

Intra-articular foreign body

Osgood-Schlatter disease

Chronic dislocation of the patella

Patellofemoral pain syndrome

Patella alta

KNEE PAIN FROM PERIARTICULAR PATHOLOGY

Bursitis

Tendinitis

Adhesive capsulitis

Joint instability

Muscle strain

Muscle sprain

Periarticular infection not involving joint space

KNEE PAIN FROM SYSTEMIC DISEASE

Rheumatoid arthritis

Collagen vascular disease

Reiter's syndrome

Gout

Other crystal arthropathies

Charcot's neuropathic arthritis

KNEE PAIN FROM SYMPATHETICALLY MEDIATED PAIN

Causalgia

Reflex sympathetic dystrophy

KNEE PAIN FROM OTHER BODY AREAS

Lumbar plexopathy

Lumbar radiculopathy

Lumbar spondylosis

Fibromyalgia

Myofascial pain syndromes

Inguinal hernia

Entrapment neuropathies

Intrapelvic tumors

Retroperitoneal tumors

Fever

Acute knee pain and fever should be considered a dangerous combination.[7] Although some acute febrile illnesses, such as streptococcal pharyngitis, may have large joint arthralgias as part of their constellation of symptoms, the clinician must rule out the septic knee joint, the collagen vascular diseases, and Lyme disease before assuming that the fever and joint pain are unrelated. In younger patients, rheumatic fever must always be considered in the differential diagnosis of knee pain in the presence of fever.

Polyarthralgias

The patient presenting with knee pain who also has pain in other joints is a cause for concern. Although in the older, otherwise healthy patient, osteoarthritis is the most common reason for this clinical presentation, the clinician should be careful to avoid jumping to this conclusion without careful consideration.[8] The

Table 111.2 Targeted History for Knee Pain

Acute or chronic

Age of patient

History of trauma

Fever

Pain in other joints

Rash

Muscle weakness

Other constitutional symptoms (e.g., malaise, anorexia)

  Recent weight gain or loss

  Addition of any new medications

  Use of anticoagulant therapy

  Recent administration of corticosteroids

  Recent tapering of corticosteroids

  Recent tick bite

connective tissue diseases, including polymyalgia rheumatic, are a common cause of polyarthralgias in older patients.[9,10] Polyarthralgias in the younger patient should point the clinician toward the diagnosis of juvenile rheumatoid arthritis, among others.

Rash

The presence of rash and knee pain should suggest a number of potentially problematic diseases, such as Lyme disease and the connective tissue diseases, especially systemic lupus erythematosus and dermatomyositis.[11] In younger patients, the rash often is a harbinger of the onset of a collagen vascular disease or rheumatic fever. Gonococcal arthritis may also present with rash as its first symptom.

Muscle Weakness

The symptom of muscle weakness should clue the physician to strongly consider the connective tissue diseases, especially polymyalgia rheumatica and polymyositis.[12,13] The paraneoplastic syndromes associated with malignancy disease can also present as large joint pain and muscle weakness. Dermatomyositis in the younger age group is another diagnostic consideration in the setting of knee pain and muscle weakness. Approximately 20% of patients with dermatomyositis have an occult malignancy disease, which could include primary or metastatic tumors that involve the knee and its related structures.[12]

Constitutional Symptoms

As with all other areas of medicine, the presence of constitutional symptoms should alert the clinician to the potential that a serious systemic illness is present. The association of constitutional symptoms and knee pain should suggest the possibility of primary tumor or metastatic disease; the connective tissue diseases, especially polymyalgia rheumatic; and hypothyroidism.[10]

Recent Weight Gain or Loss

Recent unexplained weight loss in the presence of knee pain has the same implications as the presence of constitutional

Table 111.3 Common Causes of Knee Pain in Different Age Groups

Age group	Cause		
	Intra-articular	Periarticular	Referred
Childhood (2 to 10 years)	Juvenile chronic arthritis Osteochondritis dissecans Septic arthritis Torn discoid lateral meniscus	Osteomyelitis	Perthes' disease Transient synovitis of the hip
Adolescence (10 to 18 years)	Osteochondritis dissecans Torn meniscus Anterior knee pain syndrome Patellar malalignment	Osgood-Schlatter disease Sinding-Larsen-Johansson disease Osteomyelitis Tumors	Slipped upper femoral epiphysis
Early adulthood (18 to 30 years)	Torn meniscus Instability Anterior knee pain syndrome Inflammatory conditions	Overuse syndromes Bursitis	Rare
Adulthood (30 to 50 years)	Degenerate meniscal tears Early degeneration after injury or meniscectomy Inflammatory arthropathies	Bursitis Tendinitis	Degenerative hip disease from hip dysplasia or injury
Older age (≥50 years)	Osteoarthritis Inflammatory arthropathies	Bursitis Tendinitis	Osteoarthritis of the hip

symptoms, as discussed previously. Recent weight gain may place new forces on the knee joint and exacerbate preexisting problems, such as degenerative arthritis or a torn meniscus.

Addition of New Medications

Many medications can cause joint pain as a side effect unrelated to their intended therapeutic action. In most instances, this is an idiosyncratic reaction and will abate with discontinuation of the offending drug. In some, such as procainamide and hydralazine, the drug may cause a syndrome indistinguishable from systemic lupus erythematosus.[14]

Use of Anticoagulants

Anticoagulants and knee pain spell trouble for two reasons. First, seemingly minor trauma can cause a hemarthrosis of the knee that if untreated can result in permanent knee damage. Second, the presence of anticoagulants precludes rapid surgical treatment of otherwise treatable causes of knee pain.[15]

Corticosteroids

Knee pain after treatment with the corticosteroids can be the result of the return of the inflammatory condition originally responsible for the pain or the result of pseudorheumatism.[16] The pain of pseudorheumatism can be quite severe and can also occur with the tapering of corticosteroids used to treat unrelated acute conditions, such as poison ivy, or in the chronic setting, as in the treatment of chronic obstructive pulmonary disease.

Tick Bites

Although uncommon, Lyme disease after a tick bite can cause significant knee pain.[11,17] The condition is usually associated with a specific rash known as erythema migrans that is the result of an infection with *Borrelia burgdorferi;* failure to accurately diagnose and treat this uncommon cause of knee pain can result in permanent knee damage (**Fig. 111.6**).

Targeted Physical Examination

The targeted physical examination when combined with the targeted history allows the clinician to correctly diagnose the cause of the painful knee in most instances or at least direct further radiographic and laboratory investigations. Because of the lack of soft tissue overlying the knee joint, visual inspection can provide the clinician with important clues to the cause of knee pain and dysfunction. The starting point to visual inspection of the knee is an observation of the patient both standing and walking. The degree of valgus or varus of the knee with weight bearing should be noted as should any other obvious bony deformity (**Fig. 111.7**). The clinician should then look for evidence of quadriceps wasting, which, if identified, can be quantified with careful measurement at a point 12 cm above the upper margin of the patella with the knee fully extended. The presence of rubor suggestive of infection or swelling above, below, and alongside of the patella suggestive of an inflammatory process, including bursitis and tendonitis, is also noted. The posterior knee is then inspected for presence of a popliteal fossa mass suggestive of Baker's cyst.[18]

Palpation of the Knee

Careful palpation of the knee often provides the examiner with valuable clues to the cause of the patient's knee pain and dysfunction. The examiner palpates the temperature of both knees because localized increase in temperature may indicate inflammation or infection. The presence of swelling in the suprapatellar, prepatellar, or infrapatellar regions suggestive of suprapatellar, prepatellar, or infrapatellar bursitis is then identified. Generalized joint effusion may be identified by performing the ballottement test (**Fig. 111.8**). The bony elements of the knee, including the medial and lateral femoral condyles, the patella, and the tibial tubercle, are then palpated. The patellar tendon is then palpated to identify patellar tendonitis or jumper's knee (**Fig. 111.9**). The popliteal fossa is then palpated for evidence of a mass or Baker's cyst.[18] The knee joint is then ranged through flexion, extension, and medial and lateral rotation to identify crepitus or limitation of range of motion.

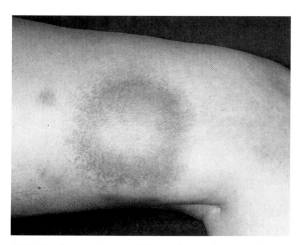

Fig. 111.6 **Erythema migrans.** This annular, erythematous lesion developed over a period of 3 weeks around the site of a tick bite. *(Reproduced with permission from McKee PH: Pathology of the skin, ed 2, London, 1996, Mosby. From Klippel JH, Dieppe PA: Rheumatology, ed 2, London, 1998, Mosby.)*

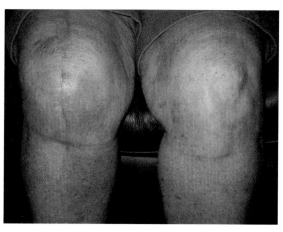

Fig. 111.7 **Visual inspection of the knee.** *(From Waldman SD: Physical diagnosis of pain: an atlas of signs and symptoms, ed 2, Philadelphia, 2010, Saunders, p 326.)*

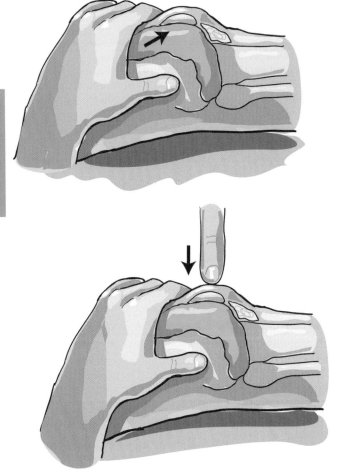

Fig. 111.8 **The ballottement test for large joint effusions.** (From Waldman SD: Physical diagnosis of pain: an atlas of signs and symptoms, ed 2, Philadelphia, 2010, Saunders, p 332.)

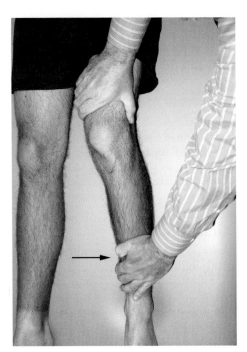

Fig. 111.10 **Valgus stress test for medial collateral ligament integrity.** (From Waldman SD: Physical diagnosis of pain: an atlas of signs and symptoms, ed 2, Philadelphia, 2010, Saunders, p 334.)

Valgus Stress Test for Medial Collateral Ligament Integrity

The valgus stress test provides the clinician with useful information regarding the integrity of the medial collateral ligaments. For the valgus stress test, the patient is placed in a supine position on the examination table with the knee flexed 35 degrees and the entire affected extremity relaxed. The examiner then places his or her hand above the knee to stabilize the upper leg. With the other hand, the examiner forces the lower leg away from the midline while observing for widening of the medial joint compartment and pain (**Fig. 111.10**). The maneuver is then repeated with the other lower extremity, and the results are compared.

Varus Stress Test for Lateral Collateral Ligament Integrity

The varus stress test provides the clinician with useful information regarding the integrity of the lateral collateral ligaments. For the varus stress test, the patient is placed in a supine position on the examination table with the knee flexed 35 degrees and the entire affected extremity relaxed. The examiner then places his or her hand above the knee to stabilize the upper leg. With the other hand, the examiner forces the lower leg forward from the midline while observing for widening of the medial joint compartment and pain (**Fig. 111.11**). The maneuver is then repeated with the other lower extremity, and the results are compared.

Anterior Drawer Test for Anterior Cruciate Ligament Integrity

The anterior drawer test is useful in helping the clinician assess the integrity of the anterior cruciate ligament. For the anterior drawer test, the patient is placed in the supine position on the examination table with the patient's head on a pillow to help

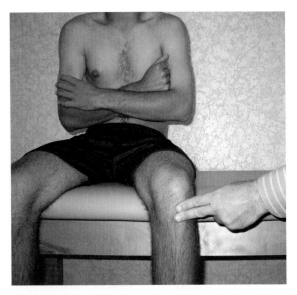

Fig. 111.9 **Palpation of the knee.** (From Waldman SD: Physical diagnosis of pain: an atlas of signs and symptoms, ed 2, Philadelphia, 2010, Saunders, p 327.)

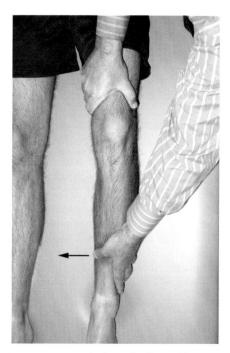

Fig. 111.11 Varus stress test for lateral collateral ligament integrity.
(From Waldman SD: Physical diagnosis of pain: an atlas of signs and symptoms, ed 2, Philadelphia, 2010, Saunders, p 335.)

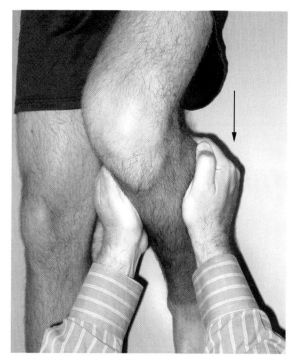

Fig. 111.12 Anterior drawer test for anterior cruciate ligament integrity. *(From Waldman SD: Physical diagnosis of pain: an atlas of signs and symptoms, ed 2, Philadelphia, 2010, Saunders, p 336.)*

relax the hamstring muscles. The patient's hip is then flexed to 45 degrees with the patient's foot placed flat on the table. The examiner then grasps the affected leg below the knee with both hands and pulls the lower leg forward while stabilizing the foot (**Fig. 111.12**). The test is considered positive if more than 5 mm of anterior motion is seen.

Posterior Drawer Test for Posterior Cruciate Ligament Integrity

The posterior drawer test is useful in helping the clinician assess the integrity of the posterior cruciate ligament. For the posterior drawer test, the patient is placed in the supine position on the examination table with the patient's head on a pillow to help relax the hamstring muscles. The patient's hip is then flexed to 45 degrees with the patient's foot placed flat on the table. The examiner then grasps the affected leg below the knee with both hands and pushes the lower leg backward while stabilizing the foot (**Fig. 111.13**). The test is considered positive if more than 5 mm of posterior motion is seen.

McMurray's Test for Torn Meniscus

The McMurray's test for torn meniscus can provide the clinician with useful information as to the whether a torn medial or lateral meniscus is responsible for the patient's knee pain. For the McMurray's test for torn meniscus, the examiner has the patient assume the supine position on the examination table with the knee maximally flexed. With the affected extremity relaxed, the examiner grasps the ankle and palpates the knee while simultaneously rotating the lower leg internally and externally and extending the knee (**Fig. 111.14**). The test is considered positive for a torn meniscus if the examiner appreciates a palpable or auditory click while rotating and extending the knee.

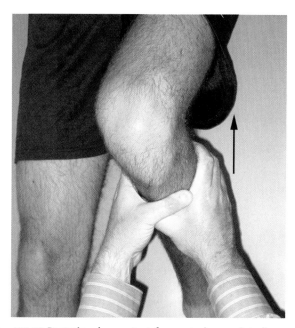

Fig. 111.13 Posterior drawer test for posterior cruciate ligament integrity. *(From Waldman SD: Physical diagnosis of pain: an atlas of signs and symptoms, ed 2, Philadelphia, 2010, Saunders, p 337.)*

Use of Testing Modalities for Evaluation of the Painful Knee

Plain radiographs are indicated in all patients who present with knee pain. On the basis of the patient's clinical presentation, additional testing may be indicated, including complete blood cell count, sedimentation rate, and antinuclear antibody testing. Magnetic resonance imaging of the knee is indicated if internal derangement is suspected. Radionuclide

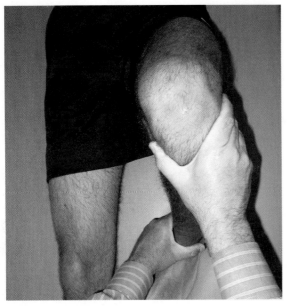

Fig. 111.14 McMurray's test for torn meniscus. *(From Waldman SD: Physical diagnosis of pain: an atlas of signs and symptoms, ed 2, Philadelphia, 2010, Saunders, p 342.)*

bone scan is indicated if metastatic disease or primary tumor involving the knee is being considered. Synovial fluid analysis should be performed in all patients suspected of having a septic joint or a crystal arthropathy. Titers for Lyme disease are indicated in patients with rash suggestive of erythema migrans or in patients with a history of tick bite who also have knee pain.[11,17]

Conclusion

The diagnosis of knee pain should be a relatively straightforward clinical endeavor as long as the clinician performs a careful targeted history and physical examination. The clinician faced with the patient with knee pain should have a relatively low threshold for the ordering of MRI, especially in the presence of trauma. A failure to heed the warning signs discussed can result in much unneeded pain and functional disability and permanent damage to the knee.

References

Full references for this chapter can be found on www.expertconsult.com.

Bursitis Syndromes of the Knee

Steven D. Waldman

Bursitis of the knee is one of the most common causes of knee pain encountered in clinical practice. The bursae of the knee are vulnerable to injury from both acute trauma and repeated microtrauma.[1] The bursae of the knee may exist as single bursal sacs or, in some patients, as a multisegmented series of sacs that may be loculated.[2] Acute injuries to the bursae of the knee frequently take the form of direct trauma to the bursa from falls or blows directly to the knee; of patellar, tibial plateau, and proximal fibular fractures; or of overuse injuries, including running on soft or uneven surfaces or from jobs that require crawling on the knees, such as laying carpet. If the inflammation of the bursae of the knees becomes chronic, calcification of the bursa may occur.[3]

Suprapatellar Bursitis

The suprapatellar bursa extends superiorly from beneath the patella under the quadriceps femoris muscle (**Figs. 112.1 and 112.2**). The patient with suprapatellar bursitis frequently has pain in the anterior knee above the patella, which can radiate superiorly into the distal anterior thigh.[4] Often, the patient is unable to kneel or walk down stairs (**Fig. 112.3**). The patient may also have a sharp, catching sensation with range of motion of the knee, especially on first arising. Suprapatellar bursitis often coexists with arthritis and tendinitis of the knee joint, and these other pathologic processes may confuse the clinical picture.[2]

Clinical Presentation

Physical examination may reveal point tenderness in the anterior knee just above the patella. Passive flexion and active resisted extension of the knee reproduce the pain. Sudden release of resistance during this maneuver markedly increases the pain.[1] Swelling in the suprapatellar region with a boggy feeling to palpation may be seen. Occasionally, the suprapatellar bursa may become infected, as evidenced by systemic symptoms including fever and malaise and local signs of rubor, color, and dolor.

Diagnosis

Plain radiographs of the knee may reveal calcification of the bursa and associated structures, including the quadriceps tendon consistent with chronic inflammation. Magnetic resonance imaging (MRI) is indicated if internal derangement, occult mass, or tumor of the knee is suspected.[5] Electromyography helps distinguish suprapatellar bursitis from femoral neuropathy, lumbar radiculopathy, and plexopathy. The injection technique described subsequently serves as a diagnostic and therapeutic maneuver. A complete blood cell count and an automated chemistry profile, including determinations of uric acid, erythrocyte sedimentation rate, and antinuclear antibody value, are indicated if collagen vascular disease is suspected. If infection is considered, aspiration, Gram stain, and culture of bursal fluid are indicated on an emergent basis.

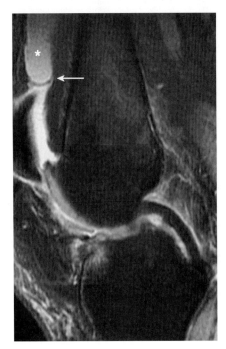

Fig. 112.1 **Suprapatellar bursa.** Sagittal proton density (3000/26) fast spin echo fat-saturated magnetic resonance imaging scan shows a suprapatellar bursa (*), which normally communicates with the joint unless the suprapatellar plica (arrow) fails to involute, thus isolating this compartment. (From Beaman FD Peterson JJ: MR imaging of cysts, ganglia, and bursae about the knee, Radiol Clin North Am 45:969, 2007.)

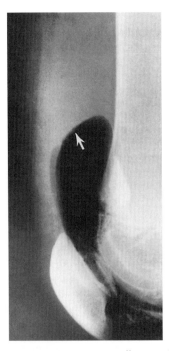

Fig. 112.2 **Noncommunicating suprapatellar pouch cyst.** A lateral view from a double-contrast knee arthrogram shows minimal extrinsic impression on the suprapatellar pouch (arrow) by an adjacent fluid-filled mass. (From Resnick D, editor: Diagnosis of bone and joint disorders, ed 4, Philadelphia, 2002, Saunders, p 284.)

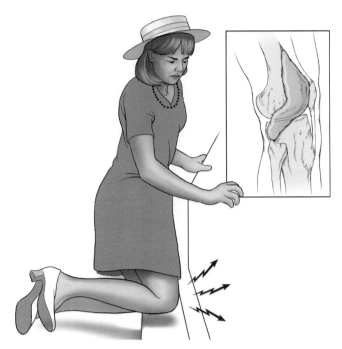

Fig. 112.3 Suprapatellar bursitis is usually the result of direct trauma to the suprapatellar bursa from either acute injury or repeated microtrauma. (From Waldman SD: Atlas of common pain syndromes, ed 2, Philadelphia, 2008, Saunders, p 255.)

Differential Diagnosis

Because of the unique anatomy of the region, not only the suprapatellar bursa but also the associated tendons and other bursae of the knee can become inflamed and confuse the diagnosis. The suprapatellar bursa extends superiorly from beneath the patella under the quadriceps femoris muscle and its tendon. The bursa is held in place by a small portion of the vastus intermedius muscle called the articularis genus muscle. Both the quadriceps tendon and the suprapatellar bursa are subject to the development of inflammation after overuse, misuse, or direct trauma. The quadriceps tendon is made up of fibers from the four muscles that comprise the quadriceps muscle: the vastus lateralis, the vastus intermedius, the vastus medialis, and the rectus femoris. These muscles are the primary extensors of the lower extremity at the knee. The tendons of these muscles converge and unite to form a single exceedingly strong tendon. The patella functions as a sesamoid bone within the quadriceps tendon, with fibers of the tendon expanding around the patella forming the medial and lateral patella retinacula that help strengthen the knee joint. These fibers are called expansions and are subject to strain, and the tendon proper is subject to the development of tendinitis (**Fig. 112.4**). The suprapatellar, infrapatellar, and prepatellar bursae may also concurrently become inflamed with dysfunction of the quadriceps tendon. Remember that anything that alters the normal biomechanics of the knee can result in inflammation of the suprapatellar bursa.

Treatment

A short course of conservative therapy consisting of simple analgesics, nonsteroidal anti-inflammatory drugs (NSAIDs), or cyclooxygenase-2 (COX-2) inhibitors and a knee brace to prevent further trauma is a reasonable first step in the treatment of patients with suprapatellar bursitis. If the patient does not have rapid improvement, the following injection technique is

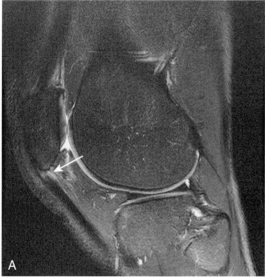

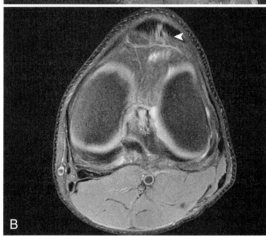

Fig. 112.4 **Moderate patellar tendinopathy.** A, Sagittal T2 fat-saturated image shows focal increased signal in the deep posterior portion of the proximal patellar tendon *(arrow)* and indistinct posterior margins of the tendon at this point. B, Axial proton density fat-saturated image of the same patient shows focal high signal in the tendon extending into the retropatellar fat *(arrowhead)*. *(From O'Keeffe SA, Hogan BA, Eustace SJ, et al: Overuse injuries of the knee,* Magnetic Resonance Imaging Clin North Am *17:725, 2009.)*

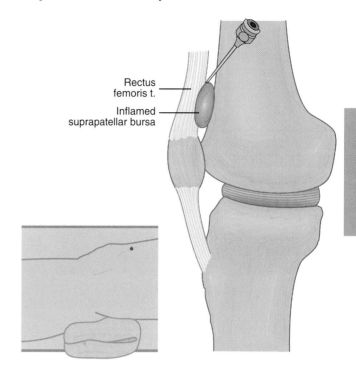

Fig. 112.5 **Injection technique for relief of the pain from suprapatellar bursitis.** *(From Waldman SD:* Atlas of pain management injection techniques, ed 2, *Philadelphia, 2007, Saunders, p 452.)*

dressing and ice pack are placed at the injection site. Physical therapy to restore function is a reasonable next step after the acute pain and swelling has subsided after injection with local anesthetic and corticosteroid.

Prepatellar Bursitis

The prepatellar bursa is vulnerable to injury from both acute trauma and repeated microtrauma. The prepatellar bursa lies between the subcutaneous tissues and the patella (**Fig. 112.6**).[1,7] This bursa may exist as a single bursal sac or, in some patients, as a multisegmented series of sacs that may be loculated. Acute injuries frequently take the form of direct trauma to the bursa from falls directly onto the knee or from patellar fractures and from overuse injuries, including running on soft or uneven surfaces. Prepatellar bursitis may also result from jobs that require crawling on the knees, such as laying carpet or scrubbing floors; hence, the other name for prepatellar bursitis is housemaid's knee (**Fig. 112.7**). It has also been reported in break dancers.[8] If the inflammation of the prepatellar bursa becomes chronic, calcification of the bursa may occur.

Clinical Presentation

The patient with prepatellar bursitis frequently has pain and swelling in the anterior knee over the patella that can radiate superiorly and inferiorly into the area surrounding the knee.[9] Often, the patient is unable to kneel or walk down stairs. The patient may also have a sharp, catching sensation with range of motion of the knee, especially on first arising. Prepatellar bursitis often coexists with arthritis and tendinitis of the knee joint, and these other pathologic processes may confuse the clinical picture.

a reasonable next step.[6] The goals of this injection technique are explained to the patient. The patient is placed supine with a rolled blanket underneath the knee to gently flex the joint. The skin overlying the medial aspect of the knee joint is prepared with antiseptic solution. A sterile syringe containing the 2.0 mL of 0.25% preservative-free bupivacaine and 40 mg of methylprednisolone is attached to a 1.5-inch 25-gauge needle with strict aseptic technique. The superior margin of the medial patella is identified. Just above this point, the needle is inserted horizontally to slide just beneath the quadriceps tendon (**Fig. 112.5**). If the needle strikes the femur, it is then withdrawn slightly and redirected in a more anterior trajectory. When the needle is in position just below the quadriceps tendon, the contents of the syringe are then gently injected. Little resistance to injection should occur. If resistance is encountered, the needle is probably in a ligament or tendon and should be advanced or withdrawn slightly until the injection proceeds without significant resistance. The needle is then removed, and a sterile pressure

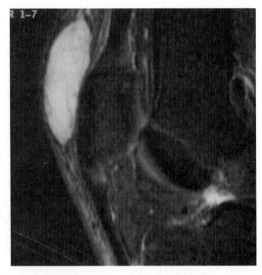

Fig. 112.6 **Prepatellar bursitis.** A sagittal short tau inversion recovery (TR/TE, 5300/30; inversion time, 150 ms) magnetic resonance imaging scan shows fluid and synovial tissue in the prepatellar bursa. *(From Resnick D, editor: Diagnosis of bone and joint disorders, ed 4, Philadelphia, 2002, Saunders, p 4257.)*

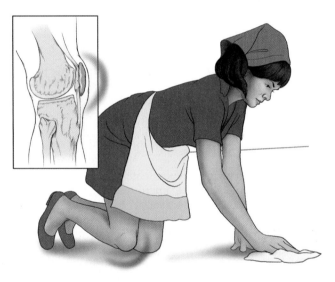

Fig. 112.7 Prepatellar bursitis is also known as housemaid's knee because of its prevalence in people whose work requires prolonged crawling or kneeling. *(From Waldman SD: Atlas of common pain syndromes, ed 2, Philadelphia, 2008, Saunders, p 312.)*

Diagnosis

Plain radiographs of the knee may reveal calcification of the bursa and associated structures, including the quadriceps tendon consistent with chronic inflammation. MRI is indicated if internal derangement, occult mass, or tumor of the knee is suspected. Electromyography helps distinguish prepatellar bursitis from femoral neuropathy, lumbar radiculopathy, and plexopathy. The injection technique described in the section on treatment serves as a diagnostic and therapeutic maneuver. Testing for antinuclear antibody is indicated if collagen vascular disease is suspected. If infection is considered, aspiration, Gram stain, and culture of bursal fluid are indicated on an emergent basis.

Differential Diagnosis

Because of the unique anatomy of the region, not only the prepatellar bursa but also the associated tendons and other bursae of the knee can become inflamed and confuse the diagnosis. The prepatellar bursa lies between the subcutaneous tissues and the patella. The bursa is held in place by the ligamentum patellae. Both the quadriceps tendon and the prepatellar bursa are subject to the development of inflammation after overuse, misuse, or direct trauma. The quadriceps tendon is made up of fibers from the four muscles that comprise the quadriceps muscle: the vastus lateralis, the vastus intermedius, the vastus medialis, and the rectus femoris. These muscles are the primary extensors of the lower extremity at the knee. The tendons of these muscles converge and unite to form a single, exceedingly strong tendon. The patella functions as a sesamoid bone within the quadriceps tendon, with fibers of the tendon extending around the patella forming the medial and lateral patella retinacula, which help strengthen the knee joint. These fibers are called expansions and are subject to strain, and the tendon proper is subject to the development of tendinitis. The suprapatellar, infrapatellar, and prepatellar bursae may also concurrently become inflamed with dysfunction of the quadriceps tendon. Remember that anything that alters the normal biomechanics of the knee can result in inflammation of the prepatellar bursa.

Treatment

A short course of conservative therapy consisting of simple analgesics, NSAIDs, or COX-2 inhibitors and use of a knee brace to prevent further trauma is a reasonable first step in the treatment of patients with prepatellar bursitis. If the patient does not have rapid improvement, the following injection technique is a reasonable next step.[5] The patient is placed supine with a rolled blanket underneath the knee to gently flex the joint. The skin overlying the patella is prepared with antiseptic solution. A sterile syringe containing the 2.0 mL of 0.25% preservative-free bupivacaine and 40 mg of methylprednisolone is attached to a 1.5-inch 25-gauge needle with strict aseptic technique. Then the center of the medial patella is identified (**Fig. 112.8**). Just above this point, the needle is inserted horizontally to slide subcutaneously into the prepatellar bursa. If the needle strikes the patella, it is then withdrawn slightly and redirected in a more anterior trajectory. When the needle is in position in proximity to the prepatellar bursa, the contents of the syringe are then gently injected. Little resistance to injection should occur. If resistance is encountered, the needle is probably in a ligament or tendon and should be advanced or withdrawn slightly until the injection proceeds without significant resistance. The needle is then removed, and a sterile pressure dressing and ice pack are placed at the injection site.

Complications and Pitfalls

Failure to identify primary or metastatic distal femur or joint disease that is responsible for the patient's pain may yield disastrous results. The major complication of this injection technique is infection. This complication should be exceedingly rare if strict aseptic technique is adhered to. Approximately 25% of patients have a transient increase in pain after injection of the suprapatellar bursa of the knee; patients should

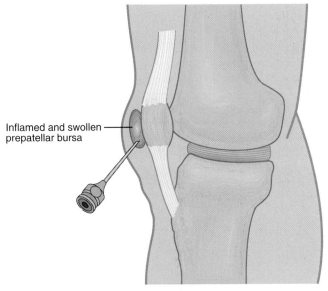

Inflamed and swollen prepatellar bursa

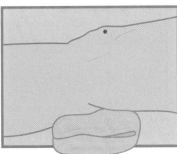

Fig. 112.8 **Injection technique for relief of the pain from prepatellar bursitis.** *(From Waldman SD: Atlas of pain management injection techniques, ed 2, Philadelphia, 2007, Saunders, p 455.)*

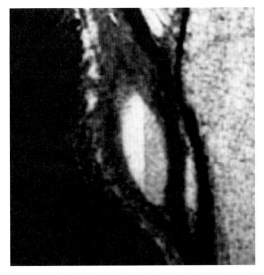

Fig. 112.9 **Superficial infrapatellar bursitis.** A fluid level within the bursa is evident on a sagittal fast spin echo (TR/TE, 2600/22) magnetic resonance imaging. *(From Resnick D, editor: Diagnosis of bone and joint disorders, ed 4, Philadelphia, 2002, Saunders, p 4257.)*

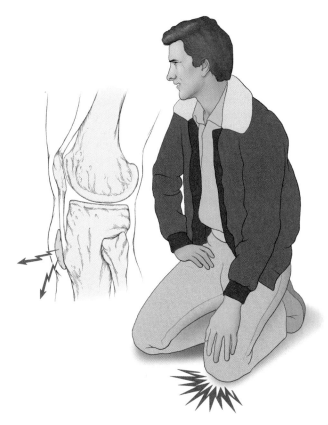

Fig. 112.10 Superficial infrapatellar bursitis is a common cause of inferior knee pain. *(From Waldman SD: Atlas of common pain syndromes, ed 2, Philadelphia, 2008, Saunders, p 314.)*

be warned of such. The use of physical modalities including local heat and gentle range-of-motion exercises should be introduced several days after the patient undergoes this injection technique for prepatellar bursitis pain. Vigorous exercises should be avoided because they exacerbate the patient's symptoms.

Superficial Infrapatellar Bursitis

The superficial infrapatellar bursa is vulnerable to injury from both acute trauma and repeated microtrauma. The superficial infrapatellar bursa lies between the subcutaneous tissues and the upper part of the ligamentum patellae (**Fig. 112.9**).[1] The deep infrapatellar bursa lies between the ligamentum patellae and the tibia. These bursae may exist as single bursal sacs or, in some patients, as a multisegmented series of sacs that may be loculated. Acute injuries frequently take the form of direct trauma to the bursa from falls directly onto the knee or from patellar fractures and from overuse injuries, including running on soft or uneven surfaces and break dancing.[1,10] Superficial infrapatellar bursitis may also result from jobs that require crawling on the knees, such as laying carpet or scrubbing floors (**Fig. 112.10**). If the inflammation of the superficial infrapatellar bursa becomes chronic, calcification of the bursa may occur.

Clinical Presentation

The patient with superficial infrapatellar bursitis frequently has pain and swelling in the anterior knee over the patella that can radiate superiorly and inferiorly into the area surrounding the knee.[10] Often, the patient is unable to kneel or walk down stairs. The patient may also have a sharp, catching sensation with range of motion of the knee, especially on first arising.

Superficial infrapatellar bursitis often coexists with arthritis and tendinitis of the knee joint, and these other pathologic processes may confuse the clinical picture.

Diagnosis

Plain radiographs of the knee may reveal calcification of the bursa and associated structures, including the quadriceps tendon consistent with chronic inflammation. MRI is indicated if internal derangement, occult mass, or tumor of the knee is suspected. Electromyography helps distinguish superficial infrapatellar bursitis from femoral neuropathy, lumbar radiculopathy, and plexopathy. The injection technique described in the section on treatment serves as a diagnostic and therapeutic maneuver. Testing for antinuclear antibody is indicated if collagen vascular disease is suspected. If infection is considered, aspiration, Gram stain, and culture of bursal fluid are indicated on an emergent basis.

Differential Diagnosis

Because of the unique anatomy of the region, not only the superficial infrapatellar bursa but also the associated tendons and other bursae of the knee can become inflamed and confuse the diagnosis. Both the quadriceps tendon and the superficial infrapatellar bursa are subject to the development of inflammation after overuse, misuse, or direct trauma. The quadriceps tendon is made up of fibers from the four muscles that comprise the quadriceps muscle: the vastus lateralis, the vastus intermedius, the vastus medialis, and the rectus femoris. These muscles are the primary extensors of the lower extremity at the knee. The tendons of these muscles converge and unite to form a single, exceedingly strong tendon. The patella functions as a sesamoid bone within the quadriceps tendon, with fibers of the tendon extending around the patella forming the medial and lateral patella retinacula, which help strengthen the knee joint. These fibers are called expansions and are subject to strain, and the tendon proper is subject to the development of tendinitis. The suprapatellar, infrapatellar, and superficial infrapatellar bursae may also concurrently become inflamed with dysfunction of the quadriceps tendon. Remember that anything that alters the normal biomechanics of the knee can result in inflammation of the superficial infrapatellar bursa.

Treatment

A short course of conservative therapy consisting of simple analgesics, NSAIDs, or COX-2 inhibitors and use of a knee brace to prevent further trauma is a reasonable first step in the treatment of patients with superficial infrapatellar bursitis. If the patient does not have rapid improvement, the following injection technique is a reasonable next step.[11] For injection of the superficial infrapatellar bursa, the patient is placed in the supine position with a rolled blanket underneath the knee to gently flex the joint. The skin overlying the patella is prepared with antiseptic solution. A sterile syringe containing 2.0 mL of 0.25% preservative-free bupivacaine and 40 mg of methylprednisolone is attached to a 1.5-inch 25-gauge needle with strict aseptic technique. The center of the lower pole of the patella is identified. Just below this point, the needle is inserted at a 45-degree angle to slide subcutaneously into the superficial infrapatellar bursa (**Fig. 112.11**). If the needle strikes the

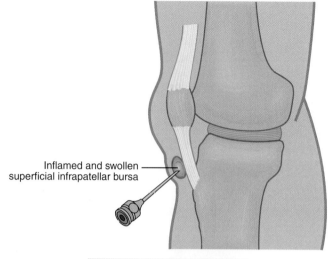

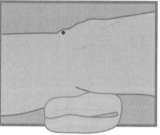

Inflamed and swollen superficial infrapatellar bursa

Fig. 112.11 Injection technique for relief of the pain from infrapatellar bursitis. *(From Waldman SD:* Atlas of pain management injection techniques, *ed 2, Philadelphia, 2007, Saunders, p 459.)*

patella, it is then withdrawn slightly and redirected in a more inferior trajectory. When the needle is in position in proximity to the superficial infrapatellar bursa, the contents of the syringe are then gently injected. Little resistance to injection should occur. If resistance is encountered, the needle is probably in a ligament or tendon and should be advanced or withdrawn slightly until the injection proceeds without significant resistance. The needle is then removed, and a sterile pressure dressing and ice pack are placed at the injection site. The use of physical modalities including local heat and gentle range-of-motion exercises should be introduced several days after the patient undergoes this injection technique for prepatellar bursitis pain. Vigorous exercises should be avoided because they exacerbate the patient's symptoms.

Pes Anserine Bursitis

The pes anserine bursa lies beneath the pes anserine tendon, which is the insertional tendon of the sartorius, gracilis, and semitendinous muscles to the medial side of the tibia (**Fig. 112.12**).[1] This bursa may exist as a single bursal sac or, in some patients, may exist as a multisegmented series of sacs that may be loculated. Patients with pes anserine bursitis present with pain over the medial knee joint and increased pain on passive valgus and external rotation of the knee (**Fig. 112.13**).[12] Activity, especially involving flexion and external rotation of the knee, makes the pain worse, with rest and heat providing some relief. Often, the patient is unable to kneel or walk down stairs.

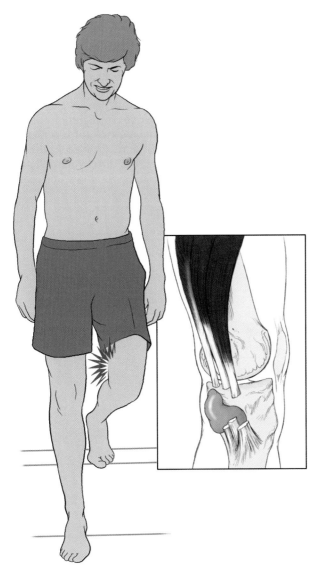

Fig. 112.12 Patients with pes anserine bursitis frequently have medial knee pain that is made worse with kneeling or walking down stairs. *(From Waldman SD: Atlas of uncommon pain syndromes, ed 2, Philadelphia, 2008, Saunders, p 290.)*

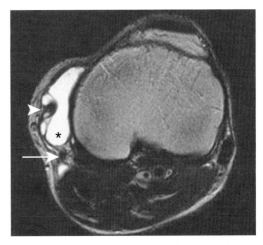

Fig. 112.13 **Pes anserine bursitis.** Axial proton density image. A homogenous high signal intensity fluid collection *(*)* is seen deep to the tendons of the pes anserinus. The tendons of sartorius *(arrowhead)* and semitendinosus *(arrow)* are visualized. *(From O'Keeffe SA, Hogan BA, Eustace SJ, et al: Overuse injuries of the knee,* Magnetic Resonance Imaging Clin North Am *17:725, 2009.)*

Clinical Presentation

The pain of pes anserine bursitis is constant and characterized as aching. The pain may interfere with sleep. Coexistent bursitis, tendinitis, arthritis, or internal derangement of the knee may confuse the clinical picture after trauma to the knee joint. Frequently, the medial collateral ligament is also involved if the patient has sustained trauma to the medial knee joint. If the inflammation of the pes anserine bursa becomes chronic, calcification of the bursa may occur.

Physical examination may reveal point tenderness in the anterior knee just below the medial knee joint at the tendinous insertion of the pes anserine.[12] Swelling and fluid accumulation surrounding the bursa are often present. Active resisted flexion of the knee reproduces the pain. Sudden release of resistance during this maneuver markedly increases the pain. Rarely, the pes anserine bursa becomes infected in a manner analogous to infection of the prepatellar bursa.

Diagnosis

Plain radiographs of the knee may reveal calcification of the bursa and associated structures, including the pes anserine tendon consistent with chronic inflammation. MRI is indicated if internal derangement, occult mass, or tumor of the knee is suspected. Electromyography helps distinguish pes anserine bursitis from neuropathy, lumbar radiculopathy, and plexopathy. The injection technique described subsequently serves as a diagnostic and therapeutic maneuver.

Differential Diagnosis

The pes anserine bursa is prone to the development of inflammation after overuse, misuse, or direct trauma. The medial collateral ligament also often is involved if the medial knee has been subjected to trauma. The medial collateral ligament is a broad, flat bandlike ligament that runs from the medial condyle of the femur to the medial aspect of the shaft of the tibia where it attaches just above the groove of the semimembranosus muscle. It also attaches to the edge of the medial semilunar cartilage. The medial collateral ligament is crossed at its lower part by the tendons of the sartorius, gracilis, and semitendinosus muscles. Because of the unique anatomic relationships of the medial knee, accurate determination of which anatomic structure is responsible for the patient's pain is often difficult on clinical grounds. MRI helps sort things out and rule out lesions such as tears of the medial meniscus that may need surgical intervention. Remember that anything that alters the normal biomechanics of the knee can result in inflammation of the pes anserine bursa.

Treatment

A short course of conservative therapy consisting of simple analgesics, NSAIDs, or COX-2 inhibitors and a knee brace to prevent further trauma is a reasonable first step in the treatment of patients with pes anserine bursitis. If the patient does not have rapid improvement, the following injection technique is a reasonable next step.[13]

For injection of the pes anserine bursa, the patient is placed in the supine position with a rolled blanket underneath the knee to gently flex the joint. The skin just below the medial knee joint is prepared with antiseptic solution. A sterile syringe containing 2.0 mL of 0.25% preservative-free bupivacaine and 40 mg of methylprednisolone is attached to a 1.5-inch, 25-gauge needle with strict aseptic technique. With strict aseptic technique, the pes anserine tendon is identified by having the patient strongly flex his or her leg against resistance. The point distal to the medial joint space at which the pes anserine tendon attaches to the tibia is the location of the pes anserine bursa. The bursa usually is identified with point tenderness at that spot. At this point, the needle is inserted at a 45-degree angle to the tibia to pass through the skin and subcutaneous tissues and into the pes anserine bursa (**Fig. 112.14**). If the needle strikes the tibia, it is then withdrawn slightly into the substance of the bursa. When the needle is in position in proximity to the pes anserine bursa, the contents of the syringe is then gently injected. Little resistance to injection should occur. If resistance is encountered, the needle is probably in a ligament or tendon and should be advanced or withdrawn slightly until the injection proceeds without significant resistance. The needle is then removed, and a sterile pressure dressing and ice pack are placed at the injection site. The use of physical modalities including local heat and gentle range-of-motion exercises should be introduced several days after the patient undergoes this injection technique for pes anserine bursitis pain. Vigorous exercises should be avoided because they exacerbate the patient's symptoms.

Deep Infrapatellar Bursitis

The deep infrapatellar bursa is vulnerable to injury from both acute trauma and repeated microtrauma. The superficial infrapatellar bursa lies between the subcutaneous tissues and the upper part of the ligamentum patellae. The deep infrapatellar bursa lies between the ligamentum patellae and the tibia (**Fig. 112.15**).[1,14] These bursae may exist as single bursal sacs or, in some patients, as a multisegmented series of sacs that may be loculated in nature. Acute injuries frequently take the form of direct trauma to the bursa via falls directly onto the knee (**Fig. 112.16**)[14] or from patellar fractures and from overuse

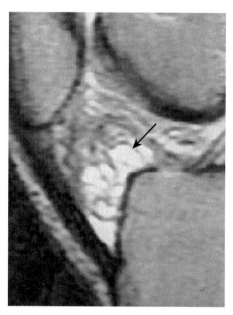

Fig. 112.15 Deep infrapatellar bursitis. Sagittal, T2-weighted, spin echo magnetic resonance imaging shows fluid of high signal intensity *(arrow)* in the deep infrapatellar bursa.

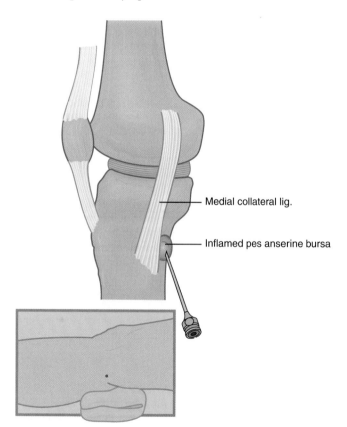

Fig. 112.14 Injection technique for relief of the pain from pes anserine bursitis. *(From Waldman SD:* Atlas of pain management injection techniques, *ed 2, Philadelphia, 2007, Saunders, p 4670.)*

Medial collateral lig.

Inflamed pes anserine bursa

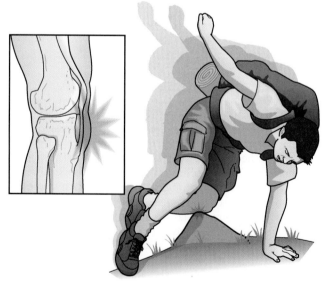

Fig. 112.16 Deep infrapatellar bursitis commonly presents as inferior knee pain accompanied by a catching sensation, especially on rising from a sitting position. *(From Waldman SD:* Atlas of common pain syndromes, *ed 2, Philadelphia, 2008, Saunders, p 316.)*

injuries, including running on soft or uneven surfaces. Deep infrapatellar bursitis may also result from jobs that require crawling and kneeling on the knees, such as carpet laying or scrubbing floors. If the inflammation of the superficial infrapatellar bursa becomes chronic, calcification of the bursa may occur.

Clinical Presentation

The patient with deep infrapatellar bursitis frequently has pain and swelling in the anterior knee below the patella that can radiate inferiorly into the area surrounding the knee. Often, the patient is unable to kneel or walk down stairs. The patient may also have a sharp, catching sensation with range of motion of the knee, especially on first arising. Infrapatellar bursitis often coexists with arthritis and tendinitis of the knee joint, and these other pathologic processes may confuse the clinical picture.

Physical examination may reveal point tenderness in the anterior knee just below the patella. Swelling and fluid accumulation surrounding the lower patella are often present. Passive flexion and active resisted extension of the knee reproduce the pain. Sudden release of resistance during this maneuver markedly increases the pain. The deep infrapatellar bursa is not as susceptible to infection as the superficial infrapatellar bursa.

Diagnosis

Plain radiographs of the knee may reveal calcification of the bursa and associated structures, including the quadriceps tendon, consistent with chronic inflammation. MRI is indicated if internal derangement, occult mass, or tumor of the knee is suspected. Electromyography helps distinguish deep and superficial infrapatellar bursitis from femoral neuropathy, lumbar radiculopathy, and plexopathy. The following injection technique serves as a diagnostic and therapeutic maneuver. Antinuclear antibody testing is indicated if collagen vascular disease is suspected. If infection is considered, aspiration, Gram stain, and culture of bursal fluid are indicated on an emergency basis.

Differential Diagnosis

Because of the unique anatomy of the region, not only the deep infrapatellar bursa but also the associated tendons and other bursae of the knee can become inflamed and confuse the diagnosis. Both the quadriceps tendon and the deep and superficial infrapatellar bursae are subject to the development of inflammation after overuse, misuse, or direct trauma. The quadriceps tendon is made up of fibers from the four muscles that compose the quadriceps muscle: the vastus lateralis, the vastus intermedius, the vastus medialis, and the rectus femoris. These muscles are the primary extensors of the lower extremity at the knee. The tendons of these muscles converge and unite to form a single exceedingly strong tendon. The patella functions as a sesamoid bone within the quadriceps tendon, with fibers of the tendon expanding around the patella to form the medial and lateral patella retinacula, which help strengthen the knee joint. These fibers are called expansions and are vulnerable to strain, and the tendon proper is subject to the

development of tendinitis. The suprapatellar, prepatellar, and superficial infrapatellar bursae may also concurrently become inflamed with dysfunction of the quadriceps tendon. Remember that anything that alters the normal biomechanics of the knee can result in inflammation of the deep infrapatellar bursa.

Treatment

A short course of conservative therapy consisting of simple analgesics, NSAIDs, or COX-2 inhibitors and a knee brace to prevent further trauma is a reasonable first step in the treatment of patients with deep infrapatellar bursitis. If the patient does not have rapid improvement, the following injection technique is a reasonable next step.[15]

For injection of the deep infrapatellar bursa, the patient is placed in the supine position with a rolled blanket underneath the knee to gently flex the joint. The skin overlying the medial portion of the lower margin of the patella is prepared with antiseptic solution. A sterile syringe containing 2.0 mL of 0.25% preservative-free bupivacaine and 40 mg methylprednisolone is attached to a 1.5-inch 25-gauge needle with strict aseptic technique. With strict aseptic technique, the medial lower margin of the patella is identified. Just below this point, the needle is inserted at a right angle to the patella to slide beneath the ligamentum patellar into the deep infrapatellar bursa. If the needle strikes the patella, it is then withdrawn slightly and redirected in a more inferior trajectory. When the needle is in position in proximity to the deep infrapatellar bursa, the contents of the syringe are then gently injected. Little resistance to injection should occur. If resistance is encountered, the needle is probably in a ligament or tendon and should be advanced or withdrawn slightly until the injection proceeds without significant resistance. The needle is then removed, and a sterile pressure dressing and ice pack are placed at the injection site.

Complications and Pitfalls in the Treatment of Bursitis of the Knee

Coexistent bursitis, tendinitis, arthritis, and internal derangement of the knee may also contribute to the patient's pain and may necessitate additional treatment. The simple analgesics and NSAIDs are a reasonable starting place in the treatment of bursitis of the knee. If these agents are ineffective, the injection of the inflamed bursa with a local anesthetic and corticosteroid is a reasonable next step. The previously described injection techniques are generally safe procedures if careful attention is paid to the clinically relevant anatomy in the areas to be injected. The use of physical modalities including local heat and gentle range-of-motion exercises should be introduced several days after the patient undergoes the injection techniques. Vigorous exercises should be avoided because they exacerbate the patient's symptoms. The clinician should remember that failure to identify infection or primary or metastatic tumors of the distal femur, joint, or proximal tibia and fibula that may be responsible for the patient's pain may yield disastrous results (**Fig. 112.17**).[16]

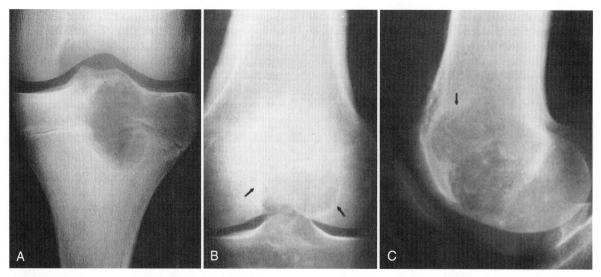

Fig. 112.17 Chondroblastoma: radiographic abnormalities of long tubular bones. A, Tibia. Note the radiolucent lesion involving the metaphysis and epiphysis of the proximal portion of the tibia. **B** and **C,** Frontal and lateral radiographs of the femur in a 22-year-old man show a large epiphyseal and metaphyseal lesion *(arrows)* that contains foci of calcification. An unusual degree of periostitis is apparent in the metaphysis and diaphysis. *(From Resnick D, editor:* Diagnosis of bone and joint disorders, *ed 4, Philadelphia, 2002, Saunders, p 3856.)*

References

Full references for this chapter can be found on www.expertconsult.com.

Baker's Cyst of the Knee

Steven D. Waldman

A common cause of knee pain, Baker's cyst is the result of an abnormal accumulation of synovial fluid in the medial aspect of the popliteal fossa.[1] Overproduction of synovial fluid from the knee joint results in the formation of a cystic sac. This sac often communicates with the knee joint with a one-way valve effect, causing a gradual expansion of the cyst.[2] Often a tear of the medial meniscus or a tendinitis of the medial hamstring tendon is the inciting factor responsible for the development of Baker's cyst.[3] Patients with rheumatoid arthritis are especially susceptible to the development of Baker's cysts.[4]

Clinical Presentation

Patients with Baker's cysts have a feeling of fullness behind the knee.[5] Often, they notice a lump behind the knee that becomes more apparent when they flex the affected knee (**Fig. 113.1**).[1,5] The cyst may continue to enlarge and may dissect inferiorly into the calf (**Fig. 113.2**).[6] Occasionally, the dissection may be so significant as to cause a lower extremity compartment syndrome.[7] Patients with rheumatoid arthritis are prone to this phenomenon.[4] The pain associated with dissection into the calf may be confused with thrombophlebitis and inappropriately treated with anticoagulants.[8,9] The pain of ruptured Baker's cyst that has been misdiagnosed as thrombophlebitis has been called pseudothrombophlebitis.

On physical examination, the patient with Baker's cyst has a cystic swelling in the medial aspect of the popliteal fossa. Baker's cysts can become quite large, especially in patients with rheumatoid arthritis. Activity, including squatting or walking, makes the pain of Baker's cyst worse; rest and heat provide some relief. The pain is constant, is characterized as aching, and may interfere with sleep. Baker's cyst may spontaneously rupture, and rubor and color in the calf may mimic thrombophlebitis.[7,8] Homan's sign is negative, and no cords are palpable.

Diagnosis

Plain radiographs are indicated in all patients who present with Baker's cyst. Ultrasound scan aids in diagnosis in patients whose body habitus makes accurate palpation of the popliteal fossa difficult (**Fig. 113.3**). On the basis of the patient's clinical presentation, additional testing may be indicated, including complete blood cell count, erythrocyte sedimentation rate, and antinuclear antibody testing. Magnetic resonance imaging (MRI) of the knee is indicated

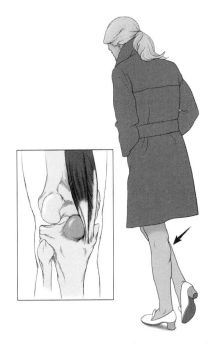

Fig. 113.1 The patient with Baker's cyst often has a sensation of fullness or a lump behind the knee. *(From Waldman SD:* Atlas of common pain syndromes, *ed 2, Philadelphia, 2008, Saunders, p 319.)*

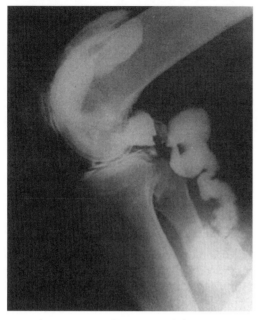

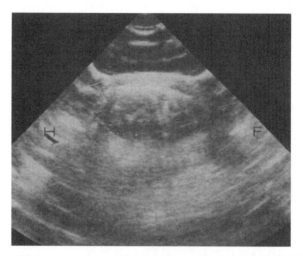

Fig. 113.3 Ultrasound scan of popliteal fossa. Baker's cyst is marked. No evidence of rupture is seen, although it contains debris. *H*, Head; *F*, feet. *(From Chaudhuri R, Salari R: Baker's cyst simulating deep vein thrombosis,* Clin Radiol *41:400, 1990.)*

Fig. 113.2 **Arthrogram revealing a typical downward rupture of Baker's cyst.** *(From Chaudhuri R, Salari R: Baker's cyst simulating deep vein thrombosis,* Clin Radiol *41:400, 1990.)*

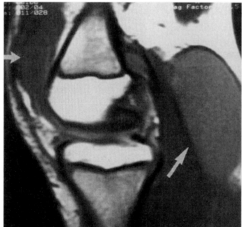

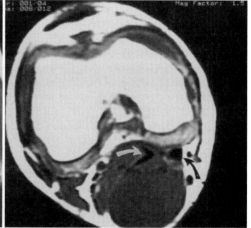

Fig. 113.4 Magnetic resonance imaging of the knee is useful in confirming the presence of Baker's cyst. *(From Haaga JR, Lanzieri CF, Gilkeson RC:* CT and MR imaging of the whole body, *ed 4, Philadelphia, 2003, Mosby, p 1808.)*

if internal derangement or occult mass or tumor is suspected and is also useful in confirming the presence of Baker's cyst (**Fig. 113.4**).

Differential Diagnosis

As mentioned previously, Baker's cyst may rupture spontaneously and may be misdiagnosed as thrombophlebitis. Occasionally, tendinitis of the medial hamstring tendon may be confused with Baker's cyst, as may injury to the medial meniscus. Primary or metastatic tumors in the region, although rare, must be considered in the differential diagnosis (**Fig. 113.5**).

Treatment

Although surgery is often necessary to successfully treat Baker's cyst, conservative therapy consisting of an elastic bandage combined with a short trial of nonsteroidal anti-inflammatory

drugs or cyclooxygenase-2 inhibitors is warranted. If these conservative treatments fail, the following injection technique represents a reasonable next step.[10]

For injection of a Baker's cyst, the patient is placed in the prone position with the anterior ankle resting on a folded towel to slightly flex the knee. The middle of the popliteal fossa is identified, and at a point 2 fingers' breath medial and two fingersbreath below the popliteal crease, the skin is prepped with antiseptic solution. A syringe containing 2.0 mL of 0.25% preservative-free bupivacaine and 40 mg of methylprednisolone is attached to a 2-inch, 22-gauge needle.

The needle is then carefully advanced through the previously identified point at a 45-degree angle from the medial border of the popliteal fossa directly toward the Baker's cyst (**Fig. 113.6**). With continuous aspiration, the needle is advanced very slowly to avoid trauma to the tibial nerve or popliteal artery or vein. When the cyst is entered, synovial fluid suddenly is aspirated into the syringe. At this point, if is no paresthesia is elicited in

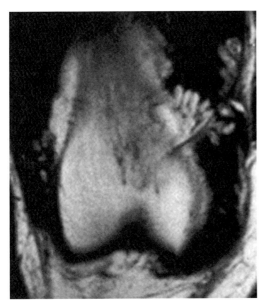

Fig. 113.5 Lipoma arborescens. Magnetic resonance image showing diffuse fatty infiltration of the synovium. *(From: Nielsen GP, O-Connell JX: Tumors of synovial tissue bone and soft tissue pathology, Philadelphia, 2010, Saunders, pp 255–275.)*

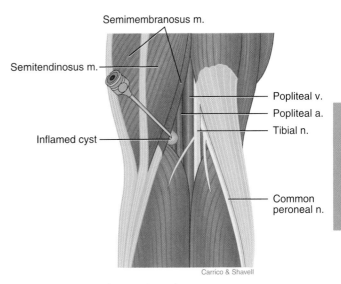

Fig. 113.6 Technique for injecting Baker's cyst. *(From Waldman SD: Atlas of pain management injection techniques, ed 2, Philadelphia, 2007, Saunders, p 485.)*

the distribution of the common peroneal or tibial nerve, the contents of the syringe are then gently injected. Minimal resistance to injection should be felt. A pressure dressing is then placed over the cyst to prevent reaccumulation of fluid.

Failure to diagnose primary knee pathology (e.g., tears of the medial meniscus) may lead to further pain and disability. MRI should help in identification of internal derangement of the knee. The proximity to the common peroneal and tibial nerves and to the popliteal artery and vein makes it imperative that this procedure be carried out only by those well versed in the regional anatomy and experienced in performing injection techniques. Many patients also have a transient increase in pain after this injection technique. Although rare, infection may occur if careful attention to sterile technique is not followed.

Conclusion

When bursae become inflamed, they may overproduce synovial fluid, which can become trapped in saclike cysts as a result of a one-way valve phenomenon. This occurs commonly in the medial aspect of the popliteal fossa and is called Baker's cyst. The injection technique described is extremely effective in the treatment of pain and swelling from this disorder. Coexistent semimembranosus bursitis, medial hamstring tendinitis, or internal derangement of the knee may also contribute to knee pain and may necessitate additional treatment with more localized injection of local anesthetic and depot corticosteroid.

References

Full references for this chapter can be found on www.expertconsult.com.

Chapter 114

Quadriceps Expansion Syndrome

Steven D. Waldman

The quadriceps expansion syndrome is an uncommon cause of anterior knee pain encountered in clinical practice. This painful condition is characterized by pain at the superior pole of the patella.[1] It is usually the result of overuse or misuse of the knee joint, such as running marathons or direct trauma to the quadriceps tendon from kicks or head butts during football. The quadriceps tendon is also subject to acute calcific tendinitis, which may coexist with acute strain injuries. Calcific tendinitis of the quadriceps tendon has a characteristic radiographic appearance of whiskers on the anterosuperior patella.

The quadriceps tendon is made up of fibers from the four muscles that comprise the quadriceps muscle: the vastus lateralis, the vastus intermedius, the vastus medialis, and the rectus femoris (**Fig. 114.1**). Fibers of the quadriceps tendon expanding around the patella form the medial and lateral patella retinacula, which help strengthen the knee joint. These fibers are called expansions and are subject to strain, and the tendon proper is subject to the development of tendinitis.

Patients with quadriceps expansion syndrome present with pain over the superior pole of the sesamoid, more commonly on the medial side. The patient notes increased pain on walking down slopes or down stairs (**Fig. 114.2**). Activity of the knee makes the pain worse; rest and heat provide some relief. The pain is constant, is characterized as aching, and may interfere with sleep.

Clinical Presentation

On physical examination, patients with quadriceps expansion syndrome have tenderness under the superior edge of the patella that occurs more commonly on the medial side.[2] Patients exhibit a positive knee extension test on active resisted extension of the knee that reproduces the pain (**Fig. 114.3**). Coexistent suprapatellar and infrapatellar bursitis, tendinitis, arthritis, or internal derangement of the knee may confuse the clinical picture after trauma to the knee joint.[3]

Diagnosis

Plain radiographs of the knee are indicated in all patients who present with quadriceps expansion syndrome pain. On the basis of the patient's clinical presentation, additional testing may be indicated, including complete blood cell count, erythrocyte sedimentation rate, and antinuclear antibody testing. Magnetic resonance imaging (MRI) of the knee is indicated if tendinosis, tendon rupture, internal derangement, or occult mass or tumor is suspected (**Fig. 114.4**). Ultrasound scan may be useful in identification of disruption of the quadriceps tendon (**Fig. 114.5**). Bone scan may be useful in identification of occult stress fractures that involve the joint, especially if trauma has occurred.

Differential Diagnosis

The most common cause of anterior knee pain is arthritis of the knee. This should be readily identifiable on plain radiographs of the knee and may coexist with quadriceps expansion syndrome. Another common cause of anterior knee pain that may mimic or coexist with quadriceps expansion syndrome is suprapatellar or prepatellar bursitis.[3] Internal derangement of the knee and a torn medial meniscus may also confuse the clinical diagnosis but should be readily identifiable on MRI of the knee.

Treatment

Initial treatment of the pain and functional disability associated with quadriceps insertion syndrome should include a combination of the nonsteroidal anti-inflammatory agents or cyclooxygenase-2 inhibitors and physical therapy. Local application of heat and cold may also be beneficial. For patients who do not respond to these treatment modalities, injection of the quadriceps expansion, as described subsequently, with a local anesthetic and a corticosteroid may be a reasonable next step.[4]

For injection of the quadriceps expansion, the patient is placed supine with a rolled blanket underneath the knee to gently flex the joint. The skin overlying the medial aspect of the knee joint is prepped with antiseptic solution. A sterile syringe containing the 2.0 mL of 0.25% preservative-free bupivacaine and 40 mg of methylprednisolone is attached to a 1.5-inch 25-gauge needle with strict aseptic technique. The medial edge of the superior patella is identified (**Fig. 114.6**). At this point, the needle is inserted horizontally toward the medial edge of

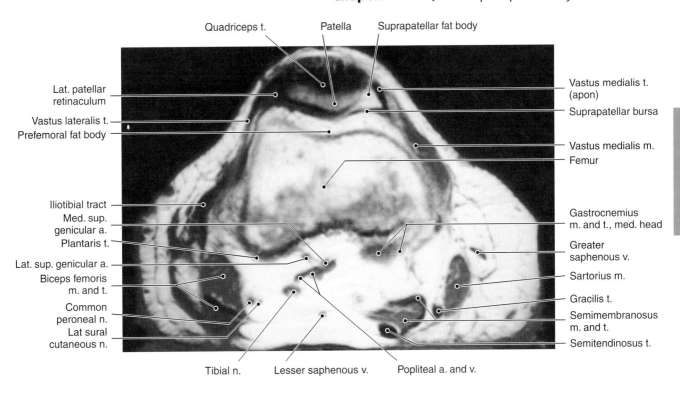

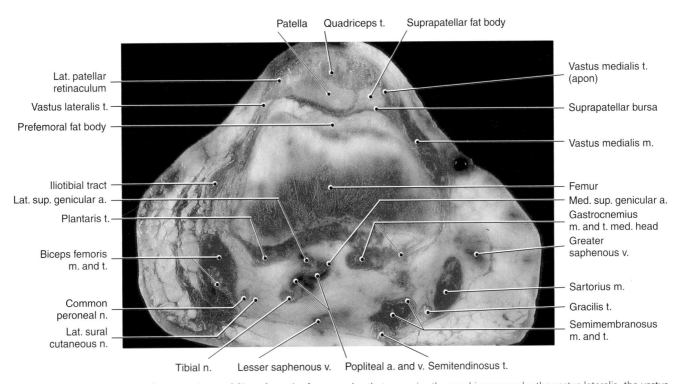

Fig. 114.1 The quadriceps tendon is made up of fibers from the four muscles that comprise the quadriceps muscle: the vastus lateralis, the vastus intermedius, the vastus medialis, and the rectus femoris. *(From Kang HS, Ahn JM, Resnick D, et al, editors: MRI of the extremities, ed 2, Philadelphia, 2002, Saunders, p 315.)*

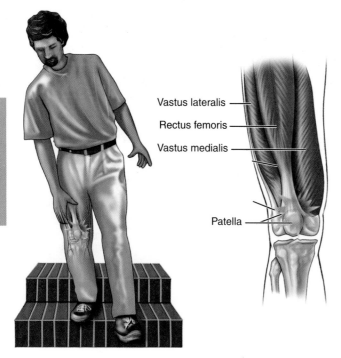

Fig. 114.2 Patients with quadriceps expansion syndrome present with pain over the superior pole of the sesamoid, more commonly on the medial side. *(From Waldman SD: Atlas of uncommon pain syndromes, Philadelphia, 2003, Saunders, p 216.)*

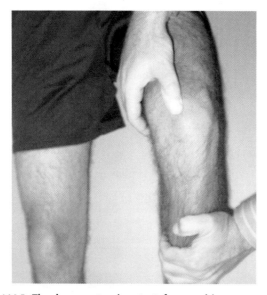

Fig. 114.3 **The knee extension test for quadriceps expansion syndrome.** *(From Waldman SD: Physical diagnosis of pain: an atlas of signs and symptoms, Philadelphia, 2010, Saunders.)*

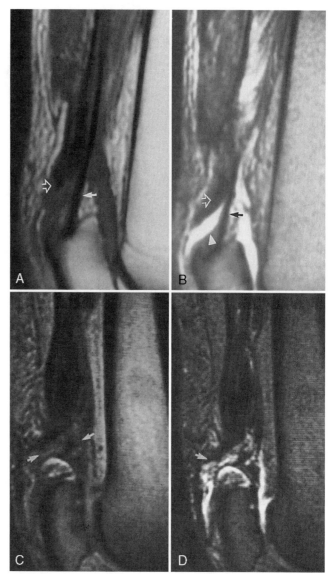

Fig. 114.4 **Partial and complete tears of the quadriceps tendon.** A and B, Partial tear. Sagittal intermediate-weighted (TR/TE, 2500/20; A) and T2-weighted (TR/TE, 2500/80; B) spin-echo magnetic resonance images (MRIs) show disruption of the normal trilaminar appearance of the quadriceps tendon. The tendon *(solid arrows)* of the vastus intermedius muscle appears intact. The other tendons have retracted *(open arrows).* Note the high signal intensity at the site of the tear *(arrowhead)* and in the soft tissues and muscles in B. C and D, Complete tear. Sagittal intermediate-weighted (TR/TE, 2500/30; C) and T2-weighted (TR/TE, 2500/80; D) spin-echo MRIs show a complete tear *(arrows)* of the quadriceps tendon at the tendo-osseous junction. Note the high signal intensity at the site of the tear in D. The patella is displaced inferiorly. *(From Resnick D, editor: Diagnosis of bone and joint disorders, ed 4, Philadelphia, 2002, Saunders, p 3229.)*

the patella. The needle is then carefully advanced through the skin and subcutaneous tissues until it impinges on the medial edge of the patella. The needle is withdrawn slightly out of the periosteum of the patella, and the contents of the syringe are then gently injected. Little resistance to injection should

be felt. If resistance is encountered, the needle is probably in a ligament or tendon and should be advanced or withdrawn slightly until the injection proceeds without significant resistance. The needle is then removed and a sterile pressure dressing and ice pack are placed at the injection site.

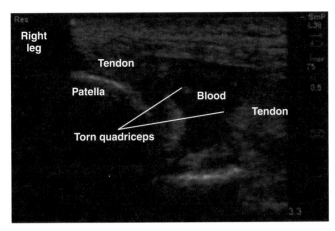

Fig. 114.5 Two-dimensional ultrasound scan of patient's right knee showing disrupted quadriceps tendon and an acute bleed. *(From LaRocco BG, Zlupko G, Sierzenski P:* Ultrasound diagnosis of quadriceps tendon rupture, *J Emerg Med 35:293, 2008.)*

The major complication of this injection technique is infection. This complication should be exceedingly rare if strict aseptic technique is adhered to. Approximately 25% of patients have a transient increase in pain after injection of the quadriceps tendon of the knee; patients should be warned of such. The clinician should also identify coexisting internal derangement of the knee, primary and metastatic tumors, and infection, which if undiagnosed may yield disastrous results.

References

Full references for this chapter can be found on www.expertconsult.com.

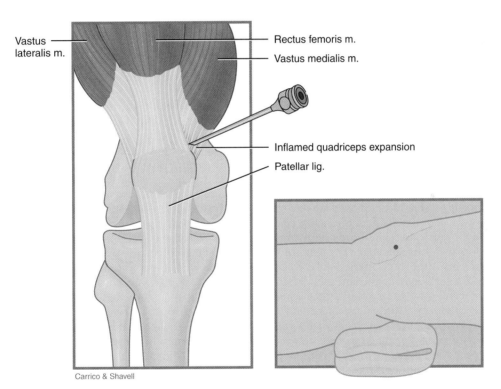

Fig. 114.6 Injection technique for relieving the pain from quadriceps expansion syndrome. *(From Waldman SD:* Atlas of pain management injection techniques, *Philadelphia, 2000, Saunders, p 266.)*

Chapter **115**

Arthritis of the Ankle and Foot

Saima Chohan

The foot and the ankle have many functions, providing a base for standing, a lever for forward propulsion, and a shock absorber for the body's weight. The ankle is probably the most commonly injured joint in athletics because of the forces it withstands and the mass it supports. Painful disorders of the ankle and foot are a common presentation in general, rheumatologic, and orthopedic practices. The pain may arise from the bones and joints of the ankle and foot, periarticular structures (tendon sheaths, tendon insertions, or bursae), plantar fascia, nerve roots and peripheral nerves, or vascular system or be referred from the lumbar spine or knee joint.[1,2] A classification of painful disorders of the ankle and foot, based on the site of origin and predominant location of the pain, is outlined in **Table 115.1**. Static disorders from inappropriate footwear, foot deformities, and weak intrinsic muscles account for most painful foot conditions. Precise diagnosis depends on knowledge of anatomy, a detailed history, and an assessment of the joints, periarticular soft tissue structures, nerve and blood supply, and lumbar spine. Diagnostic studies include routine laboratory tests, synovial fluid analysis, nerve conduction studies, vascular (Doppler) studies, bone scintiscan, sonography, plain radiographs, computed tomographic (CT) scan, and magnetic resonance imaging (MRI). Special radiographic views, arthrography, arteriography, gait analysis, and footprint studies are occasionally necessary.[1,2]

Etiology and Clinical Presentation

The main causes of arthritis of the ankle and subtalar and other joints of the foot include rheumatoid arthritis, psoriatic arthritis, gout, trauma, and osteoarthritis.

The foot and ankle can be viewed in three functional parts: forefoot (metatarsal bones, sesamoids, and phalanges), midfoot (navicular, cuboid, and three cuneiform bones), and hindfoot (talus and calcaneus). Similarly, the foot has four major joints: ankle, subtalar, midtarsal, and midfoot.

The ankle or talocrural joint (mortise) is a hinge joint between the distal ends of the tibia and fibula and the trochlea of the talus that provides plantarflexion and dorsiflexion movement. The synovial cavity does not normally communicate with other joints, adjacent tendon sheaths, or bursae. Tendons that cross the ankle region are invested for part of their course in tenosynovial sheaths (**Figs. 115.1 and 115.2**). Posteriorly, the common tendon of the gastrocnemius and soleus (Achilles tendon) is inserted into the posterior surface of the calcaneus.[1-3] The retrocalcaneal bursa is located between the Achilles tendon insertion and the posterior surface of the calcaneus. It is surrounded anteriorly by Kager's fat pad. The bursa serves to protect the distal Achilles tendon from frictional wear against the posterior calcaneus. The retroachilleal bursa lies between the skin and the Achilles tendon and protects the tendon from external pressure. The subcalcaneal bursa is located beneath the skin over the plantar aspect of the calcaneus. Two bursae, the medial and lateral subcutaneous malleolar or "last" bursae, are located near the medial and lateral malleoli, respectively (see Figs. 115.1 and 115.2).[1,3]

The subtalar (talocalcaneal) joint lies between the talus and the calcaneus. It permits about 30 degrees of foot inversion (sole of the foot turned inward) and 10 to 20 degrees of eversion (sole turned outward). Subtalar arthritis is associated with painful restriction of inversion and eversion, diffuse swelling, and tenderness in the subtalar region, but direct palpation of the joint is difficult.

The midtarsal (transverse tarsal) joint comprises the combined talonavicular and calcaneocuboid joints and serves to demarcate the hindfoot from the midfoot.[1,3] The cuboid and navicular are usually joined by fibrous tissue, but a synovial cavity may exist between them. The midtarsal joint contributes to inversion (supination) and eversion (pronation) movements at the subtalar joint. It also allows 20 degrees of adduction (foot turned toward the midline) and 10 degrees of abduction (foot turned away from the midline). Arthritis of the transverse tarsal joint is associated with painful restriction of inversion and eversion, diffuse tenderness, and swelling of the midtarsal region. The midfoot joint provides stability to the body.

The other smaller joints in the foot include the intertarsal joints, the metatarsophalangeal (MTP) joints, and the interphalangeal joints. The intertarsal joints are plane gliding joints

Table 115.1 Painful Disorders of the Ankle and the Foot

Type	Example
Articular	Rheumatoid arthritis, osteoarthritis, psoriatic arthritis, gout
Toe disorders	Hallux valgus, hallux rigidus, hammertoe
Arch disorders	Pes planus, pes cavus
Periarticular	Corn, callosity
Cutaneous	Rheumatoid arthritis nodules, gouty tophi
Subcutaneous	Ingrown toenail
Plantar fascia	Plantar fasciitis Plantar nodular fibromatosis
Tendons	Achilles tendinitis Achilles tendon rupture Tibialis posterior tenosynovitis Peroneal tenosynovitis
Bursae	Bunion, bunionette Retrocalcaneal and retroachilleal bursitis Medial and lateral malleolar bursitis Hydroxyapatite pseudopodagra (first metatarsophalangeal joint)
Osseous	Fracture (traumatic and stress) Sesamoiditis Neoplasm Infection Epiphysitis (osteochondritis) Second metatarsal head (Frieberg's disease) Navicular (Kohler's disease) Calcaneus (Sever's disease) Painful accessory ossicles Accessory navicular Os trigonum (near talus) Os intermetatarseum (first to second)
Neurologic	Tarsal tunnel syndrome Interdigital (Morton's) neuroma Peripheral neuropathy Radiculopathy (lumbar disc)
Vascular	Ischemic (atherosclerosis, Buerger's disease) Vasospastic disorder (Raynaud's phenomenon) Cholesterol emboli
Referred	Lumbosacral spine Knee Reflex sympathetic dystrophy syndrome

between the navicular, cuneiforms, and cuboid that intercommunicate with one another and with the intermetatarsal and tarsometatarsal joints. The MTP joints are ellipsoid joints lined by separate synovial cavities. They lie about 2 cm proximal to the webs of the toes.[1] The transverse metatarsal ligament binds the metatarsal heads together, preventing excessive splaying of the forefoot. The intermetatarsophalangeal bursae are frequently present between the metatarsal heads. Chronic arthritis of the MTP joints is characterized by local tenderness, swelling, synovial thickening, and a painful metatarsal compression test (pain on gentle compression of the metatarsal heads together with one hand). Forefoot splaying or spread, from weakness of the transverse metatarsal ligaments, and

toe deformities are frequent. A bursa (bunion) is commonly located over the medial aspect of the first MTP joint. Less frequently, a small bursa is present over the lateral aspect of the fifth metatarsal head (bunionette or tailor's bursa). The proximal and distal interphalangeal (PIP and DIP) joints are hinge joints.[1] The digital flexor tendon sheaths enclose the long and short flexor tendons, extending proximally along the length of the toes to the distal third of the sole. Arthritis of the PIP and DIP joints is associated with tender swelling, synovial thickening, restriction of movements, and often toe deformities.

The plantar fascia is the primary aponeurosis originating on the plantar aspect of the calcaneus and attaching to the base of each of the five metatarsal heads. Inflammation of the plantar fascia can cause pain in the plantar region, especially with initiation of walking.

Ankle arthritis is characterized by a diffuse swelling, joint line tenderness, restricted movements, and synovial thickening anteriorly with obliteration of the two small depressions that are normally present in front of the malleoli. A large ankle effusion may bulge both medial and lateral to the extensor tendons and produce fluctuance; pressure with one hand on one side of the joint produces a fluid wave transmitted to the second hand placed on the opposite side of the ankle. A traumatic tear of the talofibular ligament allows forward movement of the tibia and fibula on the talus (positive anterior draw sign).[1] Ankle tenosynovitis, by contrast, presents as a linear, superficial, tender, swelling localized to the distribution of the tendon sheath and extending beyond the joint margins. Movements of the involved tendon often produce pain.

Treatment

Management of arthritis of the ankle, subtalar, midtarsal, MTP, PIP, and DIP joints of the toes depends primarily on the underlying cause. For symptomatic treatment, rest, local heat therapy, and nonsteroidal anti-inflammatory drugs are often helpful. For persistent inflammatory synovitis, corticosteroid injections are often beneficial. The ankle joint can be injected via an anteromedial approach with the joint slightly plantarflexed. The needle is inserted at a point just medial to the tibialis anterior tendon and distal to the lower margin of the tibia. The needle is directed posteriorly and laterally to a depth of 1 to 2 cm, and 20 mg of methylprednisolone acetate or similar corticosteroid is injected. For the subtalar joint, with the patient supine and the leg-foot-ankle at 90 degrees, the needle is inserted horizontally into the subtalar joint just inferior to the tip of the lateral malleolus at a point just proximal to the sinus tarsi. The midtarsal, other intertarsal, and tarsometatarsal joints cannot easily be injected without fluoroscopic or CT scan guidance. The MTP, PIP, and DIP joints can be entered via a dorsomedial or dorsolateral route. The joint space is first identified, and then a 28-gauge needle is inserted on either side of the extensor tendon to a depth of 2 to 4 mm. Slight traction on the appropriate toe facilitates entry before injection of 10 mg of methylprednisolone acetate.[4]

References

Full references for this chapter can be found on www.expertconsult.com.

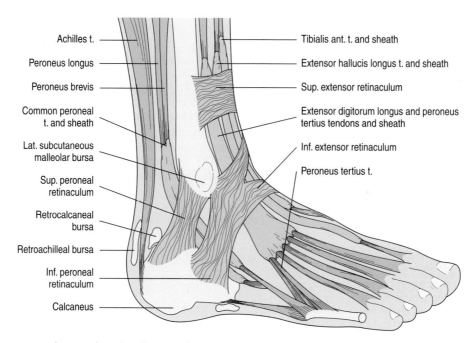

Achilles t.

Peroneus longus

Peroneus brevis

Common peroneal t. and sheath

Lat. subcutaneous malleolar bursa

Sup. peroneal retinaculum

Retrocalcaneal bursa

Retroachilleal bursa

Inf. peroneal retinaculum

Calcaneus

Tibialis ant. t. and sheath

Extensor hallucis longus t. and sheath

Sup. extensor retinaculum

Extensor digitorum longus and peroneus tertius tendons and sheath

Inf. extensor retinaculum

Peroneus tertius t.

Fig. 115.1 Bursae, tendons, and tendon sheaths of the anterior tibial (extensor) and peroneal compartments of the ankle.

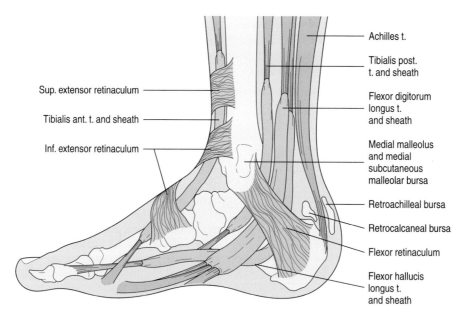

Sup. extensor retinaculum

Tibialis ant. t. and sheath

Inf. extensor retinaculum

Achilles t.

Tibialis post. t. and sheath

Flexor digitorum longus t. and sheath

Medial malleolus and medial subcutaneous malleolar bursa

Retroachilleal bursa

Retrocalcaneal bursa

Flexor retinaculum

Flexor hallucis longus t. and sheath

Fig. 115.2 Bursae, tendons, and tendon sheaths of the medial (flexor) compartment of the ankle.

Achilles Tendinitis and Bursitis and Other Painful Conditions of the Ankle

Saima Chohan

Achilles Tendinitis

Etiology

The Achilles tendon is the strongest and thickest tendon in the body; it is formed by the convergence of the gastrocnemius and soleus tendons. Injuries to the Achilles tendon are the most common lower extremity tendinous injuries. Achilles tendinitis is usually caused by repetitive trauma and microscopic tears from excessive use of the calf muscles, as in ballet dancing, distance running, track and field, jumping, and other athletic activities; from wearing faulty footwear with a rigid shoe counter; or from use of medications, including corticosteroids and fluoroquinolone antibiotics (**Fig. 116.1**).[1–7] Tendon microtears are often associated with both focal mucoid degeneration and neovascularization.[8] Insertional Achilles tendinitis, often associated with enthesopathy and retrocalcaneal bursitis, occurs frequently in patients with spondyloarthropathies, such as ankylosing spondylitis or psoriatic arthritis. The tendon is also a common site for gouty tophi, rheumatoid nodules, and xanthomas.[1]

Clinical Presentation

Tendinitis of the Achilles tendon is characterized by activity-related pain, swelling, tenderness, and sometimes crepitus over the tendon 2 to 6 cm from its insertion (**Fig. 116.2**).[1–7]

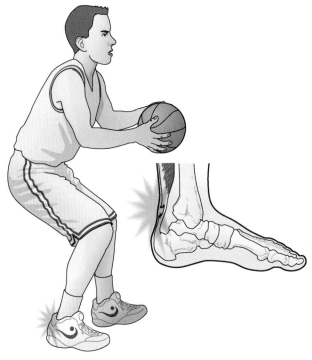

Fig. 116.1 The pain of Achilles tendinitis is constant and severe and is localized to the posterior ankle.

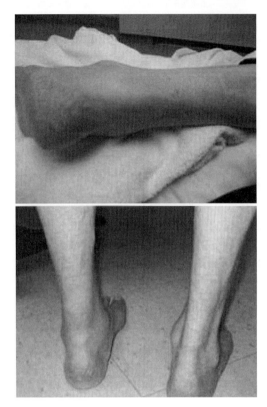

Fig. 116.2 Swelling and erythema along the left Achilles tendon in a patient receiving a fluoroquinolone. *(From Damuth E, Heidelbaugh J, Malani PN, et al: An elderly patient with fluoroquinolone-associated achilles tendinitis,* Am J Geriatr Pharmacother 6:264, 2008.)

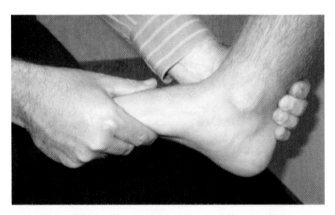

Fig. 116.3 Eliciting the creak sign for Achilles tendinitis. *(From Waldman SD: Physical diagnosis of pain: an atlas of signs and symptoms, Philadelphia, 2006, Saunders, p 377.)*

Tissues surrounding the tendon may be thick and irregular, and sometimes a palpable nodule may be present. Passive dorsiflexion of the ankle intensifies the pain, and a creak sign for Achilles tendinitis may be present (**Fig. 116.3**). The painful arc sign (movements of the tender swollen area within the tendon with dorsiflexion and plantarflexion of the ankle) and the Royal London Hospital test (tenderness on repalpating a tender swollen area within the tendon with the ankle in maximum active dorsiflexion) are often positive.[7]

Diagnosis

Abnormalities of the tendon and peritendinous tissues can be seen with both ultrasound scan[9] and magnetic resonance imaging (MRI).[3] With ultrasound scan, Achilles tendinitis is characterized by swelling and a hypoechogenic area within the substance of the tendon, with loss of the normal, well-organized, ribbon-like intratendinous echostructure. The ultrasound scan demonstration of a spindle-shaped thickening of the Achilles tendon in asymptomatic athletes may also predict those at risk of subsequent development of symptoms.[9]

Treatment

Treatment consists of a period of rest, weight reduction in obese patients, avoidance of the provocative occupational or athletic activity, shoe modification, a heel raise to reduce stretching of the tendon during walking, nonsteroidal anti-inflammatory drugs (NSAIDs), and physiotherapy, including local ice or heat application, gentle stretching exercises, and sometimes a temporary splint with slight ankle plantarflexion.[1-3] Rehabilitation is aimed at stretching the Achilles tendon, the hamstrings, and the calf muscles. Avoidance of hills and uneven running surfaces and diligent stretching before sport activities are often beneficial. Symptoms may persist for several months. The Achilles tendon is vulnerable to rupture, particularly in elderly individuals. Corticosteroid injections in or near the tendon may predispose to tendon rupture and are, therefore, strongly discouraged.[1-7,10] Surgical treatment, including open tenotomy with excision of the inflamed peritendinous tissue, open tenotomy with paratenon stripping, or percutaneous longitudinal tenotomy, is rarely necessary in conditions that do not respond to more than 6 months of nonoperative management.[1-7,11]

Achilles Tendon Rupture

Etiology

The area of the Achilles tendon, located 2 to 6 cm proximal to its calcaneal insertion, has the poorest blood supply, predisposing this region to tendinopathy and possible rupture.[6] Rupture of the Achilles tendon has increased significantly because of increased physical activity in the older population. Achilles tendon rupture occurs most commonly in active men between 30 and 50 years old, typically during a burst of unaccustomed physical activity involving forced ankle dorsiflexion. It may also result from a sharp blow, a fall, or intense athletic activities, because of repetitive microtrauma.[1-7,12,13] It may occur spontaneously or after minor trauma in elderly patients with preexisting Achilles tendinitis or retrocalcaneal bursitis, in patients with systemic lupus erythematosus or rheumatoid arthritis receiving corticosteroids, in those on long-term hemodialysis, after local corticosteroid injections in the vicinity of the tendon, and in patients treated with fluoroquinolone antibiotics.[14]

Clinical Presentation

The onset is often sudden, with pain in the region of the tendon, sometimes with a faint "pop" sound and difficulty walking or standing on the toes. Swelling, ecchymosis, tenderness, and sometimes a palpable gap are present at the site of the tear. In partial tendon rupture, active plantarflexion of the ankle may be preserved but painful. In those cases with complete rupture, active plantarflexion of the ankle with the adjacent intact flexor tendons is still possible. However, gentle squeezing of the calf muscles with the patient prone, sitting, or kneeling on a chair produces little or no ankle plantarflexion (positive Thompson calf squeeze test).[1–7,12,13] If the Thompson test is equivocal, the blood pressure cuff test can be performed. For this test, a sphygmomanometer cuff is inflated to 100 mm Hg around the calf with the patient lying prone and knee flexed 90 degrees.[13] If the tendon is intact, the pressure rises to about 140 mm Hg with passive dorsiflexion of the ankle, but it changes very little if the tendon is ruptured.[13] Rupture is typically associated with inability to perform single-leg toe raise on the affected side.

Diagnosis

Estimates are that 20% to 30% of Achilles tendon ruptures are not diagnosed on initial assessment.[6,13] The tendon defect can be disguised by hematoma, and the patient may retain some plantarflexion power because of the actions of the flexor digitorum, flexor hallucis longus, tibialis posterior, and peronei muscles. Thus, the Thompson test should be performed in all patients with suspected Achilles tendon injury. If the diagnosis is still in doubt, the extent and orientation of the rupture can be confirmed and accurately assessed with either ultrasound scan[15] or MRI.[1,3]

Treatment

Treatment for Achilles tendon rupture may be nonoperative or surgical. Nonoperative management consists of immobilization with casting to prevent dorsiflexion. Such conservative treatment is usually limited to patients at risk for surgical complications and nonathletes.[4–7,12] Immobilization is associated with a higher rerupture rate, a more prolonged recovery time, and a less favorable functional outcome.[1–7,12,16] Although open operative or percutaneous repair of the ruptured Achilles tendon is indicated in most patients, particularly in young athletes, recent literature has shown the value of minimally invasive surgery for tendionopathy, acute ruptures, and chronic tears.[1–7,13,16,17] Repair of the ruptured tendon should be done within 3 weeks to prevent atrophy of the medial gastrocnemius muscle. Surgery is followed by 6 weeks of immobilization, including 2 weeks of non–weight bearing with use of crutches. The incidence of rerupture is significantly reduced with surgical repair. Use of transforming growth factor in animal models to accelerate and improve tendon healing and improved biomechanical properties of Achilles tendon is an exciting area of research.[18]

Retrocalcaneal, Sub-Achilles, or Subtendinous Bursitis

Etiology

Retrocalcaneal bursitis usually occurs in middle-aged and elderly individuals. Known causes include rheumatoid arthritis, psoriatic arthritis, and ankylosing spondylitis.[1,2,6,19] It may also occur in association with both Haglund's deformity (abnormal prominence of the posterior superior calcaneal tubercle causing chronic irritation of Achilles tendon and bursa)[20] and Achilles tendinitis resulting from overactivity. Haglund's deformity is often associated with a varus hindfoot. When viewed from behind, it presents as a round bony swelling just lateral to the distal part of the Achilles tendon.[20]

Clinical Presentation

Retrocalcaneal bursitis is associated with posterior heel pain that is aggravated by passive dorsiflexion of the ankle.[1,2,6,19] It is often worse in the beginning of an activity, such as walking and running, and diminishes as the activity continues. Patients may present because they are unable to comfortably wear shoes. Symptoms seem to improve on weekends and during vacations. Patients may develop a limp, and wearing shoes can become painful. On examination, the bursitis is associated with tenderness and sometimes erythema on the posterior aspect of the heel at the tendon insertion. Bursal distention produces a tender swelling behind the ankle, with bulging on both sides of the tendon.[1,2,6,19] The diagnosis can be confirmed with radiography (showing obliteration of the retrocalcaneal recess, a Haglund's deformity, and sometimes calcified distal Achilles tendon), ultrasound scan,[21] or MRI.[19]

Treatment

Rest, activity modification, heat application, a slight heel elevation with a felt heel pad or cup, and NSAIDs constitute sufficient therapy for most patients.[1,2,6] A walking cast or a cautious ultrasound scan–guided corticosteroid injection into the bursa is sometimes necessary. Surgical bursectomy and resection of the superior prominence of the calcaneal tuberosity are rarely indicated.[1,2,6,20]

Retroachilleal or Subcutaneous Calcaneal Bursitis

Retroachilleal bursitis, also known as "pump bumps," produces a painful tender subcutaneous swelling overlying the Achilles tendon, usually at the level of the shoe counter.[1–4] The overlying skin may be hyperkeratotic or reddened. It occurs predominantly in women and is frequently caused and aggravated by improperly fitting shoes or pumps with a stiff, closely contoured heel counter. It may also occur in patients with bony exostoses and varus hindfoot.[1,2,4,6,20]

Treatment

Treatment consists of rest, heat application, NSAIDs, padding, and relief from shoe pressure by wearing a soft, nonrestrictive shoe without a counter. Local corticosteroid injections should be avoided. Surgical excision is rarely indicated.[1,2,6]

References

Full references for this chapter can be found on www.expertconsult.com.

Morton's Interdigital Neuroma and Other Painful Conditions of the Foot

Saima Chohan

Metatarsalgia

Etiology

Metatarsalgia, or pain and tenderness in and about the metatarsal heads or metatarsophalangeal (MTP) joints, is a common symptom of diverse causes (**Table 117.1**).[1-6] The condition often follows years of disuse and weakness of the intrinsic muscles as a result of chronic foot strain from improper footwear with the toes cramped into tight or pointed shoes.

Clinical Presentation

Metatarsalgia may either be limited to a single joint or generalized across the ball of the foot. The main clinical findings are pain in the forefoot on standing and walking and tenderness on palpation of the metatarsal heads and MTP joints (**Fig. 117.1**).[1,3-6] Prominent, dropped central metatarsal heads, plantar calluses, and clawed toes are frequently present.

Morton's Interdigital Neuroma

Historical Aspects

Detailed description of interdigital neuroma was first reported by T. G. Morton in 1876.[7]

Etiology

Morton's neuroma is commonly unilateral and occurs most often in middle-aged women. It often results from chronic foot strain and repetitive trauma caused by inappropriately fitting shoes or from mechanical foot problems such as pronated pes planus and pes cavus.[1-8] It represents an entrapment neuropathy (rather than a true neuroma) of an interdigital nerve, typically between the third and fourth metatarsal heads, although it may occasionally occur between the second and third metatarsal heads (**Fig. 117.2**). The nerve is entrapped under the transverse metatarsal ligament, causing endoneural edema, demyelination, axonal injury, and perineurial fibrosis. An intermetatarsophalangeal bursa or synovial cyst may also cause compression of the nerve.

Clinical Features

Although Morton's neuroma can be clinically silent, typical symptoms include paroxysms of lancinating, burning, or neuralgic pain in the affected interdigital cleft and occasionally paresthesia or anesthesia of contiguous borders of adjacent toes.[1-9] Hyperesthesias of the toes, numbness and tingling, and aching and burning in the distal forefoot are common symptoms. Relief of pain when the shoe is removed and the foot is massaged is characteristic. Walking on hard surfaces or wearing tight or high-heeled shoes increases the discomfort. The metatarsal arch is often depressed, and tenderness is present over the entrapped nerve between the third and fourth metatarsal heads.[1-9] The pain is made worse with compression of the metatarsal heads together with one hand while squeezing the affected web space between the thumb and index finger of the opposite hand (web space compression test). Injection of 1% lidocaine into the symptomatic interspace often temporarily relieves the pain.[1,7] Altered sensation may be found on the lateral aspect of the third toe and the medial aspect of the fourth toe. A soft tissue mass (neuroma) may be palpable between the metatarsal heads. Movements of the adjacent toes may produce a clicking sensation produced

Table 117.1 Causes of Metatarsalgia

Chronic foot strain and weakness of intrinsic muscles from improper footwear with the toes crammed into tight or pointed shoes

Altered foot biomechanics from flat, cavus, or splay foot

Interdigital (Morton's) neuroma

Attrition of the plantar fat pad in elderly patients

Painful plantar callosities, including intractable plantar keratosis (discrete or diffuse painful callus beneath one or more of the lateral metatarsals)

Plantar plate rupture with secondary metatarsophalangeal joint instability (usually the second)

Hallux valgus, hallux rigidus, hammertoes, and mallet toes

Arthritis of the metatarsophalangeal joints: osteoarthritis, rheumatoid arthritis, psoriatic arthritis, gout, trauma

Overlapping and underlapping toes

Bunion, bunionette, and intermetatarsophalangeal bursitis

Osteochondritis of the second metatarsal head (Freiberg's disease)

Metatarsal stress (march) fracture

Sesamoiditis, sesamoid fracture, or osteonecrosis

Failed forefoot surgery

Tarsal tunnel syndrome, neuropathy

Ischemic forefoot pain: peripheral vascular disease, vasospastic disorder, vasculitis

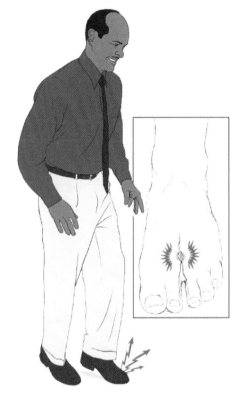

Fig. 117.2 The pain of Morton's neuroma is made worse with prolonged standing or walking.

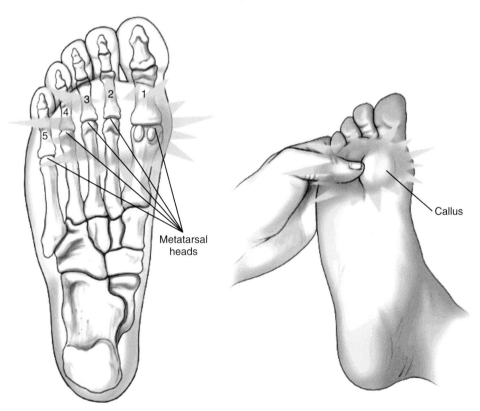

Fig. 117.1 On physical examination, pain can be reproduced with pressure on the metatarsal heads.

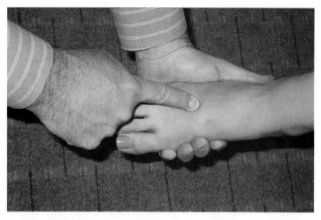

Fig. 117.3 **Eliciting the Mulder sign for Morton neuroma.** *(From Waldman SW: Physical diagnosis of pain: an atlas of signs and symptoms, ed 2, Philadelphia, 2010, Saunders, p. 348.)*

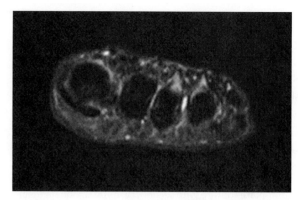

Fig. 117.4 Magnetic resonance image (STIR image) with Morton's neuroma in 3/4 intermetatarsal space. *(From George VA, Khan AM, Hutchinson CE, editor: Morton's neuroma: the role of MR scanning in diagnostic assistance, Foot 15:14, 2005.)*

by extrusion of the neuroma between the metatarsal heads as it moves beneath the transverse metatarsal ligament (Mulder's sign; **Fig. 117.3**).[1-8] The affected nerve may show slow sensory conduction velocity on electrophysiologic testing. The exact location and extent of the lesion can be determined with both magnetic resonance imaging (MRI) and sonography.[10] MRI is more sensitive and often shows a well-demarcated bulbous mass arising between the metatarsal heads on the plantar side of the transverse metatarsal ligament. The lesion shows low signal intensity on both T1-weighted and T2-weighted images.[11]

Treatment

Symptomatic management of metatarsalgia includes a metatarsal pad placed proximal to the metatarsal heads, weight reduction in obese patients, strengthening of the intrinsic muscles with toe flexion exercises, and shoe modification, including a wide toe box and, in patients with a pronated foot, an arch support.[1-9] If these measures fail, metatarsal osteotomy or metatarsal head resection is indicated. In Morton's neuroma (**Fig. 117.4**), nonoperative measures, including proper footwear, metatarsal pad, and local corticosteroid injections into the intermetatarsal space, are often helpful. Surgical excision of the neuroma (interdigital neurectomy), epineurolysis, or simple division of the transverse metatarsal ligament are necessary in patients whose conditions are refractory to conservative treatment.[1-9] After neurectomy, regeneration of the proximal cut end of the interdigital nerve, blocked by scar tissue, can result in a painful, recurrent, interdigital neuroma. This can be managed with implantation of the proximal cut end of the nerve into an intrinsic arch muscle.[12]

References

Full references for this chapter can be found on www.expertconsult.com.

Hallux Valgus, Bunion, Bunionette, and Other Painful Conditions of the Toe

Saima Chohan

Hallux Valgus

Etiology

Hallux valgus refers to lateral deviation of the first (great) toe on the first metatarsal (**Fig. 118.1**). Although the exact etiology is unknown, this deformity is likely caused by abnormal foot mechanics and anatomy, use of shoes (a lower prevalence is seen in barefoot populations), genetic influences, and female gender. It is more common in women and is aggravated by wearing short, narrow, high-heeled, or pointed shoes.[1-5] Other causes include congenital splay foot deformity, metatarsus primus varus with or without metatarsus adductus of the adjacent second and third metatarsals,[6] and arthritis of the first metatarsophalangeal (MTP) joint from rheumatoid arthritis or osteoarthritis.[1-5]

Clinical Presentation

Medial deviation and splaying of the first metatarsal (metatarsus primus varus) with an increased intermetatarsal angle of more than 9 degrees is seen. The deformity involves rotation of the great toe so that the nail faces medially. The condition is often asymptomatic, but pain may arise from wearing of improper footwear, bursitis over the medial aspect of the first MTP joint (bunion), or secondary osteoarthritis.[1-5] As the first metatarsal moves into varus at its joint with the first cuneiform, its head also moves dorsally, resulting in a transfer of weight to the second metatarsal head. This is known as transfer lesion. Altered weight bearing results in a callosity under the second metatarsal head with the second toe forced dorsally, and a hammertoe deformity develops. If the deformity is marked, the great toe may overlie or underlie the second toe and the sesamoids are displaced laterally.[1-5] The severity

of the deformity and its progression over time can be assessed radiographically with measurement of the hallux valgus angle between the first metatarsal and first proximal phalanx.[7] Structural abnormalities of metatarsal head and sesamoids and the presence of bunion bursitis can be clearly delineated with magnetic resonance imaging (MRI).[8]

Treatment

Treatment of hallux valgus consists of shoe modification to accommodate the bunion, a bunion pad, night splinting, analgesics, and, in the presence of a transfer lesion, a metatarsal pad.[1-5] Surgical correction (osteotomy of the first metatarsal base, resection of metatarsal head or base of proximal phalanx with or without distal soft tissue lateral release, and realignment of the sesamoids) is indicated in patients with severe deformity, failure with conservative management, and intractable pain.[1-5,9] Corrective osteotomies for the adduction deformities of the second and third metatarsals are often necessary to correct the metatarsus primus varus deformity in those with hallux valgus associated with metatarsus adductus.[6] Patients with symptomatic, recurrent hallux valgus after failed prior surgery may benefit from a reduction of the first to second intermetatarsal angle and arthrodesis of both the first tarsometatarsal and first to second intermetatarsal joints.[10]

Hallux Limitus and Rigidus

Etiology

Hallux limitus refers to painful limitation of dorsiflexion of the first MTP joint. In hallux rigidus, marked limitation of movement or immobility of the first MTP joint is seen,

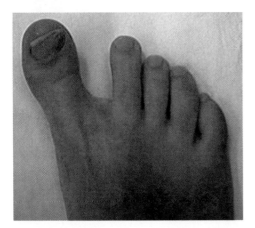

Fig. 118.1 **An AP clinical picture of a hallux varus deformity showing the medial deviation of the hallux onto the first metatarsal and the supination of the toe, particularly visible at the toenail.** *(From Devos B, Leemrijse T: The hallux varus: classification and treatment, Foot Ankle Clin North Am 14:51, 2009.)*

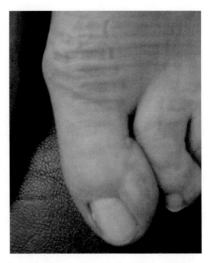

Fig. 118.2 **Valgus hallucal rotation in hallus rigidus.** *(From Beeson P, Phillipsa C, Corra S, et al: Hallux rigidus: a cross-sectional study to evaluate clinical parameters, Foot 19:80, 2009.)*

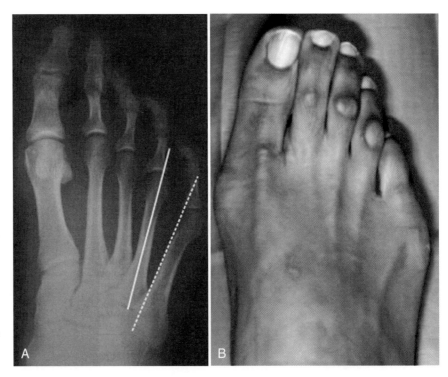

Fig. 118.3 **A,** Tailor's bunion deformity may be assessed radiographically with a lateral splaying in the distal fifth metatarsal. **B,** Clinically, the patient generally presents with symptoms that occur laterally or plantarlaterally, often with an adduction of the fifth toe. *(From Thomas JL, Blitch EL, Chaney M, et al: Clinical practice guideline: diagnosis and treatment of forefoot disorders: section 4: tailor's bunion, J Foot Ankle Surg 48: 257, 2009.)*

usually from advanced osteoarthritis, rheumatoid arthritis, or gout (**Fig. 118.2**).[1–3,8,11]

Clinical Presentation

Intermittent aching pain, joint tenderness, crepitus, osteophytic lipping, and painful limitation of movement, particularly toe dorsiflexion, are common. It usually occurs in elderly patients with osteoarthritis. A primary type is seen in younger persons; the condition may follow repetitive trauma as in ballet dancing. The "toe-off" is accomplished by the outer four toes and the distal phalanx of the great toe, thereby bypassing and protecting the first MTP joint from painful dorsiflexion. Calluses often develop beneath the second, third, and fourth metatarsal heads. In advanced stages, the first MTP joint becomes completely rigid in slight plantarflexion.[1–3,8,11]

Treatment

Treatment consists of a stiff-soled shoe with a wide toe box and a bar across the metatarsal heads to allow walking with little movement at the first MTP joint.[1–3,8,11] Intraarticular corticosteroid injections may produce temporary relief. In patients with severe pain and disability, excision of irregular osteophytic lipping that interferes with MTP movements, arthrodesis, or arthroplasty of the first MTP joint is indicated.[1–3,8,11]

Bunionette

Etiology

A bunionette (tailor's bunion) is a painful callus and an adventitious bursa that overlies a prominent, laterally deviated fifth metatarsal head and a medially deviated fifth toe.[1-3,12-15] It often occurs in conjunction with hallux valgus or splay foot deformity from an incompletely developed transverse metatarsal ligament (**Fig. 118.3**). The fourth to fifth intermetatarsal angle varies between 3 and 11 degrees, with a mean of 6.5 to 8.0 degrees. The angle is often more than 10 degrees in patients with symptomatic bunionette deformity. The fifth metatarsophalangeal angle is normally less than 14 degrees and is more than 16 degrees in those with bunionette.[12,13]

Clinical Presentation

Enlargement of the fifth metatarsal head from exostosis is commonly present. Bunionette deformity is common in athletes, especially downhill skiers. It is often asymptomatic, but patients may present with pain, tenderness, and swelling over the head of the fifth metatarsal. The pain is made worse by both activity and wearing constricting shoes. Callosity with hyperkeratosis of the skin over the fifth metatarsal head is found, and an adventitious bursa, skin ulceration, or infection may develop.[1-3,12]

Treatment

Shoe modification with a wide toe box, shaving of the callus, a bunion pad, nonsteroidal anti-inflammatory drugs, and intrabursal corticosteroid injections may reduce symptoms, particularly in those with inflamed bunionette bursitis.[1-3,12] Distal osteotomy of the fifth metatarsal,[12,14] proximal dome-shaped osteotomy of the fifth metatarsal,[15] or resection of the lateral one third of the fifth metatarsal prominence (head)[12] may be necessary in those conditions that are refractory to nonoperative treatment.

References

Full references for this chapter can be found on www.expertconsult.com.

IV

Chapter **119**

Plantar Fasciitis

Dhaneshwari Solanki

Plantar fasciitis is the most common condition treated by the orthopedist and is the most common cause of heel pain in the age group of 40 to 60 years.[1] Almost one in 10 persons will suffer from heel pain during their lifetime. It can occur in athletes and nonathletes, yet little is known about its pathophysiology. Wood in 1812 first described plantar fasciitis associated with inflammation from tuberculosis,[2] but the infectious theory was soon discredited and the association of heel spur causing this pain was popularized. This was proven not to be the case, and it is accepted that heel spurs can occur with plantar fasciitis but they do not cause it. Plantar fasciitis is presumed to be synonymous with the inflammation of the plantar fascia. But is it really an inflammatory disorder? Histologic signs of inflammation are typically absent. Histologic changes show myxoid degeneration, necrosis of the collagen, and hyperplasia of the angiofibroblasts. Microtears and presence of perifascial edema also can be seen on magnetic resonance imaging (MRI). All this evidence indicates that plantar fasciitis is not an inflammatory but a degenerative disease. Thus, the correct term to describe this condition would be plantar fasciosis.[3]

Anatomy of the Plantar Fascia

The plantar fascia is a longitudinal fibrous tissue with its origin at the medial tubercle of the calcaneus. It traverses the sole of the foot, dividing into five bands at midfoot. It is thickest at its center. Each of the five bands attaches to the proximal phalanx of the toes (**Fig. 119.1**). It is a static support for the longitudinal arch and acts as the bow string on the plantar surface of the foot (**Fig. 119.2**).[4] A normal plantar fascia has a dorsoplanar thickness of 3 mm. In plantar fasciitis, it can increase to 15 mm.[5]

Clinical Presentation

Plantar fasciitis has been reported in patients aged 7 to 85 years. It is mostly unilateral, but in one third of the cases, it could be bilateral. The skin of the heel is thicker than in other areas and is designed to deal with constant friction. Thickness of this heel pad decreases after the age of 40 years, so plantar fasciitis is more common after that age. It is also more common in women. Some of the risk factors for development of plantar fasciitis include the following:

- Obesity
- Poorly fitting shoes
- Increase in running intensity or distance
- Changes in running or walking surfaces
- Occupation that involves prolonged standing (e.g., policeman)

The foot and ankle should be examined while the patient is standing and during the gait because a pes planus or pes cavus deformity can place excess load on the plantar fascia. The pain in plantar fasciitis is located at the medial tubercle of the calcaneus, which is the origin of the plantar fascia. It is tender to palpation.

Other causes of the heel pain include heel spur, stress fracture of the calcaneum, and injury to the first branch of the lateral plantar nerve. Heel pain could also occur in patients with systemic disease, such as gout and rheumatoid arthritis. Bilateral heel pain in a young person may be from Reiter's syndrome.

Diagnosis

The diagnosis of plantar fasciitis is based on history and physical examination. No history of trauma is seen. Patients report gradually worsening heel pain. The pain is noticeably worse on awakening in the morning. Patients limp to the bathroom because weight bearing increases the pain. This pain eases after taking a few steps, decreases through the day, and gets worse toward the end of the day. The pain also worsens with prolonged standing. Rest in the evening produces pain relief. Pain of the calcaneal stress fracture worsens with walking. If the pain persists during sleep, other causes such as infection, tumors, and neuropathic pain must be sought and investigations should be done to rule out other pathologic processes that could cause the heel pain.

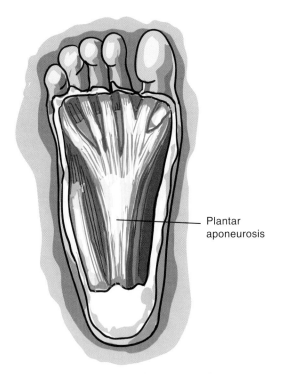

Fig. 119.1 **Anatomy of the plantar fascia.**

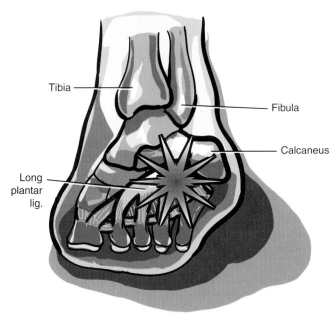

Fig. 119.2 **Increased dorsoplanar thickness of the fascia in plantar fasciitis.**

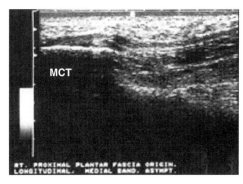

Fig. 119.3 **Ultrasound scan of normal asymtomatic plantar fascia.**

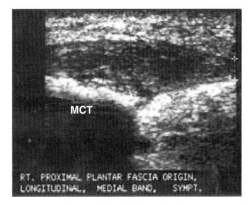

Fig. 119.4 **Ultrasound scan of the inflamed and symptomatic plantar fascia.**

The most cardinal finding is the presence of localized tenderness on the anteromedial aspect of the heel. Application of firm pressure is often necessary to determine maximum point of tenderness. Passive dorsiflexion of the toes exacerbates the pain. Tightness of the Achilles tendon is found and limits the dorsiflexion of the foot in 78% of patients. No other clinical findings in the foot or the ankle are seen. Tenderness of the posterior part of the heel may be indicative of subcalcaneal bursitis. Mediolateral tenderness on the heel is indicative of a calacaneal stress fracture. A positive Tinel's sign on the medial aspect of the heel may be the result of tarsal tunnel syndrome or the entrapment of the nerve to the abductor digiti quinti.

Investigations

Imaging has a limited role in the diagnosis of plantar fasciitis. Plain radiographs of the heel are obtained to rule out causes such as stress fracture, bony erosion from bursitis, or heel spurs that could cause heel pain. If a calcaneal stress fracture is suspected and plain radiographs are normal and the patient has not responded to 4 to 6 months of nonsurgical treatment, a triple phase bone scan should be considered. An MRI is rarely indicative, but it can define the thickness of the plantar fascia. Ultrasound scan examination shows hypoechoic thickened fascia and is as effective as bone scan and MRI. Ultrasound scan examination can be done in the office. It is inexpensive and avoids radiation exposure. Normal plantar fascia on ultrasound scan examination appears thin and hypoechoic (**Fig. 119.3**). Inflamed plantar fascia appears as a thick band yet is hypoechoic (**Fig. 119.4**).[6] A complete blood count and erythrocyte sedimentation rate should be done when the patient presents with bilateral heel pain or atypical symptoms.

Treatment

Plantar fasciitis is a self-limiting condition. The conservative treatment, if started within 6 weeks of the onset of symptoms, hastens the recovery process.[7] Conservative treatment should be tried for 12 months before surgical intervention is contemplated. Twenty-six different conservative treatments have been recommended,[8] but heel pads, orthoses, corticosteroid injections, night splints, and extracorporeal shock wave therapy (ESWT) have been evaluated with randomized control trials. The conservative treatments include:

1. Nonsteroidal anti-inflammatory drugs
2. Orthoses and insets
3. Physical therapy
4. Injections
5. ESWT

Oral nonsteroidal anti-inflammatory drugs should be used only during the acute phase. They show improved pain relief, but they have not been examined prospectively with randomized trials.

Orthoses recreate the shape of the heel, decreasing excessive pronation and stress on the plantar fascia. Pfeffer[9] compared various types of shoe inserts with a control group and found superior pain relief. Magnetic insoles were not beneficial. Pain relief with application of ice, heat, or massage is largely based on patient reports.

Patients should be taught the exercises for the Achilles tendon stretching and plantar fascia stretching. Dorsiflexion of the foot with the knee extended stretches the gastrocnemius muscle. The same movement with the knee partially flexed stretches the soleus muscle. These stretches should be done in 8 to 10 repetitions and three to five times a day. Plantar fascia stretching is done by dorsiflexing the toes while the ankle is dorsiflexed. Night splints can help because they keep the Achilles tendon in a stretched position. Patients with severe pain can benefit from a below-the-knee cast for 4 to 6 weeks; it can minimize repetitive microtrauma.

Corticosteroid injection in combination with local anesthetics has been used to treat plantar fasciitis, but hardly any evidence is found of its effectiveness. In the past, injection was done via palpation. Now, it is done with ultrasound scan to improve the accuracy of the injection site. Kane et al[10] compared the two methods and did not find any difference. In addition, complications, such as rupture of the plantar fascia and fat pad atrophy, have been reported with these injections. The Cochrane group has concluded that steroid injections are useful in the short term and to a limited degree.[8] In a case series of 20 patients, Ryan et al[11] reported pain relief in 80% of the patients when a solution of hyperosmolar dextrose and lidocaine was injected in the hypoechoic areas of the plantar fascia with ultrasound scan guidance. The hyperosmolar solution triggers proliferation of fibroblasts and collagen synthesis because of upregulation and migration of various growth factors.

ESWT has become increasingly popular for recalcitrant pain. It should be used in patients when disabling symptoms have persisted more than 6 months and other conservative therapies have failed to relieve the pain. The shockwaves are directed to the origin of the plantar fascia. The mechanism is speculative, but the hypothesis is that it produces microdisruption of the fascial tissue that starts the healing response. No consensus exists as to the use of the low-energy or high-energy waves, but randomized controlled trials have supported the use of both and no serious side effects have been reported.[12]

Surgery

Surgery should be considered only when the patient has not responded to the previously described treatment for 12 months.[9] The surgical procedures that are considered for treatment of plantar fasciitis are release of plantar fascia, calcaneal spur excision, Steindler stripping, neurolysis, and endoscopic procedures.[13] Surgery could provide relief in 50% to 60% of patients, but a possibility also exists of significant complications from such procedures.

Conclusion

Plantar fasciitis is the most common cause of heel pain. Review of the literature provides ample evidence that conservative management is the treatment of choice. In many cases, plantar fasciitis could be a self-limiting condition. Surgical intervention should only be considered when the pain and disability from plantar fasciitis persists despite adequate trial with nonsurgical therapies.

References

Full references for this chapter can be found on www.expertconsult.com.

Section V

Specific Treatment Modalities for Pain and Symptom Management

Part A

Pharmacologic Management of Pain

Chapter **120**

Simple Analgesics

Robert B. Supernaw

For most pain phenomena, pharmacotherapy represents an indispensable therapeutic tool. However, pharmacotherapy—even over-the-counter (OTC) pharmacotherapy—has the dual feature of combating the principal condition while potentially provoking undesired adverse effects. Therefore, even in cases of mild, uncomplicated pain, the best therapeutic approach is to combat the pain with physical methods (e.g., ice packs, heat, massage) if the condition is amenable to such treatment. However, the option of not employing pharmacotherapy in managing many painful conditions is not realistic. If the clinician has determined that the symptom of pain cannot be effectively treated with physical intervention, drug therapy is indicated. To determine the best pharmacotherapeutic response to pain, the nature and severity of the pain must be assessed and considered. If the pain is uncomplicated and nonpsychogenic and if the pain intensity is mild or moderate, simple analgesics, including OTC agents, represent first-line treatment options.

Even in cases of mild or moderate pain, treatment plans are formulated on the basis of the specific nature of the complaint. For example, moderate headache pain may be treated differently from moderate pain of a sprained ankle. In one case, it may be important to consider the pain of inflammation, whereas in another case inflammation may not be at the root of the pain. Unlike the basic therapeutic approach to other commonly encountered problems (e.g., hypertension, hyperlipidemia) in which drug therapy is initiated in relatively small doses and is slowly increased until the therapeutic threshold or desired outcome is achieved, the therapeutic approach to pain is predicated on the basis of matching the complete pain presentation to the appropriate agent, with a reasoned dose of the agent chosen.

In many instances, no need exists to begin drug therapy for the pain complaint with a less potent, OTC analgesic before attempting more potent drug therapy. The severe pain of a cluster headache does not respond to aspirin or acetaminophen therapy; therefore, little is gained in trying. This treatment principle underscores the need for an accurate categorization of the pain complaint. When, in the judgment of the clinician, the nature (i.e., relatively uncomplicated pain) and intensity (i.e., mild or moderate pain) of the pain complaint are deemed appropriate, first-line pharmacotherapy (i.e., simple OTC analgesics) may be initiated. These conditions include uncomplicated headache, facial pain, muscle ache, toothache, joint pain, foot pain, and uncomplicated back pain, to name a few of the more commonly encountered pain problems.

The OTC simple analgesics are the most widely used drugs for mild to moderate nociceptive pain, and sales of these agents (i.e., aspirin, acetaminophen, ibuprofen, naproxen sodium, and ketoprofen) totaled more than $2.18 billion in the United States in 2004.

Nonprescription Simple Analgesics: Overview

Mild *acute* pain is limited in its duration. Therefore, it need not be aggressively treated if it does not affect an individual's quality of life and the patient has not indicated significant or distracting discomfort. In some instances, the pain need not be treated at all. Mild *chronic* pain may prove to be more problematic in its negative impact on an individual's quality of life, family relations, and ability to work. It usually requires active treatment. If a decision is made to treat mild acute or chronic pain, the first consideration should be given to simple analgesics. These agents are available without a prescription on an OTC basis. The principal OTC simple analgesics include members of two major families of drugs—the nonsteroidal anti-inflammatory drugs (NSAIDs) and acetaminophen.

A useful categorization of the OTC NSAIDs includes two principal groupings—the salicylates and the nonsalicylates. The salicylates can be further divided into two families of drugs, the acetylated and the nonacetylated salicylates. A helpful representation of the categorization of the simple analgesics is depicted in **Figure 120.1**.

When a decision is made to treat mild to moderate nociceptive pain, consideration should be given to the nature of the pain and the patient. If the patient is not allergic to aspirin and tolerates aspirin well, then aspirin is a good first-line choice and is the most widely recommended analgesic.[1] Acetaminophen should be considered if the patient is aspirin sensitive, aspirin intolerant, or allergic to aspirin. However, as is the case with most choices in pharmacotherapy, the rules are not quite that simple. Many other factors must be taken into account before the choice of a simple analgesic can be made. These considerations are detailed in the following sections of this chapter.

Over-the-Counter Nonsteroidal Anti-Inflammatory Drugs

OTC NSAIDs are the most commonly employed of the simple analgesics. This category of drugs includes the salicylates and the propionic acids (see Fig. 120.1). The salicylates are further divided into the acetylated and the nonacetylated compounds.

Salicylates

Two forms of salicylates are available in the OTC analgesic armamentarium. The most commonly used member of the acetylated salicylate family is aspirin, including the combination products enteric-coated aspirin and buffered aspirin. The OTC nonacetylated salicylate family includes sodium salicylate.

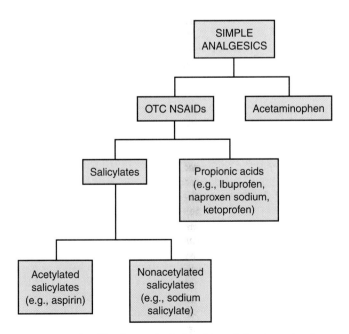

Fig. 120.1 **Classification and relationships of simple analgesics.**

Aspirin

Acetylsalicylic acid, more commonly known as aspirin, is the most commonly used simple analgesic and has been for many years. According to the Aspirin Foundation, approximately 100 billion aspirin tablets are produced annually. Aspirin represents a reasonable first choice for common mild to moderate pain, if the pain is nociceptive. The forerunner of aspirin, sodium salicylic acid, was widely used as an analgesic and antipyretic from the 1700s onward. A much improved acetyl derivative of sodium salicylic acid—acetylsalicylic acid or aspirin—was introduced commercially in the United States in 1899. By definition, aspirin is an NSAID that predates all other modern NSAIDs. Aspirin is the prototypical salicylate and, as such, has a long history of safe and effective use. However, as is the case with almost all drugs, whether OTC or prescription, aspirin is not without its risks.

The benefits of aspirin therapy are well known. It is cheap, is readily available, has a very long track record, is effective in the relief of mild to moderate nociceptive pain, improves function, and reduces inflammation, especially at higher doses. Additional benefits include its ability to reduce fever and its antiplatelet adhesion properties. Given as a 650-mg dose (two regular-strength tablets) every 4 hours, aspirin may be considered first-line drug therapy in various mild to moderate pain-related problems including chronic joint pain, minor arthritis flare-ups, common and tension-type headaches, dysmenorrhea, minor postoperative pain and inflammation, and chronic minor low back pain.

ACTION

Aspirin and the acetylated salicylates have analgesic, anti-inflammatory, antiplatelet, and antipyretic activity. These drugs are most effective for general pain, common headache pain, and especially pain of musculoskeletal origin, including arthritis and muscle pain. When peripheral tissue is insulted in trauma or when a pain-triggering event occurs, prostaglandins enhance the transmission of pain impulses and the sensitivity of the pain receptors, and an inflammatory response may ensue. Aspirin's principal mechanism of action is inhibition of prostaglandin (eicosanoid) synthesis in peripheral tissue.[2] Therefore, pain relief is not instantaneous, as eicosanoid levels dissipate. Aspirin appears to acetylate the active site of the enzyme cyclooxygenase (COX), also known as PGH synthase, which is the specific enzyme necessary for the conversion of arachidonic acid to eicosanoids. This acetylation permanently (irreversibly) deactivates the COX enzyme and thereby effectively inhibits prostaglandin production.[3] This irreversibility is an important distinction between aspirin, an acetylated salicylate, and the other NSAIDs. It is likely that aspirin also mitigates pain through central mechanisms. Investigators have hypothesized that the acetate components of aspirin pass into the brain and spinal cord and exert their activity on central nervous system prostaglandins that are involved in the perception and transmission of pain.

DOSING

Aspirin is available in 325-mg and 500-mg tablet, caplet, and effervescent tablet strengths. It is also available as an 81-mg chewable tablet and an 81-mg enteric coated tablet.

Aspirin is available in a controlled-release 800-mg oral dosage form and is embedded in chewing gum in the 228-mg strength. For rectal use, aspirin is available in 125- and 300-mg suppositories.

For administration in adult patients, for general musculoskeletal and common headache pain, aspirin is most often given orally in doses ranging from 325 to 650 mg every 3 to 4 hours as needed, not to exceed 4 g in a 24-hour period. If the condition warrants the more potent dosage form (i.e., extra strength 500 mg), the suggested dose is 500 mg every 3 to 4 hours or 1000 mg every 6 to 8 hours. For significant inflammatory processes, including arthritis, aspirin can be given in divided doses equivalent to 3.2 to 6.0 g daily, provided every 3 to 4 hours. For severe headache pain, aspirin has been demonstrated to show added analgesic activity when doses are pushed to 1000 mg.[4] For the pain and discomfort of niacin-induced flushing, 325 mg aspirin should be given before the administration of the niacin dose. Because the potential for gastrointestinal irritation is related to both a local effect and a pharmacologic effect, aspirin should always be taken with a full glass of water. Studies have also shown that doses should be slightly increased in obese patients because peak levels do not match those seen in nonobese individuals.[5]

For administration in pediatric patients who are more than of 2 years old, a 10 to 15 mg/kg/dose every 4 hours, up to 60 to 80 mg/kg per day is appropriate for general pain, discomfort, or fever. For infants and children into their teens, aspirin is contraindicated—should not be given—in cases of viral infections, including flu and chickenpox because it has been implicated in Reye's syndrome. For infants and children suffering from juvenile rheumatoid arthritis, an initial dose of 90 to 130 mg/kg per day, in divided doses every 4 to 6 hours, is appropriate for oral administration. This dose may be increased as needed to maximize anti-inflammatory efficacy to achieve a plasma salicylate level objective of 150 to 300 mg/mL.

An alternative dosing guideline for pediatric patients is based on age and weight. For children ages 2 to 11 years, a total of 64 mg/kg per day in four to six doses is appropriate. Another guideline[6,7] is as follows, if the child's weight is within normal limits:

- Children more than 11 years old (weight, greater than 43.2 kg): 650 mg every 4 hours, not to exceed 4 g per day
- Children age 11 years (weight, 32.4 to 43.2 kg): 480 mg every 4 hours
- Children age 9 to 10 years (weight, 26.9 to 32.3 kg): 400 mg every 4 hours
- Children age 6 to 8 years (weight, 21.5 to 26.8 kg): 325 mg every 4 hours
- Children age 4 to 5 years (weight, 16.0 to 21.4 kg): 240 mg every 4 hours
- Children age 2 to 3 years (weight, 10.6 to 15.9 kg): 160 mg every 4 hours
- Children younger than 2 years (up to 23 months and up to 10.5 kg in weight): aspirin not recommended

PHARMACOKINETICS

Oral aspirin is absorbed very rapidly in the stomach and upper small intestine by passive diffusion.[8] Moderate differences in absorption are noted between buffered and nonbuffered varieties. Buffered tablets are absorbed in 30 to 45 minutes, and nonbuffered tablets are absorbed within 60 minutes.[9] However, significant levels are detectable in plasma in less than 30 minutes after a single dose of aspirin.[1] In buffered aspirin, minute quantities of antacid are added to aid in the dissolution of the tablet. In theory, this would enhance absorption, but studies have not demonstrated significant differences in total absorption. Although enteric coating does delay aspirin's absorption, it does not affect total absorption or the resultant salicylate levels.[10] Taking aspirin with food or with meals does not affect its absorption.[11] Peak levels of oral aspirin occur approximately 1 hour after administration. Unlike salicylic acid, aspirin is not effectively absorbed through the skin. Percutaneous absorption is significantly less than 10% of oral absorption.[12] Rectal absorption of aspirin administered in a suppository dosage form is incomplete and variable; therefore, it is not advisable unless other routes are not feasible.[13]

The distribution of the salicylates is throughout most body tissues and depends on the patient and the drug concentration. Approximately 68% (± 3%) of the aspirin dose is available (at the initial stages after administration) as the unchanged drug, but this may be significantly different in older patients and in patients with compromised liver function.[14] Of course, aspirin (acetylsalicylic acid) is hydrolyzed to salicylic acid, which is not accounted for in this 68% figure. At usual or higher concentrations of salicylates, albumin binding varies but may approach 80%.[13] At lower concentrations, inactive binding to albumin may approach 90%. On average, at therapeutic concentrations, approximately 80% of the aspirin dosed is inactively bound.[1,13] Because of this significant albumin binding, caution is warranted when aspirin is given to a patient who is taking an oral anticoagulant (OAC) in that the OAC is approximately 97% albumin bound. The aspirin binding will displace some of the OAC, and this displacement will augment the active dose (drug level) of the OAC and significantly increase bleeding time. If as little as 3% of the OAC is displaced by the aspirin, the effective dose of the OAC will be doubled. The process of inactive albumin binding can saturate the system; therefore, high doses of aspirin (e.g., single doses greater than 650 mg) will saturate the binding system and lead to very high blood levels. In other words, increasing the dose of aspirin to more than 650 mg will increase the blood levels of aspirin in a disproportionate manner and will significantly increase the half-life of the drug. The volume of distribution of aspirin is 0.15 L/kg (±0.03 L/kg).[1] Aspirin crosses the placental barrier and is not advised in the third trimester of pregnancy (pregnancy category C/D).

Aspirin is hydrolyzed in circulation and in the liver to form salicylate and acetic acid. Within 30 minutes, only 27% of the orally administered dose remains as acetylsalicylic acid; the active remainder is salicylate.[1] As with all salicylates, aspirin is metabolized in the liver by esterases. The major metabolite of salicylates is salicyluric acid.

Salicylates are excreted in the urine, and alkalinization of the urine increases the rate of excretion.[13] Aspirin exhibits a two-compartment half-life. It has a half-life of 15 minutes as aspirin (acetylsalicylic acid) and 3 to 5 hours as its salicylate metabolite. Therefore, although normally the half-life of pure aspirin is 15 minutes, and 3 to 5 hours for salicylate, when the inactive albumin binding system is saturated, the half-life may increase up to threefold of normal (e.g., 3 to 5 hours for dosing at 600 mg daily versus 12 to 16 hours for dosing at 3.6 g daily for significant anti-inflammatory effects).[13] Only approximately

10% of aspirin is excreted as free salicylic acid; 75% is excreted as salicyluric acid.[1] Because aspirin is excreted in breast milk, the drug is unsafe to use in breast-feeding mothers.

INDICATIONS IN PAIN

As a nonselective COX-1 and COX-2 inhibitor, aspirin is indicated for the treatment of general complaints of pain associated with inflammatory processes, menstruation (e.g., dysmenorrhea), dental pain, headache, joint pain, muscle pain, and integumentary pain. It is less effective in treating visceral pain. In synovial fluid, aspirin reaches approximately 78% of plasma concentrations,[15,16] thus making it a good option for treating arthritis pain and, at higher doses, inflammation.

CAUTIONS

Aspirin should never be given to children or teenagers who exhibit symptoms of influenza or chickenpox. In these cases, aspirin administration has been associated with Reye's syndrome, which, although rare, is associated with mortality rates up to 30% and severe brain damage in patients who survive.

Ringing in the ears may indicate toxicity. Any complaints of such a symptom indicate the basis for discontinuation of aspirin. Dizziness may also indicate the onset of toxicity. Because of its irreversible antiplatelet effects, aspirin should be discontinued at least 7 days before surgery to preclude the chance of aspirin-induced postoperative bleeding.

Caution is warranted with the use of aspirin in asthmatic patients. Bronchospasms occur in up to 19% of these patients. As with all drugs metabolized in the liver, caution is warranted in patients with compromised liver function. Aspirin should not be considered in the third trimester of pregnancy and should not be administered to lactating mothers who are breast-feeding.

Because of local and pharmacologic induced gastrointestinal irritation, aspirin should be used with caution in patients who complain of gastrointestinal burning and in those with ulcers. Rectal bleeding and fecal blood loss should be monitored. When plasma concentration monitoring is possible, the therapeutic range should not exceed 300 mg/mL (30 mg/dL). Acidification of the urine increases plasma levels, and alkalinizing the urine decreases levels. Aspirin has also been implicated in blood-related problems including decreased white blood cell and platelet counts and hemolytic anemia.

Clinicians should warn patients to discard aspirin that has an odor of vinegar; this indicates that the aspirin has undergone chemical degradation. Extra caution is indicated if the patient (1) is taking an OAC; (2) is taking an oral antidiabetic agent; (3) has a history of peptic ulcer disease; (4) has systemic lupus erythematosus; (5) is pregnant or is contemplating pregnancy; (6) is scheduled for surgery; (7) is receiving a new prescription; or (8) experiences a new significant adverse effect.

Analgesic effects result from plasma levels approaching 10 mg/dL. Anti-inflammatory effects result from plasma levels from 10 to 40 mg/dL. Ringing in the ears occurs at approximately 50 mg/dL. Toxicity occurs as a function of levels higher than 50 mg/dL, and doses leading to levels higher than 160 mg/dL are lethal.[17]

Aspirin interacts with several other drugs and chemical entities. Alcohol increases the risk of gastrointestinal irritation. Ascorbic acid acidifies the urine and decreases the excretion of aspirin. Antacids and urinary alkalinizers increase the excretion of aspirin and thereby decrease the effects of aspirin. OAC levels are increased with the concomitant use of aspirin because of inactive binding displacement. Aspirin and other NSAIDs exhibit additive gastrointestinal irritative effects. Aspirin decreases the antihypertensive effects of angiotensin-converting enzyme inhibitors (ACE inhibitors) and beta blockers. Aspirin and the salicylates antagonize the action of uricosuric agents, and salicylates should not be given with methotrexate.

Sodium Salicylate

Sodium salicylate is the "other" nonprescription salicylate. Its characteristics are similar to those of aspirin, with one major exception: sodium salicylate is not acetylated. As such, it does not have a two-compartment half-life, as does aspirin. In other words, although aspirin has a "first" half-life as acetylsalicylic acid that is approximately 15 minutes, followed by an active metabolite, salicylate, with a half-life of 3 to 5 hours, sodium salicylate has a single compartment active drug half-life of 3 to 5 hours, but that half-life can be prolonged up to 19 hours.[13] The second major difference between aspirin and sodium salicylate is that aspirin acetylates and irreversibly blocks COX. Therefore, platelet aggregation is effectively inhibited for the life of the platelet with aspirin, whereas the antiplatelet adhesion effect is only temporary with the nonacetylated salicylates.

Sodium salicylate is considered somewhat less effective in reducing pain when compared with aspirin. However, some patients who are hypersensitive to aspirin may tolerate sodium salicylate. The dose of sodium salicylate is the same as for aspirin—325 to 650 mg every 4 hours, as needed.

Propionic Acids
Ibuprofen

Ibuprofen is available as an OTC analgesic in modest doses of 200 mg per tablet. For a complete description of the NSAIDs used in pain management, please see Chapter 121. Although OTC doses of ibuprofen are effective in mild to moderate pain, the drug at this low dose does not have anti-inflammatory effects. Ibuprofen is marketed generically and as Motrin, Nuprin, and Advil. It is relatively safe to give to children.

The children's OTC doses are as follows:

- 50 mg every 6 to 8 hours for children weighing 12 to 17 pounds (not more than four doses per day)
- 75 mg every 6 to 8 hours for children weighing 18 to 23 pounds (not more than four doses per day)
- 100 mg every 6 to 8 hours for children weighing 24 to 35 pounds (not more than four doses per day)
- 150 mg every 6 to 8 hours for children weighing 35 to 47 pounds (not more than four doses per day)
- 200 mg every 6 to 8 hours for children weighing 48 to 59 pounds (not more than four doses per day)
- 250 mg every 6 to 8 hours for children weighing 60 to 71 pounds (not more than four doses per day)
- 300 mg every 6 to 8 hours for children weighing 72 to 95 pounds (not more than four doses per day)

Children age 12 and older may be dosed at 200 mg every 4 to 6 hours, with a maximum 24-hour total dose of 1200 mg. The recommended OTC dose for patients who are more than

16 years old and who have mild to moderate pain is 200 to 400 mg every 4 to 6 hours as needed up to a maximum of 1200 mg in a 24-hour period. Absorption is approximately 85%, but it is 90% to 99% albumin bound. The time to peak concentrations is 1 to 2 hours, and the drug's half-life is 2 to 4 hours. In OTC doses (i.e., 200 mg), this medication is safe to use in older patients, with caution.

Naproxen Sodium

Naproxen sodium is available as an OTC analgesic in modest doses of 220 mg per tablet. For a complete description of NSAIDs used in pain management, please see Chapter 121. Although OTC doses of naproxen sodium are effective in mild to moderate pain, the drug at this low dose does not have anti-inflammatory effects. It is marketed on an OTC basis as Aleve. This drug should not be given to children less than 12 years old. The recommended OTC dose for mild to moderate pain in patients who are more than 12 years old is two tablets initially (440 mg), followed by one tablet (220 mg) every 8 to 12 hours. For individuals who are more than 65 years old, the recommended OTC dose is one tablet every 12 hours. The drug is virtually completely absorbed, but it is highly albumin bound. The time to peak concentrations is 1 to 4 hours, and its duration of action is approximately 12 hours. Therefore, naproxen sodium is an excellent choice when an OTC NSAID is indicated and extended duration of action is desired.

Ketoprofen

Ketoprofen is available as an OTC analgesic in modest doses of 12.5 mg per tablet. For a complete description of the NSAIDs used in pain management, please see Chapter 121. Although OTC doses of ketoprofen are effective in mild to moderate pain, the drug at this low dose does not have anti-inflammatory effects. It is marketed for OTC use as Orudis KT. Ketoprofen should not be given to children. The recommended OTC dose for mild to moderate pain in adults who are more than 16 years old is 12.5 mg every 4 to 6 hours as needed up to a maximum of six tablets in a 24-hour period.It is virtually completely absorbed, but it is highly albumin bound. The time to peak concentrations is 30 minutes up to 2 hours, and its half-life is 2.5 hours. In OTC doses, this medication is safe to use in older patients.

Acetaminophen

Acetaminophen is *not* an NSAID. It has a mechanism of action different from that of the NSAIDs, and it has little anti-inflammatory and no antiplatelet activity. However, it is a very good OTC analgesic and has significantly less potential for gastrointestinal irritation when compared with aspirin and the other NSAIDs. On an equivalent-dose basis, acetaminophen is comparable to aspirin in its analgesic abilities. However, acetaminophen has come under fire for its dose-related adverse effects, specifically those associated with liver damage.

Acetaminophen is *N*-acetyl-aminophenol. (The last three letters of ace*tyl* and the last four letters of aminoph*enol* have lent themselves to the naming of the most popular trade-named acetaminophen product, Tylenol.) Acetaminophen is an active metabolite of phenacetin. Analogues of acetaminophen were used in the late 1800s. Although these analogues exhibited good analgesic and antipyretic effects, most had significant adverse effects. Acetaminophen was used sparingly from 1893 until 1950. In 1951, research revealed that acetaminophen was as effective as aspirin for temporary pain relief and fever reduction. McNeil Pharmaceuticals then marketed acetaminophen as an aspirin alternative in 1953 and as an elixir for children in 1955.

Today, acetaminophen is available generically and as brand-named products including Tylenol, Acephen, Aspirin Free Anacin, Tempra, Panadol, Genipap, Liquiprin, and Datril, to name but a few.

Action

The mechanism of acetaminophen's analgesic action has not been fully determined. However, research indicates that acetaminophen inhibits prostaglandin synthesis in a manner somewhat similar to that of aspirin. Although aspirin clearly nonselectively blocks the COX-1 and COX-2 enzymes to inhibit prostaglandin synthesis, it appears that acetaminophen only partially blocks the COX-1 and, perhaps, COX-2 enzymes. Most likely, acetaminophen inhibits specific prostaglandin synthesis associated with the newly identified COX-3 enzyme, as well as a subtype of the COX-1 enzyme.[18] Other researchers have opined that the COX-3 enzyme is a subtype of the COX-2 enzyme.[19] Regardless of the nature of the COX-3 entity, blocking the activity of this newly discovered enzyme provides a reasonable explanation that accounts for acetaminophen's ability to inhibit or diminish pain impulse transmission and perception while having little effect on inflammation and platelet aggregation and not diminishing the production of the prostaglandin that protects the gastrointestinal tract lining.

Dosing

Acetaminophen is available in tablet, capsule, extended-release dosage forms, chewable tablets, rectal suppositories, and liquid elixir for oral pediatric use. The recommended OTC dose for adults is similar to that of aspirin—325 to 650 mg every 4 hours as needed, up to 1 g every 6 hours or 1300 mg every 8 hours. At these higher doses, the self-medicating patient should be carefully reviewed by the physician if the condition does not improve within 10 days. It is essential not to exceed 4 g of acetaminophen per day. The accumulation of the drug causes hepatotoxicity.[20] Initial symptoms of liver damage include nausea, vomiting, and significantly diminished appetite, often mistaken for symptoms of the flu. In June of 2009, an advisory committee to the United States Food and Drug Administration (FDA) recommended that labeling include recommendations that the single adult dose of acetaminophen be limited to no more than 650 mg, a dose significantly less than the 1000 mg currently consumed when a patient takes two 500-mg tablets or capsules. The panel also recommended that the 24-hour dose of acetaminophen be limited to a dose less than the current 24-hour limit of 4000 mg (4 g). The panel cited 56,000 emergency room visits, 26,000 hospitalizations, and 458 deaths annually, according to studies spanning the 1990s. The FDA has yet to act on these recommendations. Another recommendation of the advisory committee that has yet to be acted on is that of eliminating the acetaminophen contained in prescription analgesics (e.g., Vicodin, Percocet, Darvocet). This recommendation was more contentious, given that the affirmative panel vote was 20 to 17.

Dosing in children should be guided by the following formula: 1.5 g per day, in divided doses, for each square meter of body surface. Alternatively, a more convenient guideline[21] was developed by McNeil Laboratories:

- Infants up to 3 months old: 40 mg every 4 hours orally as needed
- Infants 4 to 14 months old: 80 mg every 4 hours orally as needed
- Children 1 to 2 years old: 120 mg every 4 hours orally as needed
- Children 2 to 4 years old: 160 mg every 4 hours orally as needed
- Children 4 to 6 years old: 240 mg every 4 hours orally as needed
- Children 6 to 9 years old: 320 mg every 4 hours orally as needed
- Children 9 to 11 years old: 320 to 400 mg every 4 hours orally as needed
- Children 11 to 12 years old: 320 to 480 mg every 4 hours orally as needed

It is recommended that children up to the age of 12 years receive no more than five doses in any 24-hour period. For children, liquid dosage forms are preferred; however, instructions to parents and caregivers on the dosage calibration when administering liquids using teaspoons or droppers must be clear.

Pharmacokinetics

Acetaminophen is rapidly and almost completely absorbed when it is taken orally.[22,23] Absorption may be decreased if the drug is taken following a meal high in carbohydrates. Rectal absorption is variable and depends largely on the vehicle base. After oral administration, peak levels are reached in 30 to 60 minutes.[22,23] The plasma half-life is approximately 2 hours, and the agent's duration of action is approximately 4 hours. The drug is widely distributed, and it is approximately 20% to 50% plasma protein bound. Acetaminophen does appear in breast milk, but only reaches levels of 10 to 15 mg/mL approximately 1 to 2 hours after administration of a 650-mg dose. The metabolism of acetaminophen occurs primarily in the liver. One of the metabolites may accumulate when the system is saturated; this metabolite is hepatotoxic and nephrotoxic. With doses up to 650 mg, plasma concentrations will reach levels of 5 to 20 mg/mL. Elimination is by the renal pathway; approximately 3% of the dose is excreted unchanged.

Indications in Pain

Acetaminophen is an excellent OTC analgesic drug to be considered in place of aspirin in patients who are sensitive to aspirin or aspirin-like medications; in patients who have ulcers; in patients who experience pain without an inflammatory process; in patients who should not receive antiplatelet drug therapy, including those who are receiving anticoagulant therapy; and in patients receiving uricosuric agents. Although acetaminophen has little or no anti-inflammatory capability and should not be considered in rheumatoid arthritis, it can be used in patients who have mild osteoarthritis. In fact, acetaminophen is recommended as a first-line agent for the treatment of pain associated with osteoarthritis of the hip and knee by the American College of Rheumatology, Subcommittee on Osteoarthritis Guidelines.[24] Additionally, acetaminophen is widely used and is effective in treating general complaints of pain associated with menstruation (e.g., dysmenorrhea), dental pain, headache, joint pain, muscle pain, and integumentary pain. It is less effective in treating visceral pain.

Cautions

The metabolites of acetaminophen are toxic and may accumulate when high doses are employed and when the drug is taken by in liver-impaired individuals. Special concern should be exercised in alcoholic patients, patients with eating disorders, and patients who are fasting.

Acute hepatotoxicity may occur when a single dose of 10 to 15 g or more is taken (150 to 250 mg/kg).[22,23] Doses of 20 to 25 g or more can be fatal.[22,23] Long-term daily use of 4 g or more for extended periods may also lead to serious toxicity. Symptoms of chronic toxicity include significant gastrointestinal disturbance.

If an acute toxic dose is detected within 4 hours, gastric lavage is indicated.[22,23] For many poison control centers, N-acetylcysteine (Mucomyst) is the treatment of choice if it can be administered less than 36 hours after acetaminophen ingestion. However, it is most effective if it is given within 10 hours after acetaminophen ingestion.[25] Treatment consists of 140 mg/kg orally (loading), followed by 70 mg/kg every 4 hours for 17 doses. In any cases of acetaminophen overdose or suspected toxicity, the caregiver should immediately call a poison control center and emergency services. While awaiting recommendations, activated charcoal may be administered. It is effective in binding acetaminophen in cases of acute toxicity.

The therapeutic effects of acetaminophen may be decreased when the drug is given concomitantly with barbiturates, carbamazepine, hydantoins, rifampin, and sulfinpyrazone, which may decrease the drug's analgesic effects. Cholestyramine may decrease acetaminophen absorption, so it is prudent to separate concomitant dosing of acetaminophen and cholestyramine by at least 1 hour.

Barbiturates, carbamazepine, hydantoins, isoniazid, rifampin, and sulfinpyrazone, when given concomitantly with acetaminophen, may have additive effects that increase their cumulative hepatotoxic potential. The effects of warfarin may also be enhanced when given to a patient taking acetaminophen. Consuming alcohol while taking acetaminophen may increase the risk of hepatotoxicity, as will the concomitant use of NSAIDs and acetaminophen.

References

Full references for this chapter can be found on www.expertconsult.com.

Nonsteroidal Anti-Inflammatory Drugs and Cyclooxygenase-2 Inhibitors

Steven D. Waldman

The nonsteroidal anti-inflammatory drugs (NSAIDs) are among the most widely used drugs in the world. This heterogeneous group of drugs includes aspirin, the nonacetylated salicylates, and an ever-increasing number of chemically diverse nonsalicylate compounds commonly referred to as the NSAIDs, a subclass of which is known as the cyclooxygenase-2 (COX-2) inhibitors. All these drugs have become an integral part of the routine treatment of numerous painful conditions.

Although investigators initially assumed that the pain-relieving properties of the NSAIDs could be attributed solely to their inhibition of prostaglandins, more recent research suggested that many of the NSAIDs may exert an antinociceptive effect that is separate from their anti-inflammatory properties and may be useful in the treatment of pain that is not inflammatory in origin. This chapter focuses on the pharmacology, mechanisms of action, adverse effects, and clinical use of NSAIDs. It also provides the clinician with a practical framework for the safe and optimal use of this class of drugs.

Prostaglandin Synthesis and the Analgesic Effects of the Nonsteroidal Anti-Inflammatory Drugs

Investigators initially believed that the pain-relieving properties of the NSAIDs were primarily the result of the ability of these drugs to inhibit the peripheral formation of prostaglandins.[1] Further understanding of the way in which the NSAIDs

produce both beneficial and harmful effects led to the concept that this class of drugs most likely works by inhibition of the enzyme COX. Currently, at least two forms of the enzyme are known to exist. These have been named COX-1 and COX-2.[2] COX-1 activation leads to the production of prostacyclin, which exhibits antithrombogenic and gastric cytoprotective properties. COX-2 is induced by inflammatory stimuli and cytokines and exhibits an anti-inflammatory response. The anti-inflammatory actions of the NSAIDs appear to result from inhibition of COX-2, whereas many of the unwanted side effects, such as gastrointestinal bleeding, result from inhibition of COX-1. Therefore, in theory, drugs that have the highest COX-2 activity and a more favorable ratio of COX-2 to COX-1 activity should have a potent anti-inflammatory activity with fewer side effects than drugs with a less favorable ratio of COX-2 to COX-1 activity. Although this conclusion was the logical result of years of basic science research and led to the development of newer NSAIDs with this seemingly desirable profile, the withdrawal of rofecoxib and valdecoxib from the market in response to unwanted cardiovascular side effects called this line of reasoning into question. At the very least, it pointed to our incomplete understanding of the way in which the NSAIDs affect the various organ systems.[3]

Although the foregoing discussion explains the mechanism by which NSAIDs can relieve pain mediated by the inflammatory response, it does not fully explain the antinociceptive properties of this group of drugs in the treatment of acute pain from a single noxious stimulus on otherwise healthy tissue. This apparent disparity between the relative anti-inflammatory and antinociceptive effects is termed *dissociation*.[4] The proposed reasons for dissociation include the following: (1) NSAIDs produce pain relief in the absence of the physicochemical changes induced by inflammation; (2) NSAIDs appear to exert some central modulation of pain by attenuation of the phenomenon of central sensitization independent of peripheral events including prostaglandin synthesis; and (3) little correlation exists between the efficacy of a given NSAID to relieve pain and the drug's ability to inhibit prostaglandin synthesis.[4] The clinical importance of these findings is the subject of much clinical research.

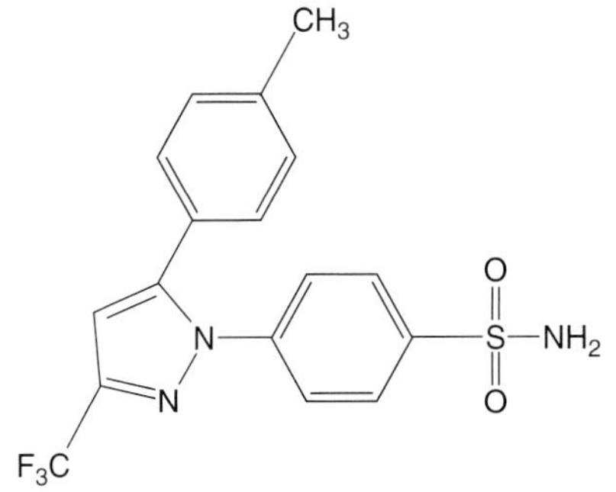

Body's Response to Inflammation

Inflammation is the body's response to tissue injury. Many of the major events in the inflammatory process have been identified, but the reasons for these events and the roles of the different chemical mediators in this process remain unclear. Factors such as the severity of tissue injury and the patient's ability to mount an inflammatory response determine the intensity of inflammation in each individual case.[5] Histamine mediates the initial inflammatory response by producing a transient period of vasoconstriction. Subsequently, vasodilation and increased permeability of blood vessels constitute a process sustained by prostaglandins.[5] In addition to these vascular events, cellular events contribute to the production of inflammation. At the site of inflammation, complement activation causes the release of chemotactic peptides called *leukotrienes*. These peptides diffuse into the adjoining capillaries and cause passing phagocytes to adhere to the endothelium. This process is *pavementing*. The phagocytes insert pseudopods between the endothelial cells and dissolve the basement membrane (diapedesis). The neutrophils then pass out of the blood vessel and move up the concentration gradient of the chemotactic peptides toward the site of inflammation.[4,6] The result of this phagocytic process is the eventual destruction of the neutrophil. When this occurs, intracellular free radicals and lysosomal enzymes are released from the cell into the extracellular space. These substances cause further tissue damage.[6]

As the process continues, other chemical mediators, including complement fragments and interleukin-1, stimulate increased release of leukocytes from the bone marrow.[7] As leukocytes, leukocyte fragments, damaged tissue, and plasma accumulate in the area of injury, an exudate (pus) forms.[6,7] These events characterize acute inflammation. When the precipitating stimulus is removed or destroyed, inflammation resolves. If, however, the precipitating stimulus cannot be eliminated by these body defenses, inflammation will progress from an acute to a chronic state.[5,8,9]

Individual Characteristics of Various Nonsteroidal Anti-Inflammatory Drugs

Salicylates

Aspirin (acetylsalicylic acid) is the prototype of the nonopioid anti-inflammatory drugs (**Fig. 121.1**). Aspirin and aspirin-like drugs are most often administered as analgesics, antipyretics, and inhibitors of platelet aggregation.[10] To achieve anti-inflammatory activity, doses of aspirin greater than 3.6 g per

Fig. 121.1 **Chemical structure of aspirin.**

day are necessary.[10] The serum half-life of salicylates ranges from 2 hours for analgesic doses to more than 20 hours for anti-inflammatory doses.[10]

Orally administered salicylates are rapidly absorbed from the small intestine and, to a lesser extent, from the stomach. No conclusive evidence indicates that sodium bicarbonate given with aspirin (buffered aspirin) results in a faster onset of action, greater peak intensity, or longer analgesic effect. Aspirin available in buffered effervescent preparations, however, undergoes more rapid systemic absorption and achieves higher plasma concentrations than the corresponding tablet formulations. These effervescent preparations also cause less gastrointestinal irritation.[11] Food delays the absorption of salicylates.

Aspirin, by acetylating COX, decreases the formation of both thromboxane (a potent vasoconstrictor and stimulant of platelet aggregation) and prostacyclin (a potent vasodilator and inhibitor of platelet aggregation). Low doses of aspirin, 60 to 100 mg daily, selectively suppress the synthesis of platelet thromboxane without inhibiting the production of endothelial prostacyclin.[9] This selective suppression may explain the favorable effect of low doses of aspirin in preventing coronary artery thrombosis.[12] Aspirin-induced platelet dysfunction seen with higher doses of aspirin lasts for the normal life span of platelets, which is 8 to 11 days.

The decreased platelet aggregation observed with aspirin is not seen with the nonacetylated salicylate products such as choline magnesium trisalicylate (Trilisate) and salsalate (Disalcid).[13,14] These nonacetylated salicylates are a much safer alternative in patients with a bleeding disorder or in those patients scheduled to undergo a surgical procedure.[14] Aspirin should be avoided in patients with severe hepatic dysfunction, vitamin K deficiency, hypoprothrombinemia, or hemophilia because platelet inhibition in such patients can result in hemorrhage.[13] Aspirin should also be avoided in children with chickenpox and flulike illnesses, because the drug has been implicated as a possible causative or contributory factor in the evolution of Reye's syndrome. Patients with asthma and nasal polyposis should also avoid aspirin and aspirin-like drugs because acute allergic reactions may result.

Salicylates may cause gastric irritation and ulceration by a reduction in prostaglandins, which normally inhibit gastric acid secretion and the ability to inhibit COX-1.[14] Alcohol ingestion may exacerbate the problem. To minimize these effects, the salicylates should be taken with food or milk or administered with cytoprotection agents. Being highly bound to albumin (80% to 90%), aspirin and aspirin-like drugs may displace other drugs such as warfarin, oral hypoglycemics, and methotrexate from protein-binding sites.[13]

Diflunisal

Diflunisal (Dolobid) is a difluorophenyl derivative of salicylic acid. This drug has pharmacodynamic and pharmacokinetics profiles similar to those of the other salicylates. Diflunisal has been used primarily for musculoskeletal pain. It is less likely to cause the tinnitus associated with higher doses of aspirin. The initial loading dose for diflunisal is 1000 mg, followed by 250 to 500 mg every 8 to 12 hours.

Nonacetylated Salicylates

Choline magnesium trisalicylate (Trilisate) and salsalate (Disalcid) are two nonacetylated salicylate derivatives that appear to lack many of the side effects of the other members of the salicylate family. These drugs exert significantly fewer effects on platelets and cause fewer gastrointestinal side effects.[15] These unique qualities are especially useful in the oncology patient who may have chemotherapy-induced clotting abnormalities. Both drugs appear to exert analgesic and anti-inflammatory effects similar to those of the acetylated salicylates. Choline magnesium trisalicylate is available in a liquid form, thus making it useful for those patients who are unable to swallow pills.

Other Nonsteroidal Anti-Inflammatory Drugs

Although technically the salicylates and *para*-amino-phenol derivatives (acetaminophen) are included in this class of drugs, the term *nonsteroidal anti-inflammatory drug* has gained common acceptance as a descriptor for the chemically heterogeneous group of drugs that exhibit aspirin-like analgesic and anti-inflammatory properties. NSAIDs provide analgesic effects at lower doses and anti-inflammatory effects at higher doses. The NSAIDs are all antipyretic. Many NSAIDs from several chemical classes are available. More products are in various phases of clinical testing in Europe and the United States. Although the drugs referred to in common parlance as the COX-2 inhibitors are also technically NSAIDs, in this chapter they are considered separately and are discussed later.

In general, the NSAIDs are indicated after simple analgesics have failed to relieve pain, toxic effects have developed, or inflammation is present.[13] All NSAIDs appear to be as effective as aspirin in terms of analgesia or anti-inflammatory properties and may cause fewer gastrointestinal complaints than aspirin, although this relationship may be dose dependent.[13,14] These characteristics have encouraged many physicians to select NSAIDs before aspirin in spite of the increased cost to the patient.

The pharmacokinetic properties of all individual NSAIDs are similar.[16] All these drugs are well absorbed after oral administration, are highly protein bound (>90%), and have a low volume of distribution (<0.21/kg). The NSAIDs readily penetrate synovial fluid in concentrations approximately one half of those found in blood. Elimination depends on hepatic biotransformation to inactive metabolites (except for sulindac, which is metabolized to an active form), with renal excretion of less than 5% of the unchanged drug.[16]

Drug Selection

Many NSAIDs are available. Busy clinicians need not be familiar with each drug, but they should have a working knowledge of one or two agents in each class of drugs. The comparative pharmacologic features of the NSAIDs are summarized in **Table 121.1**. For each drug, physicians should be aware of the need for a loading dose, time from onset of activity to peak effect, routes of administration, cost, and side effect profile. In addition, efficacy may be enhanced by choosing a drug that can be given by a nonoral route (e.g., rectal administration of indomethacin, intramuscular administration of ketorolac tromethamine, topical application of diclofenac). By capitalizing on the unique properties of each drug, physicians can tailor a treatment plan to meet each patient's needs. Practical suggestions for choosing an NSAID are offered in **Table 121.2**.

Because of the great variation in dosage ranges and dosing frequency of NSAIDs, physicians should carefully review the properties of the agent chosen. In general, dosing should be started at the low end of the recommended range and be titrated upward as therapeutic response and side effects dictate. A loading dose should be used if indicated, especially when treating acute pain syndromes.[16,17] Extreme caution should be exercised whenever the recommended ceiling dose is exceeded.[18]

Patients' responses to NSAIDs are typically variable and highly individual.[19,20] Therefore, it is reasonable to try other NSAIDs in a selective manner after an adequate trial (2 to 3 weeks) at an adequate dose (either anti-inflammatory or analgesic).[16,21] Patients should always be instructed that a trial with more than one drug may be necessary and that compliance with the scheduled regimen is important in evaluating effectiveness. Combination of one NSAID with other NSAIDs or aspirin increases toxic effects while providing no added benefit.[20] If additional analgesic effects are needed, a narcotic analgesic may be used during the acute phase of the pain problem.

Side Effects

Considering their diversity in chemical structure, NSAIDs are extremely well tolerated. When compared with all the other nonopioid drugs currently used to treat acute pain, NSAIDs have among the most favorable risk-to-benefit ratios. However, as with all medications, these drugs can cause side effects ranging from minor annoyances (e.g., dyspepsia, diarrhea, constipation) to life-threatening conditions (e.g., gastrointestinal hemorrhage, hepatic dysfunction, renal insufficiency).[22,23] Consequently, physicians need to anticipate the potential for side effects and use this important group of drugs appropriately. **Table 121.3** summarizes the potential side effects of the NSAIDs.

NSAIDs have also been shown to cause numerous renal complications, including peripheral edemas, transient acute renal insufficiency, tubulointerstitial nephropathy, hyperkalemia, and renal papillary necrosis.[23] Piroxicam, tolmetin, and especially sulindac are considered less likely to have renal side effects. Higher incidences of adverse effects on kidney function have been seen with indomethacin, ibuprofen, fenoprofen, mefenamic acid, naproxen, and diclofenac.[24] Prostaglandin-mediated renal effects are usually reversible on discontinuation of therapy if the toxicity is identified early. Identifying a patient

Table 121.1 Nonsteroidal Anti-Inflammatory Drugs: Comparative Pharmacology

Drug	Proprietary Names (Not All-inclusive)	Average Oral Analgesic Dose (mg)	Dose Interval (hr)	Maximal Daily Dose (mg)	Analgesic Efficacy Compared with Standards	Plasma Half-Life (hr)	Comments
PROPIONIC ACIDS							
Ibuprofen	Motrin, Rufen, Nuprin, Advil, Medipren, others	200–400	4–6	2,400	Superior at 200 mg to aspirin 650 mg	2.0–2.5	Most commonly used NSAID in United States; available without prescription
Naproxen	Naprosyn Naprelan	500 initially, 250 subsequently	6–8	1,500	Superior at 400 mg to aspirin 325 mg with codeine 30 mg	12–15	Better tolerated than indomethacin and aspirin
Naproxen sodium	Anaprox	550 initially, 275 subsequently	6–8	1,650	275 mg comparable to aspirin 650 mg, with slower onset and longer duration; 550 mg superior to aspirin 650 mg		
Naproxen sodium Fenoprofen Ketoprofen Ketoprofen OTC Oxaprozin	Aleve Nalfon Orudis Actron, Orudis-K+ Daypro	220 200 25–50 12.5–25 600	8–12 4–6 6–8 4–6 12–24	— 1,000 300 300 1,200	Comparable with aspirin; superior at 25 mg to aspirin 650 mg	3–1.5 24–69	— SR preparation available
PYRROLACETIC ACIDS							
Ketorolac	Toradol	30 or 60 IM or 30 IV initially, 15 or 30 IV or IM subsequently	6	150 first day, 120 thereafter	In the range of 6–12 mg of morphine	6	Limit treatment to 5 days; may precipitate renal failure in dehydrated patients; average dose in older patients, 10–15 IM/IV q6h
INDOLEACETIC ACIDS							
Indomethacin	Indocin Indocin SR Indochron ER				Comparable with aspirin 650 mg	2	Not routinely used because of high incidence of GI and CNS side effects; rectal and SR oral forms available for adults
SALICYLATES							
Acetylated							
Aspirin	Numerous	500–1,000	4–6	4,000		0.25	Because of risk of Reye's syndrome, do not use in children <12 yr with possible viral illness; rectal suppository available for children and adults; SR preparation available
Modified							
Diflunisal	Dolobid	1,000 initially, 500 subsequently	8–12	1,500	500 mg superior to aspirin 650 mg, with slower onset and longer duration; an initial dose of 1,000 mg significantly shortens time to onset	8–12	Dose in older patients of 500–1,000 mg/day does not yield salicylate

Continued

Table 121.1 Nonsteroidal Anti-Inflammatory Drugs: Comparative Pharmacology—cont'd

Drug	Proprietary Names (Not All-inclusive)	Average Oral Analgesic Dose (mg)	Dose Interval (hr)	Maximal Daily Dose (mg)	Analgesic Efficacy Compared with Standards	Plasma Half-Life (hr)	Comments
Salicylate Salts							
Choline magnesium	Trilisate	1,000–1,500	12	2,000–3,000	Longer duration of action than aspirin 650 mg	9–17	Unlike aspirin and other NSAIDs, does not increase bleeding time
Trisalicylate	Tricosal						
Sulindac	Clinoril	150	12	400		7.8 active metabolite = 16	
Etodolac	Lodine	300–400	8–12	1,000	More potent than sulindac and naproxen; less potent than indomethacin		
Tolmetin	Tolectin	200–600	8	1,800		5	
ANTHRANILIC ACIDS							
Mefenamic acid	Ponstel	500 initially, 250 subsequently	6	1,500	Comparable with aspirin 650 mg	2	In United States, use restricted to interval of 1 wk
PHENYLACETIC ACIDS							
Diclofenac potassium	Cataflam	50	8	150	Superior in efficacy and analgesic duration to aspirin 650 mg		More selective for COX-2 than COX-1
ENOLIC ACIDS							
Meloxicam	Mobic	7.5–15	24	15	Equivalent to 200 mg ibuprofen	15–20	10-fold selective for COX-2
Piroxicam	Feldene	20–40	24	40	Equivalent to 50 mg aspirin	50	
NAPHTHYLALKANONE							
Nabumetone	Relafen	1,000 initially, 500–750 subsequently	8–12	2,000	Pain relief equal to aspirin, indomethacin, naproxen, and sulindac	24	Fewer GI side effects
COX-2 SELECTIVE							
Celecoxib	Celebrex	200–400	12–24	400	Anti-inflammatory and analgesic effect similar to naproxen	11	Only COX-2 selective not withdrawn from US market.

CNS, central nervous system; COX, cyclooxygenase; ER, extended release; GI, gastrointestinal; IM, intramuscularly; IV, intravenously; NSAIDs, nonsteroidal anti-inflammatory drugs; OTC, over the counter; SR, sustained release.

with borderline renal function purely on clinical grounds is often impossible. For this reason, a baseline measurement of the serum creatinine level should be obtained before NSAID therapy is begun. This determination alerts the physician to preexisting renal problems that may be exacerbated by NSAID use and enables the physician to attribute correctly any changes in renal function that occur during NSAID therapy in patients who had normal function before treatment.[25]

In general, NSAIDs should be taken with food to minimize gastrointestinal side effects. A past history of dyspepsia and gastrointestinal upset may indicate the need for the concurrent use of gastric cytoprotective agents. A past history of gastric ulceration or hemorrhage requires that NSAIDs be used only after medications that are free of gastrointestinal side effects have failed to control the pain adequately. In this event, histamine-blocking and cytoprotective agents should be given concurrently with NSAIDs, and patients should be carefully monitored for occult gastrointestinal blood loss. NSAID therapy should be discontinued at the first sign of gastrointestinal difficulties.[22] The concurrent use of two or more NSAIDs increases the risk of side effects (as may the concurrent use of an NSAID and a simple analgesic such as acetaminophen). Thus, patients with acute pain must be carefully questioned about their use of over-the-counter agents.

Table 121.2 Guidelines for Choosing an Optimal Nonsteroidal Anti-Inflammatory Drug

Assess the patient's renal status, hepatic and cardiovascular status, and history of peptic ulcer disease before starting the drug.

Determine the best route of administration.

Identify the drugs that are appropriate for the route of administration desired.

Select a familiar agent among these drugs whose time between onset of activity and peak effect is appropriate for the pain syndrome being treated.

Table 121.3 Potential Side Effects of Nonsteroidal Anti-Inflammatory Drugs

Cardiovascular	NSAIDs: Hypertension, decreased effectiveness of antihypertensive medications, inhibition of platelet activation, propensity for bruising and hemorrhage COX-2 inhibitors: Myocardial infarction, stroke, thromboembolic events
Gastrointestinal	Ulcers, anemia, gastrointestinal hemorrhage, perforation, diarrhea, nausea, anorexia, abdominal pain
Renal	Deterioration of kidney function, analgesic nephropathy, salt and water retention, edema, decreased effectiveness of diuretic medication, decreased urate excretion, hyperkalemia
Central nervous system	NSAIDs: Headache, dizziness, vertigo, confusion, depression Salicylates: Lowering of seizure threshold, hyperventilation
Hypersensitivity	Vasomotor rhinitis, asthma, urticaria, flushing, hypotension, shock

COX-2, cyclooxygenase-2; NSAIDs, nonsteroidal anti-inflammatory drugs.

Cyclooxygenase-2 Inhibitors

With increased understanding of the role of the enzyme COX in the efficacy and side effects of the NSAIDs, investigators thought that most side effects associated with this clinically useful class of drugs resulted from inhibition of COX-1. Investigators believed that developing drugs with increased affinity for COX-2 would lead to drugs with better clinical efficacy and fewer side effects. This logic was somewhat correct, and a new subclass of NSAIDs with fewer gastrointestinal side effects was developed, the COX-2 inhibitors.[2] The first of these drugs in widespread clinical use was celecoxib (Celebrex). It became an enormous commercial success and encouraged the development and release of similar drugs. With widespread clinical use, it became apparent that, although these drugs did produce fewer gastrointestinal side

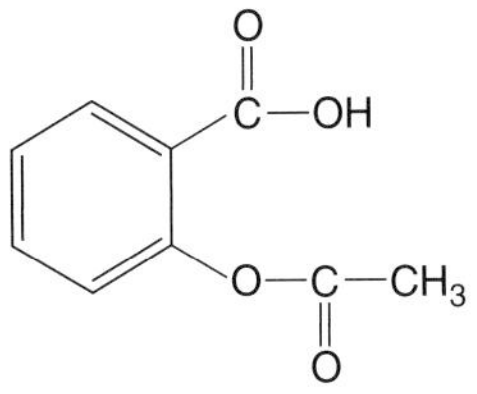

Fig. 121.2 **Chemical structure of celecoxib.**

effects, the COX-2 inhibitors appeared to increase the risk of cardiovascular side effects, including an increased risk of myocardial infarction.[26] As a consequence, several COX-2 inhibitors were withdrawn from the US market. The actual risk profile of this class of drugs has yet to be elucidated fully, and whether these drugs should remain available to patients suffering from inflammatory arthritides and connective tissue diseases remains to be answered.

Celecoxib

One of the first COX-2 inhibitors available for clinical use, celecoxib (Celebrex), found widespread acceptance as an analgesic and anti-inflammatory drug (**Fig. 121.2**). The initial promise of decreased gastrointestinal side effects, although not absolute, represented a positive advance for patients and prescribing physicians alike.[27] Supplied as 100-mg, 200-mg, and 400-mg tablets, celecoxib should be started at 100 mg twice a day by mouth or as a single 200-mg dose by mouth. The dose may be increased carefully while one observes for hepatic, renal, gastrointestinal, or cardiovascular side effects, to a maximum daily dose of 400 mg. Higher doses have been used for the treatment of familial polyposis, but they are not generally recommended for pain management indications.

Clinical experience with celecoxib has been positive, but the increased incidence of stroke and cardiac abnormalities led the US Food and Drug Administration to mandate a "black box" warning to ensure that the patients and prescribing physicians were aware of these potentially fatal side effects. Whether the risk of these side effects warrants the discontinuation of this drug in patients who have tolerated it is unclear, nor is it certain whether these drugs should be used as first-line analgesic or anti-inflammatory agents at all.

Conclusion

The NSAIDs are a heterogeneous group of compounds that have been shown to be effective in the management of numerous acute and chronic painful conditions. The clinician must understand the basic pharmacokinetic data of each NSAID prescribed, to optimize pain relief and avoid side effects.

References

Full references for this chapter can be found on www.expertconsult.com.

Opioid Analgesics

Dhanalakshmi Koyyalagunta and Steven D. Waldman

Opioid analgesics remain important agents for the treatment of most pain syndromes. Morphine is the prototypic opioid and is the standard against which all opioids are compared. Morphine and its related compounds act at the opioid receptor much like the naturally occurring substances—endogenous opioid peptides. The basic biology of this endogenous opioid system and of the available opioids has been well studied. Opioids are associated with side effects including tolerance, addiction, and abuse. Research is ongoing to discover an efficacious opioid that has minimal side effects and no potential for abuse. Current evidence supporting genetic polymorphism at the mu (μ) receptor has been implicated in variability in response to opioid analgesics and drug addiction.

The medicinal use of opium and morphine in different cultures and ancient civilizations is well documented. Primitive human beings, while experimenting with various plants to ascertain what was edible, probably discovered the value of some of these plants in relieving pain. The pharmacologic effects of opium were well documented 5000 years ago when, at the dawn of history, the Sumerians mentioned the poppy in their pharmacopoeia and called it "*HU GIL*," the plant of joy.[1] The Ebers Papyrus, written in 1552 BC, describes early Egyptian formulas, some of which contain opium.

The first reference to opium dates back to third century BC, in the writings of Theophrastus.[2] Scribonius Largus, in his *Compositiones Medicamentorum* (40 AD), described the method

Endogenous Opioid Peptides

The observation that electrical stimulation of certain areas in the rat brain elicits profound analgesia and that this analgesia[5] is readily reversible by the opioid antagonist naloxone[6] implies the presence of an endogenous opioid system.[7] In 1975, an endogenous, opiate-like factor was identified and named *enkephalin* (from the head).[8] Soon after, two more classes of endogenous opioid peptides were isolated—the dynorphins and the endorphins. Each of these peptide groups is derived from a distinct precursor polypeptide and has a characteristic anatomic distribution. The precursors are preproenkephalin, preprodynorphin, and preproopiomelanocortin (Pre-POMC). Each of these precursors undergoes complex cleavages and modifications to yield multiple active peptides. All the opioid peptides have a common amino-terminal sequence of Tyr-Gly-Gly-Phe- (met or leu), which has been called the *opioid motif.*[9] ß-Endorphin is derived from proopiomelanocortin (POMC), and met-enkephalin and leu-enkephalin are derived from the processing of proenkephalin and dynorphin arises from cleavage of prodynorphin. Pre-POMC is also processed into other nonopioid peptides, such as adrenocorticotropic hormone (ACTH), melanocyte-stimulating hormone (MSH), and ß-lipoprotein (ß-l-LPH). In 1995, a novel peptide was cloned by two groups of investigators and was named *orphanin FQ* (OFQ) by one group and *nociceptin (N)* by the other group. N/OFQ has behavioral and pain modulatory properties distinct from those of the classic opioid peptides. The endogenous opioids are degraded by peptidases, and their action is very short-lived.

The relative distributions of these endogenous peptides have been established by biochemical and histochemical studies. The production of ß-endorphin is relatively limited to the nervous system and is found in the pituitary, arcuate nucleus, medial basal hypothalamus, nucleus of the solitary tract, and nucleus commissuralis. The second major neuronal pathway (proenkephalin) is widespread and also includes endocrine and central nervous system (CNS) distributions. Proenkephalin peptides are present in areas of CNS that are involved in perception of pain (laminae I and II of the spinal cord, spinal trigeminal nucleus, and periaqueductal gray), modulation of affective behavior (cerebral cortex, amygdala, hippocampus, and locus ceruleus), modulation of motor control (caudate nucleus and globus pallidus), regulation of autonomic nervous system (medulla oblongata), and neuroendocrinologic functions (median eminence).[9] Proenkephalin peptides are also present in the gastrointestinal tract and the adrenal medulla. Even though prodynorphin has an anatomic distribution similar to that of proenkephalin, dynorphins are weak analgesics. The N/OFQ precursor is distributed in the hippocampus, cortex, and other sensory sites. N/OFQ has a complex pharmacologic profile and is capable of eliciting opposing actions that depend on the dose and paradigm employed.[10] It produces naloxone-sensitive analgesia and has also been shown to exhibit an antiopioid effect. Opioid peptides exert their pharmacologic effects through membrane bound G-protein–coupled receptors.

Opioid Receptors

The existence of opiate receptors was first hypothesized in 1954. The first convincing evidence regarding the existence of multiple opioid receptors was proposed by Martin et al, in 1976, based on addiction, cross-tolerance, and abstinence

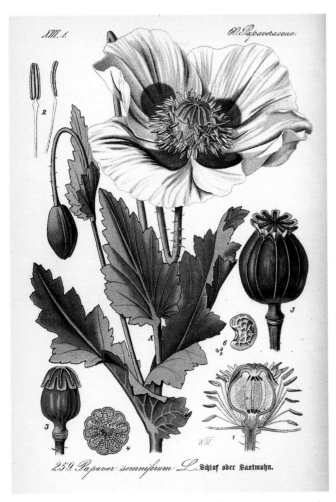

Fig. 122.1 The poppy plant (*Papaver somniferum*, Papaveraceae). *(From Prof. Dr. Otto Wilhelm Thomé: Flora von Deutschland, Österreich, und der Schweiz. Germany, 1885, Gera.)*

for procuring opium and mentioned that opium was derived from the unripe seed capsule of the poppy plant (**Fig. 122.1**).[3] Arab physicians used opium extensively and even wrote special treatises (Avicenna, 980 to 1037) on some of its preparations. Arabs introduced opium to China, where it was used to treat dysenteries. Sertuner isolated the active constituent of opium in 1805. He experimented with it on animals, himself, and his friends. He called his new discovery *principium somniferum*; in 1817 he renamed it *morphine* after Morpheus, the Greek god of dreams.

The discovery of the other alkaloids soon followed, codeine was discovered in 1832, papaverine in 1848, and the endogenous opioids in the 1970s. Some confusion still exists about the terminology used to describe these compounds. *Opiate* refers to any agent derived from opium (alkaloids), and *opioids* are all endogenous and exogenous substances with morphine-like properties.[4]

This chapter focuses on the description of the endogenous opioid system, its anatomy and diversity, the mechanism of opioid analgesia, and the pharmacokinetic and pharmacodynamic differences among opioid agonists and antagonists. A brief review of the various routes of administration is presented. The focus of the chapter is to establish a basis of understanding of the various clinically used opioid medications.

syndromes in dogs with chronic spinal transection.[11] Using receptor-binding studies and subsequent cloning, these investigators showed the existence of three main receptor types and named them based on the drugs used in their studies: μ or morphine receptor, sigma (σ) or SKF-10047 receptor, and kappa (κ) or ketocyclazocine receptor. The existence of the delta (δ; deferens) receptor was proposed by Lord et al.[12] N/OFQ receptor opioid receptor–like-1 (ORL-1) was cloned in 1994. Other subtypes include iota (ι), lambda (λ), and zeta (ζ). Subtypes of the μ receptor (μ_1 and μ_2), δ receptor (δ_1 and δ_2), and κ receptor (κ_1, κ_2, and κ_3) have been described. Several other nomenclatures have been put forth to describe these receptors. Molecular biologists have renamed the δ, κ, μ, and N/OFQ receptors DOR, KOR, MOR, and NOR, respectively. The International Union of Pharmacology (IUPHAR) has set guidelines that receptors should be named after their endogenous ligands, followed by a numeric subscript depicting the chronologic order of the demonstration of the existence of these receptors: OP_1 (δ receptor), OP_2 (κ receptor), and OP_3 (μ receptor).

Opioid receptors consist of seven transmembrane domains with conserved proline and aromatic residues, a characteristic of G-protein–coupled receptors.[13] Significant structural homology has been observed among the three opioid receptor cDNA clones. The μ receptor is 66% identical to the δ receptor and 68% identical to the κ receptor, whereas the δ and κ receptors have 58% identical amino acid sequences.[12] Charged residues located in the transmembrane domains have been implicated in the high-affinity binding of most opioid ligands. The μ receptors bind to endorphins more so than enkephalins, the δ receptors bind to enkephalins, and the κ receptors potently bind to dynorphins. N/OFQ binds to ORL-1, a protein with a structure typical of a G-protein–coupled receptor.[14]

Opioid receptors are distributed within the CNS and periphery. The μ receptors are distributed throughout the neuraxis, with the highest density in the caudate nucleus. They are also present in the neocortex, thalamus, nucleus accumbens (NAcc), hippocampus, amygdala, and superficial layers of the dorsal horn of the spinal cord.[15] Most of the spinal μ-receptor ligand binding sites are located presynaptically on the terminals of primary afferent nociceptors. The μ receptor is most strongly identified with the analgesic and addicting properties of opioid drugs. Morphine has been shown to exhibit a 50-fold higher affinity for μ than for δ receptors.[16] The μ receptor controls various physiologic functions, including nociception, respiration, cardiovascular functions, intestinal transit, feeding, learning and memory, locomotor activity, thermoregulation, hormone secretion, and immune function.[12]

δ Receptors have a more restricted distribution in the CNS. They are located in the olfactory bulb, caudate, putamen, neocortex, NAcc, thalamus, hypothalamus, and brainstem. The δ receptor is involved in analgesia, motor integration, cognitive function, mood-driven behavior, gastrointestinal motility, olfaction, and respiration. Activation of the δ receptor produces spinal analgesia without concomitant respiratory depression.

The κ receptor is involved in the regulation of nociception, diuresis, feeding, immune function, neuroendocrine function, and possibly thermoregulation. Diuresis results from inhibition of release of antidiuretic hormone. κ–Agonist application to the spinal cord produces facilitation and inhibition of the

Table 122.1 Opioid Receptors and Their Clinical Effects

Receptor	Effect
Mu (μ)	
μ_1	Supraspinal analgesia
	Spinal analgesia
	Respiratory depression
	Slowing of gastric transit
μ_2	Pruritus, nausea, vomiting
	Most cardiovascular effects
	Physical dependence
	Euphoria
Kappa (κ)	
κ_1	Spinal analgesia
	Diuresis
	Sedation
	Miosis
κ_2	Low potential for abuse
κ_3	Supraspinal analgesia
Delta (δ)	Modulation of μ-receptor activity
	Spinal analgesia
Sigma (σ)	No analgesia
	Dysphoria
	Hypertonia
	Respiratory and vasomotor stimulation
	Mydriasis

Adapted from Pasternak GW: Pharmacological mechanisms of opioid analgesics, *Clin Neuropharmacol* 16:1, 1993; and Reisine T, Pasternak G: Opioid analgesics and antagonists. In Hardman JG, Limbard LE, editors: *Goodman and Gilman's the pharmacologic basis of therapeutics,* ed 9, New York, 1996, McGraw-Hill, p 521.

C-fiber–evoked nociceptive responses.[17] Activation of κ receptors causes spinal analgesia, dysphoria, and sedation without concomitant respiratory depression.[4] Dynorphins may have a role in modulating the development of central plasticity and hyperalgesia (**Table 122.1**).

The μ-receptor mRNA is present in medium- and large-diameter dorsal root ganglion (DRG) cells, whereas the δ-receptor mRNA is found in large-diameter cells and the κ-opioid receptor mRNA is found in small- and medium-diameter cells.[18] This differential localization may be the reason for functional differences in pain modulation.

N/OFQ stimulates food intake, produces anxiolysis, and has a role in memory and information processing. Drugs interacting with the ORL-1 receptor appear to be free of abuse potential.[14]

Classification of Opioids

Three schemes are used to classify opioids. Based on their intrinsic action at the receptor site, opioids can be classified as partial agonists (buprenorphine), agonists (e.g., morphine, codeine, methadone, fentanyl), agonist-antagonists (butorphanol, nalbuphine, pentazocine, and dezocine), and antagonists (naloxone, naltrexone, cholecystokinin) (**Table 122.2**). Based on their affinity for the opioid receptor, these agents are considered weak (codeine, propoxyphene) or strong opioids. The other classification is based on how the opioids are derived: naturally occurring (morphine and codeine) or semisynthetic

Table 122.2 Classification of Opioids on the Basis of Intrinsic Activity* and Synthetic Origin

AGONISTS

Phenanthrene Alkaloids

Morphine

Codeine

Thebaine

Semisynthetic Opioids

Diacetylmorphine (heroin)

Hydrocodone

Hydromorphone

Oxycodone

Oxymorphone

Synthetic Opioids

Morphinan derivatives: levorphanol

Phenylpiperidine derivatives

Meperidine

Fentanyl

Sufentanil

Alfentanil

Propioanilide derivatives

Methadone

Propoxyphene

AGONIST-ANTAGONISTS

Semisynthetic Opioids

Buprenorphine

Nalbuphine

Synthetic Opioids

Benzomorphan derivatives: pentazocine

Morphinan derivatives: butorphanol dezocine

ANTAGONISTS

Naloxone

Naltrexone

Methylnaltrexone

Alvimopan

*Intrinsic activity refers to the intensity of the pharmacologic effect initiated by the drug-receptor complex.
From Ferrante M: Opioids. In Ferrante M, VadeBoncouer T, editors: *Postoperative pain management*, New York, 1993, Churchill Livingstone, p 145.

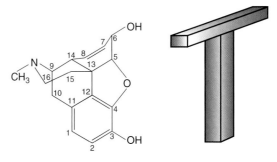

Fig. 122.2 **The T-shaped molecule of morphine.**

conforms to a "T" shape with a piperidine ring forming one crossbar and a hydroxylated aromatic ring lying in the vertical axis (**Fig. 122.2**).

Modification of functional groups on the skeleton gives rise to the semisynthetic opioids: diacetylmorphine, hydromorphone, oxymorphone, hydrocodone, and oxycodone (**Fig. 122.3**). Synthetic opioids are created by progressive reduction of the number of fused rings on the phenanthrene moiety (**Fig. 122.4**). Codeine is a methylmorphine, with the phenolic hydroxyl group possessing the methyl substitution. Thebaine has very little analgesic property but is a precursor to the strong analgesic compound oxycodone and the antagonist naloxone. Etorphine, a derivative of thebaine, is more than 1000 times as potent as morphine.

Mechanism of Action

Opioid receptors, as mentioned earlier, are widespread across the CNS and the periphery. These receptors are bivalent, with one portion (transmembrane regions) mediating signal transduction and the other (extracellular loop) determining receptor selectivity.[14] The recognition site on these receptors is specific, and only the l-isomers exhibit analgesic activity.[19] Alkaloids are small and fit at the mouth of the receptor core, whereas peptides bind to the extracellular loops and activate the common binding site by extending to the receptor core. Opioids bind to the receptors with varying affinities. The analgesic potency of an opioid is determined by its affinity to the receptor. Using various bioassay systems, the rank order of the binding affinities has been determined, with sufentanil exhibiting the highest binding affinity.[20]

The spatial orientation of the various amino acids in the transmembrane regions and the extracellular loops determine the formation of the binding pocket of the receptor. The opioid receptor is anionic, and an opioid must be in an ionic state for binding to occur.[21] Activation of the opioid receptors produces effects that are primarily inhibitory. Direct inhibitory effects of opioids are mediated by opioid receptors coupled to pertussis-sensitive G_i/G_0 proteins and direct excitatory effects through a cholera toxin–sensitive G_s protein.[22-24] Opioid agonists inhibit adenylyl cyclase and thereby decrease cyclic adenosine monophosphate (cAMP) production. They close N-type voltage-operated calcium channels and open receptor-operated potassium channels. This process results in hyperpolarization and a decrease in neuronal excitability. Nanomolar concentrations of opioids can produce excitatory effects by activating excitatory G_s proteins (**Fig. 122.5**). This antagonism of excitatory activity may explain the observation that co-treatment with extremely low doses of an antagonist can enhance the analgesic efficacy of opioid agonists.[22]

or synthetic compounds. Opium contains two distinct alkaloid types: phenanthrenes and benzylisoquinolones. The phenanthrene derivatives are morphine, codeine, and thebaine. The benzylisoquinolone alkaloids are papaverine (vasodilator, no analgesic property) and noscapine.

Opium still remains the main production source for morphine because laboratory synthesis is not possible. Morphine consists of five condensed ring systems. The morphine molecule has six chiral centers, present on the nitrogen atom and on the carbon atom 5, 6, 8, 9, and 13. The pentacyclic structure

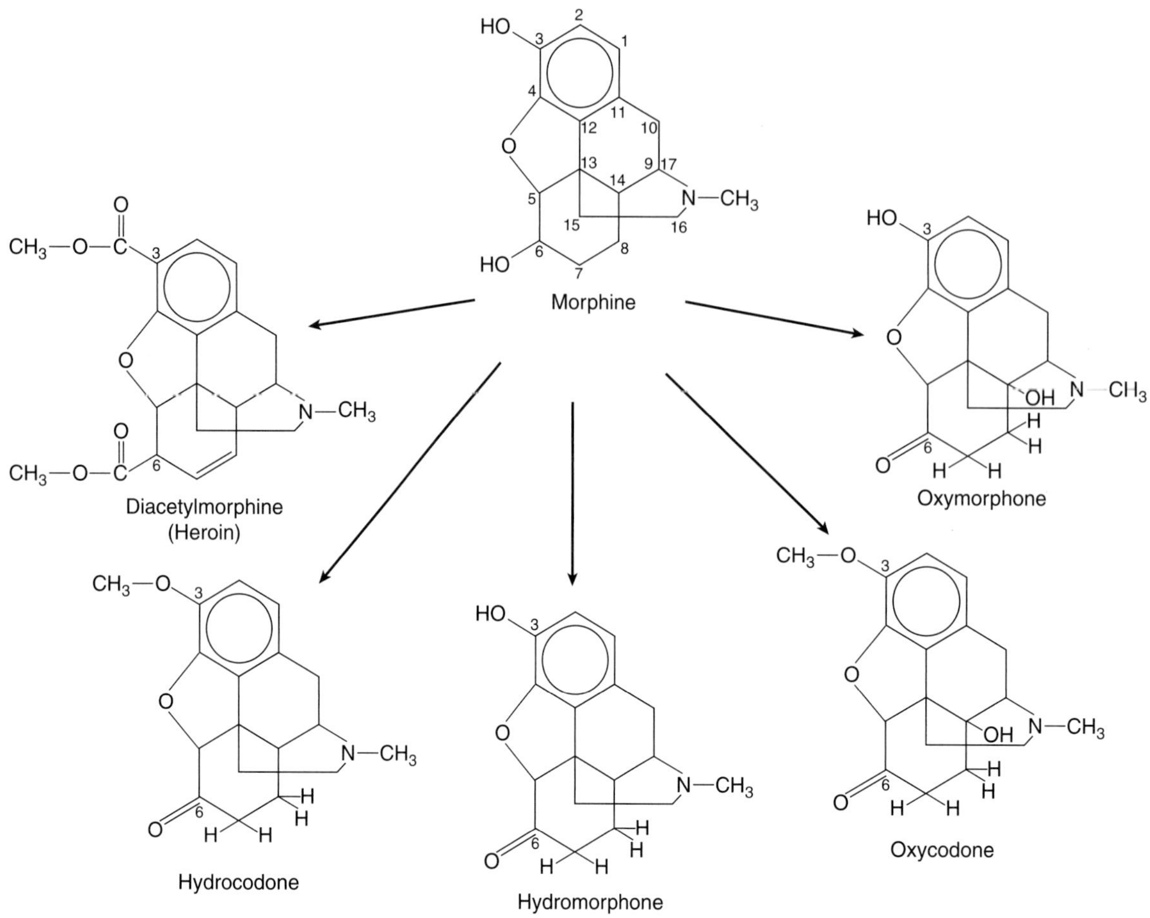

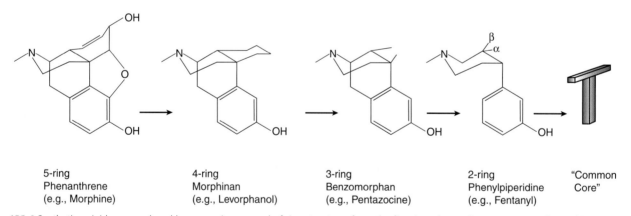

Fig. 122.3 **Chemical structure of semisynthetic opioids diacetylmorphine, hydromorphone, oxymorphone, hydrocodone, and oxycodone.** *(Adapted from Ferrante M: Opioids. In Ferrante M, VadeBoncouer T, editors:* Postoperative pain management, *New York, 1993, Churchill Livingstone, p 145.)*

Fig. 122.4 Synthetic opioids are produced by successive removal of ring structures from the five-ring phenanthrene structure of morphine. However, a common core, resembling a "T" shape, is shared by all opioids. A piperidine ring (which is believed to confer "opioid-like" properties to a compound) forms the crossbar, and a hydroxylated phenyl group forms the vertical axis. *(Adapted from Ferrante M: Opioids. In Ferrante M, VadeBoncouer T, editors:* Postoperative pain management, *New York, 1993, Churchill Livingstone, p 145.)*

Another mode of opioid action is the inhibition of γ-aminobutyric acid (GABA)-ergic transmission in a local circuit (e.g., in the brainstem, where GABA acts to inhibit pain-inhibitory neurons). The net effect of this disinhibitory action would be to excite a descending inhibitory circuit. Opioids also decrease the pain-evoked release of tachykinins from primary afferent nociceptors.[25] Opioid agonists have a peripheral analgesic effect. Opioid receptors synthesized in the DRG are transported to the peripheral tissues.[26,27] Locally released endogenous opioid compounds are up-regulated during inflammatory pain states.[28] Peripheral opioid analgesia is possibly mediated by G-protein–coupled inhibition of cAMP in peripheral terminals.[27] A single nucleotide polymorphism (SNP) at the μ receptor has been implicated in variability in response to opioid analgesics and drug addiction.[29] These genetic differences may account for unusually high doses of morphine requirement

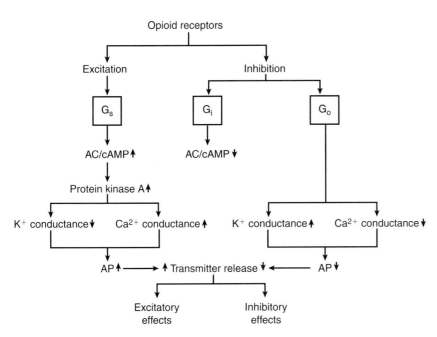

Fig. 122.5 Opioid agonists in micromolar concentrations are primarily inhibitory. They decrease the activity of adenylyl cyclase (AC), intracellular cyclic adenosine monophosphate (cAMP), and the action potential (AP), with resulting neuronal hyperpolarization. In contrast, nanomolar concentrations cause the opposite effects and increase neuronal excitability. Ca2+, calcium; K+, potassium. (*Adapted from Bovill JG: Update on opioid and analgesic pharmacology,* Anesth Analg *92[3 Suppl]:1, 2001.*)

in some patients and for intolerance to codeine administration in others.[30] Ongoing pharmacogenetic studies are investigating individual responses to various opioids further.

Pharmacodynamics

Central Nervous System

Opioids produce analgesia by mimicking the action of endogenous opioids. The drugs act to produce analgesia at several levels of the CNS. Most of the clinically used opioids cause analgesia by binding to the μ receptor and share a common spectrum of pharmacodynamic effects. δ-Receptor agonists are potent analgesics in animals and in some isolated cases in humans, but the clinical use of δ-receptor agonists is limited because these agents do not cross the blood-brain barrier.[31] κReceptor agonists produce analgesia mediated primarily at spinal sites. Some opioids (meperidine, methadone, ketobemidone, and dextropropoxyphene) have antihyperalgesic and antiallodynic effect by their *N*-methyl-d-aspartate (NMDA) antagonist properties. Preclinical studies showed that the NMDA receptor antagonists reverse or prevent the development of morphine tolerance.[32] Analgesic effects of opioids arise from the ability of these drugs to inhibit the ascending transmission of nociceptive information from the spinal cord dorsal horn and to activate the descending inhibitory pathways. Opioids, by their action on the limbic system, alter the emotional response to pain and make it bearable. In addition to central effects, opioid agonists have peripheral analgesic effects. Opioids depress the spontaneous firing of nociceptors of inflamed skin in a naloxone-reversible manner. *Equianalgesia* is the same degree of pain relief obtained by different drugs at specified doses (**Table 122.3**) and is a way of comparing the analgesic effects of drugs.

Opioids produce euphoria, tranquility, and rewarding behavior. Euphoria is mediated by μ receptors. Activation of κ receptors produces dysphoria. The dopaminergic pathways, particularly involving the NAcc, are responsible for drug-induced reward.[9] Opioid agonists with an affinity for μ and δ opioid receptors are rewarding, whereas opioid agonists with affinity for κ receptors are aversive.[33] High concentrations of

Table 122.3 Relative Potencies of Opioid Analgesics

Drug	Relative Potency IM	Relative Potency PO
Morphine	10	30
Hydromorphone	1.5	7.5
Meperidine	75	300
Methadone	10	12.5
Codeine	120	200
Levorphanol	2	4
Nalbuphine	10	
Oxycodone		30
Pentazocine	60	180

IM, intramuscularly; PO, by mouth.
From Katz JA: Opioids and nonsteroidal analgesics. In Raj PP, editor: *Pain medicine: a comprehensive review,* St Louis, 1996, Mosby, p 126.

opioid receptors and noradrenergic neurons present in the locus ceruleus are thought to play a major role in feelings of alarm, panic, fear, and anxiety. Exogenous and endogenous opioid peptides inhibit neural activity in the locus ceruleus. At high doses, opioids produce sleep; rapid alpha waves are replaced by slower delta waves on the electroencephalogram (EEG).[34]

Opioids have an antitussive effect by depressing the cough center in the medulla. No correlation exists between suppression of cough and the respiratory depressant effect of opioids. Opioids differ in their capacity to depress the cough reflex (**Table 122.4**). Suppression of coughing seems to be less sensitive to naloxone reversal.

All opioids produce some degree of nausea, as a result of direct stimulation of the chemoreceptor trigger zone for emesis in the area postrema of the medulla. The nausea also has a vestibular component caused by opioids because nausea and vomiting are more common in ambulatory patients who have

Table 122.4 Antitussive Effects of Opioids (Decreasing Order of Potency)

Diacetylmorphine = fentanyl = hydromorphone = hydrocodone
Methadone
Codeine
Morphine
Levorphanol
Meperidine = pentazocine

From Ferrante M: Opioids. In Ferrante M, VadeBoncouer T, editors: Postoperative pain management, New York, 1993, Churchill Livingstone, p 145.

Atropine   Meperidine

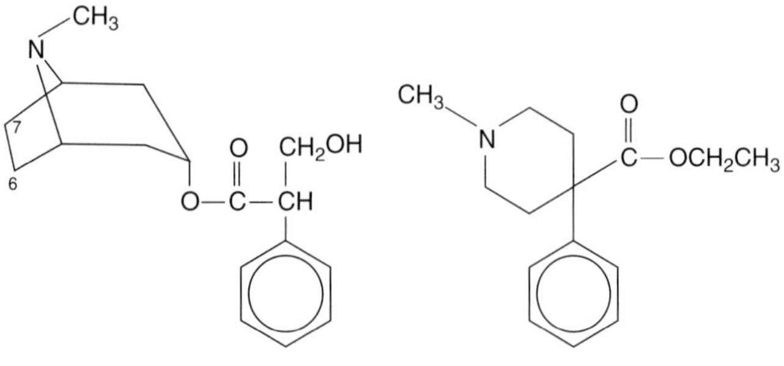

Fig. 122.6 At high doses, meperidine may cause tachycardia because of its structural resemblance to atropine. (Adapted from Ferrante M: Opioids. In Ferrante M, VadeBoncouer T, editors: Postoperative pain management, New York, 1993, Churchill Livingstone, p 145.)

received opioids. Delay in gastric transit may also contribute to the nausea produced by opioids.

Miosis is caused by stimulation of the Edinger-Westphal nucleus of the oculomotor nerve. Patients display a delayed tolerance to miosis, which is seen with most μ-receptor and κ-receptor agonist use. Pinpoint pupils are characteristic of opioid poisoning unless profound hypercarbia is associated with the respiratory depression.

Morphine and related compounds at high doses cause convulsions by stimulating neurons, especially in the hippocampal pyramidal cells. The morphine-3-glucuronide (M3G) metabolite may play a part in EEG spiking and epileptiform discharges.[35] Smith et al showed seizure-like activity in humans with no EEG evidence and concluded that what was demonstrated was muscular rigidity.[35a] Normeperidine (a metabolite of meperidine) and norpropoxyphene (a metabolite of propoxyphene) are known to cause CNS excitation.

High doses and rapid injection of intravenous opioids are notorious for causing muscular rigidity, which is more common in the older population (>60 years). The exact mechanism for muscular rigidity is not known, but it is postulated to be centrally located in the striatum, which is known to be rich in opioid binding sites.[36] The rigidity of the striatal muscles is characterized by increased muscle tone, which may progress to severe stiffness. In particular, thoracic and abdominal muscles are involved, resulting in the so-called wooden chest, which impedes ventilation.

Respiratory System

All μ-receptor agonists produce dose-dependent respiratory depression. The agonist-antagonists also depress respiration but have a ceiling effect. Opioids primarily cause respiratory depression by reducing brainstem respiratory center responsiveness to carbon dioxide (CO_2). They also depress the respiratory centers in the pons and medulla, which are involved in regulating respiratory rhythmicity.[37] The resting CO_2 increases, and the CO_2 response curve shifts to the right. Equianalgesic doses of μ-receptor agonists produce the same degree of respiratory depression. A decrease in respiratory rate is characteristic of μ-receptor agonist–induced respiratory depression. Some compensatory increase occurs in the minute volume, which is incomplete, as evidenced by an increase in the partial pressure of CO_2 ($Paco_2$). Patients must rely on hypoxic drive to stimulate ventilation. Pain is an effective antagonist to the respiratory depressant effects of opioids. κ-Receptor agonists produce less respiratory depression, even after administration of large doses. Opioid antagonists antagonize the respiratory

depressant effects of opioids. Central sleep apnea and ataxic breathing are observed in a dose-dependent fashion in patients using opioids on a long-term basis.[38,39] Partial opioid agonists have also been used to antagonize the respiratory depression caused by pure opioid agonists. Physostigmine also has been shown to reverse the respiratory depressant effect while preserving the analgesic effect.[40] Systemic morphine but not nebulized morphine is superior to placebo in the treatment of cancer-related dyspnea.[41]

Cardiovascular System

The cardiovascular effects of opioids not only depend on the dosage but also are also linked with the product and the prevailing vegetative basic tone of the patient. Opioids produce dose-dependent bradycardia by increasing centrally mediated vagal stimulation. Meperidine produces tachycardia because of its structural similarity to atropine (**Fig. 122.6**). Morphine and some other opioids (meperidine and codeine) provoke release of histamine, which plays a major role in producing hypotension. Naloxone does not inhibit the histamine release produced by opioids. Morphine exerts its well-known therapeutic effect in the treatment of angina pectoris by decreasing preload, inotropy, and chronotropy, thereby decreasing myocardial oxygen consumption.[9] Pentazocine and butorphanol cause an increase in systemic and pulmonary artery pressure, left ventricular filling pressure, systemic vascular resistance and a decrease in left ventricular ejection fraction. Opioids should be used with caution in patients with decreased blood volume because these agents can aggravate hypovolemic shock. Methadone can prolong the QT interval and lead to torsades de pointes and potentially lethal ventricular arrhythmias.

Gastrointestinal Tract

μ-Receptor agonists decrease gastric, biliary, pancreatic, and intestinal secretions. Even small doses decrease gastric motility and prolong gastric emptying time. Resting tone in the small and large intestine is increased to the point of spasm, and the propulsive peristaltic waves are decreased. Opioids exert their effect on the submucosal plexus, decrease the secretion by enterocytes, and inhibit the stimulatory effects of acetylcholine, prostaglandin E_2, and vasoactive intestinal peptide. These effects are mediated in large part by the release of norepinephrine and stimulation of alpha$_2$-adrenergic receptors on the enterocytes.[42] The gastrointestinal effects of opioids are primarily mediated by μ and δ receptors in the bowel. However, neuraxial application of opioids can also cause these effects as long as the extrinsic innervation of the bowel is intact. Patients usually develop very little tolerance to the constipating effects of opioids. Opioids constrict the sphincter of Oddi and raise the common bile duct pressure. Opioids in patients with biliary disease may cause severe sphincter constriction and pain. Delayed respiratory depression associated with opioids is postulated to be caused by enterosystemic circulation of opioids. Secondary peaks are often seen in plasma concentration-time graphs during pharmacokinetic studies of the more lipid-soluble opioids.[43] This phenomenon is thought to be caused by absorption of the opioids first sequestered in the acidic gastric juices and then absorbed from the small intestine.

Genitourinary System

Retention of urine, a frequent finding with opioid analgesics, increases urinary sphincter pressure and decreases the central inhibition of detrusor tone. The hypothesized site of action of opioids is in the thoracic spinal cord, where some preganglionic cell bodies are surrounded by terminals containing enkephalins and substance P.[44]

Endocrine System

μ-Receptor agonists inhibit the release of gonadotropin-releasing hormone and corticotropin-releasing hormone and thereby decrease the circulating concentrations of luteinizing hormone (LH), follicle-stimulating hormone (FSH), ACTH, and ß-endorphin. As a result of decreased pituitary trophic hormones, plasma levels of testosterone and cortisol also decrease. With long-term administration, patients develop a tolerance to these effects. κ-Receptor agonists inhibit the release of antidiuretic hormone and cause diuresis, and μ-receptor agonists tend to produce an antidiuretic effect.

Uterus

Opioids in therapeutic doses prolong labor by decreasing uterine contractions.[45] Parenteral opioids given within 2 to 4 hours of delivery can produce neonatal respiratory depression because they cross the placenta.

Skin

Morphine in therapeutic doses can cause dilation of cutaneous blood vessels. This is in part the result of histamine release and a decrease in peripheral vascular resistance. The skin of the face, neck, and upper thorax becomes flushed. Morphine- and meperidine-induced histamine release accounts for the urticaria at the site of injection; this effect is not reversed by naloxone.[9] Oxymorphone, methadone, fentanyl, and sufentanil are not associated with histamine release. Pruritus is a disabling side effect of opioid use. Pruritus is more intense with the intrathecal application of opioids,[46] and the effect appears to be mediated in large part by dorsal horn neurons.[47]

Immune System

Opioids affect host defense mechanisms in a complex manner. Acute, central immunomodulatory effects seem to be mediated by activation of the sympathetic nervous system, whereas long-term effects may involve modulation of hypothalamic-pituitary-adrenal axis function.[48] Morphine alters numerous mature immunocompetent cells that are involved in cell-mediated and humoral immune responses and also modulates the neuronal mechanism centrally. Heroin addicts have an altered and impaired immune system and also have a higher prevalence of infectious diseases than do nonaddicts.[49]

Tolerance

Tolerance refers to a phenomenon in which exposure to a drug results in the diminution of an effect or the need for a higher dose to maintain an effect. Tolerance can be innate (genetically determined) or acquired. The three types of acquired tolerance are pharmacokinetic, pharmacodynamic, and learned. *Pharmacokinetic tolerance* comes from changes in the metabolism and distribution of the drug after repeated administration (i.e., enzyme induction). *Pharmacodynamic tolerance* originates from adaptive changes (i.e., drug-induced changes in receptor density). *Learned tolerance* is a result of compensatory mechanisms that are learned.[50] Short-term tolerance probably involves phosphorylation of the μ and δ receptors through protein kinase C,[51] whereas long-term tolerance is associated with increases in adenylyl cyclase activity, a counterregulation to the decrease in cAMP levels seen after acute opioid administration.[52] In opioid tolerance, functional decoupling of opioid receptors from the G-protein–regulated cellular mechanisms occurs, in addition to down-regulation of endogenous opioids or opioid receptors and behavioral changes.[53]

Tolerances to different opioid side effects develop at different rates; this phenomenon is termed *selective tolerance*. Tolerance to nausea, vomiting, sedation, euphoria, and respiratory depression develop rapidly, whereas tolerance to constipation and miosis is minimal.[54] Repeated doses of a drug in a given category confer tolerance not only to the drug used but also to other drugs in the same structural and mechanistic category; this effect is known as *cross-tolerance*. Cross-tolerance has been shown to be incomplete in animal studies and has been reported in humans as well.[55] Incomplete cross-tolerance is frequently attributed to opioids, which have differing opioid-receptor subtype affinity.[55,56] NMDA antagonists have been shown to block the antinociceptive tolerance to morphine.[57]

Hyperalgesia

The process of increased sensitivity to pain with the short-term and long-term use of opioids is termed *opioid-induced hyperalgesia*. Multiple mechanisms for the development of this condition have been proposed. Investigators have observed activation of the central glutamatergic system, a cellular mechanism common to the development of tolerance.[58] Spinal dynorphins also have an important role in the development of opioid-induced hyperalgesia. Opioid use is associated with a rise in spinal dynorphin levels, and this increase, in turn, mediates release of spinal excitatory neuropeptides. Basically, up-regulation of the pronociceptive pathways appears to occur. Decreasing the opioid dose (40% to 50%) and adding adjuvants or a low dose of methadone can be used to treat opioid-induced hyperalgesia.[59] Ketamine, a NMDA receptor antagonist is another option for the management of this condition.

Addiction and Physical Dependence

Addiction has been defined by the World Health Organization as "a state, psychic and sometimes also physical, resulting from the interactions between a living organism and a drug, characterized by a behavioral and other responses that always include a compulsion to take the drug on a continuous or periodic basis in order to experience its psychic effects, and sometimes to avoid the discomfort of its absence. Tolerance may or may not be present." Increasing evidence implicates the mesolimbic dopamine system in the rewarding effects of drugs of abuse such as opioids; in addition, endogenous opioids may play a key role in the underlying adaptive mechanisms.[33] Opioid agonists with affinity for μ and δ receptors are rewarding, whereas opioid agonists with affinity for κ receptors are aversive. Experiments with opioid antagonists have demonstrated the presence of an endogenous opioidergic tone in the reward system. The dopaminergic mesolimbic system, originating in the ventral tegmental area of the midbrain, has been implicated in the rewarding effects seen with opioid use (**Fig. 122.7**). The D_1 subtype of dopamine receptors mediates a tonic activation of this pathway. The basal release of dopamine in the NAcc is under tonic control of both opposing opioid systems: μ-receptor (and possibly δ-receptor) activity originating from the ventral tegmental area increases and κ-receptor activity (originating from the NAcc) decreases basal activity of the mesolimbic reward system.[60] Some evidence suggests a possible genetic predisposition to the development of addiction. The term *pseudoaddiction* has been used to describe the iatrogenic syndrome of behavioral changes similar to addiction that can develop as a result of inadequate pain management. *Opiophobia* is the phenomenon of failure to administer legitimate opioid analgesics because of fear of the power of these drugs to produce addiction. Aggressive prosecution of physicians who prescribe large quantities of opioid analgesics to patients in pain has had a chilling effect on the appropriate use of opioid analgesics in pain management in many communities. Efforts by the national and international pain management community to highlight the appropriateness of the use of opioid analgesics for the management of all types of pain have helped to decriminalize such activities. Further efforts to define and codify best practices in opioid prescribing have also helped. Patient contracts and urine drug screening have also assisted in decreasing the incidence of diversion of prescribed opioids and opioid overuse.

Physical dependence is defined as the potential for an abstinence syndrome, or withdrawal, after abrupt dose reduction, discontinuation of the drug, or administration of an antagonist or agonist-antagonist drug. This is a physiologic phenomenon and is associated with disabling symptoms (**Table 122.5**). The lowest dose and shortest duration of treatment that may predispose patients to a significant abstinence syndrome are not known.[33] Clinically, the dose can be decreased by 10% to 20% every other day and eventually stopped without signs and symptoms of withdrawal.[9]

Pharmacokinetics

Pharmacokinetics is the study of drug disposition in the body (what the body does to the drug) over time, including absorption, distribution, biotransformation, and elimination. Opioids have similar pharmacodynamic properties but have widely different kinetic properties (**Tables 122.6** and **122.7**).

Absorption and Routes of Administration

Absorption refers to the rate and extent of removal of the drug from the site of administration. This process is determined by the drug's molecular shape and size, ionization constant, lipid solubility, and physicochemical properties of the membrane it must cross.[61]

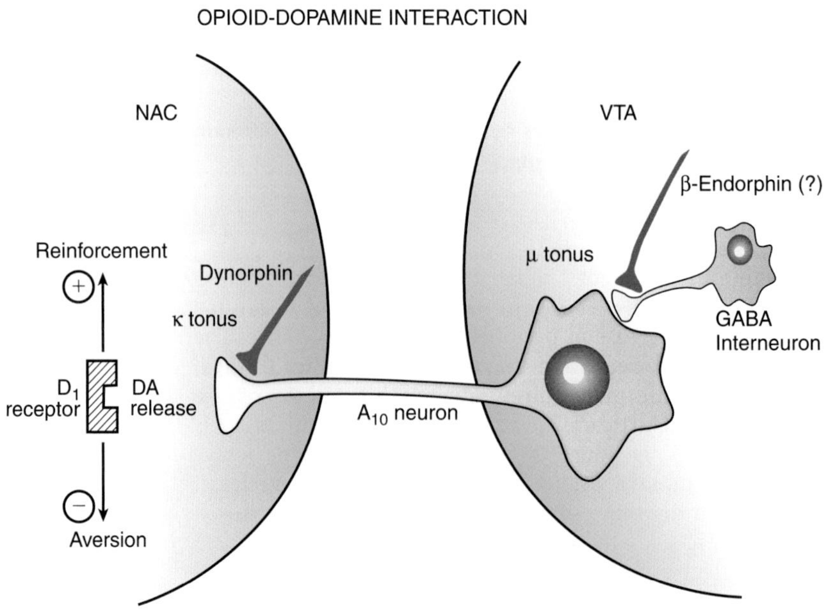

OPIOID-DOPAMINE INTERACTION

Fig. 122.7 Model for the modulation of mesolimbic A_{10} neurons by endogenous opioid systems. D_1, dopamine receptor subtype; DA, dopamine; GABA, γ-aminobutyric acid; NAC, nucleus accumbens; VTA, ventral tegmental area. *(Adapted from Spanagel R, Herz A, Shippenberg TS: Opposing tonically active endogenous opioid systems modulate the mesolimbic dopaminergic pathway, Proc Natl Acad Sci U S A 89:2046, 1992.)*

Oral Route

The oral route is the preferred route for long-term administration of opioids because it is convenient and cost effective. Most opioids are well absorbed after oral administration. Aqueous solutions are absorbed the best, followed by oily solutions, suspensions, and oral solids. Drugs absorbed from the gut are subject to first-pass metabolism in the liver and some degree of metabolism by enzymes in the intestinal wall. The onset of action is slower and variable in comparison with parenteral administration. Some opioids (e.g., codeine, oxycodone) have a high oral-to-parenteral potency ratio because they are protected from conjugation by substitution on C3 aromatic hydroxyl residue.[62] Oral opioids are available in tablet and liquid form and in immediate-release and controlled-release preparations. Morphine, oxycodone, and oxymorphone are available in controlled-release forms. The controlled-release form of hydromorphone is not available in the United States.

Table 122.5 Symptoms and Signs of Opioid Withdrawal

Symptoms	Signs
Craving for opioids	Pupillary dilatation
Restlessness	Sweating
Irritability	Piloerection
Increased sensitivity to pain	Tachycardia
Nausea	Vomiting
Abdominal cramps	Diarrhea
Myalgia	Hypertension
Dysphoria	Yawning
Insomnia	Fever
Anxiety	Rhinorrhea

From Collett BJ: Opioid tolerance: the clinical perspective, *Br J Anaesth* 81:58, 1998.

Table 122.7 Plasma Half-Life Values for Opioids and Their Active Metabolites

	Plasma Half-Life (hr)
SHORT HALF-LIFE OPIOIDS	
Morphine	2–3.5
Morphine-6-glucuronide	2
Hydromorphone	2–3
Oxycodone	2–3
Fentanyl	3.7
Codeine	3
Meperidine	3–4
Pentazocine	2–3
Nalbuphine	5
Butorphanol	2.5–3.5
Buprenorphine	3–5
LONG HALF-LIFE OPIOIDS	
Methadone	24
Levorphanol	12–16
Propoxyphene	12
Norpropoxyphene	30–40
Normeperidine	14–21

From Inturrisi CE: Clinical pharmacology of opioids for pain, *Clin J Pain* 18(Suppl 4):S3, 2002.

Table 122.6 Pharmacokinetic and Physiochemical Variables of Opioid Analgesics

Drug	Vc (L/kg)	Vd (L/kg)	Cl (mL/min/kg)	T½β	Partition Coefficient (Octanol/Water)
Morphine	0.23	2.8	15.5	134 min	1
Hydromorphone	0.34	4.1	22.7	15 min	1
Meperidine	0.6	2.6	12	180 min	21
Methadone	0.15	3.4	1.6	23 hr	115
Levorphanol		10.0	10.5	11 hr	
Alfentanil	0.12	0.9	7.6	94 min	130
Fentanyl	0.85	4.6	21	186 min	820
Sufentanil	0.1	2.5	11.3	149 min	1,750
Buprenorphine	0.2	2.8	17.2	184 min	10,000
Nalbuphine	0.45	4.8	23.1	222 min	
Butorphanol		5.0	38.6	159 min	
Dezocine		12.0	52	156 min	

Cl, clearance; T½β, elimination half-life; Vc, central volume of distribution; Vd, volume of distribution.
Adapted from Hill H, Mather L: Patient-controlled analgesic, pharmacokinetic and therapeutic considerations, *Clin Pharmacokinet* 24:124, 1993; and O'Brien JJ, Benfield P: Dezocine: A preliminary review of its pharmacodynamic and pharmacokinetic properties and therapeutic efficacy, *Drugs* 38:226, 1989.

Subcutaneous Route

In comparison with the oral route, subcutaneous adminis- tration is faster and does not have to rely on gastrointestinal function. Absorption can be variable and erratic. The subcutaneous route can be used for continuous infusion, patient-controlled analgesia, and intermittent boluses. The drawbacks are that only small volumes can be infused and that pain and necrosis may occur at the site of injection The intramuscular route is painful and inconvenient, and absorption can show some variability. As compared with the subcutaneous route, larger volumes and oil-based solutions can be used intramuscularly. The intravenous route provides the most rapid onset of analgesia, but the duration of anal- gesia after a bolus dose is shorter than with other routes. This route provides more reliable absorption and drug levels in the plasma. Intravenous drugs must be water soluble, or the oil-based solutions need to be diluted and given in larger volumes.

Rectal Route

The rectal route is an alternative when the upper gastroin- testinal tract cannot be used and the parenteral route is not available or acceptable. The rectal route is contraindicated if the patient has lesions of the anus or rectum. Absorption of medications is similar to that with the oral route. The bioavail- ability of drugs is variable; the bioavailability of morphine is 55% to 60%, a finding suggesting that this route partially avoids the first-pass metabolism.

Intranasal Route

Intranasal administration is particularly familiar to the recreational abuser of opioids. Reliable absorption across the nasal mucosa is determined by lipid solubility. This route avoids first-pass metabolism. Opioids administered by this route can be used either as a dry powder or dis- solved in water. Butorphanol is the only opioid available formulated in a metered-dose spray form. Clinical trials are ongoing to evaluate a nasal fentanyl preparation. Many opioids dissolved in water or saline solution have been investigated. Intranasal administration of opioids for acute pain settings is not superior to parenteral administration. The intranasal route may have a role in patients with dif- ficult intravenous access.

Inhalational Route

Administration of opioids by the inhalational route is a novel technique. Use of this technique has been encouraging because of the suggestion that this method may target opioid receptors in the lung. After inhalation of morphine and diamorphine, morphine has been detected in the plasma after 1 minute, with a time of maximal concentration in 10 and 6 minutes, respec- tively.[63,64] Fentanyl administered by this route achieves a time of maximal concentration in 2 minutes.[65] Inhaled opioids have been investigated for several indications: dyspnea at rest, post- operative pain, and provision of pain relief in the general pop- ulation. Nebulized morphine is not superior to placebo for treatment of dyspnea in patients with cancer.[41]

Transdermal Route

The transdermal route is used in two forms: passive sys- tem and active (iontophoresis) system. Fentanyl is the only opioid currently available in a transdermal form. Fentanyl can be used for transdermal delivery because of its physico- chemical properties: low molecular weight, high lipid solubil- ity, and high potency. Transdermal fentanyl uses the passive system. The two principal system components are a fentanyl- containing reservoir and a rate-controlling membrane. Five patch sizes are available and provide delivery of fentanyl at 12.5, 25, 50, 75, or 100 μg/hour. The transdermal system is not ideal for rapid dose titration. Transdermal fentanyl should be considered when patients have relatively constant pain with infrequent episodes of breakthrough pain. The transdermal therapeutic system used to administer fentanyl is designed to release the drug for 72 hours at a controlled rate dictated by the system, rather than by the skin.[66] Fentanyl is dissolved in ethanol, is gelled with hydroxyl cellulose, and is held in a res- ervoir between a clear occluding polyester-ethylene backing layer and a rate-controlling membrane (ethylene-vinyl acetate copolymer film) on an adhesive base (**Fig. 122.8**). The amount of fentanyl administered per hour is proportional to the sur- face area of the patch. Multiple patches must be applied if higher doses are needed. The major obstacle to diffusion is the stratum corneum, where diffusion occurs primarily through the intracellular lipid medium.[67]

Because a depot is established in the dermis, absorp- tion continues even after patch removal. After the first patch application, initial detection of fentanyl in the blood has been reported to occur at 1 to 2 hours. The plasma fentanyl

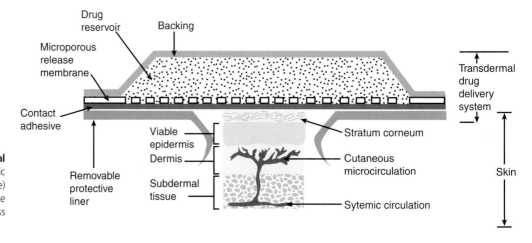

Fig. 122.8 **Fentanyl transdermal therapeutic system.** Schematic representation (not to scale) of the delivery system and the pathway of absorption across the skin.

concentration increases over 12 to 18 hours until a plateau develops. Under normal physiologic conditions, skin temperature and regional blood flow do not influence fentanyl absorption significantly.[66] Absorption rises by approximately one third with a rise in body temperature to 40°C (104°F).[68] The plasma concentration remains constant as long as the patch is changed every 72 hours. After patch removal, the plasma fentanyl concentration slowly declines, with an apparent half-life of 15 to 21 hours.[67]

A transdermal formulation of sufentanil is currently in clinical trials and may represent another option for patients who have become tolerant to the less potent drug fentanyl. A transdermal formulation of sufentanil in combination with the local anesthetic bupivacaine is also undergoing clinical trials. Buprenorphine is available as a transdermal preparation in some countries.

Iontophoresis is a method of transdermal delivery of drugs in an ionized state with the use of an electric current. Morphine has been administered using this route for postoperative analgesia.[69] The delivery of fentanyl by iontophoresis is being investigated more extensively than is that of other opioids. Iontophoresis has the advantage of achieving a rapid steady state and the ability to vary delivery rate.[70]

Neuraxial Route

Neuraxial delivery by intrathecal, epidural, and intraventricular administration of opioids has the advantage of producing profound analgesia with relatively small doses. The mechanism of analgesia produced by epidural morphine is bimodal and synergistic. During the first 20 minutes, the vascularly absorbed morphine activates the descending inhibitory system. Then, as the cerebrospinal fluid (CSF) morphine concentration increases, the spinal cord receptors are activated.[1] The short-term use of this route is most commonly advocated for postsurgical pain relief. It is indicated for long-term use when other routes do not control the pain or are associated with significant side effects. Opioids injected in the neuraxis should be free of preservatives. Duramorph (preservative-free morphine) is commercially available. Other opioids such as fentanyl, sufentanil, meperidine, methadone, and hydromorphone are used intrathecally and epidurally. Remifentanil cannot be given intraspinally; it is prepared with glycine, which can cause temporary motor paralysis.

The most common side effects are pruritus, nausea, vomiting, somnolence, urinary retention, and respiratory depression. The most worrisome side effect is delayed respiratory depression, which may occur 12 hours after the intraspinal administration of morphine. Lipophilic drugs such as fentanyl do not spread much after intrathecal administration, but hydrophilic drugs such as morphine can spread rostrally and cause delayed respiratory depression. This effect is also seen sporadically after epidural administration. Other late side effects of long-term administration of neuroaxial opioids are tolerance and the development of subarachnoid granulation tissue, which may decrease the efficacy of the opioids administered and may cause neurologic compromise. This last side effect is seen most commonly with intrathecal morphine at high doses.[71] Intraventricular opioid administration is a satisfactory analgesic method that should be reserved for patients who have intractable pain and a short life expectancy and who have exhausted other modalities of pain management. Small doses of intraventricular morphine provide satisfactory control of otherwise intractable pain in patients with terminal cancer.[72]

Distribution

After being injected into the circulation or being absorbed, opioids are distributed within the body in two phases. In the early phase, the drug is distributed to highly perfused tissues such as the heart, liver, kidney, and brain. This is a function of the cardiac output and regional blood flow. The second phase is characterized by a slow diffusion to less-perfused areas such as muscle, fat, viscera, and skin. *Volume of distribution* is the extent to which a drug is distributed within the body. The differences in distribution determine the onset of activity. A highly diffusible drug that acts on a highly diffusible organ has a very rapid onset of action. The nonionized and unbound fraction of the drug is diffusible, and this fraction leaves the circulation to be distributed. Highly protein-bound drugs are poorly diffusible and have a small volume of distribution. Lipid-insoluble drugs diffuse poorly and also have a small volume of distribution, whereas highly lipid-soluble drugs have a large volume of distribution. The measure of acid strength (pKa) determines the ionized versus the nonionized fraction at a particular pH. The clinical effects of the highly lipophilic opioids are determined by the apparent volume of distribution (tissue: blood partition coefficient). For a given opioid, the larger the volume of distribution, the lesser the concentration in the plasma will be. Alfentanil has a small volume of distribution and therefore a rapid onset of action and a short duration.

Metabolism

Opioids containing a hydroxyl group are conjugated in the liver with glucuronic acid to form opioid glucuronides that are then excreted by the kidney. Uridine 5-diphosphate-glucuronyltransferase (UGT) performs an important group of conjugation reactions.[62] UGTs are involved in metabolism of many opioid analgesics. Some natural opioids and semisynthetic opioids are metabolized by the cytochrome P-450 isoforms. The phenylpiperidine derivatives undergo oxidative metabolism. *N*-demethylation is a minor pathway for metabolism of opioids. Remifentanil undergoes rapid hydrolysis by plasma esterases.

Excretion

The kidneys excrete most polar metabolites, and a small amount is excreted unchanged. Glucuronide conjugates are also excreted in bile and may undergo enterohepatic circulation.

Phenanthrene Alkaloids

Morphine

Morphine is a naturally occurring alkaloid derived from opium, and, to date, chemical synthesis is difficult. The milky juice obtained from the unripe seed capsule of the poppy plant is dried and powdered to make powdered opium, which contains certain alkaloids: the principal phenanthrenes are morphine (10% of opium), codeine (0.5%), and thebaine (0.2%). The morphine molecule consists of five fused ring systems (see Fig. 122.2).[73] The carbon atoms are numbered 1 to 16. It has 5 asymmetrical carbon atoms,[5,6,8,9,13] resulting in strong levorotation, the l-isomer being pharmacologically active and the D-isomer inactive.[74] The pKa for the morphine base is 7.9, and at physiologic pH, it is 76% nonionized. Morphine is relatively water soluble and poorly lipid soluble because of the hydrophilic OH- groups present.[75] This poor lipid solubility limits movement of morphine across membranes and is a barrier to accessing the CNS.

Morphine is absorbed, to some extent, through all mucosa and the spinal dura. Therefore, multiple routes are available for drug administration. Protein binding of morphine in plasma is 45%. The mean elimination half-life ranges from 1.4 to 3.4 hours. After intravenous administration, morphine is rapidly distributed to tissues and organs. Within 10 minutes of administration, 96% to 98% of the drug is cleared from the plasma. Mean volume of distribution is large, ranging from 2.1 to 4.0 L/kg. Intramuscular absorption is rapid, and the peak occurs at 10 to 20 minutes.[76] Peak plasma concentrations after subcutaneous administration occur at approximately 15 minutes, and plasma levels equivalent to those obtained with the intravenous route can be achieved.[77,78] Morphine is rapidly distributed out of the plasma after intravenous administration. Intramuscular or subcutaneous injection creates a depot, which continues to release morphine into the plasma for distribution.

After oral administration, plasma levels of morphine peak at 30 to 90 minutes. Absorption is mainly from the upper small intestine; morphine is poorly absorbed from the stomach.[75] Bioavailability from the oral route is low owing to extensive first-pass metabolism in the liver. Great interindividual variability exists for bioavailability (20% to 30% reported in various studies). Low bioavailability of oral morphine is a factor in determining oral-to-parenteral conversion ratios, 1:3 in chronic pain states.[77,79,80] Peak plasma levels after controlled-release morphine occur two to three times later (at 150 minutes) than with immediate-release oral morphine preparations. Bioavailability of controlled-release morphine is 85% to 90% that of immediate-release formulations. Rectal absorption appears to be as good as or better than oral absorption. Morphine can be administered intrathecally, epidurally, or intraventricularly. Epidural morphine is rapidly absorbed into the systemic circulation and produces significant plasma levels. Plasma levels after intrathecal administration are too low to be of any clinical significance. Rostral distribution of morphine occurs in the CSF, and this causes delayed respiratory depression (12 to 18 hours).

Morphine is not suited to be administered transdermally or by the nasal route because it is poorly lipid soluble. Morphine has been delivered by iontophoresis for postoperative analgesia after total hip and knee replacement surgery.[69] Absorption after buccal and sublingual administration is similar to oral administration in terms of peak plasma level and time to peak, low bioavailability, and large degree of inter-individual variation.[80] After being absorbed, morphine is rapidly distributed throughout the body to highly perfused tissues, such as the lungs, kidney, liver, and spleen.[76,77] Morphine and its highly polar metabolites M3G and morphine-6-glucuronide (M6G) cross the blood-brain barrier to a small extent. CSF morphine levels are 4% to 60% after systemic administration.[81] The mean volume of distribution is large, ranging from 2.1 to 4.0 L/kg. It is affected by the hemodynamic status of the patient, alterations in plasma protein binding, and variations in tissue blood flow. Morphine binds to albumin and gamma globulin. Morphine is 20% to 40% protein bound.[82,83] Major changes in

binding would be required to influence plasma morphine levels because of the normally low extent of binding.

The predominant metabolic fate of morphine in humans is glucuronidation, and the liver is the predominant site for this biotransformation. Approximately 90% of injected morphine is converted into metabolites, the major metabolites being M3G (45% to 55%) and M6G (10% to 15%) (**Fig. 122.9**). Other metabolites include morphine-3,6-diglucuronide, morphine-3-ethereal sulfate, normorphine, normorphine-6-glucuronide, normorphine-3-glucoronide,[84] and codeine.[85] M3G is the major metabolite quantitatively. It has a very low affinity for the μ receptor and as a consequence has no analgesic potency. M3G was found to antagonize morphine- and M6G-induced analgesia and respiratory depression in the rat and has led to the hypothesis that M3G may influence the development of morphine tolerance.[86] M3G was shown to cause nonopioid mediated hyperalgesia and allodynia after intrathecal administration in rats. M6G has a higher affinity for μ receptors than for δ or κ receptors. M6G is poorly lipid soluble, and very little crosses the blood-brain barrier. M6G can accumulate in patients with renal insufficiency and is a likely factor in prolonged opioid effects after morphine administration. Increases in M6G levels in patients with renal failure elevate the CSF concentration and result from the mass effect of the accumulated M6G. Within the CSF, M6G is 45 to 100 times more potent than morphine in its analgesic activity and 10 times more potent in depressing ventilation.

Normorphine is produced in small amounts and is pharmacologically active. Normorphine may be neurotoxic, analogous to normeperidine.[87] Excretion of morphine is predominantly renal, by glomerular filtration of water-soluble conjugates. Up to 85% of a dose of morphine is recovered from the urine as free morphine and metabolites. Some morphine (10% to 20%) is unaccounted for by renal excretion and is presumably excreted in urine as unidentified metabolite or is excreted by other routes.[73] Enterohepatic circulation of morphine and its glucuronides accounts for the presence of small amounts of morphine in the feces and in the urine for several days after the last dose.

Morphine remains the reference against which all other opioids are compared. The clinical effects and side effects are those that are seen with all μ-receptor agonists. These effects are detailed in the previous section on the pharmacodynamics of opioids.

Clinical Uses and Preparations

Morphine is available as its sulfate and hydrochloride forms. It is the most commonly used medication for moderate to severe pain in the acute and chronic setting. Oral morphine is available as tablets and suspension in immediate-release and sustained-release forms. Immediate-release formulations have the disadvantage of frequent dosing. Various sustained-release forms are available that can be administered every 8 to 12 hours (MS Contin, Oramorph) or every 24 hours (Kapanol, MXL, Kadian, Avinza). Most sustained-release formulations adsorb morphine onto a hydrophilic polymer that is embedded in some form of a wax or hydrophobic matrix, granulated and finally compressed into tablets.[88] Following oral administration, gastric fluid dissolves the tablet surface and hydrates the hydrophilic polymer to produce a gel, the formation of which is controlled by higher aliphatic alcohols. Varying the hydrophilic polymer, the type of hydrophobic matrix, or their ratio can control the release rate.

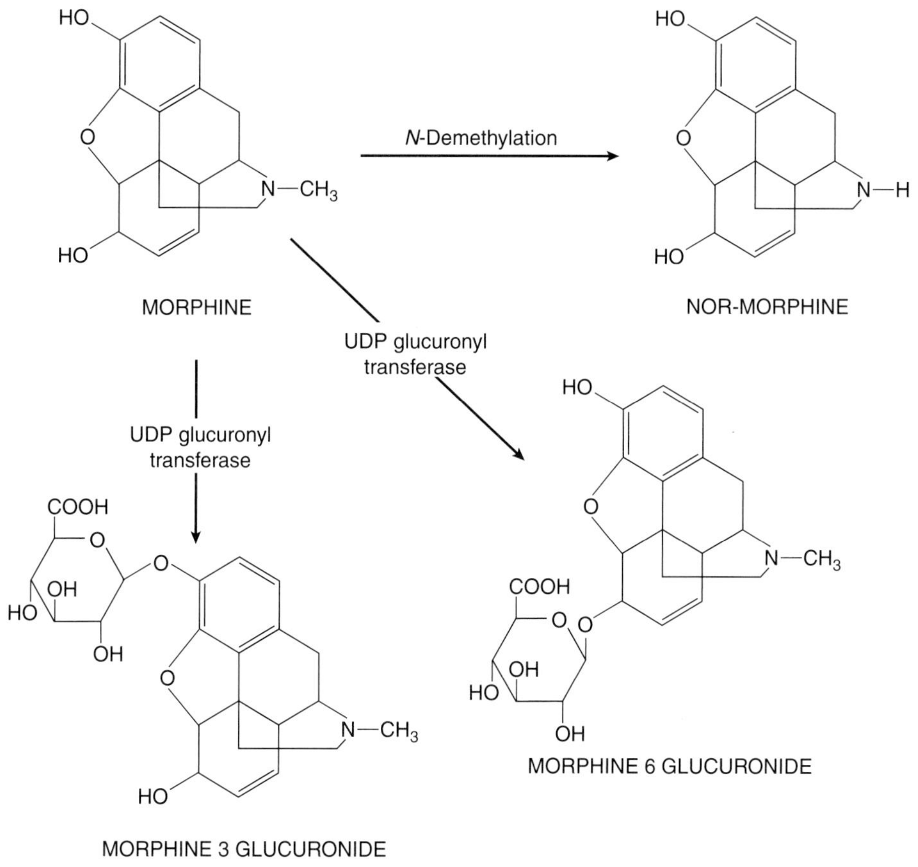

Fig. 122.9 **Metabolism of morphine.** Morphine-3-glucuronide and morphine-6-glucuronide are major metabolites. Morphine-6-glucuronide possesses significant analgesic activity and may substantially contribute to the analgesic effects of morphine. Both metabolites are excreted in the urine, and accumulation may occur after repetitive dosing in patients with renal failure. Demethylation is a minor pathway for morphine metabolism. *(Adapted from Ferrante M: Opioids. In Ferrante M, VadeBoncouer T, editors:* Postoperative pain management, *New York, 1993, Churchill Livingstone, p 145.)*

Also available is a suspension formulation, in which morphine is attached to small beads of an ion exchange resin. Rectal suppositories are available; a specific sustained-release formulation contains morphine, sodium alginate, and a calcium salt in a suitable vehicle that melts in the rectum. Parenteral formulations are available for intravenous, intramuscular, and subcutaneous use. A preservative-free formulation for intrathecal and epidural use is available. Morphine has also been used intra-articularly, with varying results.

Codeine

Like morphine, codeine is a naturally occurring alkaloid. Codeine is methylmorphine, the methyl substitution being on the phenolic hydroxyl group. With the exception of aspirin, codeine is perhaps the most widely used oral analgesic and is generally accepted as the alternative to aspirin as a standard of comparison of drugs in this category[89] (e.g., 60 mg of codeine is comparable to 600 mg of aspirin). Codeine is approximately 60% as effective orally as parenterally, both as an analgesic and as a respiratory depressant. Compared with morphine, codeine has a high oral-to-parenteral potency ratio as a result of less first-pass metabolism in the liver. Codeine is metabolized by the liver to inactive forms (90%), which are excreted in the urine. Free and conjugated forms of morphine are found in urine after codeine administration: 10% of administered codeine is O-demethylated to morphine. The cytochrome P-450 enzyme CYP2D6 effects the conversion of codeine to morphine. Ten percent of the white population has a well-characterized genetic polymorphism in the CYP2D6 enzyme, and these persons are not able to convert codeine

to morphine and thus do not attain an analgesic effect from codeine administration.

Codeine's major disadvantage is its lack of effectiveness in treating severe pain. Codeine has a low affinity for opioid receptors and is a weak analgesic; the analgesic effect is the result of its conversion to morphine. It has a limited propensity to produce sedation, nausea, vomiting, constipation, and respiratory depression. It also produces a lower incidence and degree of physical dependence than most other opioids. Codeine is used for mild to moderate pain conditions. The addictive potential of codeine is low. Codeine has an excellent antitussive effect at doses as low as 15 mg; greater cough suppression is seen at higher doses. The antitussive effects are mediated by the active metabolites depressing the cough reflex in the medulla. Distinct receptors that bind to codeine itself may exist.[61] Codeine is available in the United States in oral, subcutaneous, intramuscular, and intravenous formulations. Oral forms of codeine are formulated with acetaminophen. Parenteral forms of codeine are also available; 130 mg of codeine is equianalgesic to 10 mg of intramuscular morphine. Codeine should not be used intravenously because the histamine-releasing potency of codeine is even greater than that of morphine.[4]

Thebaine

Thebaine is a naturally occurring alkaloid derived from opium. Thebaine has little analgesic action but is a precursor to several important 14-OH agents such as oxycodone and naloxone. A few derivatives of thebaine are more than 1000 times as potent as morphine (e.g., etorphine).[9]

Semisynthetic Opioids

Heroin

Diacetylmorphine, or heroin, is derived from acetylation of morphine at the 3 and 6 positions (**Fig. 122.10**). Heroin is deacetylated to 6-monoacetylmorphine (6-MAM) and subsequently to morphine. The liver has the greatest capacity for the production of morphine from 6-MAM. In serum, the conversion to 6-MAM is mediated by a serum cholinesterase, which is present also in kidney, liver, and brain tissues and could be responsible for conversion in these organs as well.[90] Direct renal clearance of heroin is less than 1% of the administered dose.[91] Both heroin and 6-MAM are more lipid soluble than morphine and cross the blood-brain barrier more readily.

Heroin should be given orally; it is approximately 1.5 times more potent than morphine in controlling chronic pain. Given parenterally, heroin is 2 to 4 times more potent than morphine and is faster in onset of action. Heroin has a short half-life, but the effects of its active metabolites last longer. Heroin has a high addictive potential and it is not known to have any real advantage over morphine. It is banned from manufacture and medicinal use in the United States.[4]

Hydrocodone

Hydrocodone is a semisynthetic opioid with multiple actions qualitatively similar to those of codeine. It has a bioavailability of 50% and is available as oral formulations in combination with nonopioid analgesics.

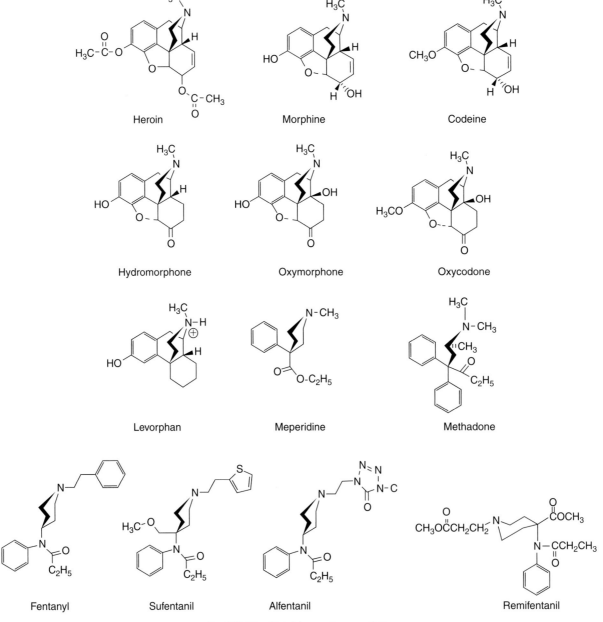

Fig. 122.10 **μ-Opioid receptor agonists.**

Hydrocodone undergoes O-demethylation, *N*-dealkylation, and 6-ketoreduction to the corresponding 6-α and 6-ß hydroxymetabolites. The O-demethylation to dihydromorphine is mediated by the polymorphically expressed cytochrome P-450 CYP2D6 enzyme. Some of the hydrocodone metabolites (dihydromorphine, dihydrocodeine, and hydromorphone) are pharmacologically active and may produce adverse effects if their excretion is impaired.[62]

Hydrocodone is considered a weak analgesic. It has excellent antitussive properties. Like other opioids, hydrocodone can cause respiratory depression, sedation, and impairment of mental and physical performance, constipation, and urinary retention. Sensorineural hearing loss associated with long-term hydrocodone use has been reported.[92,93] Drug dependence and addiction are seen with long-term use. Hydrocodone is available only for oral use in combination with acetaminophen or acetylsalicylic acid. These combinations provide a synergistic effect, and the side effects are reduced.

Hydromorphone (Dilaudid)

Hydromorphone, a direct derivative of morphine, was first synthesized in the 1920s. Like morphine, hydromorphone has a basic amino group as well as a phenolic group. However, hydromorphone is more lipophilic than morphine because its 6-alcoholic hydroxyl group has been converted to a less hydrophilic ketone group (see Fig. 122.10).[94] The global pharmacokinetic properties of hydromorphone are generally similar to those of morphine. It is six to eight times as potent as morphine; the best-accepted conversion is that 1.5 mg of hydromorphone is equianalgesic to 10 mg of morphine. Hydromorphone is easily absorbed from the gastrointestinal tract and so is effective after oral and rectal administration. It has a rapid distribution phase; approximately 90% of a specific dose is lost from the plasma in 10 minutes.[95] Hydromorphone elimination, like that of morphine, depends on tissue uptake, with subsequent slow release from tissue to plasma.

Hydromorphone has no active metabolites and therefore is a particularly useful drug in patients with renal insufficiency. The side effect profile is very similar to that of other opioids. Despite anecdotal reports of reduced incidences of nausea, vomiting, respiratory depression, urinary retention, and constipation, little evidence exists as proof.[96]

Hydromorphone is available as tablets for oral administration and as rectal suppositories. A controlled-release form for administration every 12 hours is available in some countries. Injectable preparations are available, and hydromorphone is particularly useful for subcutaneous use because of its relatively high solubility. Hydromorphone is used intrathecally and epidurally with good effect. The drug is hydrophilic: when given epidurally, its long half-life resembles that of epidural morphine, and its short latency of analgesia is similar to that of meperidine.[97]

Oxycodone

Oxycodone (14-hydroxyl-7, 8-dihydrocodeine) is derived from modification of the morphine molecule. Its pharmacokinetic and opioid-receptor binding characteristics differ from those of morphine. Oxycodone is a μ-receptor agonist and also exhibits some κ-mediated antinociceptive effects.[98] It is available in immediate-release and sustained-release forms and also in combination with nonopioid analgesics. The parenteral forms are currently not available in the United States.

The oral bioavailability, 50% to 80%, is superior to that of morphine. Bioavailability and peak plasma concentration are altered by high-fat meals; absorption is delayed, but bioavailability is improved. Normal-release oxycodone absorption is monoexponential; the mean half-life is 3.5 to 5.6 hours. Controlled-release oxycodone is absorbed in a biexponential fashion. The drug has a rapid phase with a half-life of 37 minutes and a slow phase with a half-life of 6.2 hours.[99] In uremic patients, the mean half-life of oxycodone is increased by increased volume of distribution and reduced clearance, and plasma concentrations of noroxycodone are higher.[94] Oxycodone is metabolized by the liver to the active metabolite, oxymorphone (10%), through O-demethylation by the cytochrome P-450 enzyme CYP2D6 and to the dominant nonactive metabolite, noroxycodone, through *N*-demethylation.[100] The metabolites are excreted in the urine, noroxycodone in an unchanged form and oxymorphone in the form of a conjugate. Women eliminate oxycodone 25% more slowly than do men.[101] Protein binding is low (i.e., 38% to 45%). Lipid solubility is very similar to that of morphine.

Oxycodone is a μ-receptor agonist, but part of its antinociceptive effect is mediated by κ-opioid receptors.[98] The relative potency of parenteral oxycodone is 70% that of morphine. The wide variability of oral morphine bioavailability, unequal incomplete cross-tolerance depending on the drug sequence, and delayed oxycodone clearance in women account for bioequivalent ratios between 1:1 and 2.3:1.[100] Less cross-tolerance occurs with a switch from morphine to oxycodone than from oxycodone to morphine.[102] The side effects of oxycodone are similar to those normally attributed to opioids. The incidence of constipation is higher than with morphine, but the incidence of nausea is lower. Oxycodone causes drowsiness, lightheadedness, nausea, vomiting, pruritus, constipation, and sweating. Fluoxetine and its metabolite norfluoxetine inhibit CYP2D6 and prevent O-demethylation of oxycodone to oxymorphone, processes that may lead to higher plasma oxycodone levels.[103] Presumably, sertraline does the same.

Oxymorphone

Oxymorphone is a congener of morphine with a substitution of a ketone group at the C-6 position, conferring a more rapid onset of action, greater potency, and a slightly longer duration of action than morphine.[104] Oxymorphone has a short half-life but has a prolonged duration of action owing to slow dissociation from its receptor sites.[61] It has a high affinity for μ-opioid receptors and is approximately 10 times more potent than morphine in the parenteral form and three times more potent in the oral form. Like heroin, oxymorphone has a high addictive potential. Oxymorphone and naloxone have significant structural similarities; naloxone is the N-allyl (−CH2−CH=CH2)–substituted analogue of oxymorphone.[4] The structural similarities between the μ-receptor antagonist naloxone and the agonist oxymorphone have been used to study and develop new agonists and antagonists.

Oxymorphone is available in the United States in oral, injectable, and rectal forms (Numorphan). It is available in immediate-release and sustained-release oral formulations. The adult subcutaneous or intramuscular dose is 1 to 1.5 mg every 4 to 6 hours, with a starting intravenous dose of 0.5 mg. Rectal administration is approximately one tenth as potent as intramuscular administration.

Synthetic Opioids

Levorphanol and Congeners

Levorphanol is the only commercially available opioid agonist of the morphinan series. Only the l-isomer has analgesic effect. The d-isomer (dextromethorphan) is relatively devoid of analgesic effect but may have inhibitory effects at NMDA receptors and it also has an antitussive activity. Levorphanol has activity mainly at the μ-opioid receptors and some effect at κ and δ receptors. Because of its effect on multiple receptors, levorphanol is used as a second-line agent or in patients who are tolerant to morphine.[105]

The pharmacologic profile of levorphanol closely parallels that of morphine. The analgesic effects are similar to those of morphine, but levorphanol has a lower incidence of nausea and vomiting. Levorphanol is available in forms that can be administered subcutaneously, intramuscularly, intravenously, or orally. It is less effective when given orally; the oral-to-parenteral potency ratio is comparable to that of codeine and oxycodone. Levorphanol is seven times more potent than oral morphine and five times more potent than parenteral morphine.

Levorphanol has a half-life of 12 to 16 hours, but its duration of analgesia is similar to that of morphine (i.e., 4 to 6 hours). The longer half-life may lead to systemic accumulation with repeated dosing. Levorphanol is available for oral administration in 2-mg tablets and as an injectable solution for parenteral administration.

Meperidine and Congeners

Meperidine is a synthetic phenylpiperidine opioid analgesic. The other opioids in the phenylpiperidine series are fentanyl, sufentanil, alfentanil, and remifentanil.

Oral bioavailability of meperidine is 45% to 75%, owing to extensive first-pass metabolism. Its absorption is slow and peaks at 2 hours. Meperidine is absorbed by all routes of administration, but absorption after intramuscular injection is very erratic.[106] Approximately 60% of meperidine is protein bound. Meperidine is metabolized in the liver and is *N*-demethylated to meperidinic acid and normeperidine. Normeperidine has a half-life of 15 to 40 hours. Meperidine has a half-life of 3 hours, but in patients with liver disease, the half-lives of both meperidine and normeperidine are prolonged. Patients with renal insufficiency accumulate normeperidine, with resulting systemic toxicity.

Normeperidine is an active metabolite possessing one half the analgesic potency of meperidine. It has twice the potency of the parent compound as a proconvulsant. Normeperidine has CNS stimulant effects, and toxicity may be manifested as myoclonus and seizures.[107,108] Meperidine is no longer recommended for chronic pain; use for longer than 48 hours or doses greater than 600 mg/24 hours are not advocated, according to Agency for Health Care Policy and Research in 1992.[9]

Meperidine is 7 to 10 times less potent than morphine in producing analgesia; 75 to 100 mg of meperidine is equivalent to 10 mg of morphine. The peak analgesic effect is seen 1 to 2 hours after oral administration and in less than an hour after parenteral administration. The analgesic effect lasts 2 to 3 hours, a duration shorter than that of morphine. Meperidine also produces sedation, respiratory depression, and euphoria, and a few patients experience dysphoria. Like other opioids, meperidine produces nausea and vomiting, as

well as pupillary dilation with large doses. It also affects the pituitary hormones. The accumulation of normeperidine can cause CNS excitation, which may manifest as tremors, myoclonus, and seizures. Unlike other opioids, meperidine causes tachycardia because of its structural similarity to atropine. Meperidine can cause hypotension owing to its histamine-releasing effect. In large doses, meperidine can cause a decrease in myocardial contractility and stroke volume and a rise in filling pressures.[109] No deleterious effects were seen when therapeutic doses of meperidine were given to patients with acute myocardial infarction.[110] Like other opioids, meperidine is known to cause spasm of smooth muscle but to a lesser degree. It is a preferred agent in patients with pain from renal colic and biliary spasm. Therapeutic doses of meperidine administered during active labor do not delay the birth process.

The adverse effects associated with meperidine are qualitatively similar to those produced by morphine. Meperidine is associated with a lower incidence of constipation and urinary retention. Tolerance develops to the actions of meperidine, and the drug has a high addictive potential. CNS excitation is seen with long-term use of meperidine, especially in patients with compromised renal and liver function owing to the accumulation of normeperidine. Naloxone does not reverse meperidine-induced seizures.

Meperidine administration is relatively contraindicated in patients taking monoamine oxidase inhibitors. Two types of interactions are seen. The most prominent interaction is excitatory,. It manifests as hyperthermia, hypertension or hypotension, muscular rigidity, convulsions, coma, and death.[111] This reaction is probably the result of the ability of meperidine to block neuronal reuptake of serotonin and thereby cause an increase in local serotonin activity.[112] The other type of interaction is seen as a potentiation of opioid effect resulting from inhibition of hepatic microsomal enzymes in patients taking monoamine oxidase inhibitors.

The major use of meperidine is for acute pain control. It is no longer recommended for long-term use because of its active metabolite. Meperidine in single doses is used to treat postanesthesia shivering. Congeners of meperidine, diphenoxylate and loperamide, are used to treat diarrhea. Meperidine is available for oral administration in the form of tablets and elixir. It is available for parenteral administration in varying concentrations. Intramuscular doses of 50 to 100 mg are used to treat severe pain and need to be repeated every 2 to 4 hours.

Fentanyl

Fentanyl is a synthetic opioid, a meperidine congener of the phenylpiperidine series. It is a pure opioid agonist with a high affinity for the μ receptor. It is approximately 75 to 100 times more potent than morphine as an analgesic. Fentanyl is very commonly used in anesthetic practice owing to its high potency and quick onset and offset of action.

Fentanyl is a highly lipid-soluble opioid and crosses the blood-brain barrier rapidly. The plasma level equilibrates with the CSF levels within 5 minutes. It has a rapid onset of action (30 seconds) and a short duration of action owing to redistribution to fat and skeletal muscle. The fairly rapid decline in plasma concentration reflects the redistribution. With repeated dosing or continuous infusion, however, saturation of the fat and muscle depots occurs. This leads to a prolonged effect resulting from systemic accumulation and a slower decline in the plasma concentration. Fentanyl is 50% protein bound. Fentanyl is primarily metabolized in the liver by cytochrome P-450 CYP3A4 to phenylacetic acid, norfentanyl, and small amounts of the pharmacologically active compound, *p*-hydroxyl fentanyl,[113] which are excreted in the bile and urine. A small portion (8%) is excreted unchanged in the urine. Fentanyl is the drug of choice in patients with renal disease because almost all the metabolites are inactive.

Fentanyl has a large volume of distribution, as reflected by its long (3 to 4 hours) elimination half-life.[4] As with other highly lipid-soluble opioids, the half-life of fentanyl is influenced by duration of administration, which is a function of the extent of fat sequestration. The elimination half-life is 7 to 12 hours in steady-state conditions.[113] Liver disease does not prolong the half-life, but a prolonged effect is seen in older patients.[114]

Fentanyl has a high affinity for the μ-opioid receptor, is almost 100 times more potent than morphine, and produces the same degree of respiratory depression as morphine in equianalgesic doses. Because fentanyl is highly lipid soluble, the risk of delayed respiration resulting from rostral spread of intrathecally administered drug to medullary respiratory centers is greatly reduced. When fentanyl is administered intravenously, the peak analgesic effect is seen after 5 minutes, and a quick recovery is also seen after single doses. With repeated dosing or prolonged infusions, a prolonged effect is seen. Muscle rigidity is commonly seen with intravenous fentanyl administration. Like other μ-receptor agonists, fentanyl produces nausea, vomiting, and itching. Respiratory depression is noted, and the onset is much more rapid than with morphine. As with morphine and meperidine, delayed respiratory depression seen after the use of fentanyl is possibly caused by enterohepatic circulation.[9] High doses of fentanyl can cause neuroexcitation and, rarely, seizure-like activity. Fentanyl decreases heart rate and mildly decreases blood pressure. It also causes minimal myocardial depression. Fentanyl does not release histamine and provides a marked degree of cardiovascular stability.

Fentanyl is used very commonly as an anesthetic agent because of its rapid onset and offset of action and relative cardiovascular stability. Because of its short duration of action, fentanyl is generally not the drug of choice for single-shot parenteral administration for chronic pain. It is one of the drugs of choice for intravenous patient-controlled analgesia in patients with renal disease. It is administered frequently by the epidural and intrathecal routes. Its high lipophilicity and small molecular weight make it well suited for use in a transdermal preparation. Fentanyl is not used for oral administration because of extensive first-pass metabolism and poor bioavailability (32%). It is available as a preparation for oral transmucosal use; bioavailability is 52% to 65%. This form is used for breakthrough cancer pain and is not recommended for acute postoperative pain. Transdermal fentanyl has a lower incidence of constipation than do oxycodone and morphine.[115]

Alfentanil

Alfentanil and remifentanil were developed in search of analgesics with a more rapid onset of action and predictable termination of effects.[111] Alfentanil is 5 to 10 times less potent than fentanyl and has a shorter duration of effect.

Alfentanil has a rapid onset (1 to 2 minutes) of analgesic effect after intravenous administration. This is because 90% of the drug is nonionized at physiologic pH as a result of a low pKa value. Alfentanil has a smaller volume of distribution, lower lipid solubility, and slightly greater protein binding compared with fentanyl.[116] Its analgesic effect is terminated rapidly as a result of redistribution. Hepatic metabolism accounts for most of the elimination of alfentanil. A small percentage (1%) is excreted unchanged in urine. The elimination half-life is 70 to 98 minutes.[117] The elimination half-life is significantly increased in patients with cirrhosis. Renal disease does not affect alfentanil clearance.

Alfentanil is used for epidural analgesia and for intravenous patient-controlled analgesia. Owing to its short duration of analgesic effect, alfentanil is not an ideal choice for patient-controlled analgesia use. It is available for injection in a concentration of 500 μg/mL.

Sufentanil

Sufentanil is a synthetic opioid that is a member of the phenylpiperidine series. Sufentanil is the most potent μ-receptor agonist available for human clinical use.[61] It is 5 to 10 times more potent than fentanyl and 1000 times more potent than morphine. It has an affinity for opioid receptors 30 times greater than that of fentanyl.[118]

Sufentanil is highly lipid soluble, more so than fentanyl and alfentanil. It rapidly crosses the blood-brain barrier, equilibrates with the CSF, and therefore has a rapid onset of action. The analgesic effect is terminated quickly as a result of rapid redistribution to fat and skeletal muscle. Sufentanil has a volume of distribution, distribution half-life, and elimination half-life that fall between those of fentanyl and alfentanil.[119] More than 90% of sufentanil is protein bound. The shorter elimination half-life is the result of a small volume of distribution and higher hepatic mobilization. Sufentanil is metabolized in the liver; products of *N*-dealkylation are inactive, and the O-demethylation product (methylsufentanil) is active. Sufentanil metabolites are excreted in the urine. The pharmacologic profile of sufentanil is very similar to that of fentanyl. Like other opioids, sufentanil produces bradycardia, respiratory depression, nausea, vomiting, itching, and smooth muscle spasm.

Sufentanil is available only in an injectable form. It is administered parenterally and by the epidural and intrathecal routes. A transdermal formulation of sufentanil is currently in clinical trials.

Remifentanil

Remifentanil is an esterase-metabolized opioid of the phenylpiperidine series. Its potency is approximately equal to that of fentanyl. The analgesic effect occurs within 1 to 1.5 minutes. Remifentanil undergoes rapid hydrolysis by nonspecific esterases in blood and tissues.[120,121] Clearance is unaffected by cholinesterase inhibition. Renal and liver disease does not alter remifentanil pharmacokinetics. Remifentanil has a distribution half-life of 2 to 4 minutes and an elimination half-life of 10 to 20 minutes.

Remifentanil is available only for parenteral administration. Its short duration of effect does not make it an ideal drug for use in intravenous patient-controlled anesthesia. It is currently formulated with glycine and is therefore not recommended for epidural or intrathecal use.

Methadone and Congeners

Methadone, a synthetic drug developed in the 1940s, is an opioid of the structural class of diphenylpropylamines. It was originally synthesized during World War II by the German pharmaceutical industry. Methadone bears no structural resemblance to morphine. Methadone is used clinically as a racemic mixture, the levorotatory (l) form being 8 to 50 times more potent than the dextrorotatory (D) form. Methadone is popular as a maintenance drug for heroin addicts and is a time-honored therapy for cancer pain.[122,123] It has excellent bioavailability and a long half-life, thus making it an ideal drug for outpatient use.[124] The oral bioavailability of methadone is high (i.e., 81% to 95%).[125] Methadone is rapidly absorbed from the gastrointestinal tract, and measurable concentrations in plasma are seen in 30 minutes,[126] but the analgesic effect peaks at 4 hours. After parenteral administration, methadone can be detected in plasma within 10 minutes, and CSF levels peak at 1 to 2 hours. Methadone is a basic and lipophilic drug subject to considerable tissue distribution.[127] The sequestration of methadone at extravascular binding sites, followed by slow release into plasma, contributes to the prolonged duration of methadone half-life in plasma. The protein (alpha$_1$-acid-glycoprotein, AAG) binding of methadone is 60% to 90%, which is double that of morphine. Methadone binds to AAG with a relatively high affinity. Methadone can be displaced from AAG by the following drugs: propranolol, chlorpromazine, prochlorperazine, thioridazine, and tricyclic antidepressants.[128]

Biotransformation and renal and fecal excretion are important determinants of the elimination of methadone. Methadone undergoes extensive metabolism in the liver by N-demethylation and cyclization to form the inactive metabolites pyrroline and pyrrolidines. These inactive metabolites are excreted in the urine and bile along with small amounts of unchanged drug. Urinary pH is an important determinant of elimination half-life of methadone; the half-life increases with rising pH. The elimination half-life of methadone after a single dose is approximately 15 hours, and with long-term administration, it is 22 hours. Methadone has a secondary half-life of more than 55 hours (from release of tissue stores).

Methadone is a μ-receptor agonist with pharmacologic properties qualitatively similar to those of morphine. Although it is a potent μ-receptor agonist, methadone also has considerable affinity for the δ-opioid receptor.[129] Methadone also has some agonist actions at the κ- and σ-opioid receptors.[130] Methadone binds with low affinity to NMDA receptors and acts as a noncompetitive NMDA receptor antagonist in the brain and spinal cord.[131,132] The analgesic potency is equal to or slightly greater than that of morphine. The duration of analgesia after a single dose of methadone is 4 to 6 hours, governed by the rapid initial absorption-distribution phase.[127,133] Methadone and many of its congeners retain a considerable degree of their effectiveness when given orally. Methadone, when given orally, is approximately 50% as effective as the same dose administered intramuscularly; the oral-to-parenteral potency ratio is 1:2.[134] With repeated dosing, cumulative effects are seen because of slow release from tissues. Dosage should be tailored accordingly; either the dose or the frequency of doses should be decreased. The occurrence of side effects with equianalgesic doses is similar for both morphine and methadone.

Therapeutic Uses and Preparations

Methadone is an excellent analgesic with good bioavailability. Its low cost and long half-life make it a good choice for outpatient use in chronic pain states. Methadone is also used for treatment of opioid abstinence syndromes and in heroin users. The NMDA blocking property of methadone makes it a choice of opioid for the treatment of neuropathic pain. Methadone may be an option in patients with opioid-induced hyperalgesia. It is available for oral administration in tablets (5 and 10 mg) and as a solution (10 mg/5 mL). Methadone is also available for parenteral administration and is used for intravenous patient-controlled analgesia. Methadone has also been used epidurally and intrathecally.

Levo-Alpha Acetyl Methadol

An alternative to methadone for individuals who are addicted to opioids, levo-alpha acetyl methadol (LAAM) is a medication that is a derivative of methadone. LAAM was first developed in 1948 by German chemists as a painkiller. In 1993, the US Food and Drug Administration (FDA) approved LAAM for use in medication therapy for opiate addiction.[135]

LAAM itself is not effective; its metabolites, nor-LAAM and dinor-LAAM, are the active agents. LAAM is ineffective through intravenous injection and therefore is not attractive for illegal use.[136] The delay occurs before the effects of LAAM can be detected, and the drug remains in the body much longer than methadone (72 hours for most people at doses of ≥80 mg). LAAM has pharmacologic cross-tolerance to other opioids and thereby blocks the euphoric effects seen with these drugs, but it still controls opiate craving. It is available for oral administration in a suspension form. Doses range from 10 to 140 mg, three times a week.[61] LAAM requires administration every 2 to 3 days and can be given at treatment centers by itself with no take-home medications.

Propoxyphene

Propoxyphene is structurally related to methadone (**Fig. 122.11**) and is a weak analgesic. The analgesic activity of the racemate was found to reside in the D-isomer, and it is this compound that is currently used as a mild analgesic. The l-isomer, which lacks analgesic activity, has been introduced as an antitussive.[89]

After oral administration, propoxyphene undergoes first-pass metabolism and has a bioavailability of 30% to 70%.[4]

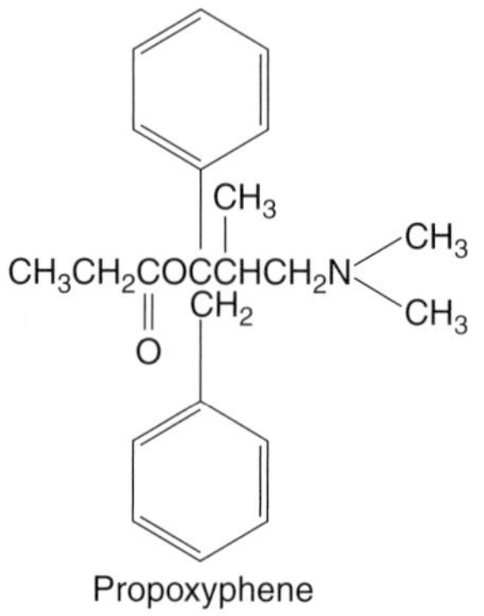

Propoxyphene

Fig. 122.11 **Chemical structure of propoxyphene.**

Plasma concentration peaks at 1 to 2 hours. Propoxyphene undergoes extensive redistribution and tissue binding because its redistribution volume (960 L) is much greater than that of the other opioid analgesics.[94] Propoxyphene is metabolized in the liver by *N*-demethylation to form norpropoxyphene. Propoxyphene has an average half-life of 6 to 12 hours, which is much longer than that of codeine. Norpropoxyphene has a half-life of approximately 30 hours, and its accumulation with repeated doses may be responsible for the toxicity seen with propoxyphene administration. Norpropoxyphene also undergoes extensive first-pass metabolism, and liver disease can enhance accumulations.

Propoxyphene is a weak analgesic, with a relative potency one half to one third that of codeine. The classic triad of physical dependence, psychological dependence, and tolerance accompanies the use of propoxyphene. Moderately toxic doses produce CNS and respiratory depression, but increasing doses cause CNS excitation, cardiotoxicity, and pulmonary edema. These toxicities are attributed to the effects of the active metabolite, norpropoxyphene.

Propoxyphene is recommended for the treatment of mild to moderate pain. A dose of 90 to 120 mg of propoxyphene is equianalgesic to 60 mg of codeine or 600 mg of aspirin. Propoxyphene hydrochloride is available in 32- and 65-mg tablets; it is formulated with acetaminophen or aspirin to give a synergistic effect. It is also available as propoxyphene napsylate in a suspension form and in 100-mg tablets.

Tramadol

Tramadol is a synthetic opioid structurally related to morphine and codeine. It is a centrally acting opioid agonist with some selectivity for the μ receptor and also binds weakly to κ and δ receptors. It also acts on the monoamine system by inhibiting the reuptake of norepinephrine and serotonin (5-hydroxytryptamine, 5-HT).[137]

Tramadol undergoes some first-pass metabolism after oral administration and has a bioavailability of 68%.[9] It is O-demethylated by the cytochrome P-450 enzyme CYP2D6 to the therapeutically active O-desmethyltramadol and is *N*-demethylated by CYP34A to the inactive *N*-desmethyltramadol. O-desmethyltramadol is two to four times more potent than tramadol itself. A significant amount (10% to 30%) of tramadol is excreted unchanged in the urine. Whereas plasma protein binding is low (20%), its apparent volume of distribution is large (2.7 L/kg), indicating considerable tissue uptake.[137] The elimination half-life for tramadol is 6 hours, and the active metabolite has a slightly longer half-life of 7.5 hours.

Tramadol produces analgesia by its opioid-like activity and also by inhibiting the reuptake of norepinephrine and serotonin. It is contraindicated in patients taking monoamine oxidase inhibitors. Tramadol produces nausea, vomiting, sedation, dizziness, dry mouth, hot flashes, and headache. It produces less respiratory depression than morphine in equianalgesic doses. The incidence of seizures in patients receiving tramadol is less than 1%. Tramadol-induced seizures are not reversed by the μ-opioid antagonist naloxone.

With its dual mode of action (opioid agonist, norepinephrine and 5-HT reuptake inhibition), tramadol is a useful drug in nociceptive and neuropathic pain. It is superior to morphine in the treatment of some neuropathic pain syndromes. Unlike other opioids, tramadol produces only a weak and clinically irrelevant respiratory depression at the recommended analgesic doses.[138] Tramadol has a low potential for drug abuse and dependence. It is available as 50-mg tablets, to be administered every 6 hours. The daily dose should not exceed 400 mg. It is also available formulated in combination with acetaminophen.

Tapentadol

Tapentadol is a centrally acting opioid agonist that has as its sites of action the μ and norepinephrine receptors. It has been approved by the FDA as an oral analgesic for moderate to severe pain. Early clinical experience suggests that tapentadol is comparable to hydrocodone and oxycodone and has a slightly more favorable side effect profile.

Tapentadol is rapidly absorbed orally and appears to have no analgesically active metabolites. The drug reaches a maximum concentration in approximately 1.5 hours. It is excreted primarily by the kidneys.

With its dual mode of action (opioid agonist and norepinephrine inhibition), tapentadol should theoretically be useful for treatment of neuropathic pain. In diabetic animal models, tapentadol showed selective inhibition of disease-related hyperalgesia with not much change in normal sensation.[139] Based on its pharmacology, tapentadol should have a relatively low potential for drug abuse and dependence, but the FDA has classified it as a schedule II opioid. It is available as 50-, 75-, and 100-mg tablets, to be administered every 4 to 6 hours. The daily dose should not exceed 600 mg.

Agonist-Antagonists

The agonist-antagonists produce opposing action at the μ and κ receptors; they are μ-receptor antagonists and κ-receptor agonists. These drugs were initially developed in search of an analgesic with less respiratory depression and addictive potential. These compounds are less efficacious than pure μ-receptor agonists in their analgesic effect and seem to have a lower potential for abuse.[61]

Pentazocine

Pentazocine is a synthetic opioid of the benzomorphan (**Fig. 122.12**) series that is a weak competitive antagonist at the μ receptor and an agonist at the $κ_1$ and possibly $κ_2$ receptors.

Pentazocine is well absorbed after oral and parenteral administration. It undergoes extensive first-pass metabolism, and only 20% of the drug enters the systemic circulation. It has a peak analgesic effect in 15 minutes to 1 hour after intramuscular injection and in 1 to 3 hours after oral administration.[9] Pentazocine has a plasma half-life of 3 to 4 hours. Its action is terminated by hepatic metabolism to inactive glucuronide conjugates and renal excretion. Less than 2% of the given dose is excreted in the bile.

Pentazocine is an agonist at the κ receptors and produces analgesia. Higher doses of pentazocine elicit psychotomimetic and dysphoric effects. The exact mechanism of these effects is not known but is thought to be caused by weak σ-receptor agonist activity[4] and activation of supraspinal κ receptors.[111] Like other agonist-antagonists, pentazocine exhibits a ceiling effect

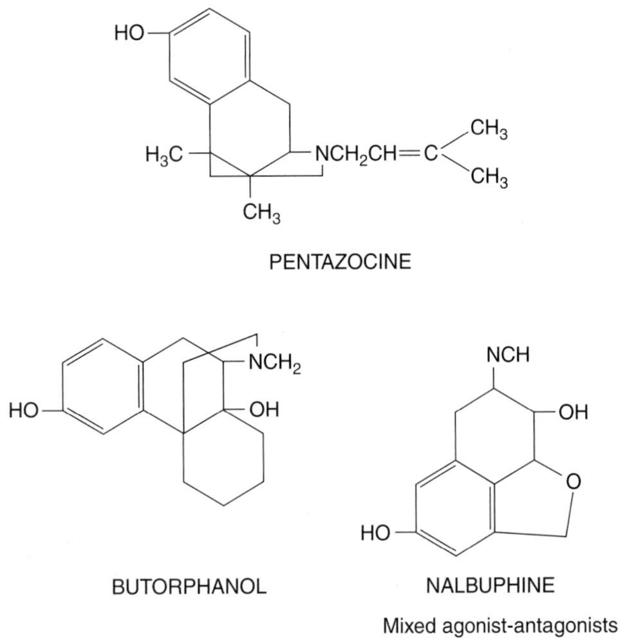

Fig. 122.12 **Chemical structure of pentazocine, butorphanol, and nalbuphine.**

for respiratory depression and analgesic effect. The ceiling effect is seen with 60 to 100 mg of pentazocine.[140] Pentazocine does not reverse the respiratory depression produced by morphine. Pentazocine may, however, precipitate withdrawal if it is given to patients taking pure μ-receptor agonists.

Unlike other opioids, pentazocine does not cause bradycardia. High doses of pentazocine increase heart rate and blood pressure. In patients with acute myocardial infarction, pentazocine produces substantial elevation in cardiac preload and afterload and thereby increases the cardiac workload.[110] In addition, an increase in systemic and pulmonary artery pressure, left ventricular filling pressure, and systemic vascular resistance and a decrease in left ventricular ejection fraction are seen. These effects may be caused by a rise in the plasma concentration of catecholamine. Pentazocine also produces smooth muscle spasm but appears to cause less of a biliary spasm than does morphine.[141] The most common adverse effects are sedation, sweating, dizziness, and nausea. With parenteral doses higher than 60 mg, psychotomimetic effects occur, manifested by anxiety, strange thoughts, nightmares, and hallucinations. With prolonged use, tolerance develops to the analgesic and subjective effects of the drug.

Pentazocine is used to treat mild to moderate pain; an oral dose of 50 mg is equianalgesic to 60 mg of codeine orally. Oral forms are available compounded with aspirin and acetaminophen. To reduce the incidence of parenteral injection, tablets for oral use are formulated with naloxone. Naloxone is completely degraded with oral administration, but if injected, the combination would have no effect because of the antagonist effects of naloxone. Abuse patterns seem to be low with the oral forms of pentazocine.

Nalbuphine

Nalbuphine is a semisynthetic mixed agonist-antagonist that is chemically related to naloxone and oxymorphone. Bioavailability of oral nalbuphine is less than 20% as a result

of extensive first-pass metabolism. It is lipophilic and has a large volume of distribution. Nalbuphine is metabolized in the liver to inactive glucuronide conjugates. Nalbuphine and its metabolites are excreted to a great extent in the feces. The elimination half-life of nalbuphine is 3 to 6 hours.[142]

Compared with pentazocine, nalbuphine is a more potent antagonist at the μ receptor. Intramuscularly administered nalbuphine produces analgesia comparable to that of morphine (potency ratio of 1:1). It exhibits a ceiling effect at approximately 0.45 mg/kg,[4] and no further respiratory depression or analgesia is obtained. In contrast to pentazocine and butorphanol, nalbuphine does not increase cardiac index, pulmonary artery pressure, or cardiac work. The systemic blood pressure does not change significantly.[111] The most common adverse effects are sedation, sweating, and headache. Higher doses can produce dysphoria and psychotomimetic effects. Nalbuphine can precipitate withdrawal symptoms in individuals taking μ-opioid receptor agonists. Nalbuphine also reverses the respiratory depression[143] associated with opioids and can be used to treat pruritus related to opioid use.[144] Long-term use of nalbuphine can cause physical dependence.

Butorphanol

Butorphanol is a synthetic mixed agonist-antagonist compound of the morphinan series. It has a profile of action similar to that of pentazocine but with greater analgesic efficacy and fewer side effects.[61]

Bioavailability after oral administration is low (5% to 17%)[145] as a result of extensive first-pass metabolism. No first-pass metabolism occurs with parenteral or transnasal administration, and these routes produce similar plasma levels.[9] Butorphanol is rapidly absorbed after parenteral administration and has a distribution half-life of 5 minutes. Transnasal administration results in rapid absorption with onset of analgesia within 15 minutes. Plasma protein binding is approximately 85%. Butorphanol is converted to the inactive metabolites hydroxybutorphanol and norbutorphanol. The plasma terminal half-life of butorphanol is 3 hours with parenteral administration and 4.5 to 5.5 hours with transnasal administration.

Butorphanol has agonistic activity at the κ receptor and antagonistic activity at the μ receptor. It also exhibits partial agonistic activity at the σ receptor.[146] A dose of 2 to 3 mg of parenteral butorphanol is equivalent to 10 mg of parenteral morphine. Like other agonist-antagonists, butorphanol has a ceiling effect for respiratory depression and analgesia. Common adverse effects of butorphanol are sedation and diaphoresis. It also causes dysphoria because of its σ-agonist activity. As with pentazocine, analgesic doses of butorphanol produce an increase in heart rate, systemic blood pressure, and pulmonary artery pressure.[147] Its effects on the biliary tract are milder than are those of morphine. Butorphanol can reverse the analgesia produced by pure μ-receptor agonists but does not reverse the respiratory depression. Physical dependence is noted with long-term use of butorphanol.

Because of its high analgesic potency, butorphanol is indicated for the treatment of moderate to severe pain. The recommended parenteral dose is 1 to 2 mg intramuscularly and 0.5 to 2 mg intravenously every 3 to 4 hours. Butorphanol is also available for intranasal administration in a spray form.

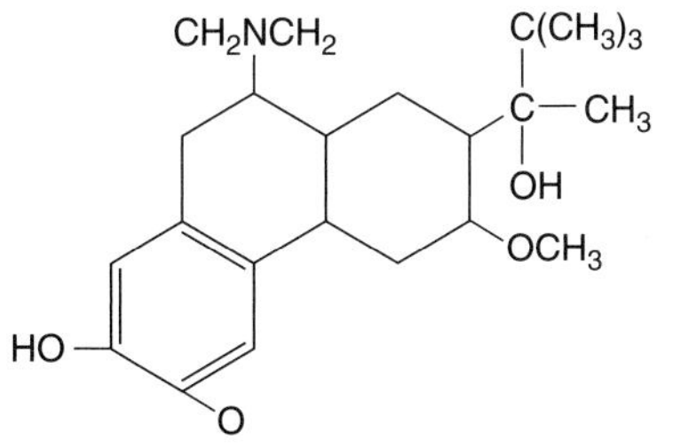

Fig. 122.13 **Chemical structure of buprenorphine.**

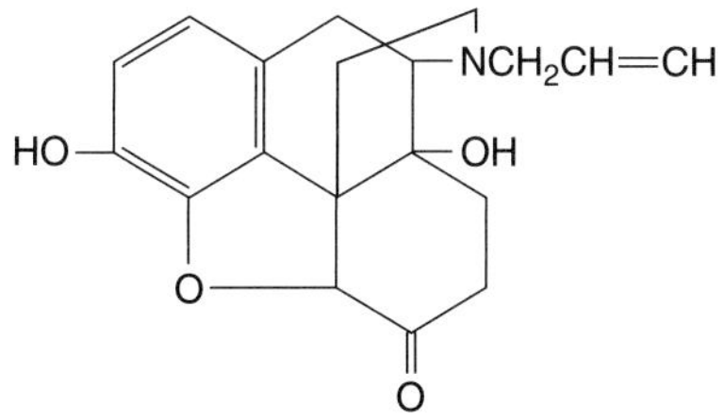

Fig. 122.14 **Chemical structure of naloxone.**

Buprenorphine

Buprenorphine is a semisynthetic, highly lipophilic opioid derived from the naturally occurring alkaloid thebaine (**Fig. 122.13**). It is 25 to 50 times more potent than morphine[111] and is a partial μ-receptor agonist.

Bioavailability after oral administration is 16% because of extensive first-pass metabolism.[148] Buprenorphine displays a bell-shaped dose-response curve, with peak antinociceptive opioid effects at approximately 0.5 mg/kg (subcutaneously) 60 minutes after the dose and a gradual decline of the effects in the dosage range of 0.5 to 10 mg/kg.[149] Buprenorphine is highly lipophilic and is approximately 96% bound to plasma proteins. After parenteral administration, the analgesic response is governed by the kinetics of receptor dissociation.[150] The half-life of dissociation from the μ receptor is 166 minutes for buprenorphine versus 7 minutes for fentanyl.[151] It has an elimination half-life of 3 to 4 hours but a prolonged duration of effect because of slow dissociation from receptor site. Information concerning the metabolism of buprenorphine is limited. In animal studies, buprenorphine disposition is by hepatic conjugation to glucuronides, eliminated in the bile (92%).

A dose of 0.3 mg of parenteral buprenorphine produces analgesia equivalent to that of 10 mg of parenteral morphine.[152] Buprenorphine acts as a partial agonist at the μ receptor and as an antagonist at the κ receptor. Buprenorphine has a less well-defined effect on respiratory function than that usually expected of opioids; it has a ceiling effect on respiratory depression with an increase in dose. The adverse effects associated with buprenorphine are sedation and nausea. Usual parenteral doses of buprenorphine can reduce the adrenocortical response after surgery.[153] Buprenorphine partially reverses the effects of large doses of μ-receptor agonists and can reverse the ventilatory depression seen with these opioids. The cardiovascular hemodynamic responses are similar to those of morphine.

Buprenorphine is used to treat moderate to severe pain conditions. Parenteral buprenorphine can be given in a dose of 0.3 mg every 6 to 8 hours. The drug may not be a good choice for intravenous patient-controlled analgesia because of its slow onset of action. Few studies have described effective analgesia with minimal respiratory depression associated with buprenorphine in intravenous patient-controlled analgesia. Sublingual buprenorphine, 0.4 mg every 8 hours, provides analgesia equivalent to 10 mg of morphine intramuscularly every 4 hours. A sublingual formulation of buprenorphine and naloxone hydrochloride dihydrate in a 4:1 ratio is also awaiting FDA approval for the treatment of pain. Transdermal buprenorphine is available for clinical use in some countries.

Antagonists

Pohl[154] developed the first opioid antagonist, N-allylnorcodeine in 1915 by making minor changes in the codeine molecule (**Fig. 122.14**).

Naloxone, Naltrexone, Methylnaltrexone, and Alvimopan

Naloxone is the first opioid antagonist to be developed that is devoid of agonist activity. Naloxone is a synthetic N-allyl derivative of oxymorphone. Naltrexone is a lipid-soluble opioid antagonist that readily crosses the blood-brain barrier. Methylnaltrexone is a quaternary derivative of naltrexone formed by addition of a methyl group at the amine ring that makes it less lipid soluble and with restricted ability to cross the blood-brain barrier.

Naloxone is rapidly absorbed after oral administration, but high presystemic metabolism makes this route unreliable. The oral-to-parenteral potency ratio has been estimated at 1:50. Effects are seen 1 to 2 minutes after an intravenous dose and 2 to 5 minutes after a subcutaneous dose. Naloxone is highly lipid soluble and is rapidly distributed throughout the body. As a result of this rapid redistribution, naloxone has a very short duration (30 to 45 minutes) of action. Supplementation of the initial dose of naloxone is usually necessary if sustained antagonism is desired. Approximately 50% of the drug is bound to plasma proteins, mainly albumin. The plasma half-life is 1 to 2 hours. Naloxone undergoes extensive biotransformation in the liver to inactive metabolites. The metabolites are, in large part, excreted in the urine.

The effects produced by naloxone are the result of antagonism of endogenous and exogenous opioids. Naloxone has no effects when administered in clinical doses to normal human volunteers. On administration to humans with pain who have not received exogenous opioids, naloxone demonstrates a biphasic response. Low doses produce analgesia, and higher doses produce hyperalgesia.[155] Naloxone reverses all the effects of exogenous opioids (i.e., analgesia, respiratory depression, pupillary constriction, delayed gastric transit, and sedation). Naloxone also reverses the analgesic effects of placebo medications and acupuncture. Small doses (0.4 to 0.8 mg) of naloxone given parenterally reverse the effects of μ-receptor agonists. Naloxone can be titrated to reverse the respiratory depression produced by opioids while maintaining some analgesic effect. Naloxone infusions of 5 μg/kg/hour have been shown to reverse the respiratory depression produced by epidural morphine and not affect the quality of analgesia.[156] Rebound release of catecholamines may cause hypertension, tachycardia, and ventricular arrhythmias. Pulmonary edema has also been observed after naloxone administration. Small doses of naloxone can precipitate a withdrawal syndrome in patients who are opioid dependent. Long-term administration of naloxone increases the density of opioid receptors and produces a temporary exaggeration of response to subsequently administered opioids.[111]

Naltrexone reverses the analgesia as well as the adverse effects associated with opioids and therefore can cause withdrawal symptoms. Methylnaltrexone, in contrast, reverses side effects of opioids that are mediated by the peripheral receptors (gastrointestinal tract) and has no effect on the analgesia.

The treatment of life-threatening consequences of known or suspected opioid overdose is the prime indication for naloxone use. Naloxone is also used in small doses to reverse some of the side effects (respiratory depression and pruritus) associated with opioid use. Oral naloxone given in a dose of 8 to 12 mg has been used to ameliorate constipation in patients taking opioids. Naloxone is also used in a formulation with oral pentazocine to prevent diversion. To reverse sedation and respiratory depression, an intravenous dose of 10 μg of naloxone (followed by increasing doses) is given. An infusion may be necessary to maintain the antagonism. Naloxone is available for parenteral administration in concentrations of 0.02, 0.4, and 1 mg/mL. Methylnaltrexone was approved in 2008 for the treatment of opioid-induced constipation in the palliative setting in patients not responsive to laxative therapy. It is available for subcutaneous injection at 8 to 12 mg (0.15 mg/kg), not to exceed one dose over a 24-hour period.

Alvimopan is a μ-receptor antagonist approved by the FDA in 2008 for the treatment of postoperative ileus. The drug antagonizes the peripheral effects of opioids (constipation) without reversing centrally mediated analgesia. The peak plasma concentration is seen approximately 2 hours after oral ingestion, and the bioavailability is 6%. Alvimopan does not cross the blood-brain barrier because of its large molecular weight and low lipophilicity. It has a terminal half-life of 10 to 18 hours. It has one active metabolite as a result of intestinal metabolism. It is approved for oral use in a hospital setting, at an initial 12-mg dose 30 minutes to 5 hours preoperatively, followed by twice daily for 7 days.

Conclusion

Since their initial discovery thousands of years ago, opioids remain important agents in the treatment of pain. They have become the drugs of choice in the management of acute perioperative pain and of moderate to severe cancer pain. The use of opioids to treat chronic noncancer pain conditions remains controversial.

Multiple preparations of various opioids are available in immediate-release and extended-release preparations. The choice of agent is based on the patient's previous response, the patient's medical condition, the degree of pain, and the physician's experience. Careful titration of drugs for pain control with vigilance about side effects is needed. Opioid use is associated with side effects, including tolerance, addiction, and abuse. Aggressive prosecution of physicians who prescribe large quantities of opioid analgesics to patients in pain has had a chilling effect on the appropriate use of opioid analgesics in pain management in many communities. Efforts by the national and international pain management community to highlight the appropriateness of the use of opioid analgesics for the management of all types of pain have helped to decriminalize such activities.

Research is ongoing to discover an efficacious opioid that has minimal side effects and does not have a potential for abuse. Tamper-resistant and nonaddictive preparations are needed. Genetic differences account in part for the individual differences in response to opioid analgesics and in the development of addiction. Pharmacogenetic studies are looking further into individual responses to various opioids and hold promise for the use of genetics in the treatment of pain.

References

Full references for this chapter can be found on www.expertconsult.com.

Role of Antidepressants in the Management of Pain

Steven D. Waldman and Corey W. Waldman

The antidepressant compounds have been used in patients suffering from a variety of painful conditions since these drugs were first released in the 1950s. The use of these agents in this clinical setting was predicated on the logical notion that most patients with unremitting pain were depressed. Not until the early 1970s, however, did Merskey and Hester[1] and other investigators put forth the notion that this group of drugs could also have analgesic properties separate and apart from their primary mood-altering purpose. This notion has stood the test of time, and the results of numerous controlled studies have confirmed it.[2] Given the widespread use of the antidepressant compounds as a first-line treatment for pain, one must wonder that if the pharmaceutical companies that first introduced these drugs as antidepressants could turn back the hands of time, they would have introduced them as analgesics. This chapter reviews the clinically relevant pharmacology of the various antidepressant compounds that are thought to be useful in the management of pain with an eye to providing the clinician with a practical roadmap on how to implement, manage, and discontinue therapy with this heterogeneous group of drugs.

Classification of Antidepressants

For the purposes of this chapter, the antidepressant compounds can be divided into the following six groups: (1) the tricyclic antidepressants (TCAs); (2) the selective serotonin reuptake inhibitors (SSRIs); (3) the serotonin and noradrenergic reuptake inhibitors (SNaRIs); (4) the noradrenergic and specific serotoninergic antidepressants (NaSSAs); (5) the noradrenergic reuptake inhibitors (NaRIs); and (6) the monoamine oxidase inhibitors (MAOIs) (**Table 123.1**). In addition, an emerging group of pharmacologically heterogeneous drugs is known as the atypical antidepressants. Although many of the characteristics of the various types of antidepressant compounds are similar to the properties of the TCAs, the unique properties of each class of drugs are discussed individually.

Tricyclic (Heterocyclic) Antidepressants

The TCAs are the prototypical antidepressant compounds in clinical use for the treatment of pain and are, by far, the most studied. Their name is derived from their molecular structure, which is composed of three rings (**Fig. 123.1**). The modification of the middle ring and the alteration of the amine group on the terminal side chain resulted in numerous clinically useful drugs. More recently, the addition of a fourth ring to the TCAs in drugs such as trazodone and amoxapine complicated the nomenclature of this class of drugs (**Fig. 123.2**). In terms of chemical structure, these drugs are now correctly referred to as *heterocyclic antidepressants;* however, the more familiar term *tricyclic antidepressants* is still used by most clinicians to indicate the amitriptyline-like drugs, regardless of their actual chemical structure, and to differentiate them from other classes of antidepressants such as the SSRIs and the MAOIs.

Mechanism of Action

The mechanism of action of the TCAs is thought to be through their ability to alter monoamine transmitter activity at the synapse by blocking the reuptake of serotonin and norepinephrine.[3] Although this pharmacologic effect begins with the first dose of the drug, most clinicians believe that clinically demonstrable improvement in the patient's pain complaints requires 2 to 3 weeks of treatment. This lag in onset of clinically demonstrable improvement suggests that more may be at play than the simple alteration of monoamine transmitter activity.[4] Some investigators have postulated that the normalization of a disturbed sleep pattern is ultimately responsible for the analgesic properties of these drugs, rather than their direct action on monoamine transmitter activity itself.

Absorption and Metabolism

The TCAs are well absorbed orally and are bound to serum proteins. This class of drugs undergoes rapid first-pass hepatic metabolism, but these agents have relatively long elimination half-lives of 1 to 4 days, owing to their lipophilic nature. Diseases that affect serum proteins or decrease liver function can alter the serum levels of these drugs. These drugs are excreted in the urine and feces.

Table 123.1 Classification of Antidepressant Compounds

Tricyclic antidepressants

Selective serotonin reuptake inhibitors

Serotonin and noradrenergic reuptake inhibitors

Noradrenergic and specific serotoninergic antidepressants

Noradrenergic reuptake inhibitors

Monoamine oxidase inhibitors

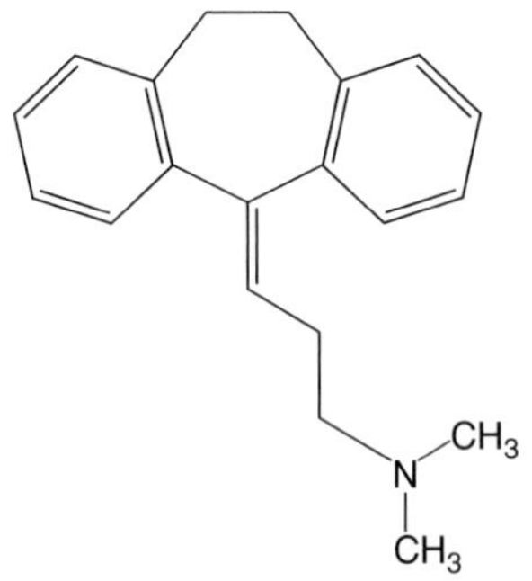

Fig. 123.1 **The chemical structure of amitriptyline, the prototypical tricyclic antidepressant.**

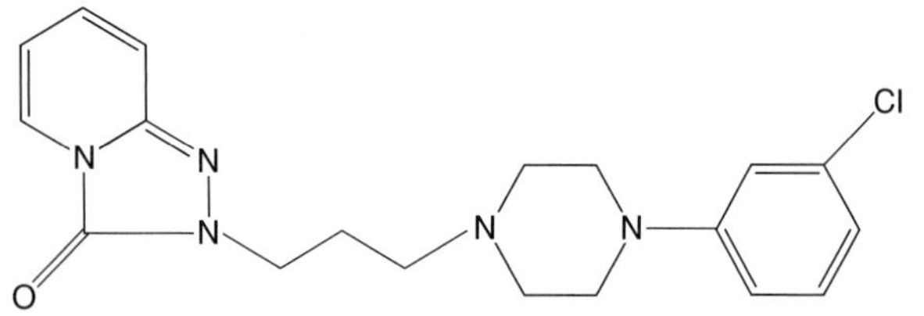

Fig. 123.2 **The chemical structure of trazodone.**

Side Effects

In addition to blocking the synaptic reuptake of serotonin and norepinephrine, the TCAs also interact with other receptors. These interactions account for the wide and varied side effect profile of TCAs (**Table 123.2**). Many of the early TCAs, as typified by amitriptyline, exert significant anticholinergic side effects through the muscarinic receptors. Such side effects include xerostomia, xerophthalmia, constipation, urinary retention, tachycardia, decreased gastric emptying, and difficulties in visual accommodation.[5]

In addition to the anticholinergic side effects of the TCAs, many of these drugs cause significant blockade of the alpha-adrenergic receptors, with resulting orthostatic hypotension. The orthostatic hypotension is most likely the result of venous blood pooling in the lower extremities and viscera. This potentially dangerous side effect can range from a mildly annoying sensation of transient light-headedness when arising to near syncopal episodes, with falling and head injury distinct possibilities.

Other side effects include the blocking of the histamine (H_2) receptors with resultant decrease in gastric acid production, as well as various psychomimetic side effects that can be most upsetting to the patient. These psychomimetic side effects include vivid "Technicolor" dreams, prolonged and intense dreaming, restlessness, and occasionally psychic activation. Some drugs in this class seem to produce increased appetite and weight gain, whereas others seem to suppress appetite. Increased and decreased libido, as well as sexual dysfunction, can occur and should be discussed with patients when assessing the efficacy of therapy with the TCA compounds. The unique side effect of priapism, which occurs in approximately 1 in 10,000 men when taking trazodone, should also be discussed when implementing treatment with this drug.

Table 123.2 Common Side Effects of the Tricyclic Antidepressants

Xerostomia

Xerophthalmia

Urinary retention

Blurred vision

Constipation

Sedation

Cardiac arrhythmias

Orthostatic hypotension

Sleep disruption

Weight gain

Headache

Nausea

Gastrointestinal disturbance/diarrhea

Abdominal pain

Inability to achieve an erection

Inability to achieve an orgasm (men and women)

Loss of libido

Agitation

Anxiety

These side effects can usually be managed by proper dosing techniques when implementing therapy with the TCAs, as discussed subsequently. However, they may necessitate switching to a drug with a different side effect profile to achieve patient compliance with the drug regimen.

Abuse Potential and Side Effects of Withdrawal of the Drug

The TCAs do not appear to interact significantly with the opioid, benzodiazepine, γ-aminobutyric acid, or beta-adrenergic receptors. No clinical evidence of addiction occurs when these drugs are discontinued. Some drugs in this class, however, have a propensity to cause various symptoms including insomnia, restlessness, lack of energy, and increased cholinergic activity as manifested by excessive salivation and occasional gastrointestinal distress. These side effects can be avoided by slowly tapering the TCA over 10 to 14 days.

Overdosage

Overdosage of significant amounts of the TCAs is a serious event that, if not aggressively managed, can result in death.[6] In general, the dosages that are required to treat pain are lower than those required to treat severe depression. However, the advent of mail order pharmacies, with their 90-day prescription requirements, has made overdose a real issue because amitriptyline doses greater than 2000 mg can be fatal—well within the amounts supplied in a 90-day prescription. Sedation progressing to coma, combined cardiac abnormalities including delays in cardiac conduction as manifested by a prolonged QT interval, and bizarre cardiac dysrhythmias can make the management of TCA overdose most challenging. Further complicating this clinical picture is the potential for grand mal seizures and a hypercholinergic state consisting of mydriasis, urinary retention, dry mouth and eyes, and delirium. Because of the potential for disastrous results of TCA overdosage, all such events should be taken seriously, and all patients suspected of overdosage should be immediately evaluated and treated in an emergency department equipped to manage the attendant life-threatening symptoms.

Some Common Tricyclic and Tetracyclic Antidepressants

AMITRIPTYLINE (ELAVIL)

Amitriptyline is the prototype of all antidepressants (see Fig. 123.1). Its efficacy as an analgesic has been studied extensively, and significant clinical experience exists in this setting.[7,8] Blocking both norepinephrine and serotonin, amitriptyline is an efficacious analgesic, but it has significant side effects including sedation, orthostasis, and most of the troublesome anticholinergic side effects. This drug should be used cautiously in patients with cardiac conduction defects owing to its propensity to cause tachycardia, and it should not be used in patients with narrow-angle glaucoma and significant prostatism. In spite of its side effect profile, amitriptyline remains a reasonable starting point for implementation of TCA therapy because of its proven efficacy, low cost, availability of liquid and parenteral formulations, ability to treat sleep disturbance, dosing flexibility, and universal availability, even for those patients on Medicaid or in managed care plans with restrictive formularies. Because of its sedative properties, amitriptyline should be given as a bedtime dose starting at 10 to 25 mg. The drug can be titrated upward as side effects allow in 10- to 25-mg doses, with care being to identify the increases in side effects as the dose is raised. In particular, orthostatic hypotension can be insidious in onset as the dose of the drug is raised and may lead to falls at night when the patient gets up to use the bathroom. If analgesia is not achieved by the time the dose is raised to 150 mg, the patient should be switched to a different antidepressant compound, preferably from another class of drugs, or another adjuvant analgesic can be added, such as gabapentin if appropriate. If the patient has partial relief of pain, this drug can be carefully titrated upward to a single bedtime dose of 300 mg.

DESIPRAMINE (NORPRAMIN) AND NORTRIPTYLINE (PAMELOR)

Both desipramine and nortriptyline are good choices for initial TCA therapy if sedation is not desired or if the sedative side effects of amitriptyline are too great (**Fig. 123.3**).[9,10] Given as a morning dose, these drugs are good first choices in those patients suffering from pain who have complained of lack of energy or who are at risk for the orthostatic side effects of amitriptyline (e.g., patients taking warfarin [Coumadin]). Dosed at 10 to 25 mg every morning and titrated upward to a maximum dose of 150 mg, pain relief is usually noted at doses of 50 to 75 mg after 2 to 3 weeks of therapy, although improvement in sleep may occur much sooner. These drugs should be used cautiously in patients with cardiac arrhythmia and in those prone to psychic activation or agitation. Such psychic activation or agitation may be exacerbated by the concomitant administration of steroids (e.g., epidural steroid injections).

TRAZODONE (DESERYL)

Although the unique side effect of priapism may limit the use of this drug in men, trazodone has the sedating characteristic of amitriptyline, which is desirable in those patients suffering from sleep disturbance as part of their pain symptoms, without the cardiac, anticholinergic, and orthostatic side effects (see Fig. 123.2).[11] The drug should be started at 75 mg at bedtime and titrated upward to 300 mg as side effects allow. Pain relief usually occurs at a dose range of 150 to 200 mg.

Selective Serotonin Reuptake Inhibitors

Although generally less efficacious than the TCAs or heterocyclic antidepressants in the treatment of pain, the SSRIs have proven efficacy in this clinical setting. Their lack of side effects relative to the TCAs makes the SSRIs a good choice for those patients with pain who cannot or will not tolerate the side effects of the TCAs, albeit at greater monetary cost.[12]

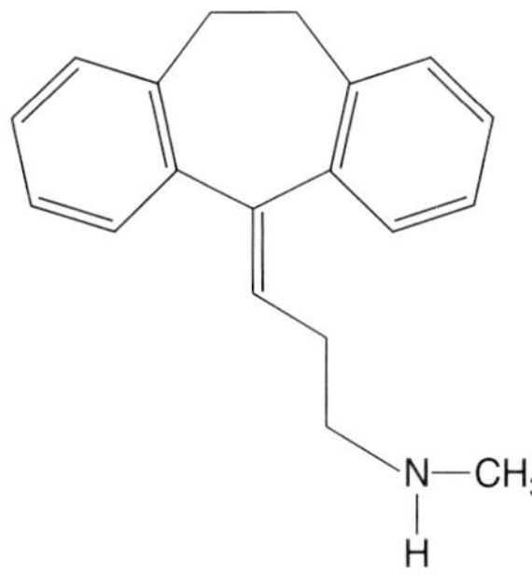

Fig. 123.3 **The chemical structure of nortriptyline.**

Mechanism of Action

The SSRIs selectively block the reuptake of serotonin by blocking the sodium/potassium adenosine triphosphate pump. The result is an increased level of serotonin at the synaptic cleft. The SSRIs also affect other serotonin receptors, most notably in the gut, a characteristic that probably accounts for the propensity of these drugs to cause gastrointestinal side effects, especially during initiation of therapy.

Absorption and Metabolism

The SSRIs are well absorbed orally. This class of drugs undergoes rapid first-pass hepatic metabolism and may compete with other drugs for these enzymes. The result is an increase in blood levels of warfarin (Coumadin) and the benzodiazepines, among others. These drugs have relatively long serum elimination half-lives, and given that many of the SSRIs have active metabolites, side effects may persist for a long time after this class of drugs is discontinued. The SSRIs are excreted in the urine and feces.

Side Effects

As mentioned, the SSRI interaction with the serotonin receptors of the gut may result in the side effects of cramping, nausea, and diarrhea, especially during the initial implementation of therapy. These symptoms are usually self-limited and actually decrease as the gut accommodates to the increased serotoninergic milieu. In addition to the gastrointestinal side effects associated with the SSRIs, side effects associated with central nervous system activation, including tremors, insomnia, and physic activation can limit the use of these drugs, as can the increased incidence of sexual side effects relative to the TCAs. These sexual side effects include alterations in libido, erectile and orgasmic difficulties, ejaculatory delay, and impotence. The allegation that the SSRI fluoxetine may cause increased suicidal ideation has not appeared to be a problem with the use of this drug as an analgesic, although the relative lack of efficacy of fluoxetine for this purpose when compared with the TCAs has. The SSRIs can interact with the MAOIs to produce a potentially life-threatening constellation of symptoms known as the *central serotonergic syndrome*. The central serotonergic syndrome is characterized by hypertension, fever, myoclonus, tachycardia, and seizures. In extreme instances, cardiovascular collapse and death may occur.[13] For this reason, these classes of drugs should never be used together, and a long, drug-free period of at least 10 half-lives should be implemented when stopping the SSRI and starting the MAOIs. This class of drugs also appears to interact with St. John's wort, and hypertensive crises have been reported when the drugs are taken together.

Abuse Potential and Side Effects on Withdrawal of the Drug

Like the TCAs, the SSRIs do not appear to interact significantly with the opioid, benzodiazepine, γ-aminobutyric acid, or beta-adrenergic receptors. No clinical evidence of addiction occurs when these drugs are discontinued, but some drugs in this class have a propensity to cause various symptoms including lack of energy and decreased serotoninergic activity, as manifested by constipation. These side effects can be avoided by slowly tapering the SSRI over 10 to 14 days.

Overdosage

In general, overdosage with the SSRIs is much less serious than is overdosage with the TCAs.[14] Remarkably few fatal overdoses have been reported in the literature or to the US Food and Drug Administration involving ingestion only of an SSRI. Moderate overdoses of up to 30 times the daily dose are associated with minor or no symptoms, whereas ingestions of greater amounts typically result in drowsiness, tremor, nausea, gastrointestinal disturbances, and vomiting. At very high doses of greater than 75 times the common daily dose, the more serious adverse events, including seizures, electrocardiogram changes, and decreased consciousness may occur. SSRI overdoses in combination with alcohol or other drugs are associated with increased toxicity, and almost all fatalities involving SSRIs have involved co-ingestion of other substances.

Some Common Selective Serotonin Reuptake Inhibitors

FLUOXETINE (PROZAC, SERAFEM)

Fluoxetine is available in capsule, tablet, and liquid forms, which are usually taken once a day in the morning or twice a day, in the morning and at noon. In addition, a fluoxetine delayed-relayed capsule is usually taken once a week (**Fig. 123.4**). Because the side effect profile is minimal, it is usually possible to start this drug at the lower range of the doses thought to provide analgesia 20 mg, and titrate upward to 60 mg as side effects allow and efficacy demands. The onset of analgesic action of fluoxetine usually occurs within 2 to 3 weeks.[15]

PAROXETINE (PAXIL)

Well tolerated by most patients, paroxetine is another reasonable choice for patients who do not tolerate the TCAs. This drug comes in both an immediate-release form and a controlled-release form. It is taken either once a day or twice a day in the morning and at noon, to minimize the side effects of tremors or irritability. Anecdotal reports indicate that paroxetine may have a lower incidence of ejaculatory side effects when compared with fluoxetine. Paroxetine should be started at a dose of 20 mg and titrated upward to 40 mg as side effects allow and efficacy dictates.

SERTRALINE (ZOLOFT)

Sertraline is available as an immediate-release tablet or capsule, as well as an oral liquid concentrate. Generally well tolerated, sertraline is take once a day as a morning dose starting at 50 mg and titrated upward to 200 mg as side effects and efficacy allow.[16] This drug may have efficacy for those patients suffering from pain who also exhibit obsessive-compulsive tendencies.

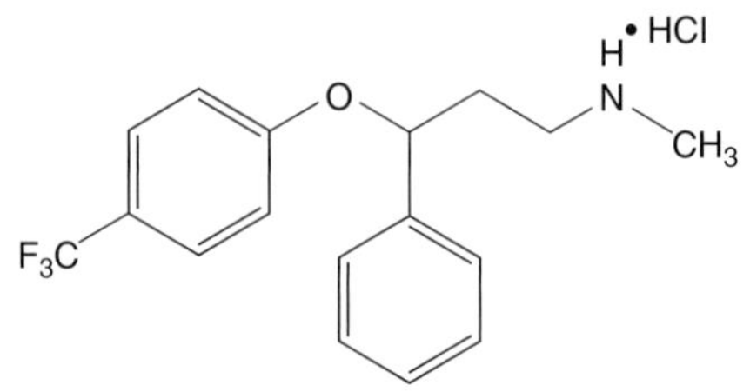

Fig. 123.4 **The chemical structure of fluoxetine.**

Serotonin and Noradrenergic Reuptake Inhibitors
Venlafaxine (Effexor)

Venlafaxine was shown to be useful as an analgesic in controlled clinical trials.[17,18] Its structure differs from that of any of the other clinically useful antidepressant compounds (**Fig. 123.5**). With a better side effect profile than the SSRIs, this drug is a good starting point for those patients who seem to have side effects with most adjuvant analgesics. Like amitriptyline, venlafaxine affects both serotonin and norepinephrine, a feature that theoretically should make it more efficacious for pain than the SSRIs. It remains to be seen whether widespread clinical use will bear out this premise. A reasonable starting dose for pain is 25 mg of venlafaxine every 12 hours, with the dose increased by 25 mg every week as side effects allow and efficacy dictates.

Noradrenergic Reuptake Inhibitors
Reboxetine (Edronax)

The newest class of antidepressants, the NaRIs are among the least studied of the antidepressant compounds in the role of analgesics.[19,20] Given that reboxetine acts primarily on the noradrenergic system, theoretically it is most useful for those patients with pain who are also suffering from significant anergia and depression and who cannot tolerate desipramine or nortriptyline (**Fig. 123.6**). Not yet unavailable in the United States but available in more than 50 countries, reboxetine is given as a 4-mg twice-daily dose titrated upward by 1 mg each week to 10 mg as side effects allow and efficacy dictates. Anecdotal reports indicate that painful ejaculation can occur at higher doses of this drug.

Monoamine Oxidase Inhibitors

Isoniazid and its derivative iproniazid were introduced in 1951 as pharmacologic treatments for tuberculosis. Investigators found that iproniazid inhibited the enzyme MAO and that patients with tuberculosis who were treated with this drug experienced an elevation of mood. This discovery, along with the introduction of the phenothiazines, ushered in the modern era of the pharmacologic treatment of psychiatric disorders. Widespread experience with this class of drugs led to an understanding that these drugs were also useful in patients suffering from chronic pain, most notably intractable headache, as well as the realization that their side effect profile limited their clinical utility.[21] The introduction of the TCAs in the early 1960s led to the almost complete abandonment of the MAOIs, except in the most severely disturbed psychiatric patients and a few recidivist patients with headache. Through the almost single-handed efforts of Diamond et al at the Diamond Headache Clinic in Chicago, the efficacy and the safety of the MAOIs in combination with the TCAs in the treatment of intractable headache were firmly established.

The MAOIs are a heterogeneous group of drugs that work by blocking the oxidative deamination of the biogenic amines at the nerve synapse.[22] This process leads to the release of a larger than normal amount of these amines by the synapse when an action potential is present. The MAOIs are well absorbed by mouth and are metabolized in the liver, primarily by acetylation. Some potential for liver damage from this class of drugs exists, and appropriate monitoring of liver function tests should be part of the patient's overall treatment plan.[23] In spite of the efficacy of the MAOIs in the treatment of intractable pain, the unpredictable and sometimes severe side effects of this class of drugs limit their use in pain management to patients in whom other, less problematic treatments have failed and who are willing and able to adhere strictly to the dietary and medication restrictions required with these drugs. These restrictions are extremely important because many drugs and foods can potentiate the adrenergic and serotonergic effects of MAOIs (**Tables 123.3** and **123.4**).[24]

Commonly used MAOIs include phenelzine, isocarboxazid, and tranylcypromine, which are nonselective MAOIs. Phenelzine is the most commonly used MAOI in pain

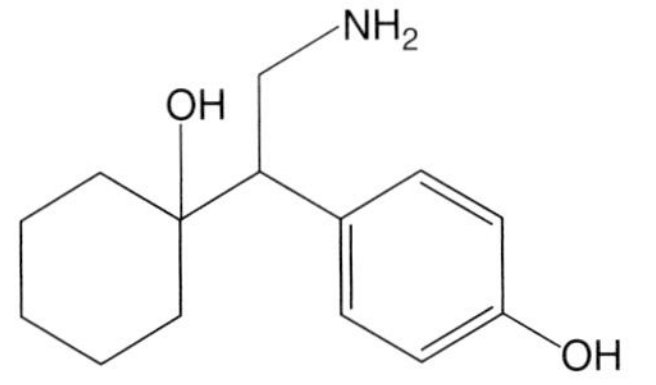

Fig. 123.5 **The chemical structure of venlafaxine.**

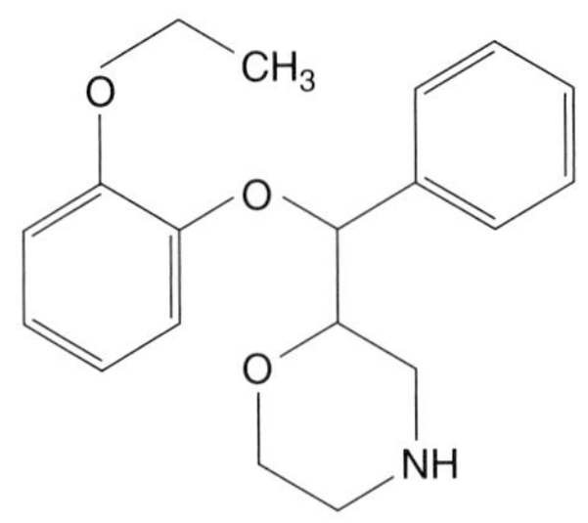

Fig. 123.6 **The chemical structure of reboxetine.**

Table 123.3 Dietary Restrictions When Taking Monoamine Oxidase Inhibitors

Aged food or meat
Overripe fruit
Fermented food
Chicken liver
Soy sauce
Smoked or pickled meat, poultry, or fish
Cold cuts, including bologna, pepperoni, salami, summer sausage
Alcoholic beverages (especially Chianti, sherry, liqueurs, and beer)
Alcohol-free or reduced-alcohol beer or wine
Anchovies
Caviar
Cheeses (especially strong or aged varieties)
Figs
Raisins, bananas
Meat prepared with tenderizers
Meat extracts

Table 123.4 Drug Interactions with Monoamine Oxidase Inhibitors

Allergy medications (including nose drops or sprays)
Amantadine (Symmetrel)
Antihistamines (e.g., Actifed DM, Benadryl, Benylin, Chlor-Trimeton, Compoz)
Antipsychotics
Appetite suppressants
Asthma drugs
Blood pressure medication
Buclizine
Bupropion (Wellbutrin)
Buspirone (BuSpar)
Carbamazepine (Tegretol)
Cocaine
Cold medications
Cyclizine (Marezine)
Cyclobenzaprine (Flexeril)
Dextromethorphan
Disopyramide (Norpace)
Flavoxate (Urispas)
Fluoxetine (Prozac) and other SSRIs
Insulin (MAOIs may change amount of insulin needed)
Ipratropium (Atrovent)
Levodopa (Dopar, Larodopa)
Maprotiline (Ludiomil)
Meclizine (Antivert)
Meperidine (Demerol; deaths have occurred when combining MAOIs and a single dose of meperidine)
Methylphenidate (Ritalin)
Other MAOIs (e.g., Norflex)
Oxybutynin (Ditropan)
Procainamide (Pronestyl)
Promethazine (Phenergan)
Quinidine (Quinidex)
Sinus medication
Tricyclic antidepressants
Tryptophan

MAOIs, monoamine oxidase inhibitors; SSRIs, selective serotonin reuptake inhibitors.

management (**Fig. 123.7**).[25] Phenelzine is started at an initial morning dose of 15 mg. The dose may be increased by 15 mg per week, with the second dose given at noon as side effects allow and as efficacy dictates to a total dose of 60 mg. If the patient has no relief of pain at this point, amitriptyline at a dose of 10 mg should be added, with careful monitoring for side effects. Phenelzine should not be abruptly discontinued; the patient should be cautioned about this, and the drug should be tapered over a 2- to 3-week period.[26]

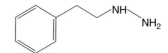

Fig. 123.7 **The chemical structure of phenelzine.**

Practical Considerations for Clinical Use of Antidepressants as Analgesics

As many ways exist to use antidepressants to treat pain as there are antidepressant drugs. The following is an approach that has proved beneficial in the management of patients with various painful conditions in numerous clinical settings.

The first step in the practical implementation of antidepressant treatment for pain is to explain to the patient that pain, not depression, is being treated as the primary symptom. Patients have an unfortunate tendency to attribute motive to the act of prescribing antidepressants, because they may feel that they are being labeled as crazy or being told that "it's all just in your head." Referring to the drugs as "tricyclic analgesics" and providing patient information sheets that reflect this nomenclature will also help. Beware that efforts by pharmacies to provide written patient information materials with each prescription may undermine the best of intentions. When the physician is treating patients who questions his or her prescribing motive, a call to the pharmacist to enlist his or her help in patient education is beneficial.

The second step in the practical implementation of antidepressant treatment for pain is to explain to the patient that the medication will not work immediately, but it will take a period of weeks for the patient to experience meaningful pain relief. The physician should explain that treatment is starting at a low dose and that an increased dosage may be needed in the future. This helps alleviate concerns that the patient is taking "too much medicine." Again, the pharmacist can be of great help in this setting.

The third step is to educate the patient with regard to normalizing sleep when treating pain. The physician should reinforce the salutary effects of normalization of the patient's sleep cycle as a benefit of most of the drugs discussed earlier. The physician should also let the patient know that this drug is not a "sleeping pill" but actually will help treat the sleep disturbance and, most importantly, the pain.

The fourth step is to discuss side effects without setting the stage for medication noncompliance. For the most part, these drugs are well tolerated because the chosen drug is started at the lower range of the dosage spectrum, and increases in dosage are done slowly. Supportive measures for early side effects such as eye drops for xerophthalmia or cough drops for xerostomia can improve compliance. Informing the patient that the "hangover" feeling that may be experienced early on will soon subside may be helpful, too.

The final step is to remain positive regarding the potential for the patient to obtain pain relief. Let the patient know that changes in dosing or even medication may occur and is a routine part of treating pain. Most importantly, the message should be one of hope, not negativity.

References

Full references for this chapter can be found on www.expertconsult.com.

Anticonvulsants

Steven D. Waldman and Corey W. Waldman

It is not surprising that with the introduction of each new anticonvulsant into clinical practice, the drug has been tried as a treatment for neuropathic pain, albeit with varying degrees of success. This chapter reviews the anticonvulsant compounds that have proven efficacy in the treatment of various painful conditions and provides the clinician with a practical step-by-step guide for their use.

What is striking about the anticonvulsants used to treat pain is their heterogenicity. Unlike the antidepressants, which can readily be grouped into classes based on their chemical structure (e.g., the tricyclic antidepressants) or their mechanism of action (e.g., the selective serotonin reuptake inhibitors), the anticonvulsants defy simple classification. However, some generalizations can be made. The anticonvulsants useful in the treatment of pain can be placed into two broad categories (**Table 124.1**). Category 1 includes those drugs whose primary mechanism of action is to modulate the function of the voltage-dependent sodium channels, whereas category 2 drugs have mechanisms other than modulation of the sodium channel.

Category 1 Anticonvulsants

Category 1 anticonvulsants modulate the voltage-dependent sodium channels. Although the exact mechanism of neuropathic pain has not been fully explained, some generalizations can be made that may help to describe how the anticonvulsants exert their analgesic effect in this clinical setting. If one begins with an assumption that neuropathic pain is the result of abnormal nerve firing, it is reasonable to assume that anything that modulates this abnormal nerve firing downward should decrease the pain, regardless of the drug's exact mechanism of action.

Conceptually, the category 1 anticonvulsant drugs exert their pain-relieving effect by raising the firing threshold required to open the sodium channel and allow the nerve to reach its action potential and fire (**Fig. 124.1**).[1] Although overly simplistic and ignoring the role of pain modulation at the spinal cord and central levels, the idea that it requires more subthreshold stimuli to elicit an action potential in the presence of Category 1 anticonvulsants and the concept of a dose-response curve that is roughly linear fit with our overall clinical observations in this setting, given the diverse nature of pain syndromes treated with the anticonvulsant drugs. Again, to attribute a solely peripheral mechanism of action to the anticonvulsants is probably incorrect given that all the drugs discussed subsequently have the ability to cross the blood-brain barrier and that many of the drugs exert other pharmacologic actions at both the peripheral and higher levels (e.g., the ability of phenytoin to modulate the calcium and potassium channels).

Phenytoin (Dilantin)

The first modern anticonvulsant drug used to treat neuropathic pain, phenytoin has seen extensive use as an adjuvant analgesic since the 1950s, with mixed results (**Fig. 124.2**). Reasonably well absorbed after oral administration, phenytoin is extensively protein bound, with only approximately 10% existing in its free state. The drug is metabolized by the liver, and only a small amount is excreted in the urine. Phenytoin is available in a large array of formulations including immediate-release and sustained-release oral products in a variety of doses, as well as liquid solutions and an injectable preparation. In clinical dosage ranges, it is relatively nonsedating and reasonably well tolerated. Side effects of phenytoin are summarized in **Table 124.2** and include nystagmus, behavioral changes, peripheral neuropathy, gingival hyperplasia (**Fig. 124.3**), gastrointestinal disturbance, osteomalacia, rash, Stevens-Johnson syndrome, liver dysfunction, blood dyscrasias, and a unique side effect of pseudolymphoma that is clinically difficult to distinguish from Hodgkin's disease. Because phenytoin is so highly protein bound, any drugs that compete with the binding sites on serum albumin have the potential to increase the free fraction of the drug and can result in toxicity.

To treat neuropathic pain with phenytoin, a dose of 100 mg at bedtime is a reasonable starting point. After 1 week, an additional 100-mg morning dose may be added. If the patient is not experiencing limiting side effects, an additional 100-mg noontime dose may be added. At this point, a complete blood count and liver function tests should be performed. If the patient is tolerating the 300-mg dosing regimen and has experienced partial pain relief, the drug may be titrated upward by 30 mg per week to a maximum dose of 400 mg as side effects allow and efficacy dictates. If at the 300-mg dose the patient is experiencing no diminution of pain, it may be reasonable to switch to another anticonvulsant. Like other anticonvulsants, this drug should be discontinued slowly to avoid any rebound effect.

Carbamazepine (Tegretol)

Particularly useful in the treatment of lancinating and neuritic pain syndromes such as trigeminal neuralgia, carbamazepine has proven efficacy in the treatment of numerous neuropathic pain syndromes including diabetic polyneuropathy, trigeminal neuralgia, glossopharyngeal neuralgia, postherpetic neuralgia, and central pain states (**Fig. 124.4**).[2-4] Many anecdotal reports

support the efficacy of carbamazepine in certain other painful conditions including neuropathic pain related to human immunodeficiency virus (HIV) infection or chemotherapy. Chemically related to the tricyclic antidepressants, carbamazepine is highly protein bound and is metabolized in the liver. After glucuronidation, it is excreted in the urine. As with phenytoin, interaction with other drugs that are protein bound, such as isoniazid and warfarin (Coumadin), can affect free fraction concentrations and lead to toxicity. In addition to raising the firing threshold of the

Fig. 124.2 **Chemical structure of phenytoin.**

Table 124.1 Classification of Anticonvulsants Based on Their Mechanism of Action

CATEGORY 1 ANTICONVULSANTS (DRUGS THAT MODULATE VOLTAGE-DEPENDENT SODIUM CHANNELS)
Phenytoin
Carbamazepine
Lamotrigine
Topiramate
CATEGORY 2 ANTICONVULSANTS (DRUGS WHOSE PRIMARY MECHANISM OF ACTION IS UNRELATED TO MODULATION OF THE VOLTAGE-DEPENDENT SODIUM CHANNEL)
Gabapentin
Tiagabine
Valproic acid
Pregabalin

Table 124.2 Side Effects Associated with Phenytoin

Nystagmus
Behavioral changes
Peripheral neuropathy
Gingival hyperplasia
Gastrointestinal disturbance
Osteomalacia
Rash
Stevens-Johnson syndrome
Liver dysfunction
Blood dyscrasias
Pseudolymphoma

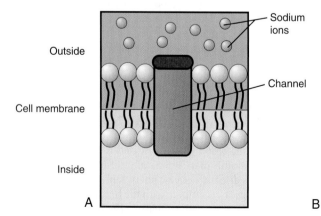
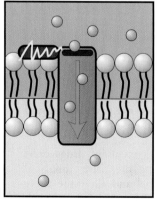
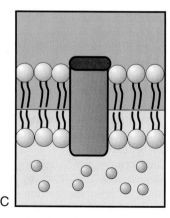

Fig. 124.1 **Modulation of voltage-gated sodium channels by category 1 anticonvulsants.** A, Voltage-gated sodium channel closed. B, Depolarization opens the voltage-gated sodium channel. C, Sodium ions inside the cell result in a positive change within the cell, and the "gate" closes.

voltage-dependent sodium channel, carbamazepine suppresses norepinephrine reuptake and, in all likelihood, exerts some of its actions centrally, given it tendency to cause sedation at the higher end of the therapeutic dosage range.

In addition to sedation, carbamazepine can cause various central nervous system (CNS) side effects including vertigo, ataxia, diplopia, dizziness, and blurred vision. Gastrointestinal side effects and rash may occur, but the most worrisome side effect of carbamazepine is its potential to cause aplastic anemia. This side effect can generally be avoided if careful and systematic monitoring of hematologic parameters is followed in *all* patients considered for treatment with this drug. **Table 124.3** provides a recommended monitoring protocol for patients who are to receive carbamazepine. Failure to monitor the carbamazepine-treated patient scrupulously can have fatal consequences. This drug should be used with extreme caution in those patients suffering from neuropathic pain who have previously undergone chemotherapy or radiation therapy for malignant disease, even if their hematologic parameters have returned to normal. These patients are extremely sensitive to the hematologic side effects of carbamazepine.

Given the reasonably high incidence of CNS side effects associated with carbamazepine therapy, this drug should be started at a low nighttime dose of 100 mg. The drug may then be increased in 100-mg increments, with the drug given on a dosing schedule of four times a day to a maximum dose of 1200 mg as side effects allow and efficacy dictates. In patients with pain emergencies such as intractable trigeminal neuralgia that is limiting the patient's ability to maintain adequate nutrition and hydration, hospitalization is recommended so more rapid upward titration may be safely accomplished. Regardless of the speed at which the drug is titrated upward, the monitoring

protocol outlined in Table 124.3 must be followed to avoid disaster. Like all other anticonvulsants, this drug should be discontinued slowly to avoid any rebound effect.

Lamotrigine (Lamictal)

Lamotrigine is another anticonvulsant whose mechanism of action involves modulation of the voltage-dependent sodium channel (**Fig. 124.5**). Useful in the treatment of various neuropathic pain states including HIV-induced polyneuropathy, trigeminal neuralgia, and poststroke pain, lamotrigine is worth a try in those patients who have lancinating or sharp neuropathic pain that has not responded to carbamazepine or in those patients in whom carbamazepine is contraindicated.[5-7] Lamotrigine is rapidly and completely absorbed following oral administration, and it reaches peak plasma concentrations (t_{max}) 1.4 to 4.8 hours after administration. When it is administered with food, the rate of absorption is slightly reduced, but the extent remains unchanged. Lamotrigine is approximately 55% bound to human plasma proteins. Unlike many of the other anticonvulsants, protein binding is unaffected by therapeutic concentrations of phenytoin, phenobarbital, or valproic acid, although valproic acid significantly increases the plasma half-life of lamotrigine. Therefore, the dose should be decreased with the concurrent use of these drugs. Lamotrigine is metabolized predominantly in the liver by glucuronic acid conjugation. The major metabolite is an inactive 2-H-glucuronide conjugate that can be hydrolyzed by beta-glucuronidase. Approximately 70% of an oral lamotrigine dose is recovered in urine as this drug metabolizes.

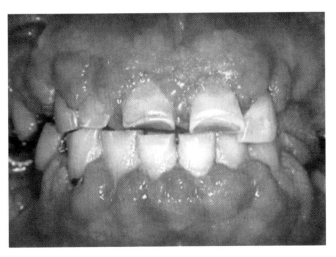

Fig. 124.3 **Gingival hyperplasia as a side effect of phenytoin.**

Table 124.3 Monitoring Protocol for Carbamazepine Use
1. Obtain baseline CBC, chemistry profile including creatinine and liver function tests, and urinalysis before the first dose of carbamazepine.
2. Repeat CBC and chemistry profile after 1 week of therapy.
3. Repeat CBC and chemistry profile after the second week of therapy.
4. Repeat CBC and chemistry profile after the fourth week of therapy.
5. Repeat CBC and chemistry profile after the sixth week of therapy.
6. Repeat CBC after the eighth week of therapy and every 2 months thereafter.
7. Stop carbamazepine immediately at the first sign of hematologic or liver function abnormalities.

CBC, complete blood count.

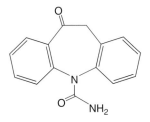

Fig. 124.4 **Chemical structure of carbamazepine.**

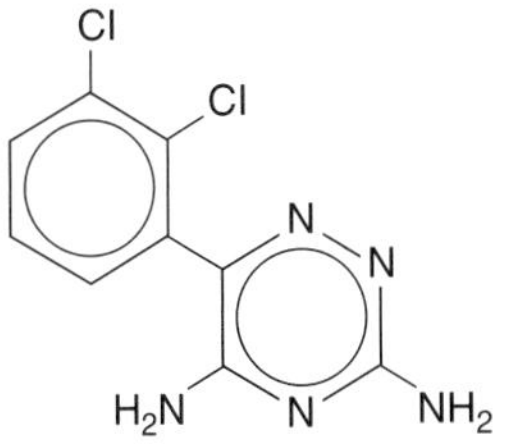

Fig. 124.5 **Chemical structure of lamotrigine.**

Side effects of lamotrigine include CNS side effects similar to those of carbamazepine, although less severe, as well as occasional gastrointestinal upset and liver function test abnormalities. Although free of the hematologic side effects associated with carbamazepine, lamotrigine has 10% of significant dermatologic side effects ranging from rash to fatal Stevens-Johnson syndrome. Severe dermatologic side effects associated with lamotrigine occur with great enough frequency that they must be carefully looked for and the drug discontinued immediately at the first sign of even the slightest rash or skin irritation. Most dermatologic side effects of lamotrigine occur within the first week of therapy. No monitoring of hematologic parameters is required with this drug.

Lamotrigine is supplied in a chewable tablet and an oral tablet formulation in a variety of dosage strengths, thus making titration of the drug reasonably easy. In treating patients suffering from neuropathic pain with lamotrigine, a reasonable starting dose is 25 mg at bedtime, with upward titration in 25-mg increments using a twice-daily dosing schedule to a maximum dose of 400 mg as side effects allow and efficacy dictates. Like other anticonvulsants, this drug should be discontinued slowly to avoid any rebound effect.

Topiramate (Topamax)

With demonstrated efficacy in the treatment of pain associated with diabetic polyneuropathy, topiramate is a reasonable next choice for those patients with neuropathic pain who have not responded to the tricyclic antidepressants, either alone or in combination with other anticonvulsants (**Fig. 124.6**).[8,9] Topiramate's mechanism of action is thought to be related to its ability to modulate the voltage-dependent sodium channel and, in part, to its ability to inhibit carbonic anhydrase. Topiramate is well absorbed orally, and its absorption is unaffected by food. Topiramate is not extensively metabolized, and approximately 70% is primarily eliminated unchanged in the urine. Available in tablet and sprinkle formulations, topiramate is dispensed in various of doses, thus making titration easy. A reasonable starting dose of topiramate is 25 mg at bedtime. The dosage is then increased in weekly intervals by 25 mg with a twice-daily dosing schedule to a maximum dose of 400 mg as side effects allow and efficacy dictates. CNS side effects similar to carbamazepine occur in approximately 15% of patients taking topiramate. Like other anticonvulsants, this drug should be discontinued slowly to avoid any rebound effect.

Category 2 Anticonvulsants

Category 2 anticonvulsants are drugs whose primary mechanism of action is unrelated to modulation of the voltage-dependent sodium channel. They include gabapentin, tiagabine, valproic acid, and pregabalin.

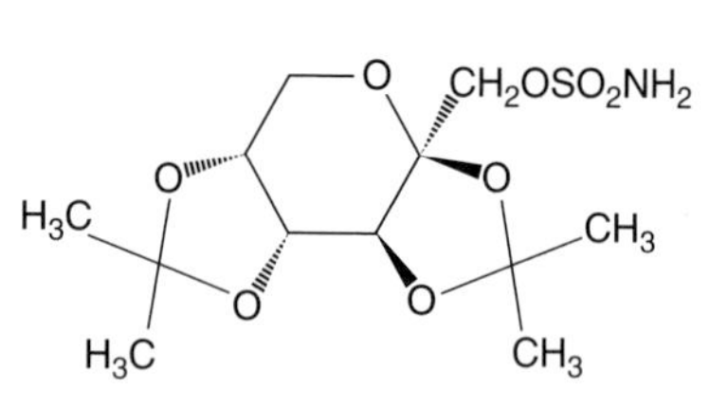

Fig. 124.6 **Chemical structure of topiramate.**

Gabapentin (Neurontin)

One of the most extensively used anticonvulsants in the management of neuropathic pain, gabapentin has proven efficacy in the management of diabetic polyneuropathy, postherpetic neuralgia, phantom limb pain, and pain following spinal cord injury (**Fig. 124.7**).[10–13] An analogue of γ-aminobutyric acid (GABA), gabapentin is thought to exert its analgesic effect by modulating high-voltage calcium channels as well as interacting at the N-methyl-D-aspartate (NMDA) receptors. Gabapentin is generally well tolerated. The drug's oral absorption is not dose dependent in that as the oral dose increases, the proportion that is absorbed decreases. Less than 3% of orally administered gabapentin is protein bound, with negligible drug metabolism. The drug is excreted unchanged in the urine. Treatment with gabapentin is begun with a 100-mg bedtime dose and is then increased on a weekly basis by 100-mg increments using a dosing schedule of four times a day. Gabapentin can be increased to a maximum dose of 3600 mg as side effects allow and efficacy dictates. CNS side effects are similar to those of the other anticonvulsants, but they are generally milder. Occasional gastrointestinal side effects including nausea and gastrointestinal upset can occur. Like other anticonvulsants, this drug should be discontinued slowly to avoid any rebound effect.

Tiagabine (Gabitril)

Anecdotal reports have suggested that tiagabine may be efficacious in the treatment of neuropathic pain (**Fig. 124.8**).[14] Tiagabine blocks *GABA uptake* into *presynaptic* neurons and permits more *GABA* to be available for *receptor* binding on the surfaces of postsynaptic cells. Some investigators have suggested that tiagabine is especially effective in preventing the wind-up phenomenon often seen in many neuropathic pain states. Although tiagabine is well absorbed orally, fatty food may decrease absorption and should be avoided when taking the drug. Like phenytoin, tiagabine is highly protein bound, and the possibility for drug-drug interactions

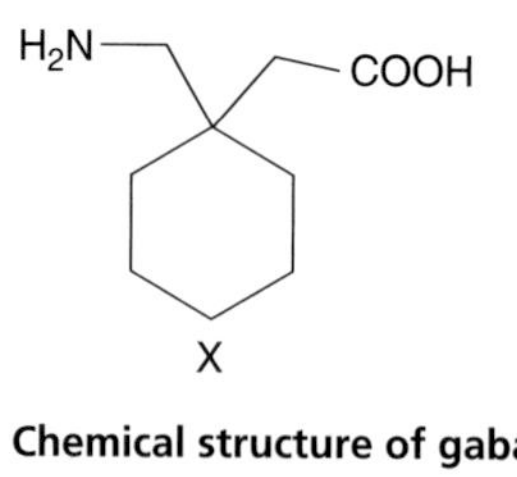

Fig. 124.7 **Chemical structure of gabapentin.**

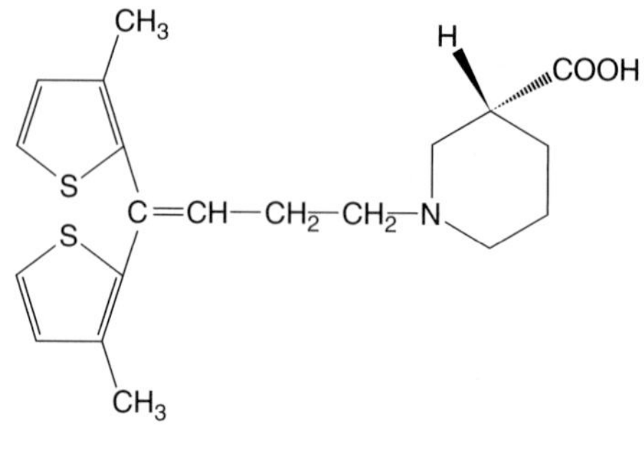

Fig. 124.8 **Chemical structure of tiagabine.**

with other highly protein-bound drugs exists. Tiagabine is partially metabolized in the liver and is excreted in the feces and urine. Therapy with tiagabine should begin with a 4-mg daily dose, with the dose increased in weekly intervals by 4 mg to a maximum dose of 56 mg as side effects allow and efficacy dictates. Side effects of tiagabine include dizziness, sedation, difficulty thinking, and gastrointestinal intolerance. Reports of painful urination and hematuria have also been associated with the use of tiagabine. Like other anticonvulsants, this drug should be discontinued slowly to avoid any rebound effect.

Divalproex Sodium (Depakote)

Divalproex sodium, which is metabolized to valproic acid in the gastrointestinal tract, has been used to treat various neuropathic pain syndromes.[15] Although the mechanism of action has not yet been established, investigators have suggested that divalproex sodium's activity is related to its ability to increase levels of GABA. Valproic acid is well absorbed orally and is rapidly distributed throughout the body. More than 90% of the drug is strongly bound to human plasma proteins, thus giving the potential for drug-drug interactions with other drugs that are highly protein bound. Divalproex sodium is metabolized in the liver and is excreted in the urine. An initial dose of 250 mg twice daily for a period of 7 to 10 days represents a reasonable starting dose. The dose may be slowly increased to a maximum of 250 mg four times daily. CNS side effects are similar to those observed with tiagabine. Fatal hepatic side effects have been reported with this drug, and patients started on divalproex sodium require careful monitoring of liver function studies throughout therapy. Like other anticonvulsants, this drug should be discontinued slowly to avoid any rebound effect.

Pregabalin (Lyrica)

Like gabapentin, pregabalin (**Fig. 124.9**) acts by binding at the alpha$_2$delta subunit of the voltage-dependent calcium

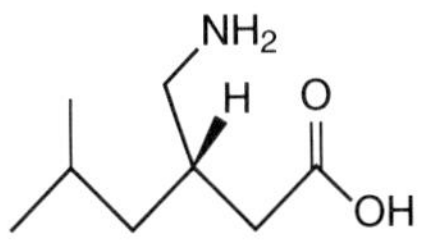

Fig. 124.9 **Chemical structure of pregabalin.**

channel in the CNS and thus reducing the influx of calcium into the nerve endings.[16] Pregabalin is believed to have a much higher affinity for the alpha$_2$delta subunit binding sites when compared with gabapentin, and this feature theoretically should make pregabalin a more effective drug in the treatment of pain.[17] Not all clinicians believe that this premise has been borne out in clinical practice. Pregabalin increases intraneuronal GABA by causing a dose-dependent increase in glutamic acid decarboxylase. Glutamic acid decarboxylase is responsible for converting glutamate into GABA. Pregabalin is well absorbed orally, and food decreases absorption. The drug is excreted unchanged by the kidneys. Drowsiness and dizziness occur in significant numbers of patients who are started on pregabalin, and these effects appear to be dose dependent when initiating therapy. Like other anticonvulsants, this drug should be discontinued slowly to avoid any rebound effect. Treatment with pregabalin is begun at a dose of 150 mg/day given in two or three divided doses, and titrated up to 300 mg/day over a 1 to 2 weeks as side effects and pain relief dictate. Side effects are for the most part dose dependent. Many clinicians believe that patients experience a faster onset of pain relief with pregabalin when compared with gabapentin.[18]

Conclusion

The anticonvulsant compounds have demonstrable efficacy in the treatment of various neuropathic pain syndromes. Much like with the antidepressants, the art of using these drugs correctly is paramount if high levels of patient compliance and satisfaction are to be achieved and potentially serious side effects are to be avoided. The admonition to "start low and go slow" is quite apt when contemplating starting a patient on an anticonvulsant drug to treat neuropathic pain. Clear and frequent communication with the patient to emphasize the "trial and error" nature of the use of this class of drugs is mandatory, to avoid noncompliance. Maintaining a positive and hopeful attitude toward the probability of success often enhances the therapeutic outcome for the patient in this challenging clinical setting.

References

Full references for this chapter can be found on www.expertconsult.com.

Centrally Acting Skeletal Muscle Relaxants and Associated Drugs

Howard J. Waldman, Steven D. Waldman, and Katherine A. Kidder

Numerous painful conditions have associated muscle spasm. These are most frequently musculoskeletal disorders (e.g., muscle strain) or central nervous system (CNS) disorders associated with spasticity. Various therapeutic interventions, including pharmacologic agents, have been used in an attempt to reduce or obliterate muscle spasm in the belief that this will secondarily alleviate pain and improve function.[1–4]

Although there is controversy regarding the efficacy of this class of drug, centrally acting skeletal muscle relaxants (SMRs) are the most frequently prescribed drugs for the treatment of muscle spasm (**Table 125.1**).[5] Studies have suggested that these drugs are effective, have tolerable side effects, and can be an adjunct in the treatment of painful musculoskeletal conditions with associated muscle spasm.[5–8] Their use is limited by somnolence[9–13] and the potential for abuse and dependency.[14–17] The SMRs should not be confused with peripherally acting SMRs (e.g., curare and pancuronium), which block neuromuscular junction function and are generally confined to use in surgical anesthesia.

Mechanism of Action

The exact mode of action of the SMRs is not known. The SMRs appear to depress polysynaptic reflexes preferentially. At higher dosages, the SMRs may influence monosynaptic reflexes. In animal studies, these drugs appear to produce their muscle relaxation effects by inhibiting interneuronal activity and blocking polysynaptic neurons in the spinal cord and descending reticular formation in the brain.[5,10,12] In humans, the SMRs do not appear to relax skeletal muscle directly. Rather, they may produce their effects through sedation, with resultant depression of neuronal activity at therapeutic doses.[6,9,12,18]

Pharmacokinetics

The SMRs are generally well absorbed after oral ingestion. They have a rapid onset of action, generally within 1 hour. Some SMRs may be administered parenterally, and this route yields a more rapid onset of action. The drugs undergo biotransformation in the liver and are excreted primarily in the urine as metabolites. Significant variability exists among individual drugs, their plasma half-lives, and their duration of action (**Table 125.2**).[10–13]

Clinical Efficacy

Numerous clinical trials of SMRs have been conducted. Unfortunately, study design deficiencies have made interpretation of results and comparisons among studies difficult. These deficiencies include ill-defined patient selection criteria, noncomparable musculoskeletal disorders studied, variability of disease severity and duration, and subjective assessment of patients' responses to therapy.[5,18–24] Despite these difficulties, certain conclusions are possible. In almost all studies, SMRs were more effective than placebo in the treatment of acute painful musculoskeletal disorders and muscle spasm. Efficacy was less consistent in the treatment of chronic disorders. When used alone, SMRs were not consistently superior to simple

Table 125.1 Commonly Used Centrally Acting Skeletal Muscle Relaxants

Generic Name	Trade Name
Carisoprodol	Soma
Chlorphenesin	Maolate
Chlorzoxazone	Paraflex, Parafon Forte DSC
Cyclobenzaprine	Flexeril
Metaxalone	Skelaxin
Methocarbamol	Robaxin
Orphenadrine	Norflex
Tizanidine	Zanaflex

Table 125.2 Skeletal Muscle Relaxant Onset of Action, Duration, and Half-Life*

Drug	Onset	Duration (hr)	Half-Life
Carisoprodol	30 min	4–6	8 hr
Chlorphenesin	30 min	NR	2.5–5 hr
Chlorzoxazone	1 hr	3–4	1–2 hr
Cyclobenzaprine	1 hr	4–6	2–3 hr
Metaxalone	30 min	NR	1–2 hr
Methocarbamol	1 hr	4–5	14 hr
Orphenadrine	1 hr	12–24	1–3 days

*Data are based on oral administration.
NR, duration of action not reported.
From Basmajian JV: Acute back pain and spasm: a controlled multicenter trial of combined analgesic and antispasm agents, Spine 14:438, 1989.

analgesics (e.g., aspirin, acetaminophen, and nonsteroidal anti-inflammatory medications) in pain relief. However, when SMRs were used in combination with an analgesic, pain relief was superior to that of either drug used alone. Comparative studies of SMR efficacy failed to document superiority of one drug over another.[25–27]

Side Effects

The most commonly reported side effect of the SMRs is drowsiness. Manufacturers of these agents warn against activities that require mental alertness (e.g., driving, operating machinery) while taking these medications. Other CNS side effects include dizziness, blurred vision, confusion, hallucinations, agitation, and headaches. Gastrointestinal (GI) side effects have also been frequently reported, including anorexia, nausea, vomiting, and epigastric distress. Allergic reactions, including skin rash, pruritus, edema, and anaphylaxis, have also been observed. SMRs are generally not recommended for use in children or in pregnant or lactating women. Because SMRs undergo hepatic metabolism and renal excretion, they must be used cautiously in patients with compromised hepatic or renal function. SMRs should be used with caution in combination with alcohol and other CNS depressants because the effects of these substances may be cumulative.[9–13] Excessive

doses of SMRs may result in significant toxicity, with CNS depression consisting of stupor, coma, respiratory depression, and even death.[14,17–28] Abrupt cessation of some SMRs may cause withdrawal symptoms similar to those seen in barbiturate or alcohol withdrawal.

Potential for Abuse

The SMRs have the potential for abuse and dependence. Although the abuse potential of the SMRs is lower than that for benzodiazepines or opioids, numerous incidences have been reported in the medical literature.[14,17,29–31]

The SMRs may be the primary drug of abuse, presumably for their sedative or mood-altering effects. More frequently, SMRs are used in combination with other CNS depressants, such as opioids or alcohol. These combinations may be taken to prolong the effect of the opioid or benzodiazepines or to achieve the same effect with a lesser amount of the primary drug of abuse. Prescriptions for the SMRs are more readily obtainable than are prescriptions for opioids or benzodiazepines, and prescriptions for SMRs elicit less suspicion when they are frequently refilled.[14,15,17] Because of the potential for abuse, investigators have recommended that SMRs be prescribed only for acute conditions and for short periods of time. The SMRs should be used cautiously in known or suspected drug abusers, especially if these patients are already using other CNS depressants.

Individual Skeletal Muscle Relaxants

Carisoprodol (Soma)

Carisoprodol is a precursor of meprobamate (Miltown and Equanil). Meprobamate is one of the three primary metabolites produced by hepatic biotransformation of carisoprodol. Meprobamate dependency secondary to carisoprodol use has been reported with associated drug-seeking behavior and withdrawal symptoms. Withdrawal symptoms are similar to those seen in withdrawal from barbiturates and include restlessness, anxiety, insomnia, anorexia, and vomiting. Severe withdrawal symptoms have included agitation, hallucinations, seizures, and, rarely, death. Because of this potential for physical dependency, carisoprodol should be tapered rather than abruptly discontinued following long-term use. Idiosyncratic adverse effects include weakness, speech disturbances, temporary visual loss, ataxia, and transient paralysis.

The onset of action of carisoprodol is 30 minutes. The plasma half-life is 8 hours, and the duration of action is 4 to 6 hours. The drug is supplied as 350-mg tablets, and the recommended dose is one tablet taken four times daily. Carisoprodol is also available in combination with aspirin (Soma Compound) or aspirin and codeine (Soma Compound with Codeine).[4,10–13]

Chlorzoxazone (Parafon Forte DSC)

Chlorzoxazone is similar to the other SMRs, except for some reported cases of significant hepatotoxicity in individuals taking this drug.[9,11,32] Chlorzoxazone has an onset of action within 1 hour and a plasma half-life of 1 to 2 hours. The duration of action is 3 to 4 hours. The drug is available in 250- and

500-mg caplets, and the recommended adult dose is 250 to 750 mg taken three to four times daily. A pediatric dose of 20 mg/kg divided into three or four doses is suggested by the manufacturer.[9,11–13]

Cyclobenzaprine Hydrochloride (Flexeril)

Cyclobenzaprine is related structurally and pharmacologically to the tricyclic antidepressants (TCAs). Like other SMRs, cyclobenzaprine produces its effects within the CNS, primarily at the brainstem level. Like the TCAs, cyclobenzaprine has anticholinergic properties and may cause dry mouth, blurred vision, increased intraocular pressure, urinary retention, and constipation. The drug should therefore be used with caution in individuals with angle-closure glaucoma or prostatic hypertrophy. As with the TCAs, cyclobenzaprine should not be used in patients with cardiac arrhythmias, conduction disturbances, or congestive heart failure or during the acute phase of recovery from myocardial infarction. Cyclobenzaprine may interact with monoamine oxidase inhibitors and should not be used concurrently or within 14 days of discontinuation of these drugs. Withdrawal symptoms consisting of nausea, headache, and malaise have been reported following abrupt cessation of cyclobenzaprine after prolonged use.[9,11–13,28]

Cyclobenzaprine has an onset of action within 1 hour. The plasma half-life is 1 to 3 days, and the duration of action is 12 to 24 hours. Cyclobenzaprine is supplied as 10-mg tablets and has a recommended dose of 10 mg three times per day. Up to 40 mg daily in divided doses may be prescribed.[9,11–13,28]

A long-acting formulation of cyclobenzaprine has been introduced and is believed by some clinicians to have a lower side effect profile than the immediate-release formulation of this drug.

Metaxalone (Skelaxin)

Metaxalone is comparable in effect to the other SMRs. Adverse effects are also similar, with the exception of drug-associated hemolytic anemia and impaired liver function. Hepatotoxicity associated with metaxalone has not been as severe as that reported with chlorzoxazone. Monitoring of liver function is recommended with long-term usage. Metaxalone has an onset of action of 1 hour, a plasma half-life of 2 to 3 hours, and a duration of action of 4 to 6 hours. This drug is supplied as 400-mg tablets and has a recommended dose of 800 mg three to four times daily.[9,11–13]

Methocarbamol (Robaxin)

Methocarbamol is available in oral and parenteral form for intravenous (IV) or intramuscular (IM) injection. Subcutaneous injection is not recommended. Taken orally, this drug is similar to the other SMRs. Parenteral use of methocarbamol has been associated with pain, sloughing of skin, and thrombophlebitis at the injection site. Additionally, overly rapid IV injection has been associated with syncope, hypotension, bradycardia, and convulsions. Because of the risk of convulsion, parenteral use of the drug is not recommended for use in patients with epilepsy.

The onset of action is 30 minutes following oral ingestion and is almost immediate following parenteral administration. The plasma half-life of the drug is 1 to 2 hours. The duration of action has not been reported. Methocarbamol is produced in 500- and 750-mg tablets and has a recommended dosage range of 4000 to 4500 mg daily in three to four divided doses. For severe conditions, a dose as high as 6 to 8 g may be given for the first 48 to 72 hours. This drug is available for IV or IM injection in 10-mL single-dose vials containing 10 mg/mL. Methocarbamol tablets are also available in combination with aspirin (Robaxisal).[9,12–15]

Orphenadrine Citrate (Norflex)

Orphenadrine is an analogue of the antihistamine diphenhydramine (Benadryl). Orphenadrine shares some of the antihistaminic and anticholinergic effects of diphenhydramine. Unlike the other SMRs, orphenadrine produces some independent analgesic effects that may contribute to its efficacy in relieving painful skeletal muscle spasm. In addition to adverse effects commonly associated with other SMRs, dry mouth, blurred vision, and urinary retention may occur as a result of the drug's anticholinergic activity. Rare instances of aplastic anemia have been reported. Like methocarbamol, orphenadrine is available for IV or IM injection. Anaphylactoid reactions have been reported following parenteral administration.

Orphenadrine has an onset of action of 1 hour following oral administration. The onset of action is approximately 5 minutes after IM injection and is almost immediate with IV administration. The drug's plasma half-life is 14 hours, and the duration of action is 4 to 6 hours. Orphenadrine is available in 100-mg tablets with a recommended dose of one tablet twice daily. Orphenadrine is available for parenteral use in 2-mL ampules containing 60 mg of the drug and is also administered once every 12 hours. Orphenadrine tablets are also produced in combination with aspirin and caffeine (Norgesic and Norgesic Forte, respectively).[9–13,31]

Tizanidine Hydrochloride (Zanaflex)

Tizanidine hydrochloride is a centrally acting alpha$_2$-adrenergic agonist. Tizanidine is thought to exert its antispasticity properties by increased presynaptic inhibition of motoneurons; this action reduces facilitation of spinal motoneuron firing. Tizanidine does not appear to have any direct effect on the neuromuscular junction or on skeletal muscle fibers. The drug is well absorbed after oral administration and has a half-life of approximately 2.5 hours. Tizanidine is metabolized by the liver, and 95% is excreted in the urine and feces. The drug is available in 2-mg and 4-mg tablets for oral administration.

Because of the drug's short half-life, it must be administered every 6 to 8 hours. Because of the common side effects of weakness and sedation, it is best to start the patient on a 2-mg bedtime dose and then titrate upward every 4 to 6 days in 2-mg doses given every 6 to 8 hours. Faster upward titration is best accomplished in an inpatient setting. The maximum daily divided dose should not exceed a total of 36 mg.

Associated Drugs Used in the Treatment of Muscle Spasm and Spasticity

Two additional drugs with muscle relaxant effects, specifically the benzodiazepine diazepam and the antispasmodic agent baclofen, may be useful in the treatment of pain. A third drug, dantrolene sodium, a peripherally acting spasmolytic agent, is limited to controlling chronic spasticity associated with upper motoneuron disorders. Finally, the cinchona alkaloid quinine sulfate may help to reduce nocturnal leg cramps. A discussion of each drug follows.

Diazepam (Valium)

Diazepam is the most frequently prescribed benzodiazepine used in the treatment of muscle spasm and pain.[33] Other available benzodiazepines have not been proven superior to diazepam for this use.[10,33] Diazepam has anxiolytic, hypnotic, and antiepileptic properties in addition to its antispasmodic actions.

The muscle relaxant effects of this drug are thought to result from enhancement of γ-aminobutyric acid (GABA)–mediated presynaptic inhibition at spinal and supraspinal sites. Numerous studies have been performed comparing diazepam with placebo and with other SMRs in the treatment of painful musculoskeletal disorders. Results have been inconsistent; in general, however, diazepam has been found to be superior to placebo, but not consistently superior to other SMRs in the relief of muscle spasm and pain.[5–21,33–35] Diazepam appears to offer greater relief of associated anxiety than the other SMRs tested.[5,6,33] Diazepam is superior, however, to other SMRs in the treatment of spasticity associated with CNS disorders such as spinal cord injury and cerebral palsy.[11,12,36,37] Efficacy is similar to that of baclofen and dantrolene sodium for CNS disorders. Diazepam's long-term use in these disorders is limited primarily by sedation, abuse potential, and dependence.[36,38]

Diazepam is well absorbed from the GI tract, although it may also be administered by IV or IM injection. The drug undergoes biotransformation in the liver and is excreted in the urine. Diazepam is highly lipid soluble and rapidly crosses the blood-brain barrier. The onset of action is rapid following oral and parenteral administration. Diazepam's plasma half-life is 20 to 50 hours, and active metabolites of the drug have plasma half-lives ranging from 3 to 200 hours. The duration of action is variable, depending on rate and extent of drug distribution and elimination.

Abuse and dependence have been reported with the use of diazepam and the other benzodiazepines. The incidence of these problems is somewhat controversial. The potential for abuse varies among individuals and also varies with doses and length of therapy.[33,39–41] Withdrawal symptoms may occur with abrupt cessation of the drug and are similar to symptoms of barbiturate or alcohol withdrawal, including anxiety, dysphoria, insomnia, diaphoresis, vomiting, diarrhea, tremor, and seizures. Diazepam may have an additive effect when taken with other CNS depressants. Diazepam may have reduced plasma clearance and an increased half-life when taken in combination with disulfiram (Antabuse) or cimetidine (Tagamet).

Diazepam's most common adverse effects are related to its CNS-depressant activity: sedation, impairment of psychomotor performance, cognitive dysfunction, confusion, dizziness, and behavioral changes. Paradoxical CNS stimulation has also been reported. Other reported adverse effects include GI complaints, skin rash, blood dyscrasias, and elevation of liver enzymes. Parenteral administration has been associated with pain and thrombophlebitis at the injection site. IV and IM administration has produced more serious side effects, especially in seriously ill or geriatric patients; these side effects include cardiopulmonary depression, apnea, hypotension, bradycardia, and cardiac arrest.

Diazepam is available in 2-, 5-, and 10-mg tablets. The recommended dose for relief of painful musculoskeletal conditions is 2 to 10 mg three to four times daily. An extended-release 15-mg capsule (Valrelease) is produced and has a daily single dose of 1 to 2 capsules. Diazepam is available for parenteral administration in 2-mL ampules or 10-mL vials with 5 mg/mL. The recommended IM or IV dose is 5 to 10 mg every 3 to 4 hours as necessary.[9–13]

Baclofen (Lioresal)

Baclofen is a chemical analogue of GABA, which is an inhibitory neurotransmitter. The drug produces its effects primarily by inhibiting monosynaptic and polysynaptic transmission in the spinal cord, although some supraspinal activity may also occur. Baclofen is used chiefly in the management of spasticity associated with CNS disorders such as spinal cord lesions and multiple sclerosis.[9–13] The drug is reported to be equal or superior in efficacy when compared with diazepam and dantrolene sodium. It is less sedating than diazepam and has fewer serious side effects than dantrolene sodium.[12,36,38,42,43] Baclofen may be administered intrathecally to manage severe spasticity in patients who are intolerant or unresponsive to oral therapy.[44–48]

Baclofen has been useful in the treatment of trigeminal neuralgia. Because the a more favorable side effect profile, some researchers consider baclofen to be the drug of first choice in the treatment of this condition. The coadministration of baclofen and carbamazepine may be more effective than either drug used singly owing to a synergistic effect; however, adverse effects may be cumulative.[33,49–51] L-Baclofen has been reported to be more effective and to have fewer side effects than racemic baclofen.[52]

Baclofen is well absorbed from the GI tract and undergoes limited hepatic biotransformation. Most of the drug is excreted unchanged in the urine. The onset of action is highly variable, ranging from hours to weeks. The drug has a plasma half-life of 2.5 to 4 hours. The onset of action following intrathecal injection is 0.5 to 1 hour.

The most frequent side effects associated with the use of baclofen are drowsiness, dizziness, weakness, confusion, nausea, and hypotension. Side effects may be minimized by starting the drug at a low dose and gradually increasing it to the desired level. Abrupt discontinuation of the drug has been associated with hallucinations, psychiatric disturbances, and seizures; therefore, the drug should be gradually withdrawn.[9,10,53] Baclofen is produced in 10- and 20-mg tablets. The recommended starting dose is 5 mg three times daily for 3 days with an incremental increase of 5 mg per dose every 3 days. The therapeutic range is 40 to 80 mg daily.[9–13]

Dantrolene Sodium (Dantrium)

Dantrolene sodium is a peripherally acting skeletal muscle relaxant that produces its effect on skeletal muscle by interfering with the release of calcium ions from the sarcoplasmic reticulum. The primary indication for this drug is reduction of spasticity associated with upper motoneuron disorders, including spinal cord injury, stroke, multiple sclerosis, and cerebral palsy. This drug is also used in the treatment of malignant hyperthermia by reducing the hypometabolic processes associated with this disorder. Dantrolene sodium is not indicated in the treatment of other painful musculoskeletal disorders.[10–13]

Dantrolene sodium is incompletely absorbed from the GI tract. It is metabolized by the liver and is excreted in the urine primarily as metabolites. The onset of action may require a week or more in the treatment of CNS-associated spasticity. The drug's plasma half-life is 8.7 hours. The most frequent side effects associated with its use are muscle weakness, drowsiness, dizziness, malaise, and diarrhea, which may be severe. Serious idiosyncratic and hypersensitive hepatocellular injury may occur that may be fulminant and fatal. This adverse effect has occurred most frequently in women more than 35 years old. The drug is supplied in 25-mg, 50-mg, and 100-mg tablets. For treatment of spasticity, the recommended starting dose is 25 mg, which is gradually increased to a maximum daily dose of 400 mg.[9–13,18]

Quinine Sulfate (Quinamm)

Quinine sulfate is a cinchona alkaloid best known for its use as an antimalarial agent. Although the use of this drug for the treatment of nocturnal leg cramps is controversial, many clinicians believe that the drug is useful in this setting.[54–57] The drug reportedly produces its effect on skeletal muscle by an increased refractory period, reduced excitability of the motor end plate to acetylcholine, and redistribution of calcium within the muscle fiber. After oral ingestion, the drug is well absorbed, metabolized by the liver, and excreted in the urine. Quinine sulfate has a plasma half-life of 4 to 5 hours.

Some individuals are hypersensitive to quinine sulfate and develop thrombocytopenic purpura, which may be life-threatening. Visual disturbances, nausea, vomiting, and skin rash have also been reported. The drug may increase plasma levels of digoxin and may potentiate the effects of neuromuscular blocking agents owing to its curariform-like effects. Cinchonism does not usually occur at doses used to treat leg cramps. The drug is supplied as 260-mg tablets, and the recommended dose is one or two tablets nightly.[9–12]

Conclusion

The SMRs are efficacious in the treatment of painful musculoskeletal disorders. They are generally more effective in combination with analgesics and may potentiate the effects of other CNS depressants. The use of these drugs may be limited by sedation and other undesirable side effects, as well as by their potential for abuse and dependence. Diazepam may also be useful as a muscle relaxant and an anxiolytic, but it also causes sedation and has potential for abuse. Baclofen is used primarily to treat spasticity resulting from CNS lesions. It is also useful in the treatment of trigeminal neuralgia and may be the drug of first choice for this condition. Dantrolene sodium is a peripherally acting agent used to treat spasticity. It is not useful in the treatment of other painful musculoskeletal disorders. Quinine sulfate is an antimalarial agent that may be useful in the treatment of nocturnal leg cramps. Numerous evaluations have failed to demonstrate clear superiority of one SMR over another. Practitioners should base their choice of an agent on careful consideration of individual variables in a given clinical situation.

References

Full references for this chapter can be found on www.expertconsult.com.

Topical and Systemic Local Anesthetics

James E. Heavner

Local anesthetics are widely used to prevent or treat acute pain—cancer, chronic, and inflammatory pain—and for diagnostic and prognostic purposes. Koller is credited with introducing local anesthetics into medical practice when he used cocaine to numb the cornea before performing eye surgery.[1] Drugs classified as local anesthetics reversibly block action potential propagation in axons by preventing the sodium entry that produces the potentials.[2] However, other actions of these drugs, such as anti-inflammatory actions by interaction with G-protein receptors,[3] also are thought to help prevent or treat pain. Nociceptive pain and neuropathic pain are targeted with this group of drugs. Any part of the nervous system, from the periphery to the brain, may be where local anesthetics act to produce a desired anesthetic or analgesic effect. Various formulations of local anesthetics, routes of administration, and methods of administration are used. The drugs are formulated according to intended route of administration or to address specific concerns or needs. This chapter provides a concise review of the pharmacology of local anesthetics. Details regarding some specific indications (e.g., dentistry) are not considered.

Chemistry

All local anesthetic molecules in clinical use have three parts: a lipophilic (aromatic) end, a hydrophilic (amine) end, and a link between the ends (**Fig. 126.1**). The link contains either an aminoester or an aminoamide bond, and local anesthetics are designated as belonging to one of two groups, the aminoester-linked local anesthetics or the aminoamide-linked local anesthetics. Procaine is the prototypic aminoester-linked local anesthetic, and lidocaine is the prototypic aminoamide-linked local anesthetic (**Fig. 126.2**). Procaine was first synthesized in 1904, and lidocaine was first synthesized in 1943. Fundamental to the development of synthetic local anesthetics was the isolation of cocaine from coca beans and the elucidation of its chemical structure. Synthesis of molecules with local anesthetic activity paved the way for "tinkering" with the molecules by systematically modifying chemical structure and testing for a desired result (e.g., reduced toxicity) to develop new local anesthetics. **Figure 126.3** presents a chronology of the introduction of local anesthetic into clinical practice. Four

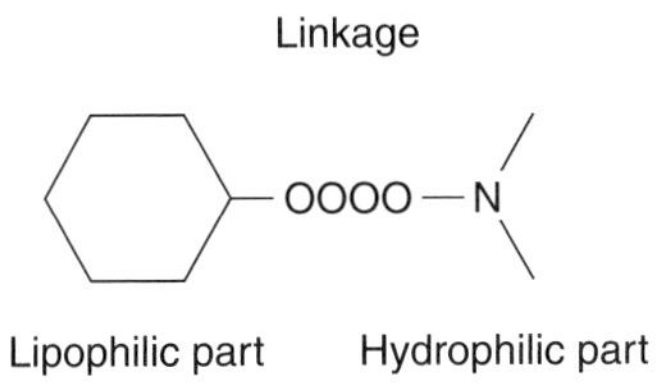

Lidocaine

Linkage

Lipophilic part   Hydrophilic part

Procaine

Fig. 126.1 All local anesthetic molecules in clinical use have three parts: a lipophilic (aromatic) end, a hydrophilic (amine) end, and a link between the ends.

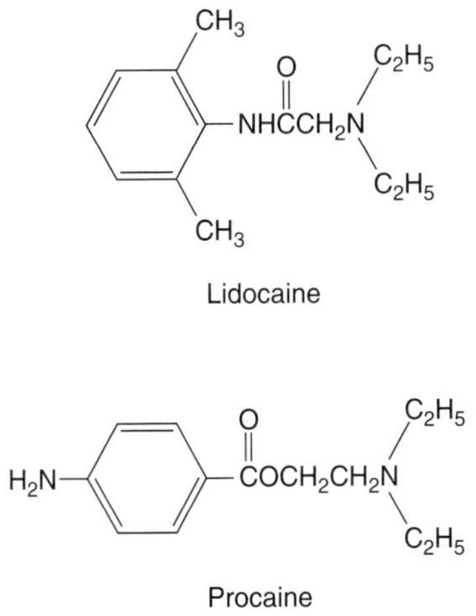

Fig. 126.2 Chemical structures of the prototypic aminoester-linked local anesthetic (procaine) and the prototypic aminoamide-linked local anesthetic (lidocaine).

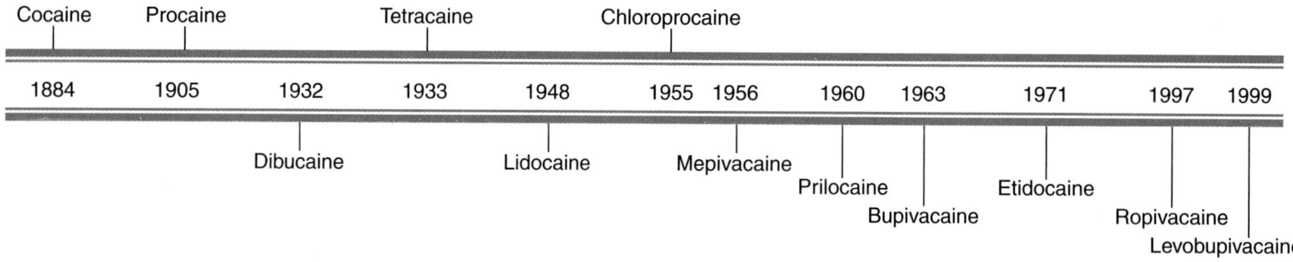

Fig. 126.3 Chronology of the introduction of different anesthetics into clinical practice. Chloroprocaine (1955) is the last aminoester-linked local anesthetic introduced that is still in clinical use. *(Courtesy of David A. Scott, Melbourne, Australia.)*

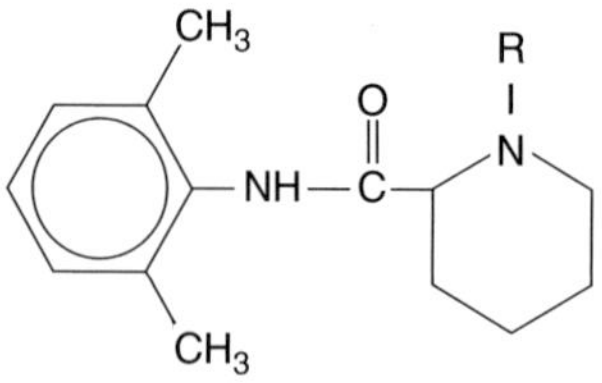

	Mepivacaine	Ropivacaine	Bupivacaine
R=	CH_3	C_3H_6	C_4H_9
Equieffective	1	0.37	0.25
Lipid/H_2O	0.8	2.8	27.5
Protein-bound (%)	77.5	94	95.6

Fig. 126.4 Results of structure alterations: amide linked. The aminoamide-linked local anesthetics mepivacaine, ropivacaine, and bupivacaine vary only by substitution at R on the basic molecule shown *at the top.* As the number of carbon atoms increases at R, potency, lipid solubility, and protein binding increase. *(Adapted from Heavner JE: Pain mechanisms and local anesthetics: scientific foundations for clinical practice. In Raj PP, editor: Textbook of regional anesthesia, New York, 2002, Churchill Livingstone, p 105.)*

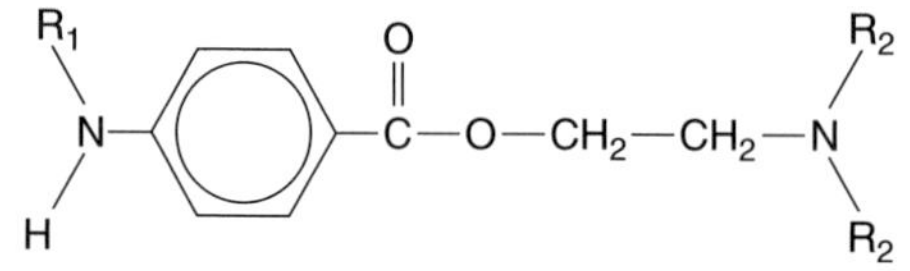

	Procaine	Tetracaine
R_1	H	C_4H_9
R_2	C_2H_5	CH_3
Hydrolysis rate (uM/ml/hr)	1.1	0.25
=potent	2	0.25
Duration (min)	50	175
LD50 (mice)	615	48

Fig. 126.5 Results of structure alterations: ester linked. The aminoester-linked local anesthetics procaine and tetracaine vary only by substitution at R1 and R2 on the basic molecule shown *above. (Adapted from Heavner JE: Pain mechanisms and local anesthetics: scientific foundations for clinical practice. In Raj PP, editor:* Textbook of regional anesthesia, *New York, 2002, Churchill Livingstone, p 105.)*

aminoester-linked local anesthetics are shown in this figure: cocaine, procaine, tetracaine, and chloroprocaine. The other local anesthetics are aminoamide-linked substances. What is evident from the figure is that, since 1955, the focus has been on the development of aminoamide—rather than aminoester-linked—local anesthetics. Reasons for this focus include the allergenic potential of aminoester-linked local anesthetics and the instability of aminoester bonds.

Testing of various modifications to the basic procaine and lidocaine structure revealed that increasing the molecular weight of the molecules by adding carbon atoms to either end of the structure or to the link generally increases lipid solubility, protein binding, duration of action and toxicity, and influences biotransformation of the molecule (**Figs. 126.4** and **126.5**). A positive correlation exists between intrinsic local anesthetic potency and lipid solubility of local anesthetics.

Most local anesthetics have a tertiary amine on the hydrophilic end. Exceptions include prilocaine, which has a secondary amine, and benzocaine, which has a primary amine. Tertiary amines have a positive charge (cation) or are uncharged (base). The ratio of cation to base is determined by the acid dissociation constant (pKa) of the local anesthetic and the pH of the solution. The "state" of the amine determines how well local anesthetic molecules move through biologic membranes. The unchanged forms of local anesthetics pass readily through cell membranes. Therefore, speed of onset of local anesthetic

block, at least theoretically, is increased by raising the concentration of uncharged local anesthetic molecules injected.

Because local anesthetics are weak bases, increasing the pH ("alkalinization") of solution increases the ratio of base to cation. The Henderson-Hasselbalch equation can be used to quantitate the ratio:

$$Log([cation]/[base]) = pKa(local\,anesthetic) - pH(solution)$$

Sodium bicarbonate is used clinically to increase the pH of local anesthetic solutions. Commercial solutions of local anesthetics are acidified, so the hydrophilic (cationic) state is favored. Overzealous alkalinization can cause local anesthetic molecules to precipitate from solution.

The newest additions to clinically available local anesthetics, ropivacaine (**Fig. 126.6**) and levobupivacaine, represent (1) the exploitation of technology that permits cost-favorable separation of racemic mixtures of local anesthetics into pure enantiomers and (2) the search for local anesthetics with greater safety margins. Simply stated, molecules with an asymmetrical carbon atom exist in forms that are mirror images (i.e., exhibit "handedness," chirality), with images (enantiomer, stereoisomers) distinguished by how they rotate light according to the orientation of the structures in three dimensions. Various terms are used to refer to the different enantiomers; this discussion uses S- and R- to designate two different enantiomers. A racemic mixture contains equal amounts of the R- and S- isomers.

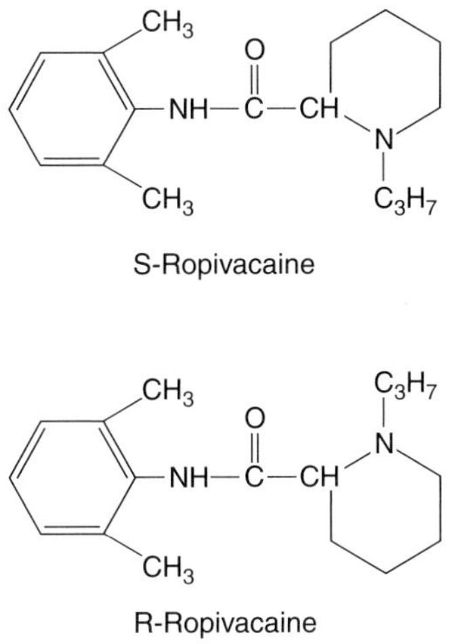

Fig. 126.6 Chisal forms of ropivacaine. The only difference between the S- and R- isomers is their spatial orientation.

Table 126.1 Anesthetic Duration and Toxicity of Local Anesthetic Isomers

Drug	Duration	Toxicity
Etidocaine	S = R	S = R
Mepivacaine	S > R	S = R
Bupivacaine	S > R	S < R
Ropivacaine	S > R	S < R

R, R-enantiomer; S, S-enantiomer.

Commercial formulations of ropivacaine and levobupivacaine contain the S- enantiomer. Levobupivacaine is the S- form of bupivacaine. The motive for marketing pure enantiomers is evidence that the S- form is less toxic, more potent, and longer acting than the R- form or the racemic mixture (**Table 126.1**).

Pharmacodynamics

Reversible block of voltage-gated sodium channels in axons is generally thought to be how a local anesthetic blocks sensory and motor function. Some evidence supporting this view includes the following: (1) action potentials do not develop in axons exposed to local anesthetics, (2) sodium currents responsible for generation of action potentials are blocked by these drugs, and (3) local anesthetics do not affect the transmembrane potential of axons. The "state" of the sodium channel (resting, open, inactivated) changes during the cycles of polarized, depolarized, and repolarized. The order of affinity of local anesthetics for different channel states is open > inactivated > resting. Many investigators have shown that the block of propagation of action potentials is a function of frequency of depolarization, a finding that supports the conclusion that the open state of the sodium channel is the primary target of local anesthetic molecules. This is referred to as *state-dependent block*.

Certain sodium channel subtypes are generally divided into those that are tetrodotoxin sensitive (TTXs) and those that are tetrodotoxin resistant (TTXr).[4] Most sensory neurons generate TTXs currents. However, TTXr currents are present in a high proportion of smaller dorsal root ganglion neurons associated with nociceptive A-delta and C fibers. Available evidence indicates that channels from both groups are involved in pain states as a result of changes in channel function and expression caused by disease or injury. Arguments have been put forth that local anesthetics may exert their pharmacologic action not only on sodium conductance, but also on other ionic conductances (e.g., potassium and calcium).[5,6]

Differential block, the block of pain perception without motor block, for example, is observed clinically, but the mechanism responsible for this is poorly understood. The clinical manifestations of differential block vary depending on the local anesthetic used.[7] For many years, differential block was ascribed to greater sensitivity of smaller axons than large ones to local anesthetics,[8] but this "size principle" was challenged.[9] Berde and Strichartz[7] cited different factors that could contribute to differential block, including anatomic factors, and the relative sensitivity of different local anesthetics for sodium and potassium channels. Oda et al[10] suggested that preferential block of TTXr sodium channels by ropivacaine in small dorsal root ganglia neurons (associated with nociceptive sensation) underlies the differential block observed during epidural anesthesia with this drug.

Using a combination of local anesthetic and another drug to produce nociceptive selective block is under investigation. For example, activating transient receptor potential vanilloid subtype 1 channels on C fibers with capsaicin to deliver the local anesthetic, QX-314, into the fibers is effective in animal models.[11] Another approach is to combine local anesthetic and α2-adrenergic agonist such as dexmedetomidine and has yielded favorable results. The mechanism for the α2-adrenergic agonist action is not known but may include direct inhibition of TTXr Na[+] channel or through hyperpolarization activated cation current.[12]

Another pharmacodynamic puzzle is the mechanism whereby systemically administered local anesthetic relieves pain. An analgesic effect has been reported following intravenous lidocaine administration in many acute and chronic conditions.[13–20] Subcutaneously injected bupivacaine reportedly produces analgesia by a systemic effect.[21] Normal or altered sodium channels located in various areas of the brain, spinal cord, dorsal root ganglia, or peripheral axons are mentioned most frequently as the action sites. Zhang et al[22] reported that in rats, systemic lidocaine delivered by implanted osmotic pump reduces sympathetic nerve sprouting in dorsal root ganglion that is associated with some neuropathic pain behaviors.

Local anesthetics have effects on other biologic processes that are potentially important pharmacodynamic actions of value in treating pain. These include inhibition of G-protein–coupled receptor signaling.[3]

Pharmacokinetics

Usual pharmacokinetic parameters (**Table 126.2**) for drugs incompletely describe important details regarding distribution of local anesthetics from application sites to target and nontarget structures. It is well established that systemic absorption of local anesthetics correlates positively with the vascularity of the injection site: intravenous > tracheal > intracostal > paracervical > epidural > brachial plexus > sciatic > subcutaneous.[23] The spinal cord meninges influence distribution of local anesthetics from the epidural and subarachnoid spaces. Intact

Table 126.2 Disposition Kinetics in Adult Male Subjects

Local Anesthetic	V_{dss} (L)	Clearance (L/min)	Half-Life (hr)	Hepatic Extraction	Lipid Solubility	Protein Binding (%)	Blood/Plasma Partitioning
Mepivacaine	84	0.78	1.9	0.40	0.8	78	0.92
Ropivacaine	59	0.73	1.8	0.40	2.8	94	0.69
Bupivacaine	73	0.58	2.7	0.51	27.5	96	0.73
Lidocaine	91	0.95	1.6	0.72	2.9	60	0.84

V_{dss}, Steady state volume of distribution.

skin is nearly a complete barrier to local anesthetic penetration. For delivery of local anesthetic through intact skin, special local anesthetic formulations (e.g., EMLA cream, a eutectic mixture of lidocaine and prilocaine) or delivery methods (e.g., electrophoresis) are employed to facilitate transcutaneous transfer. Because of the large number of different injection sites used by pain physicians (e.g., epidural, intrathecal, intrapleural, intra-articular, intramuscular, perineural, topical) and the variety of dosing methods (e.g., single injection, continuous infusion, intermittent infusion), more than a superficial discussion of the distribution kinetics of local anesthetics from injection sites is beyond the scope of this chapter.

Aminoester-linked local anesthetics are hydrolyzed by esterases in tissues and blood. Aminoamide-linked local anesthetics are biotransformed primarily in the liver by cytochrome P-450 enzymes. Metabolites may retain local anesthetic activity and toxicity potential, albeit usually at lower potency than the parent compound.

Vasoconstrictors (e.g., epinephrine 1:400,000 [2.5 mg/mL]) are used to reduce absorption of local anesthetics into the systemic circulation. The value of this practice depends on the vascularity of injection site and the tissue binding of different local anesthetics. The value of the addition of sodium bicarbonate to solutions to enhance speed of onset of local anesthetics also depends on injection site, as well as on the physiochemical properties of different local anesthetics. The addition of sodium bicarbonate increases the pH of solutions and thus increases the ratio of uncharged to charged molecules. This change raises the number of local anesthetic molecules in the form that most readily passes through biologic membranes.

Hyaluronidase (tissue spreading factor) is sometimes added to local anesthetic solutions to facilitate spread of solution at the injection site, thereby affecting speed of onset and extending a block. This seems to be useful only when local anesthetic is injected behind the eyes preparatory to ophthalmologic surgery. Hyaluronidase may be injected with local anesthetic during epidural neurolysis to treat pain, with positive benefit. An issue of *Techniques in Regional Anesthesia and Pain Medicine* (volume 8, issue 3, July 2004) discussed in detail additives to local anesthetics. Various attempts have been made to prolong the duration of action of local anesthetics by loading them into liposomes or microcapsules, but no such formulations have been approved by the US Food and Drug Administration (FDA) for marketing.

Toxicity

The toxic effects of local anesthetics can be categorized as shown in **Figure 126.7**. True allergic reactions are associated with aminoester-linked local anesthetics, not amino amide-

Localized or Systemic
Allergic reactions

Localized
Tissue toxicity

Systemic
Cardiac/vascular
Central nervous system
Methemoglobin

Fig. 126.7 Categories of local anesthetic toxic reactions.

linked ones. In a study of anaphylactic and anaphylactoid reactions ($n = 789$) occurring during anesthesia, Mertes et al[24] found no such reactions to local anesthetics. However, Mackley et al[25] reported that of 183 patients patch tested, 4 had positive reactions to lidocaine, and 2 of these patients had histories of sensitivity to local injections of lidocaine manifested by dermatitis. These investigators concluded that contact type IV sensitivity to lidocaine may occur more frequently than previously thought. It is common, but inappropriate, to refer to all adverse events as "allergic reactions." Tissue toxicity, primary myotoxicity and neurotoxicity, can be produced by all local anesthetics if "high" concentrations are used. Signs and symptoms of varying degrees of neuropathy (e.g., transient neurologic symptoms, cauda equina syndrome) have been reported following spinal anesthesia with 2% and 5% lidocaine.

A systematic review[26] compared the frequency of transcutaneous nerve stimulation (TNS) and neurologic complications after spinal anesthesia with lidocaine with TNS after other local anesthetics. These investigators found that the risk for developing TNS after spinal anesthesia with lidocaine was higher than with bupivacaine, prilocaine, procaine, or mepivacaine.[27] Symptoms in all patients disappeared spontaneously by the tenth postoperative day. The lithotomy position seems to be a predisposing factor. In 1980, Foster and Carlson[27] reported that of the local anesthetics tested, procaine produced the least severe and bupivacaine the most severe muscle injury. More recently, Zink et al[28] concluded that the myotoxic potential of ropivacaine is less than the potential of bupivacaine. However, both drugs produced morphologically identical patterns of calcified myonecrosis, formation of scar tissue, and a marked rate of muscle fiber regeneration in animals after continuous peripheral nerve blocks.[29]

Various local anesthetics reportedly may produce methemoglobinemia. Prilocaine is the local anesthetic associated with the greatest risk for this complication. As the concentration of local anesthetic in the systemic circulation increases, various cardiovascular system (CVS) and central nervous system (CNS) signs and symptoms appear (**Fig. 126.8**). The relative CVS and CNS toxicity of local anesthetics has been of interest, especially after Albright[30] reported unexpected cardiovascular toxicity of bupivacaine. In animal studies, the

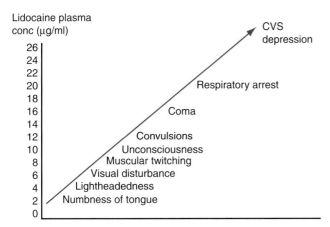

Lidocaine plasma conc (µg/ml)

CVS depression

Respiratory arrest

Coma

Convulsions
Unconsciousness
Muscular twitching
Visual disturbance
Lightheadedness
Numbness of tongue

Fig. 126.8 Cardiovascular (CVS) and central nervous system side effects of local anesthetics, depending on their concentration (conc) in systemic circulation.

Table 126.3 Generic and Trade Names of Local Anesthetics*

Generic Name	Trade Name(s)
Benoxinate (oxybuprocaine)	Dorsacaine; Novesine
Bupivacaine	Marcaine; Sensorcaine
Butacaine	Butyn
Chloroprocaine (2-chlorprocaine)	Nesacaine
Cyclomethycaine	Surfacaine
Dibucaine	Nupercaine; Percaine
Etidocaine	Duranest
Hexylcaine	Cyclaine
Levobupivacaine	Chirocaine
Lidocaine	Xylocaine; Xylotox
Mepivacaine	Carbocaine; Polocaine
Piperocaine	Metycaine
Prilocaine	Citanest
Procaine	Novocain
Proparacaine	Ophthaine
Ropivacaine	Naropin
Tetracaine	Pontocaine; Pantocaine

*These local anesthetics are administered chiefly as the chloride or sulfate salts, and it would be more accurate to specify procaine hydrochloride rather than just procaine. Because procaine is the active species, it is the commonly used term. Adapted from de Jong RH: *Local anesthetics,* St. Louis, 1994, Mosby–Year Book.

Table 126.4 Topical Local Anesthetics and Their Available Preparations

Benzocaine	**Lidocaine/prilocaine**
Cream	Cream
Ointment	**Lidocaine/tetracaine**
Topical aerosol	Patch
Benzocaine and menthol	**Pramoxine**
Lotion	Cream
Topical aerosol solution	Lotion
Butamben	**Pramoxine and menthol**
Ointment	Gel
Dibucaine	Lotion
Cream	**Tetracaine**
Ointment	Cream
Lidocaine	**Tetracaine and menthol**
Film-forming gel	Ointment
Ointment	
Patch	
Cream	

Adapted from http://www.nlm.nih.gov/medlineplus/druginfo/uspdi/202042.html

ratio of doses of bupivacaine that produced convulsive activity and cardiovascular collapse[7] was lower than for other local anesthetics such as lidocaine. Human volunteer studies of doses required to produce early features of CNS and CVS toxicity by ropivacaine and levobupivacaine demonstrated that the doses were about equal and higher than for bupivacaine.[31-33]

Brown et al[34] reviewed records of patients who had seizures while undergoing brachial plexus, epidural, and caudal regional anesthetic regimens. No adverse CVS, pulmonary, or nervous system events were associated with any of the seizures, including 16 patients who received bupivacaine blocks. Clinically, which of the usual features if systemic local anesthetic toxicity occurs, the order in which it occurs, and how soon after local anesthetic administration is quite variable.[35] This is not surprising given what is known about how various health conditions, other drugs, and rate of increase of local anesthetic concentration in systemic circulation can influence the manifestation and progression of signs and symptoms of local anesthetic toxicity.

Measures to prevent systemic toxic reactions to local anesthetics include following dose recommendations, injecting aliquots over time, avoiding inadvertent intravascular injections, and monitoring vital signs during injection. Blanket recommended doses versus block-specific recommended doses have been discussed.[36,37] Drug administration must be stopped should signs or symptoms of toxicity develop. Seizures induced by local anesthetics are usually self-limiting and require maintenance of respiratory gas exchange and control of muscle contractions (e.g., intubation, oxygenation, short-acting muscle paralysis). Drugs such as propofol, thiopental, midazolam, and diazepam are effective against these seizures.

Cardiovascular toxicity is treated according to American Heart Association guidelines, depending on the nature of the toxicity. Evidence suggests that lipid emulsion infusion may be beneficial in some instances.[38] The American Society of Regional Anesthesia and Pain Medicine now include intralipid in their recommended approach to treating local anesthetic systemic toxicity.[39]

Local Anesthetics in Clinical Use

Generic and trade names of local anesthetics are listed in **Table 126.3**. Undoubtedly, lidocaine is most commonly used to prevent procedure-related pain and for diagnostic tests. Immediate-acting to long-acting local anesthetics such as ropivacaine, levobupivacaine, and bupivacaine are used for therapy. **Table 126.4** lists topical anesthetics and their preparations. Most of the forms are available without prescription. A 5% lidocaine patch (Lidoderm) is approved by the FDA for controlling postherpetic neuralgia.

References

Full references for this chapter can be found on www.expertconsult.com.

Chapter **127**

Alternative Pain Medicine

Winston C.V. Parris and Salahadin Abdi

Pain and illness continue to be the scourge of humankind even with the tremendous strides that have been made in the cure and relief of several diseases. Since the 1990s, great progress has been made in the management of pain derived from disease, trauma, or idiopathic origin. However, pain continues to be a major problem in the very young, the very old, cancer patients, diabetic patients, poststroke patients, and almost all patients whose disorder produces unrelenting pain. Pain in the injured worker is a major problem because of the occupational, legal, emotional, economic, political, psychosocial, and societal factors that influence or modify the patient's ultimate perception of pain.

Since the advent of the pain medicine specialty, significant developments have contributed to modest success in resolving chronic pain,[1] although much remains to be done in optimizing pain control. While we await these advances, patients become disappointed, disenchanted, and at times disgusted with the inadequacy of their pain management. This disillusionment has led many people to seek nontraditional, unconventional, and at times dangerous remedies to control pain. Unfortunately, a few unscrupulous practitioners take advantage of this situation, but it is heartening to note that some of these nontraditional remedies are effective in controlling, if not eliminating, chronic pain syndromes in selected patients. This whole arena is known as *alternative medicine* or *complementary medicine.*[2] This chapter explores the role of alternative medicine in chronic pain management and examines how these methods can contribute to traditional or conventional pain medicine.

Some conventional physicians scoff at any remedy that is not well described in standard medical textbooks or is not thoroughly investigated in peer-reviewed journals and supported by placebo-controlled, randomized, scientifically conducted studies. These methods reflect the standard approach by which medical information is disseminated and passed on from teacher to student or from colleague to colleague. If a given alternative medicine practitioner proposed that snake oil is effective for migraine headaches, most traditional physicians would laugh. This reaction would be based on the fact that no Pharmacopoeia or *Physicians' Desk Reference* (PDR) or medical journal describes snake oil as a pharmacologic agent or as having any therapeutic value. Yet, if snake oil were analyzed and one of its active principles were absorbed transdermally and had a specific effect on cerebral vasculature that ultimately relieved migraine headaches, this originally preposterous idea would become a multimillion-dollar scientific breakthrough. Although this hypothetical scenario is unlikely, it is possible. The major challenge is to determine how to evaluate those "preposterous ideas" that, after all, may not have any deleterious effect on a patient and may, in fact, be beneficial.

The existing scientific, medical, and academic structure does not leave much room for this kind of investigation. Except for a few cases (e.g., The University of New Mexico in Albuquerque), most medical school administrators adhere rigidly, and in many situations blindly, to the curricula handed down by tradition. Change takes place, but most changes are insignificant and do not reflect the realities of medicine today and the needs of today's patient. Thus, although recent medical school graduates may be highly skilled in many new and sophisticated techniques of medicine, they may be relatively uninformed about the principles and practice of pain medicine. A needlessly defensive posture may be adopted when new and unconventional techniques are proposed. It takes approximately 1 to 2 decades of physician experience to allow for exploration or, at least, intelligent examination of unconventional information.

Prevalence of Alternative Medicine

The prevalence of alternative medicine in the United States was studied by Eisenberg et al,[3] and their results were published in the *New England Journal of Medicine* in 1993. These investigators found that one in three persons in the United States used unconventional or alternative medicine for various illnesses, most of which were associated with pain. This study also highlighted the cost of alternative medicine and the fact that most modalities used in alternative medicine are not subject to governmental scrutiny, regulation, or supervision. Nevertheless, many patients use alternative medicine as their main therapeutic option, and most patients use alternative medicine along with conventional medicine, occasionally with the assent of a conventional physician. Some regional bias exists, in that alternative medicine, including herbal medicine,[4] is used more commonly in the western United States and, to a lesser extent, in the southern than in the northern and eastern regions of the United States.

To address the burgeoning business of alternative medicine and its impact on citizens, the federal government of the United States, through the Department of Health and Human Services, created the Office of Alternative Medicine by congressional mandate under the 1992 National Institutes of Health (NIH) appropriations bill. The creation of this office was motivated by the groundswell from citizens who demanded that government look into the efficacy of unconventional medicine and its modalities.[5]

Toward the end of the 1980s, the Mexican herbal medicine called laetrile generated great interest. Thousands of US citizens crossed the Mexican border in search of that elusive cancer cure. Most were not successful in that search. These events, and many others like it, politicized the issue and led to the formation of the Office of Alternative Medicine. The major objective of the Office of Alternative Medicine[6] was to facilitate evaluation of alternative medical treatment modalities to determine their effectiveness in treating disease. Its congressional mandate provided for a public information clearinghouse to gather and appropriately categorize information and to fund and organize research training programs for alternative medicine.

Definition

In this chapter, *alternative medicine* may be defined as unconventional or unorthodox medical interventions not routinely taught at US medical schools or not generally available in hospitals in the United States.[7] Some alternative therapies are benign; others are invasive. Some have been used for a long time; others are more recent. Some alternative therapies are well known; others are mysterious and, on occasion, dangerous. Although some alternative therapies have sound scientific principles to recommend their use in clinical practice, they may not have been subjected to the scientifically conducted placebo-controlled randomized studies that most conventional medical therapies undergo, and they may not have been exposed to the peer review process necessary before any therapy is accepted as clinically useful. Thus, the claims of many alternative therapies are usually anecdotal. At times, inappropriate or inconsistent assumptions have been made regarding their clinical efficacy.

Alternative medicine covers a wide scope of healing philosophies, methodologic approaches, and clinical therapies. Besides not being taught in medical schools, most alternative medical practices are not reimbursed by medical insurance companies. This situation is changing slowly; for example, acupuncture services now not only are recognized as effective but also are reimbursed by several medical insurers.

Alternative medicine has been labeled "holistic medicine," and although some common areas exist, the comparison is not accurate. The term *holistic* generally implies that the health care practitioner considers the whole person, including physical, mental, emotional, and spiritual aspects. In today's health-conscious society, many therapies are labeled preventive. This label implies that the practitioner is involved primarily in educating the patient about the disease, its symptoms, its complications, and its treatment. Even more important, however, the practitioner is committed to instructing the patient regarding the techniques and methods of preventing the disease. Using the principle that prevention is better than cure, many preventive practitioners lay heavy emphasis on cessation of smoking and promotion of exercise, a healthy diet, and similar measures to prevent heart disease, metabolic disorders (e.g., diabetes), morbid obesity, and some forms of cancer.

Whereas some forms of alternative medicine are consistent with the fundamental physiologic principles involving the circulation and the central nervous system as understood by Western medicine, other approaches are based on different and unfamiliar healing systems. Gradually, some non-Western systems are being absorbed into the mainstream of Western medicine.

Classification

To a large extent, alternative medicine has not been evaluated or scrutinized according to accepted scientific principles or methods. Consequently, the architects of individual alternative modalities have been more concerned with acceptance and positive results rather than an open and unconditional evaluation of their efficacy. As a result, no consistent organization existed before the creation of the Office of Alternative Medicine,[6] and no attempts were made to classify the modalities used for alternative medicine. Under the aegis of the NIH, a task force was created to address classification issues. The result is seven categories of complementary or alternative medical practices, including the following:

1. Alternative systems of practice
2. Bioelectromagnetic applications
3. Diet, nutrition, and lifestyle changes
4. Herbal medicine
5. Manual healing methods
6. Mind-body interventions
7. Pharmacologic and biologic treatments

The task force also reported on corresponding issues, such as research methodology, research and training needs, the peer review process, and information dissemination activities.[7]

The classification of alternative medicine practices was designed primarily to facilitate the review process for grant allocation. It was not designed as an arbitrary or definitive classification of alternative medicine. A summary of the classification is listed in **Table 127.1**.

Table 127.1 Classification of Alternative Medicine Practices	
Alternative Systems of Medical Practice Acupuncture Anthroposophically extended medicine Ayurveda Community-based health care practices Environmental medicine Homeopathic medicine Latin American rural practices Native American practices Natural products Naturopathic medicine Past life therapy Shamanism Tibetan medicine Traditional Asian (Oriental) medicine **Bioelectromagnetic Applications** Blue light treatment and artificial lighting Electroacupuncture Electromagnetic fields Electrostimulation and neuromagnetic stimulation devices Low-level laser Magnetic resonance spectroscopy **Diet, Nutrition, and Lifestyle Changes** Changes in lifestyle Diet Macrobiotics Megavitamins Nutritional supplements **Herbal Medicine** *Echinacea* (purple coneflower) Ginger rhizome *Ginkgo biloba* extract Ginseng root Wild chrysanthemum flower Witch hazel Yellow wood	**Manual Healing** Acupressure Alexander technique Aromatherapy Biofield therapeutics Chiropractic medicine Feldenkrais method Massage therapy Osteopathy Reflexology Rolfing Therapeutic touch Trager method Zone therapy **Mind-Body Control** Art therapy Biofeedback Counseling Dance therapy Guided imagery Humor therapy **Hypnotherapy** Meditation Music therapy Prayer therapies Psychotherapy Relaxation techniques Support groups Virtual reality Yoga **Pharmacologic and Biologic Treatments** Antioxidizing agents Cell treatment Chelation therapy Metabolic therapy Oxidizing agents (ozone, hydrogen peroxide)

Office of Alternative Medicine

Since its inception, the Office of Alternative Medicine has served certain important functions that have helped to legitimize some modalities of alternative medicine. Most notably, it has served as an institution that compiles data and serves as a granting agency for sponsoring some of those research projects.

Other functions are outlined as follows[8]:

1. To provide and evaluate a research database. The research database program provides a framework for identifying and organizing scientific literature on alternative medical practices. This literature has grown to more than 100,000 specific citations on complementary and alternative medical topics. Currently, the program is involved in implementing a process of developing systematic reviews and meta-analyses of the alternative medicine scientific literature.
2. To serve as a clearinghouse of alternative medicine data. The agency disseminates information to the public, the media, and health care professionals to promote awareness and to provide education about alternative medical research.
3. To optimize media relations. The media relations section provides accurate coverage and subsequent follow-up of

relevant stories on alternative medicine to the news media and provides information about the Office of Alternative Medicine and its activities for mass media audiences.
4. To facilitate sponsored research. Shortly after its inception, the agency provided 30 grants to fund research applications to study different aspects of complementary and alternative medicine.
5. To create and fund alternative medicine specialty research centers. The agency has funded 10 specialty research centers designed to study complementary and alternative medicine treatments for specific health conditions.
6. To facilitate an international and professional liaison program that participates in and promotes cooperative efforts in research and education.
7. To organize intramural research training. This program allows scientists to conduct basic and clinical research in alternative medicine and supports postdoctoral training for appropriate candidates. The agency also evaluates specific alternative medical modalities by other institutes and centers within the NIH structure. Furthermore, several other governmental agencies interact with the Office of Alternative Medicine, including the Health Care Finance Agency, the Food and Drug Administration, the Agency for Health Care Policy and Research, and the Centers for Disease Control and Prevention.

Scope

In an attempt to determine prevalence, costs, and patterns of use of alternative medicine in the United States, Eisenberg et al[3] demonstrated that alternative modalities are used not only for chronic pain but also for cancer, arthritis, acquired immunodeficiency syndrome (AIDS), gastrointestinal problems, chronic renal failure, and eating disorders. Among the commonly used therapies were the following:

- Relaxation techniques
- Chiropractic manipulation
- Massage
- Imagery
- Spiritual healing
- Promotional weight loss programs
- Lifestyle diets (e.g., macrobiotics, herbal medicine, megavitamin therapy)
- Self-help groups
- Energy healing
- Biofeedback
- Hypnosis
- Magnetic therapy
- Low-power laser therapy
- Homeopathy
- Acupuncture
- Folk remedies
- Exercise
- Prayer

More than 60% of the patients who used unconventional therapy did so without medical supervision and without active consultation with a provider of either conventional or unconventional therapy. The medical conditions for which most patients sought alternative therapy included back pain, allergies, arthritis, insomnia, sprains, strains, headaches, high blood pressure, digestive problems, anxiety, and depression. Most of the medical conditions listed here are associated with some form of chronic pain.

Another criterion for considering the efficacy of alternative therapeutic modalities is based on reimbursement by either patients or third-party payers. Reimbursement for alternative therapy in 1990 was approximately $11.7 billion. Although this criterion is not a scientific index of efficacy, the magnitude of this sum of money does highlight the importance that patients placed on these modalities. Thus, unconventional or alternative medicine has a major presence in the health care system of the United States. The magnitude of this presence may be underestimated by conventional health care providers, but in 1990, approximately 22 million persons in the United States used alternative therapy modalities as a means of treating their health problems. Occasionally, these methods are used simultaneously with conventional medicine.

A satisfying observation is that most users of alternative therapy do not replace conventional therapy with alternative techniques but rather use those alternative therapy modalities as adjuncts to conventional therapy. For example, few patients use alternative therapy modalities for the treatment of high blood pressure or digestive problems. This finding suggests that patients have been satisfied with the validity and efficacy of conventional therapy for these ailments. Yet many patients do use alternative medicine for the treatment of chronic back pain, headaches, arthritis, strains, or sprains.

As a part of the medical evaluation of patients with chronic pain, an attempt should be made to determine whether the patient is receiving alternative therapy and the frequency, amount (units), or intensity with which that particular modality is used. Currently, medical students are being taught very little about unconventional alternative therapy.[9] Perhaps including some information about the subject in the medical school curriculum not only may broaden physicians' outlook on what patients are seeking but also may provide the sensitivity necessary to evaluate these modalities scientifically.

Alternative Therapy Modalities

Many unorthodox modalities may be effective in patient care. The laws of consumerism may be influential in dictating not only the popularity but also the longevity of various medical modalities directly related to their therapeutic efficacy. Thus, patients seldom seek an alternative modality for a fractured bone because the conventional orthopedic maneuvers for treating a fractured bone are associated with satisfactory results. Many conditions do not respond to conventional therapy, and, in frustration, patients are prompted to seek alternative therapy even if the therapeutic efficacy of the alternative modality is not established. Some patients with cancer pain who receive satisfactory results and for whom death is imminent may seek not only unconventional treatments but also risky ones out of desperation. Many of the alternative and unconventional therapies do not fit the Western medical paradigm. More research is needed to evaluate the most widely used modalities. Although it is impossible to describe all the modalities used in alternative medicine, a few have been arbitrarily selected and are discussed here.

Music Therapy

In a study of 30 women with chronic pain secondary to rheumatoid arthritis, Schorr[10] demonstrated that chronic pain may be effectively controlled using music as a unitary-transformative intervention. Pain measurements used in the study were obtained from the Pain Rating Index rank (PRI-R) of the McGill Pain Questionnaire. Hanser[11] also described the effective use of music as a distraction during lumbar punctures. Unfortunately, this study was a series of anecdotal reports and was not a scientifically conducted investigation. Nevertheless, it is reasonable to propose that for some patients with well-defined disorders, music therapy may not be effective by itself but can be a useful adjunct to conventional modalities for pain management.

Intercessionary Prayer and Spiritual Healing

Several claims have been made regarding the effectiveness of intercessionary prayer, spiritual healing, divine intercessions, and meditation in controlling chronic pain.[12] Certainly, it is not good medical practice for providers to be arbitrary about patients' respective spiritual or religious persuasions. In fact, those persuasions may be passively supported as long as they do not interfere with the delivery of medical care necessary for treatment. Many anecdotal reports regarding the efficacy of those modalities have been made, but few scientifically controlled studies have been done to determine efficacy.

Sundblom et al,[13] in a well-conducted clinical trial, demonstrated that spiritual healing was not only harmless but also subjectively helpful in managing patients with idiopathic chronic pain syndrome. In this study, 24 patients with idiopathic chronic pain were randomly assigned to 1 of 2 groups. One group received spiritual healing, and the other received no active treatment. All patients had passed a pretreatment psychological interview. The main outcome measures used included Visual Analog Scale, International Association for the Study of Pain (IASP) database outline, and various psychological measures. Patients were evaluated at baseline and 2 weeks after treatment and were studied over 1½ years. A final assessment was performed at 1 year after treatment using a modified IASP database outline, and it revealed a minor decrease in analgesic drug intake and an improvement in the sleep pattern in patients treated by the spiritual healer. The group exposed to spiritual healing also experienced a decrease in the feeling of hopelessness and an increased acceptance of psychological factors as reasons for pain. One half of the treated patients believed that spiritual healing gave them satisfactory pain relief. Although this therapeutic approach is not effective for everyone, for selected patients, particularly those with terminal illness, spiritual healing may be used as an adjunct to conventional treatment if the patient or the family requests it.

Relaxation Therapy

Relaxation therapy is a well-established psychogenic modality for managing chronic pain. Several variations of relaxation strategies have been used. Jacobson's progressive muscle relaxation techniques[14] have been widely used to manage chronic pain syndromes, particularly myofascial pain syndromes, including low back pain.

The use of relaxation to promote comfort and pain relief in patients suffering from advanced cancer pain was demonstrated to be effective by Sloman et al.[15] Relaxation strategies, including deep breathing, muscle relaxation, and imagery, were tested as a nursing intervention for the promotion of comfort and pain relief in a group of hospitalized cancer patients. This intervention was implemented in accordance with Oren's self-care approach to nursing practice. Sixty-seven cancer patients were randomly assigned to 1 of 3 groups to receive relaxation training by audiotapes, live relaxation training by nurses, or no relaxation training at all. The relaxation training was administered twice a week over a 3-week period. All patients were tested before and after the study using the McGill Pain Questionnaire and the Visual Analog Scale for pain. Analgesic medication administered to the patients who received relaxation training led to significant reduction in subjective pain ratings, and nonopioid, as-needed (prn) analgesic intake also decreased significantly, a probable reflection of a reduced incidence of breakthrough pain. The study suggests that relaxation techniques can be effective in management of chronic cancer pain, especially when the techniques are used concurrently with conventional modalities.

Hypnosis

Until recently, certain modalities were considered unconventional. With their widespread acceptance not only by the patient population but also by the medical establishment, these formerly unconventional modalities have now become conventional. Unfortunately, at times they have not undergone the clinical trials necessary to be considered truly conventional. Hypnosis and acupuncture may fall into this category.

Some well-established medical interventions, including surgical procedures, would not be used in clinical practice today if rigorous clinical trials had been instituted. A good example is the use of epidural steroids for chronic diskogenic back pain. The use of epidural steroids rapidly became widespread, although few well-conducted scientific studies were carried out to evaluate the efficacy of this approach.[16] Hypnosis has been used with sufficient frequency to warrant investigation. Unfortunately, some providers of hypnotic therapy are not necessarily competent in the method's principles, applications, and nuances.[17] This is precisely the danger of using a modality that has not been rigorously subjected to peer review evaluations. Hypnotherapy or hypnotic relaxation has been used as a sedative for medical procedures such as colonoscopy. Although colonoscopy is not exquisitely painful, it is associated with significant emotional and physical discomfort.

Cadranel et al[18] investigated the usefulness of hypnotic relaxation in 24 patients scheduled for colonoscopy in whom other forms of anesthesia were not available. Using hypnotic relaxation before the procedure resulted in moderate to deep sedation in 12 of the 24 patients. In the patients for whom hypnosis was successful, the pain and discomfort from the colonoscopy were less intense than in the patients for whom hypnosis was unsuccessful. All patients who received successful hypnotherapy were able to undergo colonoscopy uneventfully, whereas only 50% of the patients who did not receive hypnotic relaxation were able to undergo the procedure. All the patients in the successful group agreed to another examination under the same conditions using hypnotic relaxation, whereas only 2% of the patients in the unsuccessful group agreed to have hypnotic relaxation as the primary means of sedation after their experience. This study suggests that in a subgroup of hypnotizable patients, hypnotic relaxation may be a safe alternative to drug sedation for colonoscopy and related procedures.

Chiropractic Therapy

The use of chiropractic therapy is widespread in the United States and is legal. No doubt it has a place in the management of musculoskeletal dysfunction and various myofascial pain syndromes. This modality has continued to develop, and, properly conducted, it can be effective. Although research into chiropractic therapy is not very widespread, the method is said to be much more effective than other conservative approaches, including bed rest, medication, physical therapy, and massage therapy.

Unfortunately, in many instances chiropractic practitioners and medical practitioners have not been able to work together for the good of the patient with chronic musculoskeletal dysfunction. Indeed, inappropriately applied and incompetently administered, chiropractic therapy can be dangerous in some patients and may lead to a worsening of the patient's general condition. A classic case in point is the application of chiropractic measures for the management of back pain in a patient not recognized as having multiple myeloma or metastatic prostate cancer. By the time the misdiagnosis is recognized, major and irreversible harm may be done. In an ideal situation, chiropractic therapy would be administered to a patient in conjunction with and concurrent with conventional medical treatment.

Comfort Measures

In addition to its being a science, medicine is also an art. In today's busy practice, physicians may appear to be uncaring, arrogant, and inattentive to a patient's real needs. The application of comfort measures goes a long way toward making patients feel comfortable and optimizing their immunosuppressant mechanisms to promote rapid healing and recuperation.[19]

Buchko et al[20] demonstrated that comfort measures in breast-feeding primiparous women are very effective in treating postpartum nipple pain. This same principle may be applied to numerous relatively minor but uncomfortable procedures such as bone marrow biopsy, burn dressing changes, acquisition of vascular access, and cataract surgery. When properly applied, these comfort measures may obviate the need for pharmacologic intervention and may help to introduce a soft touch into a medical experience that may appear cold and uncaring.

Transcutaneous Electrical Nerve Stimulation

Initially, transcutaneous electrical nerve stimulation (TENS)[21] was thought of as a primitive alternative therapy modality. Its popularity increased after the publication of the gate control theory by Melzack and Wall.[22] In fact, a proposed mechanism of action is that electrical stimulation of A-alpha and A-beta fibers suppresses nociception transmitted by A-delta and C fibers. Many published studies have shown the efficacy of TENS in the management of large numbers of pain syndromes,[23] including myofascial, neuropathic, and cancer pain.[24] Today, TENS is no longer considered an alternative modality and is, in fact, well established as a conventional medical modality for the treatment of chronic pain.[25] Two other variants of TENS that have not been well studied are high-frequency external muscle stimulation (HF) and percutaneous electrical nerve stimulation (PENS).

Acupuncture

Acupuncture has been used for more than 2000 years. It is based on various Chinese scientific principles that are not understood or taught in most Western medical systems, including the United States. Many publications have attested to the efficacy of acupuncture,[26] and it is clear that acupuncture does control pain in selected patients. However, patient selection must be meticulous because some patients are more predisposed to benefit from acupuncture than are others. Many other intrinsic factors contribute to the success or failure of acupuncture.[27] The tragedy of acupuncture in the United States or in a Western context is that very few practitioners are adequately trained to use this modality effectively.

Biostimulation Techniques

Biostimulation techniques include the following:

- Acupressure
- Auriculotherapy
- Vibration therapy
- Magnetic field therapy
- Low-power laser stimulation
- Movement therapy

A major reason for the popularity of these modalities is that they are usually noninvasive and, in appropriate patients, may be beneficial adjuncts to conventional therapy. In a study of 24 patients with chronic pain, Guieu et al[28] demonstrated that TENS therapy and vibration therapy, whether used singly or jointly, were more effective in providing long-lasting analgesia as compared with sham stimulation or placebo.

Magnetic Field Therapy

First proposed by Franz Mesmer of Austria, magnetic stimuli and magnetic fields have been used medicinally since the 16th century. Mesmer's theories were investigated by a Royal Commission chaired by Lavoisier, whose recommendations were not favorable to the continued use of magnetic therapy. Since that time, magnetic field therapy has been practiced mainly by charlatans.

In the early twentieth century, orthopedic surgeons often used magnetic therapy to correct malunion of long bone fractures. At that time, it was safer to use magnetic therapy than orthopedic surgery for long bone fractures, which were usually associated with osteomyelitis. Many claims have been made regarding the efficacy of magnetic field blocks and magnetic fields,[29] but these have not been evaluated scientifically.

To determine the efficacy of magnetic fields, Parris et al[30] investigated the chronic pain animal model (rat) using the sciatic nerve ligation or chronic constriction injury. The objective was to determine whether repeated pulsating magnetic field therapy (PMFT) would affect hyperalgesia and spinal cord, brain, and plasma levels of substance P, met-enkephalin, and dynorphin after chronic constriction injury of the rat sciatic nerve. In this study, the rats were exposed daily to 180 g and 30 Hz for 1 hour. Control rats were exposed to a device in which the magnetic fields were not activated. The magnetic fields significantly increased the delay of hind paw withdrawal and decreased the duration of the evaluation on the side of the chronic constriction injury. Magnetic field therapy did not alter the behavioral pain response in sham rats. The findings also demonstrated that dynorphin levels were greatly elevated in the spinal cord on the side of the constriction injury as compared with the contralateral (unligated) side in animals with chronic constriction injury. No significant changes were noticed in met-enkephalin and substance P levels.

The study showed that magnetic field therapy reduces hyperalgesia induced by chronic constriction injury of the sciatic nerve in the rat model of chronic pain. These basic science studies are important to help investigate purported mechanisms of analgesia in various alternative modalities. Furthermore, this study suggests that magnetic field therapy may be effective in various forms of neuropathic pain.

Low-Power Laser Therapy

Parris et al,[31] using the same animal model described for magnetic field therapy, investigated the effect of low-power laser on neuropathic pain. No biochemical or behavioral changes resulted. This finding illustrated that low-power laser therapy is not effective for neuropathic pain; however, this modality has been effective for myofascial pain.[32]

Conclusion

Conventional medicine teaches that it is reasonable and prudent to reexamine and reuse old techniques and old drugs for new applications. Examples of these principles include the use of aspirin not only for the prevention of heart disease but also for the management of myocardial infarction. The use of gabapentin, an anticonvulsant and antidepressant medication, to treat chronic neuropathic pain syndrome is another example of that principle.

As investigators evaluate new techniques and new drugs, it is also appropriate to evaluate alternative medicine practices. This assessment must be done scientifically and fairly, however, not in response to commercial interests but in accordance with scientific principles. To accomplish that goal, the Office of Alternative Medicine has been invaluable, not only to the field of pain medicine but also to patients in general. Many aspects of conventional and traditional medicine possibly would be condemned if they were subjected to rigorous scientific scrutiny. The scientific evaluation of alternative medicine may reveal tremendous benefits to patients with chronic pain. It is hoped that just as regulations and safeguards exist for conventional medicine, similar governmental safeguards and regulations will govern alternative and complementary medicine. In this ideal scenario, the appropriate federal, state, and local societies, the different medical organizations, the Food and Drug Administration, and the various agencies within the Department of Health and Human Services, the Drug Enforcement Agency, and the other centers and divisions of the NIH will help to support the burgeoning field of alternative medicine using their respective expertise, to ensure that patients are not exploited but, instead, are served with some degree of efficiency and integrity. Although practitioners of alternative medicine have no rigid guidelines to follow at present, ideally some regulation will be provided under the leadership of responsible clinical organizations and with direct, or indirect, governmental oversight.

The future appears bright for alternative medicine. It is hoped that, with an unbiased, creative, and honest approach to evaluating alternative medicine modalities, beneficial agents and techniques will be promoted so that patients with chronic pain unresponsive to conventional therapeutic modalities may have the option of using approved alternative medicine modalities for pain control.

References

Full references for this chapter can be found on www.expertconsult.com.

Limitations of Pharmacologic Pain Management

Richard B. Patt and Steven D. Waldman

Risk-to-Benefit Ratio

All medical interventions are associated with risks and benefits that, when considered together, constitute that intervention's *risk-to-benefit ratio*. Alternatives exist for all interventions (including no intervention), and these alternatives also possess their own risk-to-benefit ratios. Clinical decision making involves comparing and contrasting the risk-to-benefit ratios of alternative interventions *(relative risk-to-benefit ratio)*.

The risk-to-benefit ratio is multiply determined and is usually inexact. It is, in part, intrinsic to a given therapy, and it also, in part, depends on the clinical situation for which treatment is under consideration. How the risk-to-benefit ratio is determined or interpreted is influenced by numerous factors, some of which are difficult to quantitate (e.g., provider bias, patient preference) or have an ambiguous value (e.g., cost, patient suffering). As a result, the perceived risk-to-benefit ratio may differ profoundly based on interrelated factors pertinent to the patient (e.g., age, overall health, functional status, ethnocultural and religious background), the physician (e.g., attitudes, beliefs, training, financial incentives), and the system (e.g., regulatory forces, facilities, economic factors). The risk-to-benefit ratio is not a fixed entity but instead varies as these factors and their relationships with each other change over time. This situation is further complicated when applied to the treatment of pain because as a result of the subjective nature of pain and the newness of pain management as a specialty, data regarding the outcomes of even accepted interventions are scarce. In the past, this allowed for wide latitude in decision making. However, increased scrutiny of health care costs is likely to be associated with greater constraints on decision making.

Pharmacologic Dichotomy: Cancer Pain and Chronic Nonmalignant Pain

Cultural and social forces have profound influences on therapeutic decision making regarding the treatment of pain with medications. A curious but contextually understandable dichotomy exists with respect to the treatment of pain of malignant versus nonmalignant origin with opioid analgesics.[1]

Cancer Pain

Until relatively recently, opioids were avoided for all but the most desperate medical conditions. This stigmatization was based more on cultural bias than on medical fact. Initiatives emphasizing the concept of comprehensive cancer care mandate attention to symptom control throughout the course of a malignant illness.[2] Contemporary approaches to managing pain in cancer patients emphasize earlier and more liberal use of opioids, and investigators cite a low potential for addiction and a generally favorable risk-to-benefit ratio.[3,4] A review of the literature suggests that these principles are grounded firmly in science.

Chronic Pain

Opioids were long considered taboo as treatment for chronic nonmalignant pain.[5,6] These concerns were mostly grounded in beliefs about the inevitability of addiction and typically reflected not just medical concerns but moral views as well. In light of data generated by opioid use in cancer pain, the prohibition of opioid therapy for noncancer pain has been called into question. A spectrum of opinion currently exists regarding the advisability and proper methodology for prescribing opioids in such patients. Although both proponents and detractors cite data that support opposing views, investigators agree that opioid therapy is more beneficial than harmful in a proportion of patients with chronic nonmalignant pain. Although reasonable scientific support exists for this general contention, support for guidelines to determine the risk-to-benefit ratio prospectively in individual cases remains empirical.[7,8]

Role of Invasive Procedures

In the treatment of both cancer and noncancer pain, evidence-based support of the role of interventional pain-relieving modalities is less well defined than is support for the use of drugs. The situation is analogous to that of opioids for nonmalignant pain. Although fairly widespread agreement exists that procedures sometimes possess favorable risk-to-benefit ratios, a uniformly accepted, validated methodology is lacking for prospectively determining which settings are valuable for certain procedures.

Cancer Pain

Although the use of interventional pain management modalities in the treatment of cancer pain has been well accepted in the clinical arena for decades, the more recent aggressive use of systemic opioids and adjuvant analgesics combined with the increased use of the spinal administration of opioids has reduced the frequency of neurodestructive procedures in the management of cancer pain.[9,10] Certain procedures, such as celiac plexus neurolysis, radiofrequency lesioning of intercostals nerves, transsphenoidal pituitary neurolysis, and gasserian ganglion neurolysis continue to have a significant place in cancer pain management.[11,12]

Chronic Pain

Debate over the role of interventional procedures for chronic nonmalignant pain is, if possible, even more contentious that the debate over the use of these modalities for cancer pain management. Evidence has been cited supporting diametrically opposed views, and the quality of such evidence has legitimately been questioned. Factors influencing this debate are as noted previously but also include bias (even rivalry) among specialists, third-party and governmental payers, financial stake, and opiophobia. Limited reasonable agreement remains among these parties regarding when, and in whom, certain procedures provide sufficiently meaningful and durable pain relief to justify their risks and costs. Agreement exists that the outcomes for procedures are most favorable when they are "properly" integrated within a multidisciplinary matrix, although the evidence for even this conventional wisdom is questionable. Because of the subjective nature of pain and the difficulty in blinding subjects to the administration or withholding of local anesthetics in nerve blocks, evidence-based outcomes will continue to remain elusive, although downward pressure on health care spending may make the matter moot.

Advantages of Pharmacotherapy for Cancer Pain

For various reasons, oral opioid therapy is considered the treatment of choice for uncomplicated cancer pain. These reasons include the induction of analgesia that is reversible, titratable, and suitable for different types of pain, including multiple topographically distinct pains, generalized pain, and lack of invasiveness. Furthermore, the risk-to-benefit ratio of properly administered opioid therapy in this clinical setting further promotes its use.[13] The need for specialized training is modest, and efficacy is maintained when treatment is modified to apply to individuals across cultures and over a range of ages and medical fitness.[14]

Limitations of Pharmacotherapy for Cancer Pain

In 70% or more of cancer patients, pain relief is known to be achieved with uncomplicated oral or transdermal administration of opioids, especially when combined with nonsteroidal antiinflammatory drugs (NSAIDs) and adjuvant analgesics (e.g., antidepressants, anticonvulsants). Up to 30% of all patients with cancer pain, however, require alternative interventions to achieve comfort. The construct that opioids should be administered in doses sufficient either to control cancer pain or to produce unacceptable side effects is widely accepted because this class of drugs has no ceiling effect, unlike the NSAIDs and most adjuvant analgeics.[9,13,15] Although the end points of opioid therapy (i.e., comfort and unacceptable side effects) are difficult to quantify, this view recognizes unacceptable side effects as one possible consequence of drug therapy. These side effects constitute the most important limitations of drug therapy for cancer pain.

Several investigators have attempted to identify specific clinical findings that, when identified prospectively, signal that pain relief will be difficult to achieve by pharmacologic means alone. The best validated schema, the Edmonton Staging System, suggests that the presence of a history of alcohol or drug abuse or recent tolerance, neuropathic pain, psychological distress, and movement-related pain predict a relatively poorer prognosis for controlling pain pharmacologically, whereas drug dose and the presence of delirium are not predictive.[16–18] Other investigations suggest that incident and movement-related pain (kinesophobia) is the only consistent predictor of poor outcome for pharmacotherapy.[19,20] This constitutes an extremely important area for further study, especially with methodologies that target specific clinical pain syndromes. Experience suggests that syndromes such as tumor-mediated brachial and lumbosacral plexopathy, abdominopelvic pain, and pain from the skin ulceration that accompanies fungating tumors are among other daunting syndromes in which pain often persists despite aggressive drug therapy. Although no single feature reliably predicts failure of pharmacotherapy, the presence of these features should alert the clinician that additional resources may be needed to help manage pain effectively.

Limitations of Pharmacotherapy for Noncancer Pain

The historical view that the use of opioids was prima facie undesirable for the management of chronic pain allowed for a ready determination of risk-to-benefit ratio, no matter how unscientific. Contemporary views that opioid therapy for noncancer pain is justified in selected patients call for a general reappraisal of risk-to-benefit ratio and carefully individualized decision making.[21]

The baseline limitations of drug therapy for nonmalignant pain include the same potential side effects that restrict drug use in cancer patients. Additional limitations in this population depend on the degree to which a given patient is perceived as being at risk for addiction and the degree to which the practitioner perceives opioid therapy as being potentially effective and appropriate.[22–25]

Specific Limitations
Dose-Limiting Side Effects

One set of limitations relates to the various collateral (nonanalgesic) effects of the analgesics. The most prominent side effects of the opioids are constipation, nausea, vomiting, cognitive failure (ranging from drowsiness to hallucinations), dysphoria, myoclonus, and pruritus, although other side effects such as respiratory depression occasionally supervene.[3,13,20] Similarly, treatment with the NSAIDs and other adjuvants is limited by undesirable pharmacologic side effects such as gastropathy, bleeding, renal insufficiency, masking of fever, sedation, constipation, dry mouth, dysrhythmias, cognitive failure, ataxia, hepatic insufficiency, and bone marrow depression.[15]

Drug side effects, especially opioid, can often be managed effectively.[13,20,26] Strategies for managing opioid side effects in cancer patients are depicted in **Table 128.1**. Side effects of simple analgesics, NSAIDs, and adjuvant analgesics may be more problematic and are in many cases less readily reversible.[15,27–30] Thus, an important distinction between the opioids and other analgesics is that opioids have few absolute contraindications, whereas the other analgesics often need to be avoided altogether lest complications occur (e.g., aspirin in the patient with an ulcer, hypersensitivity, or bone marrow depression).[27] Paradoxically, for long-term use, the opioids are both the most stigmatized of all analgesics and, on a physiologic basis, arguably the safest.

Specific Situations

Besides the general category of dose-limiting side effects, certain clinical situations impose specific limitations or increased risks from pharmacotherapy. Only a few such issues are cited here.

Neuropathic Pain

Somatic and visceral nociceptive pain typically responds linearly to escalating doses of opioid analgesics. In contrast, the dose-response relationship for neuropathic pain is often

Table 128.1 Strategies for Limiting the Side Effects of Opioids	
Strategy	**Comments**
Prophylaxis	This approach is used especially for constipation and sometimes for nausea
Patient education	Informed of the potential for side effects, patients are less likely to assume they are allergic and more likely to cooperate with efforts at palliation
Patience	Nausea and sedation are usually transitory and remit with time
	Slower titration may reduce troublesome side effects
Symptomatic management	Treat with antiemetics, laxatives, psychostimulants, etc.
Trials of alternative (related) analgesics	Efficacy: side effect profile of opioids is often idiosyncratic
	Trials of alternative opioids are indicated because of incomplete cross-tolerance
Trials of adjuvant analgesics	Side effects may result from reliance on opioids for a pain syndrome that is relatively nonresponsive to opioids
	Successful therapy with adjuvants may allow for a reduction in opioid dose with fewer side effects
Alternate treatment modalities	Judicious application of antitumor therapy, procedures, psychotherapy, etc., may permit dose reductions with fewer attendant side effects

blunted. Treatment in higher dose ranges is required, as a result of which side effects are more likely to be problematic. Although neuropathic pain syndromes were once considered an opioid-nonresponsive set of disorders, the range of response observed for these syndromes forms the basis for the concept of relative responsivity to opioids.[31,32] Increasingly, neuropathic pain syndromes are successfully treated by an approach that uses maintenance therapy with low-dose opioids for the induction of partial analgesia, after which sequential trials of adjuvant analgesics are conducted in an effort to gain more complete analgesia.[27–32]

Movement-Related Pain (Breakthrough or Incident Pain)

The tempo of chronic pain is most often one of continuous, unrelenting, low-grade basal pain, punctuated by episodic exacerbations that can be unpredictable but that are most often related to activity. These superimposed flares are generally referred to as *breakthrough pain*.[33] The basal component of pain is typically treated with a long-acting opioid administered on a time-contingent basis (by the clock), such as an oral controlled-release formulation of morphine or oxycodone administered every 12 hours, a transdermal preparation of fentanyl applied every 72 hours, or—less commonly—methadone. Breakthrough pain is then treated with the symptom-contingent administration of a second, short-acting oral opioid administered as needed (immediate-release morphine sulfate, hydromorphone, oxycodone, or oral transmucosal fentanyl citrate [OMFC]). The dose of long-acting medication is then titrated based on the frequency and urgency of the requirement for as-required treatment of breakthrough pain.

Breakthrough pain that has a relatively consistent temporal relationship with specific activities has come to be referred to as *incident pain*.[19,20] Breakthrough pain that occurs at predictable intervals just before the next scheduled dose of an analgesic drug is referred to as *end-of-dose failure*. Breakthrough pain that appears to be idiosyncratic and unrelated to either activity or scheduled doses of analgesics is typically referred to as either *spontaneous breakthrough pain* or *idiopathic breakthrough pain*, or simply as *breakthrough pain*.

Pain that is exacerbated with movement is among the most difficult to control with analgesics.[20] The pharmacokinetic properties of currently available drugs, even those administered intravenously, are not well matched to the often unpredictable, rapid, and wide fluctuations in severity of movement-related pain.

When incident pain is relatively unpredictable, rescue doses are provided prophylactically, approximately 30 minutes in advance of the pain-provoking activity. When unanticipated breakthrough pain occurs, the rescue dose should be taken as soon after onset as possible, independent of the timing of the basal dose. If these strategies are unsuccessful, the clinician should consider a trial of an alternative short-acting opioid or a change in the route of administration. Breakthrough pain that is predictable, infrequent, of mild or moderate intensity, or slow to develop can often be managed effectively with oral analgesics such as immediate-release (IR) morphine, hydromorphone, or oxycodone. Breakthrough pain that is severe or that occurs unpredictably, frequently, or precipitously may not be adequately relieved with currently available oral agents. Although intravenous and subcutaneous opioids are pharmacokinetically well suited for labile or severe breakthrough pain, these advantages are offset by the invasiveness of the route of administration.

OTFC, a newer formulation of the established opioid analgesic fentanyl, has been approved specifically for the treatment of breakthrough pain that arises in patients already using around-the-clock opioids.[34] A sweetened fentanyl-impregnated lozenge mounted on a stick, it is a noninvasive means of delivering a potent lipophilic opioid through the oral mucosa, thus facilitating rapid absorption into the circulation and analgesia of relatively fast onset and short duration. Extensive controlled research was conducted on the use of OTFC as a specific remedy for breakthrough pain. This research confirmed the safety of this agent and demonstrated its superior efficacy to routine oral agents in cancer patients receiving concomitant therapy with immediate-release and controlled-release oral opioids for basal pain. The onset of meaningful analgesia typically occurs within 5 minutes of beginning consumption of a unit, peaks approximately 30 minutes later, and usually lasts approximately 4 hours. The duration of analgesia is slightly prolonged because approximately one half of each fentanyl dose is inevitably swallowed and is subjected to hepatic first-pass effect. The availability of fentanyl in a lozenge form allows for easy self-administration and permits patients to titrate the dose to an effective level of analgesia without the need for injections. An intranasal formulation of fentanyl may be a reasonable alternative that may have a faster onset of action.[35]

Even with this addition to the treatment armamentarium, prominent incident pain remains a treatment challenge because opioid requirements vary dramatically over short intervals. Doses of opioids required to treat pain during periods of rest are typically inadequate when activity increases, and, conversely, doses required to ease movement-related pain may produce sedation and other side effects when the provocative activity decreases.

Narrow Therapeutic Window: Cachexia and Advanced Age

Although many patients with cancer are not candidates for curative therapy, palliative and supportive care may extend life. Pharmacologically based pain control is often more difficult to achieve in patients with advanced cancer because concomitant asthenia and cachexia increase the likelihood of side effects from opioids titrated to therapeutic effect *(narrow therapeutic window)*. The sedative effects of opioids can often be countered by the judicious use of psychostimulants, such as methylphenidate, which are usually administered at starting doses of 10 mg on awakening and 10 mg at the noon meal and can be titrated to effect.[36] Although dysrhythmias and anorexia are theoretical concerns, they are rarely problematic, although psychostimulants should be avoided in the presence of an anxiety disorder or brain metastases.

Limited epidemiologic data suggest that chronic pain is about twice as common for geriatric individuals living in residential settings than in their younger counterparts; the incidence in older persons ranges from 25% to 50%.[37] Although underrecognition and undertreatment of pain in nursing homes are so rampant that statistics are often misleading, targeted surveys reveal an incidence ranging from 45% to 80%.

Degenerative arthritis and other musculoskeletal disorders are the most prominent sources of pain in older patients, although herpes zoster, decubitus ulcers, peripheral vascular disease, temporal arteritis, and polymyalgia rheumatica are disproportionately common with advanced age.[38-40] Because the incidence of almost all malignant diseases increases with advancing age, oncologic pain is a particularly common problem in the geriatric population. It is an especially important problem because many of the factors that cause cancer pain to be undertreated in the general population are amplified in aging patients.

Although some degree of age-associated changes in organ function (including the central nervous system) are ubiquitous, with a few exceptions these changes ordinarily exert little influence on pain threshold or pain tolerance, although pharmacodynamics or pharmacokinetics may be somewhat altered. Loss of neuronal tissue and proliferation of glial cells occur with advancing age, but no evidence indicates impairment in processing pain signals unless dementia or delirium is clinically evident. Clinical lore suggesting that older patients do not experience pain as keenly as their younger counterparts is unfounded and is often no more than a rationalization for an unwillingness to spend the added time often required in assessing the older patient.

The hospice experience has demonstrated that, when appropriate time and effort are applied, pain can usually be managed effectively even in the frail, older patient. However, drug titration should be performed with considerable caution, and, when possible, polypharmacy should be avoided.[41]

Suffering

Pain is determined in multiple ways and often persists as a result of unidentified psychosocial causes. Analgesics themselves are unlikely to reduce complaints of pain that are rooted in more global suffering. Psychotropic drugs combined with psychotherapy may, however, be effective in this setting.

Abdominopelvic Pain

Factors specific to patients with abdominopelvic pain that reduce the likelihood of attaining adequate pain control with systemic analgesics alone are listed in **Table 128.2**. NSAIDs, even of the cyclooxygenase-2–selective type, may be poorly tolerated or contraindicated owing to gastropathy and to general factors such as renal insufficiency, coagulopathy, bone marrow

Table 128.2 Potential Limitations of the Pharmacologic Management of Abdominopelvic Pain

Treatment Modality	Limitations
Nonsteroidal anti-inflammatory drugs	Gastropathy Renal dysfunction Bone marrow depletion Concerns about masking fever
Oral analgesics	Xerostomia Dysphagia Malabsorption Obstruction Nausea Vomiting Coma
Transdermal analgesics	Dose requirements for opioids possibly exceeding limitations of dose form
Parenteral analgesics	Inadequate household or community support to manage infusions
Opioids	Ileus Partial obstruction Intractable constipation Reduced responsivity resulting from neuropathic component of pain Dose-limiting side effects resulting from asthenia and cachexia

suppression, and masking of fever. The oral route may be unreliable in the presence of gastrointestinal dysfunction (e.g., dysphagia, malabsorption, intestinal obstruction, nausea and vomiting, xerostomia, coma). Reduced gastrointestinal motility is a common upshot of tumor encroachment or a sequela of surgery or radiation therapy. Even with a strict bowel protocol, opioids may exacerbate ileus or partial obstruction in patients with reduced motility. In such cases, the use of opioids, except in low doses, is undesirable. Although visceral pain is relatively opioid responsive, patients often present with pain of mixed causes. Typically, pain resulting from nerve injury (neuropathic pain) is less sensitive to opioids, and thus occult microscopic deposits of perineural tumor invasion may contribute to reduced opioid responsivity. Early use of alternative routes of administration (e.g., transdermal, intranasal) may help to avoid many of the problems associated with abdominopelvic pain.[34,35] Splanchnic, celiac plexus, and hypogastric plexus blocks are especially useful in this patient population.[12,42]

Conclusion

Notwithstanding the controversy on opioids for chronic pain, data support the primary role of pharmacotherapy for managing most pain syndromes. Some patients do not derive adequate comfort from systemic drug therapy alone, however, or are not candidates for liberal use of opioids. Even for cancer pain, when addiction is less of a concern and liberal prescribing is widely endorsed, physiologic and psychological features sometimes hinder achieving an adequate pharmacologic remedy.

The most formidable limitations of drug treatment relate to their potential to produce pharmacologic side effects or complications. Careful monitoring and the use of strategies for preventing and managing drug side effects are often all that is required to maintain efficacy. Specific patient-related factors (e.g., neuropathic pain, movement-related pain, psychological distress, cachexia, alterations in gastrointestinal function) are associated with greater likelihood of limitations. The degree to which a selected drug's potential to induce habituation is an impediment to long-term use remains a topic of considerable and heated debate.

References

Full references for this chapter can be found on www.expertconsult.com.

Part B

Psychological and Behavioral Modalities for Pain and Symptom Management

Chapter **129**

Psychological Interventions

Jennifer B. Levin and Jeffrey W. Janata

A review of the understanding of pain throughout history suggests that theorists have vacillated between definitions that emphasize emotional aspects of pain and definitions that promote a more sensory, physiologic view. Aristotle believed that pain is a "passion of the soul," an affective experience. Aristotle's view was generally embraced until Descartes proposed that pain is a pure sensory phenomenon, a view that has persisted, aided by the rapid advances in medical understanding of sensory systems.[1] Currently accepted definitions of pain recognize the emotional and sensory elements; it is almost impossible to read a pain text without being reminded that the International Association for the Study of Pain defined *chronic pain* as "an unpleasant sensory and emotional experience associated with actual or potential tissue damage."[2]

Current practice often fails to adequately address these psychological aspects of chronic pain. This chapter describes the emotional and behavioral components of chronic pain. It reviews the psychotherapeutic strategies that can be combined with rehabilitative, medical, and interventional procedures. It also describes patients' obstacles to engaging in treatment and presents evidence for the effectiveness of including psychotherapy as an integral part of a comprehensive approach to the management of chronic pain.

Psychological Aspects of Chronic Pain

Pain and Depression

Pain and depression are among the most common conditions seen by practitioners. At any given time, it is estimated that 17% of patients seen in primary care complain of persistent pain.[3] Furthermore, approximately 13% of adults in the United States lose productive work time as a function of a pain problem; this problem has a $61 billion economic impact on productivity alone.[4] Depression often goes undiagnosed or is inadequately treated in this large group of patients and can impede the effective treatment of pain.[5] Experienced pain clinicians attest to the frequency with which patients with chronic pain present with concurrent depressive symptoms. Studies have shown prevalence rates for depression in chronic pain to range from 10% to 100%,[6] but most find that coexisting depression is at the higher end of probability and is the most frequent psychiatric diagnosis to accompany chronic pain.[7] Depression is more common than anxiety or personality disorders in patients who develop opioid dependency,[8] and depression has been found to play an influential role in the development of chronic pain and disability.[9]

Criteria from the *Diagnostic and Statistical Manual of Mental Disorders,* fourth edition, text revision, for diagnosing depression[10] include marked changes in mood, anhedonia, insomnia or hypersomnia, weight loss or gain, fatigue, psychomotor retardation or agitation, difficulty with concentration or indecisiveness, feelings of worthlessness and guilt, and thoughts of death and suicidal ideation. *Anhedonia* is the loss of interest in things or activities that previously were pleasurable. Anhedonia often is reported by patients with pain, who describe that the pairing of pleasurable activities with pain renders the activities far less pleasurable and, as a result, much less likely to be pursued. Lewinsohn and Gotlib[11] suggested that symptoms of depression may be related to the loss of positive reinforcement that pleasurable activities provide. Loss of activities, of interests, and of the often social context in which the activities are enjoyed may contribute to the depression experienced by patients with pain. Research evidence supports this relationship; a path analysis in an older population showed that pain contributes to activity restriction, which contributes to the development of depressive symptoms.[12]

Insomnia is a common complaint in patients with chronic pain; studies suggest that insomnia accompanies pain in 50% to 88% of patients with various pain conditions.[13,14] Patients with chronic pain often complain that their pain interferes with the quality of their sleep, and clinicians naturally may attribute sleep dysregulation solely to the painful condition and may overlook the possibility that sleep problems may be symptomatic of depression. Patients with depression and insomnia experience greater affective distress, reduced sense of control, and greater pain severity. Insomnia without concurrent depression was found to be associated with increased levels of pain,[15] and evidence indicates that sleep deprivation produces hyperalgesic changes. Sleep deprivation may impede the analgesic effects of opioids and of the serotonin reuptake inhibitor class of antidepressants.[16]

Evidence suggests that although patients complain to clinicians most prominently about pain, often their less emphasized depressive issues are causing patients the greatest distress. A study of patients with facial pain found that depressive symptoms correlated more highly with psychosocial and physical functioning than did pain.[17] This study highlights the concern that clinicians may focus on treating the pain complaints while overlooking the depressive issues. As a patient's distress persists, clinicians are at risk to escalate the use of analgesics, which are not notably effective in ameliorating depression.

The correlation of pain and depressive symptoms begs the question of which comes first: Does depression increase one's vulnerability to developing chronic pain syndrome, or does the presence of chronic pain increase one's likelihood of becoming depressed? Gamsa,[18] in a review of the literature and study of patients with chronic pain, provided support for the notion that pain is more likely to create than be created by emotional distress. Similarly, a systematic review of the literature yielded evidence that depression is more likely a consequence than an antecedent of chronic pain.[19]

Pain and Anxiety

Studies generally have shown a high incidence of anxiety disorders in patients with chronic pain. Using a structured clinical interview, one study[20] documented an overall prevalence rate of 16% to 28% in a sample of patients with various diagnoses. Dersh et al[21] summarized research suggesting that studies that have examined the lifetime prevalence of anxiety in chronic pain found rates similar to those noted in the pain-free population. Current prevalence rates are found to be significantly higher, however, in individuals with chronic pain. Among the anxiety disorders, panic disorder and generalized anxiety disorder seem to be most commonly diagnosed.

A theory of the situational specificity of anxiety in pain was developed by Lethem et al,[22] who articulated the fear-avoidance model, which has been the subject of increased research interest. The model proposes that two factors mediate pain and disability. Fear of pain and hypervigilance to painful stimuli develop as patients attach catastrophic thoughts to the experience of pain. Subsequent avoidance of activity is driven by fear that engaging in activity would worsen pain or cause physical harm. This avoidance of activity serves as negative reinforcement of the patient's fear. Fear-avoidance beliefs and fear of movement and consequent injury have been shown to predict physical performance and disability from pain.[23]

Pain and Personality Disorders

Clinicians often find that their pain populations include a disproportionate share of difficult patients and describe personality difficulties rather than medical complexities. Researchers have examined the prevalence of character disorders in patients who complain of chronic pain. In a study of 200 patients with chronic low back pain, 51% met the criteria for one or more personality disorders. Paranoid personality disorder was diagnosed in 33% of the sample; borderline (15%), avoidant (14%), and passive-aggressive traits (12%) also were identified.[24] Gatchel et al[25] reported that 24% of their sample met the criteria for a personality disorder. A study of primary care patients who presented with a range of pain problems found that 25% of the small sample ($n = 17$) met criteria for borderline personality disorder.[26] These studies suggest that Axis II disease is considerably more prevalent in patients with chronic pain than in the population as a whole. Effective pain management in patients with comorbid personality disorders may be possible, but research into the necessary treatment adaptations is lacking.

Psychotherapeutic Approaches

Evidence-based psychotherapeutic approaches that have been shown to be effective for increasing function and decreasing levels of pain and emotional distress include the following: operant conditioning (behavioral therapy), developed in the late 1960s[27]; cognitive-behavioral therapy (CBT), which emerged in the early 1980s; and a comprehensive multimodal treatment approach[28] that integrates these treatments into interdisciplinary teams.

Operant Conditioning

The operant conditioning model is based on the principles of Fordyce et al.[29–31] These investigators noted that patients with pain exhibited numerous pain behaviors, such as guarding, pain complaints, and grimacing. They also observed that patients with chronic pain exhibited passive, maladaptive behaviors, such as excessive rest, inactivity, a reduction in family and work responsibilities, and an overreliance on pain medications. The operant model assumes that individuals behave in certain ways according to reinforcement patterns. It follows that for patients with chronic pain, maladaptive pain behaviors are positively and negatively reinforced, whereas adaptive, well behaviors are ignored and extinguished. An example of positive reinforcement is attention from a spouse or coworker; examples of negative reinforcement are avoidance of household or work responsibilities and relief from pain by reliance on as-needed pain medication. As such, the treatment for such maladaptive patterns is to identify the environmental contingencies and restructure them such that the emphasis is on reinforcing active, adaptive coping skills and ignoring maladaptive behaviors until they extinguish or remit. Therapies that rely on the operant conditioning model use graded activity, social reinforcement, time-contingent medication management, and self-control skills training including self-monitoring, self-reinforcement, and relaxation training.[32]

Studies have confirmed that operant conditioning is effective for increasing activity levels, exercise, and tolerance and for reducing the intake of pain medications. The direct effects on pain are less dramatic, however.[33]

Some researchers have noted that the efficacy of operant conditioning may have an alternate explanation—that cognition may be an active ingredient in the change process. Specifically, these investigators have suggested that the changes in environmental contingencies themselves may not be accounting for the improvement, but rather the way in which the patient perceives and interprets the changes may lead to progress.[34] The reconceptualization of the operant conditioning model relies to a large degree on a broader paradigmatic shift in clinical psychology—the shift toward CBT.

Cognitive-Behavioral Therapy

Similar to behavioral therapy, CBT uses numerous procedures to modify behavior, such as graded practice, relaxation training, homework assignments, and self-reinforcement. In contrast to behavioral therapy, CBT acknowledges the relationships among behavior, thoughts, and feelings and places an emphasis on modifying maladaptive thoughts and beliefs to alleviate emotional distress and reinforce behavior change. Although both behavioral therapy and CBT manipulate environmental contingencies, the purpose and path toward change differ. In CBT, the goal of these manipulations is to provide the patient with an opportunity to identify, question, reappraise, and restructure thoughts, feelings, behaviors, and physical sensations on which their belief system is built.

CBT for chronic pain management draws to a large degree from the treatment and research literature for depression and anxiety disorders. This affinity stems from the observation that the emotional sequelae of chronic pain often include depressive symptoms related to loss of function, sleep disturbance, and a reduction in pleasurable activities. As such, the treatment of these aspects of pain symptoms employs the same techniques as those used by classic forms of CBT that have been found to be highly efficacious. These techniques include the use of pleasure schedules and identification of negative thought patterns in conjunction with cognitive restructuring. Parallels also may be drawn between the somatic focus, fear-avoidance paradigms, and attention to danger signals central to the development and maintenance of anxiety disorders and those seen in chronic pain–based disorders. As such, the behavioral interventions, such as graded exposure and relaxation training, and the cognitive components, such as behavioral experiments, cognitive restructuring, and coping self-statements, that have been found to be efficacious in the treatment of anxiety disorders[34] can be applied effectively in the management of chronic pain.

Comprehensive Multimodal Treatment

The specific procedures and interventions used in CBT should be separated from the theory behind the cognitive-behavioral approach. The theoretical underpinnings of the approach advocate an active, structured, problem-focused, time-limited, educationally based, scientific methodology that involves collaboration between the patient and the therapist. The specific CBT multidisciplinary model for pain management as outlined by Turk and Stacey[28] includes an important team rehabilitation approach. Although only the psychological components of the treatment are reviewed here, in the multimodal approach, CBT treatment goals are addressed and reinforced across disciplines. Fear of reinjury is addressed simultaneously in CBT, physical therapy, and occupational therapy and by the treating physician. In CBT, the focus is on identifying fear beliefs and understanding the relationships among the beliefs, behavior, and emotions and developing a hierarchy of fears for graded exposure. In physical therapy and occupational therapy, the patient has the opportunity to carry out the graded exposure. Finally, in the physician-patient treatment relationship, the physician (1) reinforces the patient's active approach to pain management, (2) deemphasizes the role of narcotic and other analgesic medications, (3) eliminates as-needed medication, (4) works to stabilize the patient's sleep patterns, and (5) provides information that would contribute to more evidence-based thoughts and expectancies regarding reinjury. In this model, the consistency across modalities accounts for the added efficacy above and beyond that of single modalities.[35] Keeping this idea in mind, this chapter addresses the process of CBT as it relates to pain management.

The main objective of pain management is not to reduce pain, but rather to assist patients to learn to live healthier and more satisfying lives, despite the presence of pain and discomfort. Some pain reduction is a natural byproduct of the treatment and stems from increased conditioning and a reduction in focused attention on pain. As such, secondary goals are likely to include the following: taking more responsibility for one's health care, depending less on analgesic medication, and functioning better in occupational, familial, and social settings. The primary CBT objectives in pain management as outlined by Turk and Okifuji[36] include the following: (1) facilitating a change in approach to pain and suffering from being overwhelming and "out of my control" to manageable and "within my control"; (2) teaching coping skills for the pain and problems stemming from the pain; (3) moving from a passive, helpless role to an active, resourceful role; (4) facilitating the understanding of the relationships among thoughts, feelings, and behaviors and being able to identify and modify maladaptive patterns; (5) strengthening self-confidence and taking credit for successes; and (6) facilitating the identification of problems and proactive problem solving to bring about maintenance of gains.

The dominant theme of CBT to be reinforced across disciplines is the paradigm shift from taking a passive role, which leads to negative emotional, behavioral, and physical consequences, to taking an active role in finding the wherewithal to confront the pain and in doing so to "take back their lives." The focus is on the following: (1) developing a more internal rather than external locus of control, as defined by the perception that the individual (internal management or self-management), as opposed to outside sources (external or "fix me" approach), has control over the outcomes of his or her actions[37]; and (2) increasing self-efficacy, or an individual's belief in his or her ability to influence behavior, thoughts, and feelings[38] as they relate to pain management. These two concepts, although related, are not equivalent. To be successful, patients must maintain the belief that they hold the responsibility for their pain outcomes (internal locus of control) and develop a belief in their ability to carry out what is needed to reach the desired outcomes (self-efficacy).

Although no two CBT protocols look exactly alike, the overall conceptualization of pain and of appropriate treatment interventions has some consistency. Turk and Okifuji[36] outlined six phases of CBT, including (1) assessment, (2) reconceptualization, (3) skills acquisition and consolidation, (4) rehearsal and application training, (5) generalization and maintenance, and (6) treatment follow-up. Similarly, Bradley[39] and Johansson et al[40] identified four essential components of CBT: (1) education, (2) skills acquisition, (3) behavioral rehearsal, and (4) generalization. Given that assessment, conceptualization, and skills development are part of an ongoing process in the management of chronic pain, in this chapter four fundamental treatment components are discussed: (1) assessment and initial conceptualization, (2) moving toward a new conceptualization, (3) education and skills development, and (4) generalization and relapse prevention.

Component 1:
Assessment and Initial Conceptualization

The initial assessment incorporates information collected from the patient interview, medical records, family interview when available, and validated assessment measures. Areas for assessment include the following: (1) a complete history of the pain, including its location, severity, and duration, what has and has not been effective for the relief of pain, and patterns of pain and well behaviors including activity level and medication intake; (2) the degree and type of psychological distress, including depression, anxiety, and the relationship between pain and psychological distress; (3) behavioral patterns at home, work, and in social and recreational activities; (4) specific information regarding beliefs surrounding the pain, expectations for recovery, and functional goals; (5) a detailed work history; (6) the degree and character of social support, including the possible role of significant others in the maintenance of maladaptive behavior patterns and how to integrate these significant others into the paradigm shift; (7) addiction patterns and risk for addiction; and (8) incentives and disincentives for work, pain, and treatment, including financial consequences of long-standing pain, disability incentives for work-related injury, pending litigation, drug-seeking behavior, and legitimate release from responsibilities. From the information gathered in the assessment phase, the patient-therapist team can begin to develop a conceptualization of the role of the pain for this individual, of the way in which pain affects his or her thoughts, feelings, and behavior, and of the elements that may be maintaining the system.

Component 2:
Moving Toward a New Conceptualization

This stage, comparable to Turk and Ofikuji's[36] collaborative reconceptualization of pain, flows directly from the evidence gathered during the assessment phase. During this phase, the focus is on gradually moving the patient from a passive, helpless role in search of pain relief to an active, empowered role of increasing function and satisfaction. This paradigm shift is reinforced throughout the treatment process, starting as a concept that is discussed to one that is practiced and leads to a change in underlying beliefs about pain and the patient's role in managing it. This reconceptualization is most likely to be gradually internalized by the patient when it is adopted and reinforced by the entire treatment team, including the psychologist, physician, and rehabilitation staff. This attitude can be a particular challenge given that the physician and rehabilitation staff traditionally have approached pain management from a medical and physical perspective. To accomplish this challenging task, the CBT model first must gain acceptance from the team and requires ongoing communication among health care providers. This communication is essential because the patient naturally may fall back on the long-standing belief that pain results from purely medical causes whose management must be primarily medical. This conclusion is natural, given that the patient experiences the pain physically, but it must be disproved through the sense of efficacy and control that develops from the mastery of self-management strategies introduced early in treatment.

Component 3:
Education and Skills Development

After developing a new conceptualization of pain management, one that places the patient in the driver's seat, it is important to provide the patient with the skills to manage pain successfully. The education and skills development focus on the continuous process of providing information and a forum for the learning and practicing of new skills for pain management. The emphasis is on skills to manage, rather than decrease, pain. These skills fall into the behavioral and cognitive realms. In the behavioral category, elements are likely to include positive coping skills, relaxation training exercises, pacing, graded exposure to feared situations, attention diversion techniques, and pleasant activity scheduling. In the cognitive category, elements are likely to include cognitive restructuring, or the identification and challenging of negative thought patterns that perpetuate negative emotions and subsequent self-defeating behaviors, coping skills such as positive coping self-statements, and behavioral experiments with the goal of gathering evidence to negate unfounded cognitions. Other skills that may be the focus of attention include assertiveness training, development of communication and social skills, and problem solving. These skills are individualized according to the strengths and deficits of each individual patient. Some of these skills may be best introduced and practiced in group settings because role playing and group feedback are likely to enhance the learning experience.

Component 4:
Generalization and Relapse Prevention

During the generalization phase, the focus is on practicing the skills developed and reinforced in session and across disciplines in the home and work environments. This practice is essential to the maintenance of treatment gains. Additionally, during this phase, relapse prevention is introduced. Essential elements in this phase include the following: reviewing and integrating material covered during treatment; evaluating and reinforcing treatment gains; identifying areas in need of strengthening; discussing ways to incorporate skills into one's daily routine and how to apply them to unexpected situations, stressors, and flare-ups; and addressing potential pitfalls and how to handle them should they occur. Follow-up booster sessions are carried out with increasingly longer periods between sessions. The goal of these sessions is to let the patients practice their new skills independently between sessions and self-reinforce for their efforts, yet have a place to continue to hone their skills and receive outside feedback and reinforcement. This stage is often a major factor in relapse prevention. Frequently, the more the patient improves, the more obstacles he or she must face. Return to work may require more advanced skills than increasing functionality at home. It may be only after taking "a break from treatment" that the patient can really test out how well his or her new skills work in the real world. The application of skills in a real-life situation with limited structure is in stark contrast to the highly structured rehabilitation environment.

Treatment Effectiveness

How effective are these treatments and for whom? This discussion provides a brief overview of the efficacy research in this area. For a more comprehensive review of treatment outcomes, the reader is referred to McCracken and Turk.[41] When reviewing the efficacy data, one should take into consideration the literature's limitations, which include the heterogeneity of pain syndromes studied and variable inclusion criteria, levels of specificity with regard to treatment components, and outcome measures. Studies also differ in their control of the complexity and variability of medical treatment.

Much of the early efficacy research consisted of studies of patients with back pain; these investigators reported that operant conditioning was successful in increasing activity levels and in decreasing medication use in this population.[42–45] In an attempt to tease out which aspects of operant conditioning were effective, Lindstrom and associates[33] reported that graded activity led to a quicker return to work than did traditional medical treatment. Similarly, Turner et al[46] found that graded activity was an effective component that contributed significantly to the positive outcomes of behavioral therapy. In a review of the literature, McCracken and Turk[41] identified five different studies reporting a reduction in pain levels as a function of relaxation training. More recently, Vlaeyen et al[23] studied the effectiveness of graded exposure to feared stimuli (in this case, exposure to particular physical movements previously avoided because of fear of pain), as opposed to an activation intervention. The results indicated that the graded in vivo exposure protocol was more effective in reducing pain-related fear and disability and increasing activity level than was the activation intervention. Keefe et al[47,48] provided evidence for the efficacy of spouse-assisted treatment for improvement in pain, self-efficacy, psychological disability, and marital satisfaction.

The clinical efficacy of CBT for the management of chronic pain has been supported in numerous studies with patient populations having headache, arthritis, temporomandibular pain disorders, fibromyalgia, irritable bowel syndrome, low back pain, complex regional pain syndrome, and heterogeneous chronic pain samples, among others.[36] In an early meta-analysis, Malone et al[49] reviewed nonmedical treatments, including 4 studies on cognitive therapy for various chronic pain conditions, and reported effect sizes ranging from 0.55 to 2.74. In a meta-analysis of 25 studies that met inclusion criteria, Morely et al[50] found significant effect sizes on all outcome measures compared with waitlist controls. Compared with other active treatments, CBT produced significantly greater changes on measures of the pain experience, coping, and behavioral expression of pain. Overall, strong supporting evidence indicates that CBT is effective in reducing pain behavior

and coping. Results are less clear, however, with regard to work status, medication, or health care use, given that fewer studies have evaluated these variables.[41]

A meta-analysis of 65 studies of multidisciplinary treatment for chronic pain indicated that such treatments are more efficacious than no treatment, than a waitlist control, or than componential treatments made up of an isolated discipline such as medical treatment, physical therapy, psychological treatment, or occupational therapy alone.[51] In Turk's[52] more recent review of the work in this area, he concluded that multimodal rehabilitation programs are comparable to other pain treatments with regard to pain reduction. These programs have significantly better outcomes, however, for decreasing medication and health care use and for increasing function and activity level, return to work, and closure of disability claims and with significantly fewer adverse events. Turk[52] indicated that such treatment is more cost effective than some of the more invasive medication interventions, such as spinal cord stimulation and surgery. Despite these positive outcome data, none of the existing treatments are efficacious for all patients. The following questions remain: What are the obstacles to treatment for patients who are not benefiting? Ultimately, how can treatment options for these patients be improved?

Obstacles to the Treatment of Chronic Pain

Despite the demonstrated effectiveness of these psychological and behavioral approaches to chronic pain treatment, behavioral issues that may interfere with treatment require attention. Careful clinical assessment can identify the following challenges to successful outcomes and can allow clinicians to make informed judgments before proceeding with chronic pain management.

Primary Chemical Dependency

Chronic pain complaints can mask a primary chemical dependency. Addiction affects approximately 10% of the population, and it may be overrepresented in populations with chronic pain. Although substance use disorders are beyond the scope of this chapter, clinicians should be aware that pain and addiction have many symptoms in common. Depression, sleep disturbance, anxiety, and disability in work, relationships, and activity are symptoms that are separately typical of pain and addiction.[53] As such, careful addiction assessment should be an integral part of pain management, particularly in patients with a personal or family history of addiction. Although evidence suggests that addiction does not preclude effective pain treatment, practitioners should consider suspending treatment pending a thorough evaluation of any patient whose agenda may include the acquisition of pharmaceutical-grade substances. In a study of patients who were otherwise adherent to prescribed controlled substances in a carefully controlled pain practice, 16% were identified through random urine testing to be using illicit drugs.[54]

Primary Psychiatric Disorder

Significant psychological and psychiatric issues accompany chronic pain. Patients with psychotic disorders, with significant dementia, with severe affective disorders, and, particularly, with active suicidal intent are not good candidates for aggressive pain management. Although it is true that "even schizophrenics have bad backs" and should not be cavalierly dismissed from pain treatment, severe psychopathologic conditions should be addressed psychiatrically before pain management is reconsidered. Similarly, patients experiencing overwhelming life stresses other than pain are at risk to be emotionally or pragmatically unavailable to take an active role in their treatment.

Ongoing Litigation

It has been axiomatic in chronic pain treatment that practitioners delay treating patients who have ongoing litigation or pending disability until the legal issue is resolved. Although specialty programs and clinics may have the luxury of postponing treatment, most primary care physicians do not. The concern is that patients recognize (or are told) that improvement in pain or in physical function may reduce or eliminate the monetary benefit that drives litigation and disability seeking. Many, if not most, patients who are pursuing legal remedies have honorable and conscientious motives and may cease their legal pursuits if the ability to function is restored. The difficulty the practitioner faces is in determining the motives of any particular patient. The research suggests caution. Blyth et al[55] studied the effect of litigation on pain-related disability and found that past or present pain-related litigation was correlated significantly with higher levels of disability. Long-term follow-up of patients treated with a radiofrequency procedure showed a negative correlation between outcome and litigation status.[56] Factors that mediate the relationship between pain complaints and litigation or pursuit of disability deserve considerable research attention.

Lack of Motivation

A vexing issue for practitioners is to define for individuals experiencing pain the specific behavior changes that would lead to improvement in function and decreases in pain only to have the patient resist making the suggested changes. Despite the evidence supporting the effectiveness of cognition modification, exposure to feared stimuli, and increased productive activity, some patients experiencing chronic pain do not engage successfully with treatment.[57] Prominent among the approaches to addressing this apparent lack of motivation is the application of Prochaska and DiClemente's[58] stages of change model to chronic pain. At its essence, the model proposes that individuals vary in their readiness to engage in behavior change, and that series of stages of readiness exist. In a typical variant of the model, the stages include precontemplation (in which no change is considered), contemplation (in which change is considered, but is not likely to occur in the near future), preparation (in which steps are being taken to make changes), action (in which behavior change is attempted), and maintenance (in which one works to sustain change). In addition to developing instruments to quantify readiness to change, researchers have begun to examine the utility of tailoring interventions to match specific stages.[59-61]

Conclusion

Chronic pain is maintained by biologic, psychological, and social factors. Conceptual models and treatment strategies that solely emphasize sensory and organic aspects of pain are inadequate in addressing the complex problems presented by many patients with chronic pain. Evidence-based interventions require the inclusion of behavioral approaches as a component of a comprehensive interdisciplinary strategy. As treatment strategies have demonstrably become more effective, research efforts are needed to determine which specific interventions tailored to which patients for what particular problems in what social and environmental context are most efficacious. The research efforts designed to enhance treatment effectiveness for patients who fail to engage are particularly noteworthy. These studies represent important attempts to understand behavioral and psychosocial subgroups of patients within given physical diagnoses.

References

Full references for this chapter can be found on www.expertconsult.com.

Biofeedback

Frank Andrasik and Carla Rime

Biofeedback is a process that involves receiving information *(feedback)* about the body or self *(bio)*. Applied biofeedback consists of monitoring and exerting influence to produce a change in the incoming information. Combing one's hair is an everyday example of applied biofeedback.[1] An individual receives biofeedback on his or her physical appearance by looking in a mirror. Applied biofeedback, then, would be altering one's physical appearance and reflection in the mirror. In a clinical setting, biofeedback is accomplished through specialized equipment that provides information about physiologic responses occurring within the body (e.g., muscle activity, body temperature, sweat gland activity, heart rate). Obtaining accurate information about these processes would be difficult by simply looking in the mirror. The available feedback provided by proper instrumentation would then allow an individual to monitor and influence these physiologic responses.

The term applied biofeedback, as it is used in a clinical setting, was introduced by Olson[2] and encompasses the procedural operations and goals of biofeedback. Schwartz and Schwartz[3] made some minor revisions to Olson's definition (indicated by the italic words in the following list). As a process, applied biofeedback is:

1. a group of therapeutic procedures that
2. uses electronic or electromechanical instruments
3. to measure, process, and feed back accurately, to persons *and their therapists,*
4. information with *educational and* reinforcing properties
5. about their neuromuscular and autonomic activity, both normal and abnormal,
6. in the form of analogue or binary, auditory, or visual feedback signals.
7. Best achieved with a competent biofeedback professional,

8. the objectives are to help persons develop greater awareness *of, confidence in, and an increase in* voluntary control over their physiologic processes that are otherwise outside awareness or under less voluntary control,
9. by first controlling the external signal
10. and then by using *"cognitions, sensations, or other cues to prevent, stop, or reduce symptoms."*[3]

Components 1 through 7 of this comprehensive definition depict the key procedures of biofeedback, whereas elements 8 through 10 depict the key goals of biofeedback. The primary goal of biofeedback is self-management of physiologic responses. This type of treatment emphasizes an active approach on the part of the patient to cope more effectively with pain and its associated symptoms.[4] This active involvement can reduce pain-related disability by increasing a patient's confidence in the ability to prevent, manage, and cope with pain.[5,6] In fact, patients who attribute improvements in therapy to their own efforts demonstrate better long-term maintenance than do patients who attribute their improvements to others, such as the interventions of health care providers.[7]

This chapter on biofeedback outlines historical considerations of pioneers, research, and other growing fields that contributed to the development of biofeedback. Treatment indications and the efficacy of biofeedback are then addressed. The techniques section delineates three approaches of biofeedback, practitioner and patient considerations, and typical treatment procedures. Possible complications and side effects are also discussed. Biofeedback is often used in conjunction with a host of other self-regulation approaches (e.g., guided imagery, regulated breathing, autogenic training, and progressive muscle relaxation training, which are discussed in Chapter 132).

Historical Considerations

Although yogis and other individuals from Eastern cultures have long been exerting voluntary control over their internal states, it was not considered possible in Western science until the 1960s. Before then, investigators had believed that organisms could not self-regulate visceral functions of internal organs of the digestive, respiratory, endocrine, and vascular systems because these functions were considered automatic and involuntary. In the 1960s, Dr. Barry R. Dworkin and Dr. Neal E. Miller of Yale University in Connecticut countered this idea by pursuing research on this topic in the animal laboratory.[8] Skeptics believed that so-called volitional control of an involuntary response could well be mediated by slight skeletal movements. To rule out skeletal movements as an alternative explanation for visceral reactions, much of the research was conducted on curarized rats. Curare is a paralyzing agent that prevents skeletal movement, and it was considered too dangerous for human research. Nonetheless, in the name of science, a courageous individual offered to be curarized.

As recounted in Andrasik and Lords,[1] Lee Birk, who was working with David Shapiro and Bernard Tursky at Harvard University in Massachusetts, volunteered for the risky experiment of being curarized in 1967. The outcome of such an experiment would determine whether autonomic activity could be operantly conditioned without skeletal muscle movement. The research was conducted safely, and the results were successful in indicating that human voluntary control over visceral organs was possible in the absence of skeletal movement. Later, Birk wrote, edited, and published *Biofeedback: Behavioral Medicine* (1973), the first medical book on biofeedback.[1]

The aforementioned pioneers conducted research that was considered unpopular at the time, but they were responsible for a paradigm shift regarding potential voluntary control in human physiology. While these individuals were paving the way for biofeedback, other areas of study, such as psychophysiology, behavioral therapy, biomedical engineering, and cybernetics, also contributed to the development of biofeedback.

Psychophysiology is the study of the interdependent relationships between cognitive and physiologic variables. In 1965, David Shapiro offered the first class in psychophysiology, just 2 years before the pivotal research he conducted with Lee Birk. Clinical biofeedback is often considered a form of applied psychophysiology.[9]

In the twentieth century, behavior therapy was a growing field in psychology. This area of study was based on principles of learning, and investigators contended that a learned maladaptive behavior could be unlearned. Behavioral medicine was a specialized area within behavioral therapy that emerged in light of work on stress management and the physiologic stress response. The emphasis of behavioral medicine is on health behaviors associated with medical disorders.[1,9] Many behavioral therapy techniques, such as shaping and reinforcement, are used in biofeedback.

Biomedical engineering and cybernetics are two other fields that have contributed to biofeedback. Biomedical engineering supplied instruments that made monitoring physiologic responses possible. With the proper instrumentation, one could detect and monitor muscle activity, cardiac activity, peripheral blood flow, blood pressure, sweat gland activity, and brain electrical activity. Cybernetics involves providing physiologic information, which is otherwise unavailable, to an individual in such a way that learning voluntary control of these responses can be achieved.[1,9]

Miller, Shapiro, and Birk, among many others, were early pioneers in biofeedback. The scientific approaches of psychophysiology, behavioral therapy, biomedical engineering, and cybernetics also assisted in the development of applied biofeedback. The Biofeedback Society of America was formed in 1968 by researchers dedicated to seeking empirical evidence for applied biofeedback. This organization is now called the Association for Applied Psychophysiology and Biofeedback (AAPB). It cosponsors the journal *Applied Psychophysiology and Biofeedback* (previously entitled *Biofeedback and Self-Regulation*), in which many studies on biofeedback can be found. The following section addresses the efficacy of biofeedback in terms of medical disorders.

Indications

The AAPB organized two broad reviews of evidence-based research for biofeedback applications in general. The most recent[10] used five efficacy levels, formulated by La Vaque et al,[11] to evaluate and categorize the available research support. Level 1 findings are *not empirically supported*. Level 2 indicates biofeedback as *possibly efficacious*. Level 3 findings are *probably efficacious*. Level 4 signifies *efficacious* results, and level 5 represents *efficacious and specific* findings. Table 130.1 describes the criteria for each level of efficacy. Approximately 40 conditions were examined and sorted into one of the five levels according to these criteria. In some cases, the disorders were not sufficiently investigated, whereas in others, research was conducted but some negative results were reported.

The most recent broad area review by Yucha and Montgomery[11] includes a number of conditions involving pain. Here we list (see Table 130.2) and discuss those pain disorders accorded an efficacy level of 3 and above. In addition to the broad area reviews, the AAPB, in conjunction with the International Society for Neurofeedback and Research (ISNR, formerly known as the Society for Neuronal Regulation), commissioned a series of "white paper" evidence-based reviews that are being assembled by area experts and then sent out for peer review and eventual publication. These reviews are focusing on specific disorders and thus are more comprehensive. Three such reviews have appeared to date for pain: Crider, Glaros, and Gevirtz[12] for temporomandibular disorders (TMDs), Karavidas et al[13] for Raynaud's disease, and Nestoriuc et al[14] for recurrent headache.

Thermal biofeedback and electromyography (EMG) biofeedback have been used for the treatment of chronic arthritis. Bradley[15] and Bradley et al[16] found a reduction in rheumatoid factor titer, pain behaviors, and self-reports of pain intensity with a treatment consisting of thermal biofeedback in conjunction with cognitive-behavioral therapy. This treatment was compared with participants assigned to a control condition and those who received social support only. Furthermore, another study found that EMG biofeedback decreased the duration, intensity, and quality of arthritis pain.[17] A 2.5-year follow-up of the same participants found that these beneficial effects were maintained.[18] A meta-analysis of 25 randomized controlled trials revealed similar support across several dimensions.[19]

Table 130.1 Criteria for Levels of Efficacy

Level 1: Not Empirically Supported

The reports supporting this level are anecdotal or non–peer-reviewed case studies.

Level 2: Possibly Efficacious

The reports supporting this level include at least one statistically sound study, but without random assignment for a control condition.

Level 3: Probably Efficacious

The reports supporting this level consist of multiple observations, clinical studies, controlled/wait list conditions, and within-subject replication.

Level 4: Efficacious

The reports supporting this level include studies in which the treatment under examination is statistically significant and superior in comparison with a randomly assigned no-treatment control group, a different-treatment group, or a placebo group. The inclusion criteria for a special population are reliable and operationally defined. Outcome measures associated with the problem are valid. The procedures in the study are described in such a way that other independent investigators are able to replicate the study. The superiority of the treatment under examination has been indicated in at least two independent studies.

Level 5: Efficacious and Specific

The reports supporting this level include all the criteria for level 4 in addition to indicating superior statistical significance for the treatment under examination when compared with credible placebo treatment, medication, or a different treatment in at least two independent studies.

From La Vaque TJ, Hammond DC, Trudeau D, et al: Template for developing guidelines for the evaluation of the clinical efficacy of psychophysiological interventions, *Appl Psychophysiol Biofeedback* 27:273, 2002.

Table 130.2 Efficacy Levels for Biofeedback Treatment in Pain Disorders

Level 3

Arthritis
Headache: pediatric
Vulvar vestibulitis

Level 4

Chronic pain
Headache: adult
Temporomandibular disorders

A randomized controlled investigation examined whether EMG biofeedback and cognitive-behavioral therapy were equivalent to vestibulectomy.[20] All three interventions led to significant improvements in pain, sexual function, and psychological adjustment. Although the magnitude of improvement was greatest for the surgical procedure, several patients assigned to this condition refused to participate. Two less well-controlled investigations provided similar levels of support for EMG biofeedback combined with pelvic floor exercises (with regard to pain and discomfort during sexual activity).[21,22]

Biofeedback, either alone or in combination with other procedures, has been investigated for a wide range of chronic pain conditions, including endometriosis, recurrent abdominal pain, systemic lupus erythematosus, complex regional pain syndrome, osteoarthritis, phantom limb pain, advanced cancer, whiplash, and pain of the face, head, neck, and lumbar spine. The greatest focus has been on back pain, by using EMG biofeedback to treat muscle dysfunction and resultant reflexive muscle spasms that can develop and exacerbate pain. A meta-analysis of single and combined treatments found moderate evidence for EMG biofeedback as a separate therapy.[23] EMG biofeedback has also shown equivalent benefits when compared with cognitive therapy.[24,25] Additionally, Flor and

Birbaumer[26] found that EMG biofeedback had better effects on different aspects of back pain and TMD when compared with cognitive therapy. These results remained consistent at a 2-year follow-up. Biofeedback combined with relaxation has been found to be of value in treating chronic pain in children and adolescents as well.[27]

Biofeedback as a treatment for headache, both tension-type and migraine, appears to be well validated,[14,28] with an efficacy level of 4. The white paper review by Nestoriuc et al[14] found blood volume pulse (BVP) biofeedback to be the most efficacious biofeedback procedure for remediating migraine headaches. BVP biofeedback involves monitoring blood flow in the temporal artery and providing feedback to teach patients how to decrease or constrict blood flow. This approach, as first envisioned by Friar and Beatty,[29] can be thought of as the nonpharmacologic counterpart to an abortive agent. A review by the American Academy of Neurology U.S. Consortium, consisting of a panel of experts composed of representatives of the American Academy of Family Physicians, the American Academy of Neurology, the American Headache Society, the American College of Emergency Physicians, the American College of Physicians–American Society of Internal Medicine, the American Osteopathic Association, and the National Headache Foundation, accorded grade A to thermal biofeedback combined with relaxation training and EMG biofeedback in the treatment of migraine headache (and cognitive-behavioral therapy as well).[30] Thermal biofeedback has been classified as a level 3 treatment for pediatric headache. After a review of the literature, Hermann and Blanchard[31] concluded that thermal biofeedback produces clinically significant (≥50% reduction in headache) effects in approximately two thirds of the young participants.

Thermal biofeedback is the modality most studied for Raynaud's disease (a primary condition) and Raynaud's phenomenon (a secondary condition). The most recent and largest study to date, comparing medication (nifedipine) with thermal biofeedback, EMG biofeedback, and placebo, found medication to have the greatest effect.[32] However, a close inspection of patients assigned to thermal biofeedback revealed that many patients did not acquire the necessary abilities to regulate their peripheral temperature.[33] A white paper evidence-based review, selecting studies wherein patients were adequately trained to regulate hand temperature, provided sufficient support for assigning this treatment a rating of level 4.[13]

Finally, biofeedback as a treatment for TMDs has been classified as a level 4. Efficacy has been established through research with biofeedback, either alone[34] or in combination with other treatments.[35,36] Treatment reduces pain and pain-related disability while increasing mandibular functioning. A meta-analysis conducted by Crider and Glaros[37] found that EMG biofeedback was better than no treatment or placebo control for self-reported pain. The mean improvement rate for the 13 trials in this literature review was 68.6% for biofeedback treatments compared with 34.7% for the control conditions. Another meta-analysis, included in a white paper review, analyzed 14 trials for biofeedback interventions for TMDs. This review concluded that EMG treatment and biofeedback-assisted relaxation are probably efficacious, whereas EMG in combination with cognitive-behavioral therapy is efficacious.[12]

The following section outlines the different approaches of biofeedback and addresses some of the detailed treatments discussed for the conditions in this section.

Techniques

Biofeedback, as a self-management therapy, allows an individual to exert voluntary control over physiologic responses with the use of equipment that provides accurate measures. The emphasis is on active involvement. In fact, Yucha and Montgomery[10] advised using the term biofeedback *training* in place of biofeedback *treatment,* to emphasize the active participation necessary for biofeedback therapy. This term also stresses the importance of patient education. A biofeedback practitioner (certified or appropriately trained) needs to coach the patient on what to expect and to assist the patient in reaching his or her goals with biofeedback. The two approaches to biofeedback are general and specific.[4]

General Approach

The objectives of the general approach to biofeedback are to decrease overall arousal and to enhance a state of general relaxation. Three ideas underlie the association between generalized relaxation and pain reduction, as described by Andrasik and Thorn.[38] The first idea is that a decrease in general arousal reduces peripheral sensory inputs in central processing. The second is that relaxation can reduce negative affect, which is linked to an increase in pain reports and a decrease in pain tolerance.[39] The last idea is based on the observation of the relationship between stress and prolonged cortisol levels, in which activation of the stress response can increase the subjective nature of pain.[40] A decrease in arousal thus would be beneficial for those experiencing pain. The general approach to biofeedback aims to reduce this overall arousal through the three "workhorses" of biofeedback.[1] The three most commonly used methods are EMG-assisted relaxation, skin conductance–assisted relaxation, and skin temperature–assisted relaxation. Figure 130.1 shows a therapist explaining biofeedback-assisted relaxation to a child.

Electromyography-Assisted Relaxation

Sensor placement for EMG is generally on the forehead, neck, or trapezius. A series of sensors, two active and one ground electrodes, is placed on any of these areas along the muscle fibers. The two separate circuits identify electrical activity. The resultant signal is the difference between each of the two active circuits, in which the amount subtracted out is regarded as noise. When a muscle contracts, electrochemical changes occur. The electrodes detect and process the ion exchange across the muscle membrane where the muscle action potential takes place. The raw EMG signal is transformed into an audible or visual presentation with a microvolt value. The modification of the raw signal into average time periods is necessary because EMG activity is too low in its original form, thus making the small detection difficult to discriminate. To interpret and learn how to influence the muscle activity, the signals must be represented in an understandable manner.

The power spectrum of surface EMG can range from 20 to 10,000 Hz. Some of the commercially available biofeedback equipment may have a more limited range, however. This characteristic can result in lower readings overall, and clinicians need to be aware of the band pass of their machine. Similarly, a practitioner should know that measures from one machine may not be equivalent to measures from another machine. Measurements can also be affected by sensor size and type, sensor placement, distance between sensors, and the patient's adiposity (because fat can dampen the signal).[41] Practitioners should follow consistent procedures for accurate EMG readings. The goals are to reduce muscle activity and to achieve a more relaxed state overall.

Skin Conductance–Assisted Relaxation

Historically, measures of skin resistance were obtained to aid in the understanding of hysterical anesthesias. Romain Virouroux used this method of measurement in the late 1880s.[42,43] In the 1900s, Carl Jung measured electrical activity of the skin because he believed it was a technique that could be used to in reading the mind during word association experiments.[1] Electrodermal activity, or sweating, has been long regarded as a measure associated with arousal.

Biofeedback sensors are typically positioned on the palm of the hand or the fingers, which are areas of the body densely populated with eccrine sweat glands. Perspiration is made up of salts that are conductive to electricity, more so than dry skin. The biofeedback machine sends low, undetectable voltage to the skin and records changes in skin conductivity. The sweat glands are primarily responsive to psychological variables and are associated with the sympathetic division of the autonomic nervous system.[43,44] Changes in autonomic arousal produce changes in dermal activity.

Conductance measures are favored over resistance measures (measured in micro-ohms or microsiemens) because the conductance activity has a linear relation to the amount of activated sweat glands. In clinical applications, conductivity measures are more understandable. Skin conductance increases as arousal increases, and as arousal decreases so does skin conductance. The goal of skin conductance–assisted biofeedback is to promote relaxation by means of reducing skin conductance and arousal.

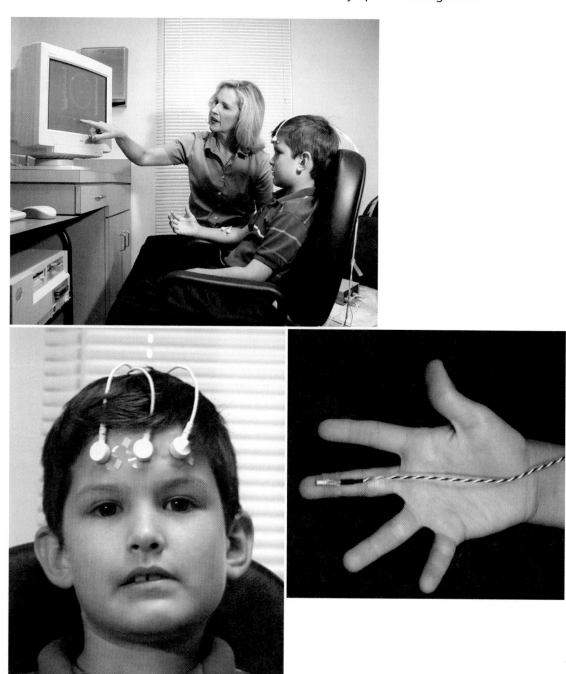

Fig. 130.1 Child receiving thermal- and electromyography (EMG)–assisted biofeedback training. In the *top panel*, the therapist is explaining the feedback modalities to the child. The vertical bars on either side of the computer monitor display EMG activity (the one to the left presents EMG activity from the forehead, whereas the one to the right is monitoring forearm muscle activity). The circle in the middle and the bar on the bottom of the monitor are providing temperature feedback (in a relative sense). Actual temperature values are provided digitally in the middle of the circle. The *bottom panel on the left* shows a typical EMG electrode array for promoting generalized relaxation. The *bottom panel on the right* shows a typical thermistor placement for monitoring surface skin temperature.

Skin Temperature–Assisted Relaxation

Skin temperature–assisted relaxation was discovered unexpectedly. During a standard evaluation at Menninger Clinic in Houston, Texas, an individual's migraine attack abruptly subsided with a flushing in the hands and a rapid increase in hand temperature.[45] Consequently, the clinicians who observed this event tested a hand-warming treatment for migraineurs. Increasing hand temperatures became a method in regulating stress and headache activity. Skin temperature is believed to provide an indirect measure of activity in the sympathetic nervous system. A reduction in arousal, or sympathetic outflow, leads to an increase in vasodilation and blood flow to the peripheral areas of the body, which is indicated by an increase in skin temperature. Conversely, an increase in arousal and sympathetic outflow constricts peripheral blood flow and results in a lower skin temperature.

Thermistors containing semiconductors, and occasionally thermocouples, are used to monitor temperature change in the skin. These temperature-sensitive sensors are placed on the fingers. Thermal-assisted biofeedback generally employs aspects of autogenic training,[46] in an effort to achieve an increase in peripheral skin temperature. When combined in this manner, the procedure has been termed autogenic feedback. While recording an individual's skin temperature activity, the practitioner needs to keep in mind that measurements may be influenced by the clinic, laboratory, outdoor temperatures, or humidity. Heat buildup on the conductive leads and sensors can also affect the accuracy of the measurements.

These three most common techniques of biofeedback—EMG, skin conductance, and skin temperature–assisted relaxation—are all designed to promote a decrease in sympathetic arousal and an overall state of relaxation. A common feature of relaxation is distraction, which has been illustrated by functional magnetic resonance imaging research to activate areas within the periaqueductal gray region.[47] This brain region has been associated with higher cortical control of pain. General relaxation-assisted biofeedback may be influencing these central mechanisms of pain.[48] For a more detailed description of relaxation therapies, including autogenic training, see Chapter 132. In many instances, a brief psychophysiologic assessment, or a psychophysiologic stress profile, is used for biofeedback-assisted relaxation. In fact, this type of assessment is prudent to include in routine practice because it helps determine psychophysiologic targets for treatment and provides another way to gauge response to subsequent treatment. A more thorough psychophysiologic assessment is used in the specific approach to biofeedback, as described in the next section. (For more information on biofeedback instrumentation, see Peek[41]).

Specific Approach

Many of the conditions listed in the section of this chapter on indications are treated through a specific approach to biofeedback. To obtain initial information about a patient's condition, a psychophysiologic assessment is conducted. This preliminary evaluation is designed to identify response modalities and physiologic dysfunction relevant to the pain disorder. Various stimulus conditions, both psychological and physical, that simulate work and rest are examined. These situations may include, for example, reclining, bending, stooping, lifting, and working a keyboard. The information gathered in this assessment guides treatment and gauges progress.

Flor[48] outlined the utility and advantages of collecting psychophysiologic data in the treatment of chronic pain: (1) it provides support for the role of psychological factors in dysfunctional physiologic functioning; (2) it justifies the use of biofeedback treatment; (3) it facilitates customized therapy for patients; (4) it makes it possible to record the efficacy, generalization, and transfer of therapy; (5) it assists in predicting treatment response; and (6) it serves as a source of motivation for the patient. This profile can help to foster self-efficacy in the patient, who comes to realize that he or she is capable of voluntarily controlling physiologic responses with his or her own cognitions and emotions. Typical phases of the psychophysiologic stress profile consist of adaptation, resting baseline, self-control baseline, reactivity, recovery, muscle scanning, and muscle discrimination.[49,50]

Adaptation

Three objectives for the adaptation phase are as follows: (1) to allow patients to become accustomed with the setting, clinician, and monitoring procedure; (2) to minimize presession effects, such as rushing to the appointment, temperature and humidity differences, and differences between the setting and areas outside of the setting; and (3) to permit habituation of the orienting response and for response stability.

During the adaptation phase, patients are instructed to sit quietly while refraining from any conscious efforts of relaxing. Even though a prebaseline period is widely accepted, the key parameters and amount of time for stability are not well researched. Generally, individuals adapt to a stable response within 5 to 20 minutes; however, some individuals do not achieve adaptation even after a 60-minute session. Practitioners are advised to extend the adaptation phase until some stability is achieved for the physiologic response of interest. Stability is defined as a minimal response or fluctuation in response for a specified period of time or a response that is going in a direction opposite to that desired. Without an appropriate amount of time for adaptation, a clinician may mistake a habituation effect for a training effect.

Baseline

After the adaptation phase, the baseline phase begins. Data collected from the baseline phase are used for the basis of comparisons with later phases. Baseline data collection also allows the therapist or researcher to gauge progress within and across subsequent treatment sessions. Again, the parameters and amount of time for collecting information in this phase are not definitive. Decisions, such as whether eyes should be open or closed, whether the patient should recline or sit upright, or whether conditions should be neutral or promote relaxation, are at the practitioner's discretion. The baseline duration generally ranges from 1 to 5 minutes, which should provide an adequate, representative sample of the patient's ordinary responses during resting states.

Often, a clinician obtains a second type of baseline. This is a particularly valuable measure for assessing biofeedback acquired skills. The practitioner instructs the patient to relax with a statement such as the following: "I would now like to see what happens when you try to relax as deeply as you can. Use whatever means you believe will be helpful. Please let me know when you are as relaxed as possible." The purpose of the second baseline is to evaluate the patient's preexisting abilities to relax and can be used to compare with future training effects.

Reactivity

The third phase of the psychophysiologic assessment examines simulated stressors that pertain to the patient's condition or similar real-world situations in which pain onset, exacerbation, and perpetuation are associated with the pain. No procedure has been empirically validated, but some common examples include the following:

- Negative imagery, wherein a patient focuses on a personally relevant unpleasant situation (these details are usually obtained during an intake interview)

- Cold exposure (e.g., for Raynaud's disease or phenomenon) or a cold pressor test (as a general physical stressor)
- Movement (e.g., sitting, walking, rising, bending, stooping)
- Load bearing (e.g., lifting or carrying an object)
- Operation of a keyboard or other office equipment

Even though baseline differences for EMG have not been reliable in distinguishing pain disorders, certain symptom responses have been found to be more consistent for specific pain conditions (for further discussion, see Flor[48]).

Travell and Simons[51] introduced a psychophysiologic model for assessing muscle reactivity. They contended that a large percentage of chronic muscle pain is an effect of trigger points. Hubbard[52] extended this view, based on the following rationale: (1) muscle tension and pain are sympathetically mediated hyperactivity of muscle spindles, or muscle stretch receptors; (2) muscle spindles are encapsulated organs that are composed of their own muscle fibers and are scattered throughout the muscle belly (hundreds of these muscle spindles are within the trapezius muscle); (3) even though muscle spindles are traditionally thought of as stretch sensors, they are now recognized as organs that can be activated by sympathetic activation and sense pain and pressure; and (4) therefore, the pain associated with trigger points actually arises in the spindle capsule.

This model is supported by research in which careful electrode placements detected high levels of EMG activity in the trigger point but minimal activity in nontender sites just adjacent (only 1 cm away) to the trigger point.[53] Additionally, when an individual is exposed to a stressful stimulus, EMG activity increases at the trigger point but not at any of the nearby sites.[54] These studies demonstrate an association between behavioral and emotional influences on muscle pain. Gevirtz, Hubbard, and Harpin[55] designed a treatment program that uses EMG biofeedback to foster muscle tension awareness in sessions and in daily life activities. This treatment also identifies stressors generating increased EMG activity and assists patients in coping with situations producing tension.

Recovery

Following the reactivity phase is the recovery phase, in which time is allotted for the patient's physiology to return to a value close to the baseline measure. Most often, the responses do not fully return to the values before the reactivity to stress phase. Therefore, a response is labeled as recovered if it returns to within a certain percentage of its initial value. If several stressful stimuli are presented to a patient, then a recovery period is suggested after each stimulus presentation.

The foregoing phases characterize the progression of a typical psychophysiologic assessment. Although used less frequently, muscle scanning and muscle discrimination are two other approaches that may be useful.

Muscle Scanning

Cram[56] designed an approach that allows a practitioner to evaluate EMG activity quickly from multiple sites and that requires only two channels. Two hand-held "post" electrodes are used to acquire brief (~2 seconds per site) sequential bilateral recordings while the patient is sitting, standing, or moving. A normative database aids the clinician in determining whether any of the measures are abnormally high or low. It also determines whether any asymmetries (right versus left side differences) exist, which may suggest bracing or favoring of a particular position or posture. The objective of biofeedback, then, is to return the aberrant recordings to a more normal state.[57] Even though this procedure may seem clear-cut, it is actually more complex because several factors may affect the measures obtained. For example, the angle and force of the applied sensors, the sensor locations used for the norming sample, and the other variables previously discussed may influence EMG readings.

Muscle Discrimination

Flor, Furst, and Birbaumer[58] found that individuals with chronic pain misperceive muscle tension, both in affected and nonaffected muscles. When patients were presented with tasks that required the production of muscle tension, they would overestimate physical symptoms, report greater pain, and rate the task as more aversive. Heightened sensitivity may account for the inability to perceive bodily states accurately. To assess muscle discrimination abilities in a clinical setting, Flor[48] recommended the following:

- Present the patient with a bar of varying height on a monitor.
- Instruct the patient to tense a muscle to the level in the height of the presented bar.
- Vary the bar height from low to high.
- Correlate the EMG measures with the actual heights of the bars.
- Define as "good" discrimination abilities with correlation coefficients greater than or equal to .80.
- Define as "bad" discrimination abilities with correlation coefficients less than or equal to .50.

The psychophysiologic assessment techniques for the specific approach to biofeedback allow a practitioner and the patient to monitor and record progress for areas associated with pain. These techniques may also be used in a more abbreviated manner for the general approach to biofeedback. Another style of biofeedback is the indirect approach.

The general and specific approaches have their own unique techniques and objectives. The general approach promotes overall relaxation, typically through EMG, thermal, or skin conductance biofeedback, which can reduce stress, tension, and pain. The specific approach can be used for precise pain sites, such as specific muscles and trigger points. A psychophysiologic assessment, or stress profile, is employed for evaluating the pain symptoms and physiologic responses. Responses to treatment may vary among individual patients. Patient considerations are discussed next.

Practitioner and Patient Considerations

The emphasis on patient education and treatment progress can establish therapy that is successful. The professional relationship between the clinician and the patient is of great importance. In fact, Taub and School[59] reviewed several experimental variables and reported that the behavior of the practitioner, as well as his or her confidence in the treatment, has the greatest effect on a patient's progress in biofeedback therapy. In addition to the clinician's expectations, the patient's expectations are also very important. Holroyd et al[60] found that the number one predictor of significant improvement for tension-type headache with EMG biofeedback is the patient's expectation about his or her ability to control the onset and course of the condition voluntarily. Similarly, beneficial treatment outcomes for headache are affected by the individual's perceived self-control.[61]

Individuals referred for biofeedback treatment may be confused about the nature of their pain condition and uncertain about their chances for improvement. Patient education offered by the practitioner is crucial in alleviating a patient's apprehension regarding biofeedback treatment. Identifying variables that may be controlled by the patient that are affecting his or her condition is often helpful for the patient's initial feelings about the therapy. Additionally, a detailed description of the treatment and a live demonstration can give the patient an idea of what to anticipate in therapy (a typical session of biofeedback is described later).

The biofeedback practitioner is regarded as a coach guiding patients in treatment. The patient is the active player learning skills of self-management. Coaching involves sharing observations for discussion ("I noticed that your EMG signal suddenly increased. It seemed you might have been clenching your teeth then. How about dropping your lower jaw and moving it a bit forward? I wonder if anything in particular was on your mind then?") The clinician also determines when breaks and encouragement may be needed. Initial attempts to lower EMG activity and skin conductance and to increase hand temperature are frequently met with the opposite effect, and this may paradoxically worsen as patients try harder and harder. These situations can be valuable in demonstrating the interaction between psychological and physiologic functioning and can illustrate how the patient's current coping strategies are actually backfiring. The coach explains how and why this happens and can alleviate the patient's frustration and get him or her back on track. The therapist also helps the patient articulate, understand, and consolidate the learning of skills. Other self-management techniques are also imparted to the patient. The discretion of the clinician is important in facilitating progress, because an overbearing coach can negatively affect treatment.[62]

The U.S. Headache Consortium[29] has summarized individuals who may be especially good candidates for biofeedback or other behavioral treatments. One or more of the following factors must be present:

- The patient prefers the approach.
- Pharmacologic treatment cannot be tolerated or is medically contraindicated.
- Pharmacologic treatment response is absent or minimal.
- The patient is pregnant, plans to become pregnant, or is nursing.
- The patient has a history of frequent or excessive use of analgesic or acute care medications.
- The patient is faced with several stressors or has deficient stress-coping skills.

Children often respond especially well to biofeedback.[63,64] Older patients usually need more time to master self-regulation skills.[65,66]

A typical biofeedback session consists of the following components:

- Sensor attachment and time for adaptation
- Initial progress review
- Resting baseline determination

- "Self-control" baseline determination (the patient's ability to regulate the target response in the desired direction in the absence of feedback, to provide a comparison with the ability to perform skills outside the treatment setting[67])
- 20 to 30 minutes of actual feedback (continuous or with breaks)
- Final resting or self-control baseline determination (assess learning within the session)
- Final progress review and assigned homework

No firm standard exists for the number of treatment sessions necessary for reaching the appropriate goals of therapy. The duration of treatment depends on the clinical response of symptom relief or the patient's adequate control of the target measure. When treatment reaches a point of diminishing returns, such as response plateaus, then the practitioner should begin to consider changing course or terminating treatment. Research on biofeedback-assisted relaxation has shown that desired goals are typically accomplished in 8 to 12 sessions. Haddock et al[68] found that patients with headache respond more quickly to treatment when homework assignments consist of detailed manuals and relaxation tapes. The treatment duration is subject to individual differences in treatment response.

Lynn and Freedman[69] outlined the following methods to increase generalization and maintenance of beneficial biofeedback skills: (1) overlearning the response and continuing to practice learned skills; (2) incorporating booster treatments; (3) fading or gradually removing feedback during treatment; (4) training under stressful situations such as during noise, distractions, and physical or mental tasks; (5) using multiple practitioners, which is possible with group treatment; (6) varying the physical setting; (7) providing portable biofeedback devices for homework assignments; and (8) supplementing biofeedback with other procedures such as cognitive and behavioral techniques. Many of these suggestions are based on learning principles of behavior therapy.

This section delineates the two approaches of biofeedback, patient considerations, coach or practitioner considerations, a typical treatment session, treatment duration, and procedures for improving the durability of the skills learned from biofeedback therapy. The next section addresses some of the side effects and complications of biofeedback treatment.

Side Effects and Complications

Even though biofeedback treatments commonly have positive outcomes, a few difficulties have been reported. A few patients may experience initial negative outcomes such as muscle cramps or disturbing sensory, cognitive, or emotional reactions. Other problems may arise that can affect adherence and practice. A few individuals may experience an abrupt increase in anxiety as they become deeply relaxed because a deep state of relaxation may be foreign to them. This condition is termed relaxation-induced anxiety, and symptoms can range from mild to moderate in intensity and may come close to a minor panic attack.[70] If this situation occurs, the practitioner must remain calm and reassure the patient that the episode will soon pass. Having the patient sit up or walk around the office usually helps. When patients are at risk for relaxation-induced anxiety, the clinician may instruct them to concentrate on the somatic aspects rather than the cognitive aspects of training.[71] See Schwartz, Schwartz, and Monastra[72] for a discussion of other problems and solutions. A more detailed description of complications for relaxation therapies can be found in Chapter 132.

Some medications may act on the central and autonomic nervous system and may thereby complicate biofeedback therapy. For example, muscle relaxants may relax target muscle groups and elicit inaccurate measures for the process of biofeedback training. Other medications, such as asthma inhalers, act on the autonomic nervous system and cause blood vessels to constrict. This may impede thermal biofeedback training by decreasing blood flow to the peripheral areas of the body. In some instances, improvement attained in biofeedback therapy may require medication adjustments. This is one of the many reasons that biofeedback clinicians should maintain a collaborative working relationship with medical associates.

Conclusion

Biofeedback treatment is a viable option for many pain disorders and accompanying symptoms. This chapter summarizes historical considerations such as early pioneers, research, and other related fields contributing to the development of biofeedback. A comprehensive AAPB evidence-based review of treatment options for arthritis, chronic pain, headache in adults and children or adolescents, vulvar vestibulitis, Raynaud's

disease and phenomenon, and TMDs is analyzed. Efficacy levels for these conditions vary, and some areas merit more research to examine outcomes with biofeedback therapy.

The section on techniques addresses the general and specific approaches of biofeedback, including the components of a psychophysiologic assessment. Furthermore, this section discusses practitioner and patient considerations, a typical biofeedback session, and treatment duration. Side effects and complications for biofeedback therapy are minimal. Relaxation-induced anxiety and medication complications are identified as infrequent occurrences. Throughout the chapter, the patient's active role and education in the therapy process are emphasized.

For more information regarding research, credential programs, or biofeedback in general, the reader may visit the following websites:

Association of Applied Psychophysiology and Biofeedback http://www.aapb.org
Biofeedback Certification International Alliance http://www.bcia.org
Biofeedback Foundation of Europe http://www.bfe.org
International Society for Neurofeedback and Research http://www.isnr.org

References

Full references for this chapter can be found on www.expertconsult.com.

Hypnosis

Howard Hall

Historical Considerations

Perhaps one of the first written descriptions of surgery on a patient under what appears to be a hypnotic trance can be found in the Bible in Genesis 2:21-22 with the creation of Eve from Adam's rib: "And the Lord God caused a *deep sleep* to fall upon Adam and he *slep*t: and he took one his ribs, and closed up the flesh instead thereof; And the rib, which the Lord God had taken from man, made he a woman, and brought her unto the man." The origin of hypnosis is associated with an 18th century Viennese physician, Franz Anton Mesmer (1734-1815; **Fig. 131.1**). Mesmer became famous in Paris for inducing a type of convulsive seizure he called a "crisis," which was apparently linked to therapeutic effects on the body. The setting for Mesmer's treatments included soft background music and a draped room in which patients would hold onto metal bars that extended from a wooden tub filled with water, ground glass, and iron filings. Mesmer developed a theory of animal magnetism that used the iron filings and magnets for healing purposes; his method later became known as "mesmerism." His theory of disease and healing involved "balancing magnetic fluids,"[1] an approach that today might be termed "energy medicine." Many of the conditions he treated with mesmerism might now be considered functional disorders, with a psychologic, rather than physical, basis. These include conversion symptoms of paralyses, seizures, and deafness and stress-related conditions, such as headaches.[2] Mesmerism generated so much attention that in 1784 Louis XVI of France formed a commission, headed by Benjamin Franklin, to examine the theory of animal magnetism. After running a series of controlled experiments to test the phenomenon, the commission concluded that Mesmer's cures were produced by the patient's imagination and not magnetism.[1] It should be noted that the commission did not find that Mesmer's results were invalid, just that they were not the results of magnetism. However, during this era of reason and enlightenment, a pronouncement of this kind was equivalent to saying that the results of magnetism therapy were not real.

One of the most important applications of mesmerism in the early 1800s in France, England, and later, the United States was as an anesthetic agent for surgical patients. Mesmerism anesthesia was used for mastectomies, amputations of legs, removal of glands and jaw tumors, and tooth extractions. In one case of tooth extraction, the patient was described as showing no apparent discomfort or reaction to the pain.[2]

Around 1840, English surgeon James Braid (1795-1860) recognized that some mesmeric phenomena were genuine but argued against the doctrine of animal magnetism. Braid put forward his own view that the phenomenon of mesmerism was related to subjective or psychologic factors.[3] He used an eye-fixation induction that he learned from a mesmerist and coined the term "hypnosis" to describe the observed trance phenomenon that he believed was an artificially induced state of sleep (Hypnos is the Greek god of sleep). Today, of course, we know hypnosis is unrelated to sleep because the two have divergent electroencephalographic (EEG) patterns.

An especially dramatic historical example of the application of hypnosis is the achievement of painless surgery in procedures performed by James Esdaile between 1845 and 1851. Esdaile, a Scottish surgeon, practiced medicine in India and performed hundreds of operations with hypnosis as the sole analgesic technique.[2] Even more impressive, more than 300 of these operations involved major surgery and

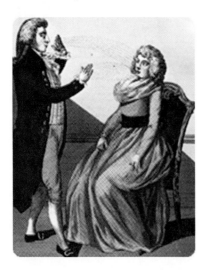

Fig. 131.1 Franz Anton Mesmer with patient.

Esdaile's mortality rate was only about 5%, as compared with the 40% to 50% death rate for conventional surgical procedures at that time. Nevertheless, the role of hypnosis as an anesthetic technique declined by the third quarter of the 19th century for several reasons. First, hypnosis provided variable and unpredictable results. A report actually cited a patient who sued for assault when she emerged from hypnotic analgesia in the middle of an operation. Second, after Liston performed the first operation with ether in England in 1846, use of chemical anesthetic agents increased.[4] Further, unprofessional and fringe practices entered the field of hypnosis, tarnishing its reputation and leading to a decline in its use.[2]

Hypnosis for the treatment of children goes back more than 200 years, but it was not until the 20th century that it emerged as a subspecialty area with novel training opportunities that emphasized pain management.[5-8] Children are generally believed to be relatively more responsive to hypnosis than adults because they have such active powers of imagination, which has important implications for successful pain management. Hypnotic induction with children also tends to be more permissive, playful, imaginative, and less structured and authoritative than the approaches used with adults. One has to be mindful of a child's developmental level with use of hypnotic approaches because techniques vary widely and must fit those developmental milestones and abilities to be effective.

Indications

Hypnosis can be used in an integrative manner as an adjunctive treatment along with traditional medical and pharmacologic approaches to pain management or as an alternative nonpharmacologic treatment. A hypnotic intervention can be used before, during, or after painful procedures or operations.

Hypnosis for Preoperative and Postoperative Pain Management

Hypnosis and other psychologic interventions applied before surgery have been associated with faster postoperative recovery, shorter hospital stays, relatively less postoperative pain

and anxiety, and reduced opioid use.[9] Other reports that indicate efficacy for hypnosis cite decreased postoperative orthopedic pain, faster surgeon-rated recovery, and in one study, no postoperative complications, versus eight instances in customary care conditions without hypnosis intervention.[10]

Hypnosis for Management of Acute Pain

Controlled trials for acute pain reduction provide good evidence that hypnosis is superior to standard care, attention controls, or other viable pain-reduction interventions.[11] Anxiety is a major contributor to distress during painful medical procedures, which becomes patently clear when children begin crying as soon as a doctor approaches them with a needle or when adults become distressed at the sound of the drill in the dentist chair. However, and more dramatically, anxiety can rise to the same level in the parking lot, before the doctor visit even begins, or in the dentist's waiting room. Hypnosis has been used within dentistry and has been helpful to reduce anxiety and pain perception during a host of medical procedures.[12] Response to hypnotic interventions for children and adolescents with cancer who undergo bone marrow aspirations varied as a function of the child's age, gender, and hypnotic susceptibility.[13] However, the relative benefit of hypnosis versus other cognitive approaches to pain management in children requires further research.[14] Hypnosis has also provided added benefit to local anesthetics, such as eutectic mixture of local anesthetics (EMLA) cream, for lumbar punctures and bone marrow aspirations with young cancer patients. This procedure has an impact on management of both pain and anticipatory anxiety.[15] An updated review of randomized controlled trials of psychologic interventions for needle-related procedural pain and distress in children and adolescents provided some insight into this issue.[16] These authors found sufficient evidence to support the efficacy of hypnosis, distraction, and combined cognitive behavioral interventions for the management of procedural pain and distress in children. The effect sizes of these psychologic interventions showed an average of more than 20% reduction of pain, compared with meta-analytic results for topical anesthetics that ranged from 20% to 50%. A recent randomized clinical trial showed that a combined multifaceted distraction intervention that included hypnotic suggestions of diminished sensation without a formal induction resulted in a significant reduction in discomfort from immunizations in children 4 to 6 years old compared with routine control conditions.[17] As these authors noted, hypnosis with young children does not necessitate a formal hypnotic induction because children easily go into natural trance states during stressful and anxiety-provoking situations such as injection.

Hypnosis for Cancer Pain Management

Hypnosis is used for the management not only of pain and anxiety of medical procedures associated with cancer, as noted previously, but also for the neuropathic pain associated with the disease itself. Often hypnosis can provide added benefits for conditions such as neuropathic cancer pain where opioids and other medical treatments have not been found to be totally effective when used alone. Emphasis is now placed on integrating hypnosis along with traditional medical treatments for chronic pain conditions.[18]

Hypnosis for Obstetric Pain

Hypnosis has been used during pregnancy for the management of nausea and vomiting, for prevention of premature labor, as an adjunctive treatment for pregnancy-induced hypertension, and as an intervention for pain and discomfort during labor and delivery.[19,20] About 20% to 35% of women are estimated to use hypnosis as the sole anesthesia during labor or delivery.[19] For other women, hypnosis can be used as adjunctive non-pharmacologic analgesia along with standard care.

Hypnosis for Emergency Treatment of Burns

Case histories of hypnotic interventions for burn victims have reported dramatic attenuation of the inflammatory response burn injury, if hypnosis is conducted during the first 2 hours after the burn.[22] However, controlled studies provide less dramatic outcomes.[23]

Hypnosis for Chronic Pain Conditions: Headaches, Fibromyalgia, Gastrointestinal Disorders, and Sickle Cell Disease

Evidence from controlled trials of chronic pain shows hypnosis to be superior to no treatment but equivalent to relaxation and autogenic training.[11] Chronic pain is a complex phenomenon and does not respond as robustly to hypnotic interventions as acute pain conditions.[11] Self-hypnosis training, however, has been associated with a reduction in pain days, disrupted or inadequate sleep, and pain medication for patients with sickle cell disease.[24] Hypnosis is also associated with a substantial reduction of the symptoms of irritable bowel syndrome in adults[25] and in children, and it is considered a well-established and efficacious treatment for recurrent headaches in children.[26] Self-hypnosis training is also associated with reduced frequency, duration, and intensity of headache symptoms in children and adolescents.[27]

Clinically Relevant Anatomy

Although views differ as to what hypnosis is and how it works for pain control,[11] hypnosis is often described in terms of an altered state of consciousness or awareness.[6] However, some consensus seems to exist as to what hypnotic pain control is not. The pain reduction effectiveness of hypnosis is not the result of simple relaxation because it does not necessarily bring about a relaxed state.[28] On the other hand, clinical hypnosis has been associated with profound relaxation effects accompanied by decreased measures of psychologic symptoms of distress and somatization scores in patients with chronic pain conditions such as irritable bowel syndrome.[29] Hypnosis does not appear to function as an opiate receptor-based analgesic because the opiate antagonist naloxone has no effect on hypnosis-induced analgesia.[11,30] The adult literature has observed that hypnotic responsiveness can be measured and predicted reliably such that individuals who score very high on these hypnotizability scales achieve robust hypnotic analgesia responses in the laboratory.[20] Hypnotic analgesia is not a placebo effect for those individuals who score very high on responsiveness scales because they show a higher pain threshold and pain tolerance under hypnotic analgesia conditions than under placebo conditions. By contrast, those who score very low on these scales show comparable response levels to pain reduction for hypnosis and placebo conditions.[31]

In highly hypnotizable individuals, hypnotic analgesia does appear to be associated with a complex ability to cognitively restructure or dissociate conscious overt pain sensation from covert experiences. In a novel set of experiments, hypnotically talented subjects who reported no overt pain to painful stimuli under hypnosis did indicate perception of pain when a covert or "hidden observer" part of their consciousness was asked about the experience.[18]

Technique

Hypnosis Technique for Preoperative and Postoperative Pain Management

The use of language plays an important role in hypnotic work and in clinical practice in general. For children in particular, and adults as well, the use of permissive and indirect language is generally preferred to authoritative approaches. For example, direct suggestions that "You will feel no pain" are avoided (especially with adults who are not highly hypnotizable). Instead, the wording to follow might be, "You may be surprised how comfortable you might feel during and after the procedure." Also, permissive suggestions can be given for the preoperative and postoperative periods. For example, the point at which the medication is administered can be a signal for the person to have a pleasant daydream; also, the area being operated on can remain soft, comfortable, and loose during the operation. A suggestion can be offered in advance that when the patients awaken in the recovery room the operation will be over, their condition relieved, and healing already under way. In addition, suggestions can be given stating how surprised they can be at how quickly recovery is likely to occur and how much easier the whole procedure was than anticipated.[32] Hypnosis for postsurgical pain management and recovery has included relaxation methods and suggestions for a smooth recovery, comfort, improved limb mobility, and success with occupational or physical therapy.[10]

Hypnosis Technique for Management of Acute Pain

Hypnoanalgesia techniques for young patients may include suggestions for feelings of numbness and glove anesthesia and numbing other body parts with that "magic" glove. Also effective are distancing suggestions such as moving pain away from self, or transferring it to another body part, or moving the self away from the pain. Yet another approach offers suggestions for feelings antithetical to pain, such as comfort, laughter, or relaxation. Distraction techniques directing attention away from the pain, adding time distortion, reframing, and suggesting amnesia are documented and effective.[6]

Hypnosis Technique for Cancer Pain Management

Hypnotic suggestions for cancer pain management may involve dissociative imagery of going to a favorite place, hypnotic analgesia suggestions of numbness or pain on-off switches (i.e., blocking pain), and sensory transformation experiences that either explore the pain or transform its intensity, color, or temperature.[18]

Hypnosis Technique for Obstetric Pain

A range of hypnotic processes and posthypnotic suggestions has been suggested for management of labor and delivery. These include simple relaxation, trance states, time distortion, redirection of attention, glove anesthesia, and transferring of numbness. A reframing approach suggests a reinterpretation of potentially negative sensations to familiar and pleasant ones (e.g., "Each contraction can be considered as a pleasing occurrence, drawing you nearer to your goal, bringing a new love for your enjoyment.").[32]

Hypnosis Technique for Emergency Treatment of Burns

Emergency situations are often traumatic and result in trance states as a natural defense against pain and fear. Thus, a formal hypnotic induction is not generally needed. When a burn patient is in a natural trance state, he or she can be told to "go to your laughing place" or be given a similar initial suggestion. Then, as the health team takes care of the injury, a hypnotic suggestion is given, alluding to a state of being "cool and comfortable."[22] This intervention is best carried out within 2 hours of the injury to reduce the inflammatory response.

Hypnosis Technique for Chronic Pain

Chronic pain is a complex phenomenon that does not respond as robustly to hypnotic interventions as acute pain conditions.[11] Thus, work with hypnosis needs to be done in an integrative fashion. Self-hypnosis practice may also facilitate clinical relaxation effects and reduce symptoms of psychologic distress for many chronic pain conditions. Attention to lifestyle factors and behavioral sleep issues may be helpful in sickle cell disease and other chronic pain conditions.[24]

Side Effects and Complications

In the hands of a practitioner with appropriate background, training, and licensure, hypnosis is generally a safe intervention. In management of pain, however, a good history and physical examination are critical to success. Karen Olness and Patricia Libbey,[33] pioneers in the field of child hypnotherapy, observed that 25% of children referred for hypnotherapy were later found to have some unrecognized organic condition that accounted for their symptoms. Of course, the most important intervention in those cases was not hypnosis but appropriate medical treatment.

The author's only negative experience with hypnosis and pain management involved a teenage boy with functional abdominal pain. This case was very early in the author's career. The author made a direct suggestion for the pain to go away (now, the author's approach is more permissive and cautious). After the induction had ended, the boy said that his pain was gone but that everything seemed upside down (i.e., he was disoriented). The author had him close his eyes and suggested that when he opened his eyes the room would be back to how it was. This approach was unsuccessful, and the patient was becoming somewhat alarmed about how he was feeling (the author was becoming concerned as well). Then, the author had him close his eyes and go back into hypnosis; the author had him "bring the pain back." He opened his eyes and said everything was back to normal, but his stomach was hurting again. Follow-up work involved weekly traditional psychotherapy and learning how to get in contact with the feelings he was somaticizing.

The patient did well and eventually learned to express his feelings in words instead of somatic symptoms. The author saw the patient again about a decade later for a different problem related to the demise of his marriage. The author and patient did a lot of talk therapy and some hypnosis with no direct suggestions of symptom removal and no complications.

The author's first-line approach to chronic pain is a thorough medical, psychologic, and lifestyle assessment, followed by permissive relaxation type of hypnotic induction with no direct suggestion for pain to go away. If the pain remains despite the lack of obvious physiologic cause and active self-hypnotic practice, hypnosis may be used to explore the meaning of the pain. A patient under hypnosis might be asked to describe the pain and ask the pain why it is there and what the pain is attempting to teach the patient. Some colleagues have children draw pictures to obtain some of this information. Another colleague encourages children to use the computer word processor to help them gain insight into psychologic factors underlying their medical symptoms.[34]

Conclusion

As noted previously, a discrepancy often exists between modest findings from experimental trials and statistically significant clinical reports for hypnotic pain control. Although this discrepancy might cast doubts on the clinical trials and case reports, one must keep in mind that clinical and experimental settings are different. Standardized protocols are often used within laboratory settings that would be of limited use in clinical situations, where one would be inclined and able to capitalize on the patient's unique interests, strengths, and preferences, especially when working with children.

Some practitioners caution against the use of hypnosis in adolescents who score low on a standard scale of hypnotizability. The author finds these scales useful in the laboratory but not as useful in a clinical setting because clinically significant improvement can be accomplished if hypnosis is used not as an isolated treatment but rather in an integrative manner. Pediatric neurologists often refer children with recurrent headaches to the author because they believe that pharmacologic treatments have limited benefit. The author's approach, after obtaining careful medical, psychologic, sleep, diet, and other lifestyle assessment, is to teach self hypnosis as a "skill and not a pill" for headache prophylaxis.[35] For hospitalized children with chronic pain, self hypnosis can be of great benefit if introduced before the administration of daily opioids with their undesirable side effects. The author's clinical success rates have been excellent, but he looks forward to more conventional analyses. In conclusion, it is the author's opinion that hypnosis can be a valuable component of a comprehensive and integrative program for pain management.

Acknowledgments

The author thanks Kenneth Spencer and Tracie Williams of the Cuyahoga County Community College Bridges to Success in the Sciences for their help in research and preparation of the manuscript for this chapter.

References

Full references for this chapter can be found on www.expertconsult.com.

Relaxation Techniques and Guided Imagery

Carla Rime and Frank Andrasik

Relaxation interventions are self-management approaches underscoring the active involvement of the patient. Relaxed breathing, progressive muscle relaxation (PMR), autogenic training (AT), meditation, yoga, and guided imagery (GI) are all forms of relaxation treatments that are reviewed in this chapter. The National Center for Complementary and Alternative Medicine, a division of the National Institutes of Health, classifies these therapies as mind-body medicine defined as "techniques designed to enhance the mind's capacity to affect bodily function and symptoms."[1] According to a 2007 survey, approximately 4 in 10 adults and 1 in 9 children in the United States had used some form of complementary or alternative medicine in that previous year.[2] The use of deep breathing exercises, meditation, and yoga had increased since the earlier survey in 2002.

The actual mechanisms contributing to the effects of relaxation techniques are unclear.[3] Theories have been put forth to account for these effects. One theory, proposed by Benson et al,[4] contends that relaxation therapies elicit a generalized *relaxation response* whereby the body undergoes a series of physiologic changes initiated by the autonomic nervous system. These changes include a decrease in respiration, oxygen consumption, carbon dioxide elimination, heart rate, and arterial blood lactate concentration. Moreover, an increase in slow alpha brain waves with intermittent theta brain waves occurs and indicates a hypometabolic, wakeful state. The *relaxation response*, which is a general increase in parasympathetic nervous system activity, competes with Cannon's *fight-or-flight response*, which is a general increase in sympathetic nervous system activity. Although Benson et al[4] asserted that relaxation

procedures are equivalent, Davidson and Schwartz[5] proposed that relaxation techniques have distinctive, *specific effects* classified primarily as cognitive, autonomic, or muscular. Despite this debate, both theories may be accurate in that many of the physiologic responses of relaxation are interconnected.

Several factors may explain the beneficial outcomes of relaxation for individuals with pain. First of all, a general decrease in arousal also diminishes the central processing of sensory stimulation.[6] Additionally, reducing the frequent activation of the autonomic stress system can decrease the pain associated with this prolonged and heightened physiologic state, which is marked by an increase in cortisol levels.[7] Distraction may also play a role in the effects of relaxation. Tracey et al[8] found, through functional magnetic resonance imaging (MRI), that distraction activates the periaqueductal gray region, a cortical area related to pain control. The anterior cingulate cortex, a structure in the limbic system, is another region of the brain implicated in pain. This region is believed to be associated with the affective and cognitive evaluation of pain.[9,10] Relaxation may result in changes of activation in the anterior cingulate cortex that reduce pain perception.[11,12]

Depression, anxiety, and fear are often a result of pain and are intricately involved in the pain–negative affect cycle.[13] A reduction in these secondary symptoms through relaxation can increase pain tolerance.[6,14,15] Relaxation may be effective in reducing symptoms by "uncoupling" pain with its affective evaluation and thus leading to better coping.[16,17] Finally, feelings of helplessness can be a consequence of an ongoing pain condition.[15,18,19] Acquiring relaxation skills may provide a sense of control through active coping of the pain. Thus, mechanisms of relaxation therapies for pain may operate on the basis of decreased sensory input, competition of the stress response, distraction, and changes in pain perception associated with the cognitive and affective evaluation of pain that may lead to a sense of control and better coping.

This chapter on relaxation techniques starts with a discussion of historical considerations of PMR, AT, meditation, yoga, and GI. The section that follows considers indications for these therapies for several pain disorders and their accompanying symptoms. Next, techniques for each of these procedures are reviewed. This chapter closes with possible side effects and precautions for relaxation procedures.

Historical Considerations

Progressive Muscle Relaxation

In the early 1900s, Edmund Jacobson studied reactions to unexpected loud noises known as the startle response. Participants who were deeply relaxed did not display this typical startle response to sudden noises. This finding prompted Jacobson to continue researching the effects of relaxation. He found that the strength, or amplitude, of knee-jerk reflexes was related to the individual's tension levels. Those who exhibited sustained chronic muscular tension had less latency and more amplitude in their knee-jerk responses. Those who practiced relaxation displayed a decrease in the amplitude of knee-jerk reflexes.[20]

Consequently, Jacobson developed PMR to aid individuals in gaining an awareness of muscle tension and muscle relaxation through physiologic introspection. He did not believe in intentionally tensing muscles to perceive the differences between relaxed and tense muscles.[21,22] Later variations of Jacobson's original PMR added the tension and release cycles and the use of suggestion for relaxation. To create slight tension, Jacobson did instruct clients to raise the arm or bend the hand. The purpose of PMR is to learn physiologic control of increasingly more subtle muscle tension. Jacobson's PMR program involves more than 100 sessions, each usually an hour in length, while focusing on specified muscle groups. It could take months or years to obtain the skill to relax through the original version of PMR.

Because of the extensive time commitment for completing Jacobson's PMR program, others developed and tested shortened versions. Joseph Wolpe[23] adapted an abbreviated version of Jacobson's PMR, called *systematic desensitization*, for the counterconditioning of fear. This therapy usually takes 10 or fewer training sessions to complete. Wolpe combined more muscle groups and included suggestions and specific instructions. Others modified Jacobson's prescribed PMR program and Wolpe's abbreviated form to fit their patients' needs. Examples of these contemporary methods are described in the section of this chapter on techniques.

Autogenic Training

Johann Schultz was a German neurologist and psychiatrist who is credited as the founder of AT. The prominent school of thought at the time was psychoanalysis. Schultz was disenchanted with this approach, and in 1924 he began implementing AT in his private practice as a therapeutic method. Schultz created formulas for AT based on brain research conducted by Oskar Vogt. Vogt had observed that his participants, through deliberate mental concentration, could self-hypnotically produce sensations of warmth and heaviness. In 1932, Schultz published a book entitled *Das Autogene Training* that described the six formulas of the AT method.[24] Wolfgang Luthe, a physician and follower of Schultz, began translating the AT formulas into English in the 1960s. Luthe, with the assistance of Schultz, wrote the six-volume *Autogenic Therapy*, which details the AT formulas. Thus began the propagation of AT in English-speaking regions.[24]

Meditation

The English word *meditation* is derived from the Latin word *meditari*, which means "to heal."[25] This implies a restoration of physical, mental, and spiritual well-being. Transcendental and mindfulness are common types of meditation.[26] Transcendental meditation involves quietly or silently repeating a mantra, which can be a syllable, word, or phrase. Mindfulness meditation requires a passive, nonjudgmental attitude while experiencing sensations and perceptions in the moment. Table 132.1 provides guidelines for practicing meditation. Meditative practices are often found in religious contexts. Merkabolism, an early form of Judaism dating back to the first century BC, has literature describing transcendental prayer sequences.[4] In Eastern cultures, Shintoism, Taoism, and Sufism use meditation. Christian writers St. Augustine and Martin Luther also applied meditation to prayers as contemplative exercises.[4] Mindfulness meditation, in contrast, has origins in Buddhist traditions dating back more than 2500 years and has become more popular in the West since the 1960s.[27]

Adiswarananda[25] explained that meditation can facilitate achieving self-knowledge and self-control by obtaining mastery over the mind through direct perception. A 12-second period of sustained focus is said to equal 1 unit of concentration. Twelve units of concentration are equal to 1 unit of meditation, and, in turn, 12 units of meditation lead to total absorption. Suffering is believed to be self-created, and meditation can awaken the mind's ability to heal. Sleep rejuvenates the body, whereas meditation rejuvenates the mind. A fatigued mind has a tendency to repeat habitual thoughts and behaviors. In contrast, a fresh mind uncovers innovative ways of meeting life's challenges, such as pain.

Table 132.1 Guidelines for Meditation

Quiet place	When starting, a quiet place with few distractions is ideal.
Specific posture	This could include sitting, standing, lying down, or walking.
Focused attention	The object of attention could be a mantra, breath, image, or sensations.
Open/passive attitude	This allows for distractions to come and go without engaging in them.

Data from Benson H, Kotch JB, Crassweller KD, et al: Historical and clinical considerations of the relaxation response, *Am Sci* 65:441, 1977; and Sood A: Mind-body medicine. *Mayo Clinic book of alternative medicine: the new approach to using the best of natural therapies and conventional medicine*, New York, 2007, Time Inc Home Entertainment, pp 87–103.

Yoga

The English word *yoke* is related to the term *yoga,* which is derived from the Sanskrit root *yuj,* meaning "to unite."[14,28] The earliest documentation of the practice of yoga dates back to 3000 BC in India.[14] Vedic science is an Indian philosophy with traditions developed in the Indus Valley by sages known as Vedas.[28] In 200 BC, sage Maharishi Patanjali expanded on this science through his writings. He wrote about the eight branches, or limbs, of yoga,[25,28] which are summarized in Table 132.2. In the ninth century, sage Adi Shankara revived the Vedic science of yoga.[28] Hatha yoga is the most commonly used form in North America, and it is based on the third branch of yoga, *asana.*[14,29]

Mindfulness meditation and Hatha yoga are key features of the Mindfulness-Based Stress Reduction (MBSR) program. This intervention draws from similar but distinct philosophies; mindfulness meditation has roots in Buddhism, and yoga has roots in Indian Ayurvedic science.[30] Dr. Kabat-Zinn[27] designed the MBSR program in 1979 at the University of Massachusetts Medical Center. The program was created to relieve suffering for medical patients, and the yoga segments were originally included to prevent disuse atrophy. It is described in more detail in the section on techniques.

Guided Imagery

It is difficult to determine who may have been the founder of GI techniques. Imagery can be traced back to Ancient Greece, however, where dreams and visions were evaluated in the Asclepian temples for medical purposes. Aristotle, Hippocrates, and Galen were all trained in this method of imagery-based healing.[31] During the behaviorist movement in the mid-1900s, imagery as a mental process was considered irrelevant for research, let alone for therapeutic purposes. When the cognitive revolution in psychology took place, imagery was reintroduced as a topic for research and treatment.

Table 132.2 The Eight Branches, or Limbs, of Yoga

Branch	Meaning/Translation
1. *Yama*	"Rules of social behavior" or restraint
2. *Niyama*	"Rules of personal behavior" or discipline
3. *Asana*	"Seat/position" or posture
4. *Pranayama*	Based on *prana,* which stands for "life force" or control of breath
5. *Pratyahara*	Based on *prati,* which means "away," and *ahara,* which means "food" and encompasses the withdrawal of the mind
6. *Dharana*	"Concentration" or the mastery of attention and intention
7. *Dhyana*	"Meditation" or the development of awareness
8. *Samadhi*	"Total absorption" or pure awareness

Data from Adiswarananda S: *Meditation and its practices,* Woodstock, Vt, 2003, Skylight Paths Publishing; and Chopra D, Simon D: *The seven spiritual laws of yoga: a practical guide to healing body, mind, and spirit,* Hoboken, NJ, 2004, John Wiley & Sons.

In the early 1900s, Edmund Jacobson and Johann Schultz discovered the therapeutic value of PMR and AT, respectively. Meditation, yoga, and imagery have a much longer history. The following section discusses the effectiveness of these techniques as they relate to pain management.

Indications

The National Institutes of Health Technology Assessment Panel[3] concluded that "...the evidence is strong for the effectiveness of [relaxation] techniques in reducing chronic pain in a variety of medical conditions." The panel further stated that "...the data are insufficient to conclude that one technique is usually more effective than another for a given condition." Baer[32] examined research on the MBSR program and acknowledged that this intervention is "probably efficacious," where the preliminary studies are promising, but more rigorous research is still needed. Relaxation techniques are often combined into a treatment package. Various investigations have been conducted in order to determine the effectiveness of these isolated or combined interventions. Relaxation procedures and GI have been applied to a wide array of acute and chronic pain conditions and their secondary symptoms. The following represents an assortment of the research regarding these procedures as treatments for arthritis, back pain, headache, carpal tunnel syndrome, cancer, ulcers, irritable bowel syndrome, and phantom limb pain.

The Arthritis Self-Management Program is a patient education intervention for the treatment of rheumatoid arthritis, osteoarthritis, and fibromyalgia. It incorporates relaxed breathing, PMR, GI, mindfulness meditation, body scan, and yoga postures, along with cognitive restructuring, problem solving, and communication skills.[33] The intervention consists of six sessions, each approximately 2 hours in length. An evaluation of the program found an average of 15% to 20% reduction from baseline in arthritis-related pain and disability.[34] A study of a modified version of the Arthritis Self-Management Program, highlighting self-efficacy, reported that reductions in pain were maintained after 4 years and that physician visits decreased by 43%; these findings suggest the long-term effectiveness of the program and a reduction in health care costs.[35]

Results of a 12-week study for rheumatic pain indicated that PMR significantly improved muscle function of the lower extremities compared with strength training.[36] Another 12-week intervention of PMR and GI for osteoarthritis led to significant decreases in pain and mobility difficulties when compared with a control group.[37] Yoga was also applied to treat osteoarthritis of the knee and resulted in enhanced flexibility, strength, and quality of life.[38] Kolasinski et al[39] found that yoga reduced pain symptoms and disability for individuals with osteoarthritis of the knee. Furthermore, they concluded that yoga is a feasible treatment for obese individuals who are more than 50 years old, because most of the participants in their study met these criteria.

Fibromyalgia, another form of arthritis, has symptoms that are difficult to treat through conventional methods.[40] A within-subjects study design found significant reductions in skin conductance levels during and after the body scan technique of the MBSR program for participants with fibromyalgia.[41] The decrease in skin conductance signifies a reduction in sympathetic nervous system activation. Another study of MBSR for fibromyalgia revealed significant improvements in pain perception, quality of life, and coping with pain for those receiving the intervention compared with patients who had an active social support condition.[42] These outcomes were sustained at a 3-year follow-up.

Relaxation procedures have also been used for the prevention and treatment of other musculoskeletal disorders, such as back pain, headache, and carpal tunnel syndrome. Yoga[43] and PMR[44] trainings have been used in corporate settings to decrease stress and the risk of injury. Chronic back pain is another disorder that is challenging to treat with conventional care.[45] In a study of MBSR, older individuals with low back pain were assessed after completing the intervention.[46] A significant increase in physical function and pain acceptance was reported for the MBSR group compared with the control group after the intervention. Approximately three fourths of the participants from the MBSR group reported a continuation of their meditation practices 3 months later. Nearly three fourths of participants reported that they had recommended the program to others, and almost half reported a reduction in pain and sleep medications. This particular study omitted the yoga and all-day retreat characteristic of the MBSR program.

A pilot study examining the effects of yoga for the treatment of chronic low back pain found that balance and flexibility improved, whereas disability and depression scores decreased for the yoga group compared with the control group. Even though the results were not statistically significant, which could be the result of the small sample size, the outcomes were in the desired direction, a finding warranting further research. Yoga, exercise, and a self-care book were compared in a study for individuals with chronic low back pain.[47] After 12 weeks, both the yoga and exercise groups were superior to the book group in terms of functional status. An analysis at the 3-month follow-up indicated that symptoms continued to improve for the yoga group only. The yoga group also reported more reductions in medication use. Similarly, a study comparing yoga and an educational control group for low back pain found a significant decrease in functional disability and medication use for the yoga group compared with the control group after the 16-week intervention.[48]

Yoga has also been used to prevent and treat carpal tunnel syndrome. Results from a study employing this method indicate that those in the yoga group had a significant increase in grip strength and a significant decrease in pain ratings compared with the control group.[49]

Meta-analytic reviews found that behavioral interventions are effective in preventing and treating tension-type and migraine headaches in both adults[50-52] and children.[53,54] These therapies include relaxation training, biofeedback, cognitive-behavioral therapy, and stress management training, either in isolation or combined. A study assessing yoga for the treatment of tension-type headache found a significant decrease in pain perception for the yoga group compared with the control group.[55] In another yoga study for tension-type headache and migraine, the yoga group displayed a significant decrease in headache activity and medication use with an improvement in coping behaviors compared with the control group.[56] Medication intake actually increased for participants in the control condition. Similarly, John et al[57] found that a yoga intervention for those with migraine significantly decreased headache frequency, intensity, duration, and medication use, in addition to reducing anxiety, depression, and pain perception

compared with the control group. Participants in the control group had an increase in all these measures except for headache duration.

Relaxation procedures have been applied to cancer pain and the side effects of chemotherapy. Syrjala et al[58] examined the following interventions for patients undergoing bone marrow transplants: (1) relaxation and imagery; (2) cognitive-behavioral treatment combined with relaxation and imagery; (3) therapist support; and (4) treatment as usual, which served as the control condition. The relaxation/imagery and cognitive-behavioral/relaxation/imagery interventions resulted in significant pain reductions on self-report measures compared with the therapist support group and treatment as usual group. Combining the cognitive-behavioral treatment to the relaxation and imagery intervention did not add incremental value.

A pilot study on yoga therapy for women with metastatic breast cancer found that, on the day of yoga practice, these women had a significant increase in invigoration and acceptance.[59] Measures taken the day after yoga practice indicated that the outcomes of increased invigoration and acceptance were still experienced, as well as an increase in relaxation and a reduction in pain and fatigue. It appears as though yoga may have immediate and long-lasting outcomes, as well as delayed effects.

Burish et al[60] investigated the utility of PMR and GI for cancer patients undergoing chemotherapy. These investigators found that patients in the treatment group had significantly less nausea and vomiting compared with the control group. Moreover, the intervention group had lower blood pressures, pulse rates, and anxiety. Campos de Carvalho et al[61] researched the use of PMR in isolation to treat the unwanted side effects of chemotherapy and found similar results.

Relaxation techniques have also been used in alleviating pain from both ulcerative colitis and irritable bowel syndrome. Shaw and Ehrlich[62] compared the pain ratings of a relaxation intervention group with an attention control group for patients with ulcers. Following the 6-week intervention, patients in the relaxation group had significant reductions in pain ratings. These results were maintained at a 6-week follow-up. Brooks and Richardson[63] found a decrease in recurrences of ulcerative symptoms over 3 years after individuals received relaxation and assertiveness training when compared with individuals in a control group. In a yoga study of adolescents with irritable bowel syndrome, investigators found that the intervention group reported significantly lower levels of gastrointestinal symptoms than the control group.[64] Participants in the experimental group found yoga therapy to be helpful for their condition.

GI has been used in the treatment of phantom limb pain. This phenomenon is believed to be caused by a remapping of the brain in the sensory and motor cortexes after amputation.[65,66] Certain pain centers in the brain may become entangled during this rewiring, and the result is pain in a nonexistent limb. MacIver et al[11] explored the use of GI in treating individuals with phantom arm pain. After participants underwent a body scan technique to induce relaxation, they were instructed to imagine movements and sensations of the phantom limb. Over the course of the seven-session intervention plus home practice, participants reported significant pain relief. Functional MRI scans denoted a reduction in cortical reorganization from the sensory, motor, and anterior cingulate cortex. Ramachandran and Blakeslee[66] noted: "It seems extraordinary to contemplate the possibility that you could use a visual illusion to eliminate pain, but bear in mind that pain itself is an illusion—constructed entirely in your brain like any other sensory experience."

The aforementioned studies in this section are just a sampling of the well-documented research in which relaxation techniques and GI had favorable outcomes. These therapies can be applied to treat various medical conditions and in some cases serve as a preventive measure for recurrent pain (e.g. headache, ulcer) or musculoskeletal pain caused by poor posture or overuse.

Techniques

This section reviews procedures for relaxed breathing, GI, AT, PMR, mindfulness meditation, and yoga. Therapists often begin with methods of deep breathing, and this topic is addressed first in this section. Next, GI techniques of pleasant imagery and pain-transforming imagery are discussed. The six formulas comprising AT are summarized. Then, an abbreviated version of Jacobson's PMR is described because the less time consuming PMR variations are more widely used in clinical settings. A relaxation treatment program usually involves more than one of these techniques, by combining and tailoring the procedures based on individual needs. An example of a treatment regimen incorporating deep breathing, GI, AT, and PMR is examined. Finally, the MBSR intervention, consisting of relaxed breathing, mindfulness meditation, and yoga, is outlined.

Relaxed Breathing

Slow diaphragmatic breathing is a commonly used technique. To minimize shallow chest breathing, the patient is directed to draw air deeply into the lungs by pushing the diaphragm downward. On average, people take 12 to 15 breaths per minute. The goal of slow diaphragmatic breathing is usually 6 to 8 breaths per minute.[67] Decelerated breathing may feel strange to an individual who has a high respiration rate (30 or more breaths per minute). Clients should be assured that these unfamiliar feelings of slow, deep breathing will soon pass.[6] The following methods demonstrate deep breathing by using the diaphragm: (1) while breathing, place one hand on the chest and the other on the upper abdomen, maximize the movement of the lower hand, and minimize movement of the upper hand; (2) hold hands straight overhead while breathing; and (3) while lying on the floor, place a moderate-weight book on the abdomen and lift and lower the book while breathing in and out.[6]

Paced respiration breathing and pursed-lip breathing are other breathing therapy techniques.[67] Paced respiration is breathing at a predetermined rate. It usually involves a metronome, an external pacing device, to coordinate the rate of respiration. Pursed-lip breathing consists of exhaling slowly while the lips are partially pursed, as if whistling. This type of therapy has been used with patients who have chronic obstructive pulmonary disease.

Slow, deep breathing is often an element of all relaxation procedures. It can be quickly and easily brought under voluntary control at any time. Patients are encouraged to use diaphragmatic breathing frequently throughout the day, especially in response to stress.[68]

Guided Imagery

Imagery sends messages from the cerebral cortex to the limbic system, an area of the brain associated with emotion.[26] Information is then relayed to the autonomic nervous system, thus influencing the immune, endocrine, nervous, cardiovascular, respiratory, and gastrointestinal systems of the body.[69] If the images are vivid enough, the body undergoes physiologic changes as if the event is actually happening.[69] The physiologic and biochemical changes that occur with imagery have been used to explain the placebo effect in untreated individuals.[31,69] The purpose of GI is to generate the healing systems of the body to reduce pain sensation and perception. GI therapies either distract from the pain or focus on it in an attempt to modulate it.[17]

Imagery with relaxing scenes is a way to distract from pain. Clients are instructed to conjure a relaxing image in the "mind's eye." Examples of pleasant imagery may include a favorite vacation spot, lying on the beach, or walking in a meadow. Images that may cause arousal (e.g., sexual content, vigorous activity) should be avoided. Other sensory modalities (auditory, olfactory, tactile, and gustatory) are included to enhance the vividness of the image.[19,70] Associating a word, such as "relax" or "calm," engages both hemispheres of the brain and can facilitate recall.[26] After practicing a relaxing image, it can be quickly and vividly evoked. Clients are encouraged to apply their personally relevant relaxing scenes in stressful situations.[6]

Imagery is also used to focus on the pain to suppress or transform it.[69] One example of symptom suppression involves a two-step approach. The first step involves inducing feelings of numbness in the hand to initiate "glove anesthesia." Patients are then instructed to place the "anesthetized" hand on painful areas in the body and to transfer this numbness where it hurts. Symptom suppression is helpful for patients who are experiencing intense discomfort and are having trouble concentrating otherwise.

Transforming the pain through symptom substitution imagery consists of mentally moving pain in the body to another area of the body where it is more tolerable. This technique is not intended to suppress the pain, but instead to move the discomfort to a less threatening area of the body.[69] For instance, a patient may be guided to move pain to his or her little finger. Another method to transform symptoms is by visualizing the pain as the color red and then imagining the color as becoming less bright, corresponding to a decrease in pain intensity.[17] Bresler[69] contended that GI draws from an individual's inner resources for coping.

Autogenic Training

Schultz created a series of six formulas for AT: (1) the heaviness experience (muscular relaxation), (2) the warmth experience (vascular dilation), (3) the regulation of the heart, (4) the regulation of breathing, (5) the regulation of visceral organs, and (6) the regulation of the head.[71] Self-suggestion is used for each stage to produce the ideal effect. Key statements are passively focused on, such as, "heavy arm," or "warm arm."[71] A patient is instructed to focus on feelings of heaviness and warmth, especially in the extremities. This peripheral warming is believed to increase blood flow, decrease arousal, and promote relaxation. It is recommended that patients personalize their own phrases for heaviness and warmth and to repeat these phrases 50 to 100 times.[72]

Progressive Muscle Relaxation

Jacobson's method[20] was adapted by Bernstein and Borkovec[73] to provide a much abbreviated version of PMR for research and clinical application. Andrasik[74] delineated a treatment therapy for PMR based on this shortened approach. Major muscle groups are systematically tensed and relaxed. Later in the therapy, muscle groups are combined for more rapid effects. The tensing and releasing of the specified muscles aid in discriminating between levels of tension. With the development of this discrimination, patients can become more aware of their tension levels during the day and can implement PMR to counteract it. Regular practice is emphasized throughout the therapy.

The patient acts out a few tension-release cycles of a specified target group. The practitioner observes these practice cycles for complete, but not excessive, tension levels of the target group only. Table 132.3 outlines the 18 steps for the sequential tensing and relaxing of 14 target muscle groups. The tension-release cycle for each target muscle group consists of 5 to 7 seconds of tensing and 20 to 30 seconds of relaxing. Each step is repeated twice, with additional practice if needed. It is important to have the previous muscle group fully relaxed before moving on to the next step. The patient is instructed to focus on the sensations of both tension and relaxation of the muscles. Muscles that are tender or causing pain are omitted from the procedure. After the patient becomes more skilled with the 18 steps of tensing and relaxing, then the muscle groups are combined into an even more abbreviated form (Table 132.4).

Relaxation Treatment Regimen

Table 132.5 describes elements of an 8-week relaxation treatment program.[74] Over the course of 10 sessions, patients are trained in diaphragmatic breathing, PMR, AT, and GI. The first session consists of an introduction and rationale for the relaxation regimen. Relaxed breathing and PMR are practiced in the first session and during every subsequent session. The specified muscle groups start with the 18 steps and progress to the combined 8 and 4 steps later in therapy (see Tables 132.3 and 132.4). Deepening exercises, such as suggestive self-statements

of warmth and heaviness that are principles of AT, are used to enhance relaxation. Another deepening exercise is having the patient count backward from 5 to 1 while imagining descending stairs or floors in an elevator and becoming more relaxed. These deepening exercises are implemented during the 20 to 30 seconds of the relaxation segment of the tense-and-release cycles. Pleasant imagery is added to treatment in the second session.

Discrimination muscle training is implemented in the third session for specific muscle groups. The patient completes a tension-release cycle for a target group and then is instructed to tense only half as much, followed by one fourth, and alternations between these values. The patient continues tensing with decreased force to learn to discriminate more subtle sensations of tension. The patient is advised to use this differential muscle tensing for problem areas. For instance, an individual who has tension-type headaches may want to focus on the forehead and neck areas.

Table 132.4 Abbreviated Target Muscle Groups

EIGHT MUSCLE GROUPS

1. Both hands and lower arms
2. Both legs and thighs
3. Abdomen
4. Chest
5. Shoulders
6. Back of neck
7. Eyes
8. Forehead

FOUR MUSCLE GROUPS

1. Arms
2. Chest
3. Neck
4. Face (with focus on eyes and forehead)

From Andrasik F: Relaxation and biofeedback for chronic headaches. In Holzman AD, Turk DC, editors: *A handbook of psychological treatment approaches,* New York, 1986, Pergamon, p 228.

Table 132.3 The 18 Steps for Tensing the Initial 14 Targeted Muscle Groups

1. Right hand and lower arm (by having the patient make a fist and simultaneously tense the lower arm)
2. Left hand and lower arm
3. Both hands and lower arms
4. Right upper arm (by having the client bring his or her hand to the shoulder and tense the biceps)
5. Left upper arm
6. Both upper arms
7. Right lower leg and foot (by having the client point his or her toe and tense the calf muscle)
8. Left lower leg and foot
9. Both lower legs and feet
10. Both thighs (by pressing the knees and thighs tightly together)
11. Abdomen (by drawing the abdominal muscles in tightly)
12. Chest (by having the client take a deep breath and hold it)
13. Shoulders and lower neck (by having the client "hunch" his or her shoulders or draw the shoulders toward the ears)
14. Back of the neck (have the client push the head backward against a headrest or chair)
15. Lips (by pressing them together very tightly but not clenching the teeth)
16. Eyes (by closing the eyes tightly)
17. Lower forehead (by having the patient frown and draw the eyebrows together)
18. Upper forehead (by having the patient wrinkle the forehead area)

From Andrasik F: Relaxation and biofeedback for chronic headaches. In Holzman AD, Turk DC, editors: *A handbook of psychological treatment approaches,* New York, 1986, Pergamon, pp 225–226.

More advanced techniques, such as relaxation by recall and cue-controlled relaxation, are introduced in the sixth and eighth sessions, respectively. Relaxation by recall involves having the patient focus on the sensations of relaxation that were created during PMR practice. The patient is then directed to reproduce these sensations without the tension and release cycles. Cue-controlled relaxation associates a word with a state of relaxation. The cue may be as simple as the word *relax*, and with the skills that have been acquired throughout the training, the body can respond to the cue accordingly. When the focus is on deep breathing, cues can be stated quietly or silently with each exhalation. It is suggested that patients use breathing, imagery, self-suggestion, and cues that are personalized. The remaining sessions further refine the learned relaxation techniques. Patients should to discover what techniques and variations are most suitable for facilitating their own relaxation. From the beginning of the program, patients are instructed to practice at home once or twice a day for 20 minutes.

An audiotape recorded during an early session can assist the patient in pacing his or her home practice. Supplementing live instruction with either commercially available or tailored audiotapes seems to promote a generalization of skills learned from the clinic to daily routines.[22] The patient is advised to use the audiotape daily until the fourth week of treatment, at which point the patient is instructed to practice both with and without the audiotape. By week 8, and the last session, the patient should be able to practice without an audiotape at all. Furthermore, patients are advised to continue practice after the treatment has been completed. The methods are designed to aid an individual in coping with daily stress and tension.

Mindfulness-Based Stress Reduction

The 8-week MBSR treatment program incorporates both meditation and yoga.[75] Mindfulness meditation is introduced in the early sessions, whereas yoga is employed later.

Kabat-Zinn[75] delineated certain attitudes that facilitate mindfulness. These include (1) nonjudging, (2) patience, (3) a beginner's mind, (4) nonstriving, (5) acceptance, and (6) letting go. Participants meet once a week for 2.5 to 3 hours and once for a full day (7 hours) of mindfulness. The first four sessions involve a 45-minute body scan meditation technique, integrating deep breathing. Lying down, an individual focuses his or her mind from the toes, slowly to the top of the head. This fosters the development of calm, sustained attention. If pain draws attention away from the focused body region, then it is suggested that the person start again at the toes and slowly move up toward the pain and then past it. The patient is instructed to experience fully every sensation in the body, including the painful areas, in a detached manner. Patients are directed to practice the body scan 6 days a week for 45 minutes in the initial 2 weeks of treatment.

The second session of the MBSR program consists of the body scan technique and sitting meditation. During sitting meditation, the focus is generally on relaxed breathing. When distracting thoughts occur, patients are encouraged to take note and return their attention to their breath. Home practice begins at 10 minutes daily and later progresses to 45 minutes at a time. In addition to an awareness of breathing, sounds, thoughts, or feelings can be the focus of meditation with the aforementioned nonjudging approach.

Two mindful yoga sequences are introduced in the third and fifth session of the MBSR program. The first yoga sequence entails postures that are all floor exercises, including the corpse, wind relieving, and locust poses. The corpse pose is similar to the position of the body during the body scan technique. The sequence begins and ends with the copse pose. The second yoga sequence consists predominantly of standing postures with a mix of floor exercises. It includes sky reaching, tree, and bent knee forward bend poses. This sequence also closes with the corpse pose. During the various postures, individuals are instructed to pay attention to their breathing and subtle sensations in the body. This attention brings awareness

Table 132.5 Relaxation Training Regimen

Week	Session	Introduction and Treatment Rationale	Number of Muscle Groups	Deepening Exercises	Breathing Exercises	Relaxing Imagery	Muscle Discrimination Training	Relaxation by Recall	Cue-Controlled Recall
1	1	X	14	X	X				
	2		14	X	X	X			
2	3		14	X	X	X	X		
	4		14	X	X	X	X		
3	5		8	X	X	X	X		
	6		8	X	X	X	X	X	
4	7		4	X	X	X	X	X	
5	8		4	X	X	X	X	X	X
6	9		4	X	X	X	X	X	X
7	None								
8	10		4	X	X	X	X	X	X

From Andrasik F: Relaxation and biofeedback for chronic headaches. In Holzman AD, Turk DC, editors: *A handbook of psychological treatment approaches*, New York, 1986, Pergamon, p 225.

Table 132.6 Yoga Asanas/Postures

Sanskrit Name	English Name	Brief Description
*Savasana	Corpse pose	Lying on the back with arms and legs extended, palms up
*Pavanamuktasana	Wind relieving pose	Starting with a corpse pose, place hands below right knee, bend and bring toward the chin, release, then repeat with the left leg, release, and then bring both legs up and gently rock forward and backward, side to side
Pranamasana	Salutation pose	Standing with feet together, bring palms together in front of chest in prayer-like fashion
*Hasta Uttanasana	Sky reaching	Starting with a salutation pose, raise arms straight above the head, palms facing forward
*Vrksasana	Tree pose	Standing with feet together, arms at sides, bring the sole of right foot up to the left thigh, then raise arms above head, palms together, release, and then repeat on left side
*Janu Sirsasana	Bent knee forward bend	Sitting upright with both legs extended in front, pull bottom of right foot into inner thigh of left leg, stretch toward left foot, release, and then repeat on other side
Bhujangasana	Cobra pose	Lying on the stomach, with palms planted under shoulders, raise chest and head up, leaving lower abdomen on floor
Parvatasana	Mountain pose	Standing with legs slightly apart and straight, place palms on the floor above the head, and lift buttocks upward, creating a triangular space below the body
Matsyendrasana	Spinal twist	Sitting upright with both legs extended in front, bend left leg with the bottom of left foot on floor next to the right thigh, place right arm around left knee and gently twist spine to the left, release, and then repeat on other side
*Salabhasana	Locust pose	Lying on the stomach with arms at sides or under abdomen, lift right leg straight up, release, then repeat with the left leg, release, and then bring both legs up, keeping knees together, release

*Yoga postures featured in the Mindfulness-Based Stress Reduction Program.[75]
From Chopra D, Simon D: *The seven spiritual laws of yoga: a practical guide to healing body, mind, and spirit*, Hoboken, NJ, 2004, John Wiley & Sons.

and acceptance of an individual's physical capabilities and limitations. Each sequence takes approximately 45 minutes to complete. In addition to the yoga group training, patients are given audiotapes to guide them through the sequences for home practice. See Table 132.6 for a list of common yoga postures and brief descriptions.

Walking meditation is practiced in the fourth session of the MBSR intervention. It can be done at any walking pace. Again, individuals are instructed to concentrate on their bodies' movements and any sensation that may arise. This technique allows one to apply meditation to a regular, daily activity. Mindfulness can also be expanded to other routine activities, such as household chores. Some patients prefer the movements of yoga and walking meditation as opposed to the stillness of the body scan and sitting meditation. Home practice is still suggested to be at least 45 minutes per day for 6 days a week, using any combination of the learned techniques.

The sixth session of the MBSR program is an all-day retreat, lasting 7 hours. The group is silent and avoids eye contact for the first 6 hours, with only the instructors talking and guiding the practices. The retreat begins with a sitting breath meditation followed by yoga. Sitting and walking meditation are alternated throughout the day. In the last hour of the retreat, participants talk about their experiences from the previous 6 hours of silence. The day of mindfulness closes with 15 minutes of sitting meditation. The remaining weeks of the intervention involve practicing and trying variations of the techniques taught in the early sessions.

Research on the effectiveness of the MBSR program typically followed this protocol, although some studies excluded the yoga segments or the all-day retreat.[12,46] Yoga, however, appears to have an important role in decreasing symptoms, increasing mindfulness, and increasing well-being when compared with the body scan and sitting meditation techniques. One study found that practice time for yoga, more than the other techniques, was significantly correlated with these outcome measures, even though yoga was practiced for fewer days and fewer minutes overall.[76]

In addition to the rationale of using relaxation in the treatment of pain, meditation and yoga techniques may also offer beneficial outcomes by enhancing mood and acceptance of the pain condition. Results from an electroencephalographic study found a significant increase in activation of the left anterior region of the brain immediately after 8 weeks of the MBSR program for the meditators compared with the control group of nonmeditators.[77] This area of the brain is believed to be associated with positive affect.[78] The changes in electroencephalographic activation endured at a 4-month follow-up, a finding signifying lasting effects of the MBSR program.[77]

The attitude of acceptance that is cultivated through the MBSR program may also apply to a level of acceptance of the pain syndrome.[32] This acceptance is not considered resignation, but rather a willingness to live in spite of the pain.[79] The perception of pain is transformed from a negative experience to just an experience.

Regular home practice is crucial in developing the techniques outlined in both the relaxation treatment regimen, using PMR, and the MBSR program. This practice requires active involvement and a commitment to treatment to acquire the skills and maximize the benefits. Individuals may respond differently to the relaxation techniques. For example, those who have migraine headaches may find peripheral warming characteristic of AT the most effective in preventing migraine attacks, whereas those who have tension-type headaches may find better results with PMR.[80] Yoga may be especially effective for those with musculoskeletal disorders, in which pain is a result of poor posture or spinal misalignment. Relaxation techniques can be used in isolation or combined with other compatible approaches. Several options are available, and no one procedure has been found to be more effective than another in inducing relaxation.[3,19] Moreover, these methods appear to be feasible and applicable for all ages including pediatric[81] and elderly[12,29,46,82] populations.

Side Effects

Relaxation techniques and GI are generally considered safe. Unwanted side effects have been reported, however. A negative phenomenon, known as *relaxation-induced anxiety* (RIA), describes a group of musculoskeletal, sensory, and cognitive effects that can result from relaxation procedures.[83] Negative musculoskeletal activity reactions include tics, spasms, restlessness; negative sensory experiences include unusual sensations, feelings of floating, and other disturbing sensations; negative cognitive and affective responses include sadness, fear, and intrusive thoughts.[84] Heide and Borkovec[83] proposed possible explanations for these paradoxical effects of RIA. First, individuals who are unfamiliar with relaxation may find the novel sensations strange or bothersome. Second, relaxation procedures emphasize a passive component, and an individual may have a fear of losing control. The fear of inactivity is another possible explanation for RIA, in which individuals have a difficult time sitting still and quietly. Other persons may find self-focused attention aversive. Finally, individuals undergoing relaxation training commonly report interfering thoughts.

RIA is uncommon and can usually be alleviated within a training session. One remedy is to change to an alternate relaxation technique.[83] For instance, if pleasant imagery is causing symptoms of RIA, then switching to PMR may be appropriate. Another remedy is to implement relaxation procedures gradually, with shorter sessions.[83] Although RIA occurs infrequently, practitioners should be aware of it and offer solutions. Even mild symptoms of RIA can influence adherence and attrition to relaxation training programs. Individuals who have pervasive or generalized anxiety seem to be more susceptible to RIA. Investigators have also found that relaxation procedures may not be beneficial for individuals with clinical depression. Support exists, however, for using relaxation techniques in individuals who have secondary depressive symptoms resulting from pain.[80]

Freeman[31] discussed certain conditions that can be exacerbated by GI. For instance, patients who have chronic severe depression may not respond favorably to GI. Individuals who have epilepsy should be carefully monitored because imagery can alter brain wave activity. Moreover, glucose levels can be affected by imagery, and patients who have unstable diabetes should also be carefully monitored.

Even though no adverse events were reported for yoga in the studies reviewed in the section on indications, certain precautions must be taken. Some yoga postures may put unneeded strain on the joints or the back. Yoga treatment for lower back pain should omit postures that involve back bending.[48] Sood[26] suggested checking with a physician before beginning a yoga regimen for individuals with neck or back pain. He also advised individuals who have high blood pressure that is difficult to treat, blood clots, certain eye conditions (i.e., glaucoma), or osteoporosis to seek a physician's approval before starting yoga. Women who are pregnant should check with their obstetrician before performing yoga. Some yoga postures that involve twisting at the waist can put pressure on the uterus. Yoga classes designed specifically for pregnant women are available.[26]

Conclusion

Relaxation techniques may generate a general *relaxation response*,[4] with a reduction in activation of the sympathetic nervous system. Additionally, *specific effects* may account for the beneficial outcomes of relaxation through cognitive and affective mechanisms.[5] This chapter begins with the rationale for the use of relaxation techniques and GI for pain conditions. Both PMR and AT were developed in the early 1900s by Jacobson and Shultz, respectively. Meditation, yoga, and GI have a much longer history, as discussed in the section on historical considerations. The section on indications discusses the way in which relaxation techniques and imagery have been successfully applied to various conditions, including arthritis, back pain, headache, carpal tunnel syndrome, cancer, ulcers, irritable bowel syndrome, and phantom limb pain. Procedures for breathing therapies, GI, AT, and PMR are outlined in the section on techniques. A treatment regimen consisting of relaxed breathing, PMR, AT, and GI and the MBSR program, consisting of deep breathing, mindfulness meditation, and yoga, is summarized. This chapter closes with the potential side effect of RIA and other patient precautions.

References

Full references for this chapter can be found on www.expertconsult.com.

Part C

Physical Modalities in the Management of Pain

Chapter 133

Therapeutic Heat and Cold in the Management of Pain

Steven D. Waldman, Katherine A. Kidder, and Howard J. Waldman

Heat and cold have been used in the treatment of pain since the time of Hippocrates. In spite of their widespread use for centuries, a search for the scientific justification for these universally accepted modalities was not undertaken until the birth of the specialty of physical medicine and rehabilitation after World War II. The knowledge that was derived from this search forms much of our rationale for the use of heat and cold in the treatment of pain. This chapter reviews common therapeutic heat and cold modalities and provides the clinician with a roadmap for their safe application.

The Physiologic Effects of Therapeutic Heat

The mechanisms by which heat exerts its analgesic effect extend beyond the simple effects of local heat on the target tissue. Locally, heat elicits the following physiologic responses: (1) increased blood flow; (2) decreased muscle spasm; (3) increased extensibility of connective tissue; (4) decreased joint stiffness; (5) reduction of edema; and most importantly, (6) analgesia (**Table 133.1**).[1] Because the sensations of temperature and pain are carried to the higher centers via the same neural pathways, imagining that heat exerts a modulating effect at the spinal and supraspinal levels is not unreasonable. In addition, the feeling of well-being associated with therapeutic heat most likely causes the release of endorphins and other neurotransmitters, further modifying the pain response. However, although the beneficial nature of therapeutic heat

cannot be denied, this treatment modality is not without side effects. The relative contraindications to the use of therapeutic heat are summarized in **Table 133.2**. Although these precautions are not absolute, special care should be taken with the decision to use therapeutic heat in these clinical settings.

Choosing a Therapeutic Heat Modality

The clinician who is considering therapeutic heat as an adjunct in the treatment of a patient's pain can choose from a variety of heating modalities (**Table 133.3**). Although the indications for the use of therapeutic heat apply to all therapeutic heating modalities discussed in this chapter, each modality has its own distinct advantages and disadvantages that can not only influence the success or failure of the therapeutic intervention but can also determine the incidence of side effects and complications if the wrong modality is chosen or if a modality is used in the incorrect clinical situation (**Table 133.4**). As a practical consideration, the failure to match the modality to the patient usually results in a less than optimal outcome.

When matching the modality to the patient, an understanding of the underlying physics of each therapeutic heat modality is essential. Each heat modality accomplishes the delivery of heat to the target tissue via a specific physical mechanism of heat transfer. For sake of organization, these mechanisms can be divided into the categories of conduction, convection, and conversion. Whereas conduction and convection provide

Table 133.1 Physiologic Effects of Therapeutic Heat

Increased blood flow

Decreased muscle spasm

Increased extensibility of connective tissue

Decreased joint stiffness

Reduction of edema

Analgesia (most important)

Table 133.2 Relative Contraindications to Therapeutic Heat

Lack of or reduced sensation

Demyelinating diseases

Acute inflammation

Bleeding disorders

Hemorrhage

Malignant disease

Inability to communicate or respond to pain

Atrophic skin

Ischemia

Scar tissue

Table 133.3 Therapeutic Heat Modalities

SUPERFICIAL HEAT MODALITIES

Modalities That Rely on Conduction

Hydrocollator packs

Circulating water heating pads

Chemical heating pads

Reusable microwavable heating pads

Paraffin baths

Modalities That Rely on Convection

Hydrotherapy

Fluidotherapy

DEEP HEAT MODALITIES

Modalities That Rely on Conversion

Ultrasound

Shortwave diathermy

Microwave diathermy

Table 133.4 Indications for the Use of Therapeutic Heat Modalities

Pain

Muscle spasm

Bursitis

Tenosynovitis

Collagen vascular diseases

Contracture

Fibromyalgia

Induction of hyperemia

Hematoma resolution

Superficial thrombophlebitis

Reflex sympathetic dystrophy

Table 133.5 Indications for Therapeutic Ultrasound

Tendinitis

Bursitis

Nonacutely inflamed arthritis

Frozen joints

Contractures

Degenerative arthritis

Fractures

Plantar fasciitis

conduction, as do heating pads, circulating water heating pads, chemical heating packs, reusable microwave heating pads, and paraffin baths. Hydrotherapy and fluidotherapy deliver superficial heat to the target tissue via convection. The deep heating modalities of ultrasound, radiant heat, shortwave diathermy, and microwave diathermy deliver heat to the target tissues via conversion. With an understanding of how each heat modality delivers heat, the clinician can use the unique characteristics of that modality to best meet patient needs. Specific heat modalities are discussed subsequently.

Superficial Heating Modalities

Modalities That Deliver Heat via Conduction

Hydrocollator Packs

As mentioned previously, the mechanism by which the various types of hot packs deliver heat to the target tissue is conduction. The amount of heat delivered via conduction is directly proportional to the following variables: (1) the area of heat delivery; (2) the length of time the heat is delivered; (3) the temperature gradient between the hot pack and the target tissue; and (4) the thermal conductivity of the surfaces.[2] The amount of heat delivered via conduction is inversely proportional to the thickness of the layers of materials and tissue through which the heat must be conducted. With alterations

primarily superficial heating, conversion has the ability to heat deep tissues. Therefore, the first question in choosing a therapeutic heat modality is whether superficial or deep heat is the desired goal.

The next step in matching the modality to the patient is an understanding of which modalities transfer heat via which mechanism (**Table 133.5**). Hot packs, the most commonly used heat modality in clinical practice, transfer superficial heat via of any of these variables, the amount of heat delivered to the target tissue can be increased or decreased as the clinical situation and patient comfort dictate.

Hydrocollator packs are flexible packs that contain a silicate gel product and are heated in a water bath to approximately 77°C (170°F) (**Fig. 133.1**). The large surface area and flexible nature make this modality ideally suited for treatment of low back and dorsal spine pain. Smaller hydrocollator packs are useful in the treatment of neck pain. The packs do not absorb significant amounts of water, but the surface is wet, which increases conduction. A terrycloth towel is placed between the patient and the hydrocollator pack, with the thickness of towels being the easiest way to control the dosimetry and allow titration of the temperature to patient comfort. The packs maintain a therapeutic temperature for approximately 20 to 30 minutes to allow for superficial heating of large surface areas. To avoid burning the patient, care must be taken to allow excess water to drain from the pack before use. The hydrocollator pack should always be placed on rather than under the patient for easy removal should the patient find the pad is too hot.

Circulating Water Heating Pads (K-Pads)

Like the hydrocollator pack, the circulating water heating pad is ideally suited for treatment of low back and dorsal spine pain. More flexible than the hydrocollator pack, the circulating water heating pad can also be used on shoulders and extremities. The circulating water pad is thermostatically controlled so that the water temperature remains constant, which allows for superficial heating of relatively large surface areas. This confers two additional benefits to this heat delivery device: (1) unlike hydrocollator packs, hot water bottles, and microwave heating pads that cool over time, the circulating water heating pads can deliver a constant temperature to the target tissue over time; and (2) the thermostatically controlled circulation system greatly decreases the risk of thermal injuries associated with traditional electric pads (**Fig. 133.2**). In spite of the increased safety of circulating water pads relative to electric heating pads, because they do not cool spontaneously, their use should be closely monitored and carefully timed.

Chemical Heating Packs

Chemical heating packs are readily available in most pharmacies. They consist of a flexible outer layer that contains inter-nally segregated chemicals. These chemicals, when mixed with squeezing or kneading of the package, cause an exothermic reaction that releases heat capable of producing superficial heating of the affected body part. Other chemical heating pads produce heat via oxidation when the chemical heating pack is exposed to air. Most chemical heating packs that rely on oxidation contain iron powder, activated charcoal, sodium chloride, and water. Although inexpensive and convenient to use, the chemical heating packs produce varying degrees of heat and have the potential to cause severe burns even when used properly.[3] The chemicals contained in the packs can cause irritation to the skin if the outer package integrity is compromised. Chemical heating packs have the advantage of being portable and not needing electricity or external heating.

Reusable Microwavable Heating Pads

The widespread use of microwave ovens has spawned a variety of new reusable heating pad products that are designed to be quickly heated in the microwave oven. These products consist of an outer bag, which may be made of cloth or plastic, and a sealed inner bag that contains gel or grains (including rice, corn, or wheat) and delivers heat via conduction to provide superficial heating of the affected tissues (**Figs. 133.3 and 133.4**). Some products add aromatic substances to provide the added theoretic benefit of aromatherapy. Although convenient and easy to use, these products have some serious drawbacks. First, as with microwave popcorn, variations in the heating abilities of microwave ovens can cause overheating or underheating. In addition, there is no simple way to verify the actual temperature of the product; and because of the nature of microwave ovens, significant inconsistencies of

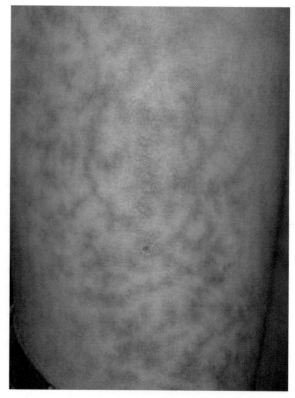

Fig. 133.2 Thermal injury of the type associated with traditional electric pads.

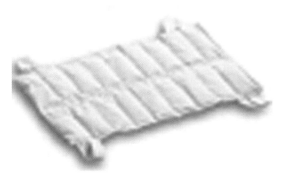

Fig. 133.1 Hydrocollator packs are flexible silicate gel packs that are heated in a water bath to approximately 77°C (170°F).

surface temperatures with "hot spots" may result in serious burns. Like hydrocollator packs and other heat delivery modalities that do not deliver a constant source of heat, cooling can be inconsistent.

Paraffin Baths

Used primarily for the treatment of hand abnormalities associated with rheumatoid arthritis, degenerative arthritis, and other collagen vascular diseases such as scleroderma, paraffin baths are a useful form of conduction-type heat therapy capable of providing superficial heating of the affected tissues.[4,5] Paraffin baths are reasonably safe as long as the temperature of the liquid paraffin is checked before extremity immersion or application. The paraffin is generally mixed with mineral oil (7 parts paraffin to 1 part of mineral oil) and placed in a thermostatically controlled heater (**Fig. 133.5**). The affected body part is dipped into the paraffin bath and then removed to allow the paraffin to solidify. This procedure is repeated up to 10 times. The affected body parts are placed under an insulating sheet for approximately 20 minutes, and then the paraffin is stripped off and returned to the thermostatically controlled heater to melt and use again. This technique is usually not undertaken with acutely inflamed joints and can be used only after anti-inflammatory drugs have begun to treat the acute inflammation.

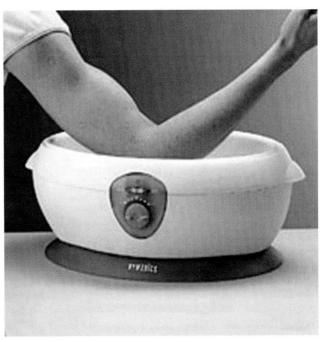

Fig. 133.5 Paraffin baths are a useful form of conduction-type heat therapy capable of providing superficial heating of the affected tissues.

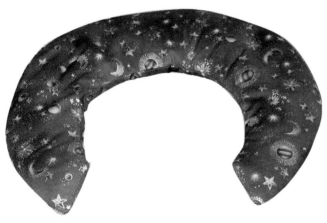

Fig. 133.3 The widespread use of microwave ovens has spawned a variety of new reusable heating pad products that are designed to be quickly heated in the microwave oven.

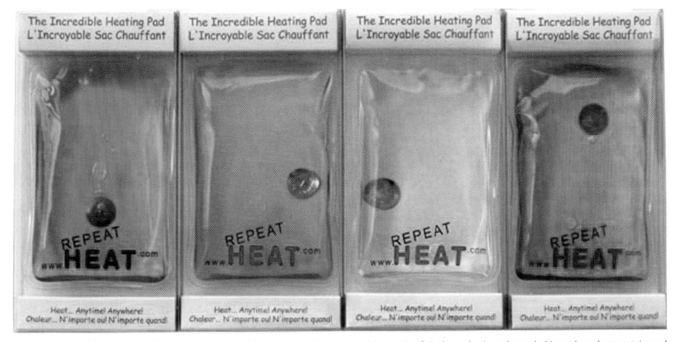

Fig. 133.4 Reusable microwavable heating pads consist of an outer bag that may be made of cloth or plastic and a sealed inner bag that contains gel or grains (rice, corn, or wheat). They deliver their heat via conduction to provide superficial heating of the affected tissues.

Modalities That Deliver Heat via Convection

Hydrotherapy

Water is an ideal medium for delivery of heat to affected tissues because of its high specific heat. Hydrotherapy uses this physical property to advantage with the agitation of a whirlpool to constantly move the layer of heated water that has cooled after contact with the skin and replace it with water heated to the correct temperature. In addition to the superficial heat delivery properties of hydrotherapy, immersion of the affected body part, or entire body in the case of Hubbard tank therapy, allows the high specific gravity of water to partially eliminate the effect of gravity, adding another potentially therapeutic sensation to the analgesic milieu (**Fig. 133.6**). The massaging effect of water can also help reduce muscle spasm and provide gentle débridement of wounds. For treatment of single limbs, immersion in waters with temperatures of 115°F (46°C) is generally well tolerated if careful monitoring is carried out. Temperatures above 102°F (39°C) should be avoided with use of total body immersion to avoid overheating. Total body immersion should not be used in patients with multiple sclerosis to avoid the triggering of neurologic deficits that may sometimes become permanent.

Fluidotherapy

Fluidotherapy uses convection as its mechanism of heat transfer. In contrast with hydrotherapy, which relies on the high specific heat of water delivered at lower temperatures, fluidotherapy relies on substances with a low affinity for heat (e.g., glass beads, pulverized corn cobs, etc) and high heat temperatures of 116°F (47°C) (**Fig. 133.7**). The result is a dry semifluid mixture that is heated with thermostatically controlled hot air. The patient is able to immerse the affected hand, foot, or portion of an extremity into the mixture. As the affected body part is heated, sweating enhances heat transfer, producing superficial heating. This treatment modality is useful in the treatment of reflex sympathetic dystrophy in that the medium used (e.g., glass beads) provides gentile tactile desensitization.

Deep Heating Modalities

Modalities That Deliver Heat via Conversion

The heat delivery modalities previously discussed have in common their ability to produce superficial heating of affected tissues. When heating of the deep tissues is desired, clinicians have several modalities at their disposal. These include three modalities in common clinical use: (1) ultrasound; (2) shortwave diathermy; and (3) microwave diathermy. These modalities all have the ability to safely heat deep tissues via the physical property of conversion of physical energy into heat when properly used.

Variables that affect the amount of heat ultimately delivered to deep tissues for each of these modalities include: (1) the pattern of relative heating; (2) the specific heat of the tissue being heated; and (3) the physiologic factors that affect the tissues being heated. Each of these variables is discussed individually.

Relative heating is the relative amount of energy that is converted into heat at any point in the tissue being heated. For sake of consistency, common reference points for the pattern of relative heating include the subcutaneous fat/muscle interface, the muscle/bone interface, and so on. The pattern of relative heating is different for each of the deep heat modalities currently in common clinical use.

The specific heat of the tissue also influences how deep heat is distributed through affected tissues. Each type of tissue being heated has its own specific heat. As each of these tissues is heated, the thermal conductivity of the tissue changes as the relative temperatures of each type of tissue reach equilibrium, thus affecting the heat exchange between warmer and cooler tissues.

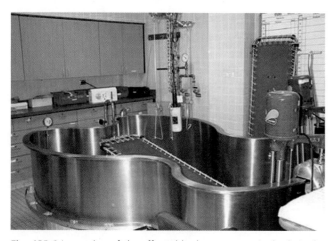

Fig. 133.6 Immersion of the affected body part, or entire body in the case of Hubbard tank therapy, allows the high specific gravity of water to partially eliminate the effect of gravity, adding another potentially therapeutic sensation to the analgesic milieu.

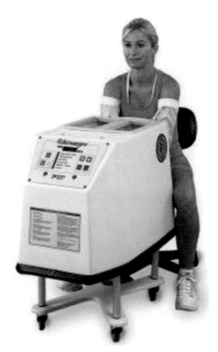

Fig. 133.7 Fluidotherapy relies on substances with a low affinity for heat (e.g., glass beads, pulverized corn cobs) and high temperatures of 47°C (116°F).

The physiologic changes induced with deep heating also influence the heat distribution by modifying the physiologic factors that existed before the deep heat was applied. For example, in normal conditions, the skin temperature is generally lower that the deeper muscle tissues. The application of a deep heating modality further raises the core temperature of the muscle being heated, thereby increasing the temperature gradient between skin and deep muscle. However, as the deep heat is applied to muscle, an increase in blood flow to the heated muscle occurs. The incoming blood is cooler than the heated muscle, so the blood with its relatively high specific heat acts as a cooling agent, carrying off excess heat and cooling the muscle.[6] The interplay of these and other physiologic factors ultimately affects the pattern of temperature distribution.

Ultrasound

Ultrasound uses sound waves to deliver energy to affected tissue. These sound waves occur at a frequency well above the upper level of human hearing (which occurs at approximately 20,000 Hz) and are produced with the use of a piezoelectric crystal that converts electrical energy into sound waves. These sound waves produce both thermal and nonthermal therapeutic effects on tissue, and manipulation of the physical properties of these effects can tailor the therapeutic response delivered—for example, high-temperature destruction of malignant liver tumors, phonophoresis (the forcing of steroids and anti-inflammatory drugs into tissues with sound), lithotripsy, and deep heating of tissues.

Although an extensive discussion of the physics involved in the therapeutic use of ultrasound is beyond the purpose of this chapter, a few general comments are useful for the clinician to understand how the modalities are used to produce deep heat for the treatment of pain and the other conditions listed in Table 133.3. For the purposes of our discussion, it is sufficient to note that the two major variables at play that determine the propagation of ultrasonic energy are: (1) the absorption characteristics of the tissues being exposed to the sound waves; and (2) the reflection of these sound waves as they impinge on tissue interfaces (e.g., muscle, bone). These two variables give ultrasound the unique characteristic of being able to heat deep tissues such as joints with little heating of overlying skin and subcutaneous tissues.[7]

Each variable can dramatically affect the amount of sound energy that is converted to heat. One example is absorption: bone absorbs almost 10 times more energy than does skeletal muscle and almost 20 times more energy than subcutaneous fat, which means that much more of the ultrasonic energy is converted into heat at the bone interface relative to the muscle or subcutaneous fat interface. Likewise, reflection of the ultrasonic energy occurs primarily at the bone interface, with very little reflection occurring at the subcutaneous fat or muscle interface. Thus, most of the sound energy delivered is able to penetrate the subcutaneous tissues and muscle, with the reflected sound waves producing much of their heating effect at the muscle-bone interface. This physical property of reflection can produce extremely high temperatures if ultrasound is accidentally used in patients with metal prosthetics or large metal surgical clips because reflection from these artificial interfaces can produce an intense increase in reflected ultrasonic energy that can cause disastrous deep thermal injury.

The admonition that ultrasound is contraindicated over metal implants should be heeded.[8]

If sound waves are to be effectively delivered to the intended tissues, coupling between the skin overlying the tissue and the ultrasound wand must be accomplished. This is accomplished with introduction of a medium called a *coupling agent*. Gel and degassed water are commonly used coupling agents. Ultrasound is usually delivered with the ultrasound wand, which has been liberally covered with coupling agent, being moved slowly over the affected area for 5 to 10 minutes. For body parts with irregular surfaces, such as the ankle, ultrasound can be delivered indirectly with immersion of the affected body part in degassed water and placement of the ultrasound wand in close proximity to the skin but not actually touching it and then slowly moved over the affected areas. This technique is known as indirect ultrasound and necessitates higher energy levels to offset the absorption of sound waves by the water to achieve similar deep heating effects when compared with direct ultrasound.

Indications for ultrasound are summarized in Table 133.5. Tendinitis and bursitis generally respond well to treatment with ultrasound, as does degenerative arthritis.[9] Although the use of ultrasound is generally avoided when a joint is acutely inflamed, it can be beneficial as the joint inflammation is resolving after intra-articular injection of steroids or the implementation of anti-inflammatory drugs. Ultrasound can be used in concert to enhance the effects of active and passive range of motion and stretching of joints that have lost normal range of motion—and in the treatment of plantar fasciitis.[10,11]

Shortwave Diathermy

Shortwave diathermy uses electromagnetic radio waves to convert energy to deep heat. As with ultrasound, shortwave diathermy is thought to exert its therapeutic effects via both thermal and nonthermal mechanisms. The primary nonthermal mechanism associated with the use of therapeutic shortwave diathermy is vibration induction of tissue molecules with exposure to radio waves. By changing the characteristics of the shortwave applicator, clinicians can target the specific type of tissue they want to heat. With use of an inductive applicator that generates a magnetically induced eddy of radio wave currents in the tissues, selective heating of water-rich tissues, such as muscle, can be obtained (**Fig. 133.8**). With use of a capacity-coupled applicator that generates heat via generation of an electrical field, selective heating of water-poor tissues, such as subcutaneous fat and adjacent soft tissues, can be accomplished.[12] With either type of shortwave diathermy, metal must be avoided; the patient must remove all jewelry, and treatment must be carried out on a nonconductive (e.g., wooden) treatment table. Implanted pacemakers, spinal cord stimulators, surgical implants, and copper-containing intrauterine devices (IUDs) should *never* be exposed to shortwave diathermy to avoid excessive heating and thermal injury. Indications for shortwave diathermy mirror those listed for ultrasound, although the ability to heat subcutaneous fat and adjacent soft tissues not reached with superficial heat modalities and less well heated with ultrasound may lead the clinician to choose shortwave diathermy for treatment of painful conditions and other pathologic processes that are thought to find their nidus in more superficial tissues.[13]

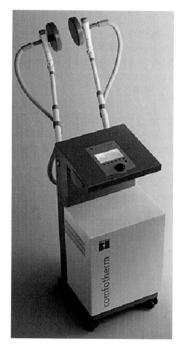

Fig. 133.8 Shortwave diathermy uses electromagnetic radio waves to convert energy to deep heat.

Table 133.6 Indications for Therapeutic Cold
Pain
Muscle spasm
Acute musculoskeletal injury
Bursitis
Tendinitis
Adjunct to muscle re-education

Table 133.7 Precautions and Contraindications with Use of Therapeutic Cold
Lack of or reduced sensation
Ischemia
Raynaud's phenomenon
Cold intolerance

Microwave Diathermy

Microwave diathermy uses electromagnetic radio waves with frequencies of 915 and 2456 MHz.[14] On the basis of the physical properties of these waves and the corresponding dimensions of the microwave antennae, microwave diathermy has two unique properties that can be used to clinical advantage. The first is that microwaves are selectively absorbed in tissues with high water content, such as muscle.[15] This makes microwave diathermy ideally suited to treatment of pathologic processes that occur in the muscles and adjacent fat.[16] The second is that microwaves are more easily focused than the short waves used in shortwave diathermy, thereby decreasing energy leakage and making heating more efficient.

Microwave diathermy also has several unique side effects of which the clinician must be aware. First, microwaves can cause cataract formation, so protective eyewear must be worn whenever microwave diathermy is used.[17] Second, in addition to the precautions and contraindications to the use of shortwave diathermy listed previously, because microwave diathermy has a selective affinity to heat water, this technique should not be used in patients with edema or blisters or in patients with hyperhidrosis because the sweat beads may become heated and cause burns to the skin.

Therapeutic Cold Modalities

The Physiologic Effects of Therapeutic Cold

The application of therapeutic cold exerts both local and remote physiologic effects.[2] Locally, the application of therapeutic cold causes vasoconstriction, which is ultimately followed by a reflex vasodilation after the vascular smooth muscles are paralyzed from the cold. Therapeutic cold decreases the metabolic activity of the treated part and decreases muscle tone. As cooling progresses, spasticity is also decreased.[18] As cooling slows nerve conduction, analgesia occurs. Indications for the use of therapeutic cold are summarized in **Table 133.6.**

Choosing a Therapeutic Cold Modality

As with the choice of heat modalities, matching of the therapeutic cold modality to the patient is paramount to the success of the treatment and to minimization of the side effects and complications associated with its use. The major determinants in the choice of therapeutic cold modalities are primarily based on two categories: (1) the body part being treated; and (2) whether the modality is administered by a qualified health care professional. As with therapeutic heat, improper use of therapeutic cold modalities can cause serious complications (**Table 133.7**).

Ice Packs and Slushes

The high specific heat capacities of ice packs and slushes allow rapid cooling of affected areas. Ice packs can be simply made with placement of melting ice and cold water in a Ziploc plastic bag. With use of crushed ice and more cold water, a slush pack can be made. Commercially available plastic gel packs, often covered with a soft fabric, may be stored in the refrigerator or freezer and are also a convenient way of therapeutic cold delivery (**Fig. 133.9**). The flexible nature of both these therapeutic cold modalities allows them to be used over joints or to cool larger areas such as the low back. The rate of cooling of the skin is rapid, and the rate of the cooling of deeper tissues is largely a function of the thickness of fat interposed between skin and muscle. When used for periods of 20 minutes or less, they packs are usually safe. The use of a towel between the ice pack or slush and the affected body part increases tolerance and compliance and decreases the incidence of thermal injury. For home use, a package of frozen peas or corn can serve as an effective and inexpensive ice pack for many painful conditions.

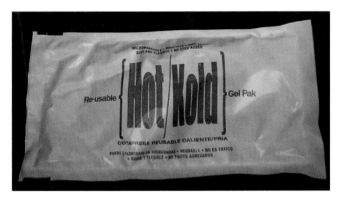

Fig. 133.9 Commercially available plastic packs, often covered with a soft fabric, that contain gel and may be stored in the refrigerator or freezer until use are a convenient way of therapeutic cold delivery.

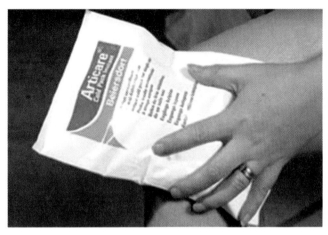

Fig. 133.10 Chemical ice packs are made of a flexible outer layer and a two-compartment inner layer.

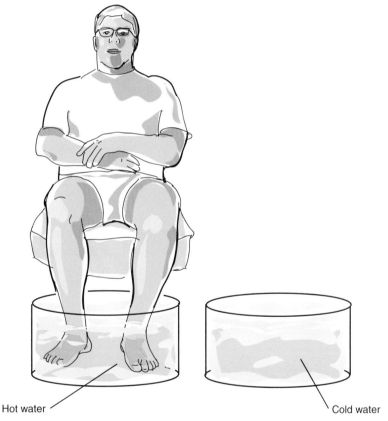

Hot water   Cold water

Fig. 133.11   Contrast baths consist of a hot and a cold bath with temperatures of 43°C (110°F) and 16°C, (60°F), respectively.

Iced Whirlpools

Used primarily for athletic injuries, the iced whirlpool can rapidly cool an injured extremity by constantly moving water that is warmed by contact with the patient's skin away and replacing it with colder water. Many patients find that the temperatures needed to adequately cool muscle are too uncomfortable to tolerate for the time necessary to achieve the intended therapeutic effect. However, some patients find the iced whirlpool more beneficial than similar heated whirlpool treatments.

Ice Rubs

Useful for application of therapeutic cold to larger surface areas such as the low back, ice rubs that use water frozen in a plastic or styrofoam cup can rapidly achieve therapeutic temperatures, with cutaneous anesthesia being achieved within 8 to 10 minutes. In addition, the rubbing action can produce a relaxing effect and aids in tactile desensitization. In healthy patients, ice rubs for periods of 20 minutes or less are usually safe.

Evaporative Cooling Spays

Useful in the treatment of trigger points associated with fibromyalgia and as an adjunct to stretching, the application of evaporative cooling sprays can be quite effective.[19] In the past, ethyl chloride spray was the agent of choice; however, the flammability and potential toxicity of the agent has led to the use of the chlorofluormethane compounds. Although effective, these compounds have been criticized as having a negative effect on the environment. For use of the evaporative sprays, the trigger point or affected muscle is identified and the agent is aimed at the target area from a distance of approximately 1 meter and applied for approximately 10 seconds. Prolonged cooling of a single point with the evaporative agents can result in thermal injury.

Chemical Ice Packs

A large number of disposable ice packs are available for home use and for clinical applications. Chemical ice packs are made of a flexible outer layer and a two-compartment inner layer (**Fig. 133.10**). One inner compartment contains water, and the other contains ammonium nitrate that, when combined with squeezing or kneading of the package, creates cooling via an endothermic reaction. These products have the advantage of needing no refrigeration, being easily moldable to joints given their flexibility, and being relatively inexpensive. As with chemical heat packs, the temperature of chemical ice packs is poorly controlled and thermal injuries or inadequate or uneven cooling may occur.[20] Exposure of the skin to the chemicals contained in the pack may cause chemical irritation.

Contrast Baths

As a combination of therapeutic heat and cold, contrast baths are useful in the treatment of reflex sympathetic dystrophy and other sympathetically maintained pain syndromes and rheumatoid arthritis.[21] Their efficacy is thought to be the result of desensitization of nerves with alternating exposure of the affected extremity to heat and cold. Contrast baths consist of a hot and a cold bath with temperatures of 43°C (110°F) and 16°C (60°F), respectively (**Fig. 133.11**). Therapeutic contrast baths begin with the soaking of the affected extremity in the warm bath for 10 minutes. The extremity is then rapidly transferred to the cold bath for a period of 3 minutes, followed by rapid transfer back to the warm bath for 5 minutes. The cycle is repeated four times. For patients with extreme allodynia, less extreme temperatures may be necessary during initiation of therapy. Contrast baths should be combined with tactile desensitization techniques if optimal results are to be obtained.

Conclusion

The use of therapeutic heat and cold represents a useful adjunct in the treatment of a variety of painful conditions. Although the modalities are relatively safe if used properly, severe injury can occur if risk factors are ignored or a specific modality is misused. The correct matching of the modality to the patient is paramount if optimal results are to be achieved and side effects and complications are to be avoided.

References

Full references for this chapter can be found on www.expertconsult.com.

Hydrotherapy

David A. Soto-Quijano and Martin Grabois

Hydrotherapy is the use of a water environment for therapeutic effects. *Aquatic rehabilitation* or *aquatic therapy* refers to the combination of healing and rehabilitation modalities in water.[1] The use of the aquatic environment to help in managing pain and increasing function through rehabilitation is rapidly increasing because of the proven physiologic and biodynamic properties of water that allow the patient with pain to rehabilitate more rapidly and safely.[2] More than 7.2 million people participated in nonswimming aquatic exercise in 2007, according to a 2008 superstudy of sports participation.[3] When used in a comprehensive therapeutic approach, aquatic exercises are designed to aid in the management and rehabilitation of patients with pain. Aquatic therapy not only promotes modification of pain and increases function but also accomplishes this in a cost-effective environment.

Historical Considerations

The use of water as a healing medium dates back many centuries, although its original use does not coincide exactly with the present perception of its use for rehabilitation purposes. The original use of water (dating back to 2400 BC) was closely connected to the mystical and religious worship of water and its perceived power of healing.[4] The Greek civilization in 500 BC began to use water more logically for specific physical treatments, and the Romans expanded the bath system. The Romans added a system of baths at various temperatures and used them not only for rest and recreational activities but also for health and exercise to heal and treat injuries.[5]

By the early Middle Ages, religious influences had led to the decline of the use of water for its healing power because this use was considered a pagan act.[6] The period from 1600 to 1800 saw a resurgence of water healing, but not for hygienic purposes, and the term *hydrotherapy* started to take hold.[7] The use of hydrotherapy continued to be primarily passive, although at about this time, spas, built around a natural spring and usually surrounded by natural beauty, were developed in Europe and then in the United States.[4]

During the early to middle 1900s, the property of buoyancy began to be used to exercise patients in water, with the development of the Bad Ragaz technique and the Hallwich method in Europe.[4] During the poliomyelitis epidemics of the early 1900s, medically supervised exercises in water began to gain popularity in the United States.[4] Finnerty and Corbitt[6] related that a young person with poliomyelitis fell from his wheelchair into a pool. While attempting to keep himself afloat, the young man discovered that he could move his paralyzed legs. This movement was not possible on land. He continued with a pool exercise program to strengthen his lower extremities and was able to progress from being wheelchair bound to ambulating independently without braces and using only a cane.

Many European rehabilitation facilities continued to maintain some type of aquatic therapy as part of an integrated rehabilitation program that was largely publicly funded. This was not the case in the United States.[4] Through the 1950s and 1960s,[7] the use of this technique declined in the United States as a result of the control of poliomyelitis, limited insurance reimbursement, and a lack of education regarding water as a therapeutic exercise medium.

In the 1980s, the use of hydrotherapy increased in the United States, but it still lagged behind Europe because of reimbursement issues, as well as lack of evidence-based efficacy studies, accepted treatment protocols, and education of practitioners.[4] This is also true of other therapeutic techniques that have withstood the test of time but lack significant evidence bases of cost effectiveness and efficacy. Morris[8] pointed out a shortage of efficacy research in aquatic physical therapy and other therapies that address patient outcomes. Currently, aquatic therapy is increasingly used in the United States. Its continued acceptance as a common modality will depend on research on cost effectiveness and efficacy, protocols of treatment, insurance coverage, and education of health care personnel.

Principles of Hydrotherapy

The practitioner must understand numerous principles of hydrotherapy to appreciate the beneficial effects of this modality in pain relief and improvement of function and to prescribe hydrotherapy in a safe, comprehensive, and effective rehabilitation program. All aquatic exercise therapy routines must address two important factors: the body's physiologic response to immersion in water and the physical properties of water.[1] Nearly all the biologic effects of immersion are related to fundamental principles of hydrodynamics, including buoyancy, hydrostatic pressure, and temperature[2] **Table 134.1** lists the principles of hydrotherapy.

Buoyancy is explained by the finding that a body submerged in water is supported by a counterforce that supports the submerged object against the downward pull of gravity. The submerged body seems to lose weight equal to the weight of the water displaced, and the results are less stress and less pressure on muscle and connective tissue.[9] Patients exercising in water feel lighter, move more easily, and feel less weight on their joints because of this buoyancy property.[10] On land, the center of gravity of a body is just in front of the sacrum at the S2 level. In the water, the center of gravity is located at the level of the lungs. The degree of partial weight bearing varies with pool depth, with buoyancy of 90% when the body is immersed up to the neck.[11] Buoyancy can be used in an assistive, resistive, or supportive manner. This force assists any movement toward the surface of the water and resists any movement away from the surface of water. These attributes of buoyancy can be enhanced through the use of flotation devices.

Hydrostatic pressure is pressure exerted by water on a submerged body. The pressure opposes the tendency of blood to pool in lower portions of the body and thus helps to increase venous return to reduce lower extremity swelling and stabilize unstable joints. Because of the property of hydrostatic pressure, patients with chronic obstructive pulmonary disease may have difficulty breathing, given that the pressure of water resists chest wall expansion of 85% immersion.[2]

Specific heat is the amount of energy necessary to increase the temperature of a substance by 1°C (34°F). Because the specific heat of water is several times that of air, heat loss is 25 times that of air at a given temperature.[12] When more heat is lost to water than is produced by muscle, the patient feels cold.[2] Vigorous exercise performed in warm water (33°C [91°F]) results in an increased core temperature (39.4°C [103°F]) and

premature fatigue.[12] The ideal temperature for vigorous exercise is 28°C (82°F) to 30°C (86°F), but for patients with pain, who perform less intense exercise, a higher pool temperature is allowed.[2]

Other properties of water to be considered in the use of hydrotherapy are viscosity and refraction. *Viscosity* is defined as the frictional resistance presented to a body moving through a fluid. Although resistance in air is negligible, in water several factors can lead to resistance proportional to effort exerted, and this property allows for the use of water for strengthening. As water temperature increases, however, the viscosity decreases and can be beneficial for stabilizing small, weak muscle.[2] *Refraction* is the deflection of light as it passes through air into water. Refraction can affect visual feedback and requires appropriate guidance for patients acquiring new skills and for coordination of movements.[1]

Physical Effects

Many profound physiologic effects are produced by immersion of the human body in water (**Table 134.2**). Additionally, the physiologic effects experienced by patients immersed in warm water depend on the posture, with the greatest physiologic changes observed in the upright posture.[13] These effects can be a problem in patients with medical conditions that limit responses to these changes. The physiologic responses experienced by the body during warm water immersion are similar to the responses of localized heat application, although they are less concentrated.[14]

Wilder et al[2] summarized the physiologic effects of immersion in water. The cardiac effects produced through immersion are profound and are probably salutary for overall health and for the rehabilitating heart. Prominent among these effects are the increases in stroke volume and cardiac output. The effects of immersion on the respiratory apparatus and the pulmonary system have been found to increase respiratory effort and work. A program of regular aquatic exercise should produce a significant training effect and should increase pulmonary functioning.

Table 134.1 Principles of Hydrotherapy

Buoyancy
Hydrostatic pressure
Specific heat
Viscosity
Refraction

Table 134.2 Physiologic Changes during Warm Water Exercise

Increased respiratory rate
Decreased blood pressure
Increased blood supply to muscle
Increased muscle metabolism
Increased superficial circulation
Increased heart rate
Increased amount of blood returned to heart
Increased metabolic rate
Decreased edema of submerged body parts*
Reduced sensitivity of sensory nerve endings
General muscular relaxation

*Because of the hydrostatic pressure at the water surface, 14.7 psi plus an increase of 0.43 psi for every 1-ft increase in depth.

The effects on the circulatory system and the autonomic nervous system and the compressive effect of water pressure dramatically alter muscle blood flow and thus increase oxygen delivery and metabolic waste product removal. These effects are salutary on healing, normal exercising muscle and ligament structures.

The aquatic environment produces renal system changes that promote removal of metabolic waste products and produce diuresis, lower the blood pressure, and assist the body in regulation of sodium and potassium. These effects persist longer than the period of immersion and may have general applicability in the management of some forms of hypertension.[2]

Therapeutic Effects

The various physiologic changes noted during warm water immersion also can offer therapeutic effects in numerous medical conditions, including chronic pain (**Table 134.3**). The relaxation response of muscles depends on how comfortable the patient is in the water. The warmth of the therapeutic pool reduces muscular tension and helps to prevent restricted joint movement.[1] Warm water also helps patients with pain to relax and feel more comfortable. The water provides support for injured limbs that allows comfortable positioning without increased pain. The stimulatory effects of warm water promote the relaxation of "tight" spastic muscles and thereby reduce muscle guarding. During warm water immersion, the sensory inputs are competing with the pain input; as a result, the patient's pain perception is blocked out or "gated." This reduction in pain is perhaps the most significant advantage of aquatic therapy. Additionally, body parts immersed in water warmer than 35°C (95°F) begin to increase in temperature toward the temperature of the core.[14] This warmth reduces abnormal muscular tone and spasticity.

The physical properties and the warmth of the water play important roles in improving or maintaining joint range of motion. The buoyancy of water decreases the compression forces on painful joints and assists movement. The water also provides support and decreases the need for splinting or guarding. The warmth of the water reduces spasticity, promotes relaxation, and helps to prepare the connective tissue for stretching. Elongated tissue has a lower risk of injury and

Table 134.3 Therapeutic Benefits of Warm Water Exercise

Promotes muscular relaxation

Reduces pain sensitivity

Decreases muscle spasm

Increases ease of joint movement

Increases muscular strength and endurance in cases of excessive weakness

Reduces gravitational forces (early ambulation)

Increases peripheral circulation (skin condition)

Improves respiratory muscles

Improves body awareness, balance, and proximal trunk stability

Improves patient morale and confidence (psychological)

of muscle soreness after exercise.[13] The water also provides greater resistance to movement than air and thus allows the joint to move more freely. In the water, movements are more consistent and are more easily graded using the principles of buoyancy without the pain of active movement. Warm water promotes relaxation of the spastic antagonists of a weak, exercising muscle. Strength training often can begin in the water before it is possible on land.[14]

Similarly, because of the reduction of gravitational forces, an injured patient can stand and begin gait training and strengthening exercises earlier on water than on land without being concerned about causing further damage to the healing structures.[15,16] Walking earlier helps to improve balance and increase muscle tone. As time goes on, a gradual reduction in the water level can help the patient retrain for the weight-bearing aspect of gait.

Circulation increases in water temperatures higher than 34°C (>93°F). The redistribution of blood during immersion augments flow to the periphery that causes an increase in the blood supply to the muscles and helps in increasing venous return.[14] Exercising injured limbs in deep water further increases circulation, and as water depth increases, so does the hydrostatic pressure exerted on the submerged body part.[14,16] In chest-deep water, the hydrostatic pressure exerted on the walls of the chest and abdominal muscles increases during breathing. The neutral warmth provided by the water relaxes spastic respiratory muscles. Aquatic activities that require an increase in respiration (e.g., swimming, aerobic exercise) or help to train the breathing component (e.g., blowing bubbles) are beneficial to patients who have respiratory problems.[17]

Warm water stimulates awareness of the moving body parts and provides an ideal medium for muscle reeducation. The supportive properties of the water give patients with poor balance time to react during falling by slowing the movement. Stabilization during exercise also can be obtained through the use of railings, parallel bars, underwater benches, submerged chairs, tubes, and other devices in water.[17] Finally, for patients with pain and patients who cannot yet exercise on land, water provides a positive medium in which to move and relax. The ease of movement allows the patient to achieve much more in water than on land and provides the patient with confidence to aid rehabilitation. In water, patients have less fear of falling or of hurting the injured or painful sites.

Techniques

As previously stated, the term *hydrotherapy* includes any use of water for healing purposes. Under that definition, hydrotherapy includes hot or cold compresses, sitz baths, steam baths, colonic irrigation, douches, enemas, shower carts, swimming, and saunas. This chapter discusses the hydrotherapy techniques most commonly used for pain management: water-based exercise, Hubbard tank, whirlpool baths, and contrast baths.

Water-Based Exercises
Indications

Water-based exercises are commonly used in the treatment of musculoskeletal ailments. The previously discussed properties of water and the physiologic effects of the water on the body allow patients with pain to enjoy the benefits of exercises in a safe and controlled environment. Water-based exercises potentially can be used in the treatment and rehabilitation of almost any musculoskeletal problem. However, most published studies are related to the treatment of knee and hip osteoarthritis, rehabilitation after joint replacement, and low back pain. Interest has also increased in the use of water-based exercise program in patients with fibromyalgia.[18,19] Other diagnoses for which water-based exercises are used include stroke,[20] lymphedema,[21] rotator cuff repair surgery,[22] and rheumatoid arthritis.[23]

Different water-based exercise programs are used for knee, hip, and back pain, depending on the severity, body characteristics, overall health status, and needs of the patient. Each patient must be evaluated by the rehabilitation team before a specific protocol is prescribed. As with land-based physical therapies, different centers and clinicians specialize in different types of programs. In addition, books of aquatic exercises for the different muscle groups can help to delineate an appropriate exercise prescription.[24]

For the treatment of joint pain, the goals of the aquatic rehabilitation program are to relieve pain, decrease muscle spasm, maintain or restore muscle strength, maintain or restore range of motion, prevent deformities, promote relaxation, and enforce a normal pattern of movement. Despite the rising popularity of aquatic rehabilitation for joint pain, more scientific studies must be published to validate its efficacy. In one study, patients awaiting joint replacement surgery of the hip or knee were enrolled in a multidimensional land-based or pool-based exercise programs for 6 weeks. When clinical outcomes were compared, both interventions were found effective in reducing pain and improving function, but the pool-based group had less pain immediately after the exercise classes.[25] The effects of gym versus hydrotherapy exercises for patients with knee or hip osteoarthritis were compared, and a similar beneficial effect on physical function was noted in both groups compared with control subjects, although the gym group gained more leg strength.[26] A review of published articles on aquatic exercises for the treatment of osteoarthritis concluded that although high-quality studies are lacking, aquatic exercises appear to have some beneficial short-term effects for patients with hip or knee osteoarthritis.[27] Studies comparing land-based and water-based exercise programs after joint replacement found comparable outcomes, with a positive effect on early recovery of hip strength in patients who received hydrotherapy.[28,29] For patients with total knee replacements, the benefits of hydrotherapy were still present 6 months after discharge.[30]

Patients with rheumatoid arthritis can also receive benefits from exercises in water. A randomized controlled trial comparing patients with rheumatoid arthritis who received hydrotherapy with patients with the same disease who received exercises on land found that the hydrotherapy group reported feeling much better or very much better more frequently than did the land exercise group.[23]

A systematic review examining the effectiveness of therapeutic aquatic exercise in the treatment of low back pain found that, although most published studies on the subject are of low methodologic quality, therapeutic aquatic exercise is potentially beneficial to patients suffering from chronic low back pain and pregnancy-related low back pain.[31] One study compared hydrotherapy with land treatment in patients with low back pain and found that both groups improved significantly in functional ability and pain levels. Overall, no significant difference was noted between the two types of treatment.[32] Based on experience with many patients, the consensus of musculoskeletal rehabilitation therapists is that water-based exercises are very helpful in the treatment of low back pain, especially in patients with severe pain that precludes any other exercise program.

Water-based exercises also have been used as part of a comprehensive treatment program for pain syndromes. Fibromyalgia is a very challenging condition to treat, and some centers use hydrotherapy as part of their multidisciplinary approach to the disease. One group of patients with fibromyalgia received group pool exercises once a week for 6 weeks, combined with an educational program. After 6 weeks, the patients showed improvements in symptom severity, walking ability, and quality of life compared with an untreated control group. A follow-up study found that improvements in symptom severity, physical function, and social function were still present 6 and 24 months after completion of the program.[18,33] A review of randomized controlled clinical trials on the efficacy of hydrotherapy in fibromyalgia syndrome found moderate evidence that hydrotherapy has short-term beneficial effects on pain and health-related quality of life in this population.[34]

Obesity is a very common health problem that is difficult to treat, especially in patients with chronic pain. Aquatic exercise programs have been used with success as a way to increase activity levels in obese patients. No good studies have been conducted to confirm the long-term effect of aquatic exercise in this population, but many patients and therapists have used this technique with success. Because of all the previously stated characteristics of the aquatic environment, obese patients are able to exercise in water without stressing their joints or exacerbating their pain. Therefore, obese patients who cannot safely tolerate physical activity on dry land can participate in exercises as part of a weight loss program. However, the long-term goal in these patients to transfer them, once they build tolerance to exercise, to a regular weight loss exercise program at home or in a gym, because studies of nonobese populations suggested that exercise in water causes less decrease in fat than does exercise on dry land.[35,36]

Patients who have had a stroke comprise another population that is sometimes difficult to enroll in an exercise program because of residual motor deficits. A relatively short program of water-based exercises, three times a week for 8 weeks, proved beneficial for the cardiovascular fitness of a group of patients with stroke who had mild to moderate residual motor deficits. The experimental group also improved in maximal workload, gait speed, and paretic lower extremity muscle strength.[20]

Equipment

Water-based exercises can be performed in any standard pool. Large rehabilitation facilities usually have an indoor, temperature-controlled pool accessible to handicapped patients. The pool at its deepest point should be deep enough to cover standard-sized patients up to their necks, although that much water is not needed to obtain the benefits of the water environment. Other features, such as ramps, grab bars, seats, or underwater treadmills, are also available. Smaller tanks can be used for water-based exercises. These special tanks can include all the features of a larger pool in a smaller space. Some tanks even include an artificial water flow system that allows the patient to swim without the need of a long pool, similar to running on a treadmill. A hydraulic motor produces an adjustable current that is used for resistance.

Special equipment can be used to enhance the effect of water-based exercises. Some aids include floating balls, web gloves, flippers, and flotation devices of different shapes. Delta bells and barbells are made of foam and are consequently weightless outside the pool. When these devices are used in water, their shape creates resistance that is used in exercise programs. An aqua jogging belt allows running-like motion and is commonly used in sports rehabilitation to keep an athlete fit while protecting weight-bearing joints.

Prescription

As previously stated, a water-based exercise prescription follows an evaluation by the physician and the therapist. Strengthening exercises are prescribed for weak muscles, and stretching and mobilization exercises are recommended for stiff joints, muscles, or segments. Exercises in water are not the same as similar exercises done on land. A complete discussion of the different exercises is beyond the scope of this chapter. Books and manuals are available that describe the different types of exercises and techniques. It is impossible to recommend a standard program that fits the needs of every patient, but the following paragraph contains a description of some aquatic exercises recommended for diskogenic pain, a common diagnosis in pain clinics.

Water walking forward (**Fig. 134.1**) helps strengthen abdominal and ambulatory muscles and promotes proper posture. *Water walking backward* (**Fig. 134.2**) helps the same muscles but emphasizes the paraspinal muscles. The *wall sit* (**Fig. 134.3**) is used to strengthen the quadriceps and hamstring

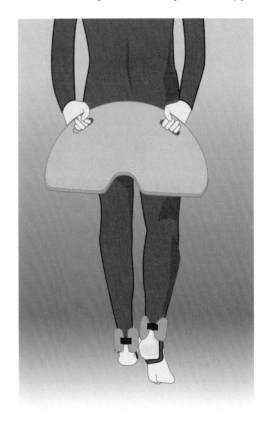

Fig. 134.2 Water walking backward.

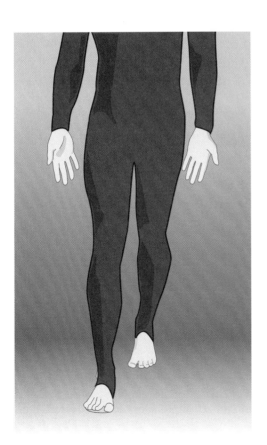

Fig. 134.1 Water walking forward.

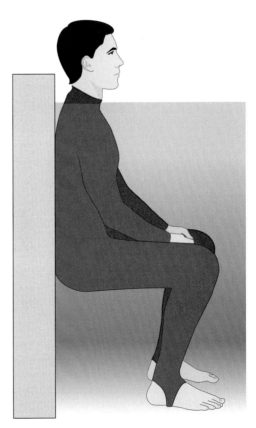

Fig. 134.3 Wall sit.

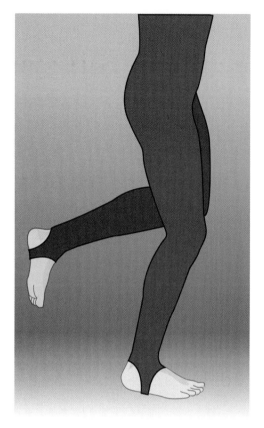

Fig. 134.4 Modified superman.

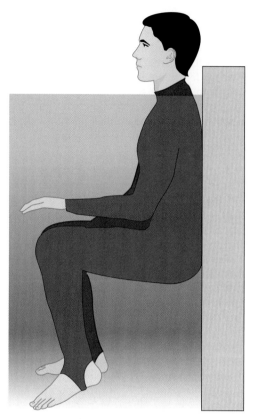

Fig. 134.6 Wall crunch.

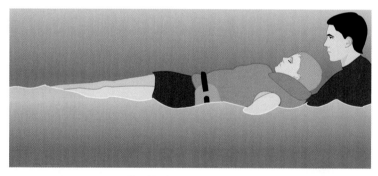

Fig. 134.5 Supine sculling.

muscles isometrically. The patient is supported by the pool wall in the vertical position while the hips and knees are kept at 90 degrees. The *modified superman* (**Fig. 134.4**) exercise requires the patient to stand vertically and hold the edge of the pool with both hands. One leg is then flexed 45 degrees at the knee. That same leg is extended to 20 degrees at the hip and is brought back to neutral repeatedly. To add difficulty, the knee is flexed to 90 degrees, or a weight or resistance is added to the ankle. This movement trains the ipsilateral hip flexor and extensor muscles, the contralateral gluteus medius, and all abdominal and paraspinal muscles. *Supine sculling* (**Fig. 134.5**) is a more complex exercise that requires the use of a flotation jacket, a flotation collar, and direct assistance from a therapist for the patient to maintain a supine position in the water. The upper extremities perform a sculling motion at the hip level, while the lower extremities execute a flutter kick. This is a good overall exercise that strengthens upper and lower extremities and paraspinal muscles. In the *wall crunch*

(**Fig. 134.6**), the patient stands with his or her back against the pool wall and attempts to flex the hip to 90 degrees with the knee flexed while the ipsilateral hand isometrically resists the movement, to maintain an isometric contraction for 5 seconds at a time. This exercise requires the use of the quadriceps, hamstring, gluteal, ipsilateral hip flexor, rotational abdominal, and paraspinal muscles. The *log roll swim* (**Fig. 134.7**) is another complex exercise, requiring the use of a mask, a snorkel, a flotation belt, and support from the therapist to keep the body in a prone position. The neck is flexed 20 degrees, the knees are flexed 25 degrees, and the patient begins a small rotatory movement of the arms under the chest. With the hips in 25 degrees of flexion, the knees initiate a small flexion-extension propulsion movement. The patient is taught a lateral rocking movement to minimize the segmental stress of the lumbar spine. The whole purpose of the exercise is to promote appropriate spine movement on ambulation while strengthening the upper and lower extremities.

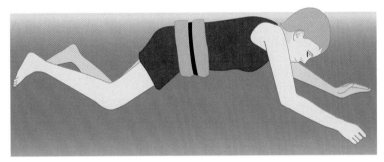

Fig. 134.7 Log roll swim.

Contraindications

When prescribing water-based exercises, the clinician must practice common sense and remember that a pool and its surroundings can be a dangerous place. Aquatic therapy should not be ordered for a patient who cannot follow basic safety rules. Difficult cases always should be discussed with the therapist before the referral. Contraindications to water-based exercises include fear of water, open wounds, bladder or bowel disorders, skin disease, and high fever. Patients with unstable angina, congestive heart failure with symptomatic low ejection fraction, frequent high-grade ectopy, or significant aortic or mitral valve problems should not participate in water programs. A cardiology evaluation and clearance usually are recommended for patients with cardiac conditions before they begin an exercise program.

Whirlpool and Hubbard Tank

Indications

The most important uses of whirlpools and Hubbard tank baths are for adjunctive treatment of degenerative arthritis and acute musculoskeletal injuries and for cleansing and débridement of burns or skin ulcerations. Patients with musculoskeletal pain (arthritis, diffuse myalgias, muscle spasm, muscle strains) can benefit from the massage created by water turbulence, the therapeutic effect of water temperature, and the decreased stress on bones and joints that the aquatic environment provides. The massage and heat effects created by the turbulence are particularly helpful for muscle pain and spasm. The agitated water causes localized and controlled joint movement that helps to improve the function of patients with arthralgias or joint stiffness. In some cases, patients are advised to move the joint actively while receiving the treatment to maximize the effect on range of motion. The movement and hydrostatic pressure of the water in whirlpool help in the mobilization of fluids and cause the resolution of edema and swelling in chronic or acute musculoskeletal injuries. The relaxation effect and the decrease in pain perception of water immersion are also beneficial.

Whirlpools and Hubbard tanks are commonly used for pressure ulcers and for wound and burn treatment. Unfortunately, little trial evidence exists to support these indications.[37] The warm, gently agitated water of the whirlpool permits comfortable solvent action and gentle débridement and aids in bandage removal. A study of patients with stage III or IV pressure ulcers compared conservative treatment with conservative treatment plus whirlpool 20 minutes per day. Conservative treatment included pressure relief measures and wound care with wet-to-wet dressings using normal saline solution. When followed up for 2 or more weeks, patients who received whirlpool treatments improved at a significantly faster rate than did patients who received conservative treatment alone.[38]

Use of a whirlpool has been mentioned as part of a multiple-intervention approach to patients with nonspecific chronic pain.[18] One study examined the effects of whirlpool therapy on pain and surgical wound healing in adults who had undergone major abdominal surgery. Measures of pain were repeated over a 3-day period. The experimental group response to verbal pain was not significant, but it did reveal an improvement in observable pain behaviors using the Pain Rating Scale. The investigators concluded that the intervention of whirlpool therapy promoted some degree of comfort and positive signs of wound healing.[39]

Equipment

Whirlpool baths and Hubbard tanks possess water pumps or turbines that agitate water and provide connective heating or cooling, massage, and gentle débridement. Whirlpool baths come in different sizes and shapes. Small, 120-L tanks are used for treatments to a single extremity or area, whereas large Hubbard tanks are used when the entire body must be immersed. The large tanks usually are equipped with a stretcher that may be fitted into an adjustable support bracket. Normally, the tank is butterfly shaped, so that the patient can move the extremities through abduction if indicated.

Prescription

Whirlpool or Hubbard tank treatments may be given daily or twice daily for acute problems and less often for more chronic problems. Treatments usually take 20 to 25 minutes. The water turbulence is directed to the involved area, unless it exacerbates pain. Depending on the affected area, a small whirlpool or a Hubbard tank is recommended. Water temperature is regulated depending on the patient's needs. Temperatures of 33°C (91°F) to 36°C (97°F) are considered neutral. If heat is indicated, water temperature can be increased to 43°C (109°F) to 46°C (115°F) in healthy patients receiving localized or single limb treatment. In full body submersion, the temperature is limited to 38°C (100°F) or less if the patient is going to exercise in the tank. Because of the water's constant motion, no insulating layer of cooling water is formed around the patient, and more vigorous heating is attained. On burns or infected areas, antiseptic conditions are preferred. Although truly sterile conditions are difficult to achieve, antibacterial solutions, such as sodium hypochlorite or povidone-iodine, may be added to the water. When large wounds or exposed organs are present, sodium chloride should be added to the water to approximate normal saline solution and to minimize fluid shift. Cases of severe hyponatremia, hyperkalemia, and prerenal uremia have been described in burn patients after they received hydrotherapy in tap water.[40]

Contraindications

A chance of drowning in a whirlpool or Hubbard tank always exists. Care should be taken with patients at risk, such as weak patients, cognitively impaired patients, and children.[41] Extreme temperatures should be avoided in patients with sensory problems, small vessel disease, affected cognition, or an inability to communicate. Hot water should not be used in patients with systemic fever or acute inflammatory conditions. Caution should be exercised when using a whirlpool in patients with motion sickness because the water movement may cause dizziness.

Epidemiologic studies suggest that the use of a hot tub or whirlpool bath during pregnancy doubles the risk of miscarriage. This risk increases with the frequency of use and with use during early gestation. This potential complication should be considered when clinicians prescribe aquatic therapy to women of childbearing age.[42,43]

Contrast Baths
Indications

Contrast baths are indicated for subacute or chronic traumatic and inflammatory conditions, impaired venous circulation, and indolent ulcers. Contrast baths also have been used for neuropathic pain, rheumatoid arthritis, chronic pain syndromes, and complex regional pain syndrome. The purpose of this technique is to cause cyclic vasodilation and vasoconstriction that produces neurologic desensitization.[44]

Equipment

Contrast baths use alternate immersion of body parts in baths. Warm water and cold water baths are used, thus causing alternate dilation and constriction of the local blood vessel. No special equipment is required for this technique. Whirlpool tanks and any other safe water container that can hold water at the required temperatures can be employed.

Prescription

After the patient has been positioned comfortably, two pails of water of a depth that covers the treated area are prepared. The cold bath is usually 13°C to 18°C (55°F to 64°F), and the hot bath is 38°C to 43°C (100°F to 109°F). The affected area is immersed in the hot bath for approximately 6 minutes and then in the cold bath for 4 minutes, or at least 1 minute if the patient cannot tolerate the cold bath. This process is repeated for approximately 30 minutes. As in the whirlpool or Hubbard tank, povidone-iodine or sodium hypochlorite can be added to the water to prevent infections.

Contraindications

Contraindications to contrast baths are the same that the contraindications to the use of whirlpools and Hubbard tanks. Extreme temperatures should be avoided in patients with sensory problems, small vessel disease, affected cognition, or an inability to communicate. Hot water should not be used in patients with systemic fever or acute inflammatory conditions.

Conclusion

Hydrotherapy has been used in the management of pain since ancient times, and more recently its use has increased again. Reduction of pain and increase in function are accomplished by using the physiologic and biodynamic properties of water. This chapter presents a basic understanding of different techniques of hydrotherapy. In addition, the physical properties of water are reviewed, including buoyancy, hydrostatic pressure, viscosity, refraction, and specific heat.

The use of water has many physiologic effects. These effects are seen in the cardiopulmonary, circulatory, autonomic, and renal systems. Most appropriate to patients with pain are the physiologic and therapeutic effects seen in patients with musculoskeletal pain. The primary therapeutic effects of hydrotherapy are the promotion of muscle relaxation with decreased muscle spasm and the increased ease of joint motion. Additionally, decreased pain sensitivity, reduced gravitational forces, increased circulation, increased muscular strength, and improved balance can be helpful in the rehabilitation of patients with chronic pain.

Water-based exercises can be used for the treatment and rehabilitation of almost any musculoskeletal problem. For patients with pain who cannot exercise on land, water provides a positive medium in which to move and relax. The ease of movement allows the patient to achieve much more benefit than on land and provides the patient with confidence to aid rehabilitation because he or she has less fear of falling or of hurting the injured or painful sites. The different water-based exercise programs are prescribed, depending on the severity, body characteristics, overall health status, and needs of the patient. Aquatic exercise programs have been proposed for the treatment of knee and hip osteoarthritis, rehabilitation after joint replacement, low back pain, fibromyalgia, stroke, lymphedema, rotator cuff repair surgery, and rheumatoid arthritis. As with other therapeutic treatment techniques, more clinical studies are needed to validate efficacy.

Whirlpool and Hubbard tank baths are used for adjunctive treatment of degenerative arthritis and acute musculoskeletal injuries, as well as for cleansing and débridement of burns or skin ulcerations. Patients with musculoskeletal pain and spasm can benefit from the massage created by water turbulence, the therapeutic effect of water temperature, and the decreased stress on bones and joints that the aquatic environment provides. This technique also is useful for resolution of edema and swelling. Antibacterial solutions such as sodium hypochlorite or povidone-iodine may be added to the water when concerns about infection exist. Contrast baths produce neurologic desensitization by alternating heat and cold cyclic vasodilation and vasoconstriction. Contrast baths have been used for subacute or chronic traumatic and inflammatory conditions, impaired venous circulation, indolent ulcers, neuropathic pain, rheumatoid arthritis, chronic pain syndromes, and complex regional pain syndrome.

References

Full references for this chapter can be found on www.expertconsult.com.

Transcutaneous Electrical Nerve Stimulation

Steven D. Waldman

Long before the gate control theory of Melzack and Wall, the use of sensory stimulation for pain relief had gained widespread acceptance. The modalities of heat and cold, massage, burning, scarification, moxibustion, cupping, and the like were the mainstays of nonpharmacologic pain relief. Reports from ancient Egypt tell of the use of electric catfish applied to the area of pain as one means of pain control. Given that these electric fish could produce a discharge of up to 400 V, one must wonder whether the patient experienced a miraculous cure just to avoid another treatment.[1]

The explanation by Melzack and Wall of how a stimulus could theoretically provide pain relief by modulating or closing a presynaptic gate that allows transmission of pain impulses to the higher centers finally gave a scientific basis for the use of what heretofore had been highly accepted but largely discounted techniques. This impetus led to renewed interest in the use of electricity as a "counter-irritant," or stimulus that could close the gate on pain. The early work by Shealy in dorsal column stimulation spurred a search for less invasive ways to deliver electricity to nerves. One of the results was transcutaneous electrical nerve stimulation (TENS), which was used initially as a noninvasive screening tool to determine whether a patient would experience pain relief with implantation of a dorsal column stimulator. The ease of use and noninvasive nature of TENS made it an instant success. These same attributes led to its overuse and, to a certain extent, to its mediocre reputation as a pain-relieving modality. This chapter discusses the scientific rationale behind TENS and provides the clinician with a practical guide to its use.

Scientific Basis of Transcutaneous Electrical Nerve Stimulation

As mentioned previously, the gate control theory was, in essence, the first unified theory of pain. Earlier theories that were largely based on the Cartesian view of peripheral nociception carried to the central nervous system could not explain how a peripheral stimulus for counter-irritative techniques (e.g., acupuncture, moxibustion, electric shock) could produce pain relief. The gate control theory changed everything. For the first time, scientists, psychologists, and physicians were presented with an elegantly simple explanation of how pain could be produced or blocked in the periphery. The theory stated that small-fiber afferent stimuli, particularly pain, entering the substantia gelatinosa can be modulated by large-fiber afferent stimuli and descending spinal pathways so that their transmission to ascending spinal pathways is blocked or gated.[2]

That the gate control theory could not explain many of the clinical observations associated with the use of TENS soon became apparent. Among these observations were the frequently seen phenomenon of anesthesia persisting hours after stimulation and the delayed onset of analgesia experienced by some patients in pain. The neurophysiologic basis of these clinical observations remains the source of much debate—with alternative explanations such as endorphin or enkephalin release currently the most popular in spite of the fact that TENS analgesia is not reversed with naloxone. This lack of a scientific rationale has not deterred TENS enthusiasts, nor has

Table 135.1 **Clinical Indications for Transcutaneous Electrical Nerve Stimulation**
Acute post-traumatic pain
Acute postoperative pain
Musculoskeletal pain
Peripheral vascular insufficiency
Functional abdominal pain (?)
Neuropathic pain (?)

it been lost on TENS critics, mainly insurance companies that do not want to pay for this popular pain-relieving technique.

Indications for Transcutaneous Electrical Nerve Stimulation

Practically every known pain syndrome has been treated with TENS because of its ease of use and lack of side effects. The true efficacy of TENS for the painful conditions discussed subsequently is complicated to ascertain because true double-blind placebo-controlled trials are difficult to conduct because of the patient's ability to perceive whether the TENS unit is delivering stimulation or not. Despite this fact, the following indications fall within the broad category of conditions in which TENS is, at least, worth considering. **Table 135.1** summarizes the current clinical applications for TENS.

Acute Pain

TENS has been shown to reduce pain and, in some cases, to reduce the need for opioid analgesics and improve pulmonary function after upper abdominal, thoracic, or orthopedic surgery and total hip or knee arthroplasty.[3,4] TENS may also be useful after traumatic rib fracture and other acute trauma.[5] Sterile electrodes allow placement of electrodes adjacent to lacerations or surgical incisions, theoretically enhancing efficacy.

Musculoskeletal Pain

TENS has been successfully used to reduce pain associated with osteoporosis-induced vertebral compression fractures, arthritis pain, and strains and sprains.[6,7] Anecdotal reports regarding the efficacy of TENS in the management of carpal tunnel syndrome suggest a positive response in some patients with failed conservative and surgical management of this entrapment neuropathy. Its benign nature and flexibility make the modality suitable for these more chronic pain reports.

Peripheral Vascular Insufficiency

Early reports suggested that TENS had the ability not only to reduce pain associated with peripheral vascular insufficiency but also to improve blood flow. Further studies have cast doubt on these claims, although many anecdotal reports are found of improvement in ulcer size and healing with the use of TENS.[8] Given the lack of treatment options for these difficult cases, TENS represents a reasonable treatment option if nothing else is working.

Abdominal and Visceral Pain

Most clinicians believe that TENS is not particularly useful in the treatment of chronic abdominal and visceral pain. Some investigators believe that, in spite of less than optimal pain relief, TENS may exert a salutary effect on bowel function and may also improve the obstipation and postoperative nausea and vomiting associated with opioid analgesics.[9,10]

Neuropathic Pain

In general, TENS has been shown to be ineffective in the treatment of most neuropathic pain states. Whether this is from lack of sensory afferent nerve function to carry the TENS impulses to the spinal cord or from other changes in the nervous system is unclear. Anecdotal reports of efficacy continue to be found in a variety of neuropathic pain states, including postherpetic neuralgia and diabetic polyneuropathy.[11]

Cancer Pain

TENS has not been a first-line treatment for pain of malignant origin. However, given the favorable side effect profile for this noninvasive, nonpharmacologic modality, it may be a reasonable option, especially in patients who experience significant side effects from pharmacologic interventions and who refuse more invasive treatments. A recent reports suggests that TENS may provide pain relief in selected patients with cancer-related bone pain.[12]

Behavioral Pain

Beyond the placebo effect, very little is found to recommend TENS in the treatment of pain without an organic basis. Initial patient enthusiasm may be quickly replaced with confounding behavior surrounding the use of TENS in this clinical setting. The use of TENS without a clear clinical indication is in most cases a fruitless endeavor.

Transcutaneous Electrical Nerve Stimulation Apparatus

The TENS unit consists of a battery-powered pulse generator that is capable of delivering a variety of different pulse characteristics and stimulation frequencies, leads, and a set of electrodes to deliver the stimulus to the affected area (**Fig. 135.1**). Most investigators prefer a monophasic square wave that is delivered by a pulse generator capable of automatically sensing and compensating for the variation in impedance caused by normal and diseased skin and less than optimal electrode contact. Stimulation frequencies between 30 and 100 Hz are most comfortable for patients. Lower frequencies, which are designed to produce what is thought to be an effect more analogous to acupuncture, are recommended by some clinicians, although many patients find this stimulation frequency too uncomfortable. This discomfort may be decreased with use of a pulse generator capable of producing a series of 8 to 10 rapid pulses of a lower frequency stimulus. Reusable electrodes that require the use of conductive gel and tape have been replaced with disposable pregelled self-sticking electrodes.

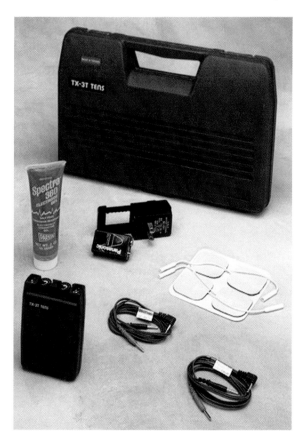

Fig. 135.1 The transcutaneous electrical nerve stimulation apparatus.

How to Use Transcutaneous Electrical Nerve Stimulation

If efficacy is to be achieved, the patient must be thoroughly familiar with the basic operation of the TENS unit and clear on how electrodes are to be placed. Although the placement of electrodes is certainly more of an art than a science, the author's experience has been that giving the patient specific parameters for electrode placement works better than telling the patient to experiment with electrode placement. The clinician should generally place the electrodes in the painful area and in most instances place the electrodes within the same dermatome whenever possible. Dual-channel units are currently the norm and allow large painful areas to be treated. A form with an anatomic outline that shows where the electrodes should be placed is helpful when instructing the patient on the use of the TENS unit.

Because electricity is involved, it may be useful for the clinician to first demonstrate the TENS unit by having the patient apply the electrodes to the clinician's forearm and then turning on the unit before placing electrodes on the patient. This increases patient confidence and lowers the anxiety regarding getting "shocked."

After proper electrode placement, the patient should be instructed to turn all settings on the pulse generator to zero before turning on the unit. This helps avoid any sudden shock sensation and allows the patient to slowly determine the sensation threshold necessary to feel the first sign of stimulation. In general, a level of 2.5 to 3 times the sensation threshold is

Table 135.2 Contraindications to Transcutaneous Electrical Nerve Stimulation
Patients with pacemakers
Patients with implantable drug delivery systems
Patients with spinal cord stimulators
Patients with significant impairment of sensation
Patients who are pregnant

most efficacious for a variety of painful conditions. A stimulus frequency of 90 to 100 Hz is generally a good starting place, and the frequency can be adjusted by the patient to comfort and efficacy, thereby giving the patient some control over one portion of the treatment. The clinician should demonstrate to the patient what TENS-induced muscle contractions look like and how adjusting the unit can make them stop.

Contraindications to Transcutaneous Electrical Nerve Stimulation

TENS is a remarkably safe treatment modality. Without the risk of thermal injury associated with heat and cold and without the side effects associated with pharmacologic, nerve block, and surgical interventions, the perception among many clinicians and third-party payers that TENS is overused is not surprising. A small group of patients remains in whom TENS may produce risk (**Table 135.2**). These patients include: (1) patients with pacemakers; (2) patients with significant sensory impairment (e.g., patients with quadriplegia, because of risk of skin breakdown; patients with implantable drug delivery systems); (3) patients with spinal cord stimulators; and (4) patients who are pregnant, because of risk of inducement of labor. Some clinicians caution against placement of TENS electrodes near the carotid sinuses or laryngeal nerves because of the risk of vasovagal syncope and laryngospasm, although this admonition may be more theoretic than real.

Conclusion

TENS as a pain-relieving modality has appeared to stand the test of time. In spite of the apparent disconnect between the enthusiastic anecdotal clinical reports and lack of demonstrable long-term efficacy of controlled studies, TENS represents a viable alternative for a variety of painful conditions. Given the favorable risk-benefit ratio and cost-benefit ratio of TENS when compared with other pain-relieving options, TENS remains a part of our armamentarium in the treatment of pain.

References

Full references for this chapter can be found on www.expertconsult.com.

Chapter 136

Osteopathic Manipulative Treatment of the Chronic Pain Patient

Kevin D. Treffer

Historical Considerations

The beginnings of what is now known as *osteopathic medicine* were first developed by Andrew Taylor Still, MD/DO, in the mid 1800s (**Fig. 136.1**). A son of an itinerant preacher/ physician, Dr. Still was trained in medicine on the prairies of Kansas by his father. This path of medical education was not unusual for the time. As Dr. Still began treating patients with the available tools of his day, he began to lose confidence in their effectiveness, believing that other options could be used to help the body help itself. In 1864, three of Dr. Still's children died of meningitis and one of pneumonia, which significantly altered his thoughts on the practice of medicine. These events caused him to be dissatisfied with the treatment methods of the day and their failures, and he began looking for a better way to approach treatment of the human body. He was a student of anatomy and had studied cadaveric specimens thoroughly, looking for the ways in which the musculoskeletal system was integrated into the body and how it could be treated to improve health. As he farmed and practiced medicine over several years, he developed his ideas of how the patient should be treated. On June 22, 1874, he first expressed his views publicly, effectively flinging the banner of osteopathy to the breeze.[1]

The Kirksville consensus report in 1953 perhaps best delineates Dr. Still's ideas for our profession; these ideas have been the standard for the tenets of osteopathic medicine (**Table 136.1**).[2] Health to Dr. Still was an optimal interaction of all body systems, communicating via neurologic, vascular, lymphatic, and hormonal means and resulting in a homeostasis (balance) between each, allowing the individual to function at an optimal capacity.[3] With this functioning, the body is able to resist environmental noxious influences and compensate for any effects of these. Disease then represents the breakdown of this homeostasis between systems, allowing symptoms to be expressed in varied patterns.

Dysfunction within the musculoskeletal system is part of the expression of disease and involves the concepts of *viscerosomatic* and *somatovisceral reflexes*. These neural reflexes involve afferent activity from either the somatic structure or a visceral structure with resulting inhibitory or excitatory effects on motor neurons (somatic or autonomic).[4] The ability to treat the musculoskeletal system effects change throughout the systems of the body by helping resolve these inappropriate neural reflexes and aiding in improving neural function to viscera associated with the spinal level in question.[5]

Osteopathic manipulative medicine then is the ultimate expression of the osteopathic philosophy. With diagnosis and treatment of dysfunction within the musculoskeletal system, abnormal function of the neurologic, vascular, hormonal, and lymphatic tissues is removed and the body is able to develop a better balance (i.e., homeostasis) between all systems. The result is a reduction of the presenting symptoms and an improvement in function of all systems: a stable state of health for the patient.

Today, osteopathic medicine consists of an integration of the original tenets along with the modern usage of all aspects of medicine (basic sciences and clinical sciences). The patient with chronic pain can be effectively treated with osteopathic manipulative treatment (OMT) within the context of the etiology of the pain, to develop an optimal balance of the patient's musculoskeletal mobility and thereby improve functional integration with all body systems.[6,7]

This chapter describes this author's osteopathic approach to the examination and treatment of the patient with chronic pain. The comprehensive evaluation and treatment presented is a unique idea that has evolved out of the osteopathic philosophy. This examination is not one that all osteopathic physicians will do for their patients. The idea of a complete evaluation is first introduced in principle in osteopathic medical schools. Although many osteopathic physicians perform manipulation, few perform an extensive approach for a variety of reasons. After several hundred patient visits, the author was not having great success with chronic pain cases. After much discussion and work with William Brooks, DO, the author modified his approach to include the grading of motion patterns and developed his version of this type of examination.[8–10] The author's personal observations have shown a better response in this patient population. A growing segment of the population is actively seeking out complementary and alternative medical treatment. The osteopathic philosophy with its use of manipulative treatment is on its way to becoming an expected standard of care within the chronic pain population.[11] This paradigm of evaluation and treatment is still evolving as further evidence-based literature is published. The physiologic basis for this paradigm, treatment modalities, and clinical problems that respond to the application of OMT are the focus of this chapter.

Somatic Dysfunction and the Nociceptive Model

In evaluation of the musculoskeletal system, the osteopathic physician looks for what is diagnosed as *somatic dysfunction*. It is defined as "the impaired or altered function of related components of the musculoskeletal system: skeletal, arthrodial, and myofascial structures, and related vascular, lymphatic, and neural elements."[12] The physician evaluates first for tissue texture changes in all aspects of the musculoskeletal system (**Table 136.2**). The next aspect is asymmetry of position and motion with palpation of bony landmarks for static position and evaluation of dynamics of motion (both active and passive motion). The physician assesses for symmetry of the joint's motion pattern, noting any restricted motion in one direction and ease of motion in the other. Palpation may also elicit tenderness at the site (*t*enderness, *a*symmetry, *r*estricted range of motion, *t*issue texture [TART] changes; **Table 136.3**).[13] With finding of TART changes in the musculoskeletal palpatory examination, somatic dysfunction can be diagnosed.

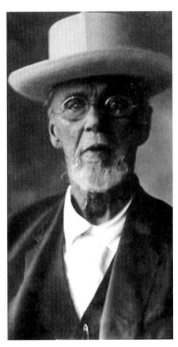

Fig. 136.1 **A. T. Still, MD, DO.**

Table 136.1 Principles Emphasized by the Philosophy of Osteopathic Medicine

The human is a dynamic unit of function

The body possesses self-regulatory mechanisms that are self healing in nature

Structure and function are interrelated at all levels

Rational treatment is based on these principles

Table 136.2 Evaluation of Tissue Texture Changes

Tissue Texture Changes	Acute	Chronic
Texture	Bogginess	Smooth
Temperature	Increased	Decreased (coolness)
Moisture	Increased	Decreased
Tension	Increased	Ropiness, tissue contraction
Tenderness	Present	Present
Edema	Present	Not generally present
Erythema	Vasodilation in tissues	Minimal

(From the Educational Council on Osteopathic Principles: *Glossary of osteopathic terminology*, Washington, DC, 2001, American Association of Osteopathic Colleges.)

Table 136.3 TART Examination

T: Tissue texture changes

A: Asymmetry of position

R: Restriction of motion

T: Tenderness

An understanding of how the body develops these TART findings and how they relate to the patient with chronic pain is important. Currently, the model for the etiology of somatic dysfunction is via nociceptive pathways. The source of the stimulation of the nociceptor varies with the variety of injuries and disease processes our patients present with. The stimulus of a peripheral nociceptor must be of sufficient strength and remain for a sufficient time to activate a cascade of events that results in the musculoskeletal effects of somatic dysfunction.[14] As the stimulus (e.g., inflammatory process) persists, the continual afferent activity into the spinal cord level affects interneurons within the cord, lowering their activation thresholds. This facilitates more efferent activity to the motor pathways, including somatic and visceral motor neurons. This is the basis of the facilitated segment concept of Korr and Denslow, developed during the mid 1900s.[15,16] These effects not only reach the somatic structures, as evidenced by the TART findings, but have consequences for visceral function (viscerosomatic and somatovisceral reflexes). The result is disruption of the body's homeostasis or system integration. The osteopathic physician recognizes this alteration in integration as a predisposition for disease processes to occur.

The facilitation changes at the spinal cord level can produce short-term effects in neuronal activity that resolve if the stimulus is short lived. If the stimulus is allowed to remain, the effects can become long term or sometimes permanent and are associated with chronic pain states and central (spinal) sensitization.[17] The nociceptive information (cause of facilitation) is then processed within the cord, brainstem, thalamus, and cortex. Spinal facilitation processes activate the brainstem arousal system that is coupled to two efferent pathways: the sympathetic nervous system (SNS) and the hypothalamic-pituitary-adrenal axis (HPA).[18] These efferent pathways are driven by norepinephrine in the SNS and cortisol in the HPA and alter bodily function (immune and neuroendocrine) to respond appropriately to a noxious stimulus. This process is referred to as *allostasis* and is a normal response by the body. However, if the stimulus is allowed to remain, the result is an increase in the allostatic load, which is detrimental to reestablishment of homeostasis. Gene expression changes allow receptors to become active at the spinal cord level, adding the modulation of central facilitation.[11] The result is the beginning of the process of allodynia (generalized lower thresholds to pain). The continual exposure to an increased allostatic load decreases the function of feedback loops meant to restore homeostasis, leaving the body "in a chronic compensatory state."[19] Osteopathic manipulative medicine as a part of the overall management plan helps to modulate the hypersympathetic tone and has been linked to pain reduction.[11]

With a chronic increased allostatic load, the response of the musculoskeletal system is continual motor output to the soma, which results in the maintenance of somatic dysfunction.[20] From a physical examination standpoint, this means maintenance of restricted ranges of motions within fascial planes, extremity joints, and spinal segments.

Allostatic load also affects visceral function by altering the outflows to the SNS and thereby affects the function of viscera innervated from the spinal segments involved in the somatic dysfunction.[19] The resulting effects do not just involve musculoskeletal tissues but potentially affect multiple organ systems and the integration of their functions.

The limbic system of the brain is responsible for the emotional component of the patient and has connections to the brainstem arousal system (SNS and HPA). The spinoreticular tracts of the brainstem arousal system can be affected by limbic system function, and emotional feelings become an important part of dealing with chronic somatic dysfunction and its resolution.[21] This reticular system also has connections to postural controls, which may explain persistent postural strain patterns observed in evaluation of patients with chronic pain.[22,23] How the patient deals emotionally with the pain or the disease process may play a role in the perpetuation of the severity of the pain and the chronicity of somatic dysfunction.

As a stimulus starts the cascade of effects within the neuroendocrine-immune axis and the spinal cord, palpable changes in the tissue textures and the decreased range of motion within the patient's musculoskeletal system can be noted. The longer this remains, the more detrimental it becomes for the patient by affecting other bodily systems, causing breakdown in function and the possibility of the disease processes to flourish. The osteopathic physician's approach to the patient with chronic pain begins with a look at the patient as a whole (all systems) and then with use of OMT to resolve somatic dysfunction. The result is a reduction in the somatic portion of inappropriate reflexes within the central nervous system (CNS) involving the SNS and HPA systems, aiding the body to reestablish a homeostasis (decreased allostatic load). The patient with chronic pain always has some form of afferent activity, and with periodic evaluation and treatment, the osteopathic physician helps the patient find health by maintaining the best homeostatic state possible, given the condition and its course.

Structural Examination of the Patient with Chronic Pain

The beginning of all patient interaction is the history and physical examination. A thorough history of the presenting symptoms, review of systems, medical history, social history, and surgical history is vital to appropriately guiding the physical examination. From an osteopathic approach, this process is no different from procedures of our other medical colleagues. The osteopathic physician does emphasize musculoskeletal, neurologic, psychosocial, and trauma histories in the approach to a patient with chronic pain but not to the exclusion of any other aspect of the history and physical examination. Because a large percentage of patients have had multiple other evaluations and treatment plans before coming for manipulative evaluation and treatment, the history of these specific evaluations and treatments and their successes and failures is important. Examination of the musculoskeletal (MS) system is of great importance to the osteopathic physician. As the MS system is evaluated, the areas of greatest restriction (the primary dysfunctions) are of particular clinical significance.

The examination begins with a postural evaluation followed by both active and passive motion patterns. How the patient's body responds to gravity may provide clues regarding the regions of the MS system that may have somatic dysfunction. A center of gravity is established to enhance ideal postural alignment because the body responds to forces from within and from without itself (**Table 136.4**). A failure of establishment of ideal posture places a strain on the myofascial and arthrodial tissues, generating inappropriate stresses to tissues that are not typically weightbearing.[23] Because the tissues respond to changing forces, the body is observed for symmetry verses asymmetry in the sagittal, coronal, and transverse planes. Surface anatomic landmarks are used to evaluate for asymmetry (**Fig. 136.2**). Some landmarks need only observation, whereas others need palpation for comparison of left versus right and anterior versus posterior.

The patient is then put through ranges of motion that involve the entire MS system. As we observe motions actively and passively, we watch for smooth and sequential motion within the myofascial and arthrodial aspects of the MS system (quantity and quality). Can the patient exhibit full range

Table 136.4 **Landmarks for the Sagittal Plane Ideal Postural Line**
External auditory meatus
Shoulders
Center of the body of L3
Greater trochanter
Lateral condyle of the femur
Just anterior to the lateral malleolus

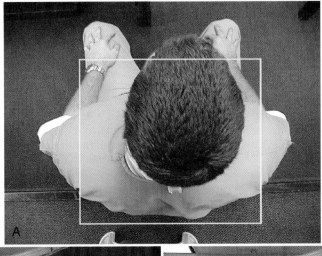

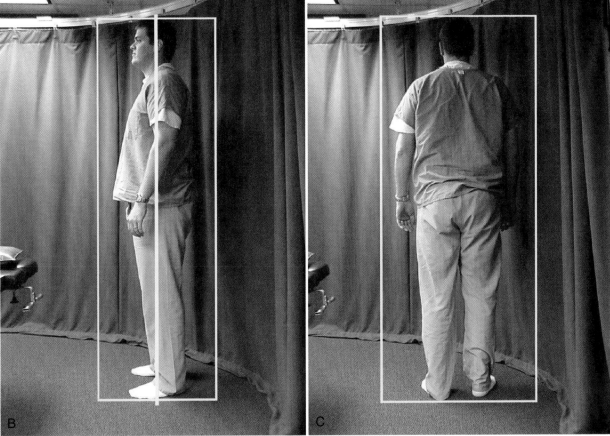

Fig. 136.2 Evaluation of posture is done in three planes. A, Transverse plane. B, Sagittal plane with ideal postural line. C, Coronal plane (anterior and posterior).

of motion actively and passively? It is important during passive evaluation to first observe where linkage to other regions of the MS system exists. For example, with the patient in the supine position with the knee and hip flexed to 90 degrees, adduction at the hip joint links into the pelvis and trunk and results in rotation of the pelvis and trunk within the transverse plane (**Fig. 136.3**). For the best assessment of the available hip joint range of motion, the physician should block this linkage with one hand while assessing the pattern of motion in question, thereby giving the clinician a truer picture of the available motion. With a restricted pattern of motion, this linkage is expected to occur early in the range of motion; how much restriction depends on this motion's significance to the overall MS system dysfunction.

As the idea of linkage is applied to each motion pattern, a grade is given for each one. The grading is done during passive motion testing. As one is passively moving part of the MS system in its range of motion, the physician can note the quality of the motion and the quantity. A patient may be able to attain the full range of motion (FROM) without causing tissue disruption but may be using a great amount of force to get to FROM. The grade should be applied when the quality of motion changes at the point in which greater force is needed to attain the FROM or linkage occurs. The grading system also provides objective evidence of the available motion within the MS system. If the motion pattern goes from 0 to 25% beyond the FROM, then the grade assigned is a +1. If the motion pattern tested achieves 100% of the expected range of motion, then FROM is documented. If the motion attained is between 75% and 100%, the grade assigned is −1. If the motion attained is between 50% and 75%, the grade is −2. If the motion is between 25% and 50%, the grade is −3; and if the motion is between starting position and 25% of expected motion, the grade is −4 (**Fig. 136.4 [online only]**).[8] This system differs slightly from the American Osteopathic Association standardized outpatient OMT form in which a 0 to 3 grading system is used. Because different postures related to the trunk and the extremities affect symptom expression, repeating the grading of motion patterns in multiple contexts is recommended.[20] The idea is to evaluate motion in the standing, seated, supine, and prone contexts to determine whether the greatest restrictions are context dependent. This becomes relevant in the planning phase of management because the area of greatest restriction should be treated in the context in which it was found to be the most restricted.[19]

After all motion patterns are graded, the physician identifies the motion pattern that has the greatest restriction. This motion pattern then should be approached by evaluating for functional pathology (i.e., somatic dysfunction) within the joints and myofascial tissues involved with that motion pattern. Once dysfunction is identified, a manipulative treatment plan can be developed and carried out to remove the restriction as much as possible given the chronicity of the cause. Another piece of information available from the grading of motion patterns is total body mobility. If the patient has a large number of −2s or −3s and very few FROM, then the patient's system is noted to be a very tight system. Contrast this with the patient with a large number of FROM and +1s; this system is considered a loose system. Most patients fall into the range of mostly FROM and a few −1s or a few +1s. Patients with a loose MS system may have pain despite a "normal" range of motion of a joint. These patients may be used to a greater than normal amount of motion and therefore may need treatment to restore them back to that range they are used to. All motion patterns are reevaluated at each visit, and the grades are compared with earlier data. This information can be used at each subsequent visit to evaluate the patient's progress and to demonstrate the success of the treatment plan. If the patient was assigned stretching exercises, then the information could be used to show the patient the benefit of the exercises. If the patient is not compliant, then the information can be used to encourage the patient to do the exercises that are essential to recovery.

The patient's symptoms may not be associated with those motion patterns with the greatest restriction. If one applies the ideas of biotensegrity, which suggests that the spinal column is not simply a stack of blocks but a structured system of continuous tension and discontinuous compression, forces are displaced throughout the MS system to find a balance of tension and force.[24] Levin explains the body as a layer of tensegrity

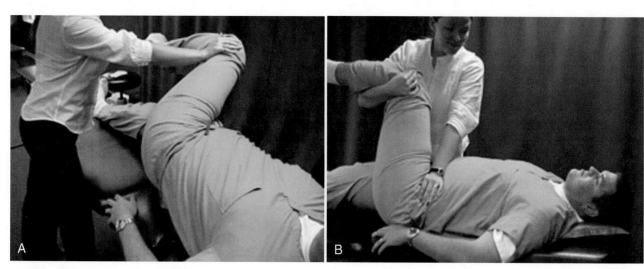

Fig. 136.3 **A,** With the hip and knee at 90 degrees, linkage within the trunk occurs with abduction at the hip. **B,** With blocking of the linkage, the true degree of available motion within the pattern is determined.

systems within tensegrity systems, thus allowing for the displacement and compensation of gravitational forces without crushing the body's tissues. The myofascial tissues are analogous to tension trusses, and the bony structures are analogous to compression structures. The icosahedral design in this system allows for instantaneous increasing or decreasing tensions and compression as loads are placed on the structure without changing overall shape.[24] The loading forces placed on the body are instantaneously displaced through all tissues and allow the body to maintain a posture in relationship to gravity, ideal or not. As disease processes and injury patterns occur in the body, a change in the distribution of force is expected, thereby changing tension within the MS system to establish a new or stable (although abnormal) posture. This is represented by somatic dysfunction and all its elements that have been discussed so far. Restriction in one motion pattern has to be compensated by another for the posture to balance. The symptomatic expression of this may be in the areas of increased mobility (prolonged functional strain) and not in the areas of greatest restriction.[11] For example, McConnell[25] notes that lack of external rotation and extension within the hip causes an increase in lumbar spine transverse plane mobility to accommodate for this restriction of motion during the gait cycle. Over time, this causes torsional strain in the annulus fibrosus portion of the intervertebral disks. Because nociceptors are found in the outer layers of the annulus fibrosus, this repetitive trauma can cause low back pain. One expects symptoms to be expressed sooner in patients with preexisting chronic dysfunction and structural pathology in the lumbar spine. The root of the problem exists within the hip muscle restriction and not in the lumbar disks. Manipulative treatment then provides a way to remove the hip rotation restriction and allow for a release in the tension/compression forces and reestablish a more normal balance in postural control and relief of low back symptoms.

After posture and motion evaluation, evaluation of the patient's gait is helpful. The patient must be observed for several full-gait cycles, with observation for symmetry in the stance and swing phases of gait. The patient's postural center of gravity is one of the determinants of how efficient the cycle is. The determinants of gait as noted by Saunders and coworkers are pelvic rotation in the transverse plane toward the stance phase side; downward pelvic tilt in the coronal plane toward the swing phase side; knee flexion during the swing phase side; combined action of the foot, ankle, and knee on the stance phase side; and the constant displacement of the center of gravity during the gait cycle.[26] Optimal mechanics of these determinants result in an efficient use of energy during the gait cycle. Evaluation of the cycle should be split into the stance and swing phases. Each phase has motions within the MS system that rely on neuromuscular and biomechanical processes to accomplish a normal cycle.

Swing phase begins with toe-off from the stance leg and ends with heel strike of the same leg. During this phase, the pelvis rotates toward the stance leg, the hip and knee are flexing, and the ankle is dorsiflexing. During the latter half of the swing phase, the knee extends; and at the end of swing phase, the foot is supinated, which combined with the remaining amount of knee flexion acts as a shock absorption during the heel strike portion of stance phase.[25,26] If dysfunction is seen within the knee (e.g., hyperextension) or the subtalar joint, an increase in pelvic rotation or coronal plane tilt is noted, resulting

in excessive motion within the lumbar spine.[25] Over time, this could lead to strain in the spine and its myofascial structures and further musculoskeletal pain. In individuals who already have significant pathology in the lumbar spine, the added strain can cause exacerbations of their pain (increased allostatic load). Manipulation of the dysfunctions to improve motion acts to decrease the allostatic load and decrease nociceptive input into the system.

Stance phase begins with heel strike and ends with toe-off. During this phase, the hip goes into extension, the knee fully extends, and the ankle and foot plantar flex and pronate to allow for toe-off at the end of the cycle.[26] The subtalar joint has great clinical significance during stance phase because dysfunction here results in a disturbance in the shock absorption on heel strike and affects lumbopelvic motion as well.[25] Physical findings are represented by abnormal areas of callus formation on the plantar surface of the foot, indicating abnormal weight-bearing.[26] Again, manipulative treatment to dysfunctional tissues involved in gait restores the necessary motions to allow a more efficient gait cycle and lessen nociceptive input. The gait efficiency shows in the stamina of patients with chronic pain in the activities of their daily lives as they try to function with a chronic problem.

The gait cycle is a total body phenomenon. To counterbalance some of the lower extremity and pelvic motions, the upper body rotates toward the swing leg side and the upper extremities swing anterior on the stance leg side. This also helps minimize head rotation, keeping the head forward. The physician should be mindful of mobility within the trunk and upper extremities that may have effects on restricting mobility within the gait cycle. Patients with chronic pain who have significant musculoskeletal structural abnormalities need to have an efficient use of energy during their gait cycle. Addressing joint function and dysfunction aids in their conservation of energy for use in other activities of daily living.

The context in which the patient is evaluated includes standing, seated, supine, and prone. Standing context includes the postural examination in three planes. Seated examination begins with simultaneous evaluation of passive right and left upper extremity flexion, extension, adduction, and abduction, blocking any linkage noted. All of these motions are done with the elbow in full extension (a so-called *straight upper extremity*). For all of these motions, the FROM is based on the practitioner's favorite reference text for motion mechanics. Hoppenfeld's *Physical Examination of the Spine and Extremities* is an excellent resource for the expected ranges of motion (**Tables 136.5 and 136.6**). Each of these patterns should be graded for available motion and documented as discussed previously.

The scapulothoracic motion is an important component of total shoulder motion, and therefore, the amount of gapping between the scapula and the thoracic cage is noted. With passive retraction of the ipsilateral shoulder girdle, the tension around the medial aspect of the scapula is loosened. The free hand then attempts to slide the fingers between the scapula and the thoracic cage. The expectation is that the fingers are able to slide up to the proximal interphalangeal joint. This is graded in the same fashion as noted before and documented. This author's experience in practice reveals that tension within the pectoralis minor muscle and subscapularis muscle commonly restricts this gapping motion, effectively locking the scapula onto the chest cage. This tension within these muscles

Table 136.5 Expected Full Range of Motion for Upper Extremity

SEATED CONTEXT

Abduction = 180 degrees
Adduction = 45 degrees
Flexion = 90 degrees
Extension = 45 degrees

SUPINE AND SEATED CONTEXT

Internal rotation = 55 degrees
External rotation = 40 to 45 degrees

From Hoppenfeld S: *Physical examination of the spine and extremities,* Norwalk, CT, 1976, Appleton and Lange, p 1.

Table 136.6 Expected Full Range of Motion for Lower Extremity

SUPINE CONTEXT

Flexion at the hip with knee flexed = 120 degrees
Flexion at the hip with the knee extended = 90 degrees
Abduction at the hip with the knee/hip flexed = 45 to 50 degrees
Adduction at the hip with the knee/hip flexed = 20 to 30 degrees
Internal rotation at the hip with the knee/hip flexed = 35 degrees
External rotation at the hip with the knee/hip flexed = 45 degrees

PRONE CONTEXT

Extension at the hip with the knee flexed = 30 degrees
External rotation at the hip with the knee flexed = 45 degrees
Internal rotation at the hip with the knee flexed = 35 degrees
Flexion at the knee = 135 degrees

From Hoppenfeld S: *Physical examination of the spine and extremities,* Norwalk, CT, 1976, Appleton and Lange, pp 143,171.

and restriction of motion of the scapulothoracic joint have been associated with atypical shoulder pain.

Supine evaluation involves motion of the upper and lower extremity motion patterns, with any linkage noted and blocked appropriately. The lower extremity flexion at the hip is noted with the knee in full extension and then in full flexion. Abduction and adduction at the hip are evaluated with the knee extended and also with the hip and knee flexed to 90 degrees. Internal and external rotation is evaluated with the hip and knee flexed to 90 degrees. The upper extremity is evaluated for internal and external rotation at the shoulder with the elbow flexed 90 degrees and glenohumeral joint abducted 90 degrees. It is important to appreciate the scapulothoracic component of internal rotation at the shoulder, which is a major portion of the normal internal rotation. Restriction within the periscapular muscles decreases this pattern of motion in combination with a decreased scapular gapping evaluation. Other muscles that cross this region may also produce restriction. The latissimus dorsi muscle takes its origin

from the lumbar aponeurosis and inserts into the shoulder, directly linking the shoulder region to the low back. Therefore, restrictions in the shoulder motions may be affected by fascial restrictions within the lumbar spine or may be from the pelvis or lower extremity because the fascial tissue is contiguous through the gluteus medius, into the posterior sacroiliac capsule, into the sacrotuberous ligament, and into the origin of the posterior thigh muscles off the ischial tuberosity. This anatomic knowledge lends credence to the idea that the area of greatest restriction may not be in the area of pain expression. Significant dysfunction from the lumbar spine or down into the feet that may manifest with upper extremity symptoms from fascial tethers within the system is entirely possible. For this reason, a thorough and comprehensive examination is the best approach to MS system chronic pain issues. For all of these motions, the FROM is based on the examiner's favorite reference text for motion mechanics.

Prone evaluation of the patient does involve both upper and lower extremity motion patterns. The lower extremity is evaluated for flexion at the knee, external rotation at the hip with the knee flexed, internal rotation with the knee flexed, and extension at the hip with the knee flexed. The upper extremity is evaluated for horizontal extension at the shoulder with the elbow fully extended. Tension with the pectoral muscles of the chest restricts this motion pattern and is associated with patients with protracted shoulder girdles (rounded shoulders) or slumping postures in today's sedentary society.

After all motion patterns are evaluated, the primary restricted patterns are noted. The muscles, fascia, and joints involved within the primary pattern are evaluated specifically for somatic dysfunction. The sequence for evaluation is variable with this approach. It may necessitate starting in the foot and ankle or in the head and neck. As the MS system is more specifically evaluated, the areas of greatest restriction are again of high clinical significance. For example, as one palpates for dysfunction of the forefoot, mid foot, and hind foot, the degree of restriction is noted and documented. This is repeated for the fibula and tibia, hip, innominates, sacrum, lumbar spine, thoracic spine, cervical spine, ribs, shoulders, clavicles, radius, ulna, carpals, and phalanges. Many osteopathic physicians practice osteopathy in the cranial field and include this portion of the examination as part of the comprehensive examination of the entire musculoskeletal system. The region with the greatest restriction should be addressed manipulatively first. The American Osteopathic Association's textbook entitled *Foundations for Osteopathic Medicine* explains how to diagnose somatic dysfunction in all of the aforementioned areas. This is by no means the only text written on this subject, and indeed, many fine texts are available to choose from.

Osteopathic Manipulative Treatment and Choosing the Treatment Modality

Once a diagnosis of somatic dysfunction is made, then a plan to relieve the restriction and restore motion is produced. The art of practicing manipulative medicine includes knowing when and where to apply a certain modality of manipulation for any given patient. First, one must be confident in the diagnosis made and that osteopathic manipulative treatment is indicated for this patient.

During the examination process, one should determine whether the source of the problem is structural pathology or functional pathology. Structural pathology generally means instability within anatomic structures that need stabilization before application of an OMT modality. Treatment of unstable structures with manipulation may cause injury and add an acute problem onto a chronic one. Most structural instabilities are associated with a hypermobility of the MS segment in question, although not all are hypermobile. For example, degenerative processes such as osteoarthritis and its associated sclerotic changes can give hypomobility to any given segment and still be unstable enough to contraindicate the use of OMT to that segment. However, this may not contraindicate the use of OMT to other MS segments within the same individual. OMT is best suited for tissues with hypomobility that are capable of responding to treatment.

One caveat should be noted: although an individual may have structural pathology, he or she possesses functional pathology in compensation for the abnormal structure. Somatic dysfunction is a component of functional pathology and is associated with hypomobility within patients with chronic pain.

If OMT is appropriate for the patient, then a decision of whether to use a direct or indirect technique needs to be addressed. With evaluation for segmental somatic dysfunction and TART findings, the physician notes the quality of the range of motion end-feel. Does it feel as if a brick wall is being encountered as the segment is being moved into the extremes of motion in one direction or another? If the range of motion for the segment is asymmetrical in one direction versus another, then a restrictive barrier is said to be present, limiting the motion. The quality of the end-feel may determine what modality is best to use for that dysfunction. A hard end-feel may be better suited for a high-velocity low-amplitude (i.e., thrusting) technique, indicating the problem is more arthrodial; a softer or tethered end-feel may respond better to muscle energy or myofascial release modality, indicating the problem is more myofascial. Patient preference of modality may make the decision easier. If a patient does not want a certain modality used, then the physician is well advised not to proceed. Comorbid diagnoses may preclude the use of some modalities.

No absolute rules have been developed for the frequency of manipulative treatments.[27] Therefore, an individualized program should be designed for each patient. Patients with very tight MS systems may need more frequent treatments at first, followed by longer periods of time between treatments. Severely affected patients may need evaluation and treatment on a weekly basis, whereas others may need only quarterly treatments. As with all patients, the ideal situation would be treatment of the patient for a short period of time, then release from care to a productive life. At times, this is a scenario that plays itself out. Given the chronicity of many MS diseases and injuries, these patients need periodic treatment to maintain the homeostasis they have achieved with their disease or injury process. OMT is not a cure for structural changes but is effective for the functional changes related to structural pathology. This author prefers to give the body a chance to adjust to changes made in the MS system and sees the patient every 4 to 6 weeks if schedules allow. Few patients need weekly treatment over extended periods of time, although there are always those small percentages that function better with weekly or biweekly treatments.

Manipulative Medicine Modalities

Multiple treatment modalities are available for the osteopathic physician in approaching the patient with chronic pain. Each has its pros and cons, and the physician must weigh the risk versus the benefit of using the modality. As discussed previously, the decision of whether the etiology of restriction originates in the arthrodial or the myofascial tissue is important. At times, the problem lies within both aspects, and multiple modalities are needed to restore motion. Sometimes, the patient may have too much tension to allow techniques to be applied to the joints, and the clinician must work on the soft tissues to ultimately treat joint motion. Osteopathic texts, such as *Foundations for Osteopathic Medicine*, describe each modality well.

Myofascial tissue modalities are effective at restoring motion restricted by soft tissue strain patterns. These modalities include soft tissue massage, myofascial release (both directly into the restrictive barrier and indirectly or away from the barrier), strain-counterstrain techniques, facilitated positional release, and spray and stretch techniques. These modalities require physicians to concentrate on tissue reaction occurring under their hands, such as palpating for tissue relaxation or stretch (tissue creep). The physician must have good proprioception skills to be successful with these modalities and be able to respond to changes within the myofascial tissues, as the treatment is applied.

Arthrodial modalities affect joint restriction more than soft tissue restriction. The realization that tissue texture changes occur with all dysfunctions is important; however, some end-feel of motion is harder, requiring different types of treatment modalities. These modalities include muscle energy, high-velocity—low-amplitude (HVLA) (i.e., thrusting techniques), articulatory, and Still's techniques. Osteopathy in the cranial field is another modality in that much of the work is done on the sutures, cranial membranes, the sphenobasilar junction, and cranial rhythmic impulse.

Manipulative medicine modalities carry some risk in performance. Most injuries come from the more forceful modalities. Thrusting techniques are popular and easy to use; however, they do have some limitations. Some patients do not care for the techniques because of fear of the popping sound or of injury. Vick et al[28] noted that HVLA techniques are safe, given several hundred million treatments done each year and only 185 reported injuries over 68 years. The reporting of injuries is probably low during the time frame of the study. The recent study from Haldeman et al[29] did not identify factors in the history and physical that accurately predict cerebral ischemia after cervical manipulation and, therefore, declared it a rare complication of this treatment approach. Although a crystal ball would be nice, the reasonable conclusion is to examine our patients thoroughly before thrusting and know that possible complications may occur. We must be aware of conditions that carry more risk than benefit from the modality. This then should be communicated to our patients before use of a thrusting technique and documented in the record.

Post–Patient Encounter Recommendations

After the examination and the treatment procedures are completed, the patient encounter is not finished without educating the patient about his or her condition. A few minutes spent explaining in simple terms the clinical findings and the plan to manage them involve the patient in the treatment plan. Recall that the grading of the motion patterns identifies restriction within patterns of motion and is useful in demonstrating the need to work on stretching exercises. The best method is to actually demonstrate the exercise and then give the patient something in writing. For the patient with chronic low back pain, exercises for the abdominal and lumbar multifidus muscles have been noted to decrease pain and increase function.[30,31] As patients return for reevaluation, the same motion patterns can be reassessed and used to show patients the success of doing the exercises; or they may be used to educate and encourage patients to perform the exercises if they are not complying. If patients report ache in the muscles for an extended time after the stretch, they potentially are using too much force in the stretch. You may want them to demonstrate how they are doing the exercise. This allows you to modify the exercise as you see fit. With stretching exercises, more can be better in this situation. Length of time in a stretch and how often patients perform the stretch are important in overcoming any myofascial recoil that may occur after stretching.

Pharmaceuticals may help the patient tolerate any pain experienced. Medications used with each patient should be individualized. Some patients may need muscle relaxants and pain medication, whereas some may just need a nonsteroidal anti-inflammatory drug. There are those who need short-term opioids, and others who need chronic opioid usage, including contracts between the doctor and patient with management of their usage. Some patients may benefit from localized epidural injections by a pain management specialist. A multidisciplinary approach is useful in the complicated chronic pain case. However, one physician coordinating the plan and prescribing the opioids is best. This physician should keep in contact with other members of the team regarding the response from the patient.

As long as the manipulative evaluations and treatments are helping the patient, they can be continued. If the patient's condition is getting worse, then the manipulative treatments should be stopped and the patient's history and physical examination should be reevaluated. Use the motion pattern grading system to evaluate progress and regression and the history. If a plateau is reached and the patient's condition is stable and comfortable, then seeing the patient every 4 to 6 months is appropriate. If a flare in symptoms or a new trauma occurs, the patient should be reevaluated sooner. Because chronic pain generally does not go away, expect the patient to return for repeat treatments. Some patients do better if they are seen on a more frequent basis. Each patient is an individual, and the frequency of treatment should be tailored to the point the patient is most functional for the longest amount of time between treatments.

Clinical Applications

Many etiologies may produce chronic pain in our patients. OMT is designed to help treat the functional pathologies that are related to the structural pathologies. Indeed, at times, only a functional pathology exists, and OMT is appropriate for treatment in this case.[32] The general principles presented in this chapter may be applied to any chronic pain case. Choice of treatment modality should be made in the context of the extent of structural pathologies present and considering the risk versus benefit ratio with each patient individually.

Low Back Pain

Low back pain is one of the most common, if not the most common, problem our patients face. Furlan and associates[33] note that 75% to 85% of the population will experience low back pain during their lives, with 10% of those with development of chronic low back pain, accounting for greater than 90% of the costs for back incapacity. Many dollars are spent in this country for low back pain, ranging from $20 billion to $50 billion annually.[34,35] Many differing approaches to the treatment of chronic low back pain are found. The approach that encompasses both structural and functional problems is the most comprehensive management plan. OMT provides an additional therapeutic option with a low risk-to-benefit ratio and a growing evidence base in the literature.[11] Chronic postural responses, as a result of structural or functional pathology, result in repetitive overuse injuries, with low back pain occurring from an abnormal increase of spinal segmental motion.[36] With the spine resembling a tensegrity tower, a response to treatment is associated with changes in motion and force displacement, thereby integrating this reaction with the rest of the extremities, head, and viscera.[37] Therefore, to use the osteopathic approach, you must be thorough in your evaluation of the musculoskeletal system to find the primary dysfunction. A broader response within the patient's musculoskeletal system is expected with this treatment approach. On the basis of a review of manipulative treatment in the literature, Mein postulates that patients with low back pain benefit most from manipulation rather than other chronic pain treatment modalities.[11]

The patient with chronic pain has increased motor output from nociceptive input that maintains the pain-spasm cycle via facilitated segments, thereby sustaining pain.[11] With central descending inhibitory pathways overwhelmed and the convergence of nociceptive and mechanoreceptor stimuli on common spinal pathways, motion can be perceived as pain.[32] Manipulative treatment is designed to decrease the facilitated segments within the cord, allowing a decrease in the motor output. The result is less muscle spasm, less pain, and more mobility to a segment and motion pattern.

Management of the patient with chronic low back pain is not complete without a psychiatric evaluation for anxiety and depression. Patients with neuropathic pain have been shown via positron emission tomography to shift acute pain activity from the sensory cortex to areas of affective/motivational control, indicating a need to evaluate for pain's impact on the mental, emotional, and spiritual functions of the patient.[11] Depression can affect the function of the descending nociceptive inhibitory pathways in the brainstem, allowing an increase in transmission of nociception.[32] With the central nociceptive connection with the limbic system, an exacerbation of the pain level can fluctuate with the mental state of the patient. Adequate treatment of depression or anxiety can go a long way in helping the patient attain homeostasis in all systems so the patient can find a state of health as defined previously. Early research in the manipulative treatment of psychiatric conditions is not detailed as to specific conditions. However, current research is pending for the role of manipulative treatment in depression. Studies show resolution of psychosomatic back pain after the patient's psychiatric issues have been resolved.[38]

Specific regions to treat depend on the findings of the examination and the associated grade applied to the dysfunctions found. The patient with routine low back pain benefits from manipulation with less medication and physical therapy.[39] Choice of manipulative treatment modality depends on the patient's structural status and personal preference. In the patient with chronic low back pain, McConnell[25] advocates restoring motion to the hips and thoracic spine and treatment of the subtalar joint motion to help decrease the lumbar compensation. This should not be understood as the only regimen for treatment. The patient with chronic needs requires a more thorough evaluation, increased frequency of treatments, medication, and counseling as needed. Addressing the stabilizing muscles (core strength), such as the multifidus, abdominal muscles, and gluteus medius, with endurance exercises aids in appropriate recruitment of muscles during desired motion patterns and helps the patient rehabilitate to the best possible homeostatic state, given the chronicity of the problem.[25]

Whiplash

Another chronic pain presentation is the whiplash injury. The symptoms associated are varied, as is the extent of injury. The typical flexion/extension inertial injury causes an S-shaped curvature in the cervical spine (flexion of upper segments and extension of lower), leading to injury. The soft tissue injury that occurs leads to changes in the mechanical function of the myofascial tissues, which may lead to a significant lowering of the thresholds of nociceptors and mechanoreceptors, resulting in the increased allostatic load and all of its effects over time.[40] If rotation of the cervical spine occurs at the time of impact, the tissue trauma may be more extensive, with involvement with the scalene muscles and the pectoralis minor muscle, resulting in a thoracic outlet syndrome presentation. The associated headache could be from the upper cervical spine because of common pathways between nociceptive inputs from C1-C3 and the spinal nucleus of the trigeminal nerve.[32] Attention to dysfunctions within the cervical spine may alleviate headache symptoms. Because of the tissue trauma that has occurred, use of modalities that may further traumatize tissue during the early stages of recovery is not recommended. For example, thrusting techniques may cause further injury to the tissues and direct muscle energy may be more painful to the patient. Indirect myofascial techniques, soft tissue massage, and articulatory, facilitated positional release, and Still's techniques are all good choices for treatment in the early stages. Giles and Muller[41] found in their comparison study that acupuncture was superior to manipulation for chronic neck pain but spinal manipulation was better for all other chronic spine pain, indicating that consideration should be given to alternative modalities in the early course of treatment. As the patient's rehabilitation progresses, other modalities may be added. Muscle strengthening exercises, along with manipulative treatment, are beneficial to helping the patient decrease pain and improve neck range of motion and muscle function.[42,43]

Migraine Cephalgia

A brief mention of migraine cephalgia and manipulation is appropriate. Head and neck injuries account for 15% of chronic daily headaches. Also, 45% of these patients have headaches 6 months after injury, 20% after 1 year.[44] The trauma is the stimulus that starts the depolarization of neurons that allows a significant potassium efflux. This leads to the release of glutamate, which subsequently activates N-methyl-D-aspartate and d-amino-3-hydorxy-5-methyl-4-isoxasolepropionic acid receptors, allowing a further efflux of potassium and calcium. These changes result in protease activation with cell damage or death, neurofilament dysfunction, increased dependence on glycolysis-generated adenosine triphosphate, and an intracellular decrease of magnesium. The culmination of these steps leads to the development of central sensitization and neuropathic pain.[45] Bronfort et al's review article found studies that show a positive effect for manipulation in tension-type headaches and for the management of migraine cephalgia.[46] By addressing the entire musculoskeletal system for dysfunction, this author has seen a decrease in severity and frequency of headache in this patient population. Use of cranial manipulation in addition to other treatment modalities, within the context of the described diagnostic approach, has been central in observation of this change. The connections of the spinal nucleus of the trigeminal nerve and the upper cervical segments may play a role in success seen.

Ankle Sprains

Many patients with chronic pain suffer falls and other MS injuries that may cause further problems for their overall homeostasis. Ankle sprains respond to manipulative treatment as long as the modality chosen does not exacerbate tissue trauma. Higher grade sprains are not effectively treated with thrusting techniques. Early intervention helps restore lymphatic flow, decrease edema, and decrease the inflammatory process.[47,48] Pellow and Brantingham[47] looked at a separation thrusting technique for the treatment of lower grade sprains with positive results. Because of compensatory changes, treatment should include a thorough evaluation and treatment of the entire extremity (attention to cuboid and fibular head), pelvis, and lumbar spine. Use the motions of gait with respect to the extremity and low back as a guide for treatment.[49] Low-grade ankle sprains are very common, and addition of manipulative treatment to the management can decrease healing time for many patients.

Scoliosis

The approach to evaluation and treatment as presented has been applied to patients with scoliosis as well. Both direct and indirect modalities can be used effectively in the management of the chronic musculoskeletal pain associated with the curvatures. With use of this comprehensive evaluation and treatment approach, Hawes and Brooks[50] showed a decrease in chest circumference inequity by more than 10 cm, an improvement in the rib cage deformity, and a 40% reduction in the Cobb angle in an idiopathic scoliotic curve that was stable for 30 years. With improvement in chest wall compliance, the respiratory function and exercise capacity improve, allowing the patient better overall body function. This may be enough change for the patient to become more active and have improved quality of life.

Fibromyalgia

Patients with fibromyalgia benefit from manipulative treatment. Soft tissue massage, myofascial release, muscle energy techniques, and counterstrain techniques are beneficial modalities to use in these patients. Manipulative treatments have been shown to reduce pain at the tender point sites, improve sleep, improve activities of daily living, and decrease depressive symptoms.[51-53] Increased physical activity increases the nociceptive threshold; therefore, with educating the patient to remain active, the long-term effect is a decrease in pain.[54]

Obstetric Application

Although pregnancy is not necessarily considered a chronic pain condition, a significant amount of postural strain contributes to multiple musculoskeletal changes over the 40 weeks. If chronic pain is defined as pain for greater than 6 months, then most of this pain by definition is chronic. Studies in the past have shown positive effects for treatment of low back pain with OMT in the pregnant patient. A recent study of 144 women was completed as a randomized, placebo-controlled trial conducted to compare usual obstetric care and osteopathic manipulative treatment, usual obstetric care and sham ultrasound treatment, and usual obstetric care only. The end point of the study included the average pain levels and the Roland-Morris Disability Questionnaire to assess back-specific functioning. The study showed that the group using OMT plus routine obstetric care had significantly less deterioration in back-specific functioning compared with the sham treatment plus routine obstetric care and routine obstetric care only. The pain of pregnancy was not shown to be significantly decreased; however, the subjects maintained better function throughout the pregnancy (effect size, 0.72; 95% confidence interval, 0.31 to 1.14; $P = .001$ versus usual obstetric care only; and effect size, 0.35; 95% confidence interval, -0.06 to 0.76; $P = .09$ versus usual obstetric care and sham ultrasound treatment).[55] The evaluation method described can be modified for the patient based on the term of the pregnancy. The study cited used a set protocol for treatment and can used as an example of a comprehensive treatment plan. The follow-up study is underway with a larger n value, and further questions are being investigated. Postpartum dysfunctions within the innominates (pubic shears or compressions) are associated with sacroiliac pain and dysfunction.[11] Multiple modalities of treatment can be used in this patient population to treat the dysfunctions safely. The effect of the pregnancy on the lumbar spine and pelvis is exaggeration of the lumbar lordosis and an anterior pelvic tilt. The thoracic spine then compensates by increasing kyphosis curvature. Because of the stress of the postural strain through the lumbar spine, pelvis, and into the lower extremity, ankle, and foot, dysfunctions can be noted.[56] The result of these dysfunctions leads to the back pain of pregnancy. Manipulative treatment did not prevent the postural changes of the developing pregnancy, but it did show an effect on how well the patient is able to compensate in a more homeostatic manner and thus maintain a higher level of function.

Conclusion

Dr. Still developed a new approach to patient care, to alleviate pain by treating the entire body and helping with function at an optimal level. His legacy and philosophy of treatment have grown over the last century. Research shows the benefits of the addition of manipulative treatment in the management of patients with chronic pain. The practitioner must be thorough in the evaluation of the MS system and be mindful of structural and functional pathology. This requires an extended amount of time during the patient encounter; however, the results are well worth the time spent. The patient must be a part of the overall management plan; the success of the treatment plan may hinge on the patient's acceptance of the plan and following through with the postevaluation instructions and exercises. If medications are used, then close monitoring of usage and effectiveness is required. If narcotics are used, a contract with the patient is recommended. As the management plan is carried out, the physician should periodically reevaluate the entire patient presentation to see whether the patient is responding to treatment and whether there is compliance with the plan.

The motion patterns observed for grading can be numerous, especially if all are done in multiple contexts. This author does a more abbreviated version of this examination, saving time in the examination room. Dr. Brooks uses a much more comprehensive evaluation for his patients. The author has found that with use of a select few motion patterns, mobility has been effectively improved in a majority of patients with chronic pain. In those individuals whose conditions do not respond, the full evaluation then becomes a better option to guide treatment.

Many patients with chronic pain have gone through multiple evaluations over the timeline of their disease process. As a result, many of them have been offered relief from the pain, but many do not get relief. For those who do not have response to medical treatment, the comprehensive evaluation and treatment plan set forth can help these patients with chronic pain find health, despite the chronicity of their problems. The emphasis in treatment of chronic pain with OMT should therefore be on removing restrictions to motion, thus decreasing nociception and central sensitization pathways. This allows our patients to return to more normal activities of daily living.[11] Much research is ongoing in this field, and the reader should be on the watch for the results of the OSTEOPATHIC Trial, which will be ending soon. This trial is a phase III randomized controlled trial of 488 subjects assessing the efficacy of OMT and ultrasound physical therapy.[57] This study, when completed in 2010, will be the largest randomized control trial involving OMT, adding much needed primary data for OMT and chronic low back pain. We welcome the addition to the evidence base so that we can find the best practice that will help our patients find "Health."

References

Full references for this chapter can be found on www.expertconsult.com.

Nociceptors, Pain, and Spinal Manipulation

Rand S. Swenson and Geoffrey M. Bove

Introduction

Spinal manipulative therapy (SMT) is among the most common of the complementary and alternative medicine therapies.[1,2] The first written description of SMT was by Hippocrates, who was quoted as saying that it was an ancient art.[3] Annually, at least 7.5% of the adult population visits a chiropractor, for a total of approximately 120 million treatments each year.[4] Most treatments are for pain in the back and neck,[5-9] but nonmusculoskeletal conditions are also treated.[10,11] The former conditions are extremely common, with approximately 18% of the population experiencing back pain that lasts more than 1 month in any given year[12] and many having significant disability.[13] Almost 95% of SMT is performed by chiropractors[14]; the remainder is performed by osteopaths, physical therapists, practitioners of Oriental Medicine, and other bodyworkers. The philosophic approach to SMT by chiropractors and osteopaths is historically similar[15,16] and seems to be based, at least in part, on observations published in the early 19th century,[17-21] although a similar philosophy was also expressed by Hippocrates.

Most of the scientific support for SMT has come from randomized clinical trials (RCTs). With the large numbers of RCTs, several efforts have been made to conduct systematic reviews and meta-analyses of this extensive literature. Most,[14,22-27] but not all,[28,29] of these evaluations have concluded some beneficial effect of SMT for low back pain when compared with no intervention or "treatment as usual." However, few studies have directly compared SMT with other treatments, and no studies have rigorously compared the many types of SMT with each other. In addition, true placebo-controlled trials, despite their importance in validation of pain therapies,[30] have proven difficult because of challenges validating of appropriate placebos for physical interventions.[31-35] Short of general anesthesia,[36] it is not clear whether completely satisfactory blinding is possible in studies of SMT.

Despite extensive clinical use of SMT, the mechanisms of effect remain elusive. Two dominant theories are used to explain these effects: the first implicates a direct effect of the manipulation on spinal biomechanics, and the second considers direct and indirect effects on neural tissue. The effects on the nervous system could be via direct alleviation of neuropathology[36] or via activation of spinal and paraspinal receptors. This latter theory implicates various central nervous system (CNS) mechanisms in the ultimate effect. In that regard, several studies have shown a short-duration (<1 minute) effect in suppressing the H-reflex.[37-40] These findings suggest that SMT may suppress muscle stretch reflex excitability in the spinal cord[41] and that this effect is segmental.[42,43] Other research with use of transcranial magnetic stimulation has shown a transient facilitation of descending motor conduction lasting up to 1 minute after SMT.[44] These findings suggest a CNS effect of such treatment.

Because SMT is predominantly used for the treatment of pain, major interest has been focused on the potential effects interactions between manipulation and pain pathophysiology. Limited evidence from several studies with psychophysiologic outcome measures suggests that SMT may have an analgesic effect.[45-51] However, these studies were unable to control completely for placebo effects. In fact, a recent study described expectation as a significant factor in analgesic responses to

SMT.[52] Studies that examined whether endogenous opioids increase after SMT have had conflicting results,[53-55] and the many questions regarding potential analgesic effects of SMT[56] await the use of more objective outcome measures and better testing methods. The development of such tests requires a detailed understanding of pain physiology. This chapter discusses the anatomy and physiology of pain in light of potential interaction with spinal manipulative procedures.

Innervation of the Spine

The spine and paraspinal tissues are innervated by the processes of motor and sensory neurons. Somatic motor neurons produce contraction of the muscles, and sympathetic motor neurons regulate blood flow through vasoconstriction. These neurons are discussed subsequently in the context of potential involvement in spinal pain conditions. All sensory neuronal cell bodies are found in the dorsal root ganglia and are pseudounipolar, meaning that they have a single axonal process that bifurcates into a central and a peripheral process (**Fig. 137.1, [online only]**). The central process extends into the spinal cord via the dorsal root, and the peripheral process extends into the peripheral nerves, providing sensory innervation to target structures (**Fig. 137.2**). The distal ends of the peripheral processes of afferent (sensory) neurons transduce, or sense, touch, nociception (pain), position, motion, and loading of tissues, such as those of the spine; these latter three sensory modalities are collectively termed proprioception. The proprioceptors, many of which are encapsulated, are associated with large-diameter, heavily myelinated, fast conducting afferent nerve fibers. These exist predominantly within ligaments (including the joint capsule)[57] and muscles of the spine[58-61] and have been implicated in discussions of the neurophysiology of spinal manipulation.[62] Proprioceptors are certainly activated by the forces applied in spinal manipulation.[63,64] The potential interactions of proprioceptors and nociceptors are discussed later in the chapter.

Evidence of nociceptors has been found in all spinal structures except the nucleus pulposis (**Fig. 137.3**). Their transductive structures are often referred to as free nerve endings, although this is an oversimplification.[65] As in other parts of the body, nociceptive nerve fibers are of small diameter, with slow conduction velocities and distinctive neurochemistry. This

latter feature allows the distribution of presumptive nociceptive fibers to be studied within the spinal and paraspinal tissues.

For an understanding of spinal pain and its treatment, consider that, although nociception and pain are usually connected, they are not identical.[66] Most pain does begin with activation of a nociceptor, which transmits information that is interpreted as pain within higher centers of the nervous system. However, not all activation of nociceptors is interpreted as pain, and the experience of pain is widely different among individuals, even with activation of similar nociceptors. The differentiation of pain and nociception is a process of the CNS, where multiple amplification and suppression mechanisms are found, many of which are considered subsequently. In addition, the experience of pain is predominantly a cerebral cortical phenomenon, where context, experience, and baseline neural functions are important to the overall experience. This is obvious in treatment of individuals with similar injuries who have different responses. Therefore, consideration of only nociception or only pain is inappropriate in a discussion of pain and its treatment.

Historically, the innervation of spinal structures has been assumed to be similar to that of the limbs, where afferent nerve fibers are easier to study. Although this is true in general terms, the study of axial innervation has revealed significant differences, and extrapolations must be made with caution. The study of axial innervation is relatively young, and the

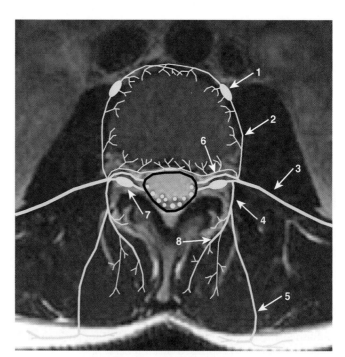

Fig. 137.3 Innervation of a mid lumbar vertebra, showing the distribution of the spinal nerve. The medial branch of the dorsal primary rami (*8*) innervates the zygapophyseal (facet) joints and continues to innervate paraspinal muscles. Branches of the sinuvertebral nerves (*6*) and grey rami communicantes (*2*) innervate the peripheral lamellae of the intervertebral disk. The sinuvertebral nerve (*6*) is involved in sensory innervation of the posterior disk and many structures of the vertebral canal and also contains sympathetic postganglionic axons. Note that the contents of the vertebral canal at this level include the nerve roots of the cauda equina surrounded by dural sac. *1,* Sympathetic ganglion; *3,* ventral primary ramus; *4,* dorsal primary ramus; *5,* lateral division of the dorsal primary ramus.

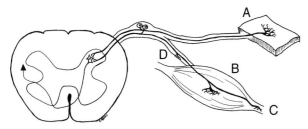

Fig. 137.2 Schematic of primary afferent neuron innervation pattern. Two neurons are depicted, one innervating skin (*A*) and the other innervating deep structures. The cutaneous neuron extends to one area of the skin, and the deep neuron branches extend to innervate muscle (*B*), tendon (*C*), and even the nerve in which it passes (*D*). Both neurons are depicted as converging to a single neuron in the dorsal horn, which is termed a wide dynamic range neuron.

following discussion highlights some of the differences with appendicular innervation and describes some of the major unknowns. Ultimately, in consideration of the physiologic basis of spinal pain syndromes and their treatment with spinal manipulation, an understanding is important of the locations of nociceptors, the mechanisms of activation of these fibers, and the pathways of transmission. In addition, appreciation is necessary of the potential mechanisms of interaction between nociceptive pathways and other neural elements, particularly proprioceptors and sympathetic neurons.

Nociceptors

Nociceptors are neurons that are involved in detecting stimuli that are likely to signal possible or actual tissue damage. Nociceptors serve a critical protective function for an organism, providing information about harmful or potentially harmful events that may cause loss of function or life. Even simple organisms have nociceptive function. For example, protochordates display the coiling reflex, a withdrawal from a noxious stimulus.[67] Through evolution, this defense mechanism has been conserved and refined, and the basic function of signaling harmful events remains unchanged. The importance of nociceptors is illustrated by the cumulative damage and short life spans of animals in whom the nerve fibers have been destroyed by neonatal treatment with capsaicin and by the rare cases in which children have been born without nociceptors.[68–70] In general, nociceptors exist where it makes sense for them to be, which is anywhere that the organism may be subjected to harmful external stimuli or internal injury.

Nociceptors of the spinal column have been studied, but not nearly to the degree that peripheral nociceptors have. Therefore, much of what is known of nociceptor function is based on study of innervation of the limbs, and mostly from skin.[71,72] The reader is referred to these excellent reviews for details on nociceptor development and neurochemistry. Here we give a general overview of nociceptor function and point out the growing evidence that spinal and other deep nociceptors differ from nociceptors that innervate skin.

Nociceptors are unmyelinated or thinly myelinated axonal processes of pseudounipolar dorsal root ganglion neurons. The unmyelinated axons are referred to as C-fibers, with conduction velocities of less than 2.5 m/sec, and the thinly myelinated axons are referred to as A-delta fibers, with conduction velocities of 2.5 m/sec to approximately 15 m/sec.[73]

Cutaneous C-nociceptors and A-delta nociceptors are often discussed as subserving slow and fast pain function, respectively. These functions may have some physiologic and clinical differences, with C-nociceptor activity more likely to give rise to burning or aching sensations and A-delta nociceptor activation to better localized, sharp, stabbing, or pricking pain. However, significant overlap in function occurs. Furthermore, this differentiation has been determined from studies of cutaneous innervation and may not apply to pain in deeper tissues, such as those of the spine. Several subcategories of nociceptors exist and are reviewed elsewhere.[71,74–77]

The portion of the nociceptor that is normally involved in detection of the noxious stimulus historically has been called a free-nerve ending. This ending consists of a brush-like distribution of small nerve processes spread over a small region of the innervated tissue, termed a receptive field. The receptive fields of cutaneous nociceptors are quite small (usually

~1 mm², and those in subcutaneous tissues have similar properties but branch more freely, thereby having more complex and larger three-dimensional receptive fields. Physiologic studies of the receptive field of paraspinal nociceptors showed that these neurons have multiple receptive fields within a given tissue, such as muscle. In addition, single nociceptive neurons may have multiple receptive fields to include muscle, tendon, nerve sheath, and occasionally, the deeper layers of the skin.[78] These complex receptive fields are predicted to make localization of deep, painful stimuli difficult (see Fig. 137.2).

Although no distinctive morphologic specializations allow morphologic characterization, the endings of nociceptors are functionally specialized to discriminate among mechanical, chemical, and thermal stimuli or may respond to a combination of these modalities. These endings have been found to manifest a growing array of specific channels that impart sensitivities to a wide range of noxious stimuli.[71] As a result of this, and because they contain specific neurotransmitters, small-caliber nerve fibers can be microscopically identified with immunohistochemical staining techniques for channel proteins and peptide neurotransmitters, such as substance P or calcitonin gene–related peptide (CGRP). These methods can be used to presumptively show the location of nociceptive terminals. In the spine, presumptive nociceptors have been identified in the outer layers of the intervertebral disks, the several ligaments of the spine, and all structures of the spinal canal,[79,80] and in facet joint capsules, including intraarticular synovial folds (meniscoids).[81]

In consideration of the location of spinal nociceptors by anatomic means, remembering that labeling of channels and transmitter is not definitive proof of function is important. Physiologic confirmation that the neuron responds to noxious stimuli (i.e., stimuli that produce or threaten tissue damage) is necessary. Unfortunately, such experiments for spinal structures are very difficult to perform, and only within the last couple of decades have spinal nociceptors been physiologically identified and characterized.[78,82,83]

The diversity of tissues that comprise the spine provides an additional challenge in the study of nociceptors. We have shown that spinal dura, muscles, nerves, joint capsules, periosteum, and ligamentous structures (including the disks) are all innervated elements of the spine (see Fig. 137.3). In addition, blood vessels are known to have a rich innervation, consisting of somatic afferent and autonomic fibers; indeed, these structures are painful when stimulated.[84] The innervation of the nerve sheaths and their accompanying blood vessels by nociceptors is a more recent finding.[85]

Nociceptor Function

Spinal nociceptors respond to noxious mechanical stimuli and also to many chemicals within the tissues. Some of these substances are directly released by damaged tissue, and others are produced by inflammatory cells or by other cells residing in the tissues. The nerves residing within the tissues provide an additional source of many of these algesic (pain-producing) compounds. The complete list of agents to which cutaneous nociceptors respond is ever growing and is beyond the scope of this chapter. Many of the agents do not directly activate nociceptors but sensitize them to other agents or stimuli. Initially, the general assumption was that intense and noxious stimuli were capable of activating nociceptive fibers simply on the basis of physical, thermal, or chemical membrane disruption. However, with the finding of specific receptors and channels on nociceptive nerve endings that are sensitive to these modalities, the concept of specificity of the afferent nociceptive response is evolving, and indeed numerous subtypes of primary afferent nociceptors have been identified.

Tissue damage or disease is capable of changing the properties of nociceptors, including their sensitivity and responsiveness to stimuli. In normal, undisturbed tissue, very few, if any, signs of activity are found in sensory neurons with slow conduction velocities (presumptive nociceptors),[86] but tissue injury can result in a change in ongoing activity, a phenomenon called sensitization. After injury or repeated activation, nociceptors also have a lowered threshold to noxious stimuli and an increase in the size of their receptive fields. This effect can occur with even a brief stimulus and can last for hours.[87] In skin, the effect is best observed in response to burns, where tissue injury produces increased sensitivity and spontaneous pain, mediated predominantly by sensitized nociceptors. Sensitization has been shown to occur in both nociceptors from cutaneous and deep tissues,[88] but the full mechanism of the process remains incompletely understood.

Stimulation of sympathetic nerves can affect nociceptors in certain situations. Normally, despite the finding that nociceptors may be sensitized by sympathetic stimulation,[89,90] sympathetic activity or the application of norepinephrine does not directly activate nociceptors.[91,92] However, during chronic inflammation or after nerve injury, sympathetic stimulation becomes able to directly activate C-fiber nociceptors.[93–96] Pain and psychologic stressors increase sympathetic discharge, leading to increased levels of norepinephrine.[97–99] This well-known response provides at least a partial explanation for the clinical observations that reduction of psychologic stress may decrease pain and facilitate a more rapid recovery.

Sensitization of nociceptors is particularly important in radiating pain syndromes, such as radicular pain. Several experiments have shown that inflammation of axons in the absence of overt damage leads to the development of mechanical sensitivity of the axon, and the appearance of spontaneous activity. The axonal mechanical sensitivity is a source of ectopic action potential generation and is perceived as an abnormal sensation (usually unpleasant) arising from the tissue in which the axon terminals reside (**Fig. 137.4**). This is the mechanism behind the commonly observed positive straight leg raise in radiating pain conditions (including lumbosacral radiculopathy) in the absence of overt nerve or axonal damage. Spontaneous activity in the injured axons is also perceived as arising from the distally innervated structure and, in this case, manifests as constant pain. The dorsal root and its attached dorsal root ganglion (DRG; the source of the afferent axons) have particular sensitivities to injury, in part because of anatomic relationships.[100,101] Experimental models of radiating pain (e.g., radiculopathy) have shown changes in gene expression and in production of cytokines and neurotransmitters associated with nociception in the DRG.[102] Furthermore, inflammatory cytokines, such as tumor necrosis factor-α (TNFα), have been implicated in hyperalgesia in some of these experimental models.[103,104] This suggests a significant degree of complexity to the process of dorsal root and DRG sensitization. A further layer is suggested by changes in the spinal cord and CNS associated with experimental radiculopathy (see subsequent).[105,106]

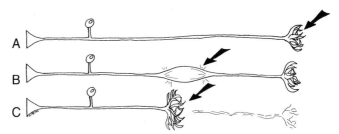

Fig. 137.4 **A,** Typical representation of primary afferent neuron, with *(right to left)* a receptor, a peripherally projecting axon, the cell body, a centrally projecting axon, and a terminal in the dorsal horn of the spinal cord. Sufficient stimuli of the receptor lead to the generation of action potentials, which are propagated along the axon to the central nervous system. **B,** The axon is an alternate source of action potential generation for slowly conducting neurons innervating deep tissues. Importantly, any sensation arising from stimulation of the axon at such a sensitive site is perceived as coming from the distal receptive area, not from the site of action potential generation. **C,** A damaged and regrowing axon is another source of action potentials. If numerous axons are cut, the regrowth can cause a mass called a neuroma. Regrowing axons are sensitive to chemical and mechanical stimuli. As in **B,** sensations arising from such stimuli are also perceived as coming from the innervated tissue.

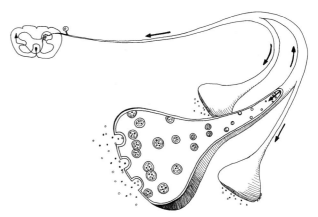

Fig. 137.5 **Release of substance P and calcitonin gene–related peptide (CGRP) by primary afferent nociceptors.** When an appropriate stimulation elicits an action potential, the action potential is propagated to the central nervous system and to other branches of the neuron *(arrows).* Simultaneously, the endings release substance P and CGRP *(small closed and open symbols)* from the terminals, which are colocalized in vesicles that are transported from the cell body. This process is thought to occur in terminals that are invaded by the action potential even when they are not directly stimulated. Substance P and CGRP cause plasma extravasation and vasodilation, respectively, which are necessary components of the inflammatory response. This process is termed neurogenic inflammation.

Neurogenic Inflammation

At the beginning of the 20th century, electrical stimulation of dorsal roots was observed to produce cutaneous vasodilation and plasma extravasation whenever the stimulus intensity was high enough to excite unmyelinated axons.[107] This response was termed the axon reflex, and the neurons responsible were found to be nociceptors.[108] Thus, when nociceptors are active, they release transmitters that are involved in the inflammatory reaction from their peripheral, and central terminals (**Fig. 137.5**). The best studied, though by no means only, transmitters involved in this process are substance P and CGRP.[109] Electrical stimulation of nociceptor axons anywhere along their course causes the release of the inflammatory mediators from distal terminals, resulting in a focal reaction, termed neurogenic inflammation (NI).[110] This function of nociceptors plays an important role in the initiation and control of inflammation; without it, animals are not able to mount a full inflammatory response, making NI critical to an organism's response to injury.[111] Because of this importance, nociceptors are also called nocifensors.[112,113]

Although the role of nociceptors in NI is undisputed, less is known about the role of the sympathetic nervous system in this process. However, sympathetic neurons are clearly important to the generation of experimental immune arthritis[111] and participate in the localized edema that occurs in certain models of chronic neuropathic pain. This participation may explain why stressful situations can exacerbate inflammatory conditions and increase pain. Sympathetic neurons have a complex physiology, releasing not only the biogenic amines such as norepinephrine, but also neuropeptide Y and adenosine triphosphate (ATP). Recently, sympathetic neurons, probably through a mechanism involving ATP release, have been shown to be essential for some of the molecular mechanisms involved in peripheral sensitization of nociceptors by capsaicin.[114] Sympathectomy blocks the upregulation of transient receptor potential receptors, CGRP, and protein kinase C (PKC) that accompanies sensitization[115] and also diminishes NI.[116] This indicates a complex peripheral interaction between the sensory and sympathetic nervous systems in the generation of NI. Indeed, recent study has shown complex interactions between the sympathetic nervous system and lymphocytes involved in the immune response.[117,118]

Differences Between Deep and Cutaneous Nociceptors

Studies of cutaneous nociceptors may not be fully applicable to deep nociceptors, with some studies showing fundamental differences between nociceptors in these two locations. For example, clinically important spinal pain conditions are not typically associated with cutaneous symptoms. Recently, the authors interviewed 25 people with diagnoses of painful lumbar radiculopathy, and none had spontaneous or evocable pain reported on their skin.[119] This finding has since been confirmed by others.[120] In the laboratory, deep nociceptor axons seem to respond differently to inflammation. During neuritis, or nerve inflammation, axons of deep nociceptors become mechanically sensitive, whereas cutaneous nociceptor axons rarely do.[121,122] In these same studies, the incidence rate of ongoing activity (equivalent to spontaneous pain) was found to be higher in deep nociceptors. After axonal damage, recordings from nociceptors in muscle nerves reveal ongoing discharge more often than is seen in recordings from cutaneous neurons.[123,124] Finally, the receptor profiles of bone-innervating and skin-innervating peptidergic (and thus possibly nociceptive) neurons[125] were shown to differ qualitatively. Taken together, these data point to fundamental differences in deep versus cutaneous nociceptor physiology.

Central Transmission and Regulation of Nociceptive Signals

An understanding of the pathways and the mechanisms involved in central processing of nociceptive signals is critical to appreciation of ways in which pain can be treated. Ultimately, the experience of pain requires participation of the CNS, and

mechanisms have been identified both for amplification and for suppression of pain. More recently, science has begun to ask questions such as "Why do two people with similar injuries have markedly different pain responses?" and "How can pain interact with cognitive processes and affect personality?" Of all of the regions of the CNS that are involved in pain processing, the best studied is the spinal cord. The spinal cord forms the most fundamental level of central processing of noxious signals. The following sections focus on this level. Briefer consideration is given to higher levels, which are no less important, if less well studied.

Spinal Cord Terminations of Nociceptors

The central processes of nociceptive DRG neurons enter the dorsolateral portion of the spinal cord. There, they branch T-wise, sending collateral branches 1 through 5 segments rostral and caudal (1 to 2 for C-fiber nociceptors; 1 to 5 for A-delta nociceptors).[126] This region of the spinal cord white matter located has been termed *Lissauer's zone* and is located immediately adjacent to the dorsal horn. C-fiber nociceptors terminate in the most dorsal part of the dorsal horn, termed *laminae I and II*,[127] whereas A-delta nociceptors additionally project more deeply in the cord (laminae V and X).[128] Nociceptors from the limbs terminate ipsilaterally. However, paraspinal tissue nociceptors project bilaterally to dorsal horn neurons.[129,130] This projection pattern is the likely explanation for the clinical observation that back pain is typically poorly localized and indicates the need for bilateral spinal examination.

Two physiologically distinct types of dorsal horn neurons are involved in the transmission of the nociceptive signals from the spinal cord to higher centers. Wide dynamic range (WDR) neurons are the most common type. These neurons respond to both noxious and innocuous peripheral stimuli, with more intense and widespread stimuli producing greater activation (see Fig. 137.2). The WDR neurons are believed to be most important to the recognition of intensity of pain. However, an extensive convergence of nociceptors from different parts of the body onto the WDR neurons[131] precludes them from signaling the precise location of the pain origin. For example, an individual WDR neuron may be activated by stimulation of paraspinal muscles, the dura, and spinal ligaments, and by noxious stimulation of a portion of the limb.[129] Therefore, when activated, these neurons are incapable of signaling the precise site of pain origin. This circuitry also provides a physiologic basis for referred pain, which is a particularly common clinical phenomenon when pain arises from the viscera and deeper somatic portions of the body. A smaller percentage of dorsal horn transmission neurons respond selectively to noxious stimuli; these are termed nociceptive specific neurons. These neurons are located in deeper layers of the dorsal horn and also layered along the most superficial laminae of the dorsal horn *(substantia gelatinosa)*. The nociceptive-specific neurons are believed to be specialized to signal the presence of pain and its precise location, rather than its intensity.

Central Neural Mechanisms for Amplification of Nociception

Many clinical phenomena cannot be adequately explained by simple neuron-to-neuron transmission along dedicated pain pathways. For example, in a classic study, Adriaensen and colleagues[132] showed that sustained pinch of the skin led to increasing reports of pain with time, whereas the neural discharge from nociceptors supplying the area actually decreased. Explaining this paradox is difficult but necessitates that the spinal cord and higher centers change their "gain" (i.e., amplify the signal) in response to the input from the nociceptors.

Substantial evidence suggests that peripheral noxious stimulation leads to changes in the CNS by various mechanisms, which are collectively called spinal cord plasticity.[133-135] Extensive research over the past two decades has gone into elucidating molecular mechanisms of this phenomenon, partially in an attempt to explain the clinical phenomena of hyperalgesia, allodynia, and chronic pain. In some conditions, activation of pain pathways has been shown to be sustained even if the sensory input from the original source is terminated. Although some experimental models, such as ligation of the sciatic nerve, readily produce long-term sensory facilitation, why certain painful stimuli produce such facilitation while others do not is not fully understood. However, once such facilitation takes place in neurons that have widespread receptive fields, allodynia and hyperalgesia may be perceived broadly from uninjured and even rather remote tissues. Indeed, these symptoms are frequently observed in patients with chronic back pain. CNS plasticity is a likely explanation for these variable presentations.

The earliest known mechanisms for sustaining and amplifying nociceptive signals include physiologic processes of wind-up and long-term potentiation (LTP). These are briefly considered here; for greater details, the reader is referred to recent reviews.[136-138] *Wind-up* is a term that was coined for the phenomenon of increasing the response of a neuron to repeated stimuli.[139,140] For example, when depolarized by a sensory input, dorsal horn neurons do not always fully recover their resting potential before the arrival of another volley from the primary afferent fiber. Therefore, the threshold for firing of the neuron is lower (i.e., the neuron is facilitated). This process typically lasts seconds to minutes.

LTP is similar to wind-up, but it lasts much longer; indeed, some consider that changes associated with LTP may be permanent. This process requires a high-frequency conditioning discharge from the primary afferent neuron[141] and results in increased synaptic efficiency mediated by activation of a specific type of glutamate receptor, the *N*-methyl-d-aspartate (NMDA) receptor. It differs from wind-up in that the increased synaptic efficiency is not related to a change in the resting membrane potential of the postsynaptic cells; rather, it involves complicated changes within the postsynaptic dorsal horn neurons that can best be considered to be a type of memory. Once established, long-term depression (LTD; discussed subsequently) is the only thing that reverses LTP.

In pain processing systems, LTP is a multistep process with many ramifications. It requires the stimulation of a nociceptor, whose central terminals release a varying combination of substance P, CGRP, neurokinin 1, and glutamate onto spinal cord neurons. The pattern and quantity of transmitter release depends on the characteristics of the actions potential activity in these neurons.[142] These transmitters activate the transmission neurons of the spinal cord but also have several other potential consequences, particularly in situations that are known to cause chronic pain (such as sciatic nerve irritation).[143] For example, the best studied of these mechanisms involves corelease of glutamate and one or more peptide transmitter from primary afferent nociceptors. This

coactivation is capable of altering the function of the NMDA receptor subtype of glutamate receptor, changing its permeability to calcium.[144] Increased intracellular calcium, in turn, is known to activate second messengers in spinal cord neurons, altering responses to subsequent stimuli. One type of change involves the phosporylation of receptors, which can alter the function of the receptor.[145] In addition, some of these second messengers can result in insertion of new receptors and ion channels in the membrane of the neuron, producing long-term changes in responsiveness to subsequent stimuli. Also, some of the second messengers are responsible for activation of early-immediate genes (such as c-*fos* and c-*jun*) within the facilitated neuron.[146-148] The proteins that are produced by these early-immediate genes can "turn on" other genes, resulting in synthesis of yet other proteins.[149,150] The net result of these changes is long-lasting alteration in physiology of the nociceptive projection neurons, which may include prolonged discharge to an innocuous stimulus. It may even result in spontaneous activity of neurons that are involved in transmitting nociceptive signals.[151] This effect is generally hypothesized to provide the physiologic substrate for hyperalgesia and chronic pain, potentially even in the absence of ongoing nociceptor activation.

Since these observations on molecular mechanisms of chronic pain, extensive study of other important mechanisms has helped explain facilitation of pain pathways and the presence of certain chronic pain states. For example, structural changes in synaptic contacts after injuries have been determined to result in chronic painful states.[138,152] These changes appear to result from activation of genes involved in synaptic spine development and maintenance, in a process that is also similar to those involved in memory formation. It is noteworthy that preliminary evidence has been found of synaptic plasticity in the spinal cord of animals with segmental spinal lesions that were designed to model aspects of lesions treated with spinal manipulation.[153]

Several additional mechanisms may be important to changes in sensitivity of spinal cord pathways in pain syndromes.[154] For example, the expression of cytokines and growth factors[155,156] by the glial cells of the spinal cord have been shown to increase during several experimental models of nerve injury.[157] Many of these cytokines are inflammatory in nature, demonstrating that the interactions between the two great communication systems in the body, the immune system and the nervous system, are substantially more complex and bidirectional than had been previously appreciated.[158,159] For example, animals genetically engineered to be deficient in one or more of these factors have diminished responses to some injuries that normally produce chronic pain.[160] One potential explanation for the observation that injury to cutaneous nerves is less likely to produce sustained pain is a lower potential for skin lesions to stimulate production of some of these growth factors.[161] Although these growth factors clearly should have significant effects on nerve function, their role in clinical phenomena of altered pain sensitivity is still under investigation.

Of course, pain is not perceived at the spinal cord level, and ascending projections through the brainstem and thalamus are responsible for the ultimate communication with higher centers of the brain. Unfortunately, less is known about the physiologic alterations that can occur at higher levels of the neuraxis. However, many of the mechanisms that alter spinal cord responses to pain have also been identified at higher centers.[162–164] Therefore, it is not a stretch to say that the plasticity involved in upregulation of pain transmission after certain types of injuries may be capable of creating a pain "memory" that contributes to excessive or prolonged pain.

Neural Mechanisms for Suppression of Nociception

The ability to perceive pain is critical to the survival and general well being of the individual. However, the ability to modulate pain is also important. An example taken from common experience is the ability to "shake off" an injury that produces severe tissue damage until any immediate threat is past. At that time, the pain may become severe or even immobilizing, although the injury itself has not changed. What, then, explains this ability to modulate pain transmission and processing? Given the importance of this function to survival of the organism, that multiple mechanisms have been identified for pain suppression should not be surprising.

Several known physiologic processes can diminish activity of neurons in the pain systems. One of these mechanisms is long-term depression.[165] LTD can be established by both high-frequency and low-frequency conditioning stimuli, and it involves a long-lasting decrease in synaptic efficacy (thus, it is the mirror image of LTP, described previously). Hypothetically, LTP is at least partially responsible for chronic pain; and the hypothesis that LTD induced by stimulating an appropriate nerve may relieve it is reasonable.[136] This mechanism may be behind the anecdotal effectiveness of various forms of clinical electrical stimulation; however, this remains to be confirmed.

Another mechanism of pain suppression relates to the demonstrated decrease in pain after stimulation of larger diameter, mechanoreceptive (mostly A-beta) afferent nerve fibers.[166] Although a neurobiologic basis for this has long been hypothesized, primarily on clinical grounds and on the fact that many types of pain feel better when mechanoreceptors are stimulated, little confirmatory experimental evidence has been found of the much cited and so-called pain "gate."[167] However, the hypothesis did spawn much research that showed complex central interactions between various sensory neuron subtypes.[168] For example, electrical stimulation of large-diameter afferent neurons has been shown to release gamma-amino butyric acid (GABA), which is capable of inhibiting nociceptive transmission in the dorsal horn.[169,170] GABA is not the only inhibitory neurotransmitter that is implicated in the inhibition accompanying stimulation of large-diameter axons. Glycine has a significant inhibitory effect at the spinal cord level with at least some of its effect from inhibition of excitatory neurotransmission through NMDA receptors.[171,172] Of note is the finding that large diameter afferent sensory input arising from deeper tissues is more potent in producing analgesic responses from electrical stimulation.[173] From a clinical perspective, recognition of the potent interaction between neurons with large-diameter axons and pain transmission neurons has led not only to the use of transcutaneous electrical nerve stimulation, which appears to be effective in suppressing pain during stimulation in acute (but not chronic) pain, but also to the more recent use of dorsal column stimulators, which probably release GABA in spinal cord[174] and supraspinal levels.[175]

Certain types of denervating nerve injuries cause chronic pain (deafferentation pain). Many such lesions are associated with a decrease in GABA in the spinal cord[176] and higher centers.[177] Presumably this causes a decrease in inhibition, amplifying nociceptive transmission through whatever afferent pathways remain.

The study of brain receptors for opiates has lead to recognition of another important pain modulating system.[178] Receptors for opiates have been found in several brain regions (notably periaqueductal gray [PAG], dorsal horn of the spinal cord, ventral medullary raphe nuclei, and basal ganglia). Depending on the subtype of opiate receptor, some are excitatory and some inhibitory. Nonetheless, electrical stimulation of most of these endogenous opiate-containing regions (notably the PAG and raphe nuclei) inhibits nociceptive responses in animals and produces analgesia in humans.[179]

Of course, the presence of these opiate receptors begs the question of why the nervous system has specific receptors for a compound (opium) derived from a Middle Eastern poppy. Investigation of this question led to the discovery of a group of transmitters contained in small interneurons. These peptides bind to opiate receptors and activate them. These "endogenous opiates" come in two types: a family of very small peptides (enkephalins) that are synthesized in small neurons of the CNS, and a larger compound (endorphin) that is found in the region of the pituitary gland and is released into the circulation. Injection of these compounds into portions of the nervous system that have opiate receptors produces powerful analgesia. In addition, enkephalins can be collected from the spinal fluid after noxious stimulation of peripheral nerves,[180,181] suggesting some effect in controlling excessive nociceptive stimulation, including within the spinal cord.

Further study has elucidated the role of enkephalins found in interneurons at other levels of the neuraxis.[182,183] Two systems of endogenous analgesia are known to use enkephalinergic interneurons to suppress pain transmission. Both of these systems involve brainstem centers that are the origin of descending pain suppression tracts. One of these systems results in widespread pain suppression in response to intense noxious stimulation anywhere in the body. This has been termed diffuse noxious inhibitory control (DNIC).[184,185] This system consists of neurons in the dorsocaudal medulla that respond to pain anywhere on that side of the body. These neurons give rise to descending tracts in the dorsolateral funiculus of the spinal cord, which terminate in the dorsal horn at all spinal levels. This pathway suppresses pain transmission diffusely, partially through activating endogenous opiate containing neurons. Essentially, DNIC diffusely suppresses pain after any intense pain stimulus.

A second descending pain suppression system uses endogenous opiates.[182] The PAG is a key center of this system, containing neurons that can be activated by many other areas of the brain, including regions involved in mood, emotions, and control of endocrine function. Enkephalinergic interneurons in the PAG activate excitatory projections to the caudal medulla. These projections, in turn, excite descending noradrenergic and serotoninergic projections to the dorsal horn. The norepinephrine and serotonin (monoamines) that are released in the dorsal horn produce complex analgesic effects. They can both directly affect pain transmission neurons and also activate other neurons at the spinal level, including small enkephalinergic interneurons. Of course, in attempting to understand the functions of this system, recognition is critical of the various roles of the brain regions that connect with the PAG. These brain regions include the frontal and insular cortex, amygdala, hypothalamus, reticular formation, locus ceruleus, and collateral branches of the spinothalamic tract. The role of these higher centers in descending pain suppression must be acknowledged.[186] This convergence of input from regions with emotional, endocrine, and autonomic effects, and from areas involved in alertness, illustrates the diverse brain systems that can play a part in regulating pain transmission.

Endogenous opiate-containing systems have become the best-known inhibitory circuits for pain modulation. They not only define the analgesic effects of exogenous opiates, such as morphine, but also explain at least some of the role that monoamine transmitters play in pain control.[187] Therefore, appreciation of this system has provided important clues in understanding of the biologic basis for some of the pharmacologic agents used in clinical practice. An understanding of antinociceptive effects of therapeutic intervention must take into account the potential impact of treatment on these mechanisms. Undoubtedly, additional descending antinociceptive systems will be identified[188] and will need to be incorporated into the model.

Psychology and Nociception

Why can two individuals be injured in exactly the same manner, with dramatically different results (at least in terms of pain and suffering)? Although some of these different results undoubtedly are caused by the differences in the peripheral pain systems and the pain transmission systems in the CNS, the experience of pain goes well beyond the mere activation of a nociceptor and the conduction of an impulse to the cerebral cortex.

Pain is defined as an unpleasant sensory and emotional experience. In addition, the issue of suffering, which is the behavioral and psychologic component that is reflected in the patient's outward affect, must be considered in any clinical discussion of pain. Patients typically describe their suffering as the consequence of the painful disorder. Although understanding of mechanisms involved in suffering and the psychologic ramifications of pain is incomplete, several lines of evidence indicate that the frontal lobes of the cerebral cortex, particularly the medial portions, are critical in this regard, with other areas playing an ancillary role.[189] The first hints of this conclusion arose from the clinical evaluation of patients with frontal lobe injuries. Such patients are able to describe the intensity of a painful stimulus, indicating that the principal transmission pathways are intact; however, they do not appear to suffer in proportion to the degree of pain. In such patients, both behavioral and autonomic responses to pain are blunted. Evidence suggests that at least a portion of the analgesic effects of some sedatives and anxiolytic drugs is from effects on the frontal lobe rather than (or in addition to) affecting pain transmission through nociceptive pathways.

Other lines of investigation have also directed attention to areas of the frontal lobe. These include experimental pain models that selectively activate portions of the frontal lobes on functional magnetic resonance imaging.[190] In addition, patients who were effectively hypnotized to block the unpleasantness, but not the intensity, of their pain showed changes in activity of the anterior cingulate cortex (i.e., a part of the medial frontal lobe).[191] An interesting note is that similar areas of the cortex are metabolically altered in affective disorders, particularly depression. On clinical grounds,

that a complex interaction exists between depression and pain is well known, suggesting at least some physiologic basis in frontal lobe physiology. Although much has been written about the capacity of depression to magnify pain, some evidence also suggests that effective treatment of chronic pain is capable of ameliorating depression,[192] an argument for a two-way interaction.

Most of the interest in cortical mechanisms of pain has focused on the issue of suffering rather than pain perception, per se. However, there is good reason to believe that psychologic factors related to the cortex can also more directly influence pain transmission. For example, several studies indicate that placebo analgesia is real and is probably mediated via endogenous opiate mechanisms.[193,194] As per the prior discussion of pain modulation, the connections between the frontal cortex and PAG (among other places) may provide a substrate for this effect, although the precise mechanisms remain unknown. Overall, there is good reason to believe that cortical mechanisms play a role in analgesia, and excellent evidence suggests that suffering is a cortical phenomenon that is largely based in the frontal lobes. These findings provide some theoretic underpinning for behavioral interventions in pain management, although they complicate many human studies of pain.

Spinal Manipulation and Pain

As more is known about the physiology of pain, consideration of the potential physiologic mechanisms for pain therapies has become increasingly important. This is certainly true for spinal manipulation, where some clinical evidence is found for an effect on pain[14,22-27] and a modest amount of evidence from physiologic psychology experiments[45-51] shows that spinal manipulation may have some antinociceptive effects. However, the nature of this interaction is far from clear, and the mechanisms for analgesic effects of spinal manipulation remain largely hypothetic.

The theories used to explain potential pain suppression have fallen into four broad categories. All of the proposed mechanisms have some limited direct or indirect support from human or animal studies or are consistent with known physiologic mechanisms. However, all remain highly speculative in nature.

Mechanism One: Direct Effect on Pain Generation

The first proposed mechanism considers the potential for SMT to decrease the generation of signals in nociceptive fibers in the pain sensitive tissue of the back. Unfortunately, consideration of this mechanism is somewhat limited by deficient knowledge of specific pain generators for most cases of back pain, as alluded to in previous sections. Therefore, any discussion must consider the various potential pain generators, including nerve roots (radiculopathy), peripheral nerves, ligaments, joints, intervertebral disks, and muscles.

Probably the best understood, but one of the less common, sources of pain is direct involvement of spinal nerves and nerve roots. Many patients with radiating pain show anatomic and physiologic evidence of direct mechanical compression of spinal nerves or nerve roots, and at least one study, which showed a return of H-reflexes in patients with radiculopathy after

SMT,[38] has suggested direct mechanical changes as a result of manipulation. Any mechanical effect on the spinal nerve root presumably also affects nociceptive fibers contained in these structures and for spinal nerves and their branches may cause mechanical irritation of nervi nervorum in the perineural and epineural coverings.[78,85,195]

In contrast to the direct involvement of nerve roots, involvement of the peripheral nerves in the spine seems to be extremely common, but not well understood. As mentioned previously, inflammation of nerves, or neuritis, causes ongoing activity and ectopic mechanical sensitivity (see Fig. 137.4),[86,121,196] at least in part caused by impaired axoplasmic transport[197] and mediated by cyclooxygenase-2.[102] Such changes are perceived in the distribution of the nerve. For instance, inflammation of the intervertebral foramen is expected to cause spontaneous and movement-induced pain perceived in the back and leg. This has been shown to occur in a rat model of nerve inflammation[198] and also to be helped with spinal manipulation.[199] Changes in the function of axons as a result of local inflammation have been shown to resolve with the inflammation.[122] Such symptoms are appropriately called ectopic nociceptive pain.

Beyond potential direct effects of SMT on nerves and nerve roots, biomechanical effects may be seen on other tissues from which pain signals arise. Perhaps the easiest to envision is the facet joint, which is known to be affected by SMT.[200] Because the facet joint capsule contains nerve fibers with presumptive nociceptive function,[58,59,201–207] facet nociceptors clearly could be influenced directly with manipulation. Furthermore, because intra-articular meniscoids are extensions of the joint capsule, manipulation of a joint may have long-lasting effects via repositioning or increasing the mobility of these joint elements. However, this hypothesis remains to be tested, largely because of inability to examine the mechanics of these meniscoids *in vivo*. Another concept is that SMT breaks innervated adhesions that form between tissues (e.g., facet joint surfaces, muscle to other muscle or fascia, connective tissue to nerve), but direct evidence for this is lacking.

Other authors have invoked direct mechanical effects on intervertebral disks.[208,209] The outer layers of the annulus fibrosis are known to be innervated with presumptive nociceptive fibers.[210,211] Despite the intuitively pleasing nature of this hypothesis, to date, no direct evidence shows that SMT produces more than a transient change in the mechanics of the intervertebral disk.

Spinal manipulative therapy has clear effects on paraspinal muscles. These muscles contain both nociceptive[130] and proprioceptive[62,212] sensory innervation, and clearly, these muscles react specifically to SMT.[213–215] Muscle responses to SMT also have been shown to be somewhat different between patients with and without back pain.[216] Furthermore, preliminary evidence shows that spinal manipulation attenuates muscle responses to noxious stimulation.[217] Spinal manipulation is also known to produce transient effects on motor system physiology, momentarily decreasing motor neuron excitability in remote muscles.[41,44] This has led some to speculate that the unique dynamics of SMT may have an effect on back pain arising from muscles either by producing relaxation of hypertonic muscles or by otherwise affecting the chemistry of painful muscles. In addition, some evidence shows a change in muscle activity[218] and function[219] that outlasts the spinal manipulative treatment period. However, what effect this may have on longer term paraspinal muscle function is still unclear.

In this regard, despite some reports to the contrary,[220] spinal manipulation is associated with a decrease in pressure pain both in painful paraspinal muscles[221–224] and in some remote symptomatic sites.[225]

Mechanism Two: Activation of Pain Suppression Mechanisms

The second proposed mechanism for an effect of SMT on pain involves activation of CNS pain suppression mechanisms. SMT-like forces clearly are capable of activating proprioceptors,[62,63,212] with which the spine is particularly well endowed. An attractive suggestion is that activation of these proprioceptors may be capable of suppressing pain signals in a manner similar to that described previously for large-diameter axon input to the spinal cord.[173] Indahl and colleagues[226] have provided some evidence for this hypothesis in a study testing interaction of facet joint proprioceptive fibers and nociceptive responses from the spine in pigs. These researchers evoked a nociceptive reflex in paraspinal muscles to electrical stimulation of outer layers of the intervertebral disk. They subsequently activated mechanoreceptors in the facet joint capsules by inflating them with saline solution. These authors reported a profound depression in the nociceptive reflexes during and, in many animals, for a prolonged period of time after the inflation of the joint. Although it is attractive to invoke direct interaction between spinal proprioceptors and nociceptive fibers in the spinal cord, the precise mechanisms for this observation are not known and presumably could result from any of the several known mechanisms for suppression of noxious reflexes in the CNS (see previous discussion). In addition, understanding of whether this effect is specific to facet joints or whether it pertains to any large-diameter proprioceptive afferent activation and whether it is applicable to other species is of theoretic importance. Nonetheless, this provides an intriguing potential mechanism for an antinociceptive effect of SMT.

Mechanism Three: Effect on Motor Output

A third potential mechanism considers the possible effects of SMT on motor output as a way of modifying pain. These motor outputs may be somatic or autonomic, and the effect of manipulation may be via the production of reflexes or via changing of ongoing patterns of motor activity. Because chronic changes in muscle activity may contribute to muscle pain and because changes in sympathetic nervous system activity can affect elements of the inflammatory reaction (see previous discussion), altered motor output is a potentially attractive mechanism of effect.

Much of this speculation has arisen from the observation by manipulative practitioners of overactive muscles in localized regions of the spine, particularly those with excessive pain sensitivity. In addition, practitioners have reported localized changes in temperature and sweating that has been taken as evidence of localized autonomic dysfunction. Despite some early experimental evidence of somatic overactivity[227–229] and abnormal autonomic activity,[230–233] little convincing evidence for this mechanism as a significant factor in spine disease has been found.

Some authors have hypothesized that localized spine pain might sensitize local proprioceptive reflexes to the point of provoking abnormal localized somatic motor reflexes, but this was not found to be the case in the one study that directly attempted to test this hypothesis.[234] Other studies have clearly shown that mechanical and noxious chemical stimulation of the spine can provoke autonomic reflexes.[235,236] However, these autonomic reflexes appear to be more generalized responses, and it is not clear how or whether they relate to spinal pathophysiology or whether they can be affected by SMT. Therefore, one has to conclude that the theories of spinal manipulative effects on motor outputs remain to be tested in a rigorous way.

Mechanism Four: Effect on Higher Centers of Processing

A fourth potential mechanism considers that SMT might have an effect at higher levels of the neuraxis. It has become increasingly clear that pain and nociception are parallel, but different, and that certain therapies may have effects on pain that are beyond the physiologic effects on nociceptive transmission pathways. Although many of these effects have been lumped under the general category of "placebo," the use of this term implies the existence of a single phenomenon and a single mechanism. It also implies that the mechanism is nonspecific and that it is not grounded in neurophysiology. This is an increasingly untenable view as changes in nervous system activity by placebo interventions can be visualized and quantified.[237–239] In addition, it is increasingly clear that there are important physiologic effects of these placebo interventions[194] and that not all placebos are created equal. Whether or not the term placebo is used, any theory of the potential effects of SMT must consider potential effects on cerebral cortical processing of nociceptive signals.

Summary of Spinal Manipulative Mechanisms

In summary, although some clinical evidence shows an effect of SMT on painful conditions and some experimental evidence shows antinociceptive effects of SMT, confirmation of any of the several potential mechanisms remains elusive. This has partially resulted from inadequate animal models of spine disease outside of a few special cases, such as radiculopathy.

It has also resulted from difficulty in study of nociception and pain from deep tissues of the spine and the important and powerful nonspecific effects of certain treatments, such as spinal manipulation.

Conclusion

Pain and nociception are related but different events. The neural events that lead to pain usually involve activation of nociceptors innervating a threatened or damaged tissue. Once activated, nociceptors transmit information to the spinal cord for processing and may also participate in the generation of the inflammatory reaction. The response properties of nociceptors are plastic, and they can become sensitized by continued stimulation and by action of other nerves and interaction with other cells in the tissues. Sensitization also occurs in the CNS, with both short-term and long-term changes in structure and function of nerve cells. These changes may explain pathologic pain sensitivity and abnormally prolonged (chronic) pain. Pain transmission can be suppressed by several mechanisms in the CNS. This has been best studied at the level of the spinal cord, although similar mechanisms probably exist at higher levels, such as the thalamus. Endogenous pain suppression mechanisms explain many of the effects of therapies that are known to suppress pain and may contribute to analgesic effects of spinal manipulation. The high degree of convergence of nociceptors from various parts of the body on spinal cord projection neurons in the pain pathway provides a substrate for referred pain. In addition, axon reflexes from nociceptive neurons are capable of contributing to neurogenic inflammation in tissues that are not involved in the initial injury. The neural basis for the affective (emotional) components of pain and suffering are localized to the frontal lobes, in areas affected by depression and anxiety disorders. This is the physiologic substrate for the common and complex clinical interaction between pain and mood.

References

Full references for this chapter can be found on www.expertconsult.com.

Acupuncture

M. Kay Garcia and Joseph S. Chiang

Public interest in complementary and alternative therapies, both for the maintenance of wellness and for the treatment of disease, has grown rapidly in the United States in recent years (**Fig. 138.1**).[1-5] In this chapter, traditional Chinese medicine (TCM) is discussed, with a focus on acupuncture for pain control. In the 2007 National Health Interview Survey, approximately 3.1 million Americans said they had used acupuncture in the past year.[6] Unfortunately, the putative mechanisms of acupuncture remain unclear, and the need for quality research for evaluation of integrative clinical practice remains.

Historical Considerations

TCM is a complete system of health care that has been practiced in China for thousands of years. According to the World Health Organization (WHO), TCM is used in treatment of at least 200 million people annually and accounts for nearly 40% of all health care provided in China. The primary disciplines within TCM include acupuncture, herbs, and food therapy; Tui na (Chinese bodywork); Tai chi (therapeutic exercise); and Qi gong (meditative/energy therapy). Acupuncture is among the most popular of these therapies and is used in at least 78 countries worldwide.[7]

In the West, acupuncture therapy has grown more common over the past few decades. In 1971, James Reston, a journalist for the *New York Times,* wrote a front-page article describing how his postoperative pain from an emergency appendectomy performed while he was traveling in Beijing was relieved with acupuncture.[8] Three months later, a group of US physicians visiting hospitals in China observed acupuncture for surgical analgesia and reported their observations in the *Journal of the American Medical Association.*[9] Growing public interest ensued, and in 1972, President Richard Nixon, accompanied by his personal physician, witnessed several surgeries that used acupuncture-assisted anesthesia.[10] The National Institutes of Health (NIH) subsequently sponsored a team of physicians to study the health care system in China.[11]

Before President Nixon's visit to China, little information about acupuncture was available in the United States. Documented evidence, however, shows the use of acupuncture in clinical practice as early as 1826, when Franklin Bache, a Philadelphia physician and grandson to Benjamin Franklin, concluded in a published report that he had found acupuncture to be an effective treatment for pain from rheumatism and neuralgia among prisoners at the Pennsylvania state penitentiary.[12] Sir William Osler also endorsed acupuncture as an effective treatment for lumbago and sciatica in *The Principles and Practice of Medicine,*[13] and interestingly, brief passages on acupuncture appeared in an American Civil War surgeon's manual and in two medical treatises written in 1876 and 1880.[14]

In the late 1970s and early 1980s, researchers showed that acupuncture analgesia was associated with the stimulation of endogenous opioid peptides and biogenic amines through the central nervous system (CNS)[15-20]; although later work has revealed multiple underlying mechanisms, these findings helped give acupuncture scientific credibility in the minds of medical professionals.[21] As a result, clinical training programs in acupuncture techniques and guidelines for education, practice, and regulation have been developed, and

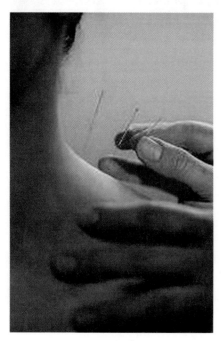

Fig. 138.1 **Example of acupuncture.**

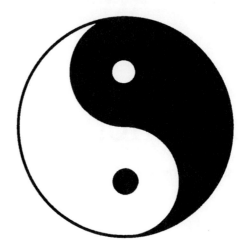

Fig. 138.2 **Yin-yang symbol.**

programs in integrative medicine are beginning to appear in medical schools, nursing schools, and hospitals throughout the United States.

Basic Principles

Acupuncturists use many different models and approaches to understand and apply treatment. These models range from a metaphysical paradigm used by those traditionally trained to a strictly neurophysiologic approach incorporated by physicians who use acupuncture exclusively for pain control. Although the former may seem untenable to the Western scientific community, it is useful in treatment of problems that are not well described by the latter. Acupuncture sometimes has effects on the body that are difficult to explain in purely scientific terms, and a symptom complex that does not easily fit a given set of diagnostic criteria may elucidate a meaningful clinical pattern when analyzed with a different model. In TCM, emphasis is placed on function, not structure. As a result, certain aspects of human physiologic functional relationships are often emphasized that are not directly addressed by Western biomedicine.

Yin-Yang Theory

Although many theoretic foundations underlie the practice of TCM and acupuncture, basic to all approaches is yin-yang theory (**Fig. 138.2**). The constructs within this framework are relatively simple, but yin-yang thinking is substantially different from the classical Aristotelian dogma underlying Western medicine. Within yin-yang conceptualization, qualities may be simultaneously opposite and complementary. Yin always possesses characteristics of yang, and vice versa. So, although opposites, yin and yang also are interdependent, can transform into each other, and can consume each other. Physiology and pathology represent variations along a continuum of health and illness. Thus, a state of

good health is determined by the dynamic balance between opposing yin-yang forces.[22]

In TCM, acupuncture is based on the premise of well-defined patterns of Qi (pronounced "chee") flow throughout the body. The concept of Qi has been discussed by Chinese philosophers throughout time, and the symbol representing Qi in the Chinese language indicates something that is simultaneously material and immaterial. Some authors define Qi as matter + energy, or "mattergy," thus expressing the same continuum of matter and energy explained by modern particle physics.[23]

In ancient Chinese thought, Qi was believed to be a fundamental and vital substance of the universe, with all phenomena produced by its changes. The many types of Qi are classified according to source, function, and distribution. It is considered one of the human body's fundamental substances, helping to maintain normal activities, permeating all parts of the body, and flowing along organized pathways known as acupuncture channels, or meridians. TCM practitioners believe that a balanced flow of Qi throughout the system is necessary for good health and imbalances can be corrected with acupuncture stimulation.[22,23]

Since the late 1950s, numerous studies have been published in the Peoples' Republic of China that hypothesize the underlying mechanisms of action for acupuncture; by the mid 1990s, compelling evidence for a neurohumoral model of acupuncture analgesia could be found in the English literature. More recently, basic scientific research has revealed that bioelectromagnetic and neurohumoral mechanisms are responsible for the effects of acupuncture on various types of health problems. The stimulation of acupuncture points is believed to cause biochemical changes that affect the body's natural healing abilities. The primary mechanisms of these changes include enhanced conduction of bioelectromagnetic signals, activation of opioid systems, and activation of the autonomic and CNS, causing the release of various neurotransmitters and neurohormones.[21]

Neurohumoral Mechanisms of Acupuncture

Awareness that acupuncture analgesia is at least partially mediated through endogenous opioids was first demonstrated in 1976. Shortly after opiate receptors were discovered in the periaqueductal gray matter, the limbic system, and the periventricular gray matter of the CNS, acupuncture analgesia was discovered to have the ability to be reversed by naloxone, a pure antagonist at all known opioid receptors.[24] Acupuncture can change concentrations of serotonin and biogenic amines, including opioid peptides, met-enkephalin, leu-enkephalin, β-endorphin, and dynorphin. These are involved in the activation of descending tracts that inhibit transmission of nociceptive information in the spinal cord and also inhibit ascending tracts transmitting nociceptive information. When large, unmyelinated A-delta fibers that sense touch and pressure are stimulated with an acupuncture needle, impulses from small, unmyelinated C-fibers transmitting ascending nociceptive information are blocked by a gate of inhibitory interneurons in the substantia gelatinosa of the spinal cord, releasing neurotransmitters such as λ-aminobutyric acid and enkephalins and resulting in the inhibition of transmission of pain impulses to the brain. A regional effect is also seen because A-delta fibers transmit cranially and caudally in the dorsolateral funiculus before entering the substantia gelatinosa to stimulate inhibitory interneurons.[25-27]

Functional magnetic resonance imaging (fMRI) studies suggest stimulation of acupuncture points can initiate multiple endogenous pathways of analgesia by the neuromodulation and integration of neurotransmitter and pain control systems at various levels. The release of serotonin, endogenous opioids, and other neurotransmitters leads to an alteration of nociceptive processing and perception, and quantifiable changes in specific areas of the human brain have been observed with fMRI after acupuncture. In patients who experienced *De Qi* sensation (see Channels and Collaterals section), unilateral needling has been shown to activate structures of the descending antinociceptive pathways and cause deactivation of multiple limbic areas subserving pain perception (i.e., activation of the hypothalamus and nucleus accumbens and deactivation of the rostral part of the anterior cingulate cortex, amygdala formation, and hippocampal complex). Superficial tactile stimulation caused a signal increase in the somatosensory cortex but did not cause signal decreases in deeper structures, as was observed with true acupuncture. When combined with fMRI studies in which brain function is localized, observations suggest that stimulation of specific points can initiate multiple endogenous pathways of analgesia through neuromodulation and integration of neurotransmitter and pain control systems at various levels of the CNS.[25,28]

Acupuncture points have also been found to have a higher temperature and a higher metabolic rate and to release more carbon dioxide than surrounding tissues.[29,30] Needle stimulation at an acupuncture point causes erythema and heat to develop, and patients often report a feeling of warmth at the site. Furthermore, unilateral stimulation can cause cutaneous skin temperatures to rise bilaterally. Local vasodilation, decreased sympathetic tone, and increased cholinergic efferent impulses may all contribute to this effect and may play an important role in relief of chronic pain.[31] Vasodilation is also mediated by the physical irritation of the needle and stimulates the release of histamine and other vasodilators.

Although acupuncture has been most widely recognized for pain control, stimulation of certain points can also affect the viscera and immune system, partially through the multifaceted role of opioids. Acupuncture promotes neuroendocrine modulation of the hypothalamus-pituitary axis, which interacts with the immune system to modulate cellular function.[25,32-36] Because opioid receptors are found on neurons and lymphocytes, they provide communication between the CNS and the immune system.

Morphogenetic Singularity Theory

A speculative but compelling theory regarding acupuncture involves developmental biology and suggests the meridian system is related to the bioelectric field in morphogenesis and growth control. According to the morphogenetic singularity theory, acupoints originate from organizing centers in morphogenesis, and channel distribution is not solely determined by nerves, muscles, or blood vessels but is the result of the morphogenesis of both internal and external structures. Although it is compatible with neurohumoral constructs, this theory explains several long-standing puzzles that the neurohumoral model cannot. For example, it helps explain indications for specific acupoints and meridians, such as the Du channel (also called the Governing vessel), whose distributions do not follow any major nerve, lymphatic vessel, or blood vessel.[37]

Clinically Relevant Anatomy

Acupuncture Points

Many studies have described acupuncture point morphology,[25,38-52] relating the so-called acupoints to areas on the skin surface with decreased electrical resistance and increased conductance. Most acupoints are palpable as a surface depression located along the cleavage between muscles. They generally correspond to peripheral, cranial, and spinal nerve endings and are often hypersensitive. According to Bossy and Sambuc,[40] they have a surface area of 1 to 5 mm^2.

In 1979, on the basis of statistical evaluation of a large number of histologic sections from rabbits, cats, mice, and human cadavers, Senelar[41] described acupoint morphology as a lymphatic trunk coupled to a large arteriole accompanied by a satellite vein. This lymph-arteriole-venous system creates a passageway between the skin and deeper tissue and is located in a vertical column of loose connective tissue surrounded by the thick, dense connective tissue of skin.[41] This sleeve of connective tissue, through which neurovascular, lymphatic, and tendinomuscular structures pass, enhances the conduction of bioelectric energy.[25] Approximately 80% of traditional acupuncture points have this morphologic organization (**Fig. 138.3**),[42] which may partially explain the effects of acupuncture in soft tissue disease.

In the 1980s, observations from both conventional light microscopy and electron microscopy confirmed a high concentration of microvesicles and perineural cells situated at the contact zones of sympathetic nerve terminations at the walls of large vessels.[42] Other studies in the 1980s described these thin-walled vascular structures as sinuous, organized in a series of closed loops, and surrounded by a web of unmyelinated cholinergic nerve fibers from the autonomic nervous system. Nerves are located proximal to the vasculature, with additional myelinated nerves woven among the blood and lymph vessels leading to superficial levels of the dermis. The epidermis thins at the acupuncture point and has a corresponding modification of collagen fibers.[43]

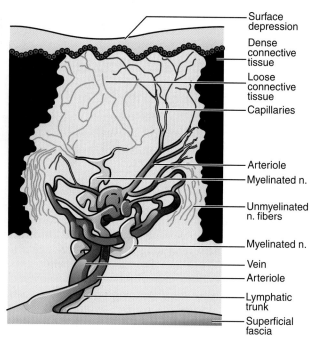

Fig. 138.3 **Acupuncture point diagram.**

Types of Acupuncture Points

Acupuncture points can be categorized in various ways.[25,38] One approach separates points according to their relationship with known neural and tendinomuscular structures. For example, type I acupoints correspond to motor points located where a nerve enters muscle. Maximal muscle contraction with minimal electrical stimulation is achieved at these points. Type II points are located on superficial nerves in the sagittal plane at dorsal and ventral midlines. Type III points are located in areas with a high density of superficial nerves and nerve plexi, and type IV points are found where tendons join muscles.

Several studies have investigated the correlation between acupuncture points and trigger points. In 1977, one group of researchers reported a 71% correlation between trigger points and acupuncture points.[53] Trigger points are hypersensitive regions in muscle tissue that can be palpated as taut bands. They are similar to acupuncture points in that they may lie within areas where referred pain is experienced or be located some distance away. The increased sensitivity of acupuncture points is not fully understood; however, hyperalgesia may arise spontaneously from local irritation or from excitation of somatic or visceral structures distant from the painful point. Stimulation of trigger points can provide long-lasting analgesia similar to that achieved through acupuncture. The high correlation between acupuncture points used to treat pain and myofascial trigger points suggests similar underlying mechanisms for analgesia.[23]

Channels and Collaterals

According to TCM theory, specific pathways known as meridians or channels carry Qi throughout the body. These pathways differ from neurovascular systems as defined by modern anatomy and physiology and comprise an infinite network linking all fundamental substances and organs. The 12 regular channels and 8 extra channels each have divergent branches and numerous divisions known as collaterals.

Channel/meridian theory assumes that blockage or disorder within the system can be identified with a systematic method of differential diagnosis and that treatment strategies can be developed on the basis of restoring orderly flow.[22]

Several attempts have been made to explain acupuncture channels in modern scientific terms, and most, but not all, channels follow the pathways of major nerves, vessels, and fascial cleavage planes.[21] During acupuncture treatment, patients frequently describe a sensation of numbness, aching, heaviness, or warmth along the channel pathway.[54] Many TCM clinicians consider this phenomenon, sometimes called *De Qi* sensation, to be essential for effective therapy and suggest it carries the therapeutic signal to the target area.[21,22,55] After needling of a point on the stomach channel in one study, fluoroscopic imaging revealed peristalsis was different among patients who experienced *De Qi* as compared with those who did not. Furthermore, gastrographs registered decreased frequency and increased amplitude of gastric contractions when the sensation was felt in the abdominal area.[56] Some studies have shown that surgical analgesia is also more effective when *De Qi* is felt.[57]

De Qi sensation has been shown to travel along channel pathways at 1 to 10 cm/sec. This rate varies depending on the subject and the type of needle stimulation but is considerably slower than visceral or somatic nerve conduction.[58,59] *De Qi* appears to be primarily a peripheral phenomenon because it can be blocked by chilling, local anesthetic, and mechanical pressure.[60,61] Some investigators, however, have stated it can travel to phantom limbs, implying participation by the CNS.[62]

Darras and colleagues[63] attempted to identify the network of acupuncture channels and collaterals by comparing the trajectory of a radioactive tracer, technetium-99m, injected into real acupuncture points with the trajectory of the tracer injected into sham points. The tracer was observed with a scintillation camera that revealed that diffusion patterns from the real acupuncture points corresponded to classically described channels, whereas a centrifugal diffusion pattern without linearity was observed at the sham points. Furthermore, radioisotope diffusion moved beyond a tourniquet that blocked surface peripheral blood circulation. Tracer injected into lymphatic vessels showed they also were distinct from acupuncture channels. Because the migration rate of the tracer did not correspond to vascular or lymphatic circulation rates, the authors concluded diffusion did not appear to be via either the vascular or the lymphatic system.

Mussat[64] evaluated the electrical propagation along traditionally defined acupuncture pathways. He concluded acupuncture channels carry a measurable charge, from lower resistance and increased conductance, that is relatively independent from surrounding tissue and that propagation of an electrical current between acupuncture points follows the organization of classical channel theory. He showed that: (1) placement of a barrier needle between needles placed at two points along the same channel can increase the resistance of the channel; (2) electrical current introduced into a channel on the upper extremity can be captured in its corresponding channel on the lower extremity; and (3) current introduced into one channel can be captured in the internally-externally related channel (as defined by TCM theory) of the same extremity after a 5-minute latent period.[64]

The following labels appear on the diagram:
- Surface depression
- Dense connective tissue
- Loose connective tissue
- Capillaries
- Arteriole
- Myelinated n.
- Unmyelinated n. fibers
- Myelinated n.
- Vein
- Arteriole
- Lymphatic trunk
- Superficial fascia

Ancient Chinese scholars were unable to identify electroionic migration patterns or discuss electron flow between needles. They were, however, able to recognize patterns and qualities of response and subjectively quantify the distribution and actions of a phenomenon they referred to as Qi. Although no single discipline can definably illustrate the presence or absence of acupuncture channels and collaterals according to classical theory, combined evidence from many different approaches can provide a basic scientific explanation for ancient Chinese conceptualizations.

In brief, the mechanical act of needling an acupuncture point stimulates a bioelectric response, initiating polarization and ionizing tissues along preferential pathways, in part because of the piezoelectrical characteristics of collagen (i.e., the property of a material that results in polarization when subjected to mechanical strain and a change in conformation when subjected to an electric field).[65] Addition of an electrical stimulus (i.e., electroacupuncture) causes further morphologic changes and alterations in the alignment of collagen fibers.[25] Increased conductance along the meridian system is further supported by a high density of gap junctions at the epithelia of acupuncture points. Gap junctions facilitate intercellular communication and increase electric conductivity through hexagonal protein complexes that form channels between adjacent cells.[66,67]

The exploration of bioelectromagnetic phenomena in living systems is an emerging area of study, and speculative theories have been proposed regarding the manipulation of the body's endogenous electromagnetic fields through acupuncture. As research in this area continues, a more comprehensive and dynamic explanation of the effects of acupuncture on physiologic functional relationships will become apparent.

Technique

Electroacupuncture

The most common acupuncture technique for pain control involves the penetration of the skin with thin, solid, metallic needles that are stimulated either manually or electrically. Electroacupuncture involves the passage of electrical energy through acupuncture points with attachment of battery-operated electronic devices to the needles. This technique allows for more accurate and uniformly regulated stimulation than can be achieved with manual stimulation of the needles alone.[68]

According to Han,[19,20,69,70] specific frequencies of electrical stimulation induce the gene expression of specific neuropeptides in the CNS. A frequency of 2 Hz induces the gene expression of endorphins in the diencephalons, which act on anxiolytic mu receptors. A frequency of 2 to 15 Hz causes the release of β-endorphin and met-enkephalin in the brain and dynorphin in the spinal cord and is more effective in relief of deep and chronic pain than is higher frequency stimulation (100 Hz), which causes the release of dynorphin alone. In the periaqueductal gray matter, the effects of acupuncture may be predominantly mediated by the enkephalins and β-endorphin. In the spinal cord, effects are predominantly from enkephalins and dynorphin.[69-72] A synergistic effect from these three types of opioids is likely to occur in response to simultaneous stimulation from acupuncture as they bind to their respective receptors.[25] Furthermore, combined or alternating low-frequency and high-frequency electrical stimulation may facilitate synaptic remodeling to pre–pain-activated microanatomy.

Although some authors state the frequency of stimulation may be of greater importance than classical rules for needle placement,[72] pain relief achieved through acupuncture treatment cannot be explained by this mechanism alone because the analgesic effect is much longer than the half-life of endorphins.

Auricular Acupuncture

Auricular acupuncture is a commonly practiced technique that involves the stimulation of specific points on the ear. Although it has long been used in China for a variety of conditions, auricular diagnosis and treatment has become a unique branch of TCM throughout other parts of the world since the late 1980s. When internal disorders occur, changes such as tenderness, decreased cutaneous electrical resistance, morphologic changes, or discoloration may appear at specific ear points.[73]

In France in the early 1950s, Paul Nogier[74-76] systematically mapped the auricular/body correspondences. His teachings spread from France to Germany, Japan, and finally, to China, where his charts were screened, verified, and refined in clinical practice. In 1960, Xu Zuolin, a physician at the Beijing Pingan hospital, published a paper that summarized the application of auricular therapy for 255 cases; and in 1970, the *Hanging Wall Chart of Acupoints*, published by the Peoples' Liberation Army (PLA) hospital in Gang Zhou, illustrated 107 auricular acupoints. Since that time, the number used in clinical practice has expanded to include points on both anterior and posterior portions of the ear.[77]

More recently, authors have discussed auriculotherapy as a reflex somatotropic microsystem.[78] Many such systems have been described in the human body and range from the very simple to the quite complex. In TCM, three primary somatotropic microsystems involve the tongue, radial pulse, and ear. The first two are used for diagnostic purposes only. Theorists have speculated that reflex somatotropic systems behave as bioholographic phenomena, with each cell containing information about the whole organism. This view reflects ancient Chinese beliefs that man is a microcosm expressing harmony of a natural order within the overall universe.[22]

In his text, *Acupuncture Energetics: A Clinical Approach for Physicians*, Helms[79] states afferent excitation arriving at a modulating center in the brain may trigger efferent impulses that change the sensitivity of the skin on surface reflex zones.[21] This may involve the reticular formation in the brainstem, which functions as a modulating intersection that activates and inhibits cranial, spinal, somatic, visceral, and autonomic neurologic impulses. This reticular unit may respond to input by patterning topographic regions of the body and subsequently activating the thalamic reticular formation involved in pain modulation, influencing somatic motor and sensory functions, and regulating viscera through the autonomic nervous system.[21]

Scalp Acupuncture

Although ancient Chinese clinicians needled acupuncture points on the scalp, Shunfa[80] first described treatment of various diseases with use of a systematic approach to scalp acupuncture in the early 1970s. Like auriculotherapy, scalp acupuncture is considered to be a microreflex system that involves needling areas directly above corresponding nerve centers.[21] It has been used to treat problems such as chronic headaches, facial paralysis, cerebrovascular disease, enuresis, vertigo, cerebral palsy, and epilepsy.[80] To date, few controlled studies evaluating the use of scalp acupuncture have been conducted in the United States.

Concomitant Therapies

In China and many parts of the world, other therapies are used as adjuncts to acupuncture. These therapies include moxibustion, cupping, gua sha or scraping, Tui na, Qi gong, Tai chi, and herbal and food therapy. The same diagnostic paradigm and treatment strategies used for acupuncture are used to develop a treatment plan with these techniques.

Moxibustion

Moxibustion (moxa) is an ancient technique that uses heat from burning preparations of the herb *Artemisia vulgaris* (mugwort) to stimulate the circulation and strengthen the immune system.[73] Moxa can be applied with a variety of direct and indirect methods. Direct moxa, which is less commonly used, involves placement of a moxa cone directly on the skin at specified acupuncture points and allowing it to burn to completion. Blistering and scarring occur at the site. A nonscarring method is also used in which the moxa cone is removed and replaced with a new one before burning to completion. With indirect moxa, the cone is insulated from the skin with slices of ginger, garlic, or salt. The type of insulating material chosen depends on the specific indication. Also with indirect moxa, the cones may be placed directly on the acupuncture needles. Finally, the indirect method may be applied with a cigar-like stick of tightly rolled moxa held near the skin at acupuncture sites. Patients are instructed to indicate when they feel warmth, and individual acupoints may be heated or groups of points warmed in succession along the channel.[73] A few studies from China and Japan have evaluated the effects of moxa on the immune system, with one reporting moxa smoke induces cytotoxicity with its pro-oxidant action[81–84]; however, its use for pain control has not been systematically evaluated.

Cupping and Scraping (Gua Sha)

Cupping is another treatment often combined with acupuncture therapy for pain control. In this technique, the inside of a small jar or cup is heated to create negative pressure. The cup is then attached to the surface of the skin with the vacuum created by the heat. In ancient times, bamboo jars were used; today, glass or plastic cups are most common. The cups may be left in place for 5 to 10 minutes or may be continuously applied and removed along the meridian pathway. Experienced clinicians may also be able to carefully slide the cup along the chosen meridian. The cups are removed with placement of a finger at its edge on the skin to release the vacuum. After removal, the area is massaged lightly for patient comfort and to further stimulate circulation. The suction from the cups may leave a painless mark on the skin,[73] and informed consent should be obtained before use of this adjunctive therapy. Although it has not been systematically evaluated, cupping is frequently combined with acupuncture to treat various pain syndromes, including myofascial pain and fibromyalgia.[21,73]

Another therapeutic approach used by TCM clinicians is scraping or gua sha. In gua sha, some form of oil or lubricant is placed on the skin, followed by scraping with a smooth-edged instrument such as a coin or porcelain spoon. Again, this is done to stimulate circulation to specific areas and is used to treat chronic pain. The procedure is somewhat uncomfortable, and a mark or bruise is left on the skin surface for 3 to 5 days. Reports have been seen in the literature of marks left from this procedure being mistaken for abuse. Physicians should be aware that it is a common practice in Asian culture and can be recognized by the pattern of the mark. Although no published randomized trials have evaluated the use of gua sha for pain, considerable anecdotal evidence shows that it mobilizes stagnant blood and body fluid, thereby relieving pain.[21] It should not be used in areas where tissue is fragile or near skin lesions of any type.

Tui Na

Tui na (Chinese bodywork) is based on the theory of meridians and collaterals and is a special form of massage that uses techniques specific to Chinese medicine. It involves stimulation of areas along specific pathways and is considered a major area of specialty within TCM.[85] In the United States, examination and certification in Chinese bodywork is provided through the National Certification Commission for Acupuncture and Oriental Medicine.[86]

Qi Gong and Tai Chi

Few randomized controlled trials evaluating the use of Qi gong or Tai chi for pain control have been published to date. The three key purposes of these exercises are to physically relax the body, to focus the mind, and to control the breath. Anecdotally, many patients have reported using these simple, behaviorally based techniques for painful conditions with good results, and further investigation is most definitely warranted.

Herbal and Food Therapy

TCM practitioners often combine acupuncture with the use of herbal or food therapy. A discussion of the topics of herbs or therapeutic dietary guidelines is not the purpose of this chapter, but the same diagnostic paradigm and treatment strategies used in acupuncture therapy are used to select herbal supplements and foods intended to correct imbalances that cause illness or pain. Many Chinese herbs have analgesic properties,[87] and further research is greatly needed to understand mechanisms and interactions.

In TCM, single herbs are rarely given. Rather, formulas that contain many plant, mineral, or animal substances are given in pill, tincture, powder, or loose herb form. Loose herbs are decocted into teas and taken in divided doses over a 24-hour period.[87] Because of the vast interest in and use of herbal supplements by the public, and especially by patients with pain, research to explore herb-drug interactions must be conducted and physicians must familiarize themselves with this growing area. Because patients are often reluctant to discuss the use of herbal supplements with their doctors, asking of questions in an open-ended, nonjudgmental way during history taking is imperative.

Outcomes

People use acupuncture to treat various types of pain, and although hundreds of clinical trials have been conducted since the 1970s, many have been poorly designed. Even today, few studies have evaluated acupuncture as it is applied in actual clinical practice.

According to the National Center for Complementary and Alternative Medicine (NCCAM),[88] acupuncture is most commonly used for back pain, followed by joint pain, neck pain, and headache. Although the evidence is good for certain types of low-back pain[89,90] and osteoarthritis of the knee,[91–94] for most other conditions, additional research is needed. Nevertheless, evidence of efficacy has reached a sufficient critical mass to draw conclusions in some areas.

A number of meta-analyses and systematic reviews[89,90,95–103] evaluating acupuncture for pain control have been published. One recent systematic review[104] of pooled data from meta-analyses found that acupuncture is more effective than placebo for commonly occurring chronic pain conditions. According to this review, for short-term outcomes, acupuncture was significantly superior to sham for back pain, knee pain, and headache. For longer term outcomes (i.e., 6 to 12 months), it was significantly more effective for knee pain and tension-type headache, but results were inconsistent for back pain. The authors suggest that now is the time to shift research priorities away from placebo-related questions toward more practical questions such as clinical significance and cost effectiveness.

Although most authors agree that methodologic rigor has been weak and further research with stronger study designs is needed, properly performed acupuncture seems to be a safe procedure and an important adjunct in the treatment of various pain-related conditions.

Acupuncture for Cancer Pain

Several studies have evaluated acupuncture for cancer pain. A randomized, blinded, controlled trial conducted in France investigated the use of auricular acupuncture for cancer pain. Ninety patients were randomly divided into three groups: one group received two courses of auricular acupuncture, one received acupuncture at placebo auricular points, and one group received auricular seeds at placebo points. Efficacy was based on a decrease in pain intensity 2 months after randomization with use of the Visual Analog Scale. At 2 months, pain intensity decreased by 36% from baseline among the treatment group versus 2% among patients in the two placebo groups ($P < .0001$).[105] A nonrandomized preliminary study of 20 subjects conducted by the same authors also revealed a significant decrease in pain intensity after auricular acupuncture. All patients had a chronic pain syndrome related to their cancer diagnosis. The authors reported improvement was not limited to a reduction in pain because some patients stated they felt better in general and wanted to interrupt analgesic treatment.[106]

Issues in Acupuncture Research

Identification of research methodologies that are scientifically sound yet sensitive to the TCM paradigm is difficult. Often, we find ourselves guilty of comparing the proverbial apples with oranges, and in many instances, application of an Eastern treatment to a Western diagnosis may be inappropriate without first understanding the relationships between Eastern and Western diagnoses. Although the fact that TCM has been used as a primary source of health care by millions of people for thousands of years provides some degree of pragmatic validity, if it is to be integrated into a Western model of health care, the two systems must merge so that the strengths of one overcome the weaknesses of the other.

Determination of an adequate study design and optimal treatment plan is extremely complex, and a number of factors must be considered beyond symptomatology and patient characteristics. For example, the specific points selected and number of points used, type of needle, depth of needle insertion, method of stimulation, duration of treatment, and number and frequency of sessions may all affect outcome. Seemingly, the art and science of practice are both important aspects of care, but this poses many problems from a researcher's perspective. Although the specific question under study determines the choice of controls, the use of sham points; penetrating sham procedures; nonpenetrating methods, such as mock transcutaneous electrical nerve stimulation (TENS) or inactivated laser to either real or sham point locations; and blinding of patients, assessors, investigators, analysts, and acupuncturists are all important considerations for ensuring the validity of findings and avoiding the misinterpretation of results, either false-positive or false-negative. Recommendations for optimizing treatments and controls have been developed,[107] but debate in this area continues.

Complications and Pitfalls

Safety and Adverse Events

In the United States, the manufacture and use of acupuncture needles is regulated by the Food and Drug Administration, and compliance with Good Manufacturing Practices and single-use standards of sterility is required. Guidelines and standards for the clean and safe clinical practice of acupuncture have been established by the National Acupuncture Foundation. This nationally accepted protocol reflects Occupational Safety and Health Administration requirements, and successful completion of a certification examination in clean-needle technique is required by most states before licensure to practice is granted.[108]

When compared with other treatments, acupuncture is considered to be relatively safe. Several publications have investigated the safety of acupuncture treatment.[109–113] One prospective survey following 34,000 consultations with professional acupuncturists (members of the British Acupuncture Council) reported no serious adverse events; serious adverse events were defined as events that necessitated hospital admission, prolonged hospital stays, permanently disabled, or resulted in death (95% confidence interval [CI], 0 to 1.1 per 10,000 treatments). Only 43 significant minor adverse events were reported (1.3 per 1000 treatments; 95% CI, 0.9 to 1.7), including severe nausea, fainting, aggravation of symptoms, pain, bruising, and psychologic and emotional reactions.[109]

Another large-scale project investigated all firsthand case reports of complications and adverse effects of acupuncture identified in the English language between 1965 and 1999. In the 35-year period, only 202 incidents were identified in reports from 22 countries. Complications from acupuncture included infections (primarily hepatitis) and organ, tissue, and nerve injury. Other minor adverse effects included cutaneous disorders, hypotension, fainting, and vomiting. Fewer adverse events have been reported since 1988 because of improvements in clinical practice, standardization of clean-needle techniques, and better training of practitioners.[110] A recent multicenter survey conducted in Norway reported that, like any treatment intervention, acupuncture has adverse effects but is safe when performed according to established guidelines.[111]

Most serious adverse events associated with acupuncture treatment occur as a result of improper needle placement from inadequate training of personnel, failure to use single-use disposable needles, or poor technique when cleaning the area before needling. In other words, most adverse events from acupuncture are from a lack of education or negligence on the part of the practitioner and are not from the treatment itself. The side effects reported when acupuncture is performed correctly by properly trained personnel are relatively minor and most commonly include fainting, nausea, vomiting, bruising, and mild pain.[109–112] For patients at higher risk (i.e., those with valvular heart disease or neutropenia), semipermanent needles should not be used because of the risk of infection.[113] Finally, electroacupuncture should not be used in patients with cardiac pacemakers or other electronic devices and should be used with caution in patients with metal implants.

Provider Credentialing

Selection of a qualified practitioner is an important decision, and guidelines have been recommended by the National Institutes of Health/NCCAM.[114] Specific requirements for credentialing of acupuncturists vary from state to state, but training programs in the United States have a standardized, clinically based curriculum and are formally accredited by the Accreditation Commission for Acupuncture and Oriental Medicine.[115] In addition, a non-profit organization, the National Certification Commission for Acupuncture and Oriental Medicine (NCCAOM), was established in 1982 to promote nationally recognized standards of competence and safety. The primary mission of NCCAOM is to protect the public interest in quality care by examining and certifying competence in the practice of acupuncture, Chinese herbology, and Asian bodywork (Tui na) through national board examinations. The first comprehensive written examination administered by NCCAOM for acupuncture was given in March 1985. Beginning in 2004, testing for competency in basic principles of biomedicine was added. Most states now require successful completion of the NCCAOM board examination for licensure to practice acupuncture.[86]

Conclusion

With an explosion of interest in complementary therapies such as acupuncture in recent years,[1–6] an understanding of their potential use in pain control is important. Acupuncture practitioners use many different approaches for diagnosing and treating patients, ranging from the purely metaphysical to the strictly neurophysiologic. Although integrating ancient concepts into a health care delivery system relying solely on modern scientific methods is difficult, it is an endeavor worthy of exploration, as certain aspects of human physiologic functional relationships are emphasized in TCM that are often not directly addressed by Western biomedicine. Thus, integration of therapies that have been shown to be empirically effective, such as acupuncture, into mainstream health care in a well-regulated environment could lead to a dramatic medical paradigm shift, benefiting the general health of the public.[116]

When properly performed, acupuncture is considered a safe procedure. The most common adverse reactions are mild pain or discomfort, fainting, nausea, and bruising. Semipermanent needles should not be used in patients with vulnerable neutropenic conditions or in patients with valvular heart disease,[113] and as a precaution, electroacupuncture should be avoided in patients with cardiac pacemakers or other implanted electronic devices.

Several promising studies are beginning to elucidate the mechanisms and efficacy of acupuncture in a variety of areas. As our understanding of how this ancient tradition works improves, our ability to optimize treatment regimens will also improve. As we endeavor to learn more about therapies such as acupuncture, our focus should not be limited to clinical medicine but should also consider the social, cultural, political, and economic contexts in which they are used.

References

Full references for this chapter can be found on www.expertconsult.com.

Prolotherapy

K. Dean Reeves and John Lyftogt

Prolotherapy Definition

Prolotherapy is injection for repair or functional restoration of soft tissue.[1] As seen in **Fig. 139.1**, soft tissue includes ligament, tendon, cartilage, and nerve. Although the term prolotherapy is from the root word *proli*, which means to regenerate (as in offspring), cells often need just restoration of function rather than multiplication. In this chapter, all solutions injected for repair or restoration of soft tissue (dextrose, sodium morrhuate, phenol, platelet rich plasma, and adult stem cells) are considered to be proliferants and their use for repair or functional restoration of soft tissue is considered prolotherapy.

Importance of Growth and Disrepair Factors and Their Balance and Teamwork

Restoration of function in soft tissue is accomplished with alteration of the balance of growth factors (GFs) and disrepair factors (DFs; **Fig. 139.2**). A GF is a complex protein (polypeptide) that changes the function of deoxyribonucleic acid (DNA), often by a change in its shape (conformation), altering genetic expression in a favorable way for its repair. This process is much like a key being placed in a lock that turns on the "engine" of the cell almost instantaneously. These GFs are produced in

our own cells. How GFs work is illustrated in a simple way in **Figs. 139.3** and **139.4**. In Fig. 139.3, the repair genes (marked with a *star)* are "covered up" and not available to transcribe. Fig. 139.4 shows the effect of a simple shift in the DNA shape, commonly used by GFs. This shift exposes the key genes for transcription, thus allowing them to be "active." Because of communication methods from the cell surface to the nuclear material, the shifts in DNA shape (conformation) that allow for cell repair or multiplication are almost instantaneous.

Types of Prolotherapy: Enthesofascial/Intra-Articular, Myofascial, and Neurofascial

Since the first edition of *Pain Management*, the concept of prolotherapy has changed considerably, in part as our understanding of pathology in soft tissue and nociceptive sources has changed. The term prolotherapy currently describes three primary approaches.

Enthesofascial/Intra-Articular Prolotherapy

Enthesofascial (EF)/intra-articular prolotherapy is the classic method of prolotherapy that has been used effectively for many years. The injection location here is onto the bony cortex or into joints. For many years, the purpose of such has been described as healing of entheses of ligament or tendon or improvement in joint health or tightening of loose structures. However, the techniques, as originally described, involved injection of regions rather than just specific spots. For this reason, some have viewed EF techniques as "excessively regional" or "not diagnosis specific." Certainly many injections that use a regional technique do not result in direct or precise injection of areas of ligament and tendon degeneration. However, regional injections infiltrate the broad end fiber territory of many individual nerve fibers that may be dysfunctional in chronic pain. Thus, the profound results on pain and function often seen with the regional approach may be on a neurogenic basis and successful proportionate to the portion of the entire umbrella of nerve endings infiltrated with dextrose or other proliferant. A neurogenic mechanism is evidenced by the rapid, almost instantaneous, improvement that many patients experience. This is far too rapid to be explained by structural repair in degenerate ligament or tendon. The term EF prolotherapy was chosen on the basis of the location of injection as distinct from intermediate depth nonenthesis structures (myofascial prolotherapy) or superficial (neurofascial prolotherapy) structures. EF prolotherapy may use ultrasound or fluoroscopic guidance for joint entry accuracy,[7] for research and treatment purposes,[8] or to target specific structures such as medial meniscus or specific portions of the sacroiliac (SI) ligament.[9] However, solution spread is substantial, rendering radiographic guidance unnecessary for the vast majority of injections. If sedation is used, an increase in the time of sedation with slowing for radiographic guidance is more problematic than helpful.

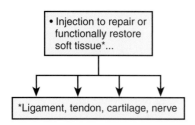

Fig. 139.1 Definition of prolotherapy.

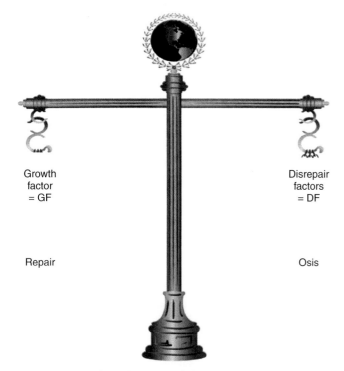

Fig. 139.2 How prolotherapy works.

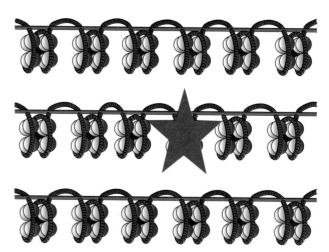

Fig. 139.3 Changing the shape of DNA to change its function: critical genes covered.

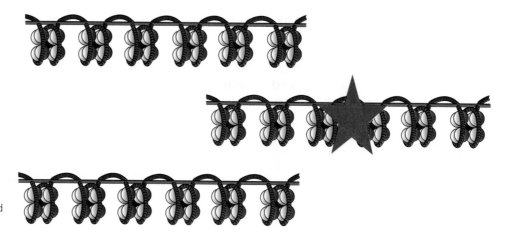

Fig. 139.4 Transcription area uncovered by growth factor effect.

Myofascial Prolotherapy

Myofascial (MF) prolotherapy is injection of specialized soft tissue off the bony cortex, outside of joints, and below the subcutaneous fascia. Targets of injection include musculotendinous degeneration, intrasubstance tendon or muscle tears, fascial defects that prevent muscle function, or other fascial areas invested with neovessels or neonerves. This type of prolotherapy is the most likely to require radiographic guidance for targeting defects. High resolution ultrasound scan (HRUS) is increasingly preferred for such guidance because of soft tissue detail provided and lack of x-ray exposure.

Neurofascial Prolotherapy

The neurofascial (NF) prolotherapy approach involves injection in the vicinity of peripheral sensory nerves and especially their points of fascial penetration where they reach a subcutaneous plane.

Born Out of Clinical Observations

NF prolotherapy began out of clinical observations. Paul Pybus, expanding on observations made by his mentor Roger Wyburn-Mason, noted that patients with chronic pain often had pain on examination over articular and sensory nerves, in particular in areas of fascial penetration. He published a text in 1989 that described a method of treatment with lidocaine injection with or without low dose steroid in which these "points" are injected.[10]

The author John Lyftogt independently noticed fascial penetration area pain with palpation and was introduced to prolotherapy, in the process noting the rapid speed of improvement after dextrose injection in some, suggesting a potential neurogenic mechanism. He then trialed the injection of a combination of dextrose and lidocaine superficially in the areas of fascial penetration as noted with anatomic guides and palpation. Sudden and striking improvement (within seconds) was noted in both pain and functional ability, with benefit that lasted far beyond the expected anesthetic period of action. Treatment at intervals with only superficial injection led to progressive improvement empirically in most patients, even through these patients presumably had a primary source of pain much deeper. Clinical benefit of prolonged nature was noted in a variety of pain conditions; and peer review collections of data, and more recently, formal clinical trials, have been published on treatment with dextrose and lidocaine of peripheral nerves.[11–14]

The definition of prolotherapy as injection for repair or functional restoration of soft tissue is met in that the result of NF prolotherapy appears to be the restoration of full function in small nerves rather than proliferation of new nerves. Although the reparative proteins (growth factors) and their teamwork in nerve repair are less well known, nerves are largely collagen-based with a good deal of overlap in component with ligament and tendon (i.e., perineureum and epineureum). Nerves must participate in repair of soft tissue defects and thus quite likely are designed to respond to a similar array of growth factors, providing rationale for why dextrose is potentially therapeutic to small nerves.

Rationale for Sensory Nerve Vulnerability at Fascial Penetration Sites

Although NF prolotherapy is a treatment founded in clinical practice, its clinical benefit is stimulating an intense search for a full neuroscientific understanding of partial nerve dysfunction. Neuropraxia, alteration of function of a nerve without damage to its axon, can account for behavior of these nerves.[15] The mechanisms by which neuropraxia can occur, and how this relates to chronic pain states, have been detailed extensively in a recent text.[16] Peripheral sensory nerves with their cell bodies (perikarya) in the dorsal root ganglion (DRG) traverse several different tissues and fascial layers before reaching their subcutaneous receptive fields. At fascial penetration points, peripheral sensory nerves are postulated to be vulnerable.

Nerves are suspected to be affected at the fascial penetration point in two major ways.

1. The first is constriction after injury. If the nerve is traumatized, small amounts of swelling occur that travel both directions. This may lead to a strangulation-type effect in an area of constriction as the nerve penetrates a fascial hole/lacunae.[17] Animal research has shown that nerve dysfunction can be created with simple contact of the sciatic nerve in a circumferential fashion (**Fig. 139.5**).[18] Although animal research began with a tie about the sciatic nerve, mere touching of the nerve all about its circumference was soon found to result in disruption of axoplasmic flow in the nerve and a "neuropraxic" state. This results in swelling of the nerve also in both directions and residual effects as seen by an hourglass-like deformity of the nerve after the circumferential contact state is removed (**Fig. 139.6**) that gradually resolves in the absence of further injury. A common clinical example of swelling of a human nerve at a point of constriction is seen in dorsal digital nerves (Morton's neuroma).

2. The second proposed mechanism of nerve dysfunction was proposed by Pybus[10] and is a change in fascial tension with function or repetitive muscle contraction about or under the opening in fascia. As a result, the

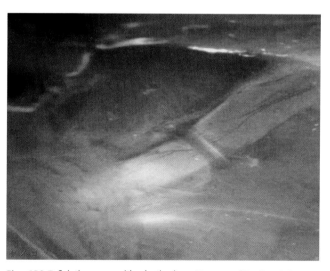

Fig. 139.5 Sciatic nerve with plastic ring. *(Courtesy of Dr Gary J. Bennett, McGill University.)*

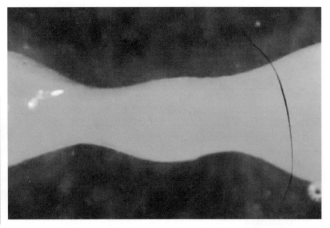

Fig. 139.6 Hourglass deformity tibial nerve after sheath removal. *(Courtesy of Dr Gary J. Bennett, McGill University.)*

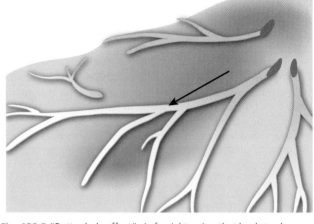

Fig. 139.8 "Buttonhole effect" via fascial tension that leads to closure of lacunae. Proposed neurogenic inflammation/degeneration cycle.

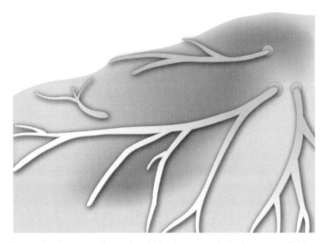

Fig. 139.7 Lacunae through which the supraclavicular nerve divisions exit. Lacunae open.

opening (lacunae) may change from a round shape (**Fig. 139.7**) into a sharp-edged buttonhole configuration (**Fig. 139.8**), which could then compress the relatively soft sensory nerve trunk.

Chronic Constriction Injury as a Site for Neurogenic Inflammation, and Key Inflammatory Proteins That Are Produced by the Nerves

The term chronic constriction injury (CCI) has been introduced to describe the areas at which neuropraxic or injury effects may occur, affecting sensory nerves.[18] The injury response of a sensory nerve has been described as a neurogenic inflammation,[17] whether the injury occurs in the trunk of the nerve from blunt or other trauma or at a point of constriction. The use of the term neurogenic inflammation is based on the findings in animal studies that different parts of the nerve complex of sensory nerves produce inflammatory proteins (peptides) when they are irritated. For example, nervi nervorum produce calcitonin gene-related peptide (CGRP) and substance P, and Schwann cells produce nitric oxide (NO).[19] A simple definition of neurogenic inflammation is the release of neuropeptides from nociceptors.[20] The ability of sensory

nerves in humans to produce degenerative neuropeptides in areas of chronic injury has been shown by Alfredson and Lorentzon.[21] Microdialysis catheter placement in small "new nerves" that develop around areas of patellar tendinosis has found greatly elevated levels of the same neuropeptides found in animal studies, that is, CGRP, substance P, NO, and vascular endothelial growth factor (VEGF).[21] Neurogenic inflammation regularly accompanies excitation of primary afferent nociceptors. It has two major components: plasma extravasation and vasodilation.[20]

Bystander Disease and Its Potential Correction
Bystander Disease: A Key Concept Related to Hilton's Law and the Importance of Stopping Neurogenic Inflammation

Pybus[10] postulated that sensory nerves can cause dystrophic changes when irritated. The production of inflammatory neuropeptides seems to be a plausible explanation for that. But how does superficial production of inflammatory neuropeptides affect distant (deeper) structures? Hilton's law states that "the nerve that supplies sensation to the skin over a joint also supplies sensation to the joint and the muscles that move that joint."[22] Thus, for example, the sensory or mixed motor and sensory nerve trunk that supplies skin sensation over a joint also sends pain fibers to the joint itself. Because neurodegenerative peptides can be transported along the axons of sensory nerves in either direction, degenerative peptides can move antegrade along the nerve to toward the spinal cord but then travel retrograde along the nerve back to a joint supplied by that nerve and have a degenerative effect there from those same neuropeptides. The mechanism of neurogenic inflammation that leads to bystander disease has been extensively detailed by Lundy and Linden.[23] **Fig. 139.9** illustrates a simplified neurogenic inflammation/degeneration cycle. CGRP, substance P, and NO are produced. CGRP is in a positive feedback loop with VEGF, which stimulates neovessel growth. Neovessels themselves can interfere with repair with a space-occupying effect and perhaps other undefined mechanisms. Matrix metalloproteinase levels such as matrix metalloproteinase-1 (MMP1; also known as collagenase) are increased as well, which can produce potent degenerative influences in cartilage,

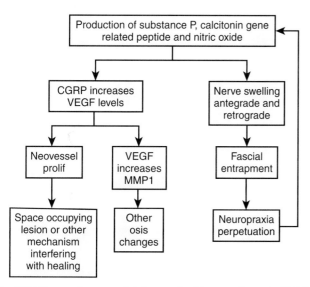

Fig. 139.9 Proposed neurogenic inflammation/degeneration cycle. (CGRP, calcitonin gene-related peptide; MMP1, matrix metalloproteinase-1; VEGF, vascular endothelial growth factor.

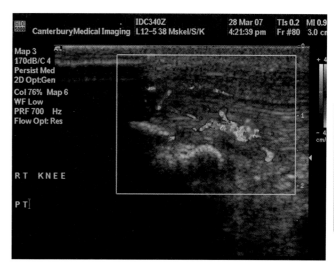

Fig. 139.10 Failed Achilles tendinosis before neurofascial prolotherapy (neovessel view).

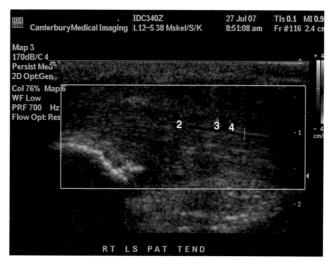

Fig. 139.11 Failed Achilles tendinosis 9 weeks after onset of neurofascial prolotherapy with same neovessel view with same PRF.

ligament, and tendon. CGRP, substance P, and NO are potent vasodilators, and CGRP increases vascular permeability. These influences, among others, lead to edema in soft tissue. The nerve swells antegrade and retrograde until it reaches a fascial penetration point. There the fascial penetration point is proposed to become a site for self-perpetuating neuropraxia.[23] This is a chronic constriction injury.

Although neuropraxia is proposed as the pathologic state present at the CCI location, it is potentially a small step with additional trauma to reach an axonotmesis state of small C fibers, which is viewed as the potential pathologic state in complex regional pain syndrome (CRPS) type I.[24]

Evidence of Ability to Correct Bystander Disease from Neurogenic Inflammation with Prolotherapy

A. MF prolotherapy: Alfredson et al,[21,25–27] who showed the dense presence of neonerves along with neovessels in areas of tendon degeneration, found that resolution of those degenerative changes occurred after injection of polidocanol targeting the areas of neovessel and neonerve density, which were identified as primarily dorsal (deep) to the tendon. Although in initial publications, the mechanism of polidocanol was described as a sclerosant, an effect on neonerves has more recently been proposed by Alfredson (personal communication) as a proliferant rather than a sclerosant effect.

B. NF prolotherapy: Preultrasound and postultrasound scan images are of much interest in NF prolotherapy because reversal of neurogenic inflammation superficially is thought to result in favorable changes in deeper structures. **Figs. 139.10** and **139.11** show preultrasound and postultrasound scan images, in a search for neovessels, in a previously supremely fit individual with chronic patellar tendinosis with failed patellar tendon debridement surgery with drilling of the tendon. The patient was treated with NF prolotherapy targeting the articular nerves about the patella. Although these longitudinal images are only 2 mm in thickness, and thus show only a small slice of the patellar tendon, a total vessel count throughout the tendon was conducted. The before (see Fig. 139.10) and after (see Fig. 139.11) images here are representative of the marked reduction in neovascularity seen over a 9-week period in this patient who experienced complete resolution of symptoms and resumption of unrestricted function. The mechanism of this improvement needs to be worked out. The proposed mechanism is that NF prolotherapy leads to a cessation of degenerative neuropeptides by the superficial sensory nerve. This, in turn, means that less degenerative neuropeptides are transported to deeper areas.

Other Related Concepts
Clinical Presentations Explainable by Neuropraxia

Neuropraxia and bystander disease have several implications. First, the "perpetuating factors" that Travell and

Simons[28] spoke of may include neurodegenerative effects on the muscle/tendon unit. Second is that neuropraxia without axonotmesis of primarily sympathetic sensory nerves provides a potential explanation for many previously poorly explained phenomenon, such as numbness in nonperipheral distributions and with negative electromyographic (EMG) findings, stocking glove–type numbness (with several nerves involved at the same time), burning pain or autonomic manifestations in the absence of dystrophy, and inhibition of muscle power development or reflexes despite good motor nerve continuity.

Relative Advantages and Combinations

Questions applicable to prolotherapy performance are many, including "Can we treat with just one type of prolotherapy and expect to affect all nociceptive sources?" Given the complete resolution of symptoms in many patients treated with EF prolotherapy over the years, and more recently, with NF prolotherapy as a single modality, the answer appears to be a qualified yes. However, the presence of pathology at several levels of the posterior rami or at different branch levels of a peripheral sensory nerve may suggest that the optimum approach is a combination of several levels of prolotherapy. For example, even if neurodegenerative peptide levels can be dropped with neurofascial prolotherapy, resulting in improvement of deeper structure healing, simultaneous treatment of the deeper structures may have advantages.

Table 139.1 summarizes several major differences between the two most common types of prolotherapy (EF and NF).

Enthesofascial/Intra-Articular: The Classic Method of Prolotherapy

EF is typically performed every 4 to 12 weeks. The original intent was described as stimulation of the inflammatory cascade for repair of degenerative change in connective tissue. GF elevations have since been shown to begin at much lower levels of dextrose, and inflammation is not required.

Table 139.1 Comparison of Treatment Advantages		
Type of Prolotherapy	**Rx Frequency**	**Advantages**
Enthesofascial, myofascial	4–12 weeks	Typical improvement in 2 treatments of comprehensive approach More practical for long-distance cases as long as a driver is available if sedation is used
Neurofascial only	Weekly	More comfortable generally than nonsedation enthesofascial or myofascial prolotherapy More exact identification of nociceptive/inhibitory sources Faster More practical for athletes

However, the basic idea was as aggressive repair as possible, and thus, some emphasis, especially in focal conditions such as a rotator cuff tear, is placed on a move to more aggressive proliferant agents as needed. With the advent of NF prolotherapy, the slow response patterns in some conditions are being viewed as resulting from the effects of degenerative neuropeptides more than simply implying a need for a more "powerful" or inflammatory proliferant. In clinical use, the cortical contact and solution spread of the classical method bathe many sensory nerves, with the expectation of calming the nociceptive contributions of nerves and correcting the underlying connective tissue lesions near enthuses directly by solution spread. The emphasis is on completeness, and the most impressive outcomes with the shortest number of treatments have been when complete pain relief is shown at the conclusion of treatment.[29] The opinion of K. Dean Reeves is that complete treatment with classic method is typically powerful enough to result in benefit with two treatments and thus an informed decision about merit of further treatment. This efficacy is particularly important in treatment of a patient from a long distance who cannot stay in the area for a prolonged period. This efficacy per treatment explains how EF prolotherapy technique has grown despite multiple injections at one time, sometimes insufficient pain control during injection because of variability between injectors, a lack of standardization of treatment, difficulty performing fully blinded research, and a nonreimbursed environment. Note that enthesofascial prolotherapy given through skin blebs can be well tolerated in regional treatment as the primary sensation with contact of the enthesis is a deep ache and with injection is a varying degree of pressure depending on volume injected with each aliquot. Tolerance is dependent on the degree of local "wind-up" present. EF prolotherapy has grown also despite a general ignorance of the difference in clinical effect between the effects of chronic inflammation, which is degenerative, and brief inflammation, which is regenerative, and a lack of awareness of methods to initiate the cascade without inflammation.

Myofascial Prolotherapy

There are those who argue convincingly that peritendinous approaches targeting neonerve/neovessel regions result in secondary healing of lesions in connective tissue and that injection directly in the visualized lesion is not necessary.[27] In contrast, there are those who continue to approach lesions intratendinously, and the two approaches may have somewhat different mechanisms of benefit.[30,31] However, defects in fascia can be critical and prevent function of the musculoskeletal system until direct repair. An example of this is shown with ultrasound images in **Figs. 139.12** and **139.13**. These illustrate the case of a female nurse in her mid 40s who was a bike racer. She suffered a wreck with a right lateral elbow contusion and had difficulty with writing and gripping brakes. Four months after the accident, she was pain free but had stopped riding because she could not brake reliably. Fig. 139.12 shows what was seen dynamically with ultrasound scan, specifically that her extensor carpi radialis (ECRL) did not expand normally during contraction. She had normal grip strength but fatigued quickly. She received one treatment with 15% dextrose into the muscle/fascial defect area and was seen 6 weeks later with no residual grip fatigue or braking difficulty. A follow-up ultrasound scan at that point (Fig. 139.13) showed an ECRL that widened normally with muscle contraction. She resumed biking and sustained improvement in a 6-year follow-up period.

MF prolotherapy, whether directed intramuscularly into a fascial repair in this case, peritendinously as per Alfredson and Lorentzon,[21] or intratendinously as per Maxwell and colleagues[30] and Ryan, Wong, and Taunton,[31] may be delivered at intervals similar to classical prolotherapy. This is because part of the intent is to allow a typical healing cycle to take place in the entire spectrum of connective tissue in the region. MF prolotherapy is not covered in detail as a separate section in this chapter, but MF prolotherapy is expected to become more common with the advent of more practically useful and available high-resolution ultrasound imaging and further understanding of mid-depth pathology. Ultimately, its frequency of performance will depend on whether such mid-depth pathology is correctible with prolotherapy at other levels, such as NF.

Neurofascial Prolotherapy

As a stand-alone treatment, this approach has unique advantages. One advantage is the ability of lidocaine to block C-fiber nociceptive sources and muscular inhibition sources within seconds. This allows the examiner to determine the exact CCI location of importance among several possibilities and which combinations act together in more complex regions, such as about the shoulder or knee. This has profound ability to educate both the practitioner and patient that the primary source of pain and impairment of function is extra-articular rather than intra-articular. The importance of this both for research protocols and clinical practice in the future is hard to overemphasize.

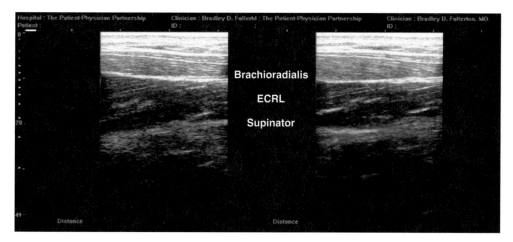

Fig. 139.12 A tear of the extensor carpi radialis longus (ECLR) resulting in a region that does not expand with attempted muscle contraction. *(Courtesy of Brad Fullerton, MD, FAAPM&R, Austin.)*

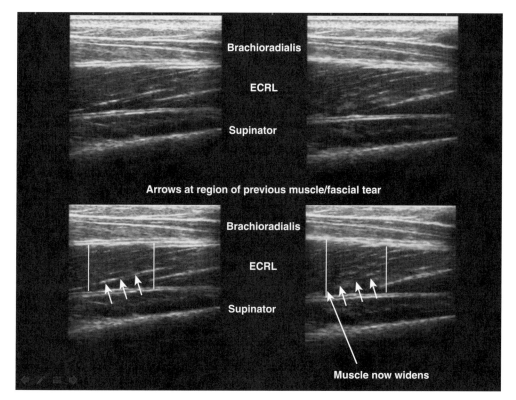

Fig. 139.13 Six weeks after one injection of dextrose 15% into the area of tear. ECLR, extensor carpi radialis longus. *(Courtesy of Bradd Fullerton, MD, FAAPM&R, Austin.)*

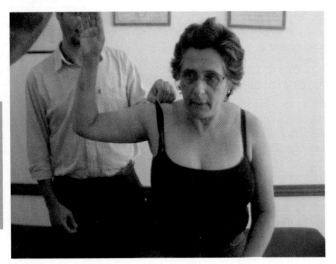

Fig. 139.14 Pain limited active range before neurofascial prolotherapy.

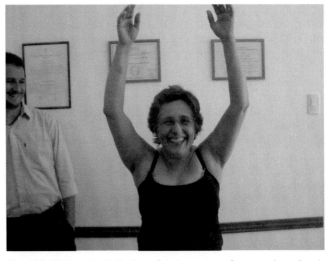

Fig. 139.16 No pain limitation of active range after complete chronic constriction injury infiltration.

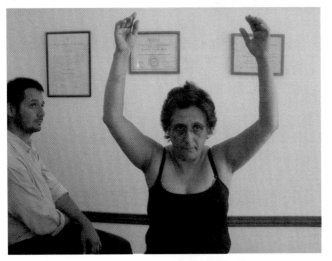

Fig. 139.15 Pain limited active range after partial neurofascial prolotherapy.

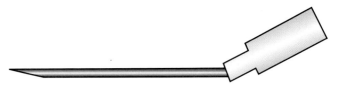

Fig. 139.17 Bevel down needle entry guaranteed with bent needle technique.

An example of how to use NF prolotherapy is shown in **Figs. 139.14, 139.15,** and **139.16.** This nurse was unable to work in nursing any longer because of pain with any loading of the shoulder or any sudden retraction, protraction, or rotational pressure on the shoulder. Despite physical therapy and dextrose proliferant injection into the glenohumeral joint and capsule and cuff, she was unable to actively elevate her arm in abduction beyond 110 degrees, with significant pain beginning at 80 degrees of abduction. Passive elevation was limited to 140 degrees, and those range limits had been present for 18 months. Note that steroid/lidocaine injection into the glenohumeral joint earlier had not reduced her pain with shoulder elevation nor allowed her to actively elevate her shoulder more than 110 degrees.

The sequence of treatment involved palpation and infiltration at the fascial exit points of the supraclavicular nerve divisions and axillary (posterior brachial cutaneous nerve) branches primarily. Subcutaneous injections of 0.5 mL of 0.1 lidocaine/12.5% dextrose were given, and 5 seconds after each injection, the patient was asked to again elevate the arm to indicate changes in function and pain; thus, the entire process can be complete in minutes with knowledge and experience

in locations and priorities of treatment of CCI locations. Fig. 139.14 shows baseline pain-limited range of motion limit for active range. Fig. 139.15, taken after subcutaneous injection of some (but not all) potential CCIs, showed active range now approximating her previous passive-only range limit. The photograph in Fig. 139.16 shows the release of pain and inhibition that is seen after the key CCI locations are infiltrated. This patient had one additional session and returned to her occupation in nursing with no functional limitations or significant pain.

General observations thus far indicate that three treatments are needed in many chronic pain cases to achieve some sustainable benefit and that the treatment frequency when injection is used alone is best performed at 1-week to 2-week intervals.

NF prolotherapy uses even smaller needles than EF prolotherapy and is generally more comfortable. To limit any needle trauma, the sharp point of the needle is best directed upward (bevel downward); one way to do so is to bend the needle as shown in **Fig. 139.17.** The needle is actually quite thin, with a 27-gauge size commonly used.

Precision NF prolotherapy is ideal for the elite athlete because benefits are typically progressive week by week and thus more swift than with EF prolotherapy. However, NF prolotherapy also typically needs more total sessions of treatment than EF prolotherapy, which can be problematic for the traveling patient. **Fig. 139.18** illustrates the most common clinical response rates and patterns seen with NF and EF prolotherapy in patients with pain for months or years. Note that, with a weekly treatment frequency, a fair approximation is an average 10% improvement per week, although the patient with neurofascial treatment may have a plateau for several weeks as activity increases or may not have improvement for several weeks at the beginning of

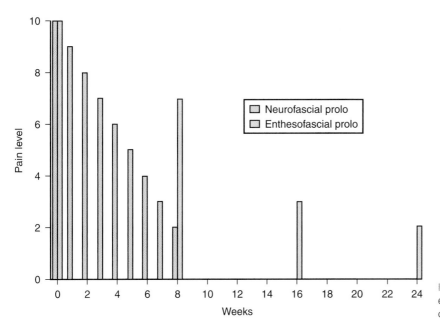

Fig. 139.18 Comparison of typical neurofascial and enthesofascial prolotherapy responses in patients with chronic pain.

treatment. Naturally, this presumes that the patient will be virtually pain free at the conclusion of each session, consistent with a comprehensive identification of CCI locations. In contrast then is the pattern typical for EF/intra-articular prolotherapy, where improvements per session depend on comprehensiveness as well, shown ideally by a pain-free state at the conclusion of the session typically, and the gain per session is more but not over as quick a time period. (In contrast, a pain-free state is not verifiable with EF prolotherapy of extensive nature as postinjection soreness is present as anesthetic effects gradually wear off.) Patients whose conditions fail to respond to NF prolotherapy may be those with deeper pathology that has reached a nonreversible state with treatment of neurogenic factors alone.

Conclusion of Research Section

Thus far, studies show that both superficial (extratendinous) and medium-depth (intratendinous) dextrose injections are effective in Achilles tendinosis,[14] along with objective evidence of neovessel changes and structural reorganization of the tendon.[30,31] The ability of dextrose prolotherapy to tighten loose structures (ACL) has been shown in pilot fashion with machine measurement.[4] Clinically significant improvements in pain and in flexibility in finger arthritis occurred with dextrose injection in a pilot RCT.[6] Golfer's elbow treated consecutively with a single injection of autologous blood showed objective radiographic and subjective clinical improvement.[32] Simple dextrose injection of painful entheses in elite rugby and soccer athletes resolved career-threatening groin pain in more than 90%, with the same speed and success for return to sport as far more expensive surgical interventions.[29,33] RCTs of knee osteoarthritis and low back pain have shown impressive sustainable improvements in functional status and pain with repetitive needling with or without proliferant solution, suggesting a need for noninjection controls in future studies.[5,34–37] Pilot studies in patellar tendinosis have resulted in favorable outcomes with both platelet-rich plasma[38] and polidocanol.[39] Plantar fascia treatment in consecutive patient fashion with ultrasound scan monitoring in a pilot study showed the ability of dextrose injection to alter ultrasound evidence of degeneration and improve clinical status.[40] A small pilot trial that compared dextrose/sodium morrhuate with saline solution in extensor tendinosis at the elbow found dextrose/sodium morrhuate to be clearly better and highly clinically effective.[41] Larger clinical trials and more RCTs are under consideration, but the largely self-funded nature of projects and minimal proprietary components have slowed research in prolotherapy, although acceleration is underway. A model design may be represented by a study pending publication on Osgood-Schlatter disease (Topol, pending), an RCT comparison of dextrose versus lidocaine injection versus an open-label usual care arm. This trial showed a marked advantage of both injection groups in speed for return to full sport over usual care exercise but clear superiority of dextrose over lidocaine in achieving complete remission of symptoms. The key ingredient in design was a usual care comparison group to avoid the usual error of interpretation that comes with a therapeutic effect of needling with lidocaine.

The Foot

The primary CCI of the distal tibial nerve (**Fig. 139.19**) with its plantar nerve and medial calcaneal nerve branches is situated at its neurofascial interface (**Fig. 139.20**) with the flexor retinaculum (distal edge primarily). In the figures, CCIs are identified with blue dots; the cutaneous nerve trunks are shown in red. Bystander disease is most commonly manifested in the plantar fascia. The author has found that a combination of neurofascial treatments and calciol (cholecalciferol) transdermal cream is effective in treatment of foot conditions such as plantar fasciitis (structures underlying medial calcaneal nerve and medial and lateral plantar nerves) and sesamoiditis (branches of medial plantar nerve). The CCI for the cutaneous deep peroneal nerve is shown in **Fig. 139.21** and is a common cause of great toe pain.

The Anterior Lower Leg and Foot

The superficial peroneal nerve (**Fig. 139.22**) is a common cause of neuropathic pain, with its CCI overlying the mid-anterior tibialis muscle. Pain and persistent swelling after

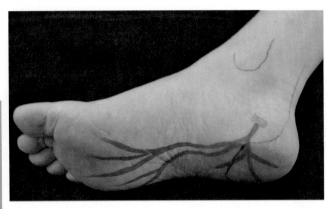

Fig. 139.19 Distal tibial nerve branches and chronic constriction injury.

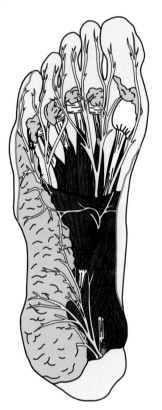

Fig. 139.20 Tibial nerve and plantar fascia. (From Spalteholz W, Spanner R: Posterior femoral cutaneous and superficial cluneal nerve branches: their relationship: 'Handatlas der Anatomy des menschen': part II: Nerven system, ed 16, Amsterdam, 1919, Scheltema & Holkema N.V, p 402.)

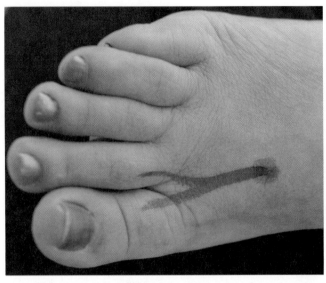

Fig. 139.21 Deep peroneal nerve chronic constriction injury location.

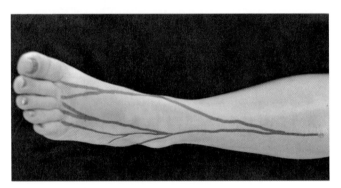

Fig. 139.22 Superficial peroneal nerve distribution.

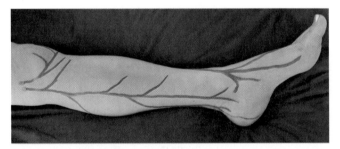

Fig. 139.23 Saphenous nerve branches to knee and lower leg and its chronic constriction injury. (Peroneal distribution is seen over the foot.)

inversion and eversion ankle sprains can be treated with targeting of the CCI and all tender swollen areas along this nerve. Other conditions associated with neuropathy of this nerve are cuboid syndrome and Morton's neuroma. A bystander disease association has been noted via elimination of anterior chronic exertional compartment syndrome (CECS) symptoms with NF prolotherapy of the superficial peroneal nerve.

The Medial Lower Leg and Foot

The main fascial CCI of the saphenous nerve of the lower leg (**Fig. 139.23**) is located medial to the mid patella in knee extension. Other anatomic narrowings are found along the course of the nerve at the level of the posterior branches to the medial gastrocnemius and Achilles tendon. A neuropathy of the gastrocnemius branch may cause "tightness" of the underlying

muscle and even a CECS. A neuropathy of the main trunk and anterior branches may lead to medial shin splints or medial tibial border stress syndrome. A lower anterior branch neuropathy may relate causally with tibial stress fractures of the lower third of the tibia.

A common place for "pinging" or "tearing" of the calf is the Achilles tendon branch where it traverses the musculotendinous junction. Here it is often felt as a cordlike tender "taut" band firmly tethered to the underlying structures. A chronic neuropathy of the Achilles branch may initially lead to "tight calves" followed months or years later by bystander disease like mid Achillodynia on the medial aspect of the tendon.

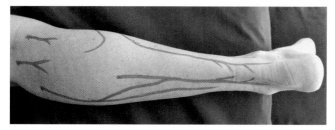

Fig. 139.24 Posterior femoral cutaneous nerve distal chronic constriction injuries to the *left*. Sural cutaneous nerve course in the posteromedial calf with its two CCIs is depicted, as is a portion of the saphenous nerve distribution medially.

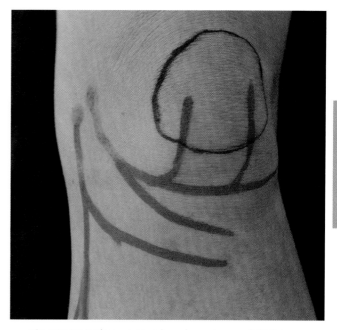

Fig. 139.26 Saphenous nerve branches anteromedial left knee.

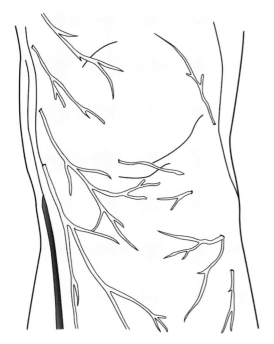

Fig. 139.25 Cutaneous branches right knee. *(Spalteholz W, Spanner R: 'Handatlas der Anatomy des menschen': part II: Nerven system, ed 16, Amsterdam, 1919, Scheltema & Holkema N.V, p 413.)*

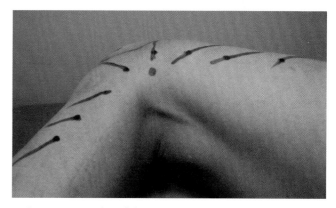

Fig. 139.27 Branches of the peroneal nerve over the lateral left leg.

The lateral aspect of the Achilles tendon is innervated by the sural nerve of the lower leg (**Fig. 139.24**). Note the posterior portion of the saphenous nerve association with the medial aspect of the Achilles tendon. Neuropathy of the lateral sural cutaneous nerve can result in muscle tightness, CECS, muscle pings, cramps, and lateral mid Achillodynia. Treatment consists of NF prolotherapy of the CCIs and tenderness and swelling along the nerves.

The Knee

Sensory innervation of the knee involves branches of the lateral femoral nerve, anterior femoral nerve, saphenous nerve, and common peroneal nerve (**Fig. 139.25**).

Peripatellar pain may arise from any neuropathies that involve the medial aspects of the saphenous patellar branches (**Fig. 139.26**), resulting in medial knee pain, infrapatellar pain, and pes anserine bursitis as bystander disease.

Neuropathy of the common peroneal nerve (**Fig. 139.27**) may lead to iliotibial band (ITB) symptoms and lateral knee pain. The central dot in the figure indicates the access point

for infiltration of the common peroneal nerve, just behind the fibular head and anterior to the biceps femoris tendon, at a depth of 1 cm. The other dots in Fig. 139.27 represent CCIs where the branches emerge through the fascia; these CCI sites are injected superficially.

According to Hilton's law, axon reflexes originating from the cutaneous neuropathies may affect the peripatellar articular nerves (**Fig. 139.28**), resulting in neurogenic inflammation of the joint, with the potential to accelerate degenerative changes.[42]

All of the mentioned conditions have been effectively treated with neurofascial prolotherapy targeting the CCIs and swollen inflamed nerves.

The Posterior Thigh and Gluteal Region

The posterior femoral cutaneous nerve (**Fig. 139.29**) is etiological in many painful conditions. It is often confused with sciatica pain in a straight leg raise (SLR) test, resulting in false-positive SLR results. The main CCI is palpated in the gluteal fold at the midline. Proximal to this CCI are usually two branches that cause inferior buttock pain and restless buttock syndrome. This uncomfortable condition is surprisingly

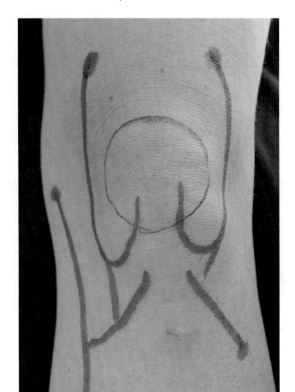

Fig. 139.28 Articular nerves of the left knee.

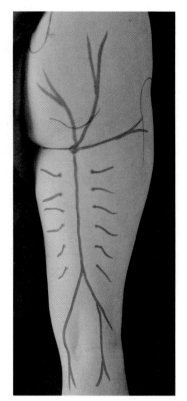

Fig. 139.29 Posterior femoral cutaneous nerve distribution and chronic constriction injury at the gluteal fold and in the thigh.

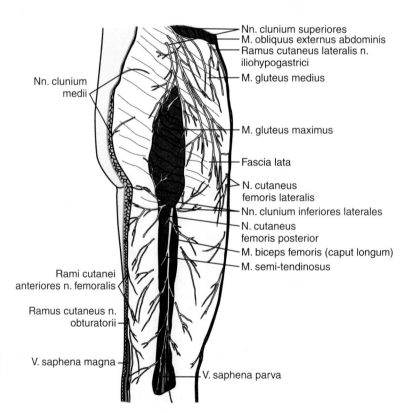

Fig. 139.30 Posterior femoral cutaneous and superficial cluneal nerve branches: their relationship. *(Spalteholz W, Spanner R: 'Handatlas der Anatomy des menschen': part II: Nerven system, ed 16, Amsterdam, 1919, Scheltema & Holkema N.V, p 413.)*

common and prohibits sitting for any length of time in cars, cinemas, lecture theaters, and dining room chairs.

The lateral branch often contributes to posterior hip pain where it networks with the distal branch of the L3 division superior cluneal nerve (**Fig. 139.30**).

The inferior branch of the posterior femoral cutaneous nerve is often traumatized by second-degree and third-degree hamstring tears. If nerve regeneration does not occur, chronic neurogenic inflammation may cause bystander disease in the form of chronic recurrent hamstring injuries and tight

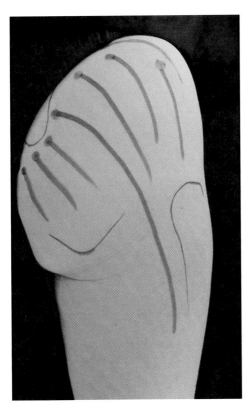

Fig. 139.31 Right superior and middle cluneal nerve chronic constriction injury (CCI) and pathways. Also shown (most lateral) is the cutaneous branch of the iliohypogastric nerve and its CCI.

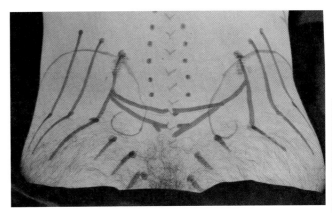

Fig. 139.32 Low back with superior and middle cluneal nerve chronic constriction injuries (CCIs) and location of CCIs for the lumbar dorsal rami.

SUPERIOR CLUNEAL NERVES

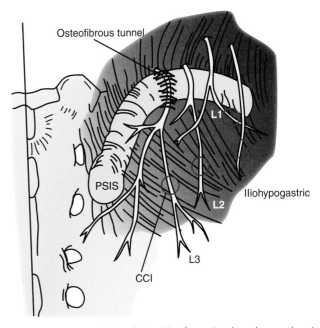

Fig. 139.33 Diagram of the relationship of superior cluneal nerve chronic constriction injuries and the osteofibrous tunnel involving the L3 portion of the superior cluneal nerve.

hamstrings. The distal branches overlie the proximal gastrocnemius tendons and may cause a degenerative tendinopathy locally. The distal CCIs are shown in Fig. 139.24. The author has noted diminution of Baker's cysts along with symptom resolution associated with treatment of these nerves and their CCIs with NF prolotherapy (unpublished).

The three superior cluneal nerves (SCNs; from posterior rami L1, L2, and L3) and middle cluneal nerves (from posterior rami S1, S2, and S3) are critically important in understanding low back pain (LBP) and buttock and hip pain (**Fig. 139.31**). Note how the superior cluneal nerve L3 extends down further and forms a sensory nerve plexus with both the lateral femoral cutaneous nerve and the posterior femoral cutaneous nerve. These branches are illustrated in Fig. 139.41. Chronic neurogenic inflammation here may cause bystander disease manifested as lateral hip stiffness, pain, and trochanteric bursitis. It is not unusual for patients to rate this pain at a VAS of 8 to 9 before treatment.

Fig. 139.32 shows the CCIs for the superior cluneal nerves (L1 to L3 portions) and the middle cluneal nerves (S1 to S3 portions). The upper CCIs shown above the iliac crest are not subcutaneous, as the cluneal nerves are actually coming up from the pelvis to cross the crest at that point. Injection with some indentation with a 1-cm needle appears to be satisfactory as an alternative to insertion to the point of crest contact, which can be 5 cm or more from the skin surface in large individuals. The CCIs for dorsal rami are shown in the figure as a row of blue dots just lateral to the midline. Again, the injections here are not subcutaneous but are with full 1-cm needle depth lateral to midline with medial inclination.

An illustration of the superior cluneal nerve divisions is shown in a different way in **Fig. 139.33**. This figure emphasizes that the L3 (medial) division passes through an osteofibrous tunnel and is particularly susceptible to injury. If a CCI develops distally, retrograde swelling of the nerve causes strangulation of the L3 nerve in the osteofibrous tunnel over the iliac crest and a classical hourglass injury.[43,44] The resultant intraneural pressure in the osteofibrous tunnel may exceed 30 mm Hg and halt anterograde and retrograde axoplasmic transport.[45]

Chronic neurogenic inflammation may result in local SI dysfunction and degeneration. It may also cause stiffness and dysfunction of the erector spinae. Whether this is associated with increased discal pressure with sudden flexion/rotation/side-bending movements and accelerated discal degeneration is unclear, but merits further investigation. The most common cause of acute, severe exacerbations of low back pain may be an intussusception or telescoping neuropraxic injury of the L3 nerve in the osteofibrous tunnel as described by Ochoa et al[46] in an animal model of intussusception injuries of peripheral nerves. With long-standing inflammation and swelling of the L3 nerve, even a trivial flexion movement may trigger an acute demyelination injury necessitating 3 to 4 weeks of repair before the worst pain settles.

Neural prolotherapy targeting all these areas of neurogenic inflammation has been shown to be highly promising.[13]

Anterior Thigh, Hip, and Lower Abdomen

Fig. 139.34 shows an overview of superficial nerves and their common CCIs in the right anterior thigh, hip, and lower abdomen; **Fig. 139.35** shows the main cutaneous branches in more detail with labels.

Injury and neurogenic inflammation of the iliohypogastric nerve is a common finding in hip and low back pain and often prevents patients from sleeping on that side. Simple entrapment of the lateral femoral nerve may cause meralgia paresthetica, but when the nerve is inflamed and entrapped in the tunnel under the inguinal ligament, pain is felt over the whole of the lateral thigh. As mentioned previously, the upper branch of this nerve forms a plexus with the L3 superior cluneal nerve and lateral branch of the posterior femoral nerve. An extensive area of neuropathic pain can be the result, stretching from the hip to the lateral knee. This condition is often experienced by midwives who were trained to place the foot of the patient on their hip during the third stage of labor to facilitate pushing. Current obstetric practice no longer teaches this technique to avoid this known complication of midwife's hip.

Failed regeneration of an injury to the femoral branches of the genitofemoral nerve may result in a mild compartment syndrome of the underlying hip flexors that causes swelling and dysfunction of the iliopsoas muscle group. The author has identified patients with marked weakness in the hip flexors and an absent tendon reflex of the quadriceps, immediately reversible after subcutaneous infiltration of CCIs of the genitofemoral nerve branches. This condition is also not

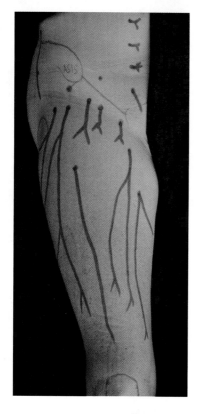

Fig. 139.34 Overview of superficial nerves and chronic constriction injuries in the anterior thigh, hip, and lower abdomen.

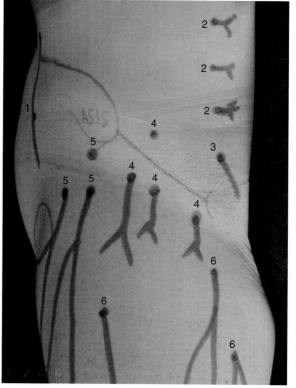

1 = Iliohypogastric nerve

2 = Cutaneous branches of intercostals

3 = Ilioinguinal nerve

4 = Femoral branches of the genitofemoral nerve

5 = Lateral femoral cutaneous nerves

6 = Anterior femoral cutaneous nerves

Fig. 139.35 Main cutaneous branches anterior thigh, hip, and lower abdomen.

uncommon in competitive cyclists, and thus, neuropraxia of the femoral branch of the genitofemoral nerve merits consideration before the common diagnosis of femoral artery obstruction is assigned.

Conditions like osteitis pubis, symphysis pubis, and kicker syndrome in soccer and rugby players are effectively treated with neural prolotherapy targeting the ilioinguinal nerve and

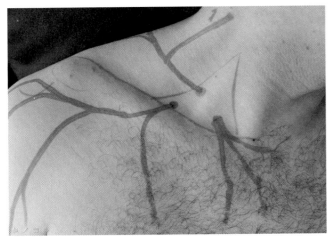

Fig. 139.36 Posterior, intermediate, and medial supraclavicular nerves.

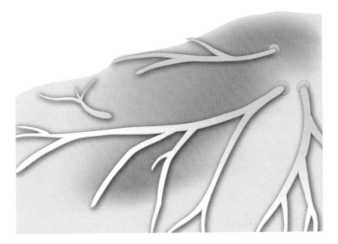

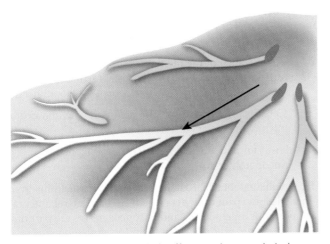

Fig. 139.37 Diagram of buttonhole effects on the supraclavicular nerve branches.

the genital branch of the genitofemoral nerve and any of the other cutaneous groin nerves tender to palpation.

Neuropathic pain caused by the anterior femoral nerves is equally responsive to neural prolotherapy.

Shoulder and Neck Region

The supraclavicular nerve (**Fig. 139.36**) arises from C3 and C4 and divides into three major portions before piercing the cervical fascial and platysmus. The medial supraclavicular nerve heads medially towards the sternoclavicular joint. The intermediate supraclavicular nerve travels laterally toward the acromion/deltoid, and the posterior supraclavicular branch is oriented toward the scapula and upper back with branches that affect the neck.

Buttonhole (neuropraxia) injuries to the supraclavicular nerve (**Fig. 139.37**) can be sudden and severe, as in whiplash injuries, or of slow onset, in either sustained neuropraxia or repetitive insult neuropraxia. The left half of the figure shows the fascia lacunae (openings) for the individual branches; the right half shows the changes in the holes with cervical fascia under tension with potential to create a buttonhole injury to the nerves.

Posterior supraclavicular nerve branches are labeled in **Figs. 139.38** and **139.39**. Neuropraxia that affects branch 1 may lead to neck stiffness in side bending and rotation. It is also a common cause of (tension) headaches. Branch 2 ends near T1 and T2 spinous processes and may result in pain, swelling, and T1–T2 dysfunction. Similarly, branch 3 ends near T3 and T4 spinous processes. A neuropathy of this branch may lead to rhomboid pain and dysfunction.

A neuropathy of branch 4 or 5 is common in hairdressers and typists, with secondary development of a CECS with

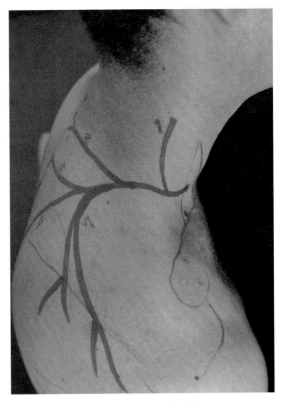

Fig. 139.38 Posterior supraclavicular nerve.

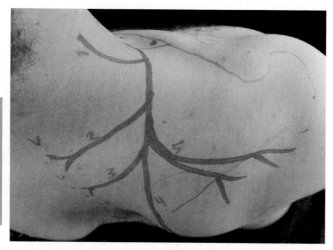

Fig. 139.39 Posterior supraclavicular nerve: a bird's eye view.

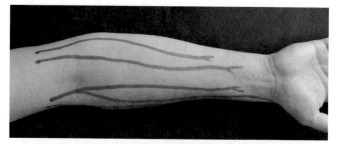

Fig. 139.41 Ventral aspect right forearm.

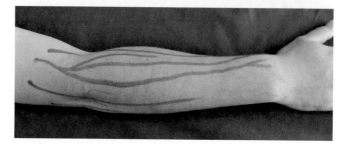

Fig. 139.42 Dorsal aspect right forearm.

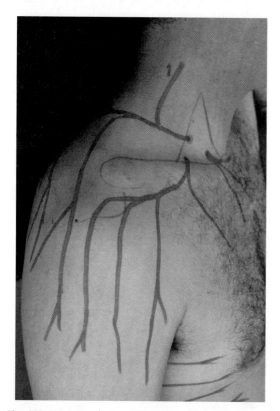

Fig. 139.40 Intermediate and anterior supraclavicular nerves.

"rock-hard trapezius and hard tender knots in the muscle. Not infrequently, thickening and hardening of these nerves may result in painful clicking of the nerves riding over the scapular spine.

A neuropathy of the intermediate supraclavicular nerve (**Fig. 139.40**) may lead to acromial pain and AC joint dysfunction. The three anterolateral branches travel distally in between the muscle bellies of the deltoid muscle. Chronic neurogenic inflammation of these nerves may result in bystander disease in the form of tendinosis of the underlying rotator cuff. In addition, alteration of sensory motor signaling as a result of neurogenic inflammation may contribute to impingement symptoms. NF prolotherapy has been

noted by this author to often completely eliminate positive O'Brien test results, supporting the view that impingement can be the result of altered rotator cuff sensorimotor function.[47] A neuropathy of the anterior branch of the intermediate supraclavicular nerve may also result in pectoralis pain and dysfunction.

The medial branch of the supraclavicular nerve reaches over the sternoclavicular joint and as far as the second costochondral joint (see Fig. 139.40). Sternoclavicular joint trauma may be slow to heal when this nerve remains chronically inflamed, with associated swelling and pain. NF prolotherapy appears to be an effective alternative before consideration of more aggressive options. The author has also observed resolution of classical presentation of Tietze's syndrome via treatment of the medial branch of the supraclavicular nerve with NF prolotherapy.

Elbow Region

Figs. 139.41 and **139.42** depict the five primary forearm sensory nerves. Fig. 139.54 shows the respective CCIs and cutaneous nerves that run down the palmar forearm; from medial to lateral, they are the:

1. Ulnar branch of the medial antebrachial nerve
2. Anterior branch of the medial antebrachial nerve
3. Lateral antebrachial nerve (from musculocutanous nerve)

Fig. 139.55 shows the dorsal forearm and also shows the lateral antebrachial cutaneous nerve and the:

4. Posterior antebrachial nerve (from radial nerve)
5. Anconeus nerve

The medial antebrachial cutaneous nerves are usually involved in medial elbow pain or golfers elbow, and the lateral antebrachial, posterior antebrachial, and anconeus nerves are part of a lateral elbow pain syndrome that includes tennis elbow.

Many other conditions are the result of a peripheral neuropathy of one or more of these cutaneous nerves. The author

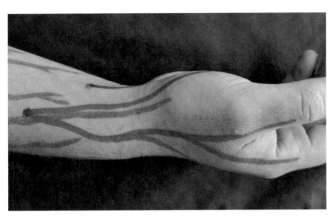

Fig. 139.43 Radial aspect right wrist.

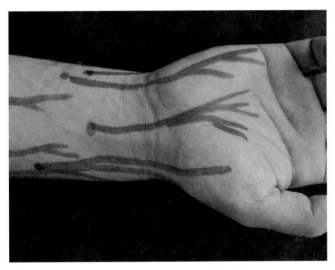

Fig. 139.44 Palmer aspect right wrist.

has successfully treated CECS of the ventral compartment in rowers, polyneuropathy of the ulnar and anterior branch from an incorrect technique on the pommel horse, and polyneuropathy from motocross racing via NF prolotherapy treatment of forearm nerves. Various degrees of severity of CECS of the flexor and extensor compartments are also an integral part of many occupational overuse syndromes or repetitive strain injuries. Focal or task-specific dystonia may also have the same underlying pathology: peripheral mononeuropathy or polyneuropathy.

Neurogenic inflammation effects are particularly pronounced in the common extensor compartment and are seen as intratendinous edema with cleavage tears, "boggy" tendons, neovascularization, or collagenolysis. The effect of MMP1 upregulation of CGRP is in a positive feedback loop with VEGF leading to neovascularization. VEGF in turn upregulates MMP1, resulting in collagenolysis.

Wrist Region

In **Figs. 139.43** and **139.44**, three cutaneous nerves of the wrist are outlined: the palmar branch of the ulnar nerve (two CCIs shown), the palmar branch of the median nerve, and the superficial branch of the radial nerve.

Neuropraxic injuries to these nerves are common occurrences of daily life. Failure of regeneration after injury may lead to peripheral neuropathies and their complications; "pins and needles" sensations, numbness, pain, and heat sensations are recognized sensory symptoms in the region. Zanette et al[48] noted proximal painful regions in more than 50% of patients with carpal tunnel syndrome. The author has identified neuropathies of these three nerves in a number of patients with carpal tunnel syndrome. Application of NF prolotherapy, along with concurrent application of calciol (cholecalciferol) transdermal cream, has empirically resolved the signs and symptoms of carpal tunnel syndrome. It is tempting to speculate that dumping of CGRP, substance P, and NO may lead to swelling and degenerative changes of the underlying carpal ligament, resulting in an encroachment of the space for the medial nerve.

Other clinical experiences have included several patients with Dupuytren's contractures, who claim that softening and easing of their contractures occurs with regular applications of calciol cream to the palmar branch of the medial nerve distribution. In addition, pain along the course of the superficial branch of the radial nerve is common and readily responds to neurofascial prolotherapy.

The definition of prolotherapy as injection to stimulate inflammation to promote healing is unacceptable, given advancement in our knowledge of the process of healing in soft tissue. In fact, the newest arm of prolotherapy, neurofascial, is intended to decrease, not stimulate, neurogenic inflammation. Neurogenic inflammation is defined simply as the release of neuropeptides from nociceptors. Neurofascial prolotherapy is aimed at eliminating degenerative neuropeptide (substance P, CGRP, and NO) release, in turn allowing healing to take place. For this reason, the definition of prolotherapy as injection to repair or functionally restore soft tissue is recommended (either through repair factor elevation or disrepair factor diminution).

Conclusion

This chapter introduced three forms of prolotherapy based on depth of injection. NF prolotherapy was emphasized because of the importance of providing rationale for, and a simple anatomic introduction to, key CCI locations and how to infiltrate them to quickly determine nociceptive sources and eliminate inhibition. Vitamin D cream use was introduced as a useful adjunct to NF and perhaps other prolotherapy types. MF prolotherapy was described as critically important in some cases and more radiographically dependent. EF prolotherapy was presented as a method where both nerve and connective tissue nociceptors are broadly and safely infiltrated in a comprehensive manner for a definite effect in two treatments. The importance of anatomic localization of deeper nociceptors was minimized in part because of the need for brevity but also because the benefits of broad infiltration for the neurologic effect of EF prolotherapy are considerable. Differences in opinion on whether lesions in ligament and tendon need to be directly injected or not were discussed. This will be the subject of much attention in the future.

Research in prolotherapy is considerable, but key factors have led to challenges in building a body of literature, such as:

1. Injections that were incorrectly considered control treatments and instead were active interventions.
2. The general pattern of lack of a usual treatment control to expose the importance of the injection "control" as an active treatment.

3. Two influential but grossly maldesigned studies (one in back pain and one for Achilles tendon treatment) with negative outcomes.
4. The large number of conditions amenable to prolotherapy treatment that have led to a limitation of concentration of studies.
5. Lack of proprietary help for funding studies on the most cost effective options.
6. Ignorance of the basic science literature about the actual pathology in soft tissue and importance of neurogenic sources of both pain and pathology.

Now the research approaches in prolotherapy need to (and want to) consider the merits of use of neurofascial approaches in study designs. This has much potential for outcome enhancement. However, it may also dilute the clinical effects in any one area.

Identification and remediation of degenerative changes in ligament, tendon, and cartilage is important in the future of pain medicine. However, identification of the actual nociceptive sources is likely more important than fascination with diagnostic radiography that shows what appears to be pathology and may have little or nothing to do with nociception. Particularly rewarding will be if the primary nociceptive sources turn out to be responsible for much or some secondary degenerative changes, and the evidence for that position is growing.

References

Full references for this chapter can be found on www.expertconsult.com.

Part D

Neural Blockade and Neurolytic Blocks in the Management of Pain

Atlanto-Occipital Block

Victor M. Taylor, Gabor B. Racz, and Miles R. Day

Historical Considerations

The upper cervical segments have been considered as a source of headache and neck pain since the early 1900s. Homes[1] reported in 1913 the existence of cervicogenic headache. Chiropractic and osteopathic manipulation of the atlanto-occipital (AO) articulation for relief of pain date to the late 1800s. Modern research has implicated the upper cervical spine as well. Bogduk[2] blocked the innervation of the atlanto-axial (AA) joint for the relief of occipital headache in the early 1980s. Later in that same decade, Busch and Wilson[3] wrote on the treatment of headache and neck pain with use of atlanto-occipital joint injection. In 1994, Dreyfus, et al[4] mapped pain patterns associated with AO joint. On the basis of a practice audit, Aprill, et al[5] estimated that 16% of the patients seen for headache in the office had symptoms attributable to the upper cervical spine.

Neck pain and headache are a significant problem for society. Estimates are that 67% of people will have neck pain at some point in life and up to 25% of the population may have pain in the cervical spine at any given time.[6] Up to 34% of people may have chronic neck pain.[7,8] Headache contributes another cause of significant morbidity in society. Fifty percent of patient with chronic neck pain have associated occipital headaches.[9] Despite the prevalence of chronic cervical pain, the contribution of the AO joint to this group of patients appears to be small.[5]

Indications for Atlanto-Occipital Joint Injection

The indications for blocking the AO joint include upper cervical spine pain and headache, with consideration given to temporomandibular joint pain or periorbital headache that resist other diagnosis.[9] Diagnostic block of the AO joint may be used to differentiate the actual pain generator in settings of upper neck pain and headache where the precise pain generator is otherwise undetermined.

Anatomy

The atlas or first cervical vertebrae is unique in structure. The atlas has no vertebral body, no associated disc, and no spinous process. The atlas consist of a ring divided into an anterior arch, which makes up approximately one fifth of the circumference, and a posterior arch that makes up about two fifths of the circumference. The arches are separated by the lateral masses that make up the bulkiest portion of the structure and form the support for the head. The superior facets of the lateral masses are elongated ellipses with a concave surface. They face cranial-medio-posterior and articulate with the occipital condyles as synovial joints. The inferior facets of the lateral masses are circular less convex and face caudal and medial to articulate as synovial joints with the superior facets of C2. The transverse processes of atlas protrude from the lateral masses. The transverse foramen allows the vertebral artery to penetrate the transverse process of atlas. The vertebral artery then winds dorsal and medially around the lateral mass in a grove on the posterior arch that cradles both the artery and the first cervical nerve. On the medial aspect of the lateral masses are found the tubercles of the transverse ligament. The transverse ligament divides the ring of the atlas into an anterior compartment housing the dens and a posterior compartment that surrounds the upper spinal cord.[10] The dens of the axis articulates with the anterior arch of atlas.

The joint is stabilized by the articular capsules bilaterally, the anterior AO membrane, the posterior AO membrane, and the cruciform ligament, tectorial membrane.[10]

Innervation of the joint is mainly from the suboccipital or first cervical nerve. The arterial supply comes from braches of the vertebral and ascending pharyngeal arteries.[10]

Motion of the joint includes flexion and extension produced by the longus capitis and rectus capitis anterior in flexion and the action of the rectus capitis posterior major and minor, obliquus capitis superior, semispinalis capitis, splenius capitis, sternocleidomastoid, and trapezius in extension. Lateral flexion is mediated by the trapezius, splenius capitis, semispinalis capitis, and sternocleidomastoid acting in concert.[10]

Examination and Workup

Thorough history is, as in any clinical situation, of paramount importance. The presenting symptom is usually localized pain or headache that can either be constant or intermittent. Trauma associated with motor vehicle accidents and sports activities can lead to undiagnosed ligamentous instability or occult bony involvement. Chronic conditions such as rheumatoid arthritis and Down syndrome are associated with instability of the upper cervical spine. Neoplasm and infection should be considered in a setting of pain at night, night sweats, chills, or recent weight loss or in a setting where pain is unremitting or worsening rapidly.[11] If infection or tumor are suspected, laboratory evaluation and diagnostic imaging should proceed immediately. Other considerations include referred pain from C2-C3 or C3-C4 facets or disc, occipital neuralgia, and myofascial pain.

Physical Findings

Examination begins with inspection, with attention to swelling and gross deformity. Atrophy of muscle groups of the upper limb indicates involvement of areas lower in the spine. Loss of lordosis is often associated with degenerative disc disease at levels below the AO joint.[8] Pathology of the upper cervical spine may be manifest as either hypomobility or hypermobility of the segments. The AO joint accounts for about 50% of flexion and extension in the neck, and the AA joint accounts for around 50% of the rotation of the neck.[12] Restriction of motion or pain in flexion and extension or side bending of the isolated AO joint indicates possible involvement as a pain generator. The joint may be isolated by retraction of the neck, thus limiting the involvement of the lower cervical segments.[13] Findings of instability with actual or potential for neurologic compromise necessitate referral to the neurosurgeon.[9]

Reflex examination for the upper cervical spine is nonspecific, but a positive response to the Shimizu or scapulohumeral reflex may indicate a disorder of the cervical cord between occiput and C4. A positive result is seen with elevation of the scapula or abduction of the humerus in response to tapping the medial aspect of the spine of the scapula and at the acromion process. (Normal result is no response, although some patients without pathology have a positive response.[14])

When considering the upper cervical spine, bear in mind possible vertebrobasilar artery symptoms, including dizziness, nausea, numbness and nystagmus, vomiting, and ataxia, among others.[15] Vascular disorders, dissections including vertebral artery[16] and carotid artery,[17,18] and aortic dissection, must be considered in a setting of a severe sudden increase in pain.[9]

The shoulder girdle and upper thoracic spine should be included in the physical examination to rule out involvement of these areas.

Physical examination should be augmented with diagnostic imaging, ranging from plain films to magnetic resonance imaging depending on the history and clinical findings.

Technique

Contraindications to the block include universal contraindications to interventional procedures, such as local infection, coagulopathy, inability of the patient to cooperate or consent, and site-specific contraindications, including mechanical instability from either ligamentous or osseous disruption and Arnold-Chiari malformation and surgical fusion of the level.

After informed written consent has been obtained, the patient is taken to the fluoroscopy suite and placed in the prone position with the head supported in a horseshoe pillow so that the neck is slightly flexed. Standard American Society of Anesthesiology monitoring is instituted, and the area over the posterior occiput and cervical spine is prepared and draped in a sterile fashion. The lateral aspect of the AO joint is identified on fluoroscopic image, and the joint is brought into crisp outline by cephalad or caudad tilt of the C-arm. A skin wheal is raised over the target site. A 22-gauge or 25-gauge spinal needle (or a blunt, curved needle through an introducer) is directed toward the target in a coaxial fashion so that the shaft of the needle exactly parallels the x-ray beam. Alternate fluoroscopic orientation from anterior-posterior to lateral is necessary as the needle progresses to stay on track (**Figs. 140.1 and 140.2**). Placement of the needle at the lateral aspect of the AO joint avoids the vertebral artery, which should be located more medially at this level. As the needle enters the joint, a pop may be felt. A lateral fluoroscopic view is obtained to confirm proper depth. Next, an arthrogram made of up to 0.5 mL of non-ionic water-soluble radiocontrast (Ominipaque 240, Isovue) is injected through an extension tubing. If venous runoff is seen, the needle is not within the joint. If arterial uptake is seen, then the needle must be repositioned or the procedure terminated. Spread of contrast within the epidural space may indicate a tear in the joint capsule. A well-placed needle into an intact joint shows a bilateral concave arthrogram on injection of contrast dye (**Fig. 140.3**). Once proper needle placement is assured and after final precautionary aspiration, 0.5 to 1 mL of local anesthetic and steroid is introduced into the joint.[13] Anecdotal reports attest to the value of viscosupplementation in the treatment of pain localized to the AO joint. Radiofrequency thermal coagulation of the nerve supply to the joints may have therapeutic benefit as well.[13]

Potential Side Effects and Complications

Side effects of blocking the AO joint include minor bruising and superficial bleeding, both of which are expected and should be included in the discussion with the patient beforehand. Muscle soreness or spasm may occur from irritation of the muscle by the passage of the block needle. Alternation of a hot water bottle applied to the area for 15 to 20 minutes every few hours helps relax the region. Ataxia, which is usually short lived, may be the result of altered proprioception

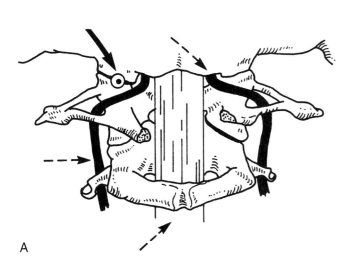

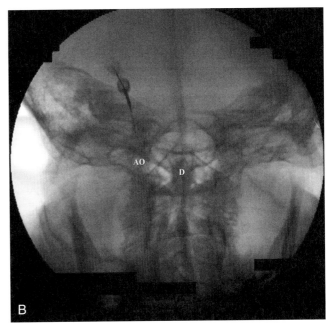

Fig. 140.1 A, A drawing of posteroranterior (oblique) view of the atlanto-occipital (AO) joint showing the needle insertion in a tunneled view. B, Posteroanterior radiographic image with a 25-gauge spinal needle in the AO joint. The dens (D) is labeled and the AO joint is just above its label. (A, From Raj P, et al: Radiographic imaging for regional anesthesia and pain management, *Philadelphia, 2003, Churchill Livingstone, p 83.*)

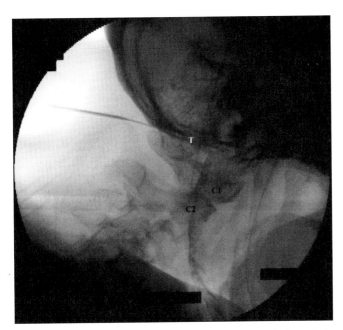

Fig. 140.2 Lateral radiographic image of the 25-gauge spinal needle in the posterior portion of the atlanto-occipital joint. *T,* Tip of needle.

from stretching of the joint capsule or anesthesia of nerves to the joint. Absorption of local anesthetic into the vertebral artery is another possible mechanism leading to ataxia.[13] More serious short-term complications include epidural or intrathecal spread of local anesthetic with possible high spinal necessitating management of the airway and cardiovascular physiology. Even small amounts of local anesthetic injected into the vertebral artery can lead to seizure. Permanent catastrophic sequelae including paralysis and death can occur from deep bleeding, infection, or embolism of air or particulate matter.[19] Resuscutative equipment should be readily available and in working condition.

Conclusion

The AO joint is anatomically unique and is positioned such that any approach must be carefully considered. Miscalculation in needle placement can lead to catastrophic consequences. Resuscitation equipment, including laryngoscope, endotracheal tubes, oxygen, and resuscitator bag, must be available. Medications to support blood pressure and heart rate must also be on hand.

No studies exist to show the long-term efficacy of AO joint injections for the treatment of either neck pain or headache. The block carries significant risk. However, in select cases, blocking of the AO joint by an expert interventionalist may provide useful diagnostic information. RFTC or pulsed radiofrequency may be useful in treatment.

References

Full references for this chapter can be found on www.expertconsult.com.

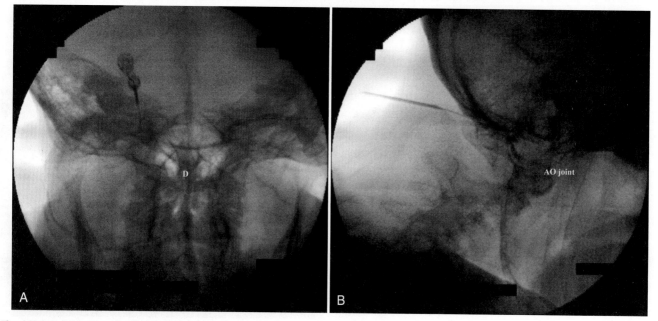

Fig. 140.3 A, Posteroanterior *(PA)* view of the atlanto-occipital (AO) joint after injection of 0.5 mL of contrast. The image is not a true PA image because two lines of contrast in the joint can be seen. **B,** Lateral view showing filling of the contrast in the AO joint.

Atlanto-Axial Block

Gabor B. Racz, Allen Dennis, and Miles R. Day

History

Cervical pathologic causes of chronic occipital headaches were first implicated by John Hilton,[1] a British surgeon, in 1860.[2] Referred pain from the upper three cervical spinal nerves, from pain generators in the upper three cervical segments, is a commonly accepted cause of cervical mediated headache.[3,4] Referred pain from the lateral atlanto-axial (AA) joint via the C2 ventral ramus is estimated as the primary pathology in up to 16% of patients with occipital headaches.[3,4] Clinical signs consistent with AA mediated headache have only a 60% predictive value for true AA involvement.[3,4] Furthermore, radiologic evaluation for cervical structural inflammation or structural changes, plain films, computed tomographic scan, and magnetic resonance imaging, has a high false-negative rate for diagnosis of AA pain generators.[5] Injection of local anesthetic and steroid into the lateral AA joint has been proposed for both diagnosis and treatment of AA mediated pain.[4]

Indications

AA pain most often stems from joint inflammation from trauma, whiplash injury, blunt head trauma, or arthritis (rheumatic or osteoarthritic) of the upper cervical spine.[5] Other causes of AA pain include intra-articular adhesions, capsular inflammation, infection, and periarticular muscle spasm.[5] Patients with suspected AA pathology often present with occipital and suboccipital neck pain, headache described as suboccipital "tightness," decreased cervical range of motion, and pain with upper cervical rotation.[4-7] When acceleration-deceleration mechanisms are the root of the AA pain source, symptoms of postconcussion syndrome or cervical spondylosis, such as dizziness, phonophobia, nausea, and unilateral blurred vision and tinnitus, may overlap with those of AA inflammation.[5,7] Because the array of symptoms of AA pain mimics multiple other conditions that have potential devastating consequences, multiple pathologies should be excluded from the patient's differential diagnoses before consideration of AA interventions (**Table 141.1**).[5]

Pain originating from the AA joint inflammation typically follows both an acute and a chronic phase.[5] The acute phase tends to last between 2 and 4 weeks after the inciting injury.[5] Treatment during this period is often conservative in nature, incorporating physical therapy with oral anti-inflammatory and muscle relaxant medications.[5] Most incidences of AA inflammatory pain resolve after the acute phase.[5] If the patient continues to have painful symptoms beyond the acute time frame, AA injection or other interventions may be necessary to allow for progression to resolution.[3-10] The AA injection with local anesthetic and steroid may be both diagnostic and therapeutic; however, most studies find the pain relief from this injection to be temporary in nature, lasting approximately 3 months.[2-6] If relief from the AA proves to be diagnostic, but temporary, other procedures to provide longer benefit, such as C2 selective nerve root pulsed radiofrequency therapy, occipital peripheral field stimulation, and upper cervical dorsal column stimulation, may be considered.[8-11] Radiofrequency thermal ablation of the C2 nerve root is ill advised because of the risk of anesthesia dolorosa.[10]

Clinically Relevant Anatomy

Several vital structures lay in close proximity to the lateral AA joint; therefore, the upper cervical anatomy must be appreciated before attempts to gain access to this joint.[3-7] The anatomy of the C1-C2 junction is unique compared with the remainder of the cervical spine. The most characteristic feature of C2 is the dens. This tooth-like prominence functions as the pivot point on which C1 rotates. The dens is not only connected to C1 but also to the occiput by the cruciate ligaments. The interaction of the dens and the arch of C1 is maintained by a synovial joint anteriorly and by the transverse ligament of the atlas (TLA). The anterior and posterior interfaces of the dens with arch of C1, combined with the bilateral biconcave lateral AA joints, allow for C1-C2 interaction along four articulations. A normal distance of 2 to 3 mm between the dens and C1 should be maintained throughout all movements. Distances that exceed this are indicative of dislocation of the dens. The lateral AA joint is a modified biconcave zygapophyseal joint.

Table 141.1 Differential Diagnoses of Occipital and Suboccipital Pain

VASCULAR
Vertebral artery aneurysm
Temporal arteritis
Basilar artery spasm (vascular migraine)
CENTRAL NERVOUS SYSTEM AND INTRACRANIAL
Dural inflammation from blood or infection
Arnold-Chari malformation
Tumor
Arteriovenous malformation
Hemorrhage
MUSCULOSKELETAL
Irritation of the C1-C3 nerve root or dorsal root ganglion
C2-C3 disk disease
Atlanto-occipital and atlanto-axial inflammatory arthropathy
C2-C3 facet arthropathy
Cervical myofascial pain

Data from Aprill C, Axinn M, Bogduk N: Occipital Headaches stemming for the lateral atlanto-axial (C1-2) joint, *Cephalagia* 22:15–22, 2002; Ogoke B: The management of the atlanto-occipital and atlanto-axial pain, *Pain Physician* 3:289–293, 2000; and Sjaastad O, Fredriksen T, Pfaffenrath V: Cervicogenic headache: diagnostic criteria, *Headache* 38:442–445, 1998.

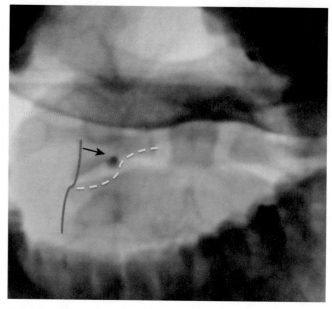

Fig. 141.1 Anterioposterior fluoroscopic view of the atlanto-axial (AA) joint. *Arrow* denotes target point for entry into the lateral AA joint. *Red solid line* denotes likely course of the vertebral artery. *Dashed yellow line* denotes anatomic location of the superior border of the C2 dorsal root ganglion.

On AP fluoroscopy, the lateral AA joint points in a caudal-lateral fashion. In the lateral plane, the biconcave nature of the lateral AA becomes evident. Here, a characteristic bowtie shape is seen.

Several vital structures lie in close proximity to the lateral AA and must be fully appreciated before attempting access to this joint. The vertebral artery courses through the transverse foramen of C1 and C2. At the level of the lateral AA, the vertebral artery lays within the posterior-lateral third of the joint. As discussed subsequently, needle placement should be targeted away from this aspect of the joint. Once the vertebral artery passes through the C1 transverse foramen, it turns medial, coursing caudal to the atlanto-occipital joint. At the level of C1-C2, the internal carotid artery lies close to the anterior aspect of the lateral AA joint.

The lateral AA joint is bordered medially by a narrow epidural space, followed by the dura and then the lower medulla.[4,5,8,9] The C2 nerve root exits the dura approximately at the level of the C1 pillar. The C2 nerve root then travels in an inferior-lateral fashion as it exits the C1-C2 neuroforamen.[4,5,8,9] This places the C2 dorsal root ganglion along the medial third of the lateral AA joint. The innervation of the lateral AA joint is complex.[8,9] The dorsal aspect of this joint receives innervation from multiple articular branches of the C2 ventral ramus.[3,4,8,9] Because of the close proximity of the meninges, the sinuvertebral nerves also play a role in the innervation of this joint.[8,9] Recently, additional ventral innervation arising from two cervical prevertebral plexuses has been described.[9] Fibers of these plexuses arise from the ventral ramus of C3 and possible C4 and run in the ventral C2 gutter, located medial to the vertebral artery along the ventral aspect of the C2 transverse process.[9]

Technique

The following materials are needed:

- 20-gauge or 22-gauge introducer needle
- 24-gauge 3.5-inch pencil-point or blunt needle (modified with a bend approximately 5 to 10 mm from the tip)
- 1 mL of local anesthetic (0.2% ropivicaine or 0.25% bupivicaine)
- 1 mL non-ionic, water-soluble radiocontrast agent, such as omnipaque
- fluoroscopy equipment

Both a lateral and a posterior approach to the AA injection have been previously described.[4,6] The posterior approach is initiated by obtaining clear views of the atlas and foramen magnum with fluoroscopy in the AP plane. Fluoroscopy is then rotated in the sagittal plane until the lateral AA joint assumes a biconcave appearance, target is then made in the skin over the lateral aspect of the AA joint (**Fig. 141.1**). The introducer needle is placed into the skin over the target point and advanced toward the middle aspect of the joint to avoid the vertebral artery as it courses the lateral border of the joint.[3] Next, the 24-gauge pencil-point or blunt needle is inserted via the introducer needle and advanced toward the posterior-lateral aspect of the inferior margin of the C1 inferior articular process to avoid the C2 nerve root and dorsal root ganglion.[3,4] After engagement with bone, the blunt needle is redirected toward the posterior-lateral aspect of the AA joint and advanced until a distinctive "pop" is felt (**Fig. 141.2**). Needle placement in the AA joint line is confirmed with fluoroscopy in the lateral plane (**Fig. 141.3**).

For the lateral approach, the patient is placed in the lateral decubitus position with the injection side up.[3,4] Fluoroscopy is initiated in the lateral plane is such a fashion that the C2 and C3 segments overlap. Next, the AA joint space is maximized by adjustments to fluoroscopy in the cephalad to

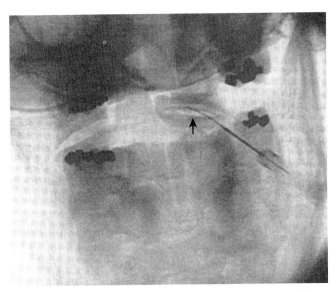

Fig. 141.2 AP fluoroscopic view of the atlanto-axial (AA) joint injection. *Arrow* denotes needle advanced into the inferior lateral aspect of the AA joint, and contrast injected outlines the AA joint.

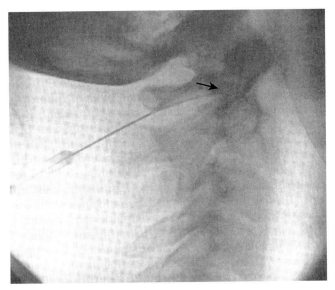

Fig. 141.3 Lateral fluoroscopic view of a needle, denoted by the *arrow*, advanced into the posterior-lateral atlanto-axial (AA) joint via the posterior approach. Injected contrast material outlines the biconcave shape of the AA joint.

caudad direction. Target is then made over the anterior third of the AA joint. The introducer needle is inserted coaxial to the fluoroscopic plane. The blunt needle is then inserted via the introducer needle and advanced toward the inferior margin of the C1 pillar in a coaxial fashion. This should allow the needle to pass posterior to the carotid artery and anterior to

the vertebral artery.[3,4] After contact with periosteum is made, the blunt needle is retracted and then advanced slightly with fluoroscopy in the AP plain. Typically a distinctive pop marks entrance into the AA joint.[3,4]

With both approaches, aspiration should be conducted after the joint is engaged to confirm the vertebral artery is not cannulated. Access into the AA joint is verified with injection of 0.2 to 0.5mL of a water-soluble contrast agent with real-time fluoroscopy.[3,4] Careful attention should be paid that the contrast spread is contained within the joint space and without epidural, intraneural, or intravascular spread. A 1-mL mixture of local anesthetic and steroid can then be injected into the joint.

Side Effects and Complications

After the AA injection is performed, the patient's headache may transiently worsen. Also, postoperative ataxia is common.[3–7] Additional complications can be predicted by the anatomic structures that lay in proximity to the joint. These include cervical epidural and intrathecal injections, injury to the surrounding venous plexus, and carotid and vertebral artery injection.[3–7] Injection of even a small amount of local anesthetic into the carotid or vertebral artery can have drastic effects.[3–7] Use of non-ionic, water-soluble contrast and nonparticulate steroid minimizes the risk of infarction if inadvertent intra-arterial injection is made. Monitoring the patient for at least half an hour after the AA injection is performed is highly advisable.

Conclusion

Injection of the AA joint is a technically challenging procedure that requires familiarity with the surrounding anatomy, the ability to assimilate two-dimensional information into a three-dimensional format, and skill with interventional techniques and equipment. Symptoms of lateral AA pain overlap with several serious conditions, which should also be explored. Although the use of the AA injection may be temporarily therapeutic, its role is primarily diagnostic for AA source of occipital and suboccipital pain. Most patients with AA pain generators show resolution after the acute phase; however, those cases that progress toward chronicity need aggressive interventional therapies to provide relief. If a positive diagnosis of AA pain generator is confirmed with AA injection, interventions with longer acting relief potential, such as C2 pulsed radiofrequency therapy and implantable stimulation devices, may be considered.[8–11] Anecdotally, Gabor Racz has used viscosupplementation (off-label use) in the past with some success in patients who experienced short-lived analgesia to intra-articular corticosteroids.

References

Full references for this chapter can be found on www.expertconsult.com.

Sphenopalatine Ganglion Block

Mark N. Malinowski and Miles R. Day

Historical Significance

Greenfield Sluder[1] was the first to identify the sphenopalatine ganglion (SPG) as a mediator of pain in the head and neck in 1908. He theorized that infection of the sinuses and tissue membranes created inflammation that irritated the SPG, resulting in a neuralgic, facial pain syndrome.[1] This syndrome was coined *Sluder's neuralgia*. Several years later, Simon Ruskin[2] stratified Sluder's neuralgia into four separate entities that together comprised the facial pain syndrome. Unlike Sluder, Ruskin believed that the SPG was involved in the pathogenesis of trigeminal neuralgia.[3] In 1940, Watts Eagle[4] presented his candidate's thesis on "Sphenopalatine Neuralgia" to the American Laryngological, Rhinological and Otological Society. He theorized that the inflammation of the SPG was primarily caused by intranasal deformities and secondarily by systemic disorders (i.e. infection).[4] In the ensuing decades, papers were sporadically published that described various applications for the blockade of the SPG, but this procedure was not considered a mainstream therapeutic interventional procedure. Within the last two decades, blockade of the SPG has found its niche in the interventional pain management algorithm for the treatment of refractory facial pain.

Indications and Contraindications

The list of indications for SPG blockade and neurolysis has expanded over the last several years. This list includes[5-11]:

- Sphenopalatine neuralgia
- Trigeminal neuralgia
- Migraine headaches
- Cluster headaches
- Persistent idiopathic facial pain (formerly atypical facial pain)
- Cancer pain arising from the tongue and floor of the mouth

Other reported, but not yet mainstream, therapeutic uses include[2-16]:

- Postherpetic neuralgia (including pain after Ramsay-Hunt syndrome)
- Vasomotor rhinitis
- Complex regional pain syndrome of the lower extremity
- Low back pain
- Post-traumatic headache

Contraindications include (*A*, absolute; *R*, relative):

- Patient refusal, A
- Local infection and sepsis, A
- Coagulopathy, A
- History of chronic nose bleeds, A
- Allergy to medication used, A & R
- Anticoagulant therapy, R
- History of facial trauma, R (intranasal technique)

Diagnosis and Pathophysiology

The SPG is a cluster of cell bodies that represent a transmission point for both motor and sensory neurons within the head and neck. Given its complex structure and anatomic arrangement, determination of whether the ganglion itself is merely a relay point or a true pain generator within this region is nearly impossible. Therefore, a primary purpose in performing a SPG block is to discern the role of the ganglion in the transmission of pain. Although Sluder and Eagle each referred to periganglionic infection and inflammation as an etiology, Ruskin believed it played a role in mediating trigeminal neuralgia. Ultimately, the true nature of its role in pain of the head and neck is still not well understood. However, two molecular mechanisms have been proposed and include: 1, a disequilibrium between sympathetic and parasympathetic tone within the SPG, resulting in the release of substance P or inhibition of the role of local enkephalins; and

2, focal demyelination of the ganglion, resulting in abnormal impulses from the afferent nociceptive C-fibers.[17] Although the etiology of SPG-mediated pain has yet to be elucidated, the proper use of the SPG block as a diagnostic and therapeutic modality should be incorporated into the clinical approach to the treatment of headache.

Precautions

As with any invasive procedure, knowledge of anticoagulation therapy should receive special consideration. The risk-to-benefit ratio must always be considered before cessation of anticoagulation therapy. Therefore, the pain physician and primary care physician must have a clear line of communication to properly coordinate the cessation and recommencement of anticoagulation therapy. As a rule, nonsteroidal anti-inflammatory drugs should be discontinued for at least 4 days before the procedure, aspirin and clopidogrel for 7 to 10 days, and ticlopidine for 10 to 14 days. Discontinuation of warfarin should be based on the indication for therapy and in consultation with the prescribing physician. A prothrombin time must be checked the morning of the procedure. The inability to stop warfarin therapy is a contraindication to the procedure. Similarly, heparin and heparinoids should receive the same consideration as warfarin, and an activated partial thromboplastin time should be obtained. Emphasis should be made that these represent guidelines and are not industry standards. Herbal and homeopathic medications should also warrant consideration for their antiplatelet and anticoagulant effects, and no recommendations regarding their cessation can be made at this time. Similarly, newer anticoagulants have recently entered the market, but limited data exist regarding their effect on interventional pain procedures and no subsequent recommendations can be made. Thus, the clinician should carefully consider the manufacturer's warnings, other published guidelines, and specialist consultation (i.e., cardiology consultation in those patients who are undergoing anticoagulation therapy after drug-eluting stent placement.)

Anatomy

The ganglion resides in the pterygopalatine fossa. The maxillary sinus borders the fossa anteriorly, the medial pterygoid plate posteriorly, the palatine bone and pterygopalatine foramen medially, and the sphenoid sinus superiorly. The pterygomaxillary fissure allows passage of a needle into the fossa from the lateral border. The ganglion resides at a level just superior to the middle turbinate. The fossa itself is approximately 1 cm wide and 2 cm high, and it assumes a V-shaped appearance on lateral fluoroscopic imaging. A large venous plexus can be found overlying the fossa. Foramen rotundum and the pterygoid canal are located on the superolateral and inferomedial aspect of the fossa, respectively. The maxillary artery and its branches also reside in the fossa.

As previously mentioned, the SPG is a complex hybrid aggregate of somatic and autonomic neural tissue. The ganglion is "suspended" from the maxillary nerve by the pterygopalatine nerves and lies medial to the maxillary nerve when viewed in the sagittal plane. Posteriorly, the SPG is connected to the vidian nerve that is formed by the deep petrosal and greater petrosal nerves. Efferent neurons leave the ganglion and form the superior posterior lateral nasal and pharyngeal nerves. Lastly, the greater and lesser palatine nerves exit the ganglion caudally.

The ganglion has somatic and autonomic components. Sensory fibers arise from the maxillary nerve, pass through the SPG and ultimately innervate the teeth and hard palate, the soft palate, nasal membranes, and some portions of the pharynx. A small number of motor nerves are believed to travel with sensory trunks.

The autonomic pathways are more complex. Preganglionic sympathetic fibers originating in the upper thoracic spinal cord form the white rami communicantes and ascend through the sympathetic chain to the superior cervical ganglion. The exiting postganglionic sympathetic fibers join the carotid plexus before branching off and traveling through the deep petrosal and vidian nerves to the SPG. These postganglionic fibers continue through the SPG en route to the lacrimal gland and the nasal and palatine mucosa. The parasympathetic preganglionic component originates in the superior salivatory nucleus and travels through a small portion of the facial nerve before forming the greater petrosal nerve. The greater petrosal nerve in turn joins the deep petrosal nerve to form the vidian nerve, which terminates in the SPG. Within the ganglion, the preganglionic fibers synapse with their postganglionic cells and continue to the nasal mucosa, with a branch traveling with the maxillary nerve to the lacrimal gland.

Evidence

Day[21] analyzed the evidence supporting the use of SPG blocks and neurolysis for a variety of accepted indications. Acceptable indications for the use of SPG blockade included trigeminal neuralgia, post-traumatic headache, cluster headache, migraine headache, sphenopalatine neuralgia, and atypical facial pain. Although blockade of the SPG can be used in complex regional pain syndrome of the lower extremity, fibromyalgia, and myofascial pain, these are not considered mainstream indications. Of the 14 articles reviewed, 10 received a grade of 1C based on the system described by Guyatt et al.[18] A grade of 1C evidence was given (low quality of evidence constituting case reports, case series, and a retrospective review), but strong recommendations were made because of the indication for which the block was performed (trigeminal neuralgia, cluster headache, posttraumatic headache, tooth pain, and head and neck cancer). The remaining three articles were graded as 2B, representing moderate quality evidence but weak recommendations based on block indications represented by low back pain, fibromyalgia, and myofascial pain of the head, neck, and shoulders (**Table 142.1**).

In spite of the predominance of lower quality studies, patients should not be denied the opportunity to undergo this procedure when conservative therapy has failed, especially in light of supporting literature for the use of SPG blockade for diagnostic purposes. SPG blockade not only decreases the overall pain level experienced by the patient but also subsequently reduces oral analgesic requirement. Therefore, the benefit of this procedure clearly outweighs the risk when performed by a properly trained pain physician.

Table 142.1 Summary of Sphenopalatine Block/Neurolysis Articles

Authors	Study Type	Diagnosis	No. of Patients	Grade of Recommendation
Gregoire et al[20]	CR	Trigeminal neuralgia	1	1C
Shah, Racz[16]	CR	Posttraumatic headache	1	1C
Yang, Oraee[21]	CR	Cluster headache	1	1C
Saade, Paige[22]	CR	Cancer	1	1C
Manahan et al[6]	CR	Trigeminal neuralgia	1	1C
Peterson et al[23]	CR	Trigeminal neuralgia, tooth pain	2	1C
Quevedo et al[14]	CR	CRPS lower extremity	2	2C
Salar et al[19]	CS	Sphenopalatine neuralgia	7	1C
Sanders et al[8]	CS	Cluster headache	66	1C
Puig et al[5]	CS	Sphenopalatine neuralgia	8	1C
Bayer et al[25]	RR	Atypical facial pain, sphenopalatine neuralgia, atypical trigeminal neuralgia, migraine headache	30	1C
Berger et al[15]	DB, PC	Low back pain	21	2B
Janzen et al[26]	DB, PC	Myofascial pain, fibromyalgia	21	2B
Ferrante et al[27]	DB, PC	Myofascial pain in head, neck, shoulders	23	2B

CR, case report; CRPS, complex regional pain syndrome; CS, case series; DB, double blind; PC, placebo controlled; RR, retrospective review.
(Recreated with permission from Backwell Publishing, Oxford, United Kingdom, 2009.)

Techniques

The intranasal and the infrazygomatic approaches are discussed in this chapter. A third technique uses an intraoral approach through the greater palatine foramen but is not discussed in this chapter.

Intranasal Approach

The intranasal SPG block is a straightforward technique and can be safely performed in an office setting. The location of the SPG in relation to the middle turbinate and the lateral nasal mucosa allows absorption of local anesthetic from a cotton-tipped applicator inserted into the nare. Cocaine 4% is the local anesthetic of choice because of its inherent vasoconstrictor property. If cocaine is unavailable or a contraindication to cocaine exists, lidocaine 1% or 2%, bupivacaine 0.25% or 0.5%, or ropivacaine 0.2% to 0.5% can be used instead. If these are chosen, the practitioner can pretreat the nare with phenylephrine to produce vasoconstriction and decrease the incidence of epistaxis.

The patient is placed in the supine position. The depth of insertion can be estimated with measurement of the distance externally from the opening of the nare to the mandibular notch. The clinician then marks the depth on the shaft of the cotton-tipped applicator. The cotton-tipped applicators are soaked in local anesthetic for several minutes. The first applicator is inserted into the nare and advanced in a line parallel to the zygoma. The tip is then angled laterally. Care should be taken so as to not advance the applicator in the cephalad direction. The endpoint should be noted as the depth previously marked on the applicator. A second applicator is then inserted into the nare with the same technique except that it is advanced approximately 0.5 to 1.0 cm deeper and superior to

the first applicator. If resistance is encountered at any time, the applicator is withdrawn and redirected. The second applicator is often not a necessity, and the nares of some patients may not accommodate them. The applicator is then left in place for 30 to 45 minutes. A successful block of the SPG demonstrates ipsilateral tearing, conjunctival injection, and nasal congestion as a result of unopposed parasympathetic activity. If the SPG is a pain generator or transmitter, analgesia should also be apparent. If after 20 to 30 minutes no signs of a block are found or the patient has not received any pain relief, additional local anesthetic may be needed; this is accomplished by trickling a small volume of local anesthetic down the shaft of the applicator. The cotton-tipped applicators should be carefully removed after 45 minutes even if no signs of a block or analgesia are found. If this is the case, the SPG may be too deep to be blocked by this technique or is not involved in the transmission of pain. Regardless, the infrazygomatic approach should be performed to rule out both of the aforementioned scenarios.

Infrazygomatic Approach

The infrazygomatic approach to SPG blockade is a technically challenging block and should not be performed by novices. This technique can be done without fluoroscopy, but fluoroscopic guidance is highly recommended because this anecdotally improves the success of the block and the speed at which it is performed and decreases potential complications. Noninvasive monitors should be used to record vital signs during this technique. Depending on the patient, light sedation with midazolam and fentanyl can be used, but on occasion, monitored anesthesia care may be necessary. Heavy sedation is sometimes needed for conventional radiofrequency lesioning of the ganglion because of discomfort. For pulsed lesioning, heavy sedation is not needed.

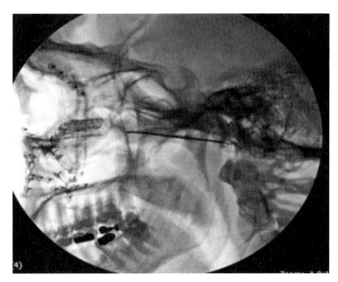

Fig. 142.1 Lateral view (left) of the pterygopalatine fissure. The pterygopalatine fissure appears as a V-shaped structure when proper alignment is obtained with lateral fluoroscopy. Note the insertion point superficial to the mandibular notch. The needle is guided in a medial, anterior, and slightly cephalad direction. The target is in the center portion of the fissure (needle tip.)

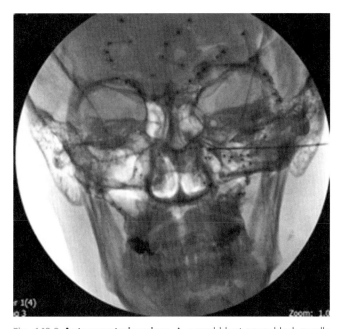

Fig. 142.2 Anteroposterior view. A curved blunt nerve block needle is inserted through an introducer. The needle is then advanced to approximate the middle turbinate.

The patient is placed in the supine position, and the side of the face where the block is to be performed is sterilely cleansed and draped. The ipsilateral eye should be left exposed, allowing the clinician to monitor for proptosis subsequent to retrobulbar hematoma formation. Beginning with the lateral fluoroscopic image (**Fig. 142.1**), the pterygopalatine fissure is visualized. However, the clinician may start with an anteroposterior (AP) image (**Fig. 142.2**) as well. The mandibular notch is palpated, and the skin overlying this area is anesthetized

with local anesthetic. If the notch is not palpable because of body habitus, the notch can be identified on lateral fluoroscopic view. The pterygopalatine fissure appears as a "V" on the lateral image by superimposition of the right and left fissure. This is accomplished by manipulating the C-arm or the head. Malinowski and Day prefer to keep the head in the midline and manipulate the C-arm.

The block can be performed with a 3.5-inch 22-gauge short-bevel spinal needle, with the distal tip bent at a 30-degree angle, or a curved blunt 10-cm 20-gauge needle. The author prefers the latter, and the description of the block reflects this choice. After the skin is anesthetized, a 1.25-inch 16-gauge angiocatheter is passed through the skin until the tip is slightly medial to the ramus of the mandible on AP view. The needle is removed, with the catheter left in place, and a blunt nerve block needle is inserted through the angiocatheter. The blunt needle is advanced medial, anterior, and slightly cephalad. A lateral image is used to check the direction of the needle. The target is the midportion of pterygopalatine fissure. An AP view is obtained such that the needle is advanced toward the middle turbinate, stopping when the tip is adjacent to the palatine bone. If resistance is encountered at any point, the needle should be withdrawn and redirected. Frequent AP and lateral images used to redirect the needle are needed given the small size of the fossa. Once within the fossa, a 0.5-mL to 1-mL aliquot of non-ionic water-soluble contrast is used to rule out intravascular spread or intranasal placement of the needle. Once correct placement of the needle has been confirmed, 2 mL of local anesthetic is injected with or without steroids.

Radiofrequency Thermocoagulation and Pulsed Lesioning

After a successful diagnostic block, therapeutic intervention can be planned. Two choices are available: conventional radiofrequency lesioning (RFTC) and pulsed electromagnetic field radiofrequency (P-EMF). An insulated radiofrequency (RF) needle with a 3-mm or 5-mm active tip is placed with the infrazygomatic approach. Once in place, sensory stimulation is performed at 50 Hz up to 1 V. If the tip of the needle is adjacent to the SPG, the patient should perceive a paresthesia at the root of the nose. Ideally, this should be obtained at less than 0.5 V. If the paresthesia is felt in the hard palate, the needle is stimulating the palatine nerves and should be redirected cephalad and medial. A paresthesia in the upper teeth indicates stimulation of the maxillary nerve, and the needle should be more caudal and medial. Motor stimulation is not necessary. After appropriate sensory stimulation is achieved, RFTC can be performed for two cycles at 67°C to 80°C (153°F to 176°F) for 90 seconds. Before lesioning, 2 to 3 mL of local anesthetic should be injected. The author also prefers to use a mixture of local anesthetic and a corticosteroid. To avoid inadvertent lesioning of the other nerves around the SPG, a 3-mm active tip is a better choice. For P-EMF, the size of the active tip is not as important because the electromagnetic field is projected from the tip of the needle and not from the shaft. With P-EMF lesioning, two to four (physician preference) 120-second lesions are performed at 40 to 42 V. Local anesthetic is not necessary for P-EMF. The choice of whether to do RFTC or P-EMF lesion after a successful block is up to the discretion of the pain practitioner.

Side Effects and Complications

Blockade of the SPG is not a benign procedure. Infection can occur if proper aseptic technique is breached. Epistaxis can occur if the practitioner is too aggressive in placing the cotton-tipped applicators into the nasal passage or the needle penetrates the lateral nasal wall during the infrazygomatic approach. Hematoma formation is possible if the venous plexus overlying the pterygopalatine fossa or the maxillary artery or one of its branches is punctured. RFTC of the ganglion can cause transient hypoesthesia or anesthesia of the palate and the pharynx.[18–19] Reflex bradycardia (also known as Konen's reflex after the physician who first reported it) has also been noted with RFTC of the ganglion.[20] Anecdotally, Malinowski and Day hvae occasionally experienced this with P-EMF of the ganglion.

KEY POINTS

- Sphenopalatine ganglion blockade has a significant role in the treatment of refractory headache and facial pain.
- Understanding the anatomy of the sphenopalatine ganglion is essential to shorten the time needed to perform the block and to reduce complications.
- The use of fluoroscopy is highly recommended.
- Sensory stimulation should produce a paresthesia at the root of the nose if the needle tip is on the sphenopalatine ganglion. This is necessary before RFTC.
- Complications and side effects are usually transient.

References

Full references for this chapter can be found on www.expertconsult.com.

Greater and Lesser Occipital Nerve Block

Steven D. Waldman

Indications

Occipital nerve block is useful in the diagnosis and treatment of occipital neuralgia.[1] This technique is also useful in providing surgical anesthesia in the distribution of the greater and lesser occipital nerves for lesion removal and laceration repair.[2,3]

Clinically Relevant Anatomy

The greater occipital nerve arises from fibers of the dorsal primary ramus of the second cervical nerve and to a lesser extent from fibers of the third cervical nerve. The greater occipital nerve pierces the fascia just below the superior nuchal ridge along with the occipital artery. It supplies the medial portion of the posterior scalp as far anterior as the vertex (**Fig. 143.1**).[4]

The lesser occipital nerve arises from the ventral primary rami of the second and third cervical nerves. The lesser occipital nerve passes superiorly along the posterior border of the sternocleidomastoid muscle, dividing into cutaneous branches that innervate the lateral portion of the posterior scalp and the cranial surface of the pinna of the ear (see Fig. 143.1).[4]

Technique

The patient is placed in a sitting position with the cervical spine flexed and the forehead on a padded bedside table (**Fig. 143.2**). A total of 8 mL of local anesthetic is drawn up in a 12-mL sterile syringe. With treatment of occipital neuralgia or other painful conditions that involve the greater and lesser occipital nerves, 80 mg of depot steroid is added to the local anesthetic with the first block and 40 mg of depot steroid is added with subsequent blocks.

The occipital artery is then palpated at the level of the superior nuchal ridge.[4,5] After preparation of the skin with antiseptic solution, a 22-gauge 1.5-inch needle is inserted just medial to the artery and is advanced perpendicularly until the needle approaches the periosteum of the underlying occipital bone. A paresthesia may be elicited, and the patient should be warned of such. The needle is then redirected superiorly, and

after gentle aspiration, 5 mL of solution is injected in a fanlike distribution, with care taken to avoid the foramen magnum, which is located medially (**Figs. 143.3** and **143.4**).

The lesser occipital nerve and a number of superficial branches of the greater occipital nerve are then blocked with the needle directed laterally and slightly inferiorly. After gentle aspiration, an additional 3 to 4 mL of solution is injected (see Figs. 143.3 and 143.5). Fluoroscopy and ultrasound scan guidance may be useful in selected patients undergoing greater and lesser occipital nerve block in whom identification of the occipital artery is difficult because of anatomic considerations (see Figs. 143.4, 143.5 and **143.6**).

Side Effects and Complications

The scalp is highly vascular, which, coupled with the fact that both nerves are in close proximity to arteries, means that the pain specialist should carefully calculate the total milligram dosage of local anesthetic that may be safely given, especially if bilateral nerve blocks are being performed. This vascularity and the proximity to the arterial supply give rise to an increased incidence of postblock ecchymosis and hematoma formation.[6] These complications can be decreased if manual pressure is applied to the area of the block immediately after injection. Despite the vascularity of this anatomic region, this technique can safely be performed in the presence of anticoagulation therapy with use of a 25-gauge or 27-gauge needle, albeit at increased risk of hematoma, if the clinical situation dictates a favorable risk-to-benefit ratio. Application of cold packs for 20-minute periods after the block also decreases the amount of postprocedure pain and bleeding the patient may experience.

As mentioned previously, care must be taken to avoid inadvertent needle placement into the foramen magnum because the subarachnoid administration of local anesthetic in this region results in an immediate total spinal anesthetic.[1,2]

Any patient with headaches severe enough to need neural blockade as part of the treatment plan should undergo a magnetic resonance imaging (MRI) scan of the head to rule out unsuspected intracranial pathology (**Fig. 143.7**). Furthermore, cervical spine x-rays should be considered to rule out congenital abnormalities such as Arnold-Chiari malformations that may be the hidden cause of the patient's occipital headaches.

References

Full references for this chapter can be found on www.expertconsult.com.

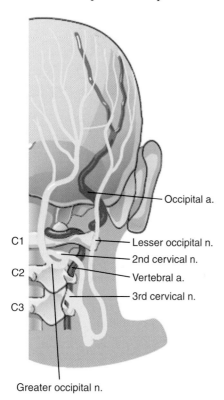

Fig. 143.1 The greater occipital nerve arises from fibers of the dorsal primary ramus of the second cervical nerve and to a lesser extent from fibers of the third cervical nerve. The greater occipital nerve pierces the fascia just below the superior nuchal ridge along with the occipital artery. It supplies the medial portion of the posterior scalp as far anterior as the vertex.

☐ Sensory distribution of greater occipital n.

☐ Sensory distribution of lesser occipital n.

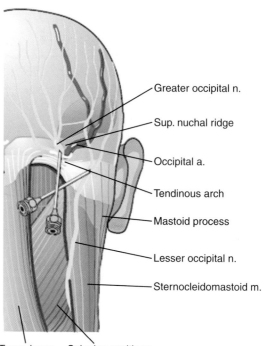

Fig. 143.3 The occipital artery is then palpated at the level of the superior nuchal ridge. After preparation of the skin with antiseptic solution, a 22-gauge 1.5-inch needle is inserted just medial to the artery and is advanced perpendicularly until the needle approaches the periosteum of the underlying occipital bone. A paresthesia may be elicited, and the patient should be warned of such. The needle is then redirected superiorly, and after gentle aspiration, 5 mL of solution is injected in a fanlike distribution, with care taken to avoid the foramen magnum, which is located medially. *(From Waldman SD: Anatomy of the greater and lesser occipital nerve. In Waldman SD, editor:* Pain review, *ed 1, Philadelphia, 2009, Saunders, p 41; Waldman SD: Greater and lesser occipital nerve block. In Waldman SD, editor:* Pain review, *ed 1, Philadelphia, 2009, Saunders, pp 393–394).*

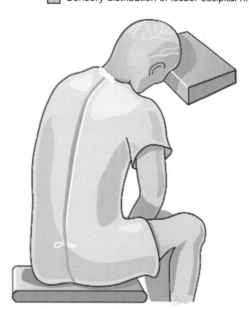

Fig. 143.2 The patient is placed in a sitting position with the cervical spine flexed and the forehead on a padded bedside table.

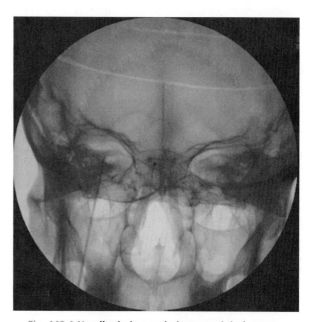

Fig. 143.4 **Needle tip in proximity to occipital nerve.**

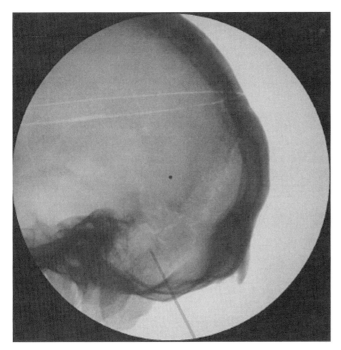

Fig. 143.5 Needle tip in proximity to lesser occipital nerve.

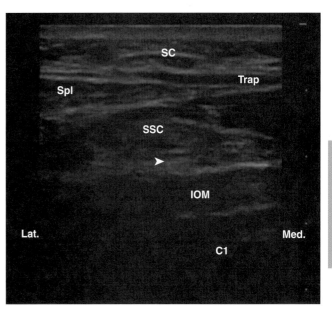

Fig. 143.6 **Ultrasound scan (US) short-axis view at C1 level showing the greater occipital nerve (GON)** *(arrowhead).* Note: At this level, the GON is more than 1 cm deep to the subcutaneous tissue (separated by the semispinalis capitis muscle). *IOM,* Inferior oblique muscle; *SSC,* semispinalis capitis; *Spl,* splenius muscle; *Tapr,* trapezius muscle; *SC,* subcutaneous tissue; *Med,* medial; *Lat,* lateral. *(From Narouze S: Ultrasonography in pain medicine: future directions,* Techniques Regional Anesthesia Pain Management *13(3):198–202, 2009.)*

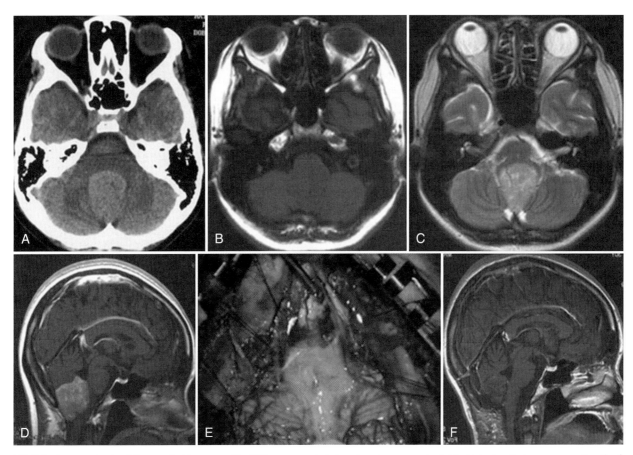

Fig. 143.7 **A,** A precontrast axial computed tomographic (CT) scan on admission showing a round, slightly high density tumor occupying the fourth ventricle. **B,** Axial T1-weighted and, **C,** T2-weighted magnetic resonance image (MRI) showing the mass occupying the lower half of the fourth ventricle and compressing the lower part of the brain stem. **D,** Sagittal T1-weighted MRI. The tumor contained a small cyst (not marked) and was homogeneously enhanced with gadolinium-diethylenetriamine penta-acetic acid (Gd-DTPA). **E,** An intraoperative photograph showing that the pinkish, soft midline tumor split the cerebellar tonsils and extended downward to the C1 lamina level. **F,** Sagittal T1-weighted MRI after intravenous injection of Gd-DTPA at 1 year after surgery showing complete remission of the tumor. *(From Akimoto J, Murakami M, Fukami S, et al: Primary medulla oblongata germinoma: an unusual posterior fossa tumors in young adults,* J Clin Neurosci *16(5):705–708, 2009.)*

Third Occipital Nerve Block

Kenneth D. Candido

Introduction

Diverse pain syndromes result from disorders of the cervical intervertebral discs and the facet joints (zygapophyseal, or Z-joints). The third occipital nerve has been implicated in chronic headache pain, primarily as attributed to cervicogenic headache. There is no doubt that syndromes related to dysfunction of the medial branch nerves of the upper cervical spine have at times been misdiagnosed as "tension-type" and other forms of headache. Undoubtedly, then, patients who have been misdiagnosed with such ultimately have failure to derive analgesic benefit from medication administration and other conservative treatment measures that were misguided.

The third occipital nerve (TON) is the superficial branch of the C3 dorsal ramus. It is the only medial branch nerve that innervates the facet joint at C2-C3 (**Figs. 144.1, 144.2,** and **144.3**). Therefore, successful blockade of the TON and the resultant block of the facet joint at C2-C3 has been associated with relief of headache pain in individuals with "third occipital headache."

Anatomic Considerations

The C2-C3 joint is the first joint of the cervical spine that possesses a true joint capsule and synovium, and this level is the first wherein an intervertebral disc exists and wherein a foramen exists to accommodate the exiting C3 nerve root. In this regard, the C2-C3 joint is distinct from the atlanto-occipital (AO; C0-C1) and atlanto-axial (AA; C1-C2) joints superior to it. This level, then, represents a sort of transitional zone between the rotational joint of the neck (AA) and the lower cervical facet joints, which function not in neck and head rotation but in neck flexion and extension.

Facet joints contain free and encapsulated nerve endings. In addition, nerves in the zygapophyseal joint (Z-joint) contain substance P and calcitonin gene-related peptide. The capsule of the Z-joint contains low threshold mechanoreceptors, mechanically sensitive nociceptors, and silent nociceptors. Each of these may respond to noxious stimulation, including moderate to severe levels of osteoarthritis, with the result being a nociceptive stimulation perceived as headache or neck pain.

The clinical anatomy of the cervical dorsal rami was described by Bogduk[1] after dissections of five adult cadavers. He pointed out in 1982 that classic textbook descriptions of the cervical dorsal rami had been limited in scope and detail up to that point. With use of the technique of dissecting the medial branches, he was able to place wires superficially and parallel to the nerves and then subject the specimens to radiographic analysis. The semispinalis capitis was noted to cover the cervical medial branches, and the lateral branches of C3-C7 to lie superficial to the tendons of origin of that same muscle. The TON penetrates the semispinalis capitis. The C3 dorsal ramus, a short nerve, was noted to arise from the C3 spinal nerve in the C2-C3 intervertebral foramen and then to curve dorsally through the intertransverse space. At this point, the C3 dorsal ramus was noted to divide into three major branches; the two medial branches, the lateral branch, and the communicating branch. In 60% of the specimens, the two medial branches of C3 were noted to arise from a common stem, and in the other specimens, they had their own respective origins. The third occipital nerve (TON) was the principal and constant medial branch of the C3 dorsal ramus.[1] After arising from the C3 dorsal ramus, the TON was found to curve dorsally and medially around the superior articular pillar of the C3 vertebral body, crossing the C2-C3 Z-joint either just below the joint itself or at the joint level. The TON runs transversely medially through the fibroadipose tissue below the obliquus inferior and dorsal to the lamina of the C2 vertebra.

A branch of the TON supplies the semispinalis capitis, which lies superficial to it. A communicating branch to the greater occipital nerve (GON) is also given off. This branch arises just above the level of the C2 spinous process. The TON then passes dorsally and pierces the semispinalis capitis and the splenius capitis, turning rostrally to pierce the trapezius, which lies over it. The more medial terminal branch supplies the skin of the rostral neck and the occiput below the external occipital protuberance. More lateral branches travel towards

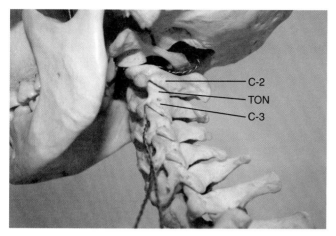

Fig. 144.1 **Lateral view of the skeletal cervical spine showing targets for third occipital nerve block.**

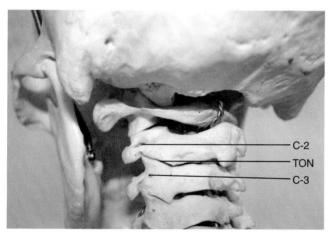

Fig. 144.2 **Close-up of lateral-oblique view of the skeletal cervical spine showing target for needle placement for third occipital nerve block.**

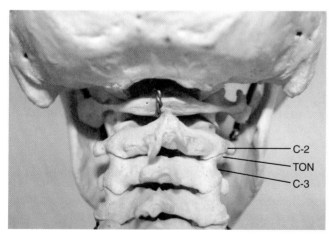

Fig. 144.3 **Posterior view of the skeletal spine showing lateral margins of the vertebral bodies as targets for third occipital nerve block needle placement.**

the mastoid process, communicating with the cutaneous rami of the GON and lesser occipital nerves (LONs). Because of the transverse direction of the GON and the TON, these two nerves may be injured by parasagittal incisions made in the upper part of the neck.

The target branch for nerve block, the TON, wraps dorsally and medially around the middle of the waist of the articular pillar of C3 (center of the bony trapezoid). As it moves more medially, the TON invests the multifidus muscle. A communicating branch typically arises from the C3 dorsal ramus, running rostromedially across the posterior part of the C2-C3 Z-joint.[1] The anatomic target for percutaneous location of the nerve, then, is use of lateral fluoroscopy to identify the waistline of the articular pillars of C2 and C3 and to advance a needle or radiofrequency cannula towards the Z-joint at C2-C3. As Bogduk[1] has stated, "needles or electrodes introduced obliquely, ventromedially onto the dorsolateral aspect of the articular pillar, will rest on the medial branch. The relationship of the nerve to bone at this site is constant, because the medial branches are bound to the periosteum by an investing fascia and are held against the articular pillar by tendons of the semispinalis capitis."[1] This target is removed both from any major arterial or vascular structure and from the exiting spinal nerve and spinal cord and is therefore both an appropriate target in terms of affording access to the medial branches and one that provides for an approach likely to minimize unwanted trespass into nontargeted tissues.

The Third Occipital Nerve and Headache Pain

Osteoarthritis of the C2-C3 Z-joint is one cause of persistent occipital or suboccipital headache pain. Because no clear-cut clinical evaluative technique or diagnostic tool exists for determination of who does, and who does not, have headache from disease of this joint (or that mediated by the TON), it is somewhat intuitive and logical that blockade of the TON should be performed in cases of persistent headache that are unresponsive to conventional medication management.[2]

Bogduk and Marsland[2] conducted fluoroscopically guided TON blocks in 10 consecutive patients with occipital or suboccipital headache. They elected to place the needles at the lower half of the silhouette of the C2-C3 Z-joint, recognizing the landmark on x-ray as a convexity arising upwards from the concavity of the C3 articular pillar, lying horizontally opposite the level of the C2 spinous process and C2-C3 disc space (see Figs. 144.1, 144.2, and 144.3). All procedures were performed with patients in the prone position and with a bolster beneath the upper chest and shoulders to permit head flexion forward towards the procedure table. A dose of 0.5 mL of 0.5% bupivacaine was injected at three distinct sites: in the middle of the Z-joint at C2-C3, at the lower end of the joint, and between the first two needle placements (for bilateral blocks, the total volume was therefore 3 mL, 1.5 mL per side). Seventy percent of patients had total pain relief that lasted the duration of the bupivacaine, after unilateral blocks.[2] The 30% of cases with failure did not have positive responses to the bilateral blocks that were performed on their behalf.[2] Bogduk and Marsland[2] stated that blockade of the medial branch nerves, particularly the TON, are easier for patients to tolerate than intraarticular injections because they are more easily performed and are associated with less pain during their performance than are the articular injections. Furthermore, local anesthetic injected into a joint may not actually stay within the joint space, potentially limiting any diagnostic information that might otherwise be derived from the procedure. Finally, markedly degenerated joints might not readily accommodate an advancing needle tip, rendering the choice of this articular approach potentially useless overall.[2]

How likely is pain in the occipital and suboccipital area to emanate from the C2-C3 Z-joint? Although no one knows for certain and various studies show greatly disparate findings, several compelling attempts at determining the incidence (a measure of the risk of development of some new condition within a specified period of time) or prevalence (the total number of cases in the population, divided by the number of individuals in the population) need to be reviewed.

One such study involved 24 consecutive patients with undiagnosed neck pain who were studied with controlled diagnostic blocks incorporating low-volume local anesthetic injections.[3] For individuals with occipital or suboccipital headache and neck pain, the lower half of the lateral margin of the C2-C3 Z-joint was selected as the injection site. Complete pain relief was considered to occur if the patients, having received the bupivacaine blocks and then going home to perform their activities of daily living, noted at least 2 hours of total analgesia. Failure to derive pain relief resulted in patients undergoing additional cervical medial branch blocks at contiguous levels. Nineteen of 24 patients had positive results, with 9 of these ultimately having pain isolated to the C2-C3 level. This represents, then, that in 47% of patients who had diagnostic block-proven cervical Z-joint pain, the TON was the nerve responsible for mediating the pain. Although this study has not been replicated, use of this information as a general rule of thumb is tempting when approaching individuals with neck pain from degenerative disease of the cervical spine and when planning nerve blocks based on the correlation of symptoms with joint pain maps.[4,5] If, in one half of cases, the level responsible for a given pain problem is known to be at the C2-C3 joint, then time, expense, and patient discomfort might be saved with rapidly moving towards ruling in or ruling out that level, and the TON, at the outset as part of the diagnostic workup. However, as noted subsequently, these figures may be overreaching in terms of the actual prevalence of C2-C3 related pain. Although TON block may be performed easily and simply, and typically is done absent the likelihood of encountering significant complications, side effects do occur commonly. Indeed, any patient with this type of procedure must be duly apprised that successful blockade of the TON (or GON) likely results in the temporary development of ataxia and some gait unsteadiness. For this reason, bilateral blocks at these levels should likely be staggered or the benefit-risk ratio significant enough that performing bilateral blocks is clearly warranted.

The subject of joint pain maps merits special mention. Multiple attempts have been made at delineating the specific cutaneous area of sensation, and hence pain, invested by each respective facet joint and medial branch.[4-8] In the report by Fukui et al,[7] the site of Z-joint intra-articular injection and electrical stimulation (selected cases) was chosen based on any focal paraspinal tenderness. They observed that with injections performed at C2-C3 ($n = 14$), symptoms were referable to the upper posterior cervical region (64%), the occipital region (50%), or the upper posterolateral cervical region (50%).[7] Windsor et al[8] electrically stimulated the cervical medial branches, including the TON, in nine patients with chronic neck pain. They used the lateral midpoint of the C2-C3 Z-joint as indicating the location of the TON. Relatively reproducible referral patterns were identified for the TON nerve distribution and for the other medial branch nerves studied.[8]

What is immediately obvious in review of these studies, however, is that considerable overlap is involved in the areas served by each of the respective segments, much more so than that observed with attempts at mapping spinal nerve dermatome distributions. This produces a diagnostic conundrum because it is entirely conceivable when approaching cervical spine pain that even perfectly performed techniques, with standardized and accepted anatomic landmarks, may result in failures to derive antinociception with the resultant confusion on behalf of the patient and treating physician.

Because both the intervertebral disc and facet joint are fairly equivalently represented as sources of neck pain (approximately 40% each as sources of neck pain, according to two separate studies), a missed diagnosis might lead a pain physician in the wrong direction in seeking to provide pain relief to a given individual.[9,10] Mapping studies may help to pinpoint discrete areas of pain referral sources that are then amenable to local anesthetic blockade or radiofrequency lesioning techniques. In one such study, joint maps were created by distending the respective joint capsules at segments from C2-C3 to C6-C7. This was done with sequential injections of contrast media, which could be subsequently identified with fluoroscopy. Each joint was noted to produce a characteristic, distinguishable pain pattern from which pain charts could be constructed.[5] Although only four total subjects comprised this evaluation, that number is not too disparate from the original small group of subjects selected to develop the original dermatome charts in neurologically impaired individuals that has persisted, largely unchallenged, for more than six decades.[11] In 10 subjects who received injections based on maps such as those derived and described previously, 90% had complete concordance of the predicted level of pain and the positive response to the blocks.[6] The C3-C4, C4-C5, and C5-C6 levels were most commonly affected, with only 10% of patients (1/10) having pain that was documented to be resultant of processes occurring at the C2-C3 (TON) level. These percentages are therefore less indicative of the possibility of the C2-C3 level being primarily involved in head and neck pain than they are of alternative levels lower in the cervical spine. However, a study by Barnsley and Bogduk[12] from 1993 did show that after cervical medial branch injections performed in 16 patients with chronic neck pain, 33% of patients (3 of 9) who had complete pain relief were patients for whom the TON was treated.[12] So, how likely the TON is to be implicated in individuals with chronic head and neck pain still remains unclear. The closest studies performed to identify the prevalence of TON-induced headache and neck pain may have been those performed by Lord et al[13] and Barnsley et al.[14] In the first study, 100 consecutive patients underwent double-blind, controlled diagnostic blocks of the TON. On two separate occasions, the nerve was blocked with either lidocaine or bupivacaine. The diagnosis of TON nerve involvement was only made if the double diagnostic blocks both relieved the symptoms, with the bupivacaine injection-induced pain relief outlasting that provided by the lidocaine. The prevalence rate of TON headache in chronic neck pain after whiplash was found to be 27%, and the prevalence rate of TON headache after whiplash was noted to be 38%.[13]

In the second study, 50 consecutive patients with chronic neck pain and whiplash injury underwent double-blind, controlled diagnostic medial branch blocks with either 0.5 mL lidocaine (2%) or bupivacaine (0.5%) in random fashion. In 12 of 27 patients (44%), the source of symptoms was identified as isolated primarily to the C2-C3 Z-joint.[14]

These findings do corroborate the impression that although substantial overlap may be found in cutaneous innervations of the central and peripheral nervous systems, these joint maps are essential tools to assist one in determining the appropriate approach to a given pain process in any individual. They also demonstrate variability in assessing the relative incidence and relative prevalence of C2-C3 Z-joint pain, depending on technique of assessment and use of varying provocation maneuvers to assess the joint and the medial branch nerve (TON).

Rationale for Blocking the Third Occipital Nerve

The TON block is useful in both the diagnostic and the therapeutic phase of treatment of cervicogenic headache. Evidence of efficacy both for local anesthetic blocks and for radiofrequency ablation of the cervical medial branches has accrued over the past several decades. Nevertheless, only relatively recently has the use of medial branch nerve blocking techniques and radiofrequency ablation techniques received scientific support in the literature. Indeed, two separate attempts at meta-analysis have shown somewhat disparate results. The first such paper, published in 2001, suggested that radiofrequency neurotomy used for treatment of pain from the cervical Z-joints after flexion-extension injury was only supported by limited scientific data.[15] However, a mere six total studies satisfied the authors' criteria for inclusion, and so it is entirely possible that the data suffer lack of suitable cohort studies to make a true assessment of its validity. The second review, performed in 2007, liberalized the inclusion criteria somewhat and found that the support for medial branch cervical block was moderate (Level III) as was the support for cervical medial branch neurotomy.[16] Here the authors relied on the criteria established by the Agency for Healthcare Research and Quality (AHRQ), which included some nonrandomized trials. They also incorporated studies from the Cochrane Musculoskeletal Review Group, which were randomized trials. One of the important points noted was that the evidence for performing cervical intraarticular facet joint injections was limited both for short-term and for long-term analgesia efficacy. This corroborates Dr Bogduk's earlier assertions that not only are medial branch techniques more likely to target the real source of pain associated with cervical degenerative facet conditions but also that articular procedures have an inherently high failure rate because no guarantee exists that injected local anesthetic remains in the confines of the joint (see previous discussion).

The rationale for blocking the TON is twofold:

1. To provide a diagnostic evaluation of the C2-C3 facet joint as being the source of pain in the occipital and suboccipital area
2. To provide an indication as to whether or not neuroablative techniques applied over that nerve might be fruitful in treatment of pain on a long-term basis

Candido suggests performing double-diagnostic blocks with 0.5 mL of local anesthetic solutions, typically 0.5% ropivacaine plain, before undertaking neurotomy of the TON. Ropivacaine is used for two major reasons. It has intrinsic vasoconstrictor properties, and therefore, no epinephrine need be added to it. It also has a cardiovascular safety profile that is superior to bupivacaine and therefore poses somewhat less of a theoretic risk for use in outpatient procedures. Unintentional injection into vascular structures, including the vertebral artery, is less likely to result in serious morbidity when ropivacaine is used, in contradistinction to bupivacaine. The further rationale for use of ropivacaine is to provide a duration of analgesia that exceeds that provided by shorter acting agents, such as lidocaine or mepivacaine. In terms of assessment of efficacy, longer acting amino-amide local anesthetics are likely to provide greater information than do shorter acting drugs because the effect of the shorter acting drugs may be so fleeting as to provide confusing or inexact clinical information.

Double-diagnostic blocks have been described for assessment of efficacy of cervical medial branch blocks.[17] Barnsley et al[17] compared single versus double-diagnostic blocks in 55 adult patients with neck pain for longer than 3 months. They used 0.5 mL of either 0.5% bupivacaine or 2% lidocaine, randomly selected. The duration of analgesia was assessed in double-blind fashion. They found that the false-positive rate (a test result that is read as positive but actually is negative; a test that shows evidence of a disease when it not present) of single blocks was 27% (16 of 60).[17] They also found that the most common positive levels were at C2-C3 and C5-C6.[17] Lord, Barnsley, and Bogduk[18] found that comparative blocks of the medial branches with either lidocaine, bupivacaine, or normal saline solution in randomized, double-blind, placebo-controlled fashion in 50 patients had a specificity (statistical probability that an individual who does not have the particular disease being tested for will be correctly identified as negative, expressed as the proportion of true-negative results to the total of true-negative and false-positive results; TN/TN + FP) of 88% but only marginal sensitivity (proportion of individuals in a population that will be correctly identified when administered a test designed to detect a particular disease, calculated as the number of true-positive results divided by the number of true-positive and false-negative results; TP/TP + FN; 54%).[18] Hence, some 46% of patients who are not placebo responders would be incorrectly labeled as placebo responders if diagnoses were based solely on comparative blocks.[18]

Slipman et al[19] retrospectively reviewed 18 patients with chronic persistent daily headaches lasting a mean of 34 months after whiplash injury who underwent intra-articular C2-C3 facet joint injections. They noted that in 61% of cases, headache frequency diminished from daily to less than three headaches a week. Although no conclusions may be drawn from this work, per se, because of its retrospective nature, the results are nevertheless compelling in demonstrating further rationale for targeting the TON in chronic headache conditions refractory to conventional conservative care and management. Furthermore, because the injections were articular and not at the medial branch (TON), the information gleaned from this report should be interpreted with some caution.

Technique for Third Occipital Nerve Block

Candido performs C2-C3 medial branch (TON) procedures with the patient in the prone position with use of continual live fluoroscopic guidance throughout the injection phase (**Figs. 144.4** and **144.5**).[20] A bolster is placed beneath the shoulders

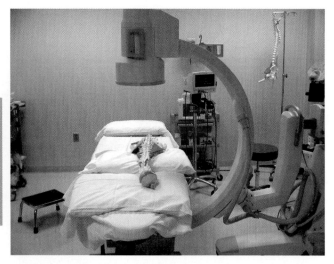

Fig. 144.4 **Anterior-posterior fluoroscopy setup with "specimen" in the prone position on the x-ray table.**

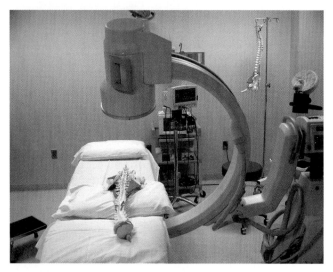

Fig. 144.5 **Cephalad tilt of the fluoroscopy unit to minimize obstruction imposed by the mandibular shadow.**

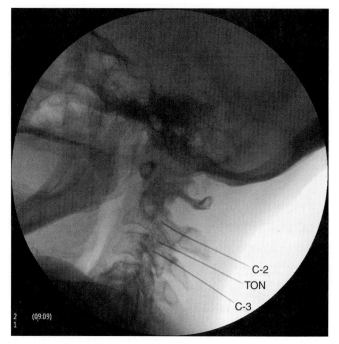

Fig. 144.6 **Needle placement for C2, third occipital nerve, and C3 medial branch blocks; lateral fluoroscopic image.**

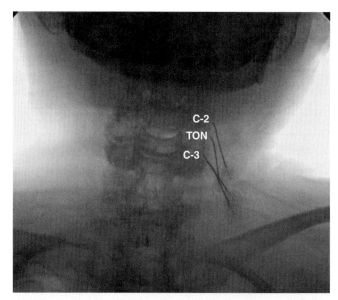

Fig. 144.7 **Anterior-posterior fluoroscopic view with needles in place for C2, third occipital nerve, and C3 medial branch blocks.**

and chest to elevate the thorax off of the table and to permit gentle head and neck flexion forward. An intravenous cannula is placed for purposes of administering resuscitative medications in the unlikely event of needing to treat either vasovagal syncope or for supportive medication administration in cases of unintentional vascular injection. Vital signs are monitored with standard American Society of Anesthesiologists (ASA) basic monitors, including pulse oximetry and noninvasive blood pressure assessment. After a sterile skin preparation is performed, scout films are obtained of the neck, with the purpose of identification of the scalloped margins of the lateral vertebral bodies. Then, skin wheals are raised over the intended target with a hypodermic needle and 1 to 3 mL of lidocaine solution with epinephrine, 1:200,000 (5 μg/mL). With short-beveled, 22-gauge, 2.5-inch to 3.5-inch needles, the targeted lateral scalloped margins of the vertebral bodies are advanced on until bony contact is made. At this point, the fluoroscopy unit is rotated laterally (**Fig. 144.6**) to assess the relationship of the advancing needle tip to the TON target, in the center of the C2-C3 Z-joint (see previous). The needle tip

must be recessed posteriorly away from the C2-C3 intervertebral foramen and from the known location of the vertebral artery. If no bony contact has been made and if 2 cm of the needle has been placed into the skin, then a reassessment of the approach and direction is undertaken while still in the anterioposterior (AP) fluoroscopy mode. Once the needle is appropriately seated, on bone at the target (see Fig. 144.4), the AP view is once again undertaken (**Fig. 144.7**) to verify that the needle is in the correct position vis-á-vis the lateral vertebral body margin. Ultrasound scan–guided approaches are rapidly gaining in popularity for all forms of interventional pain procedures but, in Candido's experience, have not yet reached the level of sophistication to supplant image intensifier use for this particular procedure. At this point, aspiration tests are performed to verify the absence of blood or cerebrospinal fluid, and the patient is queried to ascertain that no paresthesias have been elicited. If there are none and vital signs remain stable and close to baseline values, 0.5 mL of 0.5% ropivacaine is injected. No glucocorticoid is added to the solution, as Manchikanti et al[21] have shown little value if any to adding steroid to the blocks. Although this one study showed no added benefit of corticosteroid use in diagnostic or therapeutic cervical medial branch injection, versus not using steroids, many clinicians continue to use them in daily practice. It can only be stated that this is an area of some controversy, and if the risk-benefit ratio favors use of steroids in a given individual, then there may be little harm in using them in judicious doses. After completion of the injection phase, the needle is cleared and withdrawn, and a sterile dressing is applied over the injection site. The patient should be observed for no less than 30 minutes because patients quite commonly (indeed as a rule) become ataxic or unsteady of gait after successfully performed procedures. Discharge instructions should be clear and should precisely instruct patients to seek emergency medical care if any delayed onset side effects or complications from the procedure develop, as unlikely as that may be.

Radiofrequency Neurotomy

In selected patients, radiofrequency of the TON may be considered for long-term therapeutic benefit. In a study published in 1995, Lord, Barnsley, and Bogduk[22] showed efficacy of performing radiofrequency ablation (RFA) of the TON in only 40% of patients (4 of 10), with only three having long-lasting pain relief. They used 10-cm needles with either 4-mm or 6-mm exposed tips. No stimulation test was performed to ensure concordance of needle placement with the nerve; instead, the authors relied solely on fluoroscopic anatomic cannula placement. The mean duration of the C2-C3 neurotomy procedure was stated to have been 1.5 hours.[22] The rather meager success rate was in sharp contrast to the 70% success that they noted for lower cervical medial branch procedures. The authors stated that radiofrequency of the cervical medial branches "carries a high rate of technical failure."[22] In 1996, Lord et al[23] suggested that RFA of the cervical medial branches, performed in 24 patients with a median duration of pain of 34 months after motor vehicle accidents, provided a median duration of analgesia persisting 263 days. This contrasted sharply to the median analgesia of 8 days in a control group of patients. However, they excluded individuals with C2-C3 Z-joint pain based on their rather dismal results from the previous study noted. In a subsequent study published by the same group of investigators, complete pain relief was found in 71% of 28 patients after a single radiofrequency procedure, persisting a mean duration of 219 days. When failures were excluded from consideration, the mean duration extended out to 422 days (60 weeks).[24] Again, excluded from study were individuals with TON mediated C2-C3 pain. Govind et al[25] in 2003 used three large-gauge electrodes to perform RFA procedures of the TON. After controlled diagnostic blocks, 51 nerves in 40 patients were treated with RFA. Eighty-eight percent (43 of 49) had successful outcomes with this approach, with a median duration of 297 days (42 weeks). Side effects included ataxia, stated to be "slight," numbness, and temporary dysesthesias.[25] Their improved success was attributed to use of three needles and use of Ray electrodes instead of SMK electrodes (smaller) and to the assurance that each of the three lesions was made at a distance no greater than one electrode width from an adjacent lesion.[25]

Cohen et al[26] found that the only factor predicting success of RFA, defined as at least 50% pain reduction lasting at least 6 months, was paraspinal tenderness. Although the authors state that C2-C3 pain was included in this analysis, they never indicated how many individuals were treated nor what the success rate was for TON RFA.

Conclusion

Headache and neck pain are the result of diverse, often conflicting etiologies. The third occipital nerve has been implicated as one source of this, with variable incidence and prevalence. Joint maps may be useful in identification of clinical cases, and treatment consists of small-dose local anesthetic medial branch nerve blocks, followed in successful cases by the judicious use of radiofrequency neurotomy. Side effects include the development of ataxia, dysesthesias, and unsteady gait. The most productive RFA approach appears to include multiple needles, placed in tandem, surrounding the C2-C3 joint.

References

Full references for this chapter can be found on www.expertconsult.com.

Chapter **145**

Gasserian Ganglion Block

Steven D. Waldman

Historical Considerations

On December 6, 1884, Halsted and Hall reported their success in blocking the branches of the trigeminal nerve with local anesthetic in the *New York Medical Journal*.[1] Shortly after this landmark publication, these distinguished New York surgeons showed the utility of "nerve blocks" when Hall had Halsted remove a lipoma from his forehead under "painless" nerve block anesthesia.[2] One can only imagine the tremendous benefit that this clinical discovery afforded surgeons and their patients at a time when, in the absence of endotracheal intubation, muscle relaxants, and sophisticated monitoring, head and neck surgery was, at best, an extremely risky undertaking.

The effectiveness of nerve blocks was rapidly exploited for pain management. Blockades of the gasserian ganglion and distal trigeminal nerve were among the first applications of nerve blocking for pain. By 1900, blockade of these neural structures was considered one of the primary means of alleviating the pain of trigeminal neuralgia and pain from cancers of the face and head.[3] These techniques remained the mainstays of the nonsurgical treatment of trigeminal neuralgia until the introduction of carbamazepine in 1960.

The shift to the managed care paradigm has led pain management specialists to seek the most efficacious, safe, and cost-effective treatments for headache and facial pain.[4,5] This paradigm shift has led to renewed interest in gasserian ganglion block for the management of a variety of painful conditions. This chapter reviews the current indications, contraindications, and technique for blockade of the gasserian ganglion.

Indications and Contraindications

Blockade of the gasserian ganglion with local anesthetics and steroids and destruction of this neural structure via freezing, radiofrequency lesioning, neurolytic agents, compression, and other means have many applications in contemporary pain management.[6] Advances in radiographic imaging, electronics,

and needle technology have improved the efficacy and reduced the cost, complications, and adverse side effects of these useful pain management procedures.

Indications for gasserian ganglion block are summarized in **Table 145.1**. In addition to applications for surgical anesthesia, gasserian ganglion block with local anesthetics can be used as a diagnostic tool in performance of differential neural blockade on an anatomic basis for evaluation of head and facial pain.[7] This technique also is useful as a prognostic indicator of the degree of motor and sensory impairment that the patient might experience when destruction of the gasserian ganglion is being considered.[3] Gasserian ganglion block with local anesthetic may be used to palliate acute pain emergencies, including trigeminal neuralgia and cancer pain, while waiting for pharmacologic, surgical, and antiblastic methods to become effective.[8]

Destruction of the gasserian ganglion is indicated for palliation of cancer pain, including the pain of invasive tumors of the orbit, maxillary sinus, and mandible.[9] This technique also is useful in the management of the pain of trigeminal neuralgia that has been refractory to medical management or for patients who are not candidates for surgical microvascular decompression.[10] Gasserian ganglion destruction also has been used successfully in the management of intractable cluster headache and in the palliation of ocular pain from persistent glaucoma.[3,11,12]

Contraindications to blockade of the gasserian ganglion are as follows:

- Local infection
- Sepsis
- Coagulopathy
- Significantly increased intracranial pressure
- Disulfiram therapy (if alcohol is used)
- Significant behavioral abnormalities

Local infection and sepsis are absolute contraindications to gasserian ganglion block.[13] Coagulopathy and markedly increased intracranial pressure are strong contraindications.

Table 145.1 Indications for Gasserian Ganglion Block

Local Anesthetic Block	Neurolytic Block or Neurodestructive Procedure
Surgical anesthesia	Palliation of cancer pain
Anatomic differential neural blockade	Management of trigeminal neuralgia
Prognostic nerve block before neurodestructive procedures	Management of cluster headache
Palliation in acute pain emergencies	Management of intractable ocular pain

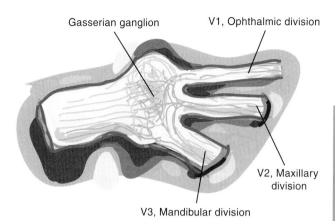

Fig. 145.1 **Gasserian ganglion and Meckel's cave.**

Because of the desperation of many patients with aggressively invasive head and face malignant diseases, however, ethical and humanitarian considerations dictate use of this procedure despite the increased risks of bleeding or cerebrospinal fluid (CSF) leak from coagulopathy or increased intracranial pressure.

Clinically Relevant Anatomy

Role of the Trigeminal System

The trigeminal nerve is the largest and the most complex of the cranial nerves, containing sensory and motor fibers.[14] Somatic afferent impulses carried by the trigeminal nerve transmit pain, light touch, and temperature sensation. Information is transmitted to the central nervous system via the trigeminal nerve from the skin of the face, the mucosal lining of the nose and mouth, the teeth, and the anterior two thirds of the tongue.[15] The trigeminal nerve also carries proprioceptive impulses and afferent impulses from stretch receptors of the teeth, oral mucosa, muscles of mastication, and temporomandibular joint to aid in mastication.

In addition to the sensory innervation just described, visceral efferent fibers help to innervate a variety of muscles of facial expression, the tensor tympani, and some muscles of mastication. Communications exist between the trigeminal nerve and the autonomic nervous system, including the ciliary, sphenopalatine, otic, and submaxillary ganglia and the oculomotor, facial, and glossopharyngeal nerves. Because of the complex structure of the trigeminal nerve, a thorough understanding of the clinically relevant anatomy is crucial to obtaining optimal results with neural blockade.

Gasserian Ganglion

The gasserian ganglion is formed from two roots that exit the ventral surface of the brainstem at the midpontine level (**Fig. 145.1**).[16] These roots pass forward and lateral in the posterior cranial fossa across the border of the petrous temporal bone. They enter a recess called Meckel's cave, which is formed by an invagination of the surrounding dura mater into the middle cranial fossa. The dural pouch that lies just behind the ganglion, called the trigeminal cistern, contains CSF. The gasserian ganglion is canoe shaped and has three sensory divisions, the ophthalmic (V_1), maxillary (V_2), and mandibular (V_3) nerves, which exit on the anterior convex aspect. A smaller motor root joins the mandibular division as it exits the cranial cavity via the foramen ovale.

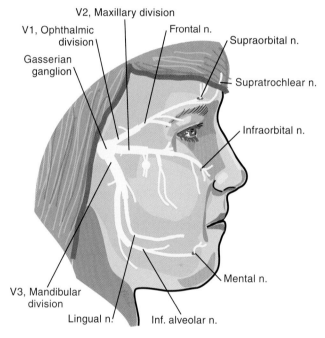

Fig. 145.2 **Trigeminal nerve and its branches.**

Ophthalmic Division

The ophthalmic branch, the smallest division of the trigeminal nerve, is purely sensory in function (**Fig. 145.2**).[17] It enters the orbit via the superior orbital fissure. The branch is divided into the frontal, nasociliary, and lacrimal nerves. The terminal cutaneous branches of the frontal nerve consist of the supraorbital and supratrochlear nerves. These terminal branches exit the orbital cavity anteriorly and provide innervation to the upper eyelid, forehead, and anterior scalp. The terminal cutaneous branches of the nasociliary nerve consist of the infratrochlear and external nasal branches, which provide cutaneous and mucosal innervation to the apex and ala of the nose and anterior nasal cavity. The lacrimal nerve continues, without any additional major branches, to innervate the lacrimal gland and outer canthus of the eye.

Maxillary Division

The maxillary division is a pure sensory nerve. It exits the middle cranial fossa via the foramen rotundum and crosses the pterygopalatine fossa (**Fig. 145.3**).[17] Passing through the

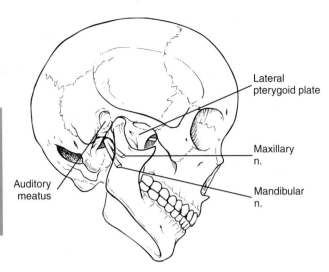

Fig. 145.3 **Major branches of the trigeminal nerve.**

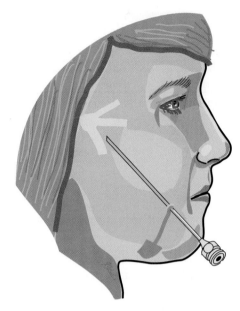

Fig. 145.4 **Needle trajectory for gasserian ganglion block.**

inferior orbital fissure, it enters the orbit, emerging on the face via the infraorbital foramen.

The branches of the maxillary nerve are divided into four regional groups. (1) The intracranial group includes the middle meningeal nerve, which innervates the dura mater of the medial cranial fossa. (2) The pterygopalatine group includes the zygomatic nerve, which provides sensory innervation to the temporal and lateral zygomatic region, and the sphenopalatine branches, which help to innervate the mucosa of the maxillary sinus, upper gums, upper molars, and mucous membranes of the cheek. (3) The infraorbital canal group comprises the anterior-superior alveolar branch, which innervates the incisors and canines, the anterior wall of the maxillary antrum, and the floor of the nasal cavity, and the middle superior branch, which supplies the premolars. (4) The infraorbital facial group consists of the inferior palpebral branch, which innervates the conjunctiva and skin of the lower eyelid; the external nasal branch, which supplies the side of the nose; and the superior labial branch, which supplies the skin of the upper lip and part of the oral mucosa (see Fig. 145.2).

Mandibular Division

The large sensory root and smaller motor root of the mandibular division leave the middle cranial fossa together via the foramen ovale.[17] They join to form the mandibular nerve (see Fig. 145.3). This combined trunk gives off two branches: (1) the nervus spinosus, which runs superiorly with the middle meningeal artery through the foramen spinosum to supply the dura mater and the mucosal lining of the mastoid sinus; and (2) the internal pterygoid, which supplies the internal pterygoid muscle and gives off branches to the otic ganglion. The mandibular nerve divides into a small anterior and a large posterior trunk (see Fig. 145.2).

Branches from the small anterior trunk are the buccinator nerve, which is purely sensory and innervates the skin and mucous membrane overlying the anterior portion of the buccinator muscle; the masseteric nerve, which provides motor innervation to the masseter muscle; the deep temporal nerves, which provide motor innervation to the temporalis muscle; and the external pterygoid nerve, which provides motor innervation to the external pterygoid muscle. The large posterior trunk comprises primarily sensory fibers but a few motor fibers as well. Branches of the posterior trunk are: (1) the auriculotemporal nerve, which provides innervation to skin anterior to the tragus and helix, the

lining of the acoustic meatus, the tympanic membrane, the posterior temporomandibular joint, the parotid gland, and the skin of the temporal region; (2) the lingual nerve, which provides sensory innervation to the dorsum and lateral aspects of the anterior two thirds of the tongue and the lateral mucous membranes of the mouth and the sublingual gland; and (3) the inferior alveolar nerve, which provides sensory innervation to the lower teeth and mandible. The terminal branch of the inferior alveolar nerve is the mental nerve, which exits the mandible via the mental foramen and provides sensory innervation to the chin and to the skin and mucous membrane of the lower lip.

Technique

The patient lies supine with the cervical spine extended over a rolled towel. Approximately 2.5 cm lateral to the corner of the mouth, the skin is carefully prepared with povidone-iodine solution, and sterile drapes are placed.[7] The skin and subcutaneous tissues are anesthetized with 1% lidocaine with epinephrine. A 13-cm 20-gauge Hinck needle is advanced through the anesthetized area, traveling perpendicular to the pupil of the eye (when the eye is in mid position) in a cephalad trajectory toward the auditory meatus (**Fig. 145.4**).[13] The needle is advanced until contact is made with the base of the skull (**Fig. 145.5**). The needle tip is withdrawn slightly and "walked" posteriorly into the foramen ovale (**Fig. 145.6**). Paresthesia of the mandibular nerve may occur as the needle enters the foramen ovale.[7]

If the procedure is performed with fluoroscopic guidance, submental and oblique views are obtained to aid in identification of the foramen ovale (**Fig. 145.7**). After the foramen ovale is entered, the stylet of the Hinck needle is removed. The operator carefully aspirates for blood. Free flow of CSF is typical. Failure to observe free flow of CSF does not mean that the needle tip does not lie within the central nervous system close to the gasserian ganglion but simply that the needle tip rests, not within the trigeminal cistern, but more anteriorly, within Meckel's cave.[13]

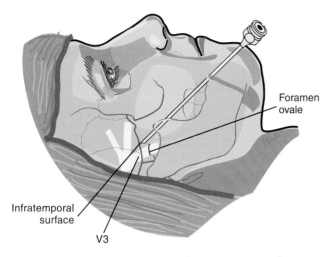

Fig. 145.5 **Needle against roof of infratemporal surface.**

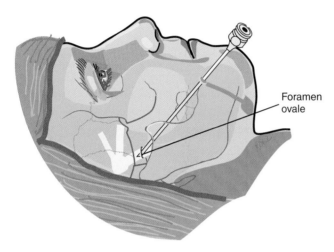

Fig. 145.6 **Needle "walked" into foramen ovale.**

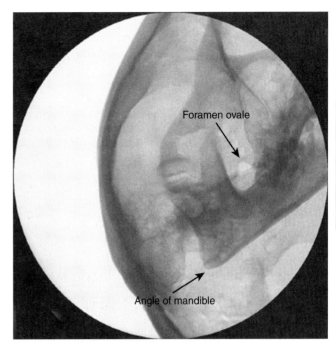

Fig. 145.7 **The foramen ovale.**

The needle position should be confirmed with radiography before any local anesthetic or neurolytic substance is injected (**Figs. 145.8 and 145.9**). After needle position is confirmed, 0.1-mL aliquots of a preservative-free local anesthetic, such as 1% lidocaine for diagnostic blocks and 0.5% bupivacaine for therapeutic blocks, or of sterile glycerol, 6.5% phenol in glycerin, or absolute alcohol may be injected.[7] An average volume of 0.4 mL of neurolytic solution is usually adequate to provide long-lasting pain relief. Because of significant interpatient variability in the size of Meckel's cave, however, careful titration of the total injected volume is indicated.

If hyperbaric neurolytic agents are used, the patient should assume a sitting position, with the chin on the chest before the injection, to ensure that the solution is placed primarily around the maxillary and mandibular divisions (**Fig. 145.10**) and to avoid the ophthalmic division. The patient should remain in the supine position when absolute alcohol is used. This approach to the gasserian ganglion may be used to place radiofrequency needles, cryoprobes, compression balloons, and stimulating electrodes (**Figs. 145.11, 145.12,** and **145.13**).

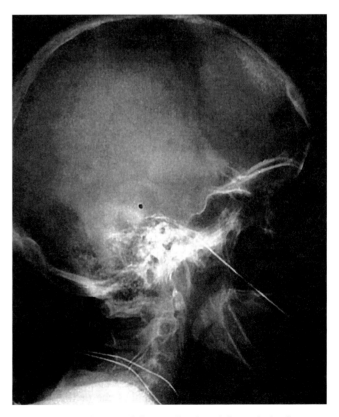

Fig. 145.8 **Lateral view of the needle placed through the foramen ovale.** *(From Waldman SD: Gasserian ganglion block. In Interventional pain management, ed 2, Philadelphia, 2001, Saunders, p 320.)*

Practical Considerations

Because of the densely vascular nature of the pterygopalatine and its proximity to the middle meningeal artery, significant hematoma of the face and subscleral hematoma of the eye are common sequelae. The patient should be warned of

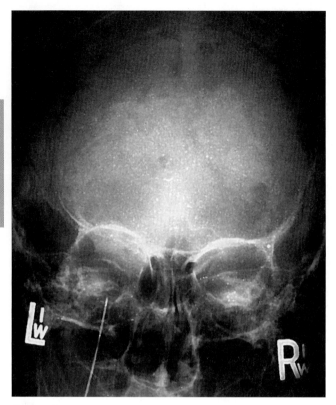

Fig. 145.9 **Anteroposterior view of the needle placed through the foramen ovale.** *(From Waldman SD: Gasserian ganglion block. In* Interventional pain management, *ed 2, Philadelphia, 2001, Saunders, p 320.)*

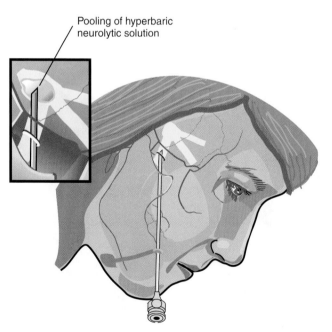

Pooling of hyperbaric neurolytic solution

Fig. 145.10 **Patient positioning for gasserian ganglion block with hyperbaric solution.**

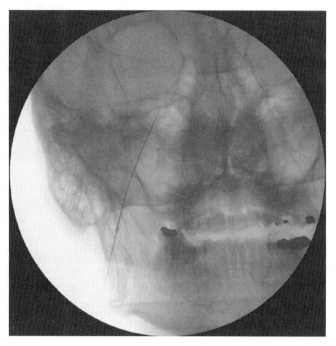

Fig. 145.11 **AP view of needle tip approaching the foramen ovale.**

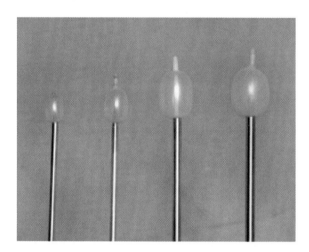

Fig. 145.12 *Left to right:* Different-sized outer cannulas with nos. 3, 4, 5, and 6 inflated Fogarty balloons. *(From Goerss SJ, Atkinson JLD, Kallmes DF: Variable size percutaneous balloon compression of the gasserian ganglion for trigeminal neuralgia,* Surg Neurol 2008. *[Epub ahead of print.])*

the probability of these complications before institution of the block. Because the ganglion lies within the CSF, small amounts of local anesthetic injected through the needle may produce total spinal anesthesia.[13] For this reason, small doses of local anesthetic must be injected incrementally, allowing time after each dose to observe its effect.[3] Chemical neurolysis and neuroablative procedures on the gasserian ganglion should be performed only by individuals familiar with the anatomy and the technique of gasserian ganglion block, and only with radiographic guidance.

Conclusion

Gasserian ganglion block is a straightforward technique with a favorable risk-to-benefit ratio when careful attention is paid to the functional anatomy, indications, and contraindications. Given the cost-effective nature of this technique, gasserian ganglion block is a reasonable next step for patients with facial pain and cluster headache who have not had a response to more conservative therapy.

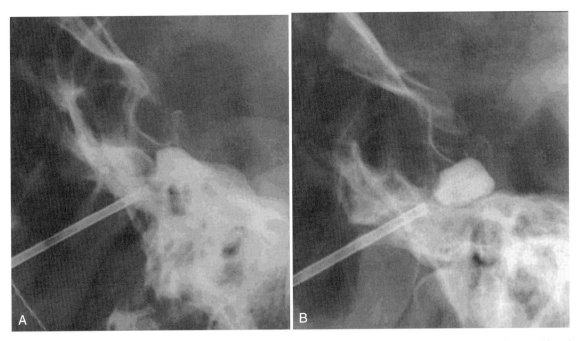

Fig. 145.13 A, Patient with a no. 4 Fogarty balloon maximally inflated for 2 minutes had failure to produce any facial hypesthesia, with early recurrence of pain 9 months later. **B,** Repeat balloon compression with a no. 5 Fogarty balloon for 1 minute with resultant perioral hypesthesia and no pain recurrence in 5 years. *(From Goerss SJ, Atkinson JLD, Kallmes DF: Variable size percutaneous balloon compression of the gasserian ganglion for trigeminal neuralgia,* Surg Neurol *2008. [Epub ahead of print.])*

References

Full references for this chapter can be found on www.expertconsult.com.

Chapter 146

Trigeminal Nerve Block

Steven D. Waldman

Indications and Contraindications

Blockade of the trigeminal nerve and its branches with local anesthetics, steroids, or neurolytic agents and destruction of these structures via freezing, radiofrequency lesioning, and other means have many applications in contemporary pain management. Technologic advances in radiographic imaging, electronics, and needle technology have improved the efficacy and decreased the cost, complications, and adverse side effects of these procedures.

The indications for blockade of the trigeminal nerve and its branches are summarized in **Table 146.1**. In addition to applications for surgical anesthesia, trigeminal nerve block with local anesthetic can be used as a diagnostic and prognostic maneuver in performance of differential neural blockade on an anatomic basis.[1] This technique can be used to treat trismus from tetanus and as an aid in awake endotracheal intubation.[2] Trigeminal nerve block with local anesthetic or steroids is an excellent adjunct to pharmacologic treatment of trigeminal neuralgia.[3] The use of this technique allows rapid palliation of pain while oral medications are being titrated to effective levels; it also may be valuable in patients with atypical facial pain.[4] Other indications for trigeminal nerve block with local anesthetic or steroids are acute pain from trauma, neoplasms of the head and face, cluster headaches refractory

to sphenopalatine ganglion block, and the pain of acute herpes zoster in the distribution of the trigeminal nerve that is not controlled with stellate ganglion block.[5,6]

Indications for destruction of the distal trigeminal nerve and its branches are similar to the indications for gasserian ganglion block.[2] Because more peripheral destruction of the trigeminal nerve results in lower incidences of unwanted motor and sensory disturbance than destruction of the gasserian ganglion (especially corneal anesthesia), this approach may be the preferred course when it is efficacious for the pain syndrome being treated.

Contraindications to blockade of the trigeminal nerve and its branches are as follows:

- Local infection
- Sepsis
- Disulfiram therapy (if alcohol is used)
- Significant behavioral abnormalities

Local infection and sepsis are absolute contraindications to all procedures.[2,7] Coagulopathy is a relative contraindication to blockade of the trigeminal nerve and its branches. Because of the desperation of many patients with aggressively invasive head and face malignant diseases, however, ethical and humanitarian considerations dictate the use of this procedure despite the increased risk of bleeding. If strong clinical

Table 146.1 Indications for Blockade of the Trigeminal Nerve and Its Branches	
Local Anesthetic Block	**Neurolytic Block or Neurodestructive Procedures**
Surgical anesthesia	Palliation of cancer pain
Anatomic differential neural blockade	Management of trigeminal neuralgia
Prognostic nerve block before neurodestructive procedures	Management of cluster headache
Treatment of trismus	
Aid to awake endotracheal intubation	
Palliation in acute pain emergencies	
Palliation of acute herpes zoster	

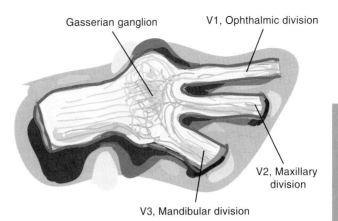

Fig. 146.1 **Gasserian ganglion and Meckel's cave.**

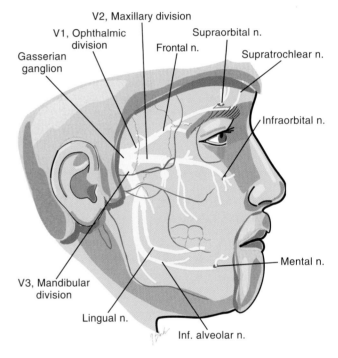

Fig. 146.2 **Trigeminal nerve and its branches.**

indications exist, blockade of the distal trigeminal nerve and its branches with a 25-gauge needle may be done in the presence of coagulopathy, albeit with increased risk of ecchymosis and hematoma formation.

Clinically Relevant Anatomy

Role of the Trigeminal System

The trigeminal nerve, the largest and the most complex of the cranial nerves, contains sensory and motor fibers.[8,9] Somatic afferent impulses carried by the trigeminal nerve transmit pain, light touch, and temperature sensation. Information is transmitted to the central nervous system via the trigeminal nerve from the skin of the face, the mucosal lining of the nose and mouth, the teeth, and the anterior two thirds of the tongue.[8] The trigeminal nerve also carries proprioceptive impulses and afferent impulses from stretch receptors of the teeth, oral mucosa, muscles of mastication, and temporomandibular joint to aid in mastication.

In addition to the sensory innervation just described, visceral efferent fibers help to innervate a variety of muscles of facial expression, the tensor tympani, and some muscles of mastication. Communications exist between the trigeminal nerve and the autonomic nervous system, including the ciliary, sphenopalatine, otic, and submaxillary ganglia and the oculomotor, facial, and glossopharyngeal nerves. Because of the complex nature of the trigeminal nerve, a thorough understanding of the clinically relevant anatomy is crucial to obtaining optimal results of neural blockade of these structures.

Gasserian Ganglion

The gasserian ganglion is formed from two roots that exit the ventral surface of the brainstem at the midpontine level (**Fig. 146.1**).[10] These roots pass in a forward and lateral direction in the posterior cranial fossa across the border of the petrous temporal bone. They enter a recess called Meckel's cave, which is formed by an invagination of the surrounding dura mater into the middle cranial fossa. The dural pouch that lies just behind the ganglion, called the trigeminal cistern, contains cerebrospinal fluid (CSF).

The gasserian ganglion is canoe shaped. Its three sensory divisions, the ophthalmic (V_1), maxillary (V_2), and mandibular (V_3) nerves, exit the anterior convex aspect of the ganglion. A smaller motor root joins the mandibular division as it exits the cranial cavity via the foramen ovale.

Ophthalmic Division

The ophthalmic branch, the smallest division of the trigeminal nerve, is purely sensory in function (**Fig. 146.2**).[11] It enters the orbit via the superior orbital fissure. The branch is divided into the frontal, nasociliary, and lacrimal nerves. The terminal cutaneous branches of the frontal nerve consist of the supraorbital and supratrochlear nerves. These terminal branches exit the orbital cavity anteriorly and provide innervation to the upper eyelid, forehead, and anterior scalp. The terminal cutaneous branches of the nasociliary nerve consist of the infratrochlear and external nasal branches, which provide cutaneous and mucosal innervation to the apex and ala of the nose and anterior nasal cavity. The lacrimal nerve continues, without additional major branches, to innervate the lacrimal gland and outer canthus of the eye.

Maxillary Division

The maxillary division is a pure sensory nerve. It exits the middle cranial fossa via the foramen rotundum and crosses the pterygopalatine fossa (**Fig. 146.3**).[8] Passing through the inferior orbital fissure, it enters the orbit, emerging on the face via the infraorbital foramen.

The branches of the maxillary nerve are divided into four regional groups. (1) The intracranial group includes the middle meningeal nerve, which innervates the dura mater of the medial cranial fossa. (2) The pterygopalatine group includes the zygomatic nerve, which provides sensory innervation to the temporal and lateral zygomatic region, and the sphenopalatine branches, which help to innervate the mucosa of the maxillary sinus, upper gums, upper molars, and mucous membranes of the cheek. (3) The infraorbital canal group comprises the anterior-superior alveolar branch, which innervates the incisors and canines, the anterior wall of the maxillary antrum, and the floor of the nasal cavity, and the middle superior branch, which supplies the premolars. (4) The infraorbital facial group consists of the inferior palpebral branch, which innervates the conjunctiva and skin of the lower eyelid; the external nasal branch, which supplies the side of the nose; and the superior labial branch, which supplies the skin of the upper lip and part of the oral mucosa (see Fig. 146.2).

Mandibular Division

The large sensory root and smaller motor root of the mandibular division leave the middle cranial fossa together via the foramen ovale.[8] They join to form the mandibular nerve (see Fig. 146.3). This combined trunk gives off two branches: the nervus spinosus, which runs superiorly with the middle meningeal artery through the foramen spinosum to supply the dura mater and the mucosal lining of the mastoid sinus, and the internal pterygoid, which supplies the internal pterygoid and gives off branches to the otic ganglion. The mandibular nerve divides into a small anterior and a large posterior trunk (see Fig. 146.2).

Branches from the small anterior trunk are the buccinator nerve, which is purely sensory and innervates the skin and mucous membrane overlying the anterior portion of the buccinator muscle; the masseteric nerve, which provides motor innervation to the masseter muscle; the deep temporal nerves, which provide motor innervation to the temporalis muscle; and the external pterygoid nerve, which provides motor innervation to the external pterygoid muscle. The large posterior trunk comprises primarily sensory fibers but also contains a few motor fibers. Branches of the posterior trunk are the auriculotemporal nerve, which provides innervation to skin anterior to the tragus and helix, lining of the acoustic meatus, tympanic membrane, posterior temporomandibular joint, parotid gland, and skin of the temporal region; the lingual nerve, which provides sensory innervation to the dorsum and lateral aspects of the anterior two thirds of the tongue and the lateral mucous membranes of the mouth and the sublingual gland; and the inferior alveolar nerve, which provides sensory innervation to the lower teeth and mandible. The terminal branch of the inferior alveolar nerve, the mental nerve, exits the mandible via the mental foramen and provides sensory innervation to the chin and to the skin and mucous membrane of the lower lip.

Technique of Blockade of the Maxillary and Mandibular Divisions of the Trigeminal Nerve via the Coronoid Approach

The patient is placed in the supine position. The coronoid notch is palpated with the patient opening and closing the mouth several times. The level of the coronoid notch is at the external auditory meatus (**Figs. 146.4** and **146.5**). After the notch is identified, the patient is asked to hold the mouth in the neutral position.[2,8]

A 3.5-inch 22-gauge styletted spinal needle is inserted just beneath the zygomatic arch, at the mid point of the coronoid notch (**Fig. 146.6**). The needle is advanced approximately 1.5 to 2 inches perpendicular to the base of the skull, until the lateral

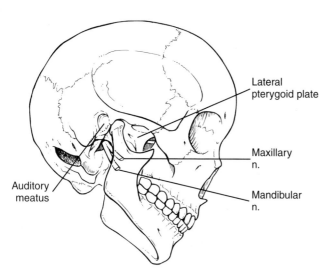

Fig. 146.3 **Major branches of the trigeminal nerve.**

Lateral pterygoid plate

Maxillary n.

Mandibular n.

Auditory meatus

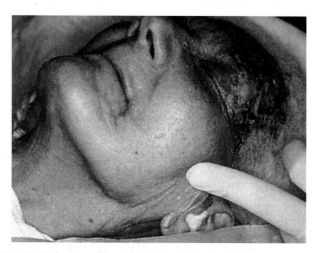

Fig. 146.4 **Palpation of the coronoid notch.** (*From Waldman SD:* Interventional pain management, *ed 2, Philadelphia, 2001, Saunders, p 323.*)

pterygoid plate is encountered (**Fig. 146.7**). At this point, if maxillary and mandibular nerve blocks are desired, the needle is withdrawn approximately 1 mm. After careful aspiration for blood, 7 to 10 mL of preservative-free local anesthetic is injected in small increments (**Fig. 146.8**).[2] During the injection procedure, the patient must be observed carefully for signs of local anesthetic toxicity. For selective maxillary nerve block, the styletted spinal needle is withdrawn and reinserted to slip just above the anterior margin of the lateral pterygoid plate (**Fig. 146.9**).[2] A maxillary paresthesia generally is produced approximately 1 cm deeper than the level at which the pterygoid plate was first encountered. After careful aspiration, 3 to 5 mL of preservative-free local anesthetic may be injected in increments.

If selective blockade of the mandibular division of the trigeminal nerve is desired, the lateral pterygoid plate is identified, and the needle is withdrawn and directed slightly farther posteriorly and inferiorly. A paresthesia in the mandibular distribution is elicited in most cases (**Fig. 146.10**).[2] After careful aspiration, 3 to 5 mL of preservative-free local anesthetic is injected in incremental doses.

For diagnostic and prognostic blocks, 1% preservative-free lidocaine is a suitable local anesthetic.[12] For therapeutic blocks, 0.5% preservative-free bupivacaine in combination with 80 mg of depot methylprednisolone (Depo-Medrol) is injected.[2] Subsequent daily nerve blocks are done in a similar manner, substituting 40 mg of methylprednisolone for the initial 80-mg dose. Five to six trigeminal nerve blocks daily may be necessary to treat the painful conditions listed

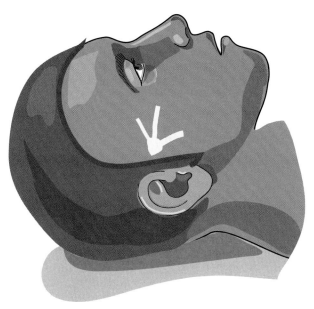

Fig. 146.5 **Patient position for maxillary and mandibular nerve block.**

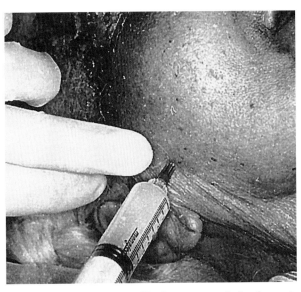

Fig. 146.7 **Needle tip positioned in the pterygopalatine fossa.** *(From Waldman SD: Interventional pain management, ed 2, Philadelphia, 2001, Saunders, p 324.)*

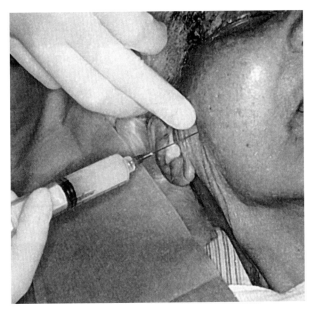

Fig. 146.6 **Correct needle position for the trigeminal nerve block via the coronoid notch.** *(From Waldman SD: Atlas of interventional pain management, ed 3, Philadelphia, 2009, Saunders, p 49.)*

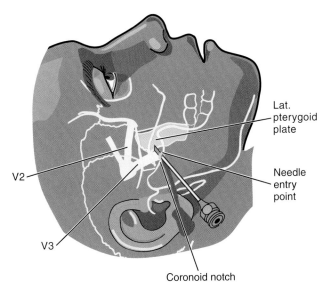

Fig. 146.8 **Correct needle placement for nonselective trigeminal nerve block via the coronoid approach.**

previously.[4] If selective neurolytic block of the mandibular or maxillary nerve is desired, incremental 0.1-mL injections of sterile glycerol, 6.5% phenol in glycerin, or alcohol to a total volume of 1 mL may be used after adequate pain relief with local anesthetic blocks is confirmed.[13]

Practical Considerations

The pterygopalatine space is densely vascular. The possibility of intravascular uptake of local anesthetic is significant with this nerve block. Careful aspiration of blood and incremental dosage with local anesthetic are important to allow early detection of local anesthetic toxicity. Careful observation of the patient during and after the nerve block is mandatory.[2]

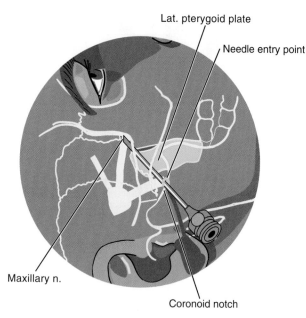

Fig. 146.9 **Selective maxillary nerve block.**

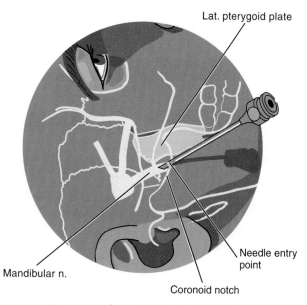

Fig. 146.10 **Selective mandibular nerve block.**

Technique of Neural Blockade of the Supraorbital and Supratrochlear Branches of the Ophthalmic Division of the Trigeminal Nerve

The patient is placed supine with the head in neutral position. The supraorbital notch is identified with palpation. The skin is prepared with povidone-iodine solution, with care taken to avoid spilling solution into the eye.

A 1.5-inch 25-gauge needle is advanced perpendicularly to the skin at the level of the supraorbital notch. To anesthetize the peripheral branches of the nerve, 3 to 4 mL of preservative-free local anesthetic is injected in a fanlike configuration (**Fig. 146.11**).[14] To block the supratrochlear nerve, the needle is directed medially from the supraorbital notch toward the apex of the nose.[8] Paresthesias are occasionally elicited.[7] If neurolytic block of the supraorbital and supratrochlear branches is desired, incremental 0.1-mL injections of sterile glycerol or 6.5% phenol in glycerin, to a total volume of 0.5 mL, may be used after adequate pain relief with local anesthetic blocks is confirmed.[13]

Practical Considerations

Because of the loose alveolar tissue of the eyelid, a gauze sponge should be used to apply gentle pressure on the eyelids and supraorbital tissues to keep the local anesthetic from dissecting into the eyelid and supraorbital tissues. This pressure is maintained after the nerve block to avoid periorbital hematoma and ecchymosis.

Technique of Neural Blockade of the Infraorbital Branch of the Maxillary Nerve

Intraoral Approach

The upper lip is folded backward, and a cotton ball soaked with 10% cocaine solution or 2% viscous lidocaine is placed in the alveolar ridge, just inferior to the intraorbital foramen

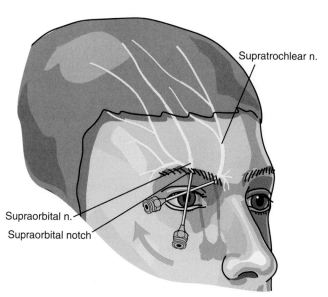

Fig. 146.11 **Supraorbital and supratrochlear block.**

(**Fig. 146.12**). After adequate topical anesthesia is obtained, a 1.5-inch 25-gauge needle is advanced through the anesthetized area superiorly toward the infraorbital foramen.[2] A paresthesia may be elicited.[2] After careful aspiration, 2 to 3 mL of preservative-free local anesthetic is injected.[3] If neurolytic block of the infraorbital nerve is desired, incremental 0.1-mL injections of sterile glycerol or 6.5% phenol in glycerin may be used after adequate pain relief with local anesthetic block is confirmed.[3]

Practical Considerations

As with the supraorbital nerve block, pressure over the inferior periorbital tissues limits dissection of the local anesthetic superiorly into the periorbital region and avoids ecchymosis and hematoma formation. The intraoral route is particularly suited to pediatric patients.

Extraoral Approach

The infraorbital ridge of the maxillary bone is identified, and the infraorbital foramen is palpated. The skin is prepared with povidone-iodine solution, with care taken to avoid spillage of the solution into the eye. A 0.5-inch 25-gauge needle is advanced at a 45-degree angle toward the foramen (see Fig. 146.12).[15] A paresthesia may be elicited. After careful aspiration of blood, 2 to 3 mL of preservative-free local anesthetic is injected. Percutaneous neurolytic block of the infraorbital nerve is performed as for the intraoral route.

Practical Considerations

Similar to the intraoral approach, pressure must be applied to the infraorbital tissues to avoid dissection of local anesthetic. When the infraorbital branch is blocked with the extraoral approach, if the needle enters the infraorbital foramen, it should be withdrawn to avoid hematoma, injection-induced compressive neuropathy, and damage to the contents of the orbit.

Technique of Neural Blockade of the Mental Branch of the Mandibular Nerve

Intraoral Approach

The lower lip is pulled downward and away from the face. A cotton ball soaked in 10% cocaine or 2% viscous lidocaine is placed in the alveolar ridge against the mucosa, just superior to the mental foramen.[2] After topical anesthesia is obtained, a 0.5-inch 25-gauge needle is advanced via the anesthetized area in a perpendicular plane (**Fig. 146.13**). Paresthesia occasionally develops. After careful aspiration of blood, 2 to 3 mL of preservative-free bupivacaine is injected.[2] If neurolytic block of the mental nerve is desired, successive 0.1-mL injections of sterile glycerol or 6.5% phenol in glycerin may be used after adequate pain relief with local anesthetic blocks is confirmed.

Extraoral Approach

An area approximately 2 cm from the midline in a plane parallel with the supraorbital and infraorbital foramina is identified. Careful palpation generally allows identification of the mental foramen. The skin is prepared with povidone-iodine solution. A 0.5-inch 25-gauge needle is advanced toward the foramen (see Fig. 146.13).[16] If the needle enters the mental foramen, it should be withdrawn to avoid injection-induced compressive neuropathy. After careful aspiration of blood, 2 to 3 mL of

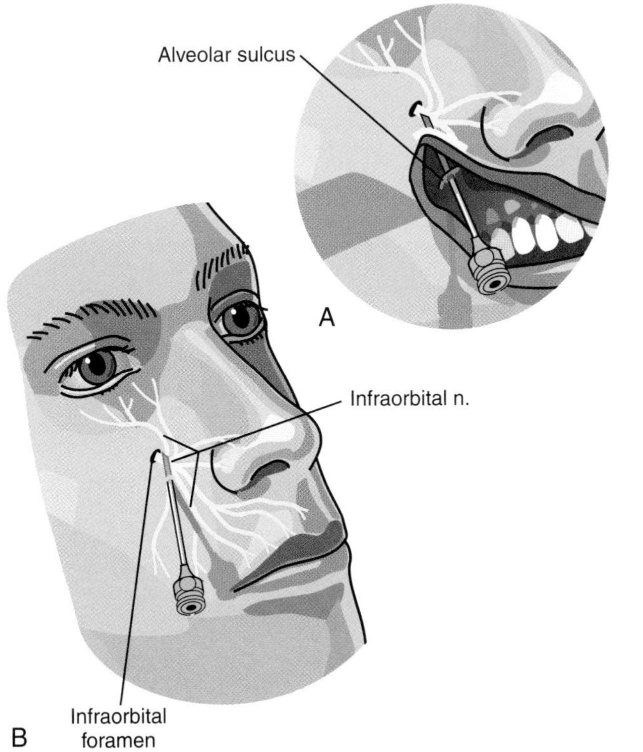

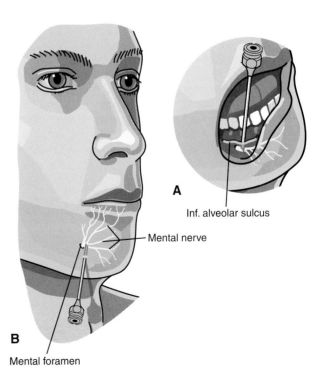

Fig. 146.12 **Approaches to infraorbital nerve block.** A, Intraoral; and B, extraoral.

Fig. 146.13 **Mental nerve block.** A, Intraoral approach. B, Extraoral approach.

preservative-free local anesthetic is injected. If neurolytic block of the mental nerve is desired, incremental 0.1-mL injections of sterile glycerol or 6.5% phenol in glycerin, to a total volume of 0.5 mL, may be given after adequate pain relief with local anesthetic blocks is confirmed.

Practical Considerations

Because of the acute angle at which the mental branch exits the mental foramen, it is susceptible to compression neuropathy. For this reason, it is advisable to avoid advancing the needle into the canal because theoretically hematoma formation or increased pressure during injection can cause compression neuropathy.

Complications and Unwanted Side Effects

The potential complications and unwanted side effects of blockade of the trigeminal nerve and its branches are as follows:

- Activation of herpes labialis and herpes zoster
- Postprocedure dysesthesias, including anesthesia dolorosa
- Abnormal motor function, including weakness
- Facial asymmetry
- Horner's syndrome
- Facial ecchymosis and hematoma
- Ocular subscleral hematoma
- Local anesthetic toxicity
- Trauma to nerves
- Infection
- Sloughing of skin and subcutaneous tissue

Although it is associated more often with procedures involving the gasserian ganglion, blockade of the trigeminal nerve and its branches may activate herpes labialis and occasionally herpes zoster in the distribution of the trigeminal nerve.

A few patients who undergo chemical neurolysis or neurodestructive procedures of the trigeminal nerve and its branches have postprocedure dysesthesias in the area of anesthesia.[17] These symptoms range from mild, uncomfortable burning or pulling sensations to severe pain. Severe postprocedure pain, called anesthesia dolorosa, may be worse than the patient's original pain symptom and often is harder to treat. Sloughing of skin and subcutaneous tissue has been associated with anesthesia dolorosa.

In addition to disturbances of sensation, neurolytic block or neurodestructive procedures of the trigeminal nerve and its branches may result in abnormal motor function, including weakness of the muscles of mastication and facial asymmetry from weakness and altered proprioception.[13] Horner's syndrome also may occur from block of the paratrigeminal sympathetic fibers.

Because of the vascular nature of the pterygopalatine space, facial ecchymosis, and hematoma, including ocular subscleral hematoma, are common.[8,18] Although generally not harmful, these unwanted side effects are distressing to the patient, so each patient should be forewarned of the possibility before the procedure. The vascularity of this anatomic region also increases the potential for local anesthetic toxicity.[18]

The terminal branches of the trigeminal nerve are susceptible to trauma from needle, hematoma, and compression during injection procedures.[2] These complications, although usually transitory, can be quite upsetting to the patient. Infection, although also uncommon, is always a possibility, especially in cancer patients with immunocompromise. Early detection of infection is crucial to avoid potentially life-threatening sequelae.

Future Directions

Continuing advances in the understanding of the basic science of pain will improve management of patients with pain. Research on the serotoninergic system and its role in the pathogenesis of headache has led to the development of a whole new class of drugs that have revolutionized the way clinicians manage acute migraine and cluster headache.[19] The search for safer local anesthetics yielded ropivacaine, which seems to have less cardiotoxicity than bupivacaine.[20] In view of the relatively high incidence rate of local anesthetic toxicity associated with this technique, such a characteristic would offer a great advantage for neural blockade of the trigeminal system. Microencapsulation of local anesthetics with lecithin seems to increase the duration of action fourfold; this advance would be beneficial for trigeminal nerve block when the lesion responsible for the pain is self limited.

References

Full references for this chapter can be found on www.expertconsult.com.

Glossopharyngeal Nerve Block

Steven D. Waldman

Historical Considerations

The early use of glossopharyngeal nerve block in pain management centered around two applications: (1) the treatment of glossopharyngeal neuralgia; and (2) the palliation of pain from head and neck malignant diseases. In the late 1950s, the clinical use of glossopharyngeal nerve block as an adjunct to awake endotracheal intubation was documented.

Weisenburg[1] first described pain in the distribution of the glossopharyngeal nerve in a patient with a cerebellopontine angle tumor in 1910. In 1921, Harris[2] reported the first idiopathic case and coined the term *glossopharyngeal neuralgia*. He suggested that blockade of the glossopharyngeal nerve might be useful in palliating this painful condition.

Early attempts at permanent treatment of glossopharyngeal neuralgia and cancer pain in the distribution of the glossopharyngeal nerve consisted principally of extracranial surgical section or alcohol neurolysis of the glossopharyngeal nerve.[3] These approaches met with limited success in the treatment of glossopharyngeal neuralgia but were useful in some patients who had cancer pain mediated via the glossopharyngeal nerve. Intracranial section of the glossopharyngeal nerve was first performed by Adson in 1925 and was subsequently refined by Dandy. The intracranial approach to section of the glossopharyngeal nerve appeared to yield better results for both glossopharyngeal neuralgia and cancer pain but was a much riskier procedure.[4] Recently, interest in extracranial destruction of the glossopharyngeal nerve with glycerol or with creation of a radiofrequency lesion has been renewed.

Indications and Contraindications

Indications for glossopharyngeal nerve block are summarized in **Table 147.1.** In addition to applications for surgical anesthesia, glossopharyngeal nerve block with local anesthetics can be used as a diagnostic tool when performing differential neural blockade on an anatomic basis in the evaluation of head and facial pain.[5] Glossopharyngeal nerve block is used to help differentiate geniculate ganglion neuralgia from glossopharyngeal neuralgia. If destruction of the glossopharyngeal nerve is being considered, this technique is useful as an indicator of the extent of motor and sensory impairment that the patient will likely experience.[6] Glossopharyngeal nerve block with local anesthetic may be used to palliate acute pain emergencies, including glossopharyngeal neuralgia and cancer pain, until pharmacologic, surgical, and antiblastic methods take effect.[7] This technique is also useful for atypical facial pain in the distribution of the glossopharyngeal nerve[8] and as an adjunct for awake endotracheal intubation.[9]

Destruction of the glossopharyngeal nerve is indicated in the palliation of cancer pain, including invasive tumors of the posterior tongue, hypopharynx, and tonsils.[10] This technique is useful in the management of the pain of glossopharyngeal neuralgia for those patients with failure to respond to medical management or those who are not candidates for surgical microvascular decompression.[11]

Contraindications to blockade of the glossopharyngeal nerve are summarized in **Table 147.2.** Local infection and sepsis are absolute contraindications to all procedures. Coagulopathy is a strong contraindication to glossopharyngeal nerve block, but because of the desperate nature of many patients with invasive head and face malignant diseases, ethical and humanitarian considerations dictate its use, despite the risk of bleeding. When clinical indications are compelling, blockade of the glossopharyngeal nerve with a 22-gauge needle may be carried out in the presence of coagulopathy, albeit with increased risk of ecchymosis and hematoma formation.

Table 147.1 Indications for Glossopharyngeal Nerve Block
Local anesthetic block
Surgical anesthesia
Anatomic differential neural blockade
Prognostic nerve block before neurodestructive procedures
Acute pain emergencies (palliation)
Adjunct to awake intubation
Neurolytic block or neurodestructive procedure
Cancer pain (palliation)
Management of glossopharyngeal neuralgia

Table 147.2 Contraindications to Glossopharyngeal Nerve Block
Local infection
Sepsis
Coagulopathy
Disulfiram therapy (if alcohol is used)
Significant behavioral abnormalities

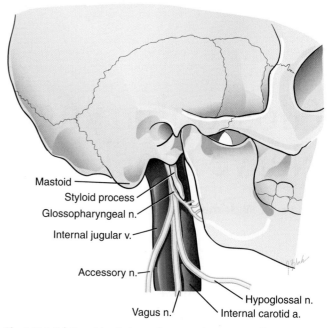

Fig. 147.1 **Relationship of glossopharyngeal, vagus, and hypoglossal nerves to artery and vein in context with skull and mandible.** *(From Waldman SD: Atlas of interventional pain management, ed 3, Philadelphia, 2009, Saunders, p 94.)*

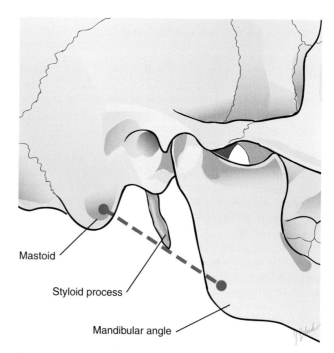

Fig. 147.2 **Close-up view of the line from mastoid to styloid.** *(From Waldman SD: Atlas of interventional pain management, ed 3, Philadelphia, 2009, Saunders, p 94.)*

Clinically Relevant Anatomy

The glossopharyngeal nerve contains both motor and sensory fibers.[10] The motor fibers innervate the stylopharyngeus muscle. The sensory portion of the nerve innervates the posterior third of the tongue, the palatine tonsil, and the mucous membranes of the mouth and pharynx. Special visceral afferent sensory fibers transmit information from the taste buds of the posterior third of the tongue. Information from the carotid sinus and body, which help to control blood pressure, pulse, and respiration, is carried via the carotid sinus nerve, a branch of the glossopharyngeal nerve.[10] Parasympathetic fibers pass via the glossopharyngeal nerve to the otic ganglion. Postganglionic fibers from the ganglion carry secretory information to the parotid gland.[12]

The glossopharyngeal nerve exits the jugular foramen near the vagus and accessory nerves and the internal jugular vein.[13] All three nerves lie in the groove between the internal jugular vein and internal carotid artery (**Fig. 147.1**). Inadvertent puncture of either vessel during glossopharyngeal nerve block can result in intravascular injection or hematoma formation. Even small amounts of local anesthetic injected into the carotid artery at this site can produce profound local anesthetic toxicity.[11]

One landmark for glossopharyngeal nerve block is the styloid process of the temporal bone. This structure is the calcification of the cephalad end of the stylohyoid ligament. Although usually easy to identify, when ossification is limited, it may be difficult to locate with the exploring needle.

Technique

The Extraoral Approach

The patient is placed in the supine position. An imaginary line is visualized running from the mastoid process to the angle of the mandible (**Fig. 147.2**).[14] The styloid process should lie

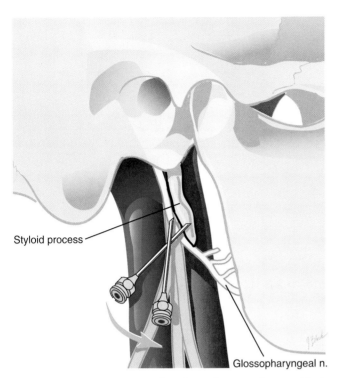

Fig. 147.3 Needle placement for glossopharyngeal nerve block. Needle is in contact with styloid process. Needle is redirected posteriorly to the glossopharyngeal nerve. *(From Waldman SD: Atlas of interventional pain management, ed 3, Philadelphia, 2009, Saunders, p 95.)*

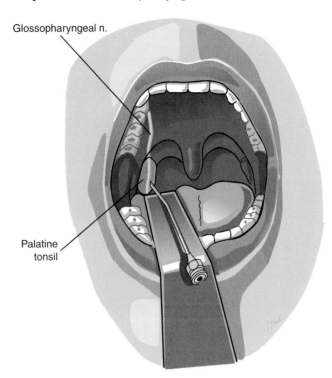

Fig. 147.4 Intraoral approach to glossopharyngeal nerve block. *(From Waldman SD: Atlas of interventional pain management, ed 3, Philadelphia, 2009, Saunders, p 98.)*

just below the midpoint of this line. The skin is prepared with antiseptic solution. A 22-gauge, 1.5-inch needle attached to a 10-mL syringe is advanced at this midpoint location in a plane perpendicular to the skin (**Fig. 147.3**). The styloid process should be encountered within 3 cm. After contact is made, the needle is withdrawn and walked off the styloid process posteriorly. As soon as bony contact is lost and careful aspiration reveals no blood or cerebrospinal fluid, 7 mL of 0.5% preservative-free lidocaine combined with 80 mg of methylprednisolone is injected in incremental doses. Subsequently, daily nerve blocks are performed in the same manner but substituting 40 mg of methylprednisolone for the first 80-mg dose. This approach may also be used for breakthrough pain in patients who previously experienced adequate pain control with oral medications.[11]

The Intraoral Approach

The tongue is anesthetized with 2.0% viscous lidocaine. With the patient's mouth open wide, the tongue is retracted downward with a tongue depressor or laryngoscope blade (**Fig. 147.4**). A 22-gauge, 3.5-inch spinal needle that has been bent approximately 130 degrees is inserted through the mucosa at the lower lateral portion of the posterior tonsillar pillar. The needle is advanced approximately 0.5 cm. After careful aspiration for blood and cerebrospinal fluid, local anesthetic or steroid, or both, is injected in a manner like that for the extraoral approach to glossopharyngeal nerve block.

Table 147.3 Complications and Unwanted Side Effects of Blockade of the Glossopharyngeal Nerve
Dysphagia
Ecchymosis and hematoma
Postprocedure dysesthesias
Anesthesia dolorosa
Weakness of trapezius muscle
Weakness of tongue
Hoarseness
Infection
Tachycardia
Local anesthetic toxicity
Trauma to nerves
Sloughing of skin and subcutaneous tissue

Potential Complications of Glossopharyngeal Nerve Block

The major complications associated with glossopharyngeal nerve block (**Table 147.3**) are related to trauma to the internal jugular and carotid artery.[10] Hematoma formation and intravascular injection of local anesthetic with subsequent toxicity are significant problems for the patient. Blockade of the motor portion of the glossopharyngeal nerve can result in dysphagia

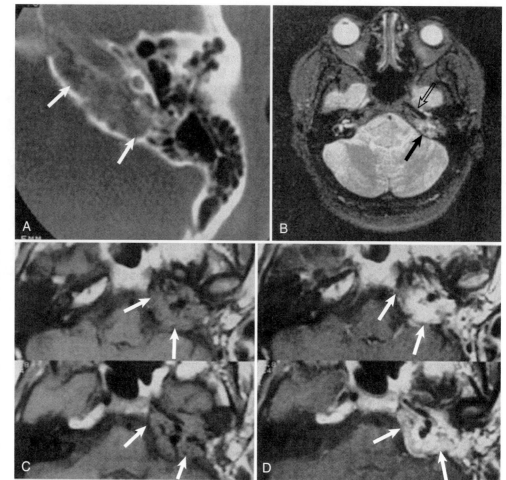

Fig. 147.5 Glomus jugulare. **A,** Computed tomographic (CT) scan shows extension of a glomus jugulare into the petrous bone *(arrows).* **B,** Axial T2-weighted magnetic resonance (MR) scan shows the tumor *(solid arrow)* and petrous portion of the internal carotid artery *(open arrow)* axial before contrast **(C)** and after contrast **(D)** MR scans showing the tumor *(arrows).* *(From Mafee MF, Raofi B, Kumar A, et al: Glomus faciale, glomus jugulare, glomus tympanicum, glomus vagale, carotid body tumors, and simulating lesions: role of MR imaging,* Radiologic Clin North Am *38:1059, 2000.)*

from weakness of the stylopharyngeus muscle.[9] If the vagus nerve is inadvertently blocked, as it often is during glossopharyngeal nerve block, dysphonia from paralysis of the ipsilateral vocal cord may occur. Reflex tachycardia from vagal nerve block is also observed in some patients.[10] Inadvertent block of the hypoglossal and spinal accessory nerves during glossopharyngeal nerve block results in weakness of the tongue and trapezius muscle.[15]

A small percentage of patients who undergo chemical neurolysis or neurodestructive procedures of the glossopharyngeal nerve experience postprocedure dysesthesias in the area of anesthesia.[16] These symptoms range from a mildly uncomfortable burning or pulling sensation to severe pain. Such severe postprocedure pain is called anesthesia dolorosa. Anesthesia dolorosa can be worse than the patient's original pain and is often harder to treat. Sloughing of skin and subcutaneous tissue has been associated with anesthesia dolorosa.

The glossopharyngeal nerve is susceptible to trauma from needle, hematoma, or compression during injection procedures. Such complications, although usually transitory, can be quite upsetting to the patient. Although uncommon, risk of infection is ever present, especially in cancer patients with immunocompromise.[6] Early detection of infection is crucial to avoid potentially life-threatening sequelae.

Neurodestructive Procedures

The injection of small quantities of alcohol, phenol, and glycerol into the area of the glossopharyngeal nerve often provides long-term relief from glossopharyngeal neuralgia and cancer-related pain that has been refractory to optimal trials of the therapies discussed previously (**Fig. 147.5**).[10,13] Destruction of the glossopharyngeal nerve can be carried out by creating a radiofrequency lesion with biplanar fluoroscopic guidance (**Fig. 147.6**).[17] This procedure is reserved for patients in whom all the treatments discussed here for intractable glossopharyngeal neuralgia have failed and whose physical status precludes more invasive neurosurgical treatments.

Microvascular Decompression of the Glossopharyngeal Root

Microvascular decompression of the glossopharyngeal root (Jannetta procedure) is the neurosurgical procedure of choice for intractable glossopharyngeal neuralgia.[18] The rationale for this operation is the theory that glossopharyngeal neuralgia is, in fact, a compressive mononeuropathy that results from a aberrant vascular loop (**Fig. 147.7**). In this operation, the glossopharyngeal root is identified close to the brainstem, and

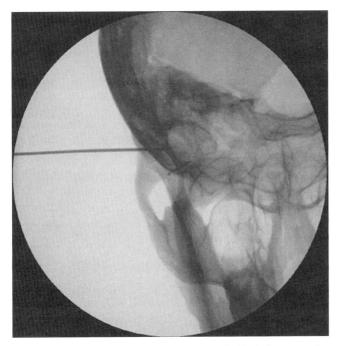

Fig. 147.6 **AP view of the needle tip just behind the posterior aspect of the styloid process.**

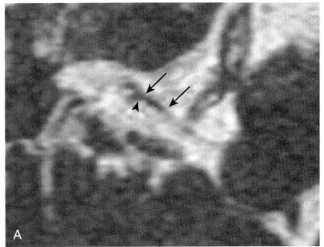

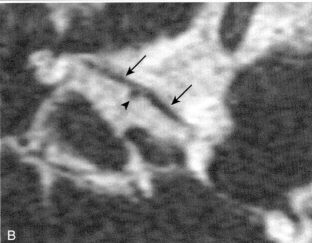

Fig. 147.7 Constructive interference in steady state (CISS) MR image successfully delineates anatomic relationship between vagoglossopharyngeal nerve root and vascular loop. A, A vascular loop *(arrowhead)* is in contact with upper vagal nerve root *(arrows).* B, Glossopharyngeal nerve root *(arrows)* is deformed by a vascular loop compression *(arrowhead). (From Karibe H, Shirane R, Yoshimoto T: Preoperative visualization of microvascular compression of cranial nerve IX using constructive interference in steady state magnetic resonance imaging in glossopharyngeal neuralgia, J Clin Neurosci 11:679, 2004.)*

the compressing blood vessel is isolated. A sponge is interposed between the vessel and nerve, affecting a cure. Intracranial section of the glossopharyngeal nerve is indicated for intractable cancer pain in the distribution of the glossopharyngeal nerve that does not respond to more conservative treatment approaches.[10]

Conclusion

The pain specialist should be aware of the clinical utility of glossopharyngeal nerve block. Correctly used, pharmacologic therapy combined with glossopharyngeal nerve block should control the pain of glossopharyngeal neuralgia and cancer-related pain in the distribution of the glossopharyngeal nerve in most cases. Surgical therapy should be considered when conservative therapy fails to provide long-lasting relief from pain mediated via the glossopharyngeal nerve.

References

Full references for this chapter can be found on www.expertconsult.com.

Chapter **148**

Vagus Nerve Block

Steven D. Waldman

Historical Considerations

Early in the history of regional anesthesia, vagus nerve block was used to treat a variety of conditions that included both pain and cardiac arrhythmias. Often combined with stellate ganglion block, blockade of the vagus nerve was a mainstay in the treatment of intractable angina and pain emanating from the esophagus, trachea, and other mediastinal structures.[1] Many of the early indications for vagus nerve block now are treated medically or surgically, but vagus nerve block remains useful for management of cancer pain in structures innervated by this nerve.

Indications

Vagus nerve block with local anesthetics can be used as a diagnostic tool when performing differential neural blockade on an anatomic basis to evaluate head and facial pain.[2] When destruction of the vagus nerve is being considered, this technique is a useful indicator of the degree of motor and sensory impairment the patient may experience. Vagus nerve block with local anesthetic can be used to palliate acute pain emergencies, including vagal neuralgia and cancer pain, while waiting for pharmacologic, surgical, or antiblastic methods to take effect.[3] Vagus nerve block is used as a diagnostic and therapeutic maneuver when vagal neuralgia is suspected. Destruction of the vagus nerve is indicated for palliation of cancer pain, including that associated with invasive tumors of the larynx, hypopharynx, and pyriform sinus and, occasionally, intrathoracic malignant diseases.[3,4]

Because of the desperate situation of many patients with aggressive head and neck malignant diseases, blockade of the vagus nerve with a 25-gauge needle may be carried out in the presence of coagulopathy or anticoagulation, albeit with increased risks of ecchymosis and hematoma formation.

Clinically Relevant Anatomy

The vagus nerve contains both motor and sensory fibers.[5] The motor fibers innervate the pharyngeal muscle and provide fibers for the superior and recurrent laryngeal nerves.

The sensory portion of the nerve innervates the dura mater of the posterior fossa, the posterior aspect of the external auditory meatus, the inferior aspect of the tympanic membrane, and the mucosa of the larynx below the vocal cords. The vagus nerve also provides fibers to the thoracic contents, including the heart, lungs, and major vessels.

The vagus nerve exits from the jugular foramen close to the spinal accessory nerve (**Fig. 148.1**). The vagus lies just caudal to the glossopharyngeal nerve and is superficial to the internal jugular vein. The vagus courses downward from the jugular foramen within the carotid sheath along with the internal jugular vein and internal carotid artery.

The technique of blockade of the vagus nerve is much like that of glossopharyngeal nerve block.[3] The key landmark for vagus nerve block is the styloid process of the temporal bone. This osseous process represents the calcification of the cephalad end of the stylohyoid ligament. Although usually easy to identify, if ossification is limited, the styloid process may be difficult to locate with the exploring needle.

Technique

The patient is placed in the supine position. An imaginary line is visualized running from the mastoid process to the angle of the mandible. The styloid process should lie just below the midpoint of this line. The skin is prepared with antiseptic solution. A 22-gauge, 1.5-inch needle attached to a 10-mL syringe is advanced at this midpoint in a plane perpendicular to the skin. The styloid process should be encountered within 3 cm (**Fig. 148.2**). After contact is made, the needle is withdrawn and "walked" off the styloid process posteriorly and slightly downward. The needle is advanced approximately 0.5 cm past the depth at which the styloid process was identified (**Fig. 148.3**). If careful aspiration reveals no blood or cerebrospinal fluid, 5 mL of 0.5% preservative-free lidocaine combined with 80 mg of methylprednisolone is injected in incremental doses. Subsequent daily nerve blocks are carried out in a similar manner, substituting 40 mg of methylprednisolone for the initial 80-mg dose. This approach may also be used for breakthrough pain in patients who previously experienced adequate pain control with oral medications.

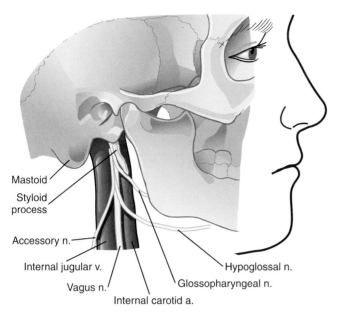

Fig. 148.1 **The vagus nerve and surrounding structures.**

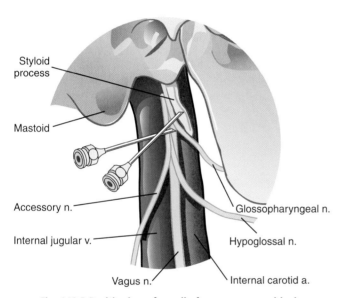

Fig. 148.2 **Positioning of needle for vagus nerve block.**

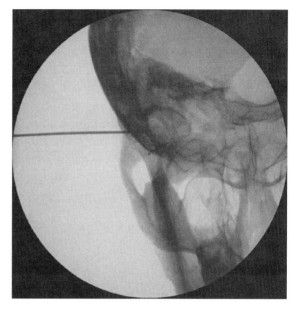

Fig. 148.3 **Needle tip just behind the posterior aspect of the styloid process in proximity to the vagus nerve.**

Side Effects and Complications

The major complications of vagus nerve block are related to trauma to the internal jugular and carotid arteries.[2,3] Hematoma formation and intravascular injection of local anesthetic (with subsequent toxicity) are not uncommon after vagus nerve block. Blockade of the motor portion of the vagus nerve can result in dysphonia and difficulty coughing from blockade of the superior and recurrent laryngeal nerves. Reflex tachycardia from vagal nerve block is also observed in some patients. Inadvertent block of the glossopharyngeal, hypoglossal, and spinal accessory nerves during vagus nerve block results in weakness of the tongue and trapezius muscle and numbness in the distribution of the glossopharyngeal nerve. Although uncommon, the risk of infection is ever present, especially in cancer patients with immunocompromise. Early detection of infection is crucial to avoid potentially life-threatening sequelae.

Clinical Pearls

Vagus nerve block should be considered in two clinical situations: (1) for vagal neuralgia; and (2) for persistent, ill-defined pain related to the cancers discussed previously that fails to respond to conservative measures. Vagal neuralgia is clinically analogous to trigeminal and glossopharyngeal neuralgia. It is characterized by paroxysms of shock-like pain into the thyroid and laryngeal areas. Pain occasionally radiates into the jaw and upper thorax. Attacks of vagal neuralgia may be precipitated by coughing, yawning, or swallowing. Excessive salivation may be present. This is a rare pain syndrome that should be considered a diagnosis of exclusion.

Neurolytic block with small quantities of alcohol, phenol, or glycerol has been shown to provide long-term relief for patients with vagus neuralgia and cancer-related pain that does not respond to more conservative treatment. The vagus nerve can also be destroyed by creating a radiofrequency lesion with biplanar fluoroscopic guidance.

The proximity of the vagus nerve to major vessels makes postblock hematoma and ecchymosis distinct possibilities. Although these complications are usually transitory, they can be upsetting to the patient. Therefore, the patient should be warned of these possibilities before the procedure. The dense vascularity of this region also increases the likelihood of inadvertent intravascular injection. Even small amounts of local anesthetic injected into the carotid artery at this level result in local anesthetic toxicity and seizures. Incremental dosing and careful monitoring of the patient for signs of local anesthetic toxicity help to avoid these complications.

References

Full references for this chapter can be found on www.expertconsult.com.

Chapter 149

Phrenic Nerve Block

Mark A. Greenfield and Steven D. Waldman

The pain management consultant may be asked to evaluate a patient for phrenic nerve block. Blockade of the phrenic nerve, like other nerve blocks, is but one component of a multifaceted approach to the patient with acute or chronic pain syndromes. It may become a useful treatment modality for patients who have no response to other therapeutic interventions.

Clinical Anatomy

The phrenic nerve, the most important branch of the cervical plexus, comprises the ventral roots of C3-C5, the principal component being the anterior primary ramus of C4. The three nerve roots join at the lateral border of the scalenus anterior muscle, and the phrenic nerve passes inferiorly between the omohyoid and sternocleidomastoid muscles.[1] In 20% to 84% of patients, an accessory phrenic nerve arises from C5 and contributes to the phrenic nerve, joining the main nerve in the root of the neck or behind the clavicle. In the phrenic nerve's course distally, it lies close to the internal mammary artery, the root of the lung, the pericardium, and the peritoneum. The superior and inferior sympathetic ganglia, the spinal accessory nerve, and the hypoglossal nerve also have communications with the phrenic nerve as it courses through the chest.

Indications

Phrenic nerve block can be useful in the diagnosis and treatment of intractable singultus (Latin for *sob* or *speech broken by sobbing*), or hiccups. Hiccups, although ubiquitous, serve no known physiologic function. Persistent hiccups are defined as an episode that lasts less than 1 month; intractable hiccups last longer than 1 month. **Table 149.1** describes some of the complications of intractable hiccups.[2] Benign and persistent or intractable hiccups have different causes (**Table 149.2**).[3] Chronic idiopathic hiccups are believed to be attributable to central and peripheral mechanisms. Chronic hiccups have been suggested to result from chronic stimulation of a central nervous system "hiccup center." The afferent limb of the hiccup reflex includes not only the phrenic nerve but

also the vagus nerve and the sympathetic chain from T6-T12.[4] This hiccup center is believed to comprise a complex association between several areas of the central nervous system, including the phrenic nerve nuclei, the brainstem, the respiratory center, the hypothalamus, and the medullary reticular formation. The primary efferent limb of this reflex is mediated by motor fibers of the phrenic nerve. Interestingly, most hiccup spasms are unilateral and usually confined to the left hemidiaphragm.[5]

The ill-defined supraclavicular or scapular pain of diaphragmatic or subdiaphragmatic cancers may be elucidated or ameliorated by phrenic nerve block. This referred pain is known as the Kerr's sign and often does not respond to direct tumor treatments.[6]

The pain management specialist must try to establish an underlying cause to guide therapeutic intervention. A targeted history and physical examination are essential first steps, followed by laboratory studies. The workup should also include magnetic resonance imaging studies of the head, especially the posterior fossa and brainstem (**Fig. 149.1**).[2,7,8] Imaging of the diaphragmatic and subdiaphragmatic regions should also be performed.

After identification and treatment of underlying causes, different therapies may be entertained. In 1932, Mayo[9] said, in reference to the myriad remedies and treatments for hiccups, "The amount of knowledge on any subject such as this can be considered as being in inverse proportion to the number of different treatments suggested and tried for it." After nonpharmacologic, noninvasive therapies have been tried and found unsuccessful, drug therapy may be used. **Table 149.3** lists several medications that have been used in treatment of hiccups.[7,10–17]

Procedure

The patient is placed supine with the head turned away from the side being blocked and is then asked to lift his or her head against resistance for identification of the sternocleidomastoid muscle. The groove between the posterior border of the sternocleidomastoid muscle and the anterior scalene muscle then

Table 149.1 Complications of Intractable Hiccups

Malnutrition

Cardiac dysrhythmias

Insomnia

Fatigue, exhaustion, dehydration

Gastroesophageal reflux

Weight loss

Death

Table 149.2 Causes of Persistent or Intractable Hiccups

Idiopathic

Psychogenic

Conversion reaction

Malingering

Hysterical neurosis

Personality disorder

Organic

Central nervous system

Neoplasm

Multiple sclerosis

Cerebrovascular accident

Trauma

Parkinson's disease

Peripheral nervous system (from phrenic or vagus nerve irritation)

Renal (uremia) or hepatic disorders
Cancer (gastric, pancreatic, pulmonary)
Pericarditis
Intestinal obstruction, gastric distention
Tumors or cysts of neck
Hiatal hernia
Drug-induced, metabolic

Intravenous steroids

Benzodiazepines, barbiturates

General anesthesia

Infection (sepsis, malaria, tuberculosis, influenza)

Electrolyte disturbances (hypocalcemia, hyponatremia)

Table 149.3 Pharmacologic Management of Hiccups

Drug	Class	Action
Chlorpromazine	Phenothiazine	Central
Haloperidol		Central
Amitriptyline	Tricyclic antidepressant	Central
Diphenylhydantoin		Central
Valproic acid	Anticonvulsant	Central
Carbamazepine		Central
Baclofen	GABA mimetic	Central
Gabapentin	Anticonvulsant	Central
Oregablin	Anticonvulsant	Central
Nifedipine	Calcium channel blocker	Central, peripheral
Nimodipine		Central, peripheral
Metoclopramide	Dopamine antagonist	Gastric emptying
Midazolam	Benzodiazepine	Central
Omeprazole	Proton pump inhibitor	Suppresses gastric acid
Cisapride	Myenteric plexus activity	Facilitates gastric emptying
Amantadine	Antiviral	Unknown

becomes palpable (**Fig. 149.2**).[1,18] At a level 1 inch above the clavicle, sterile preparation is performed. A 22-gauge, 1.5-inch block needle is inserted parallel to the scalene muscle with a slightly anterior trajectory (**Fig. 149.3**). At a depth of approximately 1 inch, and after gentle aspiration for identification of blood or cerebrospinal fluid, 8 to 10 mL of local anesthetic is incrementally injected (infiltrated) along the anterior surface of the anterior scalene muscle. This nerve block is often done in a fan-like manner. Phrenic nerve block with local anesthetic may be used in a prognostic manner to evaluate the possibility of neurodestruction of the phrenic nerve with chemical neurolysis, cryoneurolysis, radiofrequency lesioning, phrenic nerve stimulation (diaphragmatic pacing), or surgical crushing of the nerve.[19] A depot steroid may be added to the local anesthetic for inflammation-associated pain that is mediated via the phrenic nerve.[1] A nerve stimulator with stimulation as low as 0.75 mA may be useful in this block for observation of diaphragmatic contraction (via fluoroscopy or ultrasound scan).[20] The patient is then monitored closely for changes in vital signs (especially signs of respiratory compromise) and signs of local anesthetic toxicity and inadvertent subarachnoid injection.

Side Effects and Complications

The proximity of several major blood vessels to the phrenic nerve may produce local anesthetic toxicity from intravascular uptake or inadvertent intravascular injection.[1,6] In addition, the vascularity of this region may result in hematoma or ecchymosis.[1,6] Although many of these vessels may be available via direct pressure to control bleeding, bleeding of the subclavian vessels may be difficult to control. Manual pressure to the area blocked and application of ice packs after the nerve block is performed decrease bleeding or ecchymosis. Ice packs applied at 20-minute intervals may also be useful in limiting these side effects or complications.[6]

With injection of the phrenic nerve, unilateral diaphragmatic paralysis is expected. Unilateral paralysis of the diaphragm

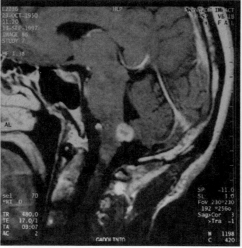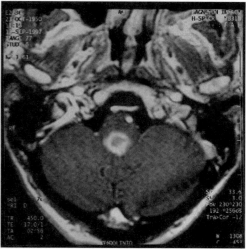

Fig. 149.1 Preoperative Magnetic resonance image. T1-weighted images on the sagittal *(left)* and axial *(right)* planes showing a well-circumscribed bleeding lesion in the dorsal aspect of the medulla oblongata, beneath the caudal floor of the fourth ventricle. *(From Musumeci A, Cristofori L, Bricolo A: Persistent hiccup as presenting symptom in medulla oblongata cavernoma: a case report and review of the literature,* Clin Neurol Neurosurg *102:13, 2000.)*

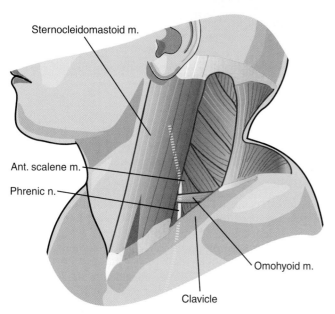
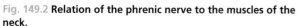

Fig. 149.2 **Relation of the phrenic nerve to the muscles of the neck.**

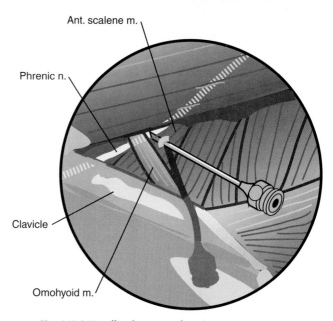

Fig. 149.3 **Needle placement for phrenic nerve block.**

may lead to a 37% reduction in total lung capacity. Maximal voluntary ventilation and vital capacity may be decreased by 20%.[21] This reduction in lung function may be exacerbated by spread of the local anesthetic solution to the recurrent laryngeal nerve and difficulty in clearing secretions as a result of vocal cord paralysis and associated hoarseness.

The phrenic nerve also lies close to central neuraxial structures. Should the needle be placed too deep, unintended subarachnoid or epidural block could result.[1] The consequences of either block could be significant sensory and motor block and marked respiratory compromise, or even cardiopulmonary arrest. Other possible complications of phrenic nerve block are infection and pneumothorax.[1,6] Horner's syndrome may be produced by spread of local anesthetic to the sympathetic ganglia. Left phrenic nerve block carries a risk of injury to the thoracic duct and, possibly, formation of a chylothorax.[1,6]

Conclusion

Phrenic nerve block is a useful diagnostic and therapeutic tool. The primary indications are chronic hiccups refractory to other nonpharmacologic and pharmacologic interventions. Phrenic nerve block may provide the pain management physician with useful information for the diagnosis and treatment of chronic shoulder or supraclavicular pain that is mediated by diaphragmatic or subdiaphragmatic processes. Careful attention to the clinically relevant anatomy should minimize side effects and complications and promote symptomatic relief.

References

Full references for this chapter can be found on www.expertconsult.com.

Cervical Plexus Block

John L. Pappas and Carol A. Warfield

History

Cervical plexus blocks were first performed by Halsted at Bellevue Hospital in New York in 1884.[1-3] Halsted performed many experiments with the new anesthetic cocaine, including an experiment showing that excellent surgical anesthesia could be obtained by injecting the nerve trunks in the neck. The first description of cervical plexus block for surgical anesthesia was published in Germany in 1912 by Kappis,[4] who advocated a posterior approach. Two years later, Heidenhein[5] introduced the lateral approach to cervical plexus block. These techniques were popularized in France by Pauchet and in the United States by Labat.[1]

The posterior approach has never achieved widespread acceptance except as an alternative to the lateral approach. Through the years, many modifications of the lateral approach have been described. Most modifications have altered the position of the primary line that connects the tip of the mastoid process to the anterior tubercle of C6. The change in position is intended to place the primary line more precisely over the tips of the cervical transverse processes.[2] Other methods of cervical plexus block have included a single-injection technique and a technique that uses the angle of the mandible and the thyroid notch as topographic landmarks to improve the success rate of the block.[1,3,6-8] The lateral and posterior approaches to cervical plexus blockade are described here.

Indications

Cervical plexus block has various indications. Because it can be performed easily in a supine patient, almost any patient is a candidate. Surgical procedures in the anterior and lateral neck and supraclavicular fossa can be performed using superficial or deep cervical plexus blocks.[3,7]

Superficial cervical plexus block provides surface anesthesia of the neck, but not muscle relaxation. Superficial cervical plexus block provides the same sensory (dermatome) anesthesia as deep cervical plexus block, which simply incorporates the motor component of the cervical plexus at the nerve roots before the sensory and motor aspects separate.[9] It is useful in procedures in which retraction of the major muscles of the neck is not required, such as cervical fat pad biopsy, lymph node biopsy, plastic procedures, and superficial surgical procedures in the neck.[8,9] Some workers have advocated superficial cervical plexus blocks for carotid artery surgery to avoid the potential complications of deep cervical plexus block.[10-12] For adequate anesthesia, however, it also may be necessary to inject local anesthetic under the carotid sheath, under the adventitia of the carotid bifurcation, and into the superior angle of the incision.

Deep cervical plexus block provides anesthesia of the deep and superficial branches of the cervical plexus because the nerve roots are anesthetized before the motor and sensory components separate. The deep block anesthetizes not only all the sensory components of the cervical plexus, but also the muscles that arise and insert on the corresponding cervical vertebrae and transverse processes of C2-4.[9]

Practically any procedure involving the anterior or lateral aspect of the neck may be performed with this technique, including the following: dissections of the neck; excision of masses, tumors, thyroglossal cysts, or branchial cysts; operations on the thyroid, parathyroid, or lymph glands; operations on the trachea and larynx; and operations on the blood vessels, including ligations of the carotid and lingual arteries and carotid endarterectomy.[1,6] Most of these procedures require only unilateral block of the deep cervical plexus. Bilateral block is advocated, however, for any operative procedure that extends to within half an inch of the midline of the neck.[1] Such procedures include thyroidectomy and excision of the lymphatic glands of the neck. During thyroidectomy, despite the depth of anesthesia after bilateral blockade, traction on the gland is felt as choking, so intravenous sedation is required.[6] In addition, bilateral blockade causes bilateral phrenic nerve paresis and carries the potential for respiratory compromise.

Carotid endarterectomies are perhaps the most common procedures performed with cervical plexus block. Most clinicians who use regional anesthetic techniques for these procedures advocate performing superficial and deep cervical plexus block to ensure a high success rate, owing to the difficulties of establishing general anesthesia and endotracheal intubation with an open wound in the neck. Several studies have compared general anesthesia with regional anesthesia for carotid endarterectomy. Most cited the value of direct assessment of central nervous system function in the awake patient and the ability to assess the need for vascular shunting as the major advantages of regional anesthesia.[13–19]

Cervical plexus blocks also are performed for relief of pain in the neck and occiput secondary to pharyngeal cancer and metastatic lesions and for occipital and posterior auricular neuralgias associated with acute inflammation or compression of the cervical plexus by tumors or aneurysms.[3,17–21] Deep cervical plexus blockade, especially bilateral blockade of the fourth cervical nerve, is useful for relief of hiccups. The success of the block may be determined during fluoroscopy, which should show bilateral diaphragmatic paresis. Although the paresis is temporary, permanent relief may be afforded by breaking the hiccup cycle.[3,6]

Contraindications

Cervical plexus block has no specific contraindications aside from contraindications to regional blocks in general, such as coagulopathy, infection at the site of the block, history of allergy to local anesthetics, and patient refusal.[7] Significant respiratory disease is a relative contraindication, especially to bilateral cervical plexus block, because of the potential for blockade of the phrenic nerve, which can cause diaphragmatic paralysis.

Anatomy of the Cervical Plexus

The cervical plexus is formed by the anterior primary division of the first four cervical nerves. The anterior and posterior roots of cervical nerves C2-4 emerge from the spinal canal through their respective intervertebral foramina.[1,8] The first cervical nerve, the suboccipital nerve, emerges between the occipital bone and the posterior arch of the atlas. The posterior sensory root of this nerve is much smaller than the anterior motor root and may be entirely absent (**Fig. 150.1**).[1]

After the mixed nerves are formed by the union of the anterior and posterior roots, they divide into anterior and posterior primary divisions. The exception is the first cervical nerve, which seldom has an anterior division. Because the first cervical nerve is composed almost exclusively of motor fibers to the muscles of the suboccipital triangle and only rarely has any significant sensory component, it is usually unnecessary to block this nerve.

After exiting the intervertebral foramina, the anterior primary rami of C2-4 pass in an anterocaudolateral direction behind the vertebral artery and vein, in the gutter formed by the anterior and posterior tubercles of the corresponding transverse processes of the cervical vertebrae (**Fig. 150.2**).[3,22] The tubercles of the transverse processes lie ½ inch (1.3 cm)

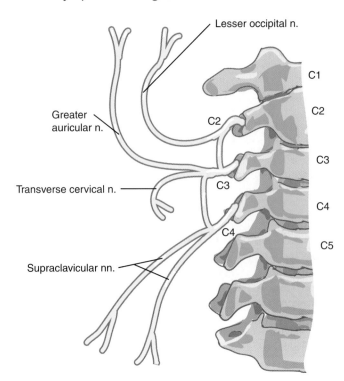

Fig. 150.1 **Formation of the cervical plexus and its branches.**

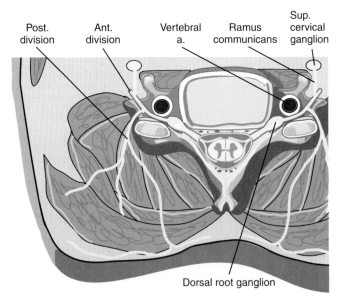

Fig. 150.2 **Cross-section of the third cervical segment.** This illustration shows the course and distribution of the posterior primary division with its medial branch passing posteriorly to supply the skin and subcutaneous structures and the lateral branch supplying the muscles. Also shown is a cross-section of the superior cervical ganglion and its connection to the nerve by the white ramus communicans. Note the vertebral vessels just anterior to the nerves.

to 1¼ inches (3.2 cm) below the skin, depending on the size of the patient and the cervical level. The lower cervical tubercles are more superficial than the tubercles of the upper cervical transverse processes.[23] The anterior tubercles are located farther cephalad and medial than the posterior tubercles.[1]

Chapter 150—Cervical Plexus Block 1093

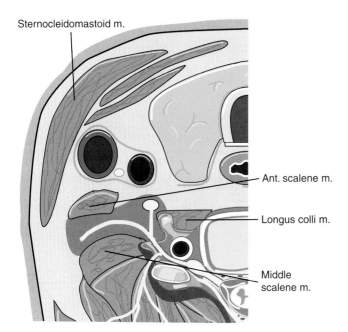

Fig. 150.3 After leaving the intervertebral foramina, the anterior primary rami of the cervical nerves pass laterally behind the vertebral artery and vein in the gutter formed by the anterior and posterior tubercles of the corresponding transverse processes of the cervical vertebrae. In this short course, each ramus actually lies in a short fibrous tunnel formed by the transverse processes superiorly and inferiorly and by the anterior and posterior intertransverse muscles (not shown here), which extend, respectively, between the anterior and posterior tubercles of the transverse processes of the contiguous cervical vertebrae. The posterior primary division leaves the anterior division just before the latter passes between the two tubercles, so that injected anesthetic solutions must move centrad into this tunnel to block the posterior division.

The first cervical nerve passes under the vertebral artery in its relationship with the posterior arch of the atlas and is held in place by a fibrous tunnel.[1] The anterior primary rami of C2-4 also are held firmly on the transverse process by a fibrous tunnel. After leaving the transverse processes, these nerves are enclosed in a perineural space formed by the muscles and tendons attached to the anterior and posterior tubercles of their respective cervical vertebrae. The muscles and tendons of the anterior tubercles are the longus colli, the longus capitis, and the scalenus anterior. The muscles and tendons attached to the posterior tubercles are the scalenus medius, the scalenus cervicis, and the longissimus cervicis.[1,2] As the prevertebral fascia moves laterally and splits to invest these muscles and tendons, it forms a closed fascial space that is a superior extension of the interscalene space (**Fig. 150.3**).[2] The fascia investing the muscles and tendons that lie anterior and posterior to the cervical plexus provides an envelope around the plexus that can serve as a perineural sheath and provides the basis for a single-injection technique to block the cervical plexus.[2]

Within the perineural sheath, the anterior primary rami of C2-4 divide into ascending and descending branches that form a series of three loops known as the *cervical plexus* (**Fig. 150.4**).[2,3,23,24] The cervical plexus, which lies lateral to the upper four cervical vertebrae and anterior to the levator scapulae muscle and the middle scalene muscle, is covered by the sternocleidomastoid muscle. Each loop gives rise to a superficial and a deep branch. This anatomic separation enables the

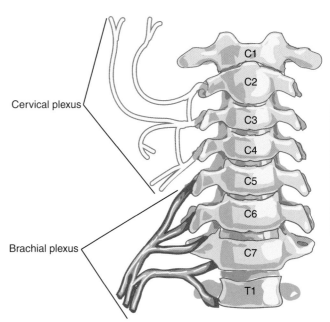

Fig. 150.4 **Cervical and first thoracic spinal nerves.** Anterior view showing the formation of the cervical and brachial plexus.

sensory branches of the cervical plexus, through the superficial branches, to be blocked selectively without any motor blockade in the neck.

The superficial branches of the cervical plexus pierce the deep fascia of the neck approximately at the middle of the posterior margin of the sternocleidomastoid muscle, just below the emergence of the accessory nerve. Then they curve around the posterior border of the muscle and proceed to supply the skin and superficial fasciae of the head, neck, and shoulder (**Figs. 150.5** and **150.6**). The ascending branches (small occipital and great auricular nerves) supply the occipitomastoid region of the head, the auricle of the ear, and the parotid gland; the transverse branch (superficial cervical) innervates the anterior part of the neck between the lower border of the jaw and the sternum; and the descending branches (suprasternal, supraclavicular, and supra-acromial) supply the shoulder and upper pectoral region (**Fig. 150.7**).[6,7,21,24]

The deep cervical plexus supplies mainly the deep structures of the anterior and lateral neck and sends branches to the phrenic nerve (**Fig. 150.8**). It also contributes to the hypoglossal loop.[3,6] One group of nerve branches, the lateral (external) group, proceeds from beneath the sternocleidomastoid muscle in a posterolateral direction toward the posterior triangle. This group provides muscular branches to the scalenus medius, sternocleidomastoid, trapezius, and levator scapulae muscles. The medial (ventral) group runs medially and forward to the anterior triangle. It provides muscular branches to the rectus capitis lateralis and rectus capitis anterior, longus capitis, and longus colli muscles and to the diaphragm through the phrenic nerve. By means of the ansa hypoglossi, it also innervates the thyrohyoid, geniohyoid, omohyoid, sternothyroid, and sternohyoid muscles (**Fig. 150.9**).[3,6,24]

The cervical plexus communicates with the sympathetic chain in the neck by means of rami communicantes. Sympathetic fibers do not accompany the spinal nerves from their origin in the cord. Instead, they are derived from the superior, middle, and inferior (stellate) cervical ganglia

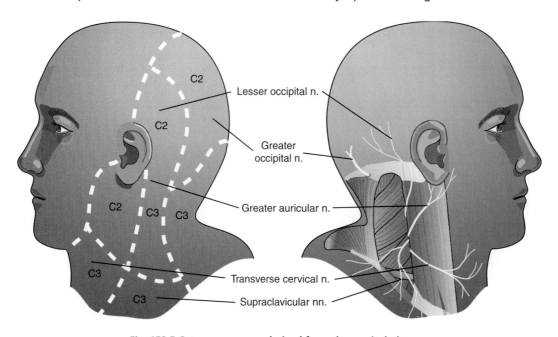

Fig. 150.5 **Cutaneous nerves derived from the cervical plexus.**

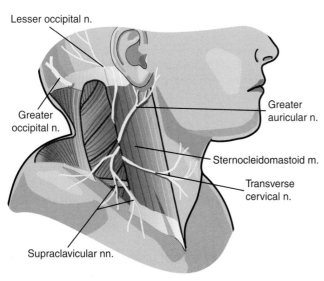

Fig. 150.6 **Superficial branches of the cervical plexus at their points of emergence on the posterior margin of the sternocleidomastoid muscle.**

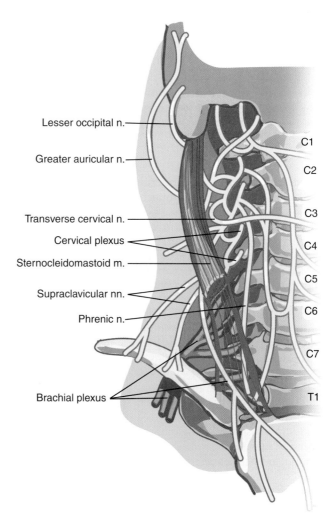

Fig. 150.7 **Semischematic representation of the cervical plexus and the phrenic nerve.** These structures are shown in relation to the transverse processes, which are threaded by the vertebral blood vessels.

(Fig. 150.10).[6,24] The cervical plexus also communicates with the vagus, hypoglossal, and accessory cervical nerves.[24] These communications may explain some of the side effects often seen with cervical plexus block.

Clinical Pearls and Tricks of the Trade

Choosing a superficial or deep cervical plexus block, or both, is based on the surgical procedure and the desired extent of anesthesia. Only one technique has been described for superficial block; multiple techniques are available for deep block.

Technique of Superficial Block

Superficial cervical plexus block provides the same sensory (dermatome) anesthesia as deep cervical plexus block, which also incorporates the motor component of the cervical plexus at the nerve roots before the sensory and motor branches separate.[9] The patient is placed in the supine position with the head turned away from the side to be blocked. The patient may be asked to raise the head slightly to outline better the border of the sternocleidomastoid muscle midway between its origin on the clavicle and its insertion on the mastoid. This is also the point where the external jugular vein crosses the posterior border of the sternocleidomastoid muscle (**Fig. 150.11**).

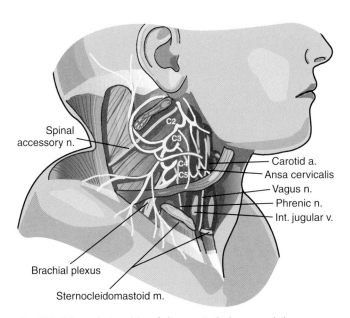

Fig. 150.8 **The relationship of the cervical plexus and the phrenic nerve.**

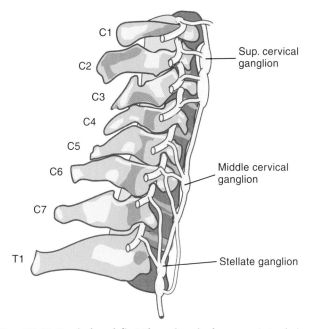

Fig. 150.10 **Cervical and first thoracic spinal nerves.** Lateral view showing the course and relation of the cervical nerves and the cervical sympathetic chain.

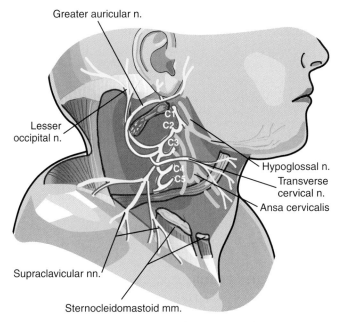

Fig. 150.9 **The branches of the cervical plexus.**

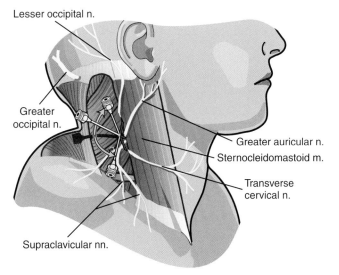

Fig. 150.11 **The technique of superficial cervical plexus block:** needle placement.

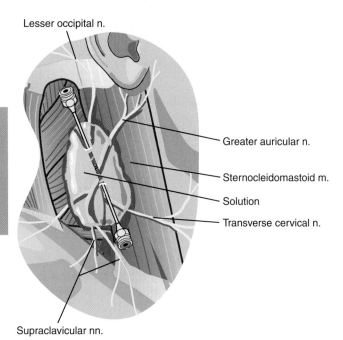

Lesser occipital n.

Greater auricular n.

Sternocleidomastoid m.

Solution

Transverse cervical n.

Supraclavicular nn.

Fig. 150.12 **The technique of superficial cervical plexus block: spread of injectatem.**

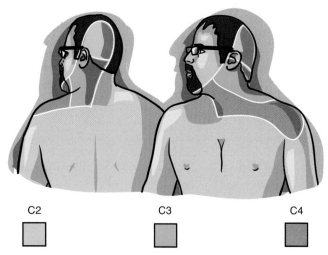

C2   C3   C4

Fig. 150.13 **Distribution of cutaneous anesthesia following superficial cervical plexus block.**

Superficial cervical plexus blockade requires a sufficient volume of local anesthetic to be effective. A 4-cm, 22-gauge or a 1-inch, 25-gauge needle is inserted subcutaneously immediately posterior and deep to the midpoint of the ster-nocleidomastoid muscle. Approximately 5 mL of local anesthetic are injected at this midpoint. The needle is redirected superiorly and inferiorly along the posterior border of the sternocleidomastoid muscle, and approximately 5 mL of local anesthetic are injected along each of these sites for a total of 15 mL of local anesthetic (**Fig. 150.12**).[8,21,22,25] Paresthesias are not sought. This injection produces cutaneous analgesia of the neck from the mandible to the clavicle anteriorly and laterally (**Fig. 150.13**).[21]

Technique of Deep Block

Deep cervical plexus block anesthetizes all the sensory components of the cervical plexus and the muscles that arise and insert on the corresponding cervical vertebrae and transverse processes of C2-4. When this deep cervical plexus is blocked close to the lateral edges of the transverse processes, the nerve roots are anesthetized before the motor and sensory components separate. This is one of the primary differences between deep and superficial cervical plexus blocks.[9] A deep cervical plexus block is a paravertebral nerve block of C2-4 as the nerves emerge from the foramina in the cervical vertebrae. The patient is in the same position as for superficial cervical plexus block.

The lateral route, also known as the Heidenhein or Labat method, is most often described because the superficial landmarks for this technique are numerous and reliable. A mark is placed on the tip of the mastoid process of the temporal bone behind the ear. A second mark is placed on the anterior tubercle of the C6 transverse process, Chassaignac's tubercle, at the level of the cricoid cartilage. The most prominent cervical transverse process, C6, may be felt by deep palpation between the trachea and carotid sheath at the level of the cricoid cartilage. A straight line, known as the *primary line*, is drawn between these two marks to indicate the position of the cervical transverse processes. Some clinicians advocate drawing this line parallel and 1 cm posterior to the first line to produce a more accurate superficial indicator of the cervical transverse processes below.[22] Other practitioners construct the primary line by connecting the mastoid process with the suprasternal notch.[25]

On this line, the transverse processes of C2-4 are palpated. The transverse process of C2 is approximately 1.5 cm caudal to the tip of the mastoid process. Points marked 1.5 and 3 cm below this first point on the primary line indicate the transverse processes of C3 and C4. The transverse process of C3 can be found at the level of the body of the hyoid bone, and the C4 transverse process is located at the level of the upper border of the thyroid cartilage (**Figs. 150.14** and **150.15**).

Skin wheals are raised at these three points with a 27-gauge needle. A 5-cm, 22-gauge or a 1-inch, 25-gauge, short beveled block needle is inserted medially and caudally to a depth of 1.5 to 2 cm, until the tip of the transverse process is contacted at the three designated points. The needle is walked laterally until it slips off the most lateral aspect of the bone, and the tip is identified again. It is important to locate the transverse processes as far laterally as possible to avoid injection into the vertebral artery.[26] A caudad direction must be maintained to avoid unintentional entry into the intervertebral foramen, which would result in epidural or subarachnoid injection (**Fig. 150.16**). Paresthesias may or may not be elicited. After careful aspiration for blood and cerebrospinal fluid (CSF), local anesthetic, 3 to 5 mL, is injected through each needle. If the needles are properly placed, the onset of analgesia occurs within 5 minutes, regardless of the agent used. The area of cutaneous anesthesia is the same as for superficial cervical plexus block, but deeper structures also are anesthetized.[3,6–8,21–23,25]

Alternative Techniques for Deep Block

Because the cervical plexus is invested in the prevertebral fascia between the anterior and middle scalene muscles, Winnie et al[2] advocated a single-injection technique for neural blockade.

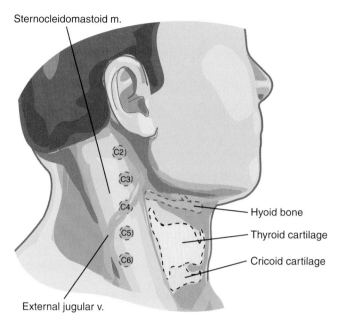

Fig. 150.14 **Position and surface landmarks for performing deep cervical plexus block.** *(From Pai U, Raj P: Peripheral nerve blocks: cervical plexus. In Raj P, editor:* Handbook of regional anesthesia, *New York, 1985, Churchill Livingstone, p 163.)*

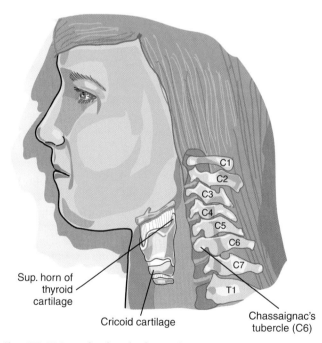

Fig. 150.15 **Bony landmarks for performing deep cervical plexus block.**

Positioning of the patient and identification of bony landmarks are as noted previously. The posterior border of the sternocleidomastoid muscle at the level of C4 is identified, and the clinician's fingers are rolled laterally until the groove between the scalenus anterior and scalenus medius muscles is palpated. A 5-cm, 22-gauge or 1-inch, 25-gauge, short, beveled block needle is inserted medially and caudally at this point until either paresthesia is elicited or the transverse process of

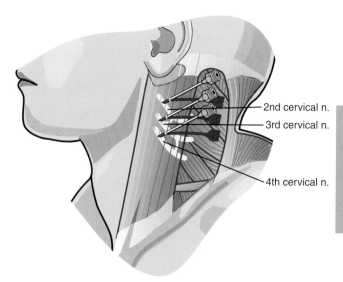

Fig. 150.16 **Needle placement for deep cervical plexus block.** The needles are noted at the sulci of the transverse processes of C2, C3, and C4.

C4 is encountered. Local anesthetic, 10 to 25 mL, is injected after aspiration to check for blood and CSF.[2,11,27] The perineural sheath provides a space that communicates freely in the cervical region, so the local anesthetic solution can spread easily to adjacent levels.[21] Finger pressure at the C5 transverse process can be used to prevent caudad spread of the anesthetic toward the brachial plexus (**Fig. 150.17**).

The single-injection technique also can be performed using a nerve stimulator to produce twitches of the neck muscles and paresthesias over the shoulder and upper arm before the blockade.[28] An 18-gauge Venflon needle connected to an electrode of the nerve stimulator is inserted as described previously; the other electrode is placed on the shoulder of interest. When appropriate twitches are obtained, local anesthetic, 10 to 15 mL, is injected after aspiration to check for blood and CSF.

Another method of using a nerve stimulator with the single-injection technique was described more recently.[29] A short, beveled needle (Stimuplex cannulas; Braun, Melsungen, Germany) is connected to a nerve stimulator and is directed into the interscalene groove at the level of the upper margin of the thyroid cartilage (C4-5). The needle is directed caudally and medially until elevation and internal rotation of the scapula is elicited (**Fig. 150.18**). This muscle-evoked response occurs because of stimulation of the levator muscle of the scapula. The tip of the needle is positioned correctly when a current intensity of less than 0.5 mA elicits this muscle response. While digital pressure is applied below the needle, a 40-mL dose of local anesthetic is injected slowly. The use of a nerve stimulator may increase the success rate of the block and improve the quality of anesthesia.

Another alternative route of deep cervical plexus block was described by Wertheim and Rovenstine (**Fig. 150.19**).[1,6] The patient is placed supine with the head midline and the chin pointing upward. The landmarks are the condyle of the mandible, the surface of the second lower molar, and the transverse processes of the cervical vertebrae. A vertical line is drawn through the condyle of the mandible, perpendicular to the operating line. The transverse processes of the cervical vertebrae are palpated, and a horizontal line is drawn along

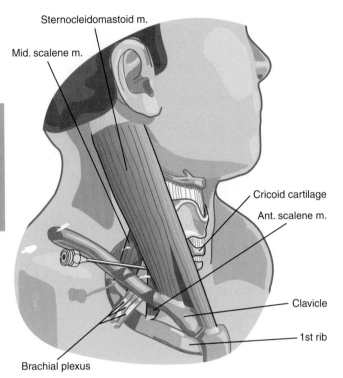

Fig. 150.17 The alternative technique of interscalene cervical plexus block. The patient is supine with the head turned slightly to the side opposite that to be blocked. The level of C4 is determined by noting the level of the upper margin of the thyroid cartilage. While the patient elevates the head to bring the sternocleidomastoid muscle into prominence, the anesthesiologist places the index and middle fingers behind (posterior to) the latter muscle at the level of C4, and the patient is asked to relax. The palpating fingers now lie upon the anterior surface of the belly of the anterior scalene muscle. The anesthesiologist now carefully rolls the fingers laterally until the groove between the anterior and middle scalene muscles is palpated. When two fingers are used for palpation, digital pressure indents the skin and decreases the distance between the skin and cervical transverse processes. An immobile needle is inserted at the level of C4 between the palpating fingers as they depress the skin over the interscalene groove. The needle is advanced perpendicular to the skin in all planes; that is, the direction is mostly mesiad but slightly dorsad and caudad. The caudal direction is critical to the safety of the technique because the advancing needle, properly directed, encounters the next cervical transverse process if paresthesias are not produced. A horizontal direction would allow a needle that has missed the cervical roots to enter the vertebral vessels or the epidural or subarachnoid space.

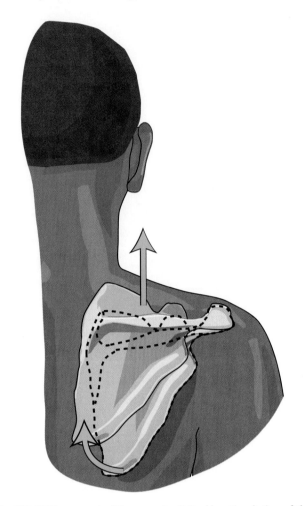

Fig. 150.18 Movement of the scapula elicited by stimulation of the cervical plexus.

Posterior Approach

A posterior approach for deep cervical plexus block also has been described. The patient lies in the lateral position with the side to be blocked placed superiorly. The head is supported with cushions to prevent distortion of the structures of the neck and to render the landmarks more accessible. The cervical spinous processes are identified, C7 being most prominent. If these structures are difficult to palpate, the spinous process of C6 can be identified by drawing a line from the cricoid cartilage to the back of the neck. The transverse processes of C5-2 are located 1.5, 3, 4.5, and 6 cm above C6.

Skin wheals are raised opposite the spinous processes of C2-4 approximately 2 cm from the midline (**Fig. 150.21**). An 8-cm, 22-gauge needle is passed through these points parallel to the sagittal plane of the neck, until its point reaches the lateral transverse processes of the vertebrae. The needle is withdrawn into the subcutaneous tissue and is redirected obliquely and outward. When the needle point rests along the lateral aspect of the vertebral arch, it is advanced 1 cm farther, and local anesthetic is injected as for the lateral approach.[6]

The posterior approach is technically difficult, and results of blockade using this technique have been poor. The landmarks are difficult to identify accurately, and the depth of

them, thus making right angles with the vertical line. A second perpendicular line is drawn that passes over the surface of the second molar. The point of intersection of this line with the horizontal line is marked, as is a point 1 cm caudal to the first point on the horizontal line. This latter point corresponds to the top of the transverse process of the second cervical vertebra. Points 2.5 and 3.5 cm caudal to the first point are marked on the skin. These points correspond to the tips of the transverse processes of C3 and C4. Four points are drawn on the horizontal line; the upper point serves only as a reference point, and the three lower points indicate sites of injection. Injection of local anesthetic for deep cervical plexus block is carried out as described for the lateral approach (**Fig. 150.20**).

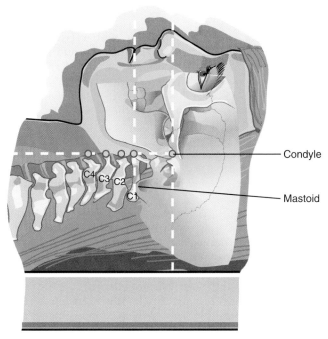

Fig. 150.19 **Cervical plexus block by an alternate route (Rovenstine and Wertheim).**

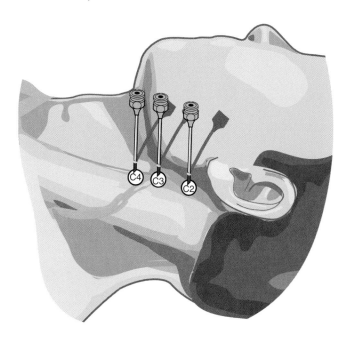

Fig. 150.20 **Cervical plexus block; site of injection by an alternate route.**

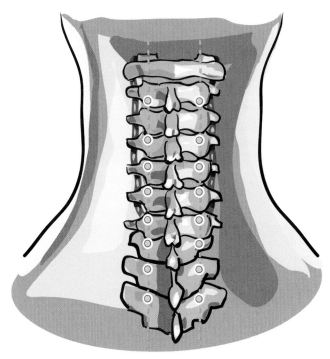

Fig. 150.21 **Cervical plexus block by the posterior route.** Superficial landmarks as viewed on the skeleton. The wheals are raised opposite the spinous processes, at a distance of 2 cm from the midline. These landmarks apply to the cervical area only.

needle insertion is greater with this technique. It is used only when the lateral approach is technically impossible (e.g., because of a tumor in the neck at the site of injection).[2]

Anesthetic Agents

Various local anesthetic agents have been used for surgical procedures under cervical plexus block.[29–35] For short procedures, 1% to 2% lidocaine or mepivacaine can be used.[32,34] For prolonged block, a 50:50 mixture of 1% to 2% lidocaine and 0.5% to 0.75% bupivacaine can be used.[35–38] Other clinicians use various concentrations of plain bupivacaine, 0.375% to 0.5%, for deep and superficial blocks.[11,27,30] Newer local anesthetics, such as ropivacaine, are used in similar volumes and concentrations and offer similar anesthesia, perhaps with a better safety profile.

Epinephrine, 1:200,000 solution, also can be used to prolong block. Because this block is used most often for carotid endarterectomies in a high-risk group of patients, the addition of epinephrine may produce undesirable cardiovascular effects.[9,39]

A total volume of 10 to 15 mL of local anesthetic usually is used for superficial cervical plexus block, and a total volume of 9 to 15 mL is used for deep cervical plexus block. The single-injection deep cervical plexus block usually requires 10 to 25 mL of local anesthetic, although greater volumes have been used.[2,11,27,29,31]

In addition to local anesthetic alone, neurolytic block using equal parts of 0.5% bupivacaine with absolute alcohol has been used to block the cervical plexus for neck pain secondary to metastatic lesions. Methylprednisolone (Depo-Medrol), 40 mg, also has been added to local anesthetics for its anti-inflammatory actions.[20]

Several studies measured the blood levels of local anesthetic and monitored side effects after cervical plexus block and found no significant degree of toxicity. One study, using lidocaine 1.5% with epinephrine 1:200,000 at 6 mg/kg, found that symptoms of lidocaine toxicity did not occur.[40] Another study, using a mixture of lidocaine and bupivacaine for cervical plexus blockade at commonly used concentrations and volumes, also failed to elicit toxic systemic effects.[33] Bupivacaine levels also were measured in a study in which patients received a combination of general anesthesia and cervical plexus block.

The mean total bupivacaine dose was 3.4 mg/kg, higher than the manufacturer's recommendation of 2 mg/kg. Nevertheless, no signs of systemic bupivacaine toxicity were noted during the procedure or in the postoperative period.[41] Although cervical plexus block is safe, the usual recommendations of multiple aspirations, slow injection, and careful needle placement must be observed.

Pitfalls

Cervical plexus block fails for many reasons. When the landmarks have been located, care should be taken to ensure that the patient does not move; otherwise, the landmarks may be misleading, and the block may fail.[23] The needle should not be inserted too deeply. The depth of the tips of the transverse processes from the skin varies from approximately 1.3 to 3.2 cm, depending on the pressure of palpation, the build of the patient, and the location of the injection. The transverse processes become more superficial as they descend.[22,23]

The needle also should be directed slightly caudad, to avoid entry into the epidural or subarachnoid space. The neck is a densely vascular area, so aspiration before injection is mandatory. Injection of a 1-mL test dose of anesthetic is prudent to detect any systemic effect. Placement of the needle should be at the lateral surface of the transverse processes before injection. When the needle lies too far posteriorly, analgesia is poor. When the needle tip is placed too far anteriorly, puncture of the carotid artery, internal jugular vein, or vertebral vessels may occur, with subsequent hematoma formation. This complication may make operating conditions difficult. Injection too far anteriorly also may cause sympathetic ganglion blockade, with resulting Horner's syndrome.[6]

If the cervical plexus block is unsuccessful and if time permits, the block may be repeated. The total dose of local anesthetic should be calculated to avoid injection of a toxic dose.[42] If partial blockade is obtained, supplementation with intravenous agents can be considered. If these techniques fail, a means providing general anesthesia should be used.[7]

Complications

Numerous complications can occur with cervical plexus block. The block is occasionally inadequate and must be supplemented by infiltration of additional local anesthetic. This complication is more common when the site of operation extends beyond the midline of the neck during unilateral blockade.[16] Surgical traction high in the neck wound, where glossopharyngeal innervation occurs, commonly requires supplementation of anesthesia.[14] Discomfort also can occur because of retraction onto the mandibular periosteum, which is innervated by branches of the mandibular division of the trigeminal nerve. Supplementation of anesthesia also may be necessary in this area.[35]

Because the neck is richly vascular, intravascular injections of local anesthetic may occur. Accidental injection into the internal and external jugular veins during superficial cervical plexus block may result in systemic toxicity, tears in the wall of the vein leading to hematoma formation, and possibly air embolism if the needle is not attached to the syringe. Ultrasound guidance in patients in whom anatomic landmarks are difficult to locate may help to avoid inadvertent intravascular injection (**Fig. 150.22**). Accidental injection of even 0.2 mL of local anesthetic into the vertebral artery, which travels through the foramina transversaria in each transverse process, can produce profound toxic effects, including convulsions, apnea, total reversible blindness, and unconsciousness. This effect results from the direct flow of the artery to the brainstem.[27,42] If colloidal materials, such as depot steroids, are added to local anesthetics for pain management, injection of this material into the vertebral artery can result in Wallenberg's syndrome or occlusion of the posterior inferior cerebellar artery (**Fig. 150.23**).[21–23,25,39] In addition, injecting a large volume of local anesthetic anterior to the transverse processes during deep cervical plexus block may compress the carotid sheath. This compression may impair blood flow to the brain, which is especially deleterious to patients with pre-existing carotid artery disease.

Local anesthetic injection into the epidural or subarachnoid spaces also is possible through penetration into dural sleeves or through the intervertebral foramina.[21,23,25,39,43,44] Another

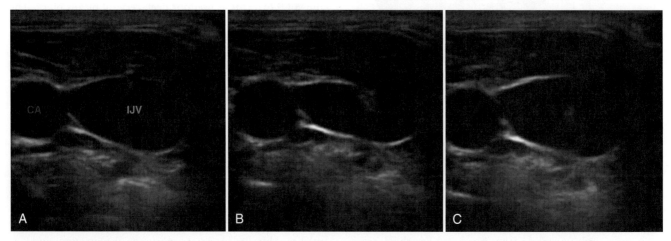

Fig. 150.22 **Cross-sectional view of right internal jugular vein (IJV) and carotid artery (CA) with needle introduced in the short axis. A,** The needle tip is seen just indenting the anterior vein wall. **B,** The needle further indents the vein wall, but the tip is still covered by vein wall, which is tented into the lumen, so no blood can be aspirated. **C,** The needle tip has passed through the vein wall to lie within lumen, vein has reexpanded, and correct position is confirmed by free aspiration of blood. *(From Flood S, Bodenham A: Central venous cannulation: ultrasound techniques,* Anaesth Intensive Care Med *11:16, 2010.)*

potential complication is injury to the spinal cord. Careful aspiration is required for any evidence of CSF. Epidural injection, in contrast to subarachnoid injection, cannot spread into the cranium. An epidural block at the cervical level results in anesthesia of the upper limbs and thorax and can cause bilateral phrenic nerve block with subsequent bilateral diaphragmatic paralysis.[9]

The recurrent laryngeal nerve is blocked in 2% to 3% of cases during unilateral cervical plexus block. This complication occurs when local anesthetic is injected too deeply along the posterior border of the sternocleidomastoid muscle. Sequelae are hoarseness, aphonia, and difficulty breathing. Also possible is blockade of the vagus nerve, which causes increased heart rate and loss of phonation. Bilateral hypoglossal nerve denervation with resultant total upper airway obstruction has been described.[37]

The phrenic nerve, arising mainly from C4 with small branches from C3 and C5, can be blocked (50% of cases) during deep cervical plexus block; this complication causes transient diaphragmatic paresis and mild hypercapnia.[45,46] If only one hemidiaphragm is paralyzed, only patients with chronic obstructive pulmonary disease seem to be at risk for significant changes in carbon dioxide concentration. Most patients describe only a "heavy chest" sensation[9]; this is usually treated by providing reassurance, administering supplemental oxygen, and elevating the patient's head.

Bilateral phrenic nerve block can be a serious hazard, especially in patients with concurrent respiratory compromise, and endotracheal intubation may be required.[31] If respiratory compromise from a paralyzed diaphragm could be a risk to a given patient, bilateral cervical plexus blocks should be avoided. If such blocks are carried out, dilute concentrations and small volumes of local anesthetic agents should be used.[21] Alternatively, the use of a superficial cervical plexus block alone may lower the risk of respiratory complications.[47]

Blockade of cranial nerves IX and X, or a combination of both, through the pharyngeal plexus also can occur during deep cervical plexus block. This complication can cause dysphagia, and patients usually complain of a sensation of fullness in the back of the throat that dissipates over time.[9]

Because the deep cervical plexus lies below the deep cervical fascia, spread of anesthetic to the cervical sympathetic chain, including the stellate ganglion, should not occur. If infiltration has spread anterior to the prevertebral fascia, the cervical sympathetic chain can be blocked, with resultant Horner's syndrome. This syndrome can manifest with ptosis, constricted pupil, unilateral anhidrosis, nasal congestion, and sometimes respiratory compromise.[37] These symptoms should be noted preoperatively, to avoid any confusion in the neurologic examination later. This complication in a failed block indicates that the injection was placed too far anteriorly and too superficially.[21] Bilateral stellate ganglion block may result in profound bradycardia that is caused by interruption of the cardioaccelerator fibers.[25]

Finally, occipital headaches have been described after some surgical procedures under cervical plexus block.[9] The cause seems to be hyperextension of the neck muscles, however, and not the block itself. Headaches also can occur after carotid endarterectomy secondary to reperfusion of the cerebral circulation.

Future Trends

Although cervical plexus block has been widely described in the literature, the use of this technique for surgical procedures has been limited. From the surgeon's standpoint, the potential for a delay in surgery because of the time required to perform the block and the potential for unsatisfactory

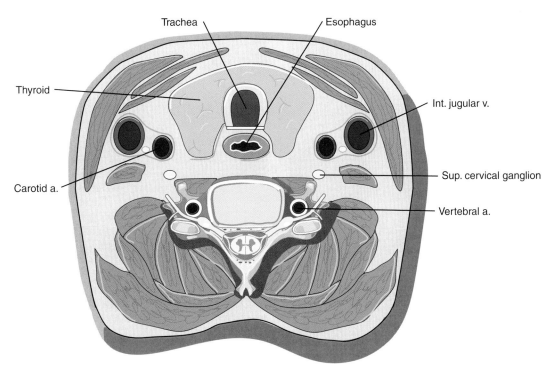

Fig. 150.23 **Cervical plexus cross-sectional anatomy: midpoint of the sternocleidomastoid muscle.**

anesthesia that would require further supplementation are deterrents to performing cervical plexus block. From the standpoint of the anesthesiologist, inexperience with performing the block and fear of complications reduce the use of this technique.[36]

The most common surgical procedure performed under cervical plexus block is carotid endarterectomy. Because enormous progress has validated the efficacy of this procedure, its use may increase.[48] A newer technique, percutaneous carotid angioplasty and stenting performed through direct common carotid access, has been done successfully with cervical plexus block.[49] This technique may broaden the indications further for this type of nerve block. As the surgical population grows older and presents with more severe systemic illnesses, regional anesthesia may prove to be the safest form of anesthesia. The use of cervical plexus block for carotid endarterectomy has many benefits over general anesthesia for this operation, among them the opportunity to monitor the patient's neurologic status during the operation. Periodic examinations of the awake patient have proved to be more accurate than electroencephalography or any other form of monitoring in assessing neurologic status. Another advantage is that regional anesthesia allows for a trial of carotid clamping and carotid stump pressure measurements while neurologic status is monitored with the patient awake. Routine shunting, which carries its own risks of morbidity and mortality, is avoided.[50]

Perioperative complications occur during carotid endarterectomy under cervical plexus block and general anesthesia. Cervical plexus block seems to be associated with greater activation of the sympathetic nervous system, which is manifested as hypertension and tachycardia, whereas general anesthesia is associated with a greater incidence of hypotension.[51,52] Postoperative blood pressure instability is less common in patients who have had cervical plexus block for the procedure.[13,16,17] A report by Corson et al[53] showed a statistically significant difference in neurologic complications between regional and general anesthesia during carotid endarterectomy—0.6% versus 4%.

Growing emphasis has been placed on cost containment by the government, third-party payers, and the public. A study by Godin et al[50] confirmed that cervical plexus block is a safe, reliable, and less costly alternative to general anesthesia in patients undergoing carotid endarterectomy. As evidence accumulates to support the use of regional anesthetic techniques for carotid endarterectomy and other procedures and conditions, facility in performing cervical plexus blocks should be encouraged. Cervical plexus block should be considered an important regional technique in the armamentarium of any anesthesiologist.

References

Full references for this chapter can be found on www.expertconsult.com.

Stellate Ganglion Block

P. Prithvi Raj

Anatomy of the Cervical Sympathetic Nerves

The cervical sympathetic nerve trunk ascends directly as far as the base of the skull. Along its course, it forms three cervical ganglia: superior, middle, and inferior. The inferior cervical ganglion, located at the C7-8 level, fuses with the first thoracic ganglion to form the cervicothoracic ganglion *(the stellate ganglion)*. These cervical ganglia produce gray communicating branches to the C1-8 and T1 nerve roots. The superior cervical ganglion also communicates with the internal carotid nerve, external carotid nerve, and superior cervical cardiac nerve (**Figs. 151.1** to **151.3**).

The deep cervical fascia envelops the muscle group that encircles the cervical spine. The deep cervical fascia is also called the *prevertebral fascia* because it envelops the prevertebral muscles (longus colli and longus capitis muscles) that attach to the cervical vertebral bodies and transverse processes. The prevertebral fascia is divided into two layers: the narrowly defined prevertebral fascia and the pterygoid fascia. The cervical sympathetic nerve trunk ascends through the prevertebral layer. The gray communicating branches of the cervical sympathetic nerve trunk penetrate the longus colli muscle anteriorly before they reach the cervical nerves. Laterally from the transverse processes of the cervical vertebrae, the brachial plexus is located between the anterior and middle scalene muscles.

The trachea, esophagus, thyroid gland, and carotid sheath are located between the prevertebral fascia and the middle cervical fascia. At the C6 level, the recurrent laryngeal nerve ascends in a path surrounded by the thyroid, esophagus, and trachea.

Origin of Sympathetic Nerve Supply to the Head and Neck

The peripheral sympathetic nerve supply to the head and neck is derived from preganglionic neurons, which have cell bodies located in the anterior lateral horn of the first and second thoracic spinal cord segment.[1,2] The axon then passes through the anterior roots of the same spinal nerve level through the rami communicantes to join the upper cervical sympathetic ganglia. These cervical ganglia are identified as the superior, middle, intermediate, and interior cervical sympathetic ganglia.[1,2]

In only 80% of the population, the inferior cervical ganglia and the first thoracic ganglia fuse to form the stellate ganglia.[1-3] From these ganglia, the postganglionic axons pass upward along the internal and external carotid and vertebral arteries to the structures within the cranium. The axon may also join the gray rami communicantes, which join the cervical nerve supply to the neck and the upper extremity (the cervical portion of the brachial plexus).

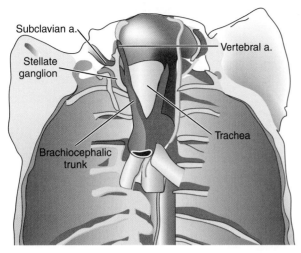

Fig. 151.1 The anatomy of the head and neck in a cadaver showing the course of the stellate ganglion and its sympathetic chain and relationship to other structures. *(From Raj PP, Lou L, Erdine S, et al:* Interventional pain management: image-guided procedures, *ed 2, Philadelphia, 2008, Saunders.)*

Indications

Stellate ganglion block (SGB) is useful in the treatment of various painful conditions, including *Raynaud's disease, arterial embolism* in the area of the arm, *accidental intra-arterial injection of drugs,* and *Meniere's disease.* SGB is beneficial also in the treatment of *acute herpes zoster of the face and lower cervical and upper thoracic dermatomes.* The technique also may be used for palliation of postherpetic neuralgia involving this anatomic area.

Some Conditions Amenable to Stellate Ganglion Block

Post-Traumatic Syndrome

Post-traumatic syndrome is often accompanied by swelling, cold sweat, and cyanosis. This condition is an ideal indication for SGB. Several clinical syndromes fall into this category, including complex regional pain syndrome (CRPS) type I (reflex sympathetic dystrophy) and type II (causalgia)[4] and Sudeck's disease. SGB is useful in the treatment of facial CRPS. For patients requiring vascular surgery of the upper extremities, SGB has diagnostic, prognostic, and, in some cases, prophylactic value. Simultaneous bilateral blocks are not advisable. Nevertheless, in rare cases of pulmonary embolism, bilateral SGB is absolutely indicated as immediate therapy.

Vasculopathies

The vasodilator effect of SGB may be used to treat acute and chronic vasculopathies. The relief of digital ischemia in children before corrective surgery has been reported.[5] SGB was shown to restore distal perfusion in a premature neonate with brachial artery insufficiency after inadvertent cannulation.[6] SGB is indicated for arteriospasm occurring after embolectomy or resulting from the inadvertent intra-arterial injection of thiopentone. It may be used to assess patients with Raynaud's phenomenon or systemic sclerosis for their suitability for surgical stellate ganglionectomy.[7]

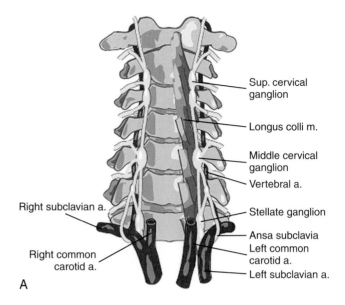

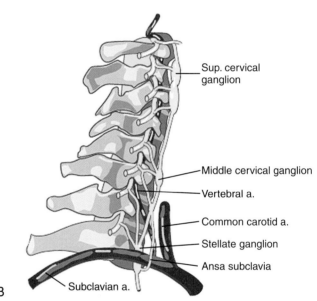

Fig. 151.2 A, Anterior view of the anatomy and relationships of the stellate ganglion. Note the connections of the stellate ganglion superiorly and its close relationship with the longus colli muscle. B, Lateral view of the anatomy of the stellate ganglion. The vertebral artery is anterior to the stellate ganglion at C7 and becomes posterior at C6.

Intractable Angina

Hammond et al[8] published evidence that left-sided SGB has a place in the treatment of refractory angina. Patients who showed evidence of cardiac denervation after left-sided SGB became pain free for approximately 5 weeks. Nitrate consumption and severity of angina, as measured by Canadian class status, were also significantly reduced. Chester[9] proposed a draft algorithm for use in the treatment of refractory angina that included left-sided SGB after multidisciplinary rehabilitation and counseling.

Herpes Zoster

SGB may have a place in treating the acute pain of herpes zoster ophthalmicus and in the management of postherpetic neuralgia.[10-12] Tenicela et al[13] demonstrated an improvement

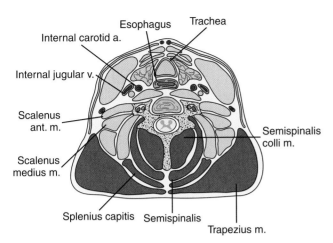

Esophagus Trachea
Internal carotid a.
Internal jugular v.
Scalenus
ant. m.
Scalenus
medius m.
Semispinalis
colli m.
Splenius capitis Semispinalis
Trapezius m.

Fig. 151.3 Transverse section of the neck showing the compartments of deep fascia of the neck. *(From Raj PP, Lou L, Erdine S, et al: Interventional pain management: image-guided procedures, ed 2, Philadelphia, 2008 Saunders, p 228.)*

in early herpes zoster in a small randomized trial. Winnie and Hartwell,[14] in a retrospective study of 122 patients, asserted that the early use of sympathetic blockade in herpes zoster infection can reduce the incidence and severity of postherpetic neuralgia. Visual acuity may be improved by SGB in herpes zoster retrobulbar optic neuritis.[15]

Miscellaneous Conditions

Visual acuity may also be improved by SGB after quinine poisoning,[16] although the authors of a review of 165 patients concluded that SGB was not effective enough to recommend its regular use.[17] The *long Q-T syndrome* is a disorder of acquired cardiac denervation that predisposes the patient to life-threatening ventricular dysrhythmias. SGB has been used in the acute situation to shorten the Q-T interval in both adults[18] and children.[19] SGB for the prevention of postoperative hypertension after coronary artery bypass grafting is now of only historical interest.[20–22] Anecdotal uses of SGB include the treatment of both thalamic lesion pain and idiopathic sensorineural hearing loss.[23,24] **Table 151.1** is an overview of indications for SGB.[25–44]

Contraindications

Absolute contraindications of SGB are as follows: (1) anticoagulant therapy, because of the possibility of bleeding if vascular damage occurs during insertion of the needle; (2) pneumothorax and pneumonectomy on the contralateral side, because of the danger of additional pneumothorax on the ipsilateral side; and (3) recent myocardial infarction, because SGB cuts off the cardiac sympathetic fibers (accelerator nerves), with possible deleterious effects in this condition. Glaucoma can be considered a relative contraindication to SGB because provocation of glaucoma by repeated SGBs has been reported.

Equipment and Drugs

Necessary equipment for SGB includes the following: a 25-gauge local infiltration needle; a 22-gauge, 1- to 2-inch block needle; a 5- or 10-cm (2- or 5-mm tip) sharp Sluijter Mehta or Racz, Finch, Kit needle (Radionics, Burlington, MA) for radiofrequency; and the radiofrequency machine. Drugs

Table 151.1 Indications for Stellate Ganglion Block

CRPS types I and II of the upper extremities[2,3,25–30]
Vascular insufficiency and occlusive vascular disorders both acute and chronic of the upper extremities including Raynaud's disease, intra-arterial embolization, and vasospasm following accidental intra-arterial injection of a drug[2,3,26–29]; possibly also vascular disease unsuitable for vascular reconstructive surgery and improvement of the blood flow following surgical graft or other vascular surgery[29,31]
Poor lymphatic drainage and local edema of the upper extremity following mastectomy[2,31]
Postherpetic neuralgia[2,3,28,29,31]
Phantom pain[2,29,31]
CRPS of the breast and pain following mastectomy[31,32]
Quinine poisoning[2,28,29]
Sudden hearing loss and tinnitus[29,33–36]
Hyperhidrosis of the upper extremity[25–27,29]
Cardiac arrhythmias including Jervell-Lang Nielson Syndrome and Ramano-Ward (idiopathic long QT syndrome), ischemic cardiac pain[2,29–31,37]
Bell's palsy and various orofacial pain syndromes, including neuropathic orofacial pain and trigeminal neuralgia[29,31,38–40]
Vascular headache, including cluster and migraine headaches and sympathetically maintained headaches[40–42] (stellate ganglion block can aggravate migraine headaches in certain conditions and more appropriate sphenopalatine ganglion block probably should be performed[41])
Neuropathic pain syndromes in cancer pain[29,31]

CRPS, complex regional pain syndrome.

used for local anesthetic blocks include 0.5% bupivacaine/ ropivacaine 0.5% (total, 8 mL) or 0.2% to 5% ropivacaine, 1% to 2% lidocaine, and steroids (optional). Phenol preparations require 3% phenol in iohexol (Omnipaque 240) (total, 6 mL) and 0.9% normal saline (total, 2 mL). Radiofrequency thermocoagulation uses the same local anesthetics as does block with steroids.

US-guided procedures typically require high-resolution, multiple-beam imaging to allow visualization of small nerves and the interface between soft tissue and bone.[43] Color Doppler is a standard feature that helps to identify neighboring blood vessels. The choice of transducer is primarily related to the anticipated target depth and size. As a rule of thumb, a broad-band, low-frequency curved-array probe is used for deep structures (e.g., lumbar spine), whereas a broad-band, high-frequency linear transducer is used for superficial targets. Use of a biopsy navigating tool has limited value because it is often necessary to rotate the transducer to verify needle position before the injection is performed. Needle choice depends on both target depth and operator preference. For instance, one operator may favor a B-beveled stimulating needle, whereas others would feel comfortable using Quincke-type spinal needle. Various needle types with improved US visibility are now available.

Patient Preparation

Ideally, proper patient preparation for SGB begins at the visit before the procedure. The patient is much more likely to remember discharge instructions and expected side effects if this information is explained during a visit when the patient is not apprehensive about the imminent procedure, possible side effects, and potential complications. Discussions of the realistic expectations of sympathetic blockade should be held before any procedure. The goals of blockade and the number of blocks in a given series differ with each pain syndrome, and these variables should be discussed, when possible, at visits before the actual blockade. Patients are much less likely to experience frustration or despair if they understand beforehand what can be expected. If the cause of pain is unclear, and the intended block is considered diagnostic, a complete explanation allows the patient to record valuable information on the effectiveness of the procedure.

Informed consent must be obtained. Potential risks, complications, and side effects should be explained in detail. The patient should share responsibility for decision making and must understand the risks and the fact that complications do occur.

Placement of an intravenous line before the block is not mandatory in all pain clinics, but it facilitates the use of intravenous sedation, when indicated, and provides access for administration of resuscitative drugs should a complication occur. In skilled hands, SGB can be performed quickly and relatively painlessly, so an intravenous line may not be necessary. All standard resuscitative drugs, suction apparatus, oxygen delivery system, cardiac defibrillators, and equipment for endotracheal cannulation must be readily accessible. For anxious patients and in teaching institutions when the operator is inexperienced or when "hands-on" teaching is expected, preblock sedation through an intravenous line is beneficial.

Physical examination should include checks for neck extension mobility, prior radical neck surgery, infection at injection site, prior thyroid surgery, and any anatomic variations related to surgery. For preoperative medications, the standard American Society of Anesthesiologists conscious sedation protocol is recommended.

The skin is antiseptically prepared, and the needle is inserted posteriorly, thus penetrating the skin at the tip of the operator's index finger. Making a skin wheal with local anesthetic is rarely necessary except in some teaching situations and in patients with obese necks (in both situations, a 5-cm needle [or a 22-gauge B-bevel needle] is used and should puncture the skin directly downward [posteriorly], perpendicular to the table in all planes). Although a smaller (e.g., 25-gauge) needle can be used, the added flexibility and smaller caliber make it more difficult to ascertain reliably when bone is encountered and then maintain the proper location for injection.

The needle passes through the underlying tissue until it contacts the C6 tubercle or the junction between the C6 vertebral body and the tubercle. The depths of these structures differ. The tubercle itself is more anterior than is the junction between body and tubercle.

Regardless of the specific location encountered at C6, if the skin is being properly displaced posteriorly by the nondominant index finger, the depth is rarely more than 2 to 2.5 cm. The important difference between the medial and lateral locations of bone at C6 relates to the presence of the longus colli muscle, which is located over the lateral aspect of the vertebral body and the medial aspect of the transverse process. It does not cover the C6 tubercle; only the prevertebral fascia that invests the longus colli muscle covers the C6 tubercle. If the needle contacts the medial aspect of the transverse process at a depth greater than expected, the operator should be prepared to withdraw the needle 0.5 cm to avoid injecting into the longus colli muscle. Injection into the muscle belly can prevent caudad diffusion of local anesthetic to the stellate ganglion. Location of the needle on the superficial tip of the C6 anterior tubercle requires withdrawal of the needle from the periosteum before injection.

The procedure is performed most easily if the syringe is attached before the needle is positioned. This prevents accidental dislodging of the needle from the bone during syringe

Techniques

Paratracheal Approach

For this blind technique, the patient is placed in the supine position with the head resting flat on the table without a pillow. A folded sheet or thin pillow should be placed under the shoulders of most patients to facilitate extension of the neck and accentuate landmarks. The head should be kept straight, with the mouth slightly open to relax the tension on the anterior cervical musculature. Hyperextension of the neck also causes the esophagus to move midline, away from the transverse processes on the left.

To ensure proper needle positioning, the operator must identify the C6 tubercle correctly. Identification is accomplished most easily by using firm pressure with the index finger (**Fig. 151.4**). In either a left-handed or a right-handed SGB, the operator's nondominant hand should be used for palpating landmarks. Patients do not tolerate jabbing; gentle but firm probing can easily define the borders of the tubercle. A single finger, the index finger, relays the most specific tactile information. An alternative approach traps the tubercle between the index and middle fingers.

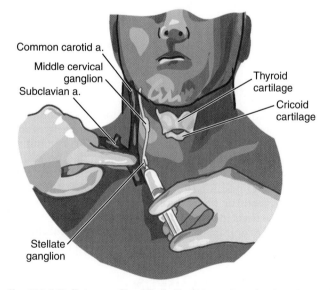

Fig. 151.4 **Stellate ganglion block.** The C6 anterior tubercle is directly beneath the operator's index finger. The carotid artery is retracted laterally when necessary. The needle is perpendicular to all skin planes and is inserted directly posterior from the point of entry.

Labels in figure: Common carotid a.; Middle cervical ganglion; Subclavian a.; Thyroid cartilage; Cricoid cartilage; Stellate ganglion attachment after the needle is placed. When bone is encountered, the palpating finger maintains its pressure, the needle is withdrawn 2 to 5 mm, and the medication is injected. Alternatively, when bone is met, the operator's palpating hand can release and fix the needle by grasping its hub, thus leaving the dominant hand free to aspirate and inject. This technique can also be performed blindly.

Fluoroscopic Technique

More often, fluoroscopy is used to confirm contrast spread (**Fig. 151.5**). With fluoroscopy, correct placement of the needle should be shown by anteroposterior and lateral views with spread of the contrast solution (**Fig. 151.6**).

When proper needle placement is confirmed, injection of medication must be done in a routine and systematic fashion. A 50:50 mix of 2% lidocaine with 0.5% ropivacaine and 1 mL of 40 mg/mL of triamcinolone may be used. An initial test dose must be injected in all cases. Less than 1 mL of solution injected intravascularly has produced loss of consciousness and seizure activity. Before any injection, careful aspiration for blood and cerebrospinal fluid must be performed. If the aspiration is negative, 0.5 to 1 mL of solution is administered, and the patient is asked to raise the thumb to indicate the absence of adverse symptoms. The patient should be informed beforehand and reminded during the blockade procedure that talking may cause movement of the neck musculature that could dislodge the needle from its proper location. To communicate during the block, the patient can be asked to point a thumb or finger upward in response to questions. After the initial test dose, the operator can inject the remainder of the solution, with carefully aspiration after each 3 to 4 mL.

During injection or needle placement, paresthesia of the arm or hand may be elicited. This finding should always be interpreted to mean that the needle has been placed deeper to the anterior tubercle, adjacent to the C6 or C7 nerve root.

Repositioning of the needle is necessary. Aspiration of blood or cerebrospinal fluid also demands repositioning of the needle. Although the needle may be in the correct position, sometimes it is necessary to confirm that the injected solution is not flowing where it is not desired. The correct total volume of solution depends on what block is desired.[44] Properly placed, 5 mL of solution will block the stellate ganglion. A skin wheal is raised over the ventrolateral aspect of the body of C7 with 1 mL of local anesthetic and a 25-gauge needle. A 22-gauge B-bevel needle is inserted through the skin wheal to contact the body of C7 in the ventrolateral aspect; this is at the junction of the transverse process with the vertebral body. Depth and direction should be confirmed with anteroposterior and lateral views. The needle tip is positioned deep to the anterior longitudinal ligament. The longus colli muscle lies lateral to the needle tip. The needle should be stabilized with a long-handled Kelly clamp or hemostat. An intravenous extension should be attached to the needle and used for injection. A dose of approximately 5 mL of water-soluble, nonirritating, nonionic, preservative-free, hypoallergenic contrast solution is injected after negative aspiration. Dye should spread around the vertebra, and intravascular, epidural, intrathecal, thyroidal, or myoneural (longus colli) uptake should be avoided.

If adequate spread of the contrast medium is visualized, a mix of local anesthetic, phenol, and steroid is injected. The total volume of 5 mL should consist of 2.5 mL of 6% phenol in saline, 1 mL of 40 mg of triamcinolone, and 1.5 mL of 0.5% ropivacaine. (The total 5-mL dose contains a final mixture of 3% phenol.) The previously injected contrast material serves as a marker for the spread of the phenol. In the anteroposterior view, the contrast solution should spread caudad to the first thoracic sympathetic ganglion, cephalad to the inferior cervical ganglion, and cephalad to the superior cervical ganglion. In the lateral view, spread should be observed in the retropharyngeal space and in front of the longus colli and anterior scalene muscles.

C7 Anterior Approach

The anterior approach to the stellate ganglion at C7 is similar to the approach described at C6. In contrast to C6, C7 has only a vestigial tubercle, so it is necessary to find Chassaignac's tubercle (C6). The palpating finger moves one fingerbreadth caudad from the inferior tip.

The advantage of blockade at C7 is manifested by the lower volume of local anesthetic needed to provide complete interruption of the upper extremity sympathetic innervation. Only 6 to 9 mL of solution will suffice. The bothersome side effect of recurrent laryngeal nerve block is less common with this approach. The technique has two drawbacks: (1) the less pronounced landmarks make needle positioning less reliable, and (2) the risk of pneumothorax increases because the dome of the lung is close to the site of entry. The use of radiographic imaging during the approach helps to avoid the complications possible with the blind technique.

New Technique

Multiple techniques have been previously reported.[45–49] In 2004, Abdi et al[50] described a newer technique. It is performed with the patient in the supine position with the neck slightly

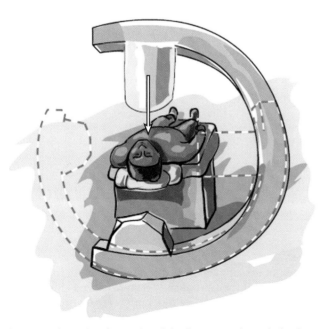

Fig. 151.5 The patient lies supine. If the fluoroscope is used, the C-arm should visualize the C6-7 vertebral region in anteroposterior and lateral views.

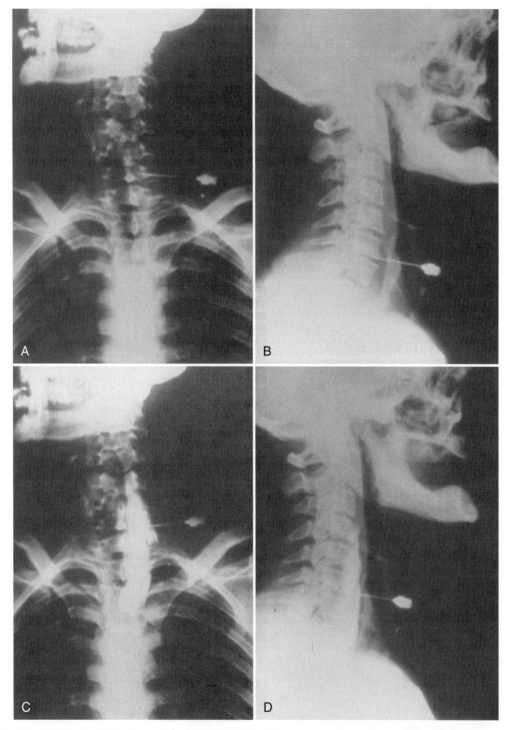

Fig. 151.6 A to **D,** Anteroposterior and lateral views of correct placement of the needle and the contrast medium spread after injection for stellate ganglion block. Anteroposterior **(A)** and lateral **(B)** views of needle placement and anteroposterior **(C)** and lateral **(D)** views of contrast medium spread. *(From Waldman SD: Stellate ganglion block. In* Interventional pain management, *ed 2, Philadelphia, 2001, Saunders, p 367.)*

extended (a pillow may be placed beneath the shoulders) and the head rotated slightly to the opposite side to be blocked. Patients are monitored with electrocardiography, pulse oximetry, and blood pressure measurement throughout the procedure. The skin temperatures are recorded in the distal portion of both the upper extremities in mirror-image locations. The procedure is performed with a sterile technique.

The fluoroscopy beam is directed in an anteroposterior direction until the C5-6 disk is well visualized (**Fig. 151.7**). This usually requires caudocranial angulations of the C-arm. The C-arm is then rotated obliquely, ipsilateral to the side where blockade is desired. The rotation must occur to allow adequate visualization of the neural foramina. A skin wheal is raised at the surface point where the junction

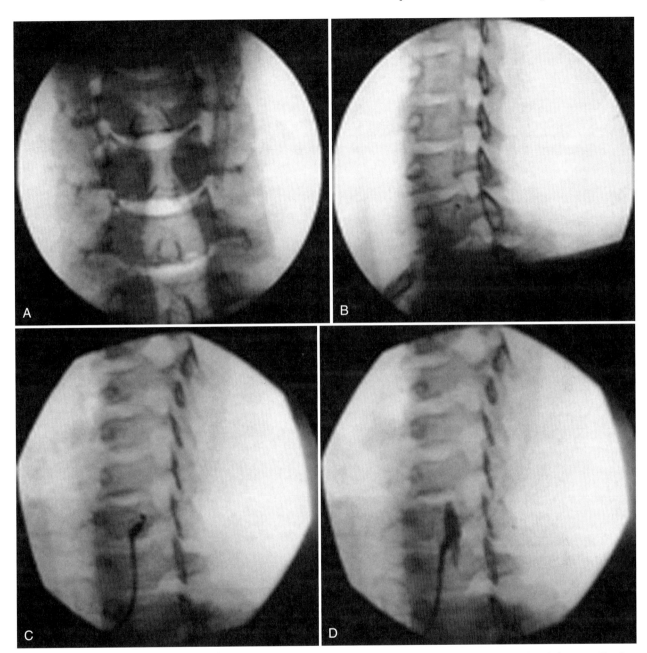

Fig. 151.7 A, The C-arm is in the anteroposterior position with caudal angulation to optimize disk view with flattened end plates. B, The C-arm is rotated in an oblique manner until the neural foramina are seen. C, Final needle placement at the base of the C7 uncinate process on the left side. D, Stellate ganglion block: final position, with contrast injection ton. *(From Abdi S, Zhou Y, Patel N, et al: A new and easy technique to block the stellate ganglion, Pain Physician 7:327, 2004.)*

of the uncinate process and the vertebral body is seen on the fluoroscope.

Under real-time imaging, a single pass is made with a 25-gauge spinal needle to contact bone at this point. Care should be exercised to avoid passage of the needle toward (1) the neural foramina and the thecal sac, which is exposed posteriorly, (2) the disk located cephalad, and (3) the esophagus, which resides medial to the ultimate target point. In its final position, the needle tip comes to rest at the junction between the uncinate process and the vertebral body. The stylet is removed, the extension set is attached, and 1 to 2 mL of radiopaque contrast is injected to visualize the

longus colli muscle. The syringe containing the contrast is exchanged with the one that contains the local anesthetic.

After ensuring that negative aspiration is performed, a 0.5-mL test dose is injected to rule out intravascular injection into the vertebral artery. The value of this test dose in providing early warning of intra-arterial injection is questionable because seizures can occur immediately, even with very small volumes of local anesthetic. This test dose is followed by slow injection of 3 to 5 mL of local anesthetic onto the ganglion. A dose of 3 to 4 mL of local anesthetic usually is adequate for caudal spread to at least the first thoracic segment. Meaningful verbal contact should be maintained, and

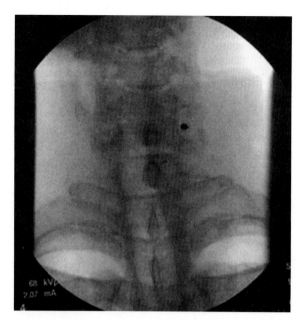

Fig. 151.8 Anteroposterior view showing the needle in the target view with the anterior paratracheal approach at C6 aiming toward the junction between the transverse process and the vertebral body at C6. *(From Narouze S, Vydyanathan A, Patel N: Ultrasound-guided stellate ganglion block successfully prevented esophageal puncture, Pain Physician 10:747, 2007.)*

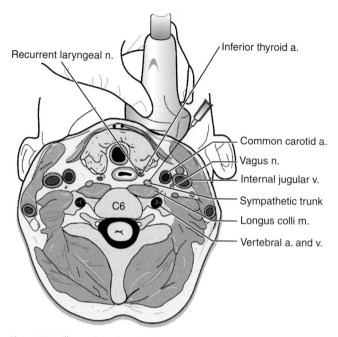

Fig. 151.9 Illustration showing the position of the ultrasound probe and the needle in the oblique path. *(From Narouze S, Vydyanathan A, Patel N: Ultrasound-guided stellate ganglion block successfully prevented esophageal puncture, Pain Physician 10:747, 2007. Reprinted with permission from the Cleveland Clinic Foundation.)*

the patient should be urged to respond verbally without moving the head or neck to allow recognition of any adverse reaction should it occur. Concomitant hemodynamic monitoring is also crucial.

Once the patient has been stable in the recovery area for 30 to 60 minutes and is tolerating clear liquids without aspiration, the patient is discharged home with an escort. Patients usually develop Horner's syndrome and Guttmann's sign, stuffy nose and increased temperature on the ipsilateral side of the block (face and upper extremity), respectively, within 5 minutes after the procedure.

Ultrasonographic Technique

Narouze et al[51] described an ultrasound (US)-guided SGB. In their technique, the patient is positioned in the supine position with the neck extended by placement of a pillow under the shoulder to stretch the esophagus and make it move medially under the trachea. Under fluoroscopic guidance, the bony target is identified at the junction of the anterolateral vertebral body with the transverse process at C6 level in the anteroposterior view, and the skin is marked. With complete aseptic technique, a 22-gauge blunt needle is used, aimed toward the identified bony target under fluoroscopic guidance (**Fig. 151.8**). After the skin and subcutaneous tissue are penetrated and the needle is stabilized, a 3- to 12-MHz linear-array probe (HD11-XL, Philips, Bothell, Wash) is used to verify the position of the needle. The needle may be shown to be aiming toward the thyroid tissue anteriorly and the esophagus posteriorly. At this point, the needle is withdrawn; it is reinserted obliquely and should then be advanced with real-time US imaging so that the needle tip will lie anterior to the longus colli muscle (anterior to C6 transverse process) (**Figs. 151.9 and 151.10**). After negative aspiration, 1 mL of contrast agent

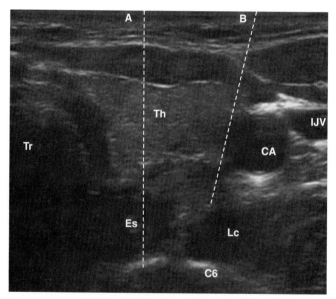

Fig. 151.10 Ultrasound imaging of the left stellate ganglion. *A,* The needle path with the anterior paratracheal approach. *B,* The needle path with ultrasound guidance. CA, carotid artery; Es, esophagus; IJV, internal jugular vein; Lc, longus colli muscle; Th, thyroid; Tr, trachea. *(From Narouze S, Vydyanathan A, Patel N: Ultrasound-guided stellate ganglion block successfully prevented esophageal puncture, Pain Physician 10:747, 2007. Reprinted with permission from the Cleveland Clinic Foundation.)*

is injected that should show adequate spread without vascular escape (**Figs. 151.11 and 151.12**). Then, 5 mL of bupivacaine 0.25% can be injected in divided doses with real-time US imaging, which should show extensive spread of the local anesthetic agent at the area of the lower cervical sympathetic chain with both cephalad and caudad spread (approximately

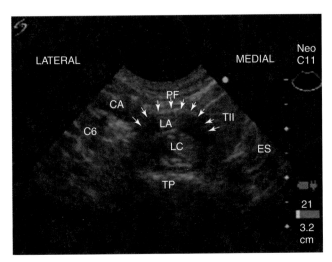

Fig. 151.11 Extent of local anesthetic spread inside the longus colli muscle and bulging of the prevertebral fascia. *(Courtesy of, Yasuyuki Shibata, MD, Aichi Medical University.)*

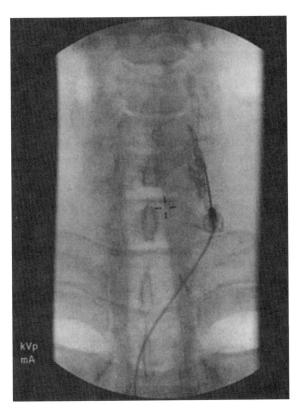

Fig. 151.12 Anteroposterior view showing the spread of the contrast agent. *(From Narouze S, Vydyanathan A, Patel N: Ultrasound-guided stellate ganglion block successfully prevented esophageal puncture, Pain Physician 10:747–752, 2007.)*

two segments each). Five minutes later, the patient should develop Horner's syndrome as well as vasodilatation of the ipsilateral upper extremity. The temperature at the left middle finger, when measured by contact thermography, should rise from 20°C (68°F) to 70°C (158°F).

Helpful Hints for Ultrasonographic Techniques

(Source: Yasuyuki S: Stellate ganglion block, Aichi Medical University: http://www.usra.ca/sb_stellate)

NERVE LOCALIZATION

The cervical sympathetic nerve trunk is within the prevertebral fascia. However, it is impossible to distinguish the sympathetic nerve trunk from the prevertebral fascia. In some patients, the middle cervical ganglion is clearly visualized within the prevertebral fascia.

NEEDLE INSERTION APPROACH

In US-guided SGB, the needle is not directed toward the stellate ganglion; rather, the cervical sympathetic nerve trunk and its gray communicating branches at the C6 level are blocked. The cervical sympathetic nerve trunk ascends through the prevertebral fascia, and their gray communicating branches penetrate the longus colli muscle from the anterior direction and communicate with the cervical nerve roots that proceed to the neck and upper limb. For that reason, it is possible to perform a C6 SGB by penetrating the prevertebral fascia with the needle and injecting local into the compartment of the longus colli muscle.

IN-PLANE APPROACH

Some investigators call this the *in-plane needle insertion approach*. The procedure is as follows:

- A 25-gauge, 1-inch long-bevel needle is used for SGB.
- A fine extension tube is connected between the needle and the syringe.
- The needle is inserted between the transducer and the trachea using an in-plane approach.
- The needle is advanced while avoiding the thyroid gland.
- The prevertebral fascia is penetrated, and the operator stops when the tip of needle reaches the inside the longus colli muscle. The tip of needle does not need to contact the transverse process of C6.
- Negative aspiration for blood is confirmed.
- The operator injects 0.5 mL of local anesthetic and checks whether the injectate has reached the longus colli muscle deep to the prevertebral fascia.
- If the spread is above the prevertebral fascia, the needle is advanced further.
- Once the needle is inside the longus colli muscle, a total of 5 to 8 mL of local anesthetic is injected.
- The extent of local anesthetic spread inside the longus colli muscle and bulging of the prevertebral fascia (see Fig. 151.11) are observed. In addition, scanning is performed cephalad and caudad to assess local anesthetic spread in the sagittal plane.

CAUTION

- One must pay particular attention to the location of the vertebral artery and the superior and inferior thyroid arteries. Color Doppler imaging is used to visualize these vascular structures.
- The vertebral artery does not always enter the C6 transverse foramen. It may bypass the C6 transverse foramen and enter the neural foramen at a higher cervical level.
- The superior thyroid artery is usually visualized on the lateral edge of the thyroid gland at the C6 level.
- The inferior thyroid artery ascends directly upward and cuts across the anterior surface of the longus colli muscle.
- These arteries are located in the path of the needle in some patients.

Chemical Neurolysis of Stellate Ganglion

The approach for chemical neurolysis is similar to that for SGB performed at C7. The patient must be positioned with the neck and head in a neutral position (see Fig. 151.4). Under direct anteroposterior fluoroscopy, the C7 vertebral body is identified. A skin wheal is raised over the ventrolateral aspect of the body of C7 with 1 mL of local anesthetic and a 25-gauge needle. A 22-gauge B-bevel needle is inserted through the skin wheal to contact the body of C7 in the ventrolateral aspect; this is at the junction of the transverse process with the vertebral body. Depth and direction should be confirmed with anteroposterior and lateral views.

The needle tip is positioned deep to the anterior longitudinal ligament. The longus colli muscle lies lateral to the needle tip. The needle should be stabilized with a long-handled Kelly clamp or hemostat. An intravenous extension should be attached to the needle and used for injection. A dose of approximately 5 mL of water-soluble, nonirritating, nonionic, preservative-free, hypoallergenic contrast solution is injected after negative aspiration. Dye should spread around the vertebra, and intravascular, epidural, intrathecal, thyroidal, or myoneural (longus colli) uptake should be avoided. If adequate spread of the contrast medium is visualized, a mix of local anesthetic, phenol, and steroid is injected. The total volume of 5 mL should consist of 2.5 mL of 6% phenol in saline, 1 mL of 40 mg of triamcinolone, and 1.5 mL of 0.5% ropivacaine. (The total 5-mL dose contains a final mixture of 3% phenol.)

The previously injected contrast material serves as a marker for the spread of the phenol. In the anteroposterior view, the contrast solution should spread caudad to the first thoracic sympathetic ganglion, cephalad to the inferior cervical ganglion, and cephalad to the superior cervical ganglion. In the lateral view, spread should be observed in the retropharyngeal space and in front of the longus colli and anterior scalene muscles. After injection, the patient remains supine with the head elevated slightly for approximately 30 minutes, to prevent spread of the phenol to other structures.[52]

Radiofrequency Neurolysis

Radiofrequency neurolysis of the stellate ganglion may be accomplished under fluoroscopic guidance. After the target area is identified as for chemical neurolysis, a 16-gauge angiocatheter is inserted through the skin wheal instead of the B-bevel needle. A 20-gauge, curved, blunt-tipped cannula with a 5-mm active tip is guided through the extracath at the superolateral aspect. The tip should rest at the junction of the transverse process and the vertebral body. The depth and direction should be confirmed with anteroposterior and lateral views. Correct placement may be confirmed conclusively with the injection of contrast medium (**Figs. 151.13** to **151.16**). A sensory (50-Hz, 0.9-V) and a motor (2-Hz, 2-V) stimulation trial must be performed owing to the location of the phrenic nerve (lateral) and the recurrent laryngeal nerve (anterior and medial) relative to the proposed lesion. While motor stimulation is performed, the patient should say "ee" to ensure preservation of motor function. A small volume of local anesthetic (0.5 mL) should be injected before lesioning. The radiofrequency is applied for 60 seconds at 80°C (176°F). The cannula is redirected to the most medial aspect of the transverse process in the same plane. Placement is in the ventral aspect of the transverse process in the same plane. Placement in the ventral aspect must be confirmed with a lateral view.

Before lesioning, the patient must be retested for sensory and motor stimulation. A repeat dose of the local anesthetic also should be given through the cannula. A third (and final) lesion should be directed at the upper portion of the junction of the transverse process and the body of C7. Potential complications include injury to the phrenic or the recurrent laryngeal nerve, neuritis, and vertebral artery injury. Side effects of SGB should be distinguished from complications. Most unpleasant side effects result from Horner's syndrome—ptosis, miosis, and nasal congestion.

Complications

Complications of SGB can be divided into technical, infectious, and pharmacologic.[53]

Technical Complications

Technical complications include injury to the nerves and nearby viscera during insertion of the needle.[2,29,31,54] These complications include injury to the brachial plexus, trauma to the trachea and esophagus (with mediastinal and surgical

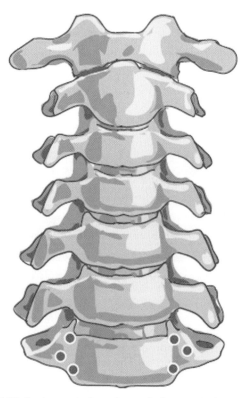

Fig. 151.13 Posteroanterior view of the cervical spine. *Dots mark the target points for radiofrequency lesioning of the cervical sympathetic nerves. These are at the junction of the medial aspect of the transverse process and the lateral aspect of its respective vertebral body.*

emphysema), injury to the pleura and lung (pneumothorax, hemothorax, which may require chest tube insertion), and bleeding and local hematoma, especially if the patient was taking anticoagulants. This situation can lead to airway compression.[55] Vasovagal attacks can also occur.

Infectious Complications

Infectious complications are possible if the aseptic barrier was breached. These complications can include local abscess, cellulitis, and osteitis of the vertebral body and transverse process.[56]

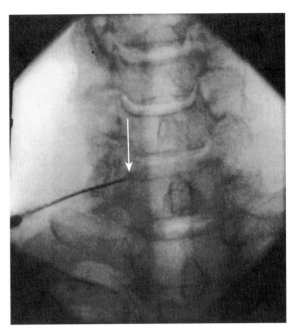

Fig. 151.15 **Posteroanterior radiograph of the cervical spine.** At the C7 level, the radiofrequency cannula rests at the junction of the lateral aspect of the vertebral body and the medial aspect of the transverse process *(arrow)*. This location represents the correct cannula position for lesioning of the C7 sympathetic fibers. *(From Raj PP, Lou L, Erdine S, et al: Stellate ganglion block. In Radiographic imaging for regional anesthesia and pain management, Philadelphia, 2003, Churchill Livingstone, p 78.)*

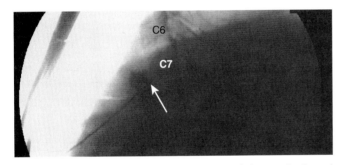

Fig. 151.14 Lateral view of correct placement of the needle *(arrow)* and the contrast spread after injection for stellate ganglion block. *(From Raj PP, Lou L, Erdine S, et al: Stellate ganglion block. In Radiographic imaging for regional anesthesia and pain management, Philadelphia, 2003, Churchill Livingstone, p 79.)*

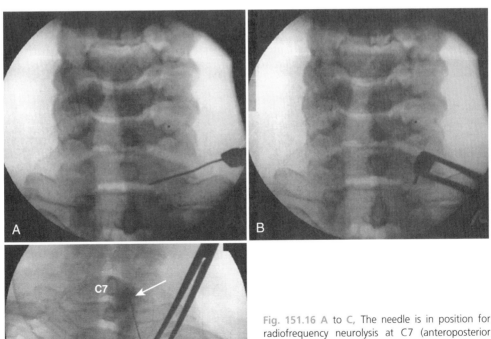

Fig. 151.16 A to C, The needle is in position for radiofrequency neurolysis at C7 (anteroposterior view). The *arrow (C)* shows the tip at the lateral border of vertebral body C7. *(From Raj PP, Lou L, Erdine S, et al: Stellate ganglion block. In Radiographic imaging for regional anesthesia and pain management, Philadelphia, 2003, Churchill Livingstone, p 79.)*

Pharmacologic Complications

Pharmacologic complications are related to the dose, volume, type of local anesthetic, and site of deposition of the solution. These complications includes hoarseness of voice because of involvement of recurrent laryngeal nerve or phrenic nerve paralysis, which leads to respiratory embarrassment, especially in the presence of contralateral dysfunction of the phrenic nerve or in patients with respiratory dysfunction (this is why bilateral SGB is contraindicated).[2,29,31] Involvement of the brachial plexus may lead to subclinical somatic blockade, which may produce the false impression that the pain is sympathetically maintained. Intra-arterial injection into the vertebral artery or the carotid artery can produce a high concentration of local anesthetic agent in the central nervous system (CNS) that leads to seizures. Intravenous injection can lead to seizure, but this is unlikely because of the low volume and dose of local anesthetic.[29] Selective nerve root spread has also been documented, epidurally of the local anesthetic, and intrathecal injection of the local anesthetic producing high spinal blockade has been reported. Horner's syndrome, the final consequence of sympathetic blockade, is really not a complication, although it can be unsightly. Air embolism has also been reported. Loss of cardioaccelerator activity may lead to various bradyarrhythmias and hypotension.[29]

Iatrogenic Postsympathectomy Syndrome

Postsympathectomy neuralgia is a poorly understood painful condition that occurs in up to 50% of all patients undergoing sympathectomy for the treatment of chronic pain.[57] This group also includes patients undergoing cervical or thoracic sympathectomy. Postsympathectomy neuralgia is proposed to be a complex neuropathic and central reafferentation and deafferentation syndrome. It depends on the transection during sympathectomy of the paraspinal somatic and visceral afferent axons, which are transmitted within the sympathetic trunk. Subsequently, cell death of many of the nociceptive axotomized afferent neurons results in central deafferentation and persistent sensitization of the spinal nociceptive neurons by the painful condition already present before the sympathectomy (viscerosomatic conversions and collateral sprouting of afferent nerves). The mechanics associated with sympathetically maintained pain are all proposed to be important factors in the development of this syndrome.

This syndrome can appear anywhere from a few days to a few weeks following chemical or surgical sympathectomy. It is characterized by deep, aching pain with superficial burning and hyperesthesia, which may or may not respond to narcotic analgesic. Postsympathectomy neuralgia is usually localized to the proximal region of the sympathectomized limb and to the trunk. This condition is sometimes confused with recurrence of CRPS type I or type II or the original disease that led to the performance of the sympathectomy. This postsympathectomy neuralgia is also sympathetically maintained. This phenomenon is explained by the finding that, when this complication occurs following sympathectomy for hyperhidrosis, it occurs only in the area of recurrence of the sweating. This syndrome has been reported in 30% to 50% of all sympathectomized patients. It is reported in only 6% of patients who have undergone sympathectomy for hyperhidrosis. This finding is in distinct contrast to the 40% to 50% incidence of postsympathectomy neuralgia following sympathectomy for CRPS type I and type II.

Bonica[31] has indicated that cardiac, esophageal, and tracheobronchial afferents that project to their target via the sympathetic trunk are removed during cervical sympathectomy (i.e., the lower part of C8-T1 [stellate ganglia] and the T1-T3 ganglia that are sometimes removed for upper-extremity sympathetically maintained pain [visceral somatic conversions theory]). Transection of these nerves during the C8-T1 or even T2-T3 sympathectomy can result in somatic referral of pain to the trunk and the proximal limb as the result of this visceral sympathetic afferent activity (deafferentation with the developing of firing ectopic neuron or because of central hypersensitization). The end result is likely to be referral of pain to the somatic tissue of the trunk and the proximal limb.[42] It has also been shown that some paraspinal somatic afferent nerves do project to their ventral spinal target tissue via the lumbar sympathetic trunk. Clearly, these nerves will be damaged during sympathectomy. This can lead to central deafferentation and central sensitization with aggravation of the pain syndrome.

As investigators understand the CNS more and more, multiple factors are recognized to aggravate this condition. They include extensive convergence of nerves within the spinal cord. The pain syndrome of postsympathectomy neuralgia may even involve a wider area of the body, including almost half of the body on the same side of the lesion. This condition can be mistaken for spread of CRPS.

Treatment of Postsympathectomy Syndrome

Treatment of postsympathectomy neuralgia depends on the symptoms. If they are the result of firing, spontaneous pain, then phenytoin, carbamazepine, or gabapentin can be helpful. Mexiletine or lidocaine given intravenously can also be helpful in patients with spontaneous pain or allodynia. Tricyclic antidepressants can also help reduce the incidence of postsympathectomy neuralgia. A discreet sympathetectomy should be produced. However, it is unavoidable that some transection of the paraspinal somatic afferent axon will occur during sympathectomy procedures.

Postsympathectomy neuralgia develops more frequently if pain is the predominant picture of the disease that requires the sympathectomy. The use of preemptive analgesia technique (i.e., continuous epidural block or continuous SGB or cervical block) can reduce the barrage of nociceptive stimulation to the CNS; this may help to reduce postsympathectomy syndrome.

During surgical sympathectomy, postsympathectomy neuralgia could be avoided if the proximal stump of the transected nerve is enclosed in an implantable sheath. This approach has been suggested to prevent centripetal transport of neurotoxic cells released from the injured tissue of the locus of the transection.

Finally, repeating the sympathetic blockade and the sympathectomy with a more complete sympathectomy procedure can also relieve this syndrome. Investigators have suggested that spinal cord stimulation or dorsal column stimulation can be of little help with this syndrome, because one of the mechanisms of action of spinal cord stimulation is through the sympathetic nervous system. The finding that these patients already have a damaged or interrupted sympathetic system may mean that they would respond poorly to a spinal cord stimulation trial. Indeed, some investigators have recommended that no sympathectomy be used for the treatment of CRPS type I and type II until a trial of spinal cord stimulator has been attempted.

Efficacy

Sympathetic interruption to the head, supplied by the stellate ganglion, can be documented easily by evidence of Horner's syndrome: miosis (pinpoint pupil), ptosis (drooping of the upper eyelid), and enophthalmos (sinking of the eyeball). Associated findings include conjunctival injection, nasal congestion, and facial anhidrosis. These signs can be present without complete interruption of the sympathetic nerves to the upper extremity.

Evidence of sympathetic blockade to the upper extremity includes visible engorgement of the veins on the back of the hand and forearm, diminution of the psychogalvanic reflex, and plethysmographic and thermographic changes. Skin temperature also increases, provided the preblock temperature did not exceed 33°C (91°F) to 34°C (93°F).

Efficacy of Chemical Neurolysis

Favorable reports of the efficiency of this procedure, as well as morbidity and mortality, have been published. The advantage of using neurolytic technique is that it covers more of the sympathetic fibers and hence produces a broader lesion and a more complete sympathectomy. The disadvantage of this method is that control of the lesion is more difficult. The radiofrequency lesion is well controlled, and the lesion cannot spread outside the 5-mm tip radius. Complications of these techniques are similar to complications produced by local anesthetic sympathetic ganglia block, with the exception of a longer-lasting block and potential neuritis.

Efficacy of Ultrasound

Kapral et al[58] described a technique for US-guided SGB in 1995. Direct visualization of the target, all nearby structures, the needle, and the spread of local anesthetic indicated that the method was safe and effective. The volume of local anesthetic required (5 mL) was significantly lower in the experimental group, compared with the blind-puncture group. Moreover, the onset of sympathetic blockade was hastened by US guidance. None of the patients in the US-guided group experienced hematoma, but this problem occurred in 3 of the 12 patients in the blind-approach group.[58] More recently, two additional articles were published. One was a case report addressing the feasibility of US-guided SGB with avoidance of esophageal penetration, which could occur during blind injection.[51] The second study considered where the local anesthetic should be injected in relation to the longus colli muscle, either subfascially or suprafascially.[59] These investigators speculated that subfascial injection could improve the spread of local anesthetic and decrease the incidence of recurrent laryngeal nerve palsy.

Notwithstanding the technical success achieved, neither technique reliably delivers local anesthetic to the stellate (cervicothoracic) ganglion. Magnetic resonance imaging has shown that the stellate ganglion is at the same level as or somewhat caudad to the head of the first rib. This position is more caudad than is commonly reported from dissections, and this finding indicates that displacement may occur during handling of anatomic material. Axial images obtained at the level of the first thoracic vertebra show that the ganglion is consistently lateral and posterior to the lateral edge of the longus colli muscle.

Efficacy of Radiofrequency

Geurts and Stolker[60] reviewed 27 cases selected from 40 patients with upper extremity reflex sympathetic dystrophy (CRPS type I) in whom these investigators performed radiofrequency lesion to the stellate ganglia. After 6 to 8 weeks' follow-up, 21 patients of the 27 were pain free, whereas 4 reported slight improvement in the pain that allowed them to participate more with physical therapy. Only 2 patients reported no benefit. During the follow-up period of 13.2 months (range, 5 to 38 months), 16 patients were still pain free without other signs of reflex sympathetic dystrophy, whereas 9 had recurrent symptoms. Seven of these patients appeared to have an underlying triggering factor, for which 6 patients required surgery. This report makes it clear that, before such a lesion is performed, it is important to select patients appropriately, to ensure that no surgically or medically treatable disease is present. After 43 radiofrequency lesions produced by this author, 4 initial technical failures, 3 minor complications, and 1 major complication resulting from irritation of the phrenic nerve that resolved after 2 weeks occurred. One of the important messages of this article is that radiofrequency lesions should be performed only in selected patients.[60]

Acknowlededgments

Some portions of this chapter were excerpted from the following sources: Raj PP, Lou L, Erdine S, et al: *Radiographic imaging for regional anesthesia and pain management*, Philadelphia, 2003, Churchill Livingstone, pp 72–80; Gofeld M: Ultrasonography in pain medicine: a critical review, *Pain Pract* 8:226, 2008; Abdi S, Zhou Y, Patel N, et al: A new and easy technique to block the stellate ganglion, *Pain Physician* 2004:7:327–331; and Narouze S, Vydyanathan A, Patel N: Ultrasound-guided stellate ganglion block successfully prevented esophageal puncture, *Pain Physician* 10:747–752, 2007.

References

Full references for this chapter can be found on www.expertconsult.com.

Chapter 152

Cervical Facet Joint Blocks

Laxmaiah Manchikanti, David M. Schultz, Frank J.E. Falco, and Vijay Singh

Historical Considerations

Chronic neck pain is common in the adult general population,[1-10] and it has a lifetime prevalence of 26% to 71%.[2,4,10] Chronic neck pain is also associated with significant economic, societal, and health impact.[10-16] Cervical intervertebral disks, cervical facet joints, atlantoaxial and atlanto-occipital joints, ligaments, fascia, muscles, and nerve root dura have been shown to be capable of transmitting pain in the cervical spine with resulting symptoms of neck pain, upper extremity pain, and headache.[1,17,18]

Based on controlled diagnostic blocks, cervical facet joints have been implicated as responsible for pain in the neck, head, and upper extremities in 36% to 67% of patients using controlled diagnostic blocks with a criterion standard of 80% pain relief and an ability to perform previously painful movements.[2,17-27]

Cervical facet or zygapophysial joints have been shown to be a source of pain in the neck and referred pain in the head and upper extremities.[28-32] Cervical facet joints are well innervated by the medial branches of the dorsal rami,[33-37] with free and encapsulated nerve endings with nociceptors and mechanonociceptors.[34,35,38-43] Studies have illustrated that 27% to 63% of patients suspected of having cervical facet joint pain present with false-positive results of diagnostic tests.[22-27,44-48]

Lumbar facet joints were identified as potential sources of back pain as early as 1911.[49] Not until 1977, however, did Pawl[31] report reproducing pain with injections of hypertonic saline into cervical facet joints in patients complaining of neck pain and headache. Bogduk and Marsland[50] studied the role of cervical facet joints in the causation of idiopathic neck pain by using diagnostic cervical medial branch blocks and facet joint injections. Dwyer et al[29] mapped out

specific locations of referred neck pain by performing facet joint injections in normal volunteers. Aprill et al[30] confirmed the accuracy of the pain chart developed by Dwyer et al[29] by anesthetizing the medial branches of the dorsal rami above and below the symptomatic joint. Fukui et al[28] studied the referred pain distribution of cervical facet joints and cervical dorsal rami, with similar results. Windsor et al[32] also studied electrical stimulation–induced cervical medial branch referral patterns.

In 1980, Sluijter and Koetsveld-Baart[51] described a technique for blocking the cervical dorsal rami near their origin and a percutaneous radiofrequency technique to coagulate these nerves. Bogduk and Marsland[50] described cervical medial branch blocks distal to the target sites used by Sluijter and Koetsveld-Baart[51] in 1980. In 1981, Okada[52] introduced intra-articular cervical facet joint blocks using a lateral approach. Later, Dory[53] described a posterior approach based on a pillar view of the cervical facet joints. Subsequently, numerous other investigators[54-57] described intra-articular cervical facet joint blocks.

Indications

As with any synovial joint, degeneration, inflammation, and injury of facet joints can lead to pain on joint motion. Pain leads to restriction of motion, which eventually produces overall physical deconditioning. Irritation of the facet joint innervation in itself also leads to secondary muscle spasm. Investigators have postulated that degeneration of the lumbar disk would lead to associated lumbar facet joint degeneration and subsequent spinal pain as the disk space loses height, with resulting excess stress on the posterior spinal elements. This process may also play a role in the cervical spine.

Diagnostic Cervical Facet Blocks
Background

- Blocks of a cervical facet joint can be performed to test the hypothesis that the target joint is the source of the patient's pain.[2,17,18–27,45–48]
- The cervical facet joints can be anesthetized with intra-articular injections of local anesthetic or by anesthetizing the medial branches of the dorsal rami that innervate the target joint.[2,17,18,45–48]
- If pain is relieved, the joint may be considered the source of pain.[45,47]
- True-positive responses are secured by performing controlled blocks, in the form of either placebo injections of normal saline solution or comparative local anesthetic blocks, in which on two separate occasions the same joint is anesthetized using local anesthetics with differing durations of action.[1,17–27]

Rationale

The rationale for using facet joint blocks for diagnosis is based on the following:

- The cervical facet joints are well innervated.[33–37]
- The cervical facet joints have been shown to be capable of causing persistent neck pain and referred pain in the head and upper extremities.[28–32]
- No reliable or valid indicator or clinical means exists to implicate cervical facet joints as the source of neck pain, headache, or upper extremity pain in a given patient.[1,17,18,45–48]
- The referral patterns described for cervical facet joints are variable.[17,18,45–48]
- A pattern of pain similar to that caused by cervical facet joints may be produced by other structures in the cervical spine, such as the disk, in the same segment.[18,45–48]
- Many of the maneuvers used in physical examinations stress multiple structures simultaneously in the cervical spine in addition to facet joints and fail to provide useful diagnostic criteria.[45–48]
- Numerous attempts by investigators to correlate neurophysiologic findings, radiologic findings, physical findings, and other signs and symptoms with the diagnosis of facet joint pain have been unsuccessful.[1]
- The reliability of cervical facet joint nerve blocks in the diagnosis of neck pain, upper extremity pain, and headaches is demonstrated by strong evidence.[1,17,18,45–48,58]
- The face validity of intra-articular injections and medial branch blocks is demonstrated by determining the spread of contrast medium after the injection of small volumes of local anesthetic under fluoroscopic visualization.[1,17,18,45–48]
- The construct validity of facet joint blocks has been demonstrated to rule out false-positive results.[1,17,18,45–48]
- The theory that evaluating a patient first with lidocaine and subsequently with bupivacaine provides a means of identifying placebo response has been tested and proven.[1,17–27,45–48]
- Significant false-positive rates with single facet joint blocks in the cervical spine have been documented (27% to 63%).[1,17–27,45–48]

Requirements

Tables 152.1 and 152.2 show indications and contraindications for diagnostic facet joint blocks. Cervical facet joint blocks are commonly performed in patients with the following:

- Neck pain, for which no cause is otherwise evident
- Pain patterns resembling that of pain evoked in normal volunteers on stimulation of the facet joints
- Lack of disk herniation or radiculopathy as the symptomatic lesion
- Lack of neurophysiologic abnormalities

Precautions

Caution must be exercised in patients receiving nonsteroidal anti-inflammatory medications. Raj et al[59] provided a detailed description of the role of anticoagulants in interventional pain management. Nonetheless, consensus is lacking on the importance of discontinuation of aspirin before facet joint injection procedures. Patients receiving warfarin therapy should be checked for prothrombin time, which should be at acceptable levels. In stopping anticoagulant therapy, the interventional pain practitioner must take into consideration the risk-to-benefit ratio and also consult with the physician in charge of anticoagulant therapy to avoid unnecessary complications and consequent liability. Thus, it may be appropriate to advise the patient to contact the

Table 152.1 Common Indications for Cervical Diagnostic Facet Joint Blocks

- Somatic or nonradicular neck or upper extremity pain
- Cervicogenic headache and upper back pain
- Lack of obvious evidence for diskogenic pain
- Lack of disk herniation or evidence of radiculitis
- Duration of pain of at least 3 months
- Failure to respond to more conservative management, including physical therapy modalities with exercise, chiropractic management, and nonsteroidal anti-inflammatory agents
- Average pain levels of greater than 5 on a scale of 0 to 10

Table 152.2 Common Contraindications for Cervical Facet Joint Blocks

- Infection
- Arnold-Chiari malformation
- Inability of the patient to understand consent, nature of the procedure, needle placement, or sedation
- Allergies to contrast material, local anesthetic, steroids, Sarapin, or other drugs
- Needle phobia
- Psychogenic pain
- Suspected diskogenic pain or disk herniation
- Anticoagulant therapy
- Nonsteroidal anti-inflammatory drug therapy (although no evidence indicates that these drugs increase the risk of serious bleeding)
- Nonaspirin antiplatelet therapy

physician in charge of anticoagulant therapy to manage this aspect of care.

Therapeutic Cervical Facet Blocks

A significant role has been described for therapeutic facet joint injections, either intra-articular or by medial branch block and medial branch neurotomy.[1,17] However, a single, randomized controlled trial demonstrated lack of efficacy for intra-articular cervical facet joint steroid injections.[1,17] Falco et al[17] reviewed the literature extensively. These investigators concluded that, except for the one negative randomized trial for intra-articular injections,[60] no other nonobservational trials qualified to be included for evidence synthesis.

In addition to intra-articular blocks, medial branch blocks have been used for therapeutic purposes in the cervical spine.[61,62] The evidence evaluating medial branch blocks for therapeutic purposes is moderate to strong.[17]

Indications and contraindications for cervical facet joint blocks are described in **Tables 152.1** and **152.2**. Therapeutic facet joint blocks are performed only in patients with a confirmed diagnosis of facet joint pain established by controlled diagnostic blocks.

Clinically Relevant Anatomy

- The cervical facet joints are paired, diarthrodial, synovial joints located between the superior and inferior articular pillars in the posterior cervical column (**Fig. 152.1**).[45]
  - The cervical facet joints extend from C2-3 to C7-T1.
  - The atlanto-occipital and atlantoaxial synovial joints are also present in the cervical spine as two paired joints but are not considered facet joints because they are anterior rather than posterior spinal structures.

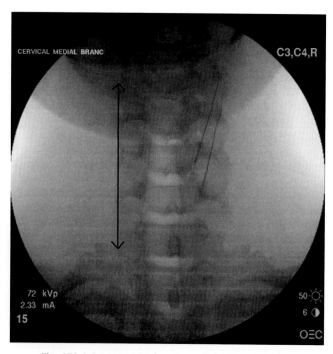

Fig. 152.1 **Anteroposterior view of the facet column.**

- The cervical facet joints are formed by the inferior articular process of the superior vertebral segment and the superior articular process of the inferior vertebral segment.
- The superior aspect of the joint faces forward and downward at 45 degrees, whereas the inferior aspect of the joint faces backward and upward at 45 degrees.
- Cervical facet joints exhibit the features of typical synovial joints.
  - The articular facets are covered by articular cartilage, and a synovial membrane bridges the margins of the articular cartilage of the two facets in each joint.
  - The cervical facet joints may contain a variety of intra-articular inclusions, the most common of which are fibroadipose meniscoids.
- The capsular recesses exist at both superior and inferior aspects, with the superior recess adjacent to the neural foramina and the dorsal root ganglia. The average joint volume is less than 1 mL.[29]
- The articular surfaces of facet joints in the cervical spine are generally flat, with only minimal concavity and convexity.[63] The obliquity of cervical facet joints averages approximately 45 degrees but is flatter at C2-3 and steeper at C6-7.[64] The C2-3 joint is more oblique in its orientation than its adjacent counterpart. Thus, the inclination of lower joints is steeper.[65]
- The cervical facet joints are well innervated by the medial branches of the dorsal rami.[33–47] The cervical facet joints below C2-3 are supplied by medial branches of the cervical dorsal rami above and below the joint, and these branches also innervate the deep paramedian muscles. The C2-3 joint is supplied by the third occipital nerve. The innervation of the atlanto-occipital and atlanto-axial joints is derived from the C1 and the C2 root, respectively.[66,67]
  - The fibrous joint capsule is richly innervated with mechanoreceptors, as well as nociceptors.[34,35,38–43]
- Each C3-7 dorsal ramus crosses the transverse process of the same segment and divides into lateral and medial branches.
  - The medial branch curves around the waist of the articular pillar of the same-numbered vertebra.
  - The medial branches are bound by fascia, held against the articular pillar, and covered by the tendinous slips of the origin of the semispinalis capitis.[68]
  - Articular branches arise as the nerve approaches the posterior aspect of the articular pillar, with an ascending branch innervating the joint above and a descending branch innervating the joint below.
  - At C7, in contrast to C3-6, the medial branch is located at a higher level owing to the transverse process. At C7, the base of the transverse process occupies most of the lateral aspect of the articular pillar pushing the medial branch higher.[21,67]
  - C4 to C7 medial branch nerves typically lack any cutaneous branches.
  - The course of the C4 and C5 medial branch nerves has been shown to be relatively constant, following the waist of their respective articular pillars in cadavers.[69]
  - C3, C6, and C7 show more variation compared with C4 and C5.[69]

- The C3 medial branch nerve with its more superior location at the upper third of the C3 articular pillar often overlaps the third occipital nerve, and the third occipital nerve is rostral to the C3 medial branch.[69] The C3 medial branch and the third occipital nerve have a common origin in the C3 dorsal ramus.
- The C6 medial branch courses around the waist of the articular pillar or above it, between the waist and the superior articular process.
- Most (70%) C7 medial branches are located high on the C7 articular pillar and cross the C6-7 facet joint. However, a few may be lower on the C7 transverse process.
- The distance between the nerves and bone varies from close proximity to separation by 2 to 3 mm.
- The C2-3 facet joint is largely innervated from the third occipital nerve, which is the superficial medial branch of the C3 dorsal ramus.
  - The deep medial branch of the C3 dorsal ramus is referred to as the *C3 medial branch.*
  - Articular branches may also arise from a communicating loop that crosses the back of the joint between the third occipital nerve and the C2 dorsal ramus.[33,67]
  - The third occipital nerve continues around the lower lateral and dorsal surface of the C2-3 joint embedded in the connective tissue that invests the joint capsule.[33,61] It also provides muscular branches to the semispinalis capitis and becomes cutaneous over the suboccipital region.
- The vertebral artery ascends through the cervical transverse foramina of C1 to C6, which are located anterolaterally.
  - The vertebral artery at C2-7 is located anterior to the facet joints from both posterior and lateral injection approaches.
  - The vertebral artery passes directly superior in the neck until it reaches the transverse process of the axis, where it courses upward and laterally to the transverse foramina of the atlas.[70]
  - The vertebral artery courses medially and superiorly from its lateral position at C1 to the medial foramen magnum. The course of the vertebral artery from the transverse foramen of the atlas to the foramen magnum may be tortuous and variable.

Technique

The cervical facet joint blockade technique has lagged behind that of lumbar facet joint block. Multiple techniques for lumbar facet joint block have been described. Cervical facet joint injections may be performed using a posterior, lateral, or anterior approach. The posterior approach is the most commonly used, followed by the lateral approach. Both approaches are described here.

Intra-Articular Blocks
Posterior Approach

The posterior approach for cervical intra-articular facet joint block can be performed with the patient in a prone position or, if required, in a sitting position. This procedure involves introducing a 22- or a 25-gauge needle into the target joint from behind, along an oblique trajectory that coincides with the plane of the joint.

- The patient is positioned in the prone position on a radiolucent fluoroscopy table with a cushion under the chest, with the head and neck completely prone or with the neck rotated to the opposite side.
- Under aseptic conditions, skin entry is achieved approximately two or more segments below the target joint. The skin entry point may be determined either by directing an imaginary line to the skin along the plane of the joint (as determined by a lateral view) or by direct visualization of the joint through a pillar view and making a skin mark along the plane of the x-ray beam into the center of the joint lucency.[71,72] The sagittal plane for skin entry is determined by identifying the sagittal plane of the facet joint column's lateral aspect under prone fluoroscopic viewing.
- The needle is passed with caution through the skin at approximately a 45-degree angle upward and ventrally through the posterior neck muscles until it makes contact with the posterior surface of the articular pillar below the target joint.
- Following this maneuver, the needle may be readjusted until it enters the joint cavity. However, this may require repeated posteroanterior and lateral fluoroscopic visualization to ensure that the needle stays on course. *Caution:* Directing the needle medially toward the interlaminar space may result in epidural or intrathecal puncture or spinal cord trauma. The depth of the needle is evaluated by a lateral view; however, repeated posteroanterior and lateral screening is used to guide the insertion until the needle strikes the back of the target joint at its midpoint.[71,72]
- After satisfactory localization of the needle in the joint, water-soluble contrast medium is injected to obtain an arthrogram and verify accurate placement. Then, local anesthetic or corticosteroid is injected for diagnostic or therapeutic purposes. *Caution:* The capacity of the joint can be assessed from the volume of the injectate of the contrast, which is typically less than 1 mL. It is important to respect the capacity of the joint because the local anesthetic and steroid may leak into the recesses and block the dorsal root ganglion.
- The C7-T1 joint may be difficult to enter with a posterior approach; therefore, a lateral approach has been suggested. However, because of the risk of pneumothorax and the proximity of other neurovascular structures, the posterior approach is preferred for the C7-T1 facet joint.[71,72] **Figure 152.2** illustrates intra-articular needle placement with a posterior approach.

Overall, the posterior approach is considered safe because the needle penetrates only the skin and posterior neck muscles. The deep cervical artery is the only structure at risk of inadvertent puncture. Further, posterior cervical arteries pose minimal risk of morbidity because they supply no major structures. However, if the needle is inserted too deeply or too aggressively, it could penetrate the anterior joint capsule and move into the neural foramen and the vicinity of the dorsal root ganglion, the cervical radicular artery, or the vertebral artery. Leakage of local anesthetic and steroid to the dorsal root ganglion may negate any diagnostic information from this injection, whereas inadvertent contact with the nerve root or anterior artery may have serious adverse consequences. In addition, the potential exists for a misplaced needle to enter the epidural space or spinal cord.

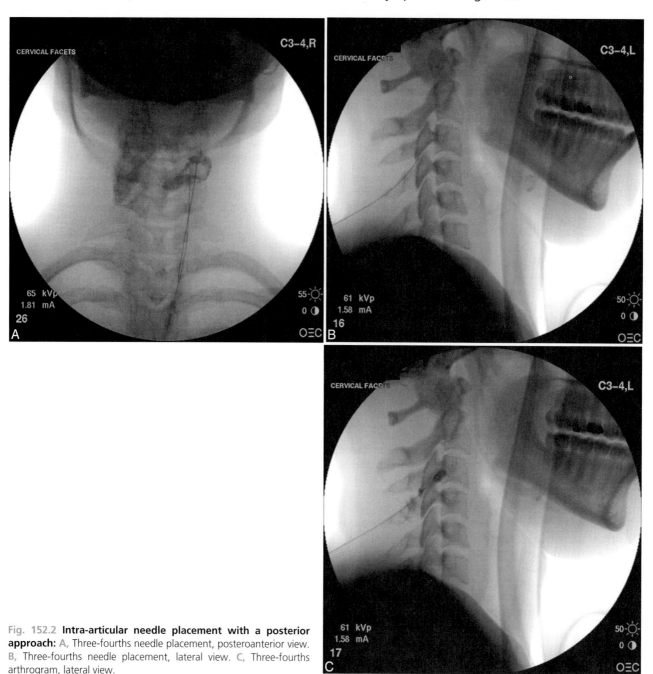

Fig. 152.2 Intra-articular needle placement with a posterior approach: A, Three-fourths needle placement, posteroanterior view. B, Three-fourths needle placement, lateral view. C, Three-fourths arthrogram, lateral view.

Lateral Approach

Proponents of the lateral approach argue that it is technically less demanding and may be performed with smaller-gauge needles.[52] These proponents also argue that the lateral approach is more comfortable for the patient because less soft tissue is traversed. Similar to the posterior approach during insertion, the risk of morbidity is minimal with the lateral approach because only the skin and posterolateral neck muscles are penetrated, and no other overlying structures are at risk of puncture. However, aggressive maneuvering or over-penetration may lead the needle into the epidural space or spinal cord. Many experts believe that the lateral technique is

more technically demanding and requires more experience. The procedure is as follows:

- The patient is positioned lying on the side with the target side upward. The patient's shoulders are pulled down to avoid obscuring the joints under fluoroscopy and are rotated slightly posterior about 25 degrees into the plane of the upper torso and shoulders.[71,72]
- The target joint is identified on lateral imaging of the neck.
  - Lateral fluoroscopic imaging must appropriately identify both joints so that the uppermost target joint is differentiated from the down-side contralateral joint (**Fig. 152.3**).

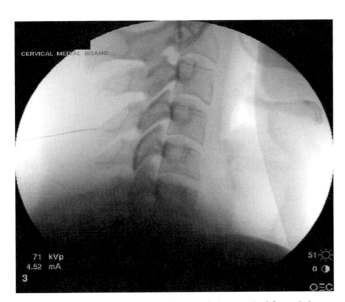

Fig. 152.3 **Lateral fluoroscopic image of the cervical facet joints.**

- The object is to identify the image of the target joint, which lies uppermost in the patient.
- The needle is introduced through the skin over the midpoint of the joint.
  - The needle is advanced deeply until it makes contact with the bone of either the superior or inferior articular process. *This technique promotes safety by providing the operator with a sense of accurate depth of insertion and prevents overinsertion.*
  - Rotation of the intensifier may help to identify both joints. It is absolutely crucial that right and left joints be identified properly so that the uppermost joint is targeted.
- Once the correct joint is clearly identified, the needle is advanced until the superior articular process is contacted just above the joint line.
  - The needle is then directed and advanced through the joint capsule.
  - The needle may be felt to pierce the capsule and to enter the joint space. Only minimal penetration is required, and the operator may also notice loss of resistance as the needle pierces the capsule.
- The appropriate position in the joint may be confirmed either by injection of a small dose of contrast medium to obtain an arthrogram or by multiple radiographic views. The facet joints in the cervical spine are more easily entered if one begins slightly superior to the joint and angles the needle inferiorly along the plane of the articular surfaces until the joint is entered.[71,72]

With the lateral approach, the needle must remain posterior to the ventral ramus and the vertebral and radicular arteries, to ensure safety. C3-4, C4-5, and C6-7 joint injections are easily performed using the lateral approach, with no disadvantages compared with the posterior approach. However, the C7-T1 joint injection may be more easily performed using the posterior approach. In patients with a large neck and shoulders, C7-T1 may not be reached from a lateral approach, and the procedure may require the posterior approach. C7-T1 may also require a much steeper

superior to inferior approach than other midcervical levels, to minimize the possibility of contact with more inferior neurovascular and pleural structures.

The C2-3 joint may be technically more difficult to visualize and enter, owing to its anatomic features. The C2-3 joint is more angulated vertically and medially and is not clearly evident on lateral views. For C2-3, the posterior approach may be modified by rotating the patient's head to bring the cavity of the C2-3 joint into view as it moves forward on the long axis of the vertebral column. Other modifications of the fluoroscopic unit can also be made. **Figure 152.4** illustrates intra-articular placement with a lateral approach.

Low volumes must be injected into the cervical facet joints in a slow and incremental fashion. If volumes greater than 1 mL are injected, or if injection is carried out rapidly or forcefully, the joint capsule may rupture, or medication may spread into nearby structures. Okada[52] showed, that in a series of 142 arthrograms, a communicating pathway existed in 80% of subjects between the facet joint and the interlaminar space, the opposite facet joint, the extradural space, or the interspinous space when volumes in excess of 1 mL were injected (**Fig. 152.5**). Even with smaller volumes, extra-articular leaks have been observed in up to 7% of cases.[52,53,55] Extra-articular spread is extremely important, specifically when diagnostic blocks are performed, because this will compromise the specificity of the block.

Cervical Medial Branch Blocks

The cervical facet joints can be anesthetized by blocking the nerves that supply them, specifically the medial branches of the cervical dorsal rami. To block the nerves supplying a cervical facet joint, two medial branches must be blocked because of each facet joint's dual innervation. **Table 152.3** illustrates the nerves to be blocked for each facet joint.

The target points for these nerves, other than the third occipital nerve, are the crossing points of the waists of the articular pillars: a point proximal to the origin of the articular branches and a point where the nerves have a constant relation to the bone.[47,71,72] These points may be reached by needles using a posterior, lateral, or anterior approach. The posterior and lateral approaches are the commonly used techniques.

Posterior Approach

- The patient is placed in the prone position with a pillow under the chest. The head may be completely prone or turned to the opposite side.
- A posteroanterior view is obtained to identify the posterior aspect of the waists of the articular pillars from C3-7.
  - In some patients, the articular pillars of the superior cervical spine (C3 and C4) may be difficult to identify, especially with the patient's head in a neutral position. Turning the head to the opposite side may facilitate visualization of the target area.
  - Asking the patient to open his or her mouth to remove the mandible from the radiologic field is an additional maneuver.
- After the waists of the articular pillars of the levels to be blocked are identified, a 22- or 25-gauge, 2- to 3-inch spinal needle is inserted through the skin and posterior neck

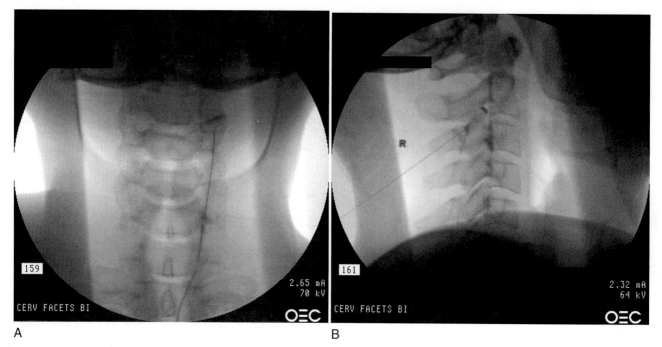

Fig. 152.4 **Intra-articular placement within C2-3 with a lateral approach.** A, Intra-articular placement of C2-3 in the posteroanterior view. B, Intra-articular placement of C2-3 with a lateral approach.

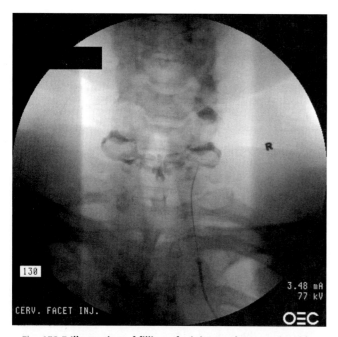

Fig. 152.5 **Illustration of filling of a joint on the opposite side.**

Table 152.3 Facet Joint Nerves to Be Blocked for Each Facet Joint in Cervical Region

Facet Joint	Facet Joint Nerves (Medial Branches) to Be Blocked	Level of Transverse Process
C2-3	Third occipital nerve or C2 and C3 medial branches	At C2-3 joint
C3-4	C3 and C4 medial branches	At C3 and C4 articular pillars
C4-5	C4 and C5 medial branches	At C4 and C5 articular pillars
C5-6	C5 and C6 medial branches	At C5 and C6 articular pillars
C6-7	C6 and C7 medial branches	At C6 and C7 articular pillars
C7-T1	C7 and C8 medial branches	At C7 articular pillar At T1 transverse process for C8

muscles. The operator aims first for the dorsal aspect of the articular pillar medial to its lateral concavity.

■ Once the needle has made contact with the bone, it is readjusted laterally to the deepest of this concavity where the C3 to C7 medial branches lie. *Caution:* Initially directing the needle medially to bone ensures that the needle is not placed too deeply. The needle is then directed laterally until the tip reaches the lateral margin of the articular pillar waist. The needle should be felt barely to slip off the bone laterally in a ventral direction at the deepest point of concavity of the articular pillar.[71,72] Thus, it is prudent to obtain lateral images to ensure that the needle tip rests at the centroid of the articular pillar. The centroid is found at the intersection of the two diagonals of the diamond-shaped pillar[71,72] (**Fig. 152.6**).

■ The C8 medial branch is blocked by placing the needle onto the transverse process of T1 and then directing it until it lies at the superolateral border of the transverse process. **Figure 152.7** illustrates medial branch blocks with the posterior approach.

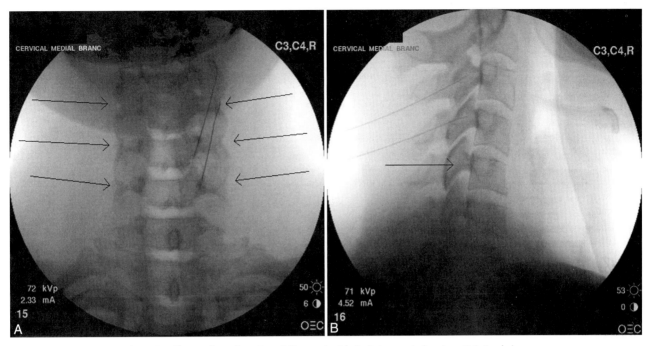

Fig. 152.6 **Illustration of center of the centroid.** A, Anteroposterior view. B, Lateral view.

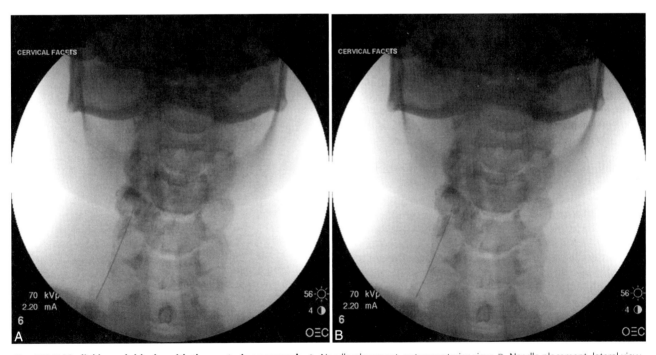

Fig. 152.7 **Medial branch blocks with the posterior approach.** A, Needle placement, anteroposterior view. B, Needle placement, lateral view.

■ Lateral viewing of needle tip location may be difficult below C6. Moving the C-arm to an oblique projection may help to identify needle depth by moving the shoulders out of the fluoroscopic beam's line.

Lateral Approach
■ The patient is positioned in the lateral position with the target side upward.
■ Articular pillars are identified by lateral fluoroscopy.

■ The uppermost articular pillar can be distinguished from the opposite side by moving the fluoroscope. *The needle will be seen to travel with the uppermost articular pillar as the two articular pillars separate on the fluoroscopic image. This approach is well suited for C3 to C6 medial branches.*[71,72]
■ The needle is directed through the skin and posterolateral neck muscles toward the centroid of the articular pillar as seen on a true lateral radiograph.[71,72]
■ To block the C7 medial branch by the lateral approach, the needle is advanced so that it stays within the confines of

the C7 superior articular process; this maneuver prevents excessive advancement into the C8 foramen and toward the vertebral artery.[71,72]

■ Once the superior articular process is contacted, anteroposterior imaging should verify that the needle lies against the lateral aspect of the superior articular process.

■ **Figure 152.8** illustrates medial branch blocks with the lateral approach.

With posterior and lateral approaches, contrast material in doses of 0.1 to 0.2 mL may be injected to confirm appropriate needle placement. However, contrast injection is not mandatory. After the needle position is confirmed, local anesthetic with or without steroid is injected incrementally around the nerve.

Cervical medial branch blocks are extremely safe. Other than general risks associated with all cervical injections, including fluoroscopic exposure, infection, and needle trauma, no specific complications have been reported. The relative safety of medial branch blocks lies in the fact that the blocks are performed on the external surface of the vertebral column, well away from any vital structures. Some investigators state that the lateral approach is advantageous because target points are clearly visible and tissue penetration is minimal. The posterior approach may require adjustment of the needle onto the lateral margin of the articular pillar with an additional step; however, with experience, this adjustment may be avoided.

Drugs

Local anesthetic for intra-articular injections, as well as for medial branch blocks, should be limited to 0.5 mL (0.3 to 0.6 mL) for a diagnostic block and approximately 1 mL (1 to 2 mL) for a therapeutic block. For diagnostic, as well as therapeutic blockade, the literature has been limited to using local anesthetic agents of different durations of action, namely, lidocaine and bupivacaine.

Side Effects and Complications

Complications of intra-articular injections or medial branch blocks in the cervical spine are exceedingly rare.[1,17,18,45–48,71–83] However, disastrous complications may occur with cervical facet joint injections. These complications include those related to placement of the needle, as well as complications related to the administration of various drugs. Proximity to the vertebral artery and spinal cord, along with nerve root ganglion, make intra-articular facet injections relatively high risk when compared with medial branch blocks. Possible complications include the following: dural puncture, spinal cord trauma, neural trauma, subdural injection, and injection into the intervertebral foramen; intravascular injection into the veins, or more seriously into vertebral or radicular arteries; infectious complications, including epidural abscess and bacterial meningitis; and side effects related to the administration of steroids, local anesthetics, and other drugs.

Other exceedingly rare but potential complications of cervical facet joint injections include vertebral artery and ventral ramus damage, embolus resulting in serious neurologic sequelae, spinal cord damage, and cerebral infarction. Minor complications include light-headedness, flushing, sweating, nausea, hypotension, syncope, pain at the injection site, and headaches. Side effects related to the administration of steroids are generally attributed to the physiologic effects of the steroids.[82] These include suppression of pituitary-adrenal access, hypocorticism, Cushing's syndrome, osteoporosis, avascular necrosis of the bone, steroid myopathy, epidural lipomatosis, weight gain, fluid retention, and hypoglycemia. However, Manchikanti et al,[83] in evaluating the effect of neuraxial steroids on weight and bone mass density, showed no significant differences in patients undergoing various types of interventional techniques, with or without steroids.

Conclusion

Cervical facet joints are commonly identified as the cause of neck pain, upper extremity pain, and headaches. Cervical facet joint blocks can be performed to test the hypothesis that the target joint is the source of the patient's pain. The rationale for using facet joint blocks for diagnosis, as well as therapy, is based on the finding that cervical facet joints have been shown to be the source of neck pain and referred pain in the head and upper extremities. Although cervical facet joint pain may not be diagnosed based on referral patterns, physical examination, history, neurophysiologic testing, or radiologic evaluation, diagnostic cervical facet joint blocks have been shown to be highly valid and specific. Because degenerative processes of the cervical spine and the origins of cervical spine pain are extremely complex, the effectiveness of many different therapeutic interventions in managing chronic pain arising from the cervical spine has not been demonstrated conclusively.

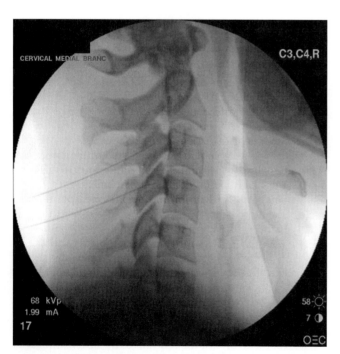

Fig. 152.8 **C3-4 medial branch blocks with a lateral approach.**

The following key points can be made:

- Cervical facet joints have been shown to be capable of causing pain in the neck and referred pain in the head and upper extremities.
- Cervical facet joints are well innervated by the medial branches of the dorsal rami.
- Based on responses to controlled diagnostic blocks of cervical facet joints, in accordance with the criteria established by the International Association for the Study of Pain, the prevalence of cervical facet joint pain has been determined to be 36% to 67%.
- To maintain the validity of diagnostic blocks, either comparative local anesthetic blocks or placebo-controlled blocks must be performed, because single blocks carry a false-positive rate of 27% to 63%.
- Multiple effective and therapeutic modalities are available for managing cervical facet joint pain.
- Adequate training and experience, proper technique, meticulous adherence to safety guidelines, and high-quality fluoroscopic imaging equipment are prerequisites for safe and effective injection of cervical structures.

References

Full references for this chapter can be found on www.expertconsult.com.

Cervical Epidural Nerve Block

Steven D. Waldman

Because cervical epidural nerve block has had a limited number of applications in surgical anesthesia, this procedure traditionally has been identified as an exotic technique of only passing historical interest. The more recent recognition of the clinical utility of cervical epidural nerve block in the management of head, face, neck, shoulder, and upper extremity pain has brought the technique into the mainstream of contemporary pain management. This chapter provides a practical overview of the indications for, technique of, and contraindications to cervical epidural nerve block.

Historical Considerations

Although the description by Pagés[1] of the paramidline approach to the lumbar epidural space in 1921 is considered the first clinically relevant report of the technique of lumbar epidural nerve block, it seems that Dogliotti[2] was the first to describe the technique of epidural block in the cervical region.[3]

Owing to the problems inherent in complete sensory blockade of the cervical nerve roots when cervical epidural nerve block is performed for surgical anesthesia, in the past many anesthesiologists believed that cervical epidural nerve block was too risky, given the general anesthetic techniques available at the time. This situation led to two persistent beliefs that colored contemporary thinking on the use of cervical epidural nerve block for pain management. The

first belief is that cervical epidural nerve block is too risky for routine clinical use. The second belief is that the procedure has a limited number of applications. Both beliefs have been refuted by the documented clinical utility of cervical epidural administration of steroids to manage cervical radiculopathy, tension-type headache, and other painful conditions, along with cervical epidural opioids to manage cancer-related pain, combined with the clinical experience of most contemporary pain specialists.

Indications and Contraindications

Indications for cervical epidural nerve block are summarized in **Table 153.1**. In addition to a few applications for surgical anesthesia, cervical epidural nerve block with local anesthetics can be used as a diagnostic tool for differential neural blockade on an anatomic basis for the evaluation of head, neck, face, shoulder, and upper extremity pain.[3-8] If destruction of the cervical nerve roots is being considered, the technique is useful as a prognostic indicator of the extent of motor and sensory impairment that the patient may experience.

Cervical epidural nerve block with local anesthetics or opioids may be used to palliate acute pain emergencies during the wait for pharmacologic, surgical, or antiblastic methods to take effect.[9,10] The technique is useful in the management of postoperative pain and pain secondary to trauma involving

Table 153.1 Indications for Cervical Epidural Nerve Block

SURGICAL, DIAGNOSTIC, PROGNOSTIC INDICATIONS

Surgical anesthesia
Differential neural blockade to evaluate head, neck, face, shoulder, and upper extremity pain
Prognostic indicator before destruction of cervical nerves

ACUTE PAIN

Palliation in acute pain emergencies
Postoperative pain
Head, face, neck, shoulder, and upper extremity pain secondary to trauma
Pain of acute herpes zoster
Acute vascular insufficiency of the upper extremities

PROPHYLACTIC AND PREEMPTIVE PAIN

Tension-type headache
Before amputation of ischemic limbs

CHRONIC BENIGN PAIN

Cervical radiculopathy
Cervical spondylosis
Cervicalgia
Vertebral compression fractures
Diabetic polyneuropathy
Postherpetic neuralgia
Reflex sympathetic dystrophy
Shoulder pain syndromes
Upper extremity pain syndromes
Phantom limb syndrome
Peripheral neuropathy
Postlaminectomy syndrome
Tension-type headache

CANCER-RELATED PAIN

Pain secondary to head, face, neck, shoulder, and upper extremity malignancies
Bony metastases to head, face, cervical spine, shoulder girdle, and upper extremity
Chemotherapy-related peripheral neuropathy

Table 153.2 Contraindications for Cervical Epidural Nerve Block

Absolute	Relative
Local infection	Hypovolemia
Sepsis	
Anticoagulant medication or coagulopathy	

the head, face, neck, and lower extremities. The pain of acute herpes zoster and cancer-related pain also are amenable to epidural administration of local anesthetics, steroids, or opioids.[11] Additionally, this technique is of value for acute vascular insufficiency of the upper extremities secondary to vasospastic and vaso-occlusive disease, including frostbite and ergotamine toxicity.[11] Evidence is increasing that the prophylactic or preemptive use of epidural nerve blocks in patients scheduled to undergo limb amputations for ischemia reduces the incidence of phantom limb pain.[12]

The administration of local anesthetics or steroids by the cervical approach to the epidural space is useful in the treatment of numerous chronic benign pain syndromes, including cervical radiculopathy, cervicalgia, cervical spondylosis, cervical postlaminectomy syndrome, tension-type headache, phantom limb pain, vertebral compression fractures, diabetic polyneuropathy, chemotherapy-related peripheral neuropathy, postherpetic neuralgia, reflex sympathetic dystrophy, and neck and shoulder pain syndromes.[7,13–15]

The cervical epidural administration of local anesthetics in combination with steroids or opioids is useful in the palliation of cancer-related pain of the head, face, neck, shoulder, upper extremity, and upper trunk.[16] This technique has been especially successful in relieving pain secondary to metastatic disease of

the spine. The long-term epidural administration of opioids has become a mainstay in the palliation of cancer-related pain.[17] The role of epidural opioids in the management of chronic benign pain syndromes is currently being evaluated.

Contraindications to the cervical epidural nerve block are listed in **Table 153.2**. Because of the potential for hematogenous spread through the epidural vasculature, local infection and sepsis represent absolute contraindications to the cervical approach to the epidural space.[18] In contrast to the caudal approach to the epidural space, anticoagulation and coagulopathy are absolute contraindications to cervical epidural nerve block because of the risk of epidural hematoma.[19] Hypovolemia is a relative contraindication to cervical epidural nerve block with local anesthetics.[20]

Clinically Relevant Anatomy

Boundaries of the Cervical Epidural Space

The superior boundary of the cervical epidural space is the point at which the periosteal and spinal layers of dura fuse at the foramen magnum.[21] These structures allow drugs injected into the cervical epidural space to travel beyond their confines if the volume of injectate is large enough. This anatomic configuration probably explains many of the early problems associated with the use of cervical epidural nerve block for surgical anesthesia, when large volumes of local anesthetics in vogue at the time were injected.

The epidural space continues inferiorly to the sacrococcygeal membrane.[22] The cervical epidural space is bounded anteriorly by the posterior longitudinal ligament and posteriorly by the vertebral laminae and the ligamentum flavum (**Fig. 153.1**). The ligamentum flavum is relatively thin in the cervical region and becomes thicker farther caudad, closer to the lumbar spine.[21] This structural characteristic has direct clinical implications, in that the loss of resistance felt during *cervical* epidural nerve block is more subtle than it is in the lumbar or lower thoracic region.

The vertebral pedicles and intervertebral foramina form the lateral limits of the epidural space (**Fig. 153.2**). The degenerative changes and narrowing of the intervertebral foramina associated with aging may be marked in the cervical region. Such changes reduce leakage of local anesthetic out of the foramina and account in part for the lower local anesthetic dose requirements of older patients undergoing cervical epidural nerve block. The distance between the ligamentum flavum and the dura is greatest at the L2 interspace, measuring 5 to 6 mm in adults.[21] Because of the enlargement of the cervical spinal cord that corresponds to the neuromeres serving the upper extremities, this distance is only 1.5 to 2 mm at

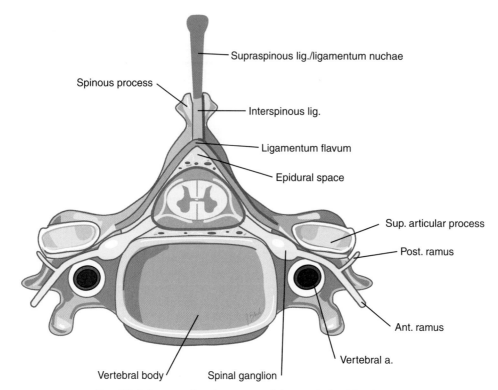

Fig. 153.1 **Cross-sectional anatomy of the cervical epidural space.**

Labels (clockwise from top):
Supraspinous lig./ligamentum nuchae
Spinous process
Interspinous lig.
Ligamentum flavum
Epidural space
Sup. articular process
Post. ramus
Ant. ramus
Vertebral a.
Spinal ganglion
Vertebral body

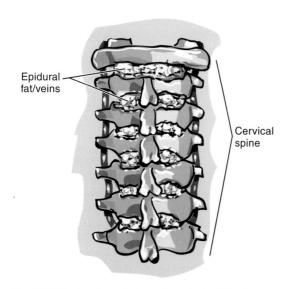

Epidural fat/veins

Cervical spine

Fig. 153.2 **Posterolateral view of cervical epidural space.**

C7 (**Fig. 153.3A**).[21] Flexion of the neck moves this cervical enlargement more cephalad and results in widening of the epidural space to 3 to 4 mm at the C7-T1 interspace (see Fig. 153.3B).[22] This situation has important clinical implications if cervical epidural block is performed with the patient in the lateral or prone position (see "Technique").

Contents of the Epidural Space
Fat

The epidural space is filled with fatty areolar tissue. The amount of epidural fat varies in direct proportion to the amount of fat stored elsewhere in the body.[21] The epidural fat is relatively vascular and seems to change to a denser consistency with aging. This change in consistency may account for the significant variations in required drug doses in adults, especially with the caudal approach to the epidural space. The epidural fat seems to perform two functions: (1) it serves as a shock absorber for the other contents of the epidural space and for the dura and the contents of the dural sac, and (2) it serves as a depot for drugs injected into the cervical epidural space. This second function has direct clinical implications for the choice of opioids for cervical epidural administration.

Epidural Veins

The epidural veins are concentrated principally in the antero-lateral portion of the epidural space.[21] These veins are valveless and transmit intrathoracic and intra-abdominal pressures. As pressure in either of these body cavities increases, owing to Valsalva's maneuver or compression of the inferior vena cava by a gravid uterus or a tumor mass, the epidural veins distend and reduce the volume of the epidural space. This decrease in volume can directly affect how much drug is needed to obtain a given level of neural blockade. Because this venous plexus serves the entire spinal column, it becomes a ready conduit for hematogenous infection.

Epidural Arteries

The arteries that supply the bony and ligamentous confines of the cervical epidural space and the cervical spinal cord enter the cervical epidural space by two routes: through the intervertebral foramina and through direct anastomoses from the intracranial portions of the vertebral arteries.[21,23] Significant anastomoses exist among the epidural arteries, most of which lie in the lateral portions of the epidural

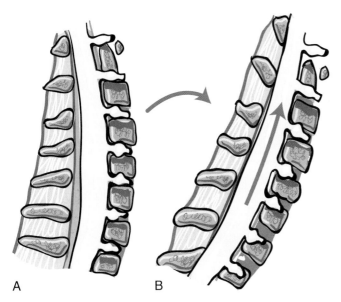

Fig. 153.3 A, Lateral view of the cervical spine in neutral position. B, Lateral view of the cervical spine flexed and moving the neuromeres cephalad.

space. Trauma to the epidural arteries can result in epidural hematoma formation and can compromise the blood supply to the spinal cord itself.

Lymphatics

The lymphatics of the epidural space are concentrated in the region of the dural roots, where they remove foreign material from the subarachnoid and epidural spaces.

Structures Encountered during Midline Insertion of a Needle into the Cervical Epidural Space

In the cervical region, after traversing the skin and subcutaneous tissues, the styletted epidural needle impinges on the ligamentum nuchae, which runs vertically between the apices of the cervical spinous processes.[22,24] The ligamentum nuchae offers some resistance to the advancing needle (**Fig. 153.4A**). This ligament is dense enough to hold a needle in position even when the needle is released.

The interspinous ligament, which runs obliquely between the spinous processes, is encountered next and offers additional resistance to needle advancement (see Fig. 153.4B). Because the interspinous ligament is contiguous with the ligamentum flavum, the operator may perceive a "false" loss of resistance when the needle tip enters the space between the interspinous ligament and the ligamentum flavum. This phenomenon is more pronounced in the cervical region than in the lumbar region because the ligaments are less well defined.

A significant increase in resistance to needle advancement signals that the needle tip is impinging on the dense ligamentum flavum. Because the ligament is composed almost entirely of elastin fibers, resistance increases as the needle traverses the ligamentum flavum because of the drag of the ligament on the needle (see Fig. 153.4C). A sudden loss of resistance occurs as

the needle tip enters the epidural space (see Fig. 153.4D). The operator should feel essentially no resistance to injection of drug into the normal epidural space.

Pitfalls in Needle Placement

A comprehensive discussion of the pitfalls of needle placement for cervical epidural block is beyond the scope of this chapter. Close attention must be paid to the site of needle entry, the needle trajectory, and the final position of the needle tip; otherwise, the block may fail. Trauma to the nerves, arteries, veins, and dural sac and its contents also may occur, possibly with disastrous results.[25]

Technique

All equipment—needles and supplies for nerve block, drugs, resuscitation equipment, oxygen supply, and suction—must be assembled and checked before the start of the cervical epidural nerve block. The patient's informed consent also must be obtained.

Positioning of the Patient

Cervical epidural nerve block may be done with the patient in the sitting, lateral, or prone position. Each position has advantages and disadvantages.

Sitting Position

The sitting position is easiest for the patient and the pain management specialist. Not only does it enhance the operator's ability to identify the midline, but also it ensures that the cervical spine is flexed, a position that widens the lower cervical epidural space. The sitting position avoids the rotation of the spine inherent in the lateral position that makes identification of the epidural space difficult. The sitting position is not always an option, as in a patient with acute vertebral compression fractures. A history of vasovagal syncope with previous needle punctures precludes the use of this position. In such situations, the lateral position is preferred, unless the patient is treated first with intravenous ephedrine.

Lateral Position

The lateral position is preferred for patients who cannot assume the sitting position or who are prone to vasovagal attacks. For the patient's comfort, the lateral position is more suitable for placement of tunneled epidural catheters or other implantable devices with an epidural terminus. If the lateral position is chosen, care must be taken to ensure that no rotation of the patient's spine occurs because spinal rotation makes epidural nerve block exceedingly difficult or impossible. Flexion of the cervical spine is mandatory to maximize the width of the epidural space.

Prone Position

The prone position is used principally for placement of tunneled epidural catheters and spinal stimulator electrodes. As with the other positions, care must be taken to flex the cervical spine to widen the epidural space. Because access to the airway is limited when the patient is in the prone position, this position should be avoided if sedation is required.

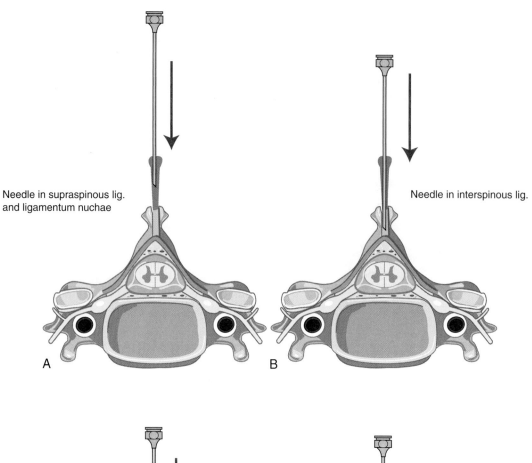

Needle in supraspinous lig. and ligamentum nuchae

Needle in interspinous lig.

A

B

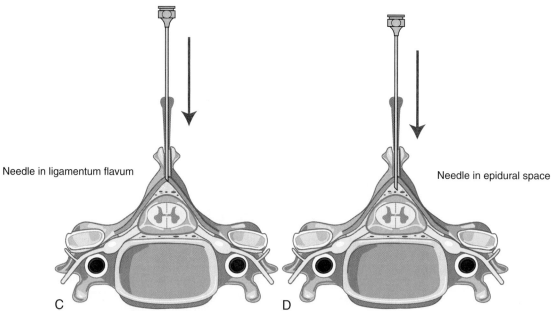

Needle in ligamentum flavum

Needle in epidural space

C

D

Fig. 153.4 Midline ligaments of the cervical epidural space. **A,** Needle in the supraspinous ligament. **B,** Needle in the interspinous ligament. **C,** Needle in the ligamentum flavum. **D,** Needle through the ligamentum nuchae with loss of resistance.

Preblock Preparation

After the patient is placed in the optimal position, the skin is prepared with an antiseptic solution, such as povidone-iodine, so that all the surface landmarks can be palpated aseptically. A fenestrated sterile drape is placed to avoid contamination by the palpating fingers. The interspace suitable for the intended epidural block is identified. At the level of this interspace, the operator's middle and index fingers are placed on either side of the spinous processes (**Fig. 153.5A**). The position of the interspace is confirmed again with palpation, by using a rocking motion in the superior and inferior planes. The midline of the selected interspace is identified by palpating the spinous processes above and below the interspace with a lateral rocking motion, to ensure that the needle entry site is exactly in the

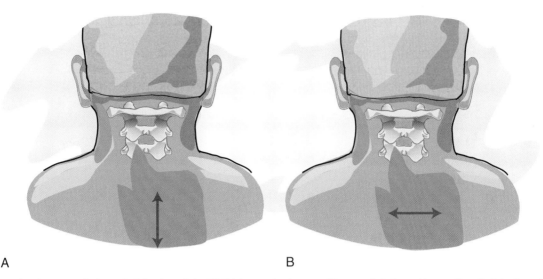

Fig. 153.5 Loss-of-resistance technique. **A,** Palpation of the C6-7 intervertebral space with superoinferior rocking motion. **B,** Palpation of the C6-7 midline with lateral rocking.

midline (see Fig. 153.5B). Failure to identify the midline accurately is the most common cause of difficulty in performing cervical epidural nerve block.

Choice of Needle

For most adult patients, a 3½-inch 18-gauge Hustead or Tuohy needle is suitable for cervical epidural block; however, with the sharper Tuohy needle, the incidence of dural punctures may be higher.[26] Many centers now use smaller, sharper, and shorter needles with equally good results. These smaller, sharper, and shorter needles decrease the amount of procedure-related and postprocedure pain and decrease the cost of the procedure.

Identification of the Epidural Space: The Translaminar Approach

The choice of technique for identifying the epidural space usually is based on the pain specialist's training and personal experience, rather than on scientific data. Most experts agree that the loss-of-resistance technique has significant advantages over the hanging-drop technique.[27] Because the hanging-drop method is associated with a 2% failure rate as compared with less than 0.5% for the loss-of-resistance technique, the hanging-drop technique cannot be recommended.

Loss-of-Resistance Technique

After careful identification of the midline at the chosen interspace using the technique described earlier, 1 mL of local anesthetic is used to infiltrate the skin, the subcutaneous tissues, and the supraspinous and interspinous ligaments. Large amounts of local anesthetic should be avoided because they disrupt the ligamentous fibers and contribute to postprocedure pain.

The styletted needle is inserted exactly in the midline in the previously anesthetized area through the supraspinous ligament into the interspinous ligament.[27] The needle stylet is removed, and a well-lubricated 5-mL glass syringe filled with preservative-free sterile saline is attached. Because saline is not compressible, it provides better tactile feedback than air. Additionally, saline avoids the risk of air embolism through the cervical epidural veins.[27]

The following instructions are written for right-handed physicians and should be reversed for left-handed physicians. The operator holds the epidural needle firmly at the hub with the left thumb and index finger. The left hand is placed firmly against the patient's neck to ensure against uncontrolled needle movements should the patient move unexpectedly (**Fig. 153.6A**). The right hand holds the syringe with the thumb exerting *continuous* firm pressure on the plunger.[28] Bromage[21] admonished, "Never advance the needle without simultaneous pressure on the plunger to tell you where you are." Ballottement of the plunger, advocated by some clinicians, should not be used because it increases the risk of inadvertent dural puncture.[29]

As constant pressure is applied to the plunger of the syringe with the thumb of the physician's right hand, the needle and syringe are continuously advanced in a slow and deliberate manner with the left hand. As the needle bevel passes through the ligamentum flavum and enters the epidural space, a sudden loss of resistance is felt, and the plunger slides effortlessly forward (see Fig. 153.6B). This loss of resistance provides the operator with visual and tactile confirmation that the needle bevel has entered the epidural space. The syringe is gently removed from the needle.

An air or saline acceptance test is done by injecting 0.5 to 1 mL of air or sterile, preservative-free saline with a well-lubricated sterile glass syringe to help confirm that the needle lies within the epidural space. The force required for injection should not exceed that necessary to overcome the resistance of the needle. Any significant pain or sudden increase in resistance during injection suggests incorrect needle placement. The injection should be stopped immediately, and the position of the needle should be reassessed. Some centers advocate the use of fluoroscopic guidance when performing cervical epidural nerve block in technically challenging situations (**Fig. 153.7**). Although not mandatory, fluoroscopic guidance can be a useful adjunct in selected patients. Ultrasound guidance has been

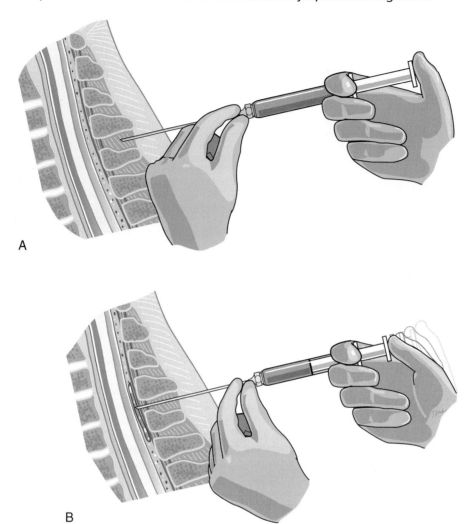

Fig. 153.6 Loss-of-resistance technique. **A,** Position of the needle and hand for the loss-of-resistance technique in the cervical region. **B,** Sudden loss of resistance.

used by some operators to avoid the radiation exposure associated with fluoroscopic guidance in technically challenging patients (**Fig. 153.8**).

Injection of Drugs

When satisfactory needle position is confirmed, a syringe containing the drugs to be injected is carefully attached to the needle. Gentle aspiration is carried out to identify cerebrospinal fluid (CSF) or blood.[28] Inadvertent dural puncture can occur with the best of operators, and careful observation for CSF is mandatory.[29] If CSF is aspirated, the epidural block may be attempted at a different interspace. In this situation, drug doses should be adjusted accordingly because subarachnoid migration of drugs through the dural rent can occur.

Aspiration of blood can result from damage to veins during insertion of the needle into the cervical epidural space or, less commonly, from intravenous placement of the needle.[28] If blood is aspirated, the needle should be rotated slightly, and the aspiration test should be repeated. If no blood is present, incremental doses of local anesthetic and other

drugs may be administered while the patient is monitored closely for signs of local anesthetic toxicity or untoward reactions to the other drugs. Injection under fluoroscopic guidance may aid in identification of inadvertent intravascular injection or injection into the subdural or subarachnoid space (**Fig. 153.9**).

Choice of Local Anesthetic

The spread of drugs injected into the cervical epidural space depends on the following factors: the volume and speed of injection; the anatomic variations of the epidural space; the extent of dilation of the epidural veins; and the position, age, and height of the patient.[30] In one study, pregnant patients required significantly less drug to achieve a given level of blockade than did nongravid controls.[31]

Local anesthetics capable of producing adequate sensory block of the cervical nerve roots when administered by the cervical epidural route include 1% lidocaine, 0.25% bupivacaine, 2% chloroprocaine, and 1% mepivacaine. Increasing the concentration of drug increases the amount of motor block and speeds the onset of action. Adding epinephrine

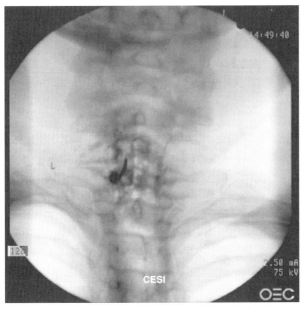

Fig. 153.7 **Loss-of-resistance technique.** The needle tip is resting in the cervical epidural space.

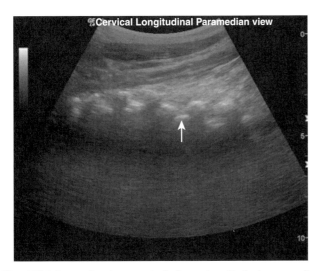

Fig. 153.8 **Loss-of-resistance technique.** Longitudinal paramedian sonographic view of the cervical spine showing the articular pillars, the lamina *(arrow)*, and the ligamentum flavum. *(From Shankar H, Zainer C: Ultrasound guidance for epidural steroid injections, Tech Reg Anesth Pain Manag 13:229, 2009.)*

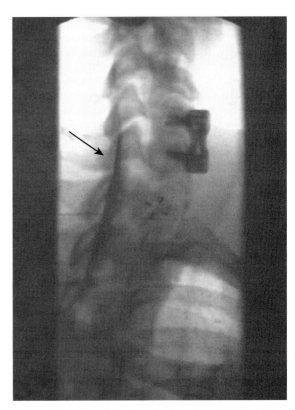

Fig. 153.9 Oblique view following injection of an additional 1.5 mL of nonionic contrast material demonstrates additional inferior flow as well as flow into the more superior cervical spinal canal *(arrow). (From Renfrew DL: Atlas of spine injection, ed 4, Philadelphia, 2004, Saunders, p 52.)*

reduces systemic absorption and slightly prolongs the duration of action.[32] Generally, 5 to 7 mL of the previously listed agents is adequate for most pain management applications in adults.[7] Significant intrapatient variability exists, however, and additional incremental doses of local anesthetic may be needed to ensure adequate anesthesia in some adult patients. All local anesthetics administered by the cervical epidural route should be formulated for epidural use.[33]

For diagnostic and prognostic blocks, 0.5% or 1% preservative-free lidocaine is a suitable local anesthetic.[8] For therapeutic blocks, 0.5% preservative-free lidocaine or 0.25%

preservative-free bupivacaine in combination with 80 mg of depot methylprednisolone (Depo-Medrol) is injected.[7,8] Subsequent nerve blocks are done in a similar manner, with 40 mg of methylprednisolone instead of the initial 80-mg dose. Daily cervical epidural nerve blocks with local anesthetic or steroid may be required to treat the acute painful conditions described earlier.[3] Chronic conditions, such as cervical radiculopathy, tension-type headache, and diabetic polyneuropathy, are treated daily, every other day, once a week, or as the clinical situation dictates.[3,4,7,13] Some centers choose to avoid the use of local anesthetic when performing therapeutic cervical epidural blocks and instead substitute preservative-free saline.

If the cervical epidural route is chosen for administration of opioids, 0.5 mg of morphine sulfate formulated for epidural use is a reasonable initial dose for opioid-tolerant patients. More lipid-soluble opioids, such as fentanyl, must be delivered by continuous infusion through a cervical epidural catheter. All opioids administered by the cervical epidural route should be formulated for epidural use.[33]

Cervical Transforaminal Epidural Block

Cervical epidural injection by the transforaminal approach with local anesthetics or corticosteroid can also be used as a diagnostic tool or treatment modality when performing differential neural blockade on an anatomic basis in the evaluation of head, neck, face, shoulder, and upper extremity pain.[34]

If destruction of the cervical nerve roots is being considered, this technique is useful as a prognostic indicator of the degree of motor and sensory impairment that the patient may experience. Although the translaminar approach described earlier is more commonly used for routine therapeutic cervical epidural nerve injection, some interventional pain management specialists believe that the transforaminal approach to the cervical epidural space is more efficacious in the treatment of painful conditions involving a single nerve root, albeit with a higher incidence of potential complications.[34] When cervical epidural injections are performed using the transforaminal approach, the goal is to place the needle just inside the posterior portion of the neural foramen of the affected nerve root[34] (**Fig. 153.10**). The operator should feel essentially no resistance to drugs injected into the normal epidural space.

Cervical epidural injection using the transforaminal approach is carried out with the patient in the supine or lateral position. Although some experienced pain practitioners perform this technique without radiographic guidance, the use of fluoroscopy is recommended to aid in needle placement and will help to avoid placing the needle too deeply into the spinal canal and unintentionally injecting into the spinal cord or misplaced intervascular structures such as the vertebral or segmental arteries. With the patient in the supine or lateral position on the fluoroscopy table, the fluoroscopy beam is rotated from a lateral to an anterior oblique position to allow visualization of the affected neural foramina at its largest diameter (**Figs. 153.11** and **153.12**). The fluoroscopy beam is then slowly moved from a cephalad to a more caudad position to also allow visualization of the affected neural foramina. When this is accomplished, the beam should be parallel to the affected nerve root.

The skin is then prepared with an antiseptic solution, and a skin wheal of local anesthetic may be placed at a point overlying the posterior aspect of the foramen just over the tip of the superior articular process of the level below the affected neural foramen. This point is approximately one third of the distance cephalad from the most posteroinferior aspect of the foramen. A 25-gauge, 2-inch needle is then placed through the previously anesthetized area and is advanced until the tip rests against the posteromedial portion of the superior articular process of the targeted neural foramen (**Figs. 153.13 to 153.15**). Failure to impinge on bone at the point should be of grave concern and may indicate that the needle has passed through the foramen and rests within the substance of the spinal cord. Failure to identify this problem can lead to disastrous results (see "Side Effects and Complications of the Cervical Approach"). After this bony landmark is identified, an anteroposterior fluoroscopic view is obtained to verify that the needle is within the nerve canal and not past the midpoint of the facetal column, to avoid placement of the needle within the dura or into the spinal cord.

After satisfactory needle position is confirmed and the needle bevel is oriented medially, 0.2 to 0.4 mL of contrast medium suitable for subarachnoid use is gently injected under active fluoroscopy. The contrast material should be seen to flow into the epidural space and distally along the affected nerve root sheath (**Fig. 153.16**). The injection of contrast medium should be stopped immediately if the patient complains of significant pain on injection. After satisfactory flow of contrast material is observed and no evidence of subdural, subarachnoid, or

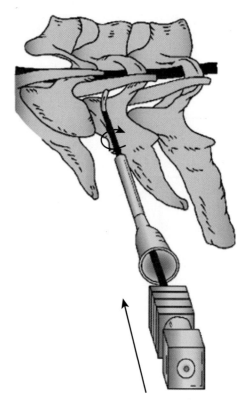

Fig. 153.10 Cervical transforaminal epidural block: proper needle position. *(From Raj PP, Lou L, Erdine S, et al: Interventional pain management: image-guided procedures, ed 2, Philadelphia, 2008, Saunders.)*

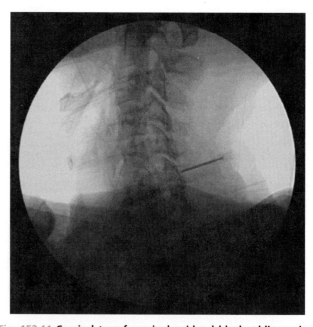

Fig. 153.11 Cervical transforaminal epidural block: oblique view with the introducer cannula. *(From Raj PP, Lou L, Erdine S, et al: Interventional pain management: image-guided procedures, ed 2, Philadelphia, 2008, Saunders.)*

intravascular spread of contrast is noted, the operator slowly injects 6 mg of betamethasone suspension or solution or 20 to 40 mg of methylprednisolone in solution or 20 to 40 mg of triamcinolone suspension with 0.5 to 1.5 mL of 2% or 4%

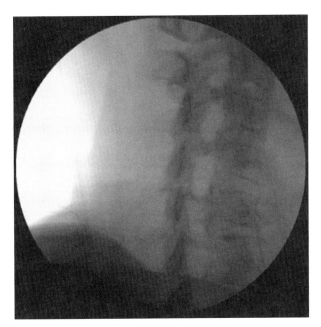

Fig. 153.12 **Cervical transforaminal epidural block: oblique view of the cervical neural foramina.**

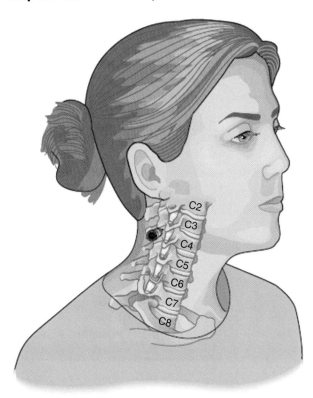

Fig. 153.14 **Cervical transforaminal epidural block.** Needle placement.

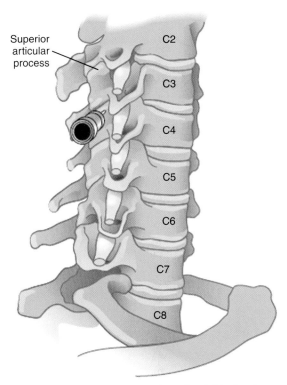

Fig. 153.13 **Cervical transforaminal epidural block.** The needle is directed toward the posteromedial portion of the superior articular process.

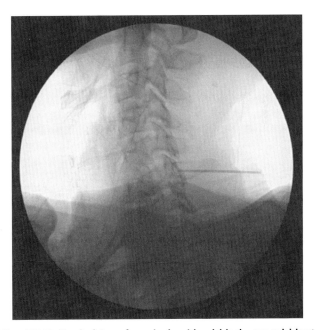

Fig. 153.15 **Cervical transforaminal epidural block: curved blunt needle advanced to bone.** *(From Raj PP, Lou L, Erdine S, et al:* Interventional pain management: image-guided procedures, *ed 2, Philadelphia, 2008, Saunders.)*

preservative-free lidocaine. Injection of the local anesthetic or steroid should be discontinued if the patient complains of any significant pain on injection. After satisfactory injection of the local anesthetic or steroid, the needle is removed, and pressure is placed on the injection site. Dr. Gabor Racz suggested that

following injection, the cervical spine should be gently flexed and then gently rotated from side to side to facilitate opening of the neural foramina to reduce epidural pressure. The technique may be repeated at additional levels as a diagnostic or therapeutic maneuver.[34]

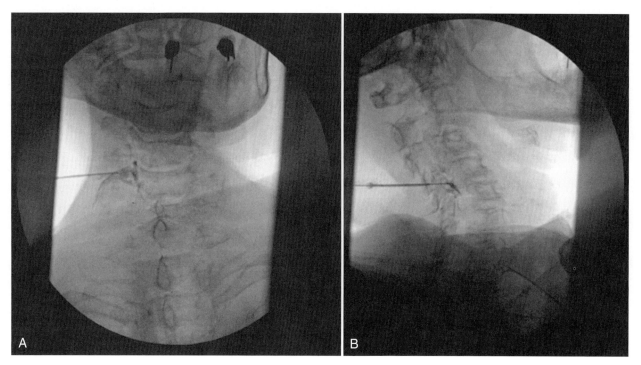

Fig. 153.16 Cervical transforaminal epidural block. Anteroposterior **(A)** and lateral **(B)** views with contrast injection. *(From Raj PP, Lou L, Erdine S, et al: Interventional pain management: image-guided procedures, ed 2, Philadelphia, 2008, Saunders.)*

Cervical Epidural Catheters

An epidural catheter may be placed into the cervical epidural space through a Hustead or Tuohy needle. The catheter is advanced approximately 2 to 3 cm beyond the needle tip. The needle is carefully withdrawn over the catheter. Under no circumstance is the catheter withdrawn back through the needle, lest shearing of the catheter occur. After the injection hub is attached to the catheter, an aspiration test is carried out for blood or CSF.[35] A test dose of 1 to 2 mL of local anesthetic is given through the catheter. The patient is observed for signs of local anesthetic toxicity and inadvertent subarachnoid injection. If no side effects are noted, a continuous infusion or intermittent boluses of local anesthetics or opioids may be administered through the catheter. Because the risk of infection limits the long-term use of percutaneous cervical epidural catheters, tunneling of the catheter is strongly recommended if the catheter is anticipated to be in place for more than 48 hours.[36]

Side Effects and Complications of the Cervical Approach

Inadvertent Dural Puncture

In the hands of an experienced pain specialist, the prevalence of inadvertent dural puncture during cervical epidural nerve block is less than 0.5%.[25,29] Although postdural puncture headache is upsetting to patient and pain specialist in and of itself, it should not result in permanent harm to the patient. Failure to recognize inadvertent dural puncture can

result in permanent harm. If an epidural needle or catheter is accidentally placed in the subarachnoid space, and the problem goes unrecognized, injection of epidural doses of local anesthetics will cause immediate total spinal anesthesia and associated loss of consciousness, hypotension, and apnea. If epidural doses of opioids are accidentally placed into the subarachnoid space, significant respiratory and central nervous system depression will result. Should either of these problems occur, immediate supportive measures must be taken to restore homeostasis.

Inadvertent Subdural Puncture

It is possible to place a needle or catheter intended for the epidural space inadvertently into the subdural space. When subdural placement goes unrecognized, and epidural doses of local anesthetics are administered, the signs and symptoms are similar to those of massive subarachnoid injection, although the resulting motor and sensory block may be spotty.[37,38] The effect of inadvertent injection of large doses of opioids into the subdural space is probably similar to that of subarachnoid injection. Massive subdural injection of local anesthetics or opioids requires immediate supportive measures, as indicated, to restore homeostasis.

Inadvertent Intravenous Needle and Catheter Placement

The cervical epidural space is densely vascular. Intravenous placement of the epidural needle complicates approximately 0.5% to 1% of lumbar epidural anesthesia procedures.[21] The prevalence of inadvertent intravenous placement of the epidural needle in the cervical epidural space is assumed to be similar. This complication is more common in patients with distended epidural veins (e.g., parturients and patients with a large intra-abdominal tumor mass and, when the transforaminal approach is used, patients with foraminal obstruction secondary to herniated nucleus pulposus or tumor). If the misplacement is unrecognized, injection of local anesthetic directly into an epidural vein will result in significant local anesthetic toxicity.[39] Damage to or injection into the segmental artery can occur with increased incidence when performing the transforaminal approach to the epidural space but is more common at the C5-7 neural foramina on the right. Careful aspiration before injection of drugs into the epidural space also is mandatory to identify this potentially serious problem. Observation of the patient during and after the injection process regardless of the approach used is necessary.

Hematoma and Ecchymosis

The epidural space is densely vascular. Needle trauma to the epidural veins may cause self-limited bleeding and postprocedure pain. Uncontrolled bleeding into the epidural space may result in compression of the spinal cord with the rapid development of neurologic deficit. Although the incidence of significant neurologic deficit secondary to epidural hematoma after cervical epidural block is exceedingly rare, this devastating complication should be considered whenever rapidly developing neurologic deficit follows cervical epidural nerve block.[40]

Infection

Although uncommon, infection in the epidural space is an ever-present possibility, especially in immunocompromised patients and in patients with cancer.[34,41,42] Because of the nature of the epidural venous system, hematogenous spread throughout the central nervous system is a possibility when epidural infection occurs.[25] Because the offending organism in epidural infections is usually *Staphylococcus aureus,* initial antibiotic treatment should be directed at this organism until culture results are available.[42] If epidural abscess occurs, emergency surgical drainage to avoid spinal cord compression and irreversible neurologic deficit is usually necessary. Early detection and treatment of infection are crucial to avoid potentially life-threatening sequelae.

Neurologic Complications

Neurologic complications of cervical nerve block are uncommon if proper technique is used. Direct trauma to the spinal cord or nerve roots usually is accompanied by pain. If significant pain occurs during placement of the epidural needle or catheter or during injection, the physician should stop immediately and ascertain the cause of the pain to avoid the possibility of additional neural trauma.[25] However, the patient may experience little or no pain with needle insertion into the spinal cord, and multiple fluoroscopic views are highly recommended when the transforaminal approach is used, to avoid this potentially devastating complication. Intravenous sedation or general anesthesia before initiation of cervical epidural nerve block renders the patient unable to provide accurate verbal feedback if the needle is misplaced. Routine use of sedation or general anesthesia before cervical epidural nerve block is discouraged because it takes away this important safeguard.[28]

Urinary Retention and Incontinence

The administration of local anesthetics and opioids into the cervical epidural space may be associated with a greater incidence of urinary retention as compared with cervical epidural block performed with local anesthetic and steroid.[34] This side effect is more common in older men and multiparous women whose bladders are ptotic. Overflow incontinence may occur when such patients are unable to void or when bladder catheterization is not used. All patients undergoing cervical epidural nerve block should be able to empty their bladder before discharge from the pain center.

Conclusion

Cervical epidural nerve block is useful in the management of various acute, chronic, and cancer-related pain syndromes. Clinical experience has shown that cervical epidural nerve block is safe as long as careful attention is paid to the technical aspects.

References

Full references for this chapter can be found on www.expertconsult.com.

Lysis of Cervical Epidural Adhesions: Racz Technique

Steven D. Waldman

Indications

Lysis of epidural adhesions has been used to treat numerous painful conditions.[1] Investigators have postulated that the common denominator in each of these pain syndromes is the compromise of spinal nerve roots as they traverse and exit the epidural space by adhesions and scarring. These adhesions and scar tissue are thought not only to restrict the free movement of the nerve roots as they emerge from the spinal cord and travel through the intervertebral foramina but also to result in dysfunction of epidural venous blood and lymph flow.[2] This dysfunction results in additional nerve root edema, which further compromises the affected nerves. Inflammation may also play a part in the genesis of pain because these nerves are repeatedly traumatized each time the nerve is stretched against the adhesions and scar tissue.

Diagnostic categories considered amenable to treatment with lysis of epidural adhesions using the Racz technique include failed cervical spine surgery with associated perineural fibrosis, herniated disk, traumatic and nontraumatic vertebral body compression fracture, metastatic carcinoma to the spine and epidural space, multilevel degenerative arthritis, facet joint pain, epidural scarring following infection, and other pain syndromes of the spine that have their basis in epidural scarring and that have failed to respond to more conservative treatments.[3]

Clinically Relevant Anatomy

The superior boundary of the cervical epidural space is the fusion of the periosteal and spinal layers of dura at the foramen magnum.[4] The epidural space continues inferiorly to the sacrococcygeal membrane. The cervical epidural space is bounded anteriorly by the posterior longitudinal ligament and posteriorly by the vertebral laminae and the ligamentum flavum. The vertebral pedicles and intervertebral foramina form the lateral limits of the epidural space. The cervical epidural space is 3 to 4 mm at the C7-T1 interspace with the cervical spine flexed. The cervical epidural space contains fat, veins, arteries, lymphatics, and connective tissue. The epidural space is subject to scarring following infection, inflammation, and surgery.[5]

Technique

Intravenous access is obtained for administration of intravenous sedation during the injection of solutions through the catheter. Sedation during injection may be necessary because of pain produced by the distraction of the nerve roots as the solution lyses the perineural adhesions. After venous access is obtained, the patient is placed in the prone position with the cervical spine placed in a flexed position that is comfortable for the patient, to allow access to the epidural space.

Preparation of a wide area of skin with antiseptic solution is then carried out so that all the landmarks can be palpated aseptically. A fenestrated sterile drape is placed to avoid contamination of the palpating fingers. At the C7-T1 interspace, the operator's middle and index fingers are placed on each side of the spinous processes. The position of the interspace is reconfirmed with palpation by using a rocking motion in the superior and inferior planes. The midline of the selected interspace is identified by palpating the spinous processes above and below the interspace by using a lateral rocking motion to ensure that the needle entry site is exactly in the midline. One milliliter of local anesthetic is used to infiltrate the skin, subcutaneous tissues, and the supraspinous and interspinous ligaments at the midline. The interspace and midline are then confirmed with fluoroscopy.

After confirmation of the interspace and midline, a 19-gauge, 3½-inch styletted needle suitable for catheter placement is inserted through the anesthetized area. The right-handed physician holds the epidural needle firmly at the hub with his or her left thumb and index finger. The left hand is placed firmly against the patient's neck to ensure against uncontrolled needle movements should the patient unexpectedly move. After a syringe containing preservative-free saline is attached, with constant pressure applied to the plunger of the syringe with the thumb of the right hand, the needle and syringe are continuously advanced in a slow and deliberate manner with the left hand. As soon as the needle bevel passes through the ligamentum flavum and enters the epidural space, the operator will feel a sudden loss of resistance to injection, and the plunger will effortlessly surge forward. If the practitioner is unsure about needle position, the syringe is gently removed from the needle, and an air or saline acceptance test is carried out by injecting 0.5 to 1 mL of air or sterile preservative-free saline with a well-lubricated sterile glass syringe to help confirm that the needle is within the epidural space (**Fig. 154.1**).

The force required for injection should not exceed that necessary to overcome the resistance of the needle. Any significant pain or sudden increase in resistance during injection suggests incorrect needle placement, and one should *stop* injecting immediately and reassess the position of the needle. Needle position should be confirmed by fluoroscopy on both anteroposterior and lateral views (**Fig. 154.2**).

After negative aspiration for blood and cerebrospinal fluid (CSF), the operator slowly injects 3 to 5 mL of a water-soluble contrast medium, such as iohexol or metrizamide, through the previously placed epidural needle under fluoroscopy (**Figs. 154.3** and **154.4**). The pain specialist should check closely for any evidence of contrast medium in the epidural venous plexus, a finding that would suggest intravenous placement of the needle or subdural or subarachnoid placement, which appears as a more concentrated centrally

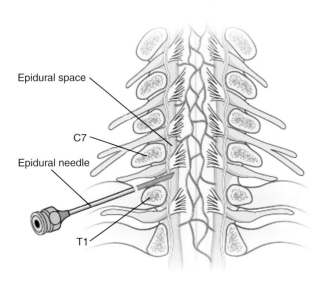

Fig. 154.1 **The needle tip in the cervical epidural space.**

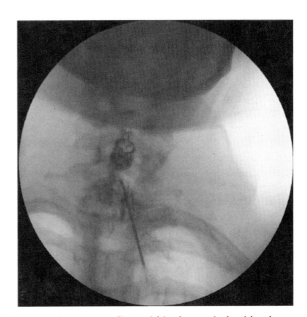

Fig. 154.3 **Contrast medium within the cervical epidural space.**

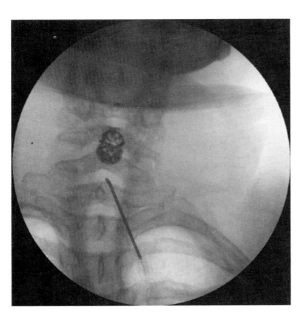

Fig. 154.2 **The needle tip in the cervical epidural space.**

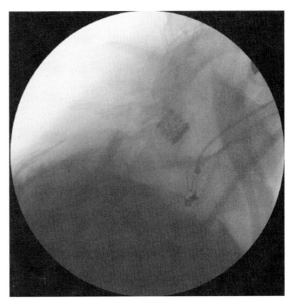

Fig. 154.4 **Contrast medium within the cervical epidural space.**

located density. When the epidural space fills with contrast medium, a "Christmas tree" shape appears as the contrast medium surrounds the perineural structures.[5] Defects in this classic appearance are indicative of epidural perineural adhesions.[3,5]

After confirming proper needle placement and ensuring that no blood or CSF can be aspirated from the needle, the operator slowly injects 3 to 4 mL of 0.25% preservative-free bupivacaine and 40 mg of triamcinolone acetate through the epidural needle while observing the fluoroscope screen. The local anesthetic forces the contrast medium around the adhesions, thus further identifying affected nerve roots.

After the area of adhesions is identified on an epidurogram, the bevel of the epidural needle is turned toward the ventrolateral aspect of the affected side. This maneuver facilitates passage of the catheter toward the affected nerves and decreases the chance of catheter breakage or shearing. The use of a wire spiral catheter such as the Racz Tun-L-Kath or Racz Brevi-XL epidural catheter (Epimed International, Johnstown, NY) further decreases the incidence of this complication.[5]

The catheter is then passed through the needle into the area of adhesions. Multiple attempts may be required to obtain placement of the catheter into the adhesions (**Figs. 154.5** and **154.6**). The Racz needle allows for the catheter to be withdrawn and repositioned and is preferred over the standard epidural needle.

After the catheter is placed within the area of adhesions, the catheter is aspirated for blood or CSF. If the aspiration test is negative, the operator slowly injects an additional 3 to 4 mL of contrast medium through the catheter. This additional contrast medium should be seen spreading into the area of the adhesion. If the contrast material is observed to flow in satisfactory position, an additional 3 mL of 0.25% bupivacaine and 40 mg of triamcinolone are injected through the catheter to lyse the remaining adhesions further. Some investigators also recommend the addition of 200 U hyaluronidase to facilitate the spread of solutions injected. Approximately 3% of the population may experience some degree of allergic reaction to this drug, and this adverse effect may limit its use.

Fifteen minutes after the second injection of bupivacaine, after negative aspiration, the pain practitioner injects 5 to 6 mL of 10% saline in small increments or by infusion pump over 20 to 30 minutes. The hyperosmolar properties of the hypertonic saline further shrink the nerve root and help to treat the perineural edema caused by the venous obstruction secondary to the adhesions. The injection of 10% saline solution into the epidural space is quite painful, and intravenous sedation may be required if the saline spreads beyond the area previously anesthetized by the 0.25% bupivacaine. This pain is transient and is generally gone within 10 minutes. After the final injection of 10% saline, the catheter is carefully secured, and a sterile dressing is placed. Intravenous cephalosporin antibiotics were recommended by Dr. Racz to prevent bacterial colonization of the catheter while it is in place.

This injection procedure of bupivacaine followed by 5% to 10% saline through the previously placed catheter is repeated the following day. Epidurograms are repeated only if a question of catheter migration exists, because the contrast medium can be irritating to the nerve roots and is quite expensive. The catheter is removed after the last injection. The patient is instructed to keep the area clean and dry and to call at the first sign of elevated temperature or infection.

Side Effects and Complications

Complications directly related to epidural lysis of adhesions are generally self-limited, although occasionally, even with the best of practitioners, severe complications can occur. Self-limited complications include pain at the injection site, transient neck pain, ecchymosis and hematoma formation over the injection site, and unintended subdural or subarachnoid injection of local anesthetic.[6] Severe complications of epidural lysis of adhesions include unintended subdural or subarachnoid injection of hypertonic saline, persistent sensory deficit in the lumbar and sacral dermatomes, paraparesis or paraplegia, persistent bowel or bladder dysfunction, sexual dysfunction, and infection.[6,7] Although uncommon, unrecognized infection in the epidural space can result in paraplegia and death.[5,7] Clinically, the signs and symptoms of epidural abscess manifest as a high temperature, spine pain, and progressive neurologic deficit.[8] If epidural abscess is suspected, blood

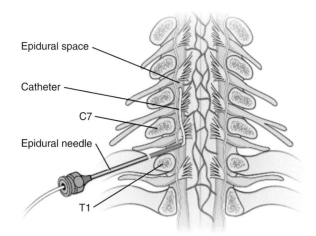

Fig. 154.5 **The Racz catheter within the cervical epidural space.**

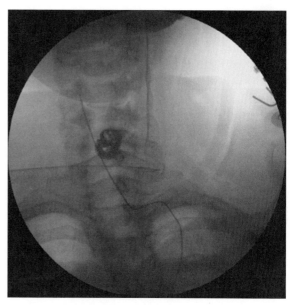

Fig. 154.6 **The Racz catheter within the cervical epidural space.**

and urine cultures should be taken, antibiotics started, and an emergency magnetic resonance imaging scan of the spine obtained to allow identification and drainage of any abscess formation before irreversible neurologic deficit occurs.[8]

Conclusion

Lysis of epidural adhesions is a straightforward technique that may provide pain relief in a carefully selected subset of patients. This technique should not be viewed as a starting point or stand-alone treatment in the continuum of pain management modalities, but instead should be carefully integrated into a comprehensive pain management treatment plan. The identification of preexisting neurogenic bowel or bladder dysfunction by the use of urodynamics and a careful neurologic examination are mandatory before performing lysis of epidural adhesions, to avoid erroneous attribution of these preexisting problems to the procedure. Careful screening for preexisting sexual dysfunction is also indicated before lysis of epidural adhesions, for the same reason.

References

Full references for this chapter can be found on www.expertconsult.com.

Brachial Plexus Block

Steven D. Waldman

Historical Considerations

Brachial plexus block was first performed by two famous surgeons—Halsted in 1884 and Crile in 1887.[1] Both surgeons first surgically exposed the brachial plexus before applying cocaine to this neural structure under direct vision. The first percutaneous brachial plexus blocks were reported in 1911 by Hirschel and Hulenkampff.[2] Over the ensuing years, numerous techniques, modifications, and advancements have made brachial plexus block one of the regional anesthetic techniques most frequently used in contemporary anesthesia practice. Work by Winnie has further elucidated the clinically relevant anatomy of the brachial plexus and has led to refinement of the technique and recognition of the role of brachial plexus block in the treatment of sympathetically maintained pain syndromes involving the upper extremity.[3]

Clinically Relevant Anatomy

A clear understanding of the clinically relevant anatomy of the brachial plexus is mandatory if the pain management specialist is to perform brachial plexus block safely and successfully, regardless of what technique is chosen. Failure to appreciate this need will increase the incidence of failed blocks and complications. The brachial plexus is formed by the fusion of the anterior rami of the C5, C6, C7, C8, and T1 spinal nerves.[4] Fibers from the C4 and T2 spinal nerves may also be contributory. The nerves that make up the plexus exit the lateral aspect of the cervical spine and pass downward and laterally in conjunction with the subclavian artery. The nerves and artery run between the anterior scalene and middle scalene muscles and pass inferiorly behind the middle of the clavicle and above the top of the first rib to reach the axilla

(**Figs. 155.1** and **155.2**). The scalene muscles are enclosed in an extension of prevertebral fascia that helps to contain drugs injected into this region.

Interscalene Block

Indications

The interscalene approach to the brachial plexus is the preferred technique for brachial plexus block when anesthesia or relaxation of the shoulder is desired.[5] In addition to applications for surgical anesthesia, interscalene brachial plexus nerve block with local anesthetics can be used as a diagnostic tool when performing differential neural blockade on an anatomic basis in the evaluation of shoulder and upper extremity pain. If destruction of the brachial plexus is being considered, this technique is useful as a prognostic indicator of the degree of motor and sensory impairment that the patient may experience. Interscalene brachial plexus nerve block with local anesthetic may be used to palliate acute pain emergencies including acute herpes zoster, brachial plexus neuritis, shoulder and upper extremity trauma, and cancer pain while the patient waits for pharmacologic, surgical, and antineoplastic methods to take effect.[6] Interscalene brachial plexus nerve block is also a useful alternative to stellate ganglion block when treating reflex sympathetic dystrophy of the shoulder and upper extremity.[5]

Destruction of the brachial plexus is indicated for the palliation of cancer pain, including invasive tumors of the brachial plexus and tumors of the soft tissue and bone of the shoulder and upper extremity[7] (**Fig. 155.3**). Because of the desperate nature of many patients' suffering from aggressively invasive tumors that have invaded the brachial plexus, blockade of the

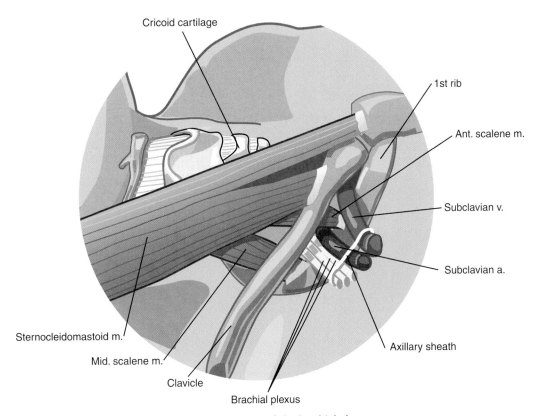

Cricoid cartilage

1st rib

Ant. scalene m.

Subclavian v.

Subclavian a.

Axillary sheath

Sternocleidomastoid m.

Mid. scalene m.

Clavicle

Brachial plexus

Fig. 155.1 **Anatomy of the brachial plexus.**

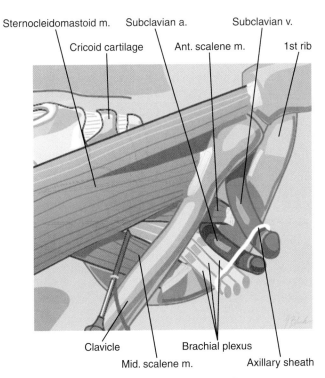

Sternocleidomastoid m.   Subclavian a.   Subclavian v.

Cricoid cartilage   Ant. scalene m.   1st rib

Clavicle   Brachial plexus

Mid. scalene m.   Axillary sheath

Fig. 155.2 **Anatomy of the brachial plexus.**

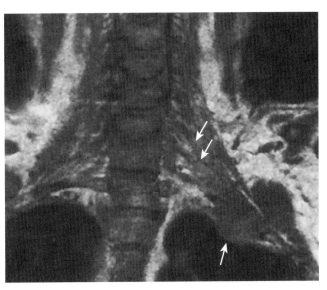

Fig. 155.3 **Pancoast's tumor (adenocarcinoma) with infiltration of the brachial plexus.** A 65-year-old man complained of severe pain in the shoulder radiating to the elbow, medial side of the forearm, and the fourth and fifth fingers in an ulnar nerve distribution. A screening coronal T1-weighted magnetic resonance image shows the brachial plexus from the region of the roots *(top arrows)* to the region of the trunks and divisions, where the patient has tumor invasion *(bottom arrow)* and loss of fat planes on the left. *(From Stark DD, Bradley WG: Magnetic resonance imaging, ed 3, St. Louis, 1999, Mosby, p 1824.)*

brachial plexus with the interscalene approach may be carried out in the presence of coagulopathy or anticoagulation by using a 25-gauge needle, albeit with increased risk of ecchymosis and hematoma formation.

Technique

The patient is placed in a supine position with the head turned away from the side to be blocked. A total of 20 to 30 mL of local anesthetic is drawn up in a 30-mL sterile syringe. For treatment of painful or inflammatory conditions that are mediated by the brachial plexus, a total of 80 mg of depot steroid is added to the local anesthetic with the first block and 40 mg of depot steroid is added with subsequent blocks.

The patient is then asked to raise his or her head against the resistance of the pain specialist's hand to help to identify the posterior border of the sternocleidomastoid muscle. In most patients, a groove can be palpated between the posterior border of the sternocleidomastoid muscle and the anterior scalene muscle. Identification of the intrascalene groove can be facilitated by having the patient inhale strongly against a closed glottis. The skin overlying this area is then prepared with antiseptic solution. At the level of the cricothyroid notch (C6) at the interscalene groove, a 25-gauge, 1½-inch needle is inserted with a slightly caudad and inferior trajectory (**Fig. 155.4**). If the intrascalene groove cannot be identified, the needle is placed just slightly behind the posterior border of the sternocleidomastoid muscle.

The needle should be advanced slowly because paresthesia is almost always produced when the needle tip impinges on the brachial plexus as it traverses the interscalene space nearly at a right angle to the needle tip. The patient should be warned that at some point paresthesia will occur and to say, "There!" as soon as it is felt. Paresthesia should be encountered at a depth

of approximately ¾ to 1 inch. After paresthesia is elicited, gentle aspiration is carried out to identify blood or cerebrospinal fluid (CSF). If the result of the aspiration test is negative and no paresthesia into the distribution of the brachial plexus persists, 20 to 30 mL of solution is slowly injected, and the patient is monitored closely for signs of local anesthetic toxicity or inadvertent subarachnoid injection. If surgical anesthesia is required for forearm or hand procedures, additional local anesthetic may have to be placed farther caudad along the brachial plexus to obtain adequate anesthesia of the lower portion of the plexus. Alternatively, specific nerves may be blocked farther distally if augmentation of the interscalene brachial plexus block is desired.[4] Studies have shown that ultrasound guidance may be useful during intrascalene brachial plexus block in patients in whom identification of the necessary anatomic landmarks presents a challenge[8] (**Figs. 155.5 to 155.7**).

Side Effects and Complications

The proximity of the brachial plexus to the subclavian artery and other large vessels suggests the potential for inadvertent intravascular injection or local anesthetic toxicity from intravascular absorption. Given the large doses of local anesthetic required for interscalene brachial plexus block, the pain specialist should carefully calculate the total milligram dose of local anesthetic that may safely be given. This vascularity also increases the incidence of postblock ecchymosis and hematoma formation. In spite of the vascularity of this anatomic region, this technique can safely be performed in the presence of anticoagulation by using a 25- or 27-gauge needle, albeit at increased risk of hematoma, if the clinical situation dictates a favorable risk-to-benefit ratio. The risk of these complications can be decreased if manual pressure is applied to the area of the block immediately after injection. Application of cold packs for 20-minute periods after the block also decreases the amount of postprocedure pain and bleeding.

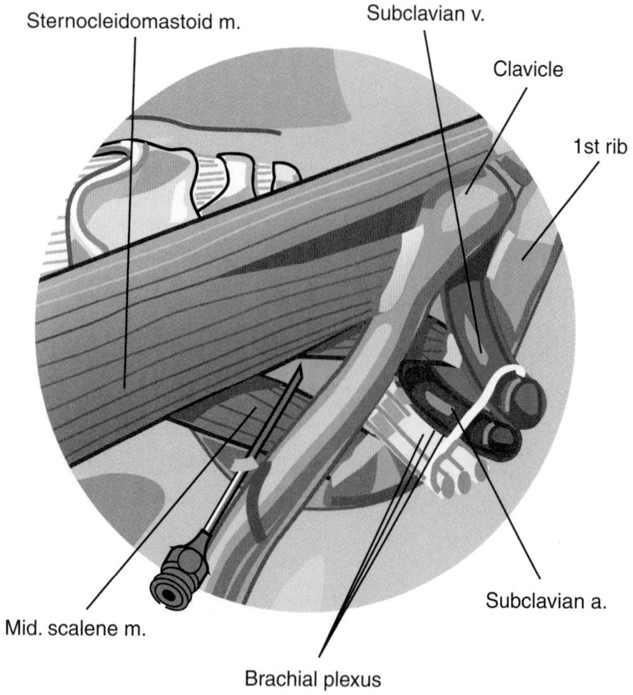

Fig. 155.4 **Needle placement for interscalene brachial plexus block.**

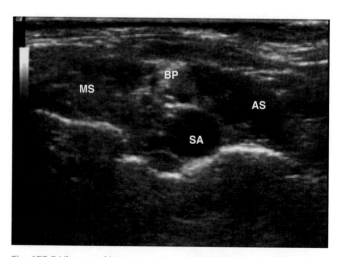

Fig. 155.5 Ultrasound image superior to the midclavicle showing a short-axis view of the subclavian artery (SA). The brachial plexus (BP) is visible in a position superficial and posterior to the artery. The middle scalene (MS) and anterior scalene (AS) muscles are also visible. *(From Davis JJ, Swenson JD, Greis PE, et al: Interscalene block for postoperative analgesia using only ultrasound guidance: the outcome in 200 patients, J Clin Anesth 21[4]:272–277, 2009.)*

In addition to the potential for complications involving the vasculature, the proximity of the brachial plexus to the central neuraxial structures and the phrenic nerve can result in side effects and complications. When the needle is placed too deeply, inadvertent epidural, subdural, or subarachnoid injection is a possibility. If the volume of local anesthetic used for this block is accidentally placed in any of these spaces, significant motor and sensory block will result. Unrecognized, these complications can be fatal. Practitioners should assume that the phrenic nerve will also be blocked during brachial plexus block using the interscalene approach, given the relationship of the phrenic nerve with the brachial plexus at this level (**Fig. 155.8**). In the absence of significant pulmonary disease, unilateral phrenic nerve block should rarely create respiratory embarrassment. However, blockade of the recurrent laryngeal nerve with its attendant vocal cord paralysis, combined with paralysis of the diaphragm, may make clearing of pulmonary and upper airway secretions difficult. Pneumothorax is also a possibility, although this complication is less likely than with the supraclavicular approach to brachial plexus block.

Clinical Pearls

The keys to the safe and successful interscalene brachial plexus block are a clear understanding of the anatomy and the careful identification of the necessary anatomic landmarks. Poking around for paresthesia without first identifying the interscalene groove is a recipe for disaster. The pain specialist should remember that the brachial plexus is quite close to the skin at the level where this block is performed. The needle should rarely be inserted more deeply than 1 inch in any but the most obese patients. Supplementation of intrascalene brachial plexus block by more peripheral block of the ulnar nerve may be required because the C8 fibers are not always adequately anesthetized with the interscalene approach. Careful neurologic examination for preexisting neurologic deficits that could later be attributed to the nerve block should be performed before beginning any brachial plexus block (see Fig. 155.2).

Supraclavicular Block

Indications

The supraclavicular approach to brachial plexus block is an excellent choice when dense surgical anesthesia of the distal upper extremity is required. This technique is less suitable for shoulder problems because it almost always requires supplementation with cervical plexus block to provide adequate cutaneous anesthesia of the shoulder.[9] In addition to applications for surgical anesthesia, supraclavicular brachial plexus nerve block with local anesthetics can be used as a diagnostic tool when performing differential neural blockade on an anatomic basis to evaluate upper extremity pain. If destruction of the brachial plexus is being considered, this technique is useful as a prognostic indicator of the degree of motor and sensory impairment that the patient may experience. Supraclavicular brachial plexus nerve block with local anesthetic may be used to palliate acute pain emergencies, including that of acute herpes zoster, brachial plexus neuritis, upper extremity trauma, and cancer while the patient waits for pharmacologic, surgical, and antineoplastic methods to take effect. Supraclavicular brachial plexus nerve block is also useful as an alternative to stellate ganglion block for treating reflex sympathetic dystrophy of the upper extremity.

Destruction of the supraclavicular brachial plexus is indicated for palliation of cancer pain, including pain arising from invasive tumors of the brachial plexus, and tumors of the soft tissue and bone of the upper extremity.[6] Because of the potential for intrathoracic hemorrhage, the interscalene approach to brachial plexus block should be used in patients who are anticoagulated only if the clinical situation dictates a favorable risk-to-benefit ratio.

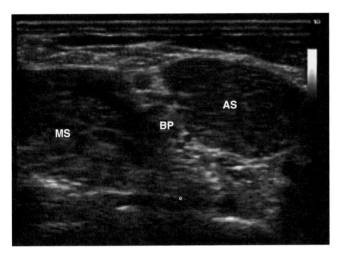

Fig. 155.6 Ultrasound image of the interscalene region at the level of the sixth cervical vertebra. The brachial plexus (BP) is visible between the anterior scalene (AS) and middle scalene (MS) muscles. *(From Davis JJ, Swenson JD, Greis PE, et al: Interscalene block for postoperative analgesia using only ultrasound guidance: the outcome in 200 patients,* J Clin Anesth *21[4]:272–277, 2009.)*

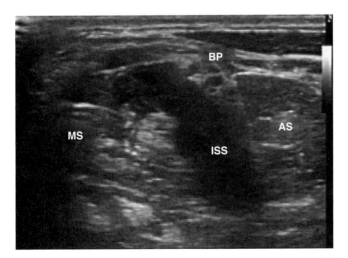

Fig. 155.7 View of the interscalene space (ISS), which has been expanded by injection of local anesthetic into the tissue plane between the anterior border of the middle scalene (MS) muscle and the brachial plexus (BP). AS, anterior scalene. *(From Davis JJ, Swenson JD, Greis PE, et al: Interscalene block for postoperative analgesia using only ultrasound guidance: the outcome in 200 patients,* J Clin Anesth *21[4]:272–277, 2009.)*

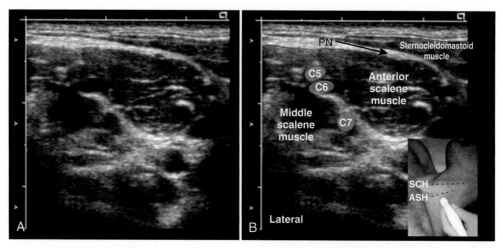

Fig. 155.8 Sonogram of the interscalene groove in the neck obtained 1 cm caudal to the cricoid cartilage (A), and the corresponding labeled image (B). The phrenic nerve (PN) is identified medial to the brachial plexus and superficial to the anterior scalene muscle (ASM), shown with the approximate probe location in the *inset*. Large tick marks are spaced 10 mm apart. The borders of the sternocleidomastoid (SCM), ASM, and middle scalene muscles are shown in red. *(From Kessler J, Schafhalter-Zoppoth I, Gray AT: An ultrasound study of the phrenic nerve in the posterior cervical triangle: implications for the interscalene brachial plexus block,* Reg Anesth Pain Med *33[6]:545–550, 2008.)*

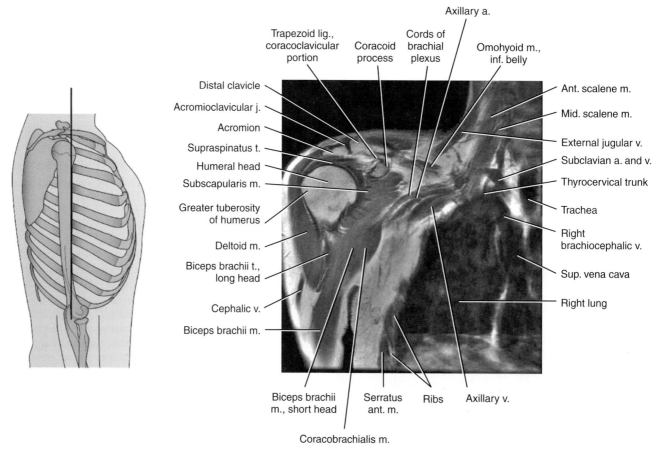

Fig. 155.9 The point at which the lateral border of the sternocleidomastoid attaches to the clavicle. *(From El-Khoury GY, Bergman RA, Montgomery WJ: Sectional anatomy by MRI and CT, ed 3, New York, 2007, Churchill Livingstone, p 27.)*

Technique

The patient is placed supine with the head turned away from the side to be blocked. A total of 10 mL of local anesthetic is drawn up in a 20-mL sterile syringe. For treatment of painful conditions that are mediated by the brachial plexus, a total of 80 mg of depot steroid is added to the local anesthetic with the first block and 40 mg of depot steroid is added with subsequent blocks.

The patient is then asked to raise his or her head against the resistance of the pain specialist's hand to aid in identifying the posterior border of the sternocleidomastoid muscle. The point at which the lateral border of the sternocleidomastoid

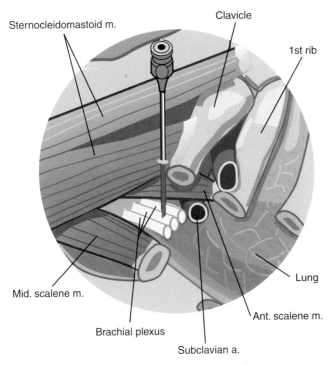

Fig. 155.10 **Needle placement for supraclavicular brachial plexus block.**

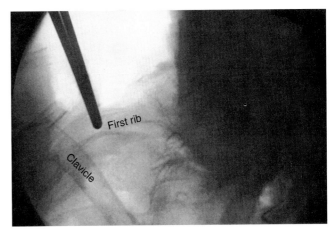

Fig. 155.11 **Radiographic supraclavicular view of the middle of the first rib.** *(From Raj PP, Lou L, Erdine S, et al: Radiographic imaging for regional anesthesia and pain management, Philadelphia, 2003, Churchill Livingstone, p 112.)*

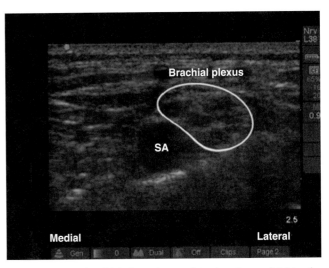

Fig. 155.12 The brachial plexus is seen lateral and superficial to the subclavian artery (SA). *(From Stone MB, Wang R, Price DD: Ultrasound-guided supraclavicular brachial plexus nerve block vs procedural sedation for the treatment of upper extremity emergencies, Am J Emerg Med 26[6]:706–710, 2008.)*

attaches to the clavicle is then identified (**Fig. 155.9**). At this point, just above the clavicle, after the skin is prepared with antiseptic solution, and a 1.5-inch needle is inserted directly perpendicular to the table top (**Fig. 155.10**). The needle should be advanced slowly because paresthesia is almost always encountered at a depth of approximately ¾ to 1 inch. The patient should be warned that paresthesia will occur and to say, "There" as soon as it is felt. If paresthesia is not elicited after the needle has been slowly advanced to a depth of 1 inch, the needle should be withdrawn and advanced again with a slightly more cephalad trajectory. This maneuver should be repeated until paresthesia is elicited. Conversely, if the first rib is encountered before paresthesia is induced, the needle should be walked laterally along the first rib until paresthesia is elicited (**Fig. 155.11**). To avoid pneumothorax, the needle should *never* be directed in a more medial trajectory.

After paresthesia is elicited, gentle aspiration is carried out to identify blood or CSF. If the aspiration result is negative and no persistent paresthesia into the distribution of the brachial plexus remains, the practitioner slowly injects 20 to 30 mL of solution, and the patient is monitored closely for signs of local anesthetic toxicity or inadvertent neuraxial injection. Studies have shown that ultrasound guidance may be useful when performing supraclavicular brachial plexus block in patients in whom identification of the necessary anatomic landmarks presents a challenge[10] (**Fig. 155.12**).

Side Effects and Complications

The proximity of the brachial plexus to the subclavian artery and other large vessels suggests the potential for inadvertent intravascular injection or local anesthetic toxicity from intravascular absorption. Given the large doses of local anesthetic required for supraclavicular brachial plexus block, the pain specialist should carefully calculate the total milligram dose

of local anesthetic that may safely be given. This vascularity also increases the risk of postblock ecchymosis and hematoma formation. These complications can be minimized if manual pressure is applied to the area of the block immediately after injection. Applying cold packs for 20-minute periods after the block also reduces the amount of postprocedure pain and bleeding the patient may experience.

In addition to the potential for complications involving the vasculature, the proximity of the brachial plexus to the central neuraxial structures and the phrenic nerve can result in side effects and complications. Although these complications occur less frequently than with interscalene brachial plexus block, inadvertent epidural, subdural, or subarachnoid injection remains a possibility. If the volume of local anesthetic used for this block is accidentally placed in any of these spaces, significant motor and sensory block will result. Unrecognized, these complications can be fatal. Practitioners should assume that the phrenic nerve will also be blocked at least 30% of the time during brachial plexus block using the supraclavicular approach. In the absence of significant pulmonary disease, unilateral phrenic nerve block should rarely create respiratory embarrassment.[7] Blockade of the recurrent laryngeal nerve with its attendant vocal cord paralysis, combined with paralysis of the diaphragm, may make clearing of pulmonary and upper airway secretions difficult. Because of the proximity of the apex of the lung, pneumothorax is a distinct possibility, and the patient should be so informed.

Clinical Pearls

The keys to performing safe and successful supraclavicular brachial plexus block are a clear understanding of the anatomy and the careful identification of the necessary anatomic landmarks. Poking around for paresthesia without first identifying the anatomic landmarks is a recipe for disaster. The pain specialist should remember that the brachial plexus is close to the surface at the level where this block is performed. The needle should rarely be inserted more deeply than 1 inch in all but the most obese patients. If strict adherence to technique is observed and the needle is never advanced medially from the lateral border of the insertion of the sternocleidomastoid muscle on the clavicle, the incidence of pneumothorax should be less than 0.5%. Careful neurologic examination to identify preexisting neurologic deficits that could later be attributed to the nerve block should be performed before beginning any brachial plexus block.

Axillary Approach to the Brachial Plexus

Indications

The axillary approach to the brachial plexus is the preferred technique for brachial plexus block when dense anesthesia of the forearm and hand is required.[11] In addition to applications for surgical anesthesia, axillary brachial plexus block with local anesthetics can be used as a diagnostic tool when performing differential neural blockade on an anatomic basis to evaluate upper extremity pain. If destruction of the brachial plexus is being considered, this technique is useful as a prognostic indicator of the degree of motor and sensory impairment that the patient may experience. Axillary brachial plexus nerve block with local anesthetic may be used to palliate acute pain emergencies including those related to acute herpes zoster, brachial plexus neuritis, shoulder and upper extremity trauma, and cancer pain while the patient waits for pharmacologic, surgical, and antineoplastic methods to take effect. Axillary brachial plexus nerve block is also useful as an alternative to stellate ganglion block for treatment of reflex sympathetic dystrophy of the upper extremity.[12]

Destruction of the brachial plexus is indicated for the palliation of cancer pain, including pain from invasive tumors of the distal brachial plexus and tumors of the soft tissue and bone of the upper extremity. Because of the desperation of many patients' suffering from aggressively invasive tumors that have invaded the brachial plexus, blockade using the axillary approach may be carried out even in the presence of coagulopathy or anticoagulation by using a 25-gauge needle, albeit with increased risk of ecchymosis and hematoma formation.

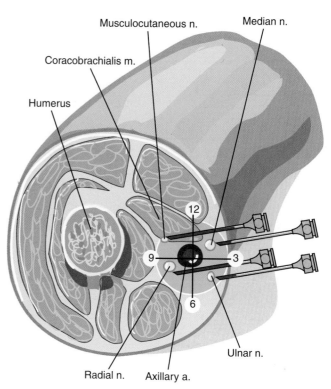

Fig. 155.13 Needle placement for the axillary approach to brachial plexus block.

Clinically Relevant Anatomy

The brachial plexus is formed by the fusion of the anterior rami of the C5, C6, C7, C8, and T1 spinal nerves. Fibers from the C4 and T2 spinal nerves may also be contributory. The nerves that make up the plexus exit the lateral aspect of the cervical spine and pass downward and laterally in conjunction with the subclavian artery. The nerves and artery run between the anterior scalene and middle scalene muscles and pass inferiorly behind the middle of the clavicle and above the top of the first rib to reach the axilla. Because the sheath that encloses the axillary artery and nerves is less consistent than the sheath that encloses the brachial plexus at the level where interscalene and supraclavicular brachial plexus blocks are performed, a single-injection technique is less satisfactory. The median, radial, ulnar, and musculocutaneous nerves surround the artery within this imperfect sheath. David Brown suggested that the position of these nerves relative to the axillary artery can best be visualized by placing them in quadrants as represented on the face of a clock with the axillary artery at the center of the clock (**Fig. 155.13**).[13] The median nerve is found in the 12- to 3-o'clock quadrant, the ulnar nerve in the 3- to 6-o'clock quadrant, the radial nerve in the 6- to 9-o'clock quadrant, and the musculocutaneous nerve in the 9- to 12-o'clock quadrant. To ensure adequate block of these nerves, drug must be injected into each quadrant to deposit it close to each of these nerves.

Technique

The patient is placed in a supine position with the arm abducted 85 to 90 degrees and the fingertips resting just behind the ear. A total of 30 to 40 mL of local anesthetic is drawn up

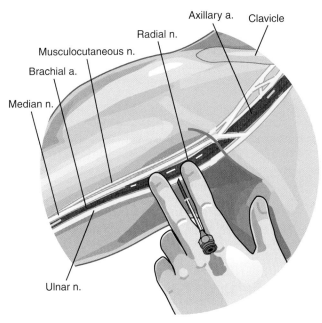

Fig. 155.14 **Relative locations of the median, radial, and ulnar nerves.**

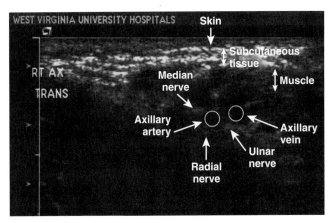

Fig. 155.15 Labeled ultrasonic view of the brachial plexus and accompanying vascular structures in the axilla just distal to the pectoralis muscle. *(From Hawkinberry DW II, Broadman LM: An introduction to ultrasonic guided axillary brachial plexus neuroblockade, Tech Reg Anesth Pain Manag 8[4]:149–154, 2004.)*

in a 50-mL sterile syringe. For treatment of painful or inflammatory conditions that are thought to be mediated by the brachial plexus, a total of 80 mg of depot steroid is added to the local anesthetic with the first block and 40 mg of depot steroid is added with subsequent blocks.

The pain specialist then identifies the pulsations of the patient's axillary artery with the middle and index fingers of the nondominant hand and traces the course of the artery distally by following the pulsations. After the skin has been prepared with antiseptic solution, a 1-inch, 25-gauge needle is inserted just below the arterial pulsations (**Fig. 155.14**). The needle should be advanced slowly because paresthesia is almost always induced as the needle tip impinges on the radial or ulnar nerve. The patient should be warned that paresthesia will occur and asked to say "There" as soon as it is felt. Paresthesia should be encountered at a depth of approximately ½ to ¾ inch. After paresthesia is elicited and its distribution is noted, gentle aspiration is carried out to identify blood or CSF. If the aspiration test result is negative and no persistent paresthesia into the distribution of the brachial plexus remains, the practitioner slowly injects 8 to 10 mL of solution, and the patient is monitored closely for signs of local anesthetic toxicity or inadvertent subarachnoid injection. If radial paresthesia is elicited, the needle is withdrawn slightly into the 3- to 6-o'clock quadrant, which contains the ulnar nerve, and, after a negative aspiration result, the practitioner injects an additional 8 to 10 mL of solution. If ulnar paresthesia is elicited, the needle is withdrawn and then slowly advanced again in a slightly more superior direction into the 6- to 9-o'clock quadrant, which contains the radial nerve, and the aspiration and injection techniques are repeated. The needle is then withdrawn and redirected above the arterial pulsation to the 12- to 3-o'clock quadrant, which contains the median nerve. If the aspiration result is negative, the practitioner

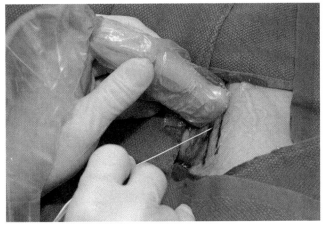

Fig. 155.16 **Close-up view of the block field.** Needle insertion is along the axis of the ultrasound beam and parallel to the axillary sheath. It will become visible on ultrasound as the tip passes into the path of the beam. The ultrasound probe is held gently against the skin, thus minimizing tissue compression and anatomic distortions. Gel in the sterile sheath and on the patient's skin produces a clear, sharp ultrasonic image. *(From Hawkinberry DW II, Broadman LM: An introduction to ultrasonic guided axillary brachial plexus neuroblockade, Tech Reg Anesth Pain Manag 8[4]:149–154, 2004.)*

injects 8 to 10 mL of solution. The needle is then directed to the 9- to 12-o'clock quadrant, which contains the musculocutaneous nerve. If the aspiration result is negative, the remaining local anesthetic is injected. Alternatively, the musculocutaneous nerve can be blocked by infiltrating the solution into the mass of the coracobrachialis muscle.[14] Studies have shown that ultrasound guidance may be useful during axillary brachial plexus block in patients in whom identification of the necessary anatomic landmarks presents a challenge[15] (**Figs. 155.15 to 155.17**).

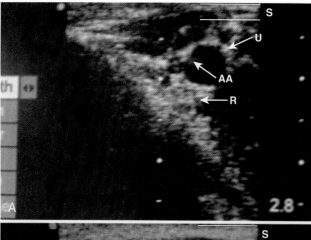

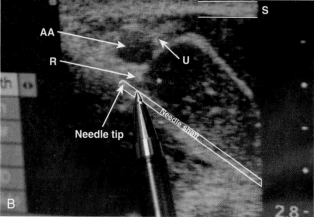

Fig. 155.17 A, Before injection. The ultrasonic image of the axillary brachial plexus is shown in the short axis (transverse view) high in the axilla just distal to the pectoralis muscle. The needle tip (indicated by the pen point) lies in close proximity to the radial nerve (R). The radial nerve (R) lies inferior to the axillary artery (AA). The ulnar nerve (U) lies caudad to the axillary artery. The skin (S) lies at the top of the photograph. **B,** After injection. The view is identical to that shown in **A,** except for the recent injection of 5 mL of local anesthetic solution, which contained a small amount of air, adjacent to the inferior border of the radial nerve (R). The ulnar nerve (U) is now obscured, and the outline of the radial nerve (R) is not quite as distinct. A fluffy white hyperechoic border circumscribes the axillary artery (AA). This border corresponds to the circumferential spread of the local anesthetic solution. *(From Hawkinberry DW II, Broadman LM: An introduction to ultrasonic guided axillary brachial plexus neuroblockade,* Tech Reg Anesth Pain Manag *8[4]:149–154, 2004.)*

Side Effects and Complications

The proximity of the nerves to the axillary artery and other large vessels carries the risk for inadvertent intravascular injection or local anesthetic toxicity from intravascular absorption.[10] Given the large doses of local anesthetic required for axillary brachial plexus block, the pain specialist should carefully calculate the total milligram dose of local anesthetic that may safely be given. The dense vascularity also increases the risk of postblock ecchymosis and hematoma formation. In spite of the vascularity of this anatomic region, this technique can safely be attempted in a patient taking an anticoagulant by using a 25- or 27-gauge needle, albeit at increased risk of hematoma, if the clinical situation dictates a favorable risk-to-benefit ratio. These complications can be reduced if manual pressure is applied to the area of the block immediately after injection. Applying cold packs for 20-minute periods after the block also reduces the amount of postprocedure pain and bleeding.

The distance of the nerves to be blocked from the neuraxis and phrenic nerve makes complications associated with injection of drugs onto these structures highly unlikely. This is an advantage of the axial approach as compared with the intrascalene and supraclavicular approaches to brachial plexus block. Because paresthesias are elicited, the potential for postblock persistent paresthesia is a possibility, and the patient should be so advised.

Clinical Pearls

The axillary approach to brachial plexus block is a safe and simple way to anesthetize the distal upper extremity. For pain above the elbow, the interscalene or supraclavicular approach is probably a better choice. Careful neurologic examination for preexisting neurologic deficits that could later be attributed to the nerve block should be performed before any brachial plexus block.

References

Full references for this chapter can be found on www.expertconsult.com.

Neural Blockade of the Peripheral Nerves of the Upper Extremity

Steven D. Waldman

Radial Nerve Block at the Humerus

Indications

Radial nerve block at the humerus is useful to supplement brachial plexus block when additional anesthesia is needed in the distribution of the radial nerve. In addition to applications for surgical anesthesia, radial nerve block at the humerus with local anesthetic can be used as a diagnostic tool during differential neural blockade on an anatomic basis in the evaluation of upper extremity pain.[1] If destruction of the radial nerve is being considered, radial nerve block at the humerus is useful as a prognostic indicator of the degree of motor and sensory impairment that the patient may experience. Radial nerve

block at the humerus with local anesthetic may be used to palliate acute pain emergencies subserved by the radial nerve while the patient waits for pharmacologic, surgical, and antiblastic methods to become effective. Radial nerve block at the humerus with local anesthetic and steroid is also useful in the diagnosis and treatment of radial tunnel syndrome.

Clinically Relevant Anatomy

The radial nerve is made up of fibers from C5-T1 spinal roots.[2] The nerve lies posterior and inferior to the axillary artery in the 6:00-o'clock–to–9:00-o'clock quadrant. Exiting the axilla, the radial nerve passes between the medial and long heads of the triceps muscle. As the nerve curves across the posterior aspect of the humerus, it supplies a motor branch to the triceps. Continuing its downward path, it gives off numerous sensory branches to the upper arm (**Fig. 156.1**). At a point between the lateral epicondyle of the humerus and the musculospiral groove, the radial nerve divides into its two terminal branches. The superficial branch continues down the arm along with the radial artery and provides sensory innervation to the dorsum of the wrist and the dorsal aspects of a portion of the thumb and index and middle fingers. The deep branch provides most of the motor innervation to the extensors of the forearm.

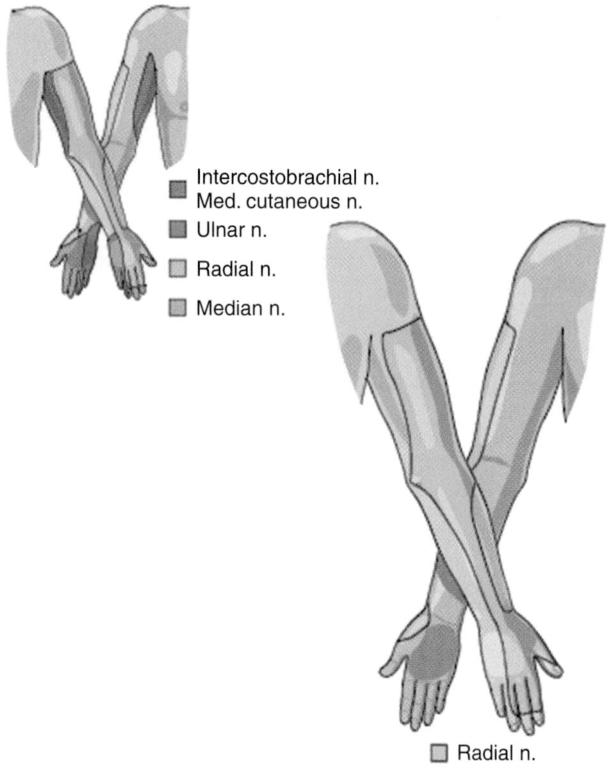

Technique

The patient is placed in a supine position with the arm abducted 35 to 45 degrees and the hand resting comfortably on the abdomen. A total of 7 to 10 mL of local anesthetic is drawn up in a 12-mL sterile syringe. For treating painful or inflammatory conditions that are mediated by the radial nerve, a total of 80 mg of depot steroid is added to the local anesthetic with the first block, and 40 mg of depot steroid is added with subsequent blocks.

The pain specialist then identifies the lateral epicondyle of the humerus, and at a point approximately inches above the epicondyle, the musculospiral groove is identified by deep palpation between the heads of the triceps muscle[2] (**Fig. 156.2**). After preparation of the skin with antiseptic solution, a 25-gauge, 1-inch needle is inserted perpendicular to the lateral aspect of the humerus and is advanced slowly toward the musculospiral groove[3] (**Fig. 156.3**). As the needle approaches the humerus, strong paresthesia in the distribution of the radial nerve is elicited. If no paresthesia is elicited and the needle contacts bone, the needle is withdrawn and is redirected slightly more anteriorly or posteriorly until paresthesia is elicited. The patient should be warned that paresthesia will occur and is asked to say "There!" as soon as the paresthesia is felt. After paresthesia is elicited and its distribution is identified, gentle aspiration is carried out to identify blood. If the aspiration test result is negative and no persistent paresthesia into the distribution of the radial nerve remains, the clinician slowly injects 7 to 10 mL of solution and closely monitors the patient for signs of local anesthetic toxicity. Studies have suggested that the use of ultrasound guidance improves the efficacy and safety of peripheral nerve blocks of the upper extremity[3] (**Fig. 156.4**).

Intercostobrachial n.
Med. cutaneous n.
Ulnar n.
Radial n.
Median n.

Radial n.

Fig. 156.1 Radial nerve block at the humerus. *(From Waldman SD: Radial nerve block at the humerus. In* Atlas of interventional pain management, *ed 3, Philadelphia, 2009, Saunders, p 212.)*

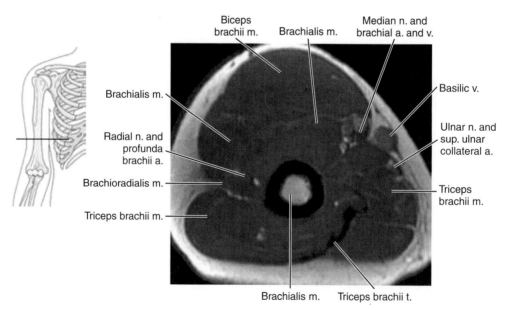

Biceps brachii m.
Brachialis m.
Median n. and brachial a. and v.
Brachialis m.
Basilic v.
Radial n. and profunda brachii a.
Ulnar n. and sup. ulnar collateral a.
Brachioradialis m.
Triceps brachii m.
Triceps brachii m.
Brachialis m. Triceps brachii t.

Fig. 156.2 Magnetic resonance imaging of the arm: axial. *(From El-houry GY, Bergman RA, Montgomery WJ, editors:* Sectional anatomy by MRI and CT, *ed 3, New York, 2007, Churchill Livingstone.)*

Side Effects and Complications

Radial nerve block at the humerus is a relatively safe block. The major complications are inadvertent intravascular injection and persistent paresthesia secondary to needle trauma to the nerve. This technique can safely be performed in the presence of anticoagulation by using a 25- or 27-gauge needle, albeit at increased risk of hematoma, if the clinical situation dictates a favorable risk-to-benefit ratio. These complications can be decreased if manual pressure is applied to the area of the block immediately after injection. Application of cold packs for 20-minute periods after the block also decreases the amount of postprocedure pain and bleeding the patient may experience.

Clinical Pearls

Radial nerve block at the humerus is a simple and safe technique. It is extremely useful in the management of radial tunnel syndrome. This painful condition is often misdiagnosed

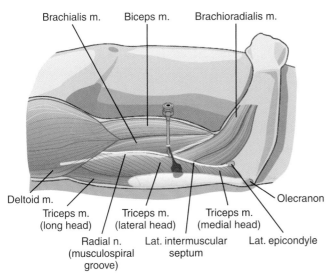

Fig. 156.3 **Radial nerve block at the humerus.** *(From Waldman SD: Radial nerve block at the humerus. In Atlas of interventional pain management, ed 3, Philadelphia, 2009, Saunders, p 212.)*

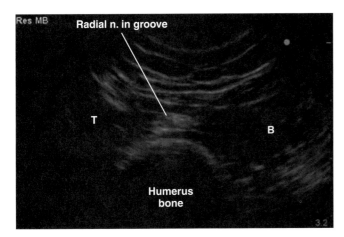

Fig. 156.4 Radial nerve is seen near shaft of humerus. It can be traced from axilla down to forearm and blocked anywhere along its course. *(From Sandhu NS: Ultrasound imaging in anesthesia: an overview of vascular access and peripheral nerve blocks, Semin Anesth Perioper Med Pain 26(4):197–209 2007.)*

as tennis elbow, and this confusion accounts for the many patients whose "tennis elbow" fails to respond to conservative measures. Radial tunnel syndrome can be distinguished from tennis elbow in that, with radial tunnel syndrome, the maximal tenderness to palpation is over the radial nerve, whereas with tennis elbow, the maximal tenderness to palpation is over the lateral epicondyle (**Fig. 156.5**). If radial tunnel syndrome is suspected, injection of the radial nerve at the humerus with local anesthetic and steroid will give almost instantaneous relief. Careful neurologic examination to identify preexisting neurologic deficits that may later be attributed to the nerve block should be performed on all patients before radial nerve block at the humerus is begun.

Median Cutaneous and Intercostobrachial Nerve Block

Indications

Median cutaneous and intercostobrachial nerve block is not commonly used as a stand-alone pain management technique. Rather, it is used to augment brachial plexus block and to provide anesthesia of the medial cutaneous surface of the arm and axilla to decrease tourniquet pain during intravenous regional anesthesia (**Fig. 156.6**).

Clinically Relevant Anatomy

The median cutaneous nerve is formed from fibers originating from the C8-T1 roots. These roots can be difficult to block adequately during brachial plexus block.[4] The fibers of the median cutaneous nerve communicate with the fibers

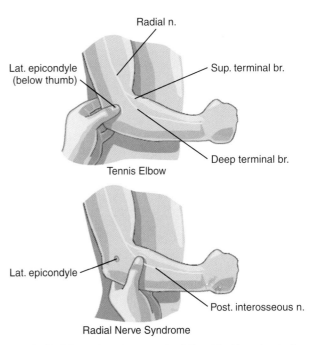

Fig. 156.5 Radial tunnel syndrome can be distinguished from tennis elbow in that with radial tunnel syndrome, the maximal tenderness to palpitation is over the radial nerve, whereas with tennis elbow, the maximal tenderness to palpation is over the lateral epicondyle. *(From Waldman SD: Radial nerve block at the humerus. In Atlas of interventional pain management, ed 3, Philadelphia, 2009, Saunders, p 213.)*

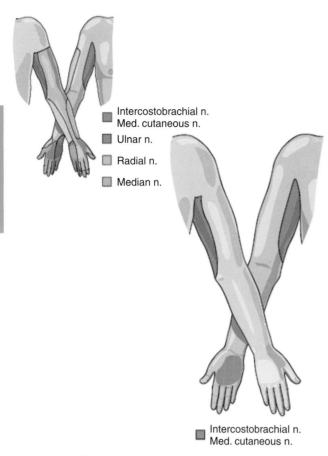

Intercostobrachial n.
Med. cutaneous n.

Ulnar n.

Radial n.

Median n.

Intercostobrachial n.
Med. cutaneous n.

Fig. 156.6 Median cutaneous and intercostobrachial nerve block. *(From Waldman SD: Median cutaneous and intercostobrachial nerve block. In Atlas of interventional pain management, ed 3, Philadelphia, 2009, Saunders Elsevier, p 216.)*

of the intercostobrachial nerve, which has its origin in the second intercostal nerve. These nerves exit the axilla outside the brachial plexus sheath and travel superficially parallel to the triceps muscle (**Fig. 156.7**). The superficial location of both these nerves makes them easily accessible for neural blockade.

Technique

The patient is placed in the supine position with the arm abducted 85 to 90 degrees in a manner analogous to positioning for axillary nerve block. A total of 8 mL of local anesthetic is drawn up in a 12-mL sterile syringe.

The superior margin of the biceps muscle is identified at the anterior axillary line. The skin at this point is prepared with antiseptic solution, and a bead of local anesthetic is placed subcutaneously from this point inferiorly in an arc from the biceps to the triceps continuing along the axillary surface of the arm[4] (**Fig. 156.8**). This technique blocks both the median cutaneous and intercostobrachial nerves.

Side Effects and Complications

This technique is relatively free of complications as long as the pain specialist keeps a subcutaneous needle tip, thus avoiding injection into the axillary artery and vein. Bruising and injection site soreness may occasionally occur.

Clinical Pearls

Medial cutaneous and intercostobrachial nerve block can turn what appears to be a failed brachial plexus block into a success. This technique should be considered prophylactically whenever intravenous regional anesthesia with prolonged tourniquet time is being considered, to decrease the incidence of tourniquet pain.

Radial Nerve Block at the Elbow

Indications

Radial nerve block at the elbow is useful for supplementing brachial plexus block when additional anesthesia is needed in the distribution of the radial nerve. In addition to applications for surgical anesthesia, radial nerve block at the elbow with local anesthetic can be used as a diagnostic tool during differential neural blockade on an anatomic basis in the evaluation of upper extremity pain below the elbow.[5] If destruction of the radial nerve is being considered, radial nerve block at the elbow is useful as a prognostic indicator of the degree of motor and sensory impairment that the patient may experience. Radial nerve block at the elbow with local anesthetic may be used to palliate acute pain emergencies subserved by the radial nerve while the patient waits for pharmacologic, surgical, and antiblastic methods to become effective.

Clinically Relevant Anatomy

The radial nerve is made up of fibers from C5-T1 spinal roots.[2] The nerve lies posterior and inferior to the axillary artery in the 6:00-o'clock–to–9:00-o'clock quadrant. Exiting the axilla, the radial nerve passes between the medial and long heads of the triceps muscle. As the nerve curves across the posterior aspect of the humerus, it supplies a motor branch to the triceps. Continuing its downward path, it gives off numerous sensory branches to the upper arm (**Fig. 156.9**). At a point between the lateral epicondyle of the humerus and the musculospiral groove, the radial nerve divides into its two terminal branches[6] (**Fig. 156.10**). The superficial branch continues down the arm along with the radial artery and provides sensory innervation to the dorsum of the wrist and the dorsal aspects of a portion of the thumb and index and middle fingers. The deep branch provides most of the motor innervation to the extensors of the forearm.

Technique

The patient is placed in a supine position with the arm fully abducted at the patient's side and the elbow slightly flexed with the dorsum of the hand resting on a folded towel. A total of 7 to 10 mL of local anesthetic is drawn up in a 12-mL sterile syringe. When the clinician is treating painful or inflammatory conditions that are mediated by the radial nerve, a total of 80 mg of depot steroid is added to the local anesthetic with the first block, and 40 mg of depot steroid is added with subsequent blocks.

The pain specialist then identifies the lateral margin of the biceps tendon at the crease of the elbow. After preparation of the skin with antiseptic solution, a 25-gauge, 1½-inch needle

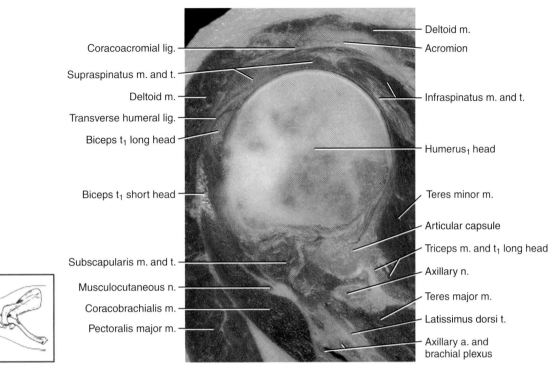

Coracoacromial lig.

Supraspinatus m. and t.

Deltoid m.

Transverse humeral lig.

Biceps t_1 long head

Biceps t_1 short head

Subscapularis m. and t.

Musculocutaneous n.

Coracobrachialis m.

Pectoralis major m.

Deltoid m.

Acromion

Infraspinatus m. and t.

Humerus$_1$ head

Teres minor m.

Articular capsule

Triceps m. and t_1 long head

Axillary n.

Teres major m.

Latissimus dorsi t.

Axillary a. and brachial plexus

Fig. 156.7 **Shoulder, sagittal.** *(From Kang HS, Ahn JM, Resnick D: MRI of the extremities: an anatomic atlas, ed 2, Philadelphia, 2002, Saunders.)*

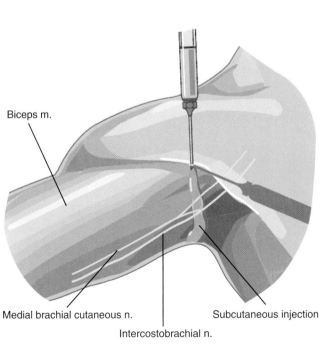

Biceps m.

Medial brachial cutaneous n.

Intercostobrachial n.

Subcutaneous injection

Fig. 156.8 The superior margin of the biceps muscle is identified at the anterior axillary line. The skin at this point is prepared with antiseptic solution, and a bead of local anesthetic is placed subcutaneously from this point inferiorly in an arc from the biceps to the triceps continuing along the axillary surface of the arm. *(From Waldman SD: Median cutaneous and intercostobrachial nerve block. In Atlas of interventional pain management, ed 3, Philadelphia, 2009, Saunders, p 216.)*

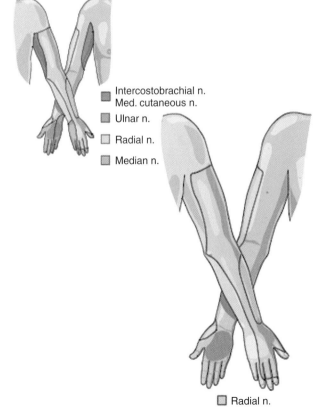

Intercostobrachial n.
Med. cutaneous n.

Ulnar n.

Radial n.

Median n.

Radial n.

Fig. 156.9 **Radial nerve.** *(From Waldman SD: Radial nerve block at the elbow. In Atlas of interventional pain management, ed 3, Philadelphia, 2009, Saunders, p 219.)*

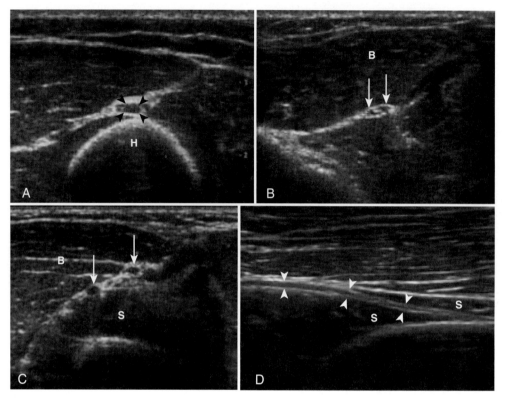

Fig. 156.10 **Radial nerve evaluation. A,** Transverse imaging relative to the humerus (H) shows the radial nerve *(arrowheads)* at the level of the radial groove. Transverse imaging distally (**B** and **C**) shows the bifurcation of the radial nerve into the superficial and deep branches *(arrows)* deep to the brachioradialis (B). S, supinator. **D,** Longitudinal imaging shows the deep branch of the radial nerve *(arrowheads)* between the two heads of the supinator muscle (S).

is inserted just lateral to the biceps tendon at the crease and is slowly advanced in a slightly medial and cephalad trajectory[5,7] (**Fig. 156.11**). As the needle approaches the humerus, strong paresthesia in the distribution of the radial nerve is elicited. If no paresthesia is elicited and the needle contacts bone, the needle is withdrawn and is redirected slightly more medially until paresthesia is elicited. The patient should be warned that paresthesia will occur and asked to say "There!" as soon as the paresthesia is felt. After paresthesia is elicited and its distribution is identified, gentle aspiration is carried out to identify blood. If the aspiration test result is negative and no persistent paresthesia into the distribution of the radial nerve remains, the clinician slowly injects 7 to 10 mL of solution and closely monitors the patient for signs of local anesthetic toxicity. Studies have suggested that the use of ultrasound guidance improves the efficacy and safety of peripheral nerve blocks of the upper extremity[8] (**Fig. 156.12**).

Side Effects and Complications

Radial nerve block at the elbow is a relatively safe block. The major complications are inadvertent intravascular injection and persistent paresthesia secondary to needle trauma to the nerve. This technique can safely be performed in the presence of anticoagulation by using a 25- or 27-gauge needle, albeit at increased risk of hematoma, if the clinical situation dictates a favorable risk-to-benefit ratio. These complications can be decreased if manual pressure is applied to the area of the block immediately after injection. Application of cold packs for 20-minute periods after the block also decreases the amount of postprocedure pain and bleeding the patient may experience.

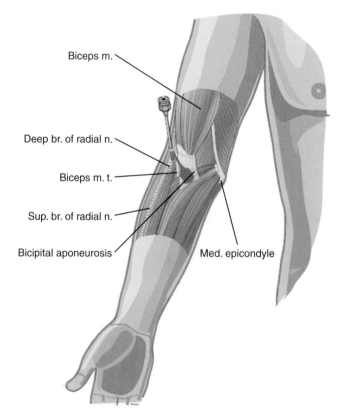

Fig. 156.11 After preparation of the skin with antiseptic solution, a 25-gauge, 1½ inch needle is inserted just lateral to the biceps tendon at the crease and is slowly advanced in a slightly medial and cephalad trajectory. *(From Waldman SD: Radial nerve block at the elbow. In* Atlas of interventional pain management, ed 3, Philadelphia, 2009, Saunders, p 220.)

Clinical Pearls

Radial nerve block at the elbow is a simple and safe technique in the evaluation and treatment of the previously mentioned painful conditions. Careful neurologic examination to identify preexisting neurologic deficits that may later be attributed to the nerve block should be performed on all patients before radial nerve block at the elbow is begun.

Median Nerve Block at the Elbow

Indications

Median nerve block at the elbow is useful in supplementing brachial plexus block when additional anesthesia is needed in the distribution of the median nerve.[9] In addition to applications for

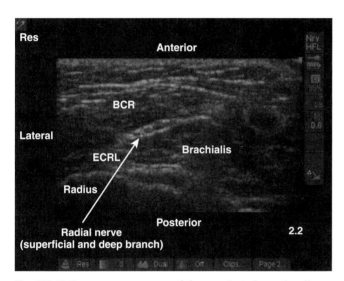

Fig. 156.12 **Transverse sonogram of the arm, just above the elbow, showing the radial nerve.** BCR, brachioradialis; ECRL, extensor carpi radialis longus. *(From Karmakar MK, Kwok WH: Ultrasound-guided regional anesthesia. In Cote CJ, Lerman J, Todres D, editors:* A practice of anesthesia for infants and children, *ed 4, Philadelphia, 2009, Saunders, pp 911–938.)*

surgical anesthesia, median nerve block at the elbow with local anesthetic can be used as a diagnostic tool during differential neural blockade on an anatomic basis in the evaluation of upper extremity pain below the elbow. If destruction of the median nerve is being considered, median nerve block at the elbow is useful as a prognostic indicator of the degree of motor and sensory impairment that the patient may experience. Median nerve block at the elbow with local anesthetic may be used to palliate acute pain emergencies subserved by the median nerve while the patient waits for pharmacologic, surgical, and antiblastic methods to become effective. Median nerve block at the elbow with local anesthetic and steroid is also useful in the palliation of pain secondary to median nerve entrapment syndromes at the elbow, including compression by the ligament of Struthers and the pronator syndrome (**Fig. 156.13**).

Clinically Relevant Anatomy

The median nerve is made up of fibers from C5-T1 spinal roots. The nerve lies anterior and superior to the axillary artery in the 12:00-o'clock–to–3:00-o'clock quadrant. Exiting the axilla, the median nerve descends into the upper arm along with the brachial artery. At the level of the elbow, the brachial artery is just medial to the biceps muscle[10] (**Fig. 156.14**). At this level, the median nerve lies just medial to the brachial artery. As the median nerve proceeds downward into the forearm, it gives off numerous branches that provide motor innervation to the flexor muscles of the forearm. These branches are susceptible to nerve entrapment by aberrant ligaments, muscle hypertrophy, and direct trauma. The nerve approaches the wrist overlying the radius. It lies deep to and between the tendons of the palmaris longus muscle and the flexor carpi radialis muscle at the wrist. The terminal branches of the median nerve provide sensory innervation to a portion of the palmar surface of the hand, as well as the palmar surface of the thumb, index and middle fingers, and the radial portion of the ring finger (**Fig. 156.15**). The median nerve also provides sensory innervation to the distal dorsal surface of the index and middle fingers and the radial portion of the ring finger.[2,10]

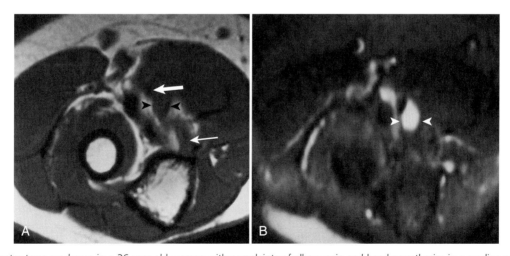

Fig. 156.13 Pronator teres syndrome in a 36-year-old woman with complaints of elbow pain and hand paresthesias in a median nerve distribution. A, Axial T1-weighted (700/18) magnetic resonance image (MRI) just proximal to the radial tuberosity shows fusiform enlargement of the median nerve that is isointense with muscle *(black arrowheads)*. The nerve projects to just medial to the brachial artery *(short white arrow)*. Enlargement is seen just proximal to the confluence of the humeral head of the pronator teres (PT) and ulnar head *(long white arrow)*. B, Axial fast spin-echo short T1 inversion recovery (STIR) (6850/45/150/16) image shows markedly increased signal intensity within the enlarged segment of the median nerve *(white arrowheads)*. *(From Stark DD, Bradley WG:* Magnetic resonance imaging, *ed 3, St. Louis, 1999, Mosby, p 764.)*

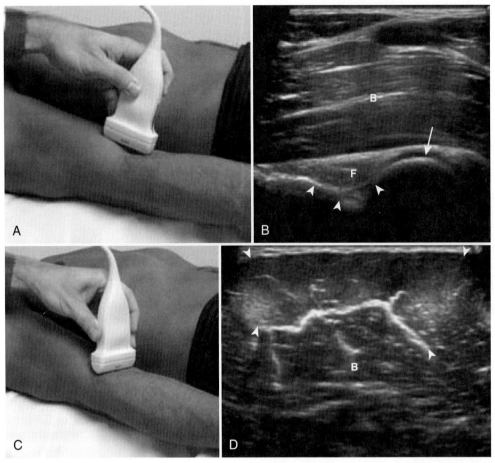

Fig. 156.14 **Biceps brachii, brachialis, anterior joint recess, and median nerve evaluation.** **A,** Sagittal imaging over the anterior elbow shows (**B**) the brachialis muscle (B), coronoid fossa *(arrowheads),* anterior elbow fat pad (F), and trochlea hyaline cartilage (arrow). **C,** Transverse imaging from superior to inferior over the anterior elbow shows (**D** to **F**) the biceps muscle *(arrowheads),* which becomes tendon lateral to the brachial artery (A), with the median artery *(arrows)* located medially. *Curved arrow,* hyaline cartilage; B, brachialis; C, capitellum; T, trochlea.

Technique

The patient is placed in a supine position with the arm fully adducted at the patient's side and the elbow slightly flexed with the dorsum of the hand resting on a folded towel. A total of 5 to 7 mL of local anesthetic is drawn up in a 12-mL sterile syringe. When treating painful or inflammatory conditions that are mediated by the median nerve, a total of 80 mg of depot steroid is added to the local anesthetic with the first block, and 40 mg of depot steroid is added with subsequent blocks.

The pain specialist then identifies the pulsations of the brachial artery at the crease of the elbow. After preparation of the skin with antiseptic solution, a 25-gauge, 1½-inch needle is inserted just medial to the brachial artery at the crease and is slowly advanced in a slightly medial and cephalad trajectory[9,11] (**Fig. 156.16**). As the needle advances approximately ½ to ¾ inch, strong paresthesia in the distribution of the median nerve is elicited. If no paresthesia is elicited and the needle contacts bone, the needle is withdrawn and is redirected slightly more medially until paresthesia is elicited. The patient should be warned that paresthesia will occur and asked to say "There!" as soon as the paresthesia is felt. After paresthesia is elicited and its distribution is identified, gentle aspiration is carried out to identify blood. If the aspiration test result is negative and no persistent paresthesia into the distribution

of the median nerve remains, the clinician slowly injects 5 to 7 mL of solution and closely monitors the patient for signs of local anesthetic toxicity. If no paresthesia can be elicited, a similar amount of solution is injected in a fanlike manner just medial to the brachial artery, with care taken not to inject into the artery inadvertently.

Side Effects and Complications

Median nerve block at the elbow is a relatively safe block. The major complications are inadvertent intravascular injection and persistent paresthesia secondary to needle trauma to the nerve. This technique can safely be performed in the presence of anticoagulation by using a 25- or 27-gauge needle, albeit at increased risk of hematoma, if the clinical situation dictates a favorable risk-to-benefit ratio. These complications can be decreased if manual pressure is applied to the area of the block immediately after injection. Application of cold packs for 20-minute periods after the block also decreases the amount of postprocedure pain and bleeding the patient may experience.

Clinical Pearls

Median nerve block at the elbow is a simple and safe technique in the evaluation and treatment of the previously mentioned painful conditions. Careful neurologic examination to identify

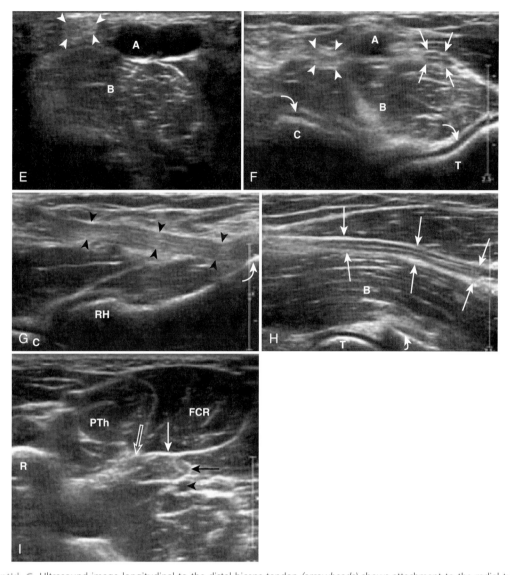

Fig. 156.14—cont'd. **G,** Ultrasound image longitudinal to the distal biceps tendon *(arrowheads)* shows attachment to the radial tuberosity *(curved arrow).* C, capitellum; RH, radial head. **H,** Ultrasound image medial to **G** shows the median nerve longitudinally *(arrows). Curved arrow,* coronoid process; B, brachialis; T, trochlea. **I,** Ultrasound image transverse to the median nerve shows the humeral head of the pronator teres (PTh), the median nerve *(open arrow),* the ulnar head of pronator teres *(arrows),* and the ulnar artery *(arrowhead).* FCR, flexor carpi radialis; R, radius.

preexisting neurologic deficits that may later be attributed to the nerve block should be performed on all patients before median nerve block at the elbow is begun.

This technique is especially useful in the treatment of pain secondary to median nerve compression syndromes at the elbow, including compression by the ligament of Struthers and the pronator syndrome. *Median nerve compression by the ligament of Struthers* manifests clinically as unexplained persistent forearm pain caused by compression of the median nerve by an aberrant ligament that runs from a supracondylar process to the medial epicondyle. The diagnosis is made by electromyography and nerve conduction velocity testing, which demonstrate compression of the median nerve at the elbow, combined with the x-ray finding of a supracondylar process. The *pronator syndrome* is characterized by unexplained persistent forearm pain with tenderness to palpation over the pronator teres muscle (**Fig. 156.17**). Positive Tinel's sign may also be present. Median nerve compression by the

ligament of Struthers and pronator syndrome must be differentiated from *isolated compression of the anterior interosseous nerve,* which occurs some 6 to 8 cm below the elbow. These syndromes should also be differentiated from *cervical radiculopathy* involving the C6 or C7 roots, which may at times mimic median nerve compression. Furthermore, cervical radiculopathy and median nerve entrapment may coexist as the so-called *double-crush syndrome.* The double-crush syndrome occurs most commonly with median nerve entrapment at the wrist or carpal tunnel syndrome.

Ulnar Nerve Block at the Elbow

Indications

Ulnar nerve block at the elbow is useful in supplementing brachial plexus block when additional anesthesia is needed in the distribution of the ulnar nerve.[12] In addition to applications

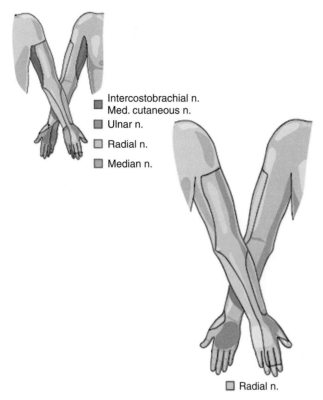

Intercostobrachial n.
Med. cutaneous n.
Ulnar n.
Radial n.
Median n.

Radial n.

Fig. 156.15 **Median nerve.** *(From Waldman SD: Median nerve block at the elbow. In* Atlas of interventional pain management, *ed 3, Philadelphia, 2009, Saunders, p 226.)*

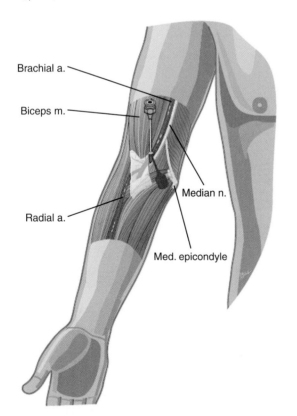

Brachial a.
Biceps m.
Radial a.
Median n.
Med. epicondyle

Fig. 156.16 The pain specialist then identifies the pulsations of the brachial artery at the crease of the elbow. After preparation of the skin with antiseptic solution, a 25-gauge 1½ inch needle is inserted just medial to the brachial artery at the crease and is slowly advanced in a slightly medial and cephalad trajectory. *(From Waldman SD: Median nerve block at the elbow. In* Atlas of interventional pain management, *ed 3, Philadelphia, 2009, Saunders, p 226.)*

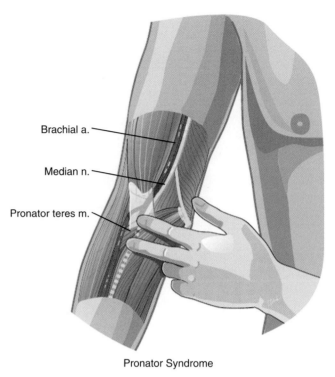

Brachial a.
Median n.
Pronator teres m.

Pronator Syndrome

Fig. 156.17 The pronator syndrome is characterized by unexplained persistent forearm pain with tenderness to palpation over the pronator teres muscle. *(From Waldman SD: Median nerve block at the elbow. In* Atlas of interventional pain management, *ed 3, Philadelphia, 2009, Saunders, p 227.)*

for surgical anesthesia, ulnar nerve block at the elbow with local anesthetic can be used as a diagnostic tool during differential neural blockade on an anatomic basis in the evaluation of upper extremity pain below the elbow. If destruction of the ulnar nerve is being considered, ulnar nerve block at the elbow is useful as a prognostic indicator of the degree of motor and sensory impairment that the patient may experience. Ulnar nerve block at the elbow with local anesthetic may be used to palliate acute pain emergencies subserved by the ulnar nerve while the patient waits for pharmacologic, surgical, and antiblastic methods to become effective. Ulnar nerve block at the elbow with local anesthetic and steroid is also useful in the palliation of pain secondary to ulnar nerve entrapment syndromes at the elbow, including cubital tunnel syndrome (**Fig. 156.18**).

Clinically Relevant Anatomy

The ulnar nerve is made up of fibers from C6-T1 spinal roots. The nerve lies anterior and inferior to the axillary artery in the 3:00-o'clock–to–6:00-o'clock quadrant. Exiting the axilla, the ulnar nerve descends into the upper arm along with the brachial artery. At the middle of the upper arm, the nerve courses medially to pass between the olecranon process and medial epicondyle of the humerus[13,14] (**Figs. 156.19** and **156.20**). The nerve then passes between the heads of the flexor carpi ulnaris muscle and continues downward, moving radially along with the ulnar artery. At a point approximately 1 inch proximal to the crease of the wrist, the ulnar nerve divides into the dorsal and palmar branches. The dorsal branch provides sensation to the ulnar aspect of the dorsum of the hand and the dorsal

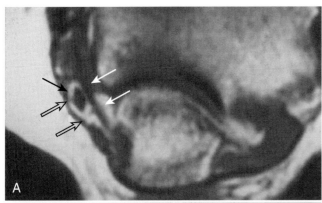

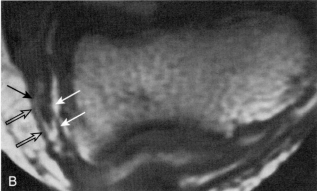

Fig. 156.18 **Dynamic configuration of the cubital tunnel with elbow flexion in a cadaver elbow.** A, Axial T1-weighted (500/15) magnetic resonance image (MRI) just distal to the medial epicondyle shows the oval configuration of the cubital tunnel defined deep by the medial capsule *(closed arrows)* and superficially by the cubital tunnel retinaculum *(open arrows)* with the elbow in extension. B, Radial T1-weighted image (500/15) perpendicular to the course of the ulnar nerve just distal to the medial epicondyle with the elbow flexed 90 degrees shows the taut contour of the borders of the cubital tunnel *(closed and open arrows same as in A)* with effaced perineural fat and a flattened configuration of the nerve. *Long black arrow,* ulnar nerve. *(From Stark DD, Bradley WG: Magnetic resonance imaging, ed 3, St. Louis, 1999, Mosby, p 762.)*

aspect of the little finger and the ulnar half of the ring finger (**Fig. 156.21**). The palmar branch provides sensory innervation to the ulnar aspect of the palm of the hand and the palmar aspect of the little finger and the ulnar half of the ring finger.

Technique

The patient is placed in a supine position with the arm abducted 85 to 90 degrees and the dorsum of the hand resting against a folded towel. A total of 5 to 7 mL of local anesthetic is drawn up in a 12-mL sterile syringe. When treating painful or inflammatory conditions that are mediated by the ulnar nerve, a total of 80 mg of depot steroid is added to the local anesthetic with the first block, and 40 mg of depot steroid is added with subsequent blocks.

The pain specialist then identifies the olecranon process and the median epicondyle of the humerus. The ulnar nerve sulcus between these two bony landmarks is then identified. After preparation of the skin with antiseptic solution, a 25-gauge, ⅝-inch needle is inserted just proximal to the sulcus and is slowly advanced in a slightly cephalad trajectory (**Fig. 156.22**). As the needle advances approximately ½ inch, strong paresthesia in the distribution of the ulnar nerve is elicited.[15] The patient should be warned that paresthesia will occur and asked

to say "there!" as soon as the paresthesia is felt. After paresthesia is elicited and its distribution is identified, gentle aspiration is carried out to identify blood. If the aspiration test result is negative and no persistent paresthesia into the distribution of the ulnar nerve remains, the clinician slowly injects 5 to 7 mL of solution and closely monitors the patient for signs of local anesthetic toxicity. If no paresthesia can be elicited, a similar amount of solution is slowly injected in a fanlike manner just proximal to the notch, with care taken to avoid intravascular injection.

Side Effects and Complications

Ulnar nerve block at the elbow is a relatively safe block. The major complications are inadvertent intravascular injection into the ulnar artery and persistent paresthesia secondary to needle trauma to the nerve. Because the nerve is enclosed by a dense fibrous band as it passes through the ulnar nerve sulcus, care should be taken to inject slowly just proximal to the sulcus to avoid additional compromise of the nerve. This technique can safely be performed in the presence of anticoagulation by using a 25- or 27-gauge needle, albeit at increased risk of hematoma, if the clinical situation dictates a favorable risk-to-benefit ratio. These complications can be decreased if manual pressure is applied to the area of the block immediately after injection. Application of cold packs for 20-minute periods after the block also decreases the amount of postprocedure pain and bleeding the patient may experience.

Clinical Pearls

Ulnar nerve block at the elbow is a simple and safe technique in the evaluation and treatment of the previously mentioned painful conditions. Careful neurologic examination to identify preexisting neurologic deficits that may later be attributed to the nerve block should be performed on all patients before ulnar nerve block at the elbow is begun because of the apparent propensity for the development of persistent paresthesia when the nerve is blocked at this level. The incidence of persistent paresthesia can be decreased by blocking the nerve proximal to the ulnar nerve sulcus and injecting slowly.

Ulnar nerve block at the elbow is especially useful in the treatment of pain secondary to ulnar nerve compression syndromes at the elbow, including cubital tunnel syndrome. Cubital tunnel syndrome is often misdiagnosed as golfer's elbow, and this confusion accounts for the many patients whose "golfer's elbow" fails to respond to conservative measures. Cubital tunnel syndrome can be distinguished from golfer's elbow in that in cubital tunnel syndrome, the maximal tenderness to palpation is over the ulnar nerve 1 inch below the medial epicondyle, whereas with golfer's elbow, the maximal tenderness to palpation is directly over the medial epicondyle (**Fig. 156.23**). If cubital tunnel syndrome is suspected, injection of the ulnar nerve at the elbow with local anesthetic and steroid will give almost instantaneous relief.

Cubital tunnel syndrome should also be differentiated from cervical radiculopathy involving the C8 spinal root, which may at times mimic ulnar nerve compression. Furthermore, cervical radiculopathy and ulnar nerve entrapment may coexist in the double-crush syndrome. The double-crush syndrome occurs most commonly with median nerve entrapment at the wrist or carpal tunnel syndrome. Pancoast's tumor invading

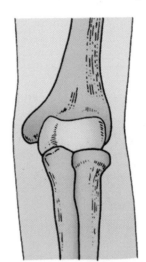

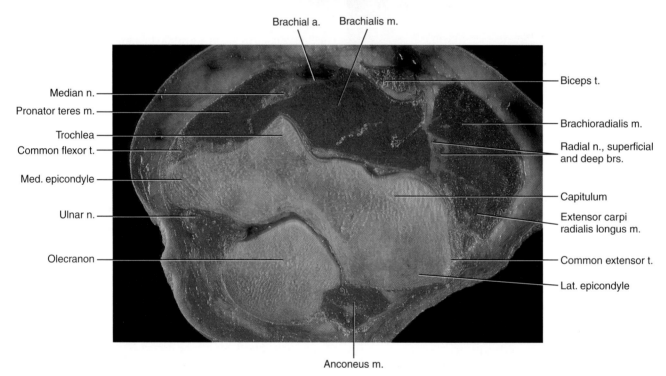

Brachial a.   Brachialis m.

Median n.
Pronator teres m.
Trochlea
Common flexor t.
Med. epicondyle
Ulnar n.
Olecranon

Biceps t.
Brachioradialis m.
Radial n., superficial and deep brs.
Capitulum
Extensor carpi radialis longus m.
Common extensor t.
Lat. epicondyle

Anconeus m.

Fig. 156.19 The ulnar nerve courses medially to pass between the olecranon process and the medial epicondyle and the humerus. *(From Kang HS, Ahn JM, Resnick D: MRI of the extremities: an anatomic atlas, ed 2, Philadelphia, 2002, Saunders, p 99.)*

the medial cord of the brachial plexus may also mimic isolated ulnar nerve entrapment and should be ruled out with an apical lordotic chest radiograph.

Radial Nerve Block at the Wrist

Indications

In contradistinction to blockade of the median and ulnar nerves at the wrist, radial nerve block at the wrist is used primarily to supplement partial brachial plexus block when additional anesthesia is needed in the distribution of the distal radial nerve.[16] Although less specific than the median and ulnar techniques, radial nerve block at the wrist is occasionally used as a diagnostic tool during differential neural block-

ade on an anatomic basis in the evaluation of upper extremity pain below the wrist. If destruction of the radial nerve is being considered, radial nerve block at the wrist is occasionally used as a prognostic indicator of the degree of motor and sensory impairment that the patient may experience. Radial nerve block at the wrist with local anesthetic may be used to palliate acute pain emergencies subserved by the radial nerve while the patient waits for pharmacologic, surgical, and antiblastic methods to become effective.

Clinically Relevant Anatomy

The radial nerve is made up of fibers from C5-T1 spinal roots. The nerve lies posterior and inferior to the axillary artery in the 6:00-o'clock to 9:00-o'clock quadrant. Exiting the axilla,

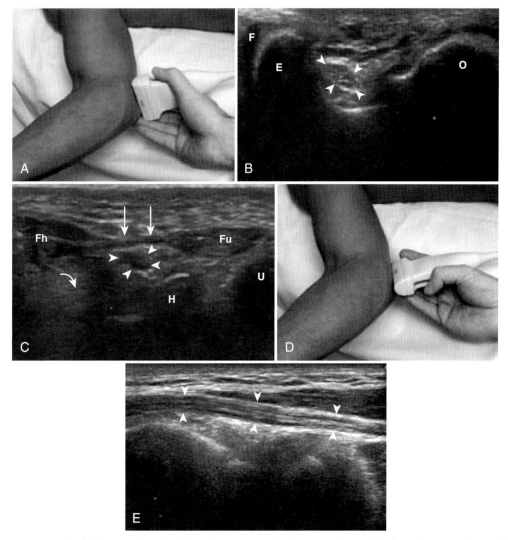

Fig. 156.20 **Ulnar nerve and cubital tunnel evaluation.** A, Transverse imaging over the medial elbow between the medial epicondyle and olecranon process (B) shows the ulnar nerve *(arrowheads)* posterior to the medial epicondyle (E). Note the common flexor tendon (F) and the olecranon process (O). C, Transverse imaging distal to B shows the ulnar nerve *(arrowheads)* in the cubital tunnel. *Arrows,* arcuate ligament; *curved arrow,* anterior band of ulnar collateral ligament; Fh, humeral head of flexor carpi ulnaris; Fu, ulnar head of flexor carpi ulnaris; H, humerus; U, ulna. D, longitudinal imaging shows (E) the ulnar nerve *(arrowheads)*. *(E From Jacobson JA: Musculoskeletal ultrasound, Philadelphia, 2007, Saunders, p. 109.)*

the radial nerve passes between the medial and long heads of the triceps muscle. As the nerve curves across the posterior aspect of the humerus, it supplies a motor branch to the triceps.[2] Continuing its downward path, it gives off numerous sensory branches to the upper arm. At a point between the lateral epicondyle of the humerus and the musculospiral groove, the radial nerve divides into its two terminal branches. The superficial branch continues down the arm along with the radial artery and provides sensory innervation to the dorsum of the wrist and the dorsal aspects of a portion of the thumb and index and middle fingers (**Fig. 156.24**). The deep branch provides most of the motor innervation to the extensors of the forearm. The major portion of the superficial branch passes between the flexor carpi radialis tendon and the radial artery. However, significant numbers of small branches ramify to provide sensory innervation of the dorsum of the hand. These small branches must also be blocked to provide complete blockade of the radial nerve.

Technique

The patient is placed in a supine position with the arm fully adducted at the patient's side and the elbow slightly flexed with the dorsum of the hand resting on a folded towel. A total of 7 to 8 mL of local anesthetic is drawn up in a 12-mL sterile syringe. When treating painful or inflammatory conditions that are mediated by the radial nerve, a total of 80 mg of depot steroid is added to the local anesthetic with the first block, and 40 mg of depot steroid is added with subsequent blocks.

The patient is instructed to flex his or her wrist to allow the pain specialist to identify the flexor carpi radialis tendon. The distal radial prominence is then identified. After preparation of the skin with antiseptic solution, a 25-gauge, 1½-inch needle is inserted in a perpendicular trajectory just lateral to the flexor carpi radialis tendon and just medial to the radial artery at the level of the distal radial prominence[17] (**Fig. 156.25**). The needle is slowly advanced. As the needle

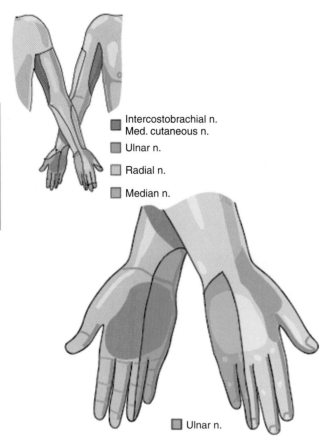

Intercostobrachial n.
Med. cutaneous n.

Ulnar n.

Radial n.

Median n.

Ulnar n.

Fig. 156.21 The dorsal branch provides sensation to the ulnar aspect of the dorsum of the hand and the dorsal aspect of the little finger and the ulnar half of the ring finger. *(From Waldman SD: Ulnar nerve block at the elbow. In* Atlas of interventional pain management, *ed 3, Philadelphia, 2009, Saunders, p 232.)*

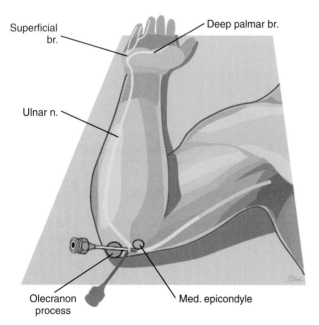

Superficial br.

Deep palmar br.

Ulnar n.

Olecranon process

Med. epicondyle

Fig. 156.22 After preparation of the skin with antiseptic solution, a 25-gauge, ⅝-inch needle is inserted just proximal to the sulcus and is slowly advanced in a slightly cephalad trajectory. *(From Waldman SD: Ulnar nerve block at the elbow. In* Atlas of interventional pain management, *ed 3, Philadelphia, 2009, Saunders, p 232.)*

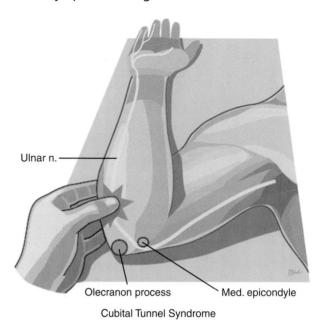

Ulnar n.

Olecranon process

Med. epicondyle

Cubital Tunnel Syndrome

Fig. 156.23 Cubital tunnel syndrome can be distinguished from golfer's elbow in that in cubital tunnel syndrome, the maximal tenderness to palpation is over the ulnar nerve 1 inch below the medial epicondyle, whereas with golfer's elbow, the maximal tenderness to palpation is directly over the medial epicondyle. *(From Waldman SD: Ulnar nerve block at the elbow. In* Atlas of interventional pain management, *ed 3, Philadelphia, 2009, Saunders, p 233.)*

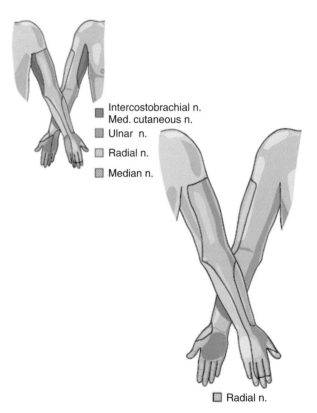

Intercostobrachial n.
Med. cutaneous n.

Ulnar n.

Radial n.

Median n.

Radial n.

Fig. 156.24 At a point between the lateral epicondyle of the humerus and the musculospiral groove, the radial nerve divides into its two terminal branches. The superficial branch continues down the arm along with the radial artery and provides sensory innervations to the dorsum of the wrist and the dorsal aspects of a portion of the thumb and index and middle fingers. *(From Waldman SD: Radial nerve block at the wrist. In* Atlas of interventional pain management, *ed 3, Philadelphia, 2009, Saunders, p 236.)*

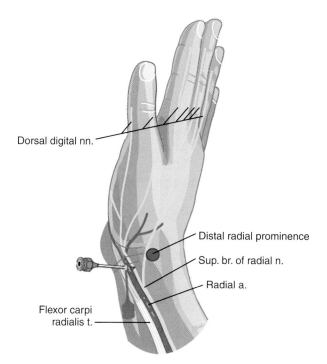

Fig. 156.25 After preparation of the skin with antiseptic solution, a 25-gauge, 1½-inch needle is inserted in a perpendicular trajectory just lateral to the flexor carpi radialis tendon and just medial to the radial artery at the level of the distal radial prominence. *(From Waldman SD: Radial nerve block at the wrist. In Atlas of interventional pain management, ed 3, Philadelphia, 2009, Saunders, p 236.)*

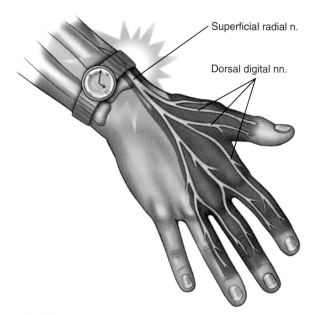

Fig. 156.26 Cheiralgia paresthetica manifests as pain, paresthesias, and numbness of the radial aspect of the dorsum of the hand to the base of the thumb. *(From Waldman SD: Atlas of uncommon pain syndromes, ed 2, Philadelphia, 2008, Saunders.)*

approaches the radius, strong paresthesia in the distribution of the radial nerve is elicited. The patient should be warned that paresthesia will occur and asked to say "there!" as soon as the paresthesia is felt. After paresthesia is elicited and its distribution is identified, gentle aspiration is carried out to identify blood. If the aspiration test result is negative and no persistent paresthesia into the distribution of the radial nerve remains, the clinician slowly injects 3 to 4 mL of solution and closely monitors the patient for signs of local anesthetic toxicity. The patient is then asked to pronate the arm, and an additional 3 to 4 mL of solution is injected in a subcutaneous bead, starting at the anatomic snuff box and carrying the injection subcutaneously to just past the midline of the dorsum of the wrist.

Side Effects and Complications

Radial nerve block at the wrist is a relatively safe block. The major complications are inadvertent intravascular injection and persistent paresthesia secondary to needle trauma to the nerve. This technique can safely be performed in the presence of anticoagulation by using a 25- or 27-gauge needle, albeit at increased risk of hematoma, if the clinical situation dictates a favorable risk-to-benefit ratio. These complications can be decreased if manual pressure is applied to the area of the block immediately after injection. Application of cold packs for 20-minute periods after the block also decreases the amount of postprocedure pain and bleeding the patient may experience.

Clinical Pearls

Radial nerve block at the wrist is a simple and safe technique. The major limitation of radial nerve block at the wrist is the difficulty of ensuring that all the nerve fibers blocked when injecting across the dorsum of the wrist in fact have their origin in the radial nerve. This difficulty limits the diagnostic and prognostic utility of this procedure. Careful neurologic examination to identify preexisting neurologic deficits, including cheiralgia paresthetica, that may later be attributed to the nerve block should be performed on all patients before radial nerve block at the wrist is begun[18] (**Fig. 156.26**).

Median Nerve Block at the Wrist

Indications

Median nerve block at the wrist is useful to supplement brachial plexus block when additional anesthesia is needed in the distribution of the distal median nerve.[19] In addition to applications for surgical anesthesia, median nerve block at the wrist with local anesthetic can be used as a diagnostic tool during differential neural blockade on an anatomic basis in the evaluation of upper extremity pain below the elbow. If destruction of the median nerve is being considered, median nerve block at the wrist is useful as a prognostic indicator of the degree of motor and sensory impairment that the patient may experience. Median nerve block at the wrist with local anesthetic may be used to palliate acute pain emergencies subserved by the median nerve while the patient waits for pharmacologic, surgical, and antiblastic methods to become effective. Median nerve block at the wrist with local anesthetic and steroid is also useful in the palliation of pain secondary to median nerve entrapment syndromes at the wrist, including carpal tunnel syndrome[19] (**Figs. 156.27** and **156.28**).

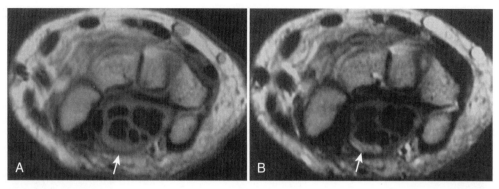

Fig. 156.27 Carpal tunnel syndrome. A, Axial protein density–weighted (2500/20) magnetic resonance image (MRI) shows the bowed flexor retinaculum *(arrow)* and flattened enlarged median nerve. **B,** Axial T2-weighted (2500/70) image shows that the median nerve is ovoid and has increased signal *(arrow)*. *(From Stark DD, Bradley WG:* Magnetic resonance imaging, *ed 3, St. Louis, 1999, Mosby, p 780.)*

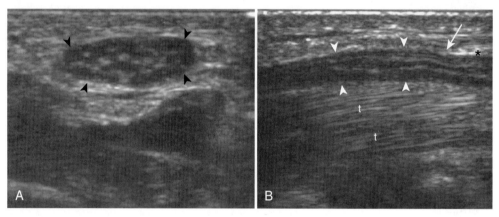

Fig. 156.28 Carpal tunnel syndrome. Ultrasound images transverse **(A)** and longitudinal **(B)** to the median nerve show hypoechoic swelling *(arrowheads)*. Note the mild deviation of the median nerve *(arrow)* as it courses beneath the flexor retinaculum *(asterisk)*. t, flexor tendons. *(From Jacobson JA:* Fundamentals of musculoskeletal ultrasound, *Philadelphia, 2007, Saunders, p 111.)*

Clinically Relevant Anatomy

The median nerve is made up of fibers from C5-T1 spinal roots. The nerve lies anterior and superior to the axillary artery in the 12:00-o'clock–to–3:00-o'clock quadrant. Exiting the axilla, the median nerve descends into the upper arm along with the brachial artery. At the level of the elbow, the brachial artery is just medial to the biceps muscle. At this level, the median nerve lies just medial to the brachial artery. As the median nerve proceeds downward into the forearm, it gives off numerous branches that provide motor innervation to the flexor muscles of the forearm. These branches are susceptible to nerve entrapment by aberrant ligaments, muscle hypertrophy, and direct trauma. The nerve approaches the wrist overlying the radius. The median nerve lies deep to and between the tendons of the palmaris longus muscle and the flexor carpi radialis muscle at the wrist[10] (**Fig. 156.29**). The median nerve then passes beneath the flexor retinaculum and through the carpal tunnel, with the nerve's terminal branches providing sensory innervation to a portion of the palmar surface of the hand, as well as the palmar surface of the thumb, index and middle fingers, and the radial portion of the ring finger[10,20] (**Fig. 156.30**). The median nerve also provides sensory innervation to the distal dorsal surface of the index and middle fingers and the radial portion of the ring finger.[10]

Technique

The patient is placed in a supine position with the arm fully adducted at the patient's side and the elbow slightly flexed with the dorsum of the hand resting on a folded towel. A total of 3 to 5 mL of local anesthetic is drawn up in a 12-mL sterile syringe. When treating painful or inflammatory conditions that are mediated by the median nerve, a total of 80 mg of depot steroid is added to the local anesthetic with the first block, and 40 mg of depot steroid is added with subsequent blocks.

The pain specialist then has the patient make a fist and at the same time flex his or her wrist to aid in identification of the palmaris longus tendon. After preparation of the skin with antiseptic solution, a 25-gauge, ⅝-inch needle is inserted just medial to the tendon and just proximal to the crease of the wrist[21] (**Fig. 156.31**). The needle is slowly advanced in a slightly cephalad trajectory. As the needle advances beyond the tendon at a depth of approximately ½ inch, strong paresthesia in the distribution of the median nerve will be elicited. The patient should be warned that paresthesia will occur and asked to say "There!" as soon as the paresthesia is felt. After paresthesia is elicited and its distribution is identified, gentle aspiration is carried out to identify blood. If the aspiration test result is negative

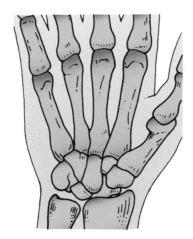

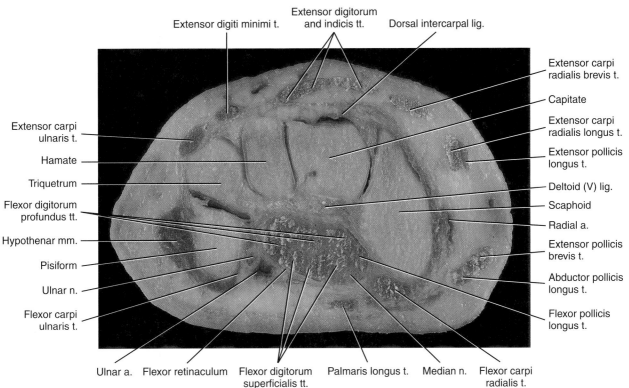

Fig. 156.29 The median nerve lies deep to and between the tendons of the palmaris longus muscle and the flexor carpi radialis muscle at the wrist. *(From Kang HS, Ahn JM, Resnick D:* MRI of the extremities: an anatomic atlas, *ed 2, Philadelphia, 2002, Saunders, p 177.)*

and no persistent paresthesia into the distribution of the median nerve remains, the clinician slowly injects 3 to 5 mL of solution and closely monitors of the patient for signs of local anesthetic toxicity. If no paresthesia is elicited and the needle tip hits bone, the needle is withdrawn out of the periosteum, and after careful aspiration, 3 to 5 mL of solution is slowly injected.

Side Effects and Complications

Median nerve block at the wrist is a relatively safe block. The major complications are inadvertent intravascular injection and persistent paresthesia secondary to needle trauma to the nerve. This technique can safely be performed in the presence of anticoagulation by using a 25- or 27-gauge needle,

albeit at increased risk of hematoma, if the clinical situation dictates a favorable risk-to-benefit ratio. These complications can be decreased if manual pressure is applied to the area of the block immediately after injection. Application of cold packs for 20-minute periods after the block also decreases the amount of postprocedure pain and bleeding the patient may experience.

Clinical Pearls

Median nerve block at the wrist is a simple and safe technique in the evaluation and treatment of the previously mentioned painful conditions. Careful neurologic examination to identify preexisting neurologic deficits that may later be attributed to the nerve block should be performed on all patients before

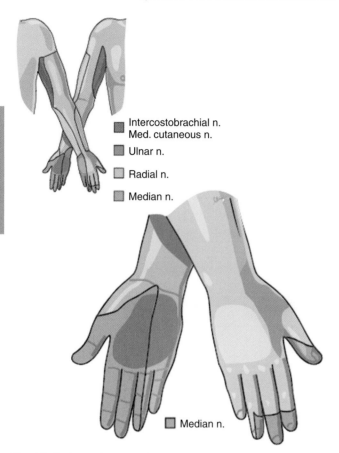

Intercostobrachial n.
Med. cutaneous n.

Ulnar n.

Radial n.

Median n.

Median n.

Fig. 156.30 The median nerve then passes beneath the flexor retinaculum and through the carpal tunnel, with the nerve's terminal branches providing sensory innervations to a portion of the palmar surface of the hand as well as the palmar surface of the thumb, the index and middle fingers, and the radial portion of the ring finger. *(From Waldman SD: Median nerve block at the wrist. In Atlas of interventional pain management, ed 3, Philadelphia, 2009, Saunders, p 241.)*

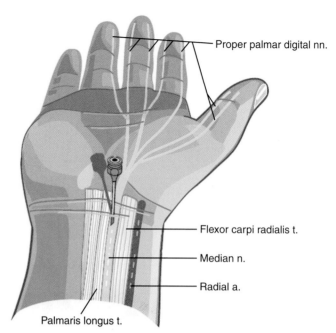

Proper palmar digital nn.

Flexor carpi radialis t.

Median n.

Radial a.

Palmaris longus t.

Fig. 156.31 After preparation of the skin with antiseptic solution, a 25-gauge, ⅝-inch needle is inserted just medial to the tendon and just proximal to the crease of the wrist. *(From Waldman SD: Median nerve block at the wrist. In Atlas of interventional pain management, ed 3, Philadelphia, 2009, Saunders, p 242.)*

median nerve block at the wrist is begun, especially in those patients with clinical symptoms to suggest carpal tunnel syndrome.[22]

This technique is useful in the treatment of pain secondary to median nerve compression syndromes at the wrist, including carpal tunnel syndrome. Care should be taken to place the needle proximal to the flexor retinaculum and to inject slowly to allow the solution to flow easily into the carpal tunnel without further compromising the median nerve. Carpal tunnel syndrome should also be differentiated from cervical radiculopathy involving the cervical nerve roots, which may at times mimic median nerve compression. Furthermore, cervical radiculopathy and median nerve entrapment may coexist in the double-crush syndrome. The double-crush syndrome occurs most commonly with median nerve entrapment at the wrist or carpal tunnel syndrome.[22]

Ulnar Nerve Block at the Wrist

Indications

Ulnar nerve block at the wrist is useful in supplementing brachial plexus block when additional anesthesia is needed in the distribution of the ulnar nerve. In addition

to applications for surgical anesthesia, ulnar nerve block at the wrist with local anesthetic can be used as a diagnostic tool during differential neural blockade on an anatomic basis in the evaluation of upper extremity pain below the elbow.[23] If destruction of the ulnar nerve is being considered, ulnar nerve block at the wrist is useful as a prognostic indicator of the degree of motor and sensory impairment that the patient may experience. Ulnar nerve block at the wrist with local anesthetic may be used to palliate acute pain emergencies subserved by the ulnar nerve while the patient waits for pharmacologic, surgical, and antiblastic methods to become effective. Ulnar nerve block at the wrist with local anesthetic and steroid is also useful in the palliation of pain secondary to ulnar nerve entrapment syndromes at the wrist, including ulnar tunnel syndrome.

Clinically Relevant Anatomy

The ulnar nerve is made up of fibers from C6-T1 spinal roots. The nerve lies anterior and inferior to the axillary artery in the 3:00-o'clock to 6:00-o'clock quadrant. Exiting the axilla, the ulnar nerve descends into the upper arm along with the brachial artery. At the middle of the upper arm, the nerve courses medially to pass between the olecranon process and medial epicondyle of the humerus.[24] The nerve then passes between the heads of the flexor carpi ulnaris muscle and continues downward, moving radially along with the ulnar artery (**Figs. 156.32** and **156.33** and **Fig. 156.34** [**online only**]). At a point approximately 1 inch proximal to the crease of the wrist, the ulnar divides into the dorsal and palmar branches. The dorsal branch provides sensation to the ulnar aspect of the dorsum of the hand and the dorsal aspect of the little finger and the ulnar half of the ring finger (**Fig. 156.35**). The palmar branch provides

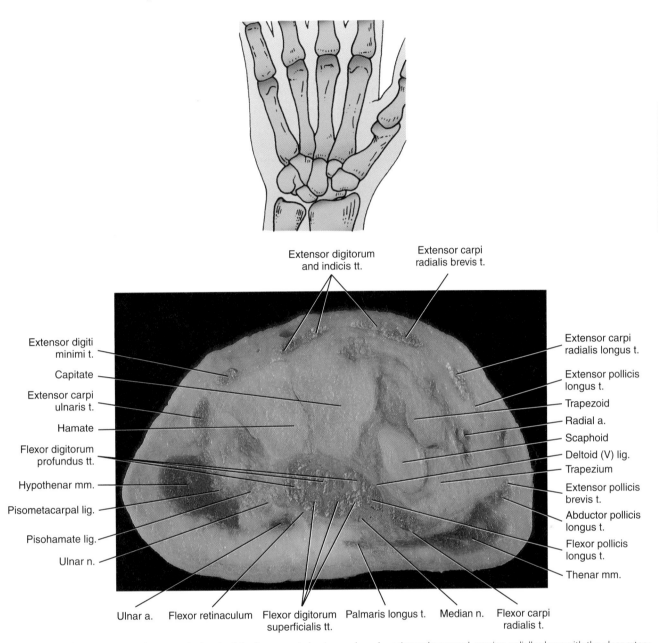

Extensor digitorum
and indicis tt.

Extensor carpi
radialis brevis t.

Extensor digiti
minimi t.

Capitate

Extensor carpi
ulnaris t.

Hamate

Flexor digitorum
profundus tt.

Hypothenar mm.

Pisometacarpal lig.

Pisohamate lig.

Ulnar n.

Extensor carpi
radialis longus t.

Extensor pollicis
longus t.

Trapezoid

Radial a.

Scaphoid

Deltoid (V) lig.

Trapezium

Extensor pollicis
brevis t.

Abductor pollicis
longus t.

Flexor pollicis
longus t.

Thenar mm.

Ulnar a.   Flexor retinaculum   Flexor digitorum   Palmaris longus t.   Median n.   Flexor carpi
                                superficialis tt.   radialis t.

Fig. 156.32 The ulnar nerve passes between the heads of the flexor carpi ulnaris muscle and continues downward, moving radially along with the ulnar artery. *(From Kang HS, Ahn JM, Resnick D: MRI of the extremities: an anatomic atlas, ed 2, Philadelphia, 2002, Saunders, p 178.)*

sensory innervation to the ulnar aspect of the palm of the hand and the palmar aspect of the little finger and the ulnar half of the ring finger.

Technique

The patient is placed in a supine position with the arm fully adducted at the patient's side and the wrist slightly flexed with the dorsum of the hand resting on a folded towel. A total of 5 to 7 mL of local anesthetic is drawn up in a 12-mL sterile syringe. When treating painful or inflammatory conditions that are mediated by the ulnar nerve, a total of 80 mg of depot steroid is added to the local anesthetic with the first block, and 40 mg of depot steroid is added with subsequent blocks.

The pain specialist then has the patient make a fist and at the same time flex his or her wrist to aid in identification of the flexor carpi ulnaris tendon. After preparation of the skin with antiseptic solution, a 25-gauge, ⅝-inch needle is inserted on the radial side of the tendon at the level of the styloid process[25] (**Fig. 156.36**). The needle is slowly advanced in a slightly cephalad trajectory. As the needle advances approximately ½ inch, strong paresthesia in the distribution of the ulnar nerve is elicited. The patient should be warned that paresthesia will occur and asked to say "There!" as soon as the paresthesia is felt. After paresthesia is elicited and its distribution is identified, gentle aspiration is carried out to identify blood. If the aspiration test result is negative and no persistent paresthesia into the distribution of the ulnar nerve

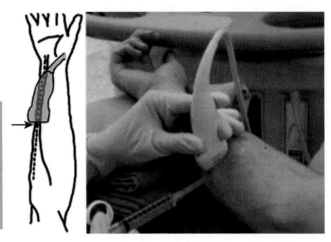

Fig. 156.33 Schematic diagram *(left)* and photograph *(right)* of the position of the transducer and the point of needle entry for ulnar nerve block in the forearm. The schematic diagram shows the approximate position of the ulnar nerve *(dashed line)*, ulnar artery *(solid line)*, ultrasound probe *(gray)*, and point of needle insertion *(arrow)*. In the photograph, the arm is supinated with the operator facing the monitoring screen on the opposite side of the armboard. For illustrative purposes, the probe is not covered, the arm is not prepared with antiseptic solution, and the needle is capped. *(From Gray AT, Schafhalter-Zoppoth I: Ultrasound guidance for ulnar nerve block in the forearm,* Reg Anesth Pain Med 28:335, 2003.)

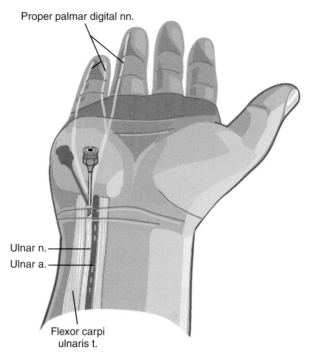

Fig. 156.36 After preparation of the skin with antiseptic solution, a 25-gauge, ⅝-inch needle is inserted on the radial side of the tendon at the level of the styloid process. *(From Waldman SD: Ulnar nerve block at the wrist. In* Atlas of interventional pain management, *ed 3, Philadelphia, 2009, Saunders, p 246.)*

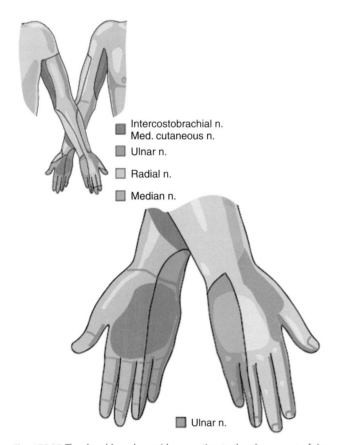

Fig. 156.35 The dorsal branch provides sensation to the ulnar aspect of the dorsum of the hand and the dorsal aspect of the little finger and the ulnar half of the ring finger. *(From Waldman SD: Ulnar nerve block at the wrist. In* Atlas of interventional pain management, *ed 3, Philadelphia, 2009, Saunders, p 245.)*

remains, the clinician slowly injects 3 to 5 mL of solution and closely monitors the patient for signs of local anesthetic toxicity. If no paresthesia can be elicited, a similar amount of solution is slowly injected in a fanlike manner just proximal to the notch, with care taken to avoid intravascular injection.

To ensure complete block of the dorsal branch of the ulnar nerve, it may be necessary to inject a bead of local anesthetic subcutaneously around the ulnar aspect of the wrist, starting from the flexor carpi ulnaris tendon to the midline of the dorsum of the hand.

Side Effects and Complications

Ulnar nerve block at the wrist is a relatively safe block. The major complications are inadvertent intravascular injection into the ulnar artery and persistent paresthesia secondary to needle trauma to the nerve. Because, like the carpal tunnel, Guyon's canal is a closed space, care should be taken to inject slowly to avoid additional compromise of the nerve. This technique can safely be performed in the presence of anticoagulation by using a 25- or 27-gauge needle, albeit at increased risk of hematoma, if the clinical situation dictates a favorable risk-to-benefit ratio. These complications can be decreased if manual pressure is applied to the area of the block immediately after injection. Application of cold packs for 20-minute periods after the block also decreases the amount of postprocedure pain and bleeding the patient may experience.

Clinical Pearls

Ulnar nerve block at the wrist is a simple and safe technique in the evaluation and treatment of the previously mentioned painful conditions. Careful neurologic examination to identify preexisting neurologic deficits that may later be attributed to the nerve block should be performed on all patients before ulnar nerve block at the wrist is begun.

Ulnar nerve block at the wrist is especially useful in the treatment of pain secondary to ulnar nerve compression syndromes at the wrist, including ulnar tunnel syndrome. Ulnar tunnel syndrome often occurs after compression of the palmar branch of the ulnar nerve proximal to Guyon's canal[26] (**Figs. 156.37** and **Fig. 156.38**). This disorder often manifests clinically after a long bicycle ride or after repeated use of pliers. The maximal tenderness to palpation is over the ulnar nerve just proximal to Guyon's canal. Injection of the ulnar nerve at the wrist with local anesthetic and steroid gives almost instantaneous relief.

Ulnar tunnel syndrome should be differentiated from cervical radiculopathy involving the C8 spinal root, which may at times mimic ulnar nerve compression. Furthermore, cervical radiculopathy and ulnar nerve entrapment may coexist in the double crush syndrome. The double crush syndrome occurs most commonly with ulnar nerve entrapment at the wrist or carpal tunnel syndrome. Pancoast's tumor invading the medial cord of the brachial plexus may also mimic an isolated ulnar nerve entrapment and should be ruled out by an apical lordotic chest radiograph.

Metacarpal and Digital Nerve Block

Indications

Metacarpal nerve block and digital nerve block are used primarily in two clinical situations: (1) to provide surgical anesthesia in the distribution of the digital nerves for laceration, tendon, and fracture repair; and (2) to provide postoperative pain relief after joint replacement or major surgical procedures on the hand.[27]

Clinically Relevant Anatomy

The common digital nerves arise from fibers of the median and ulnar nerves. The thumb also has contributions from superficial branches of the radial nerve. The common digital nerves pass along the metacarpal bones and divide as they reach the distal palm.[28] The volar digital nerves supply most of the sensory innervation to the fingers and run along the ventrolateral aspect of the finger beside the digital vein and artery. The smaller dorsal digital nerves contain fibers from the ulnar and radial nerves and supply the dorsum of the fingers as far as the proximal joints.

Technique

The patient is placed in a supine position with the arm fully abducted and the elbow slightly flexed with the palm of the hand resting on a folded towel. A total of 3 mL per digit of non–epinephrine-containing local anesthetic is drawn up in a 12-mL sterile syringe.

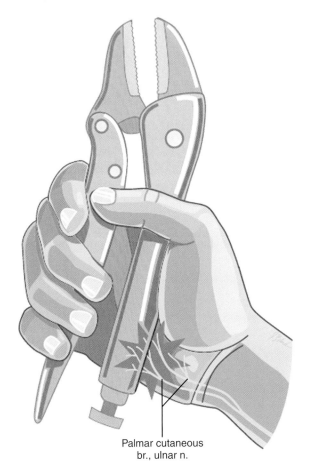

Palmar cutaneous
br., ulnar n.

Ulnar Tunnel Syndrome

Fig. 156.37 Ulnar tunnel syndrome often occurs after compression of the palmar branch of the ulnar nerve proximal to Guyon's canal. *(From Waldman SD: Ulnar nerve block at the wrist. In Atlas of interventional pain management, ed 3, Philadelphia, 2009, Saunders, p 246.)*

Metacarpal Nerve Block

After preparation of the skin with antiseptic solution, at a point proximal to the metacarpal head, a 25-gauge, 1½-inch needle is inserted on each side of the metacarpal bone to be blocked (**Fig. 156.39**). While the anesthetic is slowly injected, the needle is advanced from the dorsal surface of the hand toward the palmar surface. The common digital nerve is situated on the dorsal side of the flexor retinaculum, and thus the needle must be advanced almost to the palmar surface of the hand to obtain satisfactory anesthesia.[28] The needle is removed, and pressure is placed on the injection site to avoid hematoma formation.

Digital Nerve Block

The patient is placed in a supine position with the arm fully abducted and the elbow slightly flexed with the palm of the hand resting on a folded towel. After preparation of the skin with antiseptic solution, at a point at the base of the finger, a 25-gauge, 1½-inch needle is inserted on each side of the bone of the digit to be blocked (**Fig. 156.40**). While the anesthetic is slowly injected, the needle is advanced from the dorsal surface

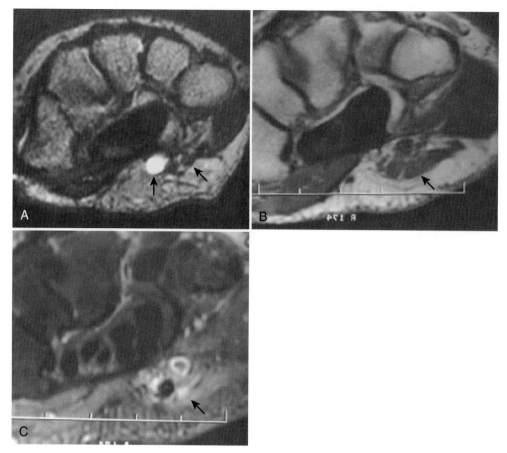

Fig. 156.38 Entrapment of the ulnar nerve: Guyon's canal syndrome (ulnar tunnel syndrome). A, Ganglion cyst. A transverse T2-weighted (TR/TE, 2000/80) spin-echo magnetic resonance image (MRI) shows a ganglion cyst (arrow) adjacent to the ulnar nerve and vessels (arrowhead). B and C, Anomalous muscle. This accessory muscle (i.e., accessory abductor digiti minimi muscle) (arrows) is well shown in transverse T1-weighted (TR/TE, 550/12) spin-echo (B) and fat-suppressed fast spin-echo (TR/TE, 3000/11); (C) MRI. Note the abnormal high signal intensity in the muscle and subjacent Guyon's canal in C. (Courtesy of D. Fanney, MD, Virginia Beach, Va; from Resnick D: Diagnosis of bone and joint disorders, ed 4, Philadelphia, 2002, Saunders, p 3527.)

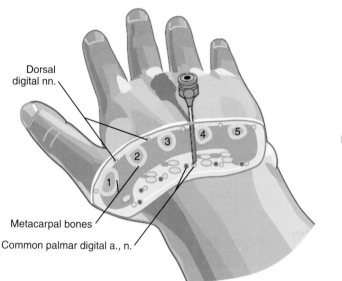

Fig. 156.39 After preparation of the skin with antiseptic solution, at a point proximal to the metacarpal head, a 25-gauge, 1½-inch needle is inserted on each side of the metacarpal bone to be blocked. (From Waldman SD: Metacarpal and digital nerve block. In Atlas of interventional pain management, ed 3, Philadelphia, 2009, Saunders, p 249.)

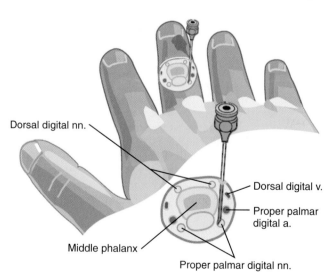

Fig. 156.40 After preparation of the skin with antiseptic solution, at a point at the base of the finger, a 25-gauge, 1½-inch needle is inserted on each side of the bone of the digit to be blocked. (From Waldman SD: Metacarpal and digital nerve block. In Atlas of interventional pain management, ed 3, Philadelphia, 2009, Saunders, p 249.)

of the hand toward the palmar surface. The same technique can be used to block the thumb.[27] The needle is removed, and pressure is placed on the injection site to avoid hematoma formation.

Side Effects and Complications

Because of the confined nature of the soft tissue surrounding the metacarpals and digits, the potential for mechanical compression of the blood supply after injection of solution must be considered. The pain specialist must avoid rapidly injecting large volumes of solution into these confined spaces, or vascular insufficiency and gangrene may occur. Furthermore, epinephrine-containing solutions should never be used, to avoid ischemia and possible gangrene.

This technique can safely be performed in the presence of anticoagulation by using a 25- or 27-gauge needle, albeit at increased risk of hematoma, if the clinical situation dictates a favorable risk-to-benefit ratio. These complications can be decreased if manual pressure is applied to the area of the block immediately after injection. Application of cold packs for 10-minute periods after the block also decreases the amount of postprocedure pain and bleeding the patient may experience.

Clinical Pearls

Digital nerve block is especially useful in the palliation of postoperative pain after total joint replacement in the hands. When digital nerve block is used for pain secondary to trauma, the pain specialist must ascertain and document the status of the vascular supply before the procedure, to avoid the erroneous attribution of subsequent vascular insufficiency to the digital nerve block, rather than to preexisting trauma to the vasculature.

References

Full references for this chapter can be found on www.expertconsult.com.

Suprascapular Nerve Block

P. Prithvi Raj

Historical Considerations

Historically, suprascapular nerve block was used as a primary treatment for conditions that limited the range of motion of the shoulder, including adhesive capsulitis and calcific tendinitis and bursitis.[1] The advent of corticosteroids allowed earlier treatment of these maladies. Subsequently, the use of suprascapular nerve block as a primary treatment modality for shoulder lesions declined. Interest in suprascapular nerve block has been renewed, however, because it allows early range of motion and rehabilitation after shoulder reconstruction or joint replacement.

Indications and Contraindications

Suprascapular nerve block with local anesthetics can be used as a diagnostic tool when performing differential neural blockade on an anatomic basis to evaluate shoulder girdle and shoulder joint pain.[2] If destruction of the suprascapular nerve is being considered, this technique is useful as a prognostic indicator of the degree of motor and sensory impairment that the patient may experience.[3] Suprascapular nerve block with local anesthetic may be used to palliate acute pain emergencies, including postoperative pain, pain secondary to trauma to the shoulder joint and girdle, and cancer pain while the patient waits for pharmacologic, surgical, or antiblastic treatment to become effective.[3] Suprascapular nerve block is also useful as adjunctive therapy for decreased range of motion of the shoulder secondary to reflex sympathetic dystrophy or adhesive capsulitis,[1,3] and it can be effective in allowing the patient to tolerate more aggressive physical therapy after shoulder reconstructive surgery.[3]

Destruction of the suprascapular nerve is indicated for palliation of cancer pain, including pain related to invasive tumors of the shoulder girdle.[3] This nerve block can be performed in patients who are taking anticoagulants, if the clinical situation dictates a favorable risk-to-benefit ratio. The procedure is contraindicated in patients with local infection, anatomic anomaly, or coagulopathies.

Equipment and Drugs

The following equipment is required for this procedure: a 3- or 5-mL syringe for local infiltration; a 5- or 10-mL syringe for local anesthetics and steroids; a 25-gauge needle for local infiltration; a 22-gauge spinal needle or a 22-gauge, 13-beveled needle for nerve block; and a 10-cm curved, blunt radiofrequency needle with a 10-mm active tip for pulsed radiofrequency.

For the block using local anesthetic, the drug preparations include the following: lidocaine 1% to 2%; bupivacaine 0.25% to 0.5%; ropivacaine 0.2% to 0.5%; and depot steroids, 40 to 80 mg. For the neurolytic block, the solution used is phenol 6%.

Ultrasound Equipment

A high-resolution ultrasound system is required to visualize the suprascapular notch and nerve. The ideal ultrasound transducer should have high-resolution capabilities between 10 and 15 MHz.[4]

Preparation and Positioning of the Patient

Physical examination should include (1) palpation of the area for needle entry and (2) examination of the shoulder motion and documentation of the range of motion for evaluating success of the block. The patient is placed in the prone position with the arms at the side. A total of 10 mL of local anesthetic is drawn up in a 10-mL sterile syringe. For treating painful conditions that are mediated by the suprascapular nerve, a total of 80 mg of depot steroid is added to the local anesthetic with the first block, and 40 mg of depot steroid is added with subsequent blocks. Medication protocol should be consistent with the American Society of Anesthesiologists conscious sedation guidelines.

Clinically Relevant Anatomy

The suprascapular nerve is formed from fibers originating from the C5 and C6 nerve roots of the brachial plexus and, in most patients, some fibers from the C4 root. The nerve passes inferiorly and posteriorly from the brachial plexus to pass underneath the coracoclavicular ligament through the suprascapular notch.[5] The suprascapular artery and vein accompany the nerve through the notch. The suprascapular nerve provides much of the sensory innervation to the shoulder joint and innervation to two of the muscles of the rotator cuff, the supraspinatus and the infraspinatus (**Fig. 157.1**).

Technique for Suprascapular Nerve Block

Blind Technique

The operator identifies the spine of the scapula and then draws a line vertically through the midpoint of the spine and parallel to the vertebral column. The upper outer quadrant so formed is bisected, and a needle is inserted at a distance of 2 cm along this line. The needle is inserted at a right angle to the skin and is advanced until the dorsal surface of the scapula is located. The needle is then "walked" along this dorsal surface until the suprascapular notch is identified. If a nerve stimulator is used, contractions of the supraspinatus and infraspinatus muscles will confirm placement. At this location, the operator injects 5 mL of local anesthetic. It is not always possible to ascertain any dermal analgesia as a result of this block. The success of block can be determined when motor-blocking concentrations of drug are used; in this situation, abduction of the arm is compromised for the first 15 degrees, before the deltoid muscle takes over (**Fig. 157.2**).

Radiographic Technique

The spine of the scapula is identified, and the pain specialist then palpates along the length of the scapular spine laterally to identify the acromion (**Figs. 157.3** and **157.4**). At the point where the thicker acromion fuses with the thinner scapular spine, the skin is prepared with antiseptic solution. At this point, the skin and subcutaneous tissues are anesthetized using a 1½-inch infiltration needle. After adequate anesthesia is obtained, a 3½-inch, 25-gauge needle or a radiofrequency needle with a previously inserted catheter is inserted with an inferior trajectory toward the body of the scapula (**Fig. 157.5**). The needle should make contact with the body of the scapula at a depth of approximately 1 inch. The needle is then gently walked superiorly and medially until the tip walks off

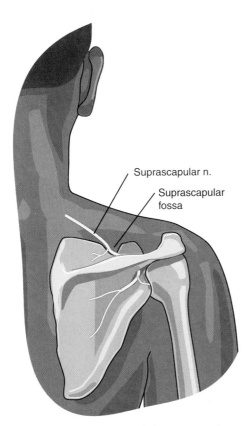

Fig. 157.1 Drawing of the anatomy of the suprascapular nerve. *(From Raj PP, Lou L, Erdine S, et al: Radiographic imaging for regional anesthesia and pain management, Philadelphia, 2003, Churchill Livingstone, p 128.)*

Suprascapular n.

Suprascapular fossa

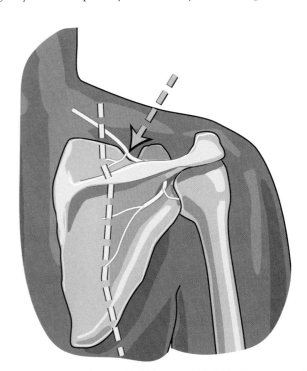

Fig. 157.2 Suprascapular nerve block. The nerve is blocked in the suprascapular fossa. The spine of the scapula is divided by a vertical line. The upper outer quadrant so formed is bisected, and a needle is introduced 2 cm along this line and is advanced to a depth of approximately 5 to 6 cm, at which point the dorsal surface of the scapula should be located. If this end point is not reached at this depth, the needle should be withdrawn and repositioned. When osseous contact is achieved, the needle is "walked" until the suprascapular notch is located, or, if an electrical stimulator is used, needle placement is confirmed by movements of the suprascapular and infrascapular muscles. At this point, the operator injects 5 mL of local anesthetic.

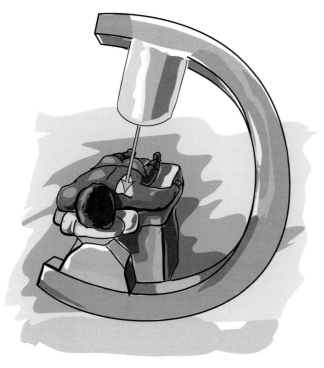

Fig. 157.3 Drawing of the patient in the prone position with the fluoroscope slightly lateral to midline at the T2-3 level with a slight cephalocaudad tilt. *(From Raj PP, Lou L, Erdine S, et al: Radiographic imaging for regional anesthesia and pain management, Philadelphia, 2003, Churchill Livingstone, p 129.)*

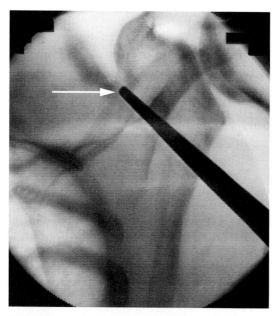

Fig. 157.4 Radiographic image of the suprascapular notch *(arrow)* emphasized by the oblique angulation of the fluoroscope. *(From Raj PP, Lou L, Erdine S, et al: Radiographic imaging for regional anesthesia and pain management, Philadelphia, 2003, Churchill Livingstone, p 130.)*

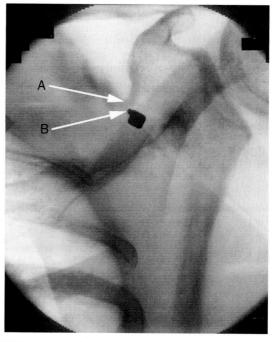

Fig. 157.5 Suprascapular nerve block with needle in place contacting bone just below the suprascapular nerve. *A,* Suprascapular notch. *B,* Curved blunt needle tip at the notch. *(From Raj PP, Lou L, Erdine S, et al: Radiographic imaging for regional anesthesia and pain management, Philadelphia, 2003, Churchill Livingstone, p 130.)*

the scapular body into the suprascapular notch. If the notch is not identified, the same maneuver is repeated, with the needle directed superiorly and laterally until the needle tip is positioned in the suprascapular notch. Paresthesia is often encountered as the needle tip enters the notch, and the patient should be warned. If paresthesia is not elicited after the needle

has entered the suprascapular notch, the needle is advanced an additional ½ inch, to place the tip beyond the substance of the coracoclavicular ligament. To avoid pneumothorax, the needle should never be advanced more deeply.

After paresthesia is elicited or the needle has been advanced into the notch as described, gentle aspiration is carried out to identify blood or air. If the aspiration test result is negative, the operator slowly injects 10 mL of solution, and the patient is monitored closely for signs of local anesthetic toxicity (**Fig. 157.6**).

Ultrasound Technique

The ultrasound technique was described by Harmon and Hearty.[4] In this report, the patient was placed in a sitting position with the right hand resting on the contralateral shoulder. The operator was positioned behind the patient with the ultrasound machine on the right side in front of the patient. This placement allowed an uninterrupted field of view of the ultrasound screen. The skin was cleaned with chlorhexidine solution. The ultrasound transducer (high-frequency linear, 6- to 13-MHz, 38-mm broadband linear-array transducer; SonoSite Micromaxx, Bothell, Wash) was inserted into a sterile sheath (CIVCO Medical Instruments, Kalona, Iowa) containing ultrasound gel. A thin layer of sterile gel was placed between the draped ultrasound transducer and the skin.

An initial scan was performed in the sagittal orientation at the superior medial border of the scapula to identify the pleura (4 cm depth). Scanning proceeded laterally with this transducer orientation. The operator noted where the scapula moved beyond the lung field. The ultrasound transducer was then placed parallel to the scapular spine (**Fig. 157.7**), to visualize that structure. By moving the transducer cephalad, the suprascapular fossa was identified. While imaging the

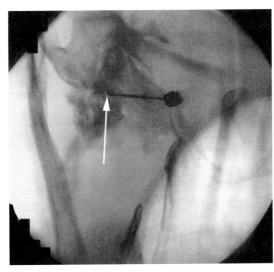

Fig. 157.6 Suprascapular nerve block with contrast medium filling the suprascapular fossa (arrow). *(From Raj PP, Lou L, Erdine S, et al:* Radiographic imaging for regional anesthesia and pain management, *Philadelphia, 2003, Churchill Livingstone, p 130.)*

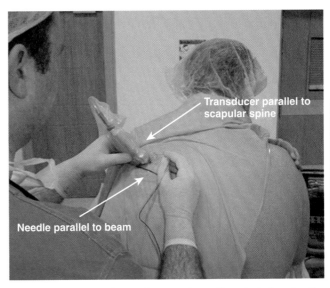

Fig. 157.7 Ultrasound transducer and needle orientation for the ultrasound-guided suprascapular block. *(From Harmon D, Hearty C: Ultrasonography in pain medicine: a critical review,* Pain Practice 8:226, 2008.)

supraspinatus muscle and the bony fossa underneath, the ultrasound transducer was slowly moved laterally (to maintain a transverse transducer orientation) to locate the suprascapular notch (see Fig. 157.2). The suprascapular nerve was seen as a round, hyperechoic structure 4 cm beneath the transverse scapular ligament in the scapular notch (**Fig. 157.8**). The nerve had an approximate diameter of 200 mm. Lung tissue in this scanning field was not seen. A 21-gauge, 50-mm B-bevel needle (Stimuplex, B. Braun, Bethlehem, Pa) was inserted along the longitudinal axis of the ultrasound beam. This needle was chosen for its good ultrasound visibility. The needle was visualized in its full course (see Fig. 157.3). The end point for injection was an ultrasound image demonstrating the needle tip in proximity to the suprascapular nerve in the suprascapular notch (**Fig. 157.9**). Electrical stimulation was not used to identify the nerve. A mixture of levobupivacaine 0.5% (4 mL) and triamcinolone (80 mg) was injected. The injection and spread of local anesthetic were visualized. The patient's pain intensity decreased to 2 out of 10 on the numeric rating scale. Shoulder movement and function improved. Sleep improved. These improvements were maintained at 12 weeks.

Technique of Neurolytic Block

After the needle is placed appropriately as described, the operator injects 3 to 4 mL of iohexol (Omnipaque). An anteroposterior radiographic image is taken. The contrast solution should fill the suprascapular notch and run toward the glenoid cavity. After the correct spread of the contrast medium is verified, a 3- to 5-mL dose of local anesthetic is injected. If no side effects occur, then a 3- to 5-mL dose of 6% phenol is injected.

Pulsed Radiofrequency of the Suprascapular Nerve

The landmarks and position are the same as described earlier. The needle chosen is a 10-cm blunt curved Racz-Finch Kit (RFK) needle with a 16-gauge introducer catheter. After the fluoroscopic view

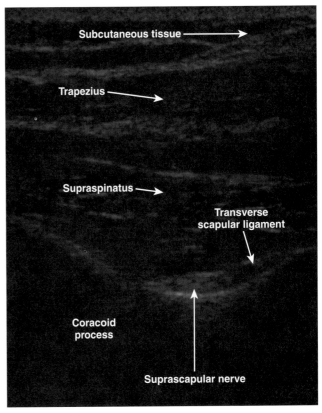

Fig. 157.8 Transverse view of suprascapular fossa and scapular notch with a SonoSite ultrasound system (Micromaxx, Bothell, Wash) and a 6- to 13-MHz linear-array transducer. *(From Harmon D, Hearty C: Ultrasonography in pain medicine: a critical review,* Pain Practice 8:226, 2008.)

of the suprascapular notch is obtained, the catheter is inserted. This insertion is performed with a "tunnel view." Following catheter insertion, the RFK needle is introduced until it reaches the suprascapular notch. Contrast solution is then injected to confirm the position of the needle on the suprascapular nerve.

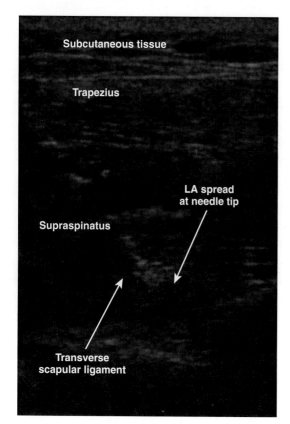

Fig. 157.9 Real-time imaging of needle insertion for the ultrasound-guided suprascapular block. Local anesthetic and steroid are injected deep to the scapular ligament. *(From Harmon D, Hearty C: Ultrasonography in pain medicine: a critical review, Pain Practice 8:226, 2008.)*

Ideally, the result of sensory stimulation at 50 Hz is positive at 0.3 to 0.6 volts to confirm proximity to the suprascapular nerve. Motor stimulation should not be more than twice the sensory stimulation voltage and at 2 Hz. Once proper placement is confirmed, the pulsating electromagnetic flow meter lesion is created at 42°C (108°F) for 120 seconds for two cycles. The needle is then removed. No local anesthetic is injected.

Complications

The proximity of the suprascapular nerve to the suprascapular artery and vein suggests the potential for inadvertent intravascular injection or local anesthetic toxicity from intravascular absorption. The pain specialist should carefully calculate the total (milligram) dose of local anesthetic that may safely be given for suprascapular nerve block. Because of the proximity of the lung, if the needle is advanced too deeply through the suprascapular notch, pneumothorax is a possibility.

Potential complications of suprascapular nerve block may be avoided through the use of ultrasound guidance. Pneumothorax has been reported following suprascapular block.[6] Pneumothorax of all origins is a significant cause of litigation in chronic pain practice, and it accounting for 4% of all claims.[7] The incidence of pneumothorax associated with suprascapular block is reported to be less than 1%.[6] Investigators have postulated that avoiding the suprascapular notch in the vertical plane will decrease this risk.[8] The pleura lies anterior to the scapula. By using a sagittal transducer orientation, the pleura can be identified deep to the superior border of the scapula at its medial aspect. By maintaining the transducer orientation, the superior border of the scapula can be traced laterally to the scapular notch.

Clinical Pearls

Suprascapular nerve block is a safe and simple regional anesthesia technique that has many pain management applications. It is probably underused as an adjunct to rehabilitation after shoulder reconstruction and for the shoulder-hand variant of reflex sympathetic dystrophy. The pain specialist must ensure that the physical and occupational therapists caring for the patient understand that suprascapular nerve block renders not only the shoulder girdle but also the shoulder joint insensate. This means that deep heat modalities and range-of-motion exercises must be carefully monitored, to avoid burns and damage to the shoulder.

Efficacy

Fluoroscopy and nerve stimulation,[9] in addition to computed tomography (CT) guidance,[10] have been described for suprascapular nerve blocks. Unlike fluoroscopy and CT, ultrasound does not expose patients and personnel to radiation. Ultrasound is also less expensive and more readily available than CT and fluoroscopy.[11]

Acknowledgment

Portions of this chapter have been excerpted from Raj PP, Lou L, Erdine S, et al: *Radiographic imaging for regional anesthesia and pain management*, Philadelphia, 2003, Churchill Livingstone, 2003.

References

Full references for this chapter can be found on www.expertconsult.com.

Thoracic Epidural Nerve Block

Somayaji Ramamurthy and Maxim Savillion Eckmann

The technique of thoracic epidural nerve block is used with increasing frequency in the practice of pain management. The presence of the spinal cord at the thoracic levels demands that the clinician have significant technical proficiency in performing epidural techniques without complications. A thorough knowledge of anatomic and physiologic changes associated with a thoracic epidural block is essential to avoiding complications. This chapter outlines the anatomy, physiologic changes, indications, applications, and complications of thoracic epidural nerve block.

Historical Considerations

The development of thoracic epidural techniques followed that of lumbar epidural techniques. Modification of the Tuohy needle with the Huber tip to facilitate insertion of the catheter further increased the utility and safety of this anesthetic technique, as did improvements in catheter material and the development of disposable, prepackaged sterile equipment. Advances in epidurally administered drugs, such as the opioids, and the ability to implant catheters for the management of cancer pain further advanced the clinical applications of thoracic epidural blocks. The addition of implantable epidural electrodes to stimulate the spinal cord in the thoracic region made this technique extremely useful for management of chronic pain.

Anatomy of the Thoracic Epidural Space

The thoracic epidural space extends from the lower margin of the C7 vertebra to the upper margin of L1.[1-5] The vertebral column in the thoracic area normally has a kyphotic curvature with its apex at approximately T6. Slight scoliosis to the right can occur, even in normal individuals. Significant scoliosis is associated with the rotation of the vertebral column, which can produce significant technical difficulty in performing this block. The inclination of the spinous processes is different at different levels of the thoracic vertebral column (**Fig. 158.1**). The spines from T1-4 have little inclination, whereas the spines of T5-8 tilt significantly downward, making a midline approach to the epidural space practically impossible. The T9-12 spines point dorsally without significant inclination, so the midline approach is possible. The ligamentum flavum is not as thick as it is in the lumbar spine, and occasionally the epidural space can be entered without encountering much resistance. The ligamentum flavum may have a gap directly in the midline, especially in the lower thoracic spine.[6] The attachment of the ligamentum flavum to the lower margin of the lamina on its inner aspect reduces the size of the epidural space, whereas the space is wider at the upper margin of the lamina because the ligamentum flavum is attached to the outer aspect of the upper margin of the lower lamina.

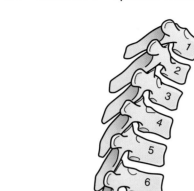

Fig. 158.1 The inclination of the T1-12 spinous processes. *(Adapted from Waldman SD: Thoracic epidural nerve block. In Interventional pain management, ed 2, Philadelphia, 2001, Saunders, p 392.)*

The epidural space is 3 to 4 mm wide in the thoracic area. The thoracic epidural space, similar to the rest of the epidural space, contains loose areolar tissue, fat, and vertebral venous plexus.

Nerve Roots

The T1 nerve root is fairly large and participates in the formation of the brachial plexus. The nerve roots at T2 and below gradually increase in size, but they are still smaller than any of the lumbar or cervical roots. The epidural space communicates through the intervertebral foramina into the paravertebral space. The spinal cord has a lumbar enlargement at T9-12. Although the nerve roots in the subarachnoid space travel caudad for significantly increasing distances below T2 before they exit the intervertebral foramina, their course in the epidural space is horizontal. The dorsal and ventral roots unite just proximal to the intervertebral foramina.

Epidural Pressure

The pressure in the thoracic epidural space is approximately −15 cm H_2O, which is very close to the pressure of the intrapleural pressure.[7] This pressure is more pronounced in the sitting position. The negative pressure in the thoracic epidural space also is considered secondary to the tenting of the dura by a blunt epidural needle.[8] In 12% of patients, the pressure is not negative.

The insignificant amount of fat in the epidural space of children younger than 5 or 6 years old makes it possible to thread a caudally introduced epidural catheter straight up into the thoracic epidural space.[9] Blanco et al[10] reported, however, that lumbar epidural catheters were successfully advanced to the T12 level only in 22% of the 199 patients. Electrically conducting catheters can be used to verify the level of the tip through stimulation and elicitation of muscle twitch.[11]

Physiologic Changes Following Thoracic Epidural Nerve Block with Local Anesthetics

Cardiovascular Effects

The cardiovascular effects of thoracic epidural nerve block depend on its level.[4,7] The preganglionic sympathetic fibers are present in all the thoracic anterior nerve roots. Levels of block to T10 produce minimal cardiovascular changes. The degree of hypotension secondary to this level of block depends on the blood volume and the position of the patient. The cardiovascular effects may be minimal because of the compensatory vasoconstriction in the upper extremities. If the local anesthetic block extends to T6, any resulting hypotension will likely be caused by peripheral vasodilation, venous pooling, or decreased right heart filling. Blocking of the fibers to the abdominal viscera, including the fibers to the adrenal medulla, can reduce the response to stress for lower abdominal and pelvic surgical procedures.

If the block extends to T1, the sympathetic fibers innervating the heart will also be affected. Block of the cardioaccelerator fibers can produce bradycardia and hypotension owing to the unopposed action of the parasympathetic fibers derived from the vagus nerve that sometimes results in cardiac standstill.[12] Studies also have shown decreased myocardial contractility.[13] The hypotension can be significant. It may respond to treatment with ephedrine initially, but patients may require aggressive treatment with epinephrine or dopamine.

Myocardial oxygen consumption is reduced by thoracic epidural block. Blomberg et al[14,15] showed that thoracic epidural analgesia can relieve the pain of angina, decrease stenosis, and reduce the oxygen requirement, thus facilitating oxygenation of the myocardium. Pulmonary hypertension[16] is decreased with thoracic epidural analgesia, and the ST-T segment changes can be reversed.

Pulmonary Effects

Weakening of the intercostal muscles can affect respiratory parameters. When a block affects all the intercostal muscles, normal ventilation and arterial partial pressure of carbon dioxide ($PaCO_2$) still can be maintained by the activity of the diaphragm because the phrenic nerve is not affected. Improved diaphragmatic shortening and tidal volume have been reported secondary to intercostal paralysis.[17] The forced vital capacity, functional residual capacity (FRC), and vital capacity (VC), notably, are decreased (up to 10% to 30%).[18] However, after surgery, even greater reductions in VC and FRC occur because of shallow breathing from thoracic or abdominal pain; therefore, thoracic epidural analgesia can provide some recovery of lost pulmonary function in that setting. Accordingly, oxygenation can improve after pain relief because of the thoracic epidural block.[19]

Horner's Syndrome

Thoracic epidural block of T1 nerve roots can result in unilateral or bilateral Horner's syndrome.[20]

Indications

Surgical Procedures

The administration of local anesthetics and opioid analgesics into the thoracic epidural space provide excellent anesthesia for surgical procedures involving the upper abdomen, thorax and intra-thoracic contents when combined with light general anesthesia.[21–27] Thoracic epidural catheters are increasingly used for providing perioperative analgesia for thoracic and abdominal surgical procedures. When compared with systemic analgesia, epidural analgesia has been associated with superior pain relief, reduced rates of pneumonia and mechanical ventilation, reduced rates of myocardial infarction, and faster recovery of bowel function.[28–33] With thoracic epidural analgesia, the physiologic stress of surgery is significantly reduced.[1–5,7] The benefits and safety of thoracic epidural analgesia for breast surgery are also well documented.[34–36]

Postoperative Analgesia

Whether thoracic epidural nerve block is indicated for postoperative analgesia has been extensively debated. Many clinicians believe that a catheter placed in the lumbar epidural space, to deliver a narcotic, can provide significant analgesia in the thoracic area without risking the complications associated with the thoracic epidural technique.[37,38] Many studies have shown the superiority of the thoracic epidural technique.[39–44] With the thoracic epidural technique, the catheter can be placed close to the nerve roots innervating the painful area; this placement becomes especially important when using any local anesthetic. Small quantities of local anesthetics can be used to provide excellent analgesia with the thoracic approach.[40–42,45] The lumbar epidural technique requires large volumes of local anesthetic to provide analgesia in the thoracic dermatomes.[37] This large volume may result in significant hypotension and significant blood levels of the local anesthetic, thus limiting the usefulness of the lumbar approach.

Even with opioids such as morphine, which ascend in the cerebrospinal fluid, the thoracic epidural technique still has advantages because the onset of analgesia is faster.[40,42] By comparison, morphine placed in the lumbar epidural space takes longer to ascend to the thoracic area and provide analgesia. With highly lipid-soluble drugs, such as fentanyl and sufentanil, the doses required to maintain analgesia are such that either epidural technique may not offer any advantages over the intravenous route of administration.[38] Patient-controlled epidural analgesia is used effectively and safely, even at thoracic levels.[46]

The thoracic epidural approach provides rapid onset of analgesia and minimizes the doses of local anesthetics and opioids needed to provide excellent analgesia. Small doses of bupivacaine with morphine do not prevent ambulation.[46] This feature is important because small quantities of local anesthetic play a significant role in reducing pain related to motion and episodic pain.[40,41,45,47] Thoracic epidural techniques also have been used in pediatric patients with good

results. The analgesia obtained from the technique has been shown to be superior to that obtained from interpleural or intravenous techniques.[48,49]

Herpes Zoster and Postherpetic Neuralgia

Herpes zoster infection is most common in the thoracic area. Pain from acute herpes zoster can be relieved by epidural administration of local anesthetic or steroids. For acute herpes zoster, the local anesthetic produces excellent pain relief and may prevent postherpetic neuralgia and limit the eruption of more vesicles.[50] An epidural catheter placed close to the involved nerve root can provide excellent analgesia with 2 to 3 mL of 0.25% bupivacaine. Usually, the catheter is left in for only 2 or 3 days. The drug is injected once or twice a day. Alternatively, single-shot epidural blocks can be performed on a daily to weekly basis with local anesthetic and steroid.

Epidural Steroids

Herniated disks are uncommon in the thoracic spine. The patient who has nerve root irritation secondary to a herniated intervertebral disk or inflammation of the nerve root secondary to cancer or radiation therapy responds extremely well to a series of epidural thoracic steroid nerve blocks. Methylprednisolone (Depo-Medrol), 80 mg, or triamcinolone (Aristocort), 25 to 50 mg, is given, alone or mixed with saline solution or local anesthetic on a daily to weekly basis as the clinical situation dictates.

Acute Pain Secondary to Trauma

Patients with multiple fractured ribs and fractured vertebrae have excellent analgesia with a properly positioned epidural catheter. Local anesthetic, such as 0.125% to 0.25% bupivacaine, opioid, or steroid can be used. Even with short-term administration of local anesthetic by the epidural route, the patient may experience prolonged pain relief after the muscle spasm and other secondary phenomena are relieved. Thoracic epidural analgesia can reduce pulmonary complications in this setting, particularly in older patients or patients with pulmonary contusions.[51,52]

Angina

Angina secondary to myocardial ischemia has been treated by the thoracic epidural technique.[1,14,15] This technique provides excellent analgesia and decreases myocardial oxygen consumption, anxiety associated with pain, and catecholamine levels. Thoracic epidural techniques also have been used for long-term home self-treatment.[53] Spinal cord stimulation with the electrode placed in the epidural space has been used to control angina,[54,55] and such stimulation does not mask the pain of acute myocardial infarction.[56]

Cancer Pain

Catheters placed in the thoracic epidural space can be used to provide long-term analgesia with opioids such as morphine or local anesthetic. Through a tunneled epidural catheter, excellent long-term analgesia can be provided. Catheters also can be completely buried under the skin, with a reservoir accessed through the skin for injection. Thoracic epidural administration of local anesthetic and steroid administered by a single-shot injection can be extremely useful in the palliation of pain secondary to bony metastatic disease. Epidural phenol[57] or alcohol[58] also has been used for analgesia in cancer patients. The catheter is placed in the area of the involved nerve roots. Alcohol is injected through the catheter in 0.5-mL increments to a maximum of 5 mL. Previous injection of local anesthetic and sedation help to reduce the pain associated with injection of the alcohol. The injection must be repeated daily for at least 3 days. More than 79% of patients report significant pain relief (50%). Phenol also has been used epidurally. The technique is similar to that of epidural alcohol: 5% phenol in dextrose or in 0.9% saline is injected slowly and repeated daily for 3 days. Both techniques have been reported to provide excellent analgesia without producing significant sensory or motor deficit. Epidural clonidine can be a useful approach in patients with various types of cancer pain or benign neuropathic pain that has failed to respond to more traditional measures.

Spinal Cord Stimulation

Electrodes for spinal cord stimulation are commonly placed through the lumbar or thoracic area and are useful in the treatment of intractable neuropathic pain. The technique is similar to that of thoracic epidural catheter insertion, except the needle is beveled so that the catheter can be gently withdrawn and redirected without shearing. The procedure uses fluoroscopic imaging. Stimulation of the cervical spinal cord is usually achieved through rostral advancement of an electrode from a high thoracic interspace. The electrode may be externalized for temporary use, or it may be anchored and connected to a subcutaneously implanted pulse generator similar in size to a cardiac pacemaker.

Acute Pancreatitis

Patients with severe pain secondary to acute pancreatitis benefit from an epidural catheter placed in the lower thoracic area to deliver local anesthetics, such as bupivacaine, or an opioid such as morphine with or without the addition of steroids.[7] The severe pain is controlled until the pancreatitis resolves. Alternatively, daily single-shot thoracic epidural blocks with local anesthetic, opioids, or steroids may be used.

Contraindications to Thoracic Epidural Nerve Block

Contraindications are the same as for any other neuraxial procedure:

- Patient refusal
- Infection in the area or septicemia
- Bleeding or clotting disorders, such as thrombocytopenia, or current anticoagulant therapy
- Uncorrected hypovolemia

Thoracic Epidural Nerve Block Technique

Midline Approach

The midline approach is applicable in the upper part of the thoracic spine between C7 and T5 and in the lower part, including T9-L1, because the spinous processes project directly posteriorly and are horizontal. The level of the spinous process corresponds to the level of the vertebra. The epidural technique is similar to that used in the lumbar areas, with a 90-degree approach. Starting at the lower part of the interspace, just above the lower spine, so that the needle is angled cephalad, facilitates insertion and advancement of the catheter.

After infiltration of a local anesthetic, such as lidocaine, intradermally with a short, 25-gauge or 27-gauge needle, injection of a local anesthetic with a slightly longer needle, such as a 1½-inch 22-gauge needle, into the paraspinal muscles on either side of the spine provides significant analgesia for the procedure by blocking the nerve fibers as they come from lateral areas toward the midline. Commonly, a 3½-inch 16- to 18-gauge Tuohy needle is used, although many pain management specialists use shorter, sharper needles. The Tuohy needle is advanced with the bevel cephalad so that the smooth part of the curvature bounces off the lamina. The needle is advanced through the skin, subcutaneous tissue, supraspinous ligament, intraspinous ligament, and ligamentum flavum. If ligament resistance is encountered, and the lamina is contacted after that, the needle is at the upper margin of the lower lamina. Intentional contact of the lamina provides an element of safety to reduce the chance of inadvertent dural puncture or entry into the spinal cord. Redirection farther cephalad facilitates entry into the epidural space.

The most common technique for identifying entry is the loss-of-resistance technique. An air or fluid-filled syringe (containing a small bubble of air to allow compression) is used. Saline solution 0.9% without preservatives is a suitable fluid choice. The hanging-drop technique has been used, especially in the thoracic area, because of the significant negative pressure. Despite a low incidence of dural puncture, the drop is sucked inward only 88% of the time. Because both hands are used to advance the needle slowly, entry into the epidural space is recognized even when the drop is not sucked inward.

Some investigators take the ability to advance the significant length of the catheters without difficulty as an indication of entry into the epidural space. If the needle is off course and enters the paraspinal muscles or a defect in the interspinous ligament, the loss of resistance can be misleading. This error can be identified by the paraspinal compression technique,[59] in which the index and middle fingers of the operator's nondominant hand compress the paraspinal tissues on either side of the needle. If the resistance that was lost reappears, the tip of the needle is superficial to the ligamentum flavum. If the external pressure does not affect pressure in the syringe, the needle is deep to the ligamentum flavum.

A catheter is advanced 3 to 4 cm. The patient may experience paresthesia if the catheter passes close to a nerve root. The catheter should not be withdrawn after it passes the tip of the needle because the catheter may be sheared off. Certain needles used for spinal cord stimulator electrode placement or epidural adhesiolysis applications are specially designed to allow for gentle withdrawal. Inserting the catheter too far may result in migration through the intervertebral foramen or epidural vein, or true knot formation. Tunneling the catheter for 5 cm with another epidural needle reduces the risk of catheter migration.[60]

The technique described by Raj[61] (**Fig. 158.2 [online only]**) for taping the catheter by using Steri-Strips (sterile strips), Mastisol (liquid adhesive), and Tegaderm (transparent dressing) provides secure fixation. This technique reduces the possibility of catheter dislodgment and facilitates maintaining the catheter for a longer time. The catheter is connected to an adapter, a filter, and an injection site and is taped over the infraclavicular area to afford easy access for reinjection. An externalized catheter can be well protected over the long term with a colostomy bag.[62]

Paramedian Lateral Approach

The paramedian lateral approach (**Fig. 158.3**) can be used at any level of the thoracic spine. Usually, the starting point is 1 to 2 cm lateral to the superior margin of the spinous process. In most patients, a 1½-inch 22-gauge needle can contact the lamina, and 1 mL of short-acting local anesthetic can be injected to decrease the pain related to "walking" on the lamina. The epidural needle is advanced at a 45- to 55-degree angle cephalad and a 15- to 30-degree angle toward the midline. Extreme angles can result in nerve root contact on the opposite side of the spine or can cause the needle to pass between the spinous processes into the paraspinal muscle without contacting the ligamentum flavum. Starting close to the midline and right next to the lateral margin of the cephalad edge of the spine minimizes the angle required

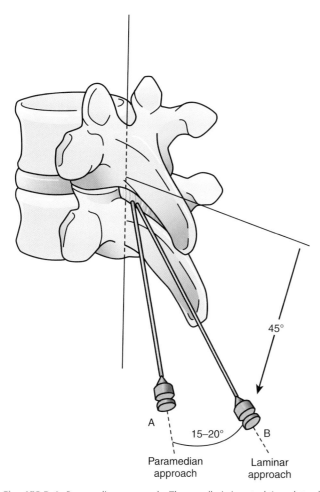

45°

A

15–20°   B

Paramedian   Laminar
approach   approach

Fig. 158.3 *A,* Paramedian approach. The needle is inserted 1 cm lateral to the midline with a 45-degree cephalad angle and a 15- to 20-degree angle in the coronal plane to enter the ligamentum flavum in the midline. *B,* Laminar (parasagittal) approach. The needle is inserted right next to the cephalad edge of the spine and is advanced straight forward without any deviation toward the midline. *(Adapted from Waldman SD: Thoracic epidural nerve block. In* Interventional pain management, *ed 2, Philadelphia, 2001, Saunders, p 393.)*

to make the puncture in the ligamentum flavum. Contact of the lamina with the epidural needle significantly increases the safety of the technique because the epidural space can be entered by walking off the superior margin of the lamina. The steep angle required to enter the epidural space in the midthoracic area also facilitates insertion of the catheter. The paramedian lateral approach is more efficient than the midline approach for gaining epidural access in the midthoracic spine due to the extreme angulation of the spinous processes in that region.

Laminar Approach

For a laminar (also known as parasagittal) approach, the starting point is the same as for the paramedian approach, but the needle is not angled toward the midline (see Fig. 158.3). Only the lateral portion of the epidural space is entered. The disadvantages of the technique are that the epidural space is narrower, and veins are more numerous in the lateral portion of the epidural space. In addition, if the starting point is too far lateral, or even has a slight lateral angle, the needle will contact the articular processes. Walking it more cephalad does not achieve entry into the epidural space. Starting right next to the cephalad margin of the spinous process minimizes the angle and thus increases the chance of entering the epidural space. The laminar approach is more useful when attempting a predominantly unilateral block, especially with epidural steroids. A small volume of injectate has a tendency to stay on one side for two to three segments.

Drugs Used for Thoracic Epidural Nerve Block

Medication similar to that used in the lumbar area is chosen, although smaller volumes of local anesthetics are needed. Placing the catheter tip at the middle of the desired segmental levels of analgesia minimizes the necessary volume. The necessary doses depend on individual factors, such as age, height, weight, intercurrent disease (e.g., diabetes), and extent of desired analgesia. Short-acting and long-acting local anesthetics and opioids have been used for single administration or infusion. Concentrations are similar to those used for lumbar epidural analgesia.

Pitfalls of Thoracic Epidural Nerve Block

1. Because the spinal cord is present at the thoracic vertebral level, a thoracic epidural technique should be attempted only by an operator who has extensive experience with lumbar epidural techniques. Bromage[4] recommended that an individual who performs a thoracic epidural procedure should have done at least 50 consecutive lumbar epidural procedures without a dural puncture or a complication.
2. Because of the inclination of the spine in the midthoracic area, the technique can be technically difficult, although it can be mastered with some practice.
3. Because high thoracic nerve roots contain the sympathetic nerves to the heart, block of these fibers can produce significant bradycardia and hypotension.

Intercostal muscle weakness resulting from thoracic epidural block can produce significant difficulty, especially in obese patients and in patients with respiratory impairment.

In a patient with impaired function of the diaphragm, chronic obstructive lung disease, or obesity, intercostal paralysis can contribute significantly to the respiratory impairment.

Complications of Thoracic Epidural Nerve Block

The complications of the thoracic epidural technique are similar to those of the lumbar epidural technique and include infection, epidural hematoma, injury to the nerve roots, intravascular injection, respiratory depression, and subdural and subarachnoid injection.[63] The presence of the spinal cord in the thoracic vertebral canal allows the possibility of spinal cord damage. The incidence of spinal cord damage owing to attempted thoracic epidural analgesia is unknown, but this complication is probably rare, and few reports have been published. In a series of 1071 postoperative patients, no long-term serious complications were reported. In a study of 4185 patients, the absence of serious neurologic complications was documented.[64] Many studies have documented the safety of the procedure and the absence of infection.[65,66]

Infection

Epidural abscess[37,67,68] secondary to a thoracic epidural catheter left in place is a possibility, especially with the increasing use of long-term catheter placement for the management of cancer pain. Some evidence indicates that the incidence of infection is higher in the thoracic area than in other areas.[37]

Pleural Puncture

Accidental pleural puncture and pleural placement of the catheter have occurred intraoperatively. Although uncommon, this complication can be life-threatening if it is not recognized.[69]

Clinical Pearls

The thoracic epidural catheter can be placed while the patient is in the sitting, lateral decubitus, or prone position. The sitting position provides better alignment of the skin midline to the spine and facilitates identification of landmarks. A patient who is anxious may have a vasovagal reaction in the sitting position, with hypotension and nausea. Because the thoracic spine has no significant flexion and extension, flexion of the patient contributes little to expanding the interlaminar space. Current safe practices in epidural catheter placement have resulted in a very low incidence of serious complications, even when most procedures are done without the assistance of imaging. Fluoroscopy is required only for spinal cord stimulator placement or for patients in whom technical considerations dictate. Verification of the position of the catheter using a nonionic contrast medium may be advisable before a neurolytic block is performed. Useful landmarks for interspace estimation by palpation include the vertebra prominens (C7), the spine of the scapula (T3), the inferior angle of the scapula (T7), and the iliac crest (L4), although commonly the provider may be in error by at least one segment.[70]

Conclusion

Thoracic epidural nerve block has become a mainstay of contemporary pain management. Careful attention to the functional anatomy of the thoracic spine increases the clinician's success rate and decreases complications.

References

Full references for this chapter can be found on www.expertconsult.com.

Intercostal Nerve Block

Steven D. Waldman

Intercostal Nerve Block with Local Anesthetic

Indications

Intercostal nerve block is useful in the evaluation and management of pain involving the chest wall and the upper abdominal wall.[1] Intercostal nerve block with local anesthetic can be used as a diagnostic tool when performing differential neural blockade on an anatomic basis in the evaluation of chest and abdominal pain. If destruction of the intercostal nerve is being considered, this technique is useful as a prognostic indicator of the degree of motor and sensory impairment that the patient may experience. Intercostal nerve block with local anesthetic may be used to palliate acute pain emergencies, including rib fractures, acute herpes zoster, and cancer pain, while the patient waits for pharmacologic, surgical, and antiblastic methods to become effective[2] (**Fig. 159.1**). This block is also useful before placement of percutaneous thoracostomy and nephrotomy tubes.[3] In addition, intercostal nerve block with local anesthetic and steroid is helpful in the treatment of postthoracotomy pain, cancer pain, rib fractures, metastatic lesions of the liver, and postherpetic neuralgia[4] (**Fig. 159.2**). Intercostal block can also be used as a primary surgical anesthesia technique for thoracic and some abdominal surgical procedures.[5,6]

Destruction of the intercostal nerve is indicated for the palliation of cancer pain, including invasive tumors of the ribs and the chest and upper abdominal wall.[7] Given the desperate nature of many patients' suffering from aggressively invasive malignant tumors, blockade of the intercostal nerve using a 25-gauge needle may be carried out in the presence of coagulopathy or anticoagulation, albeit at an increased risk of ecchymosis and hematoma formation.

Clinically Relevant Anatomy

The intercostal nerves arise from the anterior division of the thoracic paravertebral nerve. A typical intercostal nerve has four major branches[8] (**Fig. 159.3**). The first branch consists of the unmyelinated postganglionic fibers of the gray rami communicantes, which interface with the sympathetic chain. The second branch is the posterior cutaneous branch, which innervates the muscles and skin of the paraspinal area. The third branch is the lateral cutaneous division, which arises in the anterior axillary line. The lateral cutaneous division provides most of the cutaneous innervation of the chest and abdominal wall. The fourth branch is the anterior cutaneous branch, which supplies innervation to the midline of the chest and abdominal wall. Occasionally, the terminal branches of a given intercostal nerve may actually cross the midline to provide sensory innervation to the contralateral chest and abdominal wall. The 12th nerve is called the *subcostal nerve* and is unique in that it gives off a branch to the first lumbar nerve, thus contributing to the lumbar plexus.

Technique

The patient is placed in the prone position with the patient's arms hanging loosely off the side of the cart. Alternatively, this block can be performed with the patient in the sitting or lateral position. The rib to be blocked is identified by palpating its path at the posterior axillary line. The operator's index and middle fingers are then placed on the rib bracketing the site of needle insertion. The skin is prepared with antiseptic solution. A 22-gauge, 1½-inch needle is attached to a 12-mL syringe and is advanced perpendicular to the skin to aiming for the middle of the rib in between the index and middle fingers.[1] The needle should impinge on bone after being advanced approximately ¾ inch.[2] After bony contact is made, the needle is withdrawn into the subcutaneous tissues, and the skin and subcutaneous tissues are retracted with the palpating fingers inferiorly. This maneuver allows the needle to be walked off the inferior margin of the rib[2] (**Figs. 159.4 and 159.5**). As soon as bony contact is lost, the needle is slowly advanced approximately 2 mm deeper.[1] This technique places

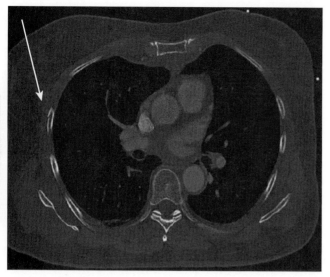

Fig. 159.1 **Rib fracture *(arrow)* on computed tomography that was not seen by radiography.** *(From Pope T, Bloem HL, Beltran J:* Imaging of the musculoskeletal system, *Philadelphia, 2008, Saunders, p 91.)*

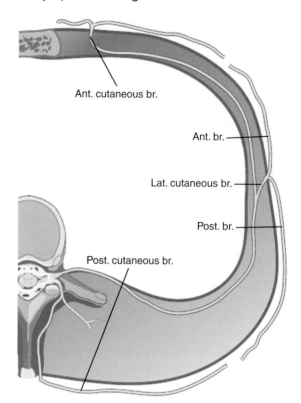

Fig. 159.3 **The four branches of a typical intercostal nerve.**

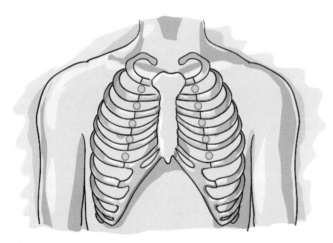

Fig. 159.2 The *circles* indicate approximate sites for parasternal block of the upper anterior intercostal nerves. This technique is an effective way to relieve pain from median sternotomy or a fractured sternum.

the needle in proximity to the costal groove, which contains the intercostal nerve as well as the intercostal artery and vein.[2] After careful aspiration reveals no blood or air, the practitioner injects 3 to 5 mL of 1.0% preservative-free lidocaine. If the pain has an inflammatory component, the local anesthetic is combined with 80 mg of methylprednisolone and is injected in incremental doses. Subsequent daily nerve blocks are carried out in a similar manner, by substituting 40 mg of methylprednisolone for the initial 80-mg dose. Because of the overlapping innervation of the chest and upper abdominal wall, the intercostal nerves above and below the nerve suspected of subserving the painful condition must be blocked. If surface landmarks are difficult to identify, fluoroscopy, ultrasound, or computed tomography guidance may be helpful[2,9] (**Figs. 159.6** and **159.7**).

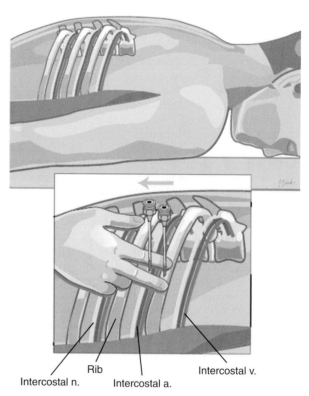

Fig. 159.4 After bony contact is made, the needle is withdrawn into the subcutaneous tissues, and the skin and subcutaneous tissues are retracted with the palpating fingers inferiorly. This maneuver allows the needle to be walked off the inferior margin of the rib.

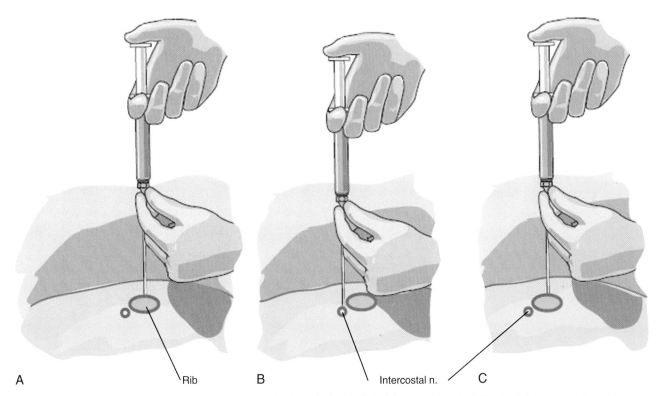

A   Rib   B   Intercostal n.   C

Fig. 159.5 **Ideal overview of a posterior intercostal block.** The right-handed physician stands on the left side of the prone patient, whose arms hang down to retract the scapulae laterally. The palpating left index finger identifies the rib to determine the depth and direction for the advancing needle. The depth of the needle is firmly controlled by the anesthesiologist's left hand, which is constantly in contact (hypothenar eminence) with the patient's back. Now the right hand is shifted to inject 3 to 5 mL of solution. The depth of the needle is controlled by the left hand. The left hand again controls return of the needle to the "safety" of osseous contact. The previous steps are repeated at the next higher rib level.

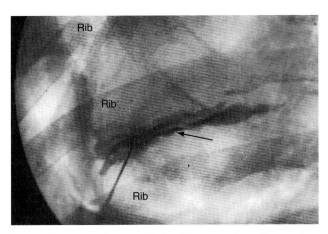

Fig. 159.6 **Intercostal nerve block with contrast medium, antero-posterior view.** The *arrow* indicates the spread of contrast in the intercostals groove. *(From Paj PP, Lou L, Staats PS, et al: Interventional pain management: image-guided procedures, ed 2, Philadelphia, 2008, Saunders, p. 250.)*

Side Effects and Complications

Given the proximity of the pleural space, pneumothorax after intercostal nerve block is a distinct possibility.[2,10] The incidence of the complication is less than 1%, but pneumothorax occurs with greater frequency in patients with chronic obstructive pulmonary disease. Because of the proximity to the intercostal nerve and artery, the pain management specialist should carefully calculate the total milligram dosage

of local anesthetic administered because vascular uptake by these vessels is high.[2,10] Given that the dura mater and the arachnoid membrane tend to fuse with the epineurium as each intercostal nerve exits vertebral foramen, it is possible to inject local anesthetic inadvertently into the epidural, subdural, or subarachnoid space when injecting in the paravertebral region[11] (**Fig. 159.8**). Although uncommon, infection remains an ever-present possibility, especially in the immunocompromised patient with cancer. Early detection of infection is crucial, to avoid potentially life-threatening sequelae.[1]

Clinical Pearls

Intercostal nerve block is a simple technique that can produce dramatic relief for patients who suffer from the previously mentioned pain complaints. Intercostal block with local anesthetic before placement of chest tubes provides a great degree of patient comfort and should routinely be used. Intercostal block with local anesthetic and steroid is useful in the palliation of the pleuritic pain secondary to lung tumors and liver tumors that are irritating the parietal peritoneum.

Neurolytic block with small quantities of phenol in glycerin or by cryoneurolysis or radiofrequency lesioning has been shown to provide long-term relief for patients suffering from post-thoracotomy and cancer-related pain who have not responded to more conservative treatments. As mentioned earlier, the proximity of the intercostal nerve to the pleural space makes careful attention to technique mandatory.

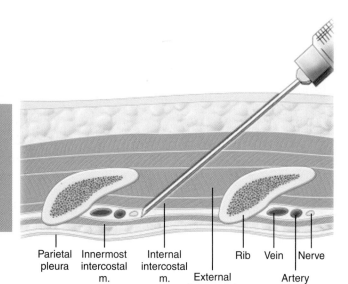

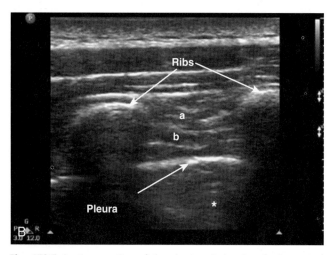

Fig. 159.7 A, Cross-section of the chest wall showing the intercostal muscles and neurovascular bundles. B, Ultrasonographic picture image corresponding to A. a, external intercostal muscle; b, internal intercostal muscle; *asterisk*, reverberation artifact. *(From Seib RK, Peng PWH: Ultrasound-guided peripheral nerve block in chronic pain management,* Tech Reg Anesth Pain Manag *13:110, 2009.)*

Intercostal Nerve Block with Radiofrequency Lesioning

Indications

Disruption of the intercostal nerve is indicated for the palliation of cancer pain, including invasive tumors of the ribs and the chest and upper abdominal wall. This technique is also used as a final step in the treatment of pain of nonmalignant origin in those patients in whom management with more conservative approaches, including adjuvant analgesics, has failed and who have experienced temporary relief with blockade of the target intercostal nerve or nerves with local anesthetic on at least two separate occasions.[7] Disruption of the intercostal nerves can be carried out by injection with neurolytic agents including phenol, cryoneurolysis, direct surgical sectioning at the time of thoracotomy, and destruction by radiofrequency

lesioning[2] (**Fig. 159.9**). Most interventional pain management specialists now favor the use of radiofrequency lesioning because of its simplicity and its acceptable level of side effects and complications compared with the other modalities currently available.[12]

Clinically Relevant Anatomy

The intercostal nerves arise from the anterior division of the thoracic spinal nerve (see Fig. 159.8). A typical intercostal nerve has four major branches. The first branch is made up of the unmyelinated postganglionic fibers of the gray rami communicantes, which interface with the sympathetic chain. The second branch is the posterior cutaneous branch, which innervates the muscles and skin of the paraspinal area. The third branch is the lateral cutaneous division, which arises in the anterior axillary line. The lateral cutaneous division provides most of the cutaneous innervation of the chest and abdominal wall (**Fig. 159.10**). The fourth branch is the anterior cutaneous branch supplying innervation to the midline of the chest and abdominal wall. Occasionally, the terminal branches of a given intercostal nerve may actually cross the midline to provide sensory innervation to the contralateral chest and abdominal wall. The twelfth nerve is called the subcostal nerve and is unique in that it gives off a branch to the first lumbar nerve and thus contributes to the lumbar plexus. The nerve travels in the subcostal groove along with the intercostal artery and vein.

Technique

The patient is placed in the prone position with the patient's arms hanging loosely off the side of the cart. Alternatively, this block can be done with the patient in the sitting or lateral position, based on the patient's ability to assume the desired position. The rib to be blocked is identified by palpating its path at the posterior axillary line or by fluoroscopy or ultrasound (see Fig. 159.10). The operator's index and middle fingers are then placed on the rib bracketing the site of needle insertion. The skin is then prepared with antiseptic solution. A 22-gauge, 54-mm radiofrequency needle with a 4-mm active tip is then advanced, perpendicular to the skin using a slight medial direction to lie as parallel as possible to the nerve, and the needle is aimed at the middle of the rib between the index and middle fingers. The needle should impinge on bone after being advanced approximately half an inch. After bony contact is made, the needle is withdrawn into the subcutaneous tissues, and the skin and subcutaneous tissues are retracted with the palpating fingers inferiorly. This maneuver allows the needle to be walked off the inferior margin of the rib[7] (see Fig. 159.10). As soon as bony contact is lost, the needle is slowly advanced approximately 2 mm more deeply. This technique places the needle in proximity to the costal groove, which contains the intercostal nerve as well as the intercostal artery and vein. After confirmation of proper needle placement with fluoroscopy, trial sensory stimulation is carried out with 2 V at 50 Hz (**Fig. 159.11**). If the needle is in the proper position, the patient should experience paresthesia in the distribution of the target intercostal nerve. If a proper stimulation pattern is identified, a pulsed radiofrequency lesion is created by heating at 40°C to 45°C for 5 minutes or by heating at 49°C to 60°C for 90 seconds. This technique (**Fig. 159.12**) is repeated for each affected nerve root.[12]

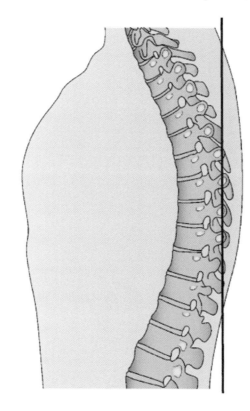

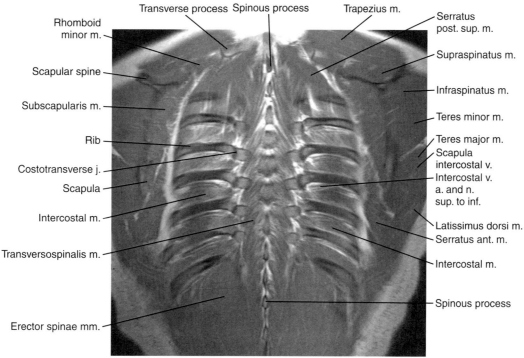

Fig. 159.8 The relationship between the intercostal nerve and the epidural, subdural, or subarachnoid space. *(From El-Khoury GY, Bergman RA, Montgomery WJ: Sectional anatomy by MRI and CT, ed 3, New York, 2007, Churchill Livingstone, p 434.)*

Side Effects and Complications

Given the proximity of the pleural space, pneumothorax after intercostal nerve block is a distinct possibility. The incidence of the complication is less than 1%, but pneumothorax occurs with greater frequency in patients with chronic obstructive pulmonary disease. Because of the proximity to the intercostal nerve and artery, the pain management specialist should carefully calculate the total milligram dosage of local anesthetic administered because vascular uptake by these vessels is high. Although uncommon, infection remains

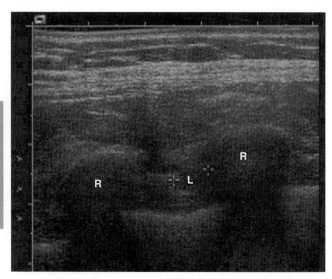

Fig. 159.9 Cryoanalgesia of an intercostal nerve. The figure shows the ice ball at the frozen tip of the cryoanalgesia probe. L, lesion produced by the ice ball; R, rib. *(From Eichenberger U, Greher M, Curatolo M: Ultrasound in interventional pain management,* Tech Reg Anesth Pain Manag *8:171, 2004.)*

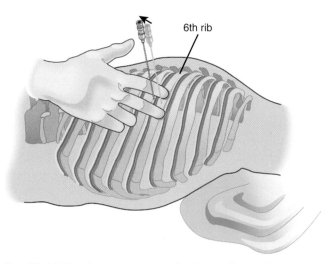

Fig. 159.11 After bony contact is made, the needle is withdrawn into the subcutaneous tissues, and the skin and subcutaneous tissues are retracted with the palpating fingers inferiorly. This maneuver allows the needle to be walked off the inferior margin of the rib.

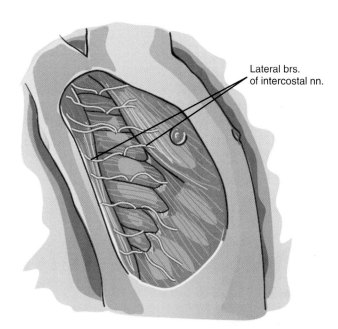

Fig. 159.10 The lateral branches of the intercostal nerves near the midaxillary line. Blocks made at or near these sites are effective and can be performed easily on the supine patient.

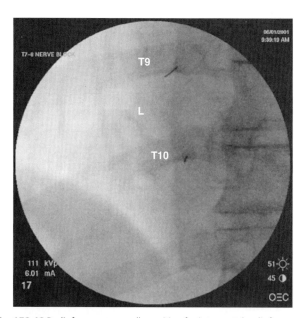

Fig. 159.12 Radiofrequency needle position for intercostal radiofrequency lesioning.

an ever-present possibility, especially in the immunocompromised patient with cancer or acquired immunodeficiency syndrome. Early detection of infection is crucial, to avoid potentially life-threatening sequelae. Even with perfect technique, postprocedure intercostal neuritis can occur, especially with increasing temperatures. In most patients, this complication responds to the injection of 40 mg of methylprednisolone and 0.5% preservative-free bupivacaine onto the affected nerve.[12] Occasionally, a short course of gabapentin is also required to manage postprocedure neuritis.

Clinical Pearls

Neurolytic block with small quantities of phenol in glycerin or by cryoneurolysis or radiofrequency lesioning has been shown to provide long-term relief for patients suffering from postthoracotomy and cancer-related pain who have not responded to more conservative treatments. As mentioned earlier, the proximity of the intercostal nerve to the pleural space makes careful attention to technique mandatory. Alcohol should be avoided as a neurolytic agent because of the high incidence of postblock intercostal neuritis.

References

Full references for this chapter can be found on www.expertconsult.com.

Splanchnic and Celiac Plexus Nerve Block

Steven D. Waldman and Richard B. Patt

Historical Considerations

In 1914, Kappis[1] introduced a percutaneous technique for blockade of the splanchnic nerves and celiac plexus with local anesthetic.*He described a posterior approach intended primarily for surgical anesthesia that used two needles, the tips of which were placed into the retroperitoneum via a retrocrural approach. He rapidly gained experience with this technique and reported on it in a series of 200 patients in 1918.[2]

The same year, Wendling[3] described a method of blocking the celiac plexus and splanchnic nerves using a single needle placed anteriorly through the liver. Judged to be riskier than Kappis's posterior approach, it rapidly fell into disfavor.

Labat, Farr, and others introduced further modifications of the Kappis technique over the ensuing 30 years.[4-6] Because of the technical demands and variable results of celiac plexus and splanchnic nerve block as a surgical anesthetic, over time, this technique was supplanted by spinal anesthesia and segmental blockade of the somatic paravertebral nerves.[7]

In the classic textbook *Conduction Anesthesia,* published in 1946, Pitkin,[8] surveying the status of the use of splanchnic nerve block for surgical anesthesia, wrote, "Posterior splanchnic block gained some popularity with a limited number of anesthetists, but because of unsatisfactory results, it was never continued beyond the experimental stage." There is no doubt that, as with many other regional anesthesia techniques, the introduction of neuromuscular blocking agents into the clinical practice of anesthesia led to the final demise of celiac plexus and splanchnic nerve block for surgical anesthesia, except at a limited number of institutions.

As celiac plexus and splanchnic nerve blocks were falling into disuse for surgical anesthesia, the clinical utility of these techniques was becoming apparent in the new specialty of pain management. In 1947, Gage and Floyd[9] described the use of celiac plexus and splanchnic nerve block in the management of pain secondary to pancreatitis. Esnaurrizar[10] and others recommended it to palliate abdominal pain secondary to a variety of causes. Recognizing the difficulty in distinguishing the somatic and visceral components of abdominal pain, Popper[11] recommended the use of splanchnic nerve block with local anesthetic as a diagnostic tool.

Alcohol neurolysis of the splanchnic nerves and celiac plexus for long-lasting relief of abdominal pain was first described by Jones[12] in 1957. Bridenbaugh et al[13] reported on the role

---

*Note: There is significant confusion about the nomenclature for the neural structures that innervate the abdominal viscera. Different investigators have used a variety of terms, including *splanchnic plexus, splanchnic nerve, solar plexus,* and *abdominal brain of Bichat,* to describe all or some of the same structures. In this chapter, we have tried to use all neuroanatomic nomenclature in an "anatomically correct" manner whenever possible.

of neurolytic celiac plexus block to treat the pain of upper abdominal malignancy. In 1965, Moore[14] further modified the original technique of Kappis and brought celiac plexus block into the mainstream of pain management practice.

In spite of these modifications over the last 80 years, the Kappis classic posterior approach to blockade of the celiac plexus and splanchnic nerves continues to serve as the basis for contemporary techniques. Interestingly, there is renewed interest in the anterior approach to celiac plexus block, using computed tomography (CT) or ultrasound to allow more accurate needle placement.[15,16]

Indications

Indications for celiac plexus block are several. Celiac plexus block with local anesthetic is indicated as a diagnostic tool to determine whether flank, retroperitoneal, or upper abdominal pain is sympathetically mediated via the celiac plexus.[17] Daily celiac plexus blocks with local anesthetic are also useful in the palliation of pain secondary to acute pancreatitis.[18,19] Clinical reports suggest that early implementation of celiac plexus block with local anesthetic and/or steroid markedly reduces the morbidity and mortality rates associated with acute pancreatitis.[20,21] Celiac plexus block is also used successfully to palliate the acute pain of arterial embolization of the liver for cancer therapy and to reduce the pain of abdominal "angina" associated with visceral arterial insufficiency.[22] Celiac plexus block with local anesthetic may be used for prognosis before performing celiac plexus neurolysis.[23]

Neurolysis of the celiac plexus with alcohol or phenol is indicated to treat pain secondary to malignancies of the retroperitoneum and upper abdomen.[24,25] Neurolytic celiac plexus block may also be useful in some chronic benign abdominal pain syndromes, including chronic pancreatitis, in carefully selected patients.[26,27] Most investigators report a lower success rate when using celiac plexus and splanchnic nerve block to treat patients suffering from chronic nonmalignant abdominal pain as compared with the rate for abdominal pain of neoplastic origin.[23]

Contraindications

Owing to the proximity to vascular structures, celiac plexus block is contraindicated in patients who are on anticoagulant therapy or who suffer from coagulopathy secondary to congenital abnormality, antiblastic cancer therapies, or liver abnormalities associated with ethanol abuse.[23,25] Local or intra-abdominal infection and sepsis represent absolute contraindications to celiac plexus block.

Because blockade of the celiac plexus results in greater bowel motility, the technique should be avoided in patients with bowel obstruction.[20] Neurolytic celiac plexus block should probably be deferred in patients who suffer from chronic abdominal pain, who are chemically dependent, or who exhibit drug-seeking behavior until these relative contraindications have been adequately addressed.[18] The use of alcohol as a neurolytic agent should be avoided in patients on disulfiram therapy for alcohol abuse.

Clinically Relevant Anatomy

To perform celiac plexus and splanchnic nerve block safely and effectively, it is necessary to understand the anatomy of the autonomic nervous system and the relationships of the

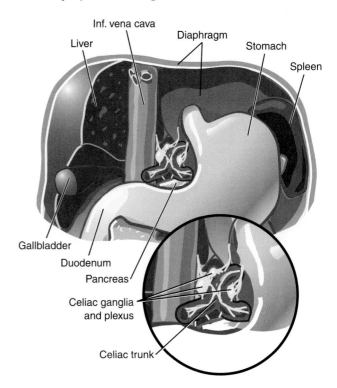

Fig. 160.1 The sympathetic innervation of the abdominal viscera.

anatomic structures surrounding the celiac plexus. CT has enhanced our understanding of the functional anatomy of the region and better documents where injected drugs are ultimately to be deposited. This information has been used to improve the efficacy and safety of celiac plexus and splanchnic nerve block.

The Autonomic Nervous System

The sympathetic innervation of the abdominal viscera originates in the anterolateral horn of the spinal cord (**Fig. 160.1**).[28] Preganglionic fibers from T5 through T12 exit the spinal cord in conjunction with the ventral roots to join the white communicating rami on their way to the sympathetic chain. Instead of synapsing with the sympathetic chain, these preganglionic fibers pass through it, ultimately to synapse on the celiac ganglia.[29]

The Splanchnic Nerves

The greater, lesser, and least splanchnic nerves provide the major preganglionic contribution to the celiac plexus (**Fig. 160.2**).[30] The greater splanchnic nerve has its origin from the T5-10 spinal roots. The nerve travels along the thoracic paravertebral border, through the crus of the diaphragm, and into the abdominal cavity, ending on the ipsilateral celiac ganglion. The lesser splanchnic nerve arises from the T10-11 roots and passes with the greater nerve to end at the celiac ganglion. The least splanchnic nerve arises from the T11-12 spinal roots and passes through the diaphragm to the celiac ganglion. It is important to note that the greater, lesser, and least splanchnic nerves are *preganglionic* structures that synapse at the celiac ganglia.[20] Blockade limited solely to these nerves is properly termed *splanchnic nerve block* (see later discussion).

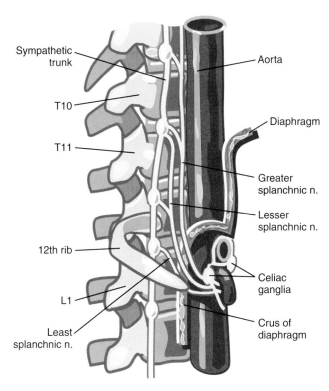

Fig. 160.2 The splanchnic nerves.

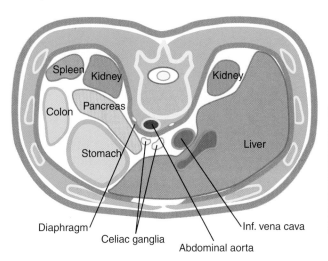

Fig. 160.3 The structures surrounding the celiac plexus.

The Celiac Ganglia

The three splanchnic nerves synapse at the celiac ganglia (see Fig. 160.2). Despite significant variability among patients of the anatomy of the celiac ganglia, the following generalizations can be drawn from anatomic studies.[31] The number of ganglia ranges from one to five and their diameters from 0.5 to 4.5 cm. The ganglia lie anterior and anterolateral to the aorta. The ganglia located on the left are uniformly farther inferior than their right-sided counterparts by as much as a vertebral level, but both groups of ganglia lie below the level of the celiac artery. In most instances, the ganglia lie approximately at the level of L1.

Postganglionic fibers radiate from the celiac ganglia along the course of the blood vessels and innervate the abdominal viscera, which are derived from the embryonic foregut[25] (i.e., much of the distal esophagus, stomach, duodenum, small intestine, ascending and proximal transverse colon, adrenal glands, pancreas, spleen, liver, and biliary system).

The Celiac Plexus

Ganglia and *plexus* are often used interchangeably, but, in point of fact, the ganglia and their respective dense network of preganglionic and postganglionic fibers constitute the celiac plexus. Anatomically, the celiac plexus arises from the preganglionic splanchnic nerves, vagal preganglionic parasympathetic fibers, sensory fibers from the phrenic nerve, and postganglionic sympathetic fibers.[28]

The celiac plexus is anterior to the diaphragmatic crura.[32] It extends in front of and around the aorta, the greatest concentration of fibers being anterior to the aorta (see Fig. 160.2). Blockade of these neural structures, which include the afferent fibers carrying nociceptive information, is properly termed *celiac plexus block*. It should be noted that the phrenic nerve also transmits nociceptive information from the upper abdominal viscera,[28] which may be perceived as poorly localized pain referred to the supraclavicular region.

Structures Surrounding the Celiac Plexus

The relation of the celiac plexus to the surrounding structures is depicted in **Figure 160.3**. The normal configuration of these structures may be dramatically distorted owing to organomegaly or tumor. The aorta lies anterior and slightly to the left of the anterior margin of the vertebral body. The inferior vena cava lies to the right of the midline, and the kidneys are posterolateral to the great vessels. The pancreas lies anterior to the celiac plexus. All of these structures lie within the retroperitoneal space.

Technique of Celiac Plexus and Splanchnic Nerve Block

The Classic Retrocrural Technique

The technique of celiac plexus block that is traditionally taught, and thus most commonly used by anesthesiologists for blocking the celiac plexus, is the retrocrural technique first described by Kappis[2] and subsequently refined and popularized by Moore.[14]

As with other techniques for celiac plexus and splanchnic nerve block, preparation includes administration of intravenous fluids to attenuate the hypotension associated with neural blockade of these structures. Evaluation for coagulopathy is especially indicated in those patients who have undergone antiblastic therapy or who have a history of significant alcohol abuse.[23] If radiographic contrast is to be used, evaluation of the patient's renal function is indicated as well.

The patient is placed in the prone position with a pillow beneath the abdomen to reverse the thoracolumbar lordosis. This position increases the distance between the costal margins and the iliac crests and between the transverse processes of adjacent vertebral bodies. For comfort, the patient's head is turned to the side, and the arms are permitted to hang freely off the sides of the table. The operative field is prepared and draped in standard aseptic manner.

Some clinicians find it beneficial to delineate the pertinent landmarks on the skin with a sterile marker. The landmarks

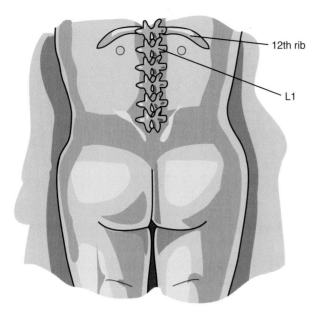

Fig. 160.4 Topographic landmarks for celiac plexus block.

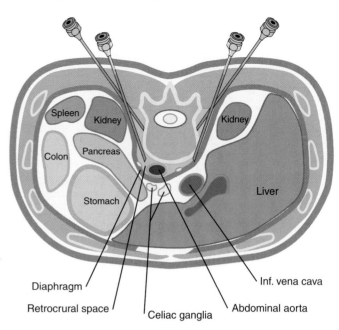

Fig. 160.5 Needle placement for "classic" celiac plexus block.

include the iliac crests, twelfth ribs, dorsal midline, vertebral bodies (T12-L2), and lateral borders of the paraspinal (sacrospinalis) muscles (**Fig. 160.4**). Moore[14] recommends that the intersection of the twelfth rib and the lateral border of the paraspinal muscles on each side (which corresponds to L2) be marked and connected with lines to each other and to the cephalic portion of the L1 spine, forming an isosceles triangle, the sides of which serve as an additional guide to needle positioning.

The skin and underlying subcutaneous tissues and musculature are infiltrated with 1.0% lidocaine at the points of needle entry, which is about four fingerbreadths (7.5 cm) lateral to the midline, just beneath the twelfth ribs. Either 20- or 22-gauge, 13 cm stylet needles are inserted bilaterally through the previously anesthetized areas. The needles are initially oriented 45 degrees toward the midline and about 15 degrees cephalad, to ensure contact with the L1 vertebral body (**Fig. 160.5**). Once contact with the vertebral body has been verified, the depth at which bone contact occurred is noted. (Some clinicians find it useful to mark this measurement on the shaft of the needle with a sterile gentian violet marker after the needle is withdrawn.)

After bone contact is made and the depth is noted, the needles are withdrawn to the level of the subcutaneous tissue and redirected slightly less mesiad (about 60 degrees from the midline) so as to "walk off" the lateral surface of the L1 vertebral body. The needles are reinserted to the depth at which contact with the vertebral body was first noted. At this point, if no contact with bone is made, the left-sided needle is gradually advanced 1.5 to 2 cm or until the pulsations emanating from the aorta and transmitted to the advancing needle are felt.[33,34] The right-sided needle is then advanced slightly farther (i.e., 3 to 4 cm past contact with the vertebral body). Ultimately, the tips of the needles should be just posterior to the aorta on the left and to the anterolateral aspect of the aorta on the right (see Fig. 160.5).

The stylets are removed, and the needle hubs are inspected for blood, cerebrospinal fluid, and urine. If radiographic guidance is being used, a small volume of contrast material is injected bilaterally and its spread is observed radiographically.

Ideally, on the fluoroscopic anteroposterior view, contrast material is confined to the midline and concentrated near the L1 vertebral body (**Fig. 160.6**). A smooth posterior contour can be observed that corresponds to the psoas fascia on the lateral view (**Fig. 160.7**).

Alternatively, if CT guidance is used, contrast material should appear lateral to and behind the aorta. If contrast material is confined entirely to the retrocrural space, the needles should be advanced to the precrural space to minimize the risk of posterior spread of local anesthetic or neurolytic agent to the somatic nerve roots (see later discussion).[35]

If radiographic guidance is not used, a local anesthetic with rapid onset and in sufficient concentration to produce motor block (such as 1.5% lidocaine or 3.0% 2-chloroprocaine) is given before administration of neurolytic agents. If the patient experiences no motor or sensory block after an adequate waiting time, it is likely that additional drugs injected through the needles will not reach the somatic nerve roots if given in similar volumes.

For diagnostic and prognostic block using the retrocrural technique, 12 to 15 mL of 1.0% lidocaine or 3.0% 2-chloroprocaine is administered through each needle.[18] For therapeutic local anesthetic block, 10 to 12 mL of 0.5% bupivacaine is administered through each needle. Owing to the potential for local anesthetic toxicity, all local anesthetics should be administered in incremental doses.[24] For treatment of the pain of acute pancreatitis, an 80-mg dose of depot methylprednisolone is advocated for the initial celiac plexus block, and 40 mg for subsequent blocks.[36]

Most investigators suggest that 10 to 12 mL of 50% ethyl alcohol or 6.0% aqueous phenol be injected through each needle for retrocrural neurolytic block. Thomson et al,[34] however, strongly recommend that 25 mL of 50% ethyl alcohol be injected via each needle.

After the neurolytic solution has been injected, each needle should be flushed with sterile saline solution. (There have been anecdotal reports of neurolytic solution being tracked posteriorly along with the needles as they are withdrawn.) Radiographic guidance, in particular CT guidance, offers the

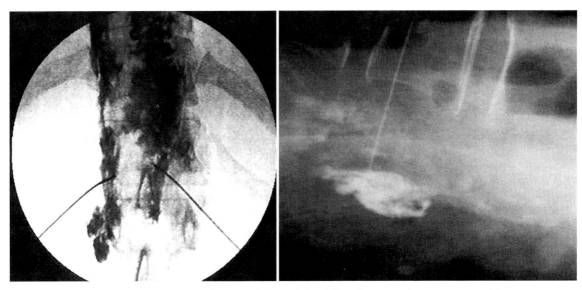

Fig. 160.6 Anteroposterior fluoroscopic view of the midline placement of contrast agent at L1.

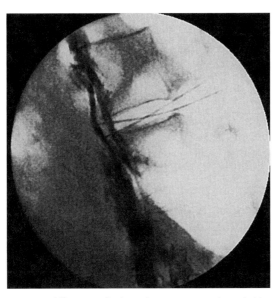

Fig. 160.7 Lateral fluoroscopic view of contrast agent bounded by psoas fascia.

pain specialist an added margin of safety when performing neurolytic celiac plexus block and thus should be used whenever possible.

Transcrural Techniques

The diaphragm separates the thoracic and abdominal cavities but permits the passage of the thoracoabdominal structures, including the aorta, vena cava, and splanchnic nerves. The diaphragmatic crura are bilateral structures that arise from the anterolateral surfaces of the upper two or three lumbar vertebrae and disks. The crura of the diaphragm serve as a barrier to effectively separate the splanchnic nerves from the celiac ganglia and plexus below.[28]

In the modified Kappis approach to celiac plexus block, described previously, the needles are behind the crura in almost all instances. That is to say, the needles and injected solution are placed posterior and cephalad to the crura of the diaphragm. On the basis of CT and cadaver studies, it has been

suggested that the classic method of retrocrural block is more likely to produce splanchnic nerve block rather than blockade of the celiac plexus. Instead of depositing injected material around and anterior to the aorta and directly onto the celiac plexus at the level of the L1 vertebral body, as was previously thought, the injectate appears to (1) concentrate posterior to the aorta and in front of and along the side of the L1 vertebral body, where it may anesthetize retroaortic celiac fibers; (2) diffuse cephalad to anesthetize the splanchnic nerve at a site rostrad to the origin of the plexus; and (3) finally encircle the aorta at the site of the celiac plexus only when a sufficient volume of drug is injected to transgress the diaphragm by diffusing caudad through the aortic hiatus.[33,37]

Although the retrocrural approach has been shown to be generally effective and safe, advocates of the transcrural approaches believe that simple modifications maximize the spread of injected solutions anterior to the aorta, where the celiac plexus is most concentrated, and minimize the risk of somatic nerve root blocks. The term *transcrural* reflects placement of needle tips and drug anterior and caudal to the diaphragmatic crura.

Singler[37] and others recommend a transcrural approach using, respectively, CT scan and fluoroscopic guidance as important modifications of the traditional retrocrural technique. Transcrural block is carried out in a manner essentially the same as that for retrocrural block, except that needles are advanced farther anteriorly. Slightly smaller volumes of local anesthetic and neurolytic agents are used for the bilateral transcrural approach. Efficacy equal to or slightly greater than that of the classic retrocrural approach is reported by most investigators.[38]

Transaortic Techniques

In 1983, Ischia et al[39] introduced a new approach to transcrural celiac plexus block that involved placing a single needle on the left side and posteriorly through the aorta, to ensure that the injected drugs are placed in the precrural space directly onto the celiac plexus. This method is, in some respects, analogous to the transaxillary approach to brachial plexus block. The safety of the transaortic approach is suggested by previous experience with both axillary block and translumbar aortograms.[40]

Despite concerns about the potential for aortic trauma and subsequent occult retroperitoneal hemorrhage with the transaortic approach to celiac plexus block, it may, in fact, be safer than the classic two-needle posterior approach.[41,42] The lower incidence of complications is thought to be due in part to the use of a single fine needle rather than two larger ones. The fact that the aorta is relatively well supported in this region by the diaphragmatic crura and prevertebral fascia also contributes to the technique's apparent relative safety.[41]

The transaortic approach to celiac plexus block has three additional advantages over the classic two-needle approach. First, it avoids the risks of neurologic complications related to posterior retrocrural spread of drugs. Second, the aorta provides a definitive landmark for needle placement when radiographic guidance is not available. Third, much smaller volumes of local anesthetic and neurolytic solutions are required to achieve efficacy equal to or greater than that of the classic retrocrural approach.[42]

Fluoroscopically Guided Transaortic Celiac Plexus Block

The fluoroscopically guided transaortic approach uses the usual landmarks for the posterior placement of a left-sided, 22-gauge, 13 cm stylet needle. Some investigators use a needle entry point 1.0 to 1.5 cm closer to the midline than that for the classic retrocrural approach, combined with a needle trajectory closer to the perpendicular, to reduce the incidence of renal trauma.

The needle is advanced with the goal of passing just lateral to the anterolateral aspect of the L1 vertebral body. If that vertebral body is encountered, the needle is withdrawn into the subcutaneous tissues and redirected in a manner analogous to that for the classic retrocrural approach. The stylet needle is gradually advanced until its tip rests in the posterior periaortic space. As the needle impinges on the posterior aortic wall, the operator feels transmitted aortic pulsations via the needle and greater resistance to its passage.

Passing the needle through the wall of the aorta has been likened to passing a needle through a large rubber band. Presence of the needle within the aortic lumen is evidenced by free flow of arterial blood when the stylet is removed. The stylet is replaced, and the needle is advanced until it impinges on the intraluminal anterior wall of the aorta. At this point, the operator again feels increased resistance to needle advancement. A pop is felt as the needle tip passes through the anterior aortic wall, indicating that it probably lies within the preaortic fatty connective tissue and the substance of the celiac plexus. A saline loss-of-resistance technique, as described earlier, may help in identification of the preaortic space.

Because the needle is sometimes inadvertently advanced beyond the retroperitoneal space into the peritoneal cavity, confirmatory fluoroscopic views of injected contrast medium are advised, especially when neurolytic blockade is to be done. On anteroposterior views, the contrast medium should be confined to the midline, with a tendency toward greater concentration around the lateral margins of the aorta. Lateral views should demonstrate a predominantly preaortic orientation extending from around T12 through L2, sometimes accompanied by pulsations.[25] Incomplete penetration of the anterior wall is indicated by a narrow longitudinal "line image."

Failure of the contrast medium to completely surround the anterior aorta may occur in the presence of extensive infiltration of the preaortic region by tumor or in patients who have undergone previous pancreatic surgery or radiation therapy. It is our experience that the chance of success is smaller when poor or irregular preaortic spread of contrast is observed. In this setting, selective alcohol neurolysis of the splanchnic nerves may provide better pain relief.

For diagnostic and prognostic block using the fluoroscopically guided transaortic technique, 10 to 12 mL of 1.5% lidocaine or 3.0% 2-chloroprocaine is administered through the needle. For therapeutic block, 10 to 12 mL of 0.5% bupivacaine is administered. Owing to the potential for local anesthetic toxicity, all local anesthetics should be administered in incremental doses. For treatment of the pain of acute pancreatitis, the same dosages of depot methylprednisolone mentioned previously for the retrocrural and transcrural techniques are indicated. Absolute alcohol or 6.0% aqueous phenol, 12 to 15 mL, is used for neurolytic block.

Computed Tomography–Guided Transaortic Celiac Plexus Block

The CT-guided transaortic celiac plexus block is probably the safest way to achieve neurolysis of the celiac plexus. CT allows the pain management physician to clearly identify the clinically relevant anatomy, including the crura of the diaphragm, aorta, vena cava, and kidneys, to ensure accurate precrural needle placement. Observation of the spread of contrast medium, as described here, enables the physician to know exactly where the injectate is deposited, and provides an added margin of patient safety in comparison with fluoroscopic or blind techniques.

The patient is prepared for CT-guided transaortic celiac plexus block just as for the techniques described earlier. After proper positioning on the CT scanning table, a scout film is obtained to identify the T12-L1 interspace (**Fig. 160.8**). A CT image is then taken through the interspace. The scan is reviewed for the position of the aorta relative to the vertebral body, the position of intra-abdominal and retroperitoneal organs, and any distortions of normal anatomy by tumor, previous surgery, or adenopathy (**Fig. 160.9**). The aorta at this level is evaluated for significant aortic aneurysm, mural thrombus, or calcifications; any of these would recommend against use of a transaortic approach.[23]

The level at which the scan was taken is identified on the patient's skin and marked with a gentian violet marker. The skin is prepared with antiseptic solution. The skin, subcutaneous tissues, and muscle at a point approximately 2.5 inches from the left of the midline are anesthetized with 1.0% lidocaine. A 13 cm, 22-gauge stylet needle is placed through the anesthetized area and is advanced until the posterior wall of the aorta is encountered, as evidenced by transmission of arterial pulsations and greater resistance to needle advancement. The needle is advanced into the lumen of the aorta. The stylet is removed, and the needle hub is observed for free flow of arterial blood (**Fig. 160.10**).

A well-lubricated 5 mL glass syringe filled with preservative-free saline is attached to the needle hub. The needle and syringe are then advanced through the anterior wall of the aorta using a loss-of-resistance technique in the same way that it is used to identify the epidural space.[43] The glass syringe is

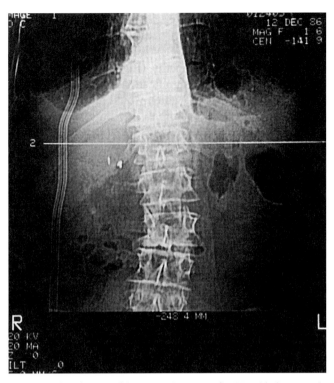

Fig. 160.8 Identification of the T12-L1 interspace for CT-guided transaortic celiac plexus block.

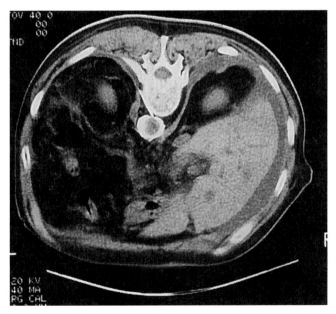

Fig. 160.9 CT scan through the T12-L1 interspace.

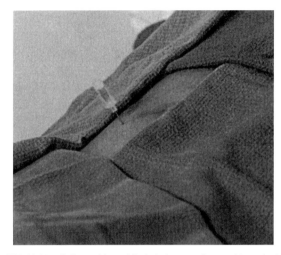

Fig. 160.10 Needle in position with tip in lumen of aorta. Note the blood in the hub of the needle.

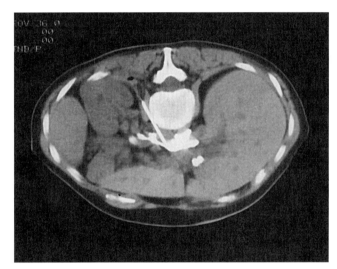

Fig. 160.11 Preaortic spread of contrast agent.

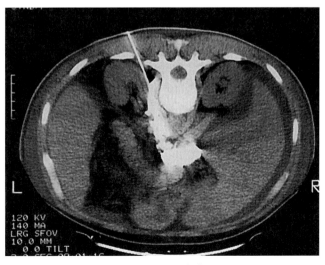

Fig. 160.12 Retrocrural spread of contrast agent.

removed, and 3.0 mL of 1.5% lidocaine in solution with an equal amount of water-soluble contrast medium is injected through the needle.

A CT scan at the level of the needle's tip is taken. The scan is reviewed for the placement of the needle and, most important, for the spread of contrast medium,[23] which should be seen in the preaortic area and surrounding the aorta (**Fig. 160.11**). No contrast medium should be observed in the retrocrural space (**Fig. 160.12**). After proper needle placement and spread of contrast medium is confirmed, 12 to 15 mL of absolute alcohol or 6% aqueous phenol is injected through the needle.[42] The needle is flushed with a small amount of sterile saline and then removed. The patient is observed carefully for hemodynamic changes, including hypotension and tachycardia secondary to the resulting profound sympathetic blockade.

Lieberman and Waldman[43] reported on the success and efficacy of transaortic celiac plexus block using the loss-of-resistance technique in a large series of patients suffering from cancer pain.[43] In this study, 91% of patients reported marked immediate pain relief after CT-guided transaortic celiac plexus block using the loss-of-resistance technique. At 6 weeks, 39% of surviving patients were pain free and did not require opioid analgesics. An additional 50% of patients reported great improvement but required adjunctive treatment with opioids. No unusual complications or side effects were encountered in this large series of patients.

Anterior Approaches to Celiac Plexus Block
Percutaneous Gangliolysis

A percutaneous anterior approach to the celiac plexus was advocated early in the twentieth century, only to be abandoned because of the high incidence of complications.[3,44] The advent of fine needles, improvements in radiologic guidance technology, and the maturation of the specialty of interventional radiology have since led to renewed interest in the anterior approach to blockade of the celiac plexus.

Extensive experience with transabdominal fine-needle aspiration biopsy has confirmed the relative safety of this approach and provides the rationale and method for the modification of this radiologic technique for anterior celiac plexus block. The anterior approach to the celiac plexus necessarily involves the passage of a fine needle through the liver, stomach, intestine, vessels, and pancreas. Surprisingly, it is associated with very low rates of complications.[45-48]

Advantages of the anterior approach to blocking the celiac plexus include its relative ease, speed, and reduced periprocedural discomfort as compared with posterior techniques.[16,25] Perhaps the greatest advantage of the anterior approach is the fact that patients are spared having to remain prone for long periods, which can be a significant problem for patients suffering from intra-abdominal pain. The supine position is also advantageous for patients with iliostomies and colostomies.

The anterior approach is probably associated with less discomfort because only one needle is used. The needle does not impinge on either periosteum or nerve roots or pass through the bulky paraspinous musculature. Because needle placement is precrural, there is less risk of accidental neurologic injury related to retrocrural spread of drug to somatic nerve roots or epidural and subarachnoid spaces.

Potential disadvantages of the anterior approach to celiac plexus block include the risks of infection, abscess, hemorrhage, and fistula formation.[46] Although preliminary findings indicate that these complications are exceedingly rare, further experience is needed to draw a definitive conclusion. By the same token, although preliminary data suggest the efficacy of the anterior approach, further experience is needed to permit adequate comparisons with better-established techniques.

The anterior technique can be carried out under CT or ultrasound guidance. Patient preparation is similar to that for posterior approaches to celiac block. The patient is placed in the

supine position on the CT or ultrasound table. The skin of the upper abdomen is prepared with antiseptic solution. The needle entry site is identified 1.5 cm below and 1.5 cm to the left of the xyphoid process (**Fig. 160.13**).[45] At that point, the skin, subcutaneous tissues, and musculature are anesthetized with 1.0% lidocaine. A 22-gauge, 15 cm needle is introduced through the anesthetized area perpendicular to the skin and advanced to the depth of the anterior wall of the aorta, as calculated using CT or ultrasound guidance (**Figs. 160.14** and **160.15**).

If CT guidance is being used, 4 mL of water-soluble contrast in solution with an equal volume of 1.0% lidocaine is injected to confirm needle placement (**Fig. 160.16**). If ultrasound guidance is being used, 10 to 12 mL of sterile saline can be injected to help confirm needle position (**Fig. 160.17**).[16] After satisfactory needle placement is confirmed, diagnostic and prognostic

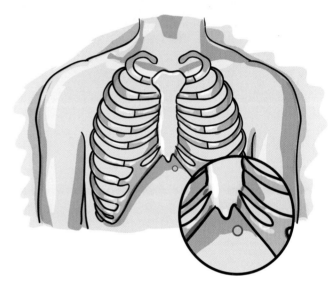

Fig. 160.13 Needle entry site for anterior celiac plexus block. *Inset,* The site is located 1.5 cm below and 1.5 cm to the left of the xyphoid process.

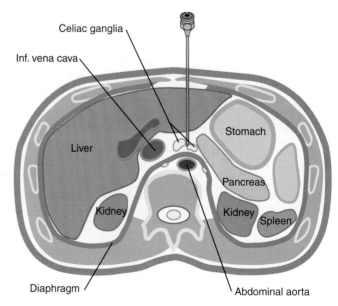

Fig. 160.14 Needle placement for anterior celiac plexus block.

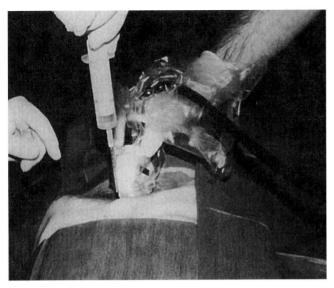

Fig. 160.15 Anterior celiac plexus block.

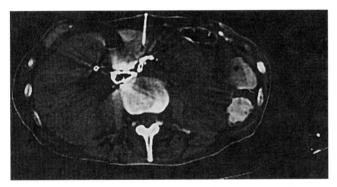

Fig. 160.16 Computed tomography scan confirms proper needle placement for anterior celiac plexus block.

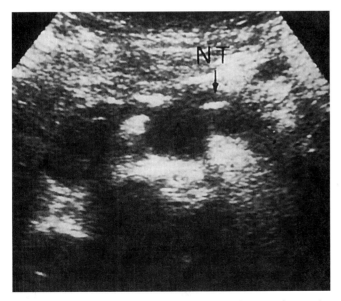

Fig. 160.17 Ultrasonogram confirms proper needle placement for anterior celiac plexus block.

block is carried out using 15 mL of 1.5% lidocaine or 3.0% 2-chloroprocaine. Therapeutic block is performed with an equal volume of 0.5% bupivacaine. Owing to the potential for local anesthetic toxicity, all local anesthetics should be administered in incremental doses.

Matamala et al[16] recommend 35 to 40 mL of 50% ethyl alcohol for neurolytic blocks of the celiac plexus via the anterior approach. Other investigators have had equally good results using 15 to 20 mL of absolute alcohol.

An alternative technique uses fluoroscopy to guide the passage of a single needle just to the right of the center of the L1 vertebral body, after which it is withdrawn 1 to 3 cm.[45] Important precautions for the anterior approach to celiac plexus block include the administration of prophylactic antibiotics and the use of needles no larger than 22 gauge to minimize the risks of infection and trauma to the vasculature and viscera.

Intraoperative Gangliolysis

The intraoperative anterior approach to the blockade of the celiac plexus and splanchnic nerves was first advocated by Braun[4] in 1921 as a means to provide intraoperative visceral anesthesia. This technique was used in combination with field block of the abdominal wall. Braun's approach involved gentle retraction of the stomach and placement of a digit between the aorta and vena cava to serve as a guide to the injection of an anesthetic over the ventral surface of the L1 vertebral body. This technique enjoyed only limited acceptance for surgical anesthesia for abdominal operations.

In 1978, Kraft and associates described a similar approach to block the splanchnic nerves and celiac plexus for pain management.[49,50] They identified the origin of the celiac artery and advanced a 20-gauge spinal needle over the exploring finger. Then, 15 to 20 mL of 6% aqueous phenol was injected intraoperatively.

The main advantage of intraoperative celiac block is the elimination of a separate procedure for pain control. In addition, intraoperative celiac block provides an opportunity to prophylactically treat the patient with only mild or no pain who is known to have an intra-abdominal malignancy that in all likelihood will produce pain as it progresses.

Disadvantages of intraoperative anterior celiac plexus neurolysis include the unfamiliarity of most surgeons with (1) the functional regional anatomy, (2) injection techniques, and (3) the use of neurolytic agents required for the block.[25] Furthermore, safe access to the specified injection site may be prohibited by bulky intra-abdominal disease and phlegmon. Because intraoperative dissection may result in leakage of the injected solution out of the intended injection site, the risk of neurologic injury is increased and the overall efficacy is decreased.[25] Concurrent general anesthesia renders a test dosing with local anesthetic invalid and further raises the patient's risk, because of the patient's inability to report untoward reactions to the local anesthetic.

Given the current availability of effective percutaneous methods of achieving celiac block, intraoperative celiac plexus block cannot be recommended except when laparotomy is already planned for exploration or bypass of the gastrointestinal or biliary tract.[49] Even in these cases, the efficacy and relative safety of the technique are controversial. A valuable alternative in such cases is placement of surgical clips in the vicinity of the celiac axis to facilitate postoperative neural blockade.[51]

Catheter Techniques

Anecdotal reports documenting the efficacy and safety of temporary periaortic catheters to facilitate daily celiac nerve blocks have been presented.[52,53] A percutaneous polytetrafluoroethylene periaortic catheter was in place for 14 days in a patient with pancreatitis, during which time serial injections of local anesthetic were administered before a definitive neurolytic block was performed.[54] Fluoroscopy and CT performed 13 days after placement revealed no catheter migration and no perivascular erosion or pleural reaction. A second report, documenting a single case of intraoperative placement of a percutaneously tunneled epidural catheter that was used after surgery to produce neurolysis, suggests another potential treatment option.[55] In a third report, after a temporary periaortic catheter was placed percutaneously, the patient had persistent hematuria, and evidence of transrenal catheter placement was obtained. This case suggests that CT guidance may be advisable during placement of percutaneous catheters for celiac plexus block.[28]

At present, indications for periaortic catheterization are ill-defined. If shown to be safe and efficacious, this approach may ultimately prove beneficial in patients with chronic nonmalignant conditions.

Splanchnic Nerve Block

The recognition that splanchnic nerve block may provide relief of pain in a subset of patients who fail to obtain relief from celiac plexus block has renewed interest in this technique.[25,56] The splanchnic nerves transmit the majority of nociceptive information from the viscera.[28] These nerves are contained in a narrow compartment made up by the vertebral body and the pleura laterally, the posterior mediastinum ventrally, and the pleural attachment to the vertebra dorsally. This compartment is bounded caudally by the crura of the diaphragm. Abram and Boas[56] have determined that the volume of this compartment is approximately 10 mL on each side.

The technique for splanchnic nerve block differs little from the classic retrocrural approach to the celiac plexus, except that the needles are aimed more cephalad so as to rest ultimately at the anterolateral margin of the T12 vertebral body (**Fig. 160.18**). It is imperative that both needles be placed medially against the vertebral body to reduce the incidence of pneumothorax.

An alternative approach to splanchnic nerve block uses 22-gauge, 3.5-inch spinal needles.[57] The needles are placed 3 to 4 cm lateral to the midline, just below the twelfth ribs. Their trajectory is slightly mesiad, so that the tips come to rest at the anterolateral margin of the T12 body.

Abram and Boas[56] have described a simplified technique for splanchnic nerve block that uses a paravertebral transthoracic approach. Standard 22-gauge, 3.5-inch spinal needles are introduced bilaterally 6 cm from the midline through the eleventh intercostal space (see Fig. 160.18). The needle is advanced to rest against the anterolateral aspect of the T11 vertebral body. Precautions include attendance to a medial entry point and observation of the lower limit of the lung, which during quiet breathing is generally observed to lie one segment higher in the costophrenic angle. These precautions allow the needles to safely traverse the transpleural spaces. If experience eventually demonstrates that this simplified technique is comparable in

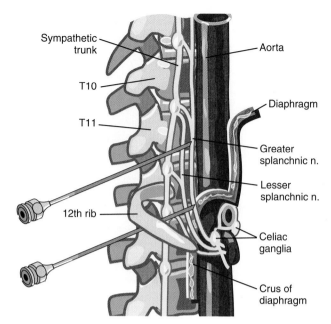

Fig. 160.18 Splanchnic nerve block.

safety and efficacy to the more difficult classic technique, it will clearly become the procedure of choice for splanchnic nerve block.

For diagnostic and prognostic splanchnic nerve block, 7 to 10 mL of 1.5% lidocaine or 3.0% 2-chloroprocaine is administered through the needle; for therapeutic block, 7 to 10 mL of 0.5% bupivacaine. Owing to the potential for local anesthetic toxicity, all local anesthetics should be administered in divided doses. A 10 mL volume of absolute alcohol or 6.0% aqueous phenol is used for neurolytic block.

The risks of splanchnic nerve block are similar to those of celiac plexus block. Additionally, the rates of pneumothorax, thoracic duct injury, and inadvertent spread of injected drugs to the somatic nerve roots are higher than those for transcrural approaches to celiac plexus block.[56] Because of the need for accurate needle placement, it is advisable to perform splanchnic nerve block under fluoroscopic or CT guidance.

Choice of Agent, Volume, Needle, Radiographic Guidance, and Technique

Choice of Agent

Investigators tend to disagree about the ideal volume, concentration, or drug for celiac plexus and splanchnic nerve blocks. Diagnostic and prognostic celiac plexus and splanchnic nerve blocks should be performed with a local anesthetic that has rapid onset and is sufficiently concentrated to produce sensory and motor block. For the classic two-needle retrocrural approach, a total volume of 20 to 25 mL of 1.0% lidocaine or 3.0% 2-chloroprocaine is appropriate. A volume of 12 to 15 mL is adequate for a single-needle transcrural approach to the celiac plexus block. Splanchnic nerve block is performed with 7 to 10 mL of 1.5% lidocaine or 3.0% 2-chloroprocaine. Similar volumes (as specified for each technique) of longer-acting local anesthetics such as 0.5% bupivacaine are used for therapeutic nerve block. Owing to the potential for local anesthetic toxicity, all local anesthetics should be administered in incremental doses. For the pain of inflammatory conditions such as pancreatitis, depot preparations of methylprednisolone may be administered in an initial dose of 80 mg and subsequent doses of 40 mg.

Neurolytic blockade of the celiac plexus and splanchnic nerves may be carried out with either ethyl alcohol or aqueous phenol. Because of limitations associated with the classic retrocrural technique, some authors have advocated 50 mL of 50% ethyl alcohol. Others have used concentrations of alcohol (25% to 100%) in volumes ranging from 20 to 80 mL without apparent differences in efficacy or side effects.[27,58,59] Smaller volumes (12 to 15 mL) of absolute alcohol are recommended for single-needle transcrural techniques.

Many investigators believe that as a neurolytic agent, alcohol is superior to phenol in duration of neural blockade; however, alcohol has the disadvantage of producing transient severe pain on injection. Furthermore, alcohol is not miscible with contrast medium. Unless alcohol is accidentally injected into a vessel, actual alcohol intoxication should not occur. Susceptible patients undergoing alcohol neurolysis may be subject to acetaldehyde syndrome, a relatively innocuous side effect (see discussion of complications).[34,60,61] Alcohol should be avoided in patients on disulfiram therapy for alcohol abuse.

Several workers have recommended 6% to 10% phenol for celiac plexus and splanchnic nerve block.[25,49,50] An advantage of phenol over alcohol is that it can be combined with contrast medium. The combination allows radiographic documentation of the distribution of neurolytic solution during and after injection, instead of relying on verification of needle placement before injection of neurolytic solution, as is necessary for alcohol injection. Mixtures of 10% phenol and iodinated contrast medium (Conray 420 or Renografin 76) remain stable up to 3 months.[62] The fact that phenol is not commercially available and must be prepared for each patient by a pharmacist is a practical disadvantage of this agent. The apparently greater affinity of phenol for vascular, rather than neurologic, tissue also represents a theoretical disadvantage, in view of the vascularity of the region surrounding the celiac plexus and splanchnic nerves.[63] Some investigators believe that phenol produces a block of shorter duration than that produced by alcohol, making it a less desirable agent for the intractable and progressive pain of cancer. It is important to note that controlled comparisons between alcohol and phenol for this application have not been conducted but they appear to be equally safe and efficacious.

Choice of Needles

Both 20- and 22-gauge needles have been advocated for celiac plexus and splanchnic nerve block. Moore[58] notes that the resistance to injection provided by a long 22-gauge needle interferes with the appreciation of differences in tissue compliance, which can provide much useful information about needle position. In addition, owing to the greater flexibility of 22-gauge needles, it is more difficult to maintain a straight trajectory during placement.[28] If 22-gauge needles are used, it is advisable to rely on radiologic guidance to confirm needle placement. A 22-gauge needle is preferred for anterior and transaortic approaches.[64]

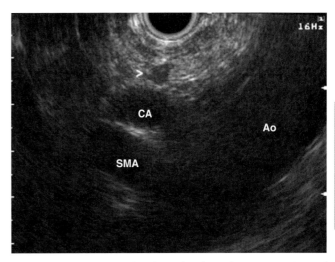

Fig. 160.19 A celiac ganglion (*arrowhead*) can be seen anterior and cephalad to the origin of the celiac artery (*CA*). *Ao,* aorta; *SMA,* superior mesenteric artery. *(From Penman ID, Gilbert D: Basic technique for celiac plexus block/neurolysis,* Gastrointest Endosc 69[2 suppl 1]:S163, 2009.)

Choice of Radiographic Guidance

The use of radiologic guidance for celiac plexus and splanchnic nerve block was once very controversial. Today, it is in favor. Provided that proper precautions are observed, celiac plexus and splanchnic nerve block with local anesthetic can safely be accomplished by experienced practitioners relying on topographic guidance alone.[34] In our opinion, and that of others, radiologic guidance is virtually mandatory for neurolytic celiac plexus and splanchnic nerve block.[23,35] Interestingly, when large series of cases are compared, it is not clear that the use of fluoroscopy actually reduces the incidence of complications.[64] It does appear, however, that CT guidance may add a margin of safety as compared with fluoroscopy, although a small number of serious complications have been reported when CT has been used for celiac plexus block.[43,64] It is our strong belief that the use of radiographic guidance must still be encouraged on practical, empirical, and medicolegal grounds.

It is clear that even sophisticated radiologic guidance by itself does not ensure against complications. Routine application of simple precautionary measures, including careful serial aspiration and incremental injections of local anesthetic, is essential to minimize the likelihood of an adverse outcome. CT permits visualization of not only bony structures, but also vascular and soft tissue elements (including diaphragmatic crura and tumor spread). It is particularly useful when anterior and transcrural approaches are planned. The disadvantages of CT include limited availability in some areas, the need for specialized support personnel, and the slightly higher cost relative to fluoroscopy.[28] Ultrasound guidance has recently been employed with greater frequency, especially for anterior and endoscopic approaches (**Fig. 160.19**).

Choice of Technique

Numerous techniques have been advocated to achieve celiac plexus and splanchnic nerve block. Most of the experience is with the classic retrocrural technique, which, as a result, is regarded as the standard against which other techniques are compared. It is anticipated that the newer techniques for celiac plexus and splanchnic nerve block will gain greater acceptance as experience accrues because they appear to be safe and efficacious and offer certain practical and theoretical advantages. The transaortic approach is particularly attractive, because it requires only a single needle—the position of which is easily verifiable—ensuring anterior deposition of the drug.[43] The anterior approach, although it requires CT or ultrasound guidance, is quick and relatively painless. It is an excellent option for patients who cannot assume the prone position.[16] The transcrural approach, with or without CT, is theoretically more desirable than retrocrural techniques, because injectate spreads reliably around the aorta, thereby avoiding the somatic nerves.[28] Ultimately, the choice of technique should be individualized to the facility, the patient's physical status, the extent of tumor spread, and the clinician's experience and preparation. As this debate continues, gastroenterologists have become advocates of celiac plexus block, which can be performed under echoendoscopic guidance[65] (see Fig. 160.19). This technique is performed by placing an echoendoscopic probe near the posterior lesser curve of the gastric fundus via oral scope placement to visualize the aorta and the celiac artery and plexus. The needle tip is advanced to the deepest point within the ganglia, and the neurolytic solution is then injected.

Complications

In the hands of the skilled clinician, serious complications should rarely occur from celiac plexus and splanchnic nerve block.[66] However, because of the proximity of other vital structures, coupled with the use of large volumes of neurolytic drugs, the following side effects and complications may be seen:

- Hypotension
- Paresthesia of lumbar somatic nerve
- Intravascular injection (venous or arterial)
- Deficit of lumbar somatic nerve
- Subarachnoid or epidural injection
- Diarrhea
- Renal injury
- Paraplegia
- Pneumothorax
- Chylothorax
- Vascular thrombosis or embolism
- Vascular trauma
- Perforation of cysts or tumors
- Injection of the psoas muscle
- Intradiskal injection
- Abscess
- Peritonitis
- Retroperitoneal hematoma
- Urinary tract abnormalities
- Failure of ejaculation
- Pain during and after procedure
- Failure to relieve pain

Hypotension, Altered Gastrointestinal Motility, and Pain

Hypotension[67] and increased gastrointestinal motility occur to some extent in most patients following celiac plexus and splanchnic nerve block. The high frequency of these side effects dictates that they should be anticipated with either prophylactic treatment or a well-conceived management plan. Hypotension occurs as a result of regional vasodilation and pooling of blood within the splanchnic vessels. This side effect is more likely to occur in patients who are elderly, debilitated, and chronically or acutely dehydrated. Without prophylaxis, clinically significant hypotension can be expected in 30% to 60% of patients but may be prevented by administration of 500 to 1000 mL of balanced salt solution intravenously before the procedure.[58] Small increments of intravenous ephedrine are occasionally required, in addition to intravenous fluids, to maintain an adequate blood pressure. Careful monitoring of blood pressure during the procedure and the recovery period is mandatory. A gradual return to a sitting position is indicated to allow early identification and treatment of unrecognized orthostatic hypotension.

Gastrointestinal hypermotility may occur as a result of unopposed parasympathetic activity. It occasionally manifests as diarrhea, except in cancer patients, who tend to be chronically constipated from high doses of opioids. For them, the hypermotility improves bowel habits. Self-limited diarrhea lasting 36 to 48 hours has been reported in as many as 60% of patients after alcohol celiac block.[39] Unrecognized, this side effect can be life threatening.[67]

Although not a complication per se, pain can occur during and after celiac plexus and splanchnic nerve block. The interval to maximal pain relief after the procedure is variable. In the majority of patients, relief is immediate and complete; in others, it develops over a few days.[59] It is not uncommon for a patient to experience transient self-limited back or pleuritic pain after the procedure.[55]

Neurologic and Vascular Complications

Among 3000 cases of celiac plexus and splanchnic nerve block, Moore[58] reported 18 episodes of dural puncture (0.006%). In all but one case, it was manifested as the appearance of clear fluid in the needle hub.[58] In the majority of these cases, radiographic guidance was not used. The results of a more contemporary series suggest that this complication can be avoided by consistent use of radiographic guidance, as can epidural puncture. One case of unilateral paraplegia was reported in a patient who, because of obesity and ascites, was positioned laterally.[34] No form of radiologic guidance was used in that case. It is probable that paraplegia was the result of unrecognized injection of the psoas muscle that accidentally produced neurolysis of lumbar somatic nerve roots.

With the classic retrocrural technique, the anesthetic may track posteriorly (even when "correct" needle placement has been confirmed) and be deposited near somatic nerve roots. The consequent neurologic injury may manifest as numbness over the anterior thigh and lower abdominal wall and quadriceps weakness.[26] This complication is less likely when transcrural techniques are used.[37,43]

Another potential mechanism of neurologic injury is disruption of or accidental injection into the small nutrient vessels of the spinal cord (i.e., the artery of Adamkiewicz).[28] This mechanism was postulated to be responsible for the rapid development of persistent paraplegia after celiac plexus block with 6 mL of 6% aqueous phenol in a patient with carcinoma of the pancreas.[68] Neither test doses of local anesthetic nor radiologic guidance was used in this case. To avoid this serious complication, preneurolysis test doses of local anesthetic and either fluoroscopy to detect "vascular runoff" or CT guidance should be used to confirm exact needle placement.[69] It is not uncommon for larger vessels to be entered, either by accident or by intention.[43,64] An obvious and essential precaution, intermittent aspiration is not entirely reliable for detecting intravascular placement. Giving test doses of local anesthetics and using radiographic guidance decrease the incidence of this potentially lethal complication. Clinically significant bleeding and hematoma formation have not been reported in the literature, even after transaortic blocks. It is essential that each patient's coagulation status be investigated and, if necessary, optimized before the procedure.

Visceral Injury

The advent of CT guidance for celiac plexus and splanchnic nerve block revealed that perforation of adjacent viscera, including the kidney, occurred more often than had been appreciated. Renal puncture is characteristically a self-limited complication suggested by the appearance of transient hematuria. Accidental injection of an appreciable volume of neurolytic drug into the renal parenchyma, however, may produce serious injury and renal infarction. Moore[58] believes that renal puncture is more likely when (1) needles are inserted farther than 7.5 cm from the midline; (2) the needle tip comes to rest too far lateral to the vertebral body; and (3) a relatively higher vertebral body (T11) is targeted.

Careful attention to technique reduces the incidence of perforation of the viscera. The risk can be further reduced by using CT guidance. An obvious advantage of CT is the ability to visualize the anatomic relationships of visceral structures before and during needle placement.[36] This practice is particularly useful in patients whose normal anatomy is distorted because of a bulky tumor or a previous surgical insult.

Pneumothorax and Pleural Effusion

Pneumothorax may occur as a result of celiac plexus and splanchnic nerve block, even when the operator has radiologic guidance. This complication may or may not require tube thoracostomy. Pleural effusion after celiac plexus neurolysis has also been reported.[70,71] The proposed mechanism of pleural effusion is diaphragmatic irritation resulting from overflow of alcohol into the subdiaphragmatic space. Other suggested mechanisms include acute pancreatitis and hemorrhage. Chylothorax, an occasional complication of translumbar aortography, has been reported to have occurred on one occasion after phenol celiac plexus block.[72,73] Ejaculatory failure has also been reported after celiac plexus neurolysis.[74]

Metabolic Complications

Although accidental intravascular injection of alcohol could conceivably produce intoxication, several investigators have measured serum ethanol levels after celiac block and have determined that circulating levels are insufficient to produce systemic effects.[61,68,75] After 50 mL of 50% alcohol administered via the classic retrocrural approach, peak serum ethanol levels ranged from 21 to 39 mg/dL. These levels are well below the legally defined levels for intoxication.

Accumulation of high levels of acetaldehyde has been observed in persons with an atypical phenotype for the enzyme aldehyde dehydrogenase. This genetic defect, which is more common in Asians, has been implicated in facial flushing, palpitations, and hypotension in susceptible persons.[60] Such patients report a history of facial flushing after ingesting small amounts of alcoholic beverages, which represents potentially useful data. The use of alcohol as a neurolytic agent should also be avoided in patients undergoing disulfiram therapy for alcoholism.

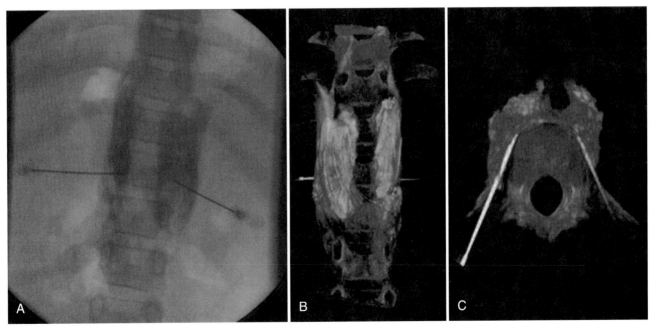

Fig. 160.20 A, Standard fluoroscopic needle placement confirmation. B, Final injection, 3-dimensional rotational angiography (3DRA) imaging, anteroposterior view. Note spread of injectate along 5 vertebral bodies. C, Final injection, 3DRA imaging, sagittal view. Note that in conjunction with B, retrocrural space is completely filled. *(From Goldschneider KR, Racadio JM, Weidner NJ: Celiac plexus blockade in children using a three-dimensional fluoroscopic reconstruction technique: case reports,* Reg Anesth Pain Med *32:510, 2007.)*

The finding that amylase levels measured before and after celiac plexus block remained normal in a series of 20 patients suggests that pancreatic injury does not typically occur with this procedure.[75] Alterations in creatine phosphokinase (CPK) levels were minimal in most of the patients studied, suggesting absence of significant skeletal muscle injury. Interestingly, the only two patients with significantly elevated CPK levels (4242 and 1640 IU/L) also experienced side effects consistent with damage to nearby muscle tissue (bilateral L1 neuritis and back pain). A single case of a generalized seizure and transient loss of consciousness has been reported after apparent accidental intravascular injection of phenol.[76]

Future Directions

Further technologic advances in radiology should produce continued improvements in the efficacy and safety of celiac plexus and splanchnic nerve blocks. Faster image acquisition and higher resolution will continue to make CT guidance a more attractive option for celiac plexus and splanchnic nerve block.[77] Three-dimensional image reconstruction may also provide the pain specialist a better understanding of the functional clinical anatomy and allow further refinement of these neurolysis techniques[78] (**Fig. 160.20**). As more experience is gained with ultrasound, it will play a role in the evolution of the anterior approach. The development of safer and longer-acting local anesthetics and neurolytic agents would be a welcome advance for the pain management specialist who performs celiac plexus and splanchnic nerve block.

References

Full references for this chapter can be found on www.expertconsult.com.

Lumbar Epidural Injections

Laxmaiah Manchikanti, Sairam Atluri, and Sukdeb Datta

Historical Considerations

Epidural administration of corticosteroids is one of the commonly used interventions in managing chronic low back pain.[1–15] Approaches available to access the lumbar epidural space include the caudal, interlaminar, and transforaminal routes. Reports of epidural corticosteroid effectiveness of have varied from 18% to 90%.[1] Numerous publications over the years have described in detail the administration of lumbar epidural steroid injections by various routes.[1–15]

In 1901 Sicard,[16] a radiologist, was the first to describe treating patients suffering from severe intractable sciatic pain or lumbago by injecting dilute cocaine solutions through the sacral hiatus (the caudal route) into the epidural space. One week later, but independently, Cathelin,[17] a urologist, described caudal administration of local anesthetic for surgical procedures and also injection of cocaine for relief of pain due to inoperable carcinoma of the rectum. Pasquier and Leri,[18] also in 1901, independently reported the use of caudal epidural injection for the relief of sciatic pain. The extension of this technique to the treatment of sciatica is attributed to Caussade and Queste[19] in 1909, Viner[20] in 1925, Evans[21] in 1930, Ombregt and Ter Veer[22] and Cyriax[23] from 1937 to the 1970s, and Brown[24] in 1960.

However, some consider that the first to use epidural anesthesia was Corning, a neurologist whose intentions were to treat some neurologic disorders by using cocaine spinally (**Fig. 161.1 [online only]**).[25,26] In the October 1885 issue of the *New York Medical Journal*, a case report by Corning[26] was based on two subjects: one a dog and the other a patient who suffered from spinal weakness and seminal incontinence.

The description of the para-midline approach to the lumbar epidural space was proposed by Pagés[27] in 1921. This is considered the first clinically relevant report of the technique of lumbar epidural injection. Multiple modifications were suggested to the technique described by Pagés.[28] In 1933

Dogliotti[29] introduced the loss-of-resistance technique into clinical practice. Gutierrez,[30] also in 1933, suggested that the negative pressure of the epidural space might be used to identify the epidural space and described the hanging-drop technique. In 1936 Rovenstein[31] established a nerve block service. By the 1950s, many nerve block clinics were in operation.[32,33]

The 1949 clinical introduction of cortisone, a purified glucocorticoid preparation, revolutionized the medical care of patients with a host of diseases and provided life-sustaining physiologic replacement in patients with acute or chronic adrenal insufficiency.[34,35] Soon after that, Robecchi and Capra[36] reported the first use of steroids in epidural injections; however, the first report of the use of epidural steroid injections has been attributed by various authorities to Lievre et al[37] in 1953. The initial American reports of epidural steroid injections by Goebert et al[38] appeared in 1961.

Indications

Tissues in the lower back capable of transmitting pain include the disk, nerve root dura, muscle, ligament, fascia, and facet joint.[39] Pain from lumbar disk herniation can arise from nerve root compression and stimulation of nociceptors in the annulus or posterior longitudinal ligament. In 1934 Mixter and Barr[40] described intervertebral disk herniation, which led many practitioners to assume that intervertebral disk herniation is the most common cause of back problems. However, modern evidence implicates intervertebral disk herniation in only a small percentage of back complaints.[1,41–43] Thus a simple compression or mass effect cannot be the mechanism of pain caused by disk disease. In fact, several studies evaluating the progress of disk herniation have shown that, even though the resolution of symptoms tends to be associated with diminution of a disk herniation's size, it is not always the case because compression may continue in spite of symptomatology resolution.[43–46]

In addition, it is also well known that disk herniations that are evident on computed tomography (CT) axial scan or magnetic resonance imaging (MRI) scan can be asymptomatic.[47,48] Various proposed mechanisms for radicular pain include partial axonal damage, neuroma formation, and focal demyelination[49]; intraneural edema[50–53]; and impaired microcirculation.[52,53] The other explanation surrounds the theory of chemical irritation and inflammation around the disks and nerve roots, which is considered a pain generator in conjunction with or without mechanical factors.[54]

Rationale

The philosophy of epidural steroid injections is based on the premise that the corticosteroid delivered into the epidural space attains higher local concentrations over an inflamed nerve root and will be more effective than a steroid administered either orally or by intramuscular injection.[1–6,8–15]

Target site concentration of steroids depends on multiple injection variables, including the route of administration. Steroids may be prevented from migrating from the posterior epidural space to the anterior or ventral epidural space by the presence of epidural ligaments or scar tissue, either with caudal or interlaminar administration. Interlaminar lumbar epidural injections are alleged to be superior to caudal epidural injections by some because of the requirement of the apparently smaller volume. Interlaminar epidural injections are also considered more target specific than caudal epidural injections. However, among the many disadvantages of interlaminar epidural injections, the extradural placement of the needle, which may go unrecognized without fluoroscopic guidance, is crucial.[1–3,55–57] Other interlaminar approach disadvantages include erroneous placement of the needle, which may miss the targeted interspace without fluoroscopic guidance[56,57]; preferential cranial flow of the solution in the epidural space[58,59]; deviation of the needle to the nondependent side[60]; difficulty entering the epidural space and delivery of injectate below L5 for S1 nerve root involvement[1,2,56]; potential risk of dural puncture and post–lumbar puncture headache[5]; and the rare, but serious, risk of spinal cord trauma.[61] Disadvantages of various types of epidural administration of drugs are listed in **Table 161.1**.[2]

Similar to interlaminar epidural injections, transforaminal epidural injections also have some disadvantages, which include intravascular penetration of the needle, neural penetration, spinal cord trauma, and paraplegia.[55,62] In addition to lumbar radiculitis or chronic low back pain, lumbar epidural injections with local anesthetics, opioids, or steroids may be used in multiple other chronic painful conditions, as well as acute painful conditions.

The present clinical rationale for steroid usage in epidurals is primarily based on the benefits, which include pain relief outlasting—by hours, days, and sometimes weeks—the pharmacologic action of steroids and local anesthetics.[63] However, appropriate explanations for such benefits continue to lack scientific validity. Additional explanations include alteration or interruption of nociceptive input, reflex mechanism of the afferent limb, self-sustaining activity of the neuronal pools in the neuraxis, and the pattern of central neural activities by neural blockade, including caudal epidural steroids.[64] The basis for these explanations is twofold. First, it is postulated that corticosteroids reduce inflammation either by inhibiting

Table 161.1 Disadvantages of Caudal, Lumbar, Interlaminar, and Transforaminal Epidural Injections

TRANSFORAMINAL

Intraneural injection

Neural trauma

Technical difficulty in presence of fusion and/or hardware

Intravascular injection

Spinal cord trauma

CAUDAL

Requirement of substantial volume of fluid

Dilution of the injectate

Extra-epidural placement of the needle

Intravascular placement of the needle

Atypical anatomy

Dural puncture

INTERLAMINAR

Dilution of the injectate

Extra-epidural placement of the needle

Intravascular placement of the needle

Preferential cranial flow of the solution

Preferential posterior flow of the solution

Difficult placement in postsurgical patients

Difficult placement below L4-5 interspace

Deviation of needle to nondependent side

Dural puncture

Trauma to spinal cord

From Manchikanti L, Singh V, Kloth D, et al: Interventional techniques in the management of chronic pain: part 2.0, *Pain Physician* 4:24, 2001.

the synthesis or release of a number of proinflammatory substances or by causing a reversible local anesthetic effect.[63–76] Second, administration of epidural solutions clears or dilutes the chemical irritants. Corticosteroids are postulated to exert their effect by multiple modes, including membrane stabilization, inhibition of neural peptide synthesis or action, blockade of phospholipase A_2 activity, prolonged suppression of ongoing neuronal discharge, and suppression of sensitization of dorsal horn neurons.[63]

Interlaminar epidural steroid injections are indicated in patients with chronic low back pain who have failed to respond to conservative modalities of treatments. Patients should have a strong radicular component or diskogenic pain, or at the least, they must not have facet joint pain or sacroiliac joint pain. Patients with combined pain generators with diskogenic pain and facet joint pain may also receive interlaminar epidural steroid injections.

In the past, a multitude of investigators have attempted to identify outcome predictors for epidural injections, as well as facet joint injections. However, these have been proven to be futile; hence, no such recommendations are made in this review. Various contraindications include the patient's inability to be in the prone position, contraindications for fluoroscopy, local or

Table 161.2 Nonsurgical Indications for Interlaminar Lumbar Epidural Block

Acute pain

Herpes zoster and postherpetic neuralgia

Ischemic pain syndromes

Renal colic

Preemptive analgesia before amputation

Complex regional pain syndromes I and II

Lumbar radiculopathy

Lumbar disk herniation

Lumbar spinal stenosis

Post–lumbar laminectomy syndrome

Lumbar degenerative disk disease

Chronic low back pain

Vertebral compression fractures

Diabetic polyneuropathy

Pelvic pain syndromes

Phantom limb syndrome

Peripheral neuropathy

Metastatic pain

systemic infection, abnormalities of the sacrum, and allergy to any of the drugs used. Multiple indications for interlaminar epidural injections are illustrated in **Table 161.2**. These indications are related to anesthesia other than surgical or obstetric.

Clinically Relevant Anatomy

The epidural space extends from the base of the skull to the end of the dural sac at S2. It is a cylindric structure enveloping the dura. The epidural space exists between the dura and ligamentum flavum.[77] The actual size of epidural spaces varies greatly. The distance from the skin to the epidural space in normal adults usually ranges from 3 to 5 cm. In the midlumbar region, the depth of the posterior epidural space is about 5 to 6 mm, and it gradually decreases to 2 mm at the S1 level. The epidural space is widest in the midline below the junction of the lamina; it narrows laterally. Laterally, the ligamentum flavum joins with the facet joint capsule. The posterior epidural space is divided by the plica mediana dorsalis and additional transverse connective tissue planes, providing a compartmentalized nature. The ligamentum flavum is also 5 to 6 mm in the lumbar region.

The epidural space contains fat, veins, spinal arteries, and lymphatics. The epidural veins are a part of the large internal vertebral venous plexus, which communicates with the occipital, sigmoid, and basilar sinuses superiorly in the cranium. If needle placement in the epidural veins is not recognized, it may result in the injectate's reaching the cranial sinuses. The spinal arteries enter the epidural space through the intervertebral foramen laterally. During the performance of the interlaminar lumbar epidural steroid injection, it is important to make sure that the needle is not too lateral in the epidural space because of the possibility of injury to the spinal artery, which is entering the epidural space laterally through the

intervertebral foramen. The largest of the spinal arteries is the artery of Adamkiewicz. This artery provides the major arterial supply to the lumbar spine. It enters the spinal canal through a single intervertebral foramen anywhere between T8 and L3 and is located on the left side 78% of the time.

The spinal cord ends in most people at the L1 or L2 level. Epidurals done above this level can result in cord trauma if the needle is inadvertently advanced too far. The dural sac terminates at S2.

Technique

Lumbar epidural injection is performed either with fluoroscopy or blindly without fluoroscopy. For all chronic pain settings, specifically for low back pain, fluoroscopic epidural is recommended.

Fluoroscopic Technique

All necessary protection against radiation should be used to avoid complications.[78–80]

Positioning

The patient should be placed in the prone position with a pillow under the abdomen. Sterile preparation should be carried out extensively. The desired interlaminar space must be identified, which should be in the middle of the viewing monitor in the anteroposterior (AP) view. The C-arm may be rotated toward the patient's right side or left side until the spinous process is exactly equidistant from the right and the left pedicle (**Fig. 161.2**). The cranial (C-arm is angled toward the patient's head) or caudal (C-arm is angled toward the patient's feet) angulation is done until the desired interlaminar space is maximally opened. Sometimes no cranial or caudal angulation is necessary, especially if the L5-S1 space is chosen. Typically the L5-S1 space is the widest, and the interspaces get smaller as one goes superior to L4-5 and L3-4. T12-L1 and L1-2 are again easily accessible.

Procedure

If the patient is having unilateral pain, the needle entry point should be on that side of the interlaminar space (**Fig. 161.3**). If the patient is having bilateral pain, the needle entry should be in the midline of the interlaminar space. The epidural needle is placed on the patient horizontally and adjusted with the help of fluoroscopy until the needle tip is at the site of needle entry. Extreme lateral placement of the needle in the interlaminar space should be avoided to minimize the risk of nerve injury and to stay away from vascular structures.

A skin wheal is raised, preferably with a 25- to 30-gauge needle, with 1% lidocaine at the needle entry site. This is done at the tip of the needle. Deeper infiltration with local anesthetic can be done. Again, using fluoroscopic guidance, the needle is adjusted so that it is seen as a "dot" (see Fig. 161.3). The dot must be in the interlaminar space and on the intended right or left side if the patient is having right or left radiculopathy, and it must be midline if the patient is suffering from bilateral radiculopathy. In this case, it was placed on the right side, as the patient was having right-sided radiculopathy. The stylet is removed. The loss-of-resistance syringe (plastic or glass) is attached to the Touhy needle. The needle is advanced straight in, inline with the x-ray beam. For the right-handed operator,

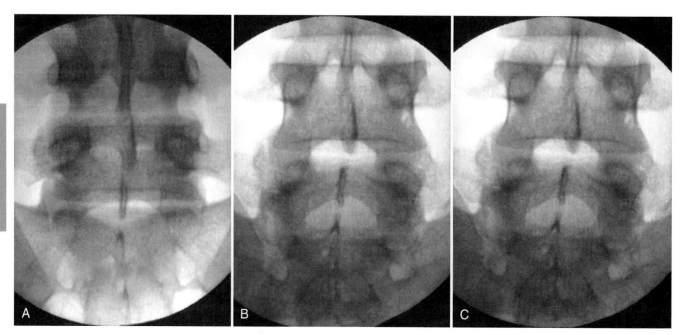

Fig. 161.2 Positioning for lumbar interlaminar epidural. **A,** The interlaminar spaces are not optimally visualized. **B,** The C-arm is at an oblique angle about 10 degrees to the right so that the spinous process is equidistant from both pedicles. **C,** Cranial or caudal maneuvering may be required to maximally open the interlaminar space.

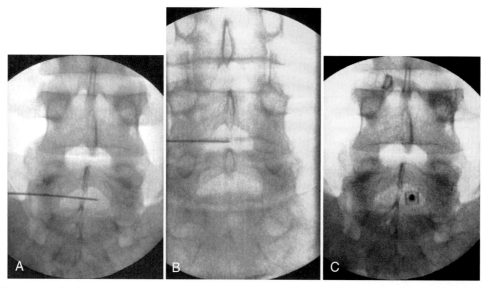

Fig. 161.3 Needle placement under fluoroscopic visualization. **A,** The needle tip is in the right side of the interlaminar space. Skin wheal is done at the tip of the needle. **B,** The tip of the needle is in the midline in the interlaminar space. **C,** The needle is pulled back almost to the skin and readjusted so that it appears as a dot.

the needle hub is held with the left thumb and index finger; this hand should rest on the patient's back to provide stability. Continuous pressure is applied on the syringe plunger with the other hand, and the needle is advanced. There is increased bounce or pressure in the syringe, especially when the needle enters the ligamentum flavum. As the needle passes through the ligament and enters the epidural space, this pressure or bounce is suddenly lost. This is the loss-of-resistance or bounce technique. Live fluoroscopy is not necessary during advancement, but occasional spot pictures may be helpful to make sure that the needle is not off course. It is important to realize that because the Touhy needle has a curved tip, the principle

of bevel control comes into play. It is possible to use this feature to advantage. Turning the bevel to the side of the intended direction results in the needle's going in that direction as it is advanced. This is analogous to the curved-needle technique that is commonly used in other spinal procedures. Getting false loss of resistance is not uncommon even in experienced hands. It cannot be emphasized enough that, if one is not sure where the needle is, the immediate course of action should be to check the lateral view. Inadvertent advancement without the knowledge of needle position can result in unnecessary dural puncture and even possibly spinal cord damage if lumbar epidural steroid injection is performed at the L1 or L2 level or higher.

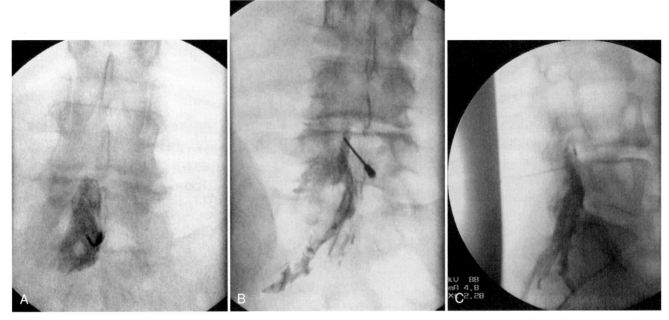

Fig. 161.4 Contrast injection under fluoroscopy. A, The areolar appearance of the contrast is noted on the left side of the epidural space. B, The contrast is seen surrounding the L5 and S1 nerves. C, The contrast is in the confines of the spine and not posterior to the spine.

Once one is convinced that the epidural space is found with loss of resistance, make sure that aspiration is negative for cerebrospinal fluid (CSF) or blood. Inject non-ionic contrast (Omnipaque or Isovue) and look for the typical contrast spread to confirm. Epidural contrast spread can have one or all of the following patterns, which can help confirm correct needle placement:

1. Contrast has a smooth, continuous flow during injection. The contrast quickly moves away (runs off) from the tip of the needle as it is injected. Usually this flow is superior to the needle tip, but inferior spreads are also seen. If one gets a false loss of resistance and is posterior to the epidural space, a "blob" or "cotton ball" appearance is commonly seen. At this time it will be useful to use live fluoroscopy to visualize the contrast flow and spread. By using small extension tubing during contrast injection, the physician's hand can be spared from radiation.
2. Areolar appearance (small bubbles within the contrast spread) is often seen (**Fig. 161.4A**).
3. Sometimes contrast can be seen surrounding the nerves, giving the typical appearance of the radiculogram (see **Fig. 161.4B**).

On the lateral view, the needle must be clearly in the spinal column and posterior to the neural foramen. In the lateral view, the contrast should be in the confines of the spinal canal. The contrast should not be posterior to the spine (see **Fig. 161.4C**). If the needle tip is posterior to the spine, it is posterior to the epidural space. If the needle tip is at the neural foramen or anterior to the foramen, it may be in the intrathecal space. Contrast spread can be checked in both the AP view and lateral view. As more experience is obtained, watching the contrast spread in the AP view will suffice.

Because the spine is a cylindric structure, if needle entry is in the midline of the interlaminar space in the AP view, the needle tip will be barely in the spine. But if the needle entry is on the right or left side of the interlaminar space in the AP view, the needle tip will be clearly within the spine in the lateral view, and it will be posterior to the intervertebral foramen. If one is using the midline technique and in the lateral view, or if one is not sure if the needle is in the epidural space because the needle tip is barely at the posterior edge of the spine, the only way to confirm this is by injecting contrast and watching its spread. In the lateral view, it should be within the spine and not posterior to the spine (see Fig. 161.4C). In the AP view, the typical epidural contrast spread should be seen.

The compliance of the epidural space is very low; therefore, after the contrast is injected, it is common to see the contrast flowing back subtly (dripping back) through the needle (but with negative aspiration). This can be an additional assurance that the needle is in the correct place. Obvious flowback of the fluid, especially with aspiration, indicates dural puncture.

It is not uncommon for the patient to feel a brief jolt or pain when the needle first enters the epidural space. This is probably from the sudden decompression of air or saline from the loss-of-resistance syringe into the epidural space. This decompression irritates the already sensitized and inflamed spinal canal structures.

There should be no resistance during the injection. If there is resistance to injection, a simple turn of the bevel will resolve the problem. Many patients may feel radicular pain during injection; if this pain is concordant to their pain, it is an additional confirmation that the steroid is reaching the desired inflamed nerve root. Severe and excruciating pain should alert the practitioner to the possibility of intraneural injection, which can cause nerve damage and obviously must be avoided. In such situations, the injection should be stopped immediately and the needle position reexamined (is it too lateral in the interlaminar space?).

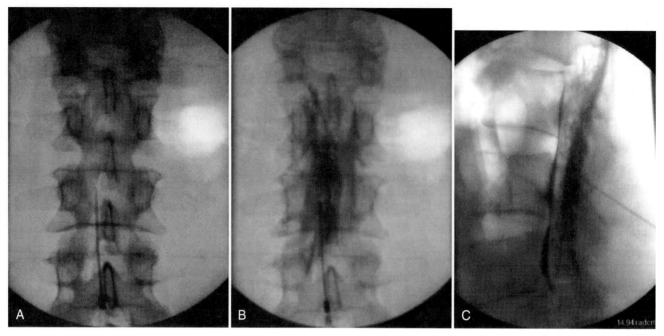

Fig. 161.5 Left-sided interlaminar approach to the epidural space under fluoroscopy with epidural filling pattern. **A,** Posteroanterior view with needle placement. **B,** Posteroanterior view with contrast injection. **C,** Lateral view with excellent ventral filling of epidural space.

Getting false loss of resistance is not uncommon, even in experienced hands. False loss of resistance is obtained commonly with the following:

1. The needle is posterior to the epidural space (not deep enough). This problem cannot be identified in the AP view. A lateral view must be checked. It is not uncommon to have a false loss of resistance. If one is not sure or if one is a beginner, the only way to confirm entry in the epidural space is to check the lateral view. When contrast is injected, it will be posterior to the spine. If the needle and/or contrast is posterior to the epidural space, reattach the syringe to the needle and resume the loss of resistance until the needle position and contrast spread are appropriate as described (see Fig. 161.4C).
2. The needle is in the epidural space. When one injects the contrast, the typical spread in the AP view can be seen. In the lateral view, the needle is in the spine (not posterior to the spine) and the contrast is in the spinal canal (not posterior to the spine). Aspiration is negative for CSF or heme. No vascular spread of the contrast is seen. Frequently, it may be difficult to visualize the needle tip in the lateral view, especially in obese patients. This problem can be offset by using epidural needles with a metal stylet.
3. The needle is in the intrathecal space (the needle is in too deep). Clear fluid (CSF) is obtained on aspiration. It is impossible to tell on the AP view if the needle is in the epidural space or the intrathecal space and also difficult to see in the lateral view. Injecting contrast into the intrathecal space will show a myelogram pattern that is clearly distinct from the epidurogram. If one is not sure about this spread, the radiology department in the hospital should be able to furnish myelogram films for review. If one thinks the needle is deep enough and

there is no loss of resistance, or if one is not sure where the needle is, check the lateral view before further needle advancement to avoid dural puncture.

Figures 161.5 and **161.6** also indicate the interlaminar approach to the epidural space under fluoroscopy with epidural filling pattern showing multiple nerve roots and ventral epidural filling. Botwin et al[80,81] described epidural filling patterns with fluoroscopic interlaminar epidural steroid injections. They showed that among 25 epidurograms, all had contrast in the dorsal epidural space. Further, 36% of the patients had contrast visualized in the ventral epidural space. They also noted that contrast patterns showed unilateral flow in 84% of the patients, whereas bilateral contrast pattern was seen in only 16%. The mean caudad spread of contrast from the injection site was recorded and found to be a mean of 0.88 levels, in contrast to cephalad spread of 1.28 levels (**Fig. 161.7**). They also noted higher levels of cephalad flow in herniated disk patients with a lower level of caudad flow with means of 1.12 and 0.96 levels, respectively. Cephalad flow was also noticed to be higher in stenosis patients (**Table 161.3**).

Blind Technique

The blind technique may be performed with the patient in the sitting, lateral, or prone position with a midline or paramedian approach.

Sitting Position

The sitting position is preferred for obese patients because it facilitates the identification of the midline. In obese patients, other bony landmarks may not be palpable. Preferably, the patient should bend forward, with the knees close to the abdomen, or rest the legs on a stool, to abolish lumbar lordosis and widen the posterior interspinous space. Following the appropriate

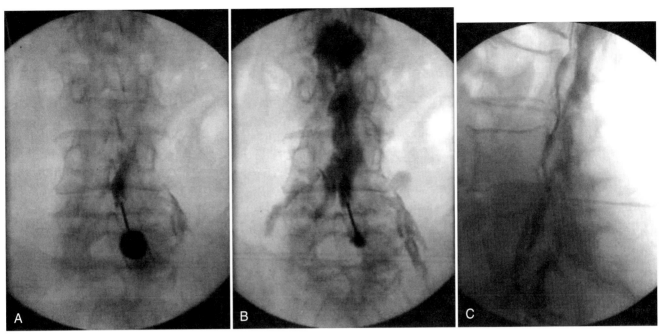

Fig. 161.6 Right-sided interlaminar approach to the epidural space. A, Posteroanterior view with needle placement. B, Posteroanterior with contrast injection. C, Lateral view with excellent ventral filling of epidural space.

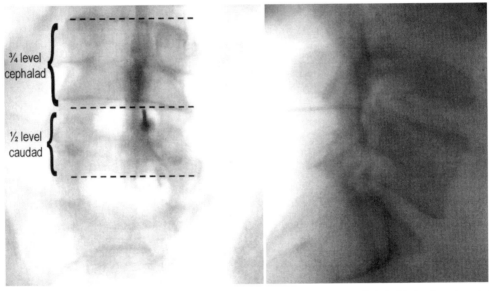

¾ level cephalad

½ level caudad

Fig. 161.7 Anteroposterior radiograph *(left)* of interlaminar injection at L4-5. Note contrast flow cephalad of ¾ levels and caudad contrast flow of ½ levels. Lateral radiograph *(right)* reveals contrast flow in dorsal epidural space. *(From Botwin KP, Natalicchio J, Hanna A: Fluoroscopic guided lumbar interlaminar epidural injections: a prospective evaluation of epidurography contrast patterns and anatomical review of the epidural space, Pain Physician 7:77, 2004.)*

Table 161.3 Mean Levels of Contrast Flow from Injection Site in 25 Injections

	HNP Injection (*n* =13)	LSS Injection (*n* =12)	Total (*n* =25)	*P* Value
Caudad	0.96 ± 0.43 (0.5–2.0)	0.79 ± 0.26 (0.5–1.0)	0.88 ± 0.36 (0.5–2.0)	0.249
Cephalad	1.12 ± 0.46 (0.5–2.0)	1.46 ± 0.58 (0.5–2.0)	1.28 ± 0.54 (0.5–2.0)	0.120
P value	0.390	0.002	0.004	

From Botwin KP, Natalicchio J, Hanna A: Fluoroscopic guided lumbar interlaminar epidural injections: a prospective evaluation of epidurography contrast patterns and anatomical review of the epidural space, *Pain Physician* 7:77, 2004.
HNP, herniated nucleus pulposus; LSS, lumbosacral spine.
Values in parentheses indicate range.
One level is defined as being from the middle of the intervertebral disk from where the injection was performed to the vertebral disk cephalad or caudad.

sterile preparation and a skin wheal, an 18- or 20-gauge epidural needle is inserted and the posterior part of the spinous process may be identified. Following this, the epidural needle is slightly withdrawn and directed more cephalad in the sagittal plane and "walked off" the spinous process with identification of a clear pathway. At this point, or immediately after identification of the interspinous process, the stylet from the needle may be removed and a syringe with air or saline solution is attached to the hub of the needle. The epidural needle is advanced slowly with a two-handed technique stabilizing it so that unwanted movements and subdural puncture are prevented. Once the ligamentum flavum is reached, the operator will feel resistance followed by sudden loss of resistance to air or saline. Once the epidural space is identified, aspiration should be carried out, which should be negative not only for CSF, but also for blood.

The paramedian approach for the sitting position is carried out in the same fashion by preparing the overlying skin. By introducing the needle approximately 1 inch lateral to the spinous process below the space to be entered, infiltration may be carried out copiously into the skin, as well as the deeper tissues along the intended pathway. An 18- or 20-gauge epidural needle is inserted cephalad and medially so that it makes a 15-degree angle to the sagittal plane. After the needle is advanced 3 to 4 cm, the stylet should be removed and a syringe containing air or saline solution should be attached to the hub of the needle. At this time, the needle is advanced slowly with the same steps as in the sitting position until the loss of resistance to air or saline solution is felt and the epidural space is identified. Once again, negative aspiration should be confirmed.

Lateral Position

Preparation for this procedure is similar to the sitting position for both midline and paramedian approach. The advantage of the lateral approach is the avoidance of hypotension. As a cautionary note, it is ideal in pain management to perform these procedures under fluoroscopic visualization for managing chronic low back pain or other related conditions.

Side Effects and Complications
Corticosteroid-Related Side Effects

Most of the side effects reported are minor and transient.[63] They are related to systemic absorption and include insomnia, erythema, nausea, rash, and pruritus. Depression of plasma cortisol levels and the pituitary-hypothalamic axis can occur for about 2 weeks, but it normalizes by 3 weeks. Patients can develop Cushing's syndrome, but it is extremely rare. Diabetic patients can commonly have temporary elevations in blood-sugar levels for up to 3 to 7 days. In rare cases, fluid retention can occur, which can precipitate congestive heart failure in the susceptible. Weight gain is rare.

Local Anesthetic–Related Side Effects

Unrecognized intrathecal injection of the local anesthetic will result in spinal anesthesia. Venous injection of local anesthetic may or may not produce any symptoms; this once again depends on the local anesthetic dose. The symptoms can range from minor transient manifestations such as dizziness, disorientation, tinnitus, metallic taste in the mouth, circumoral numbness, and muscle twitching, to

life-threatening seizures, unconsciousness, coma, and cardiovascular collapse. Arrhythmias resulting from local anesthetic overdose are usually refractory to the advanced cardiac life support protocol and are extremely difficult to treat. Central nervous system symptoms precede cardiovascular collapse. If the patient is having muscle twitching, benzodiazepines (Versed or Valium) should be used immediately. If seizures occur, intravenous thiopental sodium must be given along with the necessary ventilatory support. Fortunately, these complications are rare during lumbar epidural steroid injection because high doses of local anesthetics are rarely needed. If aspiration for blood is negative and there is no vascular runoff during contrast injection, venous injection is extremely rare. Higher concentrations of local anesthetics can lead to hypotension secondary to sympathetic blockade. This condition can be easily resolved with intravenous fluids and vasopressors such as ephedrine or phenylephrine hydrochloride (Neo-Synephrine).

Procedure-Related Side Effects

Some of the reported complications include vasovagal reactions, spinal headache, and spinal block. Subdural injection can result if the needle is between the dural membrane and the arachnoid membrane. The block resembles that of a spinal block, but it is patchy. Management is similar to spinal block. Fortunately, subdural needle placement is extremely rare. Nerve damage can occur, and any severe pain during placement of the needle or injection should alert the operator to potential neural injury. The procedure must be stopped immediately, and the needle position reevaluated. The patient must be able to report severe radicular pain in the case of intraneural injection; for this reason, the patient should *never* be oversedated.

Spinal cord injury can occur by two mechanisms: first, by direct injury to the cord with the epidural needle; second, by a rare mechanism, either by traumatizing the artery of Adamkiewicz with the needle or by injecting particulate steroid-like methylprednisolone acetate into it. This artery provides the major arterial supply to the lumbar spinal cord. It enters the spinal canal through a single intervertebral foramen anywhere between T8 and L3 and is located on the left side 78% of the time. Injury to this artery or any spinal artery can be avoided by making sure that the needle is not too lateral in the interlaminar space in the AP view.

Epidural abscess is a serious event, but if meticulous attention is paid to sterility, this complication will not be a problem, especially if the patient is not having any systemic or local infection. The most common offending agent is *Staphylococcus aureus*. The incubation period is 7 to 10 days before signs or symptoms are noted. Patients complain of severe back pain, fevers with chills, and localized tenderness; they have leukocytosis with elevated erythrocyte sedimentation rate and C-reactive protein. If not diagnosed early and treated, they may develop neurologic deficits. Treatment can range from intravenous antibiotics to urgent laminectomy and débridement. Because the epidural veins communicate directly with the cranial sinuses, this infection can spread to the central nervous system. Meningitis has also been reported, possibly from the aforementioned mechanism.

Epidural hematoma is a rare event in patients with normal clotting mechanisms. It can lead to rapidly progressing neurologic deficits secondary to compression of the spinal cord, and it is very important to recognize it early because deficits can be reversed if the hematoma is evacuated soon enough. If not, the consequences can be disastrous. Some patients have increased pain after lumbar epidural steroid injection, but in a majority of the cases it is transient.

Conclusion

Lumbar epidural steroid injections are the most commonly used interventional modality for management of low back pain; however, the differentiation between caudal and lumbar is not available statistically. Although the rationale for lumbar epidural steroid injections is the logical presumption that delivery of the steroids as close as possible to the inflamed nerve root results in high concentration of the steroid, the results of randomized trials showing the effectiveness of interlaminar epidural steroids is disappointing.

References

Full references for this chapter can be found on www.expertconsult.com.

Subarachnoid Neurolytic Blocks

Alon P. Winnie and Kenneth D. Candido

Dogliotti[1] first described the technique of subarachnoid chemical neurolysis using alcohol for the treatment of sciatic pain almost 80 years ago. In the same year, Suvansa[2] described intrathecal carbolic acid for the treatment of tetanus. A quarter of a century later, Maher,[3,4] in two landmark articles, described his experience with hyperbaric phenol and silver nitrate for subarachnoid neurolysis, stating, "It is easier to lay a carpet than to paper a ceiling." Over the ensuing years, however, lack of experience with either technique and fear of the anticipated complications resulted in underuse of this valuable modality. Better understanding and increased use of neuraxial opiates for cancer pain since the 1980s have decreased the use of subarachnoid chemical neurolysis even further. Nonetheless, because of the physical separation of the sensory and motor roots of spinal nerves within the spinal canal, intrathecal dorsal rhizotomy (more appropriately called *rhizolysis*) is the only neurolytic procedure that allows sensory block without concomitant motor block. Because of this and because of the relative precision with which the affected nerve roots can be blocked, the technique is particularly useful for treating cancer pain in an extremity, where preservation of motor function is so important. In short, the physical separation of motor and sensory fibers in the subarachnoid space preserves forever a small but unique role for subarachnoid neurolysis in the management of cancer pain in carefully selected patients.

Selection Criteria

Because the duration of action of neurolytic agents in the subarachnoid space is finite but unpredictable, great care must be exercised in choosing appropriate candidates for the procedure. Neurolytic blockade by this route is especially suited to patients in whom conventional treatment regimens have failed, who have prohibitive side effects from opioid analgesics, and who have a short life expectancy, usually less than 1 year.

As with all neurolytic procedures, patients must be completely apprised of the possibility of debilitating side effects and other serious associated complications that can follow even a successful block, most notably, motor weakness, paralysis, and incontinence. The selection criteria for subarachnoid neurolysis include the following:

- The diagnosis is well established.[5]
- The patient's life expectancy is short, usually 6 to 12 months.
- The patient's pain is unresponsive to antineoplastic therapy (chemotherapy, radiation).
- The patient's pain has failed to respond to adequate trials of analgesic agents and adjunctive drugs.
- The pain is localized to two or three dermatomes.
- The pain is predominantly somatic in origin.
- The pain is unilateral (neurolytic blocks for bilateral pain should be staggered).[6]

Informed Consent

It is crucial that not only the patient but also the patient's family fully understand the anticipated procedure, its potential risks, the alternative forms of therapy available, and, most important, the possibility of serious complications, up to and including death. It is important that the patient and family understand that the procedure does not simply "take away pain," but rather substitutes numbness (loss of sensation) for the pain. So important is this concept that, with rare exceptions, before the decision is made to proceed with a subarachnoid neurolytic block, a prognostic subarachnoid block should be carried out using a local anesthetic so that the patient can experience the pain relief that may be anticipated after a neurolytic block and the accompanying sensory block. Although an occasional patient may decide that he or she cannot tolerate the numbness, most patients prefer this lack of sensation to the pain and choose to proceed with the neurolytic procedure.

Technique

Because unfamiliarity with the details of this technique has been a major obstacle to its use, and because proper execution of the technique determines its success and safety, the focus of the present discussion is on the technical aspects of subarachnoid neurolysis. First, because of the "permanence" of the complications of this technique, subarachnoid neurolysis should be attempted only after careful review of a dermatome chart to determine precisely which nerve or nerves are subserving the patient's pain (**Fig. 162.1**). If the patient's pain is due to one or more metastases to bone, it may be useful to refer to a sclerotome chart because the innervation of some parts of the appendicular skeleton differs from that of the overlying soft tissues (**Fig. 162.2**).

Second, because a neurolytic subarachnoid block must be carried out at the level where the dorsal root to be blocked leaves the spinal cord (to spare motor function), it is essential to determine which interlaminar foramen affords access to that root. Although the cervical nerves exit at a level higher than their respective vertebral bodies, all the other nerves exit at a level below their respective vertebral bodies because of the differential growth of the spinal cord and vertebral column in utero and for the first few years of life (**Fig. 162.3**).[7] Finally, a choice must be made before the procedure is undertaken to determine whether a hyperbaric (phenol in glycerin) or hypobaric (absolute alcohol) technique is more appropriate. No controlled studies have compared the outcomes with subarachnoid alcohol and phenol, but in our experience hypobaric alcohol has been the technique of choice in most cases because most patients with severe, intractable pain cannot lie on the painful side, a requirement when using hyperbaric phenol.

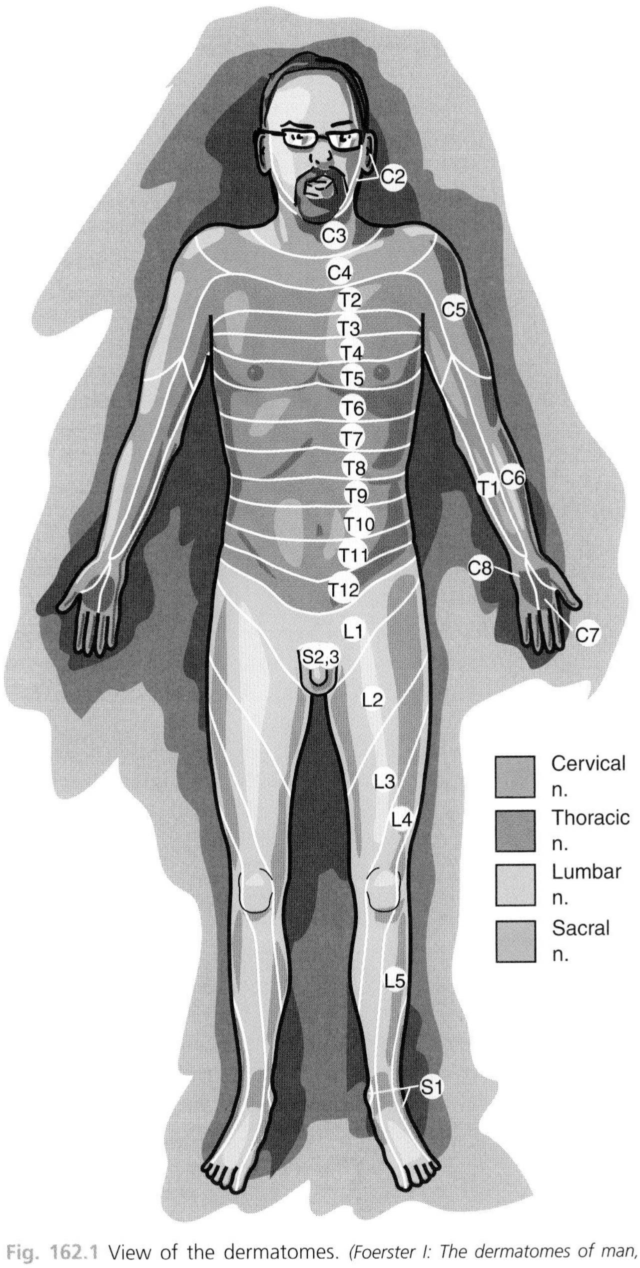

Fig. 162.1 View of the dermatomes. *(Foerster I: The dermatomes of man, Brain 56:1–39, 1993.)*

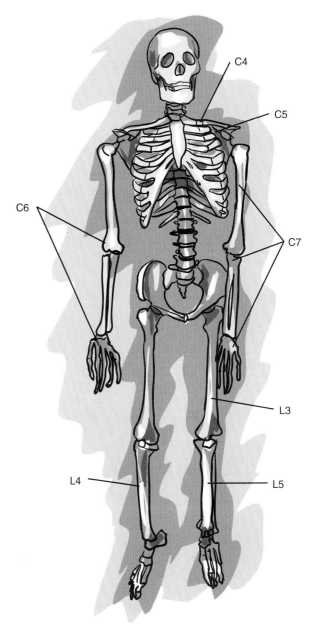

Fig. 162.2 Innervation of the skeleton by spinal segments from the anterior aspect. The various scelerotomes are indicated by the different styles of shading. *(Modified from Déjerine J: Séminologie du système nerveux, Paris, 1914, Masson.)*

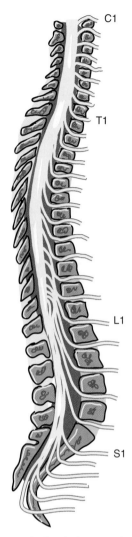

Fig. 162.3 The alignment of spinal segments with vertebrae. The bodies and spinous processes of the vertebrae are shown, and the spinal segments and their respective nerves are indicated by Arabic numbers. The cervical nerves exit through intervertebral foramina above their respective vertebral bodies, and the other nerves issue below those bodies.

Although at one time clinicians believed that phenol might exert a preferential effect on the small fibers subserving pain, it has been determined that neither alcohol nor phenol is a selective neurolytic agent, eliminating this as a rationale for choosing phenol over alcohol.[8–10]

Subarachnoid Neurolysis with Alcohol

Because absolute alcohol is extremely hypobaric, when this agent is used, the patient is first placed in the lateral decubitus position with the painful site uppermost and is then rolled anteriorly approximately 45 degrees to place the dorsal (sensory) root uppermost (**Fig. 162.4**).[11] The patient is stabilized with straps and made as comfortable as possible with pillows because he or she needs to remain in this position throughout the procedure. An assistant is mandatory to stabilize the patient and to allay anxiety. After the patient has been positioned properly, and the

patient's role in the procedure has been reviewed, a 22-gauge pencil-point spinal needle is inserted and advanced through the interlaminar space at the level of the dorsal root to be blocked. If the procedure is being carried out at a thoracic level, because of the long, caudally sloping spinous processes, a paravertebral approach is usually easier than a midline approach; whatever the approach, the needle tip should penetrate the dura in the midline. Needles smaller than 22 gauge should not be selected for this technique because the free flow of cerebrospinal fluid (CSF) is essential, and because post–dural puncture headache is extremely rare after subarachnoid alcohol neurolysis. A prognostic block with local anesthetic should already have been carried out to determine whether the pain can be relieved by the technique, and, equally important, whether the patient can tolerate the numbness.

Contrary to the recommendation in many texts, a test dose of local anesthetic should *not* be given when the needle is in place for a neurolytic block. The reason is that none of the available local anesthetics can be made as hypobaric as absolute alcohol, so a hypobaric local anesthetic "test dose" would not find its way to and block the same nerve root as the much more hypobaric alcohol, resulting in misinformation as to the placement of the neurolytic solution. Also, contrary to the recommendation in most textbooks, a local anesthetic should not be administered before the injection of the alcohol because the pain produced by the injection of the alcohol is an essential indicator that enhances the accuracy and effectiveness of the procedure. Instead of preventing the burning pain caused by the alcohol, the physician must tell the patient to *expect* severe, localized, burning pain, *but only for a fraction of a second* after each injection, and to *focus attention* on whether that burning occurs *at, above,* or *below* the level of the pain. The patient also is instructed to report any other sensations, such as tingling, warmth, or numbness.

Subarachnoid alcohol neurolysis is a precise procedure, and to ensure efficacy and safety, the alcohol should be injected in 0.1 mL aliquots using a tuberculin syringe. The syringe containing the alcohol should not be attached to the needle until the free flow of CSF indicates that the needle is definitely in the subarachnoid space. When the syringe has been attached to the needle, aspiration should *not* be carried out to verify proper needle placement because alcohol causes the CSF to form a white coagulum within the syringe. When the syringe has been attached to the needle, the subjective experience of each injection and the importance of the brief burning sensation to the success of the technique are reiterated one more time, after which sequential injection of 0.1 mL increments of alcohol begins. The operator asks the patient the same questions about the presence and location of the burning after each aliquot. The first one or two increments of alcohol usually do not produce the expected burning pain simply because this volume is just enough to fill the hub and shaft of the spinal needle. The third or fourth 0.1 mL increment invariably produces the expected burning, however, and it reassures the patient as to how short-lived it is.

More important, the level at which the burning is perceived in relation to the location of the pain serves as an indicator as to whether the needle has been placed at the proper level. If the burning occurs at precisely the level of the patient's pain, a total volume of absolute alcohol not greater than 0.7 mL is injected in 0.1 mL increments; after about the fifth or sixth increment, there should be little or no additional burning. If the burning

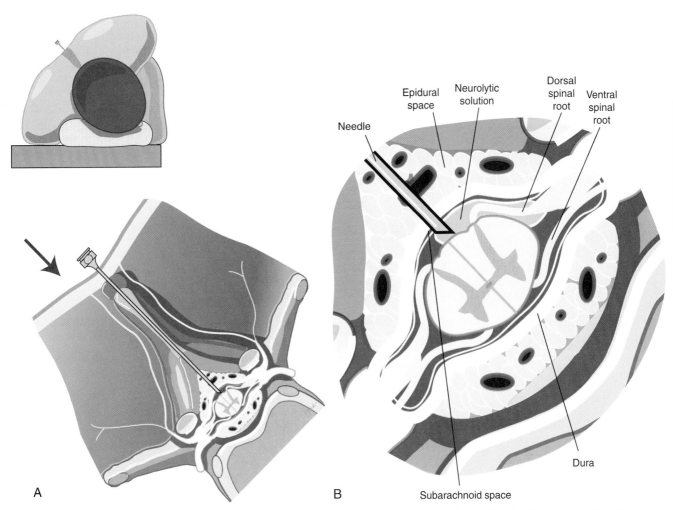

Fig. 162.4 A and **B,** Proper positioning of the patient with left-sided pain for intrathecal injection of alcohol. Note the 45-degree anterior tilt, intended to bathe the posterior (sensory) nerve roots with hypobaric alcohol, while sparing the anterior (motor) roots. *(From Lumbar subarachnoid neurolytic block. In Waldman SD:* Atlas of interventional pain management, *ed 2, Philadelphia, 2004, Saunders, pp 529–530.)*

produced by the third or fourth increment of alcohol occurs *above* the site of the patient's pain, injections through that needle are discontinued, although the needle is left in place (and is restyletted) as a marker. A second needle (and if necessary even a third) must be inserted through progressively lower interspaces until the burning produced by the incremental injection of alcohol corresponds *exactly* to the distribution of the patient's pain. Likewise, if the initial injection of alcohol produces burning pain *below* the level of the patient's pain, a second needle (and if necessary a third) must be inserted through progressively higher interspaces until the injection of the 0.1 mL increments of alcohol produces burning in the precise distribution of the pain (i.e., "concordant pain response"). At this point, the entire 0.7 mL is injected in 0.1 mL increments to produce the desired neurolysis. When the total volume of alcohol has been injected through each needle, the stylet is replaced, and the needle is left in place until the entire procedure has been completed.

When a nerve subserving a patient's pain has been identified and blocked by this process, and a total of 0.7 mL of alcohol has been injected, the process is repeated above or below (or above *and* below) the level of the initial full injection to abolish the pain completely. No more than three or four nerves should ever be blocked at one session, but as indi-

cated in the selection criteria, this procedure is best reserved for patients with pain limited to two or three dermatomes. In contrast to subarachnoid injections of local anesthetics for surgical anesthesia, the injection of alcohol for subarachnoid neurolysis must be made through a separate needle to block each nerve root. The reason that alcohol cannot be "floated" to a higher or lower level through a single needle, as is done when performing a hypobaric spinal for surgery, is that alcohol "fixes" too quickly and would not float far enough to block the adjacent dermatomes. The fila radicularia, small fimbriated structures that number 8 to 12 at each segment and that tether the respective dorsal nerve root to the spinal cord, provide a rather substantial surface area for the absorption of alcohol, which binds there rather rapidly. Matsuki et al[12] showed that the CSF concentration of alcohol is rapidly reduced after intrathecal injection, a finding that implies rapid uptake by nerve tissue. In short, for best results, a separate needle *must* be placed at the level of each nerve root to be blocked. When the injections through the appropriate three or four needles are completed, and before each needle is withdrawn (including needles placed at inappropriate levels), 0.2 to 0.3 mL of air should be injected to clear the shaft and hub of alcohol to minimize the possibility that alcohol trickling from the needle as it is withdrawn from dura to skin will form a durocutaneous fistula. Experience indicates that the 0.1 to 0.2 mL of alcohol injected at levels that turned out to be inappropriate does not cause any demonstrable neurologic damage.

Subarachnoid Neurolysis with Phenol

Intrathecal phenol in glycerin may be used as an alternative to alcohol for subarachnoid neurolysis. The technique is similar to that described earlier except that the patient must be positioned with the painful side down because phenol in glycerin is a *hyperbaric* solution. Because most patients with pain of malignant origin have difficulty lying on the painful side, in our experience alcohol remains the neurolytic of choice in most patients. If phenol neurolysis is appropriate for a particular patient, however, the technique is similar to that used for alcohol neurolysis except that the patient is positioned with the dorsal root lowermost and with the head of the bed slightly elevated (**Fig. 162.5**).[11]

The patient must be tilted posteriorly with the back as close to the edge of the bed as possible, using bolsters, straps,

or pillows to maintain the patient securely in position. The presence of an assistant to hold the patient securely and to provide emotional and physical reassurance is mandatory. For this technique, a 22-gauge (or even better, a 20-gauge) pencil-point spinal needle should be used because of the viscosity of the phenol-glycerin mixture. In a manner essentially opposite to the technique of subarachnoid alcohol neurolysis, the bevel of the spinal needle should be directed inferiorly (laterally toward the table). Because of the viscosity of phenol in glycerin, it takes significant pressure applied to the plunger of the syringe to force the phenol into the subarachnoid space, so the injection must be done slowly and carefully to prevent the escape of phenol from the syringe and onto the skin of the patient or the practitioner. Warming the phenol lessens its viscosity and makes it easier to inject. Because phenol has local anesthetic properties, its injection into the subarachnoid space is not accompanied by the burning pain produced by alcohol, although the patient may feel warmth, tingling, or even mild dysesthesias in the distribution of the nerve being injected. Similar to alcohol, the concentration of phenol in the CSF declines rapidly after the initial injection, implying rapid absorption by neural tissues.[13] This has important implications as to how long *after* the neurolytic agent has been injected

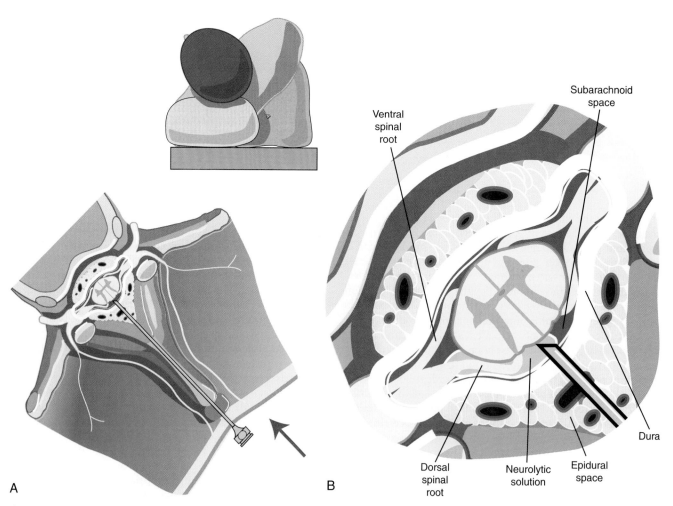

A

B

Ventral spinal root

Subarachnoid space

Dura

Dorsal spinal root

Neurolytic solution

Epidural space

Fig. 162.5 A and B, Proper positioning of the patient with left-sided pain for intrathecal injection of phenol in glycerin. Note the 45-degree posterior tilt, intended to bathe the posterior (sensory) nerve roots with hyperbaric phenol, while sparing the anterior (motor) roots. *(From Waldman SD: Lumbar subarachnoid neurolytic block. In Atlas of interventional pain management, ed 2, Philadelphia, 2004, WB Saunders, pp 531–532.)*

patients must remain as originally positioned. Traditionally, they have been kept in these (obviously uncomfortable) positions for at least 30 minutes after the neurolytic injection, but probably patients can be allowed to assume a more comfortable posture after 15 to 20 minutes, keeping in mind the relative position of the dorsal roots in the spinal canal when doing so. As with alcohol, after the subarachnoid injection of phenol in glycerin, 0.1 to 0.3 mL of air is injected to flush the lytic solution from each needle before it is removed.

Success and Complication Rates

Careful patient selection and equally careful technique are essential for successful subarachnoid neurolysis and for the prevention of complications. Although subarachnoid neurolysis may be attempted at cervical, thoracic, or lumbosacral levels, the success rates and the incidence of complications vary, depending on the level of injection, primarily because of the anatomic differences at different levels. The distance between the origins of nerve roots decreases progressively in the lumbosacral area so that the lower an injection is made, the more difficult it becomes to block a single nerve root without involving adjacent roots. Yet cervical subarachnoid neurolytic blocks seem to be less successful than similar blocks carried out at thoracic or even lumbosacral levels.[14] Penetration of the spinal cord by the needle is a concern whenever these techniques are undertaken, especially at cervical or thoracic levels. This is a rare occurrence, but when it does occur, Perese[15] reported that no permanent injury results, only transient pain, which warns the clinician of the position of the needle and prevents subsequent injection into the cord.

From the point of view of complications, neurolytic subarachnoid blocks may be safest when undertaken in the midthoracic region because this region is relatively distant from the fibers that subserve limb, bowel, and bladder function,[16] so any motor loss would be of little consequence. Conversely, in the lumbosacral region, owing to the proximity of sensory and motor fibers to each other (because of the decreasing size of the conus medullaris, the dorsal and ventral roots are very close together) and to the proximity of both to the autonomic fibers subserving bowel and bladder function, lumbar subarachnoid neurolysis usually is reserved strictly for select individuals in whom the risk-to-benefit ratio has been clearly delineated. For patients who already have compromised sphincter function, lumbosacral subarachnoid phenol neurolysis has been advocated for rectal and pelvic malignancies because of the tendency of phenol to spare motor function.[17]

It is difficult to compare the success rates achieved with subarachnoid neurolysis by various investigators because of the different methods used to quantify pain and pain relief, but it would seem that one should expect a "beneficial effect" in about 75% of the patients, "excellent results" in 50%, and "fair results" in another 25%.[16] A review of the literature seems to indicate that the success rate is slightly greater with alcohol than with phenol, whereas the complication rate is slightly greater with phenol than with alcohol.[3,4,17–31] In assessing the success of a subarachnoid neurolytic procedure, even if a block produces only moderate pain relief, it may be sufficient to allow analgesic agents that could not control the pain previously to render the patient pain free, or at least to make the patient comfortable. One should not consider a neurolytic block to be successful *only* if the patient is rendered pain free

without any supplemental analgesics, although such success is very rewarding.

The impact of a complication, even a serious complication, on a patient and his or her family depends to a large extent on whether the patient has significant pain relief from the neurolytic procedure. If the patient and family have been properly apprised of all of the possible serious complications that can follow a subarachnoid neurolytic procedure, many find even the most serious and unexpected complications acceptable *if* the patient is pain free or at least comfortable as a result of the procedure. If the patient and family are not told of the possible complications, even a fairly minor complication may upset them inordinately (but understandably), particularly if the block fails to produce the desired relief. Most complications of neurolytic subarachnoid blocks are transient. Gerbershagen[32] reviewed reports that provided data on the duration of 303 complications of subarachnoid neurolytic procedures and found that 51% of them disappeared within 1 week, 21% within 1 month, and 9% within 4 months, with only 18% lasting longer than 4 months. Although post–dural puncture headache can follow any subarachnoid block, it is less frequent after neurolytic subarachnoid blocks than after subarachnoid blocks with local anesthetics for surgery, despite the fact that larger needles are used for neurolytic subarachnoid blocks.[33] Similarly, aseptic meningitis (and even septic meningitis) can develop after any subarachnoid block; it also is exceedingly rare after subarachnoid neurolytic blocks, presumably because the neurolytic solutions are self-sterilizing.

A novel technique, recently published, describes the use of a transforaminal approach for injecting phenol into the *epidural space* in an individual who was unable to assume a lateral decubitus position required for using a subarachnoid interlaminar technique with either alcohol or phenol.[34] It remains to be seen whether or not this newly described modality supplants the use of conventional approaches detailed previously, but it demonstrates the ingenuity of pain practitioners who, faced

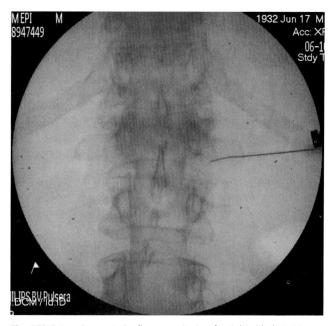

Fig. 162.6 Anterior-posterior fluoroscopic view for right-sided L1-2 transforaminal phenol injection.

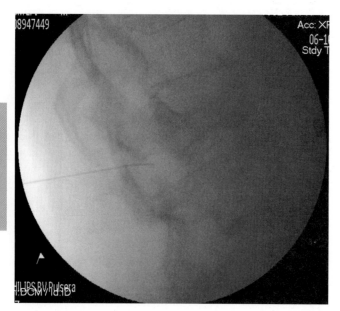

Fig. 162.7 Lateral fluoroscopic view of right-sided L1-2 transforaminal phenol injection; needle in place.

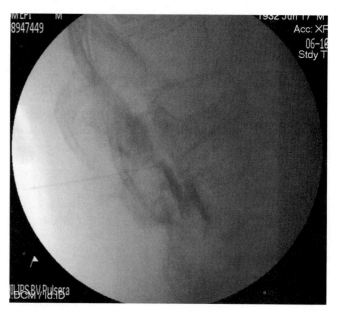

Fig. 162.9 Lateral fluoroscopic view of contrast injection at L1-2 on the right side before phenol injection for neurolysis using the transforaminal approach.

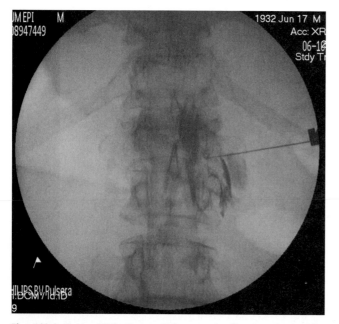

Fig. 162.8 Contrast injection; anterior-posterior fluoroscopic view for transforaminal neurolytic phenol injection, right-sided L1-2.

with an intractable and recalcitrant pain scenario, were able to utilize the principles and foundations described earlier and combine them with contemporary approaches to the spinal canal for accomplishing chemical neurolysis under fluoroscopic guidance (**Figs. 162.6** through **162.9**).

Conclusion

Because of the physical separation of the sensory and motor nerve roots in the spinal canal, intrathecal chemical dorsal rhizotomy is the only neurolytic procedure that allows sensory block without concomitant motor block. For this reason subarachnoid neurolysis is a unique, effective modality for the management of cancer pain in certain patients. If the patients are carefully selected, and the technique is carefully carried out, pain relief can be provided in most cases without an excessive rate of complications.

References

Full references for this chapter can be found on www.expertconsult.com.

Lumbar Facet Joint Blocks

Laxmaiah Manchikanti, David M. Schultz, Sukdeb Datta, and Vijay Singh

Historical Considerations

In 1911 Goldthwait[1] recognized lumbar facet joints as potential sources of back pain and explained facet joints as a cause of many cases of lumbago, sciatica, and paraplegia. Some 20 years later in 1933, Ghormley[2] coined the term *facet syndrome*, and defined it as lumbosacral pain with or without sciatic pain, particularly occurring suddenly after a twisting or rotatory strain of the lumbosacral region. In 1941 Badgley[3] suggested that facet joints themselves could be a primary source of pain separate from spinal nerve compression pain and made a plea for continuing focus on facet joints in order to explain the large numbers of patients with low back pain whose symptoms were not caused by a ruptured disk. Hirsch et al[4] demonstrated that low back pain distributed along the sacroiliac and gluteal areas with radiation to the greater trochanter could be induced by injecting hypertonic saline into the region of the facet joints.

Mooney and Robertson[5] and McCall et al[6] used fluoroscopic technique to inject hypertonic saline into the facet joints of asymptomatic volunteers and demonstrated causation of back and lower extremity pain. Marks[7] and Fukui et al[8] also described the pattern of pain caused by facet joint stimulation and confirmed the findings of previous researchers. Windsor et al[9] also confirmed that lumbar facet joints can be a source of pain in the low back. Mooney and Robertson[5] and McCall et al[6] showed that stimulation of the facet joints produced back pain and somatic-referred pain identical to that commonly seen in patients; Kaplan et al[10] and Dreyfuss et al[11] showed that this pain can be relieved by anesthetizing the facet joints responsible for low back pain.

Indications

The prevalence of persistent low back pain secondary to the involvement of lumbosacral facet joints has been described in controlled studies as varying from 21% to 41% based on the types of population and settings studied,[12-19] based on 80% relief with controlled diagnostic blocks.

Blocks of facet or zygapophysial joints can be performed for therapeutic purpose or to test the hypothesis that the target joint is the patient's pain source. Facet joints can be anesthetized by intra-articular injection of local anesthetic or by blocking the medial branches of the dorsal rami that innervate the target joint.

Lumbar facet joint blocks are useful in the diagnosis, as well as the therapeutic management, of chronic low back pain.[12,20-23] Indications for diagnostic facet joint blocks include low back pain for which no cause is otherwise evident and for which pain patterns resemble those evoked in normal volunteers on stimulation of the facet joints. Imaging studies, physical examination, and history cannot determine independently if a particular structure is painful.[24-28]

Diagnostic Facet Blocks

Background

Lumbosacral facet joints can be anesthetized either with intra-articular injection of local anesthetic or by anesthetizing the medial branches of the dorsal rami that innervate the target joint.[12,20-23] The joint may be considered to be the source of pain if the pain is relieved by joint blockade. Steps need to be taken to ensure that the observed response is not a false-positive result. True-positive responses are secured by performing controlled blocks, either in the form of placebo injections of normal saline, or by using comparative local anesthetic blocks (blocks of the same joint performed on two separate occasions, using local anesthetics with different durations of action).

Rationale

The rationale for using lumbosacral facet joint blocks for diagnosis is based on the following:

- The lumbar facet joints have abundant innervation.[29–37]
- The lumbar facet joints have been shown to be capable of being a source of low back pain and referred pain in the lower limb in normal volunteers.[5–9]
- There are no historical or clinical features that are either indicative or diagnostic of facet joint pain.[12,20–28,38–43]
- Referral patterns described for various joints are variable.[5–9]
- A pattern of pain similar to that of facet joint pain is produced by many other structures in the lumbosacral spine.
- Most maneuvers used in physical examination are likely to simultaneously stress several structures, including disks, muscles, and facet joints.
- The diagnosis of facet joint pain lacks correlation with demographic features, pain characteristics, physical findings, and specific signs or symptoms.[12,15,16,26–28,38–41]
- Imaging technologies have not provided valid or reliable means of identifying symptomatic lesions.[40–42]
- The use of controlled local anesthetic facet joint blocks for the diagnosis of chronic low back pain has been reviewed and validated.[12,20–23,44–49]

Thus placebo-controlled blocks or, more commonly in the United States, comparative local anesthetic blocks using two different local anesthetics are the only means of confirming the diagnosis of facet joint pain.

Validity

The face validity of intra-articular facet injections and medial branch blocks has been established by injecting small volumes of local anesthetic into the joint or onto the sensory nerves of the joint.[11] The construct validity of facet joint blocks has been established.[20] The placebo effect of facet joint injections may be controlled by using strict criteria for determining positive response to blockade.[20] The theory that testing a patient first with lidocaine and subsequently with bupivacaine will identify placebo responders has been tested and proven.[50,51] The specificity of controlled diagnostic blocks has been demonstrated in multiple controlled trials. Pain provocation response of facet joint injections has been shown to be unreliable.[42] The false-negative rate for diagnostic facet joint blocks has been shown to be approximately 8% as a result of unrecognized intravascular injection of local anesthetic.[11] Confounding psychologic factors,[46,47] prior opioid exposure,[52] sedation,[48,49] and previous surgery[53] were shown to lack influence on the validity of comparative, controlled diagnostic local anesthetic blocks of facet joints in the lumbar spine. False-positive rates for facet joint blockade have been evaluated in multiple investigations and are reported to be 17% to 49% in the lumbar spine.[12–19,54–58] The indications and contraindications for diagnostic facet joint blocks are described in **Tables 163.1** and **163.2**.

Table 163.1 Indications for Lumbar Diagnostic Facet Joint Blocks

Somatic or nonradicular low back and/or lower extremity pain

Lack of evidence, either for diskogenic or sacroiliac joint pain

Lack of disk herniation or evidence of radiculitis

Duration of pain of at least 3 months

Failure to respond to more conservative management, including physical therapy modalities with exercises, chiropractic management, and NSAIDs.

Average pain levels of greater than 5 on a scale of 0 to 10

Intermittent or continuous pain causing functional disability

Negative provocative diskography and sacroiliac joint blocks

Contraindications or inability to undergo physical therapy, chiropractic management, or inability to tolerate NSAIDs.

NSAIDs, nonsteroidal anti-inflammatory drugs.

Table 163.2 Contraindications for Lumbosacral Facet Joint Blocks

Infection

Inability of the patient to understand consent, nature of the procedure, needle placement, or sedation

Allergies to contrast, local anesthetic, steroids, Sarapin, or other drugs

Needle phobia

Psychogenic pain

Suspected diskogenic, sacroiliac joint, or myofascial pain

Anticoagulant therapy

Nonsteroidal anti-inflammatory drug therapy

Non-aspirin antiplatelet therapy

Precautions

Relative contraindications to facet injection have been described in patients receiving treatment with nonsteroidal anti-inflammatory medications (especially aspirin) because of concerns that these agents may compromise coagulation.[58] Raj et al[58] have provided a detailed description of the role of anticoagulants in interventional pain management. The importance of discontinuing aspirin before lumbar facet joint injection procedures lacks consensus. Patients on warfarin therapy should have prothrombin time (PT) checked and documented to be at acceptable levels before spinal injection. In stopping anticoagulant therapy, one should take into consideration the risk-benefit ratio of the procedure and also consult with the physician in charge of anticoagulant therapy before a decision to proceed. It is prudent to advise the patient to contact the physician in charge of anticoagulant therapy and let him or her make the decision as to the date to stop and for how long.

Therapeutic Facet Blocks

There is a paucity of literature on the role of therapeutic facet joint injections. However, it is well accepted that facet joint pain may be successfully managed by intra-articular injections of steroid, medial branch blockade, and/or neurolysis of medial branch nerves.

Therapeutic benefit has been reported with the injection of corticosteroids, local anesthetics, or normal saline into the facet joints. The literature describing the effectiveness of these interventions is abundant.[12,26,56] Manchikanti et al,[26] in developing evidence-based practice guidelines for interventional techniques in managing chronic spinal pain, reviewed the available literature. They were unable to find any studies meeting inclusion criteria, even though the literature included multiple randomized and observational reports. A widely referenced randomized trial not meeting the inclusion criteria showed negative results.[59]

Multiple clinical trials evaluated the therapeutic role of medial branch blockade.[60–62] Based on the earlier definition (short-term <6 months and long-term ≥6months), data on medial branch blockade provide strong evidence for short-term pain relief and moderate evidence for long-term pain relief of lumbar facet joint origin.[12]

Indications and contraindications for therapeutic lumbar facet joint injection are the same as for diagnostic blockade, except that a negative response to diagnostic facet joint block is a contraindication for therapeutic facet joint injection.

Clinically Relevant Anatomy

The lumbar facet joints are formed by the articulation of the inferior articular process of one lumbar vertebra with the superior articular process of the next vertebra. The lumbar joints exhibit the features typical of synovial joints: (1) the articular facets are covered by articular cartilage, and a synovial membrane bridges the margins of the articular cartilages of the two facets in each joint[29]; and (2) surrounding the synovial membrane is a joint capsule that attaches to the articular processes a short distance beyond the margin of the articular cartilage.

The lumbar facet joints are well innervated. Lumbar facet joint capsules are richly innervated with encapsulated and unencapsulated free nerve endings.[29–32] The lumbar facet joints are appropriately equipped with sensory apparatus to transmit nociceptive and proprioceptive information. Nerve fibers and nerve endings also occur in the subchondral bone of the facet joints.[30] Nerve fibers and nerve endings are present in erosion channels extending from the subchondral bone to the articular cartilage.[33] These fibers may provide a pathway for nociception from these joints other than from the capsules.[30] Nerve fibers are distributed to the intra-articular inclusions of the facet joints.[34–36] Even though these fibers are known to contain substance P,[33] it is unclear whether these nerves are nociceptive[35] or predominantly vasoregulatory.[37] Interspinous ligaments are also richly innervated with nociceptive fibers and contain free nerve endings.[63–66] Each lumbar facet joint has dual innervation, being supplied by two medial branch nerves. Multiple variations have been described in the number and nature of lumbar dorsal rami branches that innervate the lumbar facet joints. The occasional origin of an articular branch from the dorsal ramus proper and atypical innervation of the ventral aspect of the adjacent joint have been described.[67] Various other descriptions of innervation also exist, but none has been confirmed.[30]

The L1-4 dorsal rami are short nerves that arise at nearly right angles from the lumbar spinal nerves.[68] Each nerve measures approximately 5 mm in length[69] with the dorsal ramus directed backward to the upper border of the subjacent transverse process.[30] The L5 dorsal ramus differs from the other lumbar dorsal rami in that it is longer and travels over the top of the ala of the sacrum.[69] The L1-4 dorsal rami divide into two or three branches as they approach their transverse processes. A medial branch and a lateral branch are always represented at every level. Although always represented, a variable third branch, termed an *intermediate branch*, frequently arises from the lateral branch instead of the dorsal ramus itself.[69] The L5 dorsal ramus forms only a medial branch and a branch that is equivalent to the intermediate branches of the other lumbar dorsal rami.

The medial branches are of paramount clinical importance and relevance because they provide sensory innervation to the facet joints. The medial branches of the L1-4 dorsal rami run across the top of their respective transverse processes and pierce the dorsal leaf of the intertransverse ligament at the base of the transverse process.[30] Subsequently, each nerve runs along bone at the junction of the transverse process root, with the root of the superior articular process hooking medially around the base of the superior articular process, covered by the mamilloaccessory ligament. Finally, the medial branch crosses the vertebral lamina, where it divides into multiple branches that supply the multifidus muscle, the interspinous muscle and ligament, and two facet joints.

Each medial branch supplies the facet joints above and below its course.[10,11,30,31,67–71] The medial branch of the L5 dorsal ramus has a different course and distribution than those of the L1-4 dorsal rami in that, instead of crossing a transverse process, it crosses the ala of the sacrum. The medial branch of the L5 dorsal ramus runs in the groove formed by the junction of the ala and the root of the superior articular process of the sacrum before hooking medially around the base of the lumbosacral facet joint.[30] It sends an articular branch to the facet joint before ramifying within the multifidus muscle.

The muscular distribution of the medial branches of the lumbar dorsal rami is very specific—each medial branch supplies only those muscles that arise from the lamina and spinous process of the vertebra with the same segmental number as the nerve.[69,72] This relationship indicates that the principal muscles that move a particular segment are innervated by the nerve of that segment.[30]

The lateral branches of the lumbar dorsal rami are principally distributed to the iliocostalis lumborum muscle, but those from the L1, L2, and L3 levels can emerge from the dorsal lateral border of this muscle to become cutaneous. The intermediate branches of the lumbar dorsal rami have only a musculature distribution—to the lumbar fibers of the longissimus muscle—and within this muscle they form an intersegmental plexus. The intermediate branch of the L5 dorsal ramus supplies the most caudal fibers of the longissimus, which arise from the L5 transverse process and attach to the medial aspect of the iliac crest.[30]

Technique

Lumbar Facet Joint Intra-Articular Injections

The patient is placed in the prone position on the fluoroscopy table. A towel roll or pillow can be placed under the abdomen, for easier entry into the joint. As with any lumbar intervention, a baseline anteroposterior (AP) fluoroscopic view of the lumbar spine is obtained and the fluoroscope is oriented. Facet joints may or may not be visible on AP fluoroscopy depending on the specific anatomy of the patient (**Fig. 163.1**).

Fluoroscopic views of the target joint are obtained. The fluoroscopy beam is rotated from the AP view toward the oblique view until the target facet joint is visible. The upper lumbar facet joints are typically aligned toward the sagittal plane and may be visible on AP imaging, whereas the lower joints are typically oriented increasingly toward the coronal plane so that oblique imaging is necessary to identify joint lines.[73,74] The target joint is then visualized under fluoroscopic guidance and the skin is marked.

A 22- to 25-gauge, 3½ inch spinal needle is then inserted through the anesthetized area. The needle is directed downward and obliquely (from lateral to medial) toward the selected joint under direct fluoroscopic visualization. Contact is made with the inferior articular processes. The needle is then withdrawn slightly and redirected to enter the target facet joint. As the needle is felt to penetrate the joint, advancement is stopped to prevent any potential damage to the articular cartilage.

If there is difficulty in obtaining capsular penetration, one may try to access the articular recesses by redirection of the needle just off the margins of the inferior articular processes. Another method of gaining intracapsular entry is to redirect the needle slightly medial or lateral to the posterior joint line so that the needle gains access via its medial placement to the insertion of the capsule on the articular process.[60,75]

When the needle is in an appropriate position, 0.2 to 0.5 mL of contrast is then injected into the joint to confirm proper placement. An arthrographic image should then be visualized.[76] During contrast, the injection outline of the oval-shaped joint capsule should be visualized with lack of vascular uptake and/or epidural spread. After contrast confirmation of intra-articular needle tip placement, the joint is injected with an anesthetic agent to complete a diagnostic block or in combination with a steroid for therapeutic injection.[73,75] **Figure 163.2** illustrates intra-articular placement of needles and injection of contrast.

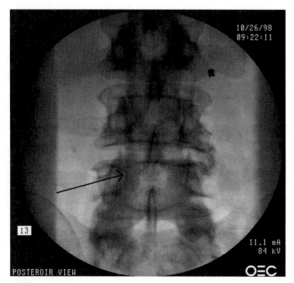

Fig. 163.1 Facet joints may or may not be visible on anteroposterior fluoroscopy depending on the specific anatomy of the patient.

Medial Branch Blocks

To block the sensory innervation to a lumbar facet joint, it is necessary to block the two medial branch nerves that supply the joint. **Table 163.3** illustrates the nerves to be blocked for each facet joint in the lumbar region. It is simple to remember which nerves need to be blocked to anesthetize a particular joint:

- Block the medial branch at the transverse process at the same level as the joint.
- Block the medial branch at the level below the joint.

Thus, to anesthetize the L3-4 facet joint, block the L2 medial branch at the transverse process of L3 and the L3 medial branch at the transverse process of L4. Similarly, to anesthetize the L5-S1 facet joint, block the L4 medial branch at the L5 transverse process and the L5 dorsal ramus at the sacral ala. For the L5-S1 facet joint, it has been suggested that additional innervation may be supplied by the communicating branch from the dorsal ramus of S1, which may be blocked just above the exit from the S1 posterior foramen.[73,74] However, it is has been demonstrated that blockade of the L4 medial branch and the L5 dorsal ramus alone adequately anesthetizes the L5-S1 facet joint from an experimental stimulus without the need for blockade of a potential ascending branch from S1.[10]

L1-4 Medial Branch Blocks

Dreyfuss et al[11] described that the nerves should be blocked proximal to the mamillo-accessory ligament and notch for the L1-4 medial branches. They described that the target location for the L1-4 medial branches is at the junction of the superior articular process and the transverse process where the nerve crosses, midway between the superior border of the transverse process and the location of the mamillo-accessory notch. In their opinion, L1-4 medial branch blocks at this location were not associated with inadvertent spread of injectate into the intervertebral foramen or epidural space. They also described that on oblique views, the target point lies high on the "eye" of the "Scottie dog" (**Fig. 163.3**). Placement more superior at the most superior junction of the superior articular process and transverse process as previously recommended apparently leads to an unacceptable incidence of spread into the neuroforamen. Dreyfuss et al[11] validated a slightly superior-to-inferior and lateral-to-medial needle approach to medial branch blocks. However, if an inferior-to-superior needle approach is used, the injected anesthetic theoretically might spread toward the spinal nerve root or the sinuvertebral nerve, thereby substantially decreasing the specificity of the block. For all medial branch blocks a 22- or 25-gauge spinal needle may be used.

Prone Position—Oblique: L1-4 Medial Branch Blocks

The patient is positioned in the prone position with a pillow under the abdomen. Fluoroscopic imaging is obtained. The C-arm must be adjusted to an oblique position. To maximally visualize the landmarks of the "Scottie dog," an approximate 25- to 30-degree angle is necessary depending on the specific level from the L1-4 medial branches. The needle is advanced toward the dorsal aspect of the transverse process root to ensure safe needle depth away from the ventral ramus. Using

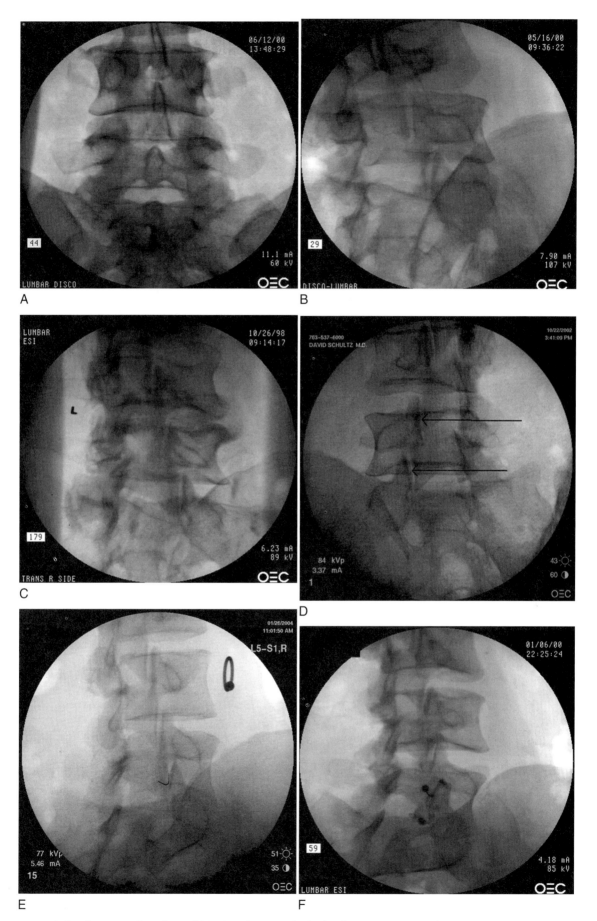

Fig. 163.2 Intra-articular placement of needles and injection of contrast for lumbar facet joint intra-articular injections. A, Anteroposterior image of lumbar spine with coronally oriented facet joints. B, Oblique view with joint lines visible, L4-5, L5-S1. C, Oblique view with joint lines visible at L3-4, L4-5, and L5-S1. D, With "down the beam" needle placement the skin insertion point is directly over the target. E, A 25-gauge spiral needle curving into L5-S1 facet joint. F, L4-5 arthrogram.

Table 163.3 **Facet Joint Nerves Required to Be Blocked for Each Facet Joint in Lumbar Region**

Facet Joint	Facet Joint Nerves to Be Blocked (Medial Branches or L5 Dorsal Ramus)	Level of Transverse Process or Sacral Ala
L1-2	T12 and L1 medial branches	At L1 transverse process for T12
		At L2 transverse process for L1
L2-3	L1 and L2 medial branches	At L2 transverse process for L1
		At L3 transverse process for L2
L3-4	L2 and L3 medial branches	At L3 transverse process for L2
		At L4 transverse process for L3
L4-5	L3 and L4 medial branches	At L4 transverse process for L3
		At L5 transverse process for L4
L5-S1	L4 medial branch L5 dorsal ramus	At L5 transverse process for L4 medial branch at sacral groove for L5 dorsal ramus

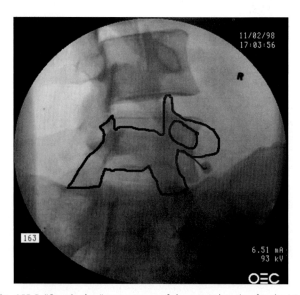

Fig. 163.3 "Scottie dog" appearance of the target location for the L1-4 medial branches.

an oblique view with the "Scottie dog" identified, the needle is advanced "down the beam" toward the target using a slightly superior starting position to the final target.

The needle will be directed anterior, medial, and caudad to reach the target location, using a "Scottie dog" view (see Fig. 163.3). Needles are typically placed down to contact with the bony end point using oblique fluoroscopic imaging. Before

injection, however, final needle tip position must be confirmed using both AP and lateral imaging to ensure that the needle tip is neither too deep nor too medial. On AP imaging, the needle tip should be at least in line with the lateral margin of the silhouette of the superior articular process and, if possible, medial to this margin.[73] On lateral imaging, the needle tip should be within the confines of the shadow of the dorsal elements and not protruding into the foramen. The superior articular process frequently bulges laterally, overlapping the target point dorsally. If the needle appears lateral to this point, it has contacted a thick transverse process instead of the superior articular process. In this case, the needle usually needs to be adjusted dorsally until correct position is obtained on both AP and oblique or lateral views.

Before injection, the bevel opening should be medial and slightly inferior to reduce lateral and superior flow to the intervertebral foramen, especially if the needle is placed inadvertently higher than the target position. **Figure 163.4** illustrates medial branch blocks with oblique approach.

Prone Position—Posteroanterior: L1-4 Medial Branch Blocks

The patient is positioned in the prone position with a pillow under the abdomen and fluoroscopic imaging is obtained. The C-arm must be adjusted straight anteroposterior from the skin entry point laterally using AP imaging, which is usually just above the tip of the target transverse process. The needle is advanced toward the back of the root of the transverse process to ensure safe needle depth away from the ventral ramus. The needle will be directed anterior, medial, and caudad to reach the target location. On AP imaging, the tip of the needle should be at least in line with the lateral margin of the silhouette of the superior articular process and, if possible, medial to this margin.[73]

The superior articular process frequently bulges laterally, overlapping the target point dorsally. If the needle appears lateral to this point, it has contacted a thick transverse process instead of the superior articular process. In this case, the needle usually needs to be adjusted dorsally until correct position is obtained. Before injection, the bevel opening should be medial and slightly inferior to reduce lateral and superior flow to the intervertebral foramen, especially if the needle is placed inadvertently higher than the target position.

L5 Dorsal Ramus Blocks

Position the patient in the prone position with a pillow under the abdomen. Begin with an AP view of the L5-S1 segment. Rotate the fluoroscope approximately 10 to 15 degrees oblique toward the side to be blocked to view the junction of the sacral ala and the superior articular process of S1. Further obliquity usually places the medial iliac crest in front of the trajectory to the target position. If the ilium obscures the target point view as the C-arm is rotated obliquely, cephalad tilt of the C-arm will usually bring the target into clear view by moving the ilium caudad within the fluoroscopic image. An angled needle tip will allow for adequate steering of the needle to the target despite a cephalad to caudad needle trajectory.

When a clear path to the target point for the L5 dorsal ramus is identified, a skin insertion point is chosen. The target point is recognized as a notch between the sacral ala

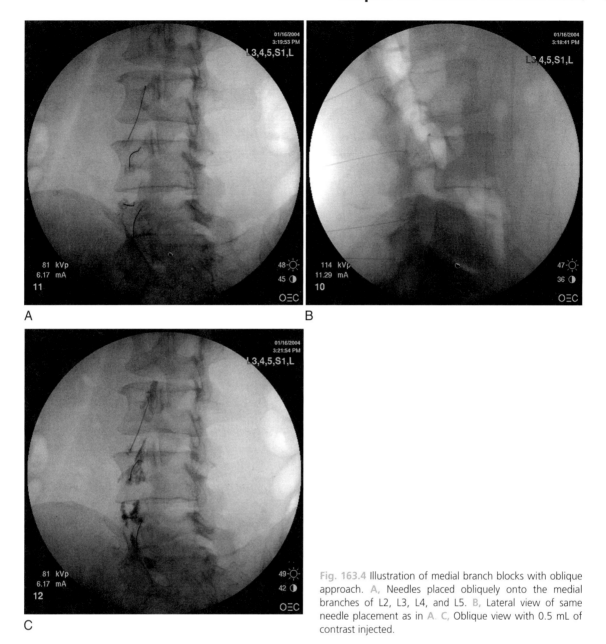

A

B

C

Fig. 163.4 Illustration of medial branch blocks with oblique approach. A, Needles placed obliquely onto the medial branches of L2, L3, L4, and L5. B, Lateral view of same needle placement as in A. C, Oblique view with 0.5 mL of contrast injected.

and the superior articulating process of S1. The target point lies opposite the middle of the superior articular process base and is slightly below the silhouette at the top of the sacral ala. Higher placement is associated with spread into the L5-S1 epidural space and lower placement with spread to the S1 posterior sacral foramen. The needle is advanced directly "down the beam" to the target position. AP imaging is then obtained to verify that the needle is placed at, or preferably medial to, the lateral silhouette of the S1 superior articular process. Lateral imaging should confirm that the needle tip lies within the shadow of the posterior spinal elements and does not protrude into the L5-S1 neuroforamen. After the needle tip is confirmed to be in the proper location, the bevel opening should be rotated medial. This has been shown to reduce inadvertent spread to the S1 posterior foramen or the L5 vertebral foramen.[11,73] **Figure 163.5** illustrates medial branch blocks with prone posteroanterior approach.

Drugs

Local anesthetic injection should be limited to 0.4 to 0.6 mL for a diagnostic block and approximately 1 mL of 1% lidocaine or 0.25% bupivacaine for a therapeutic block.

For diagnostic and therapeutic blocks, the literature has been limited to using local anesthetic agents of different durations of action, namely, lidocaine and bupivacaine. However, Manchikanti et al[62] have shown that the validity of diagnostic blocks is maintained with addition of adjuvant agents such as Sarapin and methylprednisolone, along with provision of a therapeutic benefit of much longer duration than with local anesthetic alone.

Side Effects and Complications

Complications from facet joint nerve blocks or intra-articular injections in the lumbar spine are exceedingly rare.[73,77,78] The most common complications of this technique are related to

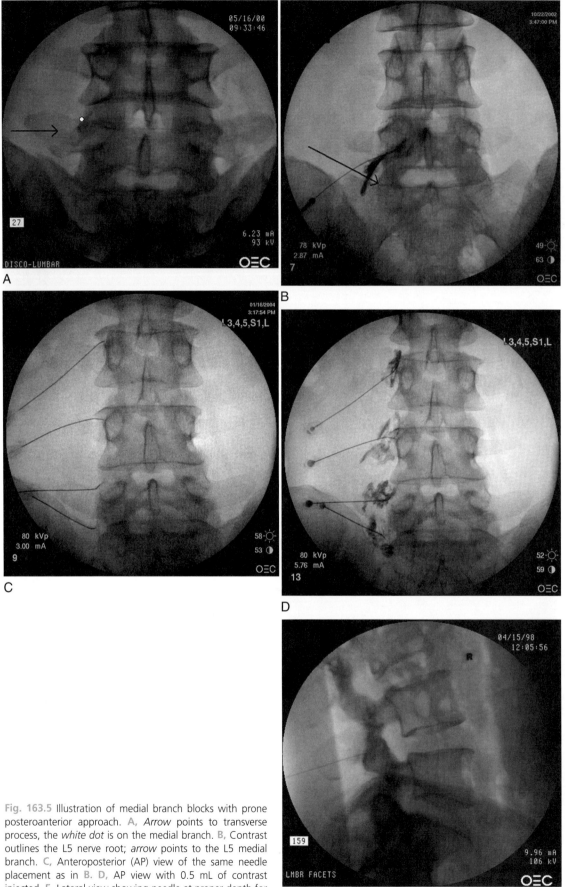

Fig. 163.5 Illustration of medial branch blocks with prone posteroanterior approach. **A,** *Arrow* points to transverse process, the *white dot* is on the medial branch. **B,** Contrast outlines the L5 nerve root; *arrow* points to the L5 medial branch. **C,** Anteroposterior (AP) view of the same needle placement as in **B. D,** AP view with 0.5 mL of contrast injected. **E,** Lateral view showing needle at proper depth for medial branch block of L4.

needle placement and drug administration. Most problems, such as local swelling, pain at the site of the needle insertion, and pain in the low back, are short-lived and self-limited. More serious complications may include dural puncture, spinal cord trauma, subdural injection, neural trauma, injection into the intervertebral foramen, and hematoma formation; infectious complications, including epidural abscess and bacterial meningitis; and side effects related to the administration of steroids, local anesthetics, and other drugs.[77–89] Thomson et al[87] reported instances of chemical meningitis after two-level facet joint injections and a one-level medial branch block from penetration of the dural cuff leading to subarachnoid placement of medication. However, large volumes of injectate were used, and the descriptions of the needle placement and contrast flow under fluoroscopic imaging before injection were not discussed. Berrigan[88] also reported chemical meningeal irritation. With the use of fluoroscopy with or without contrast, damage to a spinal nerve root or needle placement into the epidural or subarachnoid spaces should be exceedingly rare. Spinal anesthesia following lumbar facet joint injections also has been reported.[79,80] Infection associated with facet joint injections has been reported.[81,82,84]

Other minor complications may include light-headedness, flushing, sweating, nausea, hypotension, syncope, and nonpostural headaches. Some of these side effects may be related to the systemic uptake of injected steroids.[89] The major theoretical complications of corticosteroid administration include suppression of pituitary-adrenal axis, hypocorticism, Cushing syndrome, osteoporosis, avascular necrosis of bone, steroid myopathy, epidural lipomatosis, weight gain, fluid retention, and hypoglycemia. However, Manchikanti et al,[90] in evaluating the effect of neuraxial steroids on weight and bone mass density, showed no significant differences in patients undergoing various types of interventional techniques with or without steroids.

Conclusion

Lumbar facet joints are sources of local and referred pain in patients with low back and lower extremity pain in approximately 40% of cases. The definitive diagnosis of facet joint pain relies on properly performed, controlled, comparative local anesthetic or placebo-controlled blocks. These techniques provide an important diagnostic and potentially therapeutic role in the low back pain management. They should not be used in isolation but rather in the context of other diagnostic and therapeutic methodologies. The role of therapeutic facet joint nerve blocks is emerging; however, many questions remain regarding their clinical utility and role in daily interventional pain management practice. Further research is required to better define the role of diagnostic and therapeutic facet joint nerve blocks, as well as other interventional techniques, in the management of chronic low back pain.

References

Full references for this chapter can be found on www.expertconsult.com.

Chapter 164

Lumbar Sympathetic Nerve Block and Neurolysis

Michael Stanton-Hicks

Lumbar sympathetic ganglion block (LSB) is useful for the evaluation and management of sympathetically mediated pain in the kidneys, ureters, intestine, genitalia, and lower extremities. Included in this category are phantom limb pain, complex regional pain syndrome types I and II, and a variety of peripheral neuropathies. It is also useful in the palliation of pain secondary to vascular insufficiency of the lower extremity, including pain from frostbite, atherosclerosis, Buerger disease, and arteritis in collagen diseases. An LSB maximizes blood flow after vascular procedures on the lower extremities. A local anesthetic can be used for diagnosis when performing differential neural blockade on an anatomic basis in the evaluation of flank, pelvic, and lower extremity pain. Similarly, a local anesthetic is useful in the treatment of acute herpes zoster and postherpetic neuralgia involving the lumbar and sacral dermatomes. Neurolysis of the lumbar sympathetic chain may be indicated for the palliation of pain syndromes that have responded to LSB with local anesthetic.

Historical Considerations

The first report of lumbar sympathetic block was by Brunn and Mandl,[1] who, in a 1924 article, described Seiheim's technique of injecting the lumbar sympathetic nerves as a component of his paravertebral approach to blocking the mixed spinal outflow in the lumbar region. Eighteen years after Novocain was released in 1905, Kappis[2] described the technique for sympathetic block and surgical resection of the lumbar sympathetic nerves. During the 1920s various authors described a number of approaches.[3-8] During the l950s the importance of LSB, in relation to the treatment of causalgia and post-traumatic reflex dystrophies in servicemen after World War II, received

considerable attention.[9-11] The technique described by Mandl[4] in 1926 (the "classic" approach) remains one of the most popular approaches to the lumbar sympathetic trunk. Reid et al,[12] in a large series published in 1970, described a more lateral approach that avoids contact with the transverse process. This chapter describes both the classic and lateral approaches.

Indications

The indications for lumbar sympathetic block may be divided into three broad categories: (1) circulatory insufficiency in the leg, including arteriosclerotic vascular disease, diabetic gangrene, Buerger disease, Raynaud phenomenon and disease, and reconstructive vascular surgery after arterial embolic occlusion; (2) pain from renal colic, reflex sympathetic dystrophy, or causalgia (chronic regional pain syndrome types I and II), intractable urogenital pain, amputation stump pain, phantom pain, and frostbite; and (3) other conditions, such as hyperhidrosis, phlegmasia alba dolens, erythromelalgia, acrocyanosis, and trench foot. The rationale for sympathetic blocks in the treatment of pain is based on the observation that pain, under certain conditions, is potentiated or mediated by sympathetic activity. Laboratory evidence has shown that the sympathetic postganglionic neuron may act not only at its effector terminal, but also on the primary afferent neuron in certain pathologic conditions. It has been shown to communicate with the primary afferent neuron at other sites (direct and indirect coupling).[13,14] Although the mechanism is unclear, blocks of the sympathetic nervous system may have two actions: (1) interruption of preganglionic and postganglionic sympathetic efferents may influence function of the primary afferent neuron,[15-17] or (2) visceral afferents, from deep visceral structures in the leg that travel with the sympathetic nerves, may be blocked.[17] More recent work by Ali et al[18] demonstrated sensitization of C fibers to alpha$_1$-adrenergic agonists and development of spontaneous activity in C-fiber nociceptors. Acquisition of functional alpha$_1$-adrenergic receptors by nociceptors,[19] as a diagnostic and prognostic tool, sympathetic blocks are helpful in determining the nature of the pain (i.e., whether it is sympathetically maintained or whether it is independent of sympathetic function). Such procedures are always used to test the effects of destructive (neurolytic, chemical) sympatholysis or surgical sympathectomy.

Contraindications

Contraindications to sympathetic blocks are a bleeding diathesis, local infection, and certain anatomic anomalies. They may be considered relative contraindications if they are likely to render the procedure difficult or hazardous.

Functional Anatomy

The general anatomy of the sympathetic nervous system consists of central and peripheral components. The central components are the hypothalamus, midbrain, pons, medulla, and lateral columns of the spinal cord extending from TI to L2. Peripherally, the sympathetic nervous system consists of preganglionic and postganglionic efferent fibers that innervate deep somatic structures, skin, and viscera. The two paravertebral sympathetic trunks are connected segmentally by preganglionic neurons, whose cell bodies are situated in the lateral horn, intermediate nucleus, and paracentral nuclei of the thoracolumbar cord. The cell bodies responsible for vasoconstriction in the lower limbs are in the lower three thoracic and first three lumbar segments. The preganglionic fibers pass, by way of their corresponding nerves, as white rami communicantes, which communicate with considerable convergence in the paravertebral ganglia, with postganglionic efferents and in the prevertebral ganglia by postganglionic efferents to the pelvic viscera. A small percentage of postganglionic fibers pass directly to ganglia in the aortic plexus and the superior and inferior hypogastric plexus. The postganglionic fibers leave the sympathetic trunk as gray rami communicantes. Some pass to the L1 nerve to contribute to the iliohypogastric and genitofemoral nerve territories, some to the L2-5 nerves, and some to the upper three sacral nerves, where they pass on to their respective destinations in the lumbosacral plexus. Intermediate ganglia found in the psoas and iliacus muscles also communicate with postganglionic fibers that pass through the segmental lumbar and sacral nerves. The S1 and S2 nerves contain the largest numbers of postganglionic fibers. Most of these represent gray rami communicantes that subserve vasomotor, pilomotor, and sudomotor functions. It has been determined that, although each root of the lumbosacral plexus receives one group of gray rami communicantes, the S1-3 nerves contain several (i.e., a large convergence)[20] because they innervate the blood vessels in the lower extremity. Each lumbar sympathetic chain enters the retroperitoneal space under the right and left crura, continuing inferiorly in the interval between the anterolateral aspect of the vertebral bodies and the origin of the psoas muscle to enter the pelvis at the L5-S1 disk. The periosteum overlies the vertebral bodies and the fibroaponeurotic origin of the psoas muscles and their fascial coverings. Anterior is the parietal reflection of the peritoneum, the aorta lying anteromedial to the left trunk and the vena cava anterior to the right trunk. The white and gray rami communicantes pass to their respective ganglia beneath the fibrous arcades of psoas attachments to each vertebral body. Also, they tend to pass alongside the middle of the vertebral body, an observation that is of importance to needle placement. The sympathetic ganglia of the lumbar sympathetic chains vary in number and position. Rarely are five ganglia found on each side in the same individual.[21] In most cases, only four are found. There tends to be fusion of L1 and L2 ganglia in most patients, and ganglia are aggregated at the L2-3 and L4-5 disks. Also, there is considerable variability in the size of the ganglia, some being fusiform and 10 to 15 mm long and others being round and approximately 5 mm long.[22] Because of this aggregation and the fact that the right crus extends to L3 and the left to L2, sympathetic blockade is more efficacious when performed at the L3, L4, or L5 level, rather than at the L2 vertebral body, as is most common. Although most postganglionic sympathetic efferents join spinal nerves that form the lumbar plexus and pass distally as components of the femoral, sciatic, and obturator nerves, their branches distribute segmentally to their respective vessels in the lower limb. Block of L2-3 ganglia should interrupt most of the efferent sympathetic supply to the lower limb. In patients whose sympathetic pathways bypass the sympathetic chain and make synapses with their respective postganglionic efferents in somatic spinal nerves, complete sympathetic interruption is not achieved after surgical sympathectomy.[23] Important branches of the lumbar sympathetic trunk contain postganglionic efferents, visceral afferents, and lumbar somatic afferents that supply the axial skeleton and musculoskeletal structures in the hip and the lower limbs. With this understanding, there can be no "pure" sympathetic block. Some component of somatosensory block, if only a small one, always is present with every sympathetic blocking procedure.

Technique

Although the "classic" or paramedian technique describes the insertion of three needles from L2 to L4, this method has been modified to one using only two needles at L2 and L4,[24] or, in a later publication, a single-needle technique at either L2 or L3.[25] When a neurolytic procedure is to be undertaken, it is important to use at least two needles, if not three, to prevent too much local pressure developing at the injection sites with the potential for tracking toward the neural foramen. An image intensifier (fluoroscopy) or computed tomography (CT) scan should always be used to facilitate needle placement for LSB. Although the prone position is most convenient, patient comfort (e.g., pregnancy), pain, or anatomic deformity may make it necessary to place the patient in a left or right lateral decubitus position.

Classic or Traditional Technique

After sterile preparation of the skin and draping of the area, wheals are made 5 to 6 cm lateral to the spinous processes and on lines that are drawn through the upper margins of the second, third, or fourth lumbar spinous processes.[26] This placement can be verified by anteroposterior fluoroscopy (**Fig. 164.1**). With an 8-cm, 22-gauge needle, a local anesthetic solution is infiltrated down to the respective transverse processes, forming tracts through which the 15 cm, 20-gauge

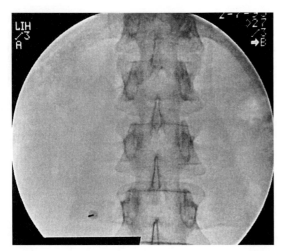

Fig. 164.1 Anteroposterior view of the needle seen end-on after being introduced to the transverse process of L3.

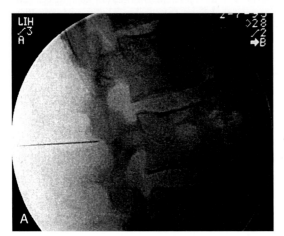

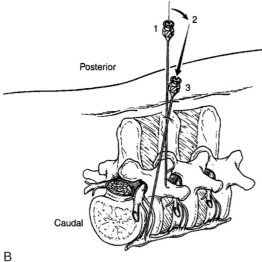

Fig. 164.2 A, Lateral radiograph shows proper needle position. B, Lateral view shows the needle tip and alignment on the inferior aspect of the transverse process of L3.

sympathectomy needle and stylet can be introduced. Each sympathectomy needle is introduced at an angle of 5 to 10 degrees from the parasagittal plane and is advanced so as to contact the transverse process (**Fig. 164.2**). At this point, a lateral view with the image intensifier is taken to observe the alignment,

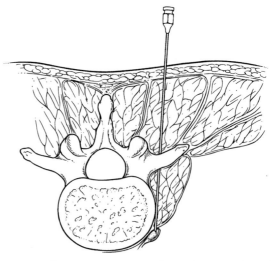

Fig. 164.3 Needle tip in correct portion for lumbar sympathetic block.

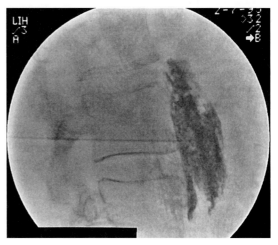

Fig. 164.4 Lateral image shows the needle at the anterolateral aspect of the vertebral body with the retroperitoneal space identified by longitudinal spread of contrast material.

and any small adjustments necessary are made to set up the proper angle so that the needle reaches the anterolateral aspect of the vertebral body (**Fig. 164.3**). The latter view is obtained by "looking down the needle" with the image intensifier. The needle is introduced by following the axis of the image intensifier camera, and an imaginary line is subtended to reach the anterolateral aspect of the vertebral body of interest. The needle depth can be determined by taking a lateral view (**Fig. 164.4**). Care should be taken when the needle is passed below the transverse process because it may contact the posterior or anterior primary rami at that level. Should the needle contact the vertebral body, medial pressure on the paraspinous muscle usually induces sufficient bend in the needle to deflect it from the side of the vertebral body and allow it to pass forward through the psoas muscle and its investing fascia to reach the retroperitoneal space (**Fig. 164.5**).[27] With a loss-of-resistance syringe and light percussion with the tip of a finger, the retroperitoneal space may be identified (**Fig. 164.6**).[28] The position of the needle tip can verified by injection of a small amount of air to produce an "airogram" or non-ionizable, water-soluble contrast material.[29,30] The technique just described is repeated

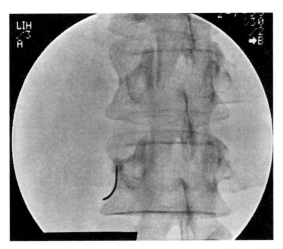

Fig. 164.5 Oblique (and slightly inclined) view of the spine shows deflection of the needle produced by lateral pressure on the trunk and slight curving of the needle to allow it to pass alongside the vertebral body.

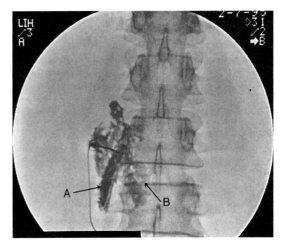

Fig. 164.7 Compound figure shows the correct position of the needle, and contrast is depicted in two tissue planes. *A,* The striated linear spread is within the psoas fascia and is incorrect. *B,* The "vacuolated" appearance is retroperitoneal. and the spread of contrast material is in the correct plane.

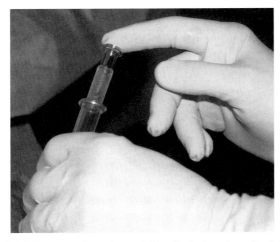

Fig. 164.6 The retroperitoneal space is identified using a loss-of-resistance syringe and light percussion with the tip of the finger.

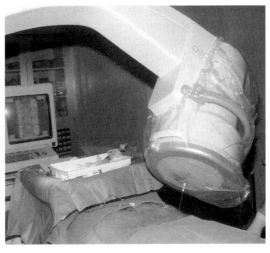

Fig. 164.9 View of the image intensifier positioned to "look down" the needle during the Reid or lateral approach.

at each additional level. If the needles have been placed in the correct space (retroperitoneal), the injected contrast material should confluent at each vertebral level (**Fig. 164.7B**; see Fig. 164.4). If the contrast material has been placed within the substance of the psoas or just beneath its fascia, the appearance is as shown in **Figure 164.7A**. This position produces incomplete sympatholysis.

Lateral Technique

The lateral technique is favored over the paramedian technique because it causes less discomfort for the patient, does not require contact with the transverse process, is unlikely to encounter a segmental nerve, and provides a direct path and optimal position to contact the lumbar sympathetic trunk and its ganglia.[12] This technique requires only two needles, and, with experience, a single-needle technique can be used successfully in almost 80% of cases.[30] It is unnecessary to measure the point of needle insertion; rather, this point is determined by using the fluoroscope's C-arm as a sighting

device (**Fig. 164.8 [online only]** and **Fig. 164.9**). Distance from the midline, depending on the girth of the patient, is 8 to 12 cm. After a skin wheal is raised, a tract of local anesthetic can be infiltrated using a 22-gauge spinal needle. The 15 cm, 20-gauge sympathetic block needle is introduced at an angle that allows it to arrive at the anterolateral aspect of the vertebral body margin. The axis of the C-arm camera, when positioned to look down the needle (**Fig. 164.10 [online only]**), should facilitate insertion of the needle into the retroperitoneal space (**Fig. 164.11**). Using a lateral view to check its depth (**Fig. 164.12**), the final few millimeters of the needle's travel can be undertaken by the loss-of-resistance syringe until the retroperitoneal space is reached. If the needle contacts the side of the vertebral body, the needle may be deflected from this position by first being withdrawn 2 to 3 cm and then being passed alongside the vertebral body by medial pressure on the paraspinous musculature (see Fig. 164.5). Correct alignment of the needle and its position

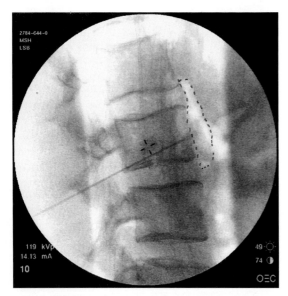

Fig. 164.11 Transverse view shows position of the needle tip at the sympathetic trunk using the Reid or lateral approach.

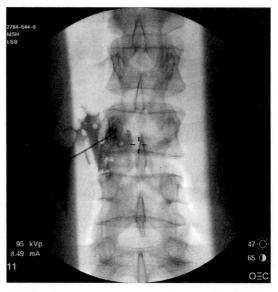

Fig. 164.13 Anteroposterior projection of contrast spread in patient shown in Figure 164.12.

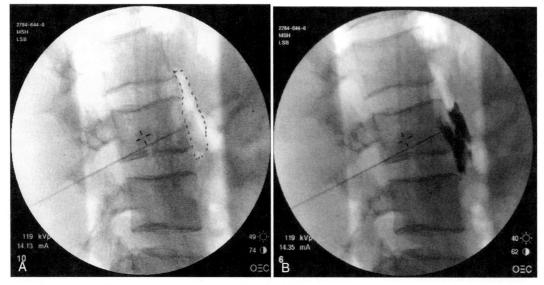

Fig. 164.12 A, Lateral image of needle in position with "airogram" obtained after injection of 2 mL of air. B, Lateral image of needle in the same patient after the injection of 2 mL of radiopaque contrast material.

in the retroperitoneal space can be determined by injecting either a small amount of air to produce an "airogram"(see Fig. 164.12A) or non-ionizable, water-soluble contrast medium (**Fig. 164.13;** see also Fig. 164.12B). Use of CT as an aid to needle placement is shown in **Fig. 164.14**.

Comment

When determining loss of resistance, it is necessary to ballotte the plunger of the syringe gently with a finger because the thumb is too insensitive in most cases to feel the small change in pressure as the needle tip enters the retroperitoneal space. Sometimes, as a result of previous retroperitoneal surgery, peritoneal inflammatory disease, or neurolytic sympatho-

lysis, the retroperitoneal space is obliterated, and no loss of resistance is recognizable. Under such circumstances, it may be necessary to place the needle tip anatomically in relation to the vertebral body, taking advantage of biplanar views, and to dissect the space by injection of saline and contrast material. Injection of any therapeutic or diagnostic solutions should be monitored by continuous imaging. Movement of the contrast tracer confirms its correct dispersion and alerts the observer to any anomalous spread. Injected solutions may enter a lymphatic, vein, or artery and may spread in an unwanted tissue plane, such as alongside the rami communicantes to the lateral foramen. Imaging time should be kept to a minimum. Bonica[9] suggested that, in the presence of an unexpectedly poor sympatholysis, it may be necessary to undertake

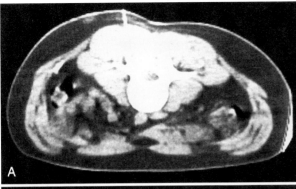

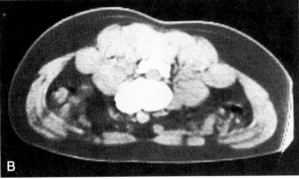

Fig. 164.14 A, CT-guided needle placement for lumbar sympathetic block. B, Proper spread of contrast medium outlining the sympathetic chain.

prognostic blocks of the lower thoracic sympathetic ganglia in addition to the lumbar ganglia, in case postganglionic fibers have taken routes other than the lumbar trunk to reach the lower extremities.

Medications Employed for Sympatholysis

Although short-acting local anesthetics are commonly used for prognostic and therapeutic sympathetic blocks, a long-acting agent, such as bupivacaine, is advantageous for therapy and prognosis. It provides the patient a longer time to evaluate the effects of sympatholysis and any effect this might have on the pain. A concentration of 0.375% bupivacaine gives optimal duration without the need for an added vasoconstrictor. The disadvantage of bupivacaine is its relatively long latency (5 to 8 minutes). It may be shortened by mixing 2% chloroprocaine and 0.75% bupivacaine in equal proportions. Alternatively, a 5 mL/test injection of 2% chloroprocaine can precede the injection of bupivacaine, thereby shortening the time of onset. A solution of 10% to 16% phenol in diatrizoate sodium (Renografin) is suitable for neurolysis. Although an "older" ionized contrast material, it is the only solution that has undergone stability testing, and it has a long shelf life.[31]

Evaluation of Sympathetic Blocks

Evidence of sympatholysis is indicated by a rise in temperature of the limb. An end-temperature measurement of greater than 34.5°C (94°F) is an indication that over 90% of the sympathetic supply to the limb has been interrupted. In the absence of severe peripheral vascular disease, only such an end point can be used to determine whether a patient has sympathetically maintained pain or sympathetically independent pain. Although there are other tests of sympathetic block, including a skin conductance test, cold pressor test, and skin potential response, these are impractical for clinical purposes. It should also be remembered that reflex activity in sympathetic vasoconstrictor fibers to muscles is independent of the activity in cutaneous vasoconstrictor neurons and therefore might not be totally blocked by sympathetic blocks, an aspect that places into question the specificity of sympatholysis for SMP.

Complications

Similar to all regional anesthetic blocks, sympatholysis may result in intravascular injection; however, the chance of intravenous injection should be negligible if fluoroscopic guidance is used throughout the injection.[32,33] The most common complication associated with lumbar sympatholysis is neuralgia of the genitofemoral nerve, particularly for the lateral approach.[34] The incidence of genitofemoral neuralgia has been reported to be 15%, but it may be only 4% with a single-needle technique. Most cases are transient and resolve with nonprescription analgesics, but the condition may last 6 weeks. A repeat local anesthetic sympathetic block commonly produces immediate remission. Similarly, intravenous lidocaine may be used in a dose of 1 to 2 mL/kg, or transcutaneous nerve stimulation may be employed over the thigh for genitofemoral neuralgia. Other complications are necrosis of the psoas muscle and sloughing of the ureter (D. Reed, personal communication, 1985). Bleeding may occur in a patient with a clotting deficiency, which, in any case, would be a contraindication to sympathetic block. Otherwise, any bleeding from needle puncture should be self-limiting. Patients should be warned that they may have some hypotension immediately after sympatholysis, and men should be apprised that they may experience impotence or failure of ejaculation, particularly if a neurolytic procedure is undertaken. No incidence has been established for this latter complication.

Interpretation of and Responses to Lumbar Sympathetic Block

It is important to understand the patient's personality when interpreting the subsequent effects of sympatholysis. Although evidence of sympatholysis—vasodilation, increased temperature, and reduction of edema—is important, the qualitative effect on the preexisting symptoms, for example, continuous pain, hyperalgesia, or touch-evoked pain such as allodynia, requires careful assessment after sympatholysis. Technical failure may be the cause of therapeutic failure, even on repeated occasions. A placebo response is normal and may merely be the response of a grateful patient to the fact that something fundamental has been done to unravel a particular medical condition. The amount of local anesthetic used for sympatholysis, as the result of its own uptake, may affect multisynaptic pathways in the central nervous system, producing central inhibition of nociception, an effect that erroneously may be attributed to sympatholysis.[35,36] Lumbar sympatholysis is associated with few complications and is normally a reproducible technique when carried out with proper imaging guidance. Appropriate knowledge of anatomy and good technique are required to minimize the risk of harm to the patient, and the procedure is valuable in the management of a comparatively small but treatment-refractory group of painful conditions. Treede et al[37] have questioned the efficacy and reproducibility of sympathetic block (as did Bonica[9]), particularly in relation to pain relief, as a response. Nevertheless, carefully performed, sympathetic block is a useful and important therapeutic diagnostic procedure.

References

Full references for this chapter can be found on www.expertconsult.com.

Ilioinguinal-Iliohypogastric Nerve Block

Vimal Akhouri and Carol A. Warfield

Historical Considerations

Ponka[1] was one of the first to describe a technique of ilioinguinal, iliohypogastric, and twelfth intercostal nerve block. Several modifications of this technique have been created, which vary mainly in the choice of local anesthetics and the injection sites. In 1978 a major article in the surgical literature propounded the broad use of this nerve block in adult herniorrhaphy.[2] In 1987 the value of this procedure gained further importance in the diagnosis of ilioinguinal and genitofemoral entrapment neuralgia when Starling et al[3] described a series of patients for whom an ilioinguinal block was essential in diagnosing postherniorrhaphy neuralgia. Since 1980 the anesthetic and analgesic efficacies of the block have been studied in combination with or in comparison with other regional techniques, including spinal anesthesia, instillation, and infiltration techniques.[4-7] Various approaches have also examined the efficacy of this nerve block combined with sedation or general anesthesia. This block seems to have gained wide acceptance by anesthesiologists and surgeons, especially for outpatient groin surgery. In particular, an article by Song et al[8] showed the cost effectiveness of this anesthetic technique when combined with monitored anesthesia care with respect to speed of recovery, patient comfort, and associated incremental cost.

Indications

Diagnostic Use

Neuropathic groin, testicular, or medial thigh pain in the distribution of the ilioinguinal and iliohypogastric nerves is caused by chronic inflammation or entrapment of the nerve following surgery, blunt abdominal trauma, or other pathologic processes.[3,9] Because of considerable overlap in their anatomic locations and courses, the ilioinguinal and iliohypogastric nerves are frequently referred to as the *ilioinguinal-iliohypogastric (INIH) nerve*. INIH nerve block with local anesthetic is used diagnostically in differentiating localized entrapment from other lumbosacral causes of neuropathic pain.[2,3] Because of the overlap of the INIH neuralgia sensory distribution with that of lumbar radiculopathy, ineffective ilioinguinal block suggests other causes of neuropathy. A differential diagnostic list may include involvement of the genitofemoral nerve, L1 lumbar radiculopathy, lumbar plexus lesions, infection, malignant disease invading the lumbar plexus, epidural or vertebral metastatic disease at T12-L1, referred pain, myofascial pain, and central causes.[3,9] Lumbosacral spine disease must be suspected, especially in patients whose groin pain occurs without a history of hernia or previous herniorrhaphy.[10] Electromyography and magnetic resonance imaging of the lumbar plexus are indicated in this patient population. If neurolysis or destruction of the nerve is to be performed, the ilioinguinal nerve block may be useful as a prognostic indicator of the degree of motor and sensory impairment.

Clinical Diagnosis

INIH neuralgia may be suspected when pain occurs after groin surgery or trauma. Besides pain in the peripheral nerve distribution over the groin, hemiscrotum, labia majora, and Scarpa's triangle, the patient may have associated paresthesia, hypoesthesia, hyperesthesia, and radiating pain. Frequently, patients report exacerbation of pain on stooping or walking and a decrease in pain by keeping the hip flexed. Tapping on the abdominal wall medial to the anterior-superior iliac spine (ASIS) may elicit the pins and needles sensation known as *Tinel's sign.*

Analgesic Use

Whether a diagnosis is made clinically or by differential nerve blockade, palliative INIH nerve block can be used as an adjunct to pharmacologic methods of pain relief. In the acute setting, the INIH nerve block has been used with variable success after inguinal herniorrhaphy, cesarean section, abdominal hysterectomy, appendectomy, varicocelectomy, and hydrocelectomy.[4,11,12] Following cesarean section, ilioinguinal nerve block may prolong the time to administration of morphine.[7] Another randomized controlled trial showed similar results with an intraoperative block.[4] No evidence indicates that combining INIH nerve block with neuraxial anesthesia provides any benefit. For example, in one randomized study, no additional benefits 6 hours postoperatively were found in patients receiving both INIH block and spinal anesthesia for herniorrhaphy.[13] In contrast, an alternative approach involving local wound instillation or infiltration[6,14,15] following inguinal herniorrhaphy was shown to be effective for postoperative analgesia in children and may be especially useful in uncooperative children who are afraid of needles.[6,16] Except for postherniorrhaphy pain, however, one systematic review of wound infiltration for various abdominal operations showed no conclusive benefits.[11,12]

Persistent or chronic pain in the groin and testicular areas is a difficult problem. The frequency of chronic pain after inguinal herniorrhaphy may be as high as 54%.[17] No reliable, standardized treatments for persistent or chronic groin pain and orchialgia exist, however. Persistent or chronic pain may be caused by inflammation, entrapment, or deafferentation from infection or trauma. Once neuralgia has been specifically attributed to either the ilioinguinal nerve or the iliohypogastric nerve, or both, a solution of local anesthetic with steroid is usually injected directly onto the nerve.[18] The use of an indwelling catheter for repeated INIH blocks into an interabdominis plane has been described,[19] and it may promote further research into devices for continuous infusion. Radiofrequency lesioning of the ilioinguinal nerve for postherniorrhaphy pain and orchialgia was successful in a small, anecdotal series of three patients in whom pain relief was 100% at 6-month follow-up.[20] This technique is particularly promising for having the longest duration of analgesia, but more definitive randomized trials are needed to evaluate its efficacy and safety. Randomized studies of cryoanalgesic ablation of the ilioinguinal nerve have not shown any benefits.[21,22]

Anesthesia

For surgical anesthesia, the INIH nerve block may be used separately or in combination with the genitofemoral nerve block, depending on the extent of the operation. The most widely accepted use of this anesthetic block in the United States is for groin surgery. However, reports exist in the literature on common uses in lower abdominal surgery, pelvic surgery with the Pfannenstiel incision (cesarean section, hysterectomy, myomectomy, Burch), varicocelectomy, hydrocelectomy, and orchidopexy.[23–25] Based on the preferences of the patient, the anesthesiologist, or the surgeon, the INIH block can be used as part of a regional technique with or without sedation or as a supplement to general anesthesia. Many studies have attempted to evaluate the efficacy of the INIH block at various perioperative stages. Currently, no conclusive

evidence of efficacy of analgesia favoring either preoperative, intraoperative, or postoperative INIH blockade is available.[26,27] The INIH nerve block is commonly used in pediatric outpatient surgery because of quicker recovery and decreased postoperative analgesic requirements.[28] Contraindications are common to any regional blockade and include patient refusal, local anesthetic allergy, severe coagulation disorders, and local infection.

Clinically Relevant Anatomy

The ilioinguinal nerve (**Fig. 165.1**) branches from the L1 nerve root, with some contribution from T12. The nerve runs obliquely across the quadratus lumborum muscle and the iliacus posterior to the kidney. It continues anteriorly at the level of the ASIS to perforate the transversus abdominis muscle. The nerve may interconnect with the iliohypogastric nerve, where it continues inferiorly and medially along the spermatic cord, through the superficial inguinal ring, and into the inguinal canal. Its lateral branch pierces the muscle of the lateral abdominal wall to supply the skin over the lateral gluteal region. In general, the sensory distribution includes the superomedial thigh, the root of the penis and upper scrotum in male patients, or the mons pubis and lateral labium majus in female patients (**Fig. 165.2**). Overlap can exist with the sensory distribution of the iliohypogastric nerve, which may interconnect with the ilioinguinal nerve.

The iliohypogastric nerve branches from the L1 nerve root, with some contribution from T12 (see Fig. 165.1). The nerve runs obliquely across the quadratus lumborum and iliacus and perforates the transversus abdominis muscle to lie between it and the oblique muscle. An anterior branch pierces the external oblique muscle to provide cutaneous sensory innervation to the abdominal skin above the pubis (**Fig. 165.3**). A lateral branch provides cutaneous sensory innervation to the posterolateral gluteal region.

Techniques

Anesthetic Technique

The patient is placed in the supine position with a pillow under the knees. A line is drawn between the ASIS and the umbilicus, and an injection site is located approximately 2 inches superomedial to the ASIS (**Fig. 165.4**). Another line is drawn between the ASIS and the pubic symphysis; the injection site is approximately 2 inches inferomedial to the ASIS.

After sterile preparation, a 25-gauge, short-bevel needle is inserted at a 45-degree angle to the skin, in a caudal direction toward the pubic symphysis (see Fig. 165.4). The bevel is kept parallel to the plane. After passing through the skin and subcutaneous tissue, the needle meets the firm resistance of the external oblique sheath. The needle is pushed to penetrate this sheath with a definite snap. From 5 to 7 mL of local anesthetic solution is injected in a fanlike manner into the plane deep to the external oblique aponeurosis. Attention should be paid when piercing the fascia of the external oblique muscle to avoid entering the peritoneal cavity. For additional anesthesia of the distal portion of the INIH nerve, another 5 mL of anesthetic solution is injected into the subcutaneous region at the pubic spine.

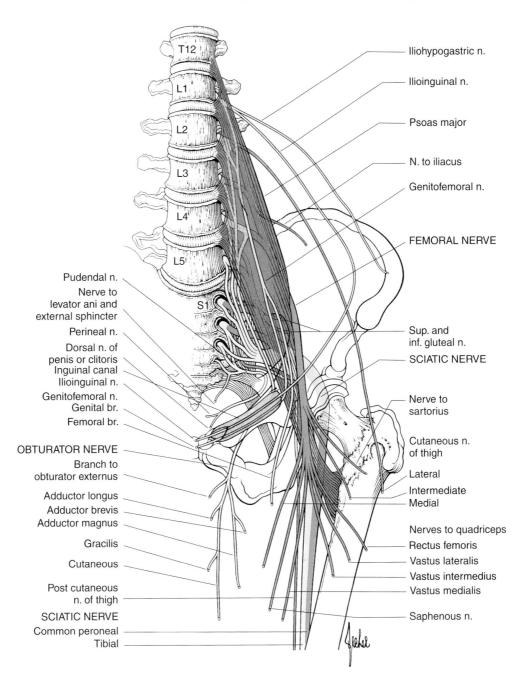

Pudendal n.
Nerve to
levator ani and
external sphincter
Perineal n.
Dorsal n. of
penis or clitoris
Inguinal canal
Ilioinguinal n.
Genitofemoral n.
Genital br.
Femoral br.
OBTURATOR NERVE
Branch to
obturator externus
Adductor longus
Adductor brevis
Adductor magnus
Gracilis
Cutaneous
Post cutaneous
n. of thigh
SCIATIC NERVE
Common peroneal
Tibial

Iliohypogastric n.
Ilioinguinal n.
Psoas major
N. to iliacus
Genitofemoral n.
FEMORAL NERVE
Sup. and
inf. gluteal n.
SCIATIC NERVE
Nerve to
sartorius
Cutaneous n.
of thigh
Lateral
Intermediate
Medial
Nerves to quadriceps
Rectus femoris
Vastus lateralis
Vastus intermedius
Vastus medialis
Saphenous n.

Fig. 165.1 **Anatomic location and course of the ilioinguinal and iliohypogastric nerves.**

Supplemental infiltrations of the spermatic cord may also be performed. Separate blockade of the iliohypogastric nerve is difficult because of its close approximation to the ilioinguinal nerve, but it may be possible by choosing an injection site 1 inch medial and inferior to the ASIS.[18] After the block, pressure may be applied to the injection site to prevent ecchymosis and hematoma formation.[18] For longer blocks lasting up to 12 hours, ropivacaine 0.5% may be used.[29] Injections of 0.25 mL/kg of ropivacaine result in safe plasma concentrations of ropivacaine that peak at 30 to 45 minutes.[30,31] In pediatric regional anesthesia, ropivacaine and levobupivacaine may be favored because of their safer pharmacokinetic properties of longer absorption times and lower peak plasma concentrations.[30–32]

Ultrasound-Guided Technique

The advent of portable ultrasound machines increased their use in identifying tissue planes more accurately, thus increasing precision and success in regional anesthesia. The ilioinguinal and iliohypogastric nerves can be visualized medial to the ASIS as it traverses between the transverses abdominis and internal oblique abdominal muscles. The patient is placed in the supine position, and a line is drawn between the ASIS and the umbilicus. An ultrasound probe (8 to 15 MHz) is placed on this line close to the ASIS and is moved medially on this line for better visualization (**Fig. 165.5**). In this position, the three muscle planes are clearly identified, with the nerves lying between the internal oblique and transverses abdominis (**Fig. 165.6**). If the nerves are not visualized, however, then the

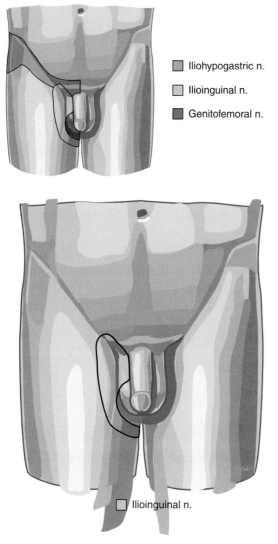

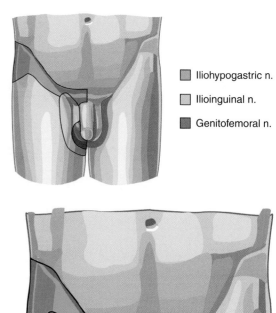

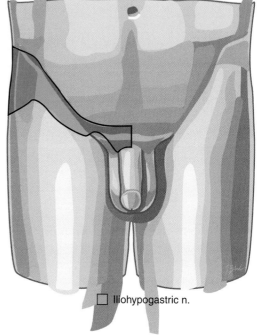

Fig. 165.2 **Sensory distribution of the ilioinguinal nerve.**

Fig. 165.3 **Sensory distribution of the iliohypogastric nerve.**

branch of deep circumflex iliac artery, which traverses parallel to ilioinguinal nerve in the same plane, can be visualized using Doppler imaging. The needle is introduced in plane from the lateral side to the fascial layer between the muscles. The needle can be more precisely placed and the deposition of medication clearly visualized. After testing for intravascular placement, the clinician injects 5 to 15 mL of local anesthetic with or without steroids. Direct sonographic visualization improves success and decreases the risk of complications.

Analgesic or Diagnostic Technique

The analgesic technique is much simpler. A single injection site is located 2 cm medially and inferiorly from the ASIS. At a 45-degree angle, and staying parallel to the plane of the aponeurosis, a 25-gauge, short-bevel needle is advanced inferiorly and medially toward the symphysis pubis while the clinician aspirates for blood, until a snap marks the piercing of the external oblique aponeurosis. At this time, after standard testing against intravascular injection, the clinician injects 5 to 15 mL of local anesthetic with or without steroids in a fanlike manner in the layer between the internal and external oblique muscles.

Side Effects and Complications

Complications of INIH nerve blockade are rare, but they can be devastating. Precautions that are common to regional anesthesia techniques should be taken throughout the procedure. Intravascular injection of bupivacaine can be catastrophic, and particular care should be taken to aspirate before any volume is injected. The safety of the local anesthetic again may depend on the agent used. In particular, avoidance of toxicity may be observed in both adults and pediatric patients by using ropivacaine or levobupivacaine instead of bupivacaine.[19–23,29–33] Higher plasma concentrations of bupivacaine occur in smaller children after ilioinguinal block.[34] Similarly, hematoma and ecchymosis can be prevented by constant aspiration of the needle on entry into the interabdominis area.

Penetration of the peritoneum and perforation of viscera are rare, but potentially disastrous, often requiring surgical repair. A few cases have been reported, mainly involving children.[33,35,36] Use of a short, blunt-bevel needle may reduce the risk of accidental visceral puncture, although caution regarding the depth of needle penetration should still

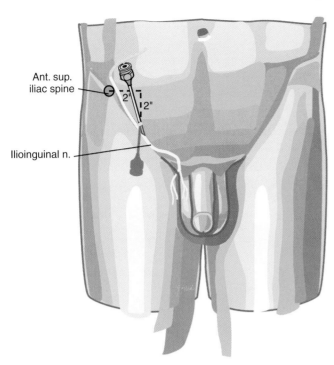

Fig. 165.4 **Injection technique for ilioinguinal-iliohypogastric nerve block.**

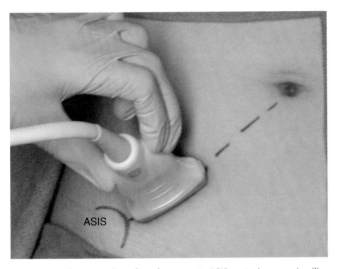

Fig. 165.5 **Ultrasound probe placement.** ASIS, anterior-superior iliac spine.

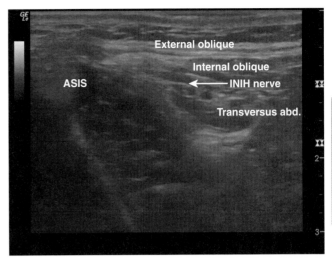

Fig. 165.6 **Ultrasound image of ilioinguinal-iliohypogastric nerve.** ASIS, anterior-superior iliac spine; abd, abdominis; INIH, ilioinguinal-iliohypogastric.

be maintained because one report noted visceral puncture with this type of needle.[36] Femoral nerve palsy is a benign complication, which is self-resolving,[33,35,36] but it may delay recovery and outpatient surgery discharge.[36–38] The mechanism for this palsy was well described by Rosario et al[37] and suggests that femoral nerve palsy may occur more commonly than has been reported. The local anesthetic may diffuse in the plane connecting the transversalis fascia and the iliacus fascia, which contains the femoral nerve. Studies may be needed to evaluate the incidence of palsy with different volumes of injectate.

Conversely, failed blockade may occur if the needle position is too superficial. When a block fails in the awake patient, a supplemental dose of local anesthetic may be injected or infiltrated into the surgical site, such as the hernia orifice and spermatic cord. Overall, ilioinguinal nerve blockade is a safe procedure. As with any regional technique, the operator should pay careful attention to technique, anatomy, proper equipment, and appropriate testing against intravascular injection.

Conclusion

The INIH nerve block is a simple regional block with minimal adverse effects. The block is easily performed, effective, and safe in both adults and children who require anesthesia or analgesia. Used as an individual regional technique or with monitored anesthesia care, this block improves outpatient surgery efficiency with minimal risks. In eliciting temporary neurotomy, it serves as a minimally invasive method for the differential diagnosis of chronic groin and testicular pain and may save patients from unnecessary groin reexploration after herniorrhaphy and from neurectomy, which may potentially worsen the condition.[20] Improvements are needed to extend the duration of the therapeutic use of this technique for patients with chronic pain. Current modalities for neurolysis hold future promise but require further investigation.

References

Full references for this chapter can be found on www.expertconsult.com.

Chapter 166

Lateral Femoral Cutaneous Nerve Block

David P. Bankston and Steven D. Waldman

Historical Considerations

Lateral femoral cutaneous neuropathy is one of the first reported entrapment neuropathies, having been initially described in Germany in 1895 by W. K. Roth and M. Bernhardt. Bernhardt coined the phrase *meralgia tica,* meaning thigh pain. Five years later, Harvey Cushing reported operating on a patient with meralgia paresthetica who transiently improved but ultimately became worse than preoperatively. Sigmund Freud had meralgia paresthetica. Freud initially believed it to be psychogenic, although he subsequently altered his thoughts.

Indications

1. The procedure may be used to block sensation to skin graft donor sites on the thigh.[1]
2. It may be used in combination with sciatic and femoral blocks for surgical procedures performed on the lower extremities.
3. Perhaps the most common application of the lateral femoral cutaneous block is to treat meralgia paresthetica, a compressive disorder of the nerve[2] (**Fig. 166.1** and **Table 166.1**).
4. If a neurolytic block is contemplated, the block may be used for prognostic value to determine the degree of impairment that may be present after destruction of the lateral femoral cutaneous nerve.[3]

Clinically Relevant Anatomy

The lateral femoral cutaneous nerve originates from the posterior divisions at L2 and L3 nerve roots.[4] The nerve pierces the psoas muscle, traveling inferior-lateral until it runs inferior or occasionally invades the ilioinguinal ligament[1,2] just medial to the anterior superior iliac spine. The nerve is prone to compression at this spot[2,4,5] (**Fig. 166.2**). It then divides into anterior and posterior branches under the fascia lata. The anterior branch supplies sensation to the anterior lateral thigh, whereas the posterior branch supplies the lateral thigh from above the greater trochanter to the knee.

Technique

Place the patient supine and identify the anterior superior iliac spine. A point 2 to 3 cm medial and 2 to 3 cm inferior to the spine, depending on the patient's size, is then marked. A 25-gauge 1½-inch needle is passed perpendicular to the skin until a fascial pop is felt or paresthesia is obtained[1,3] (**Fig. 166.3**). An injection of 10 to 15 mL of local anesthetic together with 80 mg of Depo-Medrol or Kenalog should be made in a fanlike manner. If the iliac crest is contacted, injection can continue more medially. Care should be taken not to advance the needle too far, especially in a thin patient, to avoid the peritoneal cavity and possible visceral perforation, as illustrated in **Figure 166.4**. Ultrasound guidance may help the clinician perform lateral femoral cutaneous nerve block in those patients in whom anatomic landmarks are difficult to identify[6,7] (**Fig. 166.5**). After injection, pressure may be applied to the injection site to decrease the possibility of bleeding or ecchymosis, which is more likely to occur in anticoagulated patients.

Assessing the Adequacy of the Block

The lateral femoral cutaneous nerve is purely sensory with no motor fibers. These sensory nerves innervate the lateral thigh and buttock. The block can be considered successful if the patient is unable to feel a pinch high on the lateral thigh (**Fig. 166.6**).[8]

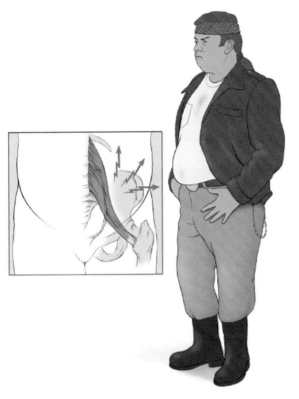

Fig. 166.1 Obesity and the wearing of wide belts may compress the lateral femoral cutaneous nerve, resulting in meralgia paresthetica.

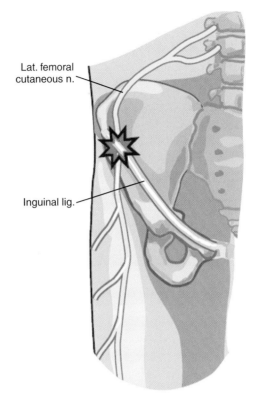

Fig. 166.2 Meralgia paresthetica is caused by compression of the lateral femoral cutaneous nerve by the inguinal ligament as it passes through or under the inguinal ligament.

Table 166.1 Causes and Differential Diagnosis of Meralgia Paresthetica

CAUSES

Abdominal or pelvic tumors (may cause compression)
Anterior pelvic surgery
Backpacks
Cardiac catheterization
Hip extension
Iliac crest bone harvest
Intramuscular injection
Jogging
Obesity
Pregnancy
Self-retaining retractors (surgical)
Spine surgery
Tight garments
Tool belts
Trauma (the nerve is superficial)

DIFFERENTIAL DIAGNOSIS

Abdominal pathology
Trochanteric bursitis
Diabetes mellitus
Lumbar radialopathy (including disk pathology)
Peripheral neuropathy
Retroperitoneal tumors

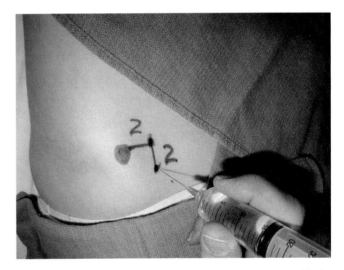

Fig. 166.3 Injection technique for lateral femoral cutaneous nerve block.

Side Effects and Complications

Complications include nerve damage, bleeding, infection, and local anesthetic toxicity. In addition, the proximity of the peritoneal cavity makes contact with visceral structure (i.e., the intestine) a possibility if the needle is inserted too deeply.[1,3]

Conclusion

The lateral femoral cutaneous nerve block is a simple, easily performed peripheral nerve block, which is not commonly associated with complications. It is most frequently used to treat entrapment neuropathy meralgia paresthetica. Lateral femoral cutaneous nerve block may be used for diagnostic purposes and also may offer extended relief when several

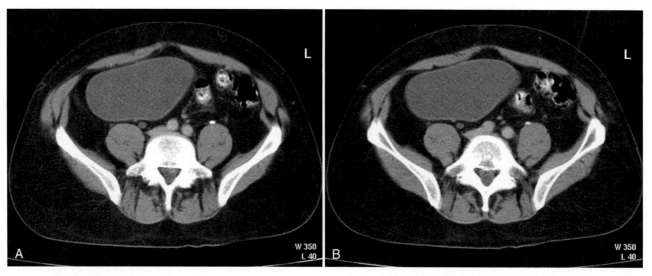

Fig. 166.4 These magnetic resonance images depict structures underlying the injection site for lateral femoral cutaneous nerve block that may be at risk if the needle is inserted too deeply. **A,** Axial view at the level of the anterior superior iliac spine. **B,** View 2 cm inferior to **A.**

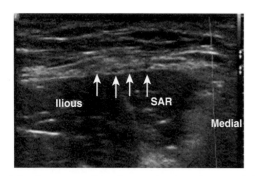

Fig. 166.5 Ultrasonographic picture showing the lateral femoral cutaneous nerve (*solid arrows*), which has already branched into smaller nerves and appears as hypoechoic structures. SAR, sartorius muscle. (*From Seib RK, Peng PWH: Ultrasound-guided peripheral nerve block in chronic pain management,* Techniques Reg Anesth Pain Manage *13:110, 2009.*)

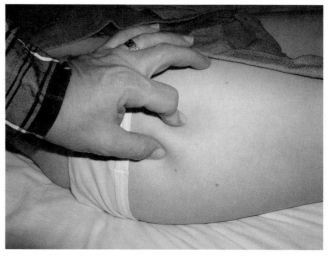

Fig. 166.6 Assessing the adequacy of lateral femoral cutaneous nerve block.

blocks are administered in short intervals. Lateral femoral cutaneous nerve block is also a valuable tool for skin grafting procedures or may be combined with other lower extremity nerve blocks (i.e., sciatic, obturator, femoral) for surgical anesthesia.

References

Full references for this chapter can be found on www.expertconsult.com.

Obturator Nerve Block

Somayaji Ramamurthy and Manuel Ybarra

Blockade of the obturator nerve is a clinically useful technique in the management of hip and lower extremity pain and spasticity. The increased use of ultrasound and nerve stimulators to aid in correct needle placement has significantly improved the success of the obturator nerve block and has made it less uncomfortable for the patient.[1] Results of blind paresthesia techniques used before the days of the nerve stimulator or the multiple reinsertion and the infiltration technique were extremely unpredictable and could be very painful for the patient.

Clinically Relevant Anatomy

The obturator nerve originates from anterior primary rami of L2-3 and L4 lumbar nerve roots. The contribution of L3 is the most predominant; contributions from L2 and L4 are small. The nerve passes through the psoas major muscle, emerging at its lateral border. It travels posterior to the iliac vessels and reaches the undersurface of the superior ramus of the pubis.[2] It passes through the obturator internus and externus muscles to emerge from the obturator foramen (**Fig. 167.1**). Shortly thereafter, it divides into anterior and posterior branches. The anterior branch innervates the anterior adductor muscles and gives a branch to innervate the hip joint. The posterior branch innervates mainly the adductor magnus muscle. It travels inferiorly and communicates with the saphenous branch of the femoral nerve. It travels along the femoral vessels to the popliteal fossa and gives a branch to innervate the knee joint. The innervation of both the hip joint and the knee joint by the obturator nerve can explain why a patient with a lesion in the hip joint sometimes complains of pain in the knee and vice versa. The obturator nerve is almost entirely a motor nerve. Sensory contribution to dermatomal distribution to the lower medial aspect of the thigh is variable and could be nonexistent in some patients.

Indications

Surgical Anesthesia

The obturator nerve has to be blocked for any procedure above the knee or when a pneumatic tourniquet is placed over the thigh. It is blocked along with the femoral, lateral femoral cutaneous, and sciatic nerves for this purpose.[3] One of the most important surgical indications is due to the anatomic relationship of the obturator nerve as it runs close to the neck of the bladder and the prostate.[4-7] Because of the proximity of the nerve to the prostate, this nerve can be electrically stimulated during the transurethral resection. This stimulation can produce significant contraction of the adductors, which can interfere with the surgical procedure, and on occasion can even result in the perforation of the bladder. This can occur even with adequate spinal analgesia that blocks the nerve roots proximal to the site of stimulation. Local anesthetic block of the obturator nerve has been well documented to abolish the spasms and facilitate the prostatic surgery.

Acute Pain

Blockade of the obturator nerve with local anesthetics such as ropivacaine is useful in the management of acute hip and lower medial thigh pain following pelvic trauma, total hip replacement surgery, and other acute pain emergencies. Because compromise or irritation of the obturator nerve may produce significant spasm in addition to pain, this technique can be extremely useful in providing symptomatic relief to allow the patient to comfortably undergo radiographic studies, magnetic resonance imaging, or computed tomographic scanning of the hip or pelvic bones.

Chronic Pain

Because the hip joint derives significant innervation from the obturator nerve, blockade of this nerve was one of the main indications in patients who had degenerative hip disease.[8]

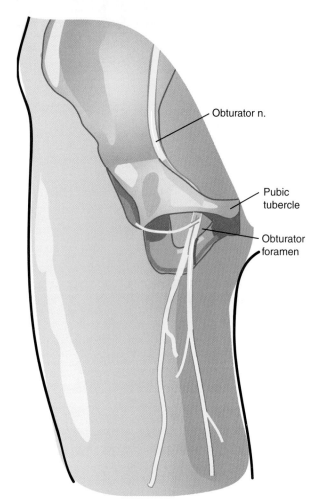

Fig. 167.1 Anatomy of obturator nerve, showing bony landmarks used in nerve block technique.

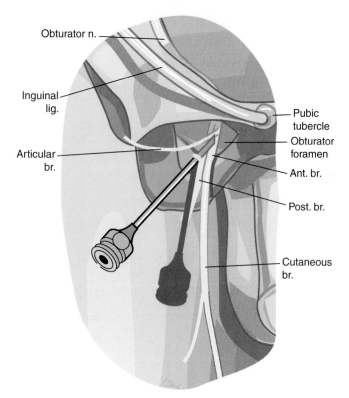

Fig. 167.2 The direct technique of obturator nerve block. (From Waldman SD, editor: Atlas of interventional pain management, ed 2, Philadelphia, 2003, Saunders, p 462)

Since the advent of total joint replacement, however, the number of patients who require this type of block has significantly decreased. It still can be of use as a diagnostic block for a complex pain problem.[9,10] Even under these circumstances, a direct hip joint injection provides more valuable diagnostic information than blockade of the obturator nerve.[11] Obturator nerve entrapment has been described in athletes[12] and after pelvic surgery.[13,14] The obturator nerve has been surgically released with good success. A diagnostic nerve block may help to make the diagnosis.

Spasticity

One of the most important nonsurgical indications was for adductor muscle spasticity. Obturator nerve block was used extensively to relieve adductor spasm to improve the personal hygiene of patients with spasticity. Oral and intrathecal dosing with baclofen has significantly reduced the use of neurolytic obturator nerve block for this purpose, but it remains a useful technique for those patients in whom pharmacologic methods are not tolerated or do not produce the desired results.

Technique

Direct Approach

The direct approach (**Fig. 167.2**) blocks the nerve as it exits the obturator foramen underneath the superior ramus of the pubis. The patient is placed in the supine position. The thigh is slightly abducted. The pubic area is sterilized with a nonirritating antiseptic such as Betadine. The pubic tubercle, the most important landmark, is identified. The entry point is 1.5 cm lateral and inferior to the pubic tubercle. The skin is anesthetized with a 25- or 27-gauge short needle and a fast-acting local anesthetic such as 1% lidocaine. A 22-gauge (8 cm) spinal needle is advanced vertically downward. The needle usually contacts the bone of the upper one third of the pubis. The negative electrode from a stimulator is attached to the needle, and the positive electrode is placed on the patient in an area where no paresthesia from the obturator nerve is expected. Over the bone 0.5 mL of 1% lidocaine is infiltrated to reduce the pain of "walking" the needle on the bone. The needle is redirected laterally and superiorly to induce contraction of the adductor muscles. When strong contractions are elicited, the nerve stimulator is adjusted until good contractions are produced with current less than 1 mA with an uninsulated needle or less than 0.5 mA with an insulated needle. A 2 mL test dose of local anesthetic should abolish the contraction, confirming proximity of the needle tip to the obturator nerve. At this point, 7 to 12 mL of local anesthetic is injected. During the lateral and superior redirection, if the pubic ramus is encountered, the needle must be walked slightly inferiorly to enter the obturator foramen. The needle should not be advanced more than 2 to 3 cm into the obturator foramen lest it enter the pelvis and damage the bladder.

An alternative approach consists of identifying the adductor longus muscle and advancing the needle underneath the proximal end of the adductor longus muscle in a medial to lateral direction and looking for contraction of the other adductor muscles with nerve stimulation.[15] A successful block can be identified when the patient is asked to adduct the thigh against resistance. The accompanying dermatomal analgesia is highly variable and can be nonexistent.

Indirect Technique

Winnie et al[16] described a three-in-one block. During this technique, the femoral nerve is identified and a volume of local anesthetic greater than 20 mL is injected, which is expected to spread to the lumbar plexus and block the obturator and the lateral femoral cutaneous nerves, in addition to the femoral nerve. This could be a significant advantage because the obturator nerve can be blocked easily without the pain of multiple injections. Whether the obturator nerve is consistently blocked is a matter of debate. The results of the three-in-one block were originally assessed by checking for cutaneous analgesia over the thigh. It was believed that analgesia over the anterior and lateral aspect of the thigh in the distribution of all three nerves indicated that the obturator nerve was also blocked. This may not be so when the obturator innervation of the skin is minimal or nonexistent. There have been cadaver studies in which injection of methylene blue indicated that the dye does not spread to the lumbar plexus or to the obturator nerve.[17] Studies compared three-in-one block with direct block of the obturator nerve with a nerve stimulator and assessed the results with motor evoked potentials.[18–21] It was clear that the three-in-one block did not produce consistent block of the obturator nerve.[18–21] Thus, if an obturator nerve block is needed to prevent abductor spasm during transurethral surgery or for neurolysis, the direct approach is preferred.

Ultrasound-Guided Technique

Ultrasound-guided obturator nerve block has been described with and without stimulation.[22,23] The patient is positioned supine with the ipsilateral thigh slightly abducted and externally rotated. The skin is prepped and draped in the usual sterile fashion and a high-frequency linear probe (>10 mHz) is used. The probe is placed in the inguinal crease to identify the femoral artery and vein. The transducer is translated medially and inferiorly along the inguinal crease to indentify pectineus, adductor longus, and adductor brevis muscles, just medial to the femoral vein (**Fig. 167.3**). The divisions of the obturator nerve are visualized with the anterior division anterior to the adductor brevis and behind the adductor longus; the posterior division lies posterior to the adductor brevis and anterior to the adductor magnus. After skin anesthesia a 50 to 100 mm insulated needle is advanced superiorly via out-of-plane technique or medially via in-plane approach. The needle tip is then placed between the pectineus and

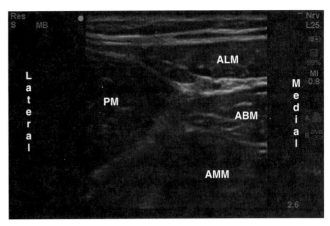

Fig. 167.3 Ultrasound image of obturator nerve branches. ABM, adductor brevis muscle; ALM, adductor longus muscle; PM, pectineus.

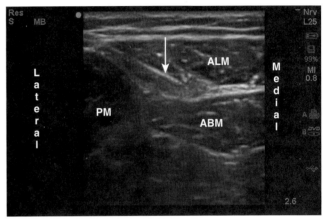

Fig. 167.4 Ultrasound image of obturator nerve block. *Arrow* shows needle placement for anterior divison obturator nerve block. ABM, adductor brevis muscle; ALM, adductor longus muscle; PM, pectineus.

adductor brevis and 5 ml of 0.5% Ropivicaine with epinephrine (1:400,000) is injected (**Fig. 167.4**). The needle is then positioned between the adductor brevis and adductor magnus and the injection is repeated. There should be interfascial spread of local anesthetic and separation of target muscles with no intramuscular swelling.

Complications

Nerve block with a local anesthetic using the landmarks and techniques described here usually does not result in serious complications. The usual complications are infection, bleeding, and pain at the site of the injection, but usually they are not serious. If the needle is advanced more than 3 cm into the pelvis, it can damage pelvic organs including the bladder. Neurolytic blockade in a patient who has normal sensation can result in neuritis, which can produce severe burning pain along the inside of the thigh.

References

Full references for this chapter can be found on www.expertconsult.com.

Caudal Epidural Nerve Block

Steven D. Waldman

Although it once seemed destined for extinction, the use of the caudal approach to the epidural space has enjoyed a remarkable resurgence in the care of the patient in pain. This resurgence has been fueled by several disparate factors: (1) an improved understanding of the functional anatomy of the sacral hiatus, sacrococcygeal ligament, and sacral canal from information gleaned from imaging (magnetic resonance imaging and computed tomography) of the region, which dispelled the commonly held belief that anatomic variations of this anatomic region made caudal block too technically challenging; (2) the increased use of sharper, shorter needles when performing other epidural blocks; and (3) the constant pressure on pain management specialists to provide pain management techniques in the most cost-effective manner possible, which placed performance of the caudal approach to the epidural space in a favorable light relative to lumbar epidural block, which required the use of more expensive Hustead or Touhy epidural needles. This renewed interest in caudal epidural block has been fueled further by studies indicating that the caudal approach to the epidural space may be more efficacious than the lumbar approach for many pain management applications. This chapter provides an overview of the current status of caudal epidural block in contemporary pain management.

Historical Considerations

Although the discovery of a practical way to administer drugs via the caudal approach to the epidural space preceded that for the lumbar approach by almost 20 years, the popularity of the caudal epidural nerve block has waxed and waned

relative to the lumbar approach to the epidural space. In 1901 Cathelin[1] published the first accurate description of the caudal approach to the epidural space. Despite the initial enthusiasm for the caudal approach after Cathelin's report, worldwide acceptance of the technique was inconsistent, at best. The reasons included lack of understanding of the clinical anatomy, overemphasis on the importance of the anatomic variations of the sacrum, and, perhaps most important, misapplication of the caudal approach for indications for which it was anatomically unsuited (i.e., to deliver drugs to the upper thoracic dermatomes). A tendency to compare the caudal epidural approach with the spinal and lumbar epidural approaches also contributed to misunderstanding of the appropriate role of this technique in surgical (and later in obstetric) anesthesia.

The description of the midline approach to the lumbar epidural space proposed by Pagés[2] in 1921 and refined by Dogliotti[3] and Gutierrez[4] in 1933 led to a further decline in use of the caudal approach. Just when it seemed that caudal nerve block was destined for extinction, in 1943 Hingson and Edwards[5] repopularized it for pain relief in childbirth. Anesthesiologists, obstetricians, and patients rapidly embraced the technique. This resurgence of interest was short-lived, however, owing in part to several widely publicized reports of fetal demise secondary to injection of local anesthetic into the fetus during caudal block and in part to the introduction of neuromuscular blocking agents in 1946. Persistent ignorance of the detailed anatomy and technique of the caudal approach to the epidural space led to reported failure rates of 5% to 7%,[6] rates that did not compare favorably with the much lower ones of spinal and general anesthesia reported at the time.

Throughout the 1950s and 1960s, the caudal approach to the epidural space was left in the hands of a few enthusiasts, who, in the words of Bromage,[7] "somewhat inexplicably, made it their hobby." The second repopularization of the caudal approach to the epidural space occurred during the 1970s and 1980s, in tandem with the increasing interest in the role of neural blockade in pain management. The growing use of the caudal approach in the pediatric population and as a route for administration of opioids in anticoagulated patients has increased use of this valuable technique further.

Indications and Contraindications

Indications for caudal epidural nerve block are summarized in **Table 168.1**. In addition to applications for surgical and obstetric anesthesia, caudal epidural nerve block with local

Table 168.1 Indications for the Caudal Approach to the Epidural Space

SURGICAL, OBSTETRIC, DIAGNOSTIC, AND PROGNOSTIC

Surgical anesthesia

Obstetric anesthesia

Differential neural blockade to evaluate pelvic, bladder, perineal, genital, rectal, anal, and lower extremity pain

Prognostic indicator before destruction of sacral nerves

ACUTE PAIN

Acute low back pain

Acute lumbar radiculopathy

Palliation in acute pain emergencies

Postoperative pain

Pelvic and lower extremity pain secondary to trauma

Pain of acute herpes zoster

Acute vascular insufficiency of the lower extremities

Hidradenitis suppurativa

CHRONIC BENIGN PAIN

Lumbar radiculopathy

Spinal stenosis

Low back syndrome

Vertebral compression fractures

Diabetic polyneuropathy

Postherpetic neuralgia

Reflex sympathetic dystrophy

Orchialgia

Proctalgia

Pelvic pain syndromes

CANCER PAIN

Pain secondary to pelvic, perineal, genital, or rectal malignancy

Bony metastases to pelvis

Chemotherapy-related peripheral neuropathy

SPECIAL SITUATIONS

Patients with previous lumbar spine surgery

Patients who are "anticoagulated" or have coagulopathy

anesthetics can be used as a diagnostic tool when differential neural blockade is performed on an anatomic basis to evaluate pelvic, bladder, perineal, genital, rectal, anal, and lower extremity pain.[8,9] If destruction of the sacral nerves is being considered, caudal epidural nerve block is useful as a prognostic indicator of the extent of motor and sensory impairment that the patient may experience.[9]

Caudal epidural nerve block with local anesthetics may be used to palliate acute pain emergencies in adults and children—postoperative pain, acute low back pain, acute radiculopathy, pain secondary to pelvic and lower extremity trauma, pain of acute herpes zoster, and cancer-related pain—during the wait for pharmacologic, surgical, or antiblastic treatment to take effect.[10,11] The technique also is valuable in patients with acute vascular insufficiency of the lower extremities secondary to vasospastic or vaso-occlusive disease, including frostbite and ergotamine toxicity.[12] Caudal nerve block also is recommended to palliate the pain of hidradenitis suppurativa of the groin.[13]

Administration of local anesthetics or steroids via the caudal approach to the epidural space is useful in the treatment of a variety of chronic benign pain syndromes, including lumbar radiculopathy, low back syndrome, spinal stenosis, postlaminectomy syndrome, vertebral compression fractures, diabetic polyneuropathy, postherpetic neuralgia, reflex sympathetic dystrophy, phantom limb pain, orchalgia, proctalgia, and pelvic pain syndromes.[14-18] Because of the simplicity, safety, and patient comfort associated with the caudal approach to the epidural space, this technique is replacing the lumbar epidural approach for these indications in some pain centers.[15]

The caudal approach to the epidural space is especially useful in patients who have previously undergone low back surgery, which may make the lumbar approach to the epidural space less efficacious.[19] The caudal approach to the epidural space can be used in the presence of anticoagulation or coagulopathy, so local anesthetics, opioids, and steroids can be administered via this route, even when other regional anesthetic techniques, including the spinal and lumbar epidural approaches, are contraindicated.[20] This fact is advantageous for patients with vascular insufficiency who are fully anticoagulated and for cancer patients who have developed coagulopathy secondary to radiation or chemotherapy.

The caudal epidural administration of local anesthetics in combination with steroids or opioids is useful in the palliation of cancer-related pelvic, perineal, and rectal pain.[21] This technique has been especially successful in the relief of pain secondary to the bony metastases of prostate cancer and the palliation of chemotherapy-related peripheral neuropathy. Another benefit is that it can be used to administer local anesthetics, opioids, or steroids despite anticoagulation or coagulopathy.

Contraindications to the caudal approach to the epidural space are the following:

- Local infection
- Sepsis
- Pilonidal cyst
- Congenital abnormalities of the dural sac and its contents

Because of the potential for hematogenous spread via Batson's plexus, local infection and sepsis are absolute contraindications to the caudal approach to the epidural space. Pilonidal cyst and congenital anomalies of the dural sac and its contents are relative contraindications.

Clinically Relevant Anatomy

Sacrum

The triangular sacrum consists of the five fused sacral vertebrae, which are dorsally convex (**Fig. 168.1**).[22] The sacrum inserts in a wedgelike manner between the two iliac bones, articulating superiorly with the L5 vertebra and caudally with the coccyx. On the anterior concave surface are four pairs of unsealed anterior sacral foramina that allow passage of the anterior rami of the upper four sacral nerves. The unsealed nature of the anterior sacral foramina allows the escape of drugs injected into the sacral canal.[23]

The convex dorsal surface of the sacrum has an irregular surface because the elements of the sacral vertebrae all fuse there. Dorsally, there is a midline crest called the *median sacral crest.* The posterior sacral foramina are smaller than their anterior counterparts. The sacrospinal and multifidus muscles effectively prevent leakage of drugs injected into the sacral canal. The vestigial remnants of the inferior articular processes project downward on each side of the sacral hiatus. These bony projections, called the *sacral cornua,* represent important clinical landmarks for caudal epidural nerve block (see Fig. 168.1).[24] Although there are gender-determined and race-determined differences in the shape of the sacrum, they are of little importance relative to the ultimate ability to perform caudal epidural nerve block successfully on a given patient.[14]

Coccyx

The triangular coccyx is composed of three to five rudimentary vertebrae (see Fig. 168.1). Its superior surface articulates with the inferior articular surface of the sacrum. Two prominent coccygeal cornua adjoin their sacral counterparts. The ventral surface of the coccyx is angulated anteriorly and superiorly. The tip of the coccyx is an important landmark for caudal epidural nerve block.[19]

Sacral Hiatus

The sacral hiatus is the result of incomplete midline fusion of the posterior elements of the lower portion of the S4 and the entire S5 vertebrae. This U-shaped space is covered posteriorly by the sacrococcygeal ligament, which is also an important clinical landmark for caudal epidural nerve block (see Fig. 168.1). Penetration of the sacrococcygeal ligament provides direct access to the epidural space of the sacral canal.[22]

Sacral Canal

A continuation of the lumbar spinal canal, the sacral canal continues inferiorly to terminate at the sacral hiatus (**Fig. 168.2**). The canal communicates with the anterior and posterior sacral foramina. The volume of the sacral canal, with all of its contents removed, averages approximately 34 mL in dried bone specimens.[14]

Contents of the Sacral Canal

The sacral canal contains the inferior termination of the dural sac, which ends between S1 and S3 (**Fig. 168.3**).[23] The five sacral nerve roots and the coccygeal nerve all traverse the canal, as does the terminal filament of the spinal cord, the filum terminale. The anterior and posterior rami of the S1-4 nerve roots exit from their respective anterior and posterior sacral foramina. The S5 roots and coccygeal nerves leave the sacral canal via the sacral hiatus. These nerves provide sensory and motor innervation to their respective dermatomes and myotomes. They also supply partial innervation to several pelvic structures, including the uterus, fallopian tubes, bladder, and prostate.[19]

The sacral canal also contains the epidural venous plexus, which generally ends at S4, but may continue caudad (see Fig. 168.3). Most of these vessels are concentrated in the anterior portion of the canal.[23] The dural sac and the epidural vessels are susceptible to trauma during cephalad advancement of needles or catheters into the sacral canal.[24] The remainder of the sacral canal is filled with fat, which is subject to age-related increase in density. Some investigators believe that this change is responsible for the higher incidence of "spotty" caudal epidural nerve blocks in adults.[6]

Technique

All equipment, including the needles and supplies for nerve block, drugs, resuscitation equipment, oxygen supply, and suction, must be assembled and checked before beginning a caudal epidural nerve block.

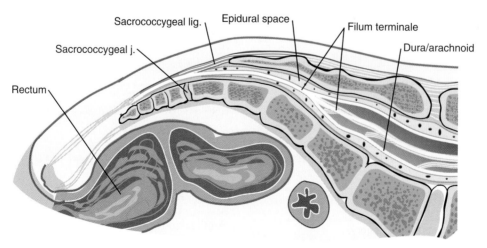

Fig. 168.1 Anatomy of the sacrum and coccyx.

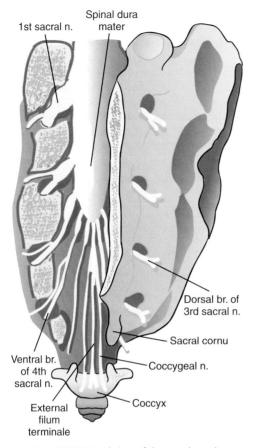

Fig. 168.2 Lateral view of the sacral canal.

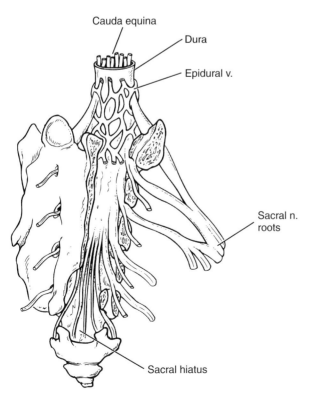

Fig. 168.3 Sacral canal and its contents.

Positioning the Patient

Caudal epidural nerve block is done with the patient in the prone or the lateral position. Each position has advantages and disadvantages. The prone position is easier for the pain management physician, but it may not be an option if the patient (1) cannot rest comfortably on the abdomen or (2) wears an ostomy appliance, such as a colostomy or ileostomy bag. The prone position limits easy access to the airway, which might be needed if problems occur during the procedure. The lateral position affords better access to the airway, but makes the approach technically more demanding.

Prone Position

The patient is placed in the prone position with the head on a pillow and turned away from the operator. Another pillow is placed under the hips, to tilt the pelvis and make the sacral hiatus more prominent. The legs and heels are abducted to prevent tightening of the gluteal muscles, which could make identification of the sacral hiatus more difficult (**Fig. 168.4**).[8]

Lateral Position

The patient is placed in the lateral position with the left side down for a right-handed pain management physician (**Fig. 168.5**). The dependent leg is slightly flexed at the hip and knee for the patient's comfort. The upper leg is flexed so that it lies over and above the lower leg and also in contact with the bed. This modified Sims position separates the buttocks, making identification of the sacral hiatus easier. Because the buttocks sag in the lateral position, the gluteal fold is usually inferior to the level of the sacral hiatus and is a misleading landmark for needle placement (see Fig. 168.5).[6]

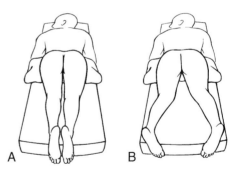

Fig. 168.4 The prone position. A, Legs-together position causes contraction of the gluteus medius muscles. B, Legs-apart position with heels rotated externally allows relaxation of the gluteus medius muscles.

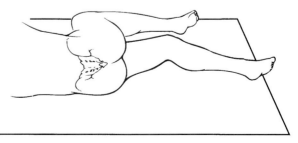

Fig. 168.5 The lateral position.

Choice of Needle

A 1½-inch 22-gauge needle is suitable for most adult patients. A ⅝-inch 25-gauge needle is indicated for pediatric applications. A 1½-inch 25-gauge needle is used when caudal epidural nerve block is performed in the presence of coagulopathy or anticoagulation.[20] The use of longer needles, as advocated by some earlier investigators, increases the incidence of complications, including intravascular injection and inadvertent dural puncture. The use of longer needles contributes nothing to the overall success of this technique.

Location of the Sacral Hiatus

A wide area of skin is prepared with an antiseptic solution such as povidone-iodine so that all landmarks can be palpated aseptically. A fenestrated sterile drape is placed to avoid contamination of the palpating finger. The middle finger of the physician's nondominant hand is placed over the sterile drape into the natal cleft with the fingertip at the tip of the coccyx (**Fig. 168.6**). This maneuver allows easy confirmation of the sacral midline and is especially important when the patient is in the lateral position.

After careful identification of the midline, the area under the physician's proximal interphalangeal joint is located (**Fig. 168.7**). The middle finger is moved cephalad from the area that was previously located under the proximal interphalangeal joint (**Fig. 168.8**). This spot is palpated using a lateral rocking motion to identify the sacral cornua. If the operator's glove size is 7.5 or 8, the sacral hiatus is found at this level. If the operator's glove size is smaller, the sacral hiatus is located just superior to the area below the proximal interphalangeal joint when the fingertip is at the tip of the coccyx. If the operator's glove size is larger, the sacral hiatus is located just inferior to the area below the proximal interphalangeal joint when the fingertip is at the tip of the coccyx (**Fig. 168.9**).

Although significant anatomic variation of the sacrum and sacral hiatus is normal, the spatial relationship between the tip of the coccyx and the location of the sacral hiatus remains amazingly constant. When the approximate position of the sacral hiatus is located by palpating the tip of the

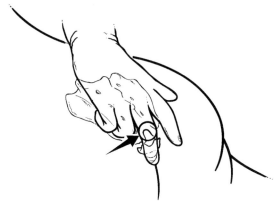

Fig. 168.7 Identification of the area under the operator's proximal interphalangeal joint (arrow).

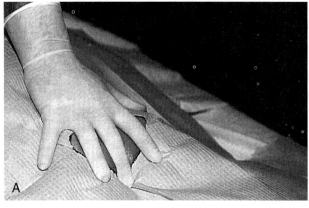

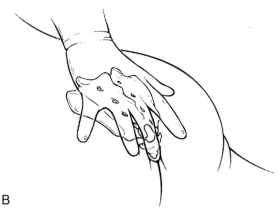

Fig. 168.6 The operator's finger identifies the tip of the coccyx. A, Photograph. B, Line drawing.

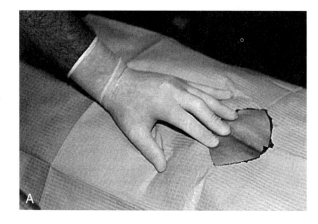

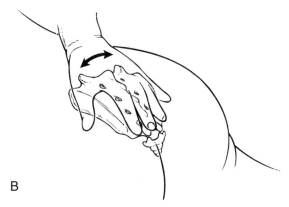

Fig. 168.8 Palpation of the sacral hiatus. A, Photograph. B, Line drawing.

coccyx, identifying the midline and locating the area under the proximal interphalangeal joint as just described, inability to identify and enter the sacral hiatus should occur in less than 0.5% of cases.

After the sacral hiatus is located, 1 mL of local anesthetic is used to infiltrate the skin, subcutaneous tissues, and sacrococcygeal ligament (**Fig. 168.10**). Large amounts of anesthetic should be avoided because the bony landmarks necessary for successful completion of this technique may be obscured. Many pain management specialists omit this technique because the pain from infiltration of local anesthetic is often greater than simply placing a 22-gauge or 25-gauge needle directly through the unanesthetized skin and subcutaneous tissues directly into the sacral canal.

The needle is inserted through the anesthetized area at a 45-degree angle into the sacrococcygeal ligament (**Fig. 168.11**). As the ligament is penetrated, the operator should feel a "pop"

or "giving way." If contact with the interior bony wall of the sacral canal occurs, the needle should be withdrawn slightly, to disengage the needle tip from the periosteum. The needle is advanced approximately 0.5 cm into the canal, to ensure that the entire needle bevel is beyond the sacrococcygeal ligament, to avoid injection into the ligament.

At this point, the needle should be held firmly in place by the bone ligament and subcutaneous tissues and should not sag if released by the pain management physician (**Fig. 168.12**). If there is any question as to whether the needle is correctly placed into the sacral canal, an air-acceptance test may performed by injecting 1 mL of air through the needle. There should be no bulging or crepitus of the tissues overlying the sacrum. The injection of air and the subsequent injection of drugs should feel to the operator like any other injection into the epidural space. The force required for injection should not exceed what was necessary to overcome the resistance of the needle. If there is initial resistance to injection, the needle should be rotated 180 degrees because it might be correctly placed in the canal while the bevel is occluded by the internal wall of the sacral canal (**Fig. 168.13**). Any significant pain or sudden increase in resistance during injection suggests incorrect needle placement; the physician should stop injecting immediately and reassess the position of the needle. If the physician encounters difficulty in placing the needle properly, fluoroscopic guidance may be used. A lateral fluoroscopic view can help ensure that the needle is within the sacral canal (**Fig. 168.14**).

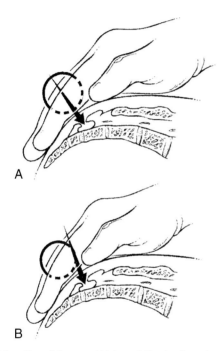

Fig. 168.9 Location of the sacral hiatus relative to glove size. A, Location of the sacral hiatus below the proximal interphalangeal joint for an operator with a size 8 glove. B, Location of the sacral hiatus above the proximal interphalangeal joint for an operator with a size 7 glove.

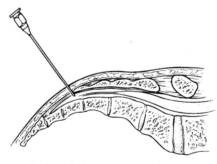

Fig. 168.11 Needle through the sacrococcygeal ligament at a 45-degree angle.

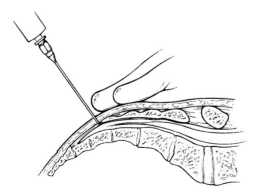

Fig. 168.10 Infiltration of the skin, subcutaneous tissues, and sacrococcygeal ligament.

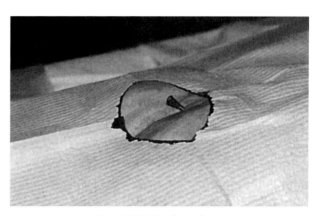

Fig. 168.12 Needle in place.

Injection of Drugs

When the needle is satisfactorily positioned, a syringe containing the drugs to be injected is attached to the needle. Gentle aspiration is carried out to identify cerebrospinal fluid (CSF) or blood (**Fig. 168.15**). Although rare, inadvertent dural puncture can occur, and careful observation for CSF must be carried out. Aspiration of blood occurs more commonly. It can be due to damage to veins during insertion of the needle into the caudal canal or, less often, to intravenous placement of the needle.

If the aspiration test is positive for either CSF or blood, the needle is repositioned, and the aspiration test is repeated.

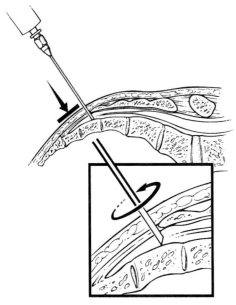

Fig. 168.13 Rotation of the needle 180 degrees away from the canal wall.

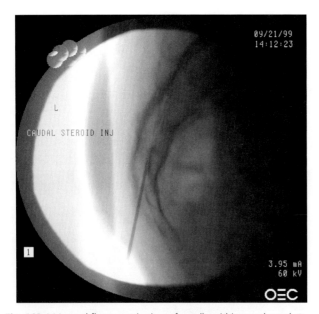

Fig. 168.14 Lateral fluoroscopic view of needle within sacral canal. *(From Waldman SD: Caudal epidural nerve block prone position. In Waldman SD: Atlas of interventional pain management, ed 2, Philadelphia, 2003, WB Saunders, p 389; courtesy of Milton Landers, DO, PhD.)*

If the repeat test is negative, subsequent injection of 0.5 mL increments of local anesthetic is done. Careful observation for signs of local anesthetic toxicity and subarachnoid spread of local anesthetic during the injection and after the procedure is indicated.

Choice of Local Anesthetic

The spread of drugs injected into the sacral canal depends on the volume and speed of injection, the anatomic variations of the bony canal, and the age and height of the patient.[14] Pregnant patients require a significantly smaller volume to achieve the same level of blockade than do nongravid controls.[6] As the injection proceeds, the drugs spread upward in the epidural space. There is a variable amount of leakage through the anterior sacral foramina, which can alter the upward spread of the injected drugs substantially. The onset of action is generally slower than with the lumbar approach to the epidural space.[14]

Local anesthetics capable of producing adequate sensory block of the sacral and lower lumbar nerve roots when administered via the caudal route include 1% lidocaine, 0.25% bupivacaine, 2% chloroprocaine, and 1% mepivacaine.[14] The addition of epinephrine decreases the amount of systemic absorption and lengthens the duration of action slightly. Increasing the concentration of drug increases the depth of motor block and speeds onset of action. A 20 mL volume of the drugs mentioned earlier, given in incremental doses, generally provides adequate sensory blockade of the sacral and lower lumbar dermatomes to allow surgical interventions in most adults.[14] Significant intrapatient variability exists, however, and additional incremental doses of local anesthetic may have to be administered to ensure adequate anesthesia in adults. All local anesthetics administered via the caudal epidural route should be formulated for epidural use.[25]

In pediatric patients, there is a much greater correlation between the dose of local anesthetic and body weight. A dose of 1 mL/kg of 0.25% bupivacaine seems to be safe in children.[14] The established maximum for the total doses of each local anesthetic always must be observed, regardless of patient age, to avoid local anesthetic toxicity. For diagnostic and prognostic blocks, 1% preservative-free lidocaine is a suitable local anesthetic.[9] For therapeutic blocks,

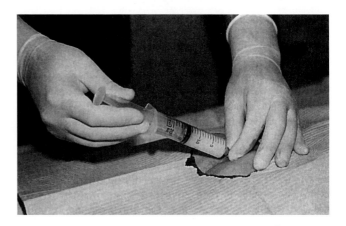

Fig. 168.15 Gentle aspiration to identify CSF or blood.

3 to 5 mL of 0.25% preservative-free bupivacaine or 0.5% preservative-free lidocaine in combination with 80 mg of depot methylprednisolone (Depo-Medrol) is injected.[10] Subsequent nerve blocks are done in a similar manner, but using only 40 mg of methylprednisolone. Daily caudal epidural nerve blocks with local anesthetic or steroid may be required to treat acute painful conditions.[10] Chronic conditions, such as lumbar radiculopathy and diabetic polyneuropathy, are treated daily to once a week, as the situation dictates.[9] Increasing clinical experience has indicated that higher volumes of local anesthetics increase side effects and complications, but add little, if anything, to the overall efficacy of caudal steroid epidural blocks if there is not a significant sympathetic component to the pain. For selective neurolytic block of an individual sacral nerve, incremental 0.1 mL injections of 6.5% phenol in glycerin or alcohol to a total volume of 1 mL may be used after the level of pain relief and potential side effects have been confirmed with local anesthetic blocks.[13]

If the caudal epidural route is chosen for administration of opioids, 4 to 5 mg of morphine sulfate formulated for epidural use is a reasonable initial dose.[20] More lipid-soluble opioids, such as fentanyl, must be delivered by continuous infusion via a caudal catheter.

Pitfalls in Needle Placement

It is possible to insert the needle incorrectly during performance of caudal epidural nerve block. The needle may be placed outside the sacral canal, resulting in the injection of air or drugs into the subcutaneous tissues (**Fig. 168.16A**). Palpation of crepitus and bulging of tissues overlying the sacrum during injection indicate needle malposition.[8] Greater resistance to injection accompanied by pain also is noted.

A second possible needle misplacement is into the periosteum of the sacral canal (**Fig. 168.16B**). This needle misplacement is suggested by considerable pain on injection, very high resistance to injection, and the inability to inject more than a few milliliters of drug.[22] A third possibility for needle malposition is partial placement of the needle bevel in the sacrococcygeal ligament (**Fig. 168.16C**). There is significant resistance to injection and significant pain as the drugs are injected into the ligament.

A fourth possible needle malposition is to force the point of the needle into the marrow cavity of the sacral vertebra, which results in very high blood levels of local anesthetic (**Fig. 168.16D**).[6] It can occur in elderly patients with significant osteoporosis. Such needle malposition is detected as initial easy acceptance of a few milliliters of local anesthetic followed by a rapid increase in resistance to injection, as the noncompliant bony cavity fills with local anesthetic. Significant local anesthetic toxicity can occur as a result of this complication.

The fifth and most serious needle malposition occurs when the needle is inserted through the sacrum or lateral to the coccyx into the pelvic cavity beyond (**Fig. 168.16E**),[23] where it could enter the rectum or the birth canal, resulting in contamination of the needle. Repositioning of a contaminated needle into the sacral canal carries with it the danger of infection. Although in competent hands this complication is exceedingly rare, some investigators believe that caudal

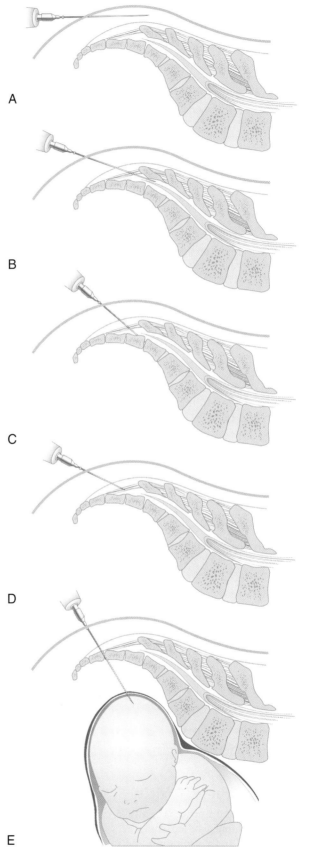

Fig. 168.16 Possible misplacements of needle. A, Outside sacral canal. B, Subperiosteal. C, In sacrococcygeal ligament. D, Into marrow cavity. E, Through sacrum into fetal cranium.

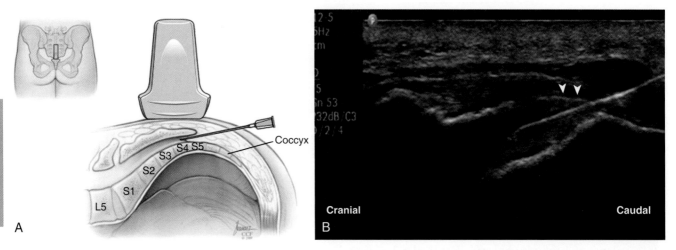

Fig. 168.17 **A,** Illustration showing the placement of the ultrasound (US) transducer in the longitudinal plane over the sacral hiatus. **B,** US longitudinal view showing the needle (in plane) inside the caudal epidural space. *Arrowheads* are pointing at the sacrococcygeal ligament. *(From Vydyanathan A, Narouze S: Ultrasound-guided caudal and sacroiliac joint injections,* Tech Reg Anesth Pain Manage *13:157, 2009.)*

analgesia for obstetric applications is inadvisable when the infant's head has entered the pelvis because inadvertent injection of local anesthetic into the head would cause fetal demise. The use of fluoroscopy or ultrasound guidance may help decrease this potential complication, especially in those patients in whom anatomic landmarks are difficult to identify (**Fig. 168.17**).

Caudal Epidural Catheters

An epidural catheter may be placed into the caudal canal through a Crawford needle, in a manner analogous to that for continuous lumbar epidural anesthesia.[6] The catheter is advanced approximately 2 to 3 cm beyond the needle tip.[26] The needle is carefully withdrawn over the catheter. To avoid shearing of the catheter, under no circumstances is the catheter withdrawn back through the needle. After the injection hub is attached to the catheter, an aspiration test is done to identify the presence of blood or CSF. A test dose of 3 to 4 mL of local anesthetic is given via the catheter. The patient is observed for signs of local anesthetic toxicity or inadvertent subarachnoid injection. If no side effects are noted, a continuous infusion or intermittent boluses of local anesthetics or opioids may be administered through the catheter. Because of proximity to the anus, the risk of infection limits the long-term use of caudal epidural catheters.[14]

Side Effects and Complications of the Caudal Approach to the Epidural Space

Local Anesthetic Toxicity

The caudal epidural space is highly vascular; the possibility of intravascular uptake of local anesthetic is significant with this technique.[14] Careful aspiration and incremental dosing with local anesthetic are important to allow early detection of toxicity. Careful observation of the patient during and after the procedure is mandatory.[9]

Hematoma and Ecchymosis

The epidural venous plexus generally ends at S4, but it may extend the entire length of the canal in some patients. Needle trauma to this plexus can result in bleeding and cause postprocedure pain. Subperiosteal injection of drugs, which also may result in bleeding, is associated with significant pain during and after injection. The chances of these two complications and the incidence of injection site eccyhmosis can be reduced by using short, small-diameter needles. Significant neurologic deficit secondary to epidural hematoma after caudal block is exceedingly rare.[14]

Infection

Although uncommon, infection remains an ever-present possibility, especially in immunocompromised cancer patients.[23] Studies comparing cultures of the skin puncture sites of patients in whom lumbar and caudal epidural catheters were placed simultaneously for obstetric anesthesia have shown consistently that the caudal sites produced a significantly larger number of positive results.[27] Early detection of infection is crucial to avoiding potentially life-threatening sequelae.

Neurologic Complications

Neurologic complications after caudal nerve block are exceedingly rare. Usually, they are associated with a preexisting neurologic lesion or with surgical or obstetric trauma, rather than with the caudal block itself.[14]

Urinary Retention and Incontinence

The application of local anesthetics and opioids to the sacral nerve roots results in a higher incidence of urinary retention.[14] This side effect of caudal epidural nerve block is seen more commonly in elderly men and multiparous women and after inguinal and perineal surgery. Overflow incontinence may occur in such patients if they are unable to void or if bladder catheterization is not used. It is advisable that all patients undergoing caudal epidural nerve block show the ability to void before discharge from the pain center.

Conclusion

Caudal epidural nerve block is a simple, safe, and effective technique for a variety of surgical anesthetic applications. It is especially useful for outpatient surgery and in pediatric patients. The ability to perform caudal epidural nerve block in the presence of anticoagulation or coagulopathy is unique among the major neuraxial regional anesthesia techniques. The utility of caudal epidural analgesia in the management of a variety of acute, chronic, and cancer-related pain syndromes makes the technique an excellent addition to the armamentarium of pain management specialists.

References

Full references for this chapter can be found on www.expertconsult.com.

Chapter 169

Lysis of Epidural Adhesions: The Racz Technique

Gabor B. Racz, Miles R. Day, James E. Heavner, and Jared Scott

Chances are relatively high that each of us will experience low back pain at some point in our lives. The usual course is rapid improvement with 5% to 10% developing persistent symptoms.[1] In the 1990s the estimated cost of low back pain to the health industry was in the billions of dollars, and with a larger proportion of our population now reported to be older, this number can only be expected to increase.[2,3] Treatment typically begins with conservative measures such as medication and physical therapy and may even include minimally and highly invasive pain management interventions. Surgery is sometimes required in patients who have progressive neurologic deficits or those who have other therapies. A quandary sometimes arises, following a primary surgery, as to whether repeat surgery should be attempted or another alternative technique should be tried. This is the exact problem that the epidural adhesiolysis procedure was designed to address. It was shown to free up nerves and to break down scar formation, deliver site-specific corticosteroids and local anesthetics, and reduce edema with the use of hyaluronidase and hypertonic saline. Epidural adhesiolysis has afforded patients a reduction in pain and neurologic symptoms without the expense and occasional long recovery period associated with repeat surgery, and often prevents the need for surgical intervention. This is the reason that epidural adhesiolysis was given an evidence rating of strong correlating to a 1B or 1C evidence level for post–lumbar surgery syndrome in the most recent American Society of Interventional Pain Physicians evidence-based guidelines. This suggests that the therapy is supported by observational studies and case series along with randomized-control trials.

Recommendation was also made that this therapy could apply to most patients in most circumstances without reservations.[4] Additionally, current procedural terminology (CPT) codes have been assigned to the two different kinds of adhesiolysis: CPT 62263 for the three-times injections over 2 to 3 days, usually done in an inpatient hospital setting, and CPT 62264 for the one-time injection series surgery-center model that may need to be repeated 3 to 3.5 times in a 12-month period.

Pathophysiology of Epidural Fibrosis (Scar Tissue) as a Cause of Low Back Pain with Radiculopathy

The etiology of low back pain with radiculopathy is not well understood. Kuslich et al[5] addressed this issue when they studied 193 lumbar spine operations on patients given local anesthesia. Their study revealed that sciatica could only be produced by stimulation of a swollen, stretched, restricted (i.e., scarred) or compressed nerve root.[5] Back pain could be produced by stimulation of several tissues, but the most common tissue of origin was the outer layer of the anulus fibrosus and the posterior longitudinal ligament. Stimulation for pain generation of the facet joint capsule rarely generated low back pain, and facet synovium and cartilage surfaces of the facet or muscles were never tender.[6]

The contribution of fibrosis to the etiology of low back pain has been debated.[7-9] There are many possible etiologies of epidural fibrosis, including surgical trauma, an annular tear, infection, hematoma, or intrathecal contrast material.[10] These etiologies have been well documented in the literature. LaRocca and Macnab[11] demonstrated the invasion of fibrous connective tissue into postoperative hematoma as a cause of epidural fibrosis, and Cooper et al[12] reported periradicular fibrosis and vascular abnormalities occurring with herniated intervertebral disks. McCarron et al[13] investigated the irritative effect of nucleus pulposus on the dural sac, adjacent nerve roots, and nerve root sleeves independent of the influence of direct compression on these structures. Evidence of an inflammatory reaction was identified by gross inspection and microscopic analysis of spinal cord sections after homogenized autogenous nucleus pulposus was injected into the lumbar epidural space of four dogs. In the control group consisting of four dogs injected with normal saline, the spinal cord sections were grossly normal. Parke and Watanabe[14] showed significant evidence of adhesions in cadavers with lumbar disk herniation.

It is widely accepted that postoperative scar renders the nerve susceptible to injury by a compressive phenomena.[9] It is natural for connective tissue or any kind of scar tissue to form fibrous layers (scar tissue) as a part of the process that transpires after disruption of the intact milieu.[15] Scar tissue is generally found in three components of the epidural space. Dorsal epidural scar tissue is formed by resorption of surgical hematoma and may be involved in pain generation.[16] In the ventral epidural space, dense scar tissue is formed by ventral defects in the disk, which may persist despite surgical treatment and continue to produce low back pain and radiculopathy past the surgical healing phase.[17] The lateral epidural space includes the epiradicular structures outside the root canals, known as the lateral recesses or "sleeves," which are susceptible to lateral disk defects, facet hypertrophy, and neuroforaminal stenosis.[18]

Although scar tissue itself is not tender, an entrapped nerve root is. Kuslich et al[5] surmised that the presence of scar tissue compounded the pain associated with the nerve root by fixing it in one position and thus increasing the susceptibility of the nerve root to tension or compression. They also concluded that no other tissues in the spine are capable of producing leg pain. In a study of the relationship between peridural scar evaluated by magnetic resonance imaging (MRI) and radicular pain after lumbar diskectomy, Ross et al[19] demonstrated that subjects with extensive peridural scarring were 3.2 times more likely to experience recurrent radicular pain.

This evidence also parallels a new study by Gilbert et al[20] in which lumbosacral nerve roots were identified as undergoing less strain than previously published during straight leg raise and in which hip motion greater than 60 degrees was determined to cause displacement of the nerve root in the lateral recess.

Radiologic Diagnosis of Epidural Fibrosis

MRI and computed tomography (CT) are diagnostic tools; sensitivity and specificity are 50% and 70%, respectively.[15] CT myelography may also be helpful, although none of the aforementioned modalities can identify epidural fibrosis with 100% reliability. In contrast, epidurography is a technique used with considerable success and it is believed that epidural fibrosis is best diagnosed by performing an epidurogram.[21–24] It can detect filling defects in good correlation with a patient's symptoms in real time.[24] A combination of several of these techniques would undoubtedly increase the ability to identify epidural fibrosis.

Current Procedural Terminology or CPT Codes

The American Medical Association has developed Current Procedural Terminology codes for epidural adhesiolysis, which include 62264 for a single infusion and 62263 for a staged three-series infusion.

Indications for Epidural Adhesiolysis

Although originally designed to treat radiculopathy secondary to epidural fibrosis following surgery, the use of epidural adhesiolysis has been expanded to treat a multitude of pain etiologies. These include the following[25]:

1. Postlaminectomy syndrome of the neck and back after surgery
2. Disk disruption
3. Metastatic carcinoma of the spine leading to compression fracture
4. Multilevel degenerative arthritis
5. Facet pain
6. Spinal stenosis
7. Pain unresponsive to spinal cord stimulation and spinal opioids

Contraindications

The following are absolute contraindications for performing epidural adhesiolysis:

1. Sepsis
2. Chronic infection
3. Coagulopathy
4. Local infection at the procedure site
5. Patient refusal
6. Syrinx formation

A relative contraindication is the presence of arachnoiditis. With arachnoiditis, the tissue planes may be adherent to one another, increasing the chance of loculation of contrast or medication. It may also increase the chance of spread of the medications to the subdural or subarachnoid space, which can increase the chance of complications. Practitioners with limited experience with epidural adhesiolysis should consider referring these patients to a clinician with more training and experience.

Patient Preparation

When epidural adhesiolysis has been deemed an appropriate treatment modality, the risks and benefits of the procedure should be discussed with the patient and informed consent obtained. The benefits are pain relief, improved physical function, and possible reversal of neurologic symptoms. Risks include, but are not limited to, bruising, bleeding, infection, reaction to medications used (i.e., hyaluronidase, local anesthetic, corticosteroids, hypertonic saline), damage to nerves or blood vessels, no or little pain relief, bowel/bladder incontinence, worsening of pain, and paralysis. Patients with a history of urinary incontinence should have a urodynamic evaluation by a urologist before the procedure to document the preexisting urodynamic etiology and pathology.

Anticoagulant Medication

Medications that prolong bleeding and clotting parameters should be withheld before performing epidural adhesiolysis. The length of time varies depending on the medication taken. A consultation with the patient's primary physician should be obtained before stopping any of these medications, particularly in patients who require chronic anticoagulation such as those with drug-eluting heart stents or prosthetic heart valves. Nonsteroidal anti-inflammatory drugs and aspirin, respectively, should be withheld 4 days and 7 to 10 days before the procedure. Although there is much debate regarding these medications and neuraxial procedures, we tend to be on the conservative side. Clopidogrel (Plavix) should be stopped 7 days before, whereas ticlopidine (Ticlid) is withheld 10 to 14 days before the adhesiolysis.[26] Warfarin (Coumadin) stoppage is variable but 5 days is usually adequate.[25] Patients on subcutaneous heparin should have it withheld a minimum of 12 hours before the procedure, whereas those on low-molecular-weight heparin require a minimum of 24 hours.[26] Over-the-counter homeopathic medications that prolong bleeding parameters should also be withheld. These include fish oil, vitamin E, gingko biloba, garlic, ginseng, and St. John's Wort. Adequate coagulation status can be confirmed by the prothrombin time, partial thromboplastin time, and a platelet function assay or bleeding time. The tests should be performed as close to the day of the procedure as possible. Tests performed only a few days after stopping the anticoagulant medication may come back elevated because not enough time has elapsed to allow the anticoagulant effects of the medication to resolve. The benefits of the procedure must be weighed against the potential sequelae of stopping the anticoagulant medication and this should be discussed thoroughly with the patient.

Preoperative Laboratory

Before the procedure, a complete blood count and a clean-catch urinalysis are obtained to check for any undiagnosed infections. An elevated white count and/or a positive urinalysis should prompt the physician to postpone the procedure and refer the patient to the primary care physician for further workup and treatment. In addition, a prothrombin time, partial thromboplastin time, and platelet function assay or bleeding time are obtained to check for coagulation abnormalities. Any elevated value warrants further investigation and postponement of the procedure until those studies are complete.

Technique

This procedure can be performed in the cervical, thoracic, lumbar, and caudal regions of the spine. The caudal and transforaminal placement of catheters will be described in

detail, whereas highlights and slight changes in protocol will be provided for cervical and thoracic catheters. Our policy is to perform this procedure under strict sterile conditions in the operating room. Prophylactic antibiotics with broad neuraxial coverage are given before the procedure. Patients will receive either ceftriaxone 1 g intravenously or Levaquin 500 mg orally in those allergic to penicillin. The same dose is also given on day 2. An anesthesiologist or nurse anesthetist provides monitored anesthesia care.

Caudal Approach

The patient is placed in the prone position with a pillow placed under the abdomen to correct the lumbar lordosis and a pillow under the ankles for patient comfort. The patient is asked to put his or her toes together and heels apart. This relaxes the gluteal muscles and facilitates identification of the sacral hiatus. After sterile preparation and draping, the sacral hiatus is identified via palpation just caudal to the sacral cornu or with fluoroscopic guidance. A skin wheal is raised with local anesthetic 1 inch lateral and 2 inches caudal to the sacral hiatus on the side opposite the documented radiculopathy. A distal approach theoretically provides some protection from meningitis as a local skin infection would be much preferred over infection closer to the epidural space. The skin is nicked with an 18-gauge cutting needle, and a 15- or 16-gauge RX Coudé (Epimed International) epidural needle is inserted through the nick at a 45-degree angle and guided fluoroscopically or by palpation to the sacral hiatus (**Figs. 169.1** and **169.2**). When the needle is through the hiatus, the angle of the needle is dropped to approximately 30 degrees and advanced. The

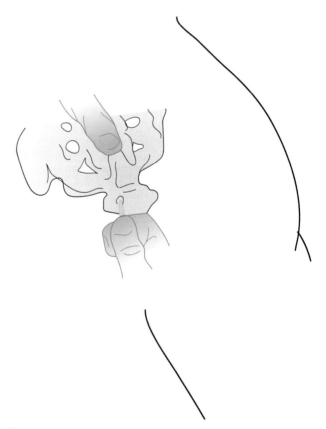

Fig. 169.1 Caudal lysis sequence—first find sacral hiatus and tip of coccyx.

advantages of the RX Coudé needle over other needles are the angled tip, which enables easier direction of the catheter, and the tip of the needle is less sharp. The back edge of the distal opening of the needle is designed to be a noncutting surface that allows manipulation of the catheter in and out of the needle. A Touhy needle has the back edge of the distal opening, which is a cutting surface and can more easily shear a catheter. A properly placed needle will be inside the caudal canal below the level of the S3 foramen on anteroposterior (AP) and later fluoroscopic images. A needle placed above the level of the S3 foramen could potentially puncture a low-lying dura. The needle tip should cross the midline of the sacrum toward the side of the radiculopathy.

An epidurogram is performed using 10 mL of a non-ionic, water-soluble contrast agent. Confirm a negative aspiration for blood or cerebrospinal fluid before any injection of the contrast or medication. Omnipaque and Isovue are the two agents most frequently used and are suitable for myelography.[27,28] Do not use ionic, water-insoluble agents such as Hypopaque or Renografin or ionic, water-soluble agents such as Conray.[29,30] These agents are not indicated for myelography. Accidental subarachnoid injections can lead to serious untoward events such as seizure and possibly death. Slowly inject the contrast agent and observe for filling defects. A normal epidurogram will have a "Christmas tree" pattern with the central canal being the trunk and the outline of the nerve roots making up the branches. An abnormal epidurogram will have areas where the contrast does not fill (**Fig. 169.3**). These are the areas of presumed scarring and typically correspond to the patient's radicular complaints. If vascular uptake is observed, the needle needs to be redirected.

After turning the distal opening of the needle ventral-lateral, insert a TunL Kath or TunL-XL (stiffer) catheter (Epimed International) with a bend on the distal tip through the needle (**Figs. 169.4** and **169.5**). The bend should be 2.5 cm from the tip of the catheter and at a 30-degree angle. The bend will enable the catheter to be steered to the target

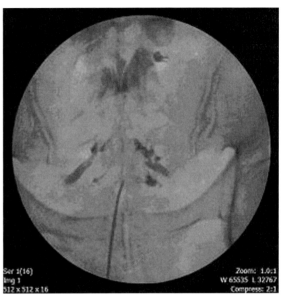

Fig. 169.3 Initial dye injection Omnipaque 240 (10 mL) showing sacral S3 runoff and filling defects at S2, S1, and right L5.

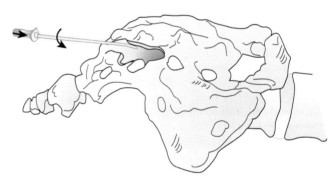

Fig. 169.4 The needle is placed through the sacral hiatus into the sacral canal and rotated in the direction of the target. Do not advance beyond the S3 foramen.

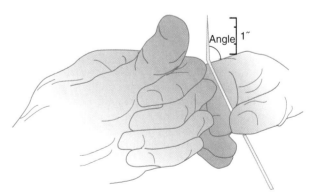

Fig. 169.5 The Epimed Racz catheter is marked for the location of the bend, or use the thumb as reference for the 15-degree angle bend.

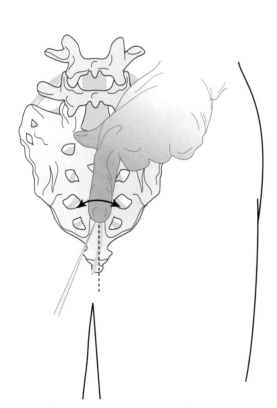

Fig. 169.2 Roll palpating index finger to identify the sacral cornua and thus the target sacral hiatus.

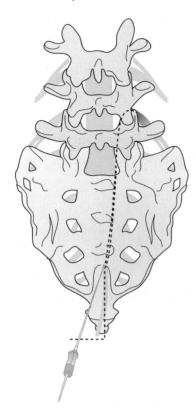

Fig. 169.6 The direction of the catheter is just near the midline; direct the curve under continuous fluoroscopic guidance to the ventral lateral target site. The needle rotation, as well as the catheter navigation, may need to be used to reach the target.

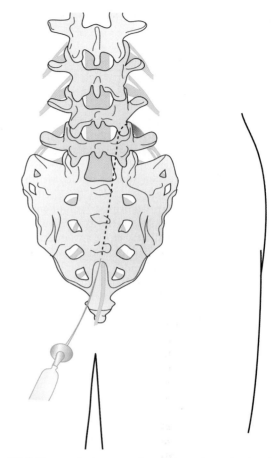

Fig. 169.7 The needle is removed, and the catheter is placed in the ventral lateral epidural space ventral to the nerve root.

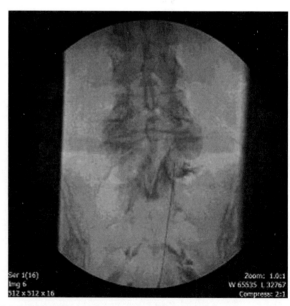

Fig. 169.8 Catheter (24xL) is threaded to lateral L5 neural foramen.

level (**Fig. 169.6**). Under continuous AP fluoroscopic guidance, advance the tip of the catheter toward the ventral-lateral epidural space of the desired level. The catheter can be steered by gently twisting the catheter in a clockwise or counterclockwise direction. Avoid "propellering" the tip (i.e., twisting the tip in circles) because this makes it more difficult to direct the catheter. Do not advance the catheter up the middle of the sacrum because this makes guiding the catheter to the ventral-lateral epidural space more difficult. Ideal location of the tip of the catheter in the AP projection is in the foramen just below the midportion of the pedicle shadow (**Figs. 169.7** and **169.8**). Check a lateral projection to confirm that the catheter tip is in the ventral epidural space.

Under real-time fluoroscopy, inject 2 to 3 mL of additional contrast through the catheter in an attempt to outline the "scarred in" nerve root (**Fig. 169.9**). If vascular uptake is noted, reposition the catheter and reinject contrast. Preferably there should not be vascular runoff, but infrequently secondary to venous congestion, an epidural pattern is seen with a small amount of vascular spread. This is acceptable as long as the vascular uptake is venous in nature and not arterial. Extra caution should be taken when injecting the local anesthetic to prevent local anesthetic toxicity. Any arterial spread of contrast always warrants repositioning of the catheter. We have never observed intra-arterial placement in 25 years of placing soft, spring-tipped catheters.

Inject 1500 U of hyaluronidase dissolved in 10 mL of preservative-free normal saline. A newer development is the use of Hylenex or human-recombinant hyaluronidase, which carries the advantage of a reportedly increased effectiveness

at the body's normal pH compared to bovine-recombinant hyaluronidase.[31] This injection may cause some discomfort, so a slow injection is preferable. Observe for "opening up"(i.e., visualization) of the "scarred in" nerve root (**Figs. 169.10** and **169.11**; see also Fig. 169.9). A 3 mL test dose of a 10 mL local

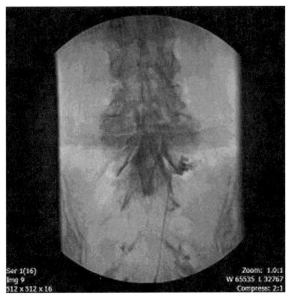

Fig. 169.9 Contrast injection Omnipaque 240, additional 5 mL opening right L5, S1, S2, and S3 perineural spaces; also left L5, S1, S2, and S3 in addition to right L4 spread in cephalad direction.

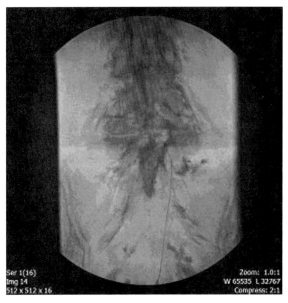

Fig. 169.11 Catheter advances to the desired symptomatic level of right L5 in the ventral lateral epidural space. Injection of contrast followed by 10 mL hyaluronidase 1,500 units opens up bilaterally L3-5, S1, S2, and S3 neural foramina.

Remove the needle under continuous fluoroscopic guidance to ensure the catheter remains at the target level (**Fig. 169.12**). Secure the catheter to the skin using nonabsorbable suture and coat the skin puncture site with antimicrobial ointment. Apply a sterile dressing and attach a 0.2 μm filter to the end of the catheter. Affix the exposed portion of the catheter to the patient with tape and transport the patient to the recovery area.

A 20- to 30-minute period should elapse between the last injection of the LA/S solution and the start of the hypertonic saline (10%) infusion. This is necessary to ensure that a subdural injection of the LA/S solution has not occurred. A subdural block mimics a subarachnoid block but it takes longer to establish, usually 16 to 18 minutes. Evidence for subdural or subarachnoid spread is the development of motor block. If the patient develops a subarachnoid or subdural block at any point during the procedure, the catheter should be removed and the remainder of the adhesiolysis canceled. The patient needs to be observed to document the resolution of the motor and sensory block and to document that 10 mL of the hypertonic saline is then infused through the catheter over 15 to 30 minutes. If the patient complains of discomfort, the infusion is stopped and an additional 2 to 3 mL of 0.2% ropivacaine is injected and the infusion is restarted. Alternatively, 50 to 75 μg of fentanyl can be injected epidurally in lieu of the local anesthetic. After completion of the hypertonic saline infusion, the catheter is slowly flushed with 2 mL of preservative-free normal saline and the catheter is capped.

Our policy is to admit the patient for 24-hour observation status and do a second and a third hypertonic saline infusion the following day. On post–catheter insertion day 2, the catheter is twice injected (separated by 4- to 6-hour increments) with 10 mL of 0.2% ropivacaine without steroid and infused with 10 mL of hypertonic saline (10%) using the same technique and precautions as the day 1 infusion. At the end of the third infusion, the catheter is removed and a sterile dressing applied. The patient is discharged home with 5 days

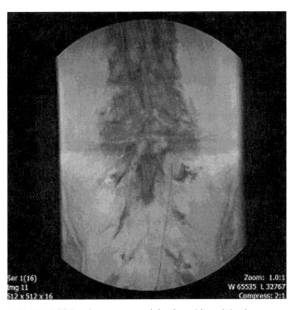

Fig. 169.10 Additional contrast and hyaluronidase injection opens up bilaterally formerly scarred areas. The Christmas tree appearance is obvious.

anesthetic/steroid (LA/S) solution is then given. Our institution used 4 mg of dexamethasone mixed with 9 mL of 0.2% ropivacaine. Ropivacaine is used instead of bupivacaine for two reasons: the former produces a preferential sensory versus a motor block, and it is less cardiotoxic than a racemic bupivacaine. Doses for other corticosteroids commonly used are 40 to 80 mg of methylprednisolone (Depo-Medrol), 25 to 50 mg of triamcinolone diacetate (Aristocort), 40 to 80 mg of triamcinolone acetonide (Kenalog), and 6 to 12 mg of betamethasone (Celestone Solu span). If, after 5 minutes, there is no evidence of intrathecal or intravascular injection of medication, inject the remaining 7 mL of the LA/S solution.

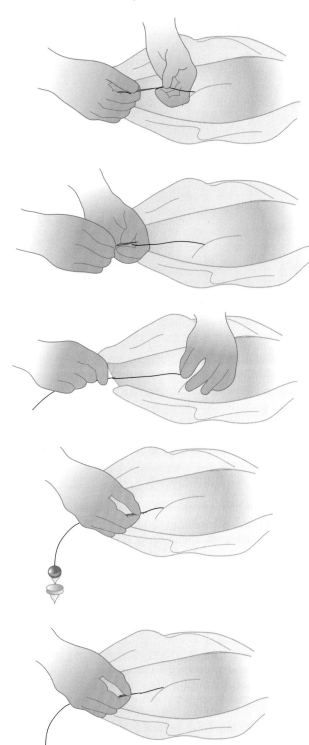

Fig. 169.12 Five picture sequence of removal of the needle to prevent dislodging the catheter from target site before suturing and application of dressing.

of oral cephalexin at 500 mg twice a day or oral levofloxacin (Levaquin) at 500 mg once a day for penicillin-allergic patients. Clinic follow-up is in 30 days.

Transforaminal Catheters

Patients with an additional level of radiculopathy or those in whom the target level cannot be reached by the caudal approach may require placement of a second catheter. The

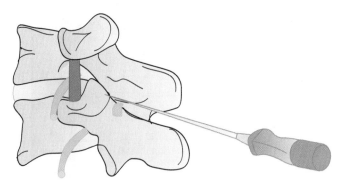

Fig. 169.13 Transforaminal lateral-oblique view. Target the SAP with the advancing RX Coude needle.

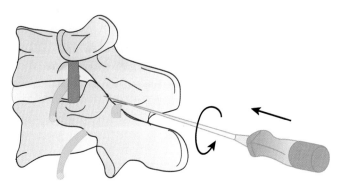

Fig. 169.14 Following bony contact with SAP. Lateral rotation of 180 degrees to allow passage toward the target.

second catheter is placed into the ventral epidural space via a transforaminal approach.

After the target level is identified with an AP fluoroscopic image, the superior endplate of the vertebra that comprises the caudal portion of the foramina is "squared," that is, the anterior and posterior shadows of the vertebral endplate are superimposed. The angle is typically 15 to 20 degrees in a caudocephalad direction. The fluoroscope is then obliqued approximately 15 degrees to the side of the radiculopathy and adjusted until the spinous process is rotated to the opposite side. This fluoroscope positioning allows the best visualization of the superior articular process (SAP) that forms the inferoposterior portion of the targeted foramen. The image of the SAP should be superimposed on the shadow of the disk space on the oblique view. The tip of the SAP is the target for the needle placement (**Fig. 169.13**). Raise a skin wheal slightly lateral to the shadow of the tip of the SAP. Pierce the skin with an 18-gauge needle and then insert a 15- or 16-gauge RX Coudé needle and advance using gun-barrel technique toward the tip of the SAP. Continue to advance the needle medially toward the SAP until the tip contacts bone. Rotate the tip of the needle 180 degrees laterally and advance about 5 mm (**Fig. 169.14**). Rotate the needle back medially 180 degrees (**Fig. 169.15**). As the needle is advanced slowly, a clear "pop" is felt as the needle penetrates the inter transverse ligament. Obtain a lateral fluoroscopic image. The tip of the needle should be just past the SAP in the posterior foramen. In the AP plane, the tip of the needle under continuous AP fluoroscopy, insert the catheter slowly into the foramen and advance until the tip should be just short of the middle of the spinal canal (**Figs. 169.16** to **169.18**). Confirm that the catheter is in the anterior epidural space with a lateral image (**Fig. 169.19**). Anatomically, the catheter is in the

3 to 5 mL of 0.25% preservative-free bupivacaine or 0.5% preservative-free lidocaine in combination with 80 mg of depot methylprednisolone (Depo-Medrol) is injected.[10] Subsequent nerve blocks are done in a similar manner, but using only 40 mg of methylprednisolone. Daily caudal epidural nerve blocks with local anesthetic or steroid may be required to treat acute painful conditions.[10] Chronic conditions, such as lumbar radiculopathy and diabetic polyneuropathy, are treated daily to once a week, as the situation dictates.[9] Increasing clinical experience has indicated that higher volumes of local anesthetics increase side effects and complications, but add little, if anything, to the overall efficacy of caudal steroid epidural blocks if there is not a significant sympathetic component to the pain. For selective neurolytic block of an individual sacral nerve, incremental 0.1 mL injections of 6.5% phenol in glycerin or alcohol to a total volume of 1 mL may be used after the level of pain relief and potential side effects have been confirmed with local anesthetic blocks.[13]

If the caudal epidural route is chosen for administration of opioids, 4 to 5 mg of morphine sulfate formulated for epidural use is a reasonable initial dose.[20] More lipid-soluble opioids, such as fentanyl, must be delivered by continuous infusion via a caudal catheter.

Pitfalls in Needle Placement

It is possible to insert the needle incorrectly during performance of caudal epidural nerve block. The needle may be placed outside the sacral canal, resulting in the injection of air or drugs into the subcutaneous tissues (**Fig. 168.16A**). Palpation of crepitus and bulging of tissues overlying the sacrum during injection indicate needle malposition.[8] Greater resistance to injection accompanied by pain also is noted.

A second possible needle misplacement is into the periosteum of the sacral canal (**Fig. 168.16B**). This needle misplacement is suggested by considerable pain on injection, very high resistance to injection, and the inability to inject more than a few milliliters of drug.[22] A third possibility for needle malposition is partial placement of the needle bevel in the sacrococcygeal ligament (**Fig. 168.16C**). There is significant resistance to injection and significant pain as the drugs are injected into the ligament.

A fourth possible needle malposition is to force the point of the needle into the marrow cavity of the sacral vertebra, which results in very high blood levels of local anesthetic (**Fig. 168.16D**).[6] It can occur in elderly patients with significant osteoporosis. Such needle malposition is detected as initial easy acceptance of a few milliliters of local anesthetic followed by a rapid increase in resistance to injection, as the noncompliant bony cavity fills with local anesthetic. Significant local anesthetic toxicity can occur as a result of this complication.

The fifth and most serious needle malposition occurs when the needle is inserted through the sacrum or lateral to the coccyx into the pelvic cavity beyond (**Fig. 168.16E**),[23] where it could enter the rectum or the birth canal, resulting in contamination of the needle. Repositioning of a contaminated needle into the sacral canal carries with it the danger of infection. Although in competent hands this complication is exceedingly rare, some investigators believe that caudal

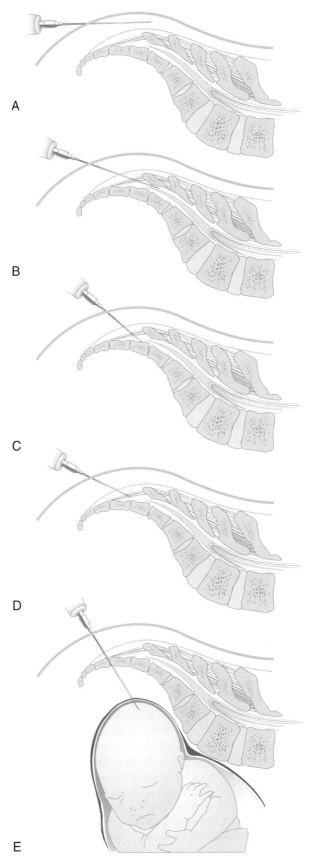

Fig. 168.16 Possible misplacements of needle. **A,** Outside sacral canal. **B,** Subperiosteal. **C,** In sacrococcygeal ligament. **D,** Into marrow cavity. **E,** Through sacrum into fetal cranium.

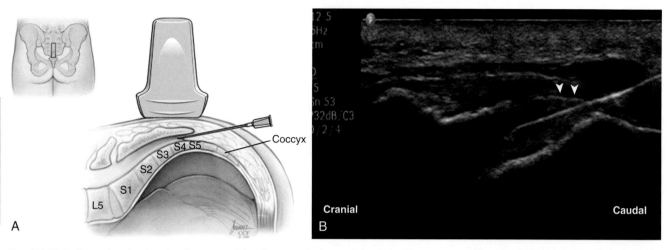

Fig. 168.17 A, Illustration showing the placement of the ultrasound (US) transducer in the longitudinal plane over the sacral hiatus. B, US longitudinal view showing the needle (in plane) inside the caudal epidural space. *Arrowheads* are pointing at the sacrococcygeal ligament. *(From Vydyanathan A, Narouze S: Ultrasound-guided caudal and sacroiliac joint injections,* Tech Reg Anesth Pain Manage *13:157, 2009.)*

analgesia for obstetric applications is inadvisable when the infant's head has entered the pelvis because inadvertent injection of local anesthetic into the head would cause fetal demise. The use of fluoroscopy or ultrasound guidance may help decrease this potential complication, especially in those patients in whom anatomic landmarks are difficult to identify (**Fig. 168.17**).

Caudal Epidural Catheters

An epidural catheter may be placed into the caudal canal through a Crawford needle, in a manner analogous to that for continuous lumbar epidural anesthesia.[6] The catheter is advanced approximately 2 to 3 cm beyond the needle tip.[26] The needle is carefully withdrawn over the catheter. To avoid shearing of the catheter, under no circumstances is the catheter withdrawn back through the needle. After the injection hub is attached to the catheter, an aspiration test is done to identify the presence of blood or CSF. A test dose of 3 to 4 mL of local anesthetic is given via the catheter. The patient is observed for signs of local anesthetic toxicity or inadvertent subarachnoid injection. If no side effects are noted, a continuous infusion or intermittent boluses of local anesthetics or opioids may be administered through the catheter. Because of proximity to the anus, the risk of infection limits the long-term use of caudal epidural catheters.[14]

Side Effects and Complications of the Caudal Approach to the Epidural Space

Local Anesthetic Toxicity

The caudal epidural space is highly vascular; the possibility of intravascular uptake of local anesthetic is significant with this technique.[14] Careful aspiration and incremental dosing with local anesthetic are important to allow early detection of toxicity. Careful observation of the patient during and after the procedure is mandatory.[9]

Hematoma and Ecchymosis

The epidural venous plexus generally ends at S4, but it may extend the entire length of the canal in some patients. Needle trauma to this plexus can result in bleeding and cause postprocedure pain. Subperiosteal injection of drugs, which also may result in bleeding, is associated with significant pain during and after injection. The chances of these two complications and the incidence of injection site ecchymosis can be reduced by using short, small-diameter needles. Significant neurologic deficit secondary to epidural hematoma after caudal block is exceedingly rare.[14]

Infection

Although uncommon, infection remains an ever-present possibility, especially in immunocompromised cancer patients.[23] Studies comparing cultures of the skin puncture sites of patients in whom lumbar and caudal epidural catheters were placed simultaneously for obstetric anesthesia have shown consistently that the caudal sites produced a significantly larger number of positive results.[27] Early detection of infection is crucial to avoiding potentially life-threatening sequelae.

Neurologic Complications

Neurologic complications after caudal nerve block are exceedingly rare. Usually, they are associated with a preexisting neurologic lesion or with surgical or obstetric trauma, rather than with the caudal block itself.[14]

Urinary Retention and Incontinence

The application of local anesthetics and opioids to the sacral nerve roots results in a higher incidence of urinary retention.[14] This side effect of caudal epidural nerve block is seen more commonly in elderly men and multiparous women and after inguinal and perineal surgery. Overflow incontinence may occur in such patients if they are unable to void or if bladder

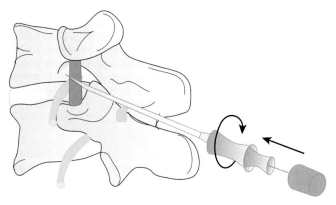

Fig. 169.15 Note the intertransverse ligament. The needle tip with the RX Coude 2 that has 1 mm protruding blunt stylet will pass through the ligament and will be less likely to damage the nerve.

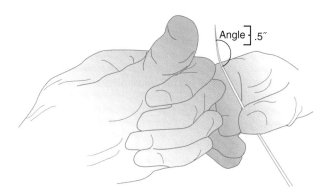

Fig. 169.16 The distal tip of the catheter may be bent 15-degrees, ¾ inch length.

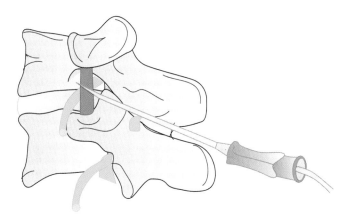

Fig. 169.17 Once the intertransverse ligament is perforated, the catheter is steered to the ventral lateral epidural space (lateral view).

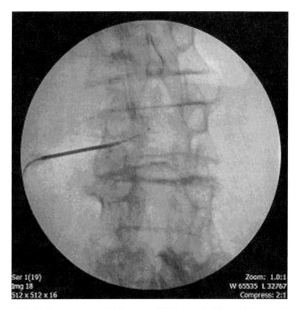

Fig. 169.18 Transforaminal 15-gauge RX-Coude 2 (Epimed International, Johnstown, NY) catheter at left L3-4 threaded almost to near *midcanal* position (anteroposterior view).

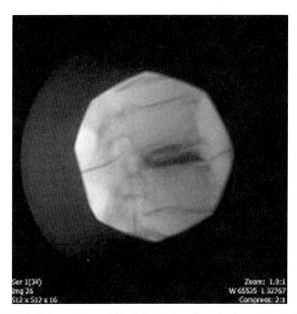

Fig. 169.19 Lateral view of Fig. 169-13. Transforaminal-ventral-anterior catheter dye spread to epidural and L3-4 intradiscal area (through annular tear).

foramen above or below the exiting nerve root (**Fig. 169.20**). If the catheter cannot be advanced, it usually means the needle is either too posterior or too lateral to the foramen. It can also indicate that the foramen is too stenotic to allow passage of the catheter. The needle can be advanced a few millimeters anteriorly in relation to the foramen, and that will also move it slightly medial into the foramen. If the catheter still will not pass, the initial insertion of the needle will need to be more lateral. Therefore the fluoroscope angle will be about 20 degrees instead of 15 degrees. The curve of the needle usually facilitates easy catheter placement. The final position of the catheter tip is just short of the midline.

Inject 1 to 2 mL of contrast to confirm epidural spread. When a caudal and a transforaminal catheter are placed, the 1500 U of hyaluronidase are divided evenly between the two catheters (5 mL of the hyaluronidase/saline solution into each). The LA/S solution is also divided evenly, but a volume of 15 mL (1 mL steroid and 14 mL 0.2% ropivicaine; of the total volume, 5 mL is transforaminal and 10 mL is caudal) is used instead of 10 mL. Remove the needle under fluoroscopic guidance to make sure the catheter does not move from the original position in the epidural space. Secure and cover the catheter as described previously. The hypertonic saline solution is infused at a volume of 4 to 5 mL per transforaminal

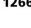

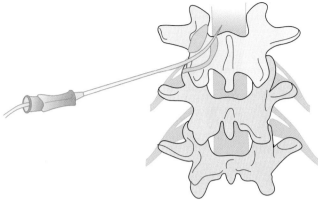

Fig. 169.20 Anteroposterior view. The catheter is in optimal position near midline via the transforaminal placement.

and 8 to 10 mL per caudal catheter over 30 minutes. The hypertonic saline injection volume should always be less than or equal to the local anesthetic volume injected to avoid pain from injection. It behooves the practitioner to check the position of the transforaminal catheter under fluoroscopy before performing the second and third infusions. The catheter may advance across the epidural space into the contralateral foramen or paraspinous muscles or more commonly back out of the epidural space into the ipsilateral paraspinous muscles. This results in deposition of the medication in the paravertebral tissue rather than in the epidural space. As with the caudal approach, remove the transforaminal catheter after the third infusion. A recent development is the R-X Coude 2 needle in which a second protruding stylet may allow closer needle placement and less chance of nerve injury.

Cervical Lysis of Adhesions

The success of the caudal approach for lysis of adhesions led to the application of the same technique to the cervical epidural space. The indications and preprocedure workup are the same as those for the caudal lysis technique, but there are a few differences in technique and volumes of medication used.

The epidural space should be entered via the upper thoracic interspaces using a paramedian approach on the contralateral side. The most common levels are T1-2 and T2-3. Entry at these levels allows for a sufficient length of the catheter to remain in the epidural space after the target level has been reached. If the target is the lower cervical nerve roots, a more caudal interspace should be selected. We place the patient in the left lateral decubitus position, but use a prone approach in larger patients.

A technique referred to as the "3-D technique" is used to facilitate entry into the epidural space. The "3-D" stands for *direction, depth,* and *direction.* Using an AP fluoroscopic image, the initial *direction* of the 15- or 16-gauge RX Coudé needle is determined. Using a modified paramedian approach with the skin entry one and a half levels below the target interlaminar space, advance and direct the needle toward the midpoint of the chosen interlaminar space with the opening of the needle pointing medial. Once the needle engages the deeper tissue planes (usually at 2 to 3 cm), check the depth of the needle with a lateral image. Advance the needle toward the epidural space and

check repeat images to confirm the *depth.* The posterior border of the dorsal epidural space can be visualized by identifying the junction of the base of the spinous process of the vertebra with its lamina. This junction creates a distinct radiopaque "straight line." Once the needle is close to the epidural space, obtain an AP fluoroscopic image to recheck the *direction* of the needle. If the tip of the needle has crossed the midline as defined by the spinous processes of the vertebral bodies, pull the needle back and redirect. The "3-D" process can be repeated as many times as is necessary to get the needle into the perfect position.

Using loss-of-resistance technique, advance the needle into the epidural space with the tip of the RX-Coudé needle pointed caudally. Once the tip is in the epidural space, rotate the tip cephalad, and inject 1 to 2 mL of contrast to confirm entry. Rotation or movement of any needle in the epidural space can cut the dura. This technique has been improved with the advent of the RX Coudé 2 needle, which has a second interlocking stylet that protrudes slightly beyond the tip of the needle and functions to push the dura away from the needle tip as it is turned 180 degrees cephalad (**Fig. 169.21A-D**). Inject an additional small volume as needed to complete the epidurogram. If there is no free flow of injected contrast, pressure may build up in the lateral epidural space. Characteristic fluid spread by the path of least resistance can be recognized as *perivenous counter spread* (PVCS). Presence of PVCS means pressure builds up in the lateral epidural space that is unable to spread laterally to decompress. The dye spread picks the path of least resistance to the opposite side. Pressure may build up and lead to ischemic spinal cord injury. Flexion and rotation of the head and neck can open up lateral runoff and release the pressure through the enlarged neural foramina (**Fig. 169.22**)[32]

As with the caudal epidurogram, look for filling defects. It is extremely important to visualize spread of the contrast in the cephalad and caudal directions. Loculation of contrast in a small area must be avoided as this can significantly increase the pressure in the epidural space and can compromise the already tenuous arterial blood supply to the spinal cord. Place a bend on the catheter as previously described for the caudal approach and insert it through the needle (**Fig. 169.21E**). The opening of the needle should be directed toward the target side. Slowly advance the catheter to the lateral gutter and direct it cephalad. Redirect the catheter as needed and once the target level has been reached, turn the tip of the catheter toward the foramen (**Fig. 169.23A**). Inject 0.5 to 1 mL of contrast to visualize the target nerve root. Make sure there is runoff of contrast out of the foramen (**Fig. 169.23B**). Slowly instill 150 U of Hylenex dissolved in 5 mL of preservative-free normal saline. Follow this with 1 to 2 mL of additional contrast and observe for "opening up" of the "scarred in" nerve root. Give a 2 mL test dose of a 6 mL solution of LA/S. Our combination is 5 mL of 0.2% ropivicaine and 4 mg of dexamethasone. If after 5 minutes there is no evidence of intrathecal or intravascular spread, inject the remaining 4 mL. Remove the needle, and secure and dress the catheter as previously described. Once 20 minutes have passed since the last dose of LA/S solution and there is no evidence of a subarachnoid or subdural block, start an infusion of 5 mL of hypertonic saline over 30 minutes. At the end of the infusion, flush the catheter with 1 to 2 mL of preservative-free normal saline and cap the catheter.

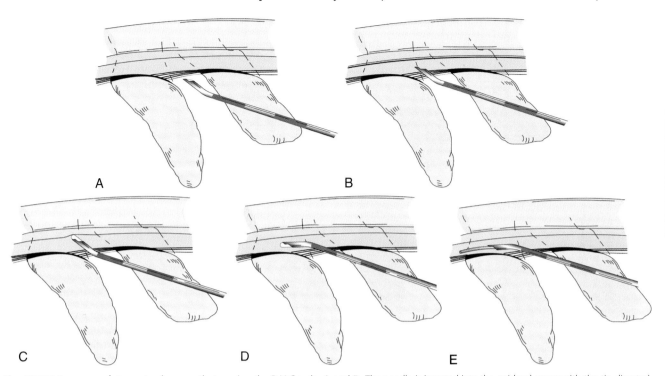

Fig. 169.21 Sequence of stages to place a catheter using the R-X Coude. **A** and **B,** The needle is inserted into the epidural space with the tip directed as shown. **C,** The protruding stylet is inserted. **D,** Then the needle is rotated so the tip is parallel to the dura. **E,** The catheter is inserted.

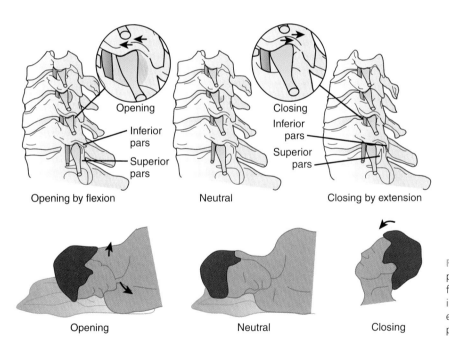

Opening

Inferior pars

Superior pars

Opening by flexion

Neutral

Closing

Inferior pars

Superior pars

Closing by extension

Opening

Neutral

Closing

Fig. 169.22 Flexion rotation, left to right regardless patient position. The neural foramen enlarges on flexion rotation and gets smaller with extension. The inferior pars slides forward over the superior pars to enlarge the foramen. This allows lateral run off and pressure release with PVCS.

The second and third infusions are performed on the next day with 6 mL of 0.2% ropivacaine without spread and 5 mL of hypertonic saline using the same technique and precautions described for the first infusion. The catheter is removed and prophylactic antibiotics are prescribed. Clinic follow-up is 30 days.

Thoracic Lysis of Adhesions

The technique for entry into the thoracic epidural space for adhesiolysis is identical to that for the cervical region. Always remember the 3-D technique. Make sure to get a true lateral when checking the depth of the needle. This can be obtained by superimposing the rib shadows on one another. The target is still the ventrolateral epidural space with the tip of the catheter in the foramen of the desired level.

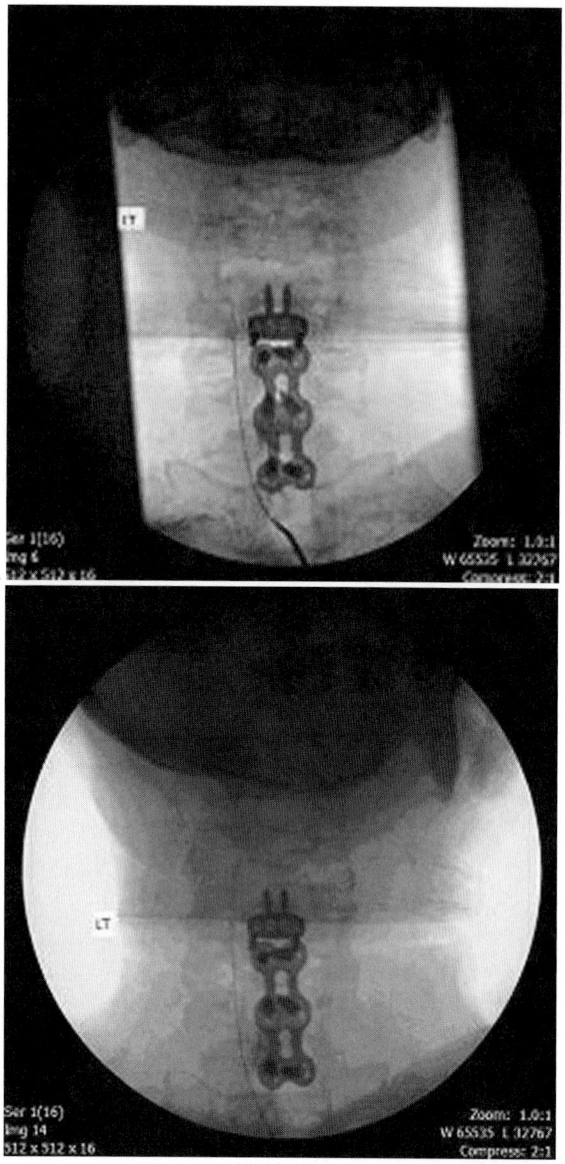

Fig. 169.23 **A** Cervical left ventral lateral catheter to the upper level of fusion C5-7. **B** Cervical-left ventral lateral catheter threaded to above level of fusion of C4. The dye injection spreads cephalad and lateral.

The major difference for thoracic lysis compared to the caudal and cervical techniques is the volumes of the various injectates. Volumes of 8 mL are used for the contrast, Hylenex, LA/S, and hypertonic saline. (**Table 169.1**) lists typical infusion volumes for epidural adhesiolysis.

Neural Flossing

The protocol for epidural adhesiolysis has been aided by neural flossing exercises that were designed to mobilize nerve roots by "sliding" them in and out of the foramen (**Fig. 169.24**). This breaks up weakened scar tissue from the procedure and prevents further scar tissue deposition. If these exercises are done effectively three to four times per day for a few months after the procedure, the formation of scar tissue will be severely restricted.

Epidural Mapping

In patients with multilevel radiculopathy and complex pain, it can be difficult to determine from where the majority of the pain is emanating. We have been using a technique that we have termed *mapping* to locate the most painful nerve root with stimulation and then carry out the adhesiolysis at that level. There are several references in the literature regarding the use of stimulation to confirm epidural placement of a catheter and for nerve root localization.[33] The TunL Kath and the TunL-XL catheter can be used as stimulating catheters to identify the nerve root(s).

After entering the epidural space, advance the catheter into the ventrolateral epidural space past the suspected target level. Make sure the tip of the catheter is pointing laterally toward the foramina, just below the pedicle. Pull the catheter stylet back approximately 1 cm. Using alligator clips, attach the cathode to the stylet and ground the anode on the needle or ground pad or a 22-gauge needle inserted into the skin. Apply electrical stimulation with a stimulator box with a rate of 50 pulses per second and a pulse width of 450 milliseconds, dialing up the amplitude until a paresthesia is perceived in small increments, usually less than 2 or 3 volts. Inquire of the patient as to whether or not the paresthesia is felt in the area of the patient's recognized greatest pain. This process is repeated at each successive level until the most painful nerve root is identified. Once identified, the adhesiolysis is carried out at that level. The mapping procedure is also useful to identify the optimal site of surgery either before the first surgery or when surgery has failed one or more times.

Table 169.1 **Typical Infusion Volumes for Epidural Adhesiolysis**				
	Contrast	**Hyaluronidase and Normal Saline**	**Local Anesthetic and Steroid**	**10% Hypertonic Saline Infusion**
Caudal	10 mL	10 mL	10 mL	10 mL
Caudal and transforaminal	5 mL in each catheter	5 mL in each catheter	5 mL in each catheter	8 mL in caudal catheter and 4 mL in transforaminal catheter
Thoracic	8 mL	8 mL	8 mL	8 mL
Cervical	5 mL	6 mL	6 mL	5 mL

Complications

As with any invasive procedure, complications are possible. These include bleeding, infection, headache, damage to nerves or blood vessels, catheter shearing, bowel/bladder dysfunction, paralysis, spinal cord compression from loculation of the injected fluids or hematoma, subdural or subarachnoid injection of local anesthetic or hypertonic saline, and reactions to the medications used. We also include on the consent form that the patient may experience an increase in pain or no pain relief at all. Although the potential list of complications is long, the frequency of complications is very rare. However, there is clearly a learning curve, and recent studies reflect this by the significantly improved long-term outcome and the very rare publications of complications and medicolegal consequences when one considers the ever-increasing clinical experience.

Subdural spread is a complication that should always be watched for when injecting local anesthetic. During the caudal adhesiolysis, particularly if the catheter is advanced along the midline, subdural catheter placement is a risk (**Figs. 169.25** and **169.26**). Identification of the subdural motor block should occur within 16 to 18 minutes. Catheters used for adhesiolysis should never be directed midline in the epidural space.

Outcomes

Initially in the early 1980s the protocol was designed to direct site-specific medication onto the dorsal root ganglion; however, after performing a number of the procedures, it was found that the dorsal root ganglion was exceptionally hard to reach secondary to developing scar tissue or adhesions. In the early days, our understanding was coming from the use of local anesthetics for surgery giving a 2- to 4-hour block for the surgeon to operate. It was a tremendous cause for excitement to see chronic pain patients get months and years of pain relief following the placement of the new steerable x-ray visible catheter. The early report in 1985 by Racz et al[34] was for the use of phenol at the dorsal root ganglion followed by an observational listing of outcomes that were clearly not as good as the latest studies on failed back surgery and spinal stenosis showing 75% to 80% improvement at 12 months' follow-up by Manchikanti.[34] Initially we were pleased to see some patients getting 3 to 4 months of relief and report seeing recovery of footdrops. This philosophy still proves to be true even in studies in 2008 by Sakai et al[35] in which they found that adhesiolysis with catheter-directed steroid and local anesthetic injection during epiduroscopy alleviated pain and reduced sensory nerve dysfunction in patients with chronic sciatica. The evolution of these findings has changed the

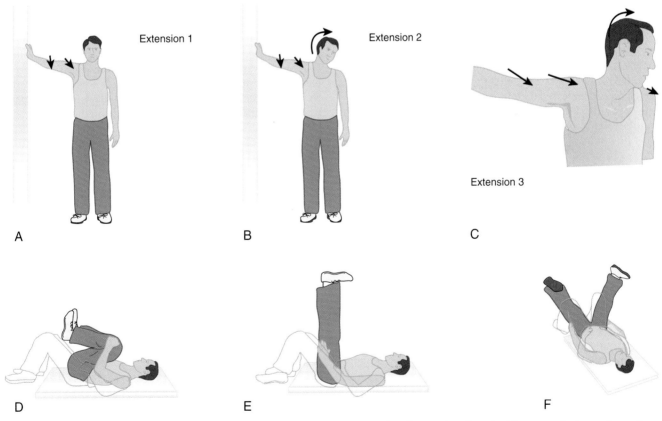

Fig. 169.24 Neural flossing exercises. A, Standing erect, firmly grasp a stable surface (e.g., a door frame) with outstretched arm. Press elbow and shoulder forward. **B,** Next, slowly tilt head in opposite direction from outstretched arm to achieve gentle tension. **C,** Finally, rotate chin toward opposite shoulder as is comfortable. Hold this final position for approximately 20 to 30 seconds. **D,** Lay down supine on an exercise mat without a pillow. Slowly bring both knees close to the chest with bent legs and hold this position for 20 seconds. Release and assume a neutral position. **E,** Again in supine position, raise both legs to 90 degrees, with knees straight while laying flat on a firm surface. Hold for 20 seconds. Assume a neutral position and rest briefly. **F,** Bring both legs to a 90-degree angle while lying supine. Slowly spread legs in a V shape, as much as is comfortable, and hold for 20 seconds.

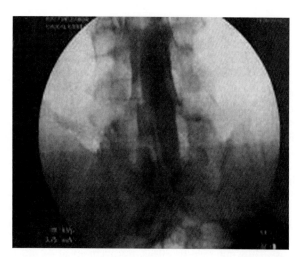

Fig. 169.25 Midline catheter placement enters subdural space. There is also some epidural dye spread. But the patient starts to complain of bilateral leg pain.

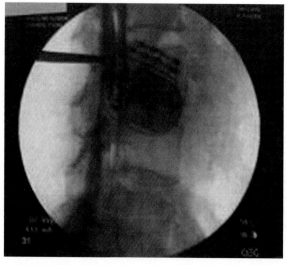

Fig. 169.26 A 22-gauge spinal needle and extension set with syringe placed in the subdural space and 12 mL fluid aspirated. The patient reported immediate reversal of bilateral leg pain. Note the dye in the extension tubing and syringe at the 7-o'clock position.

process into what it is today.[36] Racz and Holubec first reported on epidural adhesiolysis in 1989.[37] There were slight variations in the protocol compared to today's protocol, namely the dose of local anesthetic and the fact that hyaluronidase was not used. Catheter placement was lesion-specific (i.e., the tip of the catheter was placed in the foramen corresponding to the vertebral level and side of the suspected adhesions). The retrospective analysis conducted 6 to 12 months after the procedure reported initial pain relief in 72.2% of patients (N = 72) at time of discharge. Relief was sustained in 37.5% and 30.5% of patients at 1 and 3 months, respectively. Forty-three percent decreased their frequency and dosage of medication use and 16.7% discontinued their medications altogether. In total, 30.6% of patients returned to work or returned to daily functions.

At a presentation of the 7th World Congress on Pain, Arthur et al[38] reported on epidural adhesiolysis in 100 patients, 50 of whom received hyaluronidase as part of the procedure. In the hyaluronidase group, 81.6% of the participants had initial pain relief, with 12.3% having persistent relief; 68% of the no hyaluronidase group had relief of pain, with 14% having persistent relief at the end of the 3-year follow-up period from which the study sample was randomly selected.

In 1994 Stolker et al[39] added hyaluronidase to the procedure, but omitted the hypertonic saline. In a study of 28 patients, they reported greater than 50% pain reduction in 64% of patients at 1 year. They stressed the importance of the patient selection and believed that the effectiveness of adhesiolysis was based on the effect of the hyaluronidase on the adhesions and the action of the local anesthetic and steroids on the sinuvertebral nerve.

Devulder et al[40] published a study of 34 patients with failed back surgery syndrome in whom epidural fibrosis was suspected or proved with MRI.[40] An epidural catheter was inserted via the sacral hiatus to a distance of 10 cm into the caudal canal. Injections of contrast dye, local anesthetic, corticosteroid, and hypertonic saline (10%) were carried out

daily for 3 days. No hyaluronidase was used. Filling defects were noted in 30 of 34 patients, but significant pain relief was noted in only 7 patients at 1 month, 2 patients at 3 months, and no patients at 12 months. They concluded that epidurography may confirm epidural filling defects for contrast dye in patients with filling defects, but a better contrast dye spread, assuming scar lysis does not guarantee sustained pain relief. This study was criticized for lack of lesion-specific catheter placement resulting in nonspecific drug delivery.[41] The catheter was never directed to the ventral lateral epidural space where the dorsal root ganglion is located and the lateral recess scarring occurs.

Heavner et al[42] performed a prospective randomized trial of lesion-specific epidural adhesiolysis on 59 patients with chronic intractable low back pain. The patients were assigned to one of four epidural adhesiolysis treatment groups: (1) hypertonic (10%) saline plus hyaluronidase, (2) hypertonic saline, (3) isotonic (0.9%) saline, or (4) isotonic saline plus hyaluronidase. All treatment groups received corticosteroid and local anesthetic. Overall, across all four treatment groups, 83% of patients had significant pain relief at 1 month compared to 49% at 3 months, 43% at 6 months, and 49% at 12 months. The hyaluronidase and the hypertonic saline study group had a much lower incidence of additional need for pain procedures than the placebo groups, showing that site-specific catheter placement is important.

Manchikanti et al[43] performed a retrospective randomized evaluation of a modified Racz adhesiolysis protocol in 232 patients with low back pain. The study involved lesion-specific catheter placement, but the usual 3-day procedure was reduced to a 2-day (group 1) or a 1-day (group 2) procedure. Group 1 had 103 patients and group 2 had 129 patients. Other changes included changing the local anesthetic from bupivacaine to lidocaine, substituting methylprednisolone acetate or betamethasone acetate and phosphate for triamcinolone diacetate, and reduction of the volume of injectate. Of the patients in groups 1 and 2, 62% and 58% had greater than 50% pain relief at 1 month, respectively, with these percentages decreasing to 22% and 11% at 3 months, 8% and 7% at 6 months, and 2% and 3% at 1 year. Of significant interest is that the percentage of patients receiving greater than 50% pain relief after four procedures increased to 79% and 90% at 1 month, 50% and 36% at 3 months, 29% and 19% at 6 months, and 7% and 8% at 1 year for groups 1 and 2, respectively. Short-term relief of pain was demonstrated, but long-term relief was not.

In a randomized, prospective study, Manchikanti et al[44] evaluated a 1-day epidural adhesiolysis procedure against a control group of patients who received conservative therapy. Results showed that cumulative relief, defined as relief greater than 50% with one to three injections, in the treatment group was 97% at 3 months, 93% at 6 months, and 47% at 1 year. The study also showed that overall health status improved significantly in the adhesiolysis group.

In 2004 Manchikanti et al[45] published their results of a randomized, double-blind, controlled study on the effectiveness of 1-day lumbar adhesiolysis and hypertonic saline neurolysis in treatment of chronic low back pain. Seventy-five patients whose pain was unresponsive to conservative modalities were randomized into one of three treatment groups. Group 1 (control group) underwent catheterization where the catheter was in the sacral canal without adhesiolysis, followed by injection of local anesthetic, normal saline, and steroid. Group 2 consisted of catheterization with site-specific catheter placement being ventral-lateral for adhesiolysis, followed by injection of local anesthetic, normal saline, and steroid. Group 3 consisted of site-specific catheter placement for adhesiolysis, followed by injection of local anesthetic, hypertonic saline, and steroid. Patients were allowed to have additional injections based on the response, either after unblinding or without unblinding after 3 months. Patients without unblinding were offered either the assigned treatment or another treatment based on their response. If the patients in group 1 or 2 received adhesiolysis and injection and injection of hypertonic saline, they were considered withdrawn, and no subsequent data were collected. Outcomes were assessed at 3, 6, and 12 months using visual analog scale pain scores, Oswestry Disability Index, opioid intake, range-of-motion measurement, and P-3. Significant pain relief was defined as average relief of 50% or greater. Seventy-two percent of patients in group 3, 60% of patients in group 2, and 0% of patients in group 1 showed significant pain relief at 12 months. The average number of treatments for 1 year was 2.76 in group 2 and 2.16 in group 3. Duration of significant relief with the first procedure was 2.8 + 1.49 months and 3.8 + 3.37 months in groups 2 and 3, respectively. Significant pain relief (>50%) was also associated with improvement in Oswestry Disability Index, range of motion, and psychologic status.

Manchikanti et al[46,47] furthered this research using comparisons of percutaneous adhesiolysis versus fluoroscopically guided caudal epidural steroid injections. The first study involved a population of patients with chronic low back pain and known spinal stenosis. The results showed a 76% reduction in pain relief at 1 year with epidural adhesiolysis compared to 4% in the control group. The second study performed in a population of patients with post–lumbar surgery syndrome showed a reduction in pain and improvement in functional status in 73% of the epidural adhesiolysis group compared to 12% in the control group.

In 2006 a study by Veihelmann et al[48] evaluated patients with a history of chronic low back pain and sciatica. Inclusion criteria were radicular pain with a corresponding nerve root compressing substrate found on MRI or CT. All patients were randomized to receive either physiotherapy, analgesics, or lysis of adhesions. The lysis group had statistically significantly better outcome than the physical therapy treatment group.

Two other prospective evaluations by Chopra et al and Gerdesmeyer et al[49,50] evaluated patients with monosegmental radiculopathy of the lumbar spine. All the patients suffered from chronic disk herniations or failed back syndrome. All these randomized trials showed positive short-term and long-term relief. Two prospective evaluations also showed positive short- and long-term relief.[49,50]

Conclusion

Epidural adhesiolysis has evolved over the years as an important treatment option for patients with intractable cervical, thoracic, and low back and leg pain. Studies show that patients are able to enjoy significant pain relief and restoration of function. Manchikanti's studies show that the amount and duration of relief can be achieved by repeat procedures. Recent prospective randomized double-blind studies on failed back surgery and spinal stenosis show 75% and 80% improvement in visual analog scale scores and functional improvements at 12 months' follow-up. The evolution in the recognition of the site-specific importance of the catheter and medication delivery together with the fact that physicians need to aquire the skills to he able to carry out the procedure led to the improved outcomes seen in recent prospective randomized studies. Contradictory opinion usually originates from physicians who have never done the procedure or have never learned how to navigate the epidural space and quote earlier information that was published along the evolutionary trail. This is evidenced by the fact that results seen at the Texas Tech International Pain Center surpass even the strongest randomized-control trials and may be related to both patient involvement and procedure in conjunction with "neural flossing" exercises. This is due to both familiarity with the procedure itself and combining the procedure with aggressive neural flossing exercises.

Large numbers of patients have been spared unnecessary surgery or repeat surgery by the use of the percutaneous lysis procedure and at tremendous cost savings, which is based on the cost-effectiveness studies.

Endoscopy offers direct visualization of the affected nerve roots in addition to mechanical adhesiolysis, and may become more mainstream as the technique is refined.

Facet pain is commonly associated with the postlysis period or after provocative testing a month or so later if two-facet diagnostic blocks show efficacy. Radiofrequency facet denervation gives us the best long-term outcome.

More prospective, randomized, controlled studies need to be performed to further solidify the role of epidural adhesiolysis in the treatment algorithm of patients with intractable pain that is refractory to previous treatments, specifically with emphasis on the aforementioned combined facet pain.

References

Full references for this chapter can be found on www.expertconsult.com.

Hypogastric Plexus Block and Impar Ganglion Block

Steven D. Waldman

Hypogastric Plexus Block

Hypogastric plexus block continues to gain favor as a technique in the evaluation and treatment of sympathetically mediated pain emanating from the pelvic viscera. Recently repopularized by Patt and Plancarte, this useful regional anesthesia block provides the clinician with new options for patients with pelvic pain.[1] Recent advances in the use of fluoroscopic and computerized tomographic (CT) scan guidance have contributed greatly to the understanding of the functional anatomy of this anatomic region and have led to the development of several variations of the technique, including both a single-needle and a two-needle approach.[2,3]

Clinically Relevant Anatomy

In the context of neural blockade, the hypogastric plexus can simply be thought of as a continuation of the lumbar sympathetic chain that can be blocked in a manner analogous to lumbar sympathetic nerve block. The preganglionic fibers of the hypogastric plexus find their origin primarily in the lower thoracic and upper lumbar region of the spinal cord.[4] These preganglionic fibers interface with the lumbar sympathetic chain via the white communicantes. Postganglionic fibers exit the lumbar sympathetic chain and, together with fibers from the parasympathetic sacral ganglion, make up the superior hypogastric plexus. The superior hypogastric plexus lies in front of L4 as a coalescence of fibers. As these fibers descend, at a level of L5, they begin to divide into the hypogastric nerves,

following in proximity the iliac vessels (**Fig. 170.1**). As the hypogastric nerves continue their lateral and inferior course, they are accessible for neural blockade as they pass in front of the L5-S1 interspace. The hypogastric nerves pass downward from this point, following the concave curve of the sacrum and passing on each side of the rectum to form the inferior hypogastric plexus. These nerves continue their downward course along each side of the bladder to provide innervation to the pelvic viscera and vasculature.

Single-Needle Approach to Hypogastric Plexus Block

Hypogastric plexus block with the single-needle technique is useful in the evaluation and management of sympathetically mediated pain of the pelvic viscera.[2,5] Included in this category are pain from malignant disease, endometriosis, reflex sympathetic dystrophy, causalgia, proctalgia fugax, and radiation enteritis.[2] Hypogastric plexus block is also useful in the palliation of tenesmus resulting from radiation therapy to the rectum. Hypogastric plexus block with local anesthetic can be used as a diagnostic tool in performance of differential neural blockade on an anatomic basis in the evaluation of pelvic and rectal pain. If destruction of the hypogastric plexus is being considered, this technique is useful as a prognostic indicator of the degree of pain relief that the patient may experience. Hypogastric plexus block with local anesthetic is also useful in the treatment of acute herpes zoster and postherpetic neuralgia involving the sacral dermatomes. Destruction of the

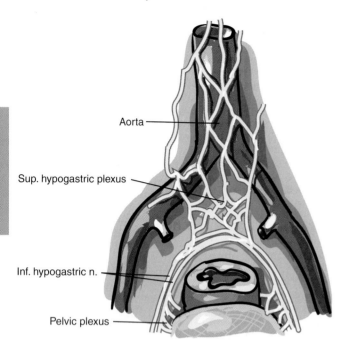

Fig. 170.1 **Clinically relevant anatomy of the hypogastric plexus.**

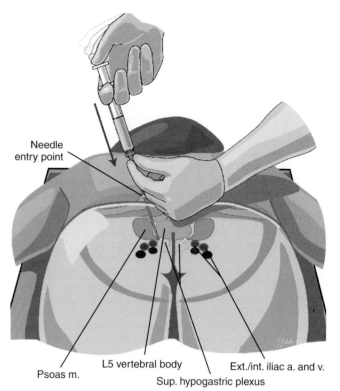

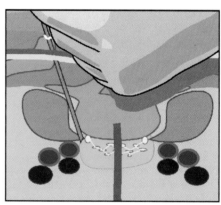

Fig. 170.2 **Blind single-needle technique for hypogastric plexus block.** *(From Waldman SD:* Atlas of interventional pain management, *ed 2, Philadelphia, 2003, Saunders, p 413.)*

hypogastric plexus is indicated for the palliation of pain syndromes that have temporarily responded to blockade of the hypogastric plexus with local anesthetic and have not been controlled with more conservative measures.[6,7]

Blind and Fluoroscopic Technique

The patient is placed in the prone position with a pillow placed under the lower abdomen to gently flex the lumbar spine and maximize the space between the transverse process of L5 and the sacral alae. The L4-L5 interspace is located by identifying the iliac crests and finding the interspace at that level. The skin at this level is prepared with antiseptic solution. A point 6 cm from the midline at this level is identified, and the skin and subcutaneous tissues are anesthetized with 1.0% lidocaine. A 20-gauge, 13-cm needle is then inserted through the previously anesthetized area and directed approximately 30 degrees caudad and 30 degrees mesiad toward the anterolateral portion of the L5-S1 interspace. If the transverse process of L5 is encountered, the needle is withdrawn and redirected slightly more caudad. If the vertebral body of L5 is encountered, the needle is withdrawn and redirected slightly more lateral until, in a manner analogous to lumbar sympathetic block, the needle is walked off the anterolateral aspect of the vertebral body.

A 5-mL glass syringe filled with preservative-free saline solution is then attached to the needle. The needle is then slowly advanced into the prevertebral space while constant pressure on the plunger of the syringe is maintained in a manner analogous to the loss-of-resistance technique used for identification of the epidural space. A "pop" and loss of resistance is felt as the needle pierces the anterior fascia of the psoas muscle and enters the prevertebral space (**Fig. 170.2**). After careful aspiration for blood, cerebrospinal fluid (CSF), and urine, 10 mL of 1.0% preservative-free lidocaine is slowly injected in incremental doses, while the patient is observed closely for signs of local anesthetic toxicity. If fluoroscopy is used, 2 to 3 mL of suitable water-soluble contrast is added to the injectate. The injectate is injected with continuous fluoroscopic guidance

(**Fig. 170.3**). If an inflammatory component to the pain is suspected, the local anesthetic is combined with 80 mg of methylprednisolone and is injected in incremental doses. Subsequent daily nerve blocks are carried out in a similar manner, substituting 40 mg of methylprednisolone for the initial 80-mg dose. The needle is then removed, and an ice pack is placed on the injection site to decrease postblock bleeding and pain.

Computed Tomography Scan–Guided Technique

The patient is placed in the prone position on the CT gantry with a pillow placed under the lower abdomen to gently flex the lumbar spine and maximize the space between the transverse process of L5 and the sacral alae. A CT scout film of the lumbar spine is taken, and the L4-L5 interspace is identified (**Fig. 170.4**). The skin overlying the L4-L5 interspace is prepared with antiseptic solution, and sterile drapes are placed.

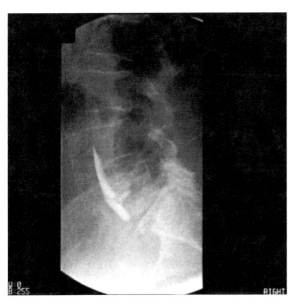

Fig. 170.3 Lateral radiograph shows verification of correct needle placement for unilateral superior hypogastric plexus block. Note smooth margins of opacity formed by contrast medium anterior to the psoas fascia, which suggests retroperitoneal placement. *(From Plancarte R, Amescua C, Patt RB: Sympathetic neurolytic blockade. In Patt RB, editor:* Cancer pain, *Philadelphia, 1993, JB Lippincott, pp 377–425.)*

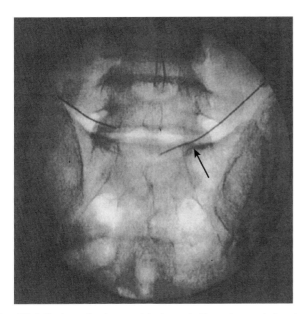

Fig. 170.4 Final needle placement is shown in the anteroposterior view. The left needle is in classic position for superior hypogastric plexus block. Blood was aspirated when the needle tip on the right side was at the point marked with the *arrow*. The right needle was advanced more medially until no blood aspirated. *(From Stevens DS, Balatbat GR, Lee FMK: Coaxial imaging technique for superior hypogastric plexus block,* Reg Anesth Pain Med *25:643, 2000.)*

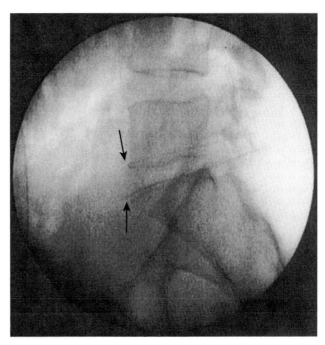

Fig. 170.5 Final needle position is shown in the lateral view. *Arrows* indicate tips of needles. The upper needle is on the left side, and the lower needle is on the right side. Both needles are located just anterior to the most anterior portion of the adjacent vertebra, which is classic position for needle placement for superior hypogastric plexus block. *(From Stevens DS, Balatbat GR, Lee FMK: Coaxial imaging technique for superior hypogastric plexus block,* Reg Anesth Pain Med *25:643, 2000.)*

vertebral body of L5 is encountered, the needle is withdrawn and redirected slightly more lateral and walked off the anterolateral aspect of the vertebral body in a manner analogous to lumbar sympathetic block. A 5-mL glass syringe filled with preservative-free saline solution is then attached to the needle. The needle is then slowly advanced into the prevertebral space while constant pressure on the plunger of the syringe is maintained. A pop and loss of resistance is felt as the needle pierces the anterior fascia of the psoas muscle (**Fig. 170.6**). After careful aspiration, 2 to 3 mL of water-soluble contrast medium is injected through the needle, and a CT scan is taken to confirm current retroperitoneal needle placement (**Fig. 170.7**). Because of contralateral spread of the contrast medium in the prevertebral space, placement of a second needle is often unnecessary, as is advocated by some pain specialists (**Fig. 170.8**). A total volume of 10 mL of 1.0% preservative-free lidocaine is then injected in divided doses after careful aspiration for blood, CSF, and urine. If adequate pain relief is obtained, incremental doses of absolute alcohol or 6.5% aqueous phenol may be injected in a similar manner after it is ascertained that the patient is experiencing no untoward bowel or bladder effects from blockade of the hypogastric plexus.

Classic Two-Needle Technique

Hypogastric plexus block with the classic two-needle technique is reserved for those patients in whom presacral tumor mass or adenopathy prevents contralateral spread of solutions injected through a single needle.[9] This technique is useful in the evaluation and management of sympathetically mediated pain of the pelvic viscera. Included in this category are pain from malignant disease, endometriosis, reflex sympathetic

At a point approximately 6 cm from midline, the skin and subcutaneous tissues are anesthetized with 1% lidocaine with a 25-gauge, 3.8-cm needle. A 20-gauge, 13-cm needle is then inserted through the previously anesthetized area and directed approximately 30 degrees caudad and 30 degrees mesiad toward the anterolateral portion of the L5-S1 interspace (**Fig. 170.5**).[8] If the transverse process of L5 is encountered, the needle is withdrawn and redirected slightly more caudad. If the

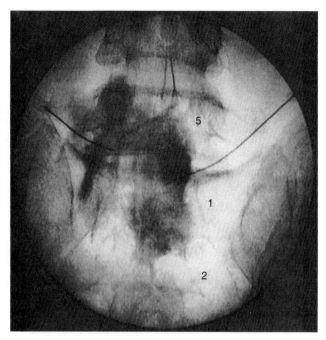

Fig. 170.6 Injection of contrast has been done on each side and is shown in the anteroposterior view. Vertebrae are marked *5* (L5), *1* (S1), and *2* (S2). The left side shows the classic pattern of contrast spread, covering all of L5 and S1 along the lateral portion of each vertebra. The right side shows coverage of the lower portion of L5, all of S1, and part of S2, but the contrast flows more medially than is usually seen. *(From Stevens DS, Balatbat GR, Lee FMK: Coaxial imaging technique for superior hypogastric plexus block,* Reg Anesth Pain Med *25:643, 2000.)*

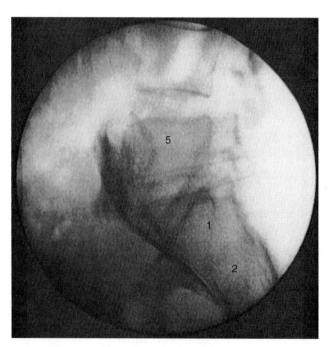

Fig. 170.7 Injection of contrast has been done on each side and is shown in the lateral view. Vertebrae are marked *5* (L5), *1* (S1), and *2* (S2). Contrast is seen to flow along the anterior aspects of L5, S1, and the upper portion of S2. The classic pattern of contrast spread for superior hypogastric plexus block is along the anterior aspect of L5 and S1, in the location of contrast shown in this figure. *(From Stevens DS, Balatbat GR, Lee FMK: Coaxial imaging technique for superior hypogastric plexus block,* Reg Anesth Pain Med *25:643, 2000.)*

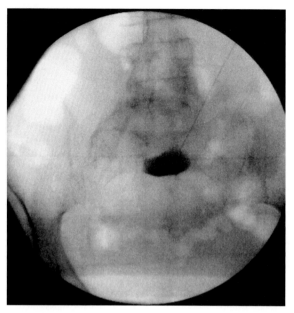

Fig. 170.8 **Anteroposterior view of the lumbosacral area with a 22-gauge Chiba needle placed at the junction of the lumbosacral vertebrae.** Notice that the injection of 3 mL of radiographic contrast was performed with a single needle to show the spread to the midline.

dystrophy, causalgia, proctalgia fugax, and radiation enteritis. Hypogastric plexus block is also useful in the palliation of tenesmus resulting from radiation therapy to the rectum. Hypogastric plexus block with local anesthetic can be used as a diagnostic tool in performance of differential neural blockade on an anatomic basis in the evaluation of pelvic and rectal pain. If destruction of the hypogastric plexus is being considered, this technique is useful as a prognostic indicator of the degree of pain relief that the patient may experience. Hypogastric plexus block with local anesthetic is also useful in the treatment of acute herpes zoster and postherpetic neuralgia involving the sacral dermatomes. Destruction of the hypogastric plexus is indicated for the palliation of pain syndromes that have temporarily responded to blockade of the hypogastric plexus with local anesthetic and have not been controlled with more conservative measures.[3,9]

Blind and Fluoroscopic Technique

The patient is placed in the prone position with a pillow placed under the lower abdomen to gently flex the lumbar spine and maximize the space between the transverse process of L5 and the sacral alae. The L4-L5 interspace is located by identifying the iliac crests and finding the interspace at that level. The skin at this level is prepared with antiseptic solution. A point 6 cm from the midline at this level is identified, and the skin and subcutaneous tissues are anesthetized with 1.0% lidocaine. A 20-gauge, 13-cm needle is then inserted through the previously anesthetized area and directed approximately 30 degrees caudad and 30 degrees mesiad toward the anterolateral portion of the L5-S1 interspace (**Fig. 170.9**). If the transverse process of L5 is encountered, the needle is withdrawn and redirected slightly more caudad. If the vertebral body of L5 is encountered, the needle is withdrawn and redirected slightly more lateral until, in a manner analogous to lumbar sympathetic block, the needle is walked off the anterolateral aspect of the vertebral body.

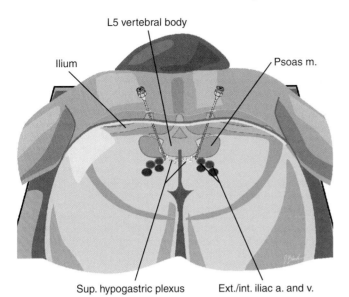

L5 vertebral body

Ilium

Psoas m.

Sup. hypogastric plexus

Ext./int. iliac a. and v.

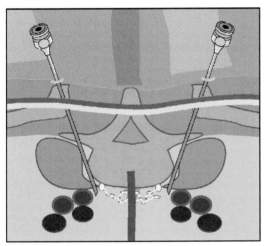

Fig. 170.9 Blind two-needle technique for hypogastric plexus block.
(From Waldman SD: Atlas of interventional pain management, ed 2, Philadelphia, 2003, Saunders, p 417.)

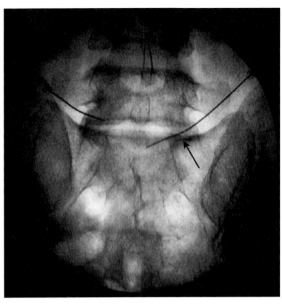

Fig. 170.10 Final needle placement is shown in the anterioposterior view. The left needle is in classic position for superior hypogastric plexus block. Blood was aspirated when the needle tip on the right side was at the point marked with an *arrow*. The right needle was advanced more medially until no blood was aspirated.

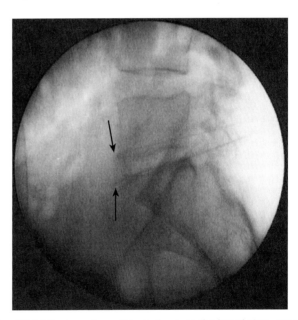

Fig. 170.11 Final needle position is shown in the lateral view. *Arrows* indicate tips of needles. The upper needle is on the left side, and the lower needle is on the right side. Both needles are located just anterior to the most anterior portion of the adjacent vertebra, which is classic position for needle placement for superior hypogastric plexus block.

A 5-mL glass syringe filled with preservative-free saline solution is attached to the needle. The needle is then slowly advanced into the prevertebral space while constant pressure on the plunger of the syringe is maintained in a manner analogous to the loss-of-resistance technique used for identification of the epidural space. A pop and loss of resistance is felt as the needle pierces the anterior fascia of the psoas muscle and enters the prevertebral space. A contralateral needle is then inserted in a similar manner with the trajectory and depth of the first needle as a guide (see Figs. 170.1, **170.10**, and **170.11**). After careful aspiration for blood, cerebrospinal fluid, and urine, 5 mL of 1.0% preservative-free lidocaine is slowly injected in incremental doses while the patient is observed closely for signs of local anesthetic toxicity. If fluoroscopy is being used, 2 to 3 mL of suitable water-soluble contrast is added to the injectate. The injectate is injected with continuous fluoroscopic guidance (**Figs. 170.12** and **170.13**). If an inflammatory component to the pain is suspected, the local anesthetic is combined with 80 mg of methylprednisolone and is injected in incremental doses. Subsequent daily nerve blocks are carried out in a similar manner, substituting 40 mg

of methylprednisolone for the initial 80-mg dose. Each needle is then removed, and an ice pack is placed on the injection site to decrease postblock bleeding and pain.

Computed Tomography Scan–Guided Technique

The patient is placed in the prone position on the CT gantry with a pillow placed under the lower abdomen to gently flex the lumbar spine and maximize the space between the transverse

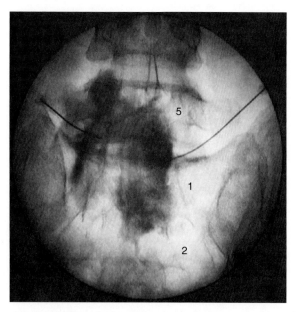

Fig. 170.12 Injection of contrast has been done on each side and is shown in the anteroposterior view. Vertebrae are marked *5* (L5), *1* (S1), and *2* (S2). The left side shows the classic pattern of contrast spread, covering all of L5 and S1 along the lateral portion of each vertebra. The right side shows coverage of the lower portion of L5, all of S1, and part of S2, but the contrast flows more medially than is usually seen.

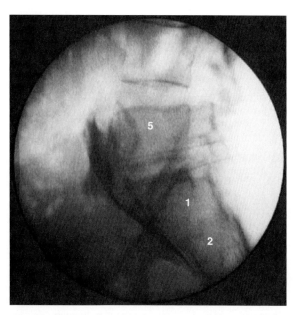

Fig. 170.13 Injection of contrast has been done on each side and is shown in the lateral view. Vertebrae are marked *5* (L5), *1* (S1), and *2* (S2). Contrast is seen to flow along the anterior aspects of L5, S1, and the upper portion of S2. The classic pattern of contrast spread for superior hypogastric plexus block is along the anterior aspect of L5 and S1, in the location of contrast shown in this figure.

process of L5 and the sacral alae. A CT scout film of the lumbar spine is taken, and the L4-L5 interspace is identified. The skin overlying the L4-L5 interspace is prepared with antiseptic solution, and sterile drapes are placed. At a point approximately 6 cm from midline, the skin and subcutaneous tissues are anesthetized with 1% lidocaine with a 25-gauge, 3.8-cm needle. A 20-gauge, 13-cm needle is then inserted through

the previously anesthetized area and directed approximately 30 degrees caudad and 30 degrees mesiad toward the anterolateral portion of the L5-S1 interspace. If the transverse process of L5 is encountered, the needle is withdrawn and redirected slightly more caudad. If the vertebral body of L5 is encountered, the needle is withdrawn and redirected slightly more lateral and walked off the anterolateral aspect of the vertebral body in a manner analogous to lumbar sympathetic block. A 5-mL glass syringe filled with preservative-free saline solution is attached to the needle. The needle is then slowly advanced into the prevertebral space while constant pressure on the plunger of the syringe is maintained. A pop and loss of resistance is felt as the needle pierces the anterior fascia of the psoas muscle. After careful aspiration, 2 to 3 mL of water-soluble contrast medium is injected through the needle, and a CT scan is taken to confirm current retroperitoneal needle placement. If no contralateral spread of the contrast medium in the prevertebral space is observed, a contralateral needle is inserted in a similar manner with the trajectory and depth of the first needle as a guide. A total volume of 5 mL of 1.0% preservative-free lidocaine is then injected in divided doses after careful aspiration for blood, cerebrospinal fluid, and urine. If adequate pain relief is obtained, incremental doses of absolute alcohol or 6.5% aqueous phenol may be injected in a similar manner after it is ascertained that the patient is experiencing no untoward bowel or bladder effects from blockade of the hypogastric plexus. Each needle is then removed, and an ice pack is placed on the injection site to decrease postblock bleeding and pain.

Transdiskal Technique

Hypogastric plexus block with the single-needle transdiskal technique is useful in the evaluation and management of sympathetically mediated pain of the pelvic viscera.[10] Included in this category are pain from malignant disease, endometriosis, reflex sympathetic dystrophy, causalgia, proctalgia fugax, and radiation enteritis. Hypogastric plexus block is also useful in the palliation of tenesmus resulting from radiation therapy to the rectum. Hypogastric plexus block with local anesthetic can be used as a diagnostic tool in performance of differential neural blockade on an anatomic basis in the evaluation of pelvic and rectal pain. If destruction of the hypogastric plexus is being considered, this technique is useful as a prognostic indicator of the degree of pain relief that the patient may experience. Hypogastric plexus block with local anesthetic is also useful in the treatment of acute herpes zoster and postherpetic neuralgia involving the sacral dermatomes. Destruction of the hypogastric plexus is indicated for the palliation of pain syndromes that have temporarily responded to blockade of the hypogastric plexus with local anesthetic and have not been controlled with more conservative measures.

Technique

Fluoroscopic Technique

The patient is placed in the prone position with a pillow placed under the lower abdomen to gently flex the lumbar spine and maximize the space between the transverse process of L5 and the sacral alae. The L5-S1 interspace is located with fluorosocopy. The skin at this level is prepared with antiseptic solution. A point 6 cm from the midline at this level is identified, and the

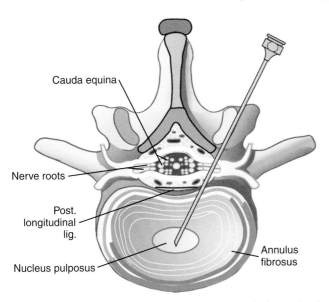

Fig. 170.14 A 20-gauge, 13-cm needle is inserted through the previously anesthetized area and directed with fluoroscopic guidance in a slightly cephalad trajectory until it enters the disk.

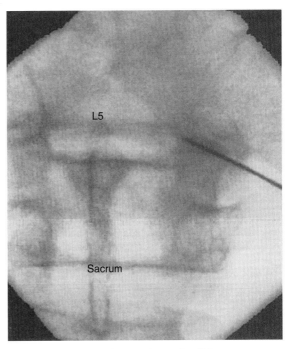

Fig. 170.16 **The needle is advanced into the disk.** *(From Raj PP, Waldman SD, Erdine S, et al:* Radiographic imaging for regional anesthesia and pain management, *ed 1, New York, 2002, Churchill Livingstone, p 235.)*

A 5-mL glass syringe filled with preservative-free saline solution is attached to the needle. The needle is then slowly advanced through the disk into the prevertebral space while constant pressure on the plunger of the syringe is maintained in a manner analogous to the loss-of-resistance technique used for identification of the epidural space. A pop and loss of resistance is felt as the needle pierces the anterior annulus of the disk and enters the prevertebral space (**Figs. 170.16 and 170.17**).[12] After careful aspiration for blood, CSF, and urine, 3 mL of water-soluble contrast medium is slowly injected in incremental doses with continuous fluoroscopic guidance to confirm bilateral spread of contrast in the prevertebral space. After proper needle placement is confirmed and aspiration for blood, cerebrospinal fluid (CSF), and urine is carried out, 5 to 7 mL of 1% preservative-free lidocaine is injected through the needle in small incremental doses while the patient is observed closely for signs of local anesthetic toxicity. If an inflammatory component to the pain is suspected, the local anesthetic is combined with 80 mg of methylprednisolone and is injected in incremental doses. Subsequent daily nerve blocks are carried out in a similar manner, substituting 40 mg of methylprednisolone for the initial 80-mg dose. The needle is then removed, and an ice pack is placed on the injection site to decrease post-block bleeding and pain. If adequate pain relief is obtained, incremental doses of absolute alcohol or 6.5% aqueous phenol may be injected in a similar manner after it is ascertained that the patient is experiencing no untoward bowel or bladder effects from blockade of the hypogastric plexus.

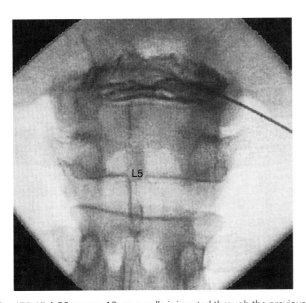

Fig. 170.15 A 20-gauge, 13-cm needle is inserted through the previously anesthetized area and directed with fluoroscopic guidance in a slightly cephalad trajectory until it enters the disk. *(From Raj PP, Waldman SD, Erdine S, et al:* Radiographic imaging for regional anesthesia and pain management, *ed 1, New York, 2002, Churchill Livingstone, p 235.)*

skin and subcutaneous tissues are anesthetized with 1.0% lidocaine. The fluoroscopy tube is the placed in the oblique position and angled 15 to 20 degrees caudad to align the inferior endplates of the adjacent vertebra and more clearly identify the disk space. A 20-gauge, 13-cm needle is then inserted through the previously anesthetized area and directed with fluoroscopic guidance in a slightly cephalad trajectory until it enters the disk (**Figs. 170.14 and 170.15**).[11] If the transverse process of L5 is encountered, the needle is withdrawn and redirected slightly more caudad. After the entry into the disk space has been confirmed on both posterioanterior and lateral views, 1 mL of contrast medium suitable for myelography is used to further confirm intradiskal placement of the needle tip.

Computed Tomography Scan–Guided Technique

The patient is placed in the prone position on the CT gantry with a pillow placed under the lower abdomen to gently flex the lumbar spine and maximize the space between the

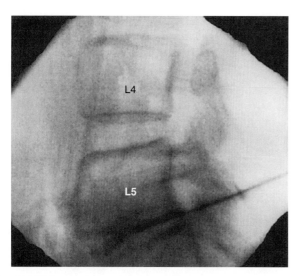

Fig. 170.17 *(From Raj PP, Waldman SD, Erdine S, et al:* Radiographic imaging for regional anesthesia and pain management, *ed 1, New York, 2002, Churchill Livingstone, p 235.)*

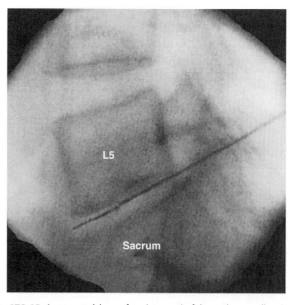

Fig. 170.19 A pop and loss of resistance is felt as the needle pierces the anterior annulus of the disk and enters the prevertebral space. *(From Raj PP, Waldman SD, Erdine S, et al:* Radiographic imaging for regional anesthesia and pain management, *ed 1, New York, 2002, Churchill Livingstone, p 235.)*

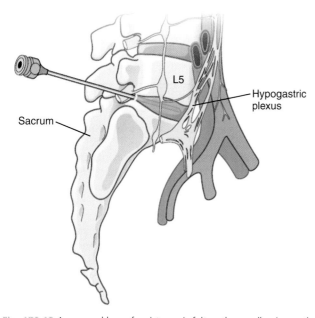

Fig. 170.18 A pop and loss of resistance is felt as the needle pierces the anterior annulus of the disk and enters the prevertebral space.

transverse process of L5 and the sacral alae. A CT scout film of the lumbar spine is taken, and the L5-S1 interspace is located with fluorosocopy. The skin at this level is prepared with antiseptic solution. A point 6 cm from the midline at this level is identified, and the skin and subcutaneous tissues are anesthetized with 1.0% lidocaine. A 20-gauge, 13-cm needle is then inserted through the previously anesthetized area and directed with CT guidance in a slightly cephalad trajectory until it enters the disk.[10] If the transverse process of L5 is encountered, the needle is withdrawn and redirected slightly more caudad. After the entry into the disk space has been confirmed on CT scan, 1 mL of contrast medium suitable for myelography is used to further confirm intradiskal placement of the needle tip (**Fig. 170.18**).

A 5-mL glass syringe filled with preservative-free saline solution is attached to the needle. The needle is then slowly advanced through the disk into the prevertebral space while constant pressure on the plunger of the syringe is maintained in a manner analogous to the loss-of-resistance technique used for identification of the epidural space (**Fig. 170.19**). A pop and loss of resistance is felt as the needle pierces the anterior annulus of the disk and enters the prevertebral space After careful aspiration for blood, cerebrospinal fluid, and urine, 3 mL of water-soluble contrast medium is slowly injected in incremental doses, and a CT scan of the prevertebral area is obtained to confirm bilateral spread of contrast in the prevertebral space.[10] After proper needle placement is confirmed and aspiration for blood, CSF, and urine is carried out, 5 to 7 mL of 1% preservative-free lidocaine is injected through the needle in small incremental doses while the patient is observed closely for signs of local anesthetic toxicity. If an inflammatory component to the pain is suspected, the local anesthetic is combined with 80 mg of methylprednisolone and is injected in incremental doses. Subsequent daily nerve blocks are carried out in a similar manner, substituting 40 mg of methylprednisolone for the initial 80-mg dose. The needle is then removed, and an ice pack is placed on the injection site to decrease postblock bleeding and pain.

If adequate pain relief is obtained, incremental doses of absolute alcohol or 6.5% aqueous phenol may be injected in a similar manner after it is ascertained that the patient is experiencing no untoward bowel or bladder effects from blockade of the hypogastric plexus.

Side Effects and Complications

The proximity of the hypogastric nerves to the iliac vessels means that the potential for bleeding or inadvertent intravascular injection remains a distinct possibility.[2,3,10,11,13] The relationship of the cauda equina and exiting nerve roots makes it imperative that this procedure be carried out only by those well versed in the regional anatomy and experienced in performing lumbar sympathetic nerve block. Given the proximity of the pelvic cavity, damage to the pelvic viscera, including the ureters, during hypogastric plexus block is a distinct possibility.[11,13] The incidence rate of this complication is decreased if care is taken to place the needle just beyond the anterolateral margin of the L5-S1 interspace. Needle placement too medial may result in epidural, subdural, or subarachnoid injections or trauma to the intervertebral disk, spinal cord, and exiting nerve roots.[2,3] Although uncommon, infection remains an ever-present possibility, especially in the cancer patient with immunocompromise. Early detection of infection, including diskitis, is crucial to avoid potentially life-threatening sequelae.[10,11]

Clinical Pearls

Hypogastric plexus block is a simple technique that can produce dramatic relief for patients with the previously mentioned pain symptoms, albeit with the increased risks of infection associated with placement of a needle through the intervertebral disk. Neurolytic block with small quantities of absolute alcohol or phenol in glycerin or with cryoneurolysis or radiofrequency lesioning has been shown to provide long-term relief for patients with sympathetically maintained pain that has been relieved with local anesthetic. As with the celiac plexus and lumbar sympathetic nerve blocks, the proximity of the sympathetic nerves to vascular structures mandates repeated careful aspiration and vigilance for signs of unrecognized intravascular injection. CT scan guidance allows visualization of the major blood vessels and their relationship to the needle, which is a significant advance over blind or fluoroscopically guided techniques. As mentioned previously, the proximity of the hypogastric plexus to the neuraxis and pelvic viscera makes careful attention to technique mandatory. Careful observation for postblock diskitis is crucial with this technique.[10]

Ganglion of Walther (Impar) Block

Ganglion of Walther (also known as the impar ganglion) block is useful in the evaluation and management of sympathetically mediated pain of the perineum, rectum, and genitalia.[14] This technique has been used primarily in the treatment of pain from malignant disease, although theoretic applications for benign pain syndromes, including pain from endometriosis, reflex sympathetic dystrophy, causalgia, proctalgia fugax, and radiation enteritis, can be considered if the pain has failed to respond to more conservative therapies.[15,16] Impar ganglion block with local anesthetic can be used as a diagnostic tool in performance of differential neural blockade on an anatomic basis in the evaluation of pelvic and rectal pain. If destruction of the impar ganglion is being considered, this technique is useful as a prognostic indicator of the degree of pain relief that the patient may experience. Destruction of the impar ganglion is indicated for the palliation of pain syndromes that have temporarily responded to blockade of the ganglion with local anesthetic and have not been controlled with more conservative measures.

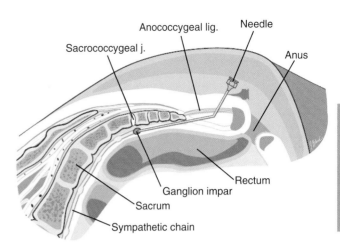

Fig. 170.20 **Needle tip against anterior surface of the sacrococcygeal junction.**

Clinically Relevant Anatomy

In the context of neural blockade, the impar ganglion can simply be thought of as the terminal coalescence of the sympathetic chain.[17] The impar ganglion lies in front of the sacrococcygeal junction and is amenable to blockade at this level. The ganglion receives fibers from the lumbar and sacral portions of the sympathetic and parasympathetic nervous system and provides sympathetic innervation to portions of the pelvic viscera and genitalia.

Blind and Fluoroscopic Technique

The patient is placed in the jackknife position to facilitate access to the inferior margin of the gluteal cleft. The midline is identified, and the skin just below the tip of the coccyx that overlies the anococcygeal ligament is prepared with antiseptic solution. The skin and subcutaneous tissues at this point are anesthetized with 1.0% lidocaine. A 3.5-inch spinal needle is then bent at a point 1 inch from its hub to a 30-degree angle to allow placement of the needle tip in proximity to the anterior aspect of the sacrococcygeal junction. The needle may be bent again at a point 2 inches from the hub to accommodate those patients with an exaggerated coccygeal curve to allow placement of the needle tip to rest against the sacrococcygeal junction.

The bent needle is then placed through the previously anesthetized area and is advanced until the needle tip impinges on the anterior surface of the sacrococcygeal junction (**Figs. 170.20** and **170.21**). If fluoroscopy is being used, after careful aspiration for blood, cerebrospinal fluid, and urine, 3 mL of water-soluble contrast medium is slowly injected in incremental doses with continuous fluoroscopic guidance to confirm bilateral spread of contrast in the prevertebral space (**Figs. 170.22** and **170.23**). After proper needle placement is confirmed and aspiration for blood, CSF, and urine is carried out, 5 to 7 mL of 1% preservative-free lidocaine is injected through the needle in small incremental doses. If an inflammatory component to the pain is suspected, the local anesthetic is combined with 80 mg of methylprednisolone and is injected in incremental doses. Subsequent daily nerve blocks are carried out in a similar manner, substituting 40 mg of

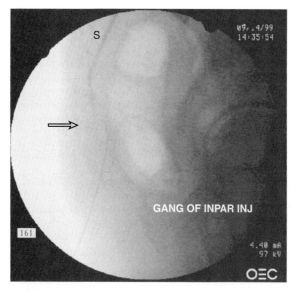

Fig. 170.21 **Needle tip against anterior surface of the sacrococcygeal junction.** *(Courtesy of Milton H. Landers, DO, PhD.)*

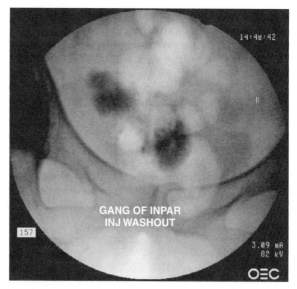

Fig. 170.23 **PA view of contrast medium anterior to the coccyx and sacrum.** *(Courtesy of Milton H. Landers, DO, PhD.)*

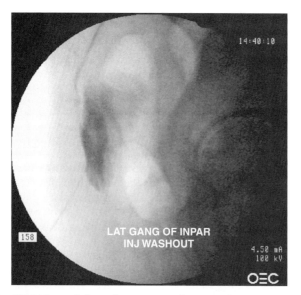

Fig. 170.22 **Lateral view of contrast medium anterior to coccyx and sacrum.**

methylprednisolone for the initial 80-mg dose. The needle is then removed, and an ice pack is placed on the injection site to decrease postblock bleeding and pain.

Computed Tomography Scan–Guided Technique

The patient is placed in the prone position on the CT gantry with a pillow placed under the pelvis to facilitate access to the inferior gluteal cleft. A CT scout film is taken, and the sacrococcygeal junction and the tip of the coccyx are identified. The midline is also identified, and the skin just below the tip of the coccyx that overlies the anococcygeal ligament is prepared with antiseptic solution. The skin and subcutaneous tissues at this point are anesthetized with 1.0% lidocaine. A 3.5-inch spinal needle is then bent at a point 1 inch from its hub to a 30-degree angle to allow placement of the needle tip in proximity to the

anterior aspect of the sacrococcygeal junction. The needle may be bent again at a point 2 inches from the hub to accommodate patients with an exaggerated coccygeal curve to allow the needle tip to rest against the anterior sacrococcygeal junction.

The needle is then placed through the previously anesthetized area and is advanced until the needle tip impinges on the anterior surface of the sacrococcygeal junction. After careful aspiration for blood, cerebrospinal fluid, and urine, 2 to 3 mL of water-soluble contrast medium is injected through the needle and a CT scan is taken to confirm the spread of contrast medium just anterior to the sacrococcygeal junction. After correct needle placement is confirmed, a total volume of 3 mL of 1.0% preservative-free lidocaine is injected in divided doses after careful aspiration for blood, cerebrospinal fluid, and urine. If adequate pain relief is obtained, incremental doses of absolute alcohol or 6.5% aqueous phenol may be injected in a similar manner, after it is ascertained that the patient is experiencing no untoward bowel or bladder effects from local anesthetic blockade of the impar ganglion. The needle is then removed, and an ice pack is placed on the injection site to decrease postblock bleeding and pain.

Transcoccygeal Technique

The transcoccygeal approach represents a reasonable alternative to the classic approach to ganglion impar block.[18] Theoretically, trauma to the rectum and pelvic viscera should be decreased. This approach is more straightforward to perform in experienced hands. Fluoroscopic or CT scan guidance should improve the safety of this technique.

Fluoroscopic Technique

The patient is placed in the jackknife position to facilitate access to the inferior margin of the gluteal cleft. The midline is identified, and the skin overlying the coccyx is prepared with antiseptic solution. The skin and subcutaneous tissues at this point are anesthetized with 1.0% lidocaine. Fluoroscopy is used to identify the sacrococcygeal and coccygeal joints. A 3.5-inch spinal needle is inserted between

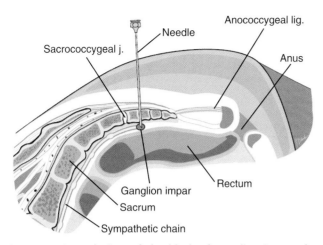

Fig. 170.24 **Lateral view of the block of ganglion impar after contrast injection.** Note the tip of the needle just anterior to the disk space between the first and second coccyx.

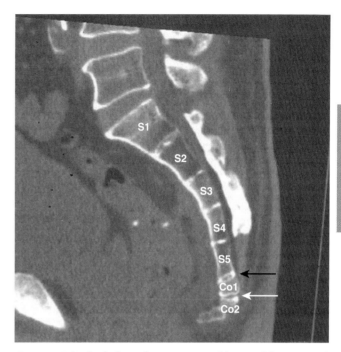

Fig. 170.26 **Sagittal view of sacrococcygeal bone with computed tomography.** Note the ossification at the sacrococcygeal joint *(black arrow)* and the conserved space between the first and second coccygeal bones *(white arrow)*. S, Sacrum; Co, coccyx. *(From Hong JH, Jang HS: Block of the ganglion impar using a coccygeal joint approach,* Reg Anesth Pain Med *31:583–584, 2006, Fig. 1.)*

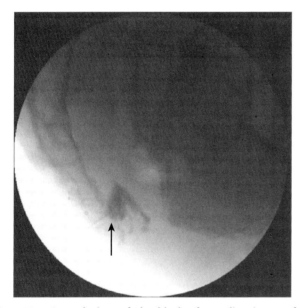

Fig. 170.25 **Lateral view of the block of ganglion impar after contrast injection.** Note the tip of the needle just anterior to the disk space between the first and second coccyx *(arrow)*. *(From Hong JH, Jang HS: Block of the ganglion impar using a coccygeal joint approach,* Reg Anesth Pain Med *31:583–584, 2006, Fig. 2.)*

the first and second coccygeal bones and slowly advanced until the needle tip rests just beyond the anterior wall of the coccyx in the precoccygeal space (**Fig. 170.24**). After careful aspiration for blood, cerebrospinal fluid, and urine, 1 mL of water-soluble iodinated contrast medium is slowly injected. After proper needle position and spread of contrast in the precoccygeal space is confirmed on both PA and lateral fluoroscopic views, 3 mL of 1.0% preservative-free lidocaine is slowly injected in incremental doses (**Fig. 170.25**). If an inflammatory component to the pain is suspected, the local anesthetic is combined with 80 mg of methylprednisolone and is injected in incremental doses. Subsequent daily nerve blocks are carried out in a similar manner, substituting 40 mg of methylprednisolone for the initial 80-mg dose. The needle is then removed, and an ice pack is placed on the injection site to decrease postblock bleeding and pain. If

adequate pain relief is obtained, 0.1-mL incremental doses of absolute alcohol or 6.5% aqueous phenol may be injected in a similar manner after it is ascertained that the patient is experiencing no untoward bowel or bladder effects from blockade of the Ganglion of Walther.

Computed Tomography Scan–Guided Technique

The patient is placed in the prone position on the CT gantry with a pillow placed under the pelvis to facilitate access to the inferior gluteal cleft. A CT scout film is taken, and the sacrococcygeal junction, coccygeal joints, and the tip of the coccyx are identified. The midline is also identified, and the skin overlying the coccyx that overlies the anococcygeal ligament is prepared with antiseptic solution. The skin and subcutaneous tissues at this point are anesthetized with 1.0% lidocaine. A 3.5-inch spinal needle is inserted between the first and second coccygeal bones and slowly advanced until the needle tip rests just beyond the anterior wall of the coccyx in the precoccygeal space (**Fig. 170.26**). After careful aspiration for blood, cerebrospinal fluid, and urine, 1 mL of water-soluble iodinated contrast medium is slowly injected. After proper needle position and spread of contrast in the precoccygeal space is confirmed with repeat CT scan, 3 mL of 1.0% preservative-free lidocaine is slowly injected in incremental doses. If an inflammatory component to the pain is suspected, the local anesthetic is combined with 80 mg of methylprednisolone and is injected in incremental doses. Subsequent daily nerve blocks are carried out in a similar manner, substituting 40 mg of methylprednisolone for the initial 80-mg dose. The needle is then removed, and an ice pack is placed on the injection site to decrease postblock bleeding and pain. If adequate pain relief is obtained,

0.1-mL incremental doses of absolute alcohol or 6.5% aqueous phenol may be injected in a similar manner after it is ascertained that the patient is experiencing no untoward bowel or bladder effects from blockade of the Ganglion of Walther.

Side Effects and Complications

The proximity of the impar ganglion to the rectum makes perforation and tracking of contaminants back through the needle track during needle removal a distinct possibility. Infection and fistula formation, especially in those patients with immunocompromise or who have received radiation therapy to the perineum, can represent a devastating and potentially life-threatening complication to this block.[17] The relationship of the cauda equina and exiting sacral nerve roots makes it imperative that this procedure be carried out only by those well versed in the regional anatomy and experienced in performing interventional pain management techniques.

Impar ganglion block is a straightforward technique that can produce dramatic relief for patients with the aforementioned pain symptoms. Given the localized nature of this neural structure when compared with the superior hypogastric plexus, neurolytic block with small quantities of absolute alcohol or phenol in glycerin or with cryoneurolysis or radiofrequency lesioning may be a reasonable choice over superior hypogastric plexus block—at least insofar as bowel and bladder dysfunction is concerned. Destruction of the impar ganglion has been shown to provide long-term relief for patients with sympathetically maintained pain that has been relieved with local anesthetic. CT scan guidance allows visualization of the regional anatomy and the relationship of the rectum to the needle. This is a significant advance over blind or fluoroscopically guided techniques.

Clinical Pearls

Ganglion of Walther block is a straightforward technique that can produce dramatic relief for patients with the previously mentioned pain symptoms. Given the localized nature of this neural structure when compared with the superior hypogastric plexus, neurolytic block with small quantities of absolute alcohol or phenol in glycerin or with cryoneurolysis or radiofrequency lesioning may be a reasonable choice over superior hypogastric plexus block, at least insofar as bowel and bladder dysfunction is concerned. Destruction of the ganglion of Walther has been shown to provide long-term relief for patients with sympathetically maintained pain that has been relieved with local anesthetic. CT scan guidance allows visualization of the regional anatomy and the relationship of the rectum to the needle. This is a significant advance over blind or fluoroscopically guided techniques.

References

Full references for this chapter can be found on www.expertconsult.com.

Injection of the Sacroiliac Joint

Steven D. Waldman

The sacroiliac joint is a diarthrodial joint that is susceptible to the development of arthritis from a variety of conditions that have in common the ability to damage the joint cartilage.[1] The sacroiliac joint is also susceptible to the development of strain from trauma or misuse. Osteoarthritis of the joint is the most common form of arthritis that results in sacroiliac joint pain. However, rheumatoid arthritis and post-traumatic arthritis are also common causes of sacroiliac pain. Less frequent causes of arthritis-induced sacroiliac pain include collagen vascular diseases, such as ankylosing spondylitis, infection, and Lyme disease. Acute infectious arthritis is usually accompanied by significant systemic symptoms, including fever and malaise, and should be easily recognized by an astute clinician and treated appropriately with culture and antibiotics rather than injection therapy. The collagen vascular diseases are generally manifested as a polyarthropathy rather than a monoarthropathy limited to the sacroiliac joint, although sacroiliac pain from the collagen vascular disease ankylosing spondylitis responds exceedingly well to the intra-articular injection technique described subsequently.[2] Occasionally, the clinician will encounter patients with iatrogenically induced sacroiliac joint dysfunction caused by overaggressive bone graft harvesting for spinal fusion.

Most patients with sacroiliac pain from strain or arthritis have pain localized around the sacroiliac joint and upper part of the leg.[3] The pain associated with sacroiliac joint strain or arthritis radiates into the posterior of the buttocks and back of the legs (**Fig. 171.1 [online only]**). The pain does not radiate below the knees.[4] Activity makes the pain worse, with rest and heat providing some relief. The pain is constant and characterized as aching. It may interfere with sleep. On physical examination, tenderness to palpation of the affected sacroiliac joint is found. The patient often favors the affected leg and exhibits a list to the unaffected side.[5] Spasm of the lumbar paraspinal musculature is often present, as is limitation of range of motion of the lumbar spine in the erect position that improves in the sitting position because of relaxation of the hamstring muscles.[6] Patients with pain emanating from the sacroiliac joint exhibit positive pelvic rock test results. The pelvic rock test is performed by placing the hands on the iliac crests and the thumbs on the anterior superior iliac spines and then

forcibly compressing the pelvis toward the midline (**Fig. 171.2**). Positive test results are indicated by the production of pain around the sacroiliac joint.

Plain radiographs are indicated in all patients with sacroiliac pain. On the basis of the patient's clinical findings, additional testing, including a complete blood count, sedimentation rate, and HLA-B27 antigen and antinuclear antibody testing, may be indicated (**Fig. 171.3**).

Clinically Relevant Anatomy

The sacroiliac joint is formed by the articular surfaces of the sacrum and iliac bones (**Fig. 171.4**). These articular surfaces have corresponding elevations and depressions that give the joints their irregular appearance on radiographs. The strength of the sacroiliac joint comes primarily from the posterior and interosseous ligaments rather than the bony articulations. The sacroiliac joints bear the weight of the trunk and

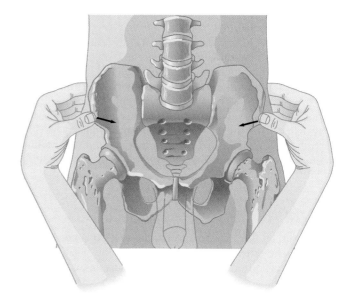

Fig. 171.2 **Pelvic rock test.** *(From Waldman SD, editor:* Atlas of interventional pain management, *ed 2, Philadelphia, 2003, Saunders, p 430.)*

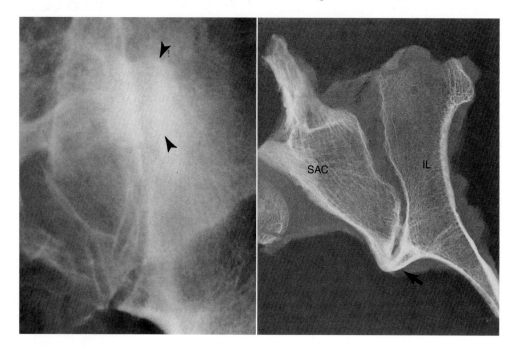

Fig. 171.3 **Ankylosing spondylitis as indicated by the *black arrows*.** *(From Resnick D: Diagnosis of bone and joint disorders, ed 4, Philadelphia, 2002, Saunders, p 1325.)*

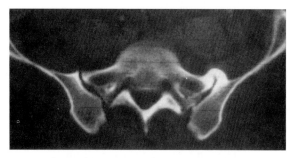

Fig. 171.4 **Radiographic anatomy of the sacroiliac joint.** *(From Waldman SD: Atlas of interventional pain management, ed 2, Philadelphia, 2003, Saunders, p 430.)*

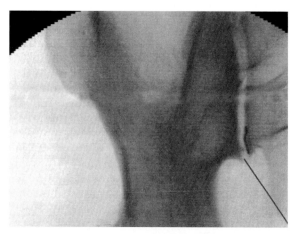

Fig. 171.5 **Sacroiliac joint enhanced fluoroscopically with oblique positioning of the C-arm.** *(From Raj PP, Lou L, Erden S, et al: Radiographic imaging for regional anesthesia and pain management, Philadelphia, 2003, Churchill Livingstone, p 243.)*

are thus subject to the development of strain and arthritis.[7] As the joint ages, the intraarticular space narrows, thus making intraarticular injection more challenging. The ligaments and the sacroiliac joint itself receive their innervation from the L3 to S3 nerve roots, with L4 and L5 providing the greatest contribution to innervation of the joint. This diverse innervation may help explain the ill-defined nature of sacroiliac pain. The sacroiliac joint has limited range of motion, and that motion is induced by changes in the force placed on the joint by shifts in posture and joint loading.

Technique

The goals of the injection technique are explained to the patient. The patient is placed in the supine position, and proper preparation with antiseptic cleansing of the skin overlying the affected sacroiliac joint space is carried out. A sterile syringe containing 4.0 mL of 0.25% preservative-free bupivacaine and 40 mg of methylprednisolone is attached to a 3.5-inch, 25-gauge needle with strict aseptic technique. Also with strict aseptic technique, the posterior superior

spine of the ilium is identified. At this point, the needle is carefully advanced through the skin and subcutaneous tissue at a 45-degree angle toward the affected sacroiliac joint (**Fig. 171.5**). If bone is encountered, the needle is withdrawn into the subcutaneous tissue and redirected superiorly and slightly more laterally.[8] After the joint space is entered, the contents of the syringe are gently injected. Little resistance to injection should occur. If resistance is encountered, the needle is probably in a ligament and should be advanced slightly into the joint space until the injection proceeds without significant resistance. Fluoroscopic guidance and the use of iodinated contrast may aid in the performance of this technique in selected patients (**Fig. 171.6**). Computed tomographic scan or ultrasound scan guidance may also be useful, especially in those patients in whom anatomic landmarks are difficult to identify (**Figs. 171.7** and **171.8**).[8,9] The needle is then removed,

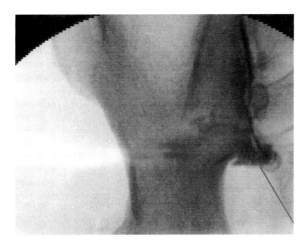

Fig. 171.6 **Sacroiliac joint fluoroscopically enhanced with contrast material.** *(From Raj PP, Lou L, Erden S, et al: Radiographic imaging for regional anesthesia and pain management, Philadelphia, 2003, Churchill Livingstone, p 244.)*

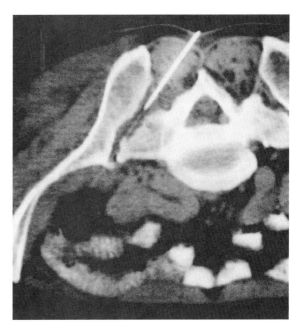

Fig. 171.7 **Sacroiliac joint injection in a 73-year-old woman with local pain without response to analgesics.** The needle is placed inside the sacroiliac joint. *(From Thanos L, Mylona S, Kalioras V, et al: Percutaneous CT guided interventional procedures in musculoskeletal system [our experience], Eur J Radiol 50:273–277, 2004, Fig. 3.)*

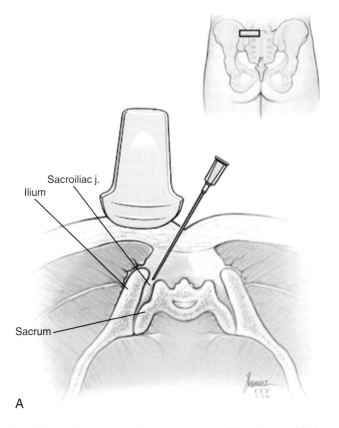

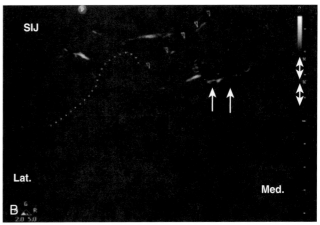

Fig. 171.8 **A,** Illustration showing the placement of the ultrasound (US) transducer in the transverse plane over the sacroiliac joint. **B,** US short-axis view showing the needle (in plane) inside the sacroiliac joint *(arrowheads).* The *dotted line* is delineating the ilium bony surface; *solid arrows* are pointing to the dorsal sacral surface. *(From Vydyanathan A, Narouze S: Ultrasound-guided caudal and sacroiliac joint injections, Techniques Regional Anesthesia Pain Manage 13:157, 2009, Fig. 2.)*

and a sterile pressure dressing and ice pack are placed at the injection site.

The major complication of intra-articular injection of the sacroiliac joint is infection. This complication should be exceedingly rare if strict aseptic technique is followed. Approximately 25% of patients have a transient increase in pain after intra-articular injection of the sacroiliac joint; patients should be warned of such. Care must be taken to avoid injection too laterally or the needle may traumatize the sciatic nerve.

References

Full references for this chapter can be found on www.expertconsult.com.

Neural Blockade of the Peripheral Nerves of the Lower Extremity

Vitaly Gordin, Sanjb Adhikary, and Ravish Kapoor

Historical Considerations

Neural blockade of the lower extremity is not a new technique. Braun[1] mentions that blockade of the lateral cutaneous femoral nerve was described by Nystrom in 1909. Läwen[2] expanded on this technique by describing the additional blockade of the anterior crural nerve, and Keppler improved both techniques by advocating the elicitation of paresthesias. Earlier, in 1887, Crile performed amputations by exposing the sciatic nerve in the gluteal fold and the femoral nerve in the inguinal fold and injecting cocaine intraneurally. Subsequently, no fewer than six other investigators advocated percutaneous approaches to the sciatic nerve alone.[3]

Many of the old techniques are still used today, although adjunct tools, such as the use of peripheral nerve stimulators and ultrasound, have evolved and have modified the older techniques. Adequate peripheral nerve blockade still hinges on a knowledge of the relevant anatomy, as emphasized by Labat:[4] "Anatomy is the foundation upon which the entire concert of regional anesthesia is built"; "landmarks are anatomic guideposts of the body which are used to locate the nerves"; "superficial landmarks are distinguished features of the surface of the body which can be easily recognized and identified by sight or palpation. Bones and their prominences, blood vessels and tendons serve as deep landmarks. Deep landmarks can be defined only by the point of the needle. They are the only reliable guide for advancing the needle in attempting to reach the vicinity of the nerve"; and "the anesthetist should attempt to visualize the anatomic structures traversed by the needle and utilize the tactile senses to determine the impulses transmitted by the point of the needle as it approaches a deep landmark (e.g., bone)."[4] Since 2000, a paradigm shift toward ultrasound use has occurred within regional anesthesia practice. This addition to the tools for performing peripheral nerve blocks has been proven advantageous by numerous clinical studies.

Although peripheral neural blockade of the lower extremity has been described for more than a century, its use is still limited in most practices when compared with blockade of the upper extremity. This limited use most likely reflects the ability to provide rapid, complete, and safe anesthesia of the lower extremity with neuraxial blockade. In addition, neural blockade of the upper extremity is accomplished with a single injection, which is not the case with the lower extremity. Despite these limitations, neural blockade of the peripheral nerves of the lower extremity does have advantages and should be considered when clinicians decide on an anesthetic technique.

Fundamentals of Ultrasound Technique

A basic comprehension of ultrasound related terminology is imperative to understand the technicalities associated with real-time ultrasound-guided nerve blocks. Although it is beyond the scope of the material presented here, deeper insight can be obtained by reviewing details pertaining to ultrasound principles in resources exclusively dedicated to such concepts.

Ultrasound beams are generally refracted as they pass through different tissues. The quality of image obtained depends on several factors, including beam angle, centering of the structure in question on the screen, and type of transducer chosen. To position the object being analyzed appropriately, the transducer (probe) is maneuvered medially or laterally, cephalad or caudad, or by adjusting the beam penetrating depth on the machine itself. Additionally, modern machines are typically able to accommodate two different types of transducers to evaluate either superficial or deeper structures. Transducer elements are generally arranged in either linear or curved arrays. Whereas linear array transducers of high frequency (HF) (6 to 13 MHz) create rectangular images of superficial structures, curved array transducers of low frequency (LF) (3 to 5 MHz) create wedge-shaped images of deeper structures. Nerves are generally imaged in short axis (cross-sectional) views or long axis (longitudinal views). Needle insertion is either performed with an out-of-plane approach in which the needle is perpendicular to the transducer or an in-plane approach in which the needle is parallel to the transducer. Both approaches have their own advantages and disadvantages; however, in any approach visualization of the needle tip is important and is highly operator dependent. It can be enhanced by injecting a small amount of fluid (1 to 2 mL) during the actual injection; this technique also helps to approximate the volume of local anesthetic required to surround the structure in question completely. Conversely, injection of air is avoided because it may cause acoustic artifacts that can hamper imaging.

Indications

Indications for neural blockade of the peripheral nerves of the lower extremity include management of acute pain and diagnostic management of chronic pain syndromes. Regional anesthesia allows the surgical site to be anesthetized without the hemodynamic instability associated with neuraxial anesthesia and also permits the provider to avoid using general anesthesia if so desired. In addition, varying approaches to neural blockade add flexibility to accommodate the surgical procedure in case of swelling or infection (e.g., performing sciatic or popliteal blocks with or without a femoral nerve block if the surgical site is a swollen or infected foot). When deciding on regional anesthesia, one must be cognizant of the site, degree, and duration of the procedure and the requirements for pain control in the postoperative period, to deliver safe and efficient anesthesia.

Sciatic Nerve Block

Indications

Blockade of the sciatic nerve is indicated for anesthesia of the distal part of the lower extremity and foot, with the exception of the medial aspect of the leg. Because of the sensory and cutaneous distribution of the sciatic nerve, few surgical procedures can be accomplished with a sciatic nerve block as the sole anesthetic. If a sciatic nerve block is combined with a saphenous nerve block, any surgical procedure below the level of the knee may be performed. Blockade of the sciatic nerve is also used to manage postoperative pain after lower extremity surgical procedures performed using general anesthesia.

Clinically Relevant Anatomy

The sciatic nerve is formed from the anterior division of the L4, L5, and S1-3 nerves. These nerves fuse and exit the pelvis through the greater sciatic notch and then pass between the greater trochanter and the ischial tuberosity.[5] The nerve becomes superficial at the lower border of the gluteus maximus muscle. From there, it courses down the posterior aspect of the thigh to the popliteal fossa, where it divides into the tibial and common peroneal nerves. The sciatic nerve is both a sensory and a motor nerve and includes some sympathetic fibers that originate in the lumbosacral plexus. It is the largest of the four major nerves supplying the leg.

Landmark Technique

The sciatic nerve can be blocked by several techniques. The least complicated, most common, and most widely recognized is the peripheral approach, also known as the *classic Labat technique.* The patient is placed in a lateral position with the operative extremity uppermost. The extremity should be flexed at the knee and should rest on the dependent extremity. The greater trochanter and the posterior-superior iliac spine (PSIS) are identified, and the midpoint between the greater trochanter and the PSIS is marked. A perpendicular line is drawn from the midpoint 4 cm caudad, and this point is marked as the entry site. The skin is cleansed with iodine solution and prepared in sterile fashion.

The skin should be anesthetized over the entry site midway between the two landmarks with 1 to 2 mL of 0.5% lidocaine injected through a 1½-inch, 25-gauge needle. A 100-mm stimulating needle is connected to a nerve stimulator (initial current, 1.5 mA, 2 Hz) and inserted perpendicular to all planes. As the needle is inserted, the gluteal muscles contract. Once these contractions disappear, the needle is advanced further, until stimulation of the sciatic nerve is achieved. The stimulation can be hamstring twitches or twitches of the tibial or common peroneal nerves. Typically, twitch of the hamstring muscles is observed first. With minimal further needle advancement, twitches of the foot are readily observed. When this maneuver fails to localize the sciatic nerve, the needle is withdrawn to the skin and is redirected 15 degrees toward the greater trochanter. If this also is unsuccessful, the needle is again withdrawn to the skin and is redirected in the opposite direction, 15 degrees toward the PSIS. The sciatic nerve is typically located at a depth of 5 to 8 cm in an average-sized adult patient. Once stimulation of the foot is achieved at 0.20 to 0.40 mA or less, 20 mL of local anesthetic is injected. The local anesthetic used is determined by the length of blockade required: 1.5% mepivacaine or 1% to 2% lidocaine for intermediate-acting effect (onset time, 5 to 15 minutes and lasting 2 to 3 hours). A combination of 0.5% bupivacaine and 1.5% mepivacaine in a 2:1 mixture can be used for quicker onset but longer duration of action. Epinephrine should not be added to this injection because of the lack of prominent blood supply to the sciatic nerve, which would increase the risk for ischemia of the nerve once vasoconstriction occurs.

An alternative approach is to identify the greater trochanter and ischial tuberosity, insert the needle as described earlier, and advance the needle until a twitch is obtained. This technique eliminates the requirements of drawing lines on the patient but may be difficult in obese patients, in whom the landmarks are not readily identified.

Ultrasound Technique

The introduction of ultrasound modified the approach to sciatic nerve in several ways. In general, when the nerve is approached from the front of the leg, it is termed the *anterior approach,* and when the nerve is approached from the back of the leg, it is termed the *posterior approach.* The posterior approach is further classified as infragluteal-parasacral or transgluteal. For simplicity, only the anterior and posterior subgluteal approaches are described here.

Anterior Approach

With the patient in the supine position, the thigh is externally rotated, and the knee is flexed. The transducer (LF) is placed transversely on the anterior thigh. After sterile skin preparation over the block area, the lesser trochanter is imaged, and the probe is moved proximally or distally along the thigh, until the nerve is imaged medial and posterior (deep) to the femur. The needle is placed in line, medial to the probe, and is advanced in a posterior-lateral direction, until the nerve is contacted or penetrated (**Fig. 172.1**). Because the nerve is usually at a depth of 6 to 10 cm, the preference is to use nerve stimulation in conjunction with ultrasound imaging with this approach. A stimulation threshold of 1 mA or less is used to identify the nerve. Once identified, local anesthetic is injected in 5-mL increments for a total of 5 to 10 mL of solution if the needle is within the nerve sheath or 10 to 20 mL if the solution is deposited

outside the nerve. A dark "halo" should be seen around the nerve if local anesthetic is deposited outside the nerve.[6]

Posterior Approach

With the patient in either the lateral or prone position, the transducer (LF) is placed between the ischial tuberosity and the greater trochanter. The nerve viewed here is a hyperechoic structure that lies deep to the gluteus maximus. Once a high-quality image is obtained on the screen (**Fig. 172.2**), the subsequent steps for performing the block are the same as in the anterior approach.

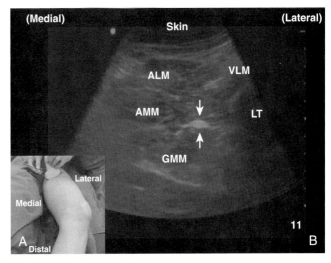

Fig. 172.1 A, Ultrasound transducer position for the anterior approach to the sciatic nerve block. B, Ultrasound image of sciatic nerve *(arrows)* obtained with transducer in short axis (transverse view). ALM, adductor longus muscle; AMM, adductor magnus muscle; GMM, gluteus maximus muscle; LT, femur (lesser trochanter); VLM, vastus lateralis muscle. *(Image courtesy of Shinichi Sakura, MD.)*

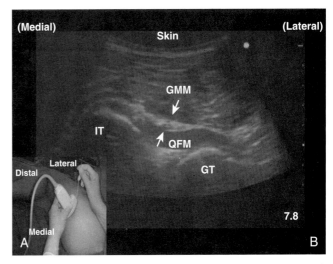

Fig. 172.2 A, Ultrasound transducer position for the posterior approach to the sciatic nerve block. B, Ultrasound image of the sciatic nerve *(arrows)* obtained with transducer using a posterior (subgluteal) approach in short axis (transverse view). GMM, gluteus maximus muscle; GT, femur (greater trochanter); IT, ischial tuberosity; QFM, quadratus femoris muscle. *(Image courtesy of Shinichi Sakura, MD.)*

Side Effects and Complications

The most common complication of sciatic nerve blockade is failure of the block. The clinician must observe stimulation of the sciatic nerve and watch for foot twitches. Foot stimulation at 0.40 mA or less greatly increases the success rate of the block. Stimulation at 0.20 mA or less indicates that needle placement is too close to the nerve, and paresthesias or intraneural injection may result. Other complications include hematoma formation in the gluteal region and local anesthesia toxicity as a result of rapid absorption. The speed of injection should not exceed 20 mL/minute because of this risk for rapid absorption. As with any injection, a risk for infection exists, and thus sterile technique should always be used.

Femoral Nerve Block

Indications

Blockade of the femoral nerve is indicated for both anesthesia and analgesia. Examples include situations in which the anterior aspect of the thigh must be anesthetized, such as for muscle biopsy or skin grafting, knee surgery such as arthroscopy or patella tendon repair, or repair of lacerations. This block also may be used to provide pain relief in patients with femoral shaft and neck fractures, as well as for postoperative pain relief after operations on the thigh, patella, and knee.[7] In addition, it is used as an adjunct to sciatic or popliteal nerve blocks to provide anesthesia to the entire lower extremity or the lower part of the leg.

Blockade of the femoral nerve was shown to be an effective adjunct to general anesthesia for knee joint surgery. Postoperative opiate administration was reduced by 80% in the recovery room and by 40% in the first 24 hours postoperatively in patients receiving nerve blocks.[8]

Clinically Relevant Anatomy

The femoral nerve is the largest branch of the lumbar plexus. It emerges through the fibers of the iliopsoas muscle and descends between the psoas major and iliacus muscles. It passes under the inguinal ligament lateral to the femoral artery. It then divides into a superficial bundle, which is primarily sensory and innervates the skin of the anterior aspect of the thigh with a motor branch to the sartorius muscle, and a deep bundle, which is primarily motor and innervates the quadriceps muscle with some sensory fibers to the knee joint and medial aspects of the lower extremity. The femoral nerve terminates as the purely sensory saphenous nerve. Therefore, the femoral nerve supplies sensation to the skin over the medial, anterior medial, and posterior medial aspects of the leg, from just above the knee to the great toe.

Landmark Technique

The patient is positioned in the supine position with the lower extremities fully extended. The femoral artery is identified, and a point immediately lateral, along the femoral crease, is marked as the entry site.[9] The skin is prepared with iodine solution and is draped in sterile fashion.

The skin overlying the entry site is anesthetized with 1 to 2 mL of 0.5% lidocaine injected through a 25-gauge, 1½-inch needle. A 22-gauge, 50-mm insulated short-beveled needle is

attached to a stimulator (initial current, 1.0 mA, 2 Hz). The needle is inserted immediately lateral to the pulse while the clinician palpates the femoral artery pulse and is advanced at a 60-degree angle posteriorly and cephalad. Contraction of the quadriceps muscle is the goal of this stimulation. The needle is redirected laterally in progressive fashion until the nerve is identified. Quadriceps contraction is not to be confused with contraction of the sartorius muscle, an error that commonly results in failure of this block. If sartorius contraction is obtained, the needle is redirected 15 degrees laterally and 1 to 2 mm deeper until the femoral nerve is identified. The ultimate goal is to achieve quadriceps muscle stimulation (patella twitches) at 0.4 mA or less. After negative aspiration for blood, the clinician injects 15 to 30 mL of local anesthetic. Local anesthetics used are 1.5% mepivacaine or 1% to 2% lidocaine for intermediate-acting effect (onset time, 5 to 15 minutes) or 0.5% to 0.75% ropivacaine or 0.5% bupivacaine for long-acting effect (onset time, 20 to 30 minutes). Again, a combination of 0.5% bupivacaine and 1.5% mepivacaine in a 2:1 mixture can be used for quicker onset but longer duration of action. Epinephrine can be added at 1:300,000 to prolong this nerve block.

Ultrasound Technique

After sterile skin preparation over the block area, the transducer (HF) is placed at a 90-degree angle to the skin and parallel to the inguinal crease. The medial side of the transducer is placed slightly caudal to the lateral side, to help in obtaining a better cross-sectional view of the nerve. Adjustments to probe positioning are then made for optimal visualization of the noncompressible, round, pulsatile, and hypoechoic femoral artery. Medial to the artery is the larger, yet compressible, femoral vein. The femoral nerve is the hyperechoic structure located just lateral and slightly deeper to the femoral artery (**Fig. 172.3**). The fascia lata and fascia iliaca are seen as linear hyperechoic structures traveling medially to laterally perpendicular to the femoral nerve and femoral artery. The fascia lata is superficial to the fascia iliaca, which is superficial to the femoral nerve. The needle is inserted at the 30 to 45 degrees lateral to the probe using an in-plane approach

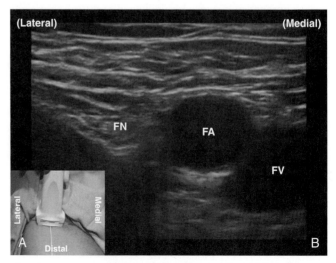

Fig. 172.3 A, Ultrasound transducer position at the inguinal crease for a femoral nerve block. **B,** Ultrasound image of the femoral nerve in short axis (transverse view). FA, femoral artery; FN, femoral nerve; FV, femoral vein.

toward the targeted structures. After the iliopsoas muscle is passed, a distinct "pop" of the fascia iliaca is felt as the triangle is entered. Here, 10 to 25 mL of local anesthetic is injected while the clinician performs intermittent aspiration, and it can be seen surrounding the femoral nerve.[10]

Side Effects and Complications

Complications of femoral nerve block may include intravascular injection, either intra-arterial or intravenous in the femoral artery or vein because of their close proximity to the femoral nerve. Care should be taken to aspirate for blood before injection of local anesthetic. Hematoma formation is also a risk associated with this injection because of the anatomic situation of the vasculature as compared with the nerve. The anesthesiologist should be alert for the presence of vascular grafts of the femoral artery, which are relative contraindications to elective femoral nerve block. Nerve injury is a possibility with intraneural injection. Needle positioning should be adjusted if stimulation is achieved at 0.2. mA or less.

Blockade of the obturator and lateral femoral cutaneous nerves may occur (three-in-one block) with femoral nerve blockade. As with any injection, a risk for infection exists, and thus sterile technique should always be used.

Lateral Femoral Cutaneous Nerve Block

Indications

Blockade of the lateral femoral cutaneous nerve is indicated in conjunction with blockade of other nerves or by itself for skin grafting sites or for the treatment of meralgia paresthetica. This procedure can also be useful for providing pain relief associated with the use of tourniquets.

Meralgia paresthetica is a pain syndrome believed to be caused by compression or injury to the lateral femoral cutaneous nerve. It causes pain emanating from the skin of the lateral aspect of the thigh. Meralgia paresthetica can be diagnosed and treated with a nerve block and neural destruction, if needed, of the lateral femoral cutaneous nerve.

Clinically Relevant Anatomy

The lateral femoral cutaneous nerve is derived from the L2-3 nerve roots and is purely a sensory nerve. It runs through the pelvis along the lateral border of the iliopsoas muscle, deep to the iliac fascia and anterior to the iliacus muscle. It emerges through the fascia inferior and medial to the anterior-superior iliac spine (ASIS) and divides into anterior and posterior branches. The anterior branch innervates the lateral aspect of the front of the thigh down to the knee. The posterior branch innervates the skin overlying the lateral portion of the buttock distal to the greater trochanter to approximately the middle of the thigh.

Landmark Technique

The patient is placed in the supine position. The ASIS is identified, and a point 2 cm medial and 2 cm inferior to the ASIS is selected as the entry site. The skin is cleansed with alcohol.

The skin is anesthetized with 1 to 2 mL of 0.5% lidocaine injected through a 25-gauge, 1½ inch needle. A 3- to 4-cm

needle is inserted perpendicular to the skin through the fascia lata. The fascia lata is identified when the operator feels a pop or a release as the needle passes through it. After careful aspiration, the clinician injects 10 to 15 mL of local anesthetic above and below the fascia in a medial-to-lateral fanlike distribution, to ensure that the nerve branches are covered. If this block is performed for surgical anesthesia, 0.5% bupivacaine or 0.5% ropivacaine is used. For treatment of meralgia paresthetica, a mixture of 5 mL of 0.5% bupivacaine, 4 mL of Sarapin (which is derived from the pitcher plant and possesses mild neurolytic action), and 40 mg of methylprednisolone (Depo-Medrol) can be used.

Ultrasound Technique

After sterile skin preparation over the block area, the transducer (HF) is placed on the skin medial and inferior to the ASIS. In this position, the sartorius muscle is seen along the lateral aspect of the probe, and the fascia lata and fascia iliaca can be identified. Using an in-plane approach, the needle can be placed either medial or lateral to the transducer. After the skin is anesthetized, the needle is advanced through the fascia iliaca until it is adjacent to the nerve. Here, the clinician injects 5 to 10 mL of local anesthetic in incremental doses. In comparative studies, the use of ultrasound resulted in a 100% success rate for lateral femoral cutaneous nerve block compared with a 40% success rate using a blind technique.[10]

Side Effects and Complications

Complications of blockade of the lateral femoral cutaneous nerve are rare. Theoretically, direct nerve injury may result from intraneural injection but is unlikely. Local hematoma may occur but is very unlikely because of the lack of large blood vessels in the area. As with any injection, a risk for infection exists, and therefore sterile technique should always be used.

Obturator Nerve Block

Indications

Obturator nerve blockade is indicated in conjunction with blockade of other nerves such as the lateral femoral cutaneous, the femoral, and the sciatic for surgical procedures on the lower extremity. This block can be used alone to prevent adductor contraction evoked by electrocautery near the bladder wall, as well as to alleviate adductor spasms of the hip and reduce pain in the hip joint. Additionally, it can be performed as a diagnostic tool for pain syndromes in the hip joint, inguinal area, or lumbar spine.

Clinically Relevant Anatomy

The obturator nerve is derived from L2-4 and travels along the medial border of the iliopsoas muscle; it is both a motor and a sensory nerve. It travels through the obturator foramen with the obturator artery and vein into the thigh. The obturator nerve divides into anterior and posterior branches. The anterior branch provides motor innervation to the superficial adductors and sensory innervation to the hip joint and medial aspect of the distal part of the thigh. The posterior branch provides motor innervation to the deep adductors and sensory innervation to the posterior knee joint.

Landmark Technique

The patient is placed in the supine position with the affected extremity slightly abducted and the knee slightly flexed. The pubic tubercle on the side to be anesthetized is identified. The entry site is 2 cm lateral and 2 cm caudal to the pubic tubercle. The skin is prepared with iodine solution and is draped in sterile fashion.

The skin overlying the entry site is anesthetized with 1 to 2 mL of 0.5% lidocaine injected through a 25-gauge, 1½- inch needle. A 22-gauge, 100-mm insulated stimulating needle is connected to a nerve stimulator (initial current, 2 to 3 mA, 2 Hz) and is inserted perpendicular to the skin until the inferior border of the superior ramus of the pubic bone is contacted at a depth of approximately 1.5 to 4 cm.

The needle is then slightly withdrawn and is redirected posteriorly and laterally to walk off the inferior margin of the superior pubic ramus. At 2 to 3 cm, the needle is in close proximity to the obturator canal. The adductor muscle twitches should be seen and felt at a current intensity of 0.5 mA or less, at which point the clinician injects 10 mL of local anesthetic. Local anesthetics used are 1.5% mepivacaine or 1% to 2% lidocaine for intermediate-acting effect (onset time, 5 to 15 minutes) or 0.5% to 0.75% ropivacaine or 0.5% bupivacaine for long-acting effect (onset time, 20 to 30 minutes). Again, a combination of 0.5% bupivacaine and 1.5% mepivacaine in a 2:1 mixture can be used for quicker onset but longer duration of action.

The following alternative approaches can also be used for an obturator nerve block:

- Interadductor approach: The patient is placed in the supine position, and a mark is made on the skin 1 to 2 cm medial to the femoral artery and immediately below the inguinal ligament to denote the direction of the needle toward the obturator canal. The adductor longus tendon is identified near its pubic insertion. A 22-gauge, 100-mm insulated stimulating needle is introduced behind the adductor longus tendon and is directed laterally, with a slight posterior-superior inclination, toward the skin mark. The needle is advanced toward the obturator canal until stimulation of the adductor muscles is still visible at a current of 0.5 mA or less.
- Three-in-one block: This block is similar to a femoral nerve block, except that digital pressure is applied distal to the site of injection and large volumes of local anesthetic (≥30 mL) are used. This results in substantial cephalad spread of local anesthetic under the fascia iliaca, and that blocks the remaining branches of the lumbar plexus: the femoral, obturator, and lateral femoral cutaneous nerves of the thigh.

Ultrasound Technique

After sterile skin preparation, an ultrasound transducer (LF) is placed as for femoral nerve block and is moved medially to scan the block area, and a short-beveled stimulating needle is advanced using an out-of-plane or in-plane technique (**Fig. 172.4**). The needle is placed at the lateral border of the probe and, under ultrasound guidance, is advanced toward the fascia between the adductor longus and adductor brevis muscles. Then the nerve stimulator is turned on. The intensity of the stimulating current is initially set to deliver 1 mA

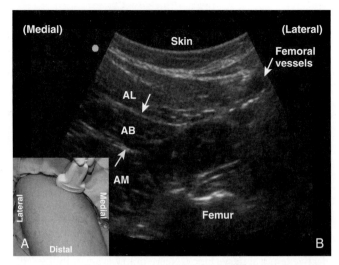

Fig. 172.4 A, Ultrasound transducer position near the inguinal crease for an obturator nerve block. **B,** Ultrasound image of branches of the obturator nerve in short axis (transverse view). AB, adductor brevis; AL, adductor longus; AM, adductor magnus; *white arrow,* anterior branch of the obturator nerve; *yellow arrow,* posterior branch of the obturator nerve.

and is gradually decreased. If a stimulating current less than 0.6 mA evokes a motor response, 3 to 5 mL of local anesthetic is injected after negative aspiration. This procedure is repeated along the fascia until the motor response is eliminated. The needle is then advanced until it contacts the posterior branch between the adductor brevis and adductor magnus muscle. After the nerve is identified by stimulation, 3 to 5 mL of local anesthetic is injected.[6] When a nerve stimulation response is not obtained, approximately 5 to 7 mL of local anesthetic should be injected along fascial planes to achieve a successful blockade.

Side Effects and Complications

Because intravascular injection into the obturator artery or vein may occur, careful aspiration should be performed before injection. Damage to the pelvic organs, such as the bladder, rectum, vagina, or spermatic cord, can occur. The depth of needle placement should be noted, and the needle should not be advanced more than 3 cm into the pelvis, to decrease the incidence of this complication. As with any injection, a risk for infection exists, and thus sterile technique should always be used.

Nerve Blocks Around the Knee

Three major nerve trunks can be blocked at the level of the knee: the posterior tibial, the common peroneal, and the saphenous. When the posterior tibial and the common peroneal nerves are blocked at the popliteal fossa, the procedure is referred to as a *popliteal block.*

Indications

Blockade of the posterior tibial, common peroneal, and saphenous nerves can be performed at the popliteal fossa to provide surgical analgesia from the knee down. Lack of access to these nerves more proximally and reduced doses of local anesthetic justify the clinician's familiarity with these valuable techniques. Many different procedures can be performed with this technique, including removal of soft and bony tumors, ankle procedures, and operations on the foot requiring a tourniquet.

Clinically Relevant Anatomy

The sciatic nerve bifurcates in the distal part of the thigh into the tibial nerve and the common peroneal nerve. The tibial nerve often arises at the upper end of the popliteal fossa, although the sciatic nerve can bifurcate more superiorly. The tibial nerve is the larger of the two terminal branches of the sciatic nerve and has both a muscular branch to the back of the leg and cutaneous branches in the popliteal fossa and down the back of the leg to the ankle. The common peroneal nerve is about half the size of the tibial nerve and provides the following: articular innervation to the knee joint; cutaneous innervation to the lateral side of the leg, heel, and ankle; and motor innervation to the muscles of the anterior lateral compartment of the lower part of the leg.[11]

The posterior tibial nerve provides motor innervation to the back of the lower part of the leg and cutaneous innervation from the popliteal fossa to the ankle, as well as the sole of the foot. The posterior tibial nerve then divides into the plantar digital nerves.

Landmark Technique

Three different approaches for performing a popliteal block have been described. The posterior approach requires the patient to be placed in the prone position. The lateral approach requires contact with periosteum but allows the patient to remain in the supine position. The lithotomy approach again allows the patient to remain in the supine position and uses the same landmarks as the posterior approach. Because none of the popliteal blocks anesthetize the saphenous nerve, this nerve must be blocked separately.

Posterior Approach

The patient is placed in the prone position with the feet extending beyond the edge of the table to allow interpretation of the twitches. The landmarks identified are the popliteal fossa crease, the tendon of the biceps femoris laterally, and the tendons of the semitendinosus and semimembranosus medially. These landmarks can easily be identified in all patients, even obese patients, by asking patients to flex the leg at the knee joint. The entry site is the midpoint between the two tendons, 7 cm above the popliteal fossa crease.[9] The skin is prepared with iodine solution and is draped in sterile fashion.

The skin overlying the entry site is anesthetized with 1 to 2 mL of 0.5% lidocaine injected through a 25-gauge, 1½- inch needle. A 22-gauge, 50-mm insulated short-beveled needle is attached to a stimulator (initial current, 1.5 mA, 2 Hz). The stimulating needle is inserted perpendicular to the skin while the clinician observes for plantar flexion or dorsiflexion of the foot with currents of 0.4 mA or less. If stimulation cannot be achieved with currents of 0.4 mA, the tibial twitch (plantar flexion) is more reliable in achieving blockade of both branches of the sciatic nerve. If no stimulation is elicited, the needle should be withdrawn and redirected laterally because a more medial insertion is less likely to result in nerve localization and carries a risk of puncturing the

popliteal artery and vein. If no stimulation is observed after redirection of the needle, the injection should be repeated through a new insertion site 5 mm laterally until the desired response is obtained. If stimulation of the biceps femoris muscle occurs, the needle is in too lateral a position, and the needle should be redirected slightly medially. Once the tibial nerve (plantar flexion) or the common peroneal nerve (dorsiflexion) is stimulated, 40 to 50 mL of local anesthetic is injected.[9] Local anesthetic used are 1.5% mepivacaine for intermediate-acting effect (onset time, 5 to 15 minutes) or 0.5% to 0.75% ropivacaine for long-acting effect (onset time, 20 to 30 minutes). Again, a combination of 0.5% bupivacaine and 1.5% mepivacaine in a 2:1 mixture can be used for quicker onset but longer duration of action. Epinephrine can be added at 1:300,000 to prolong this nerve block.

Lateral Approach

The patient is placed in the supine position. The leg is extended, and the foot is positioned at a 90-degree angle relative to the table. Landmarks include the lateral femoral epicondyle and the biceps femoris and vastus lateralis muscles. The entry site is 7 cm cephalad to the most prominent point of the lateral femoral epicondyle and in the groove between the two muscles. The skin is prepared with iodine solution and is draped in sterile fashion.

The skin overlying the entry site is anesthetized with 1 to 2 mL of 0.5% lidocaine injected through a 25-gauge, 1½-inch needle. A 100-mm insulated stimulating needle is connected to a nerve stimulator (initial current, 1.5 mA, 2 Hz) and is inserted in a horizontal plane until the shaft of the femoral bone is contacted. Once the femoral bone is contacted, the needle is withdrawn to skin and is redirected posteriorly at a 30-degree angle to the horizontal plane. Again, the operator is watching for stimulation of either the tibial or the common peroneal nerve at a current of 0.4 mA or less. If no stimulation is achieved, the needle should be redirected first 5 to 10 degrees anteriorly and then 5 to 20 degrees posteriorly through the same skin puncture. If this maneuver does not lead to nerve localization, the same technique is repeated through new skin punctures in 5-mm increments posterior to the initial insertion plane. Once the tibial nerve (plantar flexion) or the common peroneal nerve (dorsiflexion) is stimulated, 40 to 50 mL of local anesthetic is injected. Local anesthetics used are 1.5% mepivacaine for intermediate-acting effect (onset time, 5 to 15 minutes) or 0.5% to 0.75% ropivacaine for long-acting effect (onset time 20 to 30 minutes). Again, a combination of 0.5% bupivacaine and 1.5% mepivacaine in a 2:1 mixture can be used for quicker onset but longer duration of action. Epinephrine can be added at 1:300,000 to prolong this nerve block.

Lithotomy Approach

The patient is placed in the supine position. The leg is flexed at both the hip and knee joints and is supported by an assistant. Landmarks are the same as for the posterior approach: the popliteal fossa crease, the tendon of the biceps femoris laterally, and the tendons of the semitendinosus and semimembranosus medially. The entry site is the midpoint of the two tendons, 7 cm above the popliteal fossa crease. The skin is prepared with iodine solution and is draped in sterile fashion.

The skin overlying the entry site is anesthetized with 1 to 2 mL of 0.5% lidocaine injected through a 25-gauge, 1½-inch needle. A 22-gauge, 50-mm insulated short-beveled needle is attached to a stimulator (initial current, 1.5 mA, 2 Hz). The stimulating needle is inserted at a 45-degree angle cephalad while the clinician observes for plantar flexion or dorsiflexion of the foot with currents of 0.4 mA or less. If no stimulation is observed, the needle is withdrawn and is redirected 5 to 10 degrees laterally until the desired response is obtained. If no stimulation is achieved, the needle is removed and is reinserted through another entry site 5 mm lateral to the initial site. Once the tibial nerve (plantar flexion) or the common peroneal nerve (dorsiflexion) is stimulated, 40 to 50 mL of local anesthetic is injected. Local anesthetics used are 1.5% mepivacaine for intermediate-acting effect (onset time, 5 to 15 minutes) or 0.5% to 0.75% ropivacaine for long-acting effect (onset time 20 to 30 minutes). Again, a combination of 0.5% bupivacaine and 1.5% mepivacaine in a 2:1 mixture can be used for quicker onset but longer duration of action. Epinephrine can be added at 1:300,000 to prolong this nerve block.

The saphenous nerve may be blocked by injecting 5 mL of local anesthetic (any of the aforementioned mixtures) in a subcutaneous ring from the medial aspect of the tibia to the border of the patellar tendon.

Ultrasound Technique

The patient is positioned in either the prone or lateral position. After sterile skin preparation at the block site, the transducer (HF) is used to locate the tibial nerve, which is then traced just proximal to the level of its union with the peroneal nerve. The skin is anesthetized at the block site, and the needle is introduced lateral to the transducer using an in-plane approach. The nerve stimulator, if used, is switched on to a threshold of 0.7 mA while the needle approaches the nerve. Once a desired motor response is elicited, typically 20 to 25 mL of local anesthetic is injected to surround the nerve.[6] Some practitioners prefer to perform the block at the midthigh, in which case the nerve is still located at the popliteal crease and then is traced more proximally (**Fig. 172.5**).

Side Effects and Complications

Complications of these nerve blockades are extremely rare. Careful aspiration should be performed to prevent intravascular injection. Nerve injury is a possibility with intraneural injection. Needle positioning should be adjusted if stimulation is obtained at 0.20 mA or less. As with any injection, a risk for infection exists, and therefore sterile technique should always be used.

Nerve Blocks at the Ankle

Five branches of the principal nerve trunks supply the ankle and foot: the posterior tibial, sural, superficial peroneal (musculocutaneous), deep peroneal (anterior tibial), and saphenous. These nerves are relatively easy to block at the ankle.

Indications

The posterior tibial, sural, superficial peroneal, deep peroneal, and saphenous nerves can be blocked at the ankle to provide

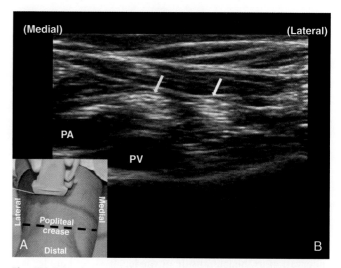

Fig. 172.5 A, Ultrasound transducer position above the popliteal crease for a sciatic nerve block at the level of the knee. **B,** Ultrasound image of caudad divisions of the sciatic nerve in short axis (transverse view). PA, popliteal artery; PV, popliteal vein; *white arrow,* peroneal nerve; *yellow arrow,* tibial nerve.

surgical analgesia of the foot for procedures such as treatment of Morton's neuroma, operations on the great toe, amputation of the midfoot and toes, and incision and drainage. An adjunct nerve block may be required if a tourniquet is used.

Clinically Relevant Anatomy

The tibial nerve is the larger of the two branches of the sciatic nerve, and it reaches the distal part of the leg from the medial side of the Achilles tendon, where it lies behind the posterior tibial artery. It divides into medial and lateral branches, with the medial branch supplying the medial two thirds of the sole and the plantar portion of the medial 3½ toes up to the nail. The lateral branch supplies the lateral third of the sole and the plantar portion of the lateral 1½ toes.[3]

The sural nerve is a cutaneous nerve that arises through the union of a branch from the tibial nerve and a branch from the common peroneal nerve. The sural nerve becomes subcutaneous distal to the middle of the leg and proceeds along with the short saphenous vein behind and below the lateral malleolus to supply the lower posterolateral surface of the leg, the lateral side of the foot, and the lateral part of the fifth toe.[3]

The common peroneal divides into the superficial and deep peroneal nerves. The superficial peroneal nerve perforates the deep fascia on the anterior aspect of the distal two thirds of the leg and runs subcutaneously to supply the dorsum of the foot and toes, except for the contiguous surfaces of the great and second toes.[3]

The deep peroneal nerve descends down the anterior aspect of the interosseous membrane of the leg and continues midway between the malleoli onto the dorsum of the foot. Here it divides into medial and lateral branches of the plantar nerves, with the medial branch dividing into two dorsal digital branches that innervate the adjacent sides of the first and second digits. At the level of the foot, the anterior tibial artery lies medial to the nerve, as does the tendon of the extensor hallucis longus muscle.[3]

The saphenous nerve, which is the sensory terminal branch of the femoral nerve, becomes subcutaneous at the lateral side of the knee joint. It then follows the great saphenous vein to the medial malleolus and supplies the cutaneous area over the medial side of the lower part of the leg, anterior to the medial malleolus and the medial part of the foot and as far forward as the midportion.[3]

Landmark Technique

The patient is placed in the supine position with the foot on a foot rest. The posterior tibial nerve is located just behind and distal to the medial malleolus. The pulse of the posterior tibial artery can be felt at this location; the nerve is just posterior to the artery. The deep peroneal nerve is located immediately lateral to the tendon of the extensor hallucis longus muscle. The pulse of the anterior tibial artery (dorsalis pedis) can be felt at this location; the nerve is immediately lateral to the artery.[9]

The superficial peroneal, sural, and saphenous nerves are located in subcutaneous tissue along a circular line stretching from the lateral aspect of the Achilles tendon across the lateral malleolus, anterior aspect of the foot, and medial malleolus to the medial aspect of the Achilles tendon.[9]

The skin of the entire foot is prepared with iodine solution and is draped in sterile fashion. This procedure should begin with the two deep nerves because subcutaneous injections for superficial blocks inevitably deform the anatomy.

Deep Peroneal Block

After palpation of the groove just lateral to the extensor hallucis longus with a finger, a 25-gauge, 1½- inch needle with 5 mL of lidocaine is inserted under the skin and is advanced until it is stopped by bone. The needle is then withdrawn 1 to 2 mm, and the previously described anesthetic is injected after a negative aspiration result.[9]

Posterior Tibial Block

A 25-gauge, 1½-inch needle with 5 mL of lidocaine is inserted in the groove behind the medial malleolus and is advanced until contact is made with bone. The needle is withdrawn 1 to 2 mm, and the aforementioned medication is injected after a negative aspiration result.[9]

Saphenous Block

A 25-gauge, 1½-inch needle with 5 mL of lidocaine is inserted at the level of the medial malleolus, and a "ring" of local anesthetic is raised from the point of needle entry to the Achilles tendon and anteriorly to the tibial ridge.[9]

Superficial Peroneal Block

A 25-gauge, 1½-inch needle with 5 mL of lidocaine is inserted at the tibial ridge and is extended laterally toward the lateral malleolus. Raising a subcutaneous wheal during injection, which indicates a proper, superficial plane, is important.[9]

Sural Block

A 25-gauge, 1½-inch needle with 5 mL of lidocaine is inserted at the level of the lateral malleolus, and the local anesthetic is infiltrated toward the Achilles tendon. The previously mentioned medication is injected in a circular fashion to raise a skin wheal.[9]

Ultrasound Technique

The superficial peroneal and sural nerves are very small and difficult to image on ultrasound. Because both nerves are superficial, most practitioners prefer to block them with skin infiltration. The deep peroneal, posterior tibial, and saphenous nerves have a round and hyperechoic appearance on ultrasound. After sterile skin preparation around the block area, the probe is applied. Use of a lateral approach, posterior approach, and anterior or posterior approach for needle insertion is preferred for the deep peroneal, posterior tibial, and saphenous nerves, respectively. As with the landmark technique, little volume is necessary to create circumferential spread of local anesthetic. Conversely, investigators have demonstrated that use of ultrasound is not very useful in blocks around the ankle, secondary to bony prominences that hinder proper maneuvering of the transducer.[12]

Side Effects and Complications

Complications of ankle blocks are rare, but residual paresthesias can result from inadvertent intraneural injection. Epinephrine-containing solutions should be avoided because of the risk for ischemia. As with any injection, a risk for infection exists, and thus sterile technique should always be used.

Digital Nerve Block of the Foot

Indications

A digital nerve block of the foot is indicated for limited procedures involving one or two digits or for postoperative pain relief.

Clinically Relevant Anatomy

Each nerve passes through the intermetatarsal space alongside each toe. The sole of the foot is innervated primarily by the posterior tibial nerve. After passing behind the medial malleolus, the posterior tibial nerve divides into the plantar digital nerves. The plantar digital nerves are larger than the dorsal digital nerves and terminally send twigs onto the dorsum of the phalanx. The digital branch of the lateral plantar nerve supplies the lateral 1½ toes. The digital branch of the medial plantar nerve supplies the medial 3½ toes. The dorsum of the foot is innervated by the superficial and deep peroneal nerves. The deep peroneal nerve divides at the extensor retinaculum into medial and lateral branches. The medial branch divides into two dorsal digital branches that innervate adjacent sides of the first and second digits. The superficial peroneal nerve innervates the dorsum of the rest of the toes.[11]

Technique

The patient is placed in the supine position, and the skin is prepared with iodine solution and is draped in sterile fashion. Skin wheals are raised over the distal intermetatarsal space. A total of 2 to 3 mL of non–epinephrine-containing local anesthetic solution such as 0.5% lidocaine or 0.25% bupivacaine is injected in a fanlike fashion subcutaneously, as well as deep to the metatarsals, to ensure blockade of both the dorsal and plantar digital nerves. Blockade can also be performed at the level of the digits by injecting skin wheals into the web space of the dorsal surface on either side of the digit to be blocked.[11]

Side Effects and Complications

Complications are extremely rare. Large volumes of solution containing local anesthetic and epinephrine should not be used, to avoid the risk of vascular compromise to the digits. As with any injection, a risk for injection exists, and therefore sterile technique should always be used.

Conclusion

Neural blockade of the lower extremity can be very useful tool for anesthesiologists. The procedure is easily accomplished, has minimal side effects, and can provide complete anesthesia of the lower extremity. To obtain adequate anesthesia during these procedures, several important facts must be kept in mind:

- When using a peripheral nerve stimulator, obtaining a nonspecific twitch at high amplitude (>1.5 to 2 mA) may result in a failed block.
- Not only the dermatomes but also the myotomes and osteotomes for the surgical procedures to be performed must be remembered.

- The local anesthetic chosen must last the duration of the procedure, and enough time must be allowed for the block to function fully before surgical intervention.

As stated earlier, peripheral blockade of the lower extremity is not a new technique. For more than a century, physicians have been anesthetizing the nerves of the lower extremity. Differences have occurred in technology and pharmacology through the years, both of which have only been improving the results of our predecessors.

Acknowledgment

Gordin et al. would like acknowledge Shinichi Sakura, MD, for permitting the use of pictures from his articles for publication.

References

Full references for this chapter can be found on www.expertconsult.com.

Part E

Neuroaugmentation and Implantable Drug Delivery Systems

Peripheral Nerve Stimulation

Matthew P. Rupert, Gabor B. Racz, and Miles R. Day

Historical Considerations

Electricity has been used to treat pain for thousands of years. In ancient times, Egyptians and Greeks were known to place electrogenic torpedo fish over painful areas in hopes of eliciting a cure. In modern times, peripheral nerve stimulation has been used to treat pain since the 1960s, in parallel with the introduction of the gate-control theory of pain, in which stimulation of larger afferent fibers diminishes the sensation from smaller pain fibers. Peripheral nerve stimulation was implemented initially with the placement of cuffed electrodes around the affected nerve.[1,2] Cuffed electrodes soon gave way to flat, paddle electrodes.[3] These electrodes were believed to be less constrictive and thereby, have potentially less risk of scarring or nerve injury.[4] This has given way to use of percutaneous cylindrical leads that can allow single-stage trialing.[5,6] This application has been broadened to include subcutaneous lead placement in proximity to a target nerve and just within the field area of pain. This chapter focuses on treatment of patients with identifiable nerve injuries who have failure with conservative and less invasive interventional therapies.

The mechanism of action of peripheral nerve stimulation is not entirely understood; both peripheral and central theories have been proposed. Campbell and Taub[7] showed a sensory loss in human subjects in the distribution of a peripherally stimulated nerve that was associated with a loss in the A-delta component of the afferent action potential. Wall and Gutnick[8] showed a reduction in the rate of spontaneous neuroma firing that outlasted a peripherally applied electrical stimulus. On the basis of a central gate-control theory, Chung et al[9] showed inhibition of spinothalamic tract transmission in primates after application of a peripheral electrical stimulation. This central response also was shown to outlast the initiating peripheral stimulus. Buonocore et al[10] have shown antidromic activation of peripheral nerves with dorsal column stimulation. Hanai[11] showed inhibition of pain pathways with peripheral stimulation of A-fiber afferents (beta and delta) in a different nerve. Advancements in the understanding of multicontact electrodes and improvements in solid-state components have allowed increasing control of the applied electrical field.[12]

Indications

Peripheral nerve stimulation is indicated for neuropathic pain in a single nerve distribution, with failed less invasive treatments. This technology was traditionally used to treat painful conditions of the median, radial, ulnar, sciatic, posterior tibial, and common peroneal nerves. It also has been used to treat neuralgias of the intercostal, ilioinguinal, occipital, superior cluneal, supraorbital, and supratrochlear nerves.[5,13] Other indications include complex regional pain syndromes, plexus avulsions, and electrical injuries.[14] Cancer pain, idiopathic pain, and nerve root injury pain have generally been found unresponsive to peripheral stimulation.[15] Treatment of mononeuropathy is more effective with peripheral nerve stimulation than with spinal cord stimulation.[16]

As with any implantable technology, patient selection is multifactorial. Ruling out correctable pathology, such as nerve entrapment, is important; however, a peripheral nerve stimulation trial might be weighed in comparison with a repeat surgery. A complete patient evaluation should include psychologic assessment, and no evidence of drug abuse should be found. A transcutaneous electrical nerve stimulation trial is suggested, although not required.[17] A positive diagnostic block of the suspected nerve with local anesthetic is likewise suggested. Temporary relief with such a block does not guarantee peripheral nerve stimulation will work, but a negative diagnostic block suggests that peripheral nerve stimulation is unlikely to help.[2] Adherence to these criteria may improve success rates. Additional interim steps before implantable trials have been suggested. Some investigators have advocated a trial of targeted needle stimulation with evidence of neuromodulation effects as an interval step.[18] Others have recommended durational failures of neurolytic procedures.[13]

Clinically Relevant Anatomy

The key to peripheral nerve stimulation implantation is correct identification of the offending peripheral nerve through history, physical examination, and diagnostic blockade. No specific limitation exists as to what nerves can be targeted for stimulation. When identified, exposure and electrode placement can be performed by a qualified physician. Physical constraints include size of electrode, anatomic restrictions, and proximity of other nerves. Hardware placement should not impinge on surrounding structures through ranges of motion. Stimulation of nontargeted nerves or surrounding musculature is undesirable. Some superficial nerves can be approached via percutaneous placement of cylindrical leads. Examples include occipital, supraorbital, supratrochlear, and superior cluneal nerves.

Technique

Peripheral nerve stimulator placement continues to change as lead design and implant techniques advance. In general, the use of the implantable devices consists of a two-stage procedure after a positive block with local anesthetic. The trial can be performed via a surgical incision or percutaneously. Both can be implanted with an extension lead for immediate conversion to a permanent lead if the trial is positive. An externalized percutaneous trial lead also can be performed so that a negative trial can be removed without a second surgery. The surgical trial and permanent pulse generator placement are described first (**Figs. 173.1** and **173.2**).

The site for electrode placement is usually proximal to the site of injury, but placement should respect surgical approach and surrounding structures. An intimate understanding of the surgical anatomy is imperative. The surgical incision and dissection are taken down to the neurovascular bundle. A 2-inch section of the nerve is freed from surrounding tissues, with care taken not to disrupt any blood supply. The selected electrode is secured with sutures immediately below the nerve, with the active leads facing the nerve. Next, a piece of fascia is sutured directly to the electrode covering the active leads (**Fig. 173.3**). This step is recommended to minimize irritation and scarring of the nerve to the electrode. The nerve is allowed to rest in its normal position, and overlying tissue is loosely secured to maintain proximity of the nerve to the electrode. The lead is connected to an extension set and secured below the skin. The limb is taken through a full range of motion to rule out impingement or increased tension before the primary incision is closed. The extension lead is externalized for trial with a temporary screening device, usually for 2 to 3 days.

If the trial is positive, the patient returns to the operating room for implantation of the permanent pulse generator. Upper extremity and occipital nerve generators can be placed on the upper chest wall. Lower extremity generators can be placed over the medial thigh or the lateral buttocks. The generator is secured to the underlying fascia with suture. A new extension set is connected from the lead to the generator through a new subcutaneous tunnel. The old extension is then removed, either by preparing and cutting it at the skin and pulling inward or by cutting at the connection and

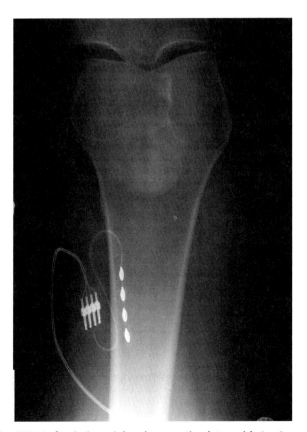

Fig. 173.1 **Left sciatic peripheral nerve stimulator with 1 × 4 array On-Point lead.** (Medtronic, Minneapolis, MN).

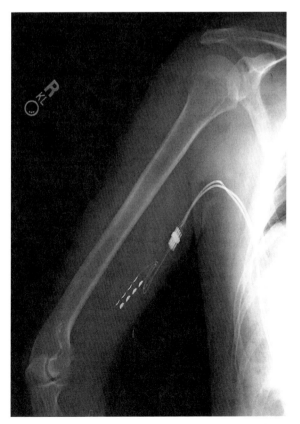

Fig. 173.2 **Right ulnar peripheral nerve stimulator with 2 × 4 array lead.**

pulling outward. If the trial is ineffective or uncomfortable, the patient needs a second surgery for hardware removal.

Percutaneous cylindrical leads can be placed as well. Initially, this placement was recommended for terminal branches of peripheral nerves. However, the increasing use of ultrasound scan guidance for peripheral nerve blocks and catheter placement has provided a natural advancement for peripheral stimulation trials.[6] The percutaneous lead can now be placed with direct visualization (**Fig. 173.4**). It can be placed with an extension as above or by itself. The advantage of a single lead wire is the ease of removal if the trial is negative. If positive, either mode necessitates a second surgery for the generator placement. Lead placement done in this fashion can be confirmed with on-table stimulation and patient affirmation.

Side Effects and Complications

Potential complications associated with peripheral nerve stimulators are similar to complications associated with other implantable technology. Infection and bioincompatibility are possible. Nerve injury, scarring, and associated

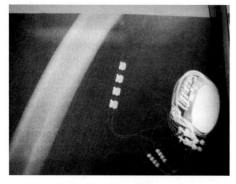

Fig. 173.3 Peripheral nerve stimulating electrode applied to the sciatic nerve above the bifurcation. Two On-Point Medtronic electrodes are sutured together in a saddle shape with nonabsorbable sutures. The active electrodes are covered with a thin layer of harvested fascia and the polytetrafluoroethylene skirt of the electrode loosely stitched around the nerve with an absorbable suture. The appropriate location of the electrodes is verified with motor or tetanic stimulation to cover the targeted tibialis or peroneal nerves.

ischemia have occurred. The use of longitudinal rather than cuffed electrodes, the placement of an overlying fascial flap, and eliminating nerve skeletalization are believed to minimize these risks. Whether percutaneous lead placement should be parallel, perpendicular, or oblique to the target nerve is unknown. Stimulation of surrounding musculature may be a concern for nonparallel placement. The patient may have no response, an uncomfortable response, or aberrant sensory or motor stimulation. The use of multicontact electrodes allows some titration of effect. Mechanical problems, such as lead fractures, electrode shorts, lead migration, and battery depletion, are possible. Implanted batteries can interfere with pacemakers and can channel electrical and magnetic fields. The units should be turned off when electrocautery or electrocardiogram is to be performed. An implanted generator is generally a contraindication for magnetic resonance imaging.

Conclusion

Peripheral nerve stimulators have shown efficacy in many clinical settings of chronic neuropathic pain in a single nerve distribution. Implantable technology is invasive and expensive; adequate conservative and less invasive methods should be tried first. Peripheral and central mechanisms of action have been postulated. Patient selection is multifactorial and should include a psychologic assessment and absence of correctable pathology. Patients should have positive screening procedures such as diagnostic nerve blockade and a period of trial stimulation before placement of permanent equipment. The use of transcutaneous nerve stimulation can be helpful but is not diagnostic or prognostic for the use of peripheral nerve stimulation. Electrode implantation is dictated by the specific nerve anatomy, which may necessitate surgical exposure or may be amenable to percutaneous placement. Advances in clinical strategies, electrode design, and neuroscience research continue to pave the road for future changes. In the modern treatment of chronic regional pain syndrome, the earlier use of neuromodulation techniques is recommended.[19,20]

References

Full references for this chapter can be found on www.expertconsult.com.

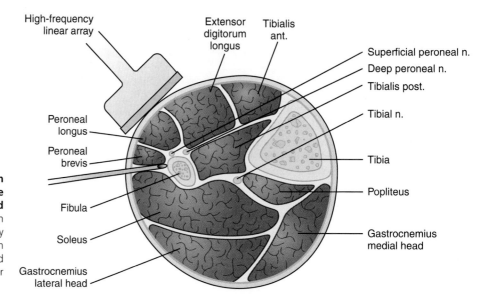

Fig. 173.4 Lateral needle access between peroneal muscles and soleus muscle to access corridor for superficial and deep peroneal nerves. Ultrasound scan visualization with high-frequency linear array probe placed anterior. Fascial separation with needle and saline solution followed by advancement of cylindrical catheter electrode.

Spinal Cord Stimulation

Danesh Mazloomdoost, Marco R. Perez-Toro, and Allen W. Burton

Spinal cord stimulation (SCS) describes the use of pulsed electrical energy near the spinal cord for control of pain.[1,2] This technique was first applied in the intrathecal space and finally in the epidural space as described by Shealy, Mortimer, and Reswick[2] in 1967. In the present day, most commonly, SCS involves the implantation of leads in the epidural space to transmit this pulsed energy across the spinal cord or near the desired nerve roots. This technique has notable analgesic properties for neuropathic pain states, anginal pain, and peripheral ischemic pain. The same technology can be applied in deep brain stimulation, cortical brain stimulation, and peripheral nerve stimulation (PNS).[3–6]

History

A bump on the head often feels better when it is vigorously rubbed. In a similar fashion, the theories on neurostimulation began when this observation was analyzed physiologically. Neurostimulation began when Melzack and Wall's[6] published the gate control theory in 1965. This theory proposed that nonpainful stimulation of large myelinated A-beta fibers could impede painful peripheral stimuli carried by C-fibers and lightly myelinated A-delta fibers. Shealy, Mortimer, and Reswick[2] designed the first spinal cord stimulator device for the treatment of chronic pain. Although this technique was noted to control pain, early devices did not garner interest for clinical application because of the impracticality of the required external power supply, which transmitted power transdermally via an internal coiled antenna.[7]

In the 1980s, implantable batteries were developed and spinal cord stimulators became a clinical option.[8] Early indications included persistent neuropathic pain, spasticity,[9] ischemic limb,[10,11] and facial pain.[12] The first rechargeable

implantable pulse generators (IPGs) became available in 2004, which dramatically increased the stimulator lifespan.[8] Deep brain stimulation was developed during the same time frame.

In 2006, 14,000 new spinal cord stimulators were reported to be implanted annually.[13] The market continues to grow rapidly.[14] Although the gate theory was initially proposed as the mechanism of action, the underlying neurophysiologic mechanisms are not clearly understood.

Mechanism of Action

Although SCS devices have existed for more than 40 years, the understanding behind the mechanism of action remains somewhat elusive. The limitations stem from the challenges of an effective model. Unlike other organ systems that can be studied on a cellular level, pain pathways depend on multicellular neural interactions; in vivo models are limited by ethical standards, and animal models can be costly or difficult to extrapolate from simple neuroanatomy because of the complexity found within humans.[15]

Current evidence suggests that an inhibitory process takes place at the dorsal horn with SCS.[15,16] As nociceptive and somatic sensory fibers enter the dorsal horn of the spinal cord, they synapse with second order neurons of the substantia gelatinosa. With SCS, the nociceptive signal is inhibited from further propagation to the sensory cortex, but the mechanism is still elusive. Some of the theories behind the mechanisms of action are listed in **Table 174.1** and include signal inhibition via interneurons or descending central fibers, modulation of neuroactive mediators, and limiting pathologic processes like antidromic inflammatory release in ischemic pain and downregulation of wind up at wide-dynamic range neurons.[13]

Table 174.1 Proposed Mechanisms of Action

Suppression of antidromic active mediators in ischemic pain
   Substance P
   CGRP

Closing gate: Blocking transmission to the spinothalamic tract at the dorsal horn
   Inhibitory effect of collateral or interneurons
   Limiting the upregulated signaling that provokes WDR neurons

Feedback loop: Activation of central inhibitory mechanisms influencing:
   Thalamocortical system
   Anterior pretectal nucleus
   WDR neurons

Autonomic: Sympathetic afferent stimulation

Neurotransmitters: Inactivation of putative neurotransmitters (e.g., glutamate, adenosine, serotonin) and activation of protective/depressant neurotransmitters (glutamate)

CGRP, calcitonin gene-related peptide; WDR, wide dynamic range.

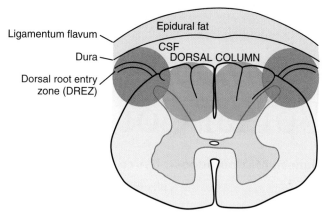

Fig. 174.1 *Green area* represents the area of desired stimulation. The *red* represents the DREZ, where the dorsal roots enter. Because of anatomic location, the DREZ has a lower threshold of stimulation than does the dorsal column. For ideal stimulation, the *green* area must be activated and the *red* area inhibited.

Technical Considerations

Anatomic Considerations

Understanding the neuroanatomic pathways involved in sensory afferents can help direct the placement, control, and modulation of SCS. Afferent fibers that relay both nociceptive and somatic sensations enter the spinal cord via the dorsal root entry zone (DREZ). After synapsing at second order neurons of the dorsal horn, nociceptive and somatic afferents respectively separate to the spinothalamic tract and the dorsal column (DC). At a single vertebral level, the DC may carry fibers from many dermatomes, whereas the DREZ holds fibers from a single dermatome.[17] Depending on the electric field, stimulation of the DC at a single level can result in paresthesia and analgesia of a wide area. Stimulation of the DREZ limits the paresthesia to a single dermatome because it relays nerves from a single dorsal root ganglion (DRG) (**Fig. 174.1**). Furthermore, because it carries somatosensory fibers and has more synaptic interactions with the musculoskeletal system, it may also induce pain or motor deficits if is set at stimulation levels intended for the DC.[8] Because of its geometry in entering the spinal canal and the impedance of the surrounding tissue, the DREZ has a lower threshold of stimulation than the DC.[17,18] Clinical evidence corroborates mathematic modeling in showing that as the electric field is moved laterally the perception threshold is reduced and area of coverage decreases.[19]

Shaping of electric fields has become a critical area of research in SCS. The tissue within the spinal column has variable conductivity: cerebrospinal fluid (CSF) > spinal cord > epidural fat.[20] This influences the electric field generated. When the distance between electrode and spinal cord is large, such as in the midthoracic level, stimulation of DC becomes challenging because the necessary electric field tends to incorporate the DREZ.[21] The electrode itself has specific influences on the tissue. Negative leads, for instance, hyperpolarize the surrounding tissue, thus inhibiting action potentials, and positive leads depolarize and propagate it. Used in combination, the resultant electric field can be maximally evoked over a designated area.[22]

Table 174.2 Locations and Lead Type Versus Dermatopic Effect[23]

C4

Unipolar
   Midline: The hand, forearm, and upperarm
   Lateral: The anterior shoulder, forearm, upper arm, and hand

Bipolar
   Midline: The hand and forearm
   Lateral: The hand, forearm, and upper arm

T10

Unipolar
   Midline: The anterior and posterior of thigh, leg, knee, ankle, and foot
   Lateral: The abdomen, anterior leg, knee, and anterior thigh

Bipolar
   Midline: The abdomen, anterior leg, knee, and anterior thigh
   Lateral: The anterior thigh, anterior leg, knee, and foot

The topographic placement of leads depends on the location of pain (**Table 174.2**).[23] Clinical data are limited, but Barolat et al[24] have provided mapping data of coverage patterns based on lead location in 106 patients.

Devices and Components

Two types of leads are used in spinal cord stimulators: paddle and percutaneous (**Fig. 174.2**). Paddle leads are flat and wide, with insulation on one side and electrical pads on the other. This has the advantage of directing current in one direction. Paddles leads must be surgically placed via laminotomy or laminectomy.[25] Percutaneous leads are cylindrical catheters placed via spinal needle. Because contacts are cylindrical, they generate an electric field circumferentially around the catheter.[8]

Percutaneous leads are less efficient in power usage because they induce an electric field 360 degrees around the electrode, whereas, because of electrode insulation, paddle leads direct the charge toward the DC. This translates into longer battery life for a paddle lead, which creates an equivalent electric field

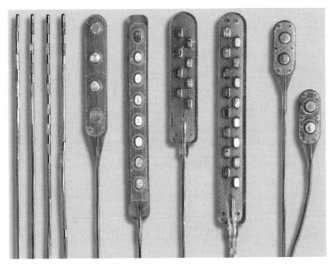

Fig. 174.2 **Neurostimulator leads *(left to right):* percutaneous type to paddle type.** *(Courtesy of St. Jude Medical, Inc.).*

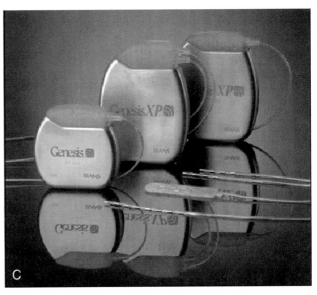

Fig. 174.3 C, Implantable pulse generator neurostimulation units with leads. *(C, Courtesy of St. Jude Medical, Inc.)*

as a percutaneous lead. Fostering a relationship between pain physician and neurosurgeon is valuable because collaboration is necessary in situations where one of these types is better suited.

Electrode selection is a complex topic with a significant amount of research on ideal lead configuration. Mathematic modeling has been used calculate electric field potentials in an effort to identify ideal lead configurations. Unipolar leads are theoretically less favorable than bipolar and tripolar leads because they provide less control over the laterality of field generation[8] and require higher pulse charges for similar field generation.[26] In clinical studies, however, these advantages are controversial, and some studies have even shown statistical disadvantage in bipolar leads.[27] The clinical data may be difficult to extrapolate generally, however, because dual-lead placement was staggered and parallel lead alignment has been shown to provide larger DC stimulation than staggered.[21] As discussed previously, tripolar lead placement theoretically stimulates the DC more selectively and shields the DREZ,[18,28] which allows for wider control of the paresthesia because the DC contains fibers from several dermatomes. Tripolar paddle leads use this property, and recently, tripolar percutaneous leads have been used in a similar fashion.[29]

Electrodes are connected to a power source, which are of two general types: an IPG or a radiofrequency unit (RF; see Fig. 174.2). RF units work by transmitting power transdermally with an external source and internal coiled wire loop. Because RFs are not limited by battery life, they can outlast IPGs and be programmed with high stimulation amplitude, rate, or pulse width, which is necessary for some patients.[30] They require an external power system with an antenna worn over the RF receiver, which is inconvenient and may irritate the skin.[8] They are generally outdated because improvements in battery technology allow for high-capacity and rechargeable systems that are internally placed.

IPGs are of two types: primary cell and rechargeable (**Fig. 174.3 A, B [online],** and **C**).

1. Primary cell devices have an average lifespan of 4 years, versus 9 years for rechargeable devices,[8] but the lifespan

is heavily dependent on usage. Primary cell devices tend to be larger but are useful for patients who need low outputs or do not recharge consistently. Small primary cell generators are available for pediatric or petite patients, but they are limited to low or infrequent currents.

2. Rechargeable IPGs contain Li-ion cells, which have a fixed number of charge-discharge cycles, with a degradation in the battery capacity over the span of multiple cycles. Most systems have a safeguard against full discharge because chemical changes can result in permanent battery failure. When patients fail to recharge the IPG, the generator fail safes to deep-discharge mode during which the device is disabled until reprogrammed.

Overall, battery life depends on the stimulation energy necessary (voltage/amplitude, number of active leads, pulse width, frequency), hours of usage (all day, during waking hours, intermittent doses), depth of discharge (interval and consistency of recharging), and battery degradation. Physicians need to understand how patients plan to use the stimulator to plan for the best generator option.

Currently, three companies produce neurostimulation equipment: Medtronic, Inc; American Neuromodulation Systems, Inc; and Advanced Bionics, Inc (**Table 174.3**). Variability is found in how the devices work, but no study has suggested superiority of one device over another. The two main differences are in how the electric field is generated. Some other differences include the following:

- Control over individual electrode versus an array of electrodes
- Fixed-current versus fixed-voltage to control the generated electric field
- Generator size and options for rechargeable or primary cell
- Options for leads

Table 174.3 Manufacturers of Neurostimulation Equipment
Medtronic Neuromodulation Patient Services: Mail Stop RCW115, 7000 Central Ave NE, Minneapolis, MN 55432-3576. (888) 638-7627. www.medtronic.com/patient-services/.
St. Jude Medical, Inc., 6901 Preston Road, Plano, TX 75024. (972) 309-8000. http://www.sjm.com/.
Boston Scientific, 25155 Rye Canyon Loop, Valencia, CA 91355. (888) 272-1001. www.bostonscientific.com/.

Table 174.4 Psychologic Testing Tools
Minnesota Multiphasic Personality Inventory–2 (MMPI-2) 567 questions (60–90 minutes) Gold standard
Millon Clinical Multiaxial Inventory–III (MCMI-III) 175 items (25–30 minutes) Correlates with DSM-IV diagnosis
Millon Behavioral Medicine Diagnostic (MBMD) 165 questions (20–25 minutes) Defined outcomes: no/relative/absolute contraindications
Oswestry Disability Index (ODI) 10 questions (10–15 minutes) Primarily for low back pain disability assessment
Pain disability index[67] Similar to ODI except applicable to any pain state

DSM-IV, *Diagnostic and statistical manual of mental disorders*, 4th ed.

Patient Selection

Patient selection is an integral factor in the overall success of neurostimulation. Failure in selection can not only yield poor outcomes from disease management but can also have numerous detrimental effects[31]:

- Increase physician demand
- Influence negative emotional outcomes for patient
- Increase cost of care
- Increase demand for medications
- Increase risk of litigation
- Contribute to disease progress

Appropriate cases for neurostimulation implant must meet the following criteria: the patient has a diagnosis amenable to this therapy; the patient has had failed conservative therapy; significant psychologic issues have been ruled out; and a trial has shown pain relief.[32]

Whereas implantable devices show improvements in pain, they lack evidence for improvements in functional outcomes.[33] Although, the reasons for this require further quantification, lack of motivation and demoralization from chronic pain may play a role. An interesting study by Olson et al[32] revealed a high correlation between many items on a complex psychologic testing battery and favorable response to trial stimulation. Few studies, however, have evaluated outcomes in combined interventional and psychobehavioral therapies on both pain and functional recovery. Early studies indicate that combining psychotherapy with implantable devices results in improved outcomes.[34]

Thus, as part of the workup for an implantable neuromodulatory device, such as a stimulator or intrathecal infusion pump, psychologic testing is recommended. A variety of testing tools are available depending on the physicians' practice; some are listed in **Table 174.4.**

To maximize the probability of improvements in functional outcomes and pain, part of the preoperative evaluation is establishment of functional goals. This evaluation reinforces to the patient that improvement in pain is not the primary endpoint; rather, the endpoint should be return to functional activity.[35] Patients are often fearful that pain is indicative of damage and that behavior may limit their rehabilitation even after pain improves.[36]

A careful trial period is advocated to avoid a failed implant. Trials of different lengths have been advocated. The main risk of a longer trial is infection, whereas the risk of too short a trial is misreading success. Mazloomdoost, Perez-Toro, and Burton use a 5-day to 7-day trial and encourage the patient to be as active as possible in the usual environment, with the exception of limiting bending and twisting movements to avoid stimulator lead migration.

Surgical Technique

The workup leading to SCS implantation takes place in two stages: (1) trial with external stimulator; and (2) internal implantation. Before implantation of a device, a trial is warranted in which leads are externally connected to a pulse generator. Trial stimulation is undertaken to attempt to "cover" the painful area with an electrically induced paresthesia. This is to avoid surgery and its associate side effects and complications in cases of poor outcome or intolerable effects from the SCS. On proven efficacy, the patient may proceed to device implantation. The procedures involved in both trial and implantation are similar except that in a trial, leads are left external, whereas for permanent implantation, leads are anchored to the supraspinous fascia and tunneled to an internal generator. Both procedures take place with fluoroscopy and with sterile conditions. Trials can be done in a sterile office-based setting, but permanent implantation requires an operative environment.

Trial

Fluoroscopic guidance is used to place stimulation leads in the posterior epidural space at the dermatome corresponding to the painful area. Insertion site for the lead is distal to the final destination of the lead to allow for steering and lead adjustment. Steering is facilitated by minimizing the catheter's angle of entry into the epidural space because it reduces the number of pivot points in the path of the catheter (**Fig. 174.4**). Thus, the second or third vertebral body caudal to the desired entry site into the epidural space is chosen for initial insertion point of the needle. Some researchers advocate making an incision before needle entry both to reduce the angle of entry and to minimize the risk of introducing skin flora into the epidural space.

A stimulator trial may be accomplished in two ways: straight percutaneous or implanted lead. In the straight percutaneous trial, the needle is withdrawn, an anchoring suture is placed into the skin, and a sterile dressing is applied. After completion of the trial, the leads must be removed and discarded *regardless* of the success of the trial. When the patient returns for implant, a new lead is placed in the location of the trial lead and connected to an implanted IPG. In the implanted lead trial, after

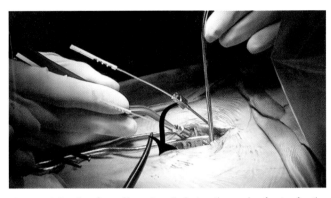

Fig. 174.4 Angle of needle entry. Reducing the angle of entry for the intrathecal (IT) needle eases steering of the catheter by reducing pivot points around which the catheter rotates.

successful positioning of the trial lead, the lead is secured, similar to a permanent placement, except a temporary extension piece is tunneled away from the back incision and out through the skin. If the trial is successful at the time of implant, the permanent lead is hooked to new extension and tunneled to an IPG. This method has the advantage of retaining the same lead position in a successful trial, reducing the probability of successful trial but failed permanent implant from new lead positioning. On the other hand, it adds an incision, which increases postoperative pain, confounding trial interpretation. Furthermore, implanted leads may have a greater risk for infection than straight percutaneous method.[37]

Most clinicians consider 50% or more pain relief to be indicative of a successful trial, although the ultimate decision should include other factors, such as activity level and medication intake. To paraphrase, some combination of pain relief, increased activity level, and decreased medication intake is indicative of a favorable trial.

Permanent Implantation

The technical challenges of permanent lead placement depend on: (1) proper fixation; and (2) lead redundancy. Consistent and reliable stimulation depends on fixing an electric field over a small area of the spinal cord. Leads have a limited capacity for stretch, and certain body movements can stretch leads significantly and prompt lead migration. Whereas sclerotic changes in the tissue surrounding the implanted system stabilize the leads over the long run, during the acute phase, proper anchoring is a major factor in successful lead placement. In the event of minor lead migration, electrode redundancy is used to accommodate for minor shifts by using alternative leads to accommodate the desired electric field.

After a successful trial, system implantation requires both reinsertion of sterile leads (because the externalize leads from trial are no longer sterile) and placement of an IPG or radiofrequency receiver. Placement of the generator requires preoperative planning because generator location, patient's operative positioning, skin preparation, and lead tunneling depend on the final destination of the generator. Sites commonly used for the generator depend on the location of the lead to minimize torque imposed by body movements. Cervical or occipital generators, for instance, may be placed between the shoulder blades lateral to spinous processes and facets. Thoracic and lumbar leads can be placed in the anterior gluteal area.

Generators are sometimes also placed anteriorly in the lower abdominal quadrants for ease of patient access during recharging. This, however, increases the risk of lead migration because twisting motions can torque the leads.

Paddle electrode implantation requires the addition of a laminotomy to slip the flat plate electrode into the epidural space. Some physicians trial the patient with the straight percutaneous approach and, if successful, send the patient to a spine surgeon for a paddle electrode implant.

Programming

Several parameters in neurostimulation may be adjusted to create stimulation paresthesias in the painful areas, thereby mitigating the patient's pain. These include amplitude, pulse width, rate, and electrode selection.[38]

- Amplitude is the intensity or strength of each individual pulse and can be controlled by voltage (V) or current (ohms). As discussed previously, various systems use either voltage or current to control the pulse charge and no evidence is found of superiority of one system over another. From a theoretic standpoint, current-control systems are more immune to changes in electrical resistance in the tissue because of sclerosis and patient positional changes. As such, mathematic modeling predicts more even paresthesia.[39] Amplitudes are variable even for an individual patient, but typical initial settings are 60% to 90% of motor threshold.[13]
- Pulse width is the duration of a pulse measured in microseconds (μsec). It is usually set between 100 and 400 μsec. Similar to increasing the amplitude, a larger pulse width delivers more energy per pulse and typically broader coverage. Common initial settings are 0.2 ms.[13]
- Rate is measured in hertz (Hz) or cycles per second, between 20 and 120 Hz. At lower rates, the patient feels more of a thumping, whereas at higher rates, the feeling is more of a buzzing. Higher frequencies (>500 Hz) are suggested to increase blood flow and decrease vascular resistance.[40]
- Electrode selection depends on the desired electrical field distribution and the breadth of dermatomes stimulated. Because much variability is seen in individual dermatomal distribution at the level of the DC, availability of more leads for future programming is advisable. Furthermore, if inadvertent lead migration is to occur, lead redundancy cephalad and caudad to the area of desired stimulation allows for compensatory programming adjustments rather than surgical revision.

The primary target is the negative cathode, from which electrons flow to the positive anode. Most patient stimulators are programmed with electrode selection changed until the patient obtains anatomic coverage; then, the pulse width and rate are adjusted for maximal comfort. The patient is left with full control of turning the stimulation off and on and the voltage up and down to comfort.

The lowest acceptable settings on all parameters are generally used to conserve battery life. Other programming modes that save battery life include a cycling mode during which the stimulator cycles full on/off at patient-determined intervals (minutes, seconds, or hours). The patient's programming may change over time, and reprogramming needs are common.

Neurostimulator manufacturing companies are helpful for clinicians with patient reprogramming assistance. Many busy pain practices designate a nurse who specializes in stimulators to handle patient reprogramming needs.

Complications

Complications with SCS range from simple problems, such as lack of appropriate paresthesia coverage, to devastating complications, such as paralysis, nerve injury, and death. Before the implantation of the trial lead, an educational session should occur with the patient and significant family members. This meeting should include a discussion of possible risks and complications. In the postoperative period, the caregiver should be involved in identifying problems and alerting the health care team.

After more than 20 years of use, overall complication rates from SCS range from 28% to 42%.[33,41] In a recent systemic review, the most common complication was found to be lead migration or breakage, which occurred in 22% of implanted cases.[42] Studies by May and Barolat reported lead revision rates from lead migration of 4.5% and 13.6% and breakage of 0% and 13.6%, respectively.[37,44] The generator can also be a source of revision if changes in body habitus affect the source position.

Three studies showed infectious rates to range from 2.5% to 7.5%,[43–45] but these infections rarely progressed into more serious infections, for an incidence rate of less than 0.1%.[33] To avoid infectious complications, the patient should be instructed on wound care and recognition of signs and symptoms indicative of infection. Many superficial infections can be treated with oral antibiotics or simple surgical exploration and irrigation. At the center of Mazloomdoost, Perez-Toro, and Burton, to avoid infection, the standard includes prophylactic intraoperative antibiotics. Although controversial, patients are commonly placed on oral antibiotics for 3 to 5 days after surgery.

If infection reaches the tissues involving the devices, in most cases, the implant should be removed. In such cases, one should have a high index of suspicion for an epidural abscess. Abscess of the epidural space can lead to paralysis and death if not identified quickly and treated aggressively. In the case of temporary epidural catheters (somewhat analogous to a percutaneous stimulator trial), Sarubbi and Vasquez[43] discovered only 22 well-described cases of complications. The mean age was 49.9 years, the median duration of epidural catheter use was 3 days, and the median time to onset of clinical symptoms after catheter placement was 5 days. Most patients (63.6%) had major neurologic deficits; 22.7% also had concomitant meningitis. *Staphylococcus aureus* was the predominant pathogen. Despite antibiotic therapy and drainage procedures, 38% of the patients continued to have neurologic deficits. These unusual but serious complications of temporary epidural catheter use necessitate efficient and accurate diagnostic evaluation and treatment because the consequences of delayed therapy can be substantial. Schuchard and Clauson[46] reported an infection with *Pasteurella* during an implanted lead trial, which necessitated explanting the system.

Outcomes

The most common use for SCS in the United States is failed back surgery syndrome (FBSS), whereas in Europe, peripheral ischemia is the predominant indication. Subdivision of clinical outcomes based on diagnosis makes sense. In a review

of the available SCS literature, most evidence falls within the level IV (limited) or level V (indeterminate) category because of the invasiveness of the modality and the inability to provide blinded treatment. Recognition must also be given to the time frame within which a study was performed because of rapidly evolving SCS technology. Basic science knowledge, implantation techniques, lead placement locations, contact array designs, and programming capabilities have changed dramatically from the time of the first implants. These improvements have led to decreased morbidity and much greater probability of obtaining adequate paresthesia coverage with subsequent improved outcomes.[44] Thus, even a level II review study, such as the one on patients with FBSS from 1966 to 1994 by Turner, Loeser, and Bell,[47] reported fewer positive outcomes than Barolat et al's[44] level IV FBSS study in 2001. The authors believe this represents the effect of improving technology.

Failed Back Surgery Syndrome

A recent systematic review that evaluated the cost efficacy of SCS found only two randomized controlled trials (RCTs) on SCS for failed back surgery.[48] North et al[49] selected 50 patients as candidates for repeat laminectomy. All the patients had undergone previous surgery and were excluded from randomization if they presented with severe spinal canal stenosis, extremely large disk fragments, a major neurologic deficit such as foot drop, or radiographic evidence of gross instability. In addition, patients were excluded for untreated dependency on opioid analgesics or benzodiazepines, major psychiatric comorbidity, the presence of any significant or disabling chronic pain problem, or a chief symptom of low back pain exceeding lower extremity pain. Crossover between groups was permitted after the 6-month follow-up interval. Of the 26 patients who had undergone reoperation, 54% (14 patients) crossed over to SCS. Of the 24 who had undergone SCS, 21% (5 patients) opted for crossover to reoperation. For 90% of the patients, long-term (3-year) follow-up evaluation has shown that SCS continues to be more effective than reoperation, with significantly better outcomes with standard measures and significantly lower rates of crossover to the alternate procedure. In addition, patients randomized to reoperation used significantly more opioids than those randomized to SCS. Other measures for assessment of activities of daily living and work status did not differ significantly.

The second RCT[50] was a multicenter international study that randomized 100 patients with FBSS and neuropathic radicular leg pain to SCS plus conventional medical management (SCS group) or conventional medical management (CMM group) for 6 months. Primary outcome was 50% or greater reduction in pain, with secondary outcome measures of quality-of-life indicators, functional capacity, pain medication use, satisfaction, and complications. Crossover was permitted at the 6-month interval with an intention-to-treat model, and patients were followed for an entire year. The results showed a statistically significant advantage of SCS over CMM for the primary ($P < 0.001$) and secondary ($P \le 0.05\%$) outcomes. After the study midpoint, 5 of 50 patients in the SCS froup crossed over to the CMM group versus 32 of 50 patients from CMM to SCS. At the study conclusion, however, 32% of patients in the SCS group had experienced device-related complications.

Three systematic review articles are found on neurostimulation.[47,48,51] Turner completed a meta-analysis from the articles related to the treatment of FBSS by SCS from 1966 to 1994.[33] Pain relief exceeding 50% was experienced by 59% of patients, with a range of 15% to 100%. On the basis of this review, however, the authors concluded that insufficient evidence was found in the literature for drawing conclusions about the effectiveness of SCS relative to no treatment or other treatments. North and Wetzel's[51] review consisted of case-control studies and two prospective control studies. They concluded that if a patient reports a reduction in pain of at least 50% during a trial, as determined with standard rating methods, and shows improved or stable analgesic requirements and activity levels, significant benefit may be realized from a permanent implant. The authors conclude the bulk of the literature appears to support a role for SCS (in neuropathic pain syndromes) but caution that the quality of the existing literature is marginal—largely case series. The review from Bala et al[48] focused more on cost efficacy and reviewed one RCT, one retrospective cohort study, and 13 case series. The conclusion was that SCS is effective for treatment of FBSS and less costly over the long term.

Complex Regional Pain Syndrome

Research of high quality regarding SCS and complex regional pain syndrome (CRPS) is limited, but existing data are overwhelmingly positive in terms of pain reduction, quality of life, analgesic usage, and function. Kemler et al[52] published a prospective, randomized, comparative trial of SCS versus conservative therapy for CRPS. Patients with a 6-month history of CRPS of the upper extremities were randomized to undergo trial SCS (and implant if successful) plus physiotherapy versus physiotherapy alone. At a 6-month follow-up assessment, the patients in the SCS group had a significantly greater reduction in pain, and a significantly higher percentage was graded as much improved for the global perceived effect. However, no clinically significant improvements were seen in functional status. The authors concluded that in the short term, SCS reduces pain and improves the quality of life for patients with CRPS involving the upper extremities.

Several important case series have been published on the use of neurostimulation in the treatment of CRPS. Calvillo et al[53] reported a series in which patients with advanced CRPS were treated with either SCS, PNS, or both. After a 3-year period, patients with SCS had a statistically significant reduction in pain score and improvement in return to work. The authors concluded that in late stages of CRPS, neurostimulation (with SCS or PNS) is a reasonable option when alternative therapies have failed. Another case series reported by Oakley and Weiner[54] is remarkable in that it used a sophisticated battery of outcomes tools to evaluate treatment response in CRPS with SCS. The study followed 19 patients and analyzed the results from the McGill Pain Rating Index, Sickness Impact Profile, Oswestry Disability Profile, Beck Depression Inventory, and Visual Analog Scale. After an average of 8 months, all scales showed statistical benefits after SCS and all patients received at least partial relief, with 30% receiving full relief. A literature review by Stanton-Hicks[55] of SCS for CRPS consisted of seven case series. These studies ranged in size from 6 to 24 patients. Results were noted as "good to excellent" in greater than 72% of patients over a time period of 8 to 40 months. The review concluded that SCS proved to be a powerful tool in the management of patients with CRPS.[55]

Even in failed, cases, evidence shows that more aggressive stimulation, only possible with RF generators, can still have a benefit. A retrospective, 3-year, multicenter study of 101 patients by Bennett et al[30] evaluated the effectiveness of SCS applied to CRPS I and compared the effectiveness of octapolar with quadripolar systems, and high-frequency and multiprogram parameters. The authors concluded that SCS is effective in the management of chronic pain associated with CRPS I. For 15% of patients, pain control was attainable only with use of dual-octapolar systems with multiple-array programming capabilities, and high-frequency stimulation (>250 Hz). These settings are not available with standard implantable devices.

Peripheral Ischemia and Angina

Cook et al[11] reported in 1976 that SCS effectively relieved pain associated with peripheral ischemia. This result has been repeated and noted to have particular efficacy in conditions associated with vasospasm, such as Raynaud disease.[56] Many studies have shown impressive efficacy of SCS in treatment of intractable angina.[57] Reported success rates are consistently greater than 80%, and these indications, already widely used outside of the United States, are certain to expand within the United States. This is an active area of research with a quickly expanding body of literature. Interested readers are encouraged to evaluate the literature because it is beyond the scope of this chapter.

Cost Effectiveness

Cost effectiveness of SCS (in the treatment of chronic back pain) was evaluated by Kumar, Malik, and Demeria[58] in 2002 and again by Bala et al[48] in 2008. Kumar, Malik, and Demeria prospectively followed 104 patients with FBSS. Of the 104 patients, 60 were implanted with an SCS with use of a standard selection criterion. Both groups were monitored over a period of 5 years. The stimulation group's annual cost was $29,000 versus $38,000 in the control group. The authors found 15% of subjects returned to work in the stimulation group versus 0% in the control group. The higher costs in the nonstimulator group were in the categories of medications, emergency center visits, radiographs, and ongoing physician visits. As discussed previously, Bala et al's group conducted a systemic review of the literature to identify RCTs (two studies found), controlled observation studies (one retrospective cohort study found), and case series with more than 50 patients and at least 1-year follow-up periods (13 qualifying case series). The beneficial effects of SCS were consistent in all studies. Of the three studies that fulfilled inclusion criteria for cost-effectiveness evaluation, all consistently showed higher initial costs, but overall long-term cost efficacy was greater than conventional medical management.

Bell, Kidd, and North[59] performed an analysis of the medical costs of SCS therapy in the treatment of patients with FBSS. The medical costs of SCS therapy were compared with an alternative regimen of surgeries and other interventions. Externally powered (external) and fully internalized (internal) SCS systems were considered separately. No value was placed on pain relief or improvements in the quality of life that successful SCS therapy can generate. The authors concluded that by reducing the demand for medical care by patients with FBSS, SCS therapy can lower medical costs and found that, on average, SCS therapy pays for itself within 5.5 years. For those patients for whom SCS therapy is clinically efficacious, the therapy pays for itself within 2.1 years.

Kemler and Furnee[60] performed a similar study by looking at "chronic reflex sympathetic dystrophy (RSD)" using outcomes and costs of care before and after the start of treatment. This essentially is an economic analysis of the Kemler et al RSD outcomes paper discussed previously. During a 12-month follow-up period, costs (routine RSD costs, SCS costs, out-of-pocket costs), and effects (pain relief with visual analog scale, health-related quality-of-life[60] improvement with a validated quality-of-life instrument) were assessed in both groups. SCS was both more effective and less costly than the standard treatment protocol. As a result of high initial costs of SCS in the first year, the treatment per patient was $4,000 more than control therapy. However, in the lifetime analysis, SCS per patient was $60,000 cheaper than control therapy. In addition, at 12 months, SCS resulted in pain relief and improved health-related quality of life (HRQL). The authors found SCS to be more effective and less expensive when compared with the standard treatment protocol for chronic RSD.

Peripheral, Cortical, and Deep Brain Stimulation

Besides stimulation of the spinal cord, neurostimulation can successfully be used at other locations in the peripheral and central nervous systems to provide analgesia. PNS was introduced by Wall and Sweet[61] in the mid 1960s. This technique has shown efficacy for peripheral nerve injury pain syndromes and CRPS, with use of a carefully implanted paddle lead with a fascial graft to help anchor the lead without traumatizing the nerve.[62]

Motor cortex and deep brain stimulation are techniques that have been explored for treatment of highly refractory neuropathic pain syndromes, including central pain, deafferentation syndromes, trigeminal neuralgia, and others.[63] Deep brain stimulation has become a widely used technique for movement disorders, and much less so for painful indications, although many case reports of utility in treatment of highly refractory central pain syndromes are found.[64]

Future

Many projected innovations will continue to make SCS an attractive option for treatment of pain. Modern implants have a lifespan of 2 to 10 years,[8] but battery capacity and microprocessor power consumption have improved rapidly, which will eventually prolong the lifespan, decrease the maintenance requirements, and reduce costs of future implantable devices. Current stimulators are contraindicated for use within magnetic resonance imaging (MRI) because of the risk of magnetically generated currents heating the leads and causing neural injury; manufacturers are developing MRI-compatible leads. Research is evolving that demonstrates synergistic effects of intrathecal medications with SCS

Table 174.5 Principles of Spinal Cord Stimulation

1. SCS mechanism of action is not completely understood but influences multiple components and levels within the central nervous system (CNS) with both interneuron and neurochemical mechanisms.
2. SCS therapy is effective for many neuropathic pain conditions. Stimulation-evoked paresthesia must be experienced in the entire painful area. No consistent evidence exists for the efficacy of neurostimulation in primary nociceptive pain conditions.
3. Stimulation should be applied with low intensity, just suprathreshold for the activation of the low-threshold, large-diameter fibers, and should be of nonpainful intensity. To be effective, SCS must be applied continuously (or in cycles) for at least 20 minutes before the onset of analgesia. This analgesia develops slowly and typically lasts several hours after cessation of the stimulation.
4. SCS has shown clinical and cost effectiveness in FBSS and CRPS. Clinical effectiveness has also been shown in peripheral ischemia and angina.
5. Multicontact, multiprogram systems improve outcomes and reduce the incidence of surgical revisions. Insulated paddle-type electrodes *probably* decrease the incidence of lead breakage, prolong battery life, and show early superiority in quality of paresthesia coverage and analgesia in FBSS as compared with permanent percutaneous electrodes.
6. Serious complications are exceedingly rare but can be devastating. Meticulous care must be taken during implantation to minimize procedural complications. The most frequent complications are wound infections (approximately 5%) and lead breakage or migration (approximately 13% each for permanent percutaneous leads and 3% to 6% each for paddle leads).

Adapted from Linderoth B, Meyerson BA: Spinal cord stimulation: mechanisms of action. In Burchiel K, editor: *Surgical management of pain*, New York, 2002, Thieme, p 505.

---

compatible leads, combined pump-stimulators. As the physiologic understanding of DC stimulation improves, newer modes of pulse waveforms and neuroanatomic distribution of currents can substantiate novel therapeutic roles. Closed-loop biofeedback innovations that record neural responses to SCS could play a role in improving the effects of SCS.[65]

Conclusion

SCS is an invasive, interventional surgical procedure. Linderoth and Meyerson[66] wrote some principles of neurostimulation that are cornerstones of SCS theory and practice (**Table 174.5**). The difficulty of randomized clinical trials in such situations is well recognized. On the basis of the present evidence with two randomized trials, one prospective trial, and multiple retrospective trials, the evidence for SCS in properly selected populations with neuropathic pain states is moderate. Clearly, this technique should be reserved for patients who have failure with more conservative therapies. With appropriate patient selection and careful attention to technical issues, the clinical results are overwhelmingly positive.

References

Full references for this chapter can be found on www.expertconsult.com.

Implantable Drug Delivery Systems: Practical Considerations

Steven D. Waldman

Spinal opioids have dramatically changed the way acute, obstetric, nonmalignant chronic pain and pain of malignant origin are managed. The development of various implantable drug delivery systems (IDDSs) has complemented and facilitated the growth of this treatment modality. With interfacing of appropriate patient selection with the unique advantages and disadvantages of each type of IDDS, improved results in terms of both pain relief and patient satisfaction can be achieved.

History

In the late 1970s, a group of cancer patients at the Mayo Clinic underwent spinal administration of morphine in the hope of finding an alternative to neurodestructive procedures for relief of intractable pain of malignant origin. This brilliant clinical application by Wang, Nauss, and Thomas[1] of the basic research of Yaksh[2] heralded a new era in the specialty of pain management. This development not only dramatically changed the management of cancer pain but also triggered an entirely new way of looking at the route of drug administration. The years since this landmark event have yielded vast clinical experience with this powerful new modality, which in turn has resulted in the publication of an extensive literature describing the use of spinal opioids in a variety of clinical situations.[3] As clinicians gained more experience in the use of spinal opioids for the management of cancer pain, they began to apply this modality to nonmalignant acute pain and experiment with the spinal administration of drugs other than opioids.

This experimentation has not been without its critics, but by and large, the use of spinal opioids for acute pain has been a great advance. Clinicians have successfully adapted this technique to relieve postoperative and other acute pain syndromes, obstetric pain, nonmalignant chronic pain, and cancer pain in thousands of patients. In tandem, the development of various IDDSs has occurred and facilitated this expanded role of spinal drugs in the palliation of pain and, more recently, spasticity.[4]

The Role of Patient Selection in Consideration of Implantable Drug Delivery Systems

Does a Spinally Administered Drug Relieve the Symptoms Being Treated?

The first factor to consider in determination of whether a patient is an appropriate candidate for implantation of an IDDS is whether spinal opioids adequately relieve the patient's pain and whether spinal administration of baclofen adequately relieves the patient's spasticity. Not all pain is relieved with spinal opioids, and not all spasticity is relieved with spinally administered baclofen.[5,6] For this reason, an IDDS should never be implanted without verification first of the ability of the intended drug to relieve the patient's pain or spasticity on at least two occasions. Failure to do so could subject the patient to implantation of a delivery system that fails to achieve the desired result—namely, pain relief.

The Preimplantation Trial

Table 175.1 outlines a suggested protocol for the preimplantation trial for spinal opioids. The expected result of the preimplantation trial of spinal opioids is adequate pain relief as perceived by the patient. This relief should be of appropriate duration for the narcotic analgesic injected.[7] Other variables that should be quantified include the level of activity, the use of narcotics via other routes, and the amount and quality of sleep. This same approach should be used to verify that spinally administered baclofen adequately relieves the patient's spasticity.

Side Effects

Side effects from spinal opioids, including pruritus, urinary retention, and respiratory depression, must be noted. Side effects from spinally administered baclofen, including weakness and sedation, must also be noted. These side effects must be acceptable to the patient before implantation can be considered. Any inconsistency in the expected versus the observed results should alert the clinician to strongly consider delaying implantation of the delivery system. Careful evaluation of the patient's ability to assess pain relief, and reevaluation of other behavioral or psychosocial factors at play, should be undertaken before implantation of an IDDS.

The Patient's Ability to Assess the Results of the Preimplantation Trial

The ability of the patient to accurately assess the adequacy of pain relief or relief of spasticity is essential to avoid the implantation of an IDDS that will be deemed useless. Impairment of this ability may be either physiologic or behavioral in origin.

Physiologic abnormalities that may impair the patient's ability to assess the adequacy of pain relief or relief of spasticity are listed in **Table 175.2**. Most occur in patients with significant multisystem disease, but occasionally, seemingly otherwise healthy patients may have significant impairment of mentation that is not obvious to the clinician. Many of these abnormalities are reversible, and every attempt should be made to correct them before a trial of spinal opioids is undertaken. Remember that the central nervous system symptoms caused by these abnormalities may be incorrectly interpreted as uncontrolled pain by the patient and clinician alike.

Behavioral factors that may affect the patient's ability to assess the adequacy of pain relief or relief of spasticity (**Table 175.3**) are often difficult to identify. They may coexist with physiologic factors, but care must be taken to not attribute inadequate pain relief solely to behavioral factors until all other reasons have been explored. A patient who received adequate pain relief during the preimplantation trial may be a candidate for implantation of an IDDS. Adequacy of patient motivation, the patient's support system, concurrent therapy,

Table 175.2 Common Physiologic Abnormalities That May Interfere with the Patient's Ability to Assess Pain Relief

Metabolic encephalopathy

Hypercalcemia

Hyponatremia

Hypoxemia

Hypercapnia

Azotemia

Hepatic encephalopathy

Paraneoplastic syndrome

Drug-induced organic brain syndrome

Narcotics

Minor tranquilizers

Barbiturates

Phenothiazine reactions

Cimetidine

Structural brain disease

Metastatic tumor

Increased intracranial pressure

Preexisting structural abnormality

Cerebral infarction

Cerebral hemorrhage

Abscess

Preexisting neurodegenerative disorders

Alzheimer's disease

Table 175.1 Protocol for Preimplantation Trials of Spinal Opioids

1. Explain the procedure, expected goals, and potential side effects to the patient and family.
2. Select an appropriate narcotic for intraspinal administration.
3. Determine the appropriate dosage and volume of diluent expected to relieve the pain.
4. Administer the intraspinal narcotic and diluent via the intended route of delivery (i.e., epidural or subarachnoid).
5. Quantify on a flow sheet the duration of pain relief, level of activity, amount of sleep, and need for additional narcotic analgesics.
6. Quantify the side effects of intraspinal narcotics.
7. Repeat the trial to quantify the results.
8. Observe 24 hours after intraspinal narcotics and requantify the variables listed in item 5 before proceeding with an implantable drug delivery system.

Table 175.3 Common Behavioral Abnormalities That May Interfere with the Patient's Ability to Assess Symptom Relief

Preexisting psychiatric illness

Preexisting chemical dependence

Use of pain as a controlling device

Use of pain to obtain more medication to alter the sensorium

Use of pain as an attention-seeking device

Patient's refusal to accept the person designated as caregiver

Patient's use of pain to punish certain caregivers within the support system systemic infection, life expectancy, and the cost of spinal opioids must also, however, be evaluated before referring a patient for implantation.

The Patient's Support System

An IDDS requires a baseline level of commitment not only from the patient but also from the support system. The person or persons designated as the patient's support system must be acceptable to the patient in the role of care provider. If such is not the case, problems may arise. This person must be available night and day to care for and, if a type I to III delivery system is used, be available to inject medication into the delivery system should the patient be unable to do so. Patients who inject narcotics into their own delivery system initially may be unable to do so later in the course of the disease. If the support system is unable or unwilling to care for the delivery system, a continuous infusion pump may be a better option; however, someone must be available to bring the patient to the pain center to have the pump refilled. Also, consider the possibility that family members may divert the patient's drugs for illicit purposes.

Unique Problems in Management of Patients with Cancer Pain

Before proceeding with implantation of an IDDS, a review of concurrent primary therapy and its potential to relieve the pain is indicated. In this author's opinion, long-term administration of spinal opioids should be reserved for patients with pain of malignant origin. Our experience with the use of spinal opioids for nonmalignant chronic pain has been disappointing. However, other clinicians have reported more satisfactory results with this group of patients. Currently, this author reserves implantation of an IDDS for the following groups of patients: (1) cancer patients in whom primary modes of tumor eradication (surgery, chemotherapy, and radiation therapy) did not relieve the pain; (2) patients with spasticity uncontrolled with aggressive oral drug therapy; and (3) rare patients with nonmalignant chronic pain whose disease process is so devastating that it is analogous to cancer pain, such as those with end-stage connective tissue disease or advanced demyelinating disease. The author's opinion is that one of two things is necessary before the use of spinal opioids for nonmalignant chronic pain can be routinely recommended: (1) a better way to identify patients who will experience long-term satisfactory results with this modality; or (2) release of new drugs suitable for spinal administration that do not cause tolerance or the myriad behavioral issues associated with the long-term use of opioids administered spinally or systemically for nonmalignant chronic pain.

In determination of whether a specific patient is suitable for the implantation of an IDDS, it should be recognized that patients with pain of malignant origin present some specific challenges. A cancer patient may have quantitative and qualitative problems with clotting that may be further compromised by chemotherapy and radiation therapy.[8] In the author's experience, this rarely presents any practical problems as long as the patient's clotting parameters are brought into acceptable range before implantation takes place. However, in a cancer patient undergoing systemic anticoagulation therapy, the risk for epidural hematoma is an ever-present possibility. In these patients, the risk-to-benefit ratio of the anticoagulants must be weighed carefully.

In a cancer patient with immunocompromise, ongoing infection is not uncommon. Epidural abscess formation, and spondylitis and diskitis, has been reported in some cases when percutaneous catheters were advanced into the epidural space without subcutaneous tunneling and left in place for as little as 6 days.[9,10] For long-term use, an IDDS that is totally implanted or subcutaneously tunneled appears to be superior to a percutaneous indwelling epidural catheter. Common sense dictates against placement of an indwelling foreign body in a patient with sepsis.

A realistic appraisal of life expectancy is necessary to determine the appropriateness of an invasive and relatively expensive procedure for pain relief. For cancer patients with limited life expectancy, simple percutaneous placement of an epidural or subarachnoid catheter with subcutaneous tunneling may be more reasonable than a more expensive type III to V system.

Cost of the Implantable Drug Delivery System, Drugs, and Supplies

In evaluation of the cost of an IDDS, consideration of the cost of both the system and the drugs to be administered through it is necessary. The hardware for an IDDS can amount to more than $10,000 for a totally implantable infusion pump, exclusive of professional fees and hospital charges. The cost of the narcotics or adjuvant drugs, or both, is not insubstantial, nor is the cost of antiseptic solutions, sterile preparation swabs, gauze, and so forth needed for patients who are self administering opioids via a type I to III system. Some patients simply cannot afford the daily expense. Cost must be considered before implantation of a delivery system that will ultimately not be used.

Classification of Implantable Drug Delivery Systems

Table 175.4 describes the five basic types of IDDS. The type I system, a simple percutaneous catheter analogous to those used for obstetric pain control, is one with which clinicians are most familiar. The type II system is simply a catheter suitable for percutaneous placement and tunneling. The type III system consists of a totally implantable injection port that is attached to a type II tunneled catheter. The type IV system is a totally implantable continuous infusion pump that is connected to a type II tunneled catheter. The type V system is

---

Table 175.4 Spinal Drug Delivery Systems

Type I: Percutaneous epidural or subarachnoid catheter

Type II: Percutaneous epidural or subarachnoid catheter with subcutaneous tunneling

Type III: Totally implanted epidural or subarachnoid catheter with a subcutaneous injection port

Type IV: Totally implanted epidural or subarachnoid catheter with an implanted infusion pump

Type V: Totally implanted epidural or subarachnoid catheter with an implanted programmable infusion pump

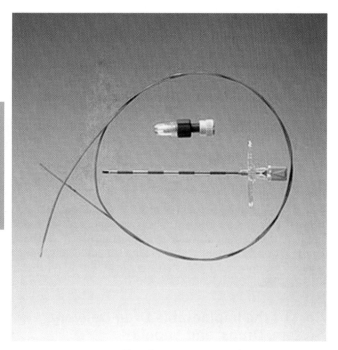

Fig. 175.1 **Type I percutaneous catheter.**

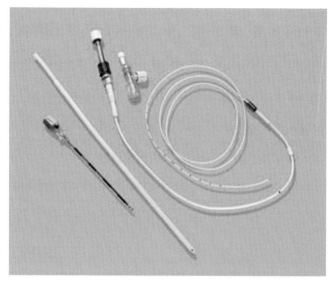

Fig. 175.2 **Type II subcutaneous tunneled catheter.**

a totally implantable programmable infusion pump attached to a type II tunneled catheter. The programmable feature of a type V IDDS allows a broad spectrum of delivery rates and modes, including occasional bolus injections.

Each of these drug delivery systems has its own unique profile of advantages and disadvantages. The clinician must be familiar with the particular merits of each system if optimal selection is to be made. In this time of increasing pressure to control the cost of health care, economic factors must also play a role in the selection of an IDDS. The cost of both the intended delivery system and the drugs to be administered through the delivery system must be considered before implantation of an IDDS. A perfectly functioning IDDS is of no value to a patient who is unable to pay for the drugs, special needles, and supplies needed to use the delivery system. Similarly, implanted systems may superimpose financial hardship on a difficult terminal course. With prior planning, the financial issues can be individualized and resolved.

Type I: Percutaneous Catheter

The type I percutaneous catheter has gained wide acceptance for the short-term administration of spinal opioids or local anesthetics, or both, for the palliation of acute pain, including obstetric and postoperative pain (**Fig. 175.1**). The type I system also has three applications in cancer pain management. The first is in the acute setting, in which the delivery of opioids into the epidural or subarachnoid space can provide temporary palliation of pain after surgery or until other concurrent treatments, such as radiotherapy, become effective. The second is in imminently dying patients too ill for more invasive procedures. The third is the use of a percutaneous catheter to administer test doses of spinal opioids before placement of a more permanent IDDS. In many centers, the use of a percutaneous catheter for the delivery of epidural and especially subarachnoid opioids is limited because of the ease with which catheters can be tunneled. The improved catheter fixation and

reduced risk for infection associated with subcutaneous tunneling, combined with the relative ease of tunneling, have led many pain specialists to tunnel the spinal catheter to the flank, abdomen, or chest wall. In view of the potentially devastating and life-threatening consequences of catheter-induced spinal infection, and the highly favorable risk-to-benefit ratio of the type II tunneled catheter, use of the type I system should, in the author's opinion, be limited solely to the acute setting.

Type II: Subcutaneous Tunneled Catheter

Subcutaneously tunneled catheters are usually selected for patients who have a finite need for spinally administered opioids (**Fig. 175.2**). Patients with pain from major trauma, such as pelvic and long bone fractures and flail chest, are appropriate candidates for a type II system, as are cancer patients with life expectancies of weeks to months who have experienced excellent palliation of symptoms with trial doses of spinal drugs.[11,12] The type II system carries significantly less risk for infection than percutaneous catheters do.[12] The simplified catheter care and the ease of injection by both medical and nonmedical personnel are also significant advantages of the type II system. The type II system can also be attached to an external continuous infusion pump.

Type III: Totally Implantable Reservoir/Port

The totally implantable reservoir is often chosen for cancer patients with life expectancies of months to years who have had excellent relief of symptoms with trial doses of spinal drugs (**Fig. 175.3**). Significantly less expensive than the type IV or V system, the type III system is a reasonable choice for patients who do not have a third party to cover the cost of a more sophisticated system.[13] The type III system is associated with potentially less risk of infection than are the type I and II systems and with a decreased risk of catheter failure.

Injection of the type III system is more difficult than with type I and II systems, and this disadvantage can have significant import when training lay people to inject and care for this system. Furthermore, removal or replacement necessitates a surgical incision.

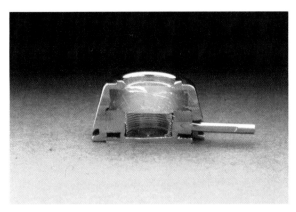

Fig. 175.3 **Type III totally implantable reservoir/port.**

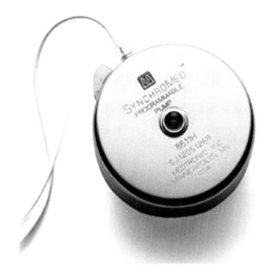

Fig. 175.5 **Type V totally implantable programmable infusion pump.**

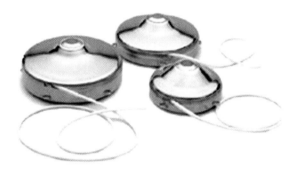

Fig. 175.4 **Type IV totally implantable infusion pump.**

Type IV: Totally Implantable Infusion Pump

The totally implantable infusion pump is also used in patients with life expectancies of months to years who obtained relief of symptoms after trial doses of spinal drugs (**Fig. 175.4**). Type IV delivery systems may also be indicated in a cancer patient with a shorter life expectancy who experiences intermittent confusion from metabolic abnormalities or systemically administered drugs. Clinical experience suggests that such patients may obtain analgesia with fewer side effects with low-dose continuous spinal opioid infusion than with repeated bolus injections into a spinal catheter. Alternatively, a type III implanted port with an external infusion pump may suffice in this situation, although such a system may be more inconvenient and require more support.

Because type IV systems require infrequent refills and run continuously, they are ideal for patients with limited medical or nonmedical family support services. The type IV system is usually selected with an auxiliary bolus injection port to take advantage of potential drug options, such as injection of local anesthetics and the ability to inject contrast to troubleshoot the system.

Advantages of the type IV system include minimal risk for infection after the perioperative period and the need to inject the pump very infrequently relative to other IDDSs (the pump

reservoir needs to be refilled approximately every 7 to 20 days). The overall high cost of the type IV system is a disadvantage and may occasionally result in the selection of a less effective or more inconvenient analgesic technique.

Type V: Totally Implantable Programmable Infusion Pump

The type V totally implantable programmable infusion pump is implanted with the same ease as the type IV system (**Fig. 175.5**).[14] These systems allow a broad spectrum of delivery rates and modes, including occasional bolus injections. Their principal application to date has been intrathecal infusion, especially for the treatment of spasticity in multiple sclerosis and patients with spinal cord injury, but the type V IDDS is also gaining increasing acceptance as the preferred type of IDDS for the long-term administration of spinal opioids.

Conclusion

The administration of spinal drugs via an IDDS is a useful addition to the armamentarium of clinicians treating patients with pain or spasticity that does not respond to conventional means. Proper selection of the patient and an appropriate delivery system are crucial if optimal results are to be achieved. The chronic administration of opioids and other drugs into the epidural or subarachnoid space is evolving. Advances in the pharmacology of spinal drugs and the development of new delivery system technology will in time no doubt expand the options available for the relief of uncontrolled pain and spasticity.[6]

References

Full references for this chapter can be found on www.expertconsult.com.

Complications of Neuromodulation

Timothy R. Deer and Matthew T. Ranson

Introduction

The physician must be vigilant to prevent, identify, and resolve complications. Even in the most talented hands, complications occur and may lead to a poor outcome. With use of careful preoperative screening and meticulous operative techniques, the outcomes of neuromodulation are improved, but complications (**Table 176.1**) persist despite the best efforts of the physician.

Overview of Complications of Spinal Cord Stimulation and Intrathecal Drug Delivery

Complications of implantable devices can range from minor problems that may go unnoticed by the physician and patient, to those treated with observation, to major adverse events that lead to paraplegia or serious neurologic injury. In this chapter, the complications are grouped into sections with consideration of the impact of each device on the potential problems that the practitioner may experience.

Complications of the Neuroaxis Bleeding

The invasion of the epidural or intrathecal space with needles, leads, and catheters can lead to major bleeding complications. In most patients, this bleeding results in no clinically apparent complication and necessitates no treatment. In some cases, this bleeding may involve an asymptomatic epidural hematoma; but in the absence, of postsurgical imaging, this normally goes unrecognized. Rarely, bleeding progresses to the development of an epidural hematoma and compresses spinal structures. If a developing epidural hematoma progresses, it can lead to numbness, back and leg pain, weakness, and eventual paraplegia. Treatment of clinically significant epidural hematoma necessitates prompt surgical evaluation and evacuation if clinically indicated. This problem must be identified early and treated within 24 hours of the development of symptoms. Patients who undergo surgical evacuation within 12 hours have been shown to have clinically better neurologic outcomes than patients who undergo decompression later than 12 hours.[1] After 24 hours from presentation, the chance of a complete recovery diminishes. Patient education is important in the early identification of this complication. The patient should be taught to watch for and report to the treating doctor any new signs of numbness, weakness, and increasing pain in the postoperative period. Weakness in the postoperative period is a red flag that should raise the suspicion of this tragic complication and warrant an immediate computed tomographic (CT) scan of the spine in the patient on a stimulator and immediate magnetic resonance imaging (MRI) with appropriate precautions in the patient on a pump.

Risk factors for development of an epidural hematoma include anticoagulation therapy, platelet-inhibiting medications, aspirin, and possibly nonsteroidal drugs. However, the role of low-dose aspirin and nonsteroidal anti-inflammatory drugs in epidural hematoma formation is controversial and has not been established. Most clinicians allow patients to remain on low-dose aspirin and nonsteroidal drugs during the perioperative period. Other factors may include

Table 176.1 Complications

Complication	Diagnosis of Problem	Treatment of Problem
Lead migration	Inability to program	Reprogramming, surgical revision
Current leak	High impedance, pain at leak site	Revision of connectors, generator, or leads
NEUROAXIS COMPLICATION		
Nerve injury	CT scan or MRI, EMG/NCS/physical examination	Steroid protocol, anticonvulsants, neurosurgery consult
Epidural fibrosis	Increased stimulation amplitude	Lead programming, lead revision
Epidural hematoma	Physical examination, CT scan, or MRI	Surgical evaluation, steroid protocol
Epidural abscess	Physical examination, CT scan or MRI, CBC, blood work	Surgical evaluation, IV antibiotics, ID consult
Postdural puncture headache	Positional headache, blurred vision, nausea	IV fluids, rest, blood patch, neurosurgery consult if evidence of CN palsy
DEVICE COMPLICATION		
Unacceptable programming	Lack of stimulation in area of pain	Reprogramming of device, revision of leads
Lead migration	Inability to program, x-rays	Reprogramming, surgical revision
Current leak	High impedance, pain at leak site.	Revision of connectors, generator, or leads
Generator failure	Inability to read device	Replacement of generator
NON-NEUROLOGIC TISSUE		
Seroma	Serosanguinous fluid in pocket	Aspiration; if no response, surgical drainage
Hematoma	Blood in pocket	Pressure and aspiration, surgical revision
Pain at generator	Pain on palpation	Lidoderm patches, injection, revision
Wound infection	Fever, rubor, drainage	Antibiotics, incision and drainage, removal

CN, cranial nerve; EMG, electromyography; ID, implantable device; IV, intravenous; NCS, nerve conduction study.

difficult percutaneous lead or catheter placement, laminotomy approach to lead placement, and revision of previously placed leads. The need to perform surgical instrumentation and create bony insult dramatically increases the risk of a significant bleed. Spine surgeons often recognize the bleed at the time of surgery and treat it without clinical significance.

The diagnosis of epidural hematoma is assisted with clinical suspicion, physical examination, and history, but the confirmatory diagnosis is made with CT scan. MRI can be obtained once the leads are removed and can be obtained in patients with intrathecal infusion systems without delay. However, given the need for prompt surgical evaluation, obtaining a CT scan may be more judicious. Epidural bleeding appears to be a much greater risk with spinal cord stimulation than with intrathecal drug delivery. The catheter is driven within the intrathecal space with pumps, and the insult to the epidural space is minimal. Intrathecal bleeding could result in arachnoid irritation, but the incidence or significance is not known.

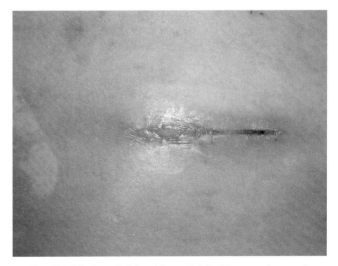

Fig. 176.1 **Early cellulitis with partial deshisance of wound.**

Infection

The other spinal compressive lesion that causes a complication of the neuroaxis associated with neuromodulation is epidural abscess. This is the most urgent infectious complication associated with implantable devices, although the implanter should be aware of the complications of superficial infections of the incision, pocket infections, diskitis, and meningitis (**Figs. 176.1** and **176.2**). The most common of these problems is superficial infection, and the risk of epidural abscess appears to be much less than one in 1000. Because of the overwhelming potential risks of epidural abscess, the implanter should have a good knowledge of this issue. Epidural abscess may present with severe pain in the area of the lead implant. This may be associated with fever, with most patients experiencing temperatures more than 38°C (101°F). Radiating pain can be severe and may develop if the abscess extends to the foramen or compresses the cord. In some patients, a progression can consist of an initial pain symptom, with an evolution to sensory loss, radicular pain, and then motor weakness and

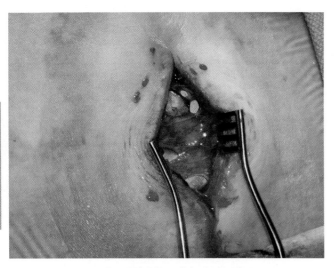

Fig. 176.2 **Infection of device pocket.**

eventual paraplegia. Risk factors for abscess include immunocompromised state, including patients with HIV infection and organ transplants, history of chronic oral steroids and immunosuppressive drugs, history of chronic skin infections, history of methicillin-resistant *Staphylococcal aureus* infection (MRSA) or colonization, chronic diseases such as poorly controlled diabetes mellitus, or local infection at the surgery site. Smoking and obesity may also lead to an increased risk of infection. Infectious complications with intrathecal catheters are uncommon and include meningitis and direct infection of the spinal cord near the catheter tip, resulting in transverse myelitis.[2] Most cases of transverse myelitis are not seen with a known infection, and the cause may be undetermined. Clinical indications of infection include the presence of a fever, elevated white blood count, elevated C-reactive protein levels, and elevated erythrocyte sedimentation rate.

Epidural abscess is diagnosed with clinical suspicion, history, and physical examination and confirmed with CT scan. MRI may be performed once the spinal cord stimulation (SCS) device is explanted or in patients with an intrathecal delivery device with proper precautions.

Direct Neurologic Trauma

Neurologic injury of the spinal cord or nerve roots is another potential risk of percutaneous lead or catheter placement. Because the spinal nerves of the cauda equina float freely within the cerebrospinal fluid (CSF) below the L1-L2 level, this problem less likely if needle entry is below this level. Lateral fluoroscopic views are especially important in percutaneous SCS lead placement because often the surgeon is advancing the needle over the conus medullaris. In addition, lead or catheter placement into the conus medullaris is possible with little production of pain in an awake patient. Injury may occur via needle trauma, lead or catheter placement and removal, or surgical manipulation during paddle lead placement.

In many patients, the injury is associated with deep sedation or general anesthesia. Monitored anesthesia care where the patient is freely arousable and communicating with the surgeon is recommended during percutaneous needle placement. In some patients, the inability to tolerate the procedure with sedation leads to the need to perform these devices with general anesthesia. This is acceptable for intrathecal catheter placement below the level of the conus but should be avoided in spinal cord stimulation unless it is done with an open laminotomy approach. In the immediate postoperative period, a neurologic injury may present in a confusing manner and may create a diagnostic dilemma. Assessment of the patient in the postanesthesia care unit and documentation of the absence of any new focal neurologic findings are advisable. CT scan may not show an abnormality, and MRI cannot be performed in the case of SCS until the device is surgically removed. With patients on a pump, an MRI is the imaging study of choice with proper precautions. An electromyogram and nerve conduction study may be helpful in determination of injury, but results may not become abnormal for several days after the insult.

The treatment of neural injury or irritation depends on the severity. In cases of cord or nerve contusion, the treatment may simply consist of observation because many of these cases often resolve with time. In the immediate postoperative period, intravenous steroids may be helpful in reducing swelling of the neural structures.

Less worrisome complications inside the neuroaxis include inadvertent dural puncture with postdural puncture headache. The literature has shown an incidence rate of up to 11% of cases, although that number appears much higher than most implanters may see in their clinical practice. This risk is increased by obesity, calcified ligaments, difficult lead or catheter placement, poor positioning from scoliosis or body habitus abnormalities, patient movement, and previous surgery at the level of needle entry. In spinal cord stimulation, the use of loss of resistance with use of fluoroscopy with an attention to the hanging drop in the syringe may reduce this risk, particularly in the midthoracic and higher levels of entry. In intrathecal catheter placement, the number of attempts is important to reducing the risk of postdural puncture headache.

CSF leak and hygroma formation are complications associated with intrathecal drug delivery systems. The use of a purse-string suture to secure the tissue around the CSF entry site may be helpful in reducing these complications. Abdominal binders in the immediate postimplant period may also be helpful, as may conservative measures such as fluid intake, caffeine, and intramuscular sumatriptan.

Spinal cord stenosis may develop over time in the vicinity of an implanted lead. This is a rare complication and develops slowly over time. The development of stenosis over the lead is diagnosed with clinical history, CT scan, or CT myelogram. This problem is unlikely with intrathecal catheters because of the compressibility of catheter material. Compression of spinal cord stimulation leads is more likely with paddle leads because of their volume. In cases of stenosis before implant, a paddle implant is the best choice because of the ability to decompress the bony structures via laminotomy before lead placement.

Intrathecal drug delivery devices pose additional risks because of the administration of intrathecal medications. Inflammatory masses surrounding the tip of the catheter were first reported in 1999.[3] The inflammatory mass appears to be a chronic fibrotic noninfectious mass that develops at the tip of the intrathecal catheter over months to years and is related to high concentrations of opioid at the catheter tip. As the inflammatory mass grows larger, patients often present with neurologic signs and symptoms that reflect direct compression of the spinal cord or other neural elements by the expanding mass.[4] Patients may present with initial loss of analgesia followed by progressive neurologic compromise. Because many

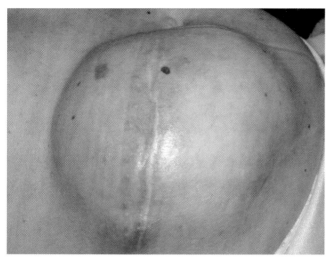

Fig. 176.3 **Gross seroma of device pocket.**

of the reported cases have been directly linked to high concentrations of morphine and hydromorphone, consensus recommendations have suggested that the concentration of morphine be limited to 30 mg/mL and the concentration of hydromorphone to 20 mg/mL. In addition, sufentanyl and fentanyl appear to have a lower risk of granuloma formation. Diagnosis is made with a T1-weighted MRI with and without gadolinium. A CT myelogram can be obtained if MRI is contraindicated.

The recommended doses and concentrations of drugs are based on the ideal clinical situation. In some cases, the risks of higher concentrations and doses are believed by the implanter to be worthwhile for a good clinical response and of greater benefit to the patient than the risk of inflammatory mass formation.

Complications Outside of the Neuroaxis

Wound infections that involve the generator, pump reservoir, tunneled area, or lead and catheter incision site can occur in 0 to 4.5% of patients based on reported incidence rates.[5] This problem is diagnosed with pain, swelling, rubor, and drainage of purulent material. An elevated white blood cell count, sedimentation rate, or C-reactive protein value should create concern regarding the infectious status of the implant. Patients whose conditions respond to antibiotics initially may have development of chronic slow-growing infections that could be subclinical for some time. Recurrent fever should lead the implanter to consider evaluation by an internal medicine specialist, family physician, or infectious disease specialist.

Seroma

In some cases, the patient may have a swollen, irritated wound develop that is not related to infectious etiology (**Fig. 176.3**). This complication, called a seroma, is caused by a buildup of serosanguineous fluid. Seroma is diagnosed with lack of fever and normal blood study evaluation of white blood count. If the diagnosis cannot be determined, incision and drainage with cultures may be necessary to make a conclusive diagnosis. In most cases, seroma can be treated without device removal. Careful dissection and attention to minimizing tissue trauma may reduce

the risk of this complication. In rare cases, fever can develop in the setting of a seroma. This is a complicated situation that can be resolved only with surgical evaluation of the wound.

Bleeding

Bleeding can occur in the generator, pump reservoir, or lead and catheter incision sites. This can lead to hematoma and necessitate drainage or wound dehiscence. The best treatment is prevention. This consists of thoughtful tissue dissection, pressure to the area of bleeding, suturing of arterial bleeding, coagulation of ongoing small-vessel hemorrhage, and careful inspection of the wound before closure. The physician should also access the patient for bleeding risks, including medications and diseases that may impact bleeding.

Painful Generator

Pain at the generator or reservoir site may occur from neuroma, tissue irritation, or bony contact with a rib or pelvic bones. Neuroma formation is rare and may be reduced with careful dissection and handling of the tissue. To avoid pain on the bony structures, the implanter should carefully access the bony landmarks. In some cases, the patient's body shape or habitus leads to difficulty in finding an ideal position for the generator. With new, smaller generators, the ability to place the pocket near the lead incision site has reduced the problem with pain at the generator in stimulation cases. The size of the pump can lead to pain even in the most carefully placed pocket. The patient with poor nutrition and minimal subcutaneous fat may have pain and pocket complications. Patients with complex regional pain syndrome are thought to be more prone to pain than other chronic pain groups. Treatment can include topical local anesthetic patches, wound injection, or surgical revision.

Complications of the Device

Loss of Appropriate Stimulation

The most commonly reported complication of SCS devices is loss of paresthesia capture over time and subsequent loss of pain reduction. These reports are often based on older studies with devices that had less ability to capture the spinal fibers and less ability to be programmed in multiple fashions to target many areas of pain generation. Common causes of loss of capture include lead migration, dead zones that do not respond to cathode activation, hypothesized tolerance to stimulation, and increased impedance from either fibrosis under and around the lead or a current leak somewhere in the system. New x-rays can be helpful in confirming any lead shift or migration. Depending on the degree of change, the physician may be able to work with technicians to reprogram the system to create an improved clinical status without the need for surgical correction. If conservative measures fail, a surgical revision may be necessary. The clinician should always be aware that new disease processes can sometimes be confused with a failure of the system and additional workup may be warranted if the history or examination changes from previous evaluations.

Lead migration has been reported as a common complication in percutaneous systems (**Fig. 176.4** and **Table 176.2**). In some studies, up to 20% or more of leads have been shown

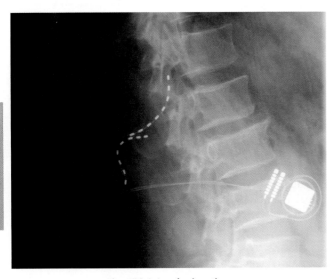

Fig. 176.4 **Lead migration.**

Table 176.2 **Migration Risks**

Migration Risk	Physician Action
Needle angle	Needle angle of 30 to 45 degrees
Needle entry	Paramedian approach
Fatty tissue at anchoring site	Débridement of fatty tissue around the needle entry site exposing fascia and ligament for proper anchoring
Anchoring to muscle	With use of an exaggerated paramedian approach, the physician should dissect medially until approaching ligament or fascia, avoiding anchoring to muscle, which may lead to migration with contraction.
Lead anchor gap	The anchor should be as close to the lead entry into the ligament or fascia as possible, avoiding room for migration distal to the anchor.
Suturing with silk	Avoid silk sutures when anchoring
Dependence on the anchor	The anchor should be seen as one component of securing the system. Total dependence on the anchor can lead to poor outcomes.
Hematoma below anchor	Hemostasis should be obtained before closing the wound. Bleeding can lead to catheter movement from hematoma compression placing pressure on the anchor.
Minimal migration changes	The catheter should be placed in an area of the spine that is not impacted by minimal migration movements. If the catheter tip is in the spinal cerebral fluid, a good outcome may be preserved even in the presence of movement.

to migrate.[6] This number is based on older data and products, with most clinicians experiencing clinical significance in less than 5% of patients with modern equipment. The problem is diagnosed with anterior-posterior and lateral films with comparison with original implant films. Treatment ranges from simple computer reprogramming to surgical lead revision. A careful attention to anchoring may reduce this complication risk but cannot prevent it from occurring. New anchors have been developed by several manufacturers and have obtained US Food and Drug Administration (FDA) approval for clinical use. The impact of these new titanium-based anchors is not yet known, but regardless of the anchor chosen, the implanter must do an adequate dissection to visualize the fascia and ligament.

Other Lead and Generator Problems

Painful stimulation or loss of stimulation can occur from current leakage or loss of system integrity. This problem is often diagnosed with computer analysis showing high impedance compared with baseline. Possible causes include lead migration, poor contacts from fluid in the contacts, or partial or total lead fracture. Lead fracture appears more common with paddle leads.

Positional stimulation can occur because of poor lead-to-tissue contact with standing, lying, or bending. This problem sometimes resolves over time but may need revision to a paddle lead that takes up more volume in the epidural space. Positional stimulation is often thought to occur because of lead movement, but physiologically, it is more likely the result of movement of the cord away from the lead and towards the lead with positional change.

Some patients experience pain from the generator or pump moving within the pocket. This problem can be reduced by anchoring the generator or pump and by using sizing templates that can be provided by the manufacturers. Proper sizing of the pocket is critical for comfort and to reduce the risk of complications. Situations in which the pocket is too small may lead to poor wound closure, pressure on the tissue, and even erosion over time. If the pocket is too large, it may lead to flipping of the device, pain from device-tissue irritation, or a seroma in the area of the pocket that is not involved in the implant. An anchoring stitch may be helpful to secure the SCS generator.

In cases of implantable pumps, suture loops can be helpful to reduce problems, but anchoring to fascia with a nonabsorbable suture is important. Polytetrafluoroethylene patches can be used to secure the pump but may lead to difficulty with future revisions because of scarring around the pocket.

Erosion of device components through the skin can lead to loss of the system. This can occur because of poor tissue health from chronic disease, weight loss, and placement of anchors in the superficial tissues. This does occur more commonly at the generator. When erythema occurs around a generator, the physician should consider surgical revision before the complete loss of tissue integrity of the dermal layers that leads to the need to remove the system. In the placement of peripheral leads, the device should be placed below the dermis. In general, the physician should determine this depth via palpation, needle placement, and observation when making an incision to secure the lead and ensuring anchoring to the thoracolumbar muscle fascia. The use of suture for securing the device without the use of a formal anchor should be considered because many cases of device erosion occur at the silastic anchor site. Erosion may be more problematic when new anchors containing harder substances, such as titanium, are used in peripheral leads.

Complications of the Intrathecal Catheters

The most common device failure in intrathecal pumps is catheter failure. Catheter failure has been reported by Follet and Naumann[7] to be 4.5% at 9 months in a prospective observation study. The most common problems associated with the catheter are migration, fracture, and kinking. Migration of the catheter may result in complications that range from lack of analgesia to severe neurologic deficits. Migration into the epidural space or out of the spinal canal produces loss of analgesia and may cause postdural puncture headaches and possibly the development of a hygroma. More worrisome migrations include erosion into the neural foramen, resulting in nerve root irritation and radicular symptoms, or erosion into the spinal cord, producing profound neurologic deficits.[8] If migration is suspected with clinical findings, a change in pump refill volumes or examination with an MRI is indicated.

Implantation of intrathecal devices with general anesthesia may result in intraparenchymal placement of the catheter. For this reason, many physicians recommend intrathecal catheter placement be performed with monitored anesthesia care with light sedation to avoid this catastrophic complication. In some cases, the patient cannot tolerate lying in the necessary position, and general anesthesia is needed. Other options include spinal anesthesia after the catheter is in position. In addition, the catheter may migrate into the subdural space, resulting in decreased efficacy from inadequate CSF distribution. Again, MRI should be performed in any patient suspected of catheter migration.

Complications Involving Intrathecal Agents

Multiple adverse reactions to intrathecal delivery of opioids have been reported and include nausea and vomiting, pruritus, edema, diaphoresis, weakness, weight gain, constipation, difficulty urinating, and decreased libido.[9,10] Peripheral edema has a reported incidence rate from 1% to 20% and appears to occur as a result of the effect of intrathecal opioids on the pituitary adrenal axis.[11] The development of intrathecal granulomas appears to result from the reaction of the infused drug and was discussed previously and seems to involve morphine more often than other medications.

Adjunctive agents commonly used in intrathecal devices include clonidine, bupivicaine, and ziconotide. Clonidine may result in somnolence and hypotension. Bupivicaine can cause muscular weakness and can result in hypotension as well. Ziconotide has many reported side effects, with the most commonly reported including nausea and vomiting, dizziness, confusion, urinary retention, and somnolence.[12]

Risk Assessment

1. Before any procedures are performed in the neuroaxis a thorough evaluation of the spinal anatomy and coagulation status of the patient is necessary. Imaging studies including MRI, CT scan, and x-rays of the patient's spinal anatomy should be reviewed to assess for critical stenosis, significant loss of disc space height, and complicating factors, such as severe scoliosis, that may make percutaneous access of the neuroaxis both difficult and dangerous.

The physician performing neuroaxial procedures must obtain a careful history, including the presence of coagulopathy and immunocompetency, before the procedure. In addition, the patient's medication list must be reviewed, and any medications that affect bleeding should be discontinued in consultation with the prescribing physician according to the latest guidelines.[13] Standard laboratory evaluation should include at a minimum prothrombin time (PT), partial thromboplastin time (PTT), international normalized ratio (INR), and complete blood count (CBC) with platelets.

2. Patients with diseases that result in immunodeficiency should undergo careful assessment, including a review of the underlying disease, preoperative laboratory evaluation, and physical examination, to identify any skin infections that may pose a risk to infection during implantation of a neuromodulation device. Coexisting diseases such as HIV infection and syndrome, neoplastic syndromes, previous MRSA infection, rheumatologic conditions that necessitate long-term steroid treatments, and brittle diabetes and conditions such as morbid obesity all place patients at risk for infection and potential catastrophic outcomes.

3. Wound infections may vary in severity from superficial infection, including frank dehiscence, to catastrophic infections, such as meningitis. Meticulous surgical technique with attention paid to proper wound closure and hemostasis can reduce the incidence of wound infection.

4. The risk of neurologic injury is low in the hands of experienced neuromodulators and is hard to quantify because of the low incidence rate. However, the presence of morbid obesity, critical stenosis, calcified ligaments, epidural fibrosis from prior surgery near the planned implant site, and spinal instrumentation increase the risk of neurologic injury and inadvertent dural puncture in SCS and nerve root injury. CSF in the epidural space can lead to difficulty obtaining adequate stimulation during a SCS trial and can result in postpuncture spinal headache that complicates or confounds the outcome of a SCS trial. The risk of neurologic injury is also increased with uncooperative patients with extensive movement during the operative procedure.

5. Significant spinal stenosis, either pre-existing or acquired after implantation, can result in severe neurologic compromise as a result of spinal compression from the implant. The neuromodulator should pay particular attention to cervical stenosis because the diameter of the spinal canal is significantly smaller that the lumbar and thoracic canals.

6. The development of seromas typically involves the generator or reservoir site and may lead to loss of the device from wound dehiscence. Inadequate hemostasis leading to hematoma formation, history of seroma formation in prior operations, and a history of connective tissues disorders such as lupus, rheumatoid arthritis, and scleroderma may predispose patients to seroma formation.

7. Pain at generator or reservoir site is commonly associated with patients that have a history of complex regional pain syndrome or fibromyalgia. However, it to prediction of which patients will develop pain in this location is impossible, and many will need revision or explantation of the device.

8. Loss of proper stimulation paresthesia or painful stimulation can occur and lead to a reduction in efficacy or increased pain with use of the SCS. Many factors may contribute to decreased efficacy of stimulation, including epidural fibrosis, migration, positional change, or other electrical stimulation factors. Patients with decreased or loss of stimulation should undergo a complete evaluation, including a physical examination, plain film evaluation, and interrogation of the device. In the case of intrathecal drug delivery devices, a dye study and MRI may be useful in determination of loss of analgesia.

9. Lead or catheter migration can lead to decreased efficacy of the device and opioid or baclofen withdrawal in intrathecal drug delivery systems. Movements such as bending at the waist, twisting, reaching overhead, and heavy lifting can all result in lead and catheter migration, particularly in the early postoperative period. Migration of the intrathecal catheter may result in movement into epidural space or completely out of the neuroaxis. Migration of the catheter or lead may occur into the neural foramen, resulting in nerve root irritation and the development of radicular symptoms.[8] Intrathecal catheter or SCS lead migration into the spinal cord is possible and may occur without the production of pain. In addition, intraparachymal placement of a catheter or lead is possible during surgical implantation. Good surgical technique during anchoring to the fascia and careful placement of needles with multiplanar fluoroscopy must be used by the surgeon.

10. Fracture of SCS leads appears to be more common in paddle leads, likely because of increased tension from the inability of the paddle to move when force is applied. Placement of a relaxing loop of the lead wires distal to the anchors is advisable and may reduce the tension forces on the paddle lead wires.

11. Improperly anchored pump reservoirs and impulse generators can result in device flipping, which can lead to inability to program or use the SCS system or to access the reservoir for refills.

12. Hardware erosion of leads, anchors, catheters, reservoirs, or generators through the skin can lead to infectious complications that necessitate the removal of the implant or an extensive revision.

13. Finally, patients with a properly functioning SCS with parethesias in the painful areas and normal impedance numbers may experience loss of pain relief.

Risk Reduction Strategies

1. Patients who are on medications that alter hemostasis, including platelet function, must discontinue these medications according to current published guidelines, with consent of the prescribing physician, before undergoing implantation of a neuromodulation device.[13] In patients who are unable to discontinue anticoagulation therapy, such as cancer patients with conditions that are hypercoaguable, may be considered for inpatient heparin infusion before surgery. This allows for limited discontinuation of anticoagulation therapy before the implantation operation and reduces, but does not eliminate, the chance of serious sequelae.

2. Perioperative antibiotics should be given at least 30 minutes before incision. Although the use of preoperative antibiotics is considered controversial by some physicians, most experienced implanters consider perioperative antibiotics standard of care. Infectious complications are further reduced with use of extensive preparation with wide draping and careful attention to standard sterile surgical techniques. Physicians with limited surgical training should be mentored by more experienced physicians before performing invasive surgical procedures. All surgical wounds should be irrigated copiously with antibiotic containing irrigation. Proper wound closure techniques are critical to prevention of infection. Patients should be seen within the first postoperative week to allow for early detection of infection, which may present with signs such as rubor, drainage, or painful incisions. Patients with these findings should be considered for incision and drainage to prevent the development serious infections that necessitate the removal of the implanted device. If the infection extends into the pocket or posterior spinal incision, the device must be explanted and an infectious disease consultation should be considered.

3. Neurologic injury can be minimized by educating the patient about movement during the surgical procedure and maintaining anesthetic levels that allow for patient cooperation without disinhibition. Proper patient positioning and fluoroscopic alignment of the spine are critical to correct needle placement. In patients who are unable to tolerate extended periods in the prone or lateral decubitus positions, referral to a spine surgeon should be considered.

4. The risk of dural puncture during SCS implantation can be minimized with use of a paramedian approach with a needle entry angle of less than 45 degrees. In addition, the use of both the hanging drop and loss resistance techniques with lateral fluoroscopic views can reduce the risk of inadvertent dural puncture.

5. Patients who have radiographic evidence of moderate to severe stenosis should be approached with caution before a trial of SCS or permanent implantation procedure. Progression of the stenosis may result in neurologic injury, especially with the addition of leads in a tight stenotic space. Consideration should be given to surgical referral for decompression and paddle lead placement. Caution is also warranted in patients with stenosis who undergo intrathecal catheter placement.

6. Seroma formation occurs as a result of inadequate hemostasis and can lead to disastrous complications, including loss of the implanted device. Although aspiration of a suspected seroma with analysis can help the physician rule out infection, careful attention to avoiding contamination of the wound must be used. Meticulous surgical technique with careful dissection and judicious use of electrocautery can reduce the risk of seroma formation. Some physicians routinely perform the generator or reservoir dissection before placing the leads or catheter and pack the wound with antibiotic-soaked sponges to allow time for tamponade of venous and arterial bleeding.

7. Pain at the generator or reservoir site can lead to patient requests for explantation. Careful planning of

the implantation site should take into consideration the patient's body habitus, location of the ilium and ribs, and placement of the away from the belt line and avoiding placement too low in the buttock. The device should be placed several centimeters below the dermis, and intramuscular placement should be avoided if at all possible. Newer devices that are significantly smaller have allowed the implantation site to be closer to the spinal incision and will likely decrease the number of revisions necessary as a result of painful device pockets.

8. Loss of paresthesia with SCS can occur over time for reasons that are not well understood. Reprogramming with a change in lead arrays, amplitudes, and pulse widths may restore paresthesias in the painful areas. In addition, the impedances of the leads should be determined through interrogation of the impulse generator. If high impedances are found, the physician may need to perform a revision or consider referral to a spine surgeon for paddle lead placement. Imaging studies should be obtained to assess for lead migration before surgical revision is considered.

9. Lead and catheter migration are often related to improper surgical techniques, either involving the anchor or the angle of needle placement. The anchors must be secured to the underlying fascia and ligaments, and in the case of SCS leads, the anchor must be secured to the leads. Needle insertion should be accomplished with a paramedian approach with an angle less than 45 degrees. Although some physicians advocate bracing, limitation of activity, and restrictions on motion, these recommendations have never been proven to be effective in a prospective fashion.

10. Migration of catheters and leads smf fracture can be avoided with use of a needle insertion angle of less than 45 degrees and placement of strain relief loops both in the spinal incision and under the implantable device.

11. Flipping of the implantable device can be minimized by securing the device to the fascia in the pocket with nonabsorbable suture. In addition, a properly sized pocket helps to prevent this complication by eliminating excess space.

12. Erosion of leads, anchors, or the implantable device may occur over time and is more common in patients with chronic disease and in patients who experience significant weight loss or gain. Erosion can be minimized with placement of the device in the subcutaneous tissue below the dermis with adequate tissue to protect the device from pressure. The risk of erosion is higher in patients who undergo peripheral stimulation, particularly in the scalp regions. Silastic anchors appear particularly prone to erosion in areas with little subcutaneous tissue, and some physicians advocate use of suture instead of these anchors.

13. The development of tolerance or severe side effects to intrathecal medications may be unavoidable even with opioid rotation and the addition of adjunct medications. Granuloma formation may necessitate removal of the device if reduction of the medication fails to resolve the inflammatory mass.

14. Loss of stimulation may occur from many factors, such as migration and fibrosis. Even in the presence of adequate stimulation in the painful areas, some patients may eventually lose pain relief and ultimately need explantation. Reprogramming may resolve some cases of loss of pain relief with the SCS. Surgical revision with paddle leads may be an option in some patients, particularly in the case of fibrosis and high impedance. However, some patients are not amenable to revision and reprogramming and ultimately need removal of the device. Neuromodulation is highly effective but may not provide permanent pain relief in all patients, despite heroic physician attempts.

Conclusion

Neuromodulation is a highly effective treatment in carefully selected patients with chronic pain. The devices continue to improve, with smaller generators with greater numbers of contacts and newer technologies that allow for greater precision in placement. Miniaturization has allowed an expanded role of SCS and will continue to lead to new treatment options in many patients. Although intrathecal drug delivery is used less commonly because of the increased efficacy of spinal cord sand peripheral stimulation, it is a viable treatment option in refractory cases. The physician must understand and identify the risks associated with these devices and treat them aggressively to prevent permanent neurologic sequelae.

References

Full references for this chapter can be found on www.expertconsult.com.

Part F

Advanced Pain Management Techniques

Neuroadenolysis of the Pituitary

Steven D. Waldman

History

Surgery has been used to palliate pain from hormone-dependent tumors since the late 1800s. Early surgical efforts were directed primarily at surgical castration.[1] The addition of adrenalectomy followed, as the importance of this gland in the secretion of sex hormones became better understood.[2] Advances in the field of endocrinology in the 1950s led to an increasing focus on the pituitary gland. To this end, transcranial hypophysectomy was performed in an effort to induce regression of hormone-dependent tumors and to palliate symptoms. Investigators became aware that pain relief was a more consistent finding than actual tumor regression.[3]

Unfortunately, transcranial hypophysectomy was a major procedure with significant surgical risk that precluded its use in many of the patients who could most benefit, namely, patients with advanced malignant disease. Consequently, less invasive means of pituitary destruction were undertaken. These attempts included radiation therapy, implantation of radon seeds, and, ultimately, chemical neurolysis of the pituitary.[4]

Neuroadenolysis of the pituitary (NALP) was first described by Moricca in 1958 as a technique to relieve pain of malignant origin with placement of multiple needles into the pituitary gland and then injection of small amounts of absolute alcohol.[5] Moricca's early reports led other investigators to adopt and modify this procedure. To date, more than 14,000 patients with intractable pain have been treated with NALP.[6]

Indications and Contraindications

Indications for NALP are summarized in **Table 177.1**.

NALP is an appropriate treatment for patients with bilateral facial or upper body cancer pain, bilateral diffuse cancer pain, intractable visceral pain, or pain from compression of neural structures after all antiblastic methods and other analgesic measures have been exhausted. When medical hormonal control of pain no longer works, patients may also benefit from the procedure.[4] Most investigators observe better results in patients whose pain is the result of hormone-dependent tumors, although the procedure is also effective for palliation of pain from hormone-unresponsive malignant diseases.[7] Contraindications to neuroadenolysis of the pituitary are summarized in **Table 177.2** Local infection, sepsis, coagulopathy, significantly increased intracranial pressure, and empty sella syndrome are absolute contraindications to NALP.[4,7] Relative contraindications to NALP include poor anesthesia risk, disulfiram therapy, and significant behavioral abnormalities. Obviously, because of the desperate circumstances of most patients considered for NALP, the risk-benefit ratio is shifted toward performing the procedure on both ethical and humanitarian grounds.

Clinically Relevant Anatomy and Technique

In an effort to improve on Moricca's original technique, Corssen et al[8] and other investigators modified it by decreasing the number of needles used. Levin et al[9] further modified the technique with use of a stereotactic head frame. Attempting to reduce the incidence of postoperative cerebrospinal fluid (CSF) leakage, these investigators suggested initial placement of an 18-gauge, 6-inch spinal needle through the floor of the sphenoidal sinus. The needle was then removed, and a smaller, 20-gauge, 6-inch spinal needle was placed through the hole left by the 18-gauge needle. The 20-gauge needle was then advanced into the sella turcica. On occasion, these investigators found it necessary to drill through the floor of the

Table 177.1 Indications for Neuroadenolysis of the Pituitary

Failure of all antiblastic treatments

Failure of all other appropriate pain-relieving measures

Bilateral facial or upper body cancer pain

Bilateral diffuse cancer pain

Intractable visceral pain

Pain from compression of neural structures

Loss of hormonal control of pain

Table 177.2 Contraindications to Neuroadenolysis of the Pituitary

Local infection

Sepsis

Coagulopathy

Increased intracranial pressure

Empty sella syndrome

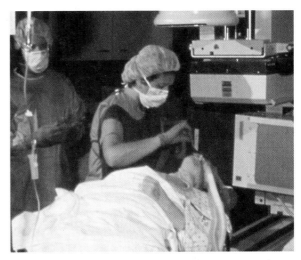

Fig. 177.1 The nose is packed to provide vasoconstriction and mucosal shrinkage.

sella turcica with a Kirschner wire because the needle would not pass through dense bone. They also noted the occasional occurrence of CSF leakage until they instituted the injection of ethyl alpha cyanomethacrylate resin through the spinal needles.

Waldman and Feldstein[10] further modified NALP with use of a needle-through-needle technique, thus eliminating the need for the stereotactic frame or drilling. These modifications made the procedure more suitable for use in the community hospital.

Phenol, cryoneurolysis, radiofrequency lesioning, and electrical stimulation in place of alcohol all have been advocated for NALP.[11–13] More experience is needed with each of these modalities to determine whether some of the theoretic advantages and disadvantages of each modification translate into clinically relevant benefits.

Preoperative Preparation

Screening laboratory tests, consisting of a complete blood cell count, chemistry profile, electrolyte determination, urinalysis, coagulation profile, chest radiography, and electrocardiography, are performed as for any other patient undergoing general anesthesia. Anteroposterior and lateral skull films are also obtained to evaluate the size and relative position of the sella turcica and to rule out sphenoidal sinus infection, which may be clinically silent.[4,10]

Preoperative treatment of all patients with an intravenous dose of a cephalosporin and aminoglycoside antibiotic 1 hour before induction of anesthesia is indicated to reduce the risk of infection in these immunocompromised patients.[10] Most investigators perform NALP with the patient under general endotracheal anesthesia, although because the procedure is relatively painless, it can be performed with local anesthesia.[14] Opioids are avoided before and during the operation to avoid pupillary miosis, which might obscure the pupillary dilatation

observed when alcohol spills out of the sella onto the oculomotor nerve (see subsequent discussion).[7,10]

Technique

With the patient intubated in the supine position on a biplanar fluoroscopy table, the nose is packed with pledgets soaked in 7.5% cocaine solution to provide vasoconstriction and shrinkage of the nasal mucosa (**Fig. 177.1**). After 10 minutes, the packs are removed and the anterior nasal mucosa and face are prepared with povidone-iodine solution. Sterile drapes are placed over the nose and face. The anterior medial mucosa and deep tissues are infiltrated with a solution of 1.0% lidocaine and 1:200,000 epinephrine. During infiltration and subsequent needle placement, care must be taken to avoid Kesselback's plexus, lest vigorous bleeding ensue. The head must be kept precisely in the midline to allow accurate needle placement.

A 17-gauge, 3.5-inch spinal needle with the stylet in place is advanced with biplanar fluoroscopic guidance, with care taken to ensure that the needle remains exactly in the midline to avoid trauma to the adjacent structures, including the carotid arteries (**Fig. 177.2**). The needle is advanced until its tip rests against the anterior wall of the sella turcica (**Fig. 177.3**). At this point, plain radiographs are taken to confirm the needle position (**Fig. 177.4**). After satisfactory positioning is verified, the stylet is removed from the 17-gauge needle. A 20-gauge, 13-cm styleted Hinck needle (Cook Incorporated, Bloomington, Ind) is placed through the 17-gauge needle and is carefully advanced through the anterior wall of the sella turcica (**Fig. 177.5**). This process feels like passing a needle through an eggshell. The Hinck needle is then further advanced with biplanar fluoroscopic guidance through the substance of the pituitary gland, until the tip rests against the posterior wall of the sella turcica (**Fig. 177.6**). Needle position is again confirmed with plain radiographs (**Fig. 177.7**).

The patient's eyes are then exposed, and alcohol in aliquots of 0.2 mL is injected as the Hinck needle is gradually withdrawn back through the pituitary gland (**Fig. 177.8**). Depending on the size of the sella, a total of 4 to 6 mL of alcohol is injected. During the injection process, the pupils are constantly monitored for dilation. Pupillary dilation indicates

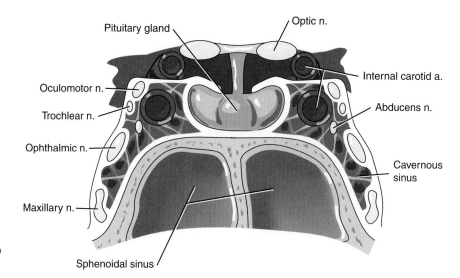

Fig. 177.2 Lateral view of the sphenoidal sinus, sella turcica, and pituitary and of the relationship of the carotid arteries and oculomotor nerve.

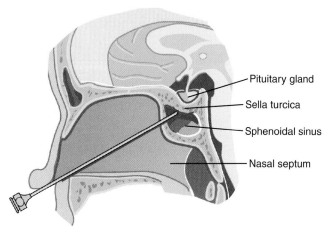

Fig. 177.3 Drawing of lateral view of the needle trajectory with the tip of a 17-gauge, 3.5-inch spinal needle against the anterior wall of the sella turcica.

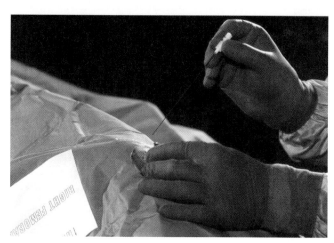

Fig. 177.5 A 20-gauge, 13-cm Hinck needle is introduced through the 17-gauge needle.

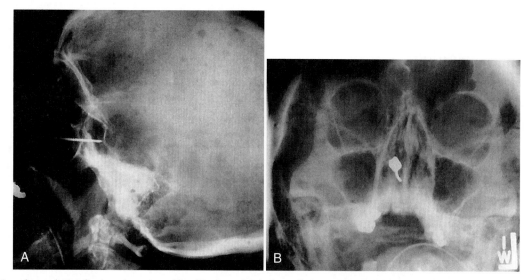

Fig. 177.4 Plain radiographs confirming placement of the 17-gauge, 3.5-inch needle in a midline position with the tip resting against the anterior wall of the sella turcica. **A,** Lateral view. **B,** Anteroposterior view. (From Waldman SD, editor: Interventional pain management, ed 2, Philadelphia, 2001, Saunders, p 679.)

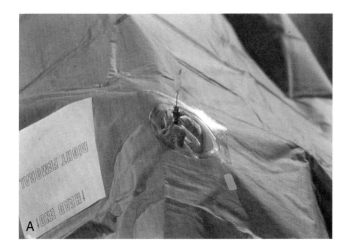

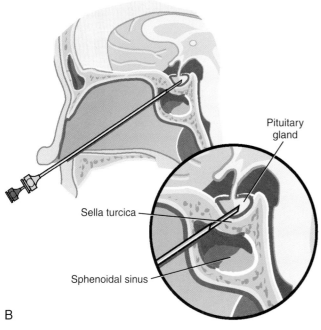

Fig. 177.6 A, The Hinck needle has been placed through the 17-gauge needle, and the Hinck needle's tip is resting against the posterior wall of the sella turcica. B, Drawing of a lateral view of the needle trajectory with the tip of the 17-gauge spinal needle against the anterior wall of the sella turcica and the Hinck needle through it into the substance of the pituitary.

Pituitary gland

Sella turcica

Sphenoidal sinus

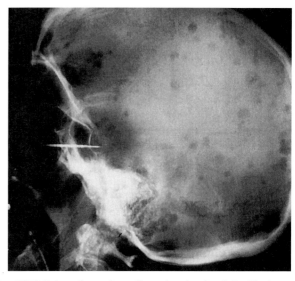

Fig. 177.7 Plain radiograph confirms that the tip of the Hinck needle is resting against the posterior wall of the sella turcica. (From Waldman SD, editor: Interventional pain management, ed 2, Philadelphia, 2001, Saunders, p 680.)

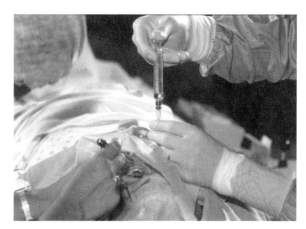

Fig. 177.8 The patient's eyes are exposed, and 0.2-mL aliquots of alcohol are injected as the Hinck needle is gradually withdrawn.

that the alcohol has spilled outside the sella turcica and has come in contact with an oculomotor nerve. If pupillary dilatation is observed, injection of alcohol is discontinued and the needle is withdrawn to a more anterior position. The injection process then resumes. In most instances, if the alcohol injection is discontinued at the first sign of pupillary dilation, any resultant visual disturbance is transitory.[15] Monitoring with visual evoked responses during alcohol injection has been suggested as a more sensitive test for visual complications than pupillary dilation.[4]

After the injection of alcohol is completed, 0.5 mL of cyanomethacrylate resin is injected via the Hinck needle to seal the hole in the sella turcica and to prevent CSF leakage. Both needles are removed. The nasal mucosa is observed for bleeding or CSF leakage. Nasal packing is not generally necessary

with this modified procedure. The patient is then extubated and taken to the recovery room. Approximately 30 minutes is needed to perform NALP.

Postoperative Care

All patients are continued on antibiotics for 24 hours. Endocrine replacement, consisting of 15 mg of prednisone and 0.15 mg of levothyroxine sodium (Synthroid) every morning, is necessary for every patient.[10]

Accurate monitoring of intake and output is mandatory because transient diabetes insipidus occurs in approximately 40% of patients undergoing NALP.[16] In most instances, the diabetes insipidus is self limited, but vasopressin administration should be considered for patients who are unable to drink as much as they excrete or whose urinary output exceeds 2.5 L/day.[4] Failure to identify and treat diabetes insipidus is the leading cause of morbidity and mortality in patients who undergo NALP.

All patients are continued on preoperative levels of oral narcotics for 24 hours, and then doses are tapered. Patients generally resume their normal diet and activities the day of the procedure.

Mechanisms of Pain Relief

Levin and Ramirez[15] and Bonica[7] have reviewed the proposed mechanisms of pain relief after NALP. Early investigators centered their theories on the concept of pain relief from elimination of the pituitary hormones responsible for enhancement of nociceptive transmission. Later, Yanagida et al[11] suggested that pain appears to be independent of the extent of pituitary damage and may be caused by reactionary hyperactivity of the hypophyseal system exerting inhibitory influences on the pain pathways of the brain. In spite of extensive research, the exact mechanism of pain relief after NALP remains unclear, as does whether the procedure produces pain relief by neurodestruction or neuroaugmentation.[13]

Results

Incidence of Pain Relief

In 1990, Bonica[7] reviewed the world literature on NALP and summarized the data and conclusions. The world literature suggests a success rate (pain relief rated complete to good) of approximately 63%. An additional 23% of patients described their pain relief as fair. Fourteen percent of patients reported poor to no relief of pain after NALP. A closer look at this patient population reveals that patients with hormone-dependent tumors experienced better pain relief than did those with non–hormone-dependent tumors.[7] Furthermore, investigators who injected larger volumes of alcohol (4 to 6 mL) or who repeated NALP when the first procedure was not successful appeared to obtain better results in terms of pain relief. In spite of the inherent limitations of analyzing data from multiple studies, NALP is obviously an effective treatment for certain patients with cancer pain.[7,10,17,18]

Complications

Complications directly related to NALP are summarized in **Table 177.3**. Virtually all patients who undergo NALP have a bilateral frontal headache that resolves spontaneously within 24 to 48 hours.[10] Diabetes insipidus develops in approximately 40% of patients who undergo the procedure. Approximately 35% of patients experience transient temperature increases up to 1.5°C (35°F) after NALP.[10,16] These temperature

Table 177.3 Complications of Neuroadenolysis of the Pituitary

Bilateral frontal headache
Diabetes insipidus
Abnormal temperature regulation
Increased pulmonary secretion
Ocular disturbances

aberrations are attributed to disturbance of the temperature-regulating mechanism of the hypothalamus.[10] About 20% of patients experience an increase in pulmonary secretions and mild orthopnea that clinically resembles congestive heart failure.[10] This problem is self limited if careful attention is paid to the patient's fluid status. This phenomenon has been postulated to be centrally mediated. Although the potential exists for serious ocular disturbances, a review of the literature suggests that transient visual disturbances, including diplopia, blurred vision, and loss of visual field, occur in fewer than 10% of patients who undergo neuroadenolysis of the pituitary gland.[4,7,16] Permanent visual disturbances occur much less often, with an average incidence rate of approximately 5%.[4,7,10,16] CSF leakage, infection, and pituitary hemorrhage develop in fewer than 1% of patients reported but are some of the most devastating complications. If they are not recognized immediately and treated, death can result.[4,7,10]

Conclusion

Neuroadenolysis of the pituitary gland is a safe, effective method for palliating diffuse cancer pain that does not respond to conservative treatment modalities. Its technical simplicity and relative safety make NALP an ideal procedure for cancer patients who have undergone a vast array of treatments. Although spinal administration of opioids has replaced NALP as the procedure of choice for many cancer pain syndromes, many cancer pain specialists believe that NALP is still underutilized today.[19] With the needle-through-needle modification described, a more favorable risk-benefit ratio is expected. As Bonica[7] has stated, "NALP is one of the most, if not the most, effective ablative procedures for the relief of severe diffuse cancer pain."

References

Full references for this chapter can be found on www.expertconsult.com.

Radiofrequency Lesioning

Richard M. Rosenthal

Radiofrequency (RF) current is used in pain medicine to make discrete therapeutic lesions in various targets throughout the nervous system.[1-6] The technique is most frequently used to block nociceptive signals from reaching the central nervous system and thereby anesthetize the source of the pain.[2] RF is implemented percutaneously by means of an insulated needle with a metal active tip that is placed in the appropriate nerve pathway. Current is then applied such that it alters the function of the nerve and blocks transmission of the painful signal.[1] Although RF current does not treat the cause of pain, its palliative effect allows the patient to return to normal daily activities and to function without pain. When appropriately applied to well-selected patients, RF current can produce profound, lasting analgesia sufficient to reverse the deleterious effects of chronic pain on the life of the patient. These effects include sleeplessness, mood disturbance, social isolation, loss of employment, and occa-

sionally loss of life. Before the introduction of modern RF equipment, various techniques (e.g., cryosurgery and chemical neurolysis) were used in an attempt to produce localized nervous system lesions; however, none have been as widely used or are as effective as RF.[6,7]

The use of electricity to treat pain was first described in 1931, when direct current was applied to the gasserian ganglion for the treatment of trigeminal neuralgia.[4,8] However, use of direct current was abandoned because it produced lesions of inconsistent size and was associated with complications. High-frequency alternating current was then introduced as a method of producing lesions of a predictable size.[9] Soon thereafter, temperature monitoring was found to enhance further the ability to make reliable, consistent lesions. Because the frequencies used (350 to 500 kHz) were also used in radio transmitters, the procedure was termed *radiofrequency*.[5] Today, the frequency used by modern RF machines (just below the AM band) is assigned by the Federal Communications Commission to prevent interference with radio transmissions.

The first reported use of RF current in the management of pain focused on percutaneous lateral cordotomy to treat malignant pain.[9] The first use for nonmalignant pain began in the 1970s for treatment of trigeminal neuralgia.[3,10] At approximately this time, Cosman and Cosman introduced an RF machine that had voltage and time settings and was also capable of monitoring temperature, impedance, and current.[11,12] Shealy[13] reported the first use of RF current for the treatment of spinal pain. He described a method of treating pain from the zygapophyseal joints (commonly referred to as facet joints or z-joints) by targeting the medial branch. Later, a modified technique was published after anatomic dissections indicated that the electrode placements described in the original paper were not actually on the medial branch.[2,14] Uematsu[11] used RF to treat radicular pain by targeting the dorsal root ganglion (DRG). His use of a large (14-gauge) electrode to heat the DRG to 75°C (167°F) resulted in nearly complete destruction of the ganglion and severe deafferent pain sequelae.[5] Because these early uses of RF for pain treatment had poor outcomes, the technique failed to gain acceptance.[3]

The widespread use of RF current for the treatment of spinal pain began in 1980, when Sluijter and Metha introduced a 22-gauge cannula through which a thermocouple probe could be inserted.[3,5] The smaller electrode meant that the procedure could be performed percutaneously on a conscious patient without causing much discomfort. This development was important because it allowed the patient to be monitored for complications. Shortly after the introduction of the Sluijter-Metha cannula (SMK) needle, a series of studies was published on the use of RF current for the treatment of facet joint pain, diskogenic pain, sacroiliac (SI) joint pain, and sympathetically mediated pain.[3,15–23] RF lesioning has since been found to be target specific, safe, and effective for the treatment of pain, and it has supplanted the use of other neurolytics (particularly chemical neurolytics), largely because of the highly focused nature of RF lesions.

This chapter is clinically focused to provide the pain practitioner with the means to treat patients. It provides an overview of the RF lesion generator and the two different types of RF lesions, continuous and pulsed. It also updates the reader on the use of RF lesioning for the most common and well-studied procedures and describes the latest, most effective methodology, based on current scientific literature and clinical experience. For example, it presents new methods of performing RF for older procedures, such as the lumbar RF procedure. RF has many other uses in varying stages of development that will expand the use of the modality in the future.

Radiofrequency Lesion Generator

An RF lesion generator is a device used to produce lesions in the nervous system or other tissue by the direct application of high-frequency current to selected sites (**Fig. 178.1**). A typical RF lesion generator has the following systems: continuous impedance monitoring; nerve stimulation; monitoring of voltage, current, and temperature; and pulsed current delivery mode.[5,6] The current flows from the electrode tip through the body to a dispersive grounding electrode. RF current alternates at a very high frequency (approximately 500 kHz). The energy is focused around the active tip of the electrode and activates charged molecules (mainly proteins) to oscillate with the rapid changes in alternating current. This produces friction in the tissue that causes heat formation directly around the active

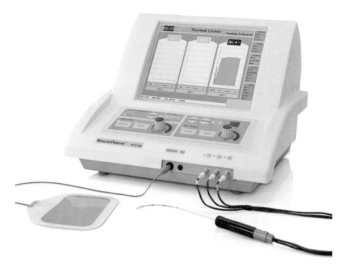

Fig. 178.1 **Image of a radiofrequency generator.**

tip. Heat is generated as a result of ionic oscillations of the charged molecules in the tissue, rather than direct heating of the electrode element itself. The formation of heat is greatest around the active tip, where the current density is largest. The grounding electrode serves to complete the circuit and to disperse heat buildup, thereby preventing a burn of the skin.[2]

RF energy can be applied as either continuous or pulsed current. Continuous RF current heats the tissue surrounding the electrode and lyses the targeted nerve. On a pathologic level, continuous RF current heats nerve fibers and results in wallerian degeneration.[24–27] On a physiologic level, continuous RF current destroys all fiber types within a nerve and is not selective for any one fiber type.[2,28,29]

Pulsed RF (PRF) was introduced in 1998. This method delivers RF current in small bursts and thus prevents the accumulation of heat around the electrode. The exact mechanism of action is not currently understood.[1,3] One of the prevailing theories postulates that the electrical field generated during a PRF procedure reversibly disrupts the transmission of impulses across small unmyelinated fibers and causes a blockade of pain signals.[1,30–32]

Continuous Impedance Monitoring

When heat lesions are made in the continuous RF mode, impedance monitoring is primarily used to confirm continuity of the electrical circuit. However, in the pulsed mode, impedance monitoring is more crucial because the strength of the electrical field is decreased when impedance is high. Thus, high impedance can reduce the efficacy of the procedure and may be a cause of treatment failure. Typically, impedance varies from 200 to 800 ohms during an RF lesion and is greatly affected by density of the tissues in which the active tip is placed. For example, impedance is high when an electrode is placed in densely packed tissue (e.g., scar tissue), whereas it is low when an electrode is placed inside a blood vessel. Both impedance and current should be noted and monitored during the creation of PRF lesions.

Nerve Stimulation

Nerve stimulation is important for both the continuous RF and the PRF modes. The two types of stimulation are sensory and motor. Sensory stimulation occurs at 50 Hz and is used to determine the distance between the electrode and the targeted nerve fiber. The minimum sensory threshold (i.e., the minimum voltage required to produce an electrical discharge of the nerve) is directly related to the distance from the nerve fiber.[5,33] Thus, sensory stimulation can be used to determine the accuracy of needle placement. This is more important in the pulsed mode than in the continuous mode, as discussed later in the chapter. Motor stimulation occurs at 2 Hz and is used to determine whether a needle is placed too close to motor fibers, typically the ventral rami of the spinal nerve root during the medial branch procedure. This type of stimulation is recommended to avoid unintended damage to neural structures.

Monitoring of Temperature, Voltage, and Current

Temperature monitoring facilitates generation of a discrete, controlled lesion of predictable size. Voltage monitoring and current monitoring are of secondary importance when producing a heat lesion, because they are automatically adjusted in accordance with the temperature setting. However, in the pulsed mode, both impedance and current are important, given that the strength of the electrical field is thought to be critical to producing the desired effect.

Voltage, impedance, and current output are related as described in the equation $V = IR$, where V is voltage, I is current, and R is impedance (defined as the electrical resistance in an alternating current circuit). Both voltage and impedance can be regulated during generation of a pulsed lesion; voltage output is adjusted using the generator; and impedance can be decreased by injection of saline solution. The goal is to adjust these variables to produce a current of approximately 200 mA. Temperature is of secondary importance, as long as it remains lower than neurolytic levels (45°C [113°F]).[34]

Sensory stimulation is helpful for two reasons. First, limited evidence indicates that increasing the proximity between the electrode and the targeted nerve can increase the duration of the effect. Second, sensory stimulation levels of less than 0.05 V are thought to indicate intraneural placement.

Types of Radiofrequency Lesioning

Figure 178.2 provides images monopolar, bipolar, and PRF lesions.

Continuous Lesioning

The heat generated in the continuous mode causes tissue coagulation in a small, discrete oval surrounding the active tip of the electrode. The largest area of damage is around the long axis of the electrode; very little energy extends distal to the tip. Therefore, to coagulate the largest area of nerve fibers reliably, the electrode must be positioned parallel to the nerve. In addition, because the area of coagulation is quite small (heat diminishes rapidly as the distance from the electrode tip increases), the electrode must be placed directly on the nerve to guarantee neurolysis. If the electrode is as much as one electrode width away from the nerve, it will fail to coagulate the nerve completely.[2,3]

Continuous RF energy causes nonselective thermal damage to the offending nerve. The size of the lesion depends on several factors:

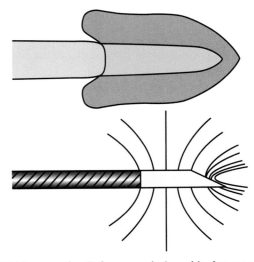

Fig. 178.2 **Images of radiofrequency lesions: bipolar, monopolar, and pulsed.**

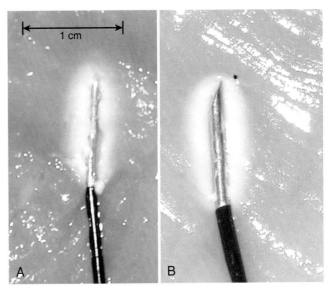

Fig. 178.3 **Image of radiofrequency lesions in meat.** A, A 20-gauge needle. B, An 18-gauge needle. *(Courtesy of Paul Dreyfuss.)*

- Tissue temperature: The volume of the lesion expands in direct proportion to the temperature surrounding the electrode, up to a maximum temperature of 90°C (194°F).[2] Temperatures higher than 90°C (194°F) risk charring of tissues, which can cause cavitation and possible sterile abscess formation.[35] In a meat model, one can observe the increased lesion size as temperatures are increased (**Fig. 178.3**).[28]
- Duration of coagulation: The volume of the lesion grows over time until it reaches its maximal size at approximately 90 seconds, after which time the lesion is stable (**Fig. 178.4**). At 60 seconds, the lesion reaches 94% of the size attained at 90 seconds. Therefore, the optimal duration of coagulation is between 60 and 90 seconds.[2]
- Gauge of electrode and length and gauge of active electrode tip: Larger-gauge electrodes and longer active tips produce a larger lesion.[5,36]

The foregoing discussion is clinically relevant. According to the guidelines of the International Spine Intervention Society (ISIS), efficacy is maximized when needle placement

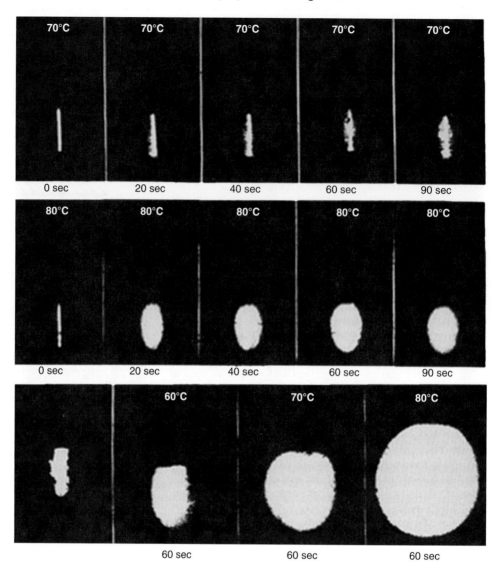

Fig. 178.4 Lesion time versus size and lesion temperature versus size.

is anatomically precise, when larger (e.g., 18- to 20-gauge) needles are used, and when multiple parallel lesions are generated (within one needle width from each other) to account for the variable nerve topography.[2] Larger lesions are created using higher temperatures, larger-gauge needles, and longer lesion times (i.e., up to 90 seconds).[28] A 60- to 90-second lesion time, at a temperature of 85°C (185°F) to 90°C (194°F) in the cervical spine and 90°C (194°F) in the lumbar spine, is recommended.

Heat decreases rapidly as the distance from the electrode tip increases. The average size of a lesion is no more than 1.6 to 2.3 electrode widths.[2] For the greatest benefit, two lesions should be made one electrode width from each other. If electrodes are positioned as little as two electrode widths away from each other or from the targeted nerve, incomplete lesioning may occur, resulting in neuritis and possibly therapeutic failure.[2] For that reason, larger, 18-gauge electrodes were developed to improve the chance of incorporating the nerve in the lesion and are recommended for use when making heat lesions.[2,37] Electrodes placed perpendicular rather than parallel to the nerve may also result in incomplete coagulation and shorter duration of relief.[2,28]

Pulsed Lesioning

In addition to generating heat, the current from RF energy also produces an intense electrical field. The therapeutic effect of PRF lesioning is thought to be the result of the electrical field, rather than of the thermal effects.[1,3]

The concept that tissue destruction was the means by which RF current produced its effect was reevaluated in light of certain findings that were inconsistent with this theory.[3–5,24,31,32,38–52] First, it was known that heat produced its effect by causing a lesion between the nociceptive focus and the central nervous system; however, Sluijter[46] had noticed that electrodes placed distally to the nociceptive focus seemed to produce a therapeutic effect. For example, treatment of radicular pain by heating the DRG seemed to produce a therapeutic effect even though the heat is applied distal to the nociceptive focus (the spinal nerve root). Second, Sluijter noticed that heat lesioning of the DRG produced only transient sensory loss, whereas pain relief lasted much longer. Finally, the role of heat was questioned when Slappendel et al[40] published a report that showed no differences in outcome when two different tip temperatures (40°C [104°F] and 67°C

[153°F]) were applied to the cervical DRG for chronic cervical radicular pain. Each of these arguments has since been brought into question. At that time, however, it seemed reasonable to attempt to deliver RF energy in a manner that did not result in the production of heat. These observations provided supporting evidence that led to the development of the PRF procedure.

The aim of PRF is to create intense electrical fields while keeping the temperature lower than neurolytic levels. This is done by delivering short bursts of energy (20 milliseconds) twice per second, followed by a quiet phase (lasting 480 milliseconds) during which no current is applied. This approach allows for heat dissipation, thus keeping the tissue temperature lower than the neurodestructive threshold of 45°C (113°F).[3] Studies in homogeneous nerve tissue suggested that irreversible conduction block occurs at temperatures greater than 45°C (113°F) to 50°C (122°F).[53-55]

Pulsing the current also allows a substantial increase in the power output of the generator. Voltage in the continuous mode is 15 to 25 V, compared with 45 V in the pulsed mode.[5] Because the electric field is strongest at the tip of the electrode, it is recommended that electrodes be placed perpendicular, rather than parallel, to the targeted nerve during creation of a PRF lesion.

PRF was originally thought to be a totally nondestructive procedure. However, experimental work indicated that this may not be the case.[38,56-58] PRF current appears to have both thermal and nonthermal effects. The thermal effects of PRF were first elucidated by Cosman and Cosman,[38] when they noticed heat spikes produced during the 20-millisecond active phase of a PRF current. It is not known whether these brief elevations in temperature have a biologic effect. A mild ablative effect in an in vitro model has also been described, but its significance in a biologic system is unknown.[38,56-58]

The nonthermal effects may be attributed to an effect on the function of voltage-gated ion channels. Central nervous system effects also appear to be direct results of the RF current.[43,45]

Convention holds that the word *lesion* should not be used when referring to a PRF procedure. However, as noted earlier, Cosman and Cosman observed heat bursts with temperatures in the neurodestructive range in a thin layer of tissue immediately surrounding the electrode.[38] Experimental evidence also indicates that PRF results in cellular damage that appears to be more pronounced for C fibers.[56,57] In a study by Erdine et al,[56] electron microscopy showed physical evidence of ultrastructural damage following exposure to PRF. Although the clinical significance of these findings is unknown, this evidence would dispute the currently held belief that PRF does not cause a lesion. *Lesion* is defined as "a localized pathologic change in a bodily organ or tissue." Sluijter and van Kleef[59] believed that a PRF procedure clearly meets this criterion. In this chapter, the word lesion is used when referring to a PRF procedure.

PRF lesioning is traditionally considered safer than continuous RF because it has no reported neurologic side effects. However, Rosenthal has direct knowledge of a case in which vocal cord paralysis lasting approximately 6 months was induced by a brief delivery of PRF current during a C3 DRG procedure. This suggests that PRF may indeed cause temporary nerve damage and supports the contention that PRF does in fact produce a lesion. However, in most cases, PRF current

delivery is a safe method of creating nervous system lesions, because no similar case reports have been published.

Although PRF does create a small lesion around the active tip, that cannot completely account for the clinical effects observed. Unfortunately, no single theory fully explains the observed effects. Despite evidence of a mild ablative effect, the current belief is that the electric field is responsible for the clinical effect. Rather than producing local effects surrounding the electrode, as with continuous RF, PRF seems to produce its effect proximal to the point where energy is applied. Indeed, changes within the central nervous system have been observed in response to PRF energy.

When PRF energy is applied to the DRG, it induces changes in gene expression within the dorsal horn of the spinal cord. The rapidly alternating current alters pain transmission by activation of a protein called C-Fos. On a cellular level, animal studies showed that exposure of the DRG to PRF current causes both early and late bilateral induction of the protein C-Fos in layers 1 and 2 of the dorsal horn. These effects are not temperature dependent and seem to occur as a result of current fluctuations, rather than tissue heating.[3,4,24,38,42,43,45,46,49,50] Other proteins are also produced in response to PRF current, although it remains unclear whether any of these changes are responsible for the observed therapeutic effect.[49,50] In addition, investigators believe that strong electrical fields alter the nerve cell membranes and thus affect nerve transmission. This theory is supported by evidence showing that PRF induces changes in synaptic transmission and causes electroporation.[46,50]

The use of the pulsed mode in clinical practice has been slow to gain widespread acceptance. The reason may be the paucity of evidence showing a clear therapeutic advantage over placebo during the early years of its use. However, since 2005 several studies have demonstrated an advantage over placebo.

The role of PRF in clinical practice has been an issue of debate. Some investigators have argued that it is unnecessary because of the availability of continuous RF, which appears to be effective according to well-designed studies. Although this argument is true for treatment of medial branches, it is not relevant when considering the use of RF current for the treatment of radiculopathies and painful peripheral neuropathies. For both these chronic and painful conditions, pain practitioners currently have little to offer these patients. When one considers the benign nature of this treatment and its possibility of real relief, little reason exists not to offer PRF as a therapeutic option. It would appear that the best use for this modality is in the treatment of these two conditions.

Clinical Applications of Radiofrequency Lesioning

Lumbar Medial Branch Radiofrequency

History

The facet joint was characterized as a source of pain as early as 1911.[60] In 1933, Ghormely coined the term *facet syndrome*.[61,62] Rees was the first to suggest a treatment.[61,63] He used a special scalpel to sever what he thought were the articular branches of the nerves. Later anatomic studies showing the correct location of the articular branches proved that the procedure as proposed was invalid.[14,61,64] The nerves were not located where Rees depicted them and were too deep to be cut by a scalpel. Shealy[13] was the first to attempt facet denervation using RF electrodes.[61,65] Unfortunately, his novel idea exceeded current knowledge of the ideal method to denervate the joints, and the procedure ultimately proved a failure. Finally, an accurate description of the anatomy was elucidated by Bogduk and Long,[14] who suggested a technique for denervating the facet joints by placing electrodes against the medial branch of the dorsal ramus (rather than against the articular branches, which are less accessible). The procedure was initially performed by placing electrodes perpendicular to the medial branches to coagulate them. However, this resulted in only short-term relief.[28,66] To understand the area of coagulation surrounding the active tip of an RF electrode more clearly, investigators performed RF lesions in experimental media.[28] These investigators found that the largest area of coagulation was around the long axis of the electrode with very little heat extending distal to the tip. They also found that larger electrodes created a larger the area of coagulation.[28,37] These facts suggested that electrodes should be oriented parallel rather than perpendicular to the nerve to coagulate that longest segment of nerve. In addition, larger-gauge (16- to 18-gauge) electrodes and more than one lesion were recommended to account for minor variations in the location of the nerves.[2,66,67] Finally, an anatomic study by Lau et al[67] recommended a technique to align electrodes better to lie parallel to the targeted nerve, to achieve maximum contact along the length of nerve. All these recommendations were incorporated into guidelines produced by the ISIS[2] that are summarized as follows:

1. Electrodes should be placed parallel to the targeted nerve to coagulate the longest segment of nerve.
2. Using standard 18- or 20-gauge electrodes, at least two lesions should be made one electrode width apart to ensure that the nerve is incorporated within the area of coagulation.
3. Lesions can be made based on accurate anatomic placement alone without the need to verify electrode placement with sensory stimulation.
4. Lesion times of 90 seconds at 85°C (185°F) produce the largest volume of coagulation without risking boiling of tissues.

Anatomy

The medial branches in the lumbar spine are located at the base of the superior articular process (SAP) at their respective vertebral levels (**Fig. 178.5**). The target is not only at the junction of the SAP and the transverse process (TP), as originally described, but also is slightly up the wall of the SAP at its neck (these points are approximately one to two needle widths apart).[67]

The nerves curve around the lateral aspect of the neck of the SAP and then give off articular branches to the z-joints at the level of origin and the level above it. The nerves at the L1-4 levels are consistently located as a result of two anatomic features. First, the nerve enters the groove between the SAP and the TP lateral to the SAP through the intertransverse ligament. Second, the nerve exits the compartment beneath the mammilloaccessory ligament (MAL).[14,68] These ligaments fix the nerve in place and allow correct anatomic positioning of an RF electrode to locate and ablate the nerve consistently.[2] The L1-4 medial branch nerves are accessible for coagulation only for a limited length. Lesions made too proximally

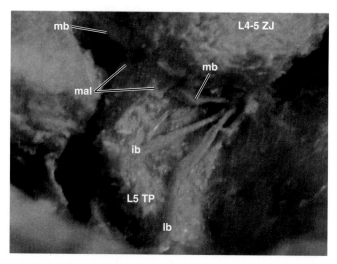

Fig. 178.5 The position of the medial branches and the mammilloaccessory ligament. *(From Lau P, Mercer S, Govind J, et al: The surgical anatomy of lumbar medial branch neurotomy (facet denervation), Pain Med 5:289–298, 2004.)*

risk coagulation of the dorsal ramus. Lesions made too distally fail to coagulate the nerve as it lies underneath the MAL. The MAL is a thick, fibrous band of tissue that protects the nerves from coagulation.[69] The nerve targeted for coagulation at the L5 level is the dorsal ramus. It is longer than the medial branch nerves and follows a rostral course from the sacral ala.[68]

To anesthetize a given facet joint, both medial branch nerves that innervated the joint must be anesthetized. This procedure requires the practitioner to know the location of the nerves. Numbering the nerves can be confusing because the vertebral segment and numbering of the medial branch do not coincide. Two medial branches innervate each facet joint or z-joint, one from the vertebral level of origin and one from the vertebral level above. For example, the L5-S1 level is innervated by a branch arising from the L4 and L5 vertebral levels. The L4-5 joint is innervated by medial branches from the L3 and L4 levels.

Symptoms and Signs of Facet Joint Pain

Patients with facet joint pain commonly present with a deep, aching sensation in the low back that refers in a nondermatomal pattern to the buttocks, the posterior or anterior thigh above the knee, the groin, and the hip (**Fig. 178.6**). These patients often report morning stiffness. Younger patients may report that the pain followed some type of trauma, but older patients report an insidious onset. The diagnosis is more common in patients older than 65 years and cannot be made solely on the basis of history, physical examination, or laboratory studies, such as radiographs.[2,5,70,71] However, certain clinical features have been found to predict a positive response to medial branch block, including pain relieved by recumbency and four of the following six characteristics: age greater than 65 years and back pain not exacerbated by forward flexion, rising from flexion, hyperextension, extension and rotation, or coughing.[2,5,70]

Mechanical pain must be distinguished from radicular pain. Radicular pain travels in a narrow band in the affected extremity. The pain is typically described as shooting or lancinating, rather than dull or aching. It has both a deep and superficial quality, in that the patient feels both a deep

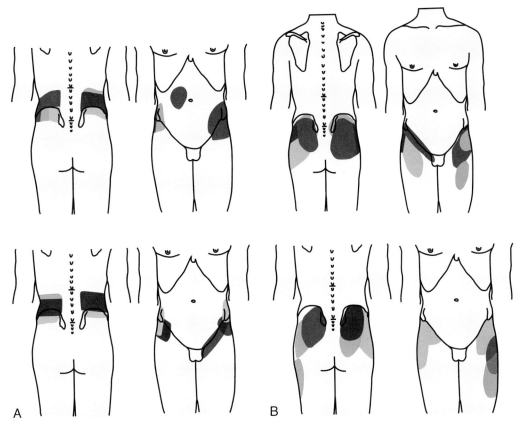

Fig. 178.6 **Lumbar zygapophyseal joint (z-joint) referral maps.**

and cutaneous sensation in the affected extremity. This pain is more often felt below rather than above the knee.[72] Lower extremity pain associated with a mechanical cause is severe only when the back pain is severe; it never occurs independent of back pain. When attempting to distinguish between these two causes of pain, it is helpful to quantify the percentage of pain in the back versus that in the lower extremity. Of the pain in the lower extremity, one must distinguish between the percentage of pain above the knee and that below it.

On physical examination, the patient may report focal tenderness over the facet joints, and extension or lateral side bending may increase the pain.[2,6,7,73–75] Patients with only facet joint pain have a normal neurologic examination. Imaging studies may show a normal-looking facet joint, although some patients show degenerative changes of the disks and facet hypertrophy.[2,6,74,75]

The diagnosis is complicated by the lack of direct correlation between clinical findings and response to medial branch block.[70,71,76,77] The outcome of an RF procedure relies on the results of a properly performed series of two medial branch blocks. The medial branch procedure involves placing a small amount (0.3 mL) of local anesthetic on the targeted nerves and quantifying the amount of pain relief reported by the patient.[2,66] Diagnoses based on single medial branch block are not considered valid because of the high false-positive response rate, which can be as high as 40%.[2] An RF procedure is indicated if the patient reports greater than 80% relief after each of two medial branch procedures, provided the pain is emanating from the facet joint alone. However, because a given patient may have more than one cause of back pain, some investigators have suggested that greater than 50% pain

relief is an adequate criterion. Other investigators have suggested that complete pain relief in a distinct topographic area is adequate to constitute a positive response.[2] The target specificity of the medial branch procedure was established by Dreyfuss et al,[78] who showed that, with properly placed needles, injected contrast dye incorporated the medial branch nerves without spread to the adjacent spinal nerve. The blocks were also shown to have both face validity and construct validity and are therefore predictive of a positive outcome for a properly performed RF procedure.

Indications

The indication for this procedure is pain that has persisted for more than 3 months and has not responded to conservative therapy. In addition, the patient must not be abusing analgesics. The patient must have responded positively on two separate occasions to medial branch blocks with greater than 80% pain relief.[2]

Technique

The patient is placed prone on the fluoroscopy table, and the back is prepared and draped in sterile fashion. A small amount of intravenous or oral sedation is administered. The patient must remain awake enough to communicate during the procedure because it is crucial that he or she report any discomfort felt. This is especially important given that the electrodes can be misplaced onto the spinal nerve and can cause coagulation of the major motor and sensory nerve to the lower extremity. An awake patient can immediately report any burning sensations in the lower extremity.

The target for the L1-4 medial branches is located proximal to the MAL but distal to the dorsal ramus. The classically described location of the nerve is at the junction of the SAP and the TP. However, the nerve can also be located at the lateral surface of the neck of the SAP.[67]

At the L5 level, a lesion is made to the dorsal ramus, instead of the medial branch. It is located at the junction of the S1 SAP and the sacral ala, and not slightly up the wall of the SAP, as at the L1-4 levels. Lau et al[67] made several recommendations that altered how the procedure is performed. First, these investigators recommended using larger-gauge needles (i.e., 16 or 18 gauge). Second, they recommended that multiple parallel lesions be made one needle width apart (the first at the base of the SAP and the second slightly up the wall), to account for the variable topography of the nerve. Third, they recommended that, for the electrode to lie parallel to the nerve, it must be inserted from an oblique, cephalocaudad trajectory. This has been referred to as a *pillar view*. The trajectory places the electrode parallel to the nerve and maximizes the length of active tip in contact with the nerve, a placement that has been shown to increase the duration of effect.[28,37,66] Fourth, Lau et al[67] recommended that needle placements be assessed in multiple views. The target zone in a pillar view is located against the lateral neck of the SAP. In an anteroposterior (AP) view, the needle should be well applied to the SAP. However, for the L1-4 levels, the needle must be passed at an angle from the sagittal plane to avoid the tip of the electrode being deflected laterally by the MAL. In a lateral view, the middle two fourths ($\frac{2}{4}$ to $\frac{3}{4}$) of the SAP are targeted. For the L5 dorsal ramus, the target zone is the middle and posterior one third of the neck of the SAP at S1.

To obtain a pillar view, first the disk space at the targeted level is visualized in an AP view. Then, the image intensifier is rotated obliquely approximately 30 degrees to the ipsilateral side or until the SAP is projected a generous one third of the way across the image of the vertebral body. A pointer is then placed approximately one vertebral level below the targeted nerve. The image intensifier is declined caudally, approximately 30 degrees, until the pointer is projected directly over the SAP at the targeted nerve level. Finally, small adjustments are made both obliquely and cephalocaudally until the lateral cortical margin of the SAP is clearly defined.[67] In this view, the nerve lies against the lateral aspect of the SAP. For example, to target the L3 medial branch, the superior end plate of L4 is squared to open the disk space between the L3 and L4 vertebral bodies. The C-arm is then rotated obliquely as described earlier. A pointer is placed over the SAP of L4 (which is the level below the targeted level), and the C-arm is moved caudally until the image of the groove between the SAP and the TP at the L3 level comes into view and overlies the pointer. Then, final adjustments are made until the lateral margin of the L3 SAP is "crisp."

The needle is passed "down the beam" until the base of the SAP is contacted at its lateral margin. The needle is then viewed in an additional three views (AP, steep oblique, and lateral), and small adjustments are made in each view. In the AP view, the needle should be seen resting tightly against the SAP and above the TP. In a steep oblique view (at least 45 degrees), the needle should be seen across the "ear" of the "Scotty dog," with the tip resting at the leading edge of the SAP. In the lateral view, the needle should cover the middle two fourths of the SAP at the L1-4 levels, whereas at the L5 level, it should cover the middle and posterior one third of the SAP. It should also

be resting on the TP, which is located posterior to the inferior aspect of the foramen. If the needle is seen above the TP (above the inferior aspect of the foramen), it is too high (cephalad) and should be adjusted inferiorly. The needle should never be located anterior to the posterior aspect of the vertebral foramen when viewed in a lateral view. The needle is too posterior if it lies posterior to the image of the SAP. In this position, the nerve lies under the MAL and is not accessible for coagulation. If the needle is seen to be anterior to the posterior aspect of the foramen, it is too ventral, and the neural foramen can be inadvertently entered.

Once the needle position is established, it is wise to check the electrical impedance to ensure the overall integrity of the RF system.[6] Traditionally, location of the targeted nerves is based on radiographic landmarks, as well as on sensory and motor stimulation. However, no comparative studies have documented the benefit of sensory stimulation over radiographic landmarks alone to determine optimal needle placement.

Motor stimulation at 1.0 V is used to confirm needle placement posterior to the DRG. Multifidus muscle contraction may be noted during this procedure and is considered normal.[6] Sensory stimulation is no longer considered necessary according to the ISIS guidelines, for the following reasons[2]:

1. Dreyfuss et al[79] showed that sensory stimulation thresholds did not correlate with improved outcome. These investigators found that correct anatomic placement of the electrode produced reliable nerve coagulation.
2. Evoked sensations may be falsely positive.
3. Electrical stimulation may cause an evoked sensation, but not necessarily close enough to coagulate the nerve.
4. Rigorous sensory testing requires testing at three different locations: at the location where the lowest sensory threshold is obtained, at a location both cephalad and caudad to the first location showing higher sensory thresholds, and at each location compared with the original location. The ISIS guidelines argue that just as many electrode placements are required in making subsequent lesions after making the initial lesion. Thus, radiographic landmarks are the primary tool to localize final needle position before lesioning.

After confirmation of correct placement with fluoroscopy and motor stimulation, 1 mL of 2% lidocaine is injected through each of the cannulas, and 30 to 60 seconds are allowed to pass while waiting for production of anesthesia. Then, the generator is turned on in the automatic mode, and lesions are created at a temperature of 85°C (185°F) applied for 60 to 90 seconds. After completion of the first lesion, a second lesion is performed one needle width cephalad to the first lesion, slightly up the wall of the SAP. The position of the second lesion is established in the same pillar view used for the initial placement of the needle.

The needle positions described earlier apply only to the lumbar medial branches from L1 to L4 (**Fig. 178.7**). At the L5 level, the anatomy is slightly different, in that the L5 dorsal ramus is much longer and more easily accessible than at typical lumbar levels. Therefore, at the L5 level, the dorsal ramus, and not the medial branch, is lesioned. The dorsal ramus runs along a groove formed between the ala of the sacrum and the base of the S1 SAP. The area exposed for lesioning is much

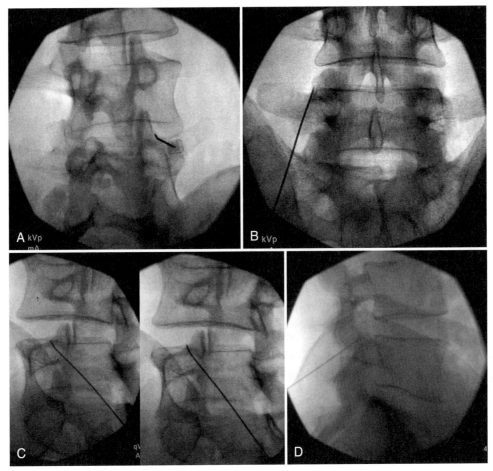

Fig. 178.7 Fluoroscopic images of medial branch (MB) radiofrequency lesioning at L1-4. A, Pillar view showing correct placement at the L3 MB. B, Anteroposterior view of correct needle position; note the needle tip above the transverse process. C, Steep oblique view showing lesion points 1 and 2. D, Lateral view showing correct needle position for L4 MB; note the needle positioned behind the foramen. *(Courtesy of Paul Dreyfuss.)*

longer than of a typical medial branch; therefore, once the first lesion is completed, the needle is repositioned caudally for a second lesion (rather than up the wall of the SAP). This procedure allows a longer length of nerve to be coagulated and thus increases the period of time before nerve regrowth.

In the lumbar spine, patients who fail to obtain relief after medial branch RF lesioning can be assessed by segmental multifidus electromyography to evaluate the technical success of the procedure (**Fig. 178.8**).[79] For patients who obtain good relief but in whom the pain recurs, the effects of the procedure can be successfully reinstated 85% of the time.[80]

Postprocedure Advice

The patient should be advised that it could take up to 3 or 4 weeks before the full effect of the procedure is experienced. During the first week following the procedure, the patient may notice increased pain, which should be treated with analgesics. During subsequent weeks, the physician may refer the patient to physical therapy for a deep muscle relaxation technique, such as deep tissue massage or augmented soft tissue manipulation, which should relieve any muscle tightness or trigger points that may have been caused by chronic inflammation associated with the facet joint syndrome. Physical therapy also facilitates healing of any small, procedure-related hematoma.

Complications

Expected procedure-related side effects are minor and self-limited. These include back pain that usually resolves within 1 to 2 weeks and neuritic pain lasting less than 2 weeks. In a review of 92 patients who received 616 lesions, neither complication had an incidence higher than 0.5%. No cases of infection or new motor or sensory deficits were reported.[81]

In a patient rendered unconscious from intravenous sedation or general anesthesia, needle placement that is inadvertently too close to the spinal nerves could result in severe injury and even permanent motor and sensory deficits. The ISIS guidelines reported just such a case, in which a patient under general anesthesia had the ventral ramus of the spinal nerve coagulated during the procedure.[2] To avoid this complication, the operator is urged to keep the patient conscious at all times during the procedure. The ISIS guidelines also described a case in which a patient suffered full-thickness burns when a spinal needle (instead of the usual dispersive grounding electrode) was used to ground the patient. This type of complication should never occur if a physician is properly trained.[2]

Efficacy

Bogduk et al[66] wrote an excellent review on the lumbar medial branch neurotomy procedure. In that review, these investigators pointed out that to evaluate the outcome of any

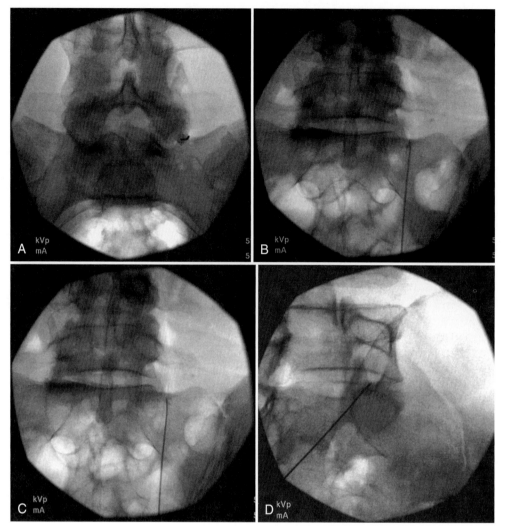

Fig. 178.8 **Lumbar L5 dorsal ramus.** **A,** Pillar view: L5 radiofrequency. **B,** Anteroposterior (AP) view: L5 lesion point 1. **C,** AP view: L5 lesion point 2. **D,** Steep oblique view: L5. *(Courtesy of Paul Dreyfuss.)*

procedure, one must first assess whether the procedure was performed properly, that is, in a manner expected to produce the desired result. They further stated that, of the six randomized controlled trials performed to date, three should not be considered as evidence, based on improper patient selection (patients not selected based on positive response to two correctly performed medial branch blocks) or improper surgical technique (electrodes not correctly aligned parallel to nerve). Although the remaining three trials were suboptimal in terms of patient selection or proper anatomic technique, all showed positive results when compared with placebo. In addition, three descriptive studies were published that used proper patient selection and anatomic technique, and all three showed positive outcomes. These investigators believed that when these results were "pooled," they presented strong evidence supporting efficacy of the procedure. In **Table 178.1**, the results of the best studies performed to date are summarized.

Five additional randomized controlled trials (Gallagher et al, 1994; van Kleef et al, 1999; Leclaire et al, 2001; van Wijk et al, 2005; and Tekin et al, 2007) had significant methodologic problems and were excluded from the table. More specifically, the studies were flawed as a result of improperly selected

patients based on the results of two medial branch blocks or appropriate positioning of the electrodes to create complete lesions of the medial branch nerves.

Lumbar Dorsal Root Ganglion Procedure
History

Uematsu[11] was the first to attempt DRG lesioning for the treatment of radicular pain by heating the DRG with the use of a large 14-gauge cannula. As expected, it caused damage to the pain fibers as well as to the motor and sensory fibers and resulted in near destruction of the spinal nerve. The procedure was quickly abandoned. DRG lesioning was reintroduced in 1980 after Sluijter developed small-diameter electrodes that fit inside a 22-gauge needle.[3] This approach permitted both smaller lesion size and less pain during the procedure. At that time, the recommended tip temperature for treatment of the DRG was 67°C (153°F). The lower temperatures and smaller lesions prevented the complications associated with the Uematsu procedure.[11] However, many patients still developed complications as a result of heating of the DRG. These complications included neuroma formation, allodynia, and

Table 178.1 Radiofrequency of the Lumbar Medial Branch

Randomized Controlled Trial

Authors	Study Design	N	Efficacy
Tekin et al, 2007[30]	Randomized controlled trial	60	Effect of RF maintained at 6 mo and 1 yr; only 40% of patients using analgesics at 1-yr follow-up
Nath et al, 2008*	Randomized controlled trial	40	Patients in treatment group reported significant improvements in pain and quality of life
van Kleef et al, 1999[†]	Randomized controlled trial	31	At 6 and 12 months after treatment, significantly more successful outcomes in RF group compared with placebo group

Prospective Uncontrolled Trials

Authors	Study Design	N	Efficacy
Dreyfuss et al, 2000[79]	Prospective audit	15	12 months after procedure, 60% of patients experienced 90% relief of pain; 87% had ≥60% relief
Gofeld et al, 2007[‡]	Prospective audit	174	68.4% had good to excellent pain relief lasting 6–24 mo
Burnham et al, 2009[§]	Prospective cohort	44	Patients reported significant improvements in pain, disability, analgesic requirement; and satisfaction; effects peaked at 6 mo after procedure

*Nath S, Nath CA, Pettersson K: Percutaneous lumbar zygapophysial (facet) joint neurotomy using radiofrequency current, in the management of chronic low back pain: a randomized double-blind trial, *Spine* 33:1291, 2008.
[†]van Kleef M, Barendse GAM, Kessels A, et al: Randomized trial of radiofrequency lumbar facet denervation for chronic low back pain, *Spine* 24:1937–1942, 1999.
[‡]Gofeld M, Jitendra J, Faclier G: Radiofrequency denervation of the lumbar zygapophysial joints: 10-year prospective clinical audit, *Pain Physician* 10:291, 2007.
[§]Burnham RS, Holitski S, Dinu I: A prospective outcome study on the effects of facet joint radiofrequency denervation on pain, analgesic intake, disability, satisfaction, cost, and employment, *Arch Phys Med Rehabil* 90:201, 2009.
RF, radiofrequency.

dysesthesias.[39] Geurts et al[82] studied the heat procedure in a double-blind, randomized, controlled trial. These investigators concluded that "lumbosacral radiofrequency lesioning of the dorsal root ganglion failed to show advantage over treatment with local anesthetics." Thus, the use of this procedure in the treatment of radicular pain was not recommended.

PRF was introduced in 1998. This method allows delivery of high-frequency electric current without the development of heat. Given the potential for nerve damage with heating of the DRG, PRF was introduced as a method of treatment for radicular pain that had the potential for therapeutic efficacy without the attendant risks. Pulsed treatment of the DRG has shown increasing evidence of efficacy in studies conducted to date. For these reasons, only PRF treatment of the DRG is presented here.

Anatomy

Five paired nerves exit their respective intervertebral foramina from L1-2 to the L5-S1 levels (**Fig. 178.9**). Just as the orientation of the lumbar z-joint differs from L1-2 to L5-S1, the lumbar nerves exit their respective foramina at different angles from L1 through L5. At L1, the nerves exit downward and forward at an acute angle, whereas at L5, the nerves exit more horizontally and at a more obtuse angle.[3,44,72] These anatomic features have important corollaries for positioning of the fluoroscope. For example, imaging the L5-S1 foramen requires much more obliquity than when imaging the L1-2 foramen. In addition, the C-arm must be tiled in a caudal direction to square the end plate at L1, whereas it should be cephalad for L5. The lumbar ventral roots find their cell bodies of origin within the spinal cord at the T9-11 vertebral level.[83] Rootlets come off the dorsal and ventral surface of the spinal cord to form the dorsal and ventral roots. The dorsal and ventral roots then join to form the spinal nerve root. The DRG contains cell bodies that provide sensation, proprioception, and pain.[44]

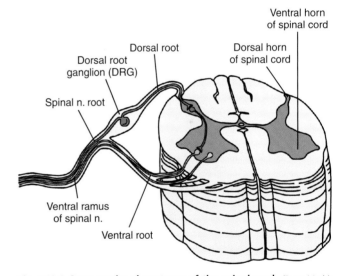

Fig. 178.9 **Cross-sectional anatomy of the spinal cord.** *(From Mathis JM, Golovac S:* Image-guided spine interventions. *New York, 2010, Springer.)*

The spinal nerve root immediately divides to form the dorsal and ventral rami. The ventral ramus is the larger branch and travels to the lower extremity. The dorsal ramus divides into three branches: medial, lateral, and intermediate. The lateral and intermediate branches supply sensation and motor function to the skin and muscles of the back, whereas the medial branch provides sensation to the z-joint and motor function to the multifidus muscles.[14]

Indications

In general, the indication for PRF is neuropathic pain that is confined to the distribution of a known nerve.[3,39,42,46] The specific indication for PRF treatment of the DRG is radicular pain or radiculopathy that is completely but temporarily relieved by transforaminal injection of local anesthetic performed on two separate occasions. The local anesthetic injections are performed diagnostically to identify the location of the origin of the pain and to confirm the nerve levels involved. The procedure has been used for both acute and chronic radicular pain and radiculopathy.[3–5,42,46,48,50–52,84–88]

Technique

PRF lesioning of the DRG requires extremely careful, precise placement of the electrode (**Fig. 178.10**). Therefore, the operator should have very soft hands (a gentle touch) and excellent needle handling skills before attempting this procedure. Although PRF lesioning of the DRG is possible at all spinal levels, this discussion is limited to the use of PRF in the lumbar spine. The discussion also focuses only on the PRF procedure, because continuous RF current applied to the DRG was found to be no more effective than control treatment with local anesthetics.[82]

The retroneural approach is the best method of needle placement to reach the DRG. It is well described in the ISIS guidelines presented in the chapter on lumbar spinal nerve block.[2] With this approach, the target lies at the intersection of two lines. In a lateral view, the first line runs longitudinally between the posterior half and the anterior half of the foramen and divides the foramen into two equal halves. The second line runs in a transverse direction between the superior one third and the inferior two thirds of the foramen. The intersection serves as a starting point for locating the DRG, however, it can lie anywhere between the midaspect and the most anterior aspect of the foramen in the AP plane.

IDENTIFY THE TARGET

For PRF to be effective, the electrode must be meticulously positioned, pointed directly perpendicular and very close to the targeted nerve. To identify the target, the operator should obtain an oblique view, similar to that used for a transforaminal procedure. More specifically, after squaring the superior end plate at the involved level, the operator should rotate the image intensifier into an oblique view until the SAP is projected one third of the distance across the image of the vertebral body (approximately 25 degrees). In this view, the starting point for the needle is slightly inferior

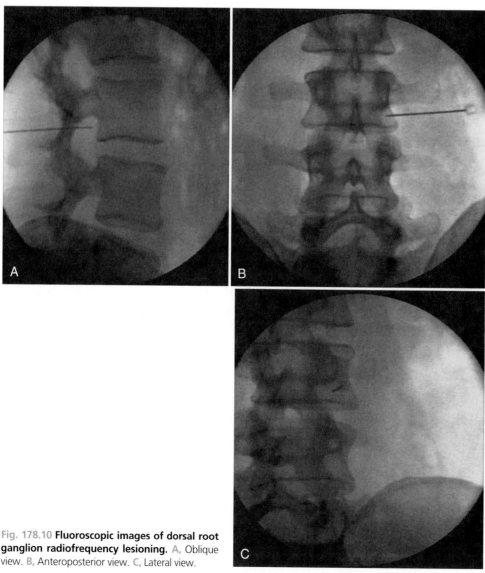

Fig. 178.10 **Fluoroscopic images of dorsal root ganglion radiofrequency lesioning.** A, Oblique view. B, Anteroposterior view. C, Lateral view.

and lateral to that used for a transforaminal injection. The target lies at a point just beneath the pedicle, one third of the way down the foramen. As the needle is advanced, the image is rotated into an AP projection to assess the depth of insertion. If further insertion is required, the image is rotated back to an oblique view and the needle continues to advance. When the needle tip approaches the lateral aspect of the vertebral body, it is best to advance further in an AP view. When the needle is advanced it must be done very slowly (only 1 mm at a time) to avoid damage to the nerve. This aim can be achieved by pinching the needle shaft at the point of skin entry. If the operator is having difficulty locating the nerve, the needle tip is usually too medial and should be corrected in an oblique view so that the tip is located directly beneath the pedicle on a line that bisects it. Because evidence indicates that a small lesion does occur around the electrode tip, it may be unwise to allow the electrode to penetrate neural tissue.

The operator should warn patients that they will feel paresthesia and should not make any sudden movements. Because the greatest current density is projected from the tip of the needle, it is best to point the needle tip directly toward nerve tissue and not against the vertebral body (i.e., the needle tip rather than the shaft should be perpendicular to the targeted nerve). Once the patient reports paresthesia, the operator places the electrode into the needle and begins testing. One must be very careful when handling the needle at this time because any movement risks spearing and damaging the nerve.

A modification of the foregoing technique is required to perform the procedure at the S1 nerve level. In the case of the S1 nerve, the procedure is performed at the level of the ventral ramus, rather than directly at the DRG, because the ventral ramus is located more proximally within the spine. The procedure is performed differently than a typical S1 transforaminal injection. First, the operator adjusts the cephalocaudal tilt in a cephalad direction to optimize the view of the foramen. The C-arm should remain in an AP view (rather than in the ipsilateral oblique position recommended for a transforaminal injection). The needle entry site is at the inferior and lateral quadrant of the foramen with the trajectory superior and medial. This follows the course of the nerve. The needle should first touch the posterior shelf of the sacrum before it enters the foramen. This technique gives a sense of depth and provides a warning before the needle enters the foramen. Once inside the foramen, the needle is advanced very slowly (1 mm at a time) toward the nerve. When contact is established, the operator performs sensory testing and proceeds as usual. If the operator is unable to locate the nerve after three or four attempts, he or she should withdraw the needle and find a new starting place. This is necessary because of the limitation in needle adjustments imposed by the foramen (i.e., the foramen confines the needle such that only a limited territory of space that can be searched).

DETERMINE PROXIMITY BETWEEN NEEDLE TIP AND NERVE

Electrical stimulation tests are used to determine proximity between the needle tip and the nerve. Adequate placement requires that the patient feel reproducible stimulation (tingling in the distribution of the stimulated dermatome) at less than 0.2 V. Two stimulation tests are conducted, once to

determine the minimum sensory threshold (the lowest voltage at which the patient can still perceive a sensation) and a second time to determine reproducibility. During stimulation the second time, the operator slowly increases the voltage by 0.05 V until the patient reports perceiving a stimulus. This should be within 0.05 V of the first stimulation test. If the patient does not feel the current at the required level of less than 0.2 V, the needle is advanced slightly (no more than 1 mm) or is repositioned altogether and retested. Values lower than 0.05 V may reflect intraneural placement, and the needle should be retracted slightly.[5] Motor stimulation is unnecessary during PRF because the modality does not damage motor fibers.

LOWER IMPEDANCE

The next step is to lower the impedance sufficiently to produce a current of 150 to 200 mA during the procedure. The maximum impedance should be less than 400 ohms and ideally less than 250 ohms. To achieve this goal, the operator injects a small amount (1 mL) of local anesthetic (0.5 mL of 0.5% lidocaine [Xylocaine]) or saline solution through the needle. When fluid is injected through the needle, the position of the needle must be secured by one hand at the skin to prohibit movement, which could cause severe pain and possible needle trauma to the nerve. If any resistance is felt during injection, the operator should stop, retract the needle slightly, inject again, and then replace the needle in its original position. Liquid should flow easily through a 20-gauge needle. The minimal stimulation threshold and impedance should be recorded before treatment.

BEGIN PULSED RADIOFREQUENCY TREATMENT

At this point, the operator turns on the power in the PRF mode, slowly increases the voltage to 45 V, and verifies that the patient feels pulsing. The needle must be close enough to the target nerve to produce a perceptible electrical discharge in the treated extremity with each pulse. The absence of a pulsing sensation may indicate that the needle is not close enough to the targeted nerve tissue to produce an effect. If this is the case, the operator repositions the needle and begins treatment again. Although no study has demonstrated that this step is necessary, it can be another useful test to verify proximity to the targeted neural tissue. If desired, this step can be performed before lesioning the nerve, because it is unlikely that the patient will feel pulsing once the nerve has been anesthetized.

The standard protocol is to proceed with PRF treatment for 3 to 4 minutes at 45 V (as long as the temperature does not exceed 42°C [108°F]), two pulses per second, with current applied for 20 milliseconds during each pulse. However, an alternative protocol is to increase the voltage as high as necessary to produce a current of at least 150 mA, which may cause additional heating around the needle. The temperature can be allowed to rise as high as 45°C (113°F), if necessary, to produce the higher current (of at least 150 mA). Because treatment protocols may vary among operators, the operator should consult the literature for other examples of lesion parameters.

Postprocedure Advice

The patient usually feels immediate relief on completion of the procedure, as a result of the injection of local anesthetic into the affected nerve. When the effect wears off, the patient may begin to feel sore. The patient should be advised that he or she may continue to feel sore for the first week and better the second week, and that the full effect can take 3 to 4 weeks to develop. During this time, the patient is not required to restrict activities except as needed to relieve pain. Deep tissue massage once a week for the first 3 weeks following the procedure may relieve soreness related to the procedure, as well as chronic trigger points that may have developed over the course of the disease.

Complications

The most common complication noted during any spinal procedure is vasovagal syncope.[89] This symptom is more common during a cervical than lumbar procedure (8% versus 1%).[90] Other complications include transient nonpositional headache, increased back pain, facial flushing (if steroids are used) and increased leg pain, ischemia of the anterior spinal artery if particulate steroid is injected, infection (epidural abscess, meningitis, diskitis), and other complications related to injected medications.[4,91,92]

A potential risk of neural trauma is associated with this procedure, but this has not been specifically studied. Certainly, with proper needle handling techniques, the complication should be rare. In Rosenthal's experience, after performance of more than 1000 procedures, no incidence of neural trauma occurred. During injection of local anesthetic to anesthetize the nerve, fluid can be inadvertently injected into the axon bundle, thus leaving the patient with persistent motor or sensory deficits. This complication should never

occur in a properly performed procedure and can be detected by resistance to flow of fluid on injection. If any resistance is encountered during injection, especially if it is accompanied by pain, the operator should stop injecting and retract the needle slightly before continuing. Hematoma may occur just under the skin or in the deeper muscle layers as a result of the procedure. Most patients report mild discomfort in the treated extremity that spontaneously resolves within approximately 3 weeks.[93] All complications have a low incidence.

Efficacy

Some investigators studied the efficacy of PRF lesioning of DRG by targeting the lumbar, thoracic, or cervical spine. Most of these studies were prospective uncontrolled trials or retrospective studies, and one was a randomized controlled trial. Each of the four prospective uncontrolled trials concluded that PRF lesioning of the DRG was a safe and effective pain treatment, and each of the five retrospective studies reported similarly positive results. These data are summarized in **Table 178.2**.

Although the foregoing studies appear promising, none included a control group, and most reported only relatively short-term efficacy. To date, only one double-blind, randomized, placebo-controlled trial of PRF lesioning has been conducted, and that trial studied 23 patients with chronic cervicobrachial pain for 6 months.[48] Patients underwent either

Table 178.2 Radiofrequency of the Dorsal Root Ganglia

Randomized Controlled Trial

Authors	N	Type of Pain	Efficacy
Van Zundert et al, 2007[48]	23	Cervical radicular	82% achieved ≥50% improvement in global perceived effect and ≥2-point reduction of VAS at 3 mo

Prospective Uncontrolled Trials

Authors	N	Type of Pain	Efficacy
Sluijter et al, 1998[31]	15	Lumbar radicular	53% achieved ≥2-point reduction of VAS at 6 mo, and 40% did so at 1 yr
Pevzner et al, 2005[163]	28	Lumbar radicular Cervicobrachial	2 patients had "excellent" pain relief, 12 had "good" pain relief, and 9 had "fair" pain relief at 3 mo
Shabat et al, 2006[93]	28	Spinal neuropathic	82% achieved ≥30% reduction of VAS at 3 mo, and 68% of did so at 1 yr
Simopoulous et al, 2008[51]	76	Lumbar radicular	Patients reported an average 4.3-point decrease in pain scores, with a 3.18-mo average duration of success

Retrospective Studies

Authors	N	Type of Pain	Efficacy
Van Zundert et al, 2003[47]	18	Cervicobrachial	72% achieved ≥50% pain relief at 2 mo, 56% did so at 3 to 11 mo, and 33% did so for >1 yr
Teixeira et al, 2005[84]	13	Lumbar radicular	92% achieved ≥5-point improvement in NRS at 1 yr
Cohen et al, 2006[164]	13	Thoracic segmental	62% achieved ≥50% pain relief at 6 wk and that 54% did so at 3 mo
Abejón et al, 2007[85]	54	Herniated disk Spinal stenosis FBSS	40% of patients with herniated disks (n = 29) and 40% of patients with spinal stenosis (n = 12) achieved "successful treatment" at 180 days after treatment; treatment not as successful in patients with FBSS (n = 13)
Chao et al, 2008[162]	154	Lumbar radicular Cervical radicular	45% of patients with lumbar pain (n = 116) and 55% of patients with cervical pain (n = 49) achieved ≥50% relief at 3 mo

FBSS, failed back surgery syndrome; NRS, numerical rating scale; VAS, Visual Analog Scale.

PRF lesioning ($n = 11$) or sham lesioning ($n = 12$) at the C5-7 nerve levels. At 3 months, significantly more patients in the treatment group (83%) than in the control group (33%) reported at least 50% improvement in global perceived effect, an effect that was also maintained at 6 months. Similarly, at 3 months, significantly more treatment-group patients (82%) than control-group patients (25%) reported at least a 20-point decrease in Visual Analog Scale (VAS) score, although the effect was not maintained. This study has been criticized because (1) recruitment challenges limited its statistical power, (2) the two study groups were not comparable in terms of average age and baseline VAS scores, and (3) the effect was not maintained at 6 months. Despite these shortcomings, this study is important because it is the first prospective controlled trial to show a treatment effect.

Martin et al[94] proposed that the efficacy of PRF lesioning of the DRG is directly related to the proximity of the RF electrode to the targeted neural structure and the amount of delivered current (**Table 178.3**). These investigators recommended using a stimulation voltage between 0.1 and 0.3 volts to position the electrode properly. They also suggested that higher current delivery (150 to 200 mA) improves outcomes.

Considering the preponderance of the evidence presented earlier, it appears that PRF does indeed have a clinical effect for the treatment of radicular pain. Further research is required to bolster the data presented here and to prove the long-term utility of the procedure. However, enough evidence currently exists to support the use of PRF lesioning in clinical practice for the treatment of radicular pain.

Cervical Medial Branch Radiofrequency
(Table 178.4)

History

Lord et al[95] published the first randomized, double-blind, placebo-controlled trial illustrating that, when performed accurately (i.e., based on results of anatomic studies), cervical medial branch RF lesioning was clearly efficacious. This land-mark research was followed by subsequent studies reporting that long-term relief of neck pain was possible and that coagulation of the third occipital nerve (TON) could relieve cervicogenic headache.[95-97]

Anatomy

Before the Lord study, Bogduk and Lord[2,29,98] dissected multiple cadavers to locate and map the positions of the cervical medial branches in each cadaver (**Fig. 178.11**). These investigators found that, unlike the location of nerves in the lumbar spine, the location of the cervical medial branches was not consistent from one cadaver to the next. Therefore, to block sensation from a particular joint completely, a region of the articular pillar (superior to inferior), rather than a specific location, must be coagulated. The region can be considered to have a volume consisting of a height, length, and width, and it must be covered with RF lesions to destroy the innervation to a particular nerve level successfully.[2]

Lord et al also found that the location of the medial branch nerves varied, depending on the vertebral level. In general, these nerves assume a curved course around the "waist" of the articular pillar. This archetypal course is exhibited at the C5 level, where the nerves run in the center of the articular pillar on a lateral view and in the waist of the articular pillar in an AP view. At the C3 level, two medial branches are present, one of which is superficial and one of which is deep. The superficial medial branch is also referred to as the *third occipital nerve* (TON) and provides sensory innervation to the C2-3 joint. Its location potentially extends from the top of the SAP of C3 to the bottom of the C2-3 intervertebral foramen (IVF). The TON is 1.5 mm in diameter, whereas the other medial branches are less than 1.0 mm, thus making it all the more difficult to destroy by RF coagulation. The deep medial branch innervates the C3-4 joint, and it is located from the joint line to the midaspect of the C3 articular pillar. The C4 and C6 medial branches are found in the upper half of the articular pillar. The location of the C7 medial branch is different, in that the nerves are pushed up by the C7 TP. Therefore, the medial branch is located significantly higher on the articular pillar than are the other nerves. The medial branch can be found on the corner formed by the junction of the C7 SAP and the root of the TP in an AP view. The anatomy of the articular pillars and their joints must be considered during an RF procedure (**Fig. 178.12**). Because the articular pillars slope caudally, the electrodes must be inserted from an inferior position heading superiorly for the electrode to lie parallel to the nerves.[2,29]

The articular branches, which innervate the joints, divide off the medial branch at the middle to posterior aspect of the articular pillar. This has clinical significance in that, if an RF lesion is performed posterior to the location where

Table 178.3 Stimulation Voltage versus Duration of Effect Based on Studies

Authors	Sensory Stimulation (V)	Duration (mo)
Simopoulos et al, 2008[51]	0.6	3.18
Teixeira et al, 2005[84]	0.22	15.8
Chao et al, 2008[162]	<0.5	3
Van Zundert et al, 2003[47]	<0.5	3

Table 178.4 Radiofrequency of the Cervical Medial Branch

Authors	Study Design	N	Efficacy
Lord et al, 1996[95]	Randomized double-blind trial	24	Median time to return of 50% of preoperative pain was 263 days
McDonald et al, 1999[96]	Observational	28	71% had complete pain relief; median duration of relief was 422 days
Govind et al, 2003[97]	Observational	49	88% achieved a successful outcome; median duration of pain relief was 297 days

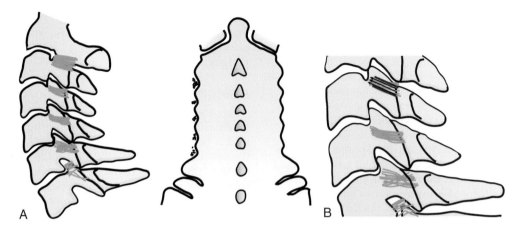

Fig. 178.11 Location of cervical medial branches. A, Images of location of medial branches of multiple cadaveric specimens. B, Location of lesions required to coagulate C3 medial branches. *(Modified from Lord SM, Barnsley L, Wallis BJ, et al: Percutaneous radio-frequency neurotomy for chronic cervical zygapophyseal-joint pain, N Engl J Med 335(23):1721–1726, 1996; and McDonald GJ, Lord SM, Bogduk N: Long-term follow-up of patients treated with cervical radiofrequency neurotomy for chronic neck pain, Neurosurgery 45(1):61–67, 1999.)*

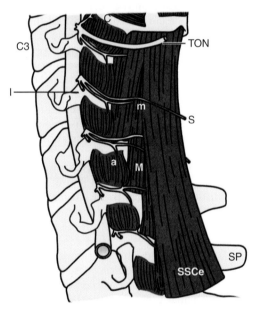

Fig. 178.12 Images of articular branches.

the articular branches divide, neurotomy of the joint has not occurred. In effect, the anterior two thirds of the articular branches must be lesioned to coagulate the nerves to the facet joints.

In the cervical spine, two nerves innervate each facet joint, one from the vertebral level above the joint and one from the vertebral level below the joint. For example, the C5 and C6 medial branches innervate the C5-6 facet joint. Because of the inconsistent and varying locations of the medial branches, Lord et al concluded that, to coagulate the nerve, multiple lesions were required at each level. To do this successfully, each lesion should be located one electrode width from the last, so that no gaps remain between the lesioned areas. In addition, careful attention must be paid to electrode placement to ensure that the most anterior aspect of the nerve is coagulated.

Patient Selection

Cervical facet joint pain is thought to result from tearing of the joint capsule, which allows microscopic movement of the joint surfaces and causes inflammation and pain.[99] The two

most commonly injured joints are the C2-3 joint and the C5-6 joint.[100] Pain emanating from the C2-3 facet joint commonly causes posterior occipital headaches. This pain is often described as a unilateral headache located at the base of the skull and sometimes radiating to the forehead. Pain in the C5-6 facet joint often radiates to the inferior aspect of the trapezius muscle and scapular area.

The goals of RF neurotomy of the cervical medial branches are to reduce afferent nociceptive signals from the facet joints and to provide palliative relief. Because pain emanating from a specific facet joint is difficult to localize, treatment is usually performed on three medial branches or two facet joints.

Patients with facet joint pain commonly present with a deep, aching sensation in the neck, punctuated by sharp shooting sensations with certain types of movements. They may complain of increased pain with flexion, extension, rotation, or lateral side bending of the head. The pain is most often bilateral, exacerbated by movement, and relieved by rest. Younger patients may report a traumatic event causing a whiplash injury, but older patients more often report an insidious onset of the pain. The pain refers in a nondermatomal pattern into the occipital area or forehead, shoulder, and upper back. Physical examination may reveal focal tenderness or spasm, with no sensory or motor deficits.[7,101]

Cervical facet joint pain cannot be definitively diagnosed by history, physical examination, or the results of imaging studies, nor is a single medial branch block considered to be a valid method of confirming the diagnosis.[2,102–104]

Dwyer et al[105,106] mapped pain referral patterns by injecting saline solution into the joints of normal volunteers (**Fig. 178.13**). Dwyer, Aprill, and Bogduk[105,106] used these data to predict the segmental location of the pain.

Indications

The indication for this procedure is pain that has persisted for more than 3 months and has not responded to conservative therapy. The patient must report relief after diagnostic blocks, but the amount of relief is controversial. Traditionally, patients must report greater than 80% pain relief on two separate occasions in response to medial

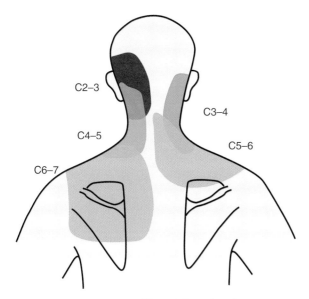

Fig. 178.13 **Images of facet joint referral maps.**

branch blocks.[2] However, a study on patients with cervical facet pain showed no difference in outcome of the RF procedure in patients reporting 50% relief and those reporting 80%.[107] Based on this study, for patients with cervical facet joint pain, 50% reduction in pain after medial branch block may be adequate.

Technique

PRONE APPROACH

The patient is positioned prone on a fluoroscopy table. It is wise to position the patient on a bolster to drop the shoulders down and away from the cervical spine and thus facilitate lateral imaging. To do this, multiple pads are placed under the patient's chest such that the area is built up enough to allow the shoulders to drop down and away from the neck. The skin is prepared and draped in the usual sterile fashion, and monitors are placed if intravenous sedation is planned. It is important that the patient remain awake and alert during the entire procedure so that any discomfort can be evaluated by the operator. A fluoroscopic image is then obtained of the targeted vertebral level. The superior end plate is squared to open the disk space. Next the C-arm is obliquely 10 to 15 degrees to the ipsilateral side to target the anterior and medial aspect of the articular pillar. A pointer is placed over the articular pillar one level inferior to the targeted medial branch and the C-arm is declined (image intensifier moved toward feet), until the targeted nerve level is directly beneath the pointer. This is referred to as a pillar view. Its purpose is to allow needle placement using a "down the beam" approach (needle parallel to x-ray beams). It also serves to align the active tip of the electrode parallel to the medial branch. A skin wheal is made slightly lateral to the targeted level at approximately the midaspect of the articular pillar. A 20-gauge needle with a 10-mm active tip is then advanced down the beam until contact with the posterior aspect of the articular pillar is made.

At this point, a lateral view is obtained, and the needle is carefully advanced to the most anterior aspect of the articular pillar. A true lateral view must be obtained to locate the tip of the needle accurately at the most anterior aspect of the articular pillar. A steep contralateral oblique view (safety view) is then obtained to confirm that the needle tip is well behind (dorsal to) the IVF. An AP view is obtained to confirm needle placement against the articular pillar (at or slightly above the waist, depending on the level targeted). It is critical that the active tip is not sciathing laterally away from the bone. This occurs if the starting place on the skin is positioned too far medially. The operator must also make certain that the active tip is in close contact with the articular pillar and not lateral to it, to coagulate the nerve and not the muscle adjacent to the nerve.

Once the correct position is established, motor testing is done at 1.0 V to confirm the proper distance from the exiting ventral ramus and the active tip of the electrode. Contraction of the paraspinal muscles of the neck is a normal finding, whereas contraction of the muscles of the arm indicates a need to reposition the needle more posteriorly. The position for needle passage for the TON is slightly different. A pillar view is not necessary for this approach because the flange of the SAP is not present, as it is at other levels. Using this approach, the starting point is at the C2-3 joint line, with the initial target the superior aspect of the SAP of C3 (as seen in a lateral view).[108]

After confirmation of correct placement with fluoroscopy and stimulation, 1 mL of 2% lidocaine is injected through each of the cannulas, and 30 to 60 seconds are allowed to pass while waiting for production of anesthesia. Then the generator is turned on in the automatic mode, and lesions are created at a temperature of 85°C (185°F) applied for 60 to 90 seconds. After completion of the first lesion, a series of subsequent lesions is performed to cover the volume of space completely where the nerves could potentially be located. This is done by retracting the needle back (while in a lateral view) no further than the posterior aspect of the articular pillar (warning: retracting the needle farther risks misplacement to the inside of the articular pillar and coagulation of the spinal cord or rootlets). The number of lesions needed to cover the prescribed volume completely varies at each level. At the C3 level, the lesion area must extend from the superior aspect of the C3 SAP to the midaspect of the C3 articular pillar, to coagulate both the superficial (TON) and deep (C3 MB) medial branches. This procedure requires five lesions, spaced one needle width apart. At the C4-6 levels, three lesions are recommended (**Figs. 178.14** to **178.17**); at C7, four lesions must be made (**Fig. 178.18**).

A modification of the technique described earlier is one in which a bipolar lesion is made at each nerve level (**Fig. 178.19**). The technique has yet to be validated but seems reasonable and provides a method of coagulating a large volume of tissue with fewer lesions.[109] In addition, because a bipolar lesion is significantly larger than a monopolar lesion, it may be more likely to incorporate the medial branch within the lesion.[109] The concept is identical to that described earlier, but instead of performing multiple lesions at each level, only one or two bipolar lesions are required per nerve level. The technique involves placing two 10-cm needles with a 10-mm active tip at the superior and inferior aspect of the prescribed lesion zone and creating a bipolar lesion between them. Bipolar lesions must be made no more than 6 mm apart (approximately three needle widths). Therefore, a single bipolar lesion would theoretically cover the lesion zone at C4-6. Two bipolar lesions should be performed at the C3 and C7 levels.

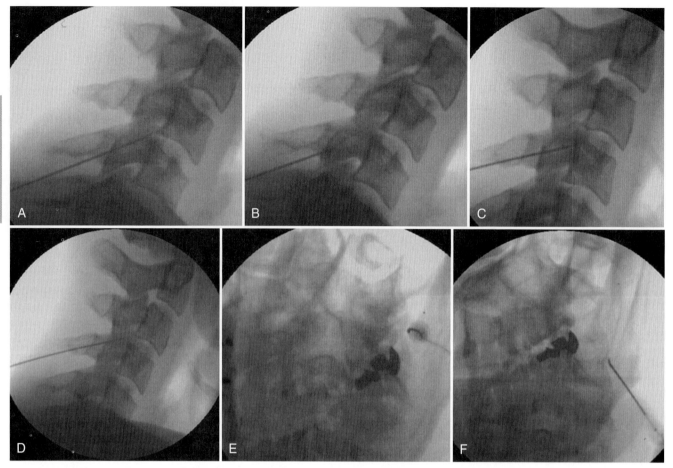

Fig. 178.14 **Fluoroscopic cervical medial branch radiofrequency lesioning: prone at C3-6.** A, Lateral view of placement at the C5 level. B, Retracting the needle no farther than the posterior articular pillar for placement at the second lesion point. C, Second lesion at the C5 level. D, Lateral view showing the third lesion point for the C5 level. E, Placement of the needle in the pillar view. F, Anteroposterior view of the needle showing placement in the superior half of the "waist" of the articular pillar at the C3 level.

POSTEROLATERAL APPROACH

Figure 178.20 shows the posterolateral approach to the cervical medial branch RF procedure.

Rationale for the Procedure

The posterolateral approach, as recommended by Sluijter, Van Kleef, Van Zundert, and others, is a second method of performing the cervical medial branch procedure. It is performed with the patient in a supine position, which is sometimes better tolerated than the prone position. Although this approach has not been as well studied as the prone approach, it can be useful in certain situations. For example, the prone approach may be difficult when a patient has a short and stout neck, which makes target visualization difficult in a lateral view. It may also be difficult when patients have severe degenerative disease and arthritic spurring, because bony wings or flanges can prevent passage of the needle to the targeted nerve. Finally, it is always wise to have more than one method of accomplishing the same task.[4,5,96,110]

For the posterolateral approach, the patient is placed supine on the operating room table with the head turned to the contralateral side. The skin is prepared and draped in the usual sterile fashion, and monitors are placed if intravenous sedation is planned. It is important that the patient be awake and alert during the entire procedure, so that any discomfort can be evaluated. A fluoroscopic image is then obtained of the target vertebral level. The C-arm is tilted slightly caudally to square the vertebral end plates and to open the disk space at the targeted level. Next, the C-arm is rotated into the oblique position on the ipsilateral side to visualize the cervical foramen at the level of interest. Observation that the pedicles on the contralateral side are projected approximately 50% of the way across the vertebral body can be used as a visual reference regarding the degree of obliquity required.[111]

The target point is the base of the SAP at or just below the most inferior aspect of the IVF. A lesion performed at this location (just distal to the dorsal ramus) is believed to provide a similar effect to a lesion performed over the entire length of the nerve, although no studies comparing both techniques have been performed.[112] The needles are not passed in a tunnel vision view. Instead, the entry point is slightly posterior and caudal to the target. The skin overlying the target is anesthetized, and a 20-gauge needle with a 10-mm active tip is advanced to the target point in the oblique or foraminal view. The needle tip must be projected over the image of the articular pillar to prevent passage posterior to the column of bone. Once bone is contacted,

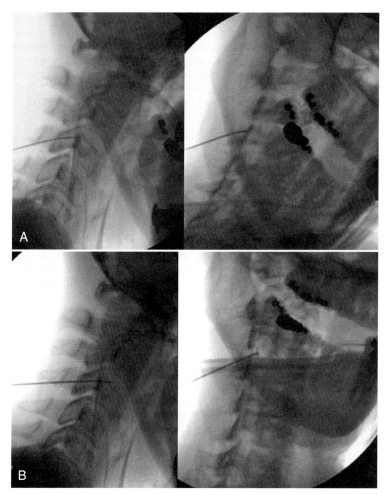

Fig. 178.15 Safety view showing location of the needle in the lateral view relative to the foramen. A, Lateral view with the needle correctly positioned. Note the location of the needle relative to the foramen in the image on the *right*. B, Lateral view with the needle advanced past the correct position. Note the location of the needle in the posterior aspect of the foramen. *(Courtesy of Aaron Calodney.)*

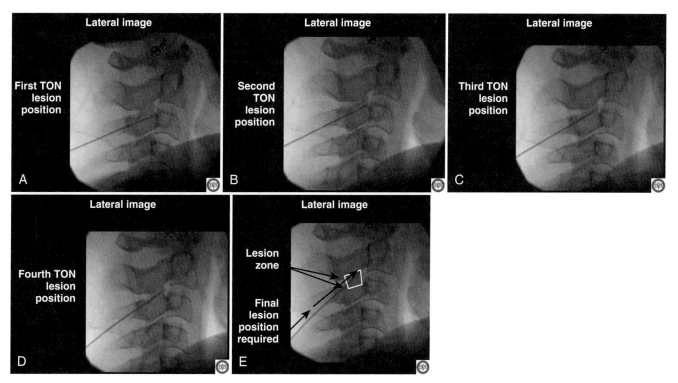

Fig. 178.16 **C3 medial branch radiofrequency lesioning showing sweeping of the needle for coagulation of multiple possible locations of C3 third occipital nerve (TON).**

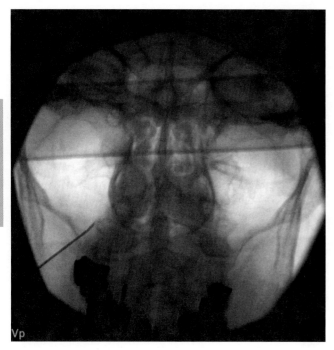

Fig. 178.17 **C3 medial branch radiofrequency lesioning: anteroposterior view.**

care must be taken to ensure that the needle tip remains behind a line created by the posterior aspect of the IVF. The needle should touch bone at a superficial depth. If bone is not immediately contacted, one should reevaluate placement in both the foraminal view and an AP view. In the AP view, the tip of the needle should be seen resting against the midaspect of the articular pillar. If it is medial to the edge of the articular pillar, one should suspect needle placement into the foramen (confirmed in an oblique view) or posterior to the articular pillar.

Once correct position is established, motor testing at 1.0 V confirms proper distance from the exiting ventral ramus. Contraction of the paraspinal neck muscles is a normal finding, whereas contraction of the arm muscles indicates a need to reposition the needle. After confirmation of correct placement with fluoroscopy and stimulation, 1 mL of 2% lidocaine is injected through each of the cannulas, and 30 to 60 seconds are allowed to pass while waiting for production of anesthesia. Then, the RF generator is turned on in the automatic mode and lesions are created at a temperature of 85°C (185°F) applied for 60 to 90 seconds. After completion of the first lesion, repeat lesions are performed both cephalad and caudad to the original needle position (as noted earlier), to coagulate the volume of space in which the medial branches may be found.

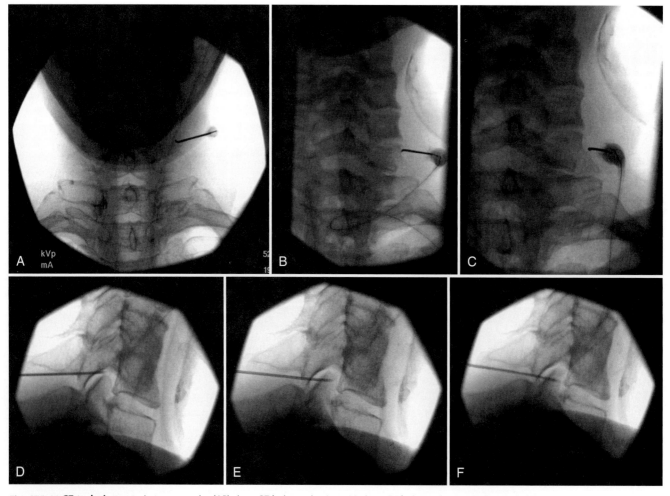

Fig. 178.18 **C7 technique.** A, Anteroposterior (AP) view: C7 lesion point 1. B, AP view: C7 lesion point 2. C, AP view: C7 lesion point 3. D, Lateral view: C7 medial branch lesion point 1. E, Lateral view: C7 lesion point 2. F, Lateral view: C7 lesion point 3. *(Courtesy of Paul Dreyfuss.)*

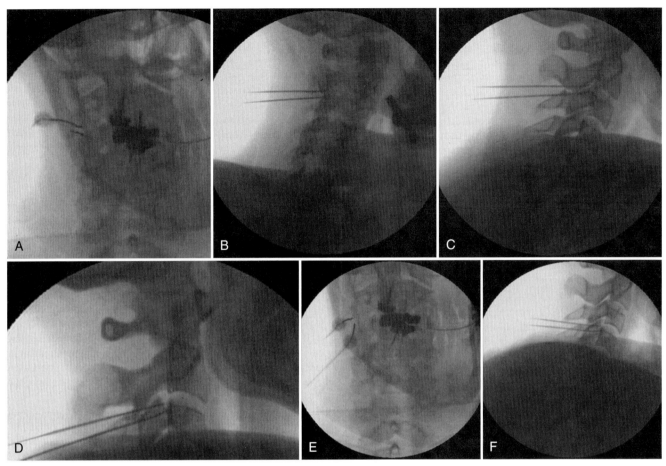

Fig. 178.19 Cervical medial branch radiofrequency (RF) lesioning: bipolar technique. A, Anteroposterior (AP) view: C3 bipolar RF. B, Oblique "safety" view: C3. C, Lateral view: needle positions for lesioning 3, third occipital nerve. D, Needle position C3, third occipital nerve position 2. E, AP view: C4 medial branch bipolar RF. F, Lateral view: C4 bipolar RF.

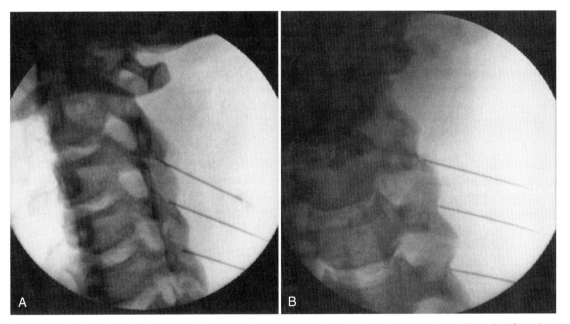

Fig. 178.20 Cervical medial branch radiofrequency (RF) posterolateral approach. A, Oblique view: cervical medial branch RF from the posterolateral approach. B, Anteroposterior view: cervical medial branch RF from the posterolateral approach.

Complications

In general, complications associated with this procedure are rare. Postprocedure pain generally lasts up to 2 weeks. Approximately 30% of patients report numbness in the cutaneous distribution of the coagulated nerves, but this is usually not disturbing to patients and does not require treatment. Twenty percent of patients may experience dysesthesias in the cutaneous distribution of the coagulated nerves that last 2 to 3 weeks. This complication usually resolves spontaneously without treatment.[2,95] Complications associated with coagulation of the TON require special mention. This nerve plays a role in proprioception such that, when coagulated, most patients experience mild transient ataxia lasting 2 to 3 weeks.[2,4,97] The symptom may be more severe if both nerves are coagulated at the same time. Patients should be cautioned not to drive or operate heavy machinery until the symptom resolves.

Other, almost universal symptoms of coagulation of the TON are hypersensitivity and dysesthesias in the cutaneous distribution of the nerve. These symptoms usually last for 1 to 4 weeks and resolve without treatment.[2,97] If treatment is required, a methylprednisolone (Medrol) dose pack or anticonvulsants are helpful. If these drugs prove ineffective, an epidural steroid injection may help to resolve the symptoms. Finally, the ISIS guidelines reported a case of spinal cord injury in a patient under general anesthesia when an electrode was passed medial to the targeted joint, through the interlaminar space, and directly onto the spinal cord and exiting nerve roots.[2] This complication is prevented by not retracting the electrode farther than the posterior aspect of the articular pillar when multiple lesions are created on a single nerve level in a lateral view. Spinal cord injury can also be easily avoided by simply checking an AP view whenever the electrode is repositioned.

Efficacy: Prone

In a double-blind, randomized, controlled study comparing cervical medial branch RF lesioning with a sham treatment, Lord et al[95] found that patients in the treatment group experienced statistically significant improvement in pain when compared with the control group (median time to recurrence of pain was 263 days and 8 days, respectively). Patients with C2-3 joint pain were excluded from the study because preliminary data indicated that RF treatment was difficult at that level. However, subsequent research demonstrated that C2-3 joint pain could be successfully treated by RF neurotomy of the TON.[97] In a follow-up to the study by Lord et al, 63% of patients reported complete pain relief for an average of 421 days.[96] Finally, a study by Schofferman and Kine[80] demonstrated that when pain recurred following RF neurotomy, repeat treatment was an effective, long-term solution.

Sacroiliac Joint Radiofrequency

History

The SI joint was first implicated as a source of pain as early as 1905.[113] It was considered the primary cause of low back pain before 1934, when Mixter and Barr suggested rupture of the intervertebral disk as the primary source of back pain.[114] Injection of anesthetic into the SI joint as a potential diagnostic and therapeutic intervention was first described in 1938, but the procedure was not guided by any sort of imaging technique.[115] Fluoroscopic guidance as a means of obtaining joint entry was first described in 1979, and the first use of contrast medium to confirm accurate spread of contrast within the joint followed in 1982.[116,117] A 1993 study determined that the volume of the SI joint is approximately 1.5 cc.[118,119] Later, pain referral patterns were studied by distending the joint with contrast medium.[120,121] An important advance in the study of SI joint pain arose from a series of studies illustrating that no valid clinical history or physical examination could reliably diagnose pain as emanating from the SI joint.[122,123] Instead, controlled intra-articular diagnostic blocks were determined to be the only reliable means of diagnosis. To date, no studies have attempted to determine whether the use of lateral branch blocks (which are analogous to the medial branch blocks used to diagnose facet joint pain) can predict the outcome of RF neurotomy. However, a cadaver study by Dreyfuss[124,125] illustrated that, when green dye was injected at three locations in close proximity to the sacral foramen, the lateral branches were stained 91% of the time, whereas when dye was injected into only one location, the lateral branches were stained only 42% of the time. This finding suggests that one must inject anesthetic at three separate locations adjacent to the sacral foramen to block the lateral branch nerves reliably. A volume of 0.4 mL must be injected at each of the three locations.

Early attempts at SI joint RF neurotomy were limited by an incomplete understanding of the anatomy of the joint. For example, investigators originally thought that the best location in which to interrupt nerve supply was directly over the surface of the joint. This prompted researchers to use a relatively ineffective "leapfrog" RF technique in which the electrodes were positioned close together and directly over the joint. Multiple lesions were sequentially made along the joint line in successive fashion, with each needle "leaping over" the former.[126] As understanding of the anatomy of the SI joint improved, better results were obtained by using a strip lesion technique in which bipolar RF lesions were created along the lateral border of the posterior sacral foramen in a continuous fashion from S1 to S3 with the addition of the L5 dorsal ramus.[127] In an effort to create an even larger lesion, cooled-probe RF ablation was introduced. This technology creates lesions that are more than twice the diameter of conventional RF probes (8 to 10 mm versus 3 to 4 mm). An extension of the strip lesion technique was introduced in 2009, when a large-diameter probe containing three electrodes became commercially available. The probe makes a long, continuous strip lesion from a single insertion site. The lesion extends from above the S1 foramen down to the S4 foramen.

Anatomy

The SI joint is a true synovial joint and the largest axial joint in the body. It is supported by a complex series of both muscles and ligaments and is covered by a fibrous capsule. The superior two thirds of the joint space is filled with fibrous cartilage. Because nociceptors are present in the joint capsule and surrounding ligaments, pain can be provoked by both distention of the joint capsule and stimulation of the ligaments.[120,121,123,128–130] When considering the origin of SI joint pain, it is helpful to remember that multiple sources of pain may lie within the SI joint complex. For example, pain caused by arthritis, infection, fracture, ligament strain, or neoplasm is treated differently than is intra-articular pain.

SI joint innervation is complex and arises from both the ventral and dorsal rami of the spinal nerve roots. Both the anterior and posterior limbs of the joint are innervated. The joint is anteriorly innervated by the ventral ramus of L5-S2 and posteriorly innervated by the dorsal ramus of L5 and the lateral branches of S1-4.[119] An anatomic study by Grob determined that the dorsal ramus of S1 makes the predominant contribution to the nerve supply of the joint with no innervation from the ventral sacral plexus. Dorsal innervation was confirmed when a similar study by Willard determined that both the S1 and S2 lateral branches provide important contributions.[119,131,132] Free nerve endings furnish sensation to the posterior and anterior capsule and the posterior ligaments. The lateral branch nerves exit the lateral border of the dorsal foramina of S1-4. The number of lateral branch nerves that exit each foramen varies from side to side, patient to patient, and level to level. Their point of exit from the foramen is unpredictable and can occur anywhere along the lateral aspect. As the nerves travel over to the joint, their anatomic course varies in both direction and depth. The nerves can be found on the sacral plate or several millimeters above it, a finding suggesting that the area of burn must not only be long but also deep to capture the nerves within it and interrupt nociceptive sensation..[132-134] One must also consider which nerves are necessary to ablate to denervate the joint adequately. Most practitioners believe it is adequate to ablate L5-S2, but lesions as large as L4-S4 can be made.

Patient Selection

Patients with SI joint pain are an important part of a pain physician's practice. The SI joint is the primary source of pain in 10% to 25% of patients presenting with back pain,[135-137] as well as in 32% of patients with lumbosacral fusion.[138,139] The symptoms of SI joint pain may be similar to those seen in patients with facet joint abnormalities (e.g., low back and buttock pain referring to the leg); however, some important differences exist. Pain originating from the SI joint is typically unilateral. It is always felt low in the back and never above the L5 vertebral level. Although pain that is felt entirely above L5 cannot be emanating from the SI joint, pain below L5 can originate from several different spinal structures because the typical radiation pattern is into the low back and buttock. For example, referral patterns from facet and diskogenic pain overlap with those from the SI joint. Pain from the SI joint can refer to the buttocks, back of the thigh, knee, and even the lateral calf and foot, thus making it difficult to distinguish SI joint pain from S1 radicular pain.

An important historical feature that can help distinguish radicular from radiating mechanical pain is that radicular pain is located almost entirely in the lower extremity and does not worsen with activity. Lower extremity pain associated with a mechanical cause is severe only when the back pain is severe; it never occurs independently of back pain. For these reasons, when taking the history of a patient complaining of back pain, one should always ask what percentage of the pain is in the back versus in the lower extremity and what percentage of the lower extremity pain is above the knee versus below it. Patients with SI joint pain typically react to abrupt movements with pain. They may also feel increased pain during lower extremity loading, such as when standing on one leg. Seemingly innocuous movements, such as turning over in bed, may also induce pain. Patients with SI joint pain may report that they unload the painful side when sitting; however, they should not report neurologic symptoms, such as paresthesias, numbness, or weakness.

Examination usually detects focal tenderness over the joint, and the findings that appear to correlate most closely with a positive diagnosis are pain below L5 and single-finger pointing by the patient to the posterior superior iliac spine when he or she is asked where the pain is located. These findings have been shown to have a positive predictive value of 60%.[119,123,140] Clinical suspicion of sacroiliac joint intra-articular or ligament pain may be confirmed by differential, fluoroscopically guided, interosseous ligament, or intra-articular injection of local anesthetic, with or without steroid.

Indications

The indications for SI joint RF lesioning are back pain below the L5 level for the past 3 months that has failed to respond to conservative therapy. The patient must report a positive response (i.e., >80% relief) to SI joint injections on two occasions to be considered a candidate for an SI joint RF procedure. Contraindications include local or systemic bacterial infection, bleeding diathesis, and possible pregnancy.

Technique

Two techniques that have emerged as having promise in the treatment of SI joint pain are strip lesion RF ablation and cooled-probe RF ablation. Because the cooled-probe RF technique requires the use of special equipment and a specific lesion generator, it is not discussed here. Instead, only the strip lesion technique is addressed because it can be performed with standard RF equipment, and no special lesion generator is required.

A strip lesion can be produced by several methods. One can create either a monopolar or a bipolar lesion, or the practitioner can use the Simplicity III device made by NeuroTherm, which contains three electrodes on a single probe. All three methods are very similar, so only the monopolar technique is discussed in detail here.

To begin the procedure, the L5-S1 disk space is opened by moving the C-arm into a cephalad tilt, to look into the L5-S1 disk space. The C-arm is then very slightly obliquely toward the ipsilateral side to visualize the groove between the sacral ala and the SAP of S1 fully. The L5 dorsal ramus is then approached in a pillar view, as previously described in the section on lumbar medial branch RF. A 10- or 15-cm needle with a 10 mm active tip is advanced directly down the beam until it contacts periosteum. Because this technique requires some manipulation of the needle as it rests against the bone, it is best to anesthetize the bone by injecting 1 to 2 mL of 2% lidocaine (Xylocaine) through the needle to prevent pain while the cannula is slid into proper position. The needle is then carefully advanced by making small back and forth twisting motions until the active tip lies in the previously described groove. Once the needle is properly located in the pillar view, the needle should be observed in three additional views: AP, lateral, and steep oblique. In the AP view, the needle should be resting against the SAP of S1; in the lateral view, it should be at the base of the SAP of S1; and in the steep oblique view, it should lie across the base of the S1 SAP. A second needle is then placed by starting on the skin at or just below the S2 foramen. The needle is carefully advanced down to periosteum, such that it touches bone slightly lateral and inferior to the S1 foramen. The needle is then carefully advanced cephalad until the needle is two active tips (10 mm) cephalad to the S1 foramen. A third needle is started on the skin inferior to the S4 foramen and advanced in similar fashion until it is located similarly against the S2 foramen.

As the nerves exit their respective foramina, they may take any path as they travel to the joint, including directly lateral, lateral and cephalad, or lateral and caudal. Therefore, one should take care to locate the needles near, but never directly in, the sacral foramen, to catch the nerves before they begin to separate significantly from one another as they travel to the joint. Once the sacral needles are in place, a lateral view is obtained. In the lateral view, the needles should

be closely applied to the posterior aspect of the sacrum, rather than located in the soft tissue above the sacrum. In addition, it is important to ensure that the needles have not entered the sacral foramina and are placed in the epidural space. Motor testing at 2 Hz and 1 V is performed to ensure that no contraction of the muscles innervated by the ventral rami has occurred. Then, 1 mL of 2% lidocaine is infiltrated through each needle, and 60 seconds are allowed to pass while the anesthetic takes effect. Finally, each nerve is ablated for 60 to 90 seconds at 80°C to 85°C (176°F to 185°F). The needles are then pulled down the length of the active tip, and second, third, and forth lesions are produced. By creating multiple lesions, the active tip of the cephalad needle is retracted caudally, 10 mm at a time, until it reaches the starting position of the needle below. This leaves a continuous strip lesion from L5 to S2 and ensures that all possible locations of the lateral branches have been burned (**Fig. 178.21**).

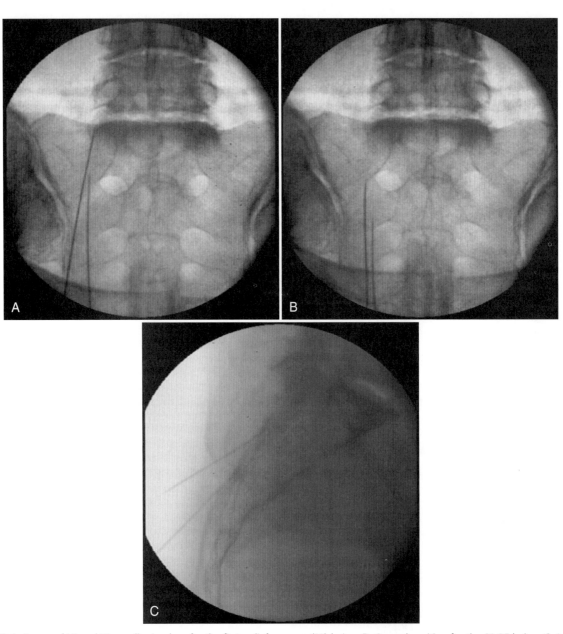

Fig. 178.21 A, Image of L5 and S1 needles in place for the first radiofrequency (RF) lesion. B, Second position for the S1 RF lesion. C, Lateral view showing S1 and S2 needles in place for the RF lesion.

A bipolar variation on this procedure uses two needles. The needles are placed as described earlier, with the caveat that the tips lie 2 to 4 mm from each other. Then, rather than pulling each needle down for successive lesions, the cephalad needle is removed and replaced as the caudad needle. A third variation on this technique involves use of the Simplicity III probe. The probe is placed from a single location just slightly below and lateral to the S4 foramen. It is then advanced to its final position at the sacral ala. Because the probe is not hollow, anesthetic must be placed using a spinal needle. For further instruction on placement of this probe, contact NeuroTherm.

Complications

Possible complications related to RF lesioning of the SI joint include those described in the section on lumbar medial branch RF. An additional risk is the possibility that the needles could enter the sacral foramina and cause heating and damage to the sacral nerve roots. Because the patient is awake and conversant during the procedure, this complication should not occur, given that the patient will feel a sensation of heating in the legs that can be communicated immediately.

Efficacy

Approaches to RF lesioning of the SI joint include intra-articular, cooled-probe RF ablation, bipolar or monopolar strip lesions, and a combination of ligamentous and neural RF ablation. This discussion focuses on cooled-probe RF ablation and bipolar or monopolar strip lesions. Cooled-probe RF ablation is a relatively new method of treating SI joint pain that can increase lesion size by a factor of 8.[134] To date, its use has been published in two papers. The first described a randomized, placebo-controlled study of 28 patients with SI joint pain confirmed by a single intra-articular diagnostic block.[141] The study compared sham and cooled-probe denervation of the S1-3 lateral branches, with conventional lesions performed at L4 and L5 medial branches. Patients in the treatment group reported significant improvement in pain (a reduction by 60%, 60%, and 57%, at 1, 3, and 6 months, respectively) compared with the patients in the placebo group, none of whom reported significant improvement. Patients in the treatment group also reported improvement in functional capacity and medication usage. The other article described a retrospective case series including 27 patients with SI joint pain confirmed using dual diagnostic blocks.[142] Thirteen of the patients (50%) reported at least a 50% decrease in pain 3 to 4 months following treatment.

Strip lesions are another relatively new method of treating SI joint pain. The technique was used in a prospective observational study that included nine patients with SI joint pain confirmed by local anesthetic joint and lateral branch nerve blocks.[127] The strip lesions were created adjacent to the lateral dorsal foraminal aperture, with conventional monopolar lesions at the L5 dorsal ramus. Eight of the nine patients were satisfied with the treatment, and 78%, 67%, 67%, 89%, and 67% reported being very satisfied at 1, 3, 6, 9, and 12 months. Median improvement in pain intensity was 4.1 on a 10-point rating scale, and reduction in disability was 17.8 on the Oswestry Disability Index.

Finally, a meta-analysis of 10 studies in which RA ablation was used to treat SI joint pain demonstrated that the procedure is an effective treatment a3 and 6 months.[143] Diminished outcomes after 6 months are likely the result of nerve regeneration and regrowth.

Thoracic Medial Branch Radiofrequency
History

When RF neurotomy was first introduced as a therapeutic modality, attention was largely focused on treatment of cervical and lumbar pain. Few studies were directed toward treatment of thoracic facet joint pain, possibly because of the lower incidence of complaints in that region. In addition, no anatomic dissections of the thoracic medial branches had been published, and poorly performed anatomic studies, described in a textbook by Hovelacque in 1927,[144] suggested that thoracic medial branch anatomy was analogous to that of the lumbar medial branches. Therefore, early attempts at thoracic facet joint RF were directed at the junction of the SAP and the TP, and outcomes were poor.[16,145,146] Despite using the same anatomic targets as earlier studies, Stolker et al[16] reported that 16 out of 36 patients (44%) were pain free 31 months after the procedure. Subsequent anatomic studies revealed that the thoracic medial branch nerve is located on distal tip of the superior aspect of the TP,[147] which redirected the target for RF procedures. Whether this change will improve efficacy remains to be seen.

Anatomy

The thoracic facet joints are innervated by the medial branches of the dorsal rami.[98,147-150] The location of the thoracic medial branches is basically the same at all levels of the thoracic spine, but their course differs slightly at the midthoracic levels. A careful anatomic study of multiple adult human cadavers found that the archetypical medial branches are located on the superior lateral aspects of the TPs and assume a consistent course.[147] On exiting the IVF, the dorsal rami immediately divide, giving off the medial, lateral, and intermediate branches. The medial branch nerves pass mostly laterally within the intertransverse space until they cross the TP at the superolateral corner. They then pass medially and inferiorly across the posterior surface of the TP before ramifying into the multifidus muscles. The exception to this pattern appears at the T4-8 levels, where the inflection point is superior to the TP. These nerves are often referred to as floating because they may be retracted into the muscles above the TP rather than actually touching the periosteum. The medial branch nerves located at the T12 and L1 vertebral levels (i.e., the T11 and T12 medial branches) are found in an analogous location to the lumbar medial branch nerves (i.e., at the junction of the SAP and the TP). The precise location of the medial branch along the TP varies from cadaver to cadaver, with some medial branches are located slightly more toward the midline than others. Thus, the target for RF lesioning is an area along the distal TP, rather than a discrete point.

The nomenclature used to identify specific nerves can be confusing. Because the spine has seven cervical vertebrae and eight cervical nerves, the C8 medial branch nerve is located at the T1 vertebra. Consequently, the nomenclature for each subsequent nerve is associated with the vertebra below it. For example, the T7 medial branch rests on the T8 TP. In addition, two nerves innervate each joint, one from the segmental level of origin and one from the level below it. For example, the T8 and T9 medial branches innervate the T8-9 joint. To ensure clear communication about any spinal procedure performed, it is necessary to specify the nerves involved, their location on the vertebral body, and the joints they innervate. For example, a report of a medial branch block could read as follows: the T7 and T8 medial branches were blocked at the T8 and T9 vertebral levels to anesthetize the T8-9 joint.[151]

Patient Selection

Midback pain is an important albeit uncommon pain complaint. Investigators have estimated that 5% to 15% of all patients referred to a typical outpatient pain clinic complain of thoracic spinal pain.[152,153] The prevalence of facet joint pain in this group of patients is 42%.

Before evaluating the origin of musculoskeletal pain in the thoracic spine, one should first exclude medical causes. This is particularly critical in the thoracic area, given the important structures that reside there. For example, thoracic pain can arise from diseases of the cardiovascular, pulmonary, or gastrointestinal systems. Serious causes of pain must also be considered such as malignant disease, infection, or impending cardiac disasters (myocardial infarction, rupturing thoracic aneurysm). Once medical causes have been excluded, the physician must differentiate between mechanical and radicular causes of pain. Thoracic radicular pain is most often of a burning, shooting, or electrical nature and radiates around to the front of the chest or abdomen. The pain is constant and not usually influenced by activity. In contrast, thoracic facet joint pain is mechanical, often manifesting as a constant ache that worsens with activity and eases with rest, and it may radiate in a nondermatomal pattern.

Once a mechanical cause is identified, it may be difficult to determine whether the pain source is a facet joint, a costovertebral joint, or a costotransverse joint, given that no clinical features allow differentiation among the three joints. Because these joints are in close proximity, sequentially anesthetizing each is the best way to determine which joint is causing the pain. A patient whose pain is relieved by a correctly performed medial branch block can be assumed to have facet disease.

An additional confounding factor in the evaluation of upper thoracic pain is that pain originating from the lower cervical facet joint refers to the upper thoracic spine. Thus, patients presenting with upper thoracic pain (e.g., pain between the shoulder blades) should first undergo a cervical medial branch block.

Indications

The indications for facet joint denervation include chronic midback pain with or without radiation in a nondermatomal pattern, focal tenderness over one or several facet joints, and positive response to a medial branch block with greater than 80% relief on two occasions. The only absolute contraindications are infection in the overlying soft tissues, systemic infection, bleeding diathesis, and possible pregnancy.

Technique

The RF techniques for thoracic medial branch neurotomy published to date have emphasized a single-needle approach. However, in the absence of definitive studies regarding an optimal approach, a two-needle bipolar technique with chemical neurolysis is presented here. The advantage of the bipolar technique is that it creates a larger burn and thus increases the likelihood of trapping the nerve between the two electrodes, a maneuver that, in turn, increases the probability of adequate neurolysis. In addition, the use of 6% phenol diluted in contrast dye may aid in achieving neurolysis, particularly of the floating nerves located at the T4-8 levels that do not rest directly on the TP.

The patient is positioned prone on the fluoroscopy table, and the back is prepared and draped in sterile fashion. If sedation is given, it should be light enough that the patient is awake and conversant throughout the procedure. The target for the medial branches is the lateral aspect of the TPs. To begin, a straight AP view with the vertebral end plates squared is obtained. The TP at the targeted level should be clearly visible. If it is not, it sometimes helpful to move the C-arm such that the TP of interest is visualized at the periphery of the screen to improve contrast and decrease the "whiteout" caused by the lungs. Once the TP is clearly visualized at the targeted levels, a skin wheal is placed slightly below the inferior aspect of the TP.

A 20-g 10-cm RFK needle with a 10-mm active tip is advanced from inferior and lateral to superior and medial toward the superior border of the lateral aspect of the TP. A second needle is then similarly advanced, slightly medial to the first, such that the needles form a V shape with the heads more lateral than the tips. This technique interference between the needle heads that can cause shifting in the location of the active tips. Once in final position, the needle tips should be separated by 2 to 4 mm or one to two needle widths. The needles are advanced from an inferior position in an attempt to place them parallel to the nerve, to provide a larger area of burn.

Sensory testing can be implemented at 0.3 to 0.5 V, although this may not have an impact on outcome.[79] One can also perform motor stimulation to ensure adequate distance from the ventral ramus by using parameters of 2 Hz and 1 V, which should not result in muscle contraction in the anterior chest wall.

Once the needles are in final position, a lateral view is obtained to confirm that the needles have not advanced off the TP. The nerves are then anesthetized by placing 0.5 mL of 2% lidocaine through each needle, and RF current is applied for 60 to 90 seconds at 80°C to 90°C (176°F to 194°F). On completion of the lesion, 0.1 to 0.2 mL of 6% phenol diluted in contrast dye is injected through each needle, so the patient receives both chemical and thermal lesions. Phenol should be used only on the T1-10 medial branches (i.e., at the T2-11 vertebral levels), where the nerves are located on the tips of the TPs (**Figs. 178.22** and **178.23**).

Efficacy

RF lesioning of the thoracic facet joints is not well studied. Only a few articles have been published, and the lesioning techniques reported are inconsistent. Some techniques incorrectly target the junction of the SAP and the TP, whereas others use the anatomically correct target.[16,147]

In an unpublished case report, the use of bipolar RF lesioning with the addition of phenol decreased a patient's pain from a 9/10 to 2/10 on a VAS. The neurotomy was performed at the distal aspect of the TPs.[109] A cadaveric study of a bipolar

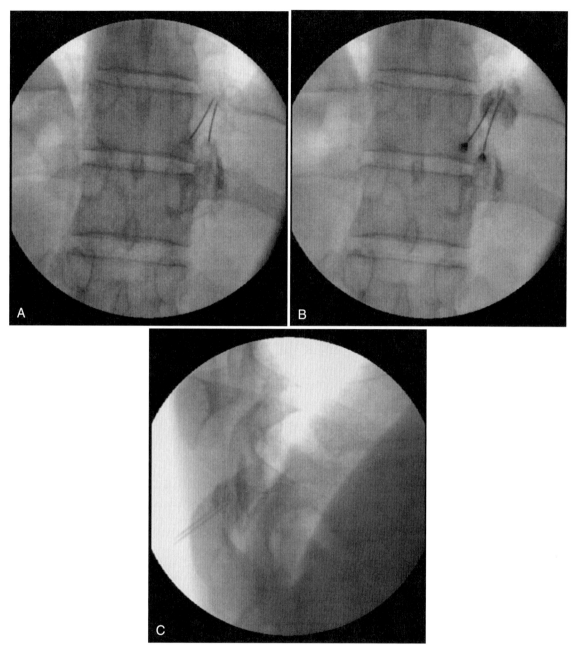

Fig. 178.22 **A,** Anteroposterior view with needles in place for thoracic bipolar radiofrequency (RF). **B,** View after injection of 6% phenol. **C,** Lateral view of needles in place for thoracic bipolar RF.

technique using interspinous ligament tissue demonstrated that heating two electrodes simultaneously appears to coagulate a wider area than a monopolar lesion and potentially produces better results in less time.[154]

Tzaan and Tasker[22] reviewed 118 cases of RF denervation performed on 90 patients. The procedures were not limited to the thoracic spine and also included cervical and lumbar procedures. The patients were followed for an average of 5.6 months, and success was defined as greater than 50% reduction in pain. Of the 17 patients who underwent thoracic RF lesioning (the exact method of lesioning was not described), 15 met the criteria for success at follow-up. The most frequent complications were sensory loss and transient neuritis in the cutaneous branches of the posterior rami.[22]

C2 Radiofrequency Treatment for Cervicogenic Headache (Table 178.5)
History
The most common cause of cervicogenic headache of spinal origin is injury to the C2-3 joint. Rarely, the C1-2 and C0-1 joints are involved. The suspicion that the upper cervical joints could be responsible for headache was first proposed in the early 1900s.[2,155] However, upper cervical joint injury as a primary cause of headaches in whiplash victims remained largely unrecognized for many years.[5] In a study by Lord et al[156] in whiplash victims who reported headache as the primary symptom, the prevalence of C2-3 joint pain was 53%.[156] In an attempt to prove the C2-3 joint as a source of

headache, Dwyer et al[105] injected contrast dye into the C2-3 joint of normal volunteers and was able to induce a characteristic headache in the occipital area.[2] Bogduk and Marsland[157,158] showed that anesthetizing the TON could relieve pain emanating from the joint. Dreyfuss et al[159] performed a similar study of the atlantoaxial joint and was able to induce pain at the base of the skull. Bogduk[2,160] described a technique of anesthetizing the C2 spinal nerve as a means of diagnosis. Later, the idea of directly anesthetizing the joint as a means of diagnosis was proposed.

Anatomy

The anatomy of the upper cervical spine is complex because several communicating branches are present among the C1, C2, and C3 dorsal rami.[5] The confusion is compounded by the trigeminal cervical system. The trigeminal nucleus descends into the upper cervical segments of the spinal cord possibly as far down as C3.[110]

Stimulation of the occipital nerves has a facilitatory influence on input from the dura. Furthermore, stimulation of muscle afferents produces more input than skin afferents, a finding suggesting that increases in cervical muscle tone may increase input into the cervical trigeminal system. This may explain why anesthetizing the occipital nerves relieves tension-type headache. For this group of patients, it may make sense to perform a PRF lesion of the C2 DRG because this is the sensory nucleus of the occipital nerve.

For those patients with headache of spinal origin, it most commonly emanates from the C1-2 or C2-3 joint (**Fig. 178.24**). The TON innervates the C2-3 joint, whereas C1-2 innervation derives from the C2 dorsal ramus. Finally, for patients with pain from occipital neuralgia caused by chronic tension headache, the greater occipital nerve derives its roots from the C2 nerve. Therefore, PRF procedures performed at the C2 and C3 levels would be expected to treat all three causes of pain.

Indications

The diagnosis of cervicogenic headache should be suspected in patients with headache pain of unknown origin. Distinguishing pain emanating from the C1-2 and C2-3 joints

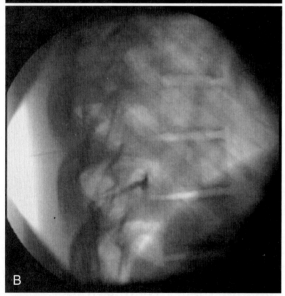

Fig. 178.23 **A,** Anteroposterior view of the course of the medial branch nerve tracking back to the dorsal ramus and spinal nerve root. **B,** Lateral view showing dye from the medial branch nerve sheath tracking into the epidural space.

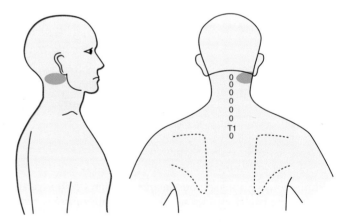

Fig. 178.24 **C1-2 joint referral pattern and C1-2 cervical facet joint referral map.**

Table 178.5 **Radiofrequency for Cervicogenic Headache**			
Authors	**Study Design**	**N**	**Efficacy**
Haspeslagh et al, 2006[161]	Randomized controlled trial	30	No difference between group treated with occipital nerve block using steroids and group treated with cervical facet joint radiofrequency and upper cervical dorsal root ganglion radiofrequency
Chao et al, 2008[162]	Retrospective analysis	49	55.10% had ≥50% pain relief at 3-mo follow-up

is difficult.[5] Patients often complain of pain at the base of the skull that sometimes radiates up the back of the head. They may report focal tenderness in the suboccipital area. The pain is often unilateral. The pain may be increased with turning of the head, axial loading, or bending toward the affected side. The pain is continuous but is often increased by activity and lessened by rest. Patients describe it as a dull aching or throbbing sensation. Neurologic symptoms are not usually associated with the pain. This pain can be extremely debilitating, and some patients give up their work or school activities to cope with it. The cause is thought to be tearing of the joint capsule surrounding one or more of the upper cervical joints.

Another cause of chronic posterior headache pain is tension-type headache. Many of these patients complain of a dull aching or a squeezing sensation bilaterally at the posterior aspect of the head that radiates into the temporal, frontal areas. The pain is usually not associated with nausea, vomiting, photophobia, or phonophobia. Patients with this type of pain can usually function in spite of it, in contradistinction to patients with migraine headache, who usually must lie down in a dark room to cope with the pain. Anecdotally, patients with tension headaches originating in the occipital area have been found to respond to treatment with an interventional procedure (described in the next subsection) at the C2 DRG level. Although no data show a clear advantage of this procedure, the theoretical basis for treatment is sound.

PRF lesioning of the C2 DRG should be undertaken only when more conservative treatment options have failed. The patient should have responded on two occasions with greater that 80% relief to diagnostic blocks (TON for C 2-3 joint pain, C2 DRG for atlantoaxial joint pain, and occipital nerve blocks for headache pain).

Technique

The patient is positioned in the lateral position on the operating room table with the head built up sufficiently that it is parallel to the operating room table and directly perpendicular to the shoulders. This position facilitates proper imaging (**Fig. 178.25**). The neck is prepared and draped in sterile fashion, and monitors are applied if intravenous sedation is planned. If intravenous sedation is given, it should be very light, to facilitate continuous communication between the patient and the operator. This serves as a monitor for any type of complication that may occur. The target point is in the anterior aspect of the dome created by the C1-2 lamina. Specifically, the point lies in the midaspect of the dome from cephalad to caudad and in the anterior aspect from dorsal to ventral. A needle placed down to this point is not expected to contact periosteum and can be placed directly through the spinal cord. Checking multiple AP views during needle insertion to assess the needle during needle placement is essential to prevent this complication.

A skin wheal overlying this target point is raised, and a 22-gauge SMK needle with a 4-mm active tip is advanced through the skin wheal directly down the beam toward the target. Caution should be taken to make certain that the needle tip is not advanced into the muscle layers until it is pointed directly toward the intended target. In addition, if the skin wheal is placed more than 3 mm off target, a new starting point should be made, and the needle should be reinserted directly over the

target. Once the needle is properly aligned, the needle is passed in a tunnel vision view down to the lamina of C2. Contact with lamina before passing the needle to the final target is done to give a sense of depth before advancing to the target. With the needle on the lamina, the operator retracts the needle slightly and redirects it toward the target. At this point, an AP view is obtained, and the needle should be seen resting on the lateral aspect of the articular pillar. If visualizing the needle tip is difficult, an open-mouth view is helpful.

The needle tip is carefully and slowly advanced toward the target. In the AP view, the target is usually directly over or slightly inferior to the midaspect of the atlantoaxial joint. When the needle approaches this area, the operator should warn the patient and advance only 0.5 mm at a time while monitoring for paresthesia. Once the patient feels mild paresthesia, needle advancement is stopped, and sensory testing is performed. With correct needle placement, the patient should

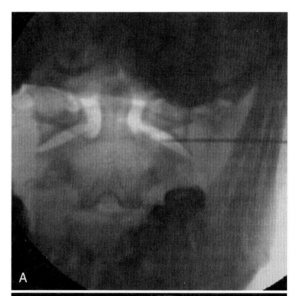

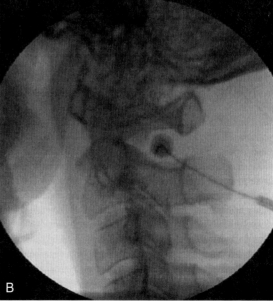

Fig. 178.25 Fluoroscopic images of a C2 dorsal root ganglion radiofrequency procedure. A, Anteroposterior view: C2 procedure. B, Lateral view: C2 procedure.

report a tingling sensation in the back of the head at less than 0.2 V. No need exists for motor stimulation during a PRF procedure. Before lesioning, one should check the final needle position in two views. In the lateral view, the needle is seen in the anterior aspect of the dome created by the C1-2 lamina and in a midposition from cephalad to caudad. In an AP view, the needle is seen at or slightly below the atlantoaxial joint in the middle aspect of the articular pillar from lateral to medial. Lesioning in the pulsed mode is done by slowly turning up the voltage while monitoring the patient. It is not uncommon to note muscle contractions during the procedure. These contractions are normal and should not cause alarm.

Efficacy

PRF lesioning of the nerves at this level of the cervical spine has not been well studied. Only one article specifically studied this issue. The study was a randomized controlled trial comparing the results of occipital nerve block with RF treatment of the upper cervical area in patients with occipital headache. Each group had 30 patients: 15 received RF treatments and 15 underwent occipital nerve blocks. The RF group first underwent RF of the C3-6 z-joints from a posterolateral approach by using 22-gauge SMK needles with a 4-mm active tip. If this procedure failed to relieve symptoms, diagnostic nerve blocks were performed at either the C2 or C3 levels followed by RF lesioning at the relevant level. The second group received an occipital nerve block. If the patient failed to obtain sufficient relief after 8 weeks, a second block was performed. Finally, if the patient remained symptomatic at 16 weeks, he or she was treated with transcutaneous electrical nerve stimulation. The results revealed no statistical difference of either treatment between the groups. The study can be criticized on multiple points. First, the RF procedure as performed would be unlikely to coagulate the TON and therefore relieve the most common cause of spinal headache. In addition, RF lesions performed at other levels (C3-6) are superfluous in the treatment of cervicogenic headache. Next, the investigators did not specify how the DRG procedure was performed. As reported in an earlier section of this chapter, PRF lesioning of the cervical DRG had an effect in relieving pain, whereas DRG performed with heat (in the lumbar spine) clearly did not.[161]

Two other small studies looked at outcomes from pulsed DRG treatment at the cervical levels. While not specifically studied, both reports included patients treated for headache with DRG lesioning at the C2 or C3 levels. The first study, reported earlier, included six patients treated at either the C2 or C3 DRG for headache. Out of six patients, three reported no effect, and three reported pain relief averaging 20 months (two patients had 18 months of relief, and one patient reported 24 months of relief). All three patients rated their pain relief at 7 on the Likert scale, a finding corresponding to greater than 75% improvement. A second study reported results of PRF lesioning at the C3-7 levels. At 1 year, 57% of patients reported satisfactory pain relief.[47,162]

Conclusion

RF treatment has been used for various painful conditions including trigeminal neuralgia, facet-mediated pain, and radicular pain syndromes. As is often the case with novel treatments for challenging medical conditions, the early use of RF current for chronic pain was fraught with problems. At first, investigators recognized the value of the modality, but did not know how to best apply it. The advent of better equipment in 1980 (in particular the SMK needle and the Cosman RF generator) prompted anatomic and clinical studies that fostered rapid advances in knowledge. Flaws in previous studies were corrected with improvements in patient selection and technique.

Thanks to pioneering studies by Bogduk, Lord, Govind, Dreyfuss, and others, proper anatomic targets for the cervical and lumbar medial branch procedures were identified and were used to devise the optimal means of destroying the nerves. This research helped to confirm the efficacy of both procedures. Through experimentation with the use of continuous RF, the PRF mode was developed, thus allowing the treatment of targets for which heat is contraindicated.

Researchers in multiple disciplines have appreciated the importance of this modality. Increasing numbers of clinical studies, when considered collectively, suggest that PRF is effective. In addition, ongoing in vitro and animal studies will bolster the evidence in this area of study. As is often the case during the development of a treatment, no single theory has been able to explain the mechanism of action for PRF fully. However, clinical data support the notion that, when PRF is properly used to treat well-selected patients, it is an effective tool for some types of chronic pain syndromes (most notably radicular pain and peripheral neuropathies). These patients in particular are often refractory to medication and, in the absence of PRF, may require more expensive and invasive treatments (e.g., spinal cord stimulation). To date, most studies show only short-term efficacy (approximately 3 months). Further research is needed to determine the best methods of applying PRF for longer-term pain relief.

This chapter summarizes best practices in the use of RF, describes new methods of RF application, and presents data on PRF to support its use in clinical practice.

References

Full references for this chapter can be found on www.expertconsult.com.

Cryoneurolysis

Lloyd R. Saberski

Cryoanalgesic therapy has widespread and diverse applications in the fields of pain management and neurosurgery. This chapter introduces the practitioner to the proper use and limitations of this relatively new technology so that appropriate clinical decisions can be made. Examples of applications are presented, but the intent is not to address all potential uses of cryoanalgesia.

Historical Considerations

Cryoanalgesia is a technique in which cold is applied to produce pain relief. The analgesic effect of cold has been known to humans for more than 2 millennia.[1] Hippocrates (460–377 BC) provided the first written record of the use of ice and snow packs applied before surgery as a local pain-relieving technique.[2] Early physicians, such as Avicenna of Persia (980–1070 AD) and Severino of Naples (1580–1656) recorded using cold for preoperative analgesia.[3,4] In 1812, Napoleon's surgeon general, Baron Dominique Jean Larrey,[5] recognized that the limbs of soldiers frozen in the Prussian snow could be amputated relatively painlessly. In 1751, Arnott[6] described using an ice-salt mixture to produce tumor regression and to obtain an anesthetic and hemostatic effect. Richardson introduced ether spray in 1766 to produce local analgesia by refrigeration; this was superseded in 1790 by ethyl chloride spray.

Contemporary interest in cryoanalgesia was sparked in 1961, after Cooper described a cryotherapy unit in which liquid nitrogen was circulated through a hollow metal probe that was vacuum insulated except at the tip. With this equipment, it was possible to control the temperature of the tip by interrupting the flow of liquid nitrogen at temperatures within the range of room temperature to −196°C (−321°F). Because the system was totally enclosed, cold could be applied to any part of the body accessible to the probe. The first clinical application of this technique was in neurosurgery for treatment of parkinsonism.[7,8] In

1967, Amoils[9] developed a simpler hand-held unit that used carbon dioxide or nitrous oxide. These devices were the prototypes for the current generation of cryoprobes used in cryoanalgesia (**Figs. 179.1** and **179.2**). The coldest temperature used today is approximately −70°C (−94°F).

Physics and Cellular Basics for Cryoanalgesia

The working principle of a cryoprobe is that compressed gas (nitrous oxide or carbon dioxide) expands. The cryoprobe consists of an outer tube and a smaller inner tube that terminates in a fine nozzle (**Fig. 179.3**). High-pressure gas (650 to 800 psi) is passed between the two tubes and is released through a small orifice into a chamber at the tip of the probe. In the chamber, the gas expands, and the substantial reduction in pressure (80 to 100 psi) results in a rapid decrease in temperature and cooling of the probe tip. (Absorption of heat from surrounding tissues accompanies expansion of any gas, according to the principles of the general gas law; this is the adiabatic principle of gas cooling and heat extraction, also known as the Joule-Thomson effect.) The low-pressure gas flows back through the center of the inner tube and back to the console, where it is vented. The sealed construction of the cryoprobe ensures that no gas escapes from the probe tip, handle, or hose.

The rapid cooling of the cryoprobe produces a tip surface temperature of approximately −70°C (−94°F). Tissue in contact with the tip cools rapidly and forms an ice ball. The ice ball varies in size, depending on probe size, freeze time, tissue permeability to water, and the presence of vascular structures (heat sink). The ice ball typically measures 3.5 to 5.5 mm in diameter. Further increase in size is prevented when thermal equilibrium is attained.

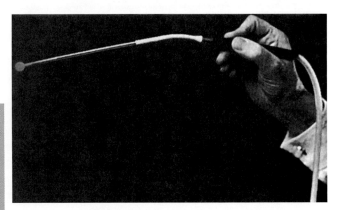

Fig. 179.1 An early hand-held cryoprobe with ice ball. *(From Holden HB: Practical cryosurgery, London, 1975, Pitman.)*

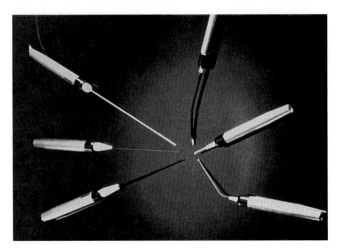

Fig. 179.2 Contemporary hand-held Lloyd cryoprobes. *(Courtesy of Westco Medical Corporation, San Diego.)*

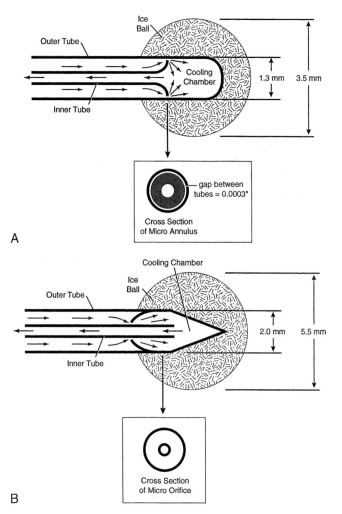

Fig. 179.3 A and **B,** Cross sections of two commonly used cryoprobe designs. High-pressure gas goes in through the outer tube at 650 to 800 psi. Low-pressure gas is vented out at 80 to 100 psi. Gas flow is at 7 to 9 L/minute. Test conditions: The tip is inserted into water at 36°C (97°F) ± 1°C (34°F). An ice ball is formed within 60 seconds.

Precise levels of gas flow through the cryoprobe are essential for maximum efficiency. Inadequate gas flow does not freeze tissue. Excessive gas flow results in freezing down the stem of the probe and the associated risk of cold skin burns. The cryoprobe console is fitted with a regulator and an indicator that are adjusted for optimal performance.

The application of cold to peripheral nerves, whether by direct cooling of localized segments or complete immersion of tissue in a cold medium, induces reversible conduction block. The extent and duration of the effect depend on the temperature attained in the tissues and the duration of exposure.[1] When nerve fibers are progressively cooled, a conduction block similar to that produced by local anesthetic develops. At 10°C, larger myelinated fibers cease conduction before unmyelinated fibers, but at 0°C (32°F), all nerve fibers entrapped in the ice ball stop conduction. Some fibers resume conduction on rewarming. To obtain a prolonged effect from a cryolesion, the intracellular contents of the nerve must be turned into ice crystals. The clinical difference is minimal as long as the temperature is less than −20°C (−4°F) for 1 minute.[10] When the nerve is frozen amid other tissues, the duration of exposure becomes more important. Within the limitations of a specific cryoprobe and its steady state of thermal equilibrium, prolonging application of the cryoprobe increases the size of the ice ball and the likelihood that the nerve will become entrapped by a cryolesion. In practice, a freeze of 2 to 3 minutes' duration produces a good result.

Prolonged exposure and repeated freeze-thaw cycles likely are beneficial with percutaneous techniques, especially when abundant surrounding soft tissue and nerve localization are poor.[1]

Histologically, the axons and myelin sheaths degenerate after cryolesioning (wallerian degeneration), but the epineurium and perineurium remain intact, thus allowing subsequent nerve regeneration. The duration of the block is a function of the rate of axonal regeneration after cryolesioning, which is reported to be 1 to 3 mm/day.[10] Because axonal regrowth is constant, the return of sensory and motor activity is a function of the distance between the cryolesion and the end organ.[1] The absence of external damage to the nerve and the minimal inflammatory reaction to freezing ensure that regeneration is exact. The regenerating axons are unlikely to form painful neuromas. (Surgical and thermal lesions interrupt perineurium and epineurium.) Other neurolytic techniques (alcohol, phenol) potentially can produce painful neuromas because the epineurium and perineurium are disrupted.

A cryolesion provides a temporary anesthetic block. Clinically, a cryoblock lasts weeks to months. The result depends on numerous variables, including operator technique and clinical circumstances. The analgesia often lasts longer than the time required for axons to regenerate.[16] The reasons are still a matter of speculation, but it is obvious that cryoanalgesia is more than just a temporary disruption of axons. Possibly, sustained blockade of afferent input to the central nervous system (CNS) has an effect on CNS windup. One report suggested that cryolesions release sequestered tissue protein or facilitate changes in protein antigenic properties.[11] The result is an autoimmune response targeted at cryolesioned tissue. The first report of such a response was from Gander et al,[12] who showed tissue-specific autoantibodies after cryocoagulation of male rabbit accessory glands. This report was followed by a parallel clinical report of regression of metastatic deposits from prostatic adenocarcinoma after cryocoagulation of the primary tumor.[13] The significance for pain management is unclear; however, it does indicate that tumor growth and regression are affected by immune function. Perhaps immune mechanisms play a role in the analgesic response after cryoablation.

Indications and Contraindications

Cryoanalgesia is best suited for clinical situations when analgesia is required for weeks or months. Permanent blockade does not usually occur because the cryoinjured axons regenerate. The median duration of pain relief is 2 weeks to 5 months.[14,15] Cryoanalgesia is suited for painful conditions that originate from small, well-localized lesions of peripheral nerves (e.g., neuromas, entrapment neuropathies, and postoperative pain).[16] Longer than expected periods of analgesia have been reported and may result from the patient's ability to participate more fully in physical therapy or from an effect of prolonged analgesia on central processing of pain (preemptive analgesic effect). Sustained blockade of afferent impulses[17–20] with cryoanalgesia may reduce plasticity (windup) in the CNS and may decrease pain permanently.[21]

Cryoablative procedures can be open or closed (percutaneous), depending on the clinical setting. Most often, open procedures are performed as part of postoperative analgesia. Under direct visualization, the operator identifies the neural structure of concern, and the cryoprobe is applied for 1 to 4 minutes, depending on tissue heat, which is a function of blood supply and distance of the probe from the nerve. Care is taken not to freeze adjacent vascular structures. The cryoprobe is withdrawn only after the tissue thaws because removing it earlier can tear tissue.

Percutaneous (closed) cryoablation is the technique of choice for outpatient chronic pain management. It has the advantages of easy application and few complications. Percutaneous (closed) cryoablative procedures have been used successfully for many benign and malignant pain syndromes. Few scientific studies have been published, however, in part because interest was minimal until more recently in pain management techniques and because of a lack of industry funding for advanced research.

Patients must give informed consent for the procedure. The consent form should describe the risk-to-benefit ratios of cryoanalgesia and of regional anesthesia. Patients should be fully aware that a cryoanalgesia procedure usually is not a permanent solution. It can ameliorate symptoms, however, and can allow the patient to participate in physical therapy more fully. In some cases, when CNS windup has occurred, cryoanalgesia may serve as a form of preemptive anesthetic and may facilitate prolonged relief. Cryoanalgesia for chronic pain syndromes always should be preceded by diagnostic or prognostic local

anesthetic injections. After a test block with local anesthetic, the examiner should inquire about the patient's tolerance to the numbness and the extent of pain reduction. If the patient's response to the test injections is inadequate, the patient will not have a good response to cryodenervation. Patients also should be aware that numbness can replace pain, and small areas of skin depigmentation can occur if the ice ball frosts skin because the probe is not deep enough or is inadequately insulated from tissues. All procedures are performed with appropriate sterile preparation. As a general rule, infected areas are avoided.

Clinically Relevant Anatomy

For any given procedure, it is essential that the provider of cryoanalgesia be aware of the regional anatomy of interest. Because cryoanalgesia has widespread applications, thorough knowledge of neuroanatomy and of regional anesthesia is required. In the next section, detailed descriptions and illustrations are provided for numerous procedures. The reader is referred to standard anatomy textbooks for more detailed discussions.

Clinical Pearls and Tricks of the Trade

Postoperative Pain Management

The postoperative use of cryoanalgesia should be widespread, but in the United States, cryoanalgesia is used routinely for postoperative patients in only a few centers. The reasons are several, among them a lack of controlled studies and physicians' reluctance to add time and costs to procedures, especially when they believe that patients already are receiving adequate care. At many institutions, cryoanalgesia is reserved for patients with special analgesia needs and patients at high risk who cannot receive standard postoperative treatment. Of the handful of studies that have been done,[22–26] most indicated significant reductions in pain and medication requirements. The use of postoperative cryoanalgesia will likely increase if investigators can show cost savings and improved long-term outcomes.

Cryoanalgesia procedures are provided intra-operatively by surgeons who have access to involved peripheral nerve and pain management specialists participating in the operative procedure. At times, pain specialists are called on to provide cryoanalgesia postoperatively, in which case they must decide whether some other alternative is more suitable than open or closed cryodenervation.

Popular Cryodenervation Techniques for Postoperative Pain Management
POST-THORACOTOMY PAIN

Intra-operative intercostal cryoneurolysis was first described by Nelson et al[27] in 1974. Since that time, a large body of literature has supported the use of cryodenervation as a component of a postoperative analgesia plan.[22–24,28] Post-thoracotomy cryoanalgesia is most effective for treating incisional pain, but it is ineffective for pain from visceral pleura supplied by autonomic fibers or for ligament pain of the chest secondary to rib retraction. Post-thoracotomy cryoanalgesia often has little effect on chest tube pain, for the same reasons. Patients treated with cryotherapy during thoracotomy have relatively less postoperative discomfort and fewer opioid requirements in the immediate postoperative period and over subsequent weeks. Only one report of neuritis has been documented as a complication of cryoneurolysis.[29] Sensory anesthesia lasts longer than 6 months along the sensory field of treated intercostal nerves.

For effective intra-operative cryoneurolysis, intercostal nerves on each side of the thoracotomy incision are lesioned. If a rib is removed, that intercostal nerve also undergoes cryolesioning. The intercostal nerves are best cryoablated just lateral to the transverse process, before the collateral intercostal nerve branches (**Fig. 179.4**). Only a small area of skin innervated by the dorsal primary ramus is missed. Care is taken to separate the intercostal nerves from the intercostal vessels, thus removing a large heat sink that would be counterproductive to cryotherapy. The vessels also are protected from cold-induced thrombosis. A cryolesion sufficient to produce visible evidence of freezing is required. In general, such a lesion takes 1 to 2 minutes. A second lesion can be placed after tissue thaws, but whether that is necessary when freezing of the first lesion is complete remains to be determined.

A retrospective study examined the medical records of patients who received percutaneous cryoanalgesia following successful intercostal nerve blockade for chronic chest pain. Sixty percent of the patients ($N = 43$) reported significant pain relief immediately following their procedure. Three months after cryoanalgesia, 50% continued to report significant pain relief. No cases of neuritis or neuroma formation were reported, and only three patients had a pneumothorax. This work provided evidence that cryoanalgesia is a safe and efficacious method of providing analgesia for chronic thoracic pain resulting from intercostal neuralgia.[30]

A comparison of epidural analgesia and intercostal nerve cryoanalgesia for post-thoracotomy pain as part of a randomized control study[31] cast some doubt on the long-term utility of cryoanalgesia for post-thoracotomy pain. The study looked at 107 adult patients, allocated randomly to thoracic epidural bupivacaine and morphine or to intercostal nerve cryoanalgesia. Acute pain scores and opioid-related side effects were evaluated for 3 postoperative days. Chronic pain information, including incidence, severity, and allodynia-like pain, was acquired on the first, third, sixth, and twelfth months postoperatively. No significant difference was noted on a numerical rating scale (NRS) at rest or on motion between the two groups during the 3 postoperative days. The patient satisfaction results were also similar between the groups. The side effects, especially mild pruritus, were reported more often in the epidural group. Both groups showed a high incidence of chronic pain (42.1% to 72.1%), with no significance between the groups. The incidence of allodynia-like pain reported in the cryoanalgesia group was higher than that in epidural group in any postoperative month, with significance on the sixth and the twelfth months postoperatively ($P < .05$). More patients rated their chronic pain intensity as moderate and severe in the cryoanalgesia group and reported that the pain interfered with daily life ($P < .05$). Both thoracic epidural analgesia and intercostal nerve cryoanalgesia produced satisfactory analgesia for post-thoracotomy acute pain. The incidence of post-thoracotomy chronic pain is high. Cryoanalgesia may be a factor that increases the incidence of neuropathic pain.

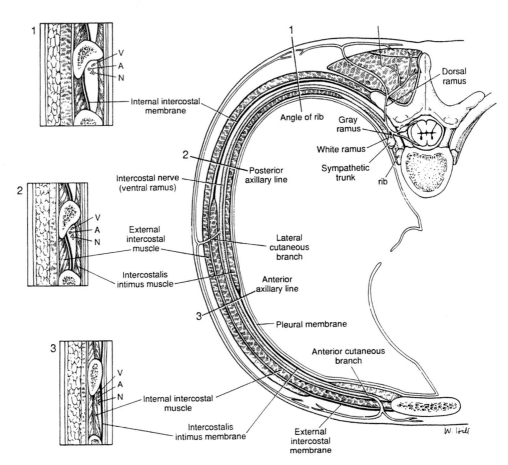

Fig. 179.4 **Cross-sectional view of intercostal nerve anatomy.** (From Chung J: Thoracic pain. In Sinatra RS, Hord AH, Ginsberg G, et al, editors: Acute pain, St. Louis, 1991, Mosby.)

POSTHERNIORRHAPHY PAIN

Cryoneurolysis after herniorrhaphy was first described by Wood et al in 1979.[32] A cryolesion of the ilioinguinal nerve reduced analgesic requirements during the postoperative period. The follow-up study in 1981 compared recovery from herniorrhaphy among three study groups: patients treated with oral analgesics, patients undergoing cryoanalgesia, and patients receiving paravertebral blockade (the last two treatments supplemented with oral analgesics as needed). The study indicated that the cryoanalgesia group not only had less pain in the postoperative period, but also used less opioid, resumed a regular diet earlier, were mobilized faster, and returned to work sooner.[25] Despite these successes, the technique is not widely used. Given its effectiveness and freedom from side effects, it is ideal for ambulatory surgery. After repair of the internal ring, posterior wall of the inguinal canal, and internal oblique muscle, the ilioinguinal nerve on the surface of the muscle is identified and mobilized. The surgeon elevates the nerve above the muscle, and an assistant performs the cryoablation.

Chronic Pain Management

For management of chronic pain, open cryoablation is avoided whenever the procedure can be performed effectively percutaneously. Before committing to cryoablation, the provider must perform a series of test blocks to determine presence of a consistent analgesic response. A favorable response before cryoablation occurs when the local anesthetic injection decreases pain, and the numbness that replaces the pain is tolerated by the patient. Care always must be taken to ensure correct positioning of the needles. When necessary, fluoroscopic guidance should be used. The smallest amount of local anesthetic required to achieve blockade must be used. A tuberculin syringe that injects 0.1 mm at a time ensures that the anesthetic does not contaminate other structures, which otherwise would make interpretation of the block difficult. This contributes to accurate localization of the primary pain generator. If the block is successful, an appropriate dermatomal representation of the analgesia is present. Subsequently, the patient is assessed for subjective changes in pain; however, this alone is insufficient to determine suitability for cryoablation. Many patients with chronic pain have suffered for a long time and are hopeful that the next procedure is going to be the long-awaited successful treatment. These patients are responsive to suggestion and placebo effect. To identify such effects, the first test injection is done with lidocaine and the second with bupivacaine. In appropriate responders, a significantly longer duration of analgesia can be found with bupivacaine, assuming that all other variables remain the same. The effects of peripheral blockade on windup and chronic pain are not clearly understood. To responsive patients, a cryoablative procedure can be offered. For patients who do not have the desired response to bupivacaine or lidocaine, further testing is necessary, including differential blockade with local anesthetics and normal saline solution and consideration of consultation with a clinical psychologist.

To perform percutaneous cryoablation successfully, the cryoprobe must be placed properly. This is a disadvantage compared with open cryoablative techniques used for postoperative pain management. The operator must ensure proper cryoprobe placement by using a combination of techniques (see later) that improve the chances that the ice ball will be made precisely on the pain generator. In addition, special care must be taken when using the cryoprobe for percutaneous procedures. Bending the probe during percutaneous introduction can distort the lumen of the low-pressure outer tube, increase the resistance pressure to the expanding nitrous oxide gas, and convert a low-pressure exhaust system to one of higher pressure. That eventuality would impede gas expansion, inhibit ice ball formation, and limit cooling of the probe. To maintain the integrity of the cryoprobe, the probe should be placed through an introducer. The preferred introducers are large-bore intravenous catheters: 12-gauge, 14-gauge, or 16-gauge catheters, depending on the size of the cryoprobe. The operator always should check to see that the cryoprobe fits through the lumen of the catheter. The depth at which the probe emerges from the distal tip of the catheter should be marked on the proximal shaft of the cryoprobe to ensure that the cryoprobe tip extends far enough beyond the catheter to create a full-sized ice ball.

Several techniques are used to enhance precise placement of the cryoprobe, as follows:

1. Careful palpation with a small blunt instrument, such as a felt-tipped pen, can help to localize a soft tissue neuroma or another palpable pain generator.
2. An image intensifier (fluoroscopy) can identify bony landmarks.
3. Contrast medium improves definition of tissue planes, capsules, and spaces. (Nonionic contrast medium should be used in areas close to neural tissue.)
4. The nerve stimulator at the tip of the cryoprobe is used to produce a muscle twitch in a mixed nerve. The stimulator is set at 5 Hz for recruitment of motor fibers. The probe is closest to the nerve when the lowest output produces a twitch response. In general, twitches should occur at 0.5 to 1.5 V. Small sensory branches contain no motor component and do not twitch with electrical stimulation. These fibers are localized by using higher-frequency (100-Hz) stimulation, which produces overlapping dysesthesia in the distribution of the small sensory nerve. This procedure may reproduce the patient's pain. Use of low-output (<0.5 to 1.5 V) stimulation ensures closer placement of the cryoprobe to the nerve in question. The operator freezes the nerve for 2 to 3 minutes. Often, the patient has discomfort initially as cooling begins, but it should dissipate quickly. If significant pain persists beyond 30 seconds, the operator should investigate whether the ice ball is in the proper position. (If the ice ball is not sufficiently close to the nerve, and only partial freezing occurs, mostly of larger myelinated fibers, unchecked unmyelinated fiber input is left. This theoretically accounts for increased pain.) The brief cooling already may have altered nerve function, in which case, if positioning of the probe depends on feedback from the patient, it could be impeded. Before moving the probe, the operator must be sure to thaw the tip to prevent tissue damage from ice ball adherence to the tissues. In general, with closed procedures, two freeze cycles of 2 minutes each, followed by thaw cycles, are sufficient. In areas with a large vascular heat sink, longer periods of cryotherapy are necessary. Pain relief should be immediate and should be assessed

subjectively and by physical examination while the patient is on the procedure table. All relevant clinical information should be recorded in the medical record. A hard-copy radiograph should be obtained for most procedures when a fluoroscope is used.

Applied Cryoanalgesia for Chronic Pain

This section provides the reader with the skills necessary to make proper clinical decisions regarding cryoanalgesia. Listing every procedure is beyond the scope of this chapter. This section reviews many of the pain syndromes that are amenable to cryodenervation and describes in detail the techniques that are requested most often. To perform cryolytic treatments correctly, the provider must be familiar with the regional anatomy and the principles of localizing pain generators described earlier.

INTERCOSTAL NEURALGIA

Percutaneous cryolesions of the intercostal nerves can be offered for various pain syndromes, including post-thoracotomy pain, traumatic intercostal neuralgia, rib fracture pain, and occasionally postherpetic neuropathy. For each of these conditions, a meticulous series of local anesthetic blocks is performed before consideration is given to cryoablation. The volume of local anesthetic should be kept to less than 3 to 4 mL to prevent tracking back into the epidural space. In addition, only two or three levels should be injected at any one time because systemic absorption could confound interpretation of the patient's response. Because the intercostal nerve runs with a large arterial and venous heat source, the use of two 4-minute cryolesions at each level is suggested. The lesions should be made proximal to the pain at the inferior border of the rib (**Fig. 179.5**). After the procedure, a chest film is obtained to check for pneumothorax. Effective blockade in some patients with postherpetic neuropathy suggests that this pain is sometimes related to peripheral afferent input, as opposed to being strictly a central neuropathy.

NEUROMAS

Typically, painful neuromas are associated with lancinating or shooting pain that is aggravated by movement or deformation of nearby soft tissues. Neurophysiologically, this phenomenon is thought to reflect lower neural thresholds and ephaptic

transmission. First-line therapy should include empirical trials of anticonvulsants, tricyclic antidepressants, steroids, and local anesthetics, including a topical local anesthetic cream or patch. These agents are thought to play a role in modulating neural thresholds. Cryoablation is considered only after careful mapping has isolated a very discrete pain generator (i.e., a neuroma). The initial injection can use a relatively larger volume of local anesthetic, but subsequent blocks should deliver small increments from a tuberculin syringe to ensure accurate interpretation. Cryoablation seems most effective when the volume of local anesthetic necessary to produce analgesia is 1 mL or less. After the block with lidocaine, the patient's response and its duration are recorded. If initial blockade is successful in decreasing the patient's symptoms, it should be followed by at least one more injection with bupivacaine. A response of longer duration may be expected with the longer-acting local anesthetic.

ILIAC CREST BONE HARVEST

The pain associated with the harvest of iliac crest bone for fusion often responds to cryoablation when more conservative therapies have failed. Such pain often is associated with deep, lancinating pain and often is attributed to periosteal neuromas. The surface area is often large, and careful diagnostic mapping is required to localize the primary pain generator as precisely as possible. When no single pain generator is found, and the periosteal surface that is the source of the pain remains large and unresponsive to other therapies (e.g., steroid injections and nonsteroidal anti-inflammatory drugs [NSAIDs]), multiple cryoablations may be necessary during one session (**Fig. 179.6**).

BIOMECHANICAL SPINE PAIN

Typically, biomechanical spine pain is exacerbated with movement, so physical therapy often is futile. In general, no neurologic deficits are present, and the pain is ascribed to numerous structures, including the articular facet nerves, the meningeal nerves, the anterior communicating ramus, and other branches of the posterior primary ramus (**Figs. 179.7** and **179.8**). Cryolesions have been used effectively for cervical and lumbar facet syndromes[33] and for pain from the interspinous ligaments.[35-37] The success of cryolesioning is a function of

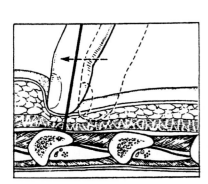
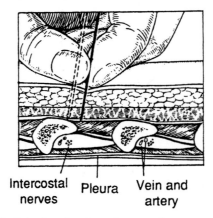
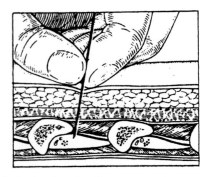

Intercostal nerves   Pleura   Vein and artery

Fig. 179.5 Percutaneous placement of a needle (introducer) onto an intercostal nerve at the inferior border of a rib. *(From Chung J: Thoracic pain. In Sinatra RS, Hord AH, Ginsberg G, et al, editors: Acute pain, St. Louis, 1991, Mosby.)*

patient selection, accurate probe placement, and follow-up rehabilitation program. For biomechanical pain of lumbar facet origin, the patient typically has pain that is exacerbated by hyperextension of the lumbar spine. The pain localizes to the lumbosacral junction and often radiates into the buttocks and the posterior aspect of the thigh, generally never below the knee. These patients have significant muscle spasm, at times extending cephalad and caudad. They complain that movement is uncomfortable and are unable to participate in lumbar physical therapy. Palpation reveals exquisite tenderness along the lumbar paravertebral margin. No significant neurologic changes are noted, but typically other biomechanical problems are present, such as pelvic obliquity, functional leg-length discrepancy, and sacroiliac joint dysfunction.

Before isolated facet arthropathy is addressed, attention should be directed to the associated biomechanical disorders. If a patient has a leg-length discrepancy and pelvic shift, a shoe orthosis should be prescribed. When a patient has severe pain from the facet arthropathy, little is gained from prescribing physical therapy. In such circumstances (which are common), denervation of the facet may enable the patient to participate

in physical therapy. A fluoroscopically guided diagnostic intra-articular facet block can be performed in patients who fulfill the aforementioned criteria. The levels chosen for injection are determined by bone scan, computed tomography, plain films, and, most important, physical examination findings.

Initial needle placement into the facet is guided by antero-posterior fluoroscopic visualization (**Fig. 179.9**) after a small skin wheal is made. Correct intra-articular placement

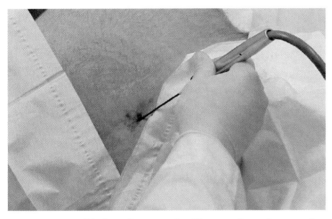

Fig. 179.6 **Cryoablation of an anterior iliac crest bone harvest site.** *(From Waldman SD: Cryoneurolysis in clinical practice. In* Interventional pain management, *ed 2, Philadelphia, 2001, Saunders.)*

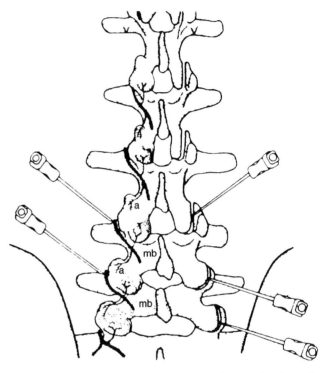

Fig. 179.8 **Dorsum of the lumbar spine.** Needles are placed into the lumbar facet joints and onto the medial branches. a, articular branch of facet; mb, medial branch of the posterior primary division. *(From Cousins M, Bridenbaugh P, editors:* Neural blockade in clinical anesthesia and management of pain, *ed 2, Philadelphia, 1994, Lippincott.)*

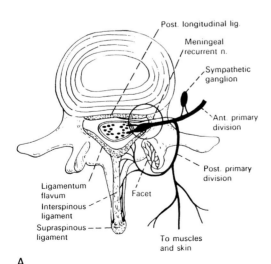

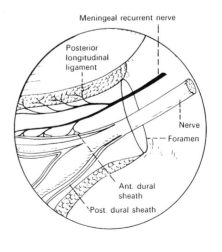

A   B

Fig. 179.7 **Cross-sectional view of innervation of the posterior motion segment, including the facet.** *(From Bonica J:* The management of pain, *Philadelphia, 1990, Lea & Febiger.)*

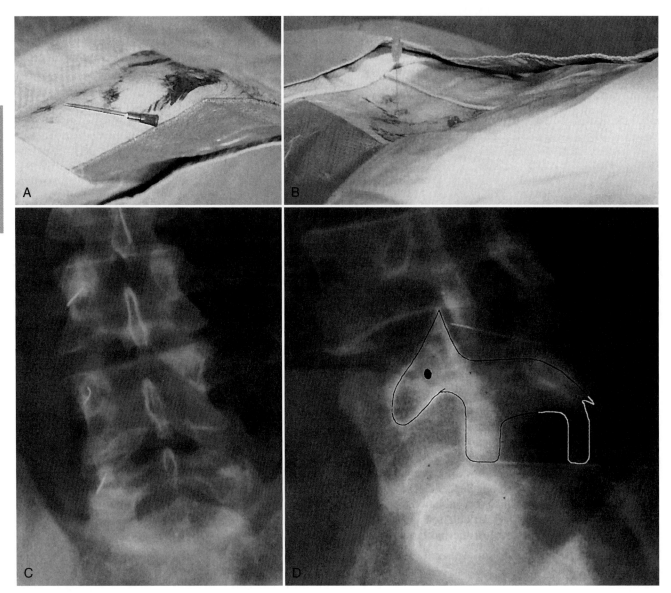

Fig. 179.9 A, Under fluoroscopic guidance, the point of a needle is placed over the lumbar facet of interest. This corresponds to the junction of the transverse process and the pedicle. B, A 22-gauge finder (spinal) needle is inserted through the skin at the point of the needle down to bone. C, Anteroposterior x-ray projection shows the needle at the junction of the transverse process and the pedicle near the facet joint. D, Using an oblique projection, the needle is manipulated into the Scottie dog's ear for intra-articular placement or into the Scottie dog's eye for the articular nerve (medial branch). *(From Waldman SD: Cryoneurolysis in clinical practice. In* Interventional pain management, *ed 2, Philadelphia, 2001, Saunders, p 233.)*

is confirmed with oblique imaging; the needle should be in the "ear" of the "Scottie dog" (see Fig. 179.9D). (Often, as the needle enters the joint space, the operator feels as though the needle is being pushed through an orange peel; that is, loss of resistance is felt.) When the needle is within the joint, 1 mL of nonionic contrast medium is injected. In patients with facet arthropathy, this is often very painful. A fluoroscopic review of the area of interest of the contrast study shows the facet capsule filled with radiodense contrast medium. In some circumstances, the capsule is deformed or leaky. At times, the capsule is large and cystic and projects into the canal. At this point, the patient is asked to consider carefully whether this is the usual pain or a different pain and to rate it on the Visual Analog Scale (VAS). If the pain reproduced is representative

of the usual pain, 1 mL of 1% lidocaine is injected. The needle is manipulated further, and the patient is asked how he or she feels and to arch the back. If the patient has a dramatic decrease in pain and improved movement, it is likely that a facet pain generator is present. If little change is noted in symptoms, an additional 4 mL of lidocaine can be injected incrementally. If the patient has no change in symptoms at the level under study, it is unlikely to be a primary pain generator. In patients who respond, a set of flexion-extension films should be made before discharge because the analgesia provided by the block should allow better motion and should help to reveal occult posterior elemental movement. If such movement is found, the patient will benefit from an orthopedic evaluation and consideration of fusion.

To confirm a facet pain generator, repeat blockade of the facet nerves can be done next. If the result is similar, it is reasonable to consider ablation. Each facet has at least dual innervation and requires at least two local anesthetic injections. A needle is placed at the junction of the transverse process and the pedicle (the Scottie dog's eye on the oblique projection; see Fig. 179.9D) at the level previously studied and the level above it. A 100-Hz nerve stimulator is used to locate the sensory nerve. Subsequently, the operator injects 2 mL of 0.25% bupivacaine. Ten minutes later, the patient is reexamined. In patients who continue to be responsive, improvement is observed on physical examination, especially with lumbar hyperextension. For these patients, a cryoablative procedure can be considered.

For the cryoablative procedure, the patient is positioned prone in the fluoroscopy suite. The lumbar spine is prepared and draped in standard sterile fashion. Superficial skin wheals are raised at the levels where cryoablations are to be performed. However, a clinical suggestion exists that contributions to facet innovation also are made from the level below. For this reason, lumbar facet cryodenervations often are performed at three levels, a technique popularized by Thomas. A 12-gauge introducer catheter (**Fig. 179.10A**) is introduced to the junction of the transverse process and the pedicle, the Scottie dog's eye. At this point, the cryoprobe is inserted into the introducer catheter (**Fig. 179.10B**). The nerve stimulator is used to locate the sensory branch. When pain is reproduced or the patient feels dysesthesia overlapping the region of the pain, motor testing is in order to ensure that the ice ball is not near a motor nerve. Two cryolesions are made, each of 2 minutes' duration. The patient is expected to have some postprocedure discomfort, but should notice improvement. In the recovery room, ice can be applied to the operative site for 30 minutes for local postoperative irritation and swelling. Application of ice may decrease swelling and facilitate mobilization. The patient should continue with outpatient lumbar strengthening programs. If the musculature is significantly deconditioned, it may be better to restart the program in water. After muscle condition improves, the patient should begin a supervised industrial rehabilitation program that offers vocational retraining and job placement. One publication demonstrated that the evidence-based information available for cryodenervation in facet denervation is indeterminate.[34,38]

CERVICAL FACET SYNDROME

Patients with cervical facet syndrome typically present with severe posterior neck pain and muscle spasm. Palpation elicits pain over cervical facets and at the midline. The pain becomes considerably worse with hyperextension and loading of the cervical spine. Cervical facet syndromes generally are not associated with long tract neurologic findings. A radionuclide bone scan and a plain film may show evidence of posterior elemental arthritic disease. Spondylolisthesis should be sought with flexion-extension films. Significant movement may be better addressed with fusion.

If these patients fail to respond to conservative therapy, a diagnostic series of injections with fluoroscopic guidance is considered. To patients who respond to local anesthetic injections with reduction in pain, cryodenervations can

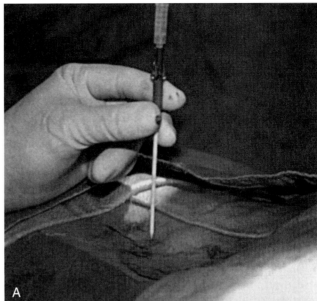
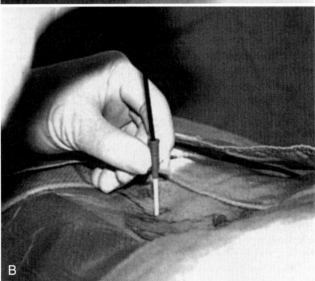

Fig. 179.10 A, For facet cryodenervation, a 12-gauge introducer catheter is placed percutaneously along the tract of the finder needle. B, The cryoprobe is then placed through the introducer catheter. The final position of the probe is determined by the patient's response to 100-Hz stimulation. The patient should have no motor response to 5-Hz stimulation. *(From Waldman SD: Cryoneurolysis in clinical practice. In* Interventional pain management, *ed 2, Philadelphia, 2001, Saunders, p 234.)*

be offered as an adjunct to comprehensive physical therapy and rehabilitation. For patients with apparent biomechanical neck pain that does not respond to local anesthetic injection, further workup is necessary to identify pain generators. One study concluded that with intra-articular facet joint injections, the evidence for short- and long-term pain relief is limited for cervical pain and moderate for lumbar pain. For medial branch blocks, the evidence is moderate for short- and long-term pain relief. For medial branch neurotomy, the evidence is moderate for short- and long-term pain relief.[38]

INTERSPINOUS LIGAMENT PAIN

Interspinous ligament pain is common after a spine operation (lumbar, thoracic, or cervical). Pain impulses from interspinous ligaments are carried by the medial branch of the posterior ramus (see Fig. 179.8). Patients report severe movement-related spine pain, identified to the midline, which is worsened with hyperextension and relieved by small volumes of local anesthetic injected into the intraspinous ligament. When cervical interspinous ligaments are involved, the patient frequently complains of posterior cervical headache. This headache often is mistaken for occipital neuralgia. Cryodenervation can be considered in local anesthetic–responsive patients. The pain relief helps the patient to complete the necessary course of physical therapy.

MECHANICAL SPINE PAIN

Anterior mechanical (diskogenic) spine pain is transmitted by different nerves, depending on the location of the injury—the sinuvertebral nerve (recurrent meningeal), small rami of the segmental nerve, rami of the communicating ramus, or sympathetic fibers.[36,37] Cryolesions have been placed successfully on rami communicantes after diagnostic local anesthetic injections have reduced the pain. Pain of sympathetic origin is not likely to respond to cryodenervation because the heat carried by the major blood vessels interferes with formation of the ice ball. Percutaneous sympathectomy is best performed with radiofrequency thermal ablation or with phenol.

COCCYGODYNIA

When coccygodynia has failed to respond to conservative therapy, including the patient's use of a donut pillow, NSAIDs, and local steroid injections, consideration can be given to coccygeal neural blockade as the coccygeal nerve exits from the sacral canal at the level of the cornu. Bilateral test injections should produce short-term analgesia before cryoablation is considered. For cryoablation of the coccygeal nerve, the probe must be inserted into the canal to make contact with the nerve. Accurate placement of the ice ball is facilitated by using the 100-Hz stimulator and gauging the patient's response. Care

should be taken to prevent bending the relatively large cryoprobe while inserting it into the canal.

PERINEAL PAIN

Pain over the dorsal surface of the scrotum, perineum, and anus that has not responded to conservative management at times can be managed effectively with cryodenervation from inside the sacral canal with bilateral S4 lesions. Test local anesthetic injections should produce a positive response before cryoablations are performed bilaterally at S4. Inserting the cryoprobe through the sacral hiatus up to the level of the fourth sacral foramen for placement of a series of cryolesions can provide good analgesia. Bladder dysfunction usually is not encountered, and analgesia lasts 6 to 8 weeks.[35] Perineal pain is difficult to treat with intrathecal neurolytic agents without risking bladder and bowel dysfunction.

ILIOINGUINAL, ILIOHYPOGASTRIC, AND GENITOFEMORAL NEUROPATHIES

Ilioinguinal, iliohypogastric, and genitofemoral neuropathies often complicate herniorrhaphy, general abdominal surgery, and cesarean section. Patients present with sharp, lancinating to dull pain radiating into the lower abdomen or groin. The pain is exacerbated by lifting and defecating. If the patient is responsive to a series of low-volume test injections, consideration can be given to cryodenervation of the appropriate nerve. Significant care and time must be spent localizing the nerve with the sensory nerve stimulator. The patient may help to localize the pain generator by pointing with one finger to the point of maximum tenderness. These nerves are difficult to localize percutaneously, and that difficulty has led to frequent misdiagnosis of the pain generator. In an effort to improve the accuracy of diagnosis, Saberski and Rosser[39] developed the *conscious pain mapping* technique. In a lightly sedated patient, a general surgeon working with a pain management specialist performs laparoscopic evaluation of the abdomen in an operating suite. The genitofemoral nerve, lateral femoral cutaneous nerve, and other structures are easily visualized (**Fig. 179.11**). Blunt probing and patient feedback help to direct the physician to the area of pain. At times, objects such as ligatures and staples are found wrapped around the nerve, in which

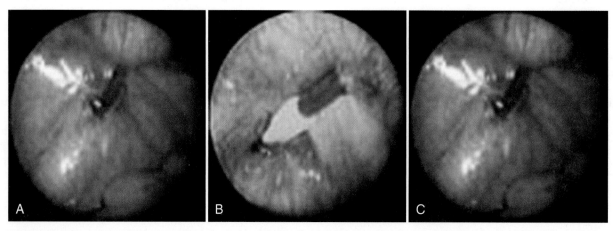

Fig. 179.11 A, Insertion of the Lloyd cryoprobe through the abdominal wall and fascia onto the genitofemoral nerve. B, Formation of the ice ball for cryodenervation of the genitofemoral nerve. C, Lloyd cryoprobe immediately after defrost. *(From Waldman SD: Cryoneurolysis in clinical practice. In In Interventional pain management, ed 2, Philadelphia, 2001, Saunders.)*

case they should be removed. If direct mechanical or electrical stimulation to the nerve reproduces the pain, cryoablation can be performed under direct vision. (Cryoablation is chosen as the appropriate test because the effect of bupivacaine does not outlast the discomfort of the perioperative period. The cryoblockade provides weeks to months of reliable analgesia and helps physicians and patients to determine whether that structure under surveillance carried the pain information.) Pain usually returns. A repeat cryoablation is possible when analgesia is long or an open surgical procedure with sectioning and burying can be performed.

Lower Extremity Pain

Many cutaneous nerve branches are responsive to cryodenervation. The clinician always must perform a complete physical examination, with careful touching of the painful area. After the primary pain generator is localized, a series of low-volume local anesthetic injections can be given. If the patient has a consistent response, cryodenervations, as outlined earlier, can be employed. Some common lower extremity nerve pain syndromes that are often amenable to cryodenervation are described next.

Neuralgia resulting from irritation of the *infrapatellar branch of the saphenous nerve* develops weeks to years after blunt injury to the tibial plateau or after knee replacement. The nerve is vulnerable as it passes superficial to the tibial collateral ligament, pierces the sartorius tendon and fascia lata, and runs inferior and medial to the tibial condyle. The clinical presentation consists of dull pain in the knee joint and achiness below the knee. Patients tend to adopt an antalgic gait. Pain with digital pressure is diagnostic. Patients are considered candidates for cryodenervation when they respond consistently to local anesthetic blocks. A 12-gauge intravenous catheter is used as the introducer, to prevent cold injury to the skin. Because prodding with a felt-tipped pen alone is sufficient to localize the pain generator, the sensory nerve stimulator does not have to be used.

Neuralgia secondary to irritation of the *deep and superficial peroneal and intermediate dorsal cutaneous nerves* can be seen weeks to years after injury to the foot and ankle. These superficial sensory nerves pass through strong ligamentous structures and are vulnerable to stretch injury with inversion of the ankle, compression injury owing to edema, and penetrating trauma from bone fragments. The intermediate dorsal cutaneous nerve runs superficial and medial to the lateral malleolus, continues superficial to the inferior extensor retinaculum, and terminates in the fourth and fifth toes. This nerve is particularly vulnerable to injury after sprains of the lateral ankle. The clinical presentation consists of dull ankle pain that is worse with passive inversion of the ankle. Disproportionate swelling, vasomotor instability, and allodynia are remarkably common. Patients tend to adjust their gait to minimize weight bearing on the lateral aspect of the foot. Pain with digital pressure in the area between the lateral malleolus and extensor retinaculum is diagnostic.

PERONEAL NERVE

Superficial and deep peroneal nerve injury often occurs in diabetic patients, who are vulnerable to compression injury from tight-fitting shoes, and is less common after blunt injury to

the dorsum of the foot. The clinical presentation consists of dull pain in the great toe that is often worse after prolonged standing. Patients tend to adjust their gait to minimize weight bearing on the anterior portion of the foot. Pain with digital pressure in the area between the first and second metatarsal heads is often diagnostic.

SUPERIOR GLUTEAL NERVE

Neuralgia resulting from irritation of the superior gluteal branch of the sciatic nerve is common after injury to the lower back and hip sustained while lifting. After exiting the sciatic notch, the superior gluteal nerve passes caudal to the inferior border of the gluteus minimus and penetrates the gluteus medius. Vulnerable as it passes in the fascial plane between the gluteus medius and gluteus minimus musculature, the superior gluteal nerve is injured as a result of shearing between the gluteal muscles on forced external rotation of the leg and with extension of the hip under mechanical load. Rarely, it is injured by forced extension of the hip, an injury that may occur in a head-on automobile collision when the foot is pressed against the floorboards with the knee in extension as the patient braces for impact. The clinical presentation consists of sharp pain in the lower back, dull pain in the buttock, and vague pain to the popliteal fossa. Pain below the knee is unusual. Patients generally experience pain with prolonged sitting, leaning forward, or twisting to the contralateral side. Often, patients describe "giving way" of the leg. They usually sit with the weight on the contralateral buttock or cross their legs to minimize pressure on the involved side. With the patient in the prone position, the medial border of the ilium is palpated. The nerve is located 5 cm lateral and inferior to the attachment of the gluteus medius. The peripheral nerve stimulator is employed to ensure that motor units are not inadvertently blocked.

Craniofacial Pain

Craniofacial nerves can be cryolesioned with a percutaneous or open technique.[40,41] Entrapment neuropathies and neuromas are more responsive to local anesthetic and cryodenervations than are neuropathies of medical causes. Meticulous diagnostic injection ensures the best outcome with cryoablation.[15] If the patient has a good analgesic response to a series of local anesthetic injections, cryodenervation is an option. The technique of cryodenervations of cranial and facial nerves is the same as that for other peripheral nerves. A nerve stimulator is used to localize the nerve. Because these areas are relatively densely vascular, injecting a few milliliters of saline solution containing 1:100,000 epinephrine is recommended before inserting the cryoprobe introducer cannula. A postprocedural ice pack applied for 30 minutes reduces pain and swelling.

Irritative neuropathy of the *supraorbital nerve* (**Fig. 179.12**) often occurs at the supraorbital notch.[41] Vulnerable to blunt trauma, this nerve often is injured by deceleration against an automobile windshield. Commonly confused with migraine and frontal sinusitis, the pain of supraorbital neuralgia often manifests as a throbbing frontal headache. At times, many of the hallmarks of vascular headache are present, including blurred vision, nausea, and photophobia. This neuralgia often worsens over time, perhaps owing to scar formation around the nerve.

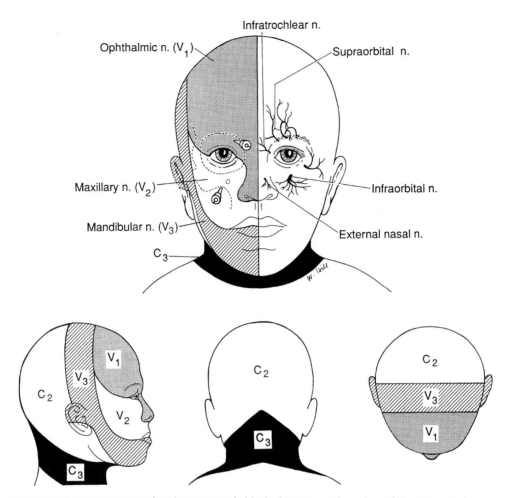

Fig. 179.12 Dermatome man showing commonly blocked cutaneous branches of the trigeminal nerve.

Neuropathic pain in the distribution of the supraorbital nerve can be addressed with an open or closed cryoablative procedure as long as appropriate conservative therapy has failed and the pain responds to a series of test local anesthetic injections. For an open procedure, the incision is buried beneath the eyebrow, so the patient has no obvious scar. For the percutaneous technique, the introducer catheter should be inserted at the eyebrow line to avoid damage to hair follicles.

The *infraorbital nerve* (see Fig. 179.12) is the termination of the second division of the trigeminal nerve. Irritative neuropathy can occur at the infraorbital foramen secondary to blunt trauma or fracture of the zygoma with entrapment of the nerve in the bony callus. Commonly confused with maxillary sinusitis, the pain of infraorbital neuralgia most often is exacerbated by smiling and laughing. Referred pain to the teeth is common, and a history of dental pain and dental procedures is typical. Cryoablation can be accomplished by an open or closed technique. The closed technique can be performed from inside the mouth through the superior buccolabial fold. In both operations, the probe is advanced until it lies over the infraorbital foramen. The intra-oral approach has cosmetic advantages only.

The *mandibular nerve* can be irritated at many locations along its path. It is often injured as the result of hypertrophy of the pterygoids secondary to chronic bruxism, but it also

can be irritated if the vertical dimension of the oral cavity is reduced owing to tooth loss or altered dentition. Pain is often referred to the lower teeth, and patients frequently undergo dental evaluations and procedures.

Injury to the *mental nerve,* the terminal portion of the mandibular nerve, frequently occurs in edentulous patients. Pain can be reproduced easily with palpation.

The *auriculotemporal nerve* can be irritated at many sites, including immediately proximal to the parietal ridge at the attachment of the temporalis muscle and, less commonly, at the ramus of the mandible. Patients often present with temporal pain associated with retro-orbital pain. Pain often is referred to the teeth. Patients frequently awaken at night with temporal headache. The pain, described as throbbing, aching, and pounding, can be bilateral, and it is commonly associated with bruxism and functional abnormalities of the temporomandibular joint, maxilla, and mandible. The clinician must rule out other medical causes for this form of headache, including temporal arteritis, before considering treatments for auriculotemporal neuralgia. Posterior auricular neuralgia often follows blunt injury to the mastoid area. It is common in abused women and usually involves the left side owing to the preponderance of right-handed abusers. The clinical presentation consists of pain in the ear associated with a feeling of "fullness" and tenderness. This syndrome often is misdiagnosed as a chronic ear infection. The posterior auricular nerve runs along the posterior border of the sternocleido-mastoid muscle, superficially and immediately posterior to the mastoid.

The *glossopharyngeal nerve* lies immediately subjacent to the tonsillar fossa (**Fig. 179.13**). This painful condition can be treated by applying the cryoprobe for two cycles of 2 minutes each after local anesthetic injections have produced the appropriate responses. This is essentially a simple procedure, but it has distinct advantages over injection of this cranial nerve at the tip of the mastoid, where injection could block the vagus nerve in addition to the spinal accessory nerves.[40]

Many other common peripheral nerve injuries are amenable to cryodenervation, including most cutaneous branches and the occipital, suprascapular, superficial radial, and anterior penetrating branches of the intercostal nerves. Applied carefully, the techniques outlined in this chapter help to achieve the safest and best possible outcomes.

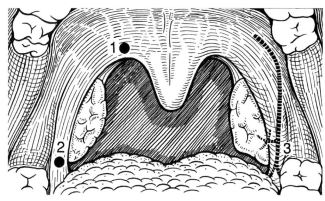

Fig. 179.13 The distal glossopharyngeal nerve subjacent to the tonsillar fossa. *1* and *2,* Locations for local anesthetic and cryodenervation. *3,* The pathway of the glossopharyngeal nerve is superficial at this site. Care must be taken to avoid entering the artery.

CASE REPORT

A 58-year-old woman sustained traumatic spondylolisthesis at L4-5 for which spinal fusion was performed.[42] Autogenous bone graft for the vertebral fusion was obtained from the left posterior iliac crest. Postoperatively, the patient continued to experience wrenching and searing pain at the iliac crest donor site (pain score 7 on the 10-point VAS). Treatment with NSAIDs for 3 weeks and transcutaneous electrical nerve stimulation for 2 weeks did not alleviate the pain (VAS = 5). The patient was referred to the pain medicine center for additional evaluation and treatment. The initial clinical assessment indicated the primary painful locus (7.5 cm × 5 cm) to be within the defect of the posterior iliac bone harvest site. The patient's symptoms—a constant, wrenching, and searing pain with radiation into the calf—were aggravated by walking and assuming the standing or sitting position and were partially relieved with rest.

A diagnosis of postoperative iliac crest pain syndrome (a new name for this symptom complex) was made. Inflammation and a post-traumatic neuroexcitatory state induced by the surgical trauma were posited to be responsible for the pain. For these reasons, the iliac crest donor site was infiltrated with a series of local anesthetic injections (10 mL of 0.5% bupivacaine), NSAID (60 mg of ketorolac), and steroid (20 mg of triamcinolone) at 2- to 3-week intervals. The first four injections contained 10 mL of 0.5% bupivacaine and 60 mg of ketorolac. The first injection relieved the patient's pain completely (VAS = 0). The pain gradually returned to pretreatment levels (VAS = 7) during the next 2 weeks, with the notable difference that the locus of pain was reduced in size (5 cm × 2.5 cm). The pain locus corresponded to the center of the graft donor site. The three subsequent injections of bupivacaine and ketorolac had minimal effect on pain scores or size of the painful locus. For the fifth injection, 10 mL of 0.5% bupivacaine was mixed with 20 mg of triamcinolone. The response to this injection was dramatic—further shrinking of the painful locus (3 cm × 2 cm) and diminution in pain scores (VAS = 1). A sixth (and final) injection at week 12 produced further diminution of the painful locus to two discrete (1 cm × 1 cm) foci. The patient nevertheless described this pain as sharp and excruciating (VAS = 7). The relatively smaller size of the painful loci prompted selection of cryodenervation as a second step of treatment. A cryoprobe that produced 0.5-cm ice balls at thermal equilibrium was selected. A grid was visualized over the area, and seven cryodenervations were performed, each

of 3 minutes' duration. The patient experienced postprocedure discomfort, but it disappeared over the first week (VAS = 0) (**Table 179.1**), and the patient resumed all previous preoperative activities after 1 month. One year after the procedure, the patient continued to have complete mobility and activity.

Discussion

The harvesting of bone has been used frequently in orthopedic surgery since 1901, when Von Eiselberg first reported autogenous cancellous bone transplantation.[43,44] The sites commonly used to

Table 179.1 Overview of Patient History

Treatment Category	VAS Reduction* (%)	Reduction in Area of Painful Locus†‡ (%)
Pretreatment (postoperative)	7 (N/A)	7.5 × 5 (N/A)
Symptomatic treatment (NSAID and TENS)	5 (28.6)	7.5 × 5 (0)
Injection Therapy		
Bupivacaine and ketorolac		
First injection	0 (100)	0 (100)
Second injection	5 (28.6)	5 × 3 (60)
Third injection	4 (4.29)	5 × 2 (73.3)
Fourth injection	5 (28.6)	4.5 × 3 (64)
Bupivacaine and triamcinolone		
Fifth injection	1 (85.7)	3 × 2 (84)
Sixth injection	6 (14.3)	1 × 1 and 1 × 1 (94.7)
Cryodenervation	1 (100)	0 (100)

* Reduction is expressed as the percentage of baseline values at the pretreatment (postoperative) stage.
† Measured by same physician using same amount of pressure for deep palpation and recorded in centimeters.
‡ One week after cryodenervation.
NSAID, nonsteroidal anti-inflammatory drug; TENS, transcutaneous electrical nerve stimulation; VAS, Visual Analog Scale score.

harvest donor bone include the iliac crests, ribs, and calvaria.[45–49] No consensus exists regarding a preferred site.[42–46] The posterior iliac crest is used for bone harvesting in many orthopedic and reconstructive procedures because of its suitability as a donor site.[45,50] The complications associated with bone graft harvesting from the posterior iliac crest include chronic pain, altered sensation at the harvest site, superior gluteal arteriovenous fistula, ureteral injury, sacroiliac joint dislocation, osteomyelitis, gluteal weakness, lumbar hernia, and injury to the sciatic and gluteal nerves.[51,52] Chronic pain is the most common postharvest complication (reported incidence, 25% to 38%).[51,53–56] The persistence of pain at the iliac crest donor site is thought to be a complication of total or partial injury to the cutaneous continuations of the lateral branches of the dorsal rami of L1-3, collectively called the *superior cluneal nerves.*[52,57] Modifying the surgical technique to avoid this complication has not altered significantly the incidence and characteristics of donor site pain.[51,58–61] Findings of a few studies have suggested the benefit of perioperative infiltration of the donor site with a local anesthetic (bupivacaine).[62–64] Other investigators have suggested giving bupivacaine through an indwelling epidural catheter for postharvest pain.[64,65] Perioperative infiltration of the donor site with a local anesthetic may alleviate the acute pain, but considering the 25% to 38% incidence of chronic pain at the donor site,[51,53,56] approximately 62% to 75% of patients receive local donor site anesthetic infiltration or intra-operative catheter treatment without any long-term benefit. This approach increases direct and indirect hospital costs because of the additional procedure, the longer hospital stay, and the increased risk of complications.

The pathophysiologic mechanisms of persistent pain at the donor site are likely to be multiple and may involve various biochemical pathways. Injury, regeneration, and remodeling of cancellous bone are thought to be associated with marked increases in osteoclastic activity that is affected by prostaglandins through many different pathways.[66,67] Harvey et al[68] used a dental model to show significant concentrations of prostaglandins in alveolar bone cysts. Inflammatory cells, macrophages, lymphocytes, and monocytes initiate degradation of connective tissue,[69] presumably through increased prostaglandin E_2 production. The plasma level of prostaglandins is of little clinical use because of the 95% clearance by the pulmonary vascular bed within 3 to 6 seconds.[70–72] Shindell et al[73] showed that injections of steroid into bone cysts reduced prostaglandin E_2 concentrations by 52% to 93%. The reduction in prostaglandin E_2 concentration has been proposed as one of the

biochemical mechanisms responsible for the effectiveness of intralesional steroid therapy.[73] Moreover, ketorolac, a direct inhibitor of cyclooxygenase, decreases prostaglandin biosynthesis and likely increases neural threshold. Prostaglandins, in addition to causing bone destruction, increase the sensitivity of peripheral nociceptors to pain mediators, including bradykinin.[74] The local anesthetic may affect the outcome by attenuating afferent input[75] and diminishing the plasticity of the CNS.

The reduction in the size of the patient's pain locus to only two discrete points most likely resulted from attenuation of afferent sensory input. This decrease in size of the painful locus made it possible to consider cryodenervation of the underlying periosteum. Cryodenervation has been used successfully for postoperative and chronic pain relief. Few long-term outcome studies on the effectiveness of cryodenervation are available. A 10-year audit of cryodenervation for trigeminal neuralgia indicated a 6-month median duration of relief and comparable pain-free intervals after repeated cryodenervations.[76] Cryoanalgesia relieves pain by producing long-lasting neurolysis combined with axonal regeneration. Freezing of nerve results in axonal disintegration and degeneration of the myelin sheaths. The perineurium and epineurium are preserved, however, and regrowth of axons occurs in the original supporting structures at the rate of 1 to 3 mm/day.[77] This obviates growth of painful neuromas, a problem associated with other neurolytic and surgical techniques, but also limits the duration of effective analgesia.[76,78,79] At present, no conclusive physiologic explanation exists for the sometimes prolonged analgesic effect because regeneration of axons seems to be completed in a matter of weeks after the procedure.[77,80] It is possible that cryoanalgesia affects the plasticity of the CNS and diminishes pain overall. The complications associated with cryotherapy are relatively minor, but they include cold injury, skin discoloration, and numbness in the distribution of the treated peripheral nerve. An important limitation is that cryoanalgesia can be applied only to sensory nerves because ablation of mixed nerves would produce temporary paralysis of the corresponding muscles. Improvement can be attributed to the additive analgesic effects of ketorolac, steroid, local anesthetic, and cryotherapy on several different nociceptive pathways. This combination may produce balanced analgesia that is likely to be more effective and to have fewer side effects than any other approach. This two-step therapeutic approach may prove to be the treatment of choice for the prolonged relief of chronic pain resulting from iliac crest bone harvest.

Future Directions

Cryotechnology offers promise for many different pain management needs. Its unparalleled track record for safety is remarkable. Its effective and safe use on sensory and mixed nerves contrasts with radiofrequency technology, which has the potential to produce deafferentation when applied to peripheral nerves. The lack of controlled studies, the lack of uniform training, and poor communication among providers have impeded widespread use of the technology. The application of

ultrasound technology may expand the use of cryoanalgesia, with visualization helping the placement of the cryoprobe on larger nerves such as the intercostal nerves.[81] The overview of contemporary cryoanalgesia in interventional pain management written by Dr. Trescott is a good source of additional information on cryoanalgesia.[82]

References

Full references for this chapter can be found on www.expertconsult.com.

Chapter **180**

V

Vertebroplasty and Kyphoplasty

Mehul Sekhadia and John Liu

Approximately 700,000 to 750,000 vertebral fractures occur each year in the United States. Up to 25% of persons who are more than 50 years old will have at least one vertebral fracture in their lifetime, and the lifetime risk of vertebral compression fractures (VCFs) in white women is 15.6%.[1,2]

Most VCFs are caused by osteoporosis, but other causes include multiple myeloma, metastatic tumor, and hemangiomas. According to Cooper et al,[3] 16% of vertebral fractures are diagnosed radiographically when the initial investigation is undertaken for another problem. The diagnosis of vertebral fracture is difficult compared with that of peripheral fractures. Decrease in height and vertebral deformities are indications of vertebral fractures. Most VCFs are asymptomatic and have no associated origin of injury.[4] However, when symptomatic, these fractures can be debilitating to the point that any movement will cause severe pain. Most fractures heal within a few months, but some patients have pain and disability and fail to respond to conservative therapy. Conservative therapy includes the use of back bracing, bed rest, and pain control with medications such as nonsteroidal anti-inflammatory drugs (NSAIDs), calcitonin, and narcotics. No absolute time frame for length of conservative therapy has been established, but adverse consequences such as deep venous thrombosis, pulmonary embolism, pneumonia, and accelerated bone loss can occur with prolonged bed rest.[5] Poor pain control can lead to chronic pain and central sensitization, which are more difficult to treat than acute pain. Other consequences of VCFs are height loss and kyphosis.

Early treatments for painful VCFs when conservative therapies had failed usually revolved around surgery,[6] but outcomes were variable secondary to inherently poor bone quality. Percutaneous vertebroplasty was first reported in 1987

by Galibert and Deramond et al[7] for the treatment of painful hemangiomas. These investigators noted that injecting polymethylmethacrylate (PMMA) into the painful vertebral body provided significant pain relief. The procedure was then performed in Europe for the treatment of pain related to multiple myeloma and metastatic neoplasms.[8] Eventually, the technique was introduced in the United States, where it has been used for the treatment of osteoporotic VCFs along with the painful hemangiomas and cancer-related VCFs.[9] Kyphoplasty was introduced in 2000 to address the additional consequences with VCFs that accompany the pain (height loss and kyphosis).[10] This procedure involves the addition of inserting and inflating a balloon in the vertebral body before the insertion of cement, to restore height and to decrease kyphosis. Some controversy exists over the potential benefits of kyphoplasty relative to its higher cost in comparison with vertebroplasty. The actual mechanism of pain relief with either procedure is still unknown.

Both vertebroplasty and kyphoplasty are performed throughout the world by radiologists, spine surgeons, anesthesiologists, and interventional pain specialists. Numerous case reports, case series, and nonrandomized and unblinded prospective studies have suggested the efficacy of vertebral augmentation in the treatment of osteoporotic fractures, but two studies that were randomized, blinded, and placebo controlled demonstrated no benefit of vertebroplasty over placebo. The data for the use of vertebral augmentation in other causes of painful VCFs are also based on retrospective and nonrandomized comparative studies. Both methods appear to have a good safety profile.

This chapter discusses the pathophysiology, diagnosis, prevention, and treatment of VCFs. Management of VCFs revolves around knowing the disease processes that cause these fractures and the appropriate steps to take in preventing further functional decline. In the current environment of health care cost conservation, practitioners must be able to determine when interventions are appropriate, safe, and efficacious. As with most interventions, appropriate patient selection and proper technique increase the likelihood that the intervention will lead to expected pain relief. The two most common techniques of vertebral augmentation are described in detail, followed by a review of the existing studies for both procedures.

Pathophysiology

VCFs are caused by the inability of the vertebra to sustain internal stresses applied from normal daily load or trauma. The inability of the vertebra to maintain its structure is related to the constant change in its composition. The primary structure of bone is distinguished by cortical, or compact, bone and trabecular bone, otherwise known as cancellous or spongy bone. Cortical bone is generally on the surface and is characterized by its dense composition without cavities. Conversely, trabecular bone has many interconnecting cavities consisting of red blood cells and yellow bone marrow composed of fat cells. Trabecular bone, found in abundant supply in vertebral bodies, is largely responsible for most of the axial forces and inherited extra-axial stress and strains. The extent of the two types of bone varies depending on its location. Bone is also composed of osteoprogenitor cells, osteoblasts, osteoclasts, osteocytes, neurovascular progenitor cells of external origin, and an array of inorganic and organic constituents. In diseases such as osteoporosis, the architecture of trabecular bone becomes altered. In multiple myeloma, an imbalance of osteoclasts and osteoblasts (increased osteoclastic activity) can cause lytic lesions in the absence of osteoporosis. This section looks at the different disease processes that lead to VCFs.

Osteoporotic Fractures

Osteoporotic fractures are more prone to occur at the hip, ribs, wrists, and vertebrae. In 2000, there were an estimated 9 million new osteoporotic fractures, of which 1.6 million were at the hip, 1.7 million were at the forearm, and 1.4 million were clinical vertebral fractures. Europe and the Americas accounted for 51% of all these fractures, whereas the Western Pacific region and Southeast Asia accounted for most of the remainder. An increased risk of mortality exists among osteoporotic patients who experience a hip fracture, and 25% of these patients die in the first year.[11-16] Of those who survive, 50% are unable to resume their previous independent lifestyle.[17] Complications such as pneumonia, blood clots in the lungs, and heart failure contribute to the morbidity of an osteoporotic hip fracture. VCFs can decrease height by up to 15 cm and can result in the "dowager's hump" kyphotic deformity. VCFs in women result in 15% higher mortality compared with women with no disruption.[18] Furthermore, VCFs increase with age and affect 40% of women in their 80s.[19]

VCFs result from the inability of the osteoporotic vertebra to sustain internal stresses applied by vertebral load from daily life or from minor or major traumatic events. Trabecular bone is largely responsible for most of the axial forces and inherited extra-axial stress and strains. With the cascade of osteoporotic effects and aging, the architecture of trabecular bone becomes altered, characterized by increased spaces, thinness, disorientation, and weakened connectivity. Although the trabecular bone network maintains its horizontal and vertical framework, decreases in density and loss of structural strength compromise the vertebra's mechanical prowess, integrity, and spinal column stability and predispose it to trabecular buckling. Therefore, alteration of trabecular bone, as seen in osteoporotic individuals and with age, is accompanied by a decrease in bone density[20-23] and a propensity for fracture.[24,25]

Multiple VCFs cause hyperkyphosis or a dowager's hump at the thoracic level, with a stooped posture that decreases the abdominal and thoracic cavities. Multiple lumbar VCFs further increase lordosis and create a protruding abdomen. Decrease in axial height is a result of reduction of intervertebral and vertebral loss of height. In addition, the stooped posture progresses to the point where ribs rest on the iliac crest, and circumferential pachydermal skin folds develop at the pelvis and ribs. When this posture becomes more severe, eating is difficult, and the patient eats less because he or she feels full and bloated. Symptoms related to the cauda equina or the spinal cord are uncommon and are secondary to other conditions, such as Paget's disease, lymphoma, primary or metastatic bone tumors, myeloma, and infection.[26] On awakening, the abdomen appears normal, only to distend throughout the day. Nonrestorative sleep or trouble getting to sleep is often the case with these patients. Lifestyle changes occur, related to difficulties driving a car or getting dressed and fear of large crowds, and depression develops. Self-esteem is also compromised as a result of a socially unacceptable body image.[27] After a second vertebral fracture, women report high levels of anxiety out of fear of future recurrences[28,29] and accompanying stress.[30,31] As the disease progresses over time osteoporotic problems continue, signs of depression develop in women.[29,32] Social support and social roles are affected by decreased function and the progressive disease-related problems of osteoporotic VCFs and deformity.

Nonosteoporotic Fractures

Multiple myeloma is are the most common primary malignant tumor of the bony spine that rarely affects the posterior elements.[33-35] These tumors are rare radiosensitive lesions occurring in 2 to 3 cases per 100,000. Diffuse multiple myeloma is manifested by recurring lesions at previously radiated levels and has a poor prognosis. Initially, patients report severe pain and disability and are unresponsive to drug treatment. The disease is usually multifocal, and surgical consolidation is not advantageous. In spite of this situation, single-level lesions are treated with vertebrectomy and strut grafting with some success. Radiation therapy alone or as an adjunct to surgery to address painful malignant lesions offers partial or complete pain relief in 90% of patients. However, pain relief is delayed for 10 to 14 days after the initial radiation therapy.[36] In addition, initiation of spine strengthening begins 2 to 4 months after the initial radiation therapy.[36,37] Thus, delayed reconstruction predisposes the spine to vertebral collapse and ensuing neural compromise. Vertebral augmentation offers an alternative route for immediate pain relief, bone strengthening, and mobility. Although vertebral augmentation goes some way to restoring the mechanical integrity of the vertebral body and provides a degree of pain relief, tumor growth is not prevented. Therefore, radiation therapy accompanying augmentation is appropriate because it does not affect the properties of the bone cement, affects tumor growth, complements pain relief, and effects spine strengthening.[38]

Hemangiomas are benign bony spine lesions whose detection is difficult because of their asymptomatic disposition. Often, hemangiomas are detected during evaluation of back pain and subsequent routine plain radiographs. Soft tissue extension of the lesion may compress the spinal cord and nerve roots and may produce neurologic symptoms and even epidural hemorrhage.[39,40] If the hemangioma grows extensively, vertebral integrity may be compromised, resulting in fracture with pain associated at the level of the lesion.[41] Hemangioma aggressiveness is determined by clinical symptoms and radiologic evaluation. Vertebral collapse, neural arch invasion, and soft tissue mass extensions are signs of the aggressive nature of hemangiomas and their candidacy for vertebral augmentation. Furthermore, lymphomas and eosinophilic granulomas are also amenable to vertebral augmentation.

Approximately 10% of patients with metastatic tumor develop malignant lesions in the spine in the Unites States.[42] Ten percent to 15% of the 120,000 new patients per year develop symptoms in the form of VCFs.[42] The most common location is the thoracic spine, but all spinal levels can be affected, and usually more than one level is involved. Every type of malignant disease has been described to spread to the spine.[42]

Prevention

Antiresorptive therapy and preventive measures are essential considerations in managing and preventing osteoporotic manifestations. An attempt to slow bone loss is of utmost concern. Bone mass is ever changing, with peak levels obtained in the mid-30s. Because more women are osteoporotic and are at greater risk for developing osteoporosis than men, various factors are at play accounting for the variable rates in bone loss. Women lose 3% to 7% of bone mineral density near the onset of menopause, followed by a 1% to 2% decline yearly in the postmenopausal period. Men also lose bone with age, but at levels similar to those of postmenopausal women. However, men seem to continue to increase cortical surface by gaining cortical bone through periosteal deposition until the age of 75 years.[2,21] Nevertheless, numerous factors must be considered before an appropriate regimen of preventative and therapeutic measures is administered to combat osteoporosis (**Table 180.1**).

Table 180.1 Potential Options for the Treatment of Osteoporosis and Prevention of Vertebral Compression Fractures

Calcium and vitamin D[25]

Bisphosphonates[26-31]

Calcitonin[32]

Selective estrogen receptor modulators[33]

Parathyroid hormone[34,35]

Sodium fluoride[36]

Exercise[37-39]

Modifiable risk factors such as cigarette smoking, excessive alcohol consumption, and treatment of potential secondary causes

---

Initial Evaluation of Painful Vertebral Compression Fractures

As in clinical medicine in general, the most important aspect of patient evaluation begins with a good clinical history and physical examination. Most VCFs are asymptomatic, with unknown origin of injury.[4,43]

Patients with symptomatic VCF typically present with acute or subacute back pain with no associated major trauma or precipitating event. The sudden onset of pain is usually described as a moderate to severe, deep ache, at a midline location, and exacerbated by any motion. More specifically, pain is experienced after standing from a seated position and during bending, lifting, and prolonged sitting or standing. Walk is sluggish, but gait is normal. Coughing, sneezing, and bowel exertion exacerbate pain. A succession of VCFs may follow the first initial fracture, with discontinued pain between each period of disruption, or the pain may be continually present. However, *cluster VCFs* are a string of fractures with severe and persistent pain. Pain may be relieved by recumbent positioning and bed rest.

Physical examination usually shows a patient in mild to severe distress, depending on the general conditioning of the patient as well as the location and type of fracture. The patient usually reports tenderness at the site of fracture in the midline, but the absence of this symptom does not rule out the presence of an unhealed fracture. Kyphosis may also be an important indicator of VCF because loss of more than 4 cm of height is associated with 15 degrees of kyphosis, although measurements of kyphosis are fraught with error.[4] Comprehensive musculoskeletal and neurological examinations are imperative to rule out other causes of symptoms, especially myelopathy, radiculopathy, and spinal stenosis.

The diagnosis of VCF is difficult compared with that of peripheral fractures. Decrease in height and vertebral deformities are indications of vertebral fractures. VCFs maintain an axis of rotation at the middle column. As a result, anterior column disruption is seen with intact middle and posterior columns. Because the neural arch remains intact, neurologic deficits are not as common. *Bioconcave VCFs* manifest as a central vertebral deformity because a crush fracture involves anterior, posterior, and central aspects. *Wedge fractures* are the most common VCFs and affect anterior elements more often than posterior. Whatever the morphology VCFs adopt, fractures occur more often at the thoracolumbar and midthoracic region.[3,44,45] The tendency of VCFs to occur at these regions could possibly be attributed to alterations in stiffness from the thoracic spine to the more mobile lumbar region and transitory curvature from kyphosis to lordosis.

Once VCF is suspected or a patient has new-onset, moderate to severe back pain that is not explained by any other cause, radiographic imaging should be ordered. The simplest, most cost-effective, initial study is a plain anteroposterior (AP) and lateral radiograph of the suspected area of the spine. However, if the clinical index of suspicion is high, it is reasonable to proceed straight to magnetic resonance imaging (MRI). MRI is useful in distinguishing acute from chronic fractures (edema on T2-weighted image), as well as determining any spinal canal compromise or tumor presence. A hypointense T1-weighted image is also suggestive of edema (**Fig. 180.1**). Short tau inversion recovery (STIR) is a type of MRI used to suppress the hyperintensive image readings of substances such as fatty

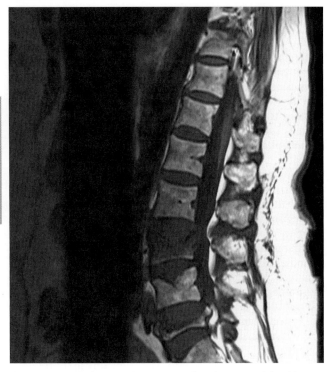

Fig. 180.1 Sagittal magnetic resonance imaging, T1-weighted image, demonstrating a hypointense area within a compression deformity of L3 suggestive of acute compression fracture. Also present is an old pars plana deformity of L5.

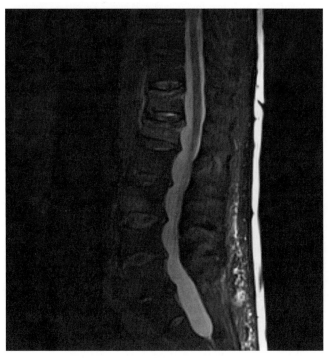

Fig. 180.2 Sagittal magnetic resonance imaging, short tau inversion recovery (STIR) sequence, demonstrating hyperintense areas along with fracture lines near the superior end plates of T12 and L1 vertebral bodies suggestive of edema.

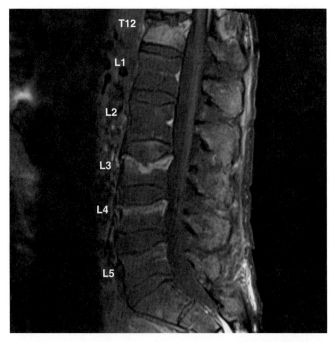

Fig. 180.3 Sagittal magnetic resonance imaging, T1-weighted image with gadolinium enhancement, demonstrating increased uptake at the superior end plates of L3 and L4 vertebral bodies and diffuse uptake at T12 vertebral body. Bone biopsy taken during the kyphoplasty procedure confirmed that these lesions were in fact hemangiomas.

tissue and cerebrospinal fluid. STIR is the most sensitive imaging sequence for visualizing edema, and edema is highly predictive of success with vertebral augmentation (**Fig. 180.2**). Finally, a T1-weighted image with gadolinium enhancement may also be used and is especially helpful in the presence of malignant disease (**Fig. 180.3**).

If MRI is contraindicated, as in patients with pacemakers, stents, or mechanically active implants, then either a bone scan or a computed tomography (CT) scan may be useful in determining the acuity of the fracture. Acute or unhealed fractures take up the injected technetium-99m methylene diphosphonate tracer in higher concentrations on bone scan. Thin-section (≤3 mm) CT is often used in conjunction with MRI reconstructions to derive the most accurate visualization of the target vertebral levels. CT has been cited specifically as the best modality for determining whether or not a fracture line has extended through the posterior wall of a vertebral body. CT can also detect fracture cavities that should be the targets (**Fig. 180.4**). Aiming the pedicle needle toward fracture cavities increases the success rate. One can also assess the size and trajectory of pedicles with three-dimensional CT. In addition, certain fracture types may be less amenable to vertebral augmentation (e.g., "butterfly"-shaped fracture).

Comprehensive evaluation of the patient should also include other causes of VCFs, as described in the previous section. Relevant diagnostic tests are listed in **Table 180.2**.

Once a determination is made that VCF is the cause of the patient's pain, steps should be taken to manage and keep the patient weight bearing and to prevent functional decline. *This is the most important consideration in the clinical decision-making process.* Approximately 2% to 10% of patients require hospital admission for pain control.[46–48] Initial modalities

include walking aids and lumbar supports, but the efficacy of lumbar supports has limited evidence, and these devices may cause more harm if they are used on a long-term basis.[49] Exercise programs have demonstrated decreased use of analgesics, improved quality of life, and increased bone mineral

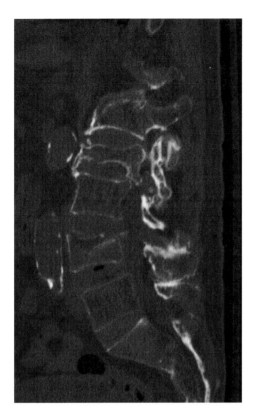

Fig. 180.4 Computed tomography scan, bone windows, demonstrating a fracture line and compression deformity of L3 vertebral body. This patient has a scoliotic deformity and did not have a compression fracture at any other level in the lumbar spine.

Table 180.2 Laboratory Investigations*

Complete blood count

Serum calcium

Serum alkaline phosphatase

Serum creatinine

Urinary calcium excretion

Serum 25-hydroxyvitamin D

Serum protein electrophoresis

Sex steroids

Serum aminotransferase

Serum thyroid-stimulating hormone

* Results should be correlated clinically. Not all tests are required in all patients.

density, along with evidence that 1% of bone loss per year in the spine and hip is prevented or reversed.[50,51] Pharmacologic therapy includes NSAIDs[52] if tolerated, short- or long-acting opioids, and possibly, calcitonin.[53] Acute pain from VCF can persist for up to 12 weeks, whereas chronic pain is secondary to vertebral deformity, paraspinal muscle spasm, or degenerative arthritis in the region of the fracture. At any point, if pain is uncontrolled to the extent that the patient cannot perform weight-bearing activities, or if the patient has side effects from analgesics, vertebral augmentation should be considered, assuming that a proper workup is completed and the VCF is the source of pain. The exact time that interventional therapies should be pursued is controversial. Some clinicians advocate immediate intervention, whereas others advocate waiting 12 weeks for bone healing.

Techniques for Vertebral Augmentation

Vertebral augmentation is a procedure that has an excellent safety profile *if* it is done properly by experienced physicians who have had appropriate training. Minimum requirements for the procedure include the following:

- Intravenous (IV) access and sedation and possibly general anesthesia are required.
- Image guidance is used, usually with fluoroscopy, possibly with CT scan, or both. Some practitioners advocate using a biplanar fluoroscope, to have AP and lateral images always visible. This approach is convenient and saves time, but it is not necessary.
- Informed consent must be obtained.
- IV antibiotic prophylaxis is with cefazolin, 1-2 g IV, or clindamycin, 600-900 mg IV, within 60 minutes of incision.
- The table is appropriately padded for prone positioning.
- Sterile precautions are taken.
- Appropriate bone biopsy needles with opacified PMMA are used.

Both vertebroplasty and balloon kyphoplasty are similar in the beginning stages of the procedure with regard to local anesthetic use and the image-guided approach to the vertebral body. Balloon kyphoplasty is approved only when performed in an operating room and not in an office-based procedure suite (as of the writing of this chapter, the procedure is not reimbursed if it is done in an office procedure suite). Two different techniques are used to place the 11- or 13-gauge needles: transpedicular and parapedicular. Proper placement with either method requires a thorough knowledge of fluoroscopic anatomy. In general, the augmentation of the lumbar and lower thoracic (below T10) spine is usually performed with a transpedicular approach, whereas upper thoracic spine (above T8) augmentation is performed with a parapedicular route. Either approach can be used at any level, but pedicle size and orientation in the upper thoracic areas usually do not allow for a transpedicular approach.

After informed consent is obtained and IV access is secured, the patient is brought to the procedure suite or operating room. IV antibiotics should be given within 60 minutes of incision. Analgesia may be required to place the patient in the prone position if local anesthetic with IV sedation is planned, as it is most of the time. Once the patient is in position and the pressure points are padded, the C-arm is brought in to identify the proper level or levels to be augmented. This level is marked, and the area is prepared and draped in the usual sterile fashion. For the transpedicular approach, two methods can be used, and they can be simply defined as the AP approach (maintaining visualization of the medial and lateral cortex of the pedicle) and the en face approach (tunnel vision). Regardless of approach, an AP image is first obtained of the appropriate level. The end plates of that level are lined up as closely as possible, but alignment may be difficult because of the deformity. If the en face approach is used, the C-arm is then angulated in an ipsilateral oblique fashion to place the pedicle in the middle of the vertebral body. Again, this may be difficult because of the deformity, in which case the AP method can be used.

For the *AP approach,* the target needle site is the superior and lateral portion of the pedicle, sometimes described as 10 o'clock or 2 o'clock for the left and right pedicle on the AP view, respectively. If the oblique view is used, then the needle should be placed in the center of the pedicle. Local anesthetic is infiltrated intradermally and subcutaneously. A 22-gauge spinal needle is then advanced coaxially to the periosteum of the pedicle. The operator injects 5 to 10 mL of either 2% lidocaine or 0.5% bupivacaine at the periosteum and during withdrawal of the spinal needle to anesthetize the tract of the larger needle. Then, a small incision is made with a No. 11 blade scalpel. The larger needle is advanced to the pedicle in the tract of the spinal needle (**Fig. 180.5**). After the needle is engaged into bone, either a screwdriver technique or gentle tapping with an orthopedic hammer is used to drive the needle into the pedicle, with frequent imaging to confirm that the needle is within the pedicle. Once the needle is properly engaged, an AP view is obtained to confirm that the medial cortex of the pedicle is not violated (**Fig. 180.6**). A lateral image is then obtained to confirm that the needle is within the pedicle and is not cephalad or caudal, in which case a disk or nerve foramen may be entered. For vertebroplasty, the needle is advanced into the anterior third of the vertebral body, whereas for kyphoplasty, the needle is advanced only into the posterior third (**Fig. 180.7**). Again, slow advancement and frequent imaging are recommended to avoid misplacement.

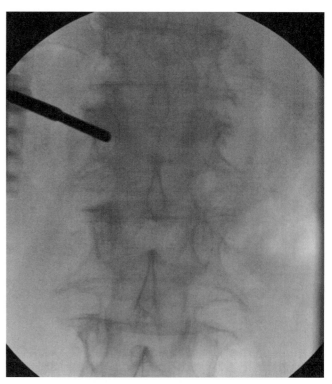

Fig. 180.6 Anteroposterior image after the needle is engaged into the pedicle. This image demonstrates that the medial cortex of the pedicle has not been traversed. The medial border can be traversed after lateral image is taken to confirm that the needle is not going through the spinal canal posteriorly.

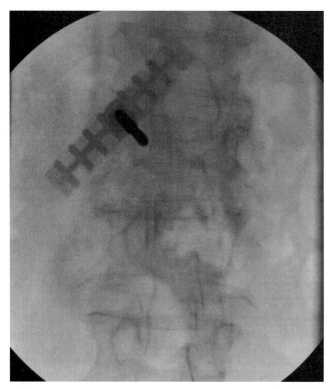

Fig. 180.5 En face (tunnel vision) approach for placement of a large needle (trocar) for kyphoplasty.

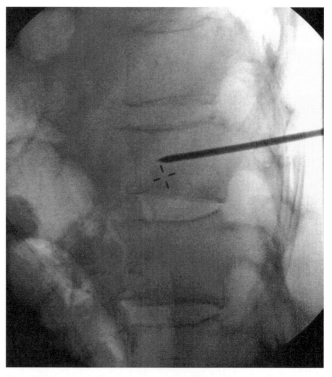

Fig. 180.7 Lateral fluoroscopic image demonstrating placement of needle for vertebroplasty. The needle tip should be in the anterior one third of the body.

The *parapedicular approach* involves placing the needle lateral to the edge of the pedicle and advancing it along the surface of the pedicle directly into the vertebral body. Initial needle placement is lateral to the lateral cortex of the pedicle. The vertebral body is entered at the junction of the pedicle, which appears more anterior on lateral imaging. This method is useful when severe collapse leads to poor visualization of the pedicle. More medial placement of the needle in the vertebral body, and thus greater likelihood of single-needle placement, may occur with this approach. This approach may be preferred for treatment of VCFs above T10 because of the smaller pedicle size.

Either one- or two-needle techniques may be used for vertebroplasty. The goal of augmentation is to fill all the fracture lines (**Figs. 180.8** and **180.9**). No absolute exists with either approach, but the procedure can begin unilaterally and then converted if needle placement is in the lateral portion of the vertebral body and bilateral filling is not likely to occur or after initial cement placement demonstrates inadequate spread to the contralateral side.

Balloon Kyphoplasty

As mentioned earlier, initial needle placement is similar to the vertebroplasty approach, except the needle is not advanced past the posterior one third of the vertebral body (**Fig. 180.10**). In addition, the introducer system is slightly larger than the vertebroplasty needles. A few different options exist for cannula placement with regard to size and tip. The introducer has a beveled or diamond tip that allows it to be gently hammered or manually pushed into the vertebral body. After entering the posterior aspect of the vertebral body, the introducer is removed, thus leaving the cannula in place. A hand-operated drill is advanced to the anterior aspect of the vertebral body, with care taken not to violate the anterior margin on lateral

imaging. Ideal placement on AP imaging is in the midline. The drill is then removed, and the deflated balloon is advanced through the cannula into the cavity created by the drill. A second introducer and balloon should be placed on the opposite side in a similar fashion. Each balloon is attached to a locking syringe that has a digital manometer, followed by slow inflation with iodinated contrast. Ideal balloon inflation is when both balloons appear to be "kissing" on the AP

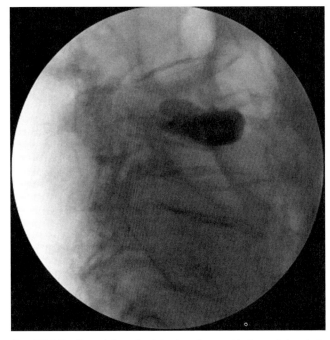

Fig. 180.9 Final lateral view after injection of cement in the vertebroplasty technique.

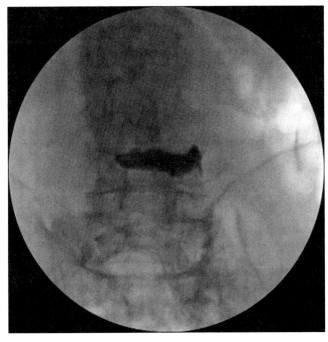

Fig. 180.8 Anteroposterior fluoroscopic image of the lumbar spine that demonstrates cement placement after vertebroplasty.

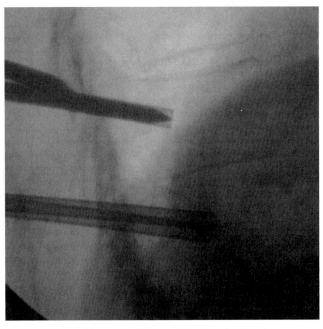

Fig. 180.10 Lateral fluoroscopic image of lumbar spine that demonstrates placement of the kyphoplasty trocar into the posterior one third of the vertebral body.

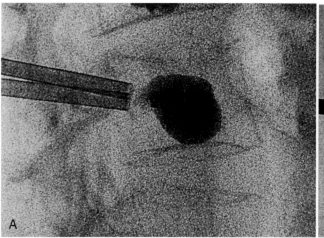

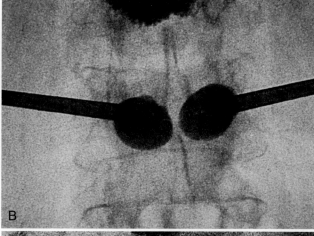

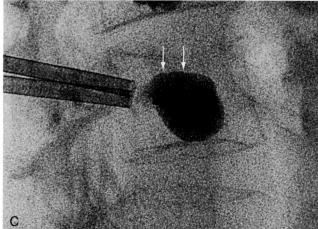

Fig. 180.11 A, Lateral image after inflation of the balloon that demonstrates excellent fracture reduction. B, Anteroposterior view after inflation of balloons that demonstrates good midline placement and cavity creation. C, Final view after cement injection into the cavities created by the balloons with minimal extension into adjacent trabecular bone (arrows).

view, thus encompassing all borders of the fractured vertebra. Both manometry and fluoroscopy are used to monitor balloon inflation (**Fig. 180.11**). The operator should continue inflating the balloon until the following occur:

1. Maximum pressure (≤400 psi) or volume is reached.
2. The balloon tamp reaches any cortical margin.
3. The kyphotic deformity is corrected.

The balloon is then deflated and removed. The extra steps act to reduce the fracture, create a cavity for the cement, and reduce the likelihood of cement extravasation (see "Evidence").

Preparation of Polymethylmethacrylate and Delivery

Some clinicians advocate of the use of a venogram at this point to look for any potential venous uptake and potential cement embolization. However, data to support this practice are limited.

Various PMMA mixing and delivery options exist for both vertebroplasty and kyphoplasty. In general, PMMA contains a sterile barium sulfate powder to provide radiographic opacity. The systems vary from a premixed powder that is combined with a liquid into a blender to a spatula and a mixing bowl. After all ingredients are mixed, the working time is usually 10 to 20 minutes, although it varies with the room temperature and formulation.

For vertebroplasty, a cannula from the cement mixer is connected to the needle, and the cement is slowly injected under live fluoroscopy in the lateral position. The injection is stopped periodically with intermittent fluoroscopy during "rest" periods to ensure proper control of cement spread and to avoid aberrant placement. Newer mixtures may allow for aspiration of the cement back into the system. The injection is stopped when the posterior one third or one fourth or any other cortical margin is reached. If any margin is not intact, a small amount of cement can be injected to the edge of the margin, followed by waiting a few minutes to allow the cement to harden and thus prevent further spread into unwanted areas. The volume of cement does not correlate with success, and complete filling of the vertebral body is not required. If midline spread of the cement does not occur, a second needle is placed on the opposite side, and a similar injection of cement is performed. The stylet must be placed into the needle to complete the injection, and the operator must not allow the cement in the lumen of the needle to track back in the needle, a situation that could cause cement leakage into the neural foramen, spinal canal, or paraspinal muscles. The stylet is placed under live or intermittent fluoroscopy, to visualize final spread of cement.

For balloon kyphoplasty, PMMA is injected using a blunt cannula under live fluoroscopy. The injection is stopped when the cavities are filled, along with any potential fracture line outside the cavity (**Figs. 180.12** and **180.13**). The needle stylet should be replaced under live fluoroscopy, to watch for cement extravasation.

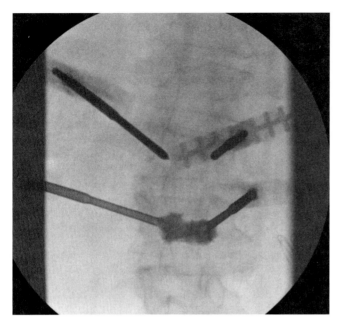

Fig. 180.12 Anteroposterior view of trocar placement for a two-level kyphoplasty, with cement already injected into cavities created by the balloons at the lower level.

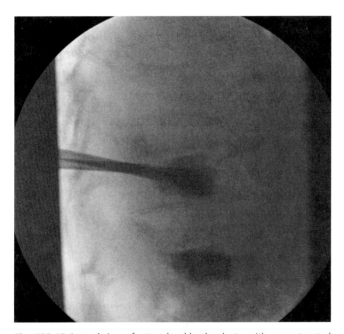

Fig. 180.13. Lateral view of a two-level kyphoplasty, with cement noted to fill cavities created by the balloons.

After the cement is injected, the delivery system is removed, and pressure is maintained on the incision sites. Sufficient time for the cement to harden must be allowed to prevent extravasation. Approximately 10 to 20 minutes should suffice, or, more objectively, the operator can place a small amount of the PMMA onto a gauze pad away from the patient, with the understanding that polymerization occurs more rapidly with higher temperatures. Thus, if the cement is firm at room temperature, it is safe to assume that it is firm at body temperature.

Table 180.3 Contraindications to Vertebral Augmentation

Absolute	Relative
Uncorrectable coagulation disorders	Inability to lie prone
Allergy to PMMA or contrast	Loss of vertebral height ≥66% (vertebroplasty)
Spinal instability myelopathy	Posterior wall destruction ≥20% retropulsion with spinal stenosis
Pregnancy	Previous spinal stenosis
Active site infection or sepsis	Vertebra plana
Fractured pedicles	Gibbus
Burst fractures Young age Pain unrelated to fracture Solid tissue or osteoblastic tumor	H shape Multiple previous surgical procedures Obesity Poor pulmonary status More than three compression fractures

PMMA, polymethylmethacrylate.

Contraindications and Complications

The contraindications to vertebral augmentation have evolved, and some are based on the potential complications seen with either procedure. Contraindications to vertebral augmentation are similar to contraindications to any neuraxial procedure (**Table 180.3**). The most common complication is cement leakage, but this complication is reduced significantly with kyphoplasty. One study reported a 3% rate of symptomatic leaks in vertebroplasty and a 0% rate with kyphoplasty.[54] Most leaks are clinically irrelevant, and further treatment is not required. Other complications include the following[54–58]:

- Osteomyelitis
- Hematoma (paraspinal or epidural)
- Rib fracture
- Sternum fracture
- Adjacent vertebral fracture
- Pedicle fracture
- Pulmonary embolus of PMMA
- Hypotension
- Spinal cord compression
- Epidural abscess
- Neurologic complications
- Allergic reaction to contrast material or PMMA

All the foregoing complications are based on analysis of numerous case series. Some of the relative contraindications can be overcome with proper vigilance and technique, whereas most of the complications can be avoided with proper interpretation of preprocedural and periprocedural imaging and patient preparation and selection. General anesthesia should be considered if the patient is unable to lie prone because of pain. Loss of vertebral height and severe VCFs such as vertebra plana, gibbus, and H shape were formerly absolute contraindications. However, Peh et al[59] retrospectively reported on 155 patients who underwent 310 vertebroplasties with any of the foregoing fractures; these investigators noted good efficacy in eliminating or reducing pain in 97% of patients without any clinically significant complications. Previous surgical procedures and obesity may cause poor visualization of landmarks, whereas patients with poor pulmonary status may not tolerate the usually asymptomatic PMMA emboli seen in 0.6% of patients who undergo vertebroplasty (0.01% in kyphoplasty). Patients with underlying, asymptomatic spinal stenosis may not tolerate any cement leakage into the epidural space. Surgical decompression may be required if any postprocedural neurologic compromise is caused by bleeding or cement leakage into the epidural or foraminal space.

Adjacent vertebral fractures are a significant concern with vertebral augmentation. A VCF causes a focal kyphotic deformity that moves the center of gravity forward, and this change increases the load onto adjacent vertebrae. Kobayashi et al[60] found that prophylactic injection of cement in adjacent, nonfractured vertebrae may prevent new VCFs in osteoporotic patients. Oakland et al[61,62] noted that, under normal physiologic loads associated with moderate physical activity, little evidence supports prophylactic augmentation of adjacent vertebrae. Eck et al[55] performed a meta-analysis and found that vertebroplasty had a slightly higher, but statistically significant, rate of adjacent fracture than did kyphoplasty (17.9% versus 14.1%). Trout et al[63] reported a 4.62 times greater risk of developing a vertebral fracture adjacent to an augmented vertebra with vertebroplasty than at a nonadjacent level. The risk of developing an additional VCF after an initial VCF secondary to osteoporosis is 4 times greater than in the population with no VCF. Therefore, the argument about whether

vertebral augmentation predisposes the patient to additional VCF needs to be studied further, and not enough evidence is available to support prophylactic augmentation of an adjacent vertebra. It appears that spinal mechanics are altered by cement extravasation into the adjacent disk, and this change, in turn, alters the load onto the adjacent vertebra.

Evidence

Vertebral augmentation has multiple outcome considerations. The clinician must take into account that vertebroplasty and kyphoplasty are different procedures. The goals of the procedures are the same, but kyphoplasty has the additional step to reduce a fracture and partially improve a kyphotic deformity. The first question is whether the procedure provides pain relief and improves quality of life when compared with placebo or conventional medical therapy. Concurrently, the potential benefits must outweigh the potential risks. Secondary outcomes include decreased opioid use, disability, cost effectiveness, and patient satisfaction. Studies have attempted to address the effects of both techniques on height restoration and on incidence of adjacent fractures. Finally, a few studies have compared the efficacy and safety of the two techniques. Two multicenter, randomized, double-blind, placebo-controlled trials were conducted to assess vertebroplasty in the treatment of painful osteoporotic vertebral fractures. No such studies exist for kyphoplasty, but one well-done, prospective, randomized, double-blind study for kyphoplasty t compared augmentation with conventional medical management (**Table 180.4**).

Table 180.4 Comparisons of Randomized Trials for Vertebroplasty and Kyphoplasty

	Kallmes et al[66]	Buchbinder et al[64]	Wardlaw et al[67]
Purpose	Efficacy and safety of VP for alleviating pain and improving physical function (1 mo)	Assessment of efficacy and safety of VP for alleviating pain (1 wk and 1, 3, and 6 mo)	Efficacy and safety of BKP for alleviating pain and improving QOL (1, 3, 6, 9, 12 and 24 mo)
Sites	11 centers (5 United States, 5 United Kingdom, 1 Australia)	4 centers (All in Australia)	**21 centers** (8 different countries)
No. patients	131 (68 VP, 63 sham)	78 (71 at 6-mo f/u) (38 VP, 40 sham)	300 (149 BKP, 151 NSM)
Inclusion criteria	≥50 yr old 1–3 painful OVCFs (T4-L5) ≥3 pain score (0–10 scale) Fx age <12 mo	≥50 yr old 1–2 recent and painful OVCFs defined as ≥grade 1 (Genant) Unhealed fx (edema and/or fx line) Fx age<12 mo	≥21 yr old 1–3 VCFs (T5-L5); at least 1 with edema and 1 with ≥15% VB height loss VCFs from osteoporosis or cancer Pain ≥4 (0–10 scale)
Exclusion criteria	Evidence of neoplasm Retropulsion of bony fragments Concomitant hip fx Active infection Uncorrectable bleeding diatheses Surgery in last 60 days Dementia	Presence of >2 fx Spinal cancer Neurologic complications VB collapse >90% Retropulsed bony fragment or impinging on spinal cord Ineligibility for ER Previous VP Likelihood of noncompliance	Previous VP Fx age >3 mo Spinal cord compression History of disabled back not from VCF Dementia Inability to walk before VCF
Primary end point	Roland Morris Disability Questionnaire disability and pain at 1 mo	Pain at 3 mo	SF-36 at 1 mo

BKP, balloon kyphoplasty; ER, emergency decompressive surgery; f/u, follow-up; fx, fracture; NSM, nonsurgical management; OVCF, osteoporotic vertebral compression fracture; QOL, quality of life; VB, vertebral; VCF, vertebral compression fracture; VP, vertebroplasty.

Vertebroplasty

Buchbinder et al[64] studied 78 patients, with 91% of participants followed up at 6 months. Study enrollment commenced in 2004 and concluded in 2008, with goal follow-up of 2 years. These investigators selected patients who had 12 months or less of back pain and who had the presence of 1 or 2 VCFs of grade 1 or higher with edema or a fracture line noted on MRI. For this study, 468 patients were screened; 248 did not meet inclusion criteria, and 141 (plus 1 death) were not willing to participate. Of the 78 patients who met inclusion criteria, 38 underwent vertebroplasty, whereas 40 underwent a sham procedure. The sham procedure involved the placement of a 13-gauge needle to the lamina, replacement of the sharp stylet with a blunt stylet, and gentle tapping to simulate vertebroplasty. These investigators also mixed the PMMA so that the smell permeated the room. All participants underwent basic testing as well as "up and go testing," which involved measuring the time required to rise from a standard arm chair, walk 3 m, turn around, return to the chair, and sit down again. Also separated were the acuity of the fractures (<6 weeks versus >6 weeks). The primary outcome was the overall pain score measured on a scale of 0 to 10, whereas secondary outcomes included quality-of-life measures, pain at rest and pain in bed at night, and Roland Morris Disability Questionnaire measures. Measurements were taken at 1 week, 1 month, 3 months, and 6 months. Mean pain reduction in the vertebroplasty and placebo groups was 2.6 ± 2.9 and 1.9 ± 3.3, respectively.

The investigators concluded that at 6 months, vertebroplasty had no beneficial effect over a sham procedure at any time point. The investigators admitted to a selection bias based on the finding that only 78 patients were enrolled, whereas 141 declined to participate. Critics[65] of the study cited multiple other flaws with the study, such as the following:

- Patients did not require edema, only a fracture line on MRI, even though the investigators stated that bone marrow edema indicated an acute fracture.
- The definition of "acute" in this study included fractures up to 1 year old, whereas most clinicians would define an acute fracture as one that occurred within the previous 4 to 6 weeks.
- The sham procedure was performed with local anesthetic at the facet joint.
- The primary outcome of pain as overall pain may not have been reflective of back pain because it was a report of overall body pain.
- The investigators did not report whether back pain was from fracture, by percussing the spinous process systematically to find a level of maximal tenderness.
- The investigators did not report pain severity and functional compromise of the patients who met criteria but who refused to enroll in the study.

Kallmes et al[66] studied 131 patients with 1 to 3 VCFs that were either fractures less than 1 year old and defined by the onset of pain and a pain score of at least 3 (0 to 10) or were fractures of uncertain age that were examined by MRI or bone scan to assess for edema. Only the patients with fractures of uncertain age underwent imaging, and those with fractures with edema were eligible for inclusion. Of the 1813 patients who were screened, 300 patients who fit criteria declined to participate. Of the 131 patients enrolled, 68 underwent

vertebroplasty, and 63 underwent a sham procedure. The sham procedure involved placement of local anesthetic at the skin and subcutaneous tissues and infiltration of the periosteum of the pedicles with 0.25% bupivacaine. Then, instead of placement of 11- or 13-gauge trocars, verbal and physical cues of pressure were given on the patient's back, and the methylmethacrylate monomer was opened.

Primary outcomes measured included modified Roland Morris Disability Questionnaire and pain scores at various times over 1 year, with the goal to evaluate the outcome at 1 month as the primary outcome. Secondary outcomes included scores on health status questionnaires, the physical and mental component summary of Short Form-36 (SF-36) version 2, and opioid use. At 1 month, the mean pain scores of the vertebroplasty and control group were 3.9 ± 2.9 and 4.6 ± 3.0, respectively. The mean Roland Morris Disability Questionnaire score was essentially the same for both groups. Forty-three percent of patients who underwent the control procedure crossed over to the vertebroplasty group, whereas only 12% did the reverse (vertebroplasty to control). No significant difference was noted in any of the secondary outcome measures, but the trend was toward more meaningful improvement in pain in the vertebroplasty group than in the control group (64% versus 48%). The investigators concluded that no significant difference existed at 1 month between the two groups, and they cited the following limitations of their study:

- Cross-over at 1 month complicated the interpretation of data.
- The study did not compare the study groups with respect to medical treatments received that could have affected outcomes.
- Persistence of pain after vertebroplasty or fracture healing may have indicated causes of pain other than the fracture.
- Vertebroplasty may be beneficial only for fractures of a certain age or healing stage, and this possibility was not taken into account.
- Kyphoplasty was not evaluated.

Critics[65] of the study cited the following weaknesses:

- Selection bias occurred.
- Patient selection criteria were poor because they did not require edema on MRI or bone scan for all patients.
- Pain severity and functional compromise of the patients who met criteria but who refused to enroll were not reported.
- The sham procedure was a facet block instead of a dry needle approach.
- The investigators did not report whether back pain was from fracture, by percussing the spinous process systematically to find a level of maximal tenderness.

The results of these studies were quite shocking to the "spine" community. Practitioners who have performed vertebral augmentation over the years have clinically seen profound relief of pain in those patients who had acute VCFs, and numerous large case series, prospective and retrospective, have demonstrated dramatic pain relief. What the studies most clearly demonstrate are the need for improvement in patient selection criteria for vertebral augmentation and the difficulties in performing randomized, double-blinded, placebo-controlled studies in patients in severe pain. Important physical examination and imaging findings need to be included, along with a comparison of the outcomes of those patients who fit criteria for inclusion but who choose not to enroll in the study. This issue may be assessed further by the investigators of the foregoing studies by retrospective review of the patients who chose not to enroll in those studies but who met inclusion criteria. Future studies should take this factor into account rather than jump to the conclusion that vertebral augmentation is no better than placebo.

Kyphoplasty

Wardlaw et al[67] studied 300 patients with VCFs by randomly assigning these patients to receive kyphoplasty or nonsurgical care (this study is also known as the FREE [Fracture REduction Evaluation] trial). These investigators used the following inclusion criteria:

- One to three VCFs from T5 to L5
- At least one fracture with edema shown by MRI
- At least one fracture associated with greater than 15% height loss
- The requirement that single fractures had to meet both criteria

The primary outcome was the change in SF-36 score from baseline to 1 month. This score showed a decrease in 7.2 points in the kyphoplasty group as opposed to 5.2 points in the nonsurgical group. These investigators also noted no difference in frequency of adverse reactions between the groups and concluded that kyphoplasty is a safe and effective procedure for patients with acute VCFs. This is the only prospective, randomized, double-blind study of kyphoplasty. The only drawback is that it has no placebo control.

Other Studies for Osteoporotic Fractures

Taylor et al[54] performed a systematic review and metaregression to compare the efficacy and safety of kyphoplasty and vertebroplasty for the treatment of VCFs and to examine the prognostic factors that predict outcome. These investigators reviewed studies that compared kyphoplasty with conventional medical therapy, vertebroplasty with conventional medical therapy, and vertebroplasty with kyphoplasty. Based on a total of 74 studies, none of which were randomized, these investigators concluded that level III evidence supports vertebral augmentation for osteoporotic fractures refractory to conventional medical therapy. The ratio of benefit over harm was favorable for both procedures, and kyphoplasty had a better adverse event profile. These investigators later followed up with a study demonstrating that patients undergoing kyphoplasty experienced superior improvements in pain, functionality, vertebral height, and kyphotic angle at least up to 3 years after the procedure. These investigators also concluded that prospective studies of low bias, with follow-up of 12 months or more, demonstrate that kyphoplasty is more effective than conventional medical management of osteoporotic VCFs and is at least as effective as vertebroplasty.

Eck et al[55] performed a meta-analysis to assess both pain relief and risk of complications associated with vertebroplasty versus kyphoplasty. These investigators included 168 studies that met inclusion criteria. They concluded that vertebroplasty caused a significantly greater improvement in Visual Analog Scale (VAS) scores compared with kyphoplasty (mean VAS decrease, 5.68 versus 4.60, respectively), but it also had a statistically greater risk of cement leakage and new fracture.

Masala et al[68] evaluated the efficacy and cost effectiveness of vertebroplasty by comparing 58 patients who accepted and underwent vertebroplasty versus 95 who refused the procedure and underwent conservative medical therapy. These investigators found that significant reduction in VAS and improvement in ambulation and activities of daily living were observed in both groups at 1 week, 3 months, and 12 months. The results were significantly superior in the vertebroplasty group at 1 week and 3 months, and vertebroplasty was more cost effective than conventional medical management with regard to VAS and activities of daily living at 1 week. By 3 months, vertebroplasty was more cost effective with regard to ambulation. However, no significant cost difference was noted at 12 months between the 2 groups.

Kyphoplasty has been touted to restore vertebral body height and sagittal alignment. Only a few retrospective reviews discuss this benefit. Hiwatashi et al[69] noted no significant difference between vertebroplasty and kyphoplasty in restoring vertebral body height and wedge angles. Kim et al[70] concluded that balloon kyphoplasty after postural reduction and intraoperative kyphotic angle correction is well tolerated and effective for treating severe osteoporotic VCFs.

Vertebral Augmentation in Multiple Myeloma and Metastases

Studies in patients with multiple myeloma and spinal metastases have also been completed. Fourney et al[71] retrospectively reviewed 56 patients who underwent vertebroplasty or kyphoplasty (total of 97 procedures) for either myeloma or metastases. These investigators reported complete pain relief in 84% and no change in 9% of patients who underwent the procedures. No patient was worse, and asymptomatic cement extravasations occurred in 9.2%. Significant improvement in pain scores was noted at 1 year, and analgesic consumption was reduced after 1 month. The CAFÉ (Cancer Patient Fracture Evaluation) study[72] randomly assigned 134 patients with various types of cancers and up to 3 painful VCFs to receive immediate kyphoplasty (n = 70) or nonsurgical supportive care (n = 64). These investigators excluded patients with primary bone tumors, osteoblastic tumors, or solitary plasmacytoma at the fracture site. The primary outcome measure was the Roland Morris Disability Questionnaire at 1 month, results of which were found to be significantly improved in the kyphoplasty group (−8.3) versus the nonsurgical care group (−0.1). Secondary measures included VAS scores, which were also improved (−4.1 versus −0.5). No significant difference was noted in serious adverse reactions between the groups. The investigators concluded that the improvements in disability and pain with kyphoplasty were both statistically and clinically significant without an increase in adverse reactions.

Pflugmacher et al[73] found that the mean VAS and Oswestry Disability Index significantly improved in patients with lumbar or thoracic VCFs secondary to metastases who underwent balloon kyphoplasty. Sixty-five patients were prospectively followed over 24 months, and sustained improvement in both scores was reported. These investigators also noted a 12% rate of cement leakage and an 8% incidence of vertebral fracture. No symptomatic cement leaks occurred.

Other retrospective reviews[74,75] have demonstrated positive results with vertebroplasty in patients with spinal metastases and multiple myeloma, with marked pain reduction and decreased analgesic consumption, along with minimal complications.

Conclusion

Osteoporosis and VCFs are significant public health concerns with high morbidity. Management of VCFs should start with prevention. In the presence of a painful VCF, all measures should be taken to keep the patient weight bearing and functional. This should start with medical management including opioids, NSAIDs, back bracing, and physical therapy. If at any time the patient cannot perform weight-bearing exercises despite appropriate medical management, interventions should be considered. A comprehensive history and physical examination, particularly neurologic and musculoskeletal examinations along with proper review of imaging studies, will help to target interventions. If the pain is determined to be related to the VCF, an experienced practitioner should determine which procedure should be done to augment the fracture.

Both vertebroplasty and kyphoplasty have excellent safety profiles when these procedures are performed appropriately. Kyphoplasty is approved only when performed in the operating room and is more expensive than vertebroplasty, which can be completed in an office based facility (with fluoroscopy). Randomized trials demonstrated that kyphoplasty is efficacious for the treatment of painful VCFs related to osteoporosis, whereas the results of vertebroplasty, although controversial, are no better than placebo. Either procedure can be performed for VCFs related to cancer. Patient selection and proper technique are the most important factors in determining whether interventional procedures will relieve pain and thus improve quality of life.

References

Full references for this chapter can be found on www.expertconsult.com.

Intradiskal Electrothermal Annuloplasty

Michael L. Whitworth

Historical Considerations

Since the mid-1990s, intradiskal radiofrequency heating has been considered for the treatment for diskogenic pain. Cadaver studies demonstrated that placement of a bipolar probe did not result in end-plate or vertebral body damage and was associated with a temperature change at the edges of the disk of 3°C (37°F) to 4°C (39°F).[1] Later experiments evaluated the thermal diffusion capacity of the intervertebral disks. Investigators discovered an age-related differential in thermal dissipation: the disk of a 32-year-old person has 250% the thermal diffusion capability of the disk of a 61-year-old person.[2] Ostensibly, this phenomenon is the result of the relatively greater aqueous content of the younger disk. Interest in diskogenic disease—and its causes—heightened after the seminal 1997 article demonstrating the presence of neural ingrowth into the inner anulus and nucleus 0% of the time in diskogram-negative disks but 57% of the time in diskogram-positive disks.[3] Additional sources of potential nociception transmission were also found in the vertebral end plate in patients with severe disk degeneration. The end plate in such cases was associated with increased sensory nerve innervation and neoangiogenesis adjacent to the end plates.[4]

Tony Yeung, a pioneer in endoscopic spine surgery, attempted to use a prototype intradiskal radiofrequency probe during endoscopic spine surgery but found that the temperatures produced in tissues were erratic. He later developed endoscopic laser annuloplasty. Interest in the radiofrequency intradiskal approach continued with subsequent clinical studies, but with disappointing results. A prospective randomized human trial using a 90-second intradiskal radiofrequency lesion at 70°C (158°F) did not produce any differences from controls.[5] A later study comparing two heating protocols of 120 and 360 seconds at 80°C (176°F) failed to produce long-term positive results. At 6 months after the procedure, Visual Analog Scale (VAS) scores had returned to baseline, although the short-term response to the procedure was statistically significant.[6]

The Saals selected a thermoresistive heating element as a means of producing sufficient heat to cause interruption in intradiskal neural transmission—if not overt intradiskal neural destruction. Although their energy source remained a radiofrequency generator, the energy was not directly imparted to the nucleus pulposus or the anulus fibrosus because the "spine wand" was insulated. Instead, unlike intradiskal radiofrequency application of energy, the radiofrequency current was used to heat a resistive coil inside the insulated intradiskal portion of the device that secondarily heated the surrounding tissues with thermal energy. An initial report on the procedure, termed *intradiskal electrothermal (IDET) annuloplasty*, was published in 1999.[7] In early 2000, a preliminary report on a 20-patient study was published with the results that 72% of patients received 50% relief.[8] A 1-year outcome study using the IDET device was published in October of 2000. The study had 62 participants with chronic low back pain and diskogram-positive findings; some improvement was found at 1 year in 71% of the patients.[9] Unfortunately, this trial was not controlled, and although the investigators cautioned that the results should be verified by placebo-controlled randomized trials, these follow-up studies were not forthcoming for several years.

A company was formed very early to market the device aggressively to physicians through training courses for them. As a result, the device had tens of thousands of uses before the first validated clinical trials were released. During a training conference in 1999, the company manufacturing the device at that time reported that reimbursement for the procedure was in the range of $3500 to $7000 and that the company had a reimbursement department for physician use. Eventually, insurers became increasingly reluctant to pay for an expensive procedure with so little clinical data and with marginal results. Insurers subsequently began to block payment for the procedure in their medical policies. At the time of this writing, in the United States, very few major insurers will cover the IDET procedure because it is considered "investigational."

Other alternatives to IDET, such as endoscopic annuloplasty, the discTRODE intra-annular radiofrequency procedure, and bipolar annuloplasty, began to appear around the turn of the millennium. However, few studies have been conducted on these procedures, and these studies have only marginal results.

Indications

The indications for and contraindications to annuloplasty are summarized in **Table 181.1**. The International Spine Intervention Society publishes *Practice Guidelines: Spinal Diagnostic and Treatment Procedures*, which represents the only validated operating guidelines for this and many other spinal procedures. These guidelines detail IDET theory, practice, and controversy. **Table 181.2** compares IDET with other forms of intradiskal therapy in common use.

Table 181.1 Indications for and Contraindications to Annuloplasty

No evidence of emergency spinal intervention indicators

No medical contraindications

Absence of radiculopathy and myelopathy

Negative Lasègue sign

MRI with no other disorders correlating to the pain production

No evidence for spinal instability or spondylolisthesis at the level of interest

No significant untreated or uncontrolled psychiatric issues

Motivated patient with realistic outcome expectations

No greater than 25% loss of disk height

Criteria for intradiskal disease satisfied:
   Disk stimulation is positive at low pressures (<50 psi)
   Disk stimulation reproduces pain of intensity (>6/10)
   Disk stimulation reproduces concordant pain
   CT diskography reveals a grade 3 or greater annular tear
   Control disk stimulation is negative in at least one adjacent disk

CT, computed tomography; MRI, magnetic resonance imaging.

Anatomy and Pathology

Painful annular radial fissures, as seen during diskography, are evidence of internal disk disruption, which is the sole indication for IDET.[10] It is known that these fissures are associated with vascular and neural ingrowth from the outer anulus, that leakage of diskal enzymes that are toxic to extradiskal materials may occur, and that mechanical changes in the disk occur with disk degeneration. The mechanism by which IDET actually works is not known but is thought to be by sealing off the fissures with thermal energy, destroying nociceptor nerve ingrowth, and stabilizing the collagen and biomechanics of the disk. Some studies of these mechanisms have been conducted in cadavers,[11-13] but clearly this model has little to do with the dynamic human intervertebral disk and the processes of tissue healing. The annular fissures are both radial and circumferential, and they split the laminar layers of the anulus. Provocative manometric diskography with a negative control disk and postdiskography computed tomography (CT) or magnetic resonance imaging (MRI) are the absolute minimum requirements for proper selection of patients for IDET. Fluoroscopic diskography may demonstrate annular fissures, but the three-dimensional location of the radial tears cannot be determined accurately with fluoroscopy. Both circumferential and radial annular tears may be visualized on postdiskography CT scans. The fissures are thought to begin peripherally and gradually expand as the degree of internal disk disruption expands to involve increasing amounts of the nucleus pulposus by cavitation.

Technique

In the United States, the acquisition cost of the SpineCath (Smith & Nephew, Inc., Andover, MA) is more than $1200, so it is prudent to select patients carefully. At times, it is impossible to advance the SpineCath into the area containing the annular tear as demonstrated on CT diskography. At other times, the SpineCath folds over on itself and becomes it utterly useless from that point on in the procedure. In such cases, a new SpineCath is required, thereby making the IDET an extremely expensive procedure to the entity purchasing

Table 181.2 Advantages and Disadvantages of Intradiskal Thermal Delivery Systems

Delivery System	Advantages	Disadvantages
LASER FIBEROPTIC		
Energy source: laser Delivery method: straight or side-firing fiberoptic catheter	Good access to disease Excellent decompression effect for radiculopathy	High expense Poor temperature control
RADIOFREQUENCY ELECTRODE		
Energy source: radiofrequency Delivery method: straight electrode	Easy intradiskal placement Cost effectiveness Safety Minimal invasiveness	Poor heating of low-water-content diskal tissues Poor decompressive effect Small treatment area Inability to reach posterior disk easily
INTRADISKAL ELECTROTHERMAL CATHETER		
Energy source: electroresistive coil Delivery method: navigable catheter	Easy intradiskal placement Broad target zone Cost effectiveness Safety Minimal invasiveness	Poor decompressive effect Inability to reach collapsed disks Poor results for radicular pain

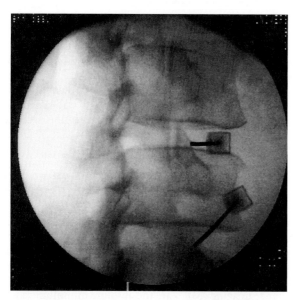

Fig. 181.1 Radiograph showing positioning of the intradiskal electro-thermal needle.

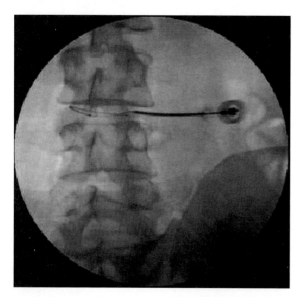

Fig. 181.2 The target for the needle tip is halfway between the end plates and just medial to the medial pedicular line, at the inner aspect of the anulus fibrosus.

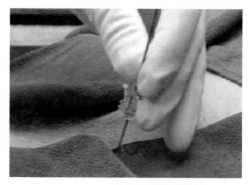

Fig. 181.3 **Technique for threading the SpineCath catheter.**

the device. A posterolateral approach is used that targets the superior articular process with a 17-gauge IDET needle with a relatively smooth beveled edge, to avoid shearing the catheter (**Fig. 181.1**). The trajectory of the needle is usually between 25 and 40 degrees to the sagittal plane, with an entry point on the contralateral side from the CT-demonstrated radial tears. The target for the needle tip is halfway between the end plates and just medial to the medial pedicular line, at the inner aspect of the anulus fibrosus (**Fig. 181.2**).

Once the needle is placed into the inner annular fibers and outer nucleus pulposus, the SpineCath is slowly inserted and, as much as possible, is "guided" into place by the flexible bent tip (**Fig. 181.3**). However, the catheter frequently lodges in irregularities in the inner anulus or travels in a circumferential annular tear or even creates its own separation of the

lamina of the anulus fibrosus (**Fig. 181.4**). In any case, the final resting place of the SpineCath tip is across the posterior anulus, to cover the CT-demonstrated location of the radial tear (**Fig. 181.5**). Frequent manipulations of the catheter may be necessary, and in some cases where excessive force would bend the catheter, a contralateral or bilateral approach is necessary with dual heatings (**Fig. 181.6**). The SpineCath has two markings—one at the tip and one more proximally—that denote the location of the thermoresistive coil, which is the active heating element. The patient must be awake enough to render feedback regarding potential nerve root heating, although this is uncommon. A manufacturer heating protocol is usually incorporated in which the temperature is gradually ramped up to 90°C (194°F) for 16.5 minutes. The safest method of catheter removal is en bloc, with the needle and catheter removed as a unit. If antibiotic is to be administered into the disk, this should be done before the catheter is introduced into the needle or, if the catheter can easily be removed through the needle, after the heating.

Controversy continues regarding the location of the catheter with respect to any circumferential fissures. Some investigators believe that the SpineCath should be placed deep into the anulus fibrosus within the circumferential tear, whereas others use the more traditional approach of the anulus-nucleus junction. Manipulation of the catheter may, at times, be very time consuming, requiring up to an hour. However, experienced physicians are usually able to place the catheter and needle carefully within several minutes.

Complications

Shortly after the first published reports of IDET, several serious complications were described in the literature. The first noted complication was cauda equina syndrome.[14] Postprocedure pain flare-ups are relatively common, and they seem to be temperature dependent.[15] Intradural migration from a broken SpineCath that ultimately required surgery for the resultant radiculopathy has been reported.[16] Osteonecrosis of the vertebral body after IDET has also been reported in the literature.[17,18] During subsequent endoscopic disk surgery, Whitworth observed charring of diskal tissues from IDET.

The complications of the procedure are divided into access issues and heating issues. Clinicians not versed in diskography may not understand the anatomic barriers to the disk, such as the furcal nerves, the iliac crest's overriding the disk space in

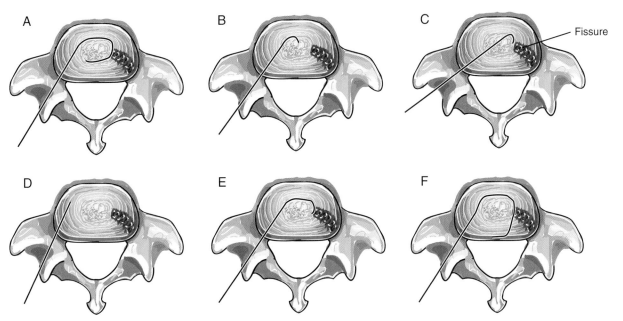

Fig. 181.4 **Problems with catheter advancement.** A, Desired catheter position. B, Needle is advanced too far, causing acute deflection. C, Deflection angle is too acute, and the catheter does not follow the anulus. D, Needle is intra-annular, and the catheter cannot be advanced. E, Catheter tip enters the annular tear, and the catheter cannot be advanced. F, Intracanal catheter placement.

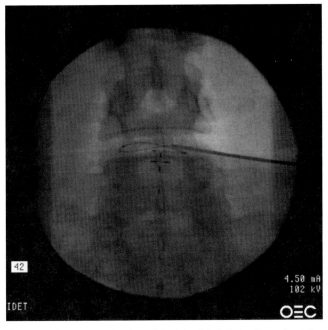

Fig. 181.5 Anteroposterior view of the intradiskal electrothermal resistive coil final position. The coil is within the L4-5 intervertebral disk and clearly away from the end plates. *(From Kapural L, Goyle A: Imaging for interventional management of chronic pain: imaging for provocative discography and minimally invasive percutaneous procedures for treatment of discogenic lower back pain,* Tech Reg Anesth Pain Manag *11:73, 2007.)*

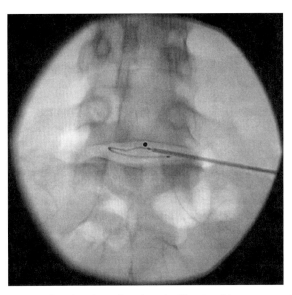

Fig. 181.6 Advancing the coil against significant resistance causes the catheter to bend within the intervertebral disk. *(From Kapural L, Goyle A: Imaging for interventional management of chronic pain: imaging for provocative discography and minimally invasive percutaneous procedures for treatment of discogenic lower back pain,* Tech Reg Anesth Pain Manag *11:73, 2007.)*

Outcome Studies

Many of the IDET studies grouped their results effectively into nonresponders and responders. Patients who did respond were then given an average VAS reduction citation. The adoption of this methodology appears to connect failure to respond with poor patient selection, inadequate technical placement of the SpineCath, or disease that was so severe that IDET with its 2-mm thermal excursion could not help. Such methodology also calls into question the validity of the technique as an effective treatment. Bogduk[19] published an excellent review

the oblique fluoroscopic rotation, the safe access zone shape and size, the potential for end-plate damage, and the risk of diskitis (septic and aseptic). The IDET catheter may travel outside the posterior anulus fibrosus into the epidural space or even into the dura or nerve roots (**Fig. 181.7**). Heating may cause radicular-type pain that cannot be readily explained in the absence of proximity to nerve roots.

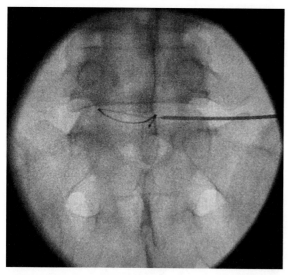

Fig. 181.7 This fluoroscopic image shows the intradiskal electrothermal catheter tip passing posteriorly through the annular fissure. Such inappropriate placement of the catheter may result in heat dissipation to the epidural space and neural elements. It is necessary to reposition the catheter and recheck it in the lateral and anteroposterior views. *(From Kapural L, Goyle A: Imaging for interventional management of chronic pain: imaging for provocative discography and minimally invasive percutaneous procedures for treatment of discogenic lower back pain, Tech Reg Anesth Pain Manag 11:73, 2007.)*

of the IDET literature and methodology. The first placebo-controlled trial demonstrated a powerful placebo effect on pain relief that suggested caution in the adaptation of IDET.[20] However, the entire effect of pain relief could not be entirely explained by placebo; therefore, IDET was believed to have a positive but modest effect. Other studies generally revealed a modest reduction in pain in the 50% responders (usually 3 points on a 10-point VAS scale), with no relief in the other 50%. A more recent evidence-based review of the literature placed IDET in a more positive light and suggested that IDET may be a reasonable "first option" in patients who have failed to respond to conservative therapy.[21]

Conclusion

Because of the lack of financial reimbursement, electrothermal annuloplasty is only occasionally practiced in the United States today. The elevation of physician and corporate avarice to a level that superseded scientific demonstration of the effectiveness of the technique has cast a pall on future use of this technique. One hopes that interventional pain practitioners will learn from this tragic episode and will become more acutely aware of their role as stewards of monetary resources available for the treatment of pain and as gatekeepers against wholesale acceptance of experimental techniques. The technique actually did work in the treatment of some patients, and practitioners should build on that knowledge to advance the potential modifications necessary to enhance effectiveness. Perhaps improvements on the IDET model could be made in the future, such as bipolar radiofrequency electrode energy applied across the posterior anulus, a more expansive heating device, or consideration of neuromodulation of the posterior anulus. Outcome studies for both discTRODE (a flexible radiofrequency catheter that splits the lamellae of the anulus circumferentially)[22,23] and intradiskal endoscopic laser annuloplasty have shown modest improvements in pain.[24] The future of the development of techniques to treat annular fissures will be partially predicated on fiscal responsibility to the medical system by demonstrating effectiveness before massive release and promotion of a product. As the understanding of the pathologic process of internal disk disruption increases, practitioners may be able to develop enhanced therapies that may include intradiskal injections along with structural support methods.

References

Full references for this chapter can be found on www.expertconsult.com.

Percutaneous Diskectomy: Automated Technique

Steven D. Waldman

Indications

Percutaneous diskectomy using the automated technique is indicated for a specialized subset of patients who are suffering from low back and radicular pain thought to be caused by contained disk protrusion[1] (**Fig. 182.1**). In this group of patients, conservative therapy consisting of a trial of simple analgesics, nonsteroidal anti-inflammatory agents or cyclooxygenase-2 inhibitors, bed rest, and epidural steroids should have failed. Some pain management specialists also recommend that a trial of transforaminal epidural steroid nerve blocks should also be attempted before percutaneous diskectomy.[2] To optimize patient selection, the ideal candidate for nucleoplasty should have magnetic resonance imaging (MRI) findings, evidence on diskography, and electromyographic changes that correlate with the patient's radicular pain pattern.

Clinically Relevant Anatomy

From a functional anatomic viewpoint, lumbar disks must be thought of as distinct from cervical disks insofar as a source of pain is concerned. Radicular symptoms originating solely from disk herniation are much more common in the lumbar region when compared with the cervical and thoracic regions.[3,4] The reason for this finding is twofold: (1) for the lumbar disk to impinge on the lumbar nerve roots, it must herniate posteriorly and laterally; the lumbar nerve roots are not protected from impingement from lumbar disk herniation by the bony wall of the facet joints, as are the cervical nerve roots; and (2) the posterior longitudinal ligament in the lumbar region is only a single layer, which is thinner and less well developed in its lateral aspects; lumbar disk herniation with impingement on exiting nerve roots is most likely to occur in this lateral region.

The nuclear material in the lumbar disk is placed more posteriorly than in its cervical counterpart. The gelatinous nucleus pulposus of the lumbar disk is surrounded by a dense, laminated fibroelastic network of fibers known as the *anulus fibrosus*.[4] The annular fibers are arranged in concentric layers that run obliquely from adjacent vertebrae. This annular layer receives sensory innervation from various sources. Posteriorly, the anulus receives fibers from the sinovertebral nerves, which also provide sensory innervation to the posterior elements, including portions of the facet joints.[4] Laterally, fibers from the exiting spinal nerve roots provide sensory innervation, with the anterior portion of the disk receiving fibers from the sympathetic chain. Whether some of or all these fibers play a role in diskogenic pain is a subject of controversy among pain specialists.

The lumbar nerve roots leave the spinal cord and travel laterally through the intervertebral foramina. If the posterior lumbar disk herniates laterally, it can impinge on the lumbar root as it travels through the intervertebral foramen and can thus produce classic radicular symptoms. If the lumbar disk herniates posteromedially, it may impinge on the spinal cord itself and produce myelopathy that may include lower extremity as well as bowel and bladder symptoms. Severe compression of the lumbar spinal cord may result in cauda equina syndrome, paraparesis, or, rarely, paraplegia.

Technique

The patient is placed in the lateral or prone position with a pillow under the abdomen to flex the lumbar spine slightly as if for a lumbar sympathetic block. Computed tomography (CT) scans or fluoroscopic views are taken through the disks to be imaged, and the relative positions of the lung, ribs, aorta, vena cava, kidneys, nerve roots, and spinal cord are noted[1] (**Fig. 182.2**). The spinous process of the vertebra just above the disk to be evaluated is palpated. At a point just below and 1½ inches lateral to the spinous process, the skin is prepared with antiseptic solution, and the skin and subcutaneous tissues are infiltrated with local anesthetic.[1] A small stab wound as made at the point of needle entry to facilitate the placement of the introducer cannula.

The stylet is placed into the introducer cannula, and the cannula is then advanced through the skin under fluoroscopic or CT guidance, with the target being the middle of the disk to be decompressed (**Figs. 182.3 to 182.5**). If fluoroscopic guidance is used, oblique images may be helpful.[1] Given the proximity of the somatic nerve roots, paresthesia in the distribution of the corresponding lumbar paravertebral nerve may be elicited. If this occurs, the needle should be withdrawn and redirected slightly more cephalad. The needle is again readvanced in incremental steps under CT or fluoroscopic guidance. Sequential imaging is always indicated to avoid advancing the needle completely through the disk and into the lower limits of the spinal cord or cauda equina.[1] The pain management

specialist must also take care not to allow the needle to track too laterally into the lower pleural or retroperitoneal space.

When the cannula is in a satisfactory position in the center of the disk, the stylet is removed, and a small amount of contrast material is injected into the disk to confirm mid-disk needle placement and to identify any significant disruption of the anulus[1] (**Fig. 182.6**). The automated disk decompressor probe is then advanced through the cannula into the center of the disk nucleus until the probe extends beyond the end of the cannula (**Fig. 182.7**). The activation switch of the device is then turned to the "on" position for 15-second increments, with the total combined time that the device is activated not to exceed 5 minutes. Under CT or fluoroscopic guidance, the device may be gently advanced toward the anterior anulus of the disk being treated, with care taken to avoid impinging on the anulus itself. Disk material will begin to appear in the clear collection chamber after approximately 1 mL of disk has been removed. After an adequate amount of disk material has been removed, the automated disk decompressor probe is removed from the cannula. A slight rotation of the probe may aid in the

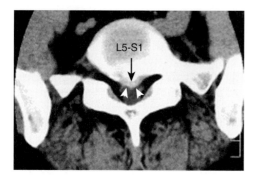

Fig. 182.1 Lumbar spine computed tomography axial image at the L5-S1 level. Note: (1) the median disk protrusion *(black arrow)* abutting the left, and particularly the right, nerve roots *(small white arrows)* and indenting the dural tube anteriorly. R, right side of the patient. *(From Giles LGF: CT versus MRI for lumbar spine intervertebral disc protrusion,* 100 challenging spinal pain syndrome cases, *ed 2, New York, 2009, Churchill Livingstone.)*

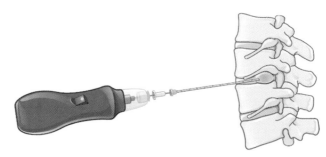

Fig. 182.3 Lateral view of the cannula within the disk. *(From Waldman SD:* Atlas of interventional pain management, *ed 3, Philadelphia, 2009, Saunders Elsevier.)*

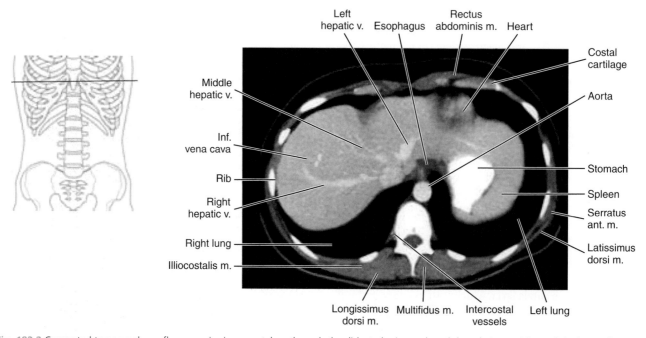

Fig. 182.2 Computed tomography or fluoroscopic views are taken through the disks to be imaged, and the relative positions of the lung, ribs, aorta, vena cava, kidneys, nerve roots, and spinal cord are noted. *(From El-Khoury GY, Bergman RA, Montgomery WJ, et al:* Sectional anatomy by MRI and CT, *ed 3, New York, 2007, Churchill Livingstone, p 492.)*

easy withdrawal of the probe. The cannula is then removed, and a sterile dressing is placed over the operative site.

After the procedure is completed, the patient is observed for 30 minutes before discharge. The patient should be warned to expect minor postprocedure discomfort, including some soreness of the paraspinous musculature. Ice packs placed on the

injection site for 20-minute time periods will help decrease these untoward effects. The patient should be instructed to call immediately if any fever or other systemic symptoms occur that could suggest infection.

Side Effects and Complications

Complications directly related to percutaneous diskectomy using the automated technique are generally self-limited, although occasionally, even with the best technique, severe complications can occur.[6] The most common severe complication of percutaneous diskectomy using the automated technique is infection of the disk, which is commonly referred to as *diskitis* (**Fig. 182.8**). Because of the limited blood supply of the disk, such infections can be extremely difficult to eradicate. Diskitis usually manifests as an increase in spine pain several days to a week after percutaneous diskectomy. Acutely, no change will be evident in the patient's neurologic examination as a result of disk infection.

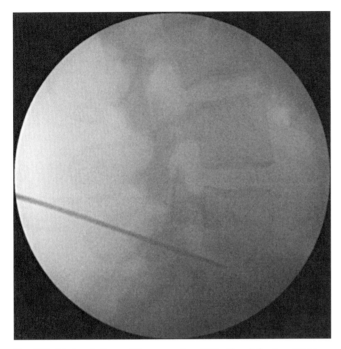

Fig. 182.4 Lateral view of the cannula within the disk. *(From Waldman SD: Atlas of interventional pain management, ed 3, Philadelphia, 2009, Saunders.)*

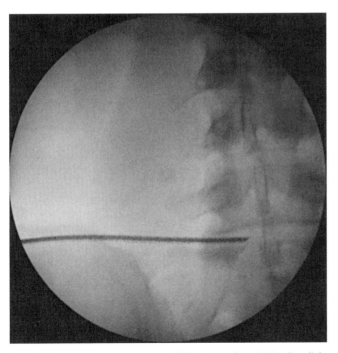

Fig. 182.5 Posteroanterior view of the cannula within the disk. *(From Waldman SD: Atlas of interventional pain management, ed 3, Philadelphia, 2009, Saunders.)*

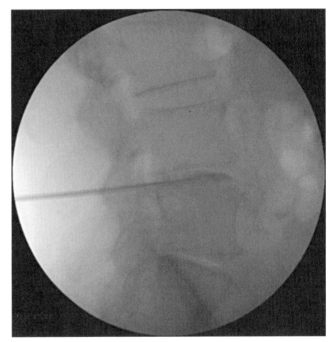

Fig. 182.6 Contrast medium is placed through the cannula into the disk.

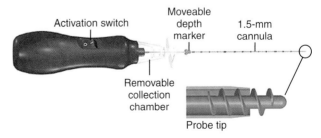

Fig. 182.7 The automated disk decompressor probe is then advanced through the cannula into the center of the disk nucleus until the probe extends beyond the end of the cannula. *(From Waldman SD: Atlas of interventional pain management, ed 3, Philadelphia, 2009, Saunders.)*

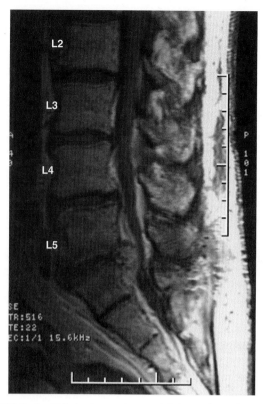

Fig. 182.8 Sagittal lumbar spine gadolinium-enhanced magnetic resonance imaging showing postoperative diskitis and complete collapse of the L5-S1 disk space. *(From Harris AE, Hennicke C, Byers K, et al: Postoperative discitis due to* Propionibacterium acnes: *a case report and review of the literature,* Surg Neurol *63:538, 2005.)*

Epidural abscess, which can rarely occur after percutaneous diskectomy, generally manifests within 24 to 48 hours. Clinically, the signs and symptoms of epidural abscess are high fever, spine pain, and progressive neurologic deficit.[5n] If either diskitis or epidural abscess is suspected, blood and urine cultures should be taken, antibiotics started, and an emergency MRI scan of the spine obtained to allow identification and drainage of any abscess formation, to prevent irreversible neurologic deficit.

In addition to infectious complications, pneumothorax may occur after percutaneous diskectomy. This complication should rarely occur if CT guidance is used during needle placement. A small pneumothorax after percutaneous diskectomy using the automated technique can often be treated conservatively, and tube thoracostomy can be avoided. Trauma to retroperitoneal structures, including the kidney, may also occur if CT guidance is not used to avoid and localize these structures.

Direct trauma to the nerve roots and the spinal cord can occur if the needle is allowed to traverse the entire disk or is placed too laterally. These complications should rarely occur if incremental fluoroscopic or CT scans are taken while the needle is advanced. Such needle-induced trauma to the lower lumbar spinal cord and cauda equina can result in deficits, including cauda equina syndrome and paraplegia.

Conclusion

Percutaneous diskectomy using the automated technique is a straightforward procedure that is a reasonable treatment option in carefully selected patients. Proper patient selection is based on correlation with the patient's symptoms and physical examination, MRI, diskogram, and electromyogram results. The use of CT guidance adds an additional measure of safety when compared with fluoroscopy, because CT allows the pain specialist to identify anatomic structures and needle position clearly. These advantages more than outweigh the possible added cost when compared with fluoroscopically guided procedures.

References

Full references for this chapter can be found on www.expertconsult.com.

Percutaneous Laser Diskectomy

Michael L. Whitworth

Historical Considerations

Since 1934, when open diskectomy was first introduced at Massachusetts General Hospital, millions of diskectomies have been performed in the United States, with the rate now approaching 500,000 operations per year. The search for a less invasive approach to laminectomy/diskectomy began in the 1960s with chymopapain—Lyman Smith in 1964;[1] microdiskectomy by Yasargil in 1968; percutaneous diskectomy introduced by Hijikata in 1975; endoscopic monitoring of disk removal by Leu in 1982; endoscopic diskectomy first used by Schreiber and Suezawa in 1986 and improved by Mayer, Brock, and Mathews; arthroscopic diskectomy by Kambin in 1983; nucleotome introduction by Onik in 1984; percutaneous nonendoscopic laser diskectomy by Ascher in 1986;[1] and Choy et al[2] in 1987 and endoscopic laser diskectomy by Mayer et al[3] in 1992 and Savitz[4] in 1994, and the subsequent refinement of endoscopic laser methods by Yeung. In 2000 to 2001, newer minimally invasive methods of diskectomy were introduced, such as coblation nucleoplasty followed by disk decompression.

Lasers were first reported to be clinically used in the intervertebral disk in 1977 as part of an open thoracic diskectomy using a CO_2 laser (**Fig. 183.1**).[5] Animal models for use of the same laser during canine anterior cervical open diskectomy did not occur until 1984.[6] In the 1980s, several lasers were available for treatment of ocular disorders including the argon, carbon dioxide, and excimer (XeCl) laser. The road to published science behind percutaneous diskectomy with a laser began in 1989 when an excimer laser was used on cadaveric disk tissue,[7] even though the first percutaneous diskectomy had occurred several years earlier in 1986. The

neodymium:yttrium/aluminum/garnet (Nd:YAG) laser was applied in laboratory applications and clinically from 1986 to 1990 and was first introduced to the scientific literature by Yonezawa et al[8] in 1990. The KTP laser (green) was used at least as far back as 1990 for diskectomy.[9] The early 1990s saw a proliferation of other laser development with the introduction of Ho:YAG, Er:YAG, and excimer lasers for widespread use in medicine and dentistry. Because of practical considerations, the Ho:YAG (**Fig. 183.2**) became the tool of choice for most physicians performing laser diskectomy.[10] This is largely due to the fact that a fiberoptic waveguide can be employed instead of a mirror system, the penetration depth into tissue is very low giving fine control of tissue modulation and ablation, and the laser output power available is very high—up to 100 watts.

Much of the history of development of lasers for diskectomy was not published until many years later, partially because of financial considerations tied to patent and technique development. The most expansive description of one author's quest to develop laser for intradiskal therapy is found in Choy's book *Percutaneous Laser Disc Decompression*.[11] Choy pioneered the development of laser coronary angioplasty with an argon laser, having performed the first such surgery in September 1983.[12] From 1984 to 1986 Choy and his colleagues worked on the basic science and animal models before introducing the laser for human diskectomy. The initial experiments, published much later, included proving the hypothesis that a minimal volumetric decompression of a pressurized disk using a laser would result in a disproportionately greater reduction in intradiskal pressure.[13] An Nd:YAG laser at 1064 nm was used to deliver 1000 J of energy to create 20 mm by 6 mm elliptical tracks in the nucleus of fresh cadaver disks loaded to 260 to 410 kPa (37 to 59 psi). Control disks were used in which the laser

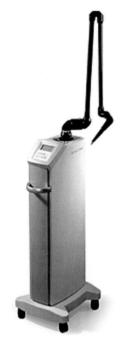

Fig. 183.1 Carbon dioxide laser.

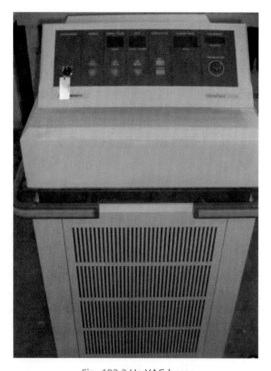

Fig. 183.2 Ho:YAG laser.

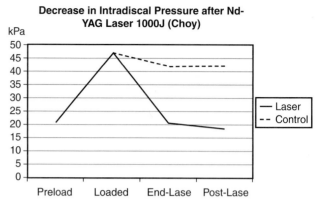

Decrease in Intradiscal Pressure after Nd-YAG Laser 1000J (Choy)

Post-lase is 9 minutes after end of laser application

Fig. 183.3 Decrease in intradiskal pressure after Nd:YAG laser at 1000 J. *(From Choy DS, Altman P: Fall of intradiskal pressure with laser ablation,* J Clin Laser Med Surg *13[3]:149, 1995.)*

was not turned on. The results are presented in **Figure 183.3**. Next, different lasers were examined as to their capability of disk ablation. At 900 J of energy, the mass of disk ablated ranged from 120 to nearly 200 mg of disk tissue. Er:YAG, Nd:YAG (1318 and 1064 nm, respectively), CO_2, argon, excimer, and Ho:YAG lasers were evaluated. The most effective in disk ablation was the pulsed CO_2 laser and erbium laser, but all other lasers were nearly as effective. However, the Ho:YAG lasers of that time were very weak compared to later lasers. For practical purposes, the Nd:YAG 1064 nm was chosen by Choy

for percutaneous laser disk decompression (PLDD) owing to the availability of fiberoptic waveguides and the high powers available with the Nd:YAG. Other experiments were conducted using bovine disks demonstrating temperature rises of less than 2°C (36°F) in the neural foramina, the anterior surface of the spinal canal, and 1 cm away from the laser tip directly in the line of fire of the laser. Next, experiments with mongrel dogs where employed under institutional research board (IRB) approval. PLDD was performed through an 18-gauge needle with 1000 J of energy delivered. The dogs were subsequently sacrificed and on autopsy, there were no extradiskal injuries. Clinical use in humans began in February 1986 in Austria, when Choy performed the first PLDD successfully. Because of bureaucratic obstacles in obtaining IRB approval, it was not until September 1988 when the first U.S. use occurred. Food and Drug Administration approval of PLDD was received in 1991, and since that time it is estimated that there have been over 100,000 users worldwide of intradiskal laser for intervertebral disk decompression.

Indications

Relative indications for this technique depend partially on the technologies employed and partially on the specific targeted pathology. In general, the major indication is the presence of a contained intervertebral disk herniation (confirmed by magnetic resonance imaging [MRI], computed tomography [CT] scan, or CT myelogram) in addition to a clinical presentation of radicular pain with or without neurologic deficits, and a minimum of 6 weeks of conservative treatment without significant improvement. Exclusion criteria are patients with foraminal or central canal stenosis, symptoms of facet syndrome, previous spinal surgery in the same region, bony deformities (such as congenital abnormalities, spondylolisthesis, and hemivertebrae), cauda equina syndrome, other symptoms of myelopathy, and pregnancy. It should be noted that a contained disk herniation is not simply a diffuse bulge, but should be less than 25% of the circumference of the anulus fibrosus and usually contacts the nerve roots or cord (for cervical or thoracic presentations). Technically, a contained disk herniation is one in which there is displaced disk tissue that is

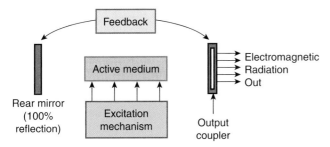

Fig. 183.4 Schematic representation of the mechanism of laser function.

wholly within an outer perimeter of uninterrupted outer anulus or capsule. Extruded disk fragments are not treatable by this technique because there is no continuity with the central nucleus pulposus.

Using the selection criteria (leg pain, positive physical findings such as motor/sensory/reflex deficits and/or straight leg raise, contained disk herniation confirmed by diskography) and exclusion criteria (normal physical examination, presence of stenosis, spondylolisthesis, extruded disk fragment, leakage of diskographic dye from the outer anulus, multiple prior lumbar surgeries), the performance of laser disk decompression resulted in a success rate of 71%, whereas those who did not meet all the section criteria were successful only 29% of the time.[14] Some authors advocate the use of disk decompression for the treatment of spinal stenosis that is primarily caused by a significant disk bulge. Intradiskal and extradiskal endoscopic diskectomy with laser assistance can be performed in the hands of experts using a posterior or posterolateral approach (foraminal).

Technical Aspects of Lasers

Laser stands for *l*ight *a*mplification through *s*timulation of *e*mitted *r*adiation and is used universally as an acronym for obvious reasons. The original equations describing its operation were developed by Albert Einstein in 1917.[15] The first optical laser was developed by Gordon Gould in 1958. Theodore Maiman developed the first solid-state laser, the ruby laser, in 1960 and was followed shortly thereafter by Ali Javan with the first gas laser (He Ne) in 1960, and the CO_2 laser by Kumar Patel in 1964. Now there are more than 100 known lasing media. Lasers produce an extremely focused monochromatic light that is virtually uniform in wavelength. The mechanism of laser function is presented in **Figure 183.4**. There is usually a primary wavelength and several secondary wavelengths of lesser amplitude produced from each laser. A resonating chamber is used (cylindrical tube) containing a lasing medium (gas, liquid, crystal) and a full mirror on one end of the tube with the other end partially mirrored. External energy is applied to the tube through the application of electricity, a flash lamp, or another laser and this causes the electrons in the lasing medium to become excited to a higher orbit. When they fall back to their baseline orbit, the electrons give off monochromatic photons, which are reflected back and forth internally until the energy of the photons is sufficient to break through the partially mirrored end. These photons are collected in a fiberoptic or mirrored waveguide and are transmitted to the target. Different lasing media produce different

wavelengths of light. The CO_2 laser generates an infrared light of 10,600 nm, whereas the Er:YAG generates 2940 nm; Ho:YAG produces 2150 nm; Nd:YAG produces wavelengths of 1318 nm and 1064 nm; KTP generates 532 nm; and the excimer laser produces 193 nm. More recently, diode lasers, especially in parallel arrays, have been shown to give wavelengths up to 2100 nm. The lasing medium is often a crystal that is doped with a rare earth impurity (holmium, neodymium, erbium) during the growth of the crystal. In reality, most lasers generate more than one wavelength of light, and in fact some, such as the CO_2 laser, generate dozens. But in most lasers, the light generated at each wavelength is *coherent* (i.e., the waves generated are all in phase with each other). Lasers are very inefficient, with usually less than 1% of the input energy being converted to the laser beam. The remainder is emitted as heat.[16] With a laser that operates at an efficiency of 2% and has an output of 80 watts, the excess heat produced is about 4000 watts. When the heat generation is excessive and cannot be diffused, the laser crystal medium may fracture. Therefore, in larger lasers, forced air or circulating water is used to dissipate heat. The efficiency of the typical YAG laser is 0.1% to 1%; the excimer laser is 2%; and CO_2 lasers have an efficiency up to 20%. Laser output power is measured in watts, whereas the tissue effect is measured in joules (watts times seconds). Pulsed lasers deliver small pulses of energy with time for thermal dissipation to occur in tissues when the pulses are far enough apart and the pulse width is narrow enough. Double-pulsed lasers can result in summation effects of thermal energy rather than permitting dissipation, thereby approximating the effect of a continuous-wave laser.

Because not all lasers are visible (e.g., Ho:YAG, Nd:YAG, Er:YAG), a second laser is used as an aiming laser through the same fiberoptic waveguide. Usually a low-power helium laser is employed (bright red) and the intensity of the aiming laser may be varied. If the aiming laser is interfering with visualization of tissue vaporization from the primary laser, the aiming laser can often be turned off.

Laser Safety

It is imperative to consider the hazards of a laser beam before engaging in laser use. Most manufacturers have laser courses designed to educate both the staff and physician about radiation hazards from the powerful laser beams. Hospitals and surgery centers usually have a "laser safety officer" who should be well versed in laser safety. Nd:YAG lasers can cause permanent retinal damage and absolutely require safety glasses. All lasers with wavelengths in the ultraviolet (UV) (excimer) or visible spectrum (KTP) and below 1.55 microns in wavelength (Nd:YAG) can seriously damage the retina by causing punctate lesions, thereby permanently reducing vision. The effect of a milliwatt laser in this wavelength range striking the eye is similar to that of staring into the sun. Laser beam energy can enter the orbit from direct beam (e.g., end of the laser fiber, disconnect in the coupling, and so on) or indirectly (reflective surfaces from needles, cannulas, instrumentation), both with devastating effects on the retina. Lasers with wavelengths longer than 1.55 m (Ho:YAG, Er:YAG) cannot reach the retina but can do damage to the cornea and skin. CO_2 lasers can be so powerful that they can cut through any tissue because they are available in output powers up to 15,000 watts. Laser glasses are designed to be specific for different laser wavelengths, and certainly for wavelengths below 1.55 microns (1550 nm). They are mandatory for everyone in the room, including the patient. The laser beam must *never ever* be pointed at a person, and when removing the laser from the patient, the laser operator must switch to standby mode. The laser may never be fired toward a paper drape or gown.

Interactions of Lasers with Intervertebral Disks

Almost immediately after the introduction of lasers, the concern regarding tissue interactions was of research interest.[17,18]

Cadaver and Animal Disk Laser Research

The search for the optimal laser for use in the intervertebral disk began in the 1980s with surveys of absorption of laser energy by intervertebral disk material.[19] It was found that the higher wavelengths such as Nd:YAG 1320 nm and mid-infrared lasers had a higher absorption than the lower-wavelength Nd:YAG 1064 nm or argon lasers. A higher amount of absorbed energy would theoretically be advantageous. However, control of the degree of heating of the disk is also necessary because with Nd:YAG 1320 nm powers above 20 W, instead of tissue shrinkage, a thermal bubble develops that ruptures tissues.[20] When intradiskal tissues reach 65°C (149°F), permanent changes are introduced to the disk, resulting in both morphology changes in the disk and also a permanently increased tension in the disk with a volume loss of 20% to 70% of the nucleus pulposus. Using an Ho:YAG laser, radial bulging is increased with low-energy level laser application whereas after 1500 J, the radial bulge and transverse disk diameter decrease.[21] One group claims that Ho:YAG lasers without cooling (as is the case with nonarthroscopic applications) cause immediate tissue damage to surrounding tissues, whereas in the case of arthroscopy there is irrigation cooling—thereby avoiding damage to surrounding tissues. The same group found that Nd:YAG lasers were much more dependent on the color of the tissue for ablation, with the highly colored tissue causing an increased absorption of energy, thereby concluding that the Nd:YAG is the superior laser for intradiskal ablation.[22] Of course, the disk material that is herniated is usually not highly colored, therefore it is perplexing why these conclusions were reached. A study of power and energy from an Ho:YAG laser with respect to ablated disk material mass and time demonstrated that temperature does not rise any more after the application of 500 J to the disk, and that the mass of ablated material was related to energy, but not to power.[23] Similarly, in another cadaver study, it was discovered that energy, not time, power, or pulse frequency, best determined the rate of disk ablation, and the rate of ablation was enhanced through suction application.[24] The same group determined that end plate damage and adjacent tissue damage is avoided if the laser remains in the middle of the disk, and that there is little tissue damage 1 cm from the tip of the laser. The amount of disk material removed with an Ho:YAG laser was determined via experiment on human cadaver spines to be 104 mg/kJ.[25] MRI correlation with histology in cadaver disks subjected to different energy pulses of Ho:YAG radiation demonstrated cavitation with end plate involvement at high pulse energies of 1 to 2 J/pulse, whereas low pulse energy of less than 1 J/pulse produced tissue modulation with end plate sparing. The overall loss of mass was determined by total

energy applied rather than pulse energy.[26] Tissue absorption and ablation of an Ho:YAG laser is limited to approximately 500 microns, which makes aggressive ablation of the disk difficult, but also reduces the likelihood of the laser contacting dura or nerve roots.

In summary, we may conclude the following from this research:

- There are different mechanisms of laser-tissue interaction at low power and high power. Low-power laser application (<20 watts) results in tissue modulation and shrinkage, whereas high power results in thermal bubble formation and tissue rupture/ablation.
- Low-energy versus high-energy application results in different responses of the disk. Low energy (<1500 J) results in an increased radial bulge and transverse disk diameter, whereas a higher energy application results in a reduction in the radial bulge, transverse diameter of the disk, and a substantially increased disk tension with a permanently altered nucleus pulposus.
- Disk ablation is influenced more by total energy than the power selected for multiple infrared lasers.
- Temperature increases do not extend more than 1 cm beyond the tip of the Nd:YAG or Ho:YAG laser and do not cause end plate damage if the tip is aimed in the center of the disk parallel to the end plates. However, with Nd:YAG lasers, high cannula temperatures may sometimes be measured, and if the laser is not moved during lasing, tissue ablation extends to 2 cm beyond the tip.
- Suction markedly increases the ablation rate.
- Ho:YAG laser ablates disk at the rate of 0.1 g/kJ disk 0.1 g of energy applied.

Live Animal Laser Research

A dog study examined the disk at several points in time after laser diskectomy and found that initially a cavity was formed, followed by growth of fibrous tissue 2 to 4 weeks later, then replacement by cartilage 12 weeks later. At no time up to 40 weeks was there any evidence of new bone formation.[27] Another dog study using a CO_2 laser demonstrated erratic amounts of nucleus pulposus ablated with 300 J of total energy and with significant damage to the end plates.[28] This implies that the CO_2 laser may not be the best choice for diskectomy. Several dog studies have been performed using Ho:YAG disk decompression prophylactically in dogs exhibiting signs of back pain, with the outcomes demonstrating good results and with relatively few complications.[29,30] One mechanism of decreased pain after laser diskectomy involves the reduction in inflammatory agents phospholipase A_2 and prostaglandin E_2,[31] which is similar to the response demonstrated with coblation nucleoplasty.

Anatomy and Pathology of Herniated Disks

The pathology of the disk herniation has been studied continuously since 1934, yet there is still much to be known about the process and initiating factors. The posterior lamellar annular layers are thinner in the posterior spine than in the anterior spine, which assists in spinal flexion and extension, but also predisposes the posterior anulus to disruption. Both trauma and internal disk derangement can lead to disk herniation, which consists of rupture of the nucleus pulposus through the anulus fibrosus. To add confusion to the picture, a disrupted outer anulus fibrosus without herniation can also be painful.[32]

The morphology of the macroscopic anulus fibrosus and the microscopic anatomy both undergo changes in disk herniation. The concavity of the disk is often reduced or inverted, whereas the cellular structure itself in the anulus fibrosus undergoes a transformation from spindle-shaped cells to rounded chondrocytes at the area of disk herniation. There are chemical changes in the wall of the herniated disks that may produce a chemical cascade from degeneration to herniation. Specifically, fibroblast growth factor–beta immunoreactivity is found in degenerative but not control disks.[33] There is a soup of inflammatory mediators that can induce neurologic symptoms of pain inside the herniated disks. These include tumor necrosis factor–alpha (TNF-α), phospholipase A$_2$, and interleukin 1–beta (IL1-β), that exist in a complex and not yet completely defined interrelationship. IL1-β induces neurologic symptoms, yet sets up a feedback loop to produce increased concentrations of cyclooxygenase-2 (induces production of inflammatory agents prostaglandin, prostacyclin, thromboxane); matrix metalloproteinase–1 (MMP1) that degrades the disk matrix, cleaves collagen type IV; dissolves the basement membrane protein fibronectin matrix metalloproteinase (MMP3) that degrades numerous extracellular matrix (ECM) substrates— including collagens III, IV, V, IX, X, and XI, laminin, elastin, entactin, fibronectin, fibrin, fibulin, link protein, osteonectin, vitronectin, and ECM proteoglycans; releases cell surface molecules such as TNF-α, EGF growth factor; and so on.[34]

Some of these agents, specifically TNF-α, are present in high concentrations in disk herniation patients,[35] but they are also present in lesser quantities in both asymptomatic juvenile and elderly disks, but not disks in middle adulthood. It has been shown that the herniated disk has the ability to disrupt the elastic capsule around the dorsal root ganglion (DRG) and permit large molecules, such as albumin, to enter the DRG within a few hours after herniation,[36] with the potential to cause endoneural edema and scarring. TNF-α has been demonstrated to have an extreme inflammatory effect on the DRG.[37] Indeed, early application of intravenous infliximab (a TNF inhibitor) has been demonstrated in human studies to produce sustained pain resolution after disk herniation.[38] Animal studies with TNF inhibitors given at the time of disk herniation demonstrate a significant reduction in damage to the DRG histologically.[39] But the TNF-α is only one of many inflammatory factors that are produced, and TNF-α does not reduce the disk herniation size, but only the inflammatory effect of TNF-α on the nerve root. Worsening of the herniation could potentially occur without depressurization of the nucleus pulposus in such situations. In a pilot study, intradiskal injection of TNF-α inhibitors into the disk did not reduce pain from disk degeneration nor did it reduce back pain associated with disk herniation. However, application of the TNF-α inhibitors on the nerve root did substantially reduce leg pain by virtually 100%.

The pathology of disk herniation is often a narrow neck of disk protruding through the annular fibers with a "mushroom" head of the nucleus pulposus compressing the nerve roots, posterior longitudinal ligament (PLL), or dura. Because the sinuvertebral nerve innervates the dura and PLL, inflammatory cytokines exuding from the exposed nucleus pulposus have the

potential to cause back pain without leg pain. Compression of the nerve root by the disk herniation often produces dermatomal numbness, dysesthesias, reflex changes, and weakness. If the nerve root is not directly mechanically compressed, there may be radicular pain from the inflammatory response of the DRG to the chemicals and enzymes from the nucleus pulposus, but without the other signs of a radiculopathy. Those with neurologic deficits demonstrated a 500% increase in blood flow after diskectomy compared to those who did not have neurologic deficits.[40] This suggests that the mechanism of neurologic deficit is partially related to vascular ischemia from compression of the nerve root. Rat studies demonstrate that application of herniated nucleus pulposus placed proximal to the DRG develops a significant decrease in blood flow compared to the control group that had muscle placed proximal to the DRG.[41] This suggests that an inflammatory response with nerve root edema is at least partially responsible for the neurologic symptoms. It has also been shown that human patients with disk herniation exhibit a marked reduction in the gliding motion of the nerve root during intra-operative straight leg raising tests with an associated significant decrease in nerve root blood flow.[42] After decompression, there is improvement in both the gliding motion and in the blood flow to the nerve.

The predisposing factors have been examined for disk herniation both in humans and in cadaver models. It appears that the sequence begins peripherally with tears in the outer anulus, which is predisposed to disruption from repeated loads plus bending and twisting.[43] A strong familial predisposition in juvenile disk herniation, with an odds ratio of 5.61, suggests that a genetic influence may be operant.[44]

Anatomic considerations for laser disk decompression include patient size, location of the disk herniation, neuroforaminal size, presence of furcal nerves, presence of an overlying annular inflammatory membrane, disk height, anatomic impediments to access (osteophytes in the neuroforamen, iliac crest morphology), and applicability to the technique selected. Using the standard foraminal posterolateral approach, the morbidly obese patient presents anatomic limitations to treatment of disk herniations. The straight anteroposterior skin-to-disk measurement may be 15 cm or more. Using a 45-degree angled insertion of a needle for laser access in a standard extrapedicular approach (as used in diskography) would require a needle length of 21 cm or more (>8 inches). Therefore depending on the access needles or cannulas available and the length of the laser wand, obese patients may not be candidates for laser diskectomy. Disk herniation location is less likely to be a significant determinant of success when most laser disk decompression techniques (intradiskal) are used. But some systems such as the Wolf YESS system use lasers to enlarge the cavity directly beneath the disk herniation with subsequent intradiskal removal of the herniation with mechanical articulating tools. A small neuroforaman predisposes to injury during disk access with large needles because of the exiting nerve root being displaced inferiorly in the neuroforamen. The safe triangle for disk access is smaller when there is significant apical foraminal impingement. The presence of osteophytes also causes some difficulties when there is zygapophyseal hypertrophy or vertebral body osteochondrosis. A calcified anulus fibrosus also causes some difficulty with disk access. The presence of a high iliac crest poses significant problems with rigid cannula or needle systems at L5-S1 because the trajectory of the disk entry will predispose to damage to the superior S1 end plate, in addition to posing problems when nonflexible instruments or lasers are used through the cannula. Curved needle systems may be advantageous in accessing the L5-S1 disk for laser decompression. A transiliac approach has been possible in cadavers,[45] but this requires drilling holes through the ilium for access. Furcal nerves are accessory nerves present in approximately 15% of the population,[46] and are found primarily at L4-5 93% of the time.[47] They traverse the foramen quite laterally, have their own separate DRG, and then exit with the L5 nerve root. Compression of the furcal nerves with a lateral disk herniation can cause both L4 and L5 symptoms. The nerves are primarily sensory nerves and, because of their anatomic location, can be injured by a needle placed across the neuroforamen into the disk. Inflammatory membranes have been described clinically by Tony Yeung during endoscopic diskectomy as a beefy red, angry membrane over the surface of the anulus fibrosus. These membranes are exquisitely sensitive to pressure, which may make posterolateral needle placement quite painful. However, they are an infrequent finding in disk herniations.

Techniques of Laser Disk Decompression

Different techniques of laser disk decompression are available, some of which have elaborate systems of instrumentation. The basic approach to all laser disk decompression is through placement of a needle or cannula via a posterior-lateral transforaminal entry into the intervertebral disk. Once the needle or cannula has entered the inner annular fibers, a laser is advanced into the disk and activated to decompress the nucleus pulposus. This may be achieved with fluoroscopic guidance, rigid endoscopic guidance, or flexible endoscopic guidance. The laser tip may be a rigid end-firing laser wand, a rigid side-firing laser wand, or a fiberoptic waveguide laser tip (polished or cross-cut). Laser choices include Ho:YAG, Nd:YAG (two wavelengths), KTP, Er:YAG, multidiode, and tunable diode. Generally, an Ho:YAG laser is preferred, although the new multidiode laser is much less expensive. After laser disk decompression, generally the needle is withdrawn, but the cannula often remains for further mechanical dissection of the disk using long instrumentation through an endoscope.

Stepwise Laser Disk Decompression

Access to the intervertebral disk is achieved by horizontal fluoroscopy beam through the intervertebral disk, and then a standard posterolateral approach is used with a needle placed onto the lateral border of the superior articular process (**Fig. 183.5**). Because the safe zone for needle placement is much larger at the superior end plate of the lower disk, it is strongly preferred to take an approach that will bring the needle tip low in the intervertebral disk. One study revealed the tolerances for error may be much less than previously thought[48]; therefore it is prudent to avoid needle placement in the mid to upper disk. The angle chosen for needle entry partially depends on the location of the disk herniation and the importance in targeting the exact area. Greater than 55 degrees oblique from the sagittal plane can cause bowel injury or dural entry. Too shallow an angle places the laser too far anterior in the disk. Therefore, if anatomically possible, the needle angle chosen is

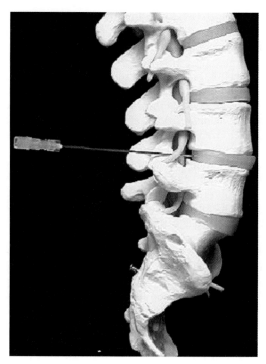

Fig. 183.5 Stepwise laser disk decompression.

usually between 40 and 55 degrees in the lumbar spine or 30 to 40 degrees in the upper lumbar and thoracic spine. Although cervical endoscopic systems do exist, the entry is at the anterior right side at approximately 20 to 30 degrees to the sagittal plane.

Laser Diskectomy Techniques

LASE System

The LASE disk access needle system consists of a straight (2.8 mm, 12 gauge) and curved needle (3.0 mm for L5-S1) (**Fig. 183.6**). The needle is inserted into the safe zone as described earlier. When the disk is contacted, a small trephine may be placed through the needle to assist with annulotomy. If the angle of the straight needle placed at L5-S1 is too acute to the sagittal plane (15 to 30 degrees), the straight needle will have its final placement too far lateral in the disk. In such cases, the beam is angled more cephalad (no longer in a direct plane with the disk) and then more lateral oblique to permit use of the 3.0 mm curved cannula. The curved cannula is advanced over the superior iliac crest; then a steep inferior angle is selected to guide the needle tip to the lateral-anterior border of the superior articular process (SAP) of S1. The needle is subsequently advanced over the trephine into the inner annular fibers and a needle-stop set screw is tightened to fix the maximum needle ingress. With the 1.7 mm diameter endoscope connected to a light source and camera (preferably CCD 3 chip), white balancing is performed. Rotor pump pressurized irrigation is turned on with an irrigant of normal saline or normal saline mixed with bacitracin 50,000 U per 3 L is infused through the irrigation port of the wand.

An Ho:YAG laser fiber (400 microns) is inserted through the flexible scope and locked into place with the tip of the fiber protruding 1 mm beyond the end of the laser. The wand is

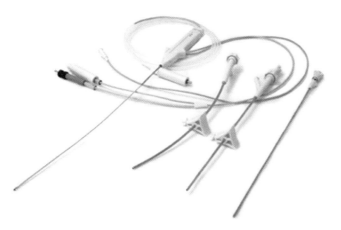

Fig. 183.6 LASE endoscope and access needles.

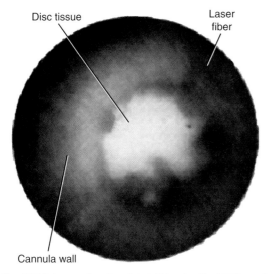

Fig. 183.7 Approach to herniated disk using the LASE wand.

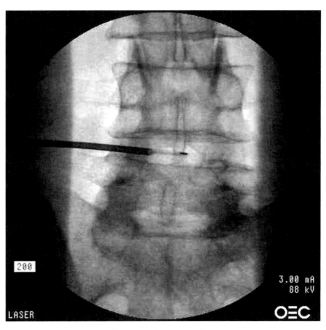

Fig. 183.8 Fluoroscopic view with LASE system.

inserted through the LASE needle until white disk material is seen. Grasping forceps or pituitary forceps are used to remove disk material in the needle and at the tip of the needle in order to advance the LASE wand just beyond the tip. It is prudent not to fire the laser inside the needle because of the potential for flashback and thermal damage to the LASE wand. The LASE wand is slowly advanced across the disk and may be curved into an area immediately anterior to the disk herniation if desired owing to the flexible guidable endoscope feature (**Fig. 183.7**).

Fluoroscopic and endoscopic guidance are used simultaneously for confirmation of intra–nucleus pulposus placement. Typically about 10,000 to 15,000 J per disk is delivered with a double-pulsed setting of 20 W. The optics of the fiberoptic scope produce modestly good visualization of tissues, and one can usually discern differences in the nucleus pulposus versus anulus fibrosus. If there is insufficient irrigation, too high a power setting (>20 W), inadequate outflow of the irrigation, or excessive lasing in one location without laser tip movement (**Fig. 183.8**), carbonization will occur and the disk tissues will become blackened; visualization will degrade with blackened fragments floating in the field of view.

It is preferred to lase for 5 seconds on, then 5 seconds off because during lasing, the cavitation obscures the optical resolution of the tissues being lased. If the tip approaches the end plate, a bright flashback can occur with reflection of the laser beam off the bone and back through the waveguide toward the laser source. This can damage the end plate (very undesirable) and potentially the laser itself if there is inadequate flashback protection built into the laser. Typically one to two disks may be treated with a single laser wand. The optics of the fiberoptic system can degrade with extended use and the tip of the laser fiber itself may degrade. If the laser fiber is not polished, it is possible to cut the laser fiber back with a special laser fiber knife and resume the LASE procedure.

After termination of the procedure, the laser wand and needles are withdrawn with local anesthetic injected in the needle track outside the neuroforamen. It is not desirable to inject local anesthesia near the DRG or exiting nerve root because if there exists a rare neurologic deficit after the termination of the procedure, the effect of the local anesthetic could muddle the diagnosis and result in significant diagnostic delay.

Nonendoscopic Laser Fiber Diskectomy (Modified Choy Technique)

The original Choy procedure used lateral decubitus patient positioning and did not employ targeting the safe operating zone of the neuroforamen. Choy used a fixed 10-cm lateral entry from the midline and an initial 45-degree angulation. Of course, in obese patients a fixed distance from the midline skin needle entry will result in a trajectory that is less than 45 degrees to the sagittal plane and potential entry into the disk at the site of exiting nerve root owing to deflection of the needle by the SAP. Very thin patients have the opposite issue with a fixed needle skin entry site and it may result in excessively posterior needle placement if the SAP is targeted and potential pithing of the exiting nerve root if a 45-degree entry angle is selected. Therefore the technique has been modified to use the standard precision "down the barrel" pain medicine method.

With the patient in the prone position, for central disk targeting the fluoroscopy beam is used to provide a horizontal trajectory across the end plates; then the beam is rotated obliquely approximately 45 degrees at L3-4 and L4-5 and 35 to 40 degrees at L1-2 and L2-3. The angle at L5-S1 is as far oblique as possible until the iliac crest overrides the superior articular process. At each level the lateral-inferior border of the SAP is targeted at the junction between the superior end plate and the disk. An aliquot of local anesthetic is infiltrated in the skin at the selected entry site, and then a 6-inch spinal needle is passed in the selected trajectory to, but not beyond, the SAP, during which time local anesthetic is infiltrated. A 20 cm, 18-gauge needle is subsequently advanced in the anesthetized track and the SAP is contacted. On advancement across the neuroforamen (*slowly*), the patient may experience some intense back pain but should not experience any radicular pain. Repositioning is necessary if there is radicular pain, which can be due to a hypersensitized DRG, furcal nerve contact, or overt contact with a displaced exiting nerve root. When annular cannulation has occurred, the end point of needle advancement is on anterior-posterior projection, halfway between the lateral border of the spinous process and the medial border of the pedicle. On lateral fluoroscopic projection, the needle tip should reside at the junction of the posterior quarter of the disk with the anterior three quarters. An Nd:YAG fiber is inserted through the needle to the tip and 1cm beyond. The needle is subsequently not moved. Lesioning at 20 W with 5 seconds between 1-second pulses is used. If a flashback is observed, the laser tip is retracted and inspected for damage. If the tip is damaged, the tip is cut and the laser reinserted. The total energy applied is 1000 J or up to 1500 J if the patient is greater than 165 cm in height. (Note: The energy used with this technique incorporating an Nd:YAG laser is only one tenth of that required with the Ho:YAG laser.) If the disks have a narrowed height, the amount of energy applied is reduced by 25%. During lasing, the patient should alert the physician of any new radicular pain. (Note: This method is completely blind and is incapable of guiding the laser tip. It also does not employ any aqueous irrigation, which can lead to charring and end plate damage. However, numerous publications attest to the safety of this procedure.)

An alternative laser source is an Ho:YAG fiber or multidiode laser, but the same limitations apply. With an Nd:YAG laser, the lesion produced is 2 cm long and 6 mm wide (**Figs. 183.9** and **183.10**).

An Ho:YAG laser produces a much smaller lesion in the disk tissue unless the laser fiber is moved; this system is not desirable because of potential laser fiber fracture within the disk.

Rigid-Scope Endoscopic Laser Diskectomy

This technique of endoscopic laser diskectomy uses a rigid scope in contrast to the LASE (flexible, steerable fiberoptic scope). The optics and visualization are much better than the fiberoptic scope and the working channels in the scope permit introduction of dissection and probing instruments. The two systems used in pain medicine are the PercScope by Clarus and the YESS scope by Wolf. The PercScope uses a 30,000-pixel fiberoptic bundle housed in a 5.2 mm rigid scope housing and

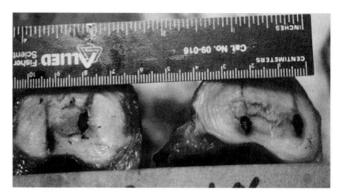

Fig. 183.9 Laser tracts formed in nucleus pulposus by 1000 J of laser energy at 1.32 µm on the left and a 1.06 µm Nd:YAG laser on the right. *(From Choy DSJ: Percutaneous laser disc decompression: history and scientific rationale,* Techniques Reg Anesth Pain Manage *9[1]:50–55, 2005.)*

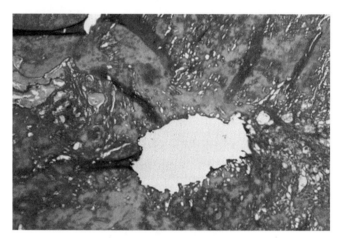

Fig. 183.10 Histologic appearance of a laser tract in the nucleus pulposus. There is a central hole surrounded by a zone of protein denaturation and then vacuoles, which are probably steam pockets. *(From Choy DSJ: Percutaneous laser disc decompression: history and scientific rationale,* Techniques Reg Anesth Pain Manage *9[1]:50–55, 2005.)*

contains a large 3.1 mm working channel. This size of working channel will permit the introduction of a variety of instruments, as depicted subsequently, that permit laser-assisted dissection. The lasers may be either a nonsteerable bare fiber, fiberoptic steerable laser, or rigid laser housing for side-firing or end-firing laser output. The Wolf system uses a 7-mm outer diameter (OD) cannula for a 6 mm OD scope. The working channel is 2.7 mm, but there are several irrigation ports. The optical system uses a rigid rod system with crystal-clear nonpixelated viewing. There is a European scope with a much larger working channel (**Fig. 183.11**), up to 4 mm, that will permit introduction of large dissection instruments and automated rotating dissectors and burrs.

Fundamentally, both systems incorporate the same basic technique of disk access and dissection. The cannula systems are so large that primary introduction is not possible without a guidewire (**Fig. 183.12**). An initial posterolateral placement of an intradiskal needle is the first step. When the disk has been entered, an injection of indigo carmine blue/iodinated

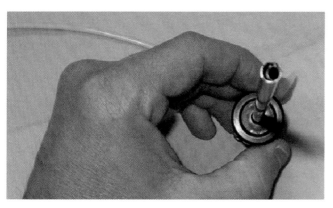

Fig. 183.11 PercScope working channel.

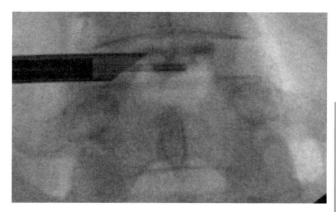

Fig. 183.13 Laser through YESS endoscope.

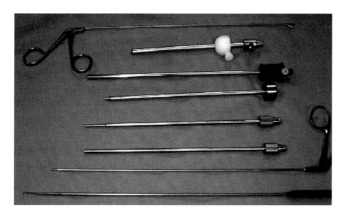

Fig. 183.12 PercScope access cannulas and surgical instruments.

contrast is rendered into the nucleus pulposus. Indigo carmine has been shown to selectively stain the degenerative/herniated parts of intervertebral disks blue.[49] A guidewire is then inserted through the needle, and the needle is removed. Next, a dilator is placed over the guidewire under fluoroscopic guidance to avert bending the guidewire. A cannula is placed over the dilator which is advanced to the external anulus fibrosus. With the cannula held in place, the external anulus is probed with the dilator for underlying nerve roots. If none are discovered, the dilator is removed and the cannula is held firmly in place; a trephine or annulotome is advanced to the anulus. If the trephine is used, the cannula is simply advanced into the intervertebral disk. However, if the annulotome is used, the dilator is replaced through the cruciate incision of the anulus, and subsequently is advanced into the nucleus pulposus. The cannula is then slid off the dilator into the nucleus pulposus. Following removal of the dilator, the endoscope is inserted with continuous saline or bacitracin containing saline irrigation flowing into the nucleus pulposus. Pituitary forceps are inserted through the endoscope to clear disk tissue from the end of the cannula. The blue-stained material is targeted with the forceps and then the laser, as this represents the herniated and severely degenerative portion of the disk (**Fig. 183.13**). An end-firing or side-firing laser wand may be placed through the working channel, and the Ho:YAG laser at 20 to 40 W is used to clear the area under the disk herniation. The usual laser energy applied is between 5000 and 25,000 J. A side-firing laser has a mirror placed at a 45-degree angle near the tip of the scope,

deflecting the laser at right angles to the wand. This has several advantages, including that a more posterior laser diskectomy may be performed. Care must be taken not to excessively weaken the posterior anulus fibrosus by firing the laser in one location onto the anulus. With the PercScope system, the procedure is terminated at this point, whereas with the Wolf system, the laser dissection is usually followed by an aggressive articulating forceps used to grasp the neck of the herniation, pulling the hernia back inside the disk and out through the cannula. At the termination of the procedure, the cannula is removed and the patient may receive steroids along the nerve root to help control postoperative periradicular edema.

Nonlumbar Systems

The cervical and thoracic areas can be approached with a laser technique for diskectomy. The lower three thoracic disks can often be accessed inferior to the transverse process, whereas the mid and upper thoracic levels may require obtuse angulations. The LASE system is ideal for these applications. Cervical diskectomy may be performed with a special cervical LASE system or a 2.5-mm cannulated system such as a Blackstone or other access system. Usually the cervical disk is approached very much like cervical diskography, except extreme care must be used in the anterior cervical spine owing to the carotid and jugular systems being in the line of the needle trajectory. It is suggested that cervical diskectomy not be performed unless the physician has immense experience with both lumbar and thoracic diskectomy and with cervical diskography.

Outcome Studies

Ho:YAG

Using 1500 J energy at 15 watts through an 18-gauge needle, one group had a 91% successful outcome rate at 18 months' follow-up.[50] Using a laser-assisted disk decompression with a side-firing laser placed through an endoscope, success was achieved on 1 year's follow-up at a 90% level[51] and at 87% at 2 years' follow-up.[52]

Nd:YAG

The results for nonendoscopic lumbar disk decompression with an Nd:YAG laser are variable, but generally range from 70% to 90% good to excellent results. A 4-year follow-up study of 200 patients with Nd:YAG 1064 nm nonendoscopic laser diskectomy produced a 74% success rate.[53] Another study used nonendoscopic Nd:YAG diskectomy in 42 patients with *thoracic* disk extrusions and protrusions, with improvement in all clinical parameters in 41 of the 42 patients.[54] Choy's experience with 389 patients using a nonendoscopic laser diskectomy with the Nd:YAG laser demonstrated a 75% success rate according to good and excellent results by the modified MacNab criteria,[55] although in his book *Percutaneous Laser Disc Decompression* he states the success rate in later cases rose to 89%.

Complications

Generally the complication rate for laser diskectomy is relatively low, around 1%. The specific complication profile for cervical, thoracic, and lumbar diskectomy are different, because of anatomic considerations, and are listed in **Table 183.1**.

Most complications are relatively mild and involve transient increases in pain caused by prone patient positioning when the patient may not have assumed that position in years, muscle spasm from the needle/cannula, and subcutaneous or intramuscular hematomas. However, on rare occasions serious complications will occur. This author has had one case of a Brown Séquard syndrome when an access cannula displaced a protruding disk herniation fragment into the cervical spinal cord, with only partial long-term neurologic recovery. Poor patient selection can lead to severe complications such as cauda equina syndrome in very rare cases.[56]

When larger cannulas are used to access the disk, a finite percentage (about 5% to 7%) will develop a transient complex regional pain syndrome type II (CRPS II) syndrome,[57] but this does not seem to occur as frequently with a needle access system. Both osteomyelitis and diskitis have been reported after laser diskectomy,[58,59] although these are rare, and most are aseptic. It is highly probable that most instances of aseptic diskitis are caused by over-reading postoperative MRI scans or mistaking end plate laser damage for diskitis. The potential for long-term disk degeneration acceleration is a very real concern when using the larger cannulas for disk access because the sheep model for long-term degeneration is coring the anulus fibrosus The use of slit lesions with a 2.5-mm device caused much less disk degeneration and instability than did the use of a box window excision of the disk,[60] which implies that if the larger cannulae are to be used, they should be preceded by an annulotome incision. Excessive removal of disk is also potentially deleterious owing to the removal of the central nucleus pulposus support with a biomechanical weight transfer to the anulus fibrosus. The anulus is not designed to hold significant weight and undergoes progressive collapse with annular bulging.

Another significant concern is the damage to the end plates that are the nutrient conduits to the avascular nucleus pulposus. The cartilaginous end plates gradually become sclerotic with subchondral bone formation because there is increased force affecting the trabecular bone when the disk is no longer serving as a hydraulic shock absorber. Additionally, Ito has demonstrated a direct correlation between calcification of the nutrient canaliculi and MRI grade of disk degeneration.[61] Adams et al[62] demonstrated that even minor damage to the vertebral end plates may lead to progressive structural changes in the adjacent disk. One study demonstrated that after endoscopic laser diskectomy, subchondral marrow abnormalities were identified in 41 of 109 patients. However, in a subset of patients examined 5 to 7 years after laser diskectomy, both back pain and marrow abnormalities improved on MRI.[63] The nature of such subchondral osteonecrosis was examined on MRI imaging and was found to include a wedge-shaped area of low signal intensity on T1 images, of high and low signal intensity on T2-weighted images, and of gadolinium-enhanced high signal intensity on T2-weighted images, respectively. The speculative causes of such changes were thought to include thermal energy and photoacoustic shock.[64] An experimental animal model of Nd:YAG laser injury to the end plates revealed an early decrease in vascularization at 1 month after laser application; however, by 2 months after laser application, the vascularization of the end plate had effectively doubled.[65] Using an experimental guinea pig model with a carbon dioxide laser fired at the end plates, as little as 300 J of energy was required to damage the end plates.[66] However, it was demonstrated by Hoogland[67] that curettage of the end plates of severely degenerative disks may later reverse some of the MRI changes of disk degeneration, including that of disk

---

Table 183.1 Potential Complications of Laser Diskectomy

	Cervical Complications	Thoracic Complications	Lumbar Complications
Disk access complications	Perforation of carotid, jugular, thyroid, esophagus, trachea	Pneumothorax, cord or nerve root penetration, chylothorax, hemothorax, CSF leak	CSF leak, nerve root injury, bowel penetration, epidural hematoma, epidural abscess, cord injury (above L2)
Laser/needle complications	Needle perforation of the end plates, cord with Brown Séquard syndrome, nerve root penetration, diskitis, CSF leak, PLL destruction, lasing the cord or nerve roots, late disk space collapse or degeneration, pseudodiskitis, epidural hematoma from lasing of epidural vessels	Lasing the cord, nerve root thermal injury, aortic/caval injury, diskitis, epidural hematoma, epidural abscess, end plate damage/pseudodiskitis	Iliac penetration, sympathetic chain injury, end plate damage/pseudodiskitis, diskitis, bowel injury, genitofemoral nerve injury, late disk degeneration, disk space collapse with increased disk bulge

CSF, cerebrospinal fluid; PLL, posterior longitudinal ligament.

desiccation. The latter finding, however, was based on limited clinical evidence; therefore the modus operandi at this juncture would invoke end plate preservation.

Conclusion

Laser diskectomy is an alternative to open or microdiskectomy for selected patients at a small fraction of the cost. Least expensive is the Choy technique, but it has the theoretical disadvantage of increased risk of end plate damage because the laser fiber angle cannot be controlled when the laser waveguide is inserted through the needle. Although the other techniques are more expensive, they provide steerability of the laser, which is useful in avoiding the end plates. The Nd:YAG laser is much more aggressive than the Ho:YAG; therefore tissue ablation will occur at a much more rapid rate. The advantage of the Ho:YAG is the safety imparted through a 500-micron controlled tissue penetration, especially when operating in a continuously irrigated field.

The major barriers to more widespread use of laser disk decompression include high cost of a laser ($50,000 to $180,000); reluctance of hospital medical staff to open laser use to pain medicine because of infrequent use by the specialty; equipment costs (endoscopes, light sources, cannula systems, video system, and flexible laser wands); lack of double-blind controlled studies; alternative, more simple solutions (coblation nucleoplasty, disk decompression); and global skill level deficits of most pain physicians in endoscopy of the spine. However, most hospitals and some surgery centers have acquired lasers (e.g., Ho:YAG lasers are often used to perform laser lithotripsy of kidney stones) and already own the video towers and cameras necessary to perform video procedures. PLDD is effective 75% to 90% of the time in selected patients at a fraction of the cost of microdiskectomy or open diskectomy.

References

Full references for this chapter can be found on www.expertconsult.com.

Percutaneous Fusion Techniques

David Petersen

Background

The TruFUSE (facet joint spinal stabilization or fusion) procedure represents a new, more biologic way of performing an established technique that has been part of the gold standard for posterior spinal fusion for many decades. In the past, the facet joints were either drilled or burred and packed with unstable chips of bone, allowing them to continue to grind until fusion occurs, causing the patient pain during recovery and allowing for the joint to settle with possibly more foraminal stenosis. Now a precision, "press-fit," stable grafting of the joint can be accomplished, relieving the patient's mechanical back pain very rapidly by separating the arthritic joint surfaces and stabilizing them immediately with a Morse tapered dowel without instrumentation and the risks/recovery and long-term issues associated with hardware (**Fig. 184.1**). The joint can also be theoretically reduced and held there for a more anatomic fusion (**Fig. 184.2**). The concept of facet angle or tropism (**Fig. 184.3**) becomes important in preoperative planning to assist in determining the opening angle for fluoroscopy and to see if there may be obstructions to graft placement (**Fig. 184.4**).

Indications

The indications for facet fusion (TruFUSE) are generally the same as those for any posterior fusion method. It is another way to perform a posterior fusion, when instrumentation is not needed. As a standalone procedure it is used for facet arthropathy or intractable mechanical low back pain unresponsive to nonoperative measures. It is often used as an adjunct after laminectomy/decompression, or with microinstability (less than 2 mm motion on lateral flexion/extension films), or after anterior spinal fusion to supplement a 360-degree fusion (posterior lumbar interbody fusion, anterior lumbar interbody fusion, extreme lateral interbody fusion, or on the contralateral side of a transforaminal lumbar interbody fusion). It has been used with several of the spinous process distraction devices (X-Stop, Aspen, and Spire plates) to fuse the decompressed level in a distracted position. It is

very useful for revision surgery to fuse an adjacent segment to avoid redoing large, old fusion constructs with additional hardware or in some cases of pseudoarthrosis (**Fig. 184.5**). Patients suffering from facet joint arthropathy whose pain is temporarily relieved with intra-articular facet joint injections and/or radiofrequency ablation procedures but in whom pain relief is not long lasting are also good candidates for TruFUSE.

Rigid constructs in spine surgery are essential for deformity correction (scoliosis), tumors (segmental loss), gross instability, and fractures and in some cases of spondylolisthesis. It makes a great deal of biologic sense to use the TruFUSE technique within rod/screw constructs to act as bleeding surface with reamed

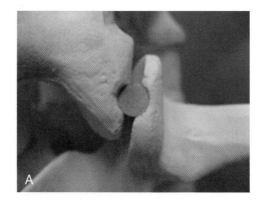

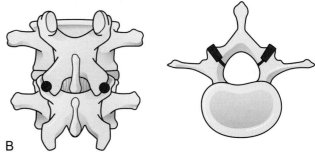

Fig. 184.1 A, Proper graft placement within the facet joint. B, Schematic drawing of proper graft placement within the facet joint.

compacted autograft and a stable allograft dowel spanning the facet joint for primary bony healing to occur across rigidly fixed segments. This is preferable to placing stress-shielded graft in the posterior lateral gutter on non–weight-bearing structures and hoping that structurally sound bone will form.

This technique does not burn bridges and allows for conversion to rod/screw stabilization surgeries without additional risk or surgical times should the patient's symptoms recur or progress following the TruFUSE posterior facet joint spinal fusion. The bone graft is a precision-cut Morse tapered allograft dowel placed into an undersized Morse tapered, press-fit, compaction reamed tunnel into the middle one third of the facet joint (**Figs. 184.6** and **184.7**).

Anatomy

Facet joints are synovial joints. They possess a joint capsule, are lined with synovium, and contain joint fluid. They are formed by the articulations of the superior and inferior

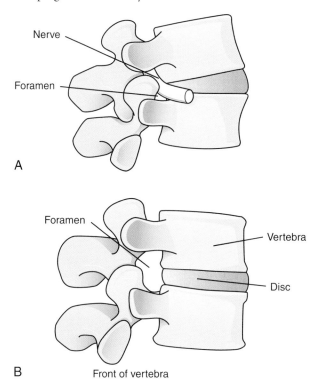

A

B

Front of vertebra

Fig. 184.2 A, Displaced degenerative facet joint. B, Reduced facet joint demonstrating positional or indirect decompression.

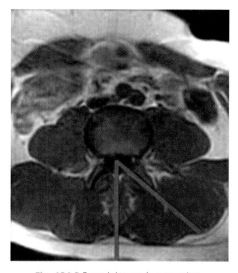

Fig. 184.3 Facet joint angle or tropism.

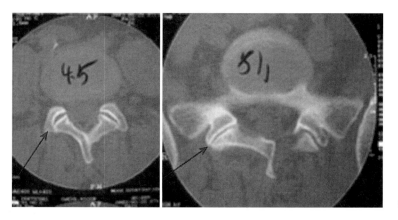

Fig. 184.4 Preoperative planning—facet approach difficulties.

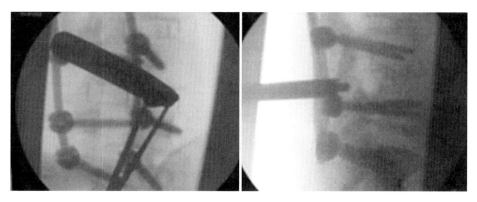

Fig. 184.5 Pseudoarthrosis—hardware "workaround."

articular processes of adjacent vertebrae. The joint capsule is richly innervated and frequently acts as a pain generator. Cervical and lumbar facet joints are more susceptible than thoracic facet joints to arthritic changes and trauma secondary to a wide variety of mechanisms. Regardless of the mechanism, damage to facet joints can result in pain secondary to synovial joint inflammation and ultimately degeneration as a final pathway (**Fig. 184.8**). Each facet joint receives innervation from up to three spinal levels. Each joint receives fibers from the dorsal ramus at the same level as the vertebra, as well as fibers from the dorsal ramus of the vertebrae above it. This is why facet-mediated pain can be difficult to localize and explains why the nerve from the level above the offending level must also be blocked, when an extra-articular block is performed, in order to provide complete pain relief, which is not the case if an intra-articular injection is performed for at least diagnostic purposes. Occasionally, a patient may experience long-lasting relief from an intra-articular injection because the inflammatory effect from the synovium decreases, at least for a time.

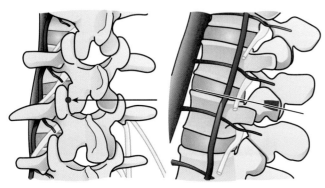

Fig. 184.6 Anatomic graft placement within the facet joint.

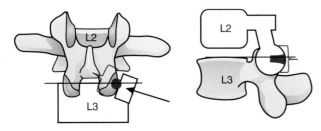

Fig. 184.7 Schematic of graft placement within the facet joint.

Technique

After the patient receives an appropriate level of anesthesia/sedation (and/or local anesthetic), the patient is placed in the prone position on a fluoroscopy table. Most patients are given prophylactic antibiotics preoperatively per routine. Longitudinal rolls or a Wilson frame (which can be adjusted for lumbar flexion with the patient prone on the frame) is placed on the fluoroscopy table before the patient. Any commonly available spine surgery adjustable fluoroscopic table will work equally well. The lumbar spine is flexed to reestablish facet joint height lost during the degenerative process. This also helps to reopen the foramina and pull the superior articular process back out of the foramina, termed *indirect decompression* (see Fig. 184.2). Alternatively, a small incision can be made over the spinous processes and a lamina spreader can be used to open the foramina during the procedure and then the lamina spreader can be removed before wound closure. The facet joint(s) to be fused are next identified on an anteroposterior (AP), lateral, and oblique fluoroscopic view, before setting up a sterile field, to be sure that adequate visualization is possible. After the patient is prepped and draped in a standard sterile fashion, a true AP x-ray view is obtained at the level to be fused. Next, the superior end plate is "flattened" by angling the fluoroscope either caudally or cranially, and then gradually increasing the oblique angle of the fluoroscope until the opening angle has been maximized. The opening angle should be measured preoperatively with either a magnetic resonance imaging (MRI) scan (coronal section) or more ideally a computed tomography (CT) scan with thin slices through the facet joint, not only to predetermine the facet angle but also to look for obstructive osteophytes and to help decide if the patient is a candidate for the procedure (see Figs. 184.3 and 184.4). Finally, the point at which the superior end plate intersects with the middle one third of the open facet joint will serve as the target (+) for the spinal needle or Steinmann pin (see Figs. 184.6 and 184.7). This approach will increase your accuracy in graft placement into the middle one third or "sweet spot" of the facet joint and will reduce the risk of nerve root injury since the nerve root will be at the top of the foramina and if the pin goes in too deep the pin will pass through the bottom of the foramina well out of the way of the exiting nerve root. After the target has been identified, a spinal needle or the Steinmann pin is then passed down through the soft tissues and into the opening of the facet joint. If a spinal needle is used, it will then need to be changed out for the Steinmann pin (**Figs. 184.9** and **184.10**).

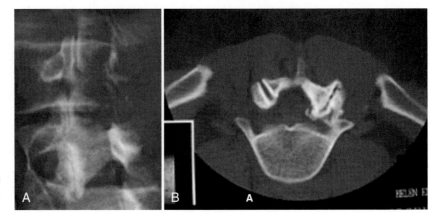

Fig. 184.8 **A,** Oblique x-ray. **B,** Computed tomography scan view of a degenerative facet joint, severe facet arthropathy.

The pin should appear as a dot on the x-ray image before it is hammered into the facet joint and fully seated (**Fig. 184.11**). The pin is then tapped with the hammer lightly into the middle one third of the facet joint approximately 1 cm until it stops when it contacts the superior articular process. The pin will slightly distract the facet joint and will confirm you are in the joint. A lateral x-ray view is checked to be sure you are not too deep, the pin should bottom out posterior to the foramina, and the pin should be directed toward the superior end plate. Following this, the contralateral pin is placed in a similar fashion. Next, a small (Wiltse approach) incision is made through the skin and subcutaneous tissues in a longitudinal fashion to free the pin up from the skin and subcutaneous tissues to allow the rest of the instruments clear passage into the

joint. The cannulated spatula is then placed over the pin and twisted over the pin repeatedly clockwise and counterclockwise (approximately 180 degrees) to gently pass the instrument thru the soft tissue and fascia down to the joint (**Fig. 184.12**). Once it is confirmed on the lateral x-ray view to be at the level of the joint, the vertical lines on the spatula are oriented in line with the facet joint plane and the blade of the spatula is advanced by impacting it slowly into the joint approximately 1 cm. Be careful not to loosen or move the pin while advancing the spatula; the pin is your guidewire at this point.

After satisfactory placement of the spatulas bilaterally (confirmed radiographically) the drill guide is placed over the spatula on one side (**Fig. 184.13**). While holding the spatula firmly with one hand to stabilize it as you would a

Video: Percutaneous technique

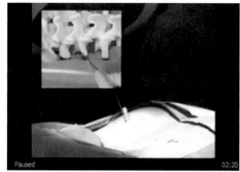

Fig. 184.9 Spinal needle is replaced by the Steinmann pin.

Video: Percutaneous technique

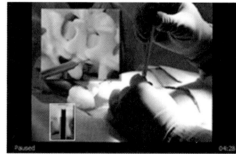

Fig. 184.12 Spatula slowly twisted over the pin through the fascia.

Video: Percutaneous technique

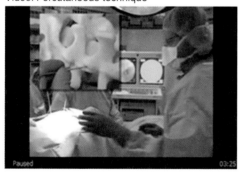

Fig. 184.10 Steinmann pin placement within the facet joint.

Video: Percutaneous technique

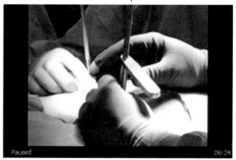

Fig. 184.13 Drill guide is inserted unilaterally.

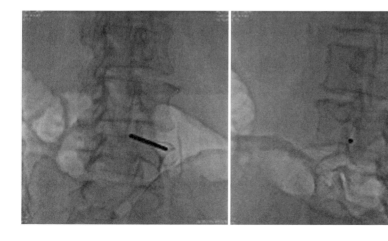

Fig. 184.11 Proper pin placement. The pin will appear as a dot in the center one third of the facet joint.

guidewire, the drill guide is rotated down through the skin, subcutaneous tissues, and fascia in a similar 360-degree clockwise and then a 360-degree counterclockwise fashion repeatedly until it gets down to the first horizontal line on the spatula (**Fig. 184.14A**). (This is similar to a warning track at a baseball field to warn the fielder that the wall is coming soon.)

Advancing the drill guide replaces the spatula with the teeth to maintain the joint separation. Now that the first line is visible, only rotate the drill guide 30 to 40 degrees back and forth (with the drill guide's handle nearly perpendicular to the patient's body) until the second line appears on the spatula (**Fig. 184.14B**), and then stop rotating the drill guide.

The lines on the top of the drill guide must be aligned with the vertical lines on the shaft of the spatula to ensure proper intra-articular placement of the drill guide teeth (**Fig. 184.15**).

Stabilize the drill guide at the patient's skin with your non-dominant hand and hold a firm downward pressure on the drill guide for the rest of the procedure, maintaining the angle of the guide during the drilling and graft placement. Now hammer the drill guide, next to the spatula (**Fig. 184.16**), down into the joint to fully seat the drill guide's teeth; stop when the third horizontal line becomes visible (**Fig. 184.14C**).

Do not release the downward pressure on the drill guide from your hand until you are completely done hammering the allograft bone into place in the joint. The Steinmann pin and spatula are then removed while maintaining the downward pressure on the drill guide with your hand. The reaming/drilling is carried out with short 2-second bursts so that the chips of the subchondral bone that are created and impacted into the facet joint are not burned. This may cause osteonecrosis, which will compromise your fusion results.

The reaming/drilling is continued until the drill has been advanced to the stop, which is in contact on the top of the drill guide (**Fig. 184.17**), a distance of 1 cm. This allows the posterior portion of the facet allograft to be countersunk approximately 2 mm below the posterior surface of the facet joint. Once the drill bit has bottomed out to the drill guide stop, ream another 2 to 3 seconds to help create a good bleeding surface on each side of the facet joint before dowel placement (the drill bit

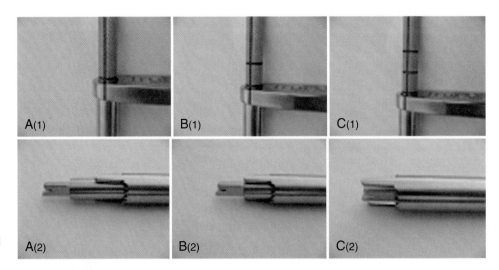

Fig. 184.14 A, First line. B, Second line. C, Third line.

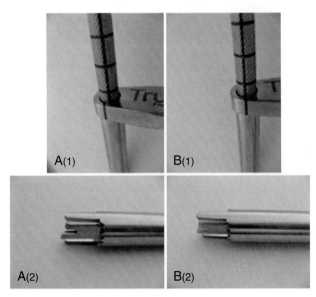

Fig. 184.15 Lining up the vertical lines of the drill guide and the spatula.

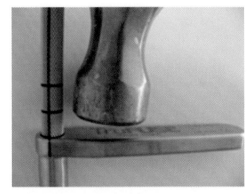

Fig. 184.16 Impacting the drill guide, close to the spatula, down into the facet joint.

has side-cutting teeth). After reaming/drilling has been completed, the TruFUSE facet fusion allograft dowel is placed into the graft holder block to ensure the graft is properly oriented so the smaller end will go into the compacted tunnel first and ensure a solid press-fit. It is then loaded into the insertion device. The TruFUSE facet fusion allograft dowel in the holder is placed down into the drill guide and then impacted into the facet joint with the impactor (**Fig. 184.18**).

When the graft is fully seated into the tunnel and countersunk 2 mm, the drill guide is carefully removed from the joint by pulling it straight out of the joint so the allograft is not dislodged by the drill guide's teeth. The same procedure is then followed for the contralateral side. The wounds are closed in layers and sterile dressings are applied. The patient is then placed in a back brace to limit flexion, extension, and lateral bending for 6 to 8 weeks.

Figure 184.19 shows an x-ray of the graft in place, and **Figure 184.20** shows a patient's recent postoperative CT scan.

Complications

Posterior spinal fusion is a salvage procedure and should always be viewed that way, regardless of the ease of this new variation of an old technique. The dura and exiting nerve roots are just beyond the bottom of the incisions, and this makes it imperative that this procedure only be performed by those well versed in the regional anatomy and experienced in performing either open or at least mini-open interventional pain management techniques. This procedure should not be performed on patients who are not cleared for surgery and who do not need rods/screws.

Clinical Pearls

The approach to L5-S1 can be very challenging and is best done similar to a diskogram angle (**Fig. 184.21**). The pin should enter the top of the joint and not the middle one third as with the other levels to ensure better bony purchase for the graft (**Fig. 184.22**).

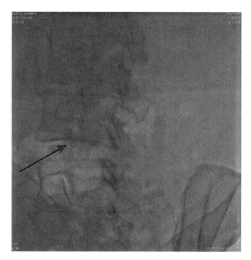

Fig. 184.19 Oblique x-ray—graft within the facet joint.

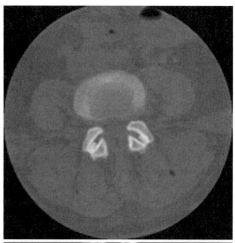

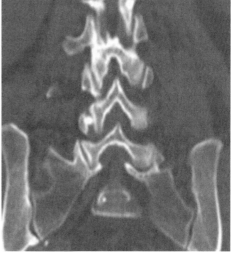

Fig. 184.20 CT scans—graft within the facet joint.

Video: Percutaneous technique

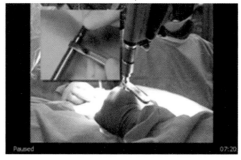

Fig. 184.17 Facet joint reaming.

Video: Percutaneous technique

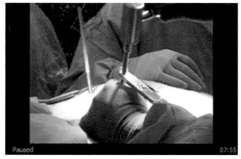

Fig. 184.18 Graft impacted and countersunk within the facet joint.

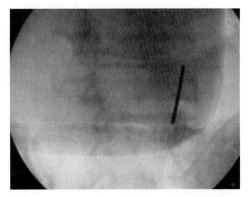

Fig. 184.21 L5-S1 approach similar to diskogram angle.

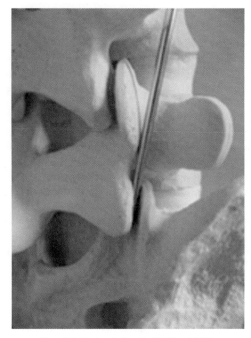

Fig. 184.22 Angle for TruFUSE at L5-S1.

The best surgical candidates are those who have experienced good, albeit transient, pain relief following intra-articular facet injections with local anesthetic and/or steroid (for localization of the pain-generating degenerative facet joint) and for those who have failed to achieve long-lasting relief with radiofrequency ablation. This technique is straight-forward when performed by those skilled in placement of needles into the facet joints. Postprocedure bracing will improve long-term outcomes and should be used in all patients undergoing posterior facet joint spinal fusion with the TruFUSE allograft dowel. Bone stimulators are medically necessary in patients with diabetes, smokers who will not stop smoking, pseudoarthrosis patients, anyone who has been on steroids recently, Down syndrome patients, and patients with multilevel fusions.

Posterior facet joint spinal fusion is a reasonable procedure for patients who suffer from intractable mechanical low back pain not relieved by nonoperative measures. It may be caused by facet joint arthropathy, adjacent segment degeneration next to long-standing hardware, or microinstability following decompressive spine surgery. The procedure is frequently used as a standalone technique or as an adjunct to other spinal fusion and/or decompression procedures.

Index

Note: Page numbers followed by *b* indicate boxes, *f* indicate figures, and *t* indicate tables.

A

Abdominal aneurysm
  aortic, femoral neuropathy due to, 826
  CT scan of, 674, 677f
  low back pain in, 699
Abdominal crunches, for sacroiliac joint
    disorders, 762
Abdominal muscles, contraction of, 674, 676f
Abdominal pain
  in acute pancreatitis, 682
  in chronic pancreatitis, 685, 685f
  in ilioinguinal neuralgia, 687
  management of
    limitations in, 945, 945t
    prolotherapy in, 1040–1041, 1040f
    transcutaneous electrical nerve stimulation
      in, 996
Abdominal wall pain, 674–681
  in anterior cutaneous nerve entrapment,
    674–677, 675f, 676f, 677f
  in liver disease, 679–681, 679f, 680f, 681f
  in slipping rib syndrome, 677–679, 678f
Abducens nerve (VI)
  evaluation of, 44t
  palsies associated with, 376, 377t
Abduction release test, resisted, for trochanteric
    bursitis, 361, 362f
A-beta fibers
  classification of, 10, 11t
  properties of, 11
Abortive therapy, for cluster headache, 446–451
Abrasions, corneal, 484, 484f
Abscess
  brain, headache in, 252, 252f, 255
  epidural. See Epidural abscess.
  iliac, femoral neuropathy due to, 826
  lung, 654, 654f
  retropharyngeal space, 500, 502f
Abused substances. See Drug abuse; *under*
    named drug.
Acetabular fracture, CT scan of, 98
Acetaldehyde accumulation, after celiac plexus
    block, 1203
Acetaminophen, 882–883
  contraindications to, 883
  dosing guidelines for, 882–883
  for cancer pain, 304, 305t
  for osteoporosis, 704
  hepatic injury caused by, 73
  indications for, 883
  mechanism of action of, 882
  pharmacokinetics of, 883
Acetazolamide
  for chronic arachnoiditis, 749
  for postoperative dural sac deformities, 785
Acetylsalicylic acid. See Aspirin.
Achilles bursitis, 367–368, 368f
Achilles tendinitis, 863–864, 863f, 864f
Achilles tendon, 860, 862f
  rupture of, 864–865
Achondroplasia (dwarfism), 78
Acoustic nerve (VIII), evaluation of, 44t
Acromioclavicular joint. See also Shoulder.
  anatomy of, 580f
  painful, 79, 579–581, 581f
    treatment of, 579–581, 581f
Action potentials, in nerve conduction, 178
Active straight leg raising test, 777, 778f
Acupuncture, 1019–1026. See also Alternative
    medicine.
  adverse effects of, 1025–1026
  anatomic aspects of, 1021–1023
  auricular, 1023
  channels and collaterals in, 1022–1023
  complications and pitfalls of, 1025–1026
  De Qi sensation in, 1022

Acupuncture *(Continued)*
  electroacupuncture, 1023
  example of, 1019, 1020f
  for cancer pain, 1025
  for chronic arachnoiditis, 749
  for low back pain, in pregnancy, 779
  for neuropathic pain, 211
  for phantom pain, 300
  for piriformis syndrome, 792
  historical considerations in, 1019–1020
  morphogenetic singularity theory and, 1021
  neurohumoral mechanisms of, 1020–1021
  outcomes of, 1025
  principles of, 1020–1021
  provider credentialing for, 1026
  safety of, 1025–1026
  scalp, 1023–1024
  techniques of, 1023–1024
  therapies concomitant with, 1024
  yin-yang theory and, 1020, 1020f
Acupuncture needles, manufacture
    and use of, 1025
Acupuncture points, 1021, 1022f
  types of, 1022
Acupuncture research, issues in, 1025
Acute chest syndrome, in sickle cell disease, 245
Acute pain
  in burn patients, 229
  management of, 216–227
    hypnosis in, 964
      technique of, 965
    narcotic analgesics in, 218–219, 218f
    neural blockade in, 219–227, 220f, 221f,
      222f, 223f, 224f, 225f, 226f, 226t.
      See also Nerve block(s), for acute/
      postoperative pain.
    nonprescription analgesics in, 878–879
    nonsteroidal anti-inflammatory drugs in,
      217–218, 217f, 217t
    prophylactic measures in, 216
    transcutaneous electrical nerve stimulation
      in, 996
  obturator nerve block for, 1245
  thoracic epidural nerve block for, 1181
Addiction, to opioids, 898, 898f
  vs. dependence, 308–309
Adductor tendinitis, 363–364, 363f, 364f
A-delta fibers, 703
  classification of, 10, 11t
  properties of, 11
Adenoma, pleomorphic, of parapharyngeal
    space, 500, 501f
Adhesions, epidural, lysis of, 1138–1141,
    1258–1272. See also Epidural adhesiolysis.
Adhesive capsulitis (frozen shoulder), 566, 567f
Adjunctive therapy
  for herpes zoster, 270–271
  for neuropathic pain, 210–211
Adson's test, for cervical radiculopathy,
    525, 526t
Adult hemoglobin (Hb A), 243
Afferent(s)
  activation of, 19–20, 20f
  dorsal horn projections of, 11t, 12, 13f
  in nerve injury
    sensitivity changes of, 26
    sprouting of, 26
  in tissue injury, 20, 20f
  primary, 10–12
    classification of, 10, 11t
    properties of, 10–12, 11f
    transmitters in, 17–18, 18f
    supraspinal projections of, 15–16, 15f, 16f
    with high thresholds, 12
Afferent line labeling, in pain processing
    system, 17

Afferent transmitter systems
  in nociception, pharmacology of, 17–18, 18f
  primary, 32f
Alanine aminotransferase (ALT), 71
Albumin, 67, 72
Alcohol
  intoxication with, 74
  neurolytic blockade with, 325–327, 325t
    subarachnoid, 1216–1218, 1217f
Alcohol use/abuse
  acute pancreatitis and, 682, 683f
  chronic pancreatitis and, 684
  triggering cluster headache, 440, 441
Alcoholism, screening for, 74
Alendronate, for complex regional pain
    syndrome, 285
Alfentanil, 907
Alkaline phosphatase (ALP), 71
Alkaloids, phenanthrene, 893t, 901–903. See also
    specific agent, e.g., Morphine.
Allergies, contrast-induced
  in diskography, 123
  in epidurography, 143
Allochiria (mirror-image pain), 8
Allodynia
  in postmastectomy pain, 662t
  tactile, 12
Alpha$_2$-adrenergic agonists, mechanism of
    action of, 30, 30f
Alpha-amino-3-hydroxy-5-methyl-4-
    isoxazolepropionic acid (AMPA)
    receptor, 31, 32f
Alternative medicine, 934–940
  acupuncture in, 936t, 939, 1019–1026. See also
    Acupuncture.
  biostimulation techniques in, 939
  chiropractic therapy in, 938–939
  classification of, 935, 936t
  comfort measures in, 939
  definition of, 935
  hypnosis in, 936t, 938, 963–966. See also
    Hypnosis.
  intercessionary prayer and, 937–938
  low-power laser therapy in, 939
  magnetic field therapy in, 939
  music therapy in, 937
  office of, 936
  relaxation therapy in, 938. See also Relaxation
    technique(s).
  scope of, 937
  spinal manipulation in, 1009–1018. See also
    Spinal manipulative therapy.
  spiritual healing and, 937–938
  transcutaneous electrical nerve stimulation
    in, 939. See also Transcutaneous electrical
    nerve stimulation (TENS).
  vs. holistic medicine, 935
Aluminum sulfate, for herpes zoster, 271
Alveolar nerve, inferior, 1070
Alvimopan, 912
Amine release, in tissue injury, 21t
Amitriptyline, 914f, 915
  for acute arachnoiditis, 748
  for cancer pain, 309
  for migraine prophylaxis, 426
  for mononeuritis multiplex, 671
  for peripheral neuropathies, 267
  for phantom pain, 297
  for postmastectomy pain, 663t
  for post-thoracotomy pain syndrome, 639
  for proctalgia fugax, 805
  for tension-type headache, 434t
  for vulvodynia, 799
Ammonium compounds, in neurolytic blockade,
    325t, 327
Amoxapine, for tension-type headache, 434t

Radiofrequency thermocoagulation
  and pulsed lesioning, after sphenopalatine
    ganglion block, 1057
  for cluster headache, 452
Radiofrequency units, in spinal cord stimulation,
  1305
Radiography, 75–84
  computed, 75
  in arachnoiditis, 745–746, 746f
  in brachial plexopathy, 539
  in cervical dystonia, 561
  in intercostal neuralgia, 640
  in lumbar osteomyelitis, 696, 696f
  in olecranon bursitis, 602, 603f
  in osteoarthritis, 388–389, 388t, 389f
  in palliative radiation therapy, 313, 313f
  in rheumatoid arthritis, 399, 399f, 400f
  in suprascapular nerve block technique,
    1175–1176, 1176f, 1177f
  of ankle, 84
  of cervical spine, 75–76, 76f
  of chondroma, in costosternal junction, 640,
    640f
  of elbow, 79–80, 80f
  of foot, 84
  of hand, 80–81
  of hip, 81–82, 82f, 83f
  of knee, 82–83, 83f
  of lumbar spine, 77–78, 77f, 78f, 79f, 80f
  of lumbosacral metastatic lesions, 697, 697f
  of pars interarticularis, 752–753, 753f
  of pelvis, 81–82
  of rotator cuff disorders, 575
  of shoulder, 78–79, 80f
    osteoarthritic, 566, 567f
  of spondylolysis, 752–754, 753f, 754t
  of thoracic spine, 77, 77f
  of thymoma, 643, 643f
  of wrist, 80–81
  traditional, 75
Radioisotope scanning. See Scintigraphy.
Radiopharmaceuticals, in palliative radiation
  therapy, 316
Radiosurgery, gamma knife
  for cluster headache, 452
  for trigeminal neuralgia, 469
Raeder's syndrome, vs. trigeminal neuralgia,
  466–467
Ramsay-Hunt syndrome, 268, 494, 496f
Ranawat's lines, 546, 546f
Range of motion, of shoulder, 572
Rapidly adapting stretch receptors (RARs), in
  respiratory system, 650, 650f, 658, 659f
Rash
  erythematous malar, in systemic lupus
    erythematosus, 403, 403f
  in dermatomyositis, 408, 408f, 409f
  in herpes zoster, 268
  knee pain with, 838
Raynaud's disease, biofeedback for, 956–957
Raynaud's phenomenon, biofeedback for,
  956–957
Reappraisal, in burn pain management,
  239–240
Rebound headache. See also Headache.
  analgesic, mechanisms of, 456, 457f
Reboxetine, 917, 917f
Rectal cancer, vs. proctalgia fugax, 804, 806,
  806f
Rectal dysfunction, in arachnoiditis, 747
Rectal examination, in sacroiliac joint disorders,
  760–761
Recurrent laryngeal nerve, inadvertent blockade
  of, in cervical plexus block, 1101
"Red back pain," 726
Red blood cell indices, 58
Referred pain
  patterns of
    from lumbar facet joints, 716–717, 717f
      to eye, 52
    to eye, 488–493. See also Ocular/periocular
      pain, referred.
Reflex(es)
  autonomic, in peripheral neuropathy, 266
  cough, 658
  deep tendon, examination of, 48–49, 48t, 49f
  H (Hoffmann), 182
  Hering-Breuer, 650
  nociceptive, in chronic tension-type headache,
    429

Reflex(es) (Continued)
  pathologic
    in cervical myelopathy, 550
    in cervical radiculopathy, 525, 525t
  somatovisceral, 998
  viscerosomatic, 998
Reflex sympathetic dystrophy. See Complex
  regional pain syndrome.
Refraction, definition of, 988
Regional anesthesia. See also Nerve block(s).
  for burn pain, 234–235
  for cancer pain, 321
    continuous, 321
    indications for, 320t
    role of, 319
  for phantom pain, 297
  for postmastectomy pain, 663–664
Regular medication scheduling, for burn pain,
  238
Rehabilitation
  aquatic, 987. See also Hydrotherapy.
  for brachial plexopathy, 539–540
  for cervical facet syndrome, 518–519
Reinforcement, positive, for burn pain, 238–239
Relaxation, cue-controlled, 973
Relaxation response, 967
Relaxation technique(s), 938, 967–975. See also
  Alternative medicine.
  anxiety in, 961–962, 975
  autogenic training, 968–969
    technique of, 971
  for acute/postoperative pain, 216
  for burn pain, 237–238
  guided imagery, 969
    technique of, 971
  historical perspectives of, 968–969
  in biofeedback. See also Biofeedback.
    electromyography-assisted, 957
    skin conductance-assisted, 957
    skin temperature-assisted, 958–959
  indications for, 969–971
  meditation, 968, 968t
  progressive muscle relaxation, 968
    technique of, 972, 972t, 973t
  regimen for, 972–975, 973t
  relaxed breathing, 971
  side effects of, 975
  techniques of, 971–975
  yoga, 969, 969t
Relaxation training regimen, 972–975, 973t
  Mindfulness Based Stress Reduction program
    in, 973–975, 974t
Relaxation-induced anxiety, 975
  in biofeedback, 961–962
Relaxed breathing, 971
Relaxin, increased levels of, during pregnancy, 776
Remifentanil, 907
Renal function tests, 69–70
Renal transplantation, femoral neuropathy
  after, 826–827
Resisted abduction release test, for trochanteric
  bursitis, 361, 362f
Resisted hip adduction test, for iliopsoas
  bursitis, 817, 818f
Respiratory dysfunction
  chest pain in, 649–659. See also Chest pain.
  opioid-induced, 896
    tolerance to, 308
Respiratory innervation, sensory, 649–650
Resurfacing procedures, for osteoarthritis, 394
Retinal migraine, 422t, 424, 424t. See also
  Migraine headache.
Retinal vein, central, occlusion of, 45, 46f
Retroachilleal bursitis, 865
Retrocalcaneal bursitis, 865
Retrocollis, 559–560
  muscles involved in, 562t
Retropharyngeal space abscess, 500, 502f
Reverse Hill-Sachs lesions, 575
Reverse Phalen maneuver, 620
Reye's syndrome, aspirin and, 880, 881
Rheumatic pain, progressive muscle relaxation
  for, 969
Rheumatoid arthritis, 396–402
  Baker's cyst in, 398, 398f
  clinical classification criteria for, 397t
  demographics of, 39t
  differential diagnosis of, 397t, 399–400, 400f

Rheumatoid arthritis (Continued)
  involving cervical spine, 546, 546f, 547f, 547t
  juvenile, 396–397
    aspirin dosing guidelines for, 880
  laboratory findings in, 398–399
  laboratory tests for, 63
  late-onset, vs. polymyalgia rheumatica, 414
  radiographic findings in, 399, 399f, 400f
  rheumatoid factor in, 398, 399
  signs and symptoms of, 397–398, 397f, 398f
  treatment of, 400–402
    anti-inflammatory agents in, 401
    assistive devices in, 402
    disease-modifying drugs in, 401
    heat and cold therapy in, 402
    immunosuppressive drugs in, 401–402
    orthotics in, 402
    surgical, 402
  vs. systemic lupus erythematosus, 404
  water-based exercises for, 990
Rheumatoid factor (RF), 63, 398, 399
Rhizotomy
  dorsal, for cancer pain, 335
  percutaneous glycerol, for trigeminal
    neuralgia, 468
  radiofrequency, for trigeminal neuralgia,
    469
Rib(s)
  cartilage abnormalities of
    in costosternal syndrome, 632, 633f
    in Tietze's syndrome, 634
  fractures of, 636–638, 637f
    intercostal nerve block for, 638, 638f
    thoracic epidural nerve block for, 1181
    treatment of, 658
  slipping, pain in, 677–679, 678f
Right upper quadrant syndrome, in sickle cell
  disease, 246
Rigid-scope endoscopic laser diskectomy,
  1404–1405, 1405f
Romberg's sign, 49
Ropivacaine
  chemistry of, 930–931, 931f, 931t
  for post-thoracotomy pain, 666
  pharmacokinetics of, 932t
Rotator cuff, anatomy of, 352, 353f
Rotator cuff disorders, 352–354, 353f,
  570–578
  angiofibroblastic hyperplasia in, 570–571
  calcific tendinosis in, 79, 80f
  clinical presentation of, 571–575
  diagnosis of, 575
  extrinsic vs. intrinsic mechanisms of,
    570–571
  historical considerations in, 570–571, 571f
  history in, 571
  magnetic resonance imaging of, 566, 568f,
    575, 576f
  overuse syndromes and, 570
  physical examination in, 571–575, 572f, 573f,
    574f
  radiographic studies of, 575
  treatment of, 576–577
    indications for, 576
    nonoperative, 576–577
    surgical, 577, 577f, 578f
  ultrasonography of, 575, 575f
Rucksack (backpack) paralysis, 535

S
"S" allele, of 5-HTTLPR gene, 205
Sacral canal
  anatomy of, 1250, 1251f
  contents of, 1250, 1251f
Sacral hiatus
  anatomy of, 1250
  localization of, in caudal epidural nerve block,
    1252–1253, 1252f, 1253f, 1254f
Sacroiliac joint
  anatomy of, 757–758, 758f
  dysfunction of, 759
  movement of, 758–759
  normal, 79f
  radiographic anatomy of, 1285–1286,
    1286f
Sacroiliac joint disorders, 1285–1288
  anatomic aspects of, 1285–1286, 1286f
  evaluation of, 760–761
  pain in, 759–760, 759f